Oral and Maxillofacial Surgery for the Clinician

Krishnamurthy Bonanthaya
Elavenil Panneerselvam • Suvy Manuel
Vinay V. Kumar • Anshul Rai
Editors

Oral and Maxillofacial Surgery for the Clinician

Volume II

Springer

Editors
Krishnamurthy Bonanthaya
Bhagwan Mahaveer Jain hospital
Bangalore
India

Suvy Manuel
Ananthapuri Hospitals & Research Institute
Kerala Institute of Medical Sciences
Trivandrum, Kerala
India

Anshul Rai
Associate Professor
Department of Dentistry
All India Institute of Medical Sciences
Bhopal, Madhya Pradesh
India

Elavenil Panneerselvam
Associate Professor
SRM Dental College, Ramapuram
Chennai, Tamil Nadu
India

Vinay V. Kumar
Department of Maxillofacial Plastic Surgery
Uppsala University Hospital
Uppsala
Sweden

Video Editors
Jimson Samson
Vice Principal
Prof & Head of Department
Department of Oral & Maxillofacial Surgery
Tagore Dental College & Hospital
Chennai, India

Nehal Patel
Director, DCKH Cleft Center
K. P. Sanghvi Hospital
Surat, India

Illustrator
Mr Brishank Pratap
Goa, India

Voice-over for Videos
Madhulaxmi Marimuthu
Professor
Saveetha Dental College
Chennai, India

Vivek Narayanan
Dean, SRM Dental College
Kaatangulathur
Chennai, India

This book is an open access publication.
ISBN 978-981-15-1345-9 ISBN 978-981-15-1346-6 (eBook)
https://doi.org/10.1007/978-981-15-1346-6

This Springer imprint is published by the registered company Springer Nature Singapore Pte Ltd.
The registered company address is: 152 Beach Road, #21-01/04 Gateway East, Singapore 189721, Singapore

Preface

An important question that always comes up when a book of this scope and extent is written is: why do we need one more?

This deserves a thoughtful answer and we shall try to do that while tracing the origin and evolution of this book from an idea. Since its inception in 1969, the *Association of Oral and Maxillofacial Surgeons of India* (AOMSI) has made steady and significant progress in terms of its vision and commitment to promote the field. The members of AOMSI have also evolved into a vibrant, multidimensional, passionate, and committed community of oral and maxillofacial surgeons who are making substantial contribution to the field in India and around the world. So it was only natural that the association decided to express its commitment to academic medicine coinciding with its 50th year in existence.

And what better way to express it than publishing an open source comprehensive textbook on oral and maxillofacial surgery. This book showcases the experts and expertise of AOMSI and has been made freely available to surgeons worldwide through generous funding from the association. We are delighted to see this open access book published for free use by worldwide community of MaxFac surgeons, especially the young surgeons and trainees in the field. This book is published with a CCBY license and we encourage associations and institutes to widely distribute the link to this book for maximum possible usage.

The AOMSI was very conscious that the development of our speciality was not an insular one. As we evolved, we looked for guidance and training from colleagues around the world, and in return, we provided our bit of experience and insights. This exchange of knowledge is extremely important for ultimately improving patient treatment methods, techniques, and outcomes. The same spirit was applied in producing this book as well' as we requested eminent clinicians and researchers from around the world along with our members to contribute to this book.

The book has contributions by society's members within India as well as 41 international authors from various countries. Thus, the extent of this makes it one of the most comprehensive textbooks on the topic. The contributors were invited by the AOMSI keeping in mind their scholastic profile while ensuring diversity and inclusiveness as well as a mix of young and experienced surgeons. All the contributors have a track record of being high-volume clinicians and educators in their field of expertise and are generally working at prestigious teaching institutions. This textbook as a scholarly venture condenses and amalgamates both the authors' personal experience as well as being in line with the current evidence-based treatment principles in the field of maxillofacial surgery. In the beginning, the heterogeneous source of knowledge did pose editorial challenges in standardization of the chapter structuring and scope. However, the final outcome has achieved a blend of evidence-based, diverse surgical practices along with cutting-edge technology for the practice of maxillofacial surgery in a fairly uniform format.

As the title suggests, this is meant to be a comprehensive resource for all clinicians, postgraduate trainees, and young surgeons in their day-to-day clinical work. Graduate students and surgeons will find this book useful in preparing for their university exams as well as board-certified exams from professional organizations. The book will help in decision-making, implementing treatment plans, and managing problems that may arise while executing these plans. Overall, the key objective is to help crystallize current evidence and provide protocols, guidelines, and recommendations to assist dealing with most clinical scenarios. Keeping this objective in mind, we have included components like case scenarios and video recordings of surgical procedures in the book.

Oral and Maxillofacial Surgery for the Clinician is a compilation of 22 sections incorporating 88 chapters dealing with the nuances in the principles and practice of cranio-maxillofacial and head and neck surgery. An important value addition is the library of 68 demonstrational videos that have been compiled to give the readers a more interactive feel with audiovisual inputs.

The book is structured in a step-ladder fashion to guide the reader through the basic principles of surgery before exposing to the full spectrum of specialty cranio-maxillofacial work. The first section is devoted to the origin and scope of oral and maxillofacial surgery as a specialty and a description of the training standards practiced globally. The next four sections are tailored to discuss the prospective patient, investigations, patient preparation, and anesthesia techniques. Subsequent sections focus on minor surgical procedures involving the practice of dento-alveolar surgery, implantology, and orofacial infections. With the above as the basis, the textbook progresses to complex surgical procedures including facial trauma, orthognathic surgery, TMJ, surgical pathology, and craniofacial and reconstructive surgery. The book also features two exclusive sections which provide the readers a perspective on practice management and research and publication.

The editors of the book would like to thank the office bearers of the AOMSI, in particular, the dynamic and effervescent secretary, Pritham Shetty, for the constant support he gave while undertaking this project.

Brishank Pratap, our tireless and innovative illustrator, needs a special mention for his superb rendition of medical and technical illustrations throughout this book.

Our publisher Springer, particularly, Naren Aggarwal and Jagjeet Kaur, deserves our gratitude for constant support and advice throughout the preparation of this book.

Last but not least, we would like to express our deep appreciation for the authors for their time, efforts, and priceless contributions.

We hope this book will be read worldwide, and we look forward to hear its critical reviews.

Bangalore, India — Krishnamurthy Bonanthaya
Chennai, India — Elavenil Panneerselvam
Trivandrum, India — Suvy Manuel
Uppsala, Sweden — Vinay V. Kumar
Bhopal, India — Anshul Rai
Chennai, India — Jimson Samson
Surat, India — Nehal Patel

Contents

List of Videos

Chapter Contributors and Video Contributors

Contributors

Avni Pandey Acharya GSR Institute of Cranio-maxillofacial & Facial Plastic Surgery, Hyderabad, Telangana, India

H. S. Adenwalla Department of Plastic Surgery, Burns and the Charles Pinto Centre for Cleft Lip, Palate and Craniofacial Anomalies, Jubilee Mission Medical College and Research Institute, Thrissur, Kerala, India

Neha Aggarwal Nair Hospital Dental College, Mumbai, Maharashtra, India

Meenakshi Cleft and Craniofacial Centre, Chennai, Tamil Nadu, India

Nisheet Anant Agni Department of Oral and Maxillofacial Surgery, SMBT Institute of Dental Sciences and Research, Nashik, India

Suman Ananathanarayana Department of Anesthesiology, Columbia Asia Referral Hospital, Yeshwantpur, Bangalore, Karnataka, India

Sonal Anchlia Department of Oral & Maxillofacial Surgery, Government Dental College & Hospital, Ahmedabad, Gujarat, India

Neelam N. Andrade Department of Oral and Maxillofacial Surgery, Nair Hospital Dental College, Mumbai, Maharashtra, India

Yashoda Ashok Department of Oral and Maxillofacial Surgery, Meenakshi Ammal Dental College and Hospitals, Chennai, Tamil Nadu, India

Prithvi S. Bachalli Department of Oral and Maxillofacial Surgery, Rangadore Memorial Hospital, Apollo Hospitals, Bangalore, Karnataka, India

Mirza Farhatullah Baig Department of Oral and Maxillofacial Surgery, Saveetha Dental College, Chennai, Tamil Nadu, India

Kannan Balaraman Department of Oral and Maxillofacial Surgery, Ganga Medical Centre and Hospitals, Coimbatore, Tamil Nadu, India

Rishi Kumar Bali Postgraduate Department of OMFS, DAV Dental College Hospital, Yamunanagar, Haryana, India

Peter A. Brennan Maxillofacial Unit, Queen Alexandria Hospital, Portsmouth, UK

Srinivasa R. Chandra Department of Head and Neck Oncology and Reconstructive Microvascular and Oral and Maxillofacial Surgery, Fred and Pamela Buffett Cancer Center, UNMC, Omaha, NE, USA

Jaideep Singh Chauhan Department of Maxillofacial Surgery, the Smile Train CHL Hospital, Indore, Madhya Pradesh, India

Aarti Chowdhary Department of Periodontology, SD Dental College and Hospital, Parbhani, Maharashtra, India

John Collin Department of Oral and Maxillofacial Surgery, University of Florida, Jacksonville, FL, USA

Ashok Dabir D. Y. Patil University School of Dentistry, Nerul, Navi Mumbai, India

Breach Candy Hospital, Mumbai, India

Abhay Datarkar Department of Oral and Maxillofacial Surgery, Government Dental College and Hospital, Medical College Premises, Nagpur, Maharashtra, India

Vijay Deshmukh Deshmukh Institute of Maxillofacial Surgery and Research Centre, Aurangabad, Maharashtra, India

JIIU'S Indian Institute of Medical Sciences, Jalna, Maharashtra, India

Amit Dhawan Department of Oral and Maxillofacial Surgery, SGRD Dental Institute, Amritsar, India

George Dimitroulis Maxillofacial Unit, St. Vincent's Hospital—University of Melbourne, Melbourne, Australia

Vikas Dhupar Department of Oral and Maxillofacial Surgery, Goa Dental College and Hospital, Bambolim, Goa, India

Supriya Ebenezer Department of Oral Surgery and Stomatology, University of Bern, Bern, Switzerland

El Mustafa Department of Oral and Maxillofacial Surgery, Queen Elizabeth Hospital, Birmingham, UK

Madan G. Ethunandan Consultant Oral and Maxillofacial/Skull Base Surgeon, Honorary Senior Clinical Lecturer, Lead, Head and Neck Cancer, University Hospital Southampton, Southampton, UK

Carlo Ferretti , Johannesburg, South Africa

Department of Maxillofacial and Oral Surgery, University of Pretoria, Pretoria, South Africa

Rui Fernandes Department of Oral and Maxillofacial Surgery, Head and Neck Oncologic Surgery and Microvascular Fellowship, University of Florida, Jacksonville, FL, USA

Rajasekhar Gaddipati Department of Oral and Maxillofacial Surgery, Mamata Dental College, Khammam, Telangana, India

Divya P. Gadre Gadre Clinic, Pune, Maharashtra, India

Kiran S. Gadre Gadre Clinic, Pune, Maharashtra, India

Department of Oral and Maxillofacial Surgery, Bharati Vidyapeeth Dental College and Hospital, Pune, Maharashtra, India

Raja Sekhar Gali Department of Oral and Maxillofacial Surgery, Narayana Dental College and Hospital, Nellore, Andhra Pradesh, India

Medicover Hospital, Nellore, Andhra Pradesh, India

Kandasamy Ganesan Department of Oral and Maxillofacial Surgery, Southend University Hospitals NHS Trust, Southend-on-Sea, UK

University of Leeds, Leeds, UK

Jaime Grant Birmingham Children's Hospital, Birmingham, UK

Beat Hammer CFC Hirslanden Kopf Zentrum, Aarau, Switzerland

Kalarikkal Mukundan Harish Department of Oral & Maxillofacial Surgery, Ragas Dental College, Chennai, Tamil Nadu, India

Velupillai Ilankovan Oral and Maxillofacial Surgery, Poole Hospital NHS Foundation Trust, Poole, UK

D' Souza Jacob Maxillofacial Unit, Royal Surrey County Hospital, Guilford, UK

Oommen Aju Jacob Department of Oral and Maxillofacial Surgery, Ananthapuri Hospitals and Research Institute, Trivandrum, Kerala, India

Kerala Institute of Medical Sciences, Trivandrum, Kerala, India

Rebecca Jacob Department of Anesthesiology, Columbia Asia Referral Hospital, Yeshwantpur, Bangalore, Karnataka, India

Anuj Jain Oral and Maxillofacial Surgeon, Department of Trauma and Emergency Medicine, All India Institute of Medical Sciences, Bhopal, Madhya Pradesh, India

B. S. Jayanth Oral and Maxillofacial Surgeon, ABMSS, Bengaluru, Karnataka, India

Samson Jimson Department of Oral and Maxillofacial Surgery, Tagore Dental College and Hospital, Chennai, Tamil Nadu, India

Bobby John Department of Oral and Maxillofacial Surgery, Government Dental College, Kottayam, Kerala, India

Kerala University of Health Sciences, Thrissur, Kerala, India

Reena Rachel John Department of Oral and Maxillofacial Surgery, Vinayaka Mission's Sankarachariar Dental College and Hospital, VMRF, DU, Salem, India

Maj Anson Jose Oral and Maxillofacial Surgery, ADC R&R, New Delhi, India

Shyamsundar K. Joshi Department of Radiology, SDM College of Medical Sciences and Hospital, Shri Dharmasthala Manjunatheshwara University, Dharwad, India

Takahiro Kanno Department of Oral and Maxillofacial Surgery, Shimane University, Faculty of Medicine, Izumo, Shimane, Japan

Taranjit Kaur Department of Oral and Maxillofacial Surgery, Government Dental College and Hospital, Jamnagar, Gujarat, India

Manal M. Khan Department of Burns and Plastic Surgery, AIIMS Bhopal, Bhopal, Madhya Pradesh, India

Rakshit Vijay Sinai Khandeparker Department of Oral and Maxillofacial Surgery, Goa Dental College and Hospital, Bambolim, Goa, India

Annie I. Kochuveettil Department of Radiology, SDM College of Medical Sciences and Hospital, Shri Dharmasthala Manjunatheshwara University, Dharwad, India

David Koppel Scottish National Craniofacial Service for Children and Young People, Royal Hospital for Children, Glasgow, UK

Shreya Krishna Oral and Maxillofacial Surgery, Rangadore Memorial Hospital, Apollo Hospitals, Bangalore, India

V. B. Krishnakumar Raja Department of Oral & Maxillofacial Surgery, SRM Dental College & Hospital, Ramapuram, Chennai, Tamil Nadu, India

B. Krishnan Department of Dentistry, Jawaharlal Institute of Postgraduate Medical Education and Research (JIPMER), Puducherry, India

Deepak G. Krishnan Oral and Maxillofacial Surgery, University of Cincinnati Medical Center, Cincinnati, OH, USA

Cincinnati Children's Hospital and Medical Center, Cincinnati, OH, USA

Balasubramanya Kumar Department of Oral and Maxillofacial Surgery, St. Marthas's Hospital, Bangalore, Karnataka, India

Bhagwan Mahaveer Jain Hospital, Vikram Hospital, Bangalore, Karnataka, India

Vinay V. Kumar Department of Maxillofacial and Plastic Surgery, Uppsala University Hospital, Uppsala, Sweden

Moni Abraham Kuriakose Cochin Cancer Research Centre, Kochi, Kerala, India

Paritkumar Ladani Swiss Cleft and Craniofacial Centre, BSES MG Hospital, Mumbai, India

Subramanyam S. Mahankali Department of Anesthesiology, Columbia Asia Referral Hospital, Yeshwantpur, Bangalore, Karnataka, India

Neelima Malik Department of Oral and Maxillofacial Surgery, Krishna Institute of Medical Sciences "Deemed to be University", Karad, Maharashtra, India

Varghese Mani Department of Oral and Maxillofacial Surgery, Mar Baselios Dental College, Kothamangalam, Kerala, India

Suvy Manuel Department of Oral and Maxillofacial Surgery, Ananthapuri Hospitals and Research Institute, Trivandrum, Kerala, India

Kerala Institute of Medical Sciences, Trivandrum, Kerala, India

Renita Maria Department of Anesthesiology, Columbia Asia Referral Hospital, Yeshwantpur, Bangalore, Karnataka, India

Madhulaxmi Marimuthu Department of Oral & Maxillofacial Surgery, Saveetha Dental College & Hospital, Chennai, Tamil Nadu, India

Paul Mathai Nair Hospital Dental College, Mumbai, Maharashtra, India

Department of Oral and Maxillofacial Surgery, Jubilee Mission Medical College & Research Institute, Thrissur, Kerala, India

Philip Mathew Department of Oral and Maxillofacial Surgery, Jubilee Mission Medical College & Research Institute, Thrissur, Kerala, India

Sainath Matsa Praseedha Clinic for Maxillofacial Cosmetic Surgery, Chennai, Tamil Nadu, India

Divya Mehrotra Department of Oral and Maxillofacial Surgery, King George's Medical University, Lucknow, India

Sushma Mehta Mazumdar Shaw Cancer Center, Bengaluru, Karnataka, India

Suresh Menon Department of Oral and Maxillofacial Surgery, Vydehi Institute of Dental Sciences and Research Centre, Bangalore, Karnataka, India

Aditya Moorthy Department of Oral and Maxillofacial Surgery, Rangadore Memorial Hospital, Apollo Hospitals, Bangalore, Karnataka, India

Mustafa. K Department of Craniofacial Surgery, Kanachur Institute of Medical Sciences, Mangalore, Karnataka, India

Veerabahu Muthusubramanian Department of Oral & Maxillofacial Surgery, Ragas Dental College, Chennai, Tamil Nadu, India

Sowjanya Nagamalla Department of Oral and Maxillofacial Surgery, Virginia Commonwealth University Medical Center, Richmond, VA, USA

Sanjiv Nair Department of Oral and Maxillofacial Surgery, Bhagwan Mahaveer Jain Hospital, Bengaluru, Karnataka, India

P. V. Narayanan Consultant Plastic Surgeon, Jubilee Mission Medical College & Research Institute, Thrissur, Kerala, India

Nasir A. Nasser Barts & London NHS Trust, Whipps Cross University Hospital, London, UK

University Hospital, Berne, Switzerland

J. Naveen Kumar Oral and Maxillofacial Surgery, Sri Ramachandra Institute of Higher Education and Research, Chennai, India

Kishore Nayak Bhagvan Jain Mahaveer Hospital, Bangalore, India

R. S. Neelakandan Department of Oral and Maxillofacial Surgery, Meenakshi Ammal Dental College and Hospital, MAHER, Chennai, Tamil Nadu, India

Rachel S. Oeppen Consultant Radiologist, University Hospital Southampton, Southampton, UK

Arun Kumar Panda Department of Oral & Maxillofacial Surgery, SD Dental College and Hospital, Parbhani, Maharashtra, India

Elavenil Panneerselvam Department of Oral and Maxillofacial Surgery, SRM Dental College, Ramapuram, Chennai, Tamil Nadu, India

Department of Orbit & Oculoplasty, Aravind Eye Hospital, Chennai, Tamil Nadu, India

Shreya Panwar Department of Oral & Maxillofacial Surgery, Meenakshi Ammal Dental College & Hospital, Chennai, Tamil Nadu, India

Ananthanarayanan Parameswaran Department of Oral and Maxillofacial Surgery, Meenakshiammal Dental College & Hospital, Chennai, Tamil Nadu, India

Department of Orbit, Oculoplasty, Reconstructive & Aesthetic Surgery, Shankara Nethralaya, Chennai, Tamil Nadu, India

Department of Orbit & Oculoplasty, Aravind Eye Hospital, Chennai, Tamil Nadu, India

Satyen Parida Department of Anesthesiology and Critical Care, Jawaharlal Institute of Postgraduate Medical Education and Research (JIPMER), Puducherry, India

Sat Parmar Department of Oral and Maxillofacial Surgery, Queen Elizabeth Hospital, Birmingham, UK

Mamatha Patil Department of Oral and Maxillofacial Surgery, Sparsh Hospital, Bangalore, Karnataka, India

George Paul Kerala University of Health Sciences, Thrissur, Kerala, India

Dr MGR Medical University, Chennai, Tamil Nadu, India

Vijay Pillai Department of Head and Neck Surgical Oncology, Mazumdar Shaw Cancer Center, Narayana Health, Bangalore, Karnataka, India

Sreedhar Reddy Pothula Oral and Maxillofacial Surgery, Pioneer advanced Hair Transplant Centre, Bengaluru, Karnataka, India

Abhinand Potturi SVS Institute of Dental Sciences, Mahabubnagar, Telangana State, India

Akhilesh Prathap Department of Oral and Maxillofacial Surgery, Pushpagiri College of Dental Sciences, Thiruvalla, Kerala, India

Prav Praveen Department of Oral and Maxillofacial Surgery, Queen Elizabeth Hospital, Birmingham NHS Foundation Trust, Birmingham, UK

Boyapati Raghu Maxillofacial Unit, Royal Surrey County Hospital, Guilford, UK

Anshul Rai Department of Dentistry, All India Institute of Medical Sciences, Bhopal, Madhya Pradesh, India

Manjunath Rai Department of OMFS, A. J. Institute of Dental Sciences, Mangalore, Karnataka, India

Faculty of Dentistry, RGUHS, Bangalore, India

Manikandhan Ramanathan Department of Oral and Maxillofacial surgery, Meenakshi Ammal Dental College and Hospital, MAHER University, Chennai, Tamil Nadu, India

Meenakshi Cleft and Craniofacial Centre, Chennai, Tamil Nadu, India

Dipesh Rao Bhagwan Mahaveer Jain Hospital, Bangalore, Karnataka, India

Latha P. Rao Department of Craniomaxillofacial Surgery, Aster Medcity, Kochi, Kerala, India

Neelam Rathod Department of Oral and Maxillofacial Surgery, Southend University Hospitals NHS trust, Southend-on-Sea, UK

Poornima Ravi Department of Oral and Maxillofacial Surgery, SRM Dental College, Ramapuram, Chennai, Tamil Nadu, India

Srinivas Gosla Reddy GSR Institute of Cranio-maxillofacial & Facial Plastic Surgery, Hyderabad, Telangana, India

N. Viveka Vardhan Reddy Oral and Maxillofacial Surgery, SVS Institute of Dental Sciences, Mahabubnagar, Telangana, India

Shravan Renapurkar Department of Oral and Maxillofacial Surgery, Virginia Commonwealth University Medical Center, Richmond, VA, USA

Christoph Renné Group Practice for Pathology Wiesbaden, Wiesbaden, Germany

Tara Renton Oral Surgery, Kings College, London, UK

Johan P. Reyneke Center for Orthognathic Surgery, Mediclinic, Cape Town, South Africa

Department of Oral and Maxillofacial Surgery, Faculty of Health Sciences, University of the Western Cape, Cape Town, South Africa

Department of Oral and Maxillofacial Surgery, University of Oklahoma, Oklahoma City, OK, USA

Sunil Richardson Richardson's Dental and Craniofacial Hospital, Nagercoil, Tamil Nadu, India

Saurabh Saigal Department of Anaesthesiology, AIIMS Bhopal, Bhopal, Madhya Pradesh, India

B. Sasikala Department of Oral and Maxillofacial Surgery, SRM Dental College, Ramapuram, Chennai, Tamil Nadu, India

Anna Sayan Poole Hospital NHS Foundation Trust, Poole, UK

Tian Ee Seah TES Clinic for Face and Jaw, Singapore, Singapore

Nallamilli V. S. Sekhar Reddy Panineeya Institute of Dental Sciences and Research Centre, Hyderabad, Telangana, India

Anjan Kumar Shah Department of Oral and Maxillofacial Surgery, Rajarajeswari Dental College, Bangalore, India

Bhagwan Mahaveer Jain Hospital, Bangalore, India

Garima Sharma Department of Anesthesiology, Columbia Asia Referral Hospital, Yeshwantpur, Bangalore, Karnataka, India

Lt Col Rohit Sharma Oral and Maxillofacial Surgery, 11 Corps Dental Unit, Jalandhar Cantt, India

Kishore Shekar Head and Neck Surgeon (OMFS), Ninewells Hospital and Dundee, University Medical School, Dundee, UK

Pritham N. Shetty Department of Oral and maxillofacial surgery, Bangalore Institute of Dental Science, Bangalore, Karnataka, India

Omkar Anand Shetye Department of Oral and Maxillofacial Surgery, Goa Dental College and Hospital, Bambolim, Goa, India

Sunil S. Shroff Department of Oral and Maxillofacial Surgery, Bhagwan Mahaveer Jain Hospital, Bengaluru, Karnataka, India

Anand Shukla Department of Oral and Maxillofacial Surgery, King George's Medical University, Lucknow, India

Deepti Simon Department of Oral and Maxillofacial Surgery, Government Dental College, Trivandrum, Kerala, India

Kerala University of Health Sciences, Thrissur, Kerala, India

Robert A. Strauss Department of Oral and Maxillofacial Surgery, Virginia Commonwealth University Medical Center, Richmond, VA, USA

Shintaro Sukegawa Division of Oral and Maxillofacial Surgery, Kagawa Prefectural Central Hospital, Takamatsu, Kagawa, Japan

Shikha Tayal Department of Oral and Maxillofacial Surgery, Government Dental College and Hospital, Medical College Premises, Nagpur, Maharashtra, India

Mary Thomas Department of Anesthesiology, Regional Cancer Centre, Medical College Campus, Thiruvananthapuram, Kerala, India

Andreas Thor Department of Maxillofacial and Plastic Surgery, Uppsala University Hospital, Uppsala, Sweden

Asha Thomson Norfolk and Norwich University Hospitals, Norfolk, UK

Benjamin Turner Department of Oral and Maxillofacial Surgery, University of Florida, Jacksonville, FL, USA

Jayesh Vahanwala Department of Oral and Maxillofacial Surgery, Vaidik Dental College & Research Centre, Nani Daman, India

Breach Candy Hospital, Mumbai, India

George Varghese Principal, Professor and Head, Department of Oral and Maxillofacial Surgery, Pushpagiri College of Dental Sciences, Tiruvalla, Kerala, India

Ravi Veeraraghavan Department of Oral and Maxillofacial Surgery, Amrita School of Dentistry, Ernakulam, India

Payal Verma Oral and Maxillofacial Surgery, University of Cincinnati Medical Center, OH, Cincinnati, USA

Christian Walter Oral and Maxillofacial Surgery—Plastic Surgery, Mediplus Clinic Mainz, Mainz, Germany

Gary Warburton Department of Oral and Maxillofacial Surgery, University of Maryland School of Dentistry, Baltimore, MD, USA

Frank Wilde Department of Oral and Plastic Maxillofacial Surgery, Armed Forces Hospital, Ulm, Germany

Department of Oral and Maxillofacial Surgery, University Hospital, Ulm, Germany

Abhilasha Yadav Department of Oral and Maxillofacial Surgery, Awadh Dental College & Hospital, Jamshedpur, Jharkhand, India

Video Contributors

Prithvi S. Bachalli Department of Oral and Maxillofacial Surgery, Rangadore Memorial Hospital, Apollo Hospitals, Bangalore, Karnataka, India

Ramdas Balakrishna Department of Oral and Maxillofacial Surgery, KLE's Institute of Dental Science and Research, Bangalore, India

Anandh Balasubramanian Department of Oral and Maxillofacial Surgery, Tagore Dental College and Hospital, Chennai, Tamil Nadu, India

Mohan Baliga Department of Oral and Maxillofacial Surgery, Manipal College of Dental Sciences, MAHE, Mangalore, Karnataka, India

Biswajit Kumar Biswas Avinash Institute of craniofacial and Reconstructive Surgery, Kolkata, India

Lokesh Bhanumurthy Department of Oral and Maxillofacial Surgery, Tagore Dental College and Hospital, Chennai, Tamil Nadu, India

Rohit Chandra Oral and Maxillofacial Surgeon, Department of Plastic Surgery, Max Hospitals, Vaishali and Noida, India

Jaideep Singh Chauhan Department of Oral and Maxillofacial Surgery, CHL Hospitals, Indore, Madhya Pradesh, India

Anil Kumar Desai Craniofacial Unit, SDM College of Dental Sciences & Hospital, Dharwad, India

Anjaneya Dube Department of Oral and Maxillofacial Surgery, Saptarshi Hospital and Cancer Centre, Jabalpur National Hospital, Jabalpur, India

Gunjan Dube Dube Surgical and Dental Hospital, Jabalpur, Madhya Pradesh, India

Shehzana Fatima Oral and Maxillofacial Surgeon, Dubai Health Authority, Dubai, UAE

S. Girish Rao Oral and Maxillofacial Surgeon, Shri Shankara Cancer Hospital and Research Center, Apollo Hospitals, Sagar Hospitals, Trustwell Hospital, NIMHANS, Bangalore, India

Charu Girotra Department of OMFS, School of Dentistry, D. Y. Patil Deemed to be University, Navi Mumbai, Maharashtra, India

Gaurav Mahesh Gupta Centre for Craniomaxillo Facial and Facial Plastic Surgery, Pushpanjali Hospital & Research Centre, Agra, Uttar Pradesh, India

Rebecca Jacob Department of Anesthesiology, Columbia Asia Referral Hospital, Yeshwantpur, Bangalore, India

Jagadish Chandra Department of OMFS, Yenepoya Dental College, Yenepoya Deemed to be University, Mangalore, India

Samson Jimson Department of Oral & Maxillofacial Surgery, Tagore Dental College & Hospital, Chennai, India

Adarsh Kudva Department of Oral and Maxillofacial Surgery, Manipal College of Dental Sciences, Mahe University, Manipal, India

Deepak Kulkarni Department of Oral and Maxillofacial Surgery, Dr D Y Patil Dental College, Pune, India

Balasubramanya Kumar Department of Oral and Maxillofacial Surgery, Bhagwan Mahaveer Jain Hospital, Vikram Hospital, Bangalore, India

Paritkumar Ladani Swiss Cleft and Craniofacial Centre, BSES MG Hospital, Mumbai, India

Ummar Mangalath Department of Oral and Maxillofacial Surgery, MES Dental College, Perinthalmanna, Kerala, India

Philip Mathew Department of Oral and Maxillofacial Surgery, Jubilee Mission Medical College and Hospital, Thrissur, Kerala, India

Sainath Matsa Praseedha Clinic for Maxillofacial Cosmetic Surgery, Chennai, Tamil Nadu, India

Aditya Moorthy Department of Oral and Maxillofacial Surgery, Rangadore Memorial Hospital, Apollo Hospitals, Bangalore, Karnataka, India

Ravindran Nair Department of Oral and Maxillofacial Surgery, Government Medical College, Manjeri, Kerala, India

Anuradha Navaneetham Department of Oral and Maxillofacial Surgery, M R Ambedkar Dental College, Rajiv Gandhi University, Bangalore, India

Nilesh Pagaria Oral and Maxillofacial Surgeon, Shrikrishna Hospital, Raipur, Chhattisgarh, India

Arun Kumar Panda Department of Oral & Maxillofacial Surgery, SD Dental College and Hospital, Parbhani, Maharashtra, India

Ananthanarayanan Parameswaran Department of Oral and Maxillofacial Surgery, Meenakshi Ammal Dental College & Hospital, Chennai, Tamil Nadu, India

Nehal Patel NuFace Maxillofacial Hospital, Surat, Gujarat, India

Kavitha Prasad Faculty of Dental Sciences, Ramaiah University of Applied Sciences, Bengaluru, India

Satish Kumaran Pugazhendi Department of Oral and Maxillofacial Surgery, M. R. Ambedkar Dental College, Bangalore, India

Gunaseelan Rajan Oral and Maxillofacial Surgeon, Rajan Dental Hospital, Chennai, Tamil Nadu, India

Rajasekhar Gaddipati Department of Oral and Maxillofacial Surgery, Mamata Dental College, Khammam, Telangana, India

Sushmitha Rajmohan Department of Dentistry & Maxillofacial Surgery, ESIC Model Hospital, Indore, India

Aasya the Clinic for Face Jaws & Teeth, Vijaynagar, Indore, MP, India

Vidya Rattan Unit of Oral & Maxillofacial Surgery, Oral Health Sciences Centre, Postgraduate Institute of Medical Education & Research, Chandigarh, India

Pothula Sreedhar Reddy Oral and Maxillofacial Surgeon, Pioneer Advanced Hair Transplant Center, Bangalore, India

Sunil Richardson Richardson's Dental and Craniofacial Hospital, Nagercoil, Tamil Nadu, India

Senthil Murugan Department of Oncology & Reconstructive Microsurgery, Saveetha Dental College, Saveetha University, Chennai, Tamil Nadu, India

DWIJAN Microsurgery Research & Training Centre, Chennai, India

Navin Shah Sunderlal Department of Oral and Maxillofacial Surgery, KM Shah Dental College, Sumandeep Vidyapeeth, A Central deemed to be University, Vadodara, Gujarat, India

Yeshaswini Thelekkat Department of Oral & Maxillofacial Surgery, Azeezia College of Dental Sciences and Research Kollam, Kollam, Kerala, India

Joji Thomas Department of Oral and Maxillofacial Surgery, Cosmopolitan Hospital Pvt Ltd, Trivandrum, Kerala, India

P. Varun Menon The Charles Pinto Centre for Cleft Lip, Palate and Craniofacial Anomalies, Jubilee Mission, Medical College & Research Institute, Thrissur, Kerala, India

Sankar Vinod Vichattu Department of OMFS, Mar Baselious Dental College, Kotamangalam, Kerala, India

B. Vikraman Department of Oral and Maxillofacial Surgery, Ragas Dental College & Hospital, Chennai, Tamil Nadu, India

Gary Warburton Department of Oral & Maxillofacial Surgery, University of Maryland Dental School, Baltimore, MD, USA

About the Editors

Krishnamurthy Bonanthaya did his postgraduate dental studies from Mangalore University, and then he obtained his MBBS from Kasturba Medical College, Manipal. He is also a fellow of the Royal College of Surgeons of England and Royal College of Surgeons of Ireland. He is currently the project director of Smile Train Project treating cleft lip and palate deformities at Bhagwan Mahaveer Jain Hospital, Bangalore. He also holds the position of professor of oral and maxillofacial surgery, Bangalore Institute of Dental Sciences, which involves undergraduate and postgraduate training and the routine mix of maxillofacial surgical management. He is the editor in chief emeritus of the *Journal of Maxillofacial and Oral Surgery* and has numerous publications to his credit.

Elavenil Panneerselvam completed her postgraduation in oral and maxillofacial surgery from the Tamil Nadu Dr. M.G.R. Government Medical University, Chennai, India. She also has a master's degree in business administration, specializing in hospital management, fellowship in Aesthetic Medicine and has been awarded Fellowship in Dental Surgery by the Royal College of Physicians & Surgeons of Glasgow. She has contributed to textbooks on oral anatomy, local anesthesia, plastic surgery, and pediatric TMJ surgery. Presently, she holds a faculty position at the SRM Dental College (Ramapuram), Chennai, as associate professor in oral and axillofacial surgery. She is a recipient of the MM Cooper Memorial Research Award from the Indian Society for Anatomists and the Ginwalla Trophy from the Association of Oral & Maxillofacial Surgeons of India.

Suvy Manuel after his postgraduation from Government Dental College, Trivandrum, University of Kerala, in 2002, gained the Diplomate of National Board in Oral & Maxillofacial Surgery, Membership from the National Academy of Medical Sciences, New Delhi, India; and Diploma of Membership in Oral surgery, Royal College of Surgeons, Edinburgh.

During his tenure in the UK, he attained the Membership of the Faculty of Dental Surgery, Royal College of Surgeons, England. Subsequently, he attained the Fellowship in Dental Surgery, Royal College of Surgeons, Edinburgh. He is the MOMS RCSEd (Diploma of Membership in Oral Surgery) Examiner for the Royal College of Surgeons of Edinburgh in the Faculty of Dental Examiners, as appointed by the Dental Examinations Committee, RCS Edinburgh.

He is former professor and postgraduate guide at the Kerala University of Health Sciences and is a reviewer for the *Journal of Maxillofacial and Oral Surgery*.

Currently, he is attached to the maxillofacial units at Ananthapuri and KIMS Hospitals, Trivandrum, India.

Vinay V. Kumar completed his master's in oral and maxillofacial surgery from Nair Hospital Dental College, Mumbai, India, in 2008. He was an ITI Scholar in the Department of Maxillofacial and Plastic Surgery in Johannes Gutenberg University (JGU) Mainz, Germany, in 2010, where he went on to complete his Doctorate of Medicine in Dentistry (2013), obtain a practicing license, and served as a visiting faculty. He completed the MD and PhD program at the University of Medicine, Rostock, Germany in 2018. He is currently a Specialist Oral and Maxillofacial Surgeon in the Department of Maxillofacial and Plastic Surgery, Uppsala University Hospital, Sweden in the Department of Maxillofacial Surgery, Uppsala University, Sweden.

Anshul Rai is an Associate Professor in Department of Dentistry at All India Institute of Medical Sciences Bhopal, MP. He has 54 publications to his credit out of which 24 belong to prestigious international journals. He has contributed as a coauthor to *Textbook of Oral and Maxillofacial Surgery* by Dr. Borle. He is a Fellow of Indian Board of Oral and Maxillofacial Surgery (FIBOMS) and a fellow of the International Board for the Certification of Specialists in Oral and Maxillofacial Surgery (FIBCSOMS). He is a reviewer for *Journal of Maxillofacial and oral surgery and Indian Journal of Dental Research.*

Jimson Samson completed his postgraduate studies at the prestigious the Tamil Nadu Dr. M.G.R. Medical University, Chennai. Since completing his MDS, he has been in academics. He is a journal reviewer and also a section editor. He has lectured at various national and international conferences. He was also a faculty at OMFS workshops.

His special interest in research has made him Vice-Principal—Research at Tagore Dental College & Hospital, Chennai. In addition, he also heads the Department of Oral and Maxillofacial Surgery. He has published in indexed journals. He is now the Hon. State Secretary of the Association of Oral and Maxillofacial Surgeons of India, Tamil Nadu and Puducherry Branch. He is also an elected member of the Executive Committee of the National Association.

He is a member of the Board of Studies for Postgraduate Studies of Oral and Maxillofacial Surgery at the Tamil Nadu Dr. M.G.R. Medical University, Chennai.

Nehal Patel completed his master's in oral and maxillofacial surgery from A.B. Shetty Institute of Dental Sciences, Mangalore. He did his fellowship in Cleft and Craniofacial Surgery from Mangalore. He did his mini residency in TMJ Arthroscopy and Total Joint replacement from the USA. He worked as consultant cleft and craniofacial surgeon in BSES MG Hospital. He is currently working as Director, ABMSS CLEFT PROJECT in Surat, Gujarat.

Part XV

Salivary Gland Pathologies

Salivary Gland Pathologies

46

Nisheet Anant Agni

46.1 Introduction

The salivary glands secrete saliva which has lubricating, immunologic, digestive, and cleansing functions. They are affected by systemic and local inflammatory conditions, obstructive pathologies, as well as neoplasms. Most of the tumors are parenchymal in origin, whereas few could be interstitial. Majority of tumors affecting major glands are benign, but those affecting minor salivary glands are more often than not, malignant. The disorders that involve these glands can either be acute or chronic inflammatory lesions, congenital abnormalities, systemic disorders, or benign and malignant tumors. However the most, common disorders affecting salivary glands are tumors and infections.

46.2 Surgical Anatomy

46.2.1 Parotid Gland

The gland lies in the retromandibular fossa bound medially by the styloid process and superiorly by external acoustic meatus and mastoid process, and it touches the medial pterygoid muscle and mandibular ramus (Fig. 46.1). A part of the gland may also cover the TMJ in front of the ear but never extends beyond the zygomatic arch. The parotid capsule is a dense, adherent fibrous condensation of deep cervical fascia which is tough and unyielding. Hence parotid space infections show minimal swelling but are severely painful. Incision and drainage is needed early on, without a frank fluctuant abscess to relieve the pressure within the capsule to prevent pressure necrosis of the parenchyma. Due to weakness in the capsule covering the deep surface of the gland, parotid abscess may spread into the lateral pharyngeal space, if not drained promptly [1]. Benign tumors grow slowly and hence take a longer time to manifest as external bulges. Parotid gland has a superficial lobe (80%) and a deep lobe (20%) connected by an isthmus with the facial nerve passing between the two lobes.

The facial nerve is related to the parotid gland in a number of ways [2].

1. (a) Superficial and deep lobes are united above, so that the gland is essentially folded over the nerve.
   (b) An isthmus uniting the two lobes.
   (c) Combination of (a) and (b)
2. The gland and nerve can also lie intertwined within superficial and deep lobes; relation will vary according to plane of section.

The intratemporal and intraparotid facial nerve has varied pattern of branching which is of immense surgical importance and might show bifurcation and trifurcation of the main trunk within the mastoid segment (Fig. 46.2). This intratemporal division of the facial nerve is associated with congenital abnormalities of the pinna or inner ear (Table 46.1).

Parotid duct or the Stensen's duct crosses the masseter about a finger breadth below the zygomatic arch. It then takes a sharp turn medially at the anterior border of the masseter further traversing through the buccal fat pad and buccinator muscle. It then runs obliquely between the buccinator and oral mucosa to open on the parotid papilla, opposite the second maxillary molar. The obliquity of the duct in between the buccinator and mucosa acts like a valve to prevent inflation of the duct while blowing air. The duct lies between the upper and lower buccal branches of the facial nerve. Its caliber is about 3 mm, but at the point where it penetrates the buccinator muscle, an isthmus narrows down the duct to 1.2 mm, and at the orifice (ostium), it is 0.5 mm.

Electronic Supplementary Material The online version of this chapter (https://doi.org/10.1007/978-981-15-1346-6_46) contains supplementary material, which is available to authorized users.

N. A. Agni (✉)
Department of Oral and Maxillofacial Surgery, SMBT Institute of Dental Sciences and Research, Nashik, India

K. Bonanthaya et al. (eds.), *Oral and Maxillofacial Surgery for the Clinician*, https://doi.org/10.1007/978-981-15-1346-6_46

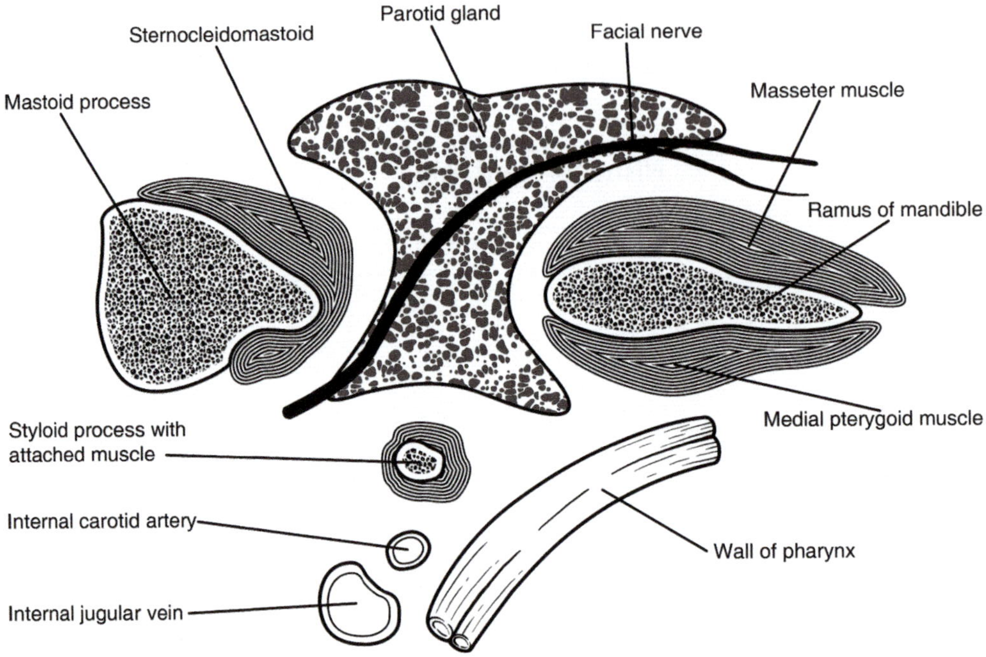

Fig. 46.1 Transverse section of parotid gland

Structures traversing the parotid gland from lateral to medial (superficial to deep) include the facial nerve, retromandibular vein, and external carotid artery. Few parotid lymph nodes are also present within the gland.

Parasympathetic secretomotor fibers from the inferior salivary nucleus of the ninth cranial nerve supply the gland. Nerve fibers pass to the otic ganglion via the tympanic branch of the glossopharyngeal nerve and the lesser petrosal nerve. Postganglionic parasympathetic fibers reach the parotid gland via the auriculotemporal nerve, which lies in contact with the deep surface of the gland. Postganglionic sympathetic fibers reach the gland as a plexus of nerves around the external carotid artery [4].

46.2.1.1 Identification of the Facial Nerve [5, 6]

The facial nerve identification can be done either proximally or distally. Proximally the main trunk of the nerve is identified before it enters the gland. Distally it is identified as branches after the nerve leaves the gland (Table 46.2).

There are four facial nerve pointers at the stylomastoid foramen. However more techniques have been added later on by various authors. They are as follows:

1. The cartilaginous pointer of Conley (1978) is created at its anterior inferior border and is the least reliable one. The backward pull on the cartilage causes the meatus to assume the shape of a horn, the curved extremity of which allegedly points to the position of the facial nerve. The nerve is located medial and inferior to the pointer (Fig. 46.3).
2. A short segment of the facial nerve lies in between the stylomastoid foramen and parotid gland and is an ideal location to identify it. It can be located in the tympanomastoid sulcus which is formed by the edge of the bony external meatus and anterior face of the mastoid process. The nerve emerges from the stylomastoid foramen some 3–4 mm deep to the outer edge of the bony external canal. The tympanomastoid sulcus is filled with fibrofatty lobules that mimic the facial nerve trunk which may lie as deep as 1 cm to this landmark.
3. The anterior superior aspect of the posterior belly of the digastric muscle is inserted just behind the stylomastoid foramen. The posterior belly of the digastric muscle lies just inferior to the nerve and is the most reliable landmark to identify the nerve (Fig. 46.4).
4. The styloid process is a confirmatory landmark. The facial nerve lies lateral to the styloid process near the styloid base. The posterior auricular artery bleeds frequently while looking for the facial nerve since it lies below and just lateral to the nerve, and hence it cannot be relied upon for identification of the nerve.
5. Borle's triangle has been recently introduced to locate the facial nerve trunk. Lines are drawn from the tip of the mastoid process, running along the superior border of the posterior belly of digastric muscle and posterior border of the ramus of the mandible. These two lines intersect with each other anteriorly, forming the apex of the triangle (angle a). The base of the triangle is marked by drawing the third line starting from the tip of the mastoid process (angle b), running anteriorly till it joins

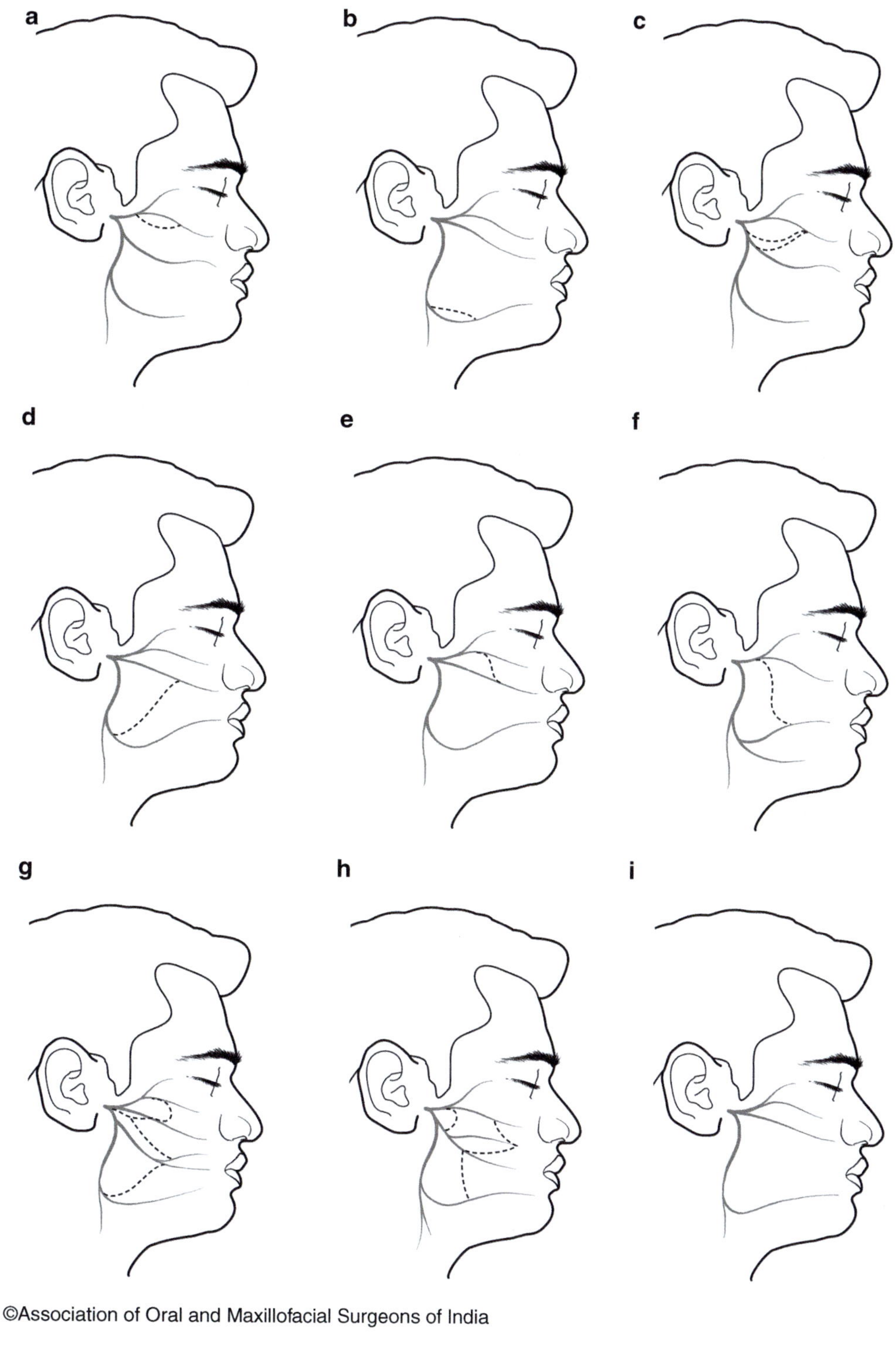

Fig. 46.2 (**a**)–(**i**) Katz-Catalano classification based on operative findings

Table 46.1 Katz-Catalano classification

Type 1	25%	Branches are separate
Type 2	14%	Buccal branch fuses with zygomatic branch
Type 3	44%	Major communicating, buccal, and other branches
Type 4	14%	Complex branching between all branches
Type 5	3%	More than one major trunk

Katz and Catalano [3], 1987

Table 46.2 Facial nerve identification

1	Anterograde approach—Direct identification of main trunk at stylomastoid foramen
2	Retrograde approach—Early identification of mandibular branch over posterior facial vein or other branches along the parotid duct
3	Supravital staining of parotid—gland is stained blue, tumor is unstained, and facial nerve is gleaming white

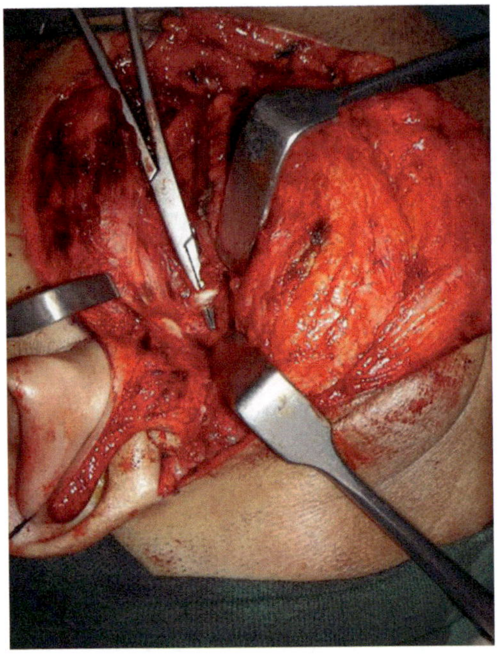

Fig. 46.3 Showing relation of cartilaginous pointer and facial nerve main trunk

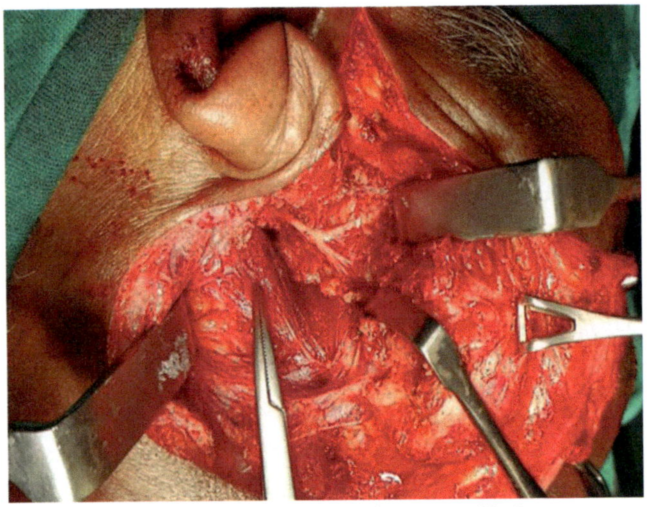

Fig. 46.4 Showing relation of the posterior belly of the digastric muscle and main trunk of the facial nerve (muscle pointed by mosquito forceps)

the second drawn line along the posterior border of the ramus (angle c). The facial nerve trunk is often found within this triangle just above the angle b formed by the first and the third line if gentle and blunt dissection is carried out at this point. The mean distance of nerve trunk from the angle b is 12.18 ± 2 mm within a range of 9–15 mm [7] [Fig. 46.5—https://www.ncbi.nlm.nih.gov/pmc/articles/PMC6126203/. doi: https://doi.org/10.1016/j.jobcr.2018.08.004. *(open access)*].

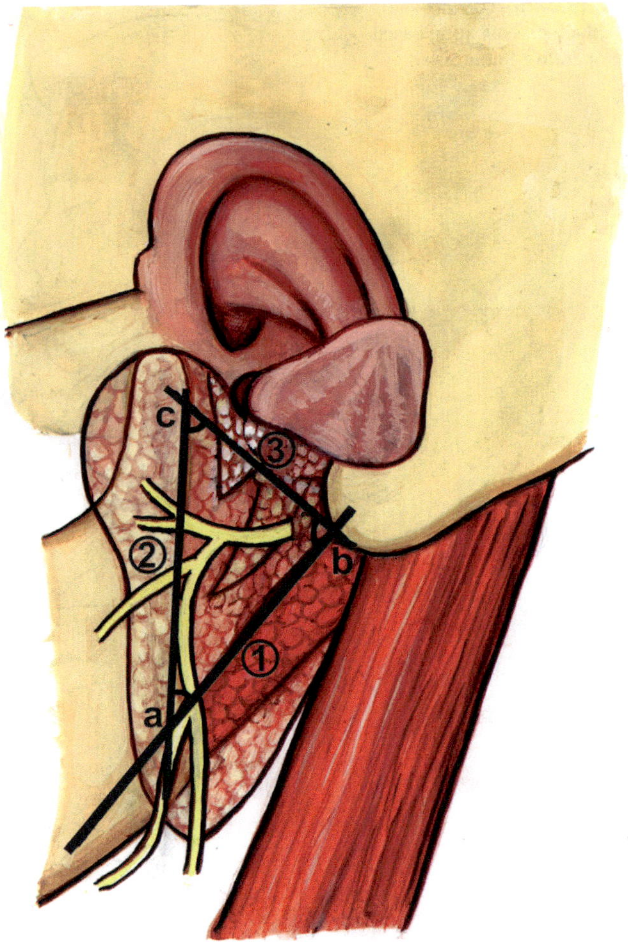

Fig. 46.5 Borle's triangle. *Line 1: Started from mastoid process tip and running along the superior border of posterior belly of the digastric muscle. Line 2: At the posterior border of ramus of the mandible. Line 3: Starts from the tip of the mastoid process running anteriorly till it joins the second line. Angle a: Lines 1 and 2 intersect with each other forming the apex of triangle. Angle b: Is the base of the triangle. Angle c: Is the angle where third line meets second line*

When identification of facial nerve trunk is difficult using the above said pointers due to distorted anatomy due to the tumor, a retrograde approach can be used by identifying a peripheral branch of the nerve and tracing it proximally. The easiest branch to locate is the marginal mandibular nerve. Baker et al. have reported that the marginal mandibular nerve is located 1–2 cm below the inferior border of the mandible. The marginal mandibular branch can be used to trace the facial nerve in a retrograde direction by identifying it at the point of emergence of the retromandibular vein and then carrying out a proximal dissection. By working backward along the nerve, the two divisions, the other branches, and the main trunk can be found [8].

Figure 46.6 represents the average distance of facial nerve pointers from the surrounding landmarks (Table 46.3).

Intraoperative facial nerve monitoring using electromyographic techniques can also be used for identification of the main branch or the peripheral branches in centripetal or retrograde approach. In pediatric population the facial nerve trunk

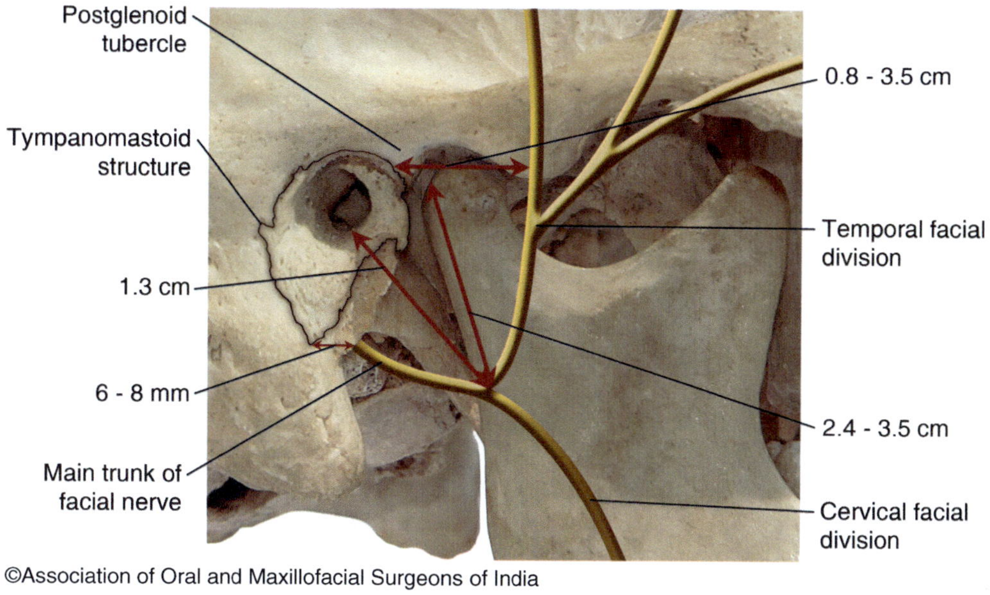

Fig. 46.6 Distance from facial nerve pointers

Table 46.3 Distance of the facial nerve pointers from the surrounding landmarks [10]

Sr. no.	Pointer	Distance in mm	Mean in mm
1	Tragal pointer	24.3–49.2	34
2	Posterior belly of the digastric muscle	9.7–24.3	14.6
3	External auditory canal	7.3–21.9	13.4
4	Tympanomastoid suture	4.9–18.6	10.0
5	Styloid process	4.3–18.6	9.7
6	Transverse process of axis	9.7–36.8	16.9
7	Angle of the mandible	25.3–48.69	38.1

exits the stylomastoid foramen and is found approximately 1 cm anterior to mastoid process and 1.5 cm posterior to the ramus of the mandible. The parotid does not extend posterior to the ramus of the mandible in the newborn infant and consequently covers only the lower distal branches of the nerve [9].

46.2.1.2 Facial Nerve Monitoring

There are two types of facial nerve monitoring:

- Electromyography
- Pressure or strain gauge sensor

Facial nerve monitoring is performed with a nerve stimulator which can either be monopolar or bipolar. The monopolar stimulator is more useful for identifying the nerve, while the bipolar is more useful if the nerve course is evident. However, a bipolar stimulator is more precise.

46.2.2 Submandibular Glands

It is a U-shaped gland with a smaller deep lobe and larger superficial lobe enveloping the mylohyoid muscle. Hence during surgical removal, the mylohyoid has to be retracted anteriorly to expose the deep lobe and the Wharton's duct. The capsule is loosely attached to the gland substance, and hence the gland can be shelled out easily.

Since the submandibular group of lymph nodes are in contact with the gland or embedded in it, it is essential to clear the nodes along with the gland during a neck dissection.

The facial artery loops around the submandibular gland. The facial artery is visualized by retracting the posterior belly of the digastric muscle inferiorly. Hence, during excision of the submandibular gland, the facial artery and vein were customarily ligated. However, during neck dissection, the current standard is to try and save it so that it can be used for anastomosis during a free flap reconstruction.

The facial artery is ligated away from the external carotid artery, so that in case the vessel retracts into the tissue, it can be located and religated and bleeding can be controlled. In case the ligature slips and the facial artery retracts, the posterior belly of the digastric muscle is divided for easy location of the bleeding vessel.

The lingual nerve passes below the duct and forms a loop around its outer aspect before inserting into the tongue mucosa. It is at risk when the deep part of the gland is being mobilized. The submandibular duct or Warton's duct is longer and has a tortous, uphill course. Thus the secretions have to be emptied against gravity, and there are increased chances of retention. Also, the mineral content of the secretion is high, especially calcium content which along with increased retention of secretions results into higher incidence of calculus formation and inflammatory pathologies in the submandibular gland and duct.

Figure 46.7a, b shows the relations of the submandibular gland.

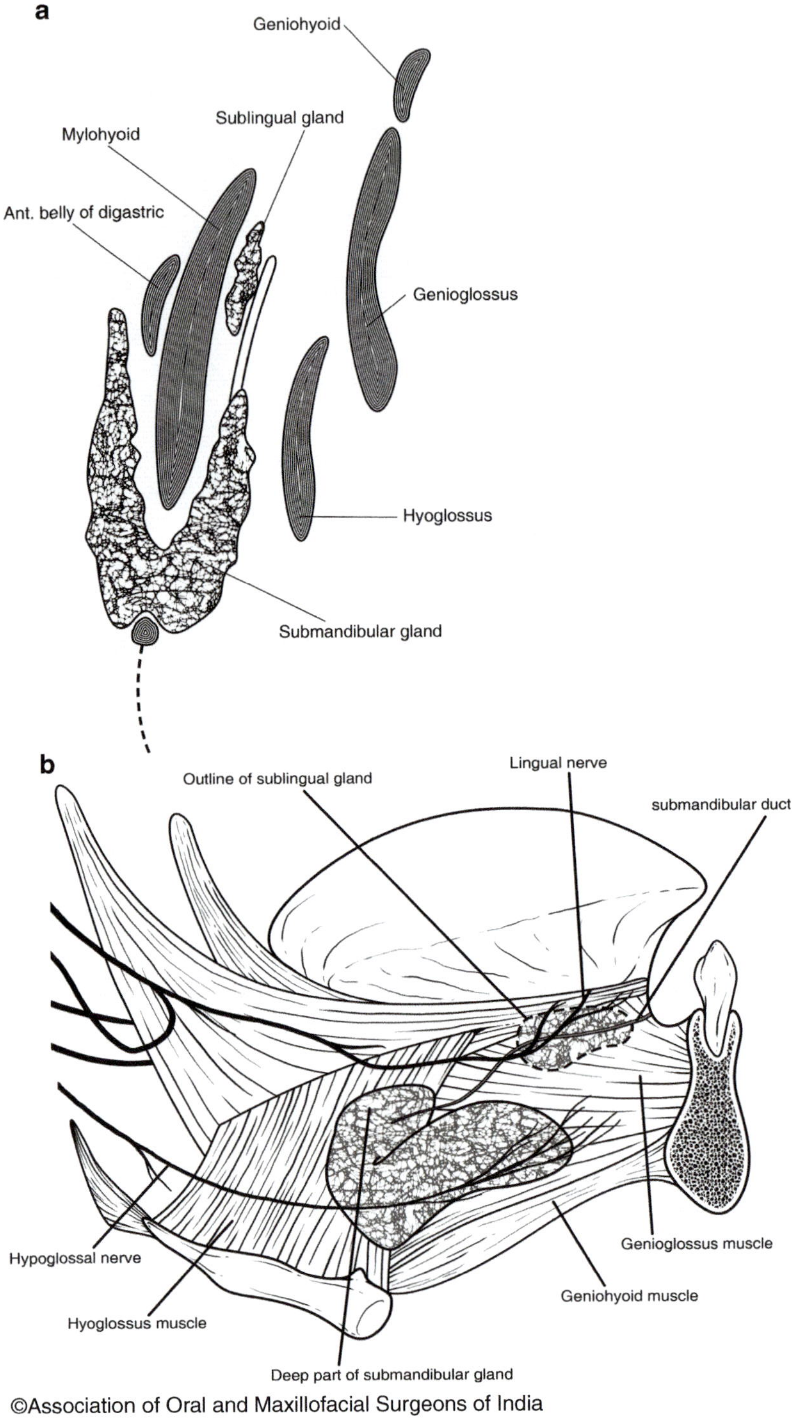

Fig. 46.7 (**a**, **b**) Relations of submandibular gland

46.2.3 Sublingual Glands

They are located beneath the mucosa of the floor of the mouth and appear as an elevation in the floor of the mouth. The excretory ducts of the sublingual glands are very superficially located and open in the floor of mouth at a superior level than the gland. Hence, they easily get damaged, and any trauma or infection of the ducts leads to salivary retention and formation of a mucous retention cyst which is called "ranula" due to its bluish color resembling the belly of a frog. The international statistical classification of diseases and related health problems shown in Table 46.4.

Table 46.4 International statistical classification of diseases and related health problems

K 11	Diseases of salivary glands
K 11.0	Atrophy of the salivary gland
K 11.1	Hypertrophy of the salivary gland
K 11.2	Sialadenitis
	Excludes epidemic parotitis and uveoparotid fever
K 11.3	Abscess of the salivary gland
K 11.4	Fistula of the salivary gland
	Excludes congenital fistula of the salivary gland
K 11.5	Sialolithiasis
	Calculus/stone of salivary gland or duct
K 11.6	Mucocele
	Mucous extravasation cyst/retention cyst
	Ranula
K 11.7	Disturbances of salivary secretion
	Hypoptyalism
	Ptyalism
	Xerostomia
	Excludes dry mouth NOS
K 11.8	Other diseases of the salivary glands
	Benign lymphoepithelial lesion of the salivary gland
	Mikulicz' disease
	Necrotizing sialometaplasia
	Sialectasia
	Stenosis/strictures of salivary ducts
	Excludes Sicca syndrome (Sjögren's syndrome)
K 11.9	Diseases of the salivary glands unspecified
	Sialoadenopathy NOS

10th Revision (Version for 2003) [11]

46.3 Diagnosis and Diagnostic Aids

A thorough history followed by meticulous examination holds the key to proper diagnosis of salivary gland pathologies. Salivary gland neoplasms are usually slow growing and non-tender. A slow-growing swelling of the salivary gland is suggestive of a neoplasm, whereas a sudden, painful swelling is suggestive of an infective pathology although it can sometimes indicate a malignant tumor with secondary infection. Nerve weakness and skin infiltration are always associated with malignant tumors which have already infiltrated the nerve or skin although the vice versa is not always true.

Major salivary glands are palpated, and secretions milked out to check flow, quantity, and quality of secretion. A turbid salivary discharge may indicate an infection, whereas reduced salivary flow could indicate either less secretion or obstruction to flow. Function of facial nerve should be checked and documented during parotid examination. On inspection submandibular gland swelling can be easily identified and compared with the contralateral side; however the submandibular glands are bimanually palpated (Figs. 46.8 and 46.9).

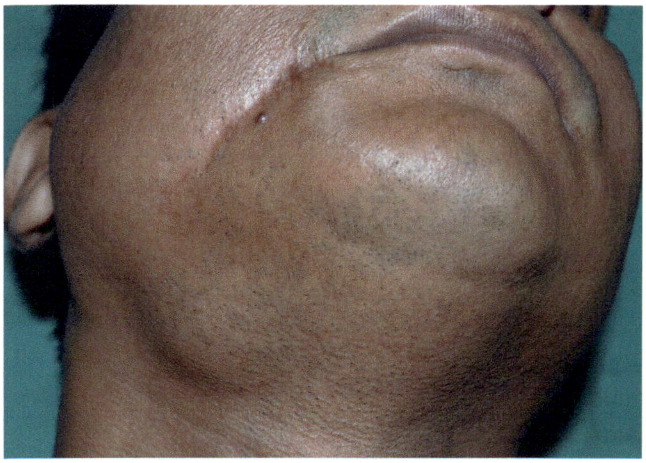

Fig. 46.8 Clinical photo showing submandibular gland enlargement, right side

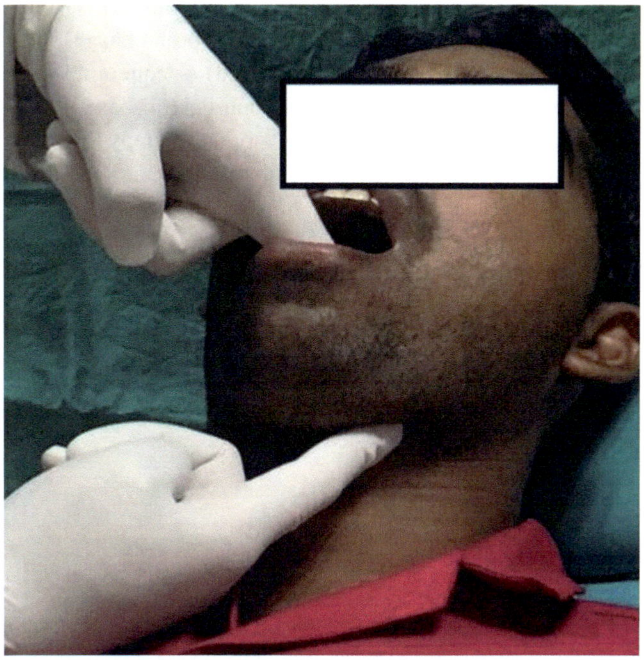

Fig. 46.9 Bimanual palpation

Various diagnostic aids for investigating salivary gland diseases are as follows:

1. Diagnostic imaging
   (a) Routine radiographs: It is useful only for diagnosing sialoliths and parenchymal calcifications. Radiopaque salivary calculi in the gland or duct can be picked up on plain films such as occlusal X-ray for submandibular gland and duct and a posteroanterior (PA) skull with blown-out cheeks for parotid calculi.

(b) Ultrasonography: Ultrasonography (USG) is a noninvasive modality that utilizes non-ionizing radiation, gives good soft tissue discrimination, has excellent sensitivity for mass lesions, and can be repeated as frequently as required. Normal gland is relatively homogenously hyperechoic than adjacent muscle, and so is cyst and tumor from parenchyma [12, 13]. It helps to distinguish a cystic lesion from a solid mass in space-occupying lesion (Fig. 46.10). USG with color Doppler is useful to rule out vascular lesions and also aids in assessing vascularity of lesions.

(c) Sialography: It assesses obstructive pathology by instillation of radiopaque contrast medium to locate obstruction in the ductal system. The technique is more or less obsolete now with the advent of MRI imaging. It is a technique which involves injection of a radiopaque dye into the ductal system of the major salivary glands and taking plain X-rays to see the pattern of the dye into the ductal systems. Most commonly the contrast dyes used are iodine based. They can either be lyophilic (oil based) or aqueous (water based or water soluble). Lyophilic (oil-based) contrast dyes include Lipiodol (iodized poppy seed oil) and Pantopaque (organic iodine compound). Aqueous contrast dyes include iothalamate (Conray) and metrizoate (Triosil). Aqueous-based dyes are most commonly preferred. Sialography is indicated to diagnose obstructive pathologies and duct anomalies, degenerative changes in the gland, chronic inflammatory conditions, and intra- and extraglandular tumors. It is contraindicated in acute infections of the gland and in case of allergies to the dye.

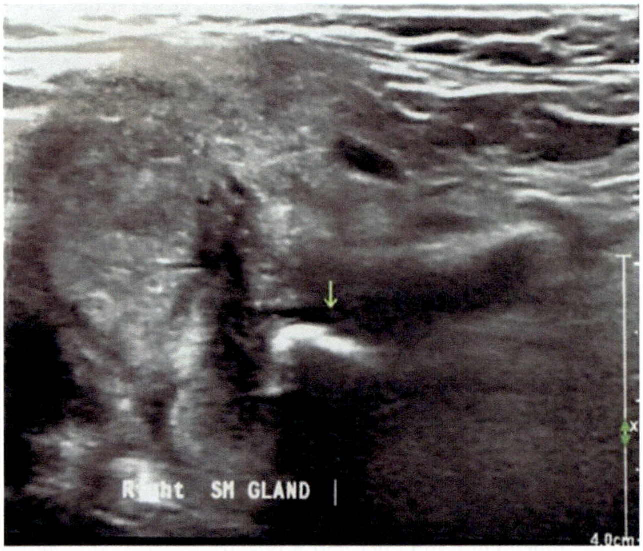

Fig. 46.10 USG of submandibular gland

Procedure: The duct orifice is enlarged using a lacrimal probe and cannulated with a 22 gauge cannula after infiltrating local anesthetic (Fig. 46.11a, b). The selected dye is injected into the ductal system using a Luer lock syringe with gentle continuous pressure with simultaneous massage of the gland. Once the patient feels some discomfort, dye injection is stopped. X-rays are taken during the filling phase and emptying phase as well.

The X-rays show different patterns:

(i) The normal parotid gland shows "tree in winter" or "leafless tree" pattern, and submandibular gland shows "bush in winter" appearance. This is because the normal acini do not allow dye to enter and it is seen only in the ducts and ductules (Fig. 46.12—normal sialography: leafless tree).
(ii) In chronic inflammation the dye enters the ductules, and the empty acini give a "blossom tree" or "leafy tree" appearance.
(iii) Sjögren's syndrome and Mikulicz' disease show a "snow storm" or "branchless fruit-laden" appearance.
(iv) Stricture in a duct is seen as a filling defect, whereas multiple strictures show a sausage string appearance.
(v) "Cannon ball" appearance is seen in intraglandular tumors, whereas extraglandular tumors show a "ball in hand" appearance.
(vi) Duct perforation and sialocele show dye spillage in the soft tissues.

(d) Radionucleotide scanning: It is used to distinguish between obstructive and nonobstructive sialadenitis. It involves both dynamic and static scanning. Radionuclide scanning is useful when a sialogram is contraindicated to distinguish between acute obstructive and nonobstructive sialadenitis [14].

(e) CT scan: It is used to evaluate masses in parotid glands and surrounding structures as it gives excellent soft tissue details (Fig. 46.13) especially when used with a contrast dye. Bony changes in the course of facial nerve like erosions, sclerotic margins, and widening of stylomastoid foramen or fallopian canal suggest involvement of nerve. Plain computed tomography (CT) scans have a major role to play for diagnosis of obstructive pathologies like a calculus.

(f) MRI scan: It allows assessment of salivary masses and early diagnosis of perineural spread due to excellent soft tissue contrast. In the case of neoplasms, it helps in demonstrating involvement of the facial nerve (Fig. 46.14).

(g) Arteriography: It assesses the vascularity and source of vascular supply of the tumors.

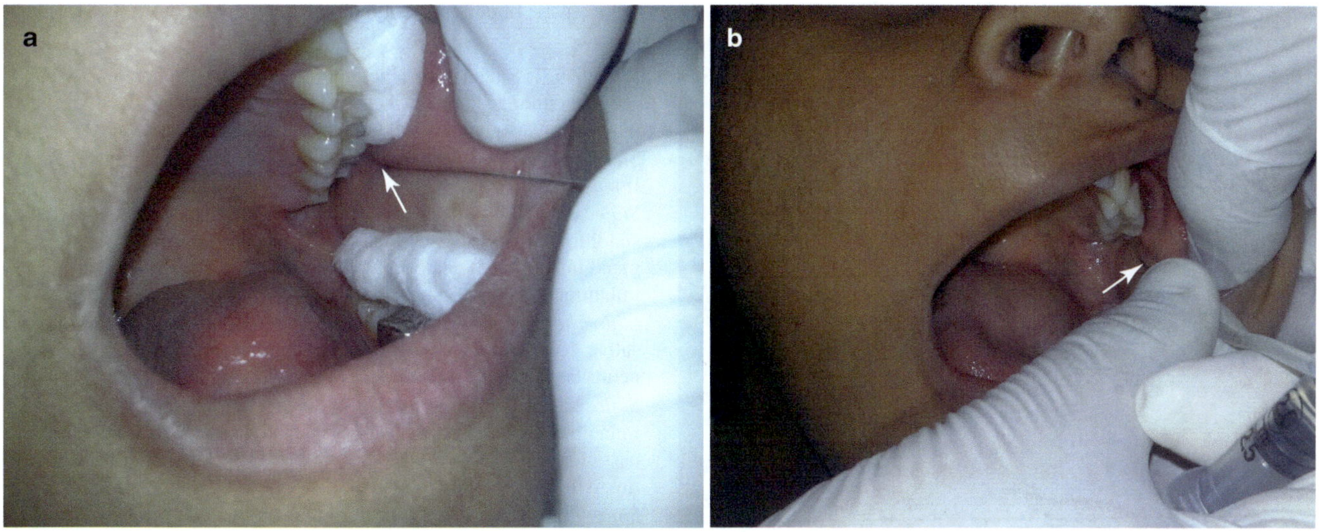

Fig. 46.11 (**a**, **b**) Sialography technique

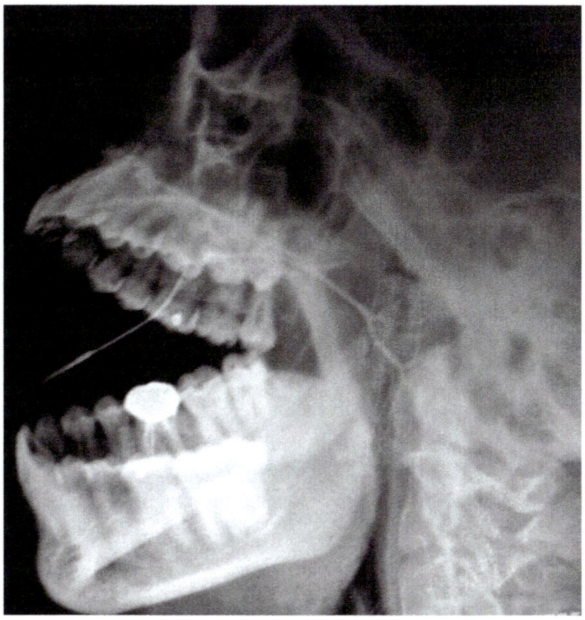

Fig. 46.12 Normal parotid gland in sialography

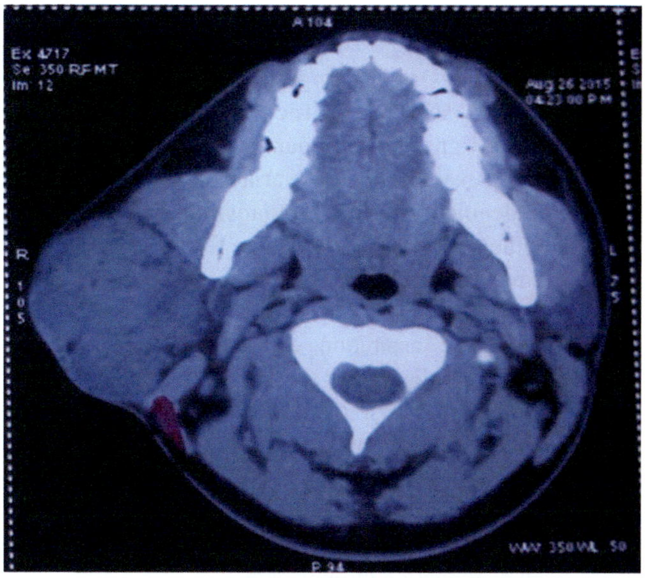

Fig. 46.13 CT scan showing parotid tumor

(h) Positron emission tomography (PET): Uptake of radiotracer fluorodeoxyglucose used with PET scans by salivary glands makes this diagnostic technique useful for salivary gland tumors. Although this is an expensive technique, measurement of metabolic activity makes it more reliable than CT and MRI scans. It can be used to diagnose recurrences, tumor hypoxia, and proliferation rates [15].

2. Histopathology: The gold standard of diagnosis for neoplasms will always be histopathology (HPE). However, as the major salivary glands are deeper structures, an FNAC (fine-needle aspiration cytology) is considered as a standard of care for diagnosis to avoid tumor seeding, which might follow an open biopsy. An open biopsy can be considered for minor salivary gland tumors or malignant tumors affecting major salivary glands with skin infiltration, needing skin excision to achieve surgical clearance. HPE for salivary gland

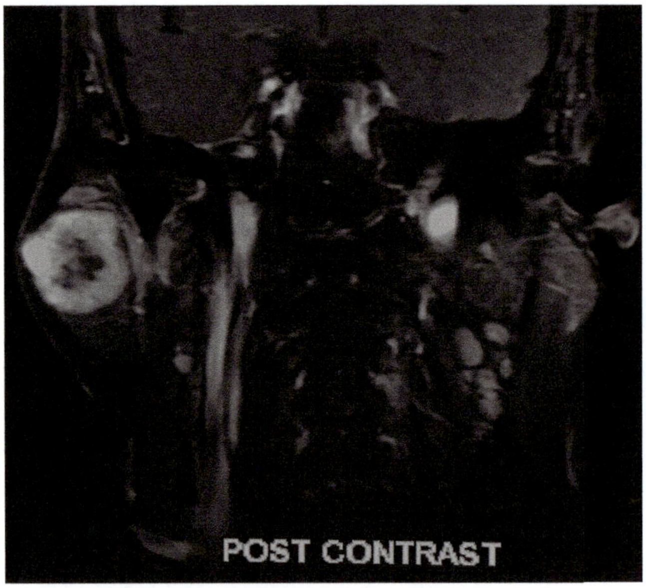

Fig. 46.14 MRI showing parotid tumor, right side

pathologies is very challenging, and hence diagnosing lesions on FNAC is more difficult. It is important to distinguish benign and malignant pathologies on FNAC even if the exact malignant variant is missed, because except adenoid cystic carcinoma which has perineurial spread, the surgery doesn't change for any other malignant tumor variant.

(a) Fine-needle aspiration cytopathology (FNAC): It shows high diagnostic accuracy both for benign and malignant tumors. Complete histological features and status of invasion can't be revealed by this technique.
(b) Incisional biopsy: It is not a reliable technique as there is high possibility of seeding of tumor cells as well as fungation through skin.

3. Frozen sections: These help in diagnosing the nature of tumor, but accurate histopathologic features can't be diagnosed.

46.4 Non-neoplastic Diseases (Table 46.5)

46.4.1 Acute Bacterial Sialadenitis

Parotitis (Fig. 46.15) occurs secondary to decreased salivary secretions, and various reasons are attributed.

Table 46.5 Important terminologies in relation to salivary gland diseases

Sialadenitis: Sialadenitis is inflammation of the gland parenchyma. It could either be suppurative (with pus) or nonsuppurative (without pus). It can also be classified as acute, subacute, or chronic.
Sialodochitis: This refers to inflammation of the salivary gland duct. It may be associated with duct strictures and/or sialoliths.
Sialectasis: This refers to cystic dilatation of the ducts due to either a sialolith or ductal strictures. It is most commonly seen in parotid gland infections. It can occur due to any condition causing chronic inflammation of the gland.
Sialorrhea: This refers to excessive secretion of saliva or drooling of saliva. It is most commonly seen in patients with cerebral palsy and neuro-degenerative disorders.
Sialosis: It is defined as an asymptomatic, non-neoplastic, non-inflammatory parenchymal salivary gland disease which manifests as persistent painless bilateral salivary gland swelling, most commonly involving the parotid gland [16].
Sialodochoplasty: It is repair of the salivary gland duct usually by translocating the ductal opening.

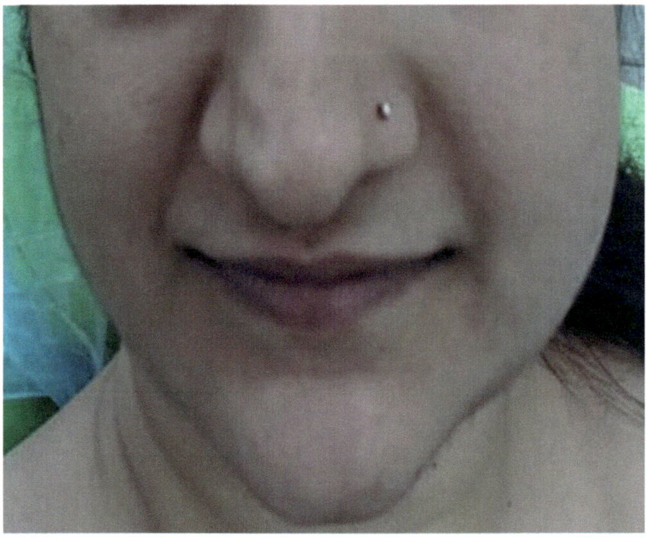

Fig. 46.15 Parotitis left side

The common etiologic factors for parotitis are reduced salivary flow due to severe dehydration, in patients with debilitating diseases, old age, post-operative patients, post radiotherapy for head and neck cancers, poor oral hygiene leading to recurrent infection, mechanical obstruction to flow, compromised host resistance due to systemic illnesses like Diabetes Mellitus, renal failure, HIV, post transplant immunosuppresants. The drugs which induce systemic dehydration such as antihypertensives, diuretics, tricyclic antidepressants , phenothiazines, barbiturates, anticholinergics and betablockers also lead to reduced salivary flow rate [17].

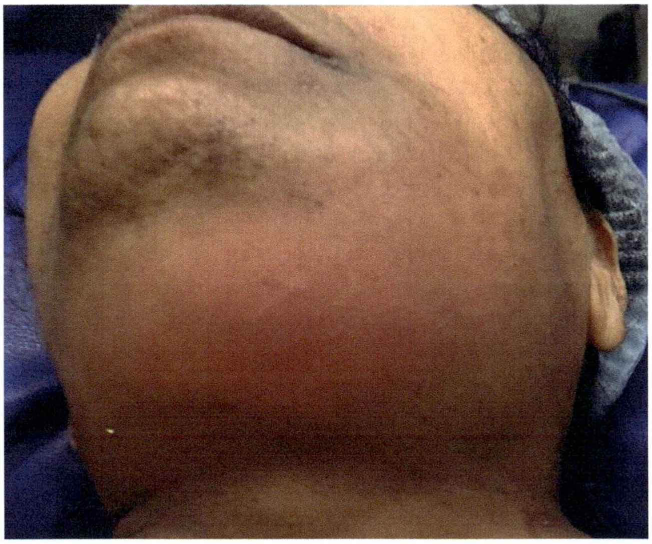

Fig. 46.16 Submandibular sialadenitis left side

It may be retrograde contamination of salivary ducts and parenchymal tissues by oral microflora providing a bacterial source of infection. Stasis of salivary flow through the ducts and parenchyma may also promote acute suppurative infection. There is a higher risk of sialolith in the submandibular duct causing secondary suppurative sialadenitis (Fig. 46.16 showing submandibular sialadenitis).

46.4.1.1 Clinical Features

- Sudden onset of pain and swelling, exacerbates with food sighting or smelling
- Generalized malaise, fever, body ache, and sometimes signs of dehydration.
- Diffuse inflammatory swelling, induration, erythema, edema, and extreme tenderness over the affected gland.
- Tense, glossy, and erythematous skin.
- Raised ear lobule is pathognomonic sign of parotid swelling.
- The duct orifices are inflamed, and milking of gland may exhibit lesser salivation or purulence.
- Systemic sepsis occurs more commonly in parotid sialadenitis as compared to submandibular sialadenitis.
- Parotid swellings are not fluctuant due to fixity of overlying investing parotideomasseteric fascia and are extremely painful due to the mounting pressure as the fascia is nonyielding. This mounting pressure leads to ischemic necrosis of the gland, and the abscess may spontaneously burst in the external auditory canal.

Routine blood count to rule out impending sepsis in addition to a plain radiograph or USG to rule out a sialolith in the duct is indicated. Sialography is contraindicated in cases of acute infections and also sialoliths. Aspiration might not yield frank pus.

46.4.1.2 Management

Treatment is managing underlying cause and adequate hydration and systemic antibiotics. If swelling doesn't subside with medical management in 2 days or shows an increasing trend, an incision and drainage is indicated. The cellulitic phase may not yield any frank pus, but toxic fluid is drained and it releases the pressure over the gland and prevents pressure necrosis of the gland parenchyma. Parotid space abscess has the tendency to spread into the pharyngeal spaces and cause respiratory distress and descending mediastinitis or burst into the auditory canal or TMJ and cause septic arthritis of the TMJ.

46.4.2 Chronic Bacterial Sialadenitis [18]

It is a recurrent sialadenitis with episodic relapsing swellings of the salivary glands, most commonly seen in the parotid gland. Salivary retention and stasis are the main predisposing factor. It might be preceded by an acute sialadenitis. Strictures may also form in the ducts leading to salivary stasis and eventually chronic sialadenitis. Generalized constitutional symptoms may be low grade, and salivary gland milking may yield scanty saliva. MRI is more specific than CT scan.

46.4.2.1 Management

Management consists of short-term corticosteroids to eliminate glandular inflammation followed by use of sialogogues to increase salivation and flush the debris. Sialoendoscopy can play a role in increasing the salivary flow.

The sialoendoscope is advanced slowly into the duct with continuous saline irrigation to help visualize the system and also dilating the strictures with help of the sialoballoon. This is followed up by placing a stent into the duct for 4 weeks.

Superficial parotidectomy with facial nerve preservation can also be considered in case of chronic pain, provided imaging studies determine the involvement of superficial lobe.

Chronic recurrent parotitis if left untreated may lead to benign lymphoepithelial lesion which can progress to lymphoproliferative disorders like non-Hodgkin's lymphoma, carcinoma, or pseudolymphoma.

46.4.3 Obstructive Disorders (Video 46.1)

Sialolithiasis or salivary calculi are most commonly seen in the submandibular gland and duct (Fig. 46.17a, b). Symptomatic calculi are much lesser in occurrence. Only those cases with superadded infection and inflammation of the gland and duct result into pain.

46.4.3.1 Etiology

Salivary stasis is a major etiologic factor for formation of sialolith. The right-angle bend of the Stenson's duct where it pierces the buccinator and the 90° bend of the Wharton's duct at the border of the mylohyoid is the common location for sialoliths. They can also result from chronic sialadenitis. Systemic abnormalities of calcium metabolism are not associated with any increased risk of salivary stone formations. Gout is the only systemic illness known to predispose to salivary stone formation [19].

Salivary stasis changes the mucoid element of saliva to a gel framework for deposition of salts and organic substances creating a stone. Unknown metabolic phenomenon increases salivary bicarbonate content altering the calcium phosphate solubility and leading to precipitation of calcium and phosphate ions [20]. Wharton's duct is longer than the Stenson's duct, and the submandibular gland is situated at a lower level than the opening of the duct. Hence the duct has to follow an uphill, tortuous course and drain against gravity. So stagnation of secretions is more common than parotid gland.

In the submandibular gland, the calculus results in sialadenitis, whereas in the parotid gland, sialadenitis causes calculus formation. In the parotid gland, stones are most commonly located at the hilum or parenchyma, whereas submandibular sialoliths develop in the duct [21]. Sometimes typically the sialolith is expelled out of the gland through the duct and is seen at the duct orifice.

46.4.3.2 Diagnosis and Management

Sialography can be used for diagnosis of sialoliths but is contraindicated if the calculus is already diagnosed on plain radiographs. Smaller stones can be expelled out through the

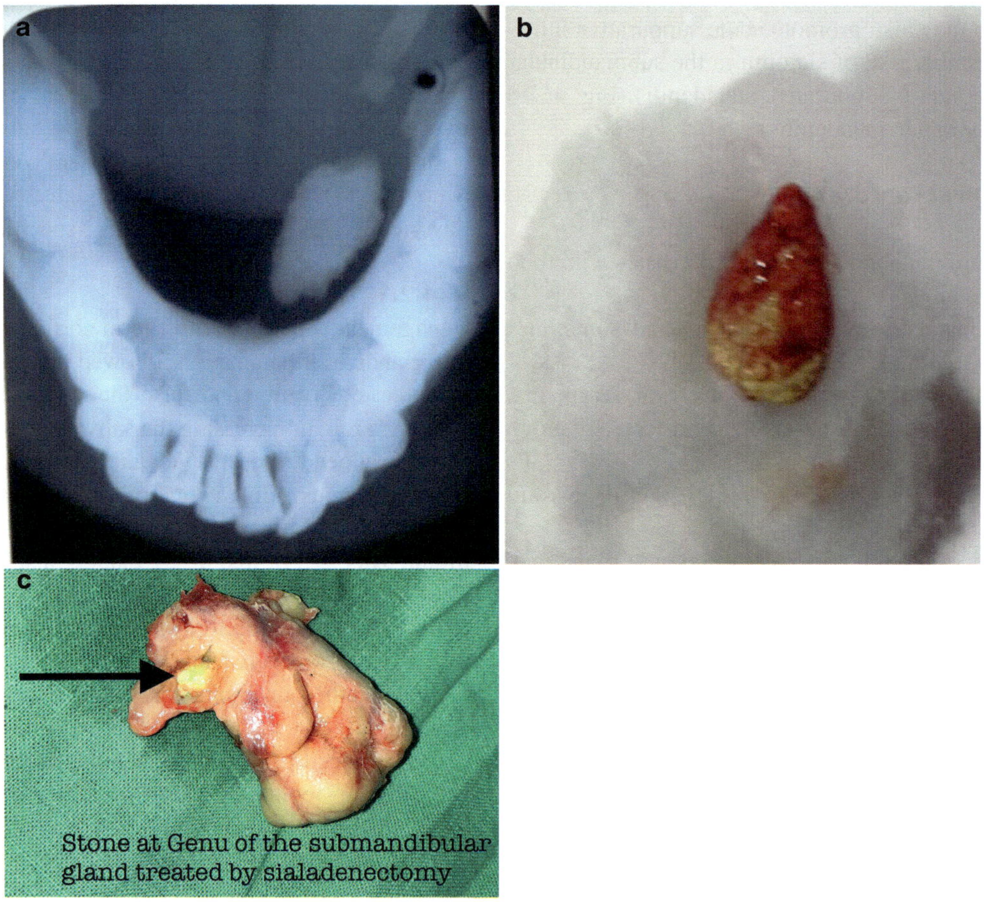

Fig. 46.17 (**a**, **b**) Left—Submandibular duct calculus (**a**). Right—Calculus after surgical removal (**b**). (**c**) Submandibular gland specimen showing calculus at the gene

duct opening using local massage, sialogogues, and adequate hydration. Larger stones are managed surgically according to its location in the duct and gland.

If the stone is palpable in the oral course of the duct, the duct is dilated with a lacrimal probe and cut open to retrieve the stone. The duct margins are sutured to the adjacent mucosa to avoid stricture formation. A stay suture can be placed around the duct proximal to the stone to avoid accidental pushing of the stone into deeper inaccessible part of the duct. In submandibular stones which are at the genu of the duct or deeper into the gland, a sialadenectomy is needed (Fig. 46.17c).

If the sialolith is posterior in the duct, a suture is placed behind the stone to prevent slippage of stone into the duct. The incision is placed over the duct to extract the stone, and the duct is left without suturing (Fig. 46.18a, b).

Sialodochoplasty is a procedure wherein the incised duct margins are sutured with adjacent mucosa leading to a translocation of duct orifice [22, 23].

In the case of parotid sialoliths, only those in the duct distal to the masseter muscle can be accessed transorally and removed. All deeper stones warrant a parotidectomy.

Extracorporeal shock wave lithotripsy and use of sialoendoscopy are newer modalities to manage sialoliths. Lithotripsy reduces calculi to small fragments that are then flushed out of the duct with spontaneous salivation or use of sialogogue [24]. The primary requirement for salivary stone lithotripsy is a functional gland which produces saliva which will clear the fragmented stone. A "gum test" which involves chewing of a sour gum can be done to test the functionality of the salivary gland. If the salivary secretions are normal, a visible swelling in the region of the gland will be noticed. If the test is negative, the patient cannot be taken up for lithotripsy.

46.5 Viral Infections of Salivary Glands

46.5.1 Mumps

Mumps is an acute nonsuppurative viral parotitis caused by paramyxovirus also known as epidemic parotitis. The term "mumps" is derived from the Danish word "Mompen" which means mumbling (like an old man) and describes the difficulty with speech because of inflammation and trismus [17].

46.5.1.1 Pathogenesis

It is an endemic disease and spreads by airborne droplet dissemination. It has an incubation of 2–3 weeks followed by 3–5-day viremia. The virus localizes to the salivary glands,

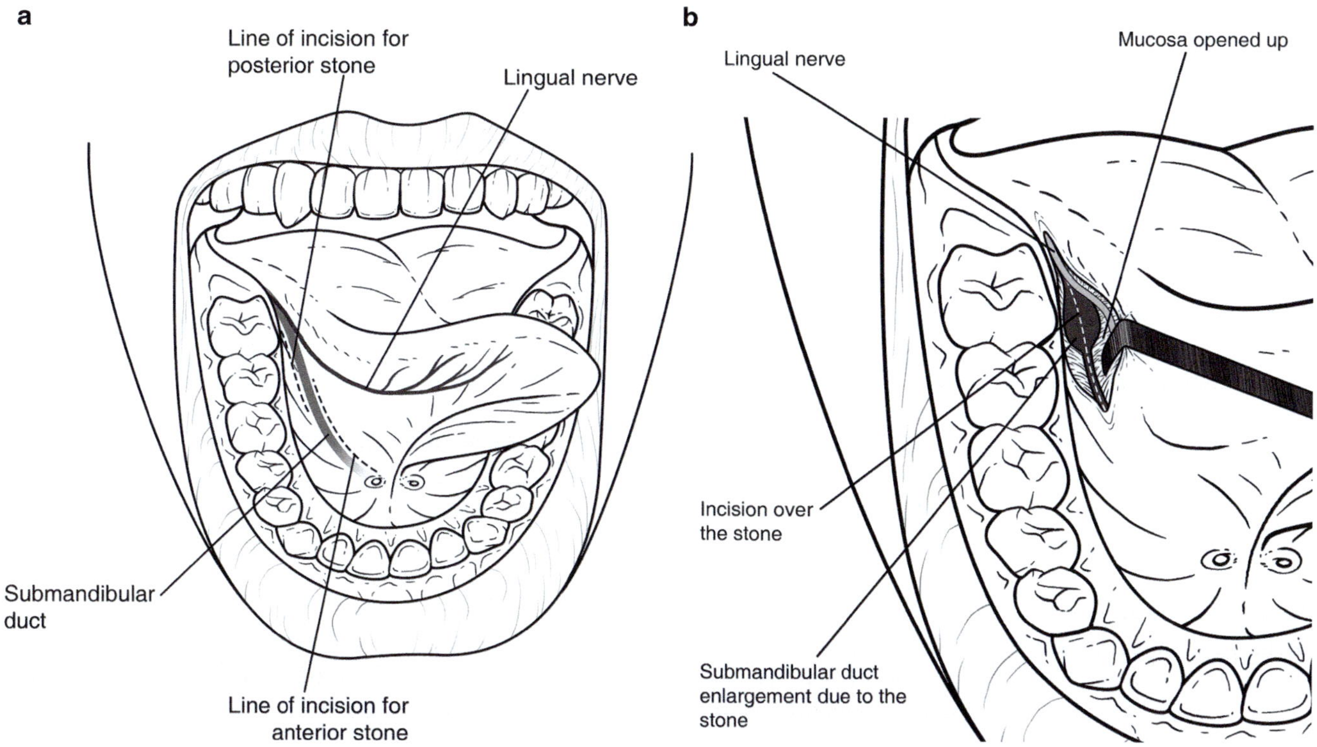

Fig. 46.18 (a, b) Technique of sialolith removal from submandibular duct

germinal tissues, and CNS [25]. The infection has a strong predilection for the parotid gland. It is highly contagious and occurs in children below 15 years of age with peak incidence being in the 4- to 6-year-old group of children [26]. Adults are rarely infected due to the immunity because of childhood exposure or due to the MMR vaccine [17].

46.5.1.2 Clinical Features

Prodromal symptoms include headache, myalgias, arthralgias, anorexia, and malaise prior to development of parotitis. It starts with an earache, pain around the gland, trismus, and dysphagia. Pain is exacerbated by salivary stimulation during meals. The parotid papilla may be inflamed and puffy. Palpation of the gland reveals a swelling of the gland which may be tense, rubbery, and firm with non-pitting-type edema. The overlying skin is tensed and shiny without erythema or increased local temperature. Swelling lasts for 1–5 days and can displace the pinna. Seventy-five percent cases result in bilateral involvement of parotid gland. However, it begins as a unilateral swelling and involves the contralateral gland after a period of 1–5 days [25].

Diagnosis is primarily clinical, but a blood count shows leukocytopenia with relative lymphocytosis. Serum amylase levels are also raised. It peaks during the first week and starts declining in the second or third week and comes back to normal later [25].

"S" or soluble antibodies directed against the nucleoprotein core of the virus appear within the first week of infection and peak within 2 weeks and disappear within 8–9 months. "V" or viral antibodies directed against the outer surface hemagglutinin appear several weeks after the "S" antibodies and persist at low levels for approximately 5 years following exposure. A fourfold rise in antibody titer is diagnostic of active infection. Mumps skin test is not useful in the diagnosis of acute infection because dermal hypersensitivity does not develop until 3 or 4 weeks following viral exposure.

46.5.1.3 Treatment

The disease is self-limiting, and treatment is primarily supportive such as rest, adequate hydration, antipyretics, and anti-inflammatory medicines.

Live attenuated Jerry Lynn vaccine is given combined with measles and rubella as MMR vaccine after 12 months of age. Immunized population is less likely to get the disease but may be infected with a nonparamyxovirus.

46.5.1.4 Complications

Orchitis and oophoritis can occur as systemic manifestations and rarely lead to complete sterility. Mastitis has been associated with decreased lactation. Aseptic meningitis occurs in 10% of cases, and asymptomatic meningeal inflammation is more common. Five percent patients are affected by acute pancreatitis, wherein serum lipase levels are also increased. Sensorineural hearing loss complicates 0.05–4% of patients and may be permanent and profound [26]. Tinnitus, aural fullness, and vertigo are associated symptoms, but they resolve over a period of few weeks. Additional complications include myocarditis, polyarthritis, hemolytic anemia, plasmacytosis, lymphocytic leukemoid reactions, and thrombocytopenia [12]. These conditions are self-limiting or resolve with or without steroid therapy.

46.5.2 HIV Parotitis

HIV-associated salivary gland disease is the term used to describe the diffuse enlargement of the salivary glands that affects HIV patients throughout all stages of the disease. In fact, HIV-SGD may be the first presenting sign of HIV. Like most of the salivary diseases, the parotid gland is the most frequently affected. Clinically, HIV-infected individuals show reduced salivary flow rates. Parotid gland enlargement is reported to occur in 1–10% of the HIV-infected population. It is usually secondary to development of benign lymphoepithelial cysts within the parotid gland [25].

46.5.2.1 Management

Antiretroviral therapy with zidovudine, maintenance of oral hygiene, and use of sialogogues form the mainstay of management.

46.6 Noninfectious Inflammatory Diseases

Mikulicz' disease and Sjögren's syndrome are closely related to each other and are autoimmune in origin, wherein the salivary tissue itself becomes antigenic [27].

46.6.1 Mikulicz' Disease

46.6.1.1 Clinical Features [28]

Middle-aged females are affected commonly. It behaves like an inflammatory as well as a neoplastic disease. Presenting symptoms may be diffuse, poorly outlined, unilateral or bilateral enlargement of the parotid or submandibular glands with an occasional increase or decrease in size of the swelling. There is mild local discomfort, occasional pain, and xerostomia. Fever, upper respiratory tract infection, tooth extraction, or some other local inflammatory disorder may precede the disease. Sometimes the lacrimal glands may be enlarged. FNAC can help diagnose the condition.

46.6.1.2 Management

Mild cases once diagnosed do not warrant any treatment. In some cases, the swelling might regress spontaneously. Persistent cases can be managed by sialadenectomy [28].

46.6.2 Sjögren's Syndrome

Sjögren's syndrome or Sicca syndrome is a chronic autoimmune disorder of the exocrine glands involving multiple extraglandular sites and can even evolve into a lymphoid malignancy. Sjögren's syndrome shows a triad of symptoms—keratoconjunctivitis sicca, xerostomia, and a systemic disease, usually but not always rheumatoid arthritis. Primary Sjögren's syndrome also known as Sicca complex presents with only dry eyes and dry mouth. Secondary Sjögren's syndrome has in addition to the above features systemic manifestations such as systemic lupus erythematosus, polyarteritis nodosa, polymyositis or scleroderma, and rheumatoid arthritis [28].

Arthritis is the most frequent first complaint, followed by ocular complaints and then xerostomia which leads to difficulty in chewing and swallowing, sore mouth, recurrent dental caries, and fungal infections in the oral cavity. The tongue appears bald with loss of filiform papillae and fissuring of tongue. The saliva is usually cloudy due to pus and abnormally viscous due to gel-like consistency. Parotid gland enlargement is seen in 25–66% cases of primary Sjögren's syndrome but is uncommon in secondary cases. Xeropthalmia leads to chronic irritation and destruction of the corneal and bulbar conjunctival epithelium, referred to as keratoconjunctivitis sicca. The patient complains of redness, itchiness, or burning sensation in the eye, rope-like secretions, dryness, and a foreign body sensation in the eye and may not be able to tolerate smoke, air draft, or light [27].

Schirmer's test is used to confirm lacrimal secretions. Patients complain of easy fatigue, general malaise, low-grade fever, myalgias, and arthralgias. Respiratory tract symptoms range from dry cough due to xerotrachea to dyspnea due to interstitial disease or even airway obstruction. High-resolution CT scan shows bronchial and peribronchial thickening, whereas transbronchial biopsies show bronchiolar lymphoid infiltrates and follicular bronchiolitis [29]. Sensorineural hearing loss is associated with Sjögren's syndrome in 21–46% of cases [30]. Dysphagia results from drying of the pharynx and esophagus. Other complications include renal disease, Raynaud's disease, inflammatory vascular disease, peripheral sensory or sensorimotor polyneuropathy or mononeuritis multiplex, skin dryness, vasculitis, and frequent allergic reactions. Labial salivary gland biopsy is used as a means of assessment of salivary pathology in Sjögren's syndrome.

46.6.2.1 Management

Xerostomia and keratoconjunctivitis sicca are managed by use of 0.5% methylcellulose artificial saliva and tears. Preventive dental care and fluoride application and maintenance of general hygiene are necessary. Eye patching and boric acid ointment can be used for corneal ulcers. Pilocarpine hydrochloride can be used as a secretagouge for management of xeropthalmia and xerostomia. Systemic corticosteroids can be used for systemic complications such as vasculitis, glomerulonephritis, and interstitial lung disease.

46.6.3 Mucoceles (Video 46.2)

Mucous retention cyst arises from ductal obstruction in a minor or accessory salivary gland due to traumatic severance of the duct due to biting of the lips, cheeks, and tongue or due to injury due to lip pinching during extraction. Majority of cases are an extravasation type of cysts which result from collection of salivary secretions in the soft tissues due to traumatic injury to the gland or duct. Lower lip was affected in 44–79% of cases. It occurs in any age with no gender predilection [31].

46.6.3.1 Clinical Features

Superficial lesions appear like a circumscribed, raised vesicle with a bluish translucent hue due to the thin overlying mucosa. However, deeper lesions being covered by normal mucosa have a normal color and texture. Mucoceles may get traumatized and rupture spontaneously and may recur later.

46.6.3.2 Management

Surgical excision of the mucocele along with a few normal minor salivary glands is the procedure of choice. Care should be taken to avoid creation of any other partially transected minor salivary glands which might give rise to the recurrent mucocele.

Mucocele can be excised by giving an elliptical incision around the lesion and closure (Fig. 46.19a–d), [32] or as the case requires, an incision may be given over the mucocele; lesion can be excised carefully without rupture and closure attained (Fig. 46.19e–h).

Huang I et al. [33] recommended use of carbon dioxide laser vaporization to treat the lower lip mucocele with good results and less complications.

46.6.4 Ranula

Ranula is a mucocele arising from the sublingual salivary gland in the floor of the mouth (Fig. 46.20). It presents as a large blue, tense vesicle in the floor of the mouth. The appearance is of that of a frog's belly, hence the term ranula (frog belongs to genus Rana). It is firm on palpation. The cyst is usually present above the mylohyoid curtain, but when it presents in the upper part of the neck, it is called as a "plunging ranula." Plunging ranulas may grow to a sufficient size so as to compromise respiration and swallowing and may also extend into mediastinum [32].

46.6.4.1 Management

Excision of the ranula and entire sublingual gland through a transoral approach is management of choice taking care to avoid damage to the lingual nerve. The incision is made through the mucosa in the lingual fold from the second molar to canine tooth. Blunt dissection is done up to the mylohyoid muscle. The gland is dissected free from the surrounding soft tissues and the Wharton's duct. The gland can be retracted using holding sutures, and blunt dissection is carried out till the lingual nerve is identified as it crosses the Wharton's duct. The gland is delivered once it is dissected free from the entire surrounding soft tissues taking care to prevent damaging the submandibular duct and lingual nerve [34].

Marsupialization can be used as an alternative modality wherein the ranula is deroofed and the mucosa sutured to the cystic lining followed by open packing of the cyst and sequentially reducing the size of the pack till it heals completely.

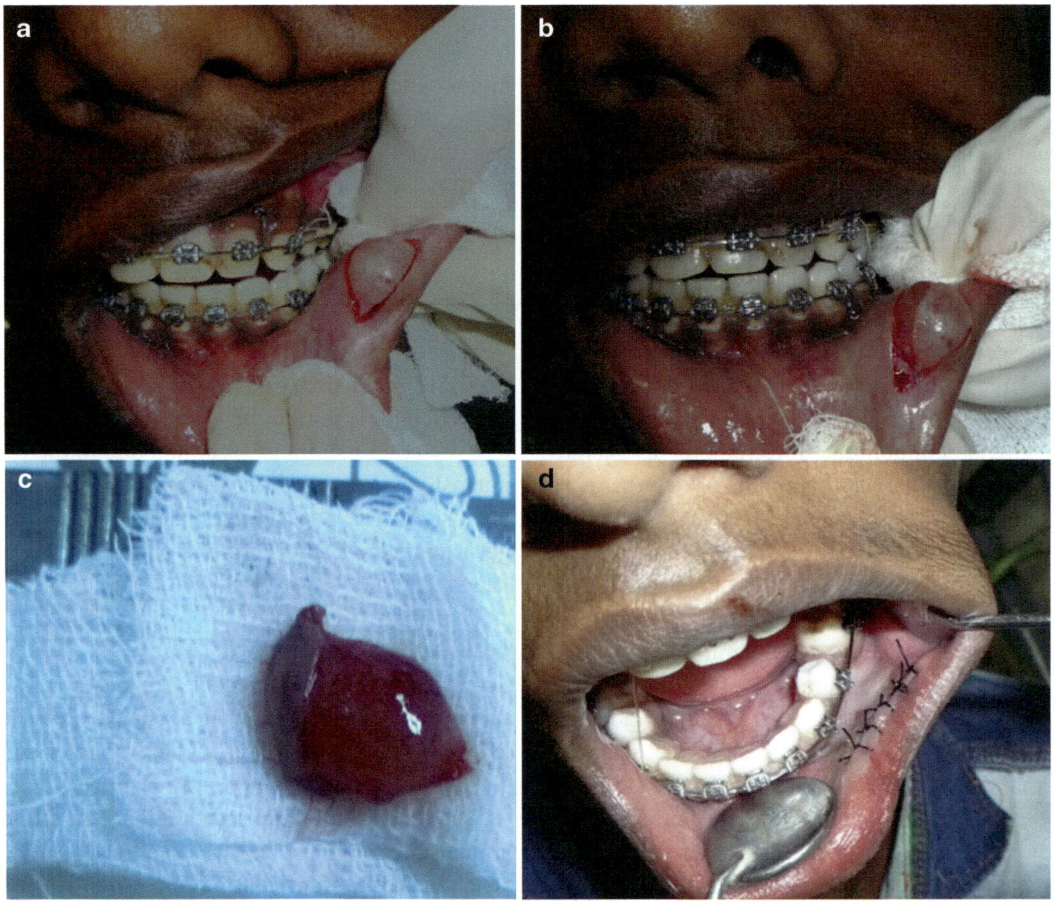

Fig. 46.19 (a)–(d) Figure showing surgical removal of mucocele by elliptical incision. (e)–(h) Figure showing excising mucocele by incision directly over the lesion

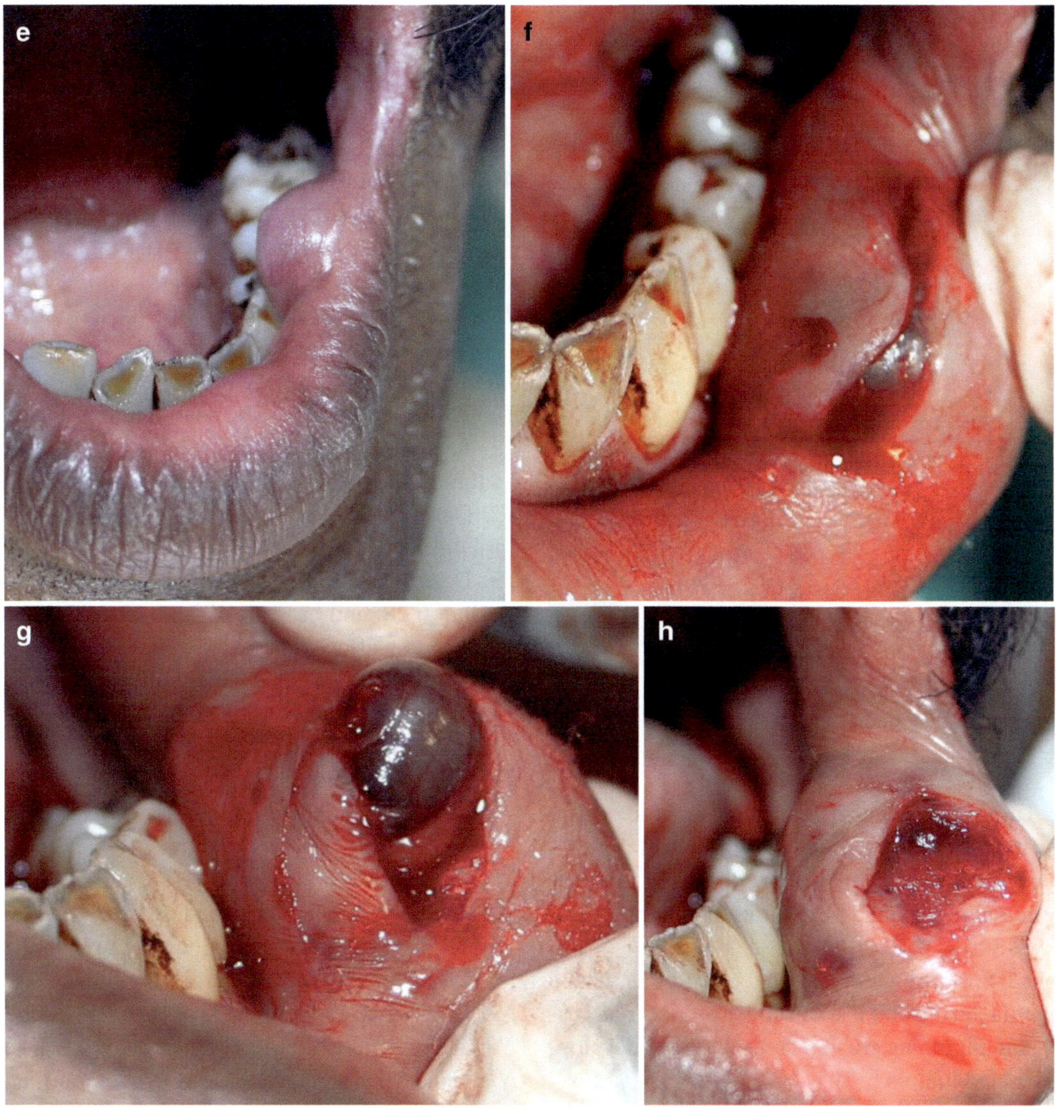

Fig. 46.19 (continued)

Higher recurrence rate (61–85%) has been reported with simple marsupialization and ranula excision. To lower the rate of recurrence, total sublingual excision is the treatment of choice [35].

Kono et al. [36] recommended an injection of sclerosing agent, OK-432 (Picibanil), as a safe and effective method of treating intraoral ranulas. The number of injections used was 1–4 (mean 1.70) in their study.

46.7 Salivary Gland Tumors

46.7.1 Etiology

Although no specific etiology has been attributed to occurrence of salivary gland tumors, its association with radiations, viruses, hormones, lifestyle, or occupation and like factors can't be denied.

- Radiation: Evidence exists regarding susceptibility of lymphoid component rather than parenchymal component of gland to low radiation and UV ray damage (140 rad) [37–39].
- Viruses: It is believed that genetic component, environment, and immunity of host play a key role in malignant transformation of salivary gland tumors. Viruses like human papillomavirus, Epstein-Barr virus, cytomegalovirus, and polyomavirus have been speculated to be responsible for occurrence of salivary gland tumors.
- Hormones: Endogenous hormones play an important role in carcinogenesis of these tumors. Patients of breast cancer are more prone to salivary gland neoplasms.

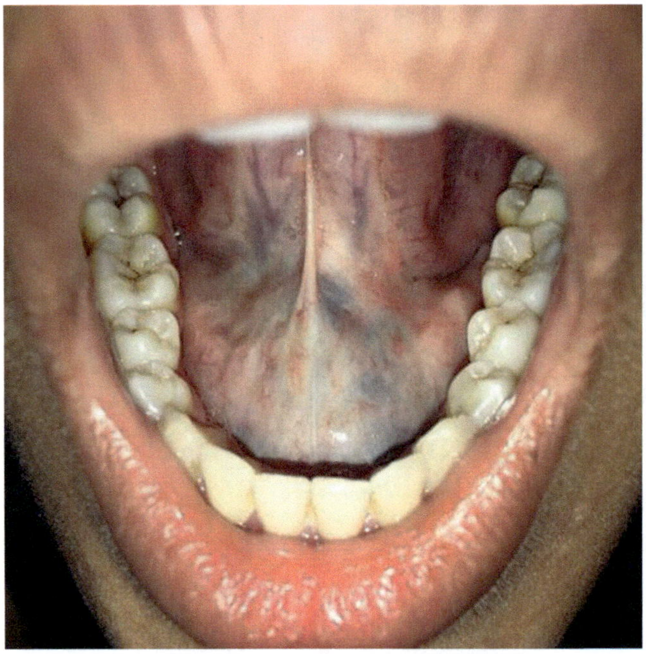

Fig. 46.20 Ranula in the floor of the mouth

- Lifestyle: Tumors like Warthin's tumor or epidermoid carcinoma have been associated with cigarette smoking. Salivary gland enlargements are observed in nutritional deficiencies, but there are no reports of malignancies [40].
- Occupation: Those who engage in occupations which involve manufacturing and use of rubber products, asbestos mining, and plumbing are at increased risk of developing salivary gland tumors [37].

46.7.2 Incidence

Salivary gland tumors occur rarely both among Indian population and around the world. Incidence of benign and malignant salivary gland tumors in major portion of the world ranges from 1 to 2 cases per 100,000 people per year [41]. There is no specific predilection of occurrence of these tumors in any particular gender, although Warthin's tumor is more common in males and acinic cell tumor in females. Site wise incidence varies for both benign and malignant tumors. Seventy-five to eighty percent of benign tumors occur in the parotid glands, 5–10% in submandibular glands, and only 1–2% in sublingual glands. Malignant tumors are more common in sublingual glands (80%) and least in parotid glands (17–20%). Benign tumors affect a mean age group of 40 years, and malignant tumors affect an age group of 55 years. Both benign and malignant tumors by large resemble each other clinically. Hence, histopathologic examination is pivotal to establish a correct diagnosis.

46.7.3 TNM Staging of Salivary Gland Tumors According to American Joint Commission on Cancer (AJCC) 2002 [42]

Tumor (T): T with a letter/number describes the location or size of the tumor

TX: Indicates the primary tumor cannot be evaluated.

T0 (T plus zero): No evidence of a tumor was found.

T1: Describes a small, noninvasive (has not spread) tumor that is 2 centimeters (cm) at its greatest dimension.

T2: Describes a larger, noninvasive tumor between 2 cm and 4 cm.

T3: Describes a tumor that is larger than 4 cm but not larger than 6 cm and has spread beyond the salivary glands but does not affect the seventh nerve, the facial nerve that controls expression, such as smiles or frowns.

T4a: The tumor has invaded the skin, jawbone, ear canal, and/or facial nerve.

T4b: The tumor has invaded the skull base and/or the nearby bones and/or encases the arteries.

Nodes (N): N is for lymph nodes. Lymph nodes of the head and neck region are regional lymph nodes, and those away from this region are distant nodes.

NX: The regional lymph nodes cannot be evaluated.

N0: There is no evidence of cancer in the regional nodes.

N1: Cancer has spread to a single node on the same side as the primary tumor, and the cancer found in the node is 3 cm or smaller.

N2: Describes any of these conditions:

- N2a: The cancer has spread to a single lymph node on the same side as the primary tumor and is larger than 3 cm but smaller than 6 cm.
- N2b: The cancer has spread to more than one lymph node on the same side as the primary tumor, and none measures larger than 6 cm.
- N2c: The cancer has spread to more than one lymph node on either side of the body, and none measures larger than 6 cm.

N3: The cancer found in the lymph nodes is larger than 6 cm.

Metastasis (M): Describes the cancer that spreads to different body parts.

MX: Indicates distant metastasis cannot be evaluated.

M0: Indicates the cancer has not spread to other parts of the body.

M1: Describes cancer that has spread to other parts of the body.

46.7.4 Classification of Salivary Gland Tumors

Salivary gland tumors were first classified by WHO in 1972. It was later modified in 1991 wherein the term "tumor" was replaced by "carcinoma" to denote acinic cell carcinoma and mucoepidermoid carcinoma [43]. It was further revised in 1997, and a greater number of entities of adenomas (myoepithelial adenoma, basal cell adenoma, canalicular adenoma) and carcinomas (acinic cell carcinoma, mucoepidermoid carcinoma, polymorphous low-grade adenocarcinoma, salivary duct carcinoma, myoepithelial carcinoma) were redefined with emphasis on the prognosis and therapy [44]. A revised classification was put forth by WHO in 2005 also. The latest classification of WHO which was given in 2017 consisted of the following changes:

- Secretory carcinoma, borderline tumor—sialoblastoma—and sclerosing polycystic adenosis were added as new entities under malignant tumors.
- Simplification of terminologies of polymorphous adenocarcinoma, clear cell carcinoma, and intraductal carcinoma was done.
- Rare entities like adenocarcinoma, NOS, canalicular adenoma, and poorly differentiated carcinoma were regrouped (Table 46.6).

Table 46.6 Revised classification of salivary gland tumors (2017) [45]

Malignant Tumors	*Benign Tumors*
Mucoepidermoid carcinoma	Pleomorphic adenoma
Adenoid cystic carcinoma	Myoepithelioma
Polymorphous adenocarcinoma	Basal Cell Adenoma
Epithelial-myoepithelial carcinoma	Warthin's tumor
Clear cell carcinoma	Oncocytoma
Basal cell adenocarcinoma	Lymphadenoma
Sebaceous adenocarcinoma	Cystadenoma
Intraductal carcinoma	Sialadenoma papilliferum
Cystadenocarcinoma	Ductal papillomas
Adenocarcinoma, NOS	Sebaceous adenoma
Myoepithelial carcinoma	Canalicular adenoma and other ductal adenomas
Carcinoma ex pleomorphic adenoma	*Other Epithelial Lesions*
Carcinosarcoma	Sclerosing polycystic adenosis
Poorly differentiated carcinoma	Nodular oncocytic hyperplasia
1) Neuroendocrine and non-neuroendocrine	Lymphoepithelial lesions Intercalated duct hyperplasia
2) Undifferentiated carcinoma	*Soft Tissue Lesions*
3) Large cell neuroendocrine carcinoma	Hemangioma
4) Small cell neuroendocrine carcinoma	
Lymphoepithelial carcinoma	Lipoma/sialolipoma
Squamous cell carcinoma	Nodular fasciitis
Oncocytic carcinoma	*Hematolymphoid Tumor*
Borderline Tumors	Extranodal marginal zone lymphoma of MALT
Sialoblastoma	

46.7.5 Pleomorphic Adenoma

"Pleomorphic adenoma" suggested by Willis closely resembles the unusual histologic pattern of the lesion [28]. The tumor derives its name from the Greek words Pleos = many and morphus = form because of the heterogeneous nature of its histologic appearance [46].

46.7.5.1 Clinical Features

Most frequently found in the superficial lobe of the parotid gland, it presents as a firm, slow-growing asymptomatic mass which is smooth, rounded, lobular, and mobile with a rubbery consistency causing ear lobule to be raised (Fig. 46.21a). If the tumor involves both the superficial and deep lobes of parotid, it is classically referred to as dumbbell tumor. Incidence of the tumor except those found in the pharynx is more in females than males, and they are often seen in the fourth and fifth decade. A bilateral tumor occurrence rate is estimated at 1 in 40,000 [47].

They are encapsulated and do not show fixity to the deeper tissues or the overlying skin in major salivary gland tumors, which can be confirmed on an MRI (Fig. 46.21b), but in the case of the minor salivary glands of the palate, it may appear to be fixed to the underlying palatal bone but does not invade or erode the bone. Pain is uncommon but 50% patients experience a pressure sensation. Accumulation of mucus can occur so that elastic swellings or frankly fluctuant cysts may form in the tumors.

In the case of the submandibular gland, palpation of the mass both extraorally and bimanually helps in localizing it and differentiating it from a lymph node, but FNAC is always needed to differentiate it from sialadenitis.

46.7.5.2 Histopathology [48]

On light microscopy morphologically complex and diverse cellular elements are seen. Both epithelial and myoepithelial elements are present. Based on cellular types, Foote and Frazel [49] have classified pleomorphic adenomas as follows:

- Principally myxoid (36%)
- Equally myxoid and cellular (30%)
- Predominantly cellular (22%)
- Extremely cellular (12%)

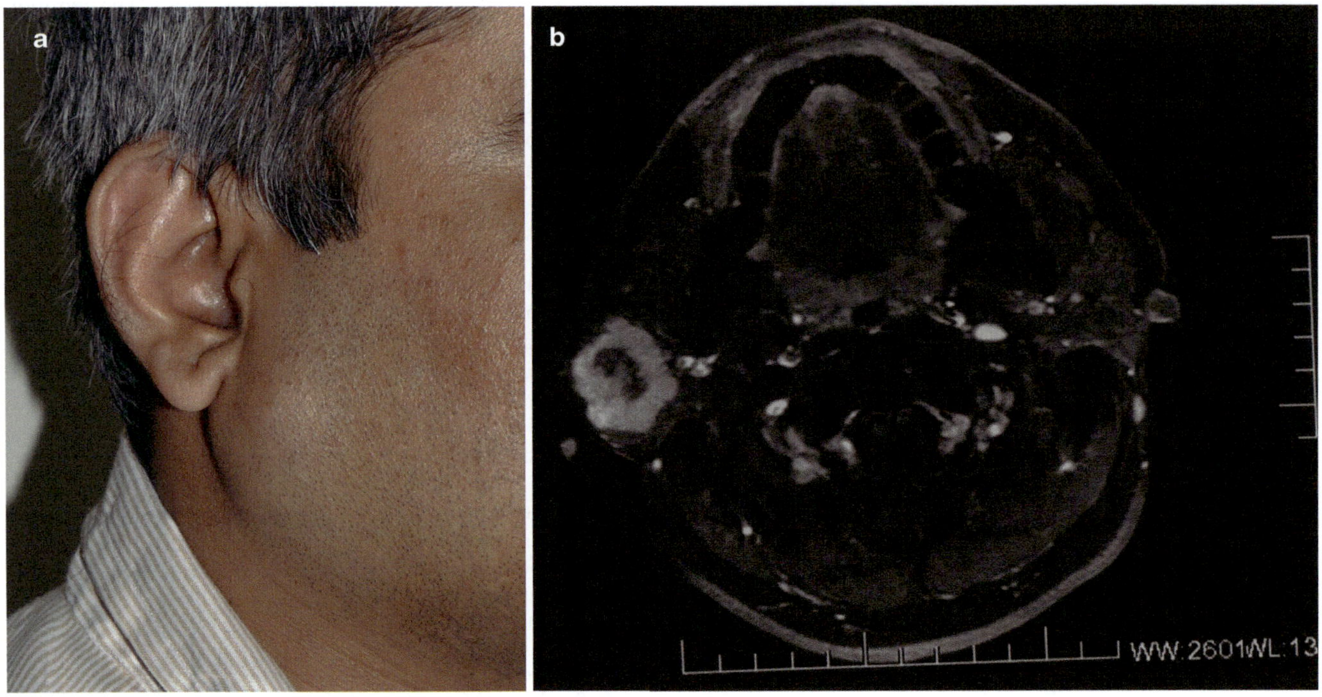

Fig. 46.21 (**a**) Parotid tumor showing elevation of ear lobule (pathognomonic sign). (**b**) MRI axial view showing the tumor

46.7.5.3 Management

Surgical excision is the treatment of choice. Historically, enucleation was practiced which resulted in inadequate surgery and recurrences [50]. Superficial parotidectomy is the most widely accepted technique in the treatment of pleomorphic adenomas in the superficial lobe of the parotid gland, and total gland excision with facial nerve preservation is carried out. Tumors of the submandibular gland are usually contained within the gland, and their resection is usually confined to the gland and surrounding fat or lymph nodes until the neoplasm is a malignant and invasive tumor. As with the parotid gland, most neoplasms are asymptomatic. Small palatal pleomorphic adenomas usually cause pressure resorption of the palate but do not invade the bone. A disk of palatal mucosa is outlined well clear of the visible swelling because the tumor is flattened owing to the toughness of the palatal tissues. The tumor along with the periosteum of the palate is excised in continuity with each other. In case the pleomorphic adenoma invades the palate or proliferates into the floor of the maxillary sinus, a partial maxillectomy or total maxillectomy depending on the extension of the tumor has to be performed.

Although pleomorphic adenoma is a benign tumor, it may cause problems in clinical management due to its tendency to recur and risk of malignant transformation.

46.7.6 Monomorphic Adenoma

The WHO classification subdivides the monomorphic adenomas into three groups [45]:

- Adenolymphoma (Warthin's tumor)
- Oxyphilic adenoma (oncocytoma)
- Others

A number of other classifications of monomorphic adenomas have been put forth, but there is no unanimity. Two main histologic patterns have evolved:

- Basal cell adenoma
- Canalicular adenoma

46.7.7 Warthin's Tumor

Warthin's tumor, also known as papillary cystadenoma lymphomatosum and adenolymphoma, is the second most common benign tumor of the salivary glands, around 5% of neoplasms [51].

It was first described by Hildebrand in 1895 as a form of congenital cyst of the neck. It is known as Warthin's tumor in recognition of the pathologist who first described it in the USA in 1929. He described two cases and also coined the term papillary cystadenoma lymphomatosum [52].

46.7.7.1 Clinical Features

The majority of the tumors arise in the parotid gland, more often bilaterally, in the elderly and occurs in the fifth and sixth decades of life. A predilection for male sex is seen, more in Caucasians. Both tumors do not occur simultaneously but are metachronous in their manifestation. A concept of multicentric and multifocal disease has been put forth to explain this. It is a solitary, nodular, slowly enlarging swelling, most commonly located in the inferior pole of the parotid next to the angle of the mandible. It varies from moderately firm to fluctuant on palpation and is asymptomatic. It is not as discrete as the mixed tumor. Very few patients present with complain of pain, pressure, or rapid increase in the tumor size. Scintigraphy may be helpful due to its increased uptake of technetium-99m pertechnetate. It appears as a smooth-margined, radiopositive "hot" nodule in contrast to the mixed tumors, nonfunctioning malignant tumors, and metastatic tumors which appear as a "cold" nodule in scintigraphy. Positive scintigraphy with ^{123}I is indicative of Warthin's tumor but may also signify presence of ectopic thyroid or metastatic thyroid tumor.

46.7.7.2 Management

Surgical removal is the established treatment for Warthin's tumor. As the tumor is superficial in the parotid gland, it is easily removed with minimal loss of glandular function and with preservation of the facial nerve.

Treatment philosophies given are:

- Tumor enucleation with resection of minimal amount of surrounding normal tissue
- Superficial parotidectomy, which is more aggressive than enucleation
- Local excision of parotid gland

Local excision of the tumor is preferred to enucleation of the tumor because lymph nodes at the posteroinferior part of the gland cannot be cleared by enucleation. Preoperative diagnosis of Warthin's tumor must be confirmed by coordinating the clinical findings with imaging and fine-needle aspiration biopsy reports before local excision is carried out. If there is associated chronic obstructive parotitis, superficial parotidectomy is essential. Similarly, if the tumor is located in front of the ear, a superficial parotidectomy is the treatment of choice.

46.7.8 Oncocytoma

An oncocytoma is a tumor characterized by large epithelial cells, i.e., oncocytes that contain a brightly eosinophilic, granular cytoplasm. The oncocyte is derived from the Greek word "onkousthai" meaning swollen or enlarged and was described in 1897 by Schaffer who observed this tumor in ductal and acinar elements of salivary glands in the tongue, pharynx, and esophagus. Jaffe was the first to introduce the term oncocytoma [53]. However, he had termed Warthin's tumor as oncocytoma. The other terminologies used to describe this tumor are oxyphilic adenoma and acidophilic adenoma.

46.7.8.1 Clinical Features

There is no race predilection for occurrence of this tumor. Oncocytoma is predominantly a tumor of the major salivary glands, parotid being the most common. Bilateral occurrence is also known. Among minor salivary glands, which are rarely affected, palatal mucosa followed by buccal mucosa and tongue is affected.

The oncocytoma is a small benign lesion which generally does not attain a great size. It most frequently presents as an indolent, single, often multi-lobulated, firm, solid, and mobile mass in the superficial lobe of the parotid gland. It can also be located in the deep lobe of the parotid gland and may be insinuated between the branches of the facial nerve. However, it does not cause any symptoms of pain or paresthesia unless the branches of the facial nerve are compromised. Tumor size varies with the duration of the lesion but generally does not increase beyond 4.0 cm. Intraoral tumors do not exhibit any special characteristic diagnostic features. However, their overlying mucosa may become ulcerated due to trauma [53].

46.7.8.2 Management

Partial parotidectomy with facial nerve preservation whenever possible is the treatment of choice. It ensures complete removal of the tumor and reduces the rate of recurrence. Curettage or simple enucleation of the tumor is to be avoided to avoid recurrence. Complete sialadenectomy is the treatment of choice in cases of submandibular gland oncocytomas. In the case of minor gland tumors, local excision of the tumor with a margin of normal tumor-free tissue is carried out. Radiation therapy after surgery has been tried but it has shown to be ineffective.

46.7.9 Basal Cell Adenoma

It was first reported as a separate entity by Kleinsasser and Klein in 1967 [28].

46.7.9.1 Clinical Features

Basal cell adenomas occur between the third and ninth decade, but the peak incidence is in the sixth decade with a slight male predilection of 5:1 [28]. They are clinically indistinguishable from mixed tumors and occur in the superficial portion of the parotid gland. They are slow-growing, painless, round or ovoid, well-circumscribed, and freely mobile masses with a smooth-surfaced capsule and a soft to moderately firm consistency. They may be mistaken for a hyperplastic lymph node because of their encapsulation, size, and color.

Clinically basal cell carcinoma of skin, ameloblastoma, pleomorphic adenoma, and adenoid cystic carcinoma can be considered in the differential diagnosis.

On the basis of histopathologic appearance, they may be divided into four subtypes:

- Solid
- Trabecular
- Tubular
- Membranous

46.7.9.2 Management

Surgical excision with a sufficient clear margin of normal tissue is the treatment of choice.

46.7.10 Canalicular Adenoma

46.7.10.1 Clinical Features

It is seen between the fourth and ninth decade, highest incidence being in the seventh decade with a female/male ratio of 1.7 to 1.0 and a higher incidence in Caucasians. It is seen more commonly in the minor salivary glands of the lip and cheek and rarely affects the major salivary gland [54].

It presents as a non-ulcerated, painless, mobile nodule that exhibits slow growth unless it is traumatized, wherein there is presence of ulceration. Clinical appearance is similar to that of a mucocele [54]. The overlying mucosa may be normal colored or bluish.

In the case of upper lip lesion, a sialolith, mucocele, mucous retention cyst, and pleomorphic adenoma can be considered in the differential diagnosis.

46.7.10.2 Management

Surgical excision, enucleation, or limited extracapsular excisions have been used as treatment modalities in these tumors with success.

46.7.11 Sialadenoma Papilleferum

First described by Abrams and Finck in 1969, it was termed sialadenoma papilleferum because of its histologic similarity to syringocystadenoma papilleferum of skin adnexal origin [55].

46.7.11.1 Clinical Features

Sialadenoma papilleferum presents as a subcentimetric, asymptomatic, exophytic, papillary surface lesion which can be confused with squamous papilloma. The most common site of occurrence is the minor salivary glands at the junction of soft and hard palate with the tumor located on one side of the midline. This tumor occurs at an average age of 56 years, cases being reported from 2 years to 87 years. Male predilection is seen in the ratio of 1.5 to 1. However, there is no racial predominance [55].

Clinically it resembles a squamous papilloma, and a differential diagnosis of verrucous carcinoma or a warty dyskeratoma needs to be considered.

46.7.11.2 Management

Being small, these tumors are easily excised usually with a clinical diagnosis of a squamous papilloma. However, recurrence is rare.

46.7.12 Inverted Ductal Papilloma

Inverted ductal papilloma is a rare tumor and was first described by White et al. in 1982 when they reported four cases [56].

46.7.12.1 Clinical Features [56]

It occurs as a firm, asymptomatic, discrete nodule of 1–1.5 cm beneath the normal mucosa which in some cases may be contiguous with a small surface pore. The mean age of occurrence is 50 years without any sex predilection. The sites usually involved are the lower lip and buccal vestibular mucosa in descending order with occasional cases reported in the upper lip, floor of mouth, and soft palate.

46.7.12.2 Treatment and Prognosis

It is treated by simple surgical excision as it is not known to recur.

46.7.13 Intraductal Papilloma

It is a rare tumor. These tumors present as asymptomatic, submucosal swellings that vary in size from less than 1 to 1.5 cm in the minor salivary glands. The ages of patients range from 29 to 77 years, with a mean age of 54 years. Men and women are equally affected.

46.7.13.1 Treatment and Prognosis

Excision is curative, and these tumors are not known to recur. In case the tumors are small, all types of papillomas of the minor salivary glands, including intraductal, inverted, and sialadenoma papilliferum, can be excised in the dental office or the clinic under local anesthesia [55].

46.7.14 Mucoepidermoid Carcinoma

Mucoepidermoid carcinoma is the most common malignant salivary gland neoplasm. They are classified as grade I (low grade) which are well differentiated, grade II (intermediate grade) which are moderately differentiated, and grade III (high grade) which are poorly differentiated tumors.

46.7.14.1 Clinical Features

Mucoepidermoid carcinomas occur more commonly in the minor salivary glands with a female predilection [57]. It occurs as a painless, circumscribed, mobile solitary enlargement of the body or tail of the parotid or the submandibular region with over a year duration generally. Pain, facial paralysis, and fixation to the overlying skin are usually suggestive of high-grade lesions [57]. Minor salivary gland lesions present as a bluish or red-purple, fluctuant, smooth-surfaced mass that is often clinically mistaken for a mucocele or hemangioma [57]. Large lesions at the base of the tongue or in the oropharynx may cause dysphagia. Aggressive tumors show ulceration. Numbness of the teeth may occur when the bone is involved. Histopathologically, mucoepidermoid carcinomas are graded as low-grade, intermediate-grade, and high-grade carcinomas. They are generally partially encapsulated and don't show adequate circumscription.

46.7.14.2 Management

Complete, adequate, and radical surgical excision is the treatment of choice for all grades of mucoepidermoid carcinomas [58]. In the case of stage I and stage II mucoepidermoid carcinomas of the parotid gland, conservative excision with preservation of the facial nerve, if possible, is recommended. The affected submandibular gland should be removed entirely. Radical neck dissection is performed in patients with clinical evidence of cervical node metastasis and is considered in any patient with a T3 lesion. In the case of facial nerve involvement, total parotidectomy with facial nerve sacrifice up to histologically tumor-negative nerve trunk is done. The 5-year disease-free rate in patients receiving this aggressive treatment was about 60% [58].

Treatment of minor salivary gland mucoepidermoid carcinomas entails a wide surgical excision with the bone if involved, to achieve a negative margin, and the wound is left to heal secondarily [59]. For small low-grade tumors in the absence of bone involvement, wide excision down to periosteum with 1 or 2 cm tumor-free lateral margins is adequate therapy [59]. High-grade and advanced stage tumors must be treated aggressively at any site. The overall recurrence rate of mucoepidermoid carcinomas is approximately 25%. Better survival is seen among younger patients and among females. Tumors in the submandibular gland and in the base of the tongue generally have a poorer outlook than those at other major and minor salivary gland sites. Also invasion into bone signifies a poorer prognosis. Survival is closely related to the clinical stage and the histologic grade.

46.7.15 Adenoid Cystic Carcinoma

Adenoid cystic carcinoma (ACC) is a highly aggressive, destructive, and clinically unpredictable tumor of the head and neck region [60]. The other terms used for ACC used in the past are cylindroma and adenomyoepithelioma. Foote and Frazell [49] proposed the currently accepted term adenoid cystic carcinoma in their classic paper in 1953 and in their fascicle on major salivary gland tumors in 1954.

46.7.15.1 Clinical Features

Adenoid cystic carcinoma occurs in adults between 50 and 70 years of age with equal prevalence in males and females [61]. The most frequent locations of this tumor are the parotid, submandibular, and palatal salivary glands [62]. They are only rarely observed in the sublingual gland [61].

Clinically adenoid cystic carcinoma manifests in the major and intraoral accessory salivary glands as a slow-growing swelling or mass. Pain and fixation to skin as well as surrounding deeper structures generally occur during the course of tumor growth. An ominous feature of adenoid cystic carcinoma of the parotid gland is paralysis of the facial nerve. Radiographic examination is valuable in assessing the extent of osseous destruction. Symptoms may have been present for months or years and are generally of longer duration than those associated with squamous carcinoma, which is the most frequent malignancy of this location. Adenoid cystic carcinomas of the maxillary antrum, nasal cavity, and ear canal produce symptoms of pain, obstruction, and deafness, respectively.

Histopathologically, ACC are classified into cribriform pattern, tubular pattern, and solid pattern. A major microscopic feature in most adenoid cystic carcinomas is the propensity for the tumor to involve peripheral nerves, reported to occur in 20–80% of the patients. Although perineural invasion is characteristic of adenoid cystic carcinoma, it is not unique to the tumor.

46.7.15.2 Management of Adenoid Cystic Carcinoma

Complete excision like all other tumors is the treatment of choice. Elective regional lymph node dissection is not indicated, because distant metastasis is more common than cervical (regional) node involvement. According to Maciejewski et al., radical surgical excision with histologically proven negative margins with postoperative radiotherapy for all cases should be the treatment of choice. Lymph node dissection is recommended only in cases of histologically proven positive lymph nodes [60]. A frozen section diagnosis to achieve tumor-free safe margins is necessary to specifically look for safe perineural margins because ACC is known to spread quickly along the nerve.

The slow biologic growth of adenoid cystic carcinoma along with a late metastasis of the disease results in relatively favorable 5-year survival rates. Factors that indicate a poor prognosis include failure to achieve clear margins at first surgery, a solid pattern histologically, recurrent disease, and distant metastasis [63].

In a study by Witten et al., local recurrences have been seen in almost 32% of the cases [63]. The risk of distant metastasis is also high, approximately 40%, and can occur in less than 8 years after treatment.

46.7.16 Clear Cell Carcinoma

Clear cell neoplasms of salivary glands have been classified as both adenomas and carcinomas [64].

46.7.16.1 Clinical Features

It occurs predominantly in the palatal minor salivary glands followed by parotid and submandibular glands without any sexual or racial predilection. It occurs between the ages of 18 and 86 years, mean 56 years. Clinical manifestation is of a swelling similar to other tumors. It may be confused with mucoepidermoid and acinic cell carcinoma as well as metastatic renal cell carcinoma. A positive reaction to mucicarmine would preclude the possibility of renal cell carcinoma.

46.7.16.2 Management

Due to their infiltrative growth and the incidence of recurrence and regional lymph node metastases, it is appropriate to consider them low-grade adenocarcinomas. Hence surgical treatment is the mainstay of management.

46.7.17 Epithelial-Myoepithelial Carcinoma

The epithelial-myoepithelial carcinoma of intercalated duct origin is a rare biphasic type of low-grade salivary gland carcinoma that constitutes less than 1% of salivary gland neoplasms.

46.7.17.1 Clinical Features

It occurs more commonly in females around 60–70 years of age. Parotid gland is the most frequently affected [65]. Patients present with an asymptomatic or painful salivary gland swelling with a history of steady increase in size over an extended period of time and may also present with facial paralysis [66]. In patients with maxillary involvement, nasal obstruction and facial deformity may be the presenting complaints. Differential diagnosis includes pleomorphic adenoma, acinic cell adenocarcinoma, adenoid cystic carcinoma, mucoepidermoid carcinoma, sebaceous carcinoma, and oncocytoma.

46.7.17.2 Management

Surgery is considered the primary mode of treatment. Total parotidectomy with facial nerve preservation is advocated for tumors in the parotid gland unless the nerve is involved by the tumor. Recurrences and distant metastasis are a known complication.

46.7.18 Carcinosarcoma

Carcinosarcoma, also known as true malignant mixed tumor, shows malignant cells in both the stromal and epithelial components [67]. When these tumors metastasize, both components metastasize together.

46.7.18.1 Clinical Features

Carcinosarcomas are rare tumors with an average incidence of 0.4% in major salivary glands and 1% in minor salivary glands. It occurs between 25 and 85 years of age (average 58.5 years) with the frequency of occurrence being more in parotid than submandibular gland and then minor glands in palate and tongue [67].

It presents as an enlarging mass with a rapid increase in size and may be associated with pain and facial nerve paralysis. Rarely, patients present with metastases or experience difficulty in swallowing or breathing. A patient with a central nervous system metastasis has been reported to present with headaches [67].

46.7.18.2 Management

The data available is insufficient to recommend one type of therapy as definitive. However radical surgical excision, together with radiation therapy and lymph node dissection for palpable disease, seems to be the most prudent form of therapy. Radiotherapy as the only means of therapy has not proved effective. Tumor metastasis is most frequent to the lungs followed by hilar and cervical lymph nodes. Distant metastasis is also rarely found [67].

46.7.19 Undifferentiated Carcinomas

This group includes three distinct entities:

1. *Lymphoepithelial carcinomas (malignant lymphoepithelial lesion):* It is more prevalent in females and occurs between fourth and fifth decade of life. The parotid gland is most commonly involved followed by submandibular gland. Painful indurated mass and occasional facial paralysis are the presenting symptoms. It might be preceded by benign lymphoepithelial lesion for many years. It is managed by wide surgical excision with or without neck dissection and may be supplemented with radiotherapy.
2. *Undifferentiated large cell carcinomas:* It occurs predominantly in older population with a male predilection. It most commonly affects the parotid followed by submandibular and minor salivary glands. Histologically it shows predominantly poorly differentiated large cell components. It carries a poor prognosis and has a higher risk of locoregional as well as distant metastasis and recurrences. The worst prognostic factor is the size of the lesion. Less than 4 cm, mean survival time was 46 months, and more than 4 cm it was reduced to 7.7 months [51].
3. *Undifferentiated small cell carcinomas*: It rarely affects the salivary glands and is primarily a pulmonary tumor. When it occurs, it shows a male preponderance and occurs between fifth and seventh decade, in the parotid mainly followed by submandibular gland. It presents as a rapidly growing mass which may or may not be painful. Management is primarily wide surgical excision with neck dissection for clinically positive neck node involvement. Chemoradiotherapy may be used as an adjunctive modality for treatment. It tends to metastasize via the hematogenous route, and hence a distant metastasis needs to be ruled out.

46.7.20 Squamous Cell Carcinoma

The diagnosis of primary squamous cell carcinoma is limited to the major glands because distinction between possible minor salivary gland primary tumors and those originating from mucosal surface epithelium is generally not possible.

46.7.20.1 Clinical Features

It occurs between 7 and 95 years of age, the mean age being 60.5 years with a male predilection of 2:1. Parotid gland is the most commonly involved followed by submandibular and sublingual glands [68]. It presents as an asymptomatic mass with occasional pain and facial nerve palsy. This tumor often replaces the entire gland with fixation to underlying structures and skin.

Ductal squamous metaplasia, high-grade mucoepidermoid carcinoma, and lymphoepithelial carcinoma should be considered in the differential diagnosis of squamous cell carcinoma of the salivary gland.

46.7.20.2 Management

Surgical management is the mainstay of treatment. Parotidectomy with or without facial nerve preservation depending on the case is needed for parotid tumors. Submandibular sialadenectomy is needed for submandibular gland tumors. A neck dissection is done in clinically positive necks at the slightest suspicion. Locoregional failure is the most significant problem, and hence a composite resection in larger submandibular malignancies might be needed. Postoperative radiotherapy when combined with surgery may improve the locoregional control [68].

46.8 Surgical Management of Parotid Tumors (Video 46.3)

The following procedures are performed:

- Local excision of the parotid gland
- Superficial parotidectomy
- Functional superficial parotidectomy
- Complete parotidectomy with facial nerve preservation
- Radical parotidectomy with or without neck dissection
- Parotidomandibulectomy
- Temporoparotidectomy

46.8.1 Skin Incisions for Parotidectomy [69]

The ideal incision should combine good exposure with the best ultimate cosmetic result. This part of the procedure is common to all the resection procedures unless skin is being excised because it is involved by the tumor.

Gutierrez (1903)—The incision had a temporal extension, a preauricular component, and a limb extending onto the neck in one of the skin creases (Fig. 46.22). The chief drawback of this incisions was esthetics in case of development of a keloid.

Redon and Vaillant and Laudenbach—The incision line is similar to that proposed by Adson (Fig. 46.23).

Adson and Ott have described a "Y"-shaped incision with a preauricular part, a postauricular part, and a cervical incision line that splits off from the site of union of the first two branches (Fig. 46.24). The advantage of this incision is improved esthetics because it lacks a temporal incision line, but the drawback is that it impairs dissection. Also, one section of the incision is located in the carotid region.

Samengo (1961)—The incision has a preauricular, a postauricular, and a neck extension in the incision line (Fig. 46.25).

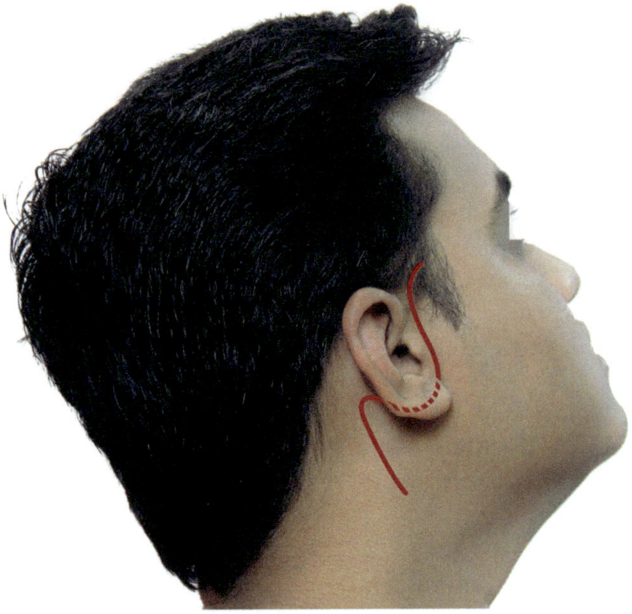

Fig. 46.22 Gutierrez incision

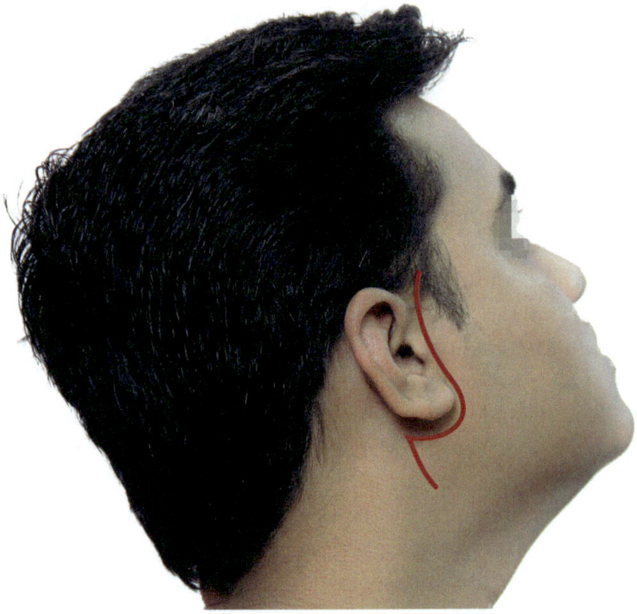

Fig. 46.23 Redon and Valliant and Laudenbach incision

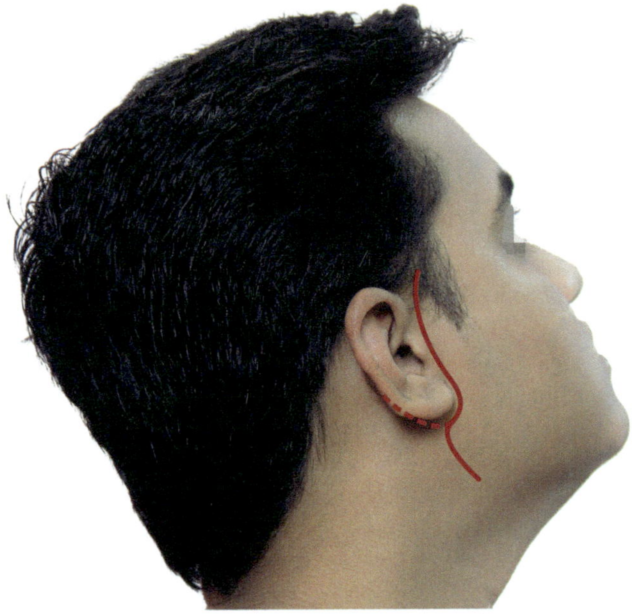

Fig. 46.24 Adson and Ott incision

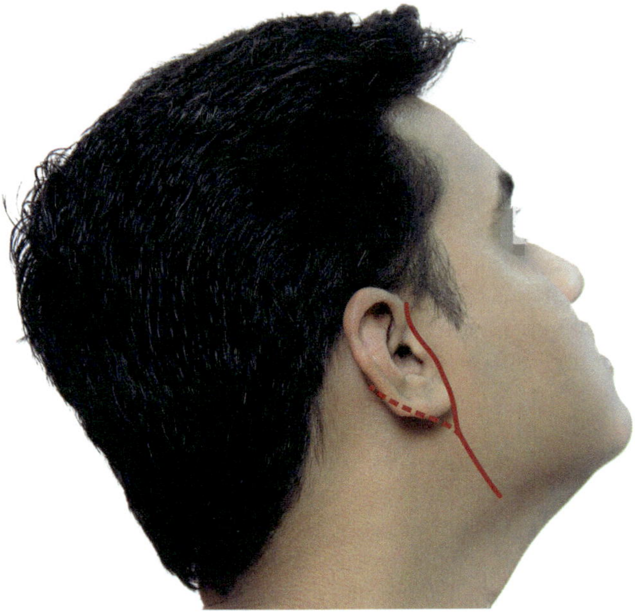

Fig. 46.25 Samengo incision

Appiani (1967)—The incision within the lower portion of the scalp is hidden by the hair instead of the vertical incision line. The benefit of this incision is better esthetics. However, the temporal extension of this incision is short, and this impairs access to the anterior portion of the gland (Fig. 46.26).

Ferreria JL et al. [69] modified Appiani's incision by extending the temporal incision line but not beyond the hairline. It provides a better access to the anterior portion of the parotid gland without compromising esthetics. Also, the angles are rounded off where the incision line changes direction reducing dehiscence and salivary fistula formation.

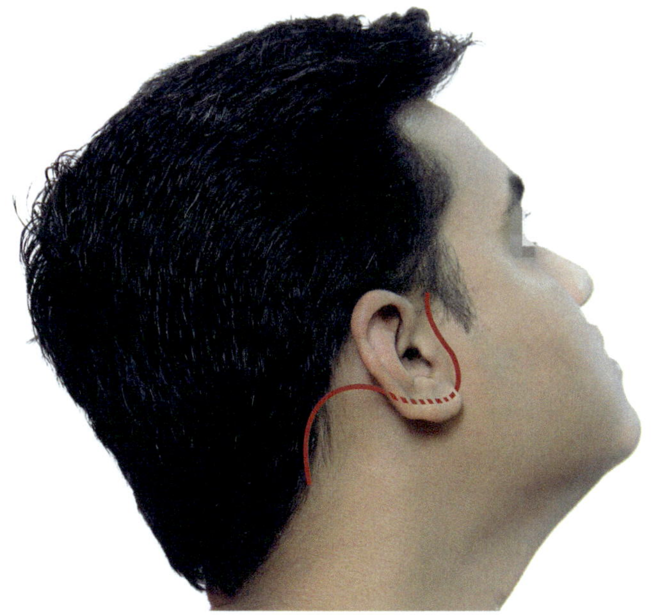

Fig. 46.26 Appiani's incision

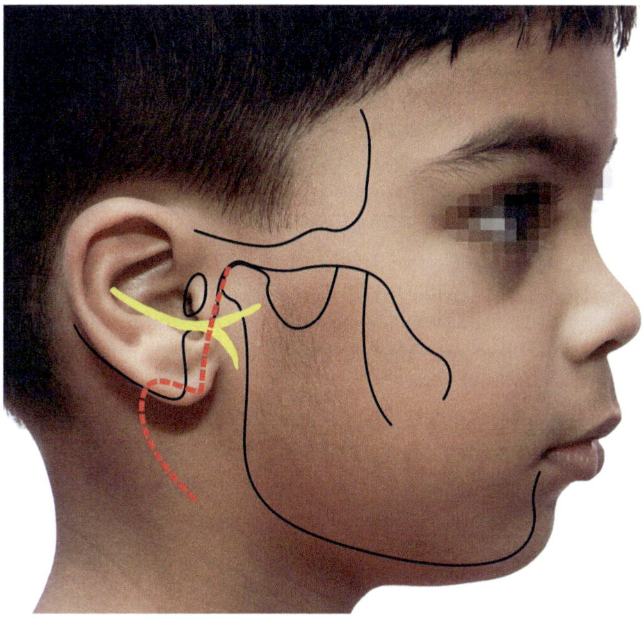

Fig. 46.27 Modified Blair incision in pediatric patient

Farrior et al. recommended a single curved incision 1.5–2.0 cm below the mandible and extending over the mastoid region 1.5 cm behind the postauricular crease in children. The preauricular crease used in adults is avoided because of the superficial location of the facial nerve and possibility of facial nerve damage during flap elevation [68] (Fig. 46.27).

The Blair incision is an S-shaped incision that starts from the preauricular region and extends in the neck. The major disadvantage of the Blair incision is a visible scar in the neck that may cause facial or cervical disfigurement causing patients dissatisfaction [70].

The standard incision is a modified Blair incision (Fig. 46.28) wherein the skin incision is placed in a preauricular crease and doesn't extend beyond the level of the root of the helix. It extends inferiorly around the ear lobule over the mastoid tip. It gently curves down along the sternocleidomastoid muscle and then slightly forward in a natural crease in the upper neck [71].

A facelift incision can be used to avoid the hollowing after parotidectomy, and the defect can be filled with SMAS advancement flap (Bananno and Casson [72], 1992). However, the SMAS-lifting technique is not a routine procedure for many surgeons [73].

Rai A et al. [74] advocated use of posterior belly of the diagastric muscle flap (PBDMF) for reconstruction of the surgical defect after superficial parotidectomy. PBDM inserts very close to stylomastoid foramen, and it is considered as an important landmark in the identification of facial nerve main trunk. The harvesting and dissection of PBDMF becomes easier as it lies in the surgical site, and no extra incision is required to harvest it. It can be used in thin and young patients with good esthetic results.

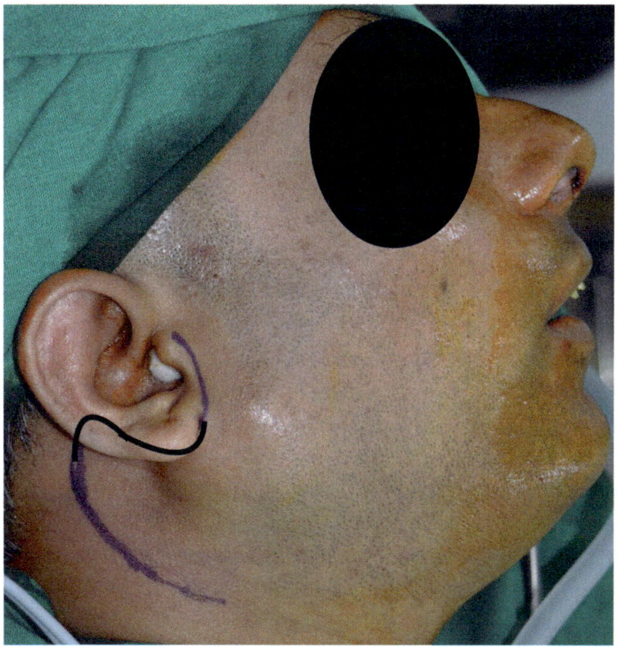

Fig. 46.28 Modified Blair incision in adults

46.8.2 Identification of the Facial Nerve

This has been previously described in the section on applied anatomy of the parotid gland.

46.8.3 Surgical Management

The selection of type of procedure for surgical management of parotid tumors depends on the site, size and clinicohistopathologic features. The various procedures are described briefly as under:

46.8.3.1 Local Excision of Parotid Gland

This technique is used for management of a small tumor in the tail of the parotid gland less than 3.5 cm. Due to small tumor size, most of the functional gland along with the duct can be preserved.

46.8.3.2 Parotidectomy with Preservation of the Facial Nerve [75]

After marking the incision, infiltration is usually done with Saline Plus 1 in 200,000 parts adrenaline instead of lignocaine with adrenaline to avoid blocking the facial nerve fibers. In case lignocaine is used, care should be taken to avoid deep injections. Care should be taken to avoid extending the incision too far posterior beneath the ear lobe to avoid persistent edema [75].

The incision in the neck crease is deepened to raise a flap in the subplatysmal plane (Fig. 46.29). The greater auricular nerve is identified and preserved. It branches over the surface of the gland where two or more branches should be followed and then divided.

Once the deep fascia has been identified, rest of the wound is deepened to this level and skin reflected forward from it. At the zygomatic bone, some subcutaneous fat should be left on the fascia to avoid damaging the branches of facial nerve which lie more superficially as they emerge from the upper part of the parotid. The main trunk of the nerve is found by first separating the lower pole of the gland from the anterior border of the sternomastoid and then from the mastoid process and the cartilaginous part of the external auditory meatus (Fig. 46.30). The wound is deepened anterior to the margin of the sternomastoid, and the lower pole is dissected free as far forward as the external jugular, uncovering the posterior belly of the digastric muscle. The vein should not be divided and tied at this stage because this will increase the venous engorgement of the parotid and the ooze from its divided tissues.

Neither should the lower pole be raised further forward because the branches of the facial nerve often pass superficial to the vein and emerge from the gland anterior to it. The parotid is retracted forward as the dissection proceeds and

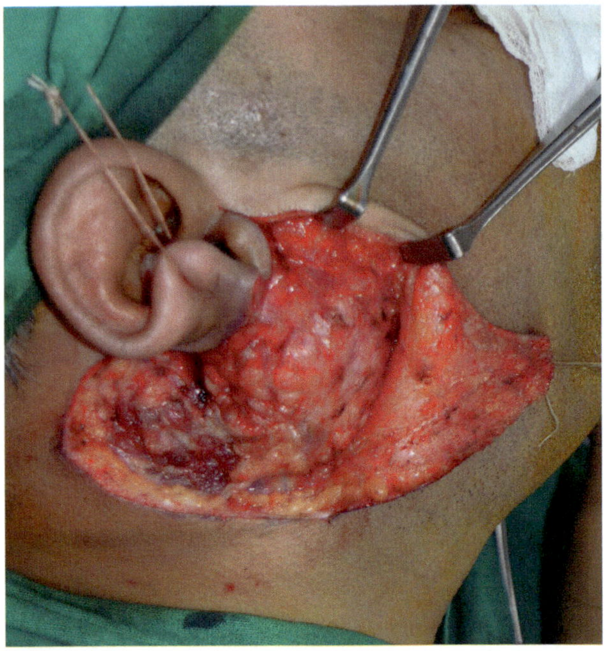

Fig. 46.29 Flap raised in the sub platysmal plane exposing the superficial surface of tumor

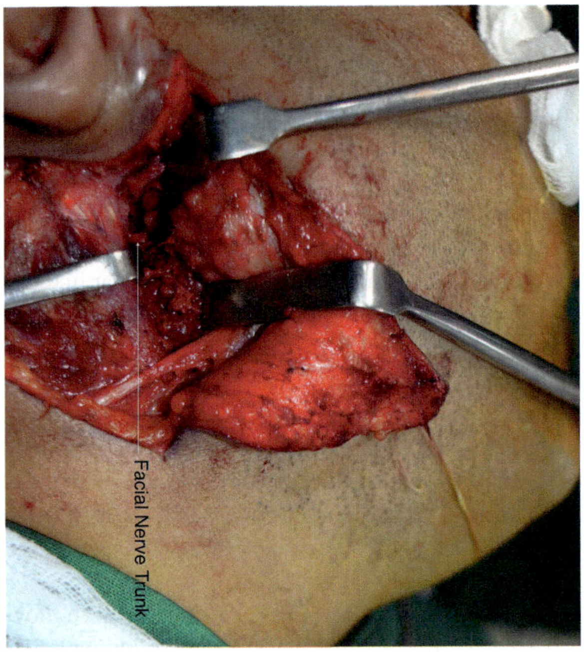

Fig. 46.30 Representing facial nerve main trunk

the pointed, lower extremity of the tragal cartilage (pointer) will be uncovered. Where possible, the edge of the fascia should be raised and the underlying tissue separated by blunt dissection until the nerve is seen as white cords some 2–3 mm thick.

The stylomastoid branch of the posterior auricular artery passes superficial to the nerve to enter the stylomastoid foramen. Damage to this vessel should be avoided as bleeding may hamper vision, and also it supplies a nutrient branch to the nerve. The curved mosquito forceps are used for dissection by opening the blades a little at a time to stretch the tissues and raise it, so as to lift the gland substance off the surface of the nerve, and then expose it by cutting through the gland with scissors. At all times when a cut is made, the adjacent nerve must be seen clearly.

Almost immediately the nerve trunk starts to travel laterally within the parotid, and just below the neck of the condyle, it splits into an upper temporofacial and a lower cervicofacial division. Follow the lower division first, and trace the cervical or the marginal mandibular branch anteriorly to a point in front of the parotid to mobilize the lower pole completely. Then by progressing upward, branch by branch further mobilization can be achieved (Fig. 46.31). Some tissue should always be left on the tumor to ensure complete removal.

In general, the nerves pass superficial to the retromandibular vein, but some may pass deep to it. Careful mobilization of both nerve and vein with division and ligation of the latter is necessary. Tiny vessels should be sealed with bipolar diathermy avoiding damage to adjacent nerves.

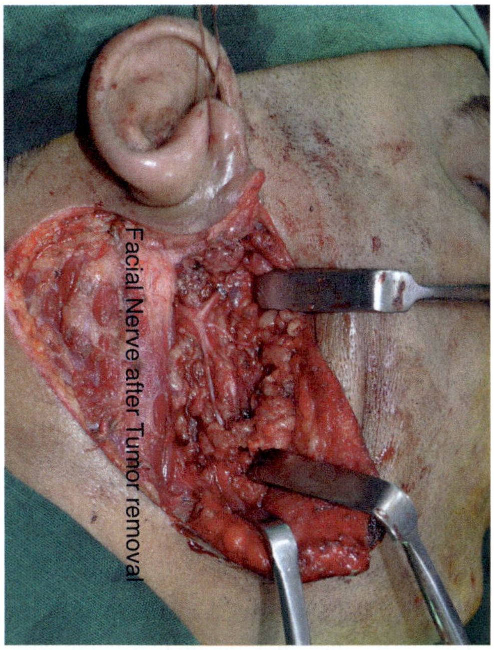

Fig. 46.31 Parotidectomy with preservation of the facial nerve

46.8.3.3 Functional Superficial Parotidectomy [76]

This is superficial parotidectomy where gland function is preserved by preservation of the Stenson's duct. If the duct is superficial to the buccal branch, its preservation is contraindicated as it will obstruct the surgical procedure. After raising the skin flap and exposing the parotid gland, the duct is identified passing on the masseter muscle. Stenson's duct is located; dissection and ligation of the duct are avoided unless it is located superficial to the buccal branches of the facial nerve. Rest of the procedure is similar to superficial parotidectomy.

Advantages

- It is a simpler surgery than conservative superficial parotidectomy.
- It preserves partial function of the parotid gland.
- It avoids the influence of subsequent gland atrophy on facial contour.

It decreases postoperative complications.

46.8.3.4 Partial Superficial Parotidectomy

This is similar to local excision of parotid gland. Maximum healthy tissue is left behind without compromising on the clearance. The advantage of this procedure over superficial parotidectomy is relatively low incidence of Frey's syndrome. The reported incidence of this complication is 4.8% [77]. In addition, better gland function is preserved due to more parenchyma that is left back [78].

46.8.3.5 Intraoral Deep Lobe Tumor Excision [79]

It is a transoral approach used in removal of few benign tumors of the deep lobe, which are easily visible displacing the superior portion of the tonsil and soft palate medially. An incision is made with cautery or knife over the most prominent aspect of the swelling in the tonsil and palate area, extending above and below the apparent location of the tumor. The constrictor muscle is identified, and dissection is continued through thinned constrictor muscle by dividing it above and below the tumor. Pressure on the neck often assists in removal of the tumor. Fascial connections from the tumor into the adjacent bed are removed with blunt dissection, and the tumor is delivered into the mouth. Any vascular connections to the tumor should be cauterized, and meticulous hemostasis should be achieved. The superior and inferior portions of the wound are closed with interrupted sutures. The middle portion of the wound is left open to heal secondarily.

Complications

- Tumor rupture
- Incomplete removal
- Uncontrolled hemorrhage

46.8.3.6 Total Parotidectomy with or Without Facial Nerve Preservation

It is usually indicated in tumors affecting the deep lobe. A neoplasm of the deep part of the parotid enters the soft palate through the interval between the styloid process and the back of the mandible and is often of dumbbell shape with the isthmus lying in this gap. After raising a skin flap, the facial nerve is identified and dissected out leaving a layer of glandular tissue on it. An access osteotomy either in the form of vertical subsigmoid or mandibular body distal to the mental foramen is used to open up the interval between the mandible and the styloid process through which the tumor has passed. The stylohyoid muscle may be divided close to the styloid process and turned forward. The external carotid artery will be encountered emerging above the muscles and should be divided. The origin of the facial artery should be identified to check the identity of the vessel.

As the parotid gland and the tumor are freed, it may be raised up between the two nerve bundles or below both bundles. Next entry is made intraorally over the tumor, and under direct vision tissues are divided to deliver the mass. Care is taken to avoid damaging the internal jugular vein and internal carotid artery which lie deep to styloid process. Following removal of the mass, the wound is irrigated, and the oral tissues closed with care using resorbable suture. The drapes are replaced over the mouth, gloves changed, and the mandibular fragments fixed together and the wound closed in the normal way.

46.8.3.7 Parotidectomy Using SMAS Plane for Dissection [73]

The advantages of this flap are that exposure of the gland is sufficient and the dissection is easy to perform. There is no donor-site morbidity, minimum additional operating time, and no extra cost. It seems to decrease the incidence of Frey's syndrome. The speed of the recovery of the facial nerve has been highlighted in the literature. It is more satisfactory from the patient's point of view.

46.8.3.8 Parotidomandibulectomy and Temporoparotidectomy [80]

Parotidomandibulectomy is indicated where there is invasion of the mandible by a malignant neoplasm.

In temporoparatidectomy, small-scale resection of the external auditory canal may be included with the excision of the pinna and overlying skin of the parotid where these structures are involved. The deficiency may be made good with a deltopectoral or other suitable flap.

46.8.4 Parotidectomy in Continuity with Neck Dissection

In the case of lymph node metastasis as stated in surgical pathology, neck dissection can be done in continuity with parotidectomy by increasing the neck skin crease incision and clearing the lymphatic structures.

46.8.5 Complications of Parotid Surgery

- Facial paresis or paralysis often results from poor technique and failure to preserve small nerve branches.
- Bleeding and hematoma formation, which can significantly compromise the airway.
- Rarely, persistent salivary leakage or sialocele formation occurs.
- Frey's syndrome.
- Skin flap necrosis.

46.9 Surgical Management of Submandibular and Sublingual Gland Tumors

Small tumors confined to the gland are treated by sialadenectomy, and tumors spreading beyond the confines of the gland are treated with a wider en bloc excision, which may include resection of the floor of mouth and mandible depending on extent of tumor. The neurotropic tumors might involve the lingual, hypoglossal, mylohyoid, and marginal mandibular nerve leading to a perineurial spread which can be confirmed on frozen section. Thickening and nodularity of the nerves may indicate perineural involvement [81].

46.9.1 Incision

For submandibular sialadenectomy, a skin crease incision below 3 cm from the lower border of mandible is taken to avoid damaging the marginal mandibular nerve which loops below the lower border of the mandible (Fig. 46.32).

For simple excision of the sublingual gland, an incision is made in the floor of the mouth lateral to the submandibular

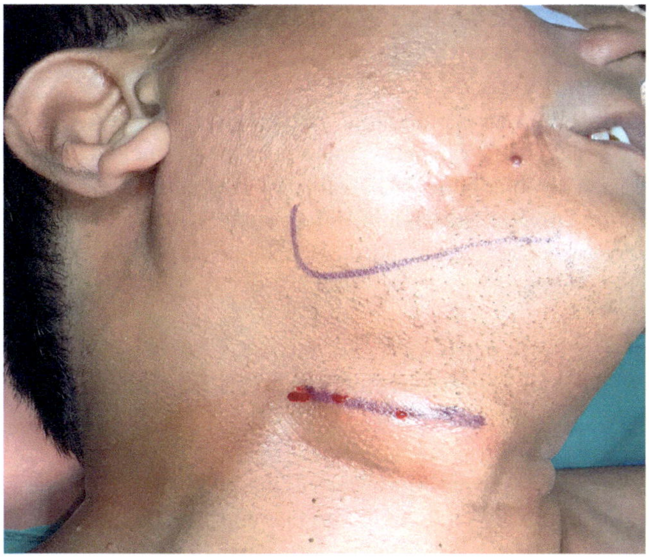

Fig. 46.32 Submandibular incision

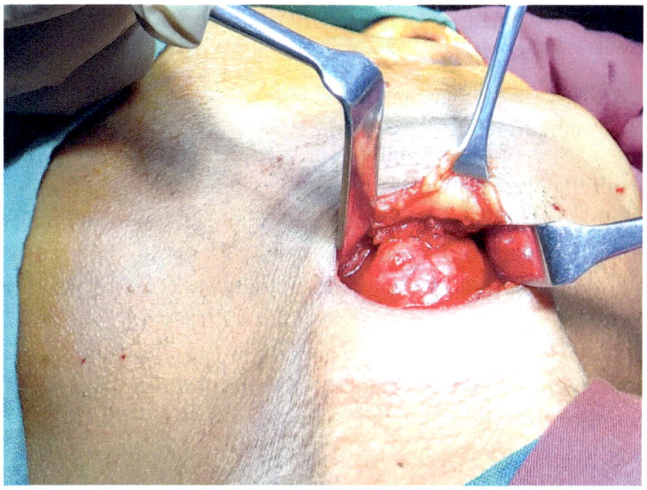

Fig. 46.33 Submandibular gland exposure with subplatysmal dissection

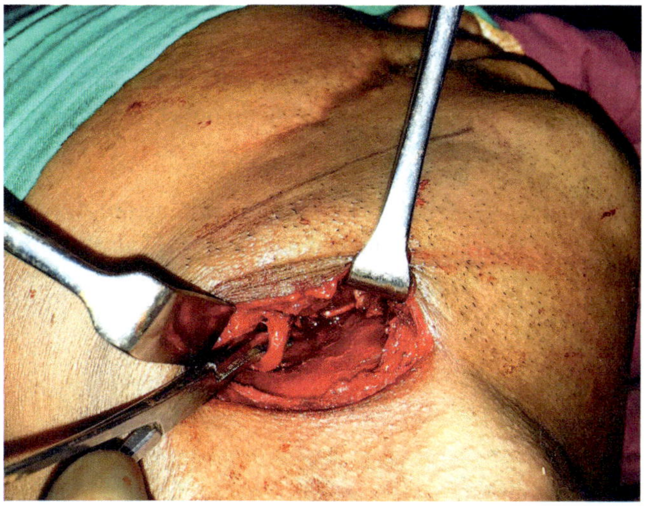

Fig. 46.34 Facial artery preservation in submandibular sialadenectomy

duct taking care to limit it up to premolar region, as at the molar region, there is a chance to damage the lingual nerve. When sublingual gland excision is necessary for a tumor, it should be removed with a wide margin including a rim resection of the mandible.

46.9.2 Extracapsular Excision of the Submandibular Salivary Gland [82]

After making an incision in the neck crease, skin flap is raised in the subplatysmal plane (Fig. 46.33). The capsule of the gland should be left intact when the sialadenectomy is being done for a tumor, which might compromise the marginal mandibular nerve. The facial artery and nerve are identified as close to the gland as possible. After transection, they are elevated superiorly to identify and reflect the marginal mandibular nerve. Nowadays the facial artery is spared during surgery to allow free flap anastomosis during oncosurgeries (Fig. 46.34). The investing fascia is then divided at the lower border of mandible, and the gland is delivered out from between the anterior and posterior bellies of the digastric muscle. Anteriorly the gland is separated from the mylohyoid muscle, and lingual nerve, hypoglossal nerve, and Wharton's duct are identified. The lingual nerve shares the same facial sheath as the gland at the upper pole. This attachment of the lingual nerve to the gland represents its parasympathetic supply. The Wharton's duct is inferior to lingual nerve and is often surrounded by sublingual glands. As fascia and gland are mobilized upward from the surface of the hyoglossus, the hypoglossal nerve is identified more inferiorly. It is accompanied by ranine vein. Posteriorly the angular tract of fascia has to be cut with scissors to allow the gland in its fascial envelope to be drawn down without grasping the gland with instruments. Where necessary the upper pole may be mobilized via the mouth. An assistant can then depress the gland toward the submandibular wound to enable the operation to be concluded.

The duct and the branch of the lingual nerve supplying the submandibular gland are ligated and transected. The duct is divided close behind the papilla. During excision for inflammatory disease, the nerve is always separated from the gland with knife or scissors. However, if the nerve appears to be involved in a tumor, it is sectioned in front of and behind the gland and the cut ends sutured. The wound is closed in layers with drainage in the usual way.

46.10 Management of Minor Salivary Gland Tumors

Surgical resection of minor salivary gland tumors depends on the site of origin and extent of disease. This may range from a wide local excision of localized low-grade tumors to more radical excision, including marginal or segmental mandibulectomy and/or partial or total resection of the hard or soft palate, partial or total maxillectomy, infratemporal fossa dissection, and/or anterior craniofacial resection for larger and/or high-grade tumors. The V2 and V3 divisions of the trigeminal nerve are at potential risk for perineural spread of minor salivary gland malignancy and may facilitate an early skull base metastasis. Resection of the cranial base may be required in some cases to eradicate the tumor and obtain negative surgical margins [81].

46.10.1 Excision of Palatal Pleomorphic Adenomas [83]

Small pleomorphic adenomas on the palate can cause pressure resorption of the bone but do not cause true bony invasion. They are managed by local excision along with the periosteum. In the case of involvement of greater palatine foramen area, the lesion is freed until it can be drawn down, and the vessels clamped and cauterized under direct vision. If not, the vessel retracts into the canal and causes irritating bleeding. The wound is left to granulate secondarily.

46.10.2 Excision of Palatal Mucoepidermoid Carcinoma [83]

Low-grade mucoepidermoid carcinomas may be treated by the excision of a full-thickness disk of palate, including palatal and alveolar bone. Nasal and oral mucous membranes are sutured together around the defect in the soft palate. Primary reconstruction is avoided and an obturator is used instead (Fig. 46.35a, b).

46.10.3 Excision of Palatal Adenoid Cystic Carcinoma [83]

Spread along the perineurial tissues makes an inadequate surgical margin very likely after surgical management of ACC. A combination of surgery and radiotherapy is best. Surgical excision should be generous. Hemimaxillectomy including the orbital floor is a minimum, unless there is very good evidence that less will be sufficient. Where the soft palate and pterygoid region are involved, extended maxillectomy approach is essential to ensure adequate excision under direct vision.

46.10.4 Excision of Neoplasms of the Cheek and Lips

A primary excision with a margin of normal adjacent tissue can be used, but if there is any doubt, it can be preceded by a biopsy. Re-operation following incomplete extirpation

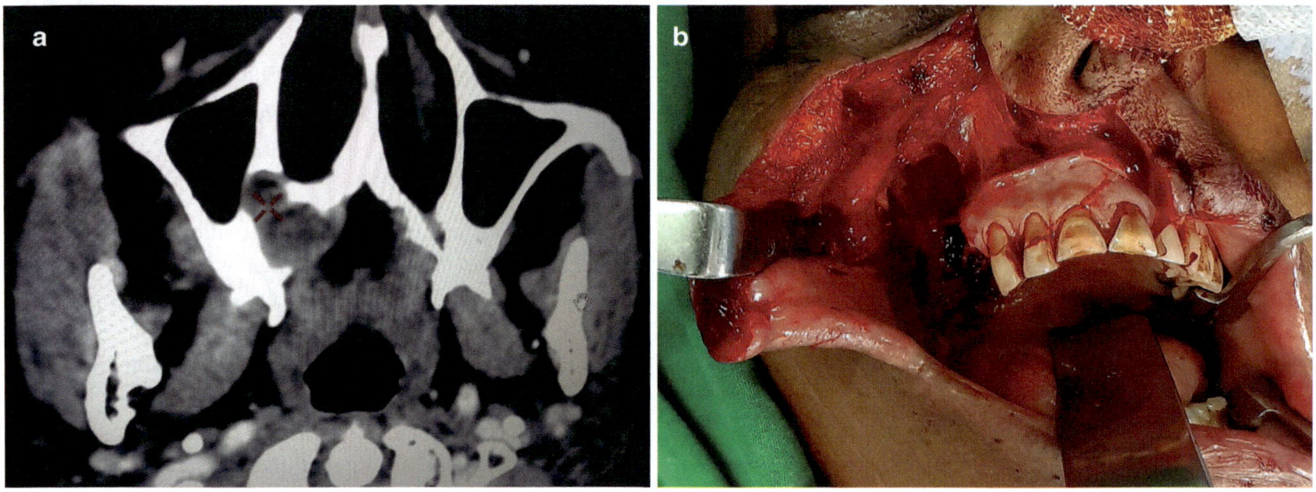

Fig. 46.35 (**a**) CT scan showing mucoepidermoid carcinoma of palate (red arrow). (**b**) Surgical excision of tumor using standard Weber-Ferguson incision

could mean the unnecessary sacrifice of tissue to ensure an adequate margin on the second occasion. Clinically aggressive neoplasms must be biopsied, since adequate treatment may involve radiotherapy and full-thickness excision and repair.

More aggressive tumors affecting the palatal salivary glands are managed by partial maxillectomy or total maxillectomy or extended maxillectomy based on the extent of disease.

46.10.5 Complications

- A hematoma may develop in the dead space after gland excision. It can be avoided by meticulous hemostasis and placement of suction drain to clear out any collection. In case a hematoma develops, it can be aspirated or sucked under aseptic precautions. However, it may not be completely effective. The patient can be just put on good antibiotic coverage, and it will resolve without getting infected.
- Trismus occurs due to masseter muscle spasm or inflammation in the TMJ. It generally resolves spontaneously and hence should be just managed symptomatically.
- Salivary fistula occurs uncommonly due to discontinuity between the residual salivary gland parenchyma and the salivary duct. In majority of cases, the problem is self-limiting. Management includes repeated aspiration, pressure dressings, wound care, an antisialogogue medication (glycopyrrolate), and patience.
- Facial nerve dysfunction results from traction injury to the facial nerve (neuropraxia) during dissection in parotid surgery. Complete recovery within a few months can be expected if nerve integrity has been maintained. In case the nerve is transected, it should be followed by immediate nerve grafting repair.
- Auriculotemporal syndrome of Frey is also called gustatory sweating. It manifests as flushing and sweating of the skin of upper cheek, temporal region, and forehead coincident with eating and smelling of food. Following damage to the auriculotemporal nerve or to communicating branches to the facial nerve, secretomotor parasympathetic nerves from the otic ganglion and also sympathetic fibers to the sweat glands traveling in the same nerve are divided. Following regeneration, fibers from otic ganglion come to supply the sweat glands. Minor's starch-iodine test is used for diagnosis [78]. It can be managed by simple treatment of antiperspirant application; 1% local application of glycopyrrolate is effective. The only effective cure is to divide the parasympathetic fibers from the glossopharyngeal nerve.

Sensory abnormalities associated with greater auricular nerve sacrifice, reflect as sensory deficit in the lower third of pinna including earlobe as well as adjacent preauricular and postauricular skin.

46.11 Recent Advances [84]

Robotic sialadenectomy of the submandibular gland has been done via a modified face lift approach. Virgilio et al. performed robotic sialadenectomy of the submandibular gland in five patients (two patients each with sialolithiasis and pleomorphic adenoma and one patient of ranula) with success. They used three robotic arms, two operative arms, and a facedown 30° endoscopic arm. The operative left arm is equipped with Maryland forceps and right arm with harmonic scalpel.

46.12 Conclusion

Salivary gland pathologies may be neoplastic, non-neoplastic, inflammatory, or non-inflammatory. Early surgical intervention after a good clinical, radiological, and histopathological diagnosis is need of an hour to minimize the postoperative complications. Early diagnosis and management with recent advanced technologies is the key factor in achieving excellent prognosis of the disease.

Acknowledgment Author wishes to thank Dr. Anshul Rai for Figs. 46.3, 46.4, 46.9, 46.13, 46.17a, b, and 46.20.

Author wishes to thank Dr. Kedar Saraf, Professor, Dept. of OMDR, SMBT Institute of Dental Sciences, Sangamner, Maharashtra, for Figs. 46.11a, b, and 46.12.

References

1. Saunders PR, Macpherson DW. Acute suppurative parotitis: a forgotten cause of upper airway obstruction. Oral Surg Oral Med Oral Pathol. 1991;72:412–4.
2. Hollinshead WH. The face. Anatomy for surgeons: Vol I. The head and neck. 3rd ed. Philadelphia: Harper and Row Publishers; 1982. p. 291–324. Chapter 6.
3. Cawson R, Gleeson M. Anatomy and physiology of the salivary glands. In: Gleeson M, editor. Scott-Brown's otolaryngology. Basic sciences. 6th ed. Great Britain: Butterworth Heinemann; 1997. Chapter 9, p. 1/9/1–1/9/18.
4. Snell RS. The head and neck. Clinical anatomy. 7th ed. Philadelphia: Lippincott Williams and Wilkins; 2004, Chapter 11, p. 719–922.
5. McGregor IA, McGregor FM. Salivary glands. Cancer of the face and mouth. Pathology and management for surgeons. Edinburgh: Churchill Livingstone; 1986. Chapter 25, p. 569–606.
6. Rankow RM, Polayes IM. Surgical anatomy and diagnosis. Diseases of Salivary glands. Philadelphia: W.B. Saunders; 1976. Chapter 7, p. 156–84.
7. Borle RM, Jadhav A, Bhola N, Hingnikar P, Gaikwad P. Borle's triangle: a reliable anatomical landmark for ease of identification of facial nerve trunk during parotidectomy. J Oral Biol Craniofac Res. 2019;9(1):33–6.

8. Wetmore SJ. Surgical landmarks for the facial nerve. Otolaryngol Clin N Am. 1991;24(3):505–30.
9. Farrior JB, Santini H. Facial nerve identification in children. Otolaryngol Head Neck Surg. 1985;93:173.
10. Pather N, Osman M. Landmark of facial nerve: implication for parotidectomy. Surg Radiol Anat. 2006;28(2):170–5.
11. http://apps.who.int/classifications/apps/icd/icd10online2003/fr-icd.htm
12. Norman JE, McGurk M. Salivary gland imaging. In: Morse MH, editor. Color atlas and text of Salivary glands – diseases, disorders and surgery. Wolfe, Spain: Mosby; 1995. p. 105–27.
13. Lowman RM, Cheng GK. Diagnostic roentgenology. In: Rankow RM, Polayes IM, editors. Diseases of salivary glands. Philadelphia: W.B. Saunders; 1976. Chapter 4, p. 54–98.
14. DelBalso A. Salivary imaging. Oral Maxillofac Surg Clin N Am. 1995;7(3):387–422.
15. Taylor & Francis. Acta Oto-Laryngologica. 1998;118 Suppl 538:214–20.
16. Kim D, Uy C, Mandel L. Sialosis of unknown origin. N Y State Dent J. 1998;64(7):38–40.
17. McQuone SJ. Acute viral and bacterial infections of the salivary glands. Otolaryngol Clin N Am. 1999;32(5):793–811.
18. Nahlieli O, Bar T, Shacham R. Management of chronic recurrent parotitis: current therapy. J Oral Maxillofac Surg. 2004;62:1150–5.
19. Work WP, Hecht DW. Inflammatory diseases of the major salivary glands. In: Papparella MM, Shumrick DF, editors. Otolaryngology, vol. 3. Philadelphia: WB Saunders; 1980. p. 2235–43.
20. Williams MF. Sialolithiasis. Otolaryngol Clin N Am. 1999;32(5):819–34.
21. Lustmann J, Regev E, Melamed Y. Sialolithiasis: a survey on 245 patients and a review of literature. Int J Oral Maxillofac Surg. 1990;19:135–8.
22. Kawaguchi K, Yamada H, Iida N, Horie A, Sato J, Seto K. Sialodochoplasty to treat sialoliths using a microsurgical technique. Br J Oral Maxillofac Surg. 2008;46(7):607–8.
23. Park JH, Kim JW, Lee YM, Oh CW, Chang HS, Lee SW. Long-term study of sialodochoplasty for preventing submandibular sialolithiasis recurrence. Clin Exp Otorhinolaryngol. 2012;5(1):34–8.
24. Arrieta AJ, McCaffrey TV. Inflammatory disorders of Salivary glands. In: Cummins Otolaryngology – head and neck surgery. 4th ed. Mosby; 2005. Part 5. Chapter 58, p. 1323–38.
25. Agni N, Borle R. Non neoplastic diseases. In: Salivary gland pathologies. Jaypee; 2013. Chapter 7, 54–89.
26. Rice DH. Salivary gland disorders: neoplastic and nonneoplastic. Med Clin N Am. 1999;83(1):197–217.
27. Mandel L. Inflammatory disorders – clinicopathologic considerations. Diseases of salivary glands. In: Rankow RM, Polayes IM, editors. Philadelphia: W.B. Saunders; 1976. Chapter 9, Part 1, p. 202–38.
28. Shafer WG, Hine MK, Levy BM. Tumors of salivary glands. A textbook of oral pathology. 4th ed. Singapore: Harcourt Asia PTE Ltd.; 1993. Chapter 3, p. 231–57.
29. Manoussakis MN, Moutsopoulos HM. Sjögren's syndrome. Otolaryngol Clin N Am. 1999;32(5):843–60.
30. Trott MS, Hughes GB, Calabrese LH. Hearing and Sjögren's syndrome. Ear Nose Throat J. 1996;75:666.
31. Yamasoba T, Tayama N, Syoji M, et al. Clinicostatistical study of lower lip mucoceles. Head Neck. 1990;12:316.
32. Marx DE, Stern D. Non-neoplastic salivary gland disease. In: Oral and maxillofacial pathology: a rationale for diagnosis and treatment. New Delhi: Quintessence Publishing; 2003. Chapter 11, p. 497–527.
33. Huang I, et al. Treatment of mucocele of the lower lip with carbon dioxide laser. J Oral Maxillofac Surg. 2007;65:855–8.
34. Baurmash HD. Mucoceles and ranulas. J Oral Maxillofac Surg. 2003;61:369–78.
35. Harrison JD. Modern management and pathophysiology of ranula: literature review. Head Neck. 2010;32:1310.
36. Kono M, et al. Evaluation of OK-432 injection therapy as possible primary treatment of intraoral ranula. J Oral Maxillofac Surg. 2017;75:336–42.
37. Schneider AB, Favus MJ, Stachura ME, et al. Salivary gland neoplasms as a late consequence of head and neck irradiation. Ann Intern Med. 1977;87(2):160–4.
38. Tsai CC, Chen CL, Hsu HC. Expression of Epstein-Barr virus in carcinomas of major salivary glands: a strong association with lymphoepithelioma-like carcinoma. Hum Pathol. 1996;27(3):258–62.
39. Sadetzki S, Oberman B, Mandelzweig L, et al. Smoking and risk of parotid gland tumors: a nationwide case-control study. Cancer. 2008;112(9):1974–82.
40. Spitz MR, Batsakis JG. Major salivary gland carcinoma. Descriptive epidemiology and survival of 498 patients. Arch Otolaryngol. 1984;110(1):45–9.
41. Van Der Waal I. Salivary gland neoplasms. In: Van Der Waal I, Prabhu SR, Wilson DF, Daftary DK, Johnson NW, editors. Oral diseases in the tropics. Delhi: Oxford University Press; 1993. Chapter 41, p. 478–86.
42. Amin MB, Edge SB, Greene FL, et al., editors. AJCC cancer staging manual. 8th ed. New York: Springer; 2017.
43. Seifert G, Sobin LH. The World Health Organization's histological classification of salivary gland tumors. A commentary on the second edition. Cancer. 1992;70(2):379–85.
44. Seifert G. Diagnosis and prognosis of salivary gland tumors. An interpretation of new revised WHO classification. Mund Kiefer Gesichtschir. 1997;1(5):252–67.
45. Seethala RR, Stenman G. Update from the 4th edition of the World Health Organization classification of head and neck tumours: tumors of the salivary gland. Head Neck Pathol. 2017;11(1):55–67.
46. Ord RA. Surgical management of Parotid tumors. Oral Maxillofac Surg Clin N Am. 1995;7(3):529–64.
47. Cornog JL, Gray SR. Surgical and clinical pathology of salivary gland tumors. In: Rankow RM, Polayes IM, editors. Diseases of salivary glands. Philadelphia: W.B. Saunders; 1976. Chapter 5, p. 99–142.
48. Waldron CA. Mixed tumor (Pleomorphic adenoma) and Myoepithelioma. In: Ellis GL, editor. Surgical pathology of the salivary glands. Philadelphia: W.B. Saunders; 1991. Chapter 10, p. 165–86.
49. Foote FW, Frazell EL. Tumours of the major salivary glands. Cancer. 1953;6:1065–133.
50. Papadogeorgakis N, Skouteris CA, Mylonas AI, Angelopoulos AP. Superficial parotidectomy: technical modifications based on tumor characteristics. J Cranio Maxillofac Surg. 2004;32:350–3.
51. Batsakis JG. Tumors of the head and neck – Clinical and pathological considerations. 2nd ed. Baltimore: Williams and Wilkins; 1979. Chapter 1.
52. Warnock GR. Papillary cystadenoma lymphomatosum (Wharton's tumor). In: Ellis GL, editor. Surgical pathology of the salivary glands. Philadelphia: W.B. Saunders; 1991. Chapter 11, p. 187–201.
53. Goode RK. Oncocytoma. In: Ellis GL, editor. Surgical pathology of the salivary glands. Philadelphia: W.B. Saunders; 1991. Chapter 13, p. 225–37.
54. Kratochvil FJ. Canalicular adenoma and Basal cell adenoma. In: Ellis GL, editor. Surgical pathology of the salivary glands. Philadelphia: W.B. Saunders; 1991. Chapter 12, p. 202–24.
55. Ellis GL, Auclair PL. Ductal papillomas. In: Ellis GL, editor. Surgical pathology of the salivary glands. Philadelphia: W.B. Saunders; 1991. Chapter 14, p. 238–51.
56. White DK, Miller AS, McDaniel RK, Rothman BN. Inverted ductal papilloma: a distinctive lesion of minor salivary gland. Cancer. 1982;49:519–24.

57. Auclair PL, Ellis GL. Mucoepidermoid carcinoma. Surgical pathology of the salivary glands. Philadelphia: W.B. Saunders; 1991. Chapter 16, p. 269–98.
58. Healey WV, Perzin KH, Smith L. Mucoepidermoid carcinoma of salivary gland origin: classification, clinical-pathologic correlation, and results of treatment. Cancer. 1970;26:368–88.
59. Olsen KD, Devine KD, Weiland LH. Mucoepidermoid carcinoma of the oral cavity. Otolaryngol Head Neck Surg. 1981;89:783–91.
60. Maciejewski A, Szymczyk C, Wierzgon J. Outcome of surgery for adenoid cystic carcinoma of head and neck region. J Cranio-Maxillofac Surg. 2002;30:59–61.
61. Tomich CE. Adenoid cystic carcinoma. In: Ellis GL, Auclair PL, Gnepp DR, editors. Surgical pathology of the salivary glands. Philadelphia: W.B. Saunders; 1991. Chapter 19, p. 333–49.
62. Kim KH, Sung MW. Adenoid cystic carcinoma of the head and neck. Arch Otolaryngol Head Neck Surg. 1994;120:721–6.
63. Witten J, Hybert F, Hansen HS. Treatment of malignant tumors in the parotid glands. Cancer. 1990;65:2515–20.
64. Auclair PL, Ellis GL. Clear cell carcinoma. In: Ellis GL, Auclair PL, Gnepp DR, editors. Surgical pathology of the salivary glands. Philadelphia: W.B. Saunders; 1991. Chapter 22, p. 379–89.
65. Corio RL. Epithelial – myoepithelial carcinoma. In: Ellis GL, Auclair PL, Gnepp DR, editors. Surgical pathology of the salivary glands. Philadelphia: W.B. Saunders; 1991. Chapter 24, p. 412–21.
66. Corio RL, Sciubba JJ, Brannon RB, Batsakis JG. Epithelial-myoepithelial carcinoma of intercalated duct origin. Oral Surg Oral Med Oral Pathol. 1982;53:280–7.
67. Gnepp D, Wenig B. Malignant mixed tumors. In: Ellis GL, Auclair PL, Gnepp DR, editors. Surgical pathology of the salivary glands. Philadelphia: W.B. Saunders; 1991. Chapter 20. p. 350–68.
68. Speight PM, Barrett AW. Salivary gland tumours. Oral Dis. 2002;8(5):229–40.
69. Ferreria JL, Maurino N, Michael E, Ratinoff M, Rubio E. Surgery of the Parotid region: a new approach. J Oral and Maxillofac Surg. 1990;48:803–7.
70. Blair VP, editor. Surgery and diseases of the mouth and jaw. 3rd ed. St Louis: Mosby; 1918.
71. Hanna EY, Lee S, Fan CY, Suen JY. Benign neoplasms of the salivary glands. In: Haughley BH, editor. Cummings otolaryngology head and neck surgery. vol. II, 4th ed. Elsevier Mosby; 2005. Chapter 60, p. 1348–77.
72. Bananno PC, Casson PR. Frey's syndrome: a preventable phenomenon. Plast Reconstr Surg. 1992;89(3):452–6.
73. Meningaud JP, Bertolus C, Bertrand JC. Parotidectomy: assessment of a surgical technique including facelift incision and SMAS advancement. J Cranio-Maxillofac Surg. 2006;34:34–7.
74. Rai A, et al. Posterior belly of digastric muscle flap for contour deformity correction after superficial parotidectomy. J Stomatol Oral Maxillofac Surg. 2018;119(4):304–6.
75. Johns M, Nachlas N. Salivary gland tumors. In: Paperella M, Shumrick D, Gluckman J, Meyerhoff W, editors. Otolaryngology. vol. 3, 3rd ed. Philadelphia: W.B. Saunders; 1991. Chapter 20, p. 2099–127.
76. Kun Z, Dao-Yi Q, Li-Min W. Functional superficial parotidectomy. J Oral Maxillofac Surg. 1994;52:1038–41.
77. Papadogeorgakis N, Skouteris CA, Mylonas AI, Angelopoulos AP. Superficial parotidectomy: technical modifications based on tumor characteristics. J Cranio Maxillofac Surg. 2004;32:350–3.
78. Yamashita T, Tomoda K, Kumazawa T. The usefulness of partial parotidectomy for benign parotid gland tumors. Acta Otolaryngol. 1993;500:113–6.
79. Oslen KD. Intraoral salivary gland tumor removal. Section I. Head and neck. In: Bailey BJ, Calhoun KH, Friedman NR, Newlands SD, Vrabec JT, editors. Atlas of head and neck surgery – Otolaryngology. 2nd ed. Philadelphia: Lippincott Williams & Wilkins. p. 6–7.
80. Shah JP. Color atlas of operative techniques in head and neck surgery. England: Wolfe Medical. p. 117–33.
81. Hanna EY, Suen JY. Malignant tumors of the salivary glands. In: Myers EN, Suen JY, Myers JN, Hanna EY, editors. Cancer of the head and neck. 4th ed. Saunders; 2003. Chapter 21, p. 475–510.
82. Seward GR. Nodular enlargement of a salivary gland. In: Moore J, editor. Surgery of the mouth and jaws. London: Blackwell Scientific; 1985. Chapter 38, p. 676–99.
83. Hanna EY, Suen JY. The Parotid neoplasm. Section 22. Controversies in otolaryngology. In: Pensak ML, editor. New York: Publication Thieme; 2001. Chapter 66, p. 348–54.
84. Virgilio DA, et al. Robotic sialoadenectomy of the submandibular gland via a modified face-lift approach. Int J Oral Maxillofac Surg. 2012;41:1325–9.

Additional Reading

Barnes L, Eveson JW, Reichart P, Sidransky D. World Health Organization classification of tumours. Pathology and genetics of head and neck tumours. vol. 9. Lyon: IARC; 2005.

Kennedy RA. WHO is in and WHO is out of the mouth, salivary glands, and jaws sections of the 4th edition of the WHO classification of head and neck tumours. Br J Oral Maxillofac Surg. 2018;56(2):90–5.

McGurk M, Combes J. Controversies in the management of salivary gland disease. 2nd ed. Oxford University Press; 2013.

Obstructive Salivary Gland Disease and Sialendoscopy

47

Prithvi S. Bachalli and Aditya Moorthy

47.1 Introduction

Salivary gland diseases have been described in the literature for centuries. From the time of Hippocrates to the descriptions of parotid tumours in the sixteenth century and the anatomical descriptions of the ductal systems of the major salivary glands in the seventeenth century, we have assimilated knowledge of anatomy and pathology of these glands [1].

The conventional approach to infections of the salivary glands is medical management, occasional expression of the stone through the papilla, marsupialisation of the duct following removal of sialolith. Failing all, removal of the involved gland [2].

Minimally invasive surgery especially those in which endoscopes are utilized has gradually become popular over the last three decades. As a whole, the trend in surgery is to improve function and hasten recovery. To achieve these ends, a combination of technology and smaller incisions has been crucial. Hence there is an increasing interest to manage salivary gland diseases endoscopically [3].

Sialendoscopy is the endoscopic management of obstructive salivary ductal disease and has rapidly become the procedure of choice for such conditions.

47.2 Obstructive Salivary Diseases

Salivary gland diseases can broadly be classified into ductal and parenchymal disorders.

Some conditions, such as Sjögren's syndrome and juvenile recurrent parotitis, tend to have an overlapping component and thus are difficult to segregate.

Ductal obstructions can be commonly attributed to-

- Sialoliths,
- Strictures within the duct or at the punctum,
- Presence of mucous plugs, and
- Retrograde bacterial infection.

The majority of obstructive salivary gland disease can be attributed to the presence of stones or sialoliths. Almost 60–70% of reported obstructive salivary disease comprises of sialolithiasis [4], which occurs in about 1.2% of the population. Amongst the major salivary glands, the submandibular is most affected (87%) , then the parotid (10%), and the sublingual (3%) to a much lesser extent [5].

Although sialolithiasis has been reported as the most common cause of salivary ductal obstructions, strictures, mucous plugs and the rare foreign body can cause significant obstruction to ductal flow.

47.3 Sialendoscopy

Sialendoscopy is a minimally invasive technique which makes use of miniature endoscopes to diagnose and treat salivary gland pathologies, including sialolithiasis, sialadenitis and strictures.

It is fast becoming the investigating procedure of choice for such conditions. Sialendoscopy has grown as a subspeciality in the last three decades, since the first attempts to retrieve salivary stones endoscopically were carried out. It is slowly gaining popularity and awareness in the last decade and a half.

Electronic Supplementary Material The online version of this chapter (https://doi.org/10.1007/978-981-15-1346-6_47) contains supplementary material, which is available to authorized users.

P. S. Bachalli (✉) · A. Moorthy
Department of Oral and Maxillofacial Surgery, Rangadore Memorial Hospital, Apollo Hospitals,
Bangalore, Karnataka, India

K. Bonanthaya et al. (eds.), *Oral and Maxillofacial Surgery for the Clinician*, https://doi.org/10.1007/978-981-15-1346-6_47

47.4 Evolution of Sialendoscopy

It took a few centuries, after the discovery of the ductal systems, for the first endoscopy to be reported. In 1990, Konigsberger et al. reported the first successful salivary endoscopy using a 0.8-mm flexible endoscope. Katz removed a stone with a flexible scope using blind passage of a basket in 1991, and for over a decade, both Nahlieli et al. and Marchal described various types of sialendoscopy instruments and approaches [3].

The last decade and a half has witnessed significant development of minimally invasive techniques for diagnosing and treating salivary ductal obstructions. Like with other surgical fields, this has led to a paradigm shift from open procedures to minimally invasive and endoscopic techniques with the emphasis on gland preservation and restoration of function. The miniaturization of endoscopes and advancing technology have made exploration and visualization of salivary ductal system possible using sialendoscopes [4].

47.5 Indications and Contraindications

As mentioned previously, sialolithiasis is the most common obstructive condition affecting the salivary duct and therefore is where sialendoscopic/sialendoscopy-assisted retrieval of sialoliths is most indicated.

Ductal strictures which may be secondary to calculi or those at the papilla opening can be very effectively treated by serial dilatation with sialendoscopes of increasing diameter [4].

Juvenile recurrent parotitis (JRP) is an inflammatory condition affecting the parotid gland and is the second most common condition in children after mumps [6, 7]. The condition affects the paediatric population primarily especially the ages between 3 and 6 years and occasionally persists in adolescence [8]. As the cause is unknown, management has generally been conservative. Anatomical aberrations, such as kinks in the duct, dehydration and possible ascending bacterial infection, have been hypothesised as causes.

Dilatation and lavage as a consequence of performing sialendoscopy has provided relief from symptoms and reduction in the frequency of attacks, even though the mechanism is not fully understood. This condition has a tendency of spontaneous cessation at puberty.

Although in Sjogren's syndrome, where the parenchyma of the parotid gland is primarily affected, there is also an associated ductal pathology, namely, strictures. Here too dilatation via sialendoscopy can provide symptomatic relief.

Acute inflammation of salivary glands and ducts is a contraindication to performing sialendoscopy. The duct is essentially a condensation of surrounding epithelium and not a rigid structure. In such an inflamed state, the risk of creating a false passage or perforating the duct is significantly higher [4].

Management in such situations is conservative, mainly with the use of appropriate antibiotics and analgesics, incision and drainage of a collection, and removal of cause, such as a sialolith, if easily visible or accessible, to allow acute symptoms to settle before a formal sialendoscopy is carried out.

Trismus is a relative contraindication to performing sialendoscopy, as naturally, reduction in mouth opening makes it both difficult to introduce and manoeuvre the scopes.

47.6 Investigations

A simple ultrasound in the hands of an experienced sonologist usually provides adequate information prior to sialendoscopy. It is a non-invasive, economical investigation which can determine the presence and size of sialoliths, strictures, dilatation or fibrosis of the duct. Alternatively a CT scan can be considered to achieve the same result.

MR sialograms are particularly useful in identifying strictures or areas of stenosis. However, like conventional sialography the papilla needs to be dilated and cannulated to inject the dye. In the hands of an inexperienced operator, damage to papilla might make performing sialendoscopy impossible.

47.7 Armamentarium

The sialendoscope can be divided very simply into two systems: the Marchal All-in-one (Fig. 47.1) and the Modular system (Fig. 47.2).

As the name suggests, the all-in-one has an irrigation port, a working channel through which various instruments can be introduced, and fibre optics in the same unit. This scope serves as both diagnostic and as an interventional tool.

The modular sialoendoscope consists only of a telescope, attached fibre-optic cable and an eyepiece. Interchangeable sheaths of various diameters are available which fit onto the basic telescope [6]. This scope with the appropriate sheaths can be used for both diagnostic and interventional purposes.

The sheaths used in the modular system make it rigid and unfortunately also bulky; thus significant dilatation of the papilla is required to introduce the scope [6].

Unlike other endoscopes, sialendoscopes come with only a zero-degree viewing angle. The all-in-one is semirigid, with a 5–15-degree angulation at the tip to facilitate manoeuvrability especially while exploring branches of the duct.

Diagnostic scopes come with only an irrigation port, whereas a working channel is also provided in therapeutic scopes to introduce instruments such as wire baskets and graspers for entrapping stones, balloons for stricture dilation

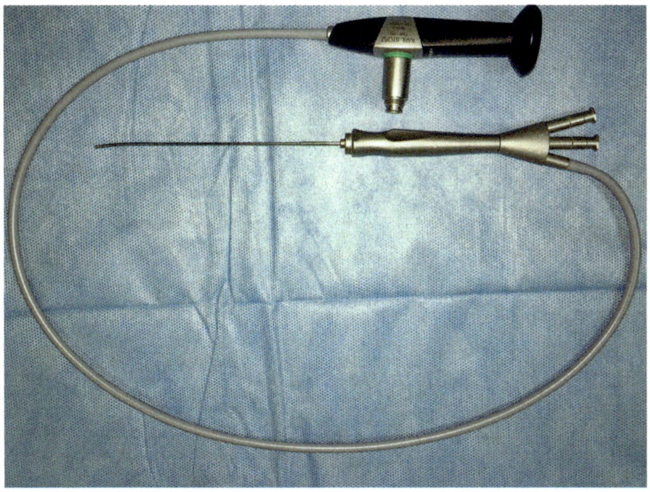

Fig. 47.1 Marchal All-in-one sialendoscope

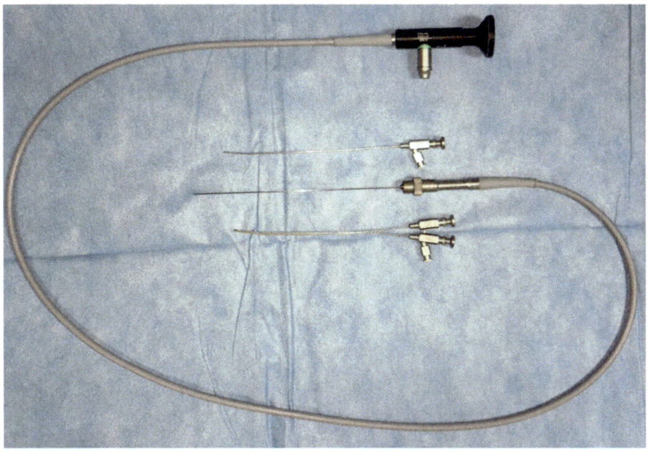

Fig. 47.2 Modular sialendoscope with sheaths

and a holmium laser fibre or a micro drill to fragment sialoliths [6].

Diameter of available scopes range from 0.9 to 1.6 mm, the smallest purely diagnostic and others having various sizes of the working channel to allow certain instruments only. This is a disadvantage of the all-in-one system in that the entire scope has to be changed if a larger instrument is required, whereas in the modular only the sheath can be changed [6].

Preliminary instruments, those that are used to dilate the papilla to facilitate the introduction of the scope, are also available. These include two types of dilators, papillotomy scissors, guide wires and hollow dilators [6] (Fig. 47.3).

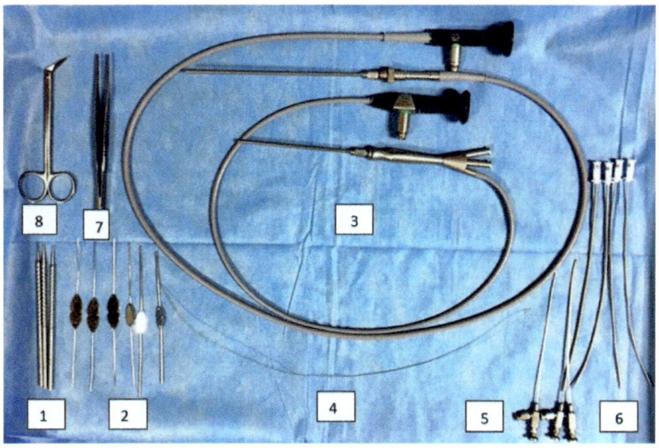

Fig. 47.3 Armamentarium. (1) Conic dilators, (2) Lacrimal probes, (3) Sialendoscopes, (4) Guide wire, (5) Sheaths for Modular sialendoscope, (6) hollow dilators, (7) vascular forceps, (8) papillotomy scissors

47.8 Anaesthesia and Technique

Anaesthetic of choice depends on the clinical and radiologically findings and the anticipated difficulty of the procedure. Local anaesthetic, with or without sedation, is usually adequate for a diagnostic procedure. In cases where sialolith retrieval is planned, either endoscopically or with a combined approach, general anaesthetic is usually preferable. Antisecretory agents like atropine and glycopyrrolate are avoided [6].

47.8.1 Positioning

Patient is placed supine with head fixed on a head rest and turned towards the surgeon. Shoulder extension is preferable. The monitor is placed opposite the surgeon. The assistant is next to the surgeon [6].

47.8.2 Identification, Cannulation and Dilatation of Punctum

The Wharton's duct punctum is comparatively more difficult to locate given the position is quite variable. There may even be a 'hood' of tissue obscuring the opening. In such situations, local anaesthetic can be infiltrated around the area which stiffens the opening, thereby aiding in location. Occasionally an incision might need to be placed on the floor of the mouth accompanied by minimal dissection to locate the duct. The Stensen's duct opening is far easier to identify. It is located on the buccal mucosa opposite upper second molar. Once the punctum is identified, the opening is serially dilated with conical dilator and probes of various sizes [6].

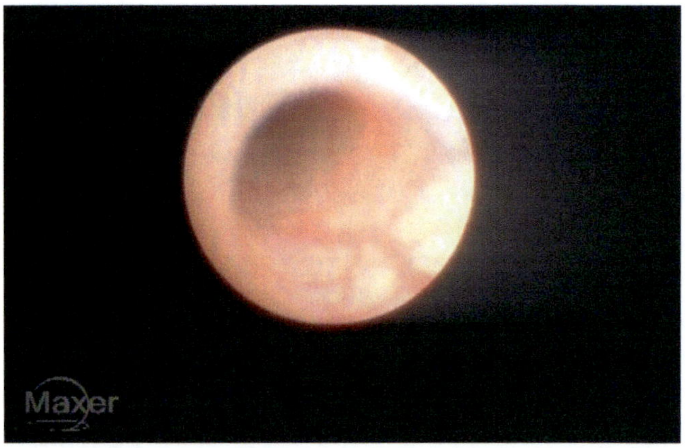

Fig. 47.4 Normal duct with vascular markings

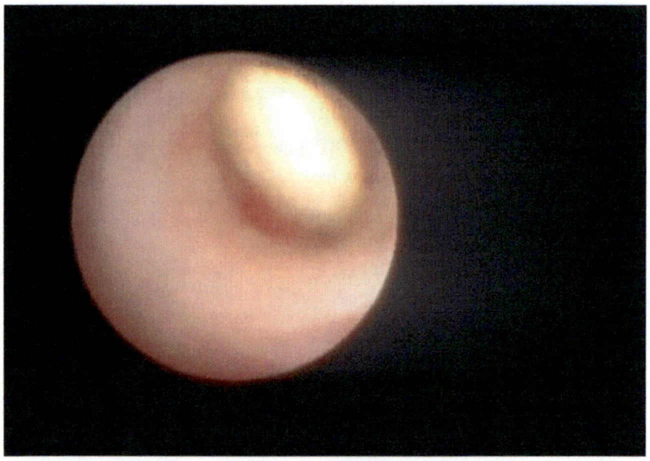

Fig. 47.5 Sialolith

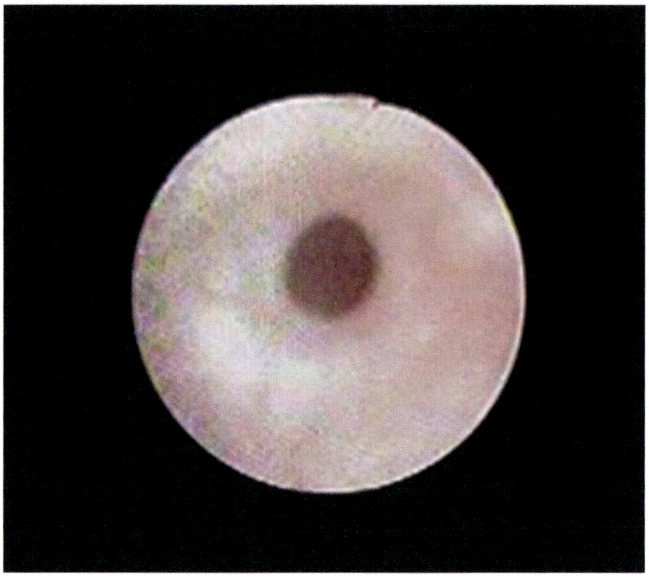

Fig. 47.6 Stricture

47.8.3 Sialendoscopic Evaluation

Once the punctum is adequately dilated, the appropriate sialendoscope is introduced into the duct. The duct is normally a collapsed structure, and irrigation fluid is required to keep the lumen open to visualise the duct and to advance the scope (Fig. 47.4). Normal saline is the preferred choice of irrigant solution and is diluted with local anaesthetic if the patient is awake for the procedure.

The irrigant also serves an additional purpose as this also performs lavage of the duct, thereby washing out debris and mucous plugs which might be accumulated [6].

The endoscope is slowly and gently passed from the punctum till branches are identified and explored if possible. This point of division of the duct is known as the hilum and is considered the end point of sialendoscopy. Alternatively, the presence of pathology such as a sialolith or stricture may prevent complete exploration of the duct (Figs. 47.5 and 47.6). It is important to note that once the pathology has been treated, the entire duct must be explored so as to ensure there are no further causes of obstruction, including the withdrawal of the scope under vision [6].

As the scope is guided through the primary and secondary ducts, the colour and texture of the mucosa are noted which are an indicator of the presence of inflammation. In relation to sialoliths, the size, shape and position need to be assessed as these will determine the method of retrieval [6].

Between the submandibular and the parotid duct, the Stensen's duct is comparatively more difficult to navigate due to the presence of the masseteric bend.

47.9 Diagnostic vs. Interventional Sialendoscopy

Indications for a diagnostic procedure include clinical symptoms, yet an unremarkable ultrasound and stricture at the papilla opening, to assess size and position of sialoliths.

Diagnostic sialendoscopy is a low morbidity, minimally invasive technique, which becomes the investigational procedure of choice for salivary duct pathologies in all age groups. Sialendoscopy has the advantage of offering a real-time ductal view. Diagnostic endoscopy is occasionally therapeutic, in minor obstructions caused by mucous plugs which can be relieved by lavage.

Interventional sialendoscopy makes use of a wide array of armamentarium including wire baskets (Fig. 47.7), balloon catheters and holmium laser to assist in sialolith retrieval (Fig. 47.8).

Sialoliths with sizes ranging between 3 and 4 mm are amenable for endoscopic retrieval. Here they may be entrapped and retrieved by use of a wire basket or dragged to the punctual opening where a small incision is placed to facilitate removal.

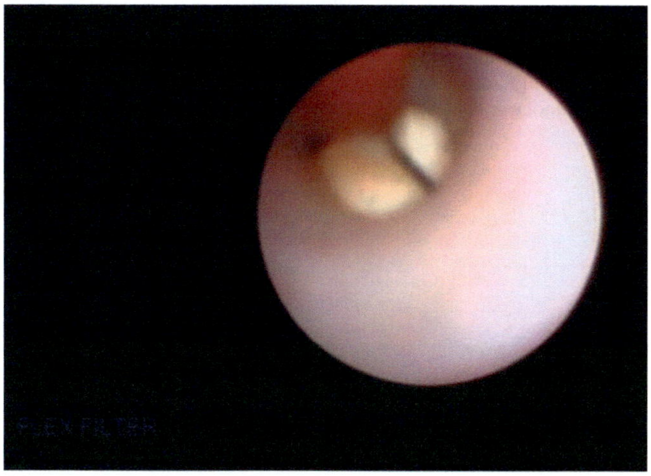

Fig. 47.7 Sialolith entrapped within wire basket

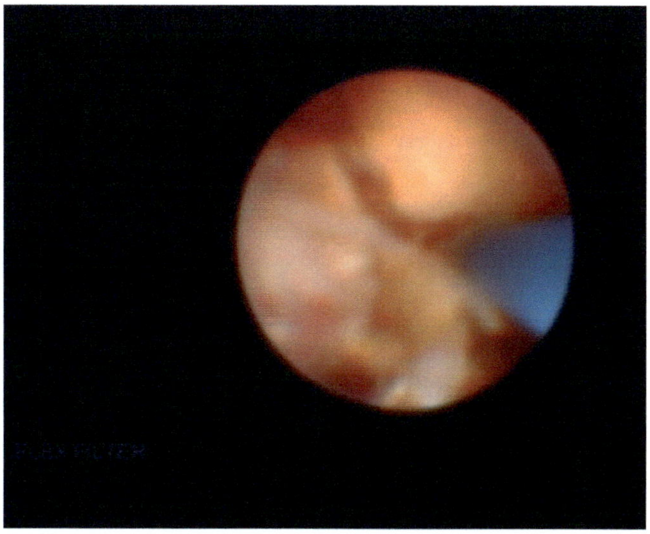

Fig. 47.8 Laser lithotripsy

Larger stones require a combined approach, whereby the position of the sialolith is identified and marked endoscopically and retrieved with an open surgical approach. The open approaches for submandibular sialoliths may be as small as a papillotomy or an extensive dissection of the floor of the mouth. The lingual nerve and iatrogenic ranula formation are important considerations when operating in this region. Large parotid stones require a SMAS flap, for the identification and protection of facial nerve branches and the duct, as well as reconstruction post-retrieval. Sialocele formation is an important consideration.

Hollow bougies of increasing diameter can threaded over a guide wire to widen strictures at the papillae. Balloons are another means of treating ductal strictures and once introduced through the working channel of the sialendoscope are inflated to dilate narrowed areas of the duct wall.

Stents are placed to maintain the patency of the duct and also to allow an incised duct to heal over with the aim of preventing stenosis. These stents are generally kept in place for up to 3 weeks. The authors have devised a salivary stent (Moorthy-Bachalli stent), made of polyurethane. These stents are available in sizes ranging from 3.5 French (diameter, 1 Fr = 0.3 mm) to 8 French and lengths from 5 to 7 cm with markings every centimetre. The stents also have a flange with prefabricated suture holes to facilitate suturing to the surrounding mucosa. An Ethilon 4-0 suture is preferred by the authors.

47.10 Complications

Like any other surgical procedure, open or endoscopic, sialendoscopy has its fair share of complications (Table 47.1).

Table 47.1 Complications of sialendoscopy

Complications	Management
Inability to locate papilla	Abort procedure/open approach to submandibular/parotid duct
False passage	If possible to locate duct-proceed, and abort procedure otherwise
Duct perforation	If possible to navigate beyond-proceed In case of floor of mouth or cheek oedema, then abort
Duct avulsion	Gland excision

47.11 Summary

When compared to other medical specialities, particularly otorhinolaryngologists, maxillofacial surgery is still in a primitive stage as far as the use of endovision is concerned. Hopefully an interest in areas like endoscopic management of salivary gland and temporomandibular joint diseases will narrow this gap.

Sialendoscopy is still in its infancy, in many parts of the world. Despite the challenges, growing awareness and the added attraction of minimally invasive surgery is steadily making it a popular choice for managing salivary ductal disease.

References

1. Marchal F. Sialendoscopy: the endoscopic approach to salivary gland ductal pathologies. Endo Press: Tuttlingen; 2012. pp 8.
2. Al-Abri R, Marchal F. New era of endoscopic approach for sialolithiasis: sialendoscopy. SQU Med J. 2010;10(3):382–7. Epub 14th Nov 10.
3. Erkul E, Gillespie MB. Sialendoscopy for non-stone disorders. Laryngoscope Investig Otolaryngol. 2016;1:140–5.
4. Singh PP, Gupta N, Goyal A, Tomar S. Interventional sialendoscopy for parotid ductal calculi: our preliminary experience. Indian J Otolaryngol Head Neck Surg. 2012;64(3):252–6.
5. Kopeć T, Szyfte W, Wierzbicka M. Sialoendoscopy and combined approach for the management of salivary gland stones. Eur Arch Otorhinolaryngol. 2013;270:219–23.
6. Singh PP, Gupta V. Sialendoscopy: introduction, indications and technique. Indian J Otolaryngol Head Neck Surg. 2014;66(1):74–8.
7. Harold D. Baurmash: chronic recurrent parotitis: a closer look at its origin, diagnosis, and management. J Oral Maxillofac Surg. 2004;62:1010–8.
8. Canzi P, Occhini A, Pagella F, Marchal F, Benazzo M. Sialendoscopy in juvenile recurrent parotitis: a review of the literature. Acta Otorhinolaryngol Ital. 2013;33:367–73.

Part XVI

Maxillofacial Traumatology

Primary Assessment and Care in Maxillofacial Trauma

48

Saurabh Saigal and Manal M. Khan

48.1 Introduction [1, 2]

Maxillofacial injuries are common in polytrauma patients, and spectrum can be minor to life-threatening injuries. Primary assessment and management can be very important. They can involve facial soft tissues, facial bones, or both. Maxillofacial injuries can be due to various causes including road traffic accidents, assaults, and fall from height, industrial injuries, animal bites, sports injuries, burns, and war injuries. Life-threatening maxillofacial injuries can complicate the initial management of a trauma patient due to presence of concomitant injuries to airway, head, or cervical spine.

The mechanism for this injury is exemplified by an unbelted automobile passenger who is thrown into the windshield and dashboard. Trauma to midface can produce fractures and dislocations that compromise the nasopharynx and oropharynx. Facial fractures can be associated with hemorrhage, increased secretion, and dislodged teeth. Fractures of mandible, especially bilateral body fractures, can cause loss of normal airway and structural support. Airway obstruction can result if the patient is in supine position.

The term "golden hour" has to be kept in mind while handling the trauma patient which indicates that the injured patient has 1 h (60 min) from the time of injury to receive definitive care. After that there will be significant increase in the morbidity and mortality of the patient. "Chances of survival of the critically injured patient will largerly determine after the first hour" [3].

Electronic Supplementary Material The online version of this chapter (https://doi.org/10.1007/978-981-15-1346-6_48) contains supplementary material, which is available to authorized users.

S. Saigal (✉)
Department of Anaesthesiology, AIIMS Bhopal, Bhopal, Madhya Pradesh, India
e-mail: saurabh.criticalcare@aiimsbhopal.edu.in

M. M. Khan
Department of Burns and Plastic Surgery, AIIMS Bhopal, Bhopal, Madhya Pradesh, India

48.2 Triage [4]

Sorting of patients based on their need for treatment and the available resources to provide the treatment is triage. This sorting may be carried out by the paramedic team at the accident scene or receiving hospital who decides what level of care is required. It may be based on which patients need immediate, lifesaving interventions, which can wait and which are, in fact, beyond saving. Depending on the urgency of treatment required, maxillofacial injuries can be broadly placed into one of four groups (Table 48.1).

Appropriate triage and prompt evaluation, using the Advanced Trauma Life Support (ATLS) system, benefit patients [5].

Box 48.1 Step-by-Step Management of a Trauma Patient in Emergency Unit

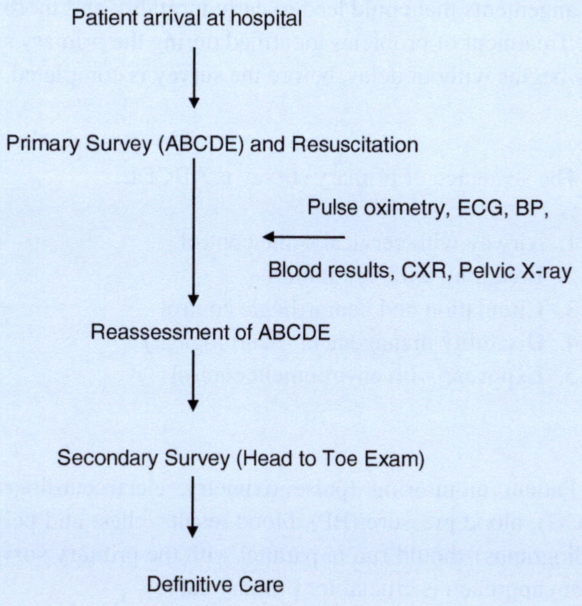

K. Bonanthaya et al. (eds.), *Oral and Maxillofacial Surgery for the Clinician*, https://doi.org/10.1007/978-981-15-1346-6_48

Table 48.1 Triage color coding

Group	Color coding	Description
Group 1	Red	Intervention required within few minutes. Immediate lifesaving management needed (airway compromise, severe uncontrolled blood loss)
Group 2	Yellow	Intervention required within few hours. Patient stable but urgent management needed (cranial fractures with open dura, contaminated wounds, and open fractures)
Group 3	Green	Intervention required within few days. Can wait a day or two (clean laceration and some fractures)
Group 4	Black	Intervention required within few weeks. Can wait for more days (most fractures)

48.2.1 Glasgow Coma Scale (Please Refer Table 7.5 in Chap. 7 of this book)

There are three variables used with the scale:

Best motor response (level of central nervous system function)
Best verbal response (ability of CNS to integrate information)
Eye opening (brainstem activity)

48.3 Primary Survey and Resuscitation [6]

The primary survey is a rapid, reproducible physical examination to evaluate every trauma patient and is designed to diagnose and treat immediately life-threatening conditions first. All patients are evaluated for physiologic or anatomic derangements that could lead to early mortality and morbidity. Treatment of problems identified during the primary survey begins without delay, before the survey is completed.

The sequence of primary survey is ABCDE:

1. **A**irway with cervical spine control
2. **B**reathing with ventilation
3. **C**irculation and hemorrhagic control
4. **D**isability management (neurological)
5. **E**xposure with environment control

Patient monitoring (pulse oximetry, electrocardiogram (ECG), blood pressure (BP), blood results, chest and pelvic radiographs) should run in parallel with the primary survey. Team approach is crucial for primary survey.

48.3.1 Airway with Cervical Spine Control

Airway assessment is first and foremost priority of primary survey. Patients with maxillofacial and head injuries are at high risk of compromised airway.

Causes of upper airway obstruction

1. Foreign body aspiration
2. Tongue fall position
3. Tracheal, laryngeal, facial, and mandibular fractures
4. Regurgitation of stomach contents

Maxillofacial injuries can cause airway obstruction because of:

– Bilateral anterior mandible fracture allows the tongue to fall posteriorly
– Downward and backward displacement of maxilla into nasopharynx, after midface fracture
– Blood clots and secretions
– Foreign bodies in the form of avulsed teeth or dentures

The chin lift or jaw-thrust maneuver is recommended to achieve patency of airway. The patient's head and neck should not be hyperextended, hyperflexed, or rotated to establish and maintain the airway. There may be associated cervical spine injury; all the cases are treated as they are having cervical spine injury unless diagnosed otherwise. Hence, cervical spine stabilization should be done.

48.3.2 Airway and Ventilatory Problems in Maxillofacial Trauma (Please Refer Chap. 7 of this book)

Early preventable deaths from airway problem after maxillofacial trauma often result from:

- Failure to identify the need for an airway intervention
- Inability to establish an airway
- Lack of backup or alternative airway plan in the setting of failed intubation attempts

- Failure to recognize an incorrectly placed airway
- Displacement of a previously established airway
- Failure to identify the need for ventilation
- Aspiration of gastric contents during dealing with airway

48.3.3 Airway and Ventilation Are the First Priorities

Airway compromise may be sudden and complete, insidious and partial, and/or progressive and recurrent. The early sign of airway or ventilator compromise is tachypnea or inability to speak words or sentences. "Talking patient" provides reassurance for that period of time that the airway is patent and not compromised. Failure to respond or an inappropriate response suggests an altered level of consciousness, airway and ventilator compromise, or both. Patient with the altered level of consciousness is at particular risk for airway compromise and aspiration, so he requires definite airway.

48.3.4 Objective Signs of Airway Obstruction

1. Observe the patient for agitation and obtundation, suggest hypercarbia, and cyanosis indicates hypoxemia due to inadequate oxygenation which can be identified by inspection of nail beds and circum-oral skin. However, cyanosis is a late finding of hypoxia. Pulse oximetry is used early in the airway assessment, to detect inadequate oxygenation prior to development of cyanosis. Look for retractions and use of accessory muscles of ventilation that, when present, provide additional evidence of airway compromise.
2. Listen for abnormal, noisy sound breathing which is usually snoring, gurgling, and crowing sound (stridor) and can be associated with partial obstruction of the pharynx or larynx. Hoarseness (dysphonia) implies functional, laryngeal obstruction.
3. Feel for location of trachea, and quickly determine whether it is in the midline position.
4. Evaluate patient behavior. Abusive and belligerent patient may in fact have hypoxia and should not be presumed to be intoxicated (suggestive of hypoxia, then only presume intoxication).

48.3.5 Airway Management [7, 8]

To assess airway patency and adequate ventilation quickly and accurately, pulse oximetry and end-tidal CO_2 measurement are essential. There are some measures to improve the oxygenation including airway maintenance techniques, definitive airway measures, or surgical airways. Because abovementioned measures include some movement of the neck, it is important to maintain cervical spine protection in all patients of trauma.

High-flow oxygen is required both before and immediately after airway management measures are instituted. A rigid suction device is essential and should be readily available. Nasal route for endotracheal route should not be chosen in patients with facial injury and midface injury. Patients who are wearing helmet and require airway management need their head and neck held in a neutral position. For this two-person procedure, one person provides manual inline stabilization from below, while the second person expands the helmet laterally and removes it from above. Then inline stabilization is re-established from above. And patient's head and neck are secured during airway management. Removal of the helmet using a cast cutter while stabilizing the head and neck can minimize cervical spine (C spine) motion in patients with known C spine injury [9].

Tracheostomy - Video 48.1.

Box 48.2 Need for Airway Protection

1. Severe maxillofacial fractures
2. Risk for obstruction
   - Neck hematoma
   - Laryngeal or trachea
   - Stridor
3. Risk for aspiration
   (i) Bleeding
   (ii) Vomiting
4. Unconscious

Box 48.3 Need for Ventilation or Oxygenation

1. Inadequate respiratory efforts
   - Tachypnea
   - Hypoxia
   - Hypercapnia
   - Cyanosis
2. Massive blood loss and need for volume resuscitation
3. Severe closed injury with need for brief hyperventilation if acute neurologic deterioration occurs
4. Apnea
   - Neuromuscular paralysis
   - Unconscious

48.3.6 Breathing with Ventilation

Next, the patient's breathing, ventilation, and oxygenation should be assessed, and any life-threatening derangements must be treated. Physical examination, pulse oximetry, and continuous end-tidal carbon dioxide monitoring should be used. For proper ventilation the lungs, chest wall, and diaphragm must all function adequately.

The most common interventions performed during the primary survey to support breathing are supplemental oxygen delivery, assisted or mechanical ventilation, and tube thoracotomy or chest tube insertion.

48.3.7 Ventilation

Sometimes it will happen that airway of the patient will be patent but ventilation will be inadequate, so look for the objective signs of inadequate ventilation. Ventilation may be compromised by airway obstruction, altered ventilatory mechanics, and central nervous system depression.

Following are the conditions where the ventilation may be compromised:

1. Direct trauma to the chest, like rib fractures, leading to severe pain during breathing and leads to shallow breathing and hypoxemia.
2. Elderly patients and other individual with pulmonary dysfunction are at significant risk for ventilator failure.
3. Intracranial injury can cause abnormal breathing patterns and compromised adequacy of ventilation.
4. Cervical spinal cord injury can result in diaphragmatic breathing and interfere with the ability to meet increased oxygen demands.
5. Complete cervical cord transection, which spares the phrenic and results in abdominal breathing paralysis of the intercostal muscles, and assisted ventilation may be required.

48.3.8 Objective Signs of Inadequate Ventilation

1. Symmetrical rise and fall of the chest and adequate chest wall excursion indicate the adequate ventilation, but asymmetrical rise and fall suggests splitting of rib cage or flail chest. Labored breathing may indicate an imminent threat to the patient's ventilation.
2. Listen for movement of air on both sides of the chest. Decreased or absent sounds over one or both hemithoraces should alert examiner to the presence of thoracic injury. Beware of rapid respiratory rate—tachypnea can indicate respiratory distress.
3. Use a pulse oximeter: This device provides information regarding patient's oxygen saturation and peripheral perfusion.

48.3.9 Circulation and Hemorrhage Control

Circulation must be assessed to determine the presence or absence of shock after addressing the highest priorities in the primary survey (airway and breathing). Shock is defined as inadequate organ perfusion and tissue oxygenation. In the trauma patient, shock is assumed to be hypovolemic/hemorrhagic, and resuscitation begins as soon as vascular access can be obtained. The possibility of neurogenic shock (e.g., spinal cord injury) or cardiogenic shock (e.g., pericardial tamponade) should also be considered. The focus of this segment of the primary survey should be assessing for the presence of shock, determining the cause (usually blood loss), and beginning resuscitation.

Signs of poor perfusion include a weak pulse, cool or clammy extremities, dry mucous membranes, pale skin, and confusion. A normal mental status examination confirms the presence of acceptable cerebral perfusion. The goal of resuscitation is to maintain tissue perfusion and homeostasis.

48.3.10 Bleeding

External or internal bleeding source should be identified. External hemorrhage is identified and controlled during the primary survey. Rapid external blood loss is managed:

- By direct manual pressure on the wound
- Tourniquets which are effective in massive exsanguinations from an extremity

Internal hemorrhage areas are chest, abdomen, retroperitoneum, pelvis, and long bones. Chest X-ray, pelvic X-ray, or focused assessment sonography in trauma (FAST) can be done to identify the source of bleeding.

48.3.11 Disability Management

The primary focus is on rapidly determining a patient's mental status and neurologic function via physical examination. The Glasgow Coma Scale (GCS) is a rapid and reliable way to quantify a patient's level of consciousness (Table 7.5). The GCS score allows for quick communication among clinicians about a patient's current mental status and can be important for decision-making. The neurologic assessment also includes an examination of the cranial nerves, pupils, and sensory and motor function.

48.3.12 Exposure with Environment Control

Exposure and environment are the final components of the primary survey. While lowering priority, they are still vital to the successful management of the trauma patient. The patients should be completely exposed so that injuries can be fully assessed. Decontamination may also be needed, depending on the nature of the trauma. Protection from hypothermia and continuous temperature monitoring are essential.

48.3.13 Monitoring of Adequacy of Oxygenation

Oxygenated inspired air is best provided via tight-fitting oxygen reservoir face mask with a flow rate of at least 11 L/min. Other methods (e.g., nasal catheter and non-breather mask) can improve the inspired oxygen concentration. Pulse oximetry is a noninvasive method of continuously measuring the oxygen saturation (O_2 sat) of arterial blood. It does not measure the partial pressure of oxygen (PaO_2), and depending upon the position of oxy-hemoglobin dissociation curve, the PaO_2 can vary widely. However a measured saturation of 95% or greater by pulse oximetry strongly suggests adequate peripheral artery oxygenation ($PaO_2 > 70$ mmHg).

Pulse oximetry requires intact peripheral perfusion and can't distinguish oxy-hemoglobin from carboxy-hemoglobin or methemoglobin, which limits its usefulness in patients with severe vasoconstriction and those with carbon monoxide poisoning. Profound anemia (Hb > 5 g/dL) and hypothermia (<30 °C) decrease the reliability of the technique. However, in most patient pulse oximetry is useful as the continuous monitoring of oxygen saturation provides an immediate assessment of therapeutic intervention.

48.3.14 Electrocardiographic (ECG) Monitoring

ECG monitoring of trauma patient is important.

Box 48.4

Injury indication	ECG changes
Blunt cardiac injury	Dysrhythmias including unexplained tachycardia, atrial fibrillation, premature ventricular contractions, and ST segment changes
Cardiac tamponade Tension pneumothorax Profound hypovolemia	Pulseless electrical activity (PEA)

48.3.15 Fluid Resuscitation

Warm resuscitation fluids should be given. IV fluid therapy with crystalloids should be initiated. A bolus of 1–2 L of an isotonic solution may be required to achieve an appropriate response in adult patient.

48.3.16 Urinary and Gastric Catheters

Urine output monitoring is important to manage the fluid therapy. Urine output reflects renal perfusion, and it is accomplished by insertion of indwelling bladder catheter.

Contraindications to the placement of Foley catheter and urethral injury should be suspected in the presence of:

1. Blood at the urethral meatus
2. Hemorrhage into the scrotum
3. High-riding prostate

A gastric tube is indicated to:

1. Reduce stomach distension
2. Decrease risk of aspiration
3. Assess for upper gastrointestinal hemorrhage from trauma

48.4 Secondary Survey [10–12]

Once the primary survey is completed, secondary survey is started. If additional personnel is available, then part of secondary survey can be conducted along with primary survey; however, it should be made sure that it does not interfere with primary survey, as primary survey is the first priority.

Secondary survey is a complete head to toe examination of the trauma patient which includes complete history taking and physical examination. During secondary survey, a complete neurologic examination is conducted. Patient's GCS score is identified, radiographs are obtained, and laboratory studies are conducted as indicated.

48.4.1 History Taking

A complete medical assessment includes history taking and understanding the mechanism of the injury. Often, patient is not in a condition to provide this history. In such cases, it should be obtained from the family members. The history taking involves identification of various allergies, present medications, past history of any illness, pregnancy, last meal taken, and the event of trauma. The mechanism of injury must be understood whether it's inflicted by a penetrating or blunt trauma or if the injury is thermal injury or due to hazardous environment.

48.4.2 Physical Examination

During physical examination in secondary survey, a sequence has to be followed, which is examination of head, maxillofacial structures, cervical spine and neck, chest, abdomen, perineum/rectum/vagina, musculoskeletal system, and neurologic system.

48.4.3 Four-Person Logroll

To examine the patient's back and remove the spine board, at least four persons are required for logrolling:

(a) Person one stands at the patient's head to control the head and C spine and two persons along the patient's sides to control the body and extremities.
(b) Three persons maintain the alignment of spine, as the patient is rolled.
(c) Fourth person examines the back and removes the board.
(d) Once the board is removed, patient is returned into the supine position while maintaining the alignment of spine.

48.4.4 Head

Secondary survey starts with examination of head which involves identification of injuries. The complete scalp should be examined for lacerations, contusions, and evidence of fractures. Other than these injuries, visual acuity, pupillary size, hemorrhage of conjunctiva and/or fundi, and ocular entrapment must be examined. These aspects must be re-evaluated once the periocular edema subsides.

Visual acuity examination must be done by asking the patient to read printed material such as handheld Snellen chart. To exclude ocular entrapment, ocular movement must be checked.

48.4.4.1 Classification of Brain Injury

Box 48.5

Severity	GCS score
Minor	13–15
Moderate	9–12
Severe	3–8

Intracranial lesions may be classified as diffuse or focal. The focal lesions include epidural hematomas, subdural hematomas, contusions, and intracerebral hematomas.

Signs of skull base fracture:

1. Hematoma or ecchymosis over the mastoid (Battle's sign)
2. CSF otorrhea or rhinorrhea
3. Hemotympanum
4. Subscleral hemorrhage

Computed tomography (CT) scan of the head should be carried out to accurately assess the neurologic injuries and detect mass lesions. CT scan helps in diagnosing:

– Intracranial hemorrhage
– Contusion
– Skull fractures
– Foreign bodies
– Brain shift
– Hydrocephalus

In a comatose patient, motor responses may be elicited by pinching the trapezius muscle or with nail bed or supraorbital pressure. Testing for doll's eye movements (oculocephalic) the caloric test with ice water (oculovestibular) and testing of corneal responses are deferred to a neurosurgeon.

48.4.5 Maxillofacial Structures

Maxillofacial examination includes examination of soft tissue, palpation of all the bony structures, checking of occlusion, and intraoral examination. Trauma to the maxillofacial region not associated with airway obstruction should be treated once the patient is stabilized after the management of life-threatening injuries.

48.4.6 Cervical Spine and Neck

Patients with maxillofacial trauma must be presumed to have an unstable cervical spine injury unless it is proven otherwise. The absence of any neurologic deficit does not exclude the presence of any C spine injury. A complete cervical spine radiographs and CT scan should be done to evaluate C spine injury. The patient wearing any kind of helmet must be removed with extreme care.

C spine injuries can result from one or a combination of the following mechanism of injury:

- Flexion
- Axial loading
- Extension
- Rotation
- Lateral bending
- Distraction

A complete examination of neck includes inspection, palpation, and auscultation. Inspection should be done to note any blunt injury over the neck. Carotid arteries should be palpated and auscultated for bruits. Penetrating injuries of neck are potentially fatal. If the wound is deep, they should not be explored in emergency department [13].

A cervical collar can be applied to the patients suspecting the cervical spinal injury. Its role is to immobilize the C spine. Cervical collars are divided into two groups: soft and rigid collars. Soft collars are generally used for whiplash injury; some surgeons prefer rigid collars. Rigid collars provide excellent immobilization in transverse and sagittal planes compared with soft collars. However patient's comfort is to be taken into consideration in selecting the collars. The Philadelphia collar is available in two pieces having front and back pieces; it is held together by Velcro straps to support the neck [14].

48.4.7 Chest

Chest examination includes inspection, palpation, percussion, and auscultation. Inspection of anterior and posterior chest can identify conditions like open pneumothorax and large flail segments. Contusions and hematoma over chest suggest occult injury. Palpation of entire rib cage, clavicle, and sternum helps in diagnosing fractures. Significant injury may present with pain, dyspnea, and hypoxia.

Auscultation of high anterior chest helps in diagnosis of pneumothorax, whereas posterior base auscultation reveals hemothorax. Cardiac tamponade can be identified by the presence of distant heart sounds and decreased pulse pressure. Presence of distended neck veins suggests cardiac tamponade and tension pneumothorax. A chest radiograph may confirm the presence of hemothorax or simple pneumothorax.

48.4.7.1 Classification of Chest Trauma

Immediate life-threatening chest injuries are to be identified and treated during primary survey.

These six life-threatening chest injuries include:

1. Open pneumothorax
2. Tension pneumothorax
3. Open pneumothorax
4. Flail chest and pulmonary contusion
5. Massive hemothorax
6. Cardiac tamponade

48.4.7.2 Managing Chest Trauma [15]

The basic principles of management remain the same with the universal sequence of airway, breathing, and circulation to be treated in that sequence.

48.4.7.3 Airway

It is necessary to recognize and address major injuries affecting the airway during the primary survey. Airway patency and air exchange should be assessed by listening for air movement at the patient's nose, mouth, and lung fields; inspecting the oropharynx for foreign body obstruction; and observing for intercostal and supraclavicular muscle retractions. Laryngeal injury can accompany major thoracic trauma. Although the clinical presentation is occasionally delayed, acute airway obstruction from laryngeal trauma is a life-threatening injury. Injury to the upper chest can create a palpable defect in the region of the sternoclavicular joint, with posterior dislocation of the clavicular head, which causes upper airway obstruction. Identification of this injury is made by listening for upper airway obstruction (stridor) or a marked change in the expected voice quality, if the patient is able to talk. Management consists of a closed reduction of the injury, which can be performed by extending the shoulders or grasping the clavicle with a pointed instrument, such as a towel clamp, and manually reducing the fracture. Once reduced, this injury is usually stable if the patient remains in the supine position.

48.4.7.4 Breathing

The patient's chest and neck should be completely exposed to allow for assessment of breathing and the neck veins. This may require temporarily releasing the front of the cervical collar following blunt trauma. In this case, cervical spine immobilization should always be actively maintained by holding the patient's head while the collar is loose. Respiratory movement and quality of respirations are assessed by observing, palpating, and listening. Important, yet often subtle, signs of chest injury or hypoxia include an increased respiratory rate and change in the breathing pattern, which is often manifested by progressively shallower respirations. Cyanosis is a late sign of hypoxia in trauma patients. However, the absence of cyanosis does not necessarily indicate adequate tissue oxygenation or an adequate airway. The major thoracic injuries that affect breathing and that must be recognized and addressed during the primary survey include tension pneumothorax, open pneumothorax (sucking chest wound), flail chest and pulmonary contusion, and massive hemothorax.

Important: After intubation, one of the common reasons for loss of breath sounds in the left thorax is a right mainstem intubation. During the reassessment, be sure to check the position of the endotracheal tube before assuming that the change in physical examination is due to a pneumothorax or hemothorax.

48.4.7.5 Tension Pneumothorax

A tension pneumothorax develops when a "one-way valve" air leak occurs from the lung or through the chest wall. Air is forced into the pleural space without any means of escape, eventually completely collapsing the affected lung. The mediastinum is displaced to the opposite side, decreasing venous return and compressing the opposite lung. Shock results from the marked decrease in venous return causing a reduction in cardiac output and is often classified as obstructive shock (Fig. 48.1). The most common cause of tension pneumothorax is mechanical ventilation with positive-pressure ventilation in patients with visceral pleural injury. However, a tension pneumothorax can complicate a simple pneumothorax following penetrating or blunt chest trauma in which a parenchymal lung injury fails to seal or after a misguided attempt at subclavian or internal jugular venous catheter insertion. Occasionally, traumatic defects in the chest wall also can cause a tension pneumothorax if incorrectly covered with occlusive dressings or if the defect itself constitutes a flap-valve mechanism. Tension pneumothorax rarely occurs from markedly displaced thoracic spine fractures. Tension pneumothorax is a clinical diagnosis reflecting air under pressure in the affected pleural space. Treatment should not be delayed to wait for radiologic confirmation.

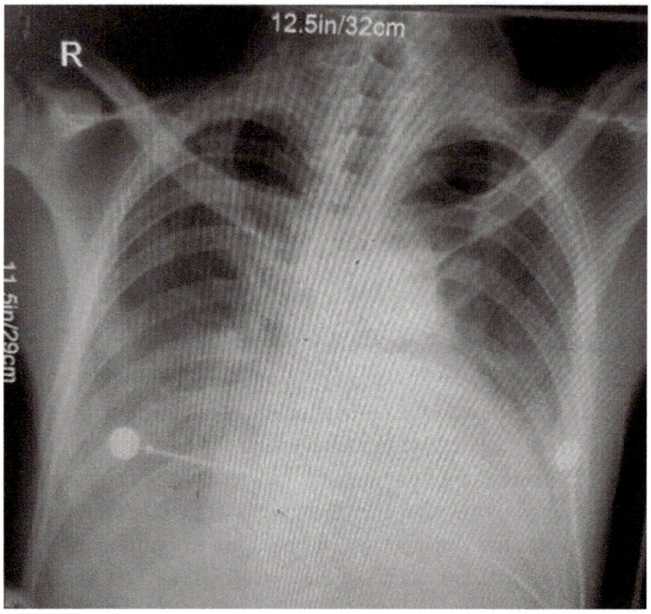

Fig. 48.1 Tension pneumothorax

Tension pneumothorax is characterized by some or all of the following signs and symptoms:

- Chest pain
- Air hunger
- Respiratory distress
- Tachycardia
- Hypotension
- Tracheal deviation away from the side of injury
- Unilateral absence of breath sounds
- Elevated hemithorax without respiratory movement
- Neck vein distention
- Cyanosis (late manifestation)

Because of the similarity in their signs, tension pneumothorax can be confused initially with cardiac tamponade. Differentiation is made by a hyper-resonant note on percussion, deviated trachea, and absent breath sounds over the affected hemithorax, which are signs of tension pneumothorax. Tension pneumothorax requires immediate decompression and may be managed initially by rapidly inserting a large-caliber needle into the second intercostal space in the midclavicular line of the affected hemithorax. However, due to variable thickness of the chest wall, kinking of the catheter, and other technical or anatomic complications, this maneuver may not be successful [16].

When successful, this maneuver converts the injury to a simple pneumothorax; however, the possibility of subsequent pneumothorax as a result of the needle stick now exists, so repeated reassessment of the patient is necessary. Chest wall thickness influences the likelihood of success with needle decompression. Recent evidence suggests that a 5 cm needle will reach the pleural space >50% of the time, whereas an 8 cm needle will reach the pleural space >90% of the time. Even with a needle of the appropriate size, the maneuver will not always be successful. Definitive treatment requires the insertion of a chest tube into the fifth intercostal space (usually at the nipple level), just anterior to the midaxillary line.

In a tension pneumothorax, air from a ruptured lung enters the pleural cavity without a means of escape. As air pressure builds up, the affected lung is compressed, and all of the mediastinal tissues are displaced to the opposite side of the chest.

48.4.7.6 Open Pneumothorax (Sucking Chest Wound)

Large defects of the chest wall that remain open can result in an open pneumothorax, which is also known as a sucking chest wound. Equilibration between intrathoracic pressure and atmospheric pressure is immediate. Air tends to follow the path of least resistance; as such, if the opening in the chest wall is approximately two-thirds of the diameter of the trachea or greater, air passes preferentially through the chest wall defect with each respiratory effort. Effective ventilation is thereby impaired, leading to hypoxia and hypercarbia. Initial management of an open pneumothorax is accomplished by promptly closing the defect with a sterile occlusive dressing. The dressing should be large enough to overlap the wound's edges and then taped securely on three sides in order to provide a flutter-type valve effect. As the patient breathes in, the dressing occludes the wound, preventing air from entering. During exhalation, the open end of the dressing allows air to escape from the pleural space. A chest tube remote from the wound should be placed as soon as possible. Securely taping all edges of the dressing can cause air to accumulate in the thoracic cavity, resulting in a tension pneumothorax unless a chest tube is in place. Any occlusive dressing (e.g., plastic wrap or petrolatum gauze) may be used as a temporary measure so that rapid assessment can continue. Subsequent definitive surgical closure of the defect is frequently required [17].

48.4.7.7 Flail Chest and Pulmonary Contusion

A flail chest occurs when a segment of the chest wall does not have bony continuity with the rest of the thoracic cage. This condition usually results from trauma associated with multiple rib fractures, that is, two or more adjacent ribs fractured in two or more places (Fig. 48.2). The presence of a flail chest segment results in disruption of normal chest wall movement. Although chest wall instability can lead to paradoxical motion of the chest wall during inspiration and expiration, this defect alone does not cause hypoxia. The major difficulty in flail chest stems from the injury to the underlying lung (pulmonary contusion). If the injury to the underlying lung is significant, serious hypoxia can result. Restricted chest wall movement associated with pain and underlying lung injury is major causes of hypoxia. Flail chest may not be apparent initially if a patient's chest wall has been splinted, in which case he or she will move air poorly and movement of the thorax will be asymmetrical and uncoordinated. Palpation of abnormal respiratory motion and crepitation of rib or cartilage fractures can aid the diagnosis. A satisfactory chest X-ray may suggest multiple rib fractures but may not show costochondral separation. Initial treatment of flail chest includes adequate ventilation, administration of humidified oxygen, and fluid resuscitation. In the absence of systemic hypotension, the administration of crystalloid intravenous solutions should be carefully controlled to prevent volume overload, which can further compromise the patient's respiratory status.

The definitive treatment is to ensure adequate oxygenation, administer fluids judiciously, and provide analgesia to improve ventilation. The latter can be achieved with intravenous narcotics or local anesthetic administration, which

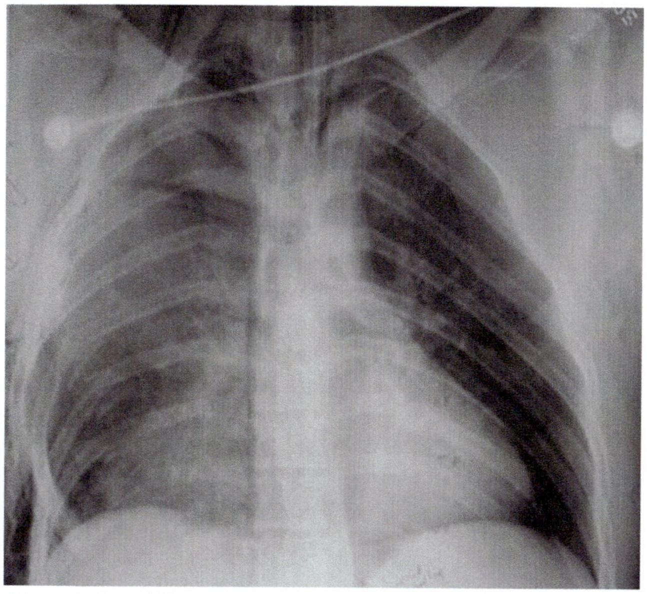

Fig. 48.2 Flail chest with pulmonary contusion

avoids the potential respiratory depression common with systemic narcotics. The options for administration of local anesthetics include intermittent intercostal nerve block(s) and intrapleural, extrapleural, or epidural anesthesia. When used properly, local anesthetic agents can provide excellent analgesia and prevent the need for intubation. However, prevention of hypoxia is of paramount importance for trauma patients, and a short period of intubation and ventilation may be necessary until diagnosis of the entire injury pattern is complete. A careful assessment of the respiratory rate, arterial oxygen tension, and work of breathing will indicate appropriate timing for intubation and ventilation [18].

48.4.7.8 Massive Hemothorax

Massive hemothorax results from the rapid accumulation of more than 1500 mL of blood or one-third or more of the patient's blood volume in the chest cavity (Fig. 48.3). It is most commonly caused by a penetrating wound that disrupts the systemic or hilar vessels. However, massive hemothorax can also result from blunt trauma. In patients with massive hemothorax, the neck veins may be flat as a result of severe hypovolemia, or they may be distended if there is an associated tension pneumothorax. Rarely will the mechanical effects of massive intrathoracic blood shift the mediastinum enough to cause distended neck veins. A massive hemothorax is suggested when shock is associated with the absence of breath sounds or dullness to percussion on one side of the chest. This blood loss is complicated by hypoxia. Massive hemothorax is initially managed by the simultaneous restoration of blood volume and decompression of the chest cavity.

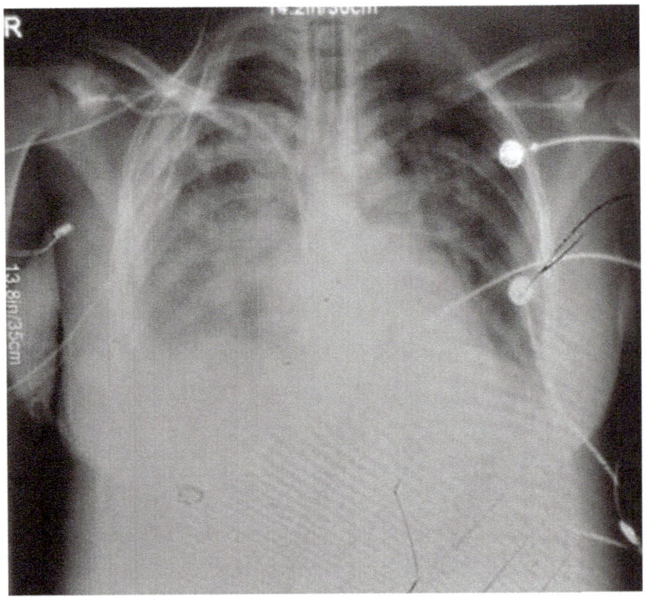

Fig. 48.3 Hemothorax

Large-caliber intravenous lines and a rapid crystalloid infusion are begun, and type-specific blood is administered as soon as possible. Blood from the chest tube should be collected in a device suitable for autotransfusion. A single chest tube (36 or 40 French) is inserted, usually at the nipple level, just anterior to the midaxillary line, and rapid restoration of volume continues as decompression of the chest cavity is completed. When massive hemothorax is suspected, prepare for autotransfusion. If 1500 mL of fluid is immediately evacuated, early thoracotomy is almost always required. Patients who have an initial output of less than 1500 mL of fluid, but continue to bleed, may also require thoracotomy. This decision is not based solely on the rate of continuing blood loss (200 mL/h for 2–4 h) but also on the patient's physiologic status. The persistent need for blood transfusions is an indication for thoracotomy. During patient resuscitation, the volume of blood initially drained from the chest tube and the rate of continuing blood loss must be factored into the amount of intravenous fluid required for replacement. The color of the blood (indicating an arterial or venous source) is a poor indicator of the necessity for thoracotomy. Penetrating anterior chest wounds medial to the nipple line and posterior wounds medial to the scapula should alert the practitioner to the possible need for thoracotomy because of potential damage to the great vessels, hilar structures, and the heart, with the associated potential for cardiac tamponade. Thoracotomy is not indicated unless a surgeon, qualified by training and experience, is present.

48.4.7.9 Cardiac Tamponade

Cardiac tamponade (Fig. 48.4) most commonly results from penetrating injuries. However, blunt injury also can cause the pericardium to fill with blood from the heart, great vessels, or pericardial vessel. The human pericardial sac is a fixed fibrous structure; a relatively small amount of blood can restrict cardiac activity and interfere with cardiac filling. Cardiac tamponade may develop slowly, allowing for a less urgent evaluation, or may occur rapidly, requiring rapid diagnosis and treatment. The diagnosis of cardiac tamponade can be difficult in the setting of a busy trauma or emergency room. Cardiac tamponade is indicated by the presence of the classic diagnostic Beck's triad: venous pressure elevation (distended neck veins), decline in arterial blood pressure, and muffled heart sounds. However, muffled heart tones are difficult to assess in the noisy examination area, and distended neck veins may be absent due to hypovolemia. Additionally, tension pneumothorax, particularly on the left side, can mimic cardiac tamponade. Kussmaul's sign (a rise in venous pressure with inspiration when breathing spontaneously) is a true paradoxical venous pressure abnormality associated with tamponade. Pulseless electrical activity (PEA) is suggestive of cardiac tamponade but can have other causes, as listed above [19]. Insertion of a central venous line with measurement of central venous pressure (CVP) may aid diagnosis, but CVP can be elevated for a

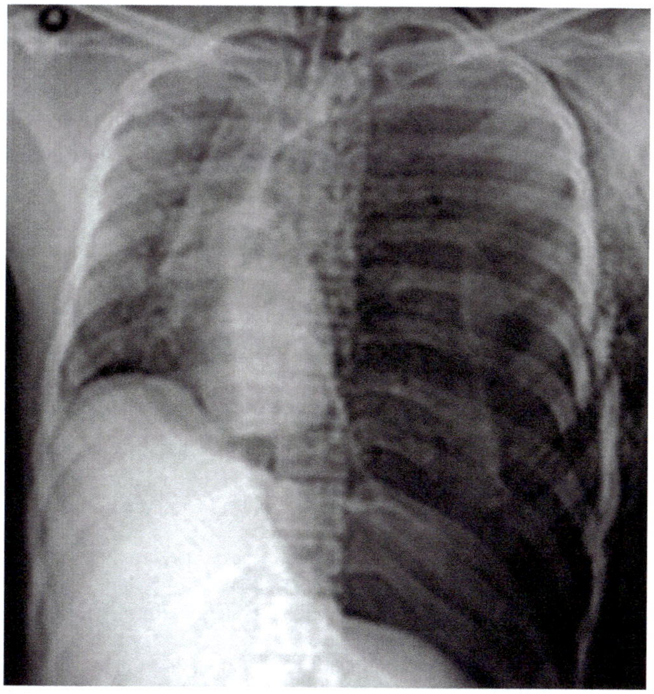

Fig. 48.4 Cardiac tamponade

variety of reasons. Additional diagnostic methods include echocardiogram, focused assessment sonography in trauma (FAST), or pericardial window. In hemodynamically abnormal patients with blunt or penetrating trauma and suspected cardiac tamponade, an examination of the pericardial sac for the presence of fluid should be obtained as part of a focused ultrasound examination performed by a properly trained provider in the emergency department (ED). FAST is a rapid and accurate method of imaging the heart and pericardium. It is 90–95% accurate for the presence of pericardial fluid for the experienced operator. Concomitant hemothorax may account for both false-positive and false-negative ultrasound exams. Prompt diagnosis and evacuation of pericardial blood are indicated for patients who do not respond to the usual measures of resuscitation for hemorrhagic shock and in whom cardiac tamponade is suspected. The diagnosis can usually be made with the FAST exam. If a qualified surgeon is present, surgery should be performed to relieve the tamponade. This is best performed in the operating room if the patient's condition allows. If surgical intervention is not possible, pericardiocentesis can be diagnostic as well as therapeutic, but it is not a definitive treatment for cardiac tamponade. However all patients with acute tamponade and a positive pericardiocentesis will require surgery to examine the heart and repair the injury. Pericardiocentesis may not be diagnostic or therapeutic when the blood in the pericardial sac has clotted. Preparation to transfer such a patient to an appropriate facility for definitive care is always necessary. Pericardiotomy via thoracotomy is indicated only when a qualified surgeon is available.

48.4.8 Abdomen [20]

Abdominal injuries must be identified and managed aggressively. It is not as important to arrive at a specific diagnosis as it is to recognize the injury which requires a surgical intervention. It is important to closely observe and re-evaluate the abdomen to identify the blunt injury. The safest management of penetrating wounds is a laparotomy.

Abdominal Trauma	
Blunt trauma	Penetrating trauma [21]
Direct blow, e.g., crushing injury to abdominal viscera and pelvis	Stab wounds commonly involve liver (40%), small bowel (30%), diaphragm (20%), and colon (15%)
Shearing injuries, e.g., laceration of the liver and spleen	Gunshot wounds commonly involve small bowel (50%), colon (40%), liver (30%), and abdominal vascular structures (25%)

The diagnostic peritoneal lavage (DPL) was used to diagnose blunt and occasionally penetrating abdominal trauma, but its use was decreased with the advancement of CT and USG. Focused assessment sonography in trauma (FAST) is very helpful to detect the presence of hemoperitoneum.

48.4.8.1 Focused Assessment Sonography in Trauma (FAST) [22]

The ultrasound machine and water-based gel are necessary to perform FAST.

Fast includes the following views:

1. **Pericardial view:** fluid within the heart should be black.
2. **Right upper quadrant view (RUQ):** diaphragm-liver interface and Morison's pouch.
3. **Left upper quadrant view (LUQ):** diaphragm-spleen interface and spleen-kidney interface
4. **Suprapubic view:** to see bladder

48.4.9 Perineum/Rectum/Vagina

Contusions, hematomas, lacerations, and urethral bleedings should be examined in the perineal area. The presence of blood at urethral meatus suggests urethral injury. Inspect the scrotum and perineum for ecchymosis or hematoma, also suggestive of injury to the urethra. In patients with perineal hematoma or high-riding prostate, Foley catheters should be avoided.

Rectal examination can be done to evaluate the presence of blood within the bowel lumen. In patients with the risk of vaginal injury, vaginal examination should be carried out. Pelvic compressions should be carried out to identify any pelvic fractures. Pelvic fractures can be suspected by the presence of ecchymosis over iliac wings, pubis, scrotum, or labia. The pelvic fracture can be divided into closed, open book, and vertical shear fracture. Hemorrhage control and fluid resuscitation will be in the initial management of major pelvic disruption associated with hemorrhage. Pelvic binder or sheet can apply sufficient stability for the unstable pelvis at the level of greater trochanters of the femur bone.

48.4.10 Musculoskeletal System

The patient must be completely undressed for adequate examination. Extremities should be inspected for deformities, abrasion, and contusions. Presence of tenderness on palpation of bones and abnormal movement helps in identification of occult fractures. Significant injuries of extremities can exist without fracture being evident. Ligament ruptures and a muscle tendon unit injury interferes with active motions. The musculoskeletal examination is incomplete without examination of the back of the patient.

Musculoskeletal injuries are a potential source of blood loss in patients with hemodynamic abnormalities. The proper splint application helps in blood loss control, reducing pain, and preventing further soft tissue injury. Splinting is required in the patients with joint dislocations.

Crush syndrome: it refers to the injured muscle which if left untreated can lead to acute renal failure. Traumatic rhabdomyolysis ranges from asymptomatic illness with elevation of creatine kinase level to a life-threatening condition associated with acute renal failure and disseminated intravascular coagulation (DIC). Early and aggressive fluid therapy protects the kidneys and prevents renal failure in patients with rhabdomyolysis.

Compartment syndrome: develops when the pressure within an osteofascial compartment of muscle causes ischemia and subsequent necrosis. Sometimes fasciotomy is required to manage the condition.

48.5 Conclusion

Management of airway is challenging in patients with maxillofacial trauma. Securing airway in these patients is dependent on the clinical status and the features of trauma. Before initiation of airway management, a series of steps are to be planned. For optimal care, one must have adequate knowledge of the specific attributes of difficult airway. Also, the expertise in techniques for managing the difficult airway, familiarity with devices, and recognition of failed airway are necessary. A multidisciplinary approach involving anesthesiologist, maxillofacial surgeon, and a trauma expert must be a practice for better outcome (please refer Chap. 7 for further reading).

References

1. Perry M. Advanced trauma life support (ATLS) and facial trauma: can one size fit all? Part 1: dilemmas in the management of the multiply injured patient with coexisting facial injuries. Int J Oral Maxillofac Surg. 2008;37:209–14.
2. Perry M, Morris C. Advanced trauma life support (ATLS) and facial trauma: can one size fit all? Part 2: ATLS, maxillofacial injuries and airway management dilemmas. Int J Oral Maxillofac Surg. 2008;37:309–20.
3. Cowley RA. A total emergency medical system for the state of Maryland. Md State Med J. 1975;45:37–45.
4. Johnson G. Trauma triage and trauma system performance. West J Emerg Med. 2016;17:331–2.
5. Ray JM, Cestero RF. Initial management of the trauma patient. Atlas Oral Maxillofac Surg Clin North Am. 2013;21(1):1–7.
6. Gondek S, Schroeder ME, Sarani B. Assessment and resuscitation in trauma management. Surg Clin North Am. 2017;97:985–98.
7. Kovacs G, Sowers N. Airway management in trauma. Emerg Med Clin North Am. 2018;36:61–84.
8. Barak M, Bahouth H, Leiser Y, Abu El-Naaj I. Airway management of the patient with maxillofacial trauma: review of the literature and suggested clinical approach. Biomed Res Int. 2015:724–32.
9. Roccia F, Cassarino E, Boccaletti R, Stura G. Cervical spine fractures associated with maxillofacial trauma: an 11-year review. J Craniofac Surg. 2007;18:1259–63.
10. Galvagno SM, Nahmias JT, Young DA. Advanced Trauma Life Support® Update 2019: Management and applications for adults and special populations. Anesthesiol Clin. 2019;37:13–32.
11. Sidwell R, Matar MM, Sakran JV. Trauma education and prevention. Surg Clin North Am. 2017;97:1185–97.
12. Rodrigues IFDC. To log-roll or not to log-roll—That is the question! A review of the use of the log-roll for patients with pelvic fractures. Int J Orthop Trauma Nurs. 2017;27:36–40.
13. Rogers WA. Fractures and dislocations of the cervical spine: An end-result study. J Bone Joint Surg Am. 1957;39-A:341–76.
14. Whitcroft KL, Massouh L, Amirfeyz R, Bannister GC. A comparison of neck movement in the soft cervical collar and rigid cervical brace in healthy subjects. J Manipulative Physiol Ther. 2011;34:119–22.
15. Saillant NN, Sein V. Management of severe chest wall trauma. J Emerg Crit Care Med. 2018;2:41.
16. Eckstein M, Suyehara D. Needle thoracostomy in the prehospital setting. Prehosp Emerg Care. 1998;2:132–5.
17. Butler FK, et al. Management of open pneumothorax in tactical combat casualty care: TCCC guidelines change 13-02. J Spec Oper Med. 2013;13:81–6.
18. Pettiford BL, et al. The management of flail chest. Thorac Surg Clin. 2007;17:25–33.

19. Spodick DH. Pathophysiology of cardiac tamponade. Chest. 1998;113:1372–8.
20. Matar ZS. The clinical profile of poly trauma and management of abdominal trauma in a general hospital in the central region of the Kingdom of Saudi Arabia. Internet J Surg. 2008;14:11.
21. Demetriades D, et al. The management of penetrating injuries of the back: a prospective study of 230 patients. Ann Surg. 1988;207:72–4.
22. Chaudhry R, Galagali A, Narayanan RV. Focused abdominal sonography in trauma (FAST). Med J Armed Forces India. 2007;63:62–3.

Management of Soft Tissue Injuries in the Maxillofacial Region

49

Abhay Datarkar and Shikha Tayal

49.1 Introduction

Soft tissue injuries are one of the most commonly encountered injuries in head and neck region and present especially in the emergency department or surgical casualty. They can be isolated soft tissue injuries, or injuries having concomitant skeletal trauma. The frequent facial soft tissue injuries include simple lacerations, abrasions, contusions, bites, avulsions, and burns. These injuries are complicated by presence of vital anatomical structures like vessels, ducts, nerves, and muscles. Presence of foreign debris and hematoma further complicates the soft tissue injuries. The face is a region of high esthetics and functional importance. Hence, there are many factors that help to manage such injuries.

Factors that guide facial soft tissue injury management are:

(i) **Recognition of nature of the injury**—Helps in logical treatment planning that ultimately results in better esthetic and functional outcomes.

(ii) **Extent of injury**—Many facial soft tissue injuries that are relatively minor are treated in emergency department by the oral and maxillofacial surgeons. These wounds are managed by thorough cleaning, irrigation, debridement, primary suturing, and cleaning whenever needed. More complex wounds require special intervention by taking the patient into operation theatre and reconstructing using various grafts and flaps.

(iii) **Timing of the injury**—Any type of injury, by default, should be attended at the earliest to maximize the prognosis. The bottom line of many past and present literature is that the wounds of face and scalp should be primarily closed as soon as they are seen and as long as active infection is not present.

To achieve this, the surgeon needs to understand the etiopathogenesis, surgical anatomy, biomechanics of tissue wound, biology of wound healing, and the art of soft tissue repair.

49.2 Etiology

The most common etiology of facial soft tissue injuries varies according to the age, sex, and geographical distribution of the population. Facial soft tissue trauma tends to occur in certain areas of the head depending on the causative mechanism. It typically includes the T-shaped area that includes forehead, nose, lips, and chin, followed by the occiput and anterior temporal areas.

(a) **Falls** are by far the most common cause, accounting for 48–51% of the injuries [1, 2]. This etiology has a trimodal distribution. The first peak is 2–3 years, when toddlers begin to walk and fall into objects. There is smaller peak during the second and third decades and then a steady rise after age of 50 years. Alcohol consumption is a major factor for soft tissue injuries due to fall between 30 and 50 years. Medical comorbidities such as epilepsy are also the causative factor for falls in old age group.

(b) **Non-fall impacts**. Approximately 16% of facial soft tissue trauma is the result of a non-fall impact with structural element such a door, wall, or window frame. Other collisions with furnishings such as tables also counted. These types of injuries peak in children younger than 5 years. The common areas include the forehead, nose, and anterior temples.

(c) **Assaults** account for 16–32% of facial soft tissue injuries [1]. The assaults are most commonly caused by fists, kicks, and blunt instruments. The injuries due to assault occurs more frequently among young men on left side of face. Alcohol consumption is a factor in two-thirds of these patients.

Disclosure: Authors have no financial conflicts to disclose.

A. Datarkar (✉) · S. Tayal
Department of Oral and Maxillofacial Surgery, Government Dental College and Hospital, Medical College Premises, Nagpur, Maharashtra, India

K. Bonanthaya et al. (eds.), *Oral and Maxillofacial Surgery for the Clinician*, https://doi.org/10.1007/978-981-15-1346-6_49

(d) **Road traffic accidents** cause 6–13% of facial trauma [2] where soft tissue injuries may occur alone or in combination with other fractures. The peak incidence is seen in young men at 15–24 years of age [3]. Impact from steering wheel, dashboard, and windshields results in most lacerations.

(e) **Sporting injuries** account for about 8% of facial soft tissue trauma [1], commonly occurring in young men. The forehead, nose, and teeth are the most likely areas to be injured. Concomitant facial fractures like nasal fractures, avulsive teeth injuries, and mandibular fractures are also common among these group of patients.

(f) **Others include occupational injuries, bites from humans or animals**, and other miscellaneous causes. Occupational injuries [3] account for 5% of facial trauma and are primarily seen in young men. The risk of dog bites is higher for children aged 5–9 years and decreases with age. The frequency of facial injuries is highest in children younger than 4 years, in whom nearly 65% of dog bite injuries involve the face. In adults, it is about 9%. Most dog bite injuries are from dogs known to person or occur near home. These injuries typically involve the cheek, lips, forehead, and nose.

49.3 Classification of Soft Tissue Injuries

Soft tissue injuries can be classified into multiple categories:

(A) **Based on mechanism of injuries**

(I) Mechanical or physical injuries:

- When injury is caused due to blunt force:
  1. Abrasions
  2. Contusions
  3. Lacerations
- When injury is caused due to sharp force:
  1. Incised wounds
  2. Chop wounds
  3. Stab/punctured wounds

(II) Thermal injuries:

- Due to excessive cold: e.g., frostbite
- Due to moist heat: e.g. burns and scald wounds

(III) Chemical injuries: Due to corrosive acids and alkalis

(IV) Miscellaneous: Electricity, lightning, etc.

(V) Explosions: Blast injuries

(B) **Legal classification**

1. **Simple**—soft tissue injuries without much tissue loss and can be managed conservatively. Heals rapidly without any permanent deformity.
2. **Grievous injuries**—described under Section 320 of Indian Penal Code as any injuries that endanger life and cause severe disfigurement or deformities like permanent hearing loss, vision loss, and severe head injuries. Tooth fracture or tooth loss following a blow in an interpersonal violence is also considered a grievous injury and penalized by the court of law. These injuries heal slowly and incompletely.
3. **Dangerous**—the grievous injuries that endanger life immediately after impact (Box 49.1).

Box 49.1 Classification of Soft Tissue Injuries

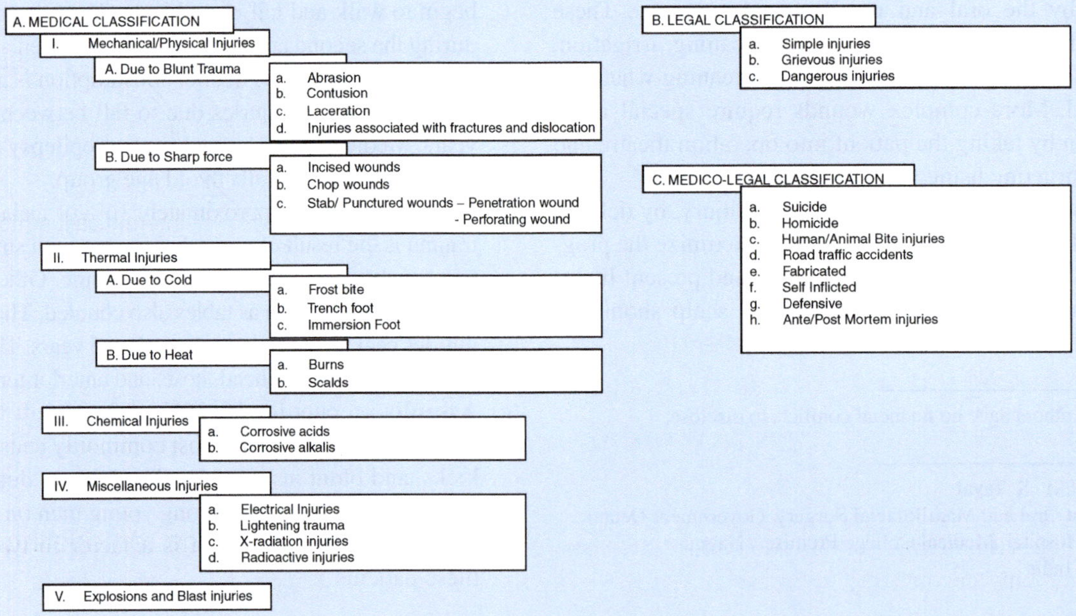

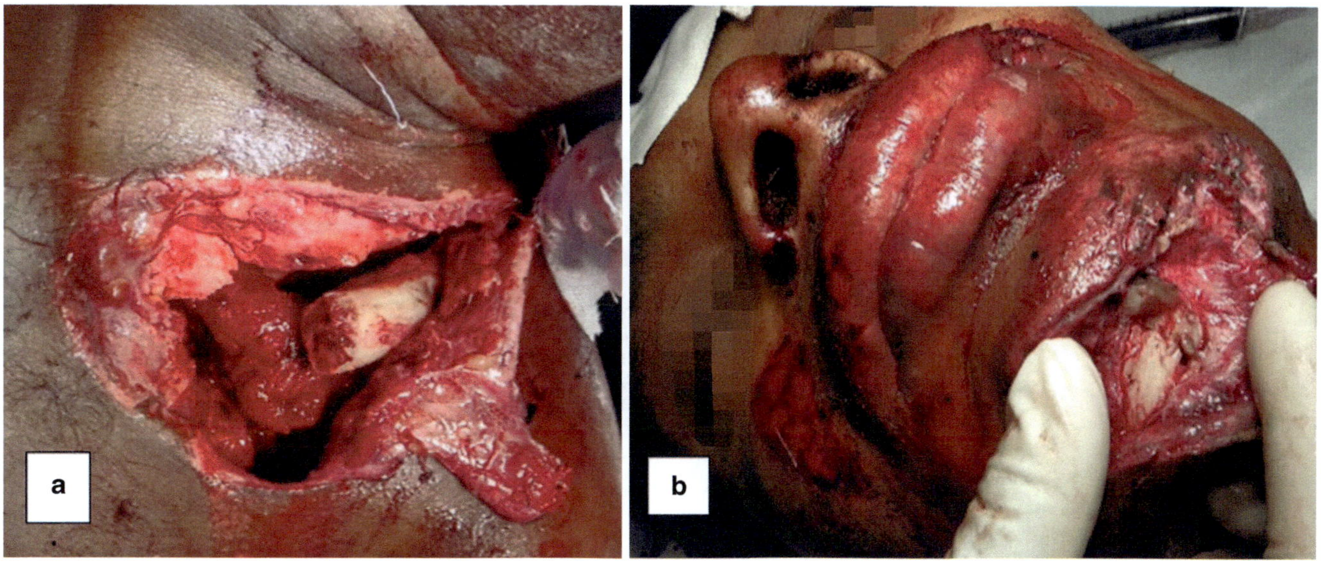

Fig. 49.1 (**a**) Showing open wound where fractured left clavicle is visible from the wound surface. (**b**) Open wound of maxillofacial region where underlying mandible is visible

(C) **Based on the communication of the injury with the external environment**

Closed wound: Only the underlying tissue and/or structures are damaged without breaking the skin. Examples of closed wounds include hematomas, contusions, and crush injuries. These types of wounds are not contaminated and, hence, heal on their own without any sequelae.

Open wounds: There is a break in the skin, which exposes the underlying structures to the external environment. Open wounds include simple and complex lacerations, avulsions, punctures, abrasions, accidental tattooing, and retained foreign body with a tendency to heal with scarring. These injuries require extensive exploration and debridement followed by a course of antibiotic regimen for uneventful healing (Fig. 49.1).

(D) **According to the facial subunit(s) involved**. The major esthetic subunits on the face are the scalp, forehead, nose, periorbital region, cheek, perioral region, auricle, and neck [4].

These major facial esthetic subunits are further divided into smaller subunits by location. The individual subunits must be reconstructed individually one by one in order to attain good esthetics (Fig. 49.2).

(E) **Based on additional injuries to the related structures**

(a) **Injuries to nerve**—The nerve injuries are most commonly encountered in cases of open wounds. The nerve injuries are further classified into neuropraxia, axonotmesis, and neurotmesis (Seddon's classification of nerve injuries [5]). Sunderland [6] further revised this classification of nerve injuries based on the histologic degree of nerve damage. There should be careful evaluation of sensory and motor components of the nerves in the involved region for proper treatment. The most commonly encountered nerve injuries in maxillofacial region are the facial nerve and trigeminal nerve.

(b) **Injuries to arteries and veins**—The face is a highly vascular region where even a small injury leads to significant bleeding. Any wound in maxillofacial region should be attended in emergency setting at the earliest due to chances of injury to the extensive vascular network which necessitates hemostasis.

(c) **Injuries to parotid duct**—Seen in cases of deep lacerations on cheek at the region of parotid duct. If undiagnosed and untreated, this injury can lead to cumbersome sequelae of parotid fistula. Parotid duct injury is suspected if the laceration involves an imaginary line joining the tragus of the ear to the upper lip. In such cases, exploration is performed to evaluate the injury, and suturing should be done using a stent to establish patency of the duct.

(F) **Rank and Wakefield classification** [7] **of wounds**

(a) **Tidy wounds**—The wounds that are inflicted by sharp instruments like surgical blades and contain

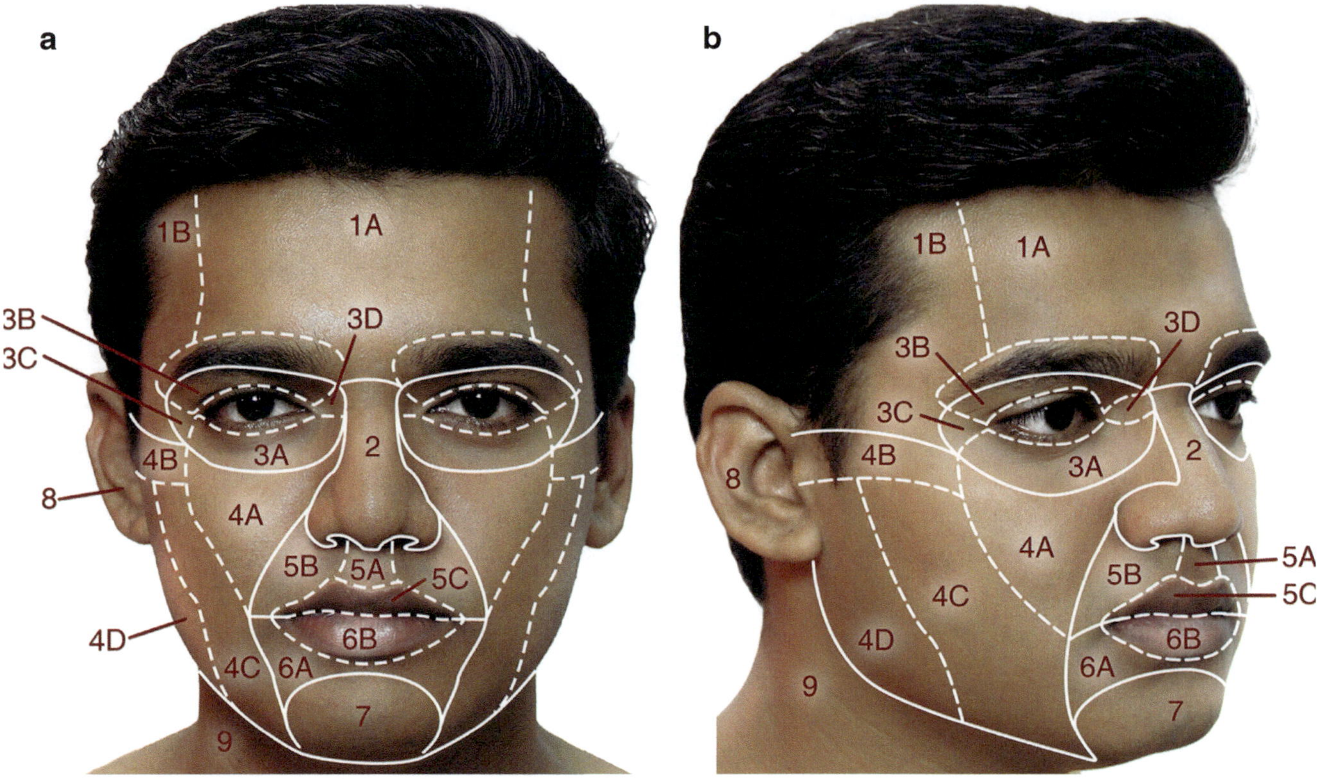

Fig. 49.2 Various facial esthetic subunits (Also see Fig. 86.3 in this book)

no devitalized tissue are called tidy. These wounds are closed primarily. Examples are surgical incisions, cuts from glass, and knife wounds.

(b) **Untidy wounds**—Untidy wounds result from crushing, tearing, avulsion, vascular injury, or burns and contain devitalized tissue. Such wounds must be managed by wound excision. The devitalized tissue is excised, and the untidy wound is converted into the tidy wound before proper closure is achieved. The chances of infection are high if inadequately managed.

(G) **CDC classification of surgical wounds**

A **surgical wound** is a wound created by incisions and placement of drains during surgeries.

Surgical wounds can be classified into four different categories depending on the bacterial load, the risk of infection, and where the wound is located on the body.

Class I: **Clean wounds**. They show no signs of infection or inflammation. They often involve the eye, skin, or vascular system. It is often due to non-penetrating (blunt) trauma.

Class II: **Clean-contaminated wounds**. Although the wound may not show signs of infection, it is at an increased risk of becoming infected because of its location. For example, surgical wounds in the respiratory tract like oropharynx and gastrointestinal tract may be at a high risk of becoming infected.

Class III: **Contaminated wound**. A surgical wound in which an outside object has come into contact with the skin and has a high risk of infection. For example, a gunshot wound may contaminate the skin around where the surgical repair occurs.

Class IV: **Dirty-contaminated or infected wounds**. The wounds that have been exposed to fecal material and have a high bacterial load.

This wound classification guides in choosing appropriate treatment as well as helps in predicting post-repair form and function.

49.3.1 Common Soft Tissue Injuries

The common clinical presentation of soft tissue injuries included abrasions, contusions, and lacerations.

1. **Abrasions**—(also known as gravel rash) (Fig. 49.3)—It is destruction of the superficial layer of skin only. It is caused by frictional forces that are light enough to erode only the superficial layer of epidermis. It can be scratches

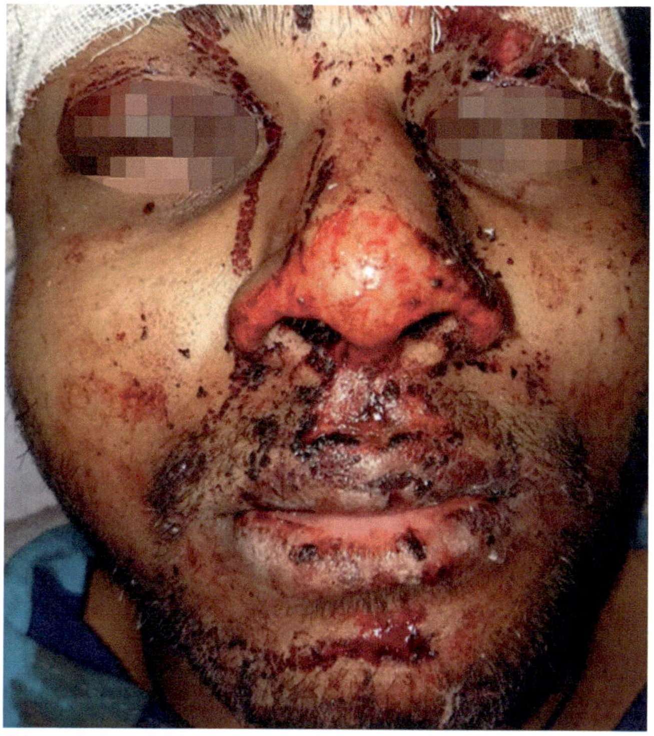

Fig. 49.3 Showing multiple abrasions over face involving the supraorbital region, nose, upper lip, and chin

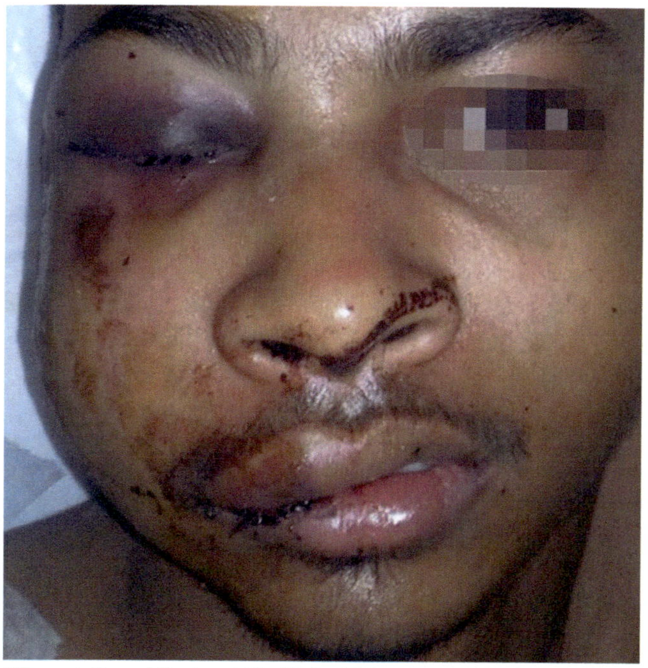

Fig. 49.4 Showing contusion wound over right cheek and periorbital ecchymosis of the right eye. The color changes can be appreciated intraorally

or linear type of abrasion, graze or sliding abrasion, pressure abrasions, and impact abrasions.

The healing of abrasions takes place from the periphery of the wound towards the center by new growth of epithelial cells. The wound is bright red in color for the first 12–24 h due to extravasation of blood which dries up to form a red scab. After 2–3 days, a reddish-brown scab is formed. After 4–7 days, epithelium grows and covers the defect under the scab, which gives it a dark brown to brownish-black appearance. After 7 days, the scab dries and ultimately falls off, leaving depigmented bright pinkish area underneath, which attains its normal pigmentation gradually over a period.

2. **Contusions (bruising)** (Figs. 49.4 and 49.5)—This is effusion of blood into the tissues, due to the rupture of small blood vessels at the site of impact. There is no destruction of the superficial layer of skin. The subtypes are (a) intradermal, (b) subcutaneous, and (c) deep.

   A bruise heals by disintegration of extravasated blood. The red cells in the wound are hemolyzed, and the hemoglobin molecule is broken down into hemosiderin, hematoidin, and bilirubin by the action of enzymes.

   This type of injury demonstrates a change in the color of the wound according to the time lapsed after injury: red at the time of injury, blue within few hours to 3 days, and

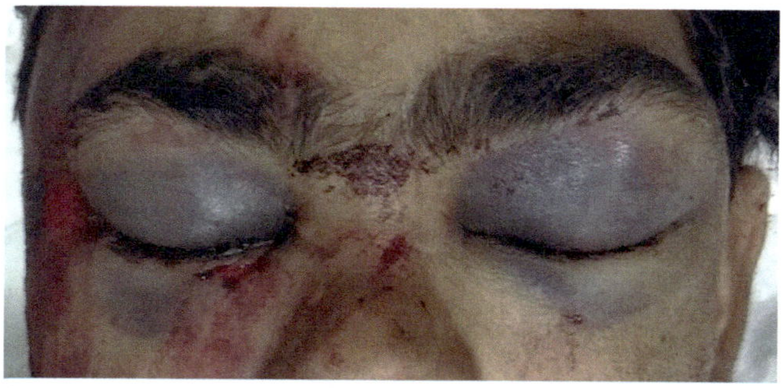

Fig. 49.5 Showing bilateral periorbital ecchymosis (raccoon eyes)

   bluish-black to brown color due to deposition of hemosiderin from the extravasated RBCs, by the 4th day. In 5–6 days, the wound appears greenish due to disintegration of hemoglobin to hemosiderin. Between 7 and 12 days, the wound appears yellow due to the presence of bilirubin which is the final disintegrated product from hemoglobin. The wound appears normal by 2 weeks. The various factors affecting the color of contusion include the depth of the bleeding, amount of extravasated blood, and overlying skin color.

3. **Lacerations**—It is the tear or split of skin, mucous membrane, muscle, or internal organs produced by the application of blunt force to a broad surface area, which

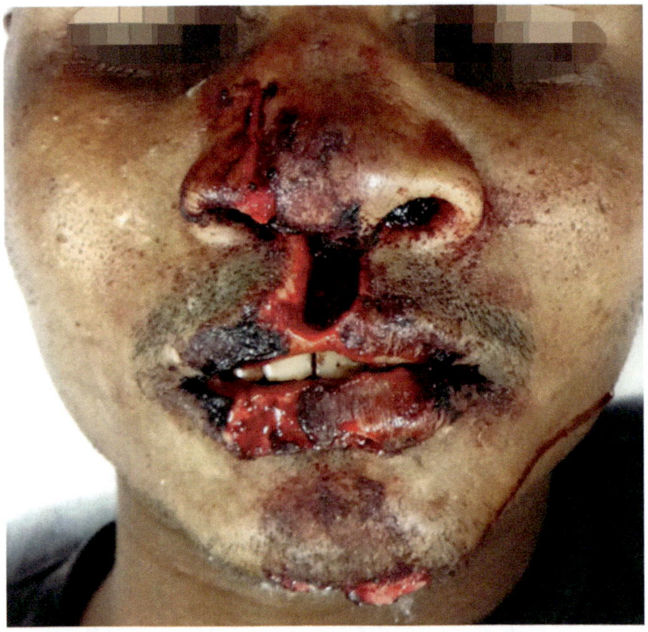

Fig. 49.6 Showing split lacerated wound over the nose, columella, lower lip, and chin

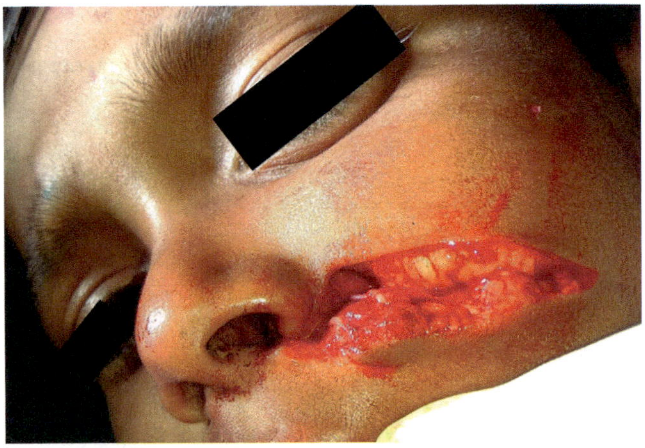

Fig. 49.7 Cut laceration having sharp clean cut edges

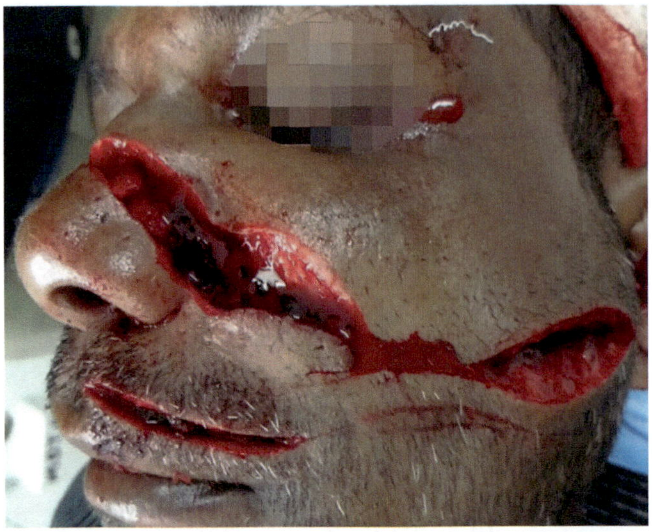

Fig. 49.8 Showing incised wound extending from dorsum of the nose till pre-auricular region; caused by knife in a case of assault

crushed or stretched tissues beyond the limits of their elasticity. They can be split lacerations (Fig. 49.6), stretch lacerations, shearing lacerations, and cut lacerations (Fig. 49.7).

4. **Incised wounds**—The wound is longer than it is deep. It is caused by the pressure and friction of any sharp object against the soft tissues (Fig. 49.8).
5. **Chop wounds (slash wounds)**—They are deep bigger wounds with gaping caused by a blow with the sharp-cutting edge of a heavy weapon, like an axe or chopper.
6. **Stab or punctured wounds**—Produced when the force is delivered along the long axis of a narrow or pointed object, such as knife, sword, chisel, scissors, nail, needle, spear, arrow, screw driver, etc. into the depths of the body. This type of wound is deeper than its length and width. These can be of the following types:
   (a) **Penetrating wounds**—When an object pierces the skin and enters a cavity of body or a viscus creating a localized path of entry leaving it an open wound (Fig. 49.9). In head and neck region, this type of injuries should be assessed for upper airway and bleeding as direct trauma to vital structures occurs along with facial bone fractures. Careful exploration of the wounds should be performed, and any impacted debris should be removed before closure.
   (b) **Perforating wounds or through-and-through puncture wounds**—Produced when the object enters the body at one surface and exits at another surface without causing much tissue loss. The wound of entry is larger with inverted edges, and the wound of exit is smaller with everted edges. They are considered to be sterile wounds (Fig. 49.10).
7. **Crush injury**—A crush injury typically occurs when the body part is crushed between two heavy blunt objects. Most severe trauma cases will have this type of injury. Crush injuries have ragged edges, varying amounts of devitalized tissue, and, sometimes, tissue loss.
8. **Avulsion injuries**—These involve significant tissue loss. Avulsion can be considered a very severe form of abrasion, wherein all layers of skin are torn off and the underlying structures are grossly exposed. The term avulsion can also mean complete loss of a small body part such as eyelid, fingertip, part of ear, etc.

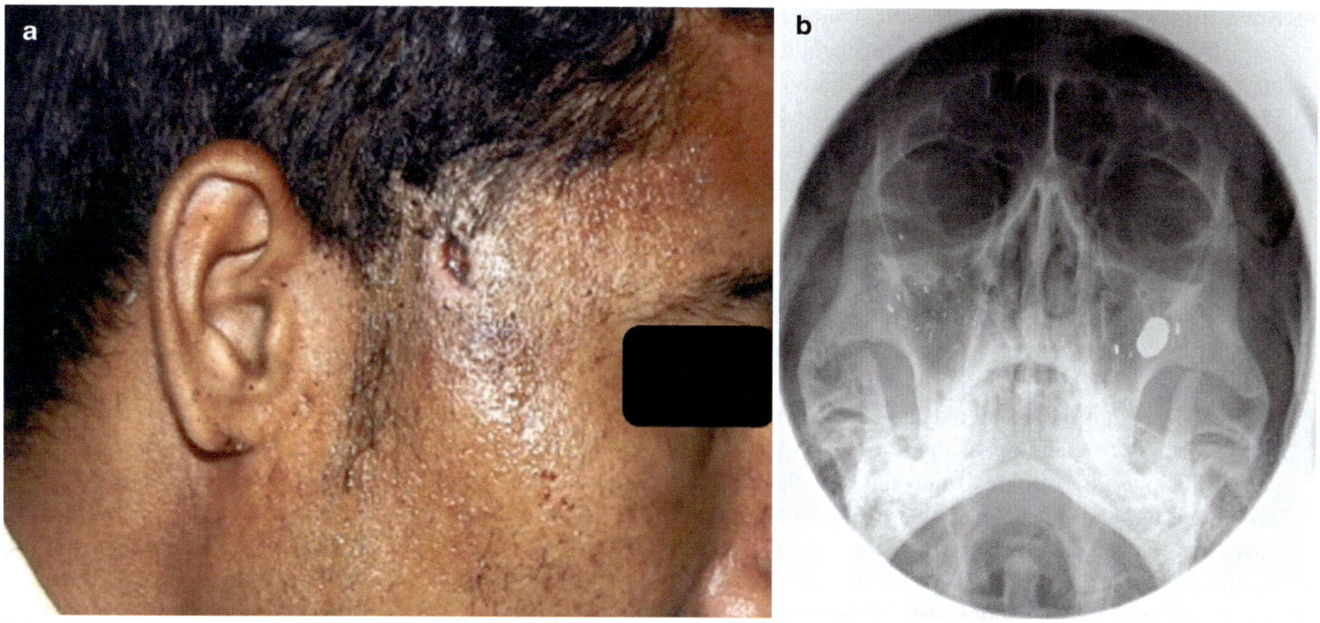

Fig. 49.9 Showing penetrating wound. (**a**) Only the entry site is seen over the right temporal region. (**b**) The object remains dislodged within the body cavities

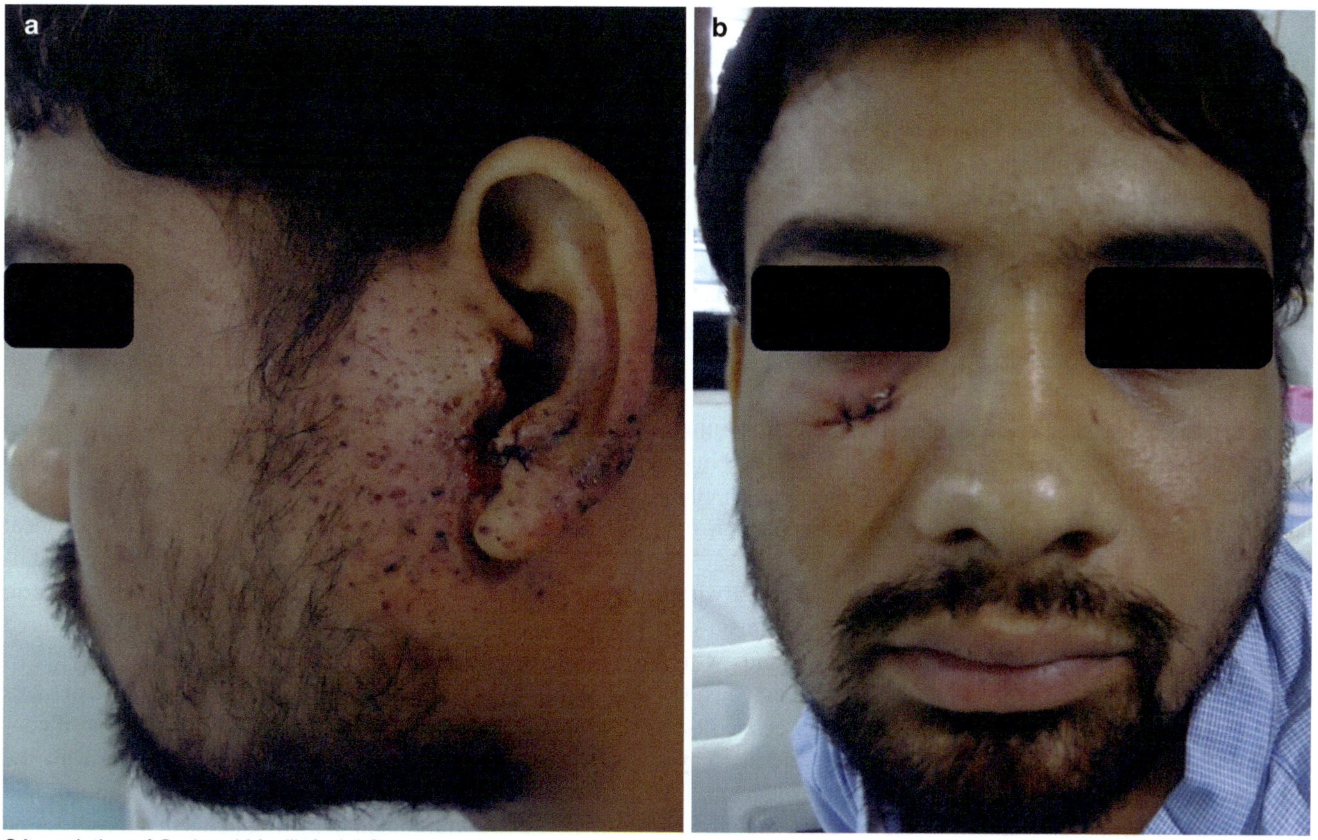

Fig. 49.10 Showing gunshot wound injuries. (**a**) Picture showing entry wound over pre-auricular region. (**b**) Showing exit wound over right infraorbital region on opposite side

9. **Burn injuries**—Burns are injuries to tissues caused by heat, friction, electricity, radiation, or chemicals. Most burns are from hot objects (including fluids) and fire. Burns cause severe skin damage where the cells die. Burns are highly painful injuries which require specific treatment as distinct from other injuries depending on the degree of burn.
   The clinical presentation of burns depends largely on the depth of injury. Superficial burns (first degree) are confined to the epidermis. They are characterized by severe pain, dryness, and redness of skin. Superficial partial-thickness (second degree) burns extend into the papillary dermis. The skin is moist and red and blanches with pressure. Blisters are common in this type of injury. Deep partial-thickness burns extend into the reticular dermis. The skin is dry and appears yellow or white with minimal blistering. Full-thickness burns extending to the entire depth of dermis are classified as 3rd degree. These are very severe injuries. The skin is stiff, leathery, and brown, but pain is not a common feature. Fourth-degree burns involve charring of skin and affect the deeper structures like fat and muscle. The skin is dry, black, and painless.

49.4 Initial Evaluation and Assessment

All trauma patients should be assessed and managed initially according to the principles of Advanced Trauma Life Support. Soft tissue injuries of the head and neck region can be accompanied by significant swelling and bleeding leading to airway compromise. The patient also should be assessed for associated ophthalmologic, intracranial, and cervical spine injuries.

49.5 History and Examination

Once the patient has been evaluated for life-threatening injuries and stabilized as necessary, a thorough and focused history and physical examination of the head and neck should be performed. History includes timing and mechanism of injury.

Early treatment of soft tissue injuries is associated with optimal esthetic outcomes. Determining the mechanism of injury may help the surgeon in managing the wounds with special consideration. For example, crush injuries may result in a larger area of compromised tissue than appreciated on initial examination. Tissue that appears healthy initially may subsequently necrose and may require serial debridement.

The site(s), depth, and nature of all wounds should be noted. Presence of nonviable tissue, gross contamination, and any foreign body like dirt and debris are important to discern.

Palpation helps to identify the presence of underlying bony injuries. Palpation can be done through the open wound itself.

49.6 Management of Soft Tissue Injuries

The principles of management of soft tissue injuries include the control of bleeding, copious irrigation of the wound, debridement of devitalized tissue, and removal of foreign bodies before closure.

(a) **Control of bleeding**—Blood loss is minimized by applying local pressure using hands and pressure dressings. The wound should be examined thoroughly with suction, irrigation, and meticulous dissection to identify the offending vessel, if any. If local pressure fails to achieve hemostasis, local hemostatic agents can be used. Local anesthesia with adrenaline helps in control of pain as well as bleeding through its vasoconstrictive action. If generalized oozing is still present which is hampering the ability of a surgeon to close the wound, systemic measures like injectable vitamin K, tranexamic acid, or ethamsylate can be given, provided the blood investigations (INR, BT, CT) are within normal limits.
(b) **Copious irrigation** serves to dilute and wash out the contamination present in a wound. All grossly contaminated wounds should be copiously irrigated with sterile saline. The fluids may be warmed to 37 °C to promote cellular activity. The cleanser should be nontoxic and have a neutral pH. Alkaline soaps are best avoided. Antiseptics are generally not recommended for cleansing. They are applied on the wound after wound cleansing. The most commonly used antiseptic is Povidone-iodine 10% solution. An alternative solution for this purpose is Cetrimide 15% in combination with chlorhexidine gluconate 1.5%.
(c) **Broad-spectrum antibiotic prophylaxis** is warranted in grossly contaminated wounds and bite wounds and in immunocompromised patients.
(d) **Tetanus vaccination** [8]—Prevention of the local wound infection especially in crushed injuries, contaminated wounds, and bite wounds is a main concern. Tetanus prophylaxis in wound management is required as per the accepted international protocols.
(e) **Wound excision** (also known as **wound debridement** or **toileting of the wound**)—Serial debridement of contaminated and untidy wounds done to remove all the necrotic tissues like devitalized muscles, tendons, and fascia and comminuted bony fragments that have lost the soft tissue cover of periosteum and are hanging within the wound, in order to aid in uneventful and optimum healing. The blunt contused margins of skin are also

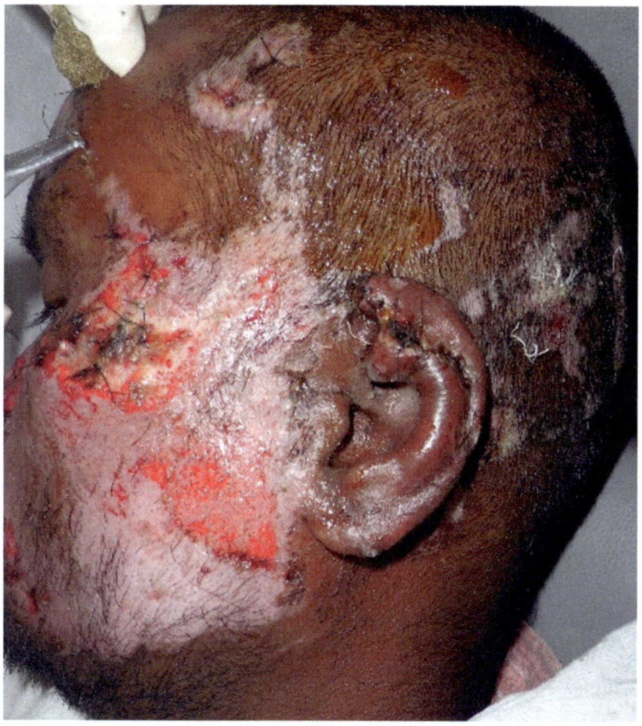

Fig. 49.11 Showing wound excision and serial debridement of an extensive untidy wound gradually healing secondarily

excised using sharp scissors, and the wound margins are freshened up. The toilet of any wound should be done in a systematic layer-wise manner from superficial to deep (Fig. 49.11).

(f) **Closure**—Ideally, facial soft tissue injuries should be closed as early as possible. Primary closure of a wound should be completed within 8 h of injury when possible [9]. Early intervention and closure decreases the risk of infection as well as optimizes the functional and cosmetic result. Basic principles of suturing should be met, which include precise approximation and eversion of the skin edges, avoidance of excessive tension, and layer-wise closure to prevent dead space and fluid accumulation.

If gaping of the lacerated margins or tissue loss is present that cannot be closed primarily, the tissue can be managed by regular dressing and allowed to heal secondarily. Revision surgeries to improve esthetics and function are performed after minimum of 9 months.

(g) **Reconstruction** [10]—Done in cases of extensive degloving injuries. There are several options for soft tissue reconstruction using flaps. Starting from local, regional, distant flaps and free microvascular flaps, depending on the type, location, and extent of the injury (Box 49.2).

Box 49.2 Reconstructive Options for the Head and Neck Region

CLASSIFICATION SCHEME OF VARIOUS RECONSTRUCTIVE FLAPS

Based on **CIRCULATION**

a. **Axial** – flap with one blood vessel. Further classified as fasciocutaneous, musculocutaneous, venous and direct. E.g. – Radial forearm flap, nasolabial flap, submental flap etc.

a. **Random** – multiple random tributes of small vessels.

According to **SOURCE OF HARVEST**

a. **Local** – area adjacent to the wound
b. **Regional** – Same region e.g. – head and neck
c. **Distant** – Region away from the wound
d. **Free Flaps** – Flaps having their own blood supply, connected to the defect using microvascular technique.

Based on the **MODE OF TRANSFER** of flap

a. **Rotational** – a semicircular type of flap pivoting onto the defect.
b. **Transpositional** – flap that moves laterally around the adjacent defect.
c. **Advancement** – Flap moved forward into the wound defect. E.g.. –VY flap
d. **Interpolational** – the flap moved laterally into the defect but not adjacent. Undermined to reach the area.

According to **THE THICKNESS** of the flap

a. **Full thickness flap** – offers better esthetics

a. **Partial thickness flap**

Based on **COMPOSITION** of the flap

a. Dermal
b. Muscle
c. Fascia
d. Tendon
e. Bone
f. Various combinations

49.7 Wound Dressings

Wound dressings are sterile pads used to cover the wounds. Lister [11] introduced antiseptic dressings by soaking gauze in carbolic acid. The dressings should be clean and provide a warm and moist environment for the successful wound healing. The dressings should be frequently changed in order to keep the wound free from bacterial load. Antibacterial ointments must be applied over the wound to keep it lubricated and free from bacteria. The dressings are selected on the basis of two concepts: occlusion and absorption. The reasons for placing a wound dressing are enumerated in Box 49.3.

Box 49.3 Purposes of Dressings

Purposes of applying dressings over wounds

(i) Protection the wound from elements of nature
(ii) Prevention of bacterial contamination
(iii) Application of compression where required
(iv) Absorption of exudate
(v) Facilitation of hemostasis
(vi) Prevention of further inadvertent trauma to wound site

In selected cases, the dressing is modified to achieve additional purposes such as

(vii) Relief of pain
(viii) Application of topical antibiotic
(ix) Removal of slough and foreign bodies from the wound

Studies [12] have demonstrated that the rate of epithelialization under a moist occlusive dressing is twice that of a wound that is left uncovered and allowed to dry. An occlusive dressing provides a mildly acidic pH and low oxygen tension on the wound surface, which is conducive for fibroblast proliferation and formation of granulation tissue.

However, wounds that produce significant amounts of exudate or have high bacterial counts require a dressing that is absorptive and prevents maceration of the surrounding skin. These dressings also need to reduce the bacterial load while absorbing the exudate produced. Placement of a pure occlusive dressing without bactericidal properties would allow bacterial overgrowth and worsen the infection.

The various types of dressings [13] can be enumerated as in Table 49.1.

49.8 Other Therapies

1. **Hyperbaric oxygen therapy**—uses oxygen as a drug and the hyperbaric chamber as a delivery system to increase PO2 at the target area. It involves inhalation of 100% oxygen at 1.9–2.5 atm, for sessions of 90–120 min each. Treatments are given once daily, five to six times per week and should be given as an adjunct to surgical or medical therapies. Clinical evidence of wound improvement should be noted after 15–20 treatments.

Table 49.1 Types of wound dressing materials

Kind of dressing	Examples	Properties	Indications
Protective	Gauze	Inexpensive, readily available Highly permeable and nonocclusive Dry dressing—can stick to the wound if used primarily	As secondary dressing over another material
	Polymeric films (Opsite, Tegaderm)	Transparent, waterproof dressing Semi-permeable, thin, highly elastic	Surgical incisions
Absorbent	Hydrogels	Mostly contain water Provide a moist and cool environment	Wounds with mild exudates Not for heavily exudating or infected wounds
	Hydrocolloids	Composed of methylcellulose, pectin, and gelatin Absorb fluids and convert them into a gel that covers the wound Provides pain relief as the gel covers nerve endings	Light to heavily exuding wounds such as burns Must not be used on infected wounds
Bioactive	Antimicrobial dressings	Soft, paraffin dressing impregnated with chlorhexidine (Bactigras) or framycetin (Sufratulle) Actively prevent bacterial contamination	Flat, shallow wounds such as skin graft donor sites, superficial burns, and abrasions
		Require a secondary dressing over it **Scarlet Red**, a relatively nonocclusive dressing that is impregnated with *O*-tolylazo-*O*-tolylazo-β-naphthol Xeroform—hydrophobic dressing containing 3% bismuth tribromophenate in a petrolatum base, which helps mask wound odors and has antimicrobial activity against *Staphylococcus aureus* and *Escherichia coli*	Skin graft harvest sites in burn care
	Collagen dressings	Activate matrix metalloproteinases and promote new collagen formation	Chronic non-healing wounds Burn wounds

Mechanism of action—HBO therapy can increase tissue PO2 ten times higher than usual. The higher PaO2 is sufficient to supply the tissue with all its metabolic requirements even in the absence of hemoglobin. This elevated level lasts for 2–4 h after termination of HBO therapy and induces synthesis of endothelial cell NO synthase as well as angiogenesis. Oxygen stimulates angiogenesis, enhances fibroblast and leukocyte function, and normalizes cutaneous microvascular reflexes, thus aiding in healing of chronic, complicated, non-healing wounds.

2. **Negative pressure-assisted wound therapy**—Argenta [14] and associates originally described the use of negative pressure to assist in wound closure in 1997. By applying subatmospheric pressure to wounds, they demonstrated removal of chronic edema, an increase in local blood flow, and stimulation of granulation tissue. This technique may be used on acute, subacute, and chronic wounds. The wound is filled with a foam substance. A drainage tube is inserted into, or laid on, the foam, and the part is then covered with impermeable film. Suction is applied at around 125 mmHg between changes of dressing.

49.9 Necrotizing Fasciitis

It is a rapidly spreading necrotizing soft tissue infection, also known as flesh-eating disease. It is one of the most challenging infections faced by the maxillofacial surgeons due to its diagnosis and management. The most common bacteria responsible for the fascial necrosis are hemolytic *Streptococcus* and *Staphylococcus*.

It is foul-smelling with loss of skin and superficial subcutaneous tissue, having patchy blackish necrosis and frank pus along with the raw surface of the wound, margins of which are pale and spreading in nature. If it involves the skin of scrotum, it is known as Fournier's gangrene.

The prompt diagnosis and aggressive treatment is the key to manage this complicated condition. Removal of the offending factors like carious tooth and infected foreign material is the prime step followed by aggressive debridement and desloughing involving the normal tissue margins under the antibiotic coverage and adequate anesthesia. Once the wound is free of the active infection, showing healing margins with no evidence of pus, it is reconstructed with the skin grafts (Fig. 49.12).

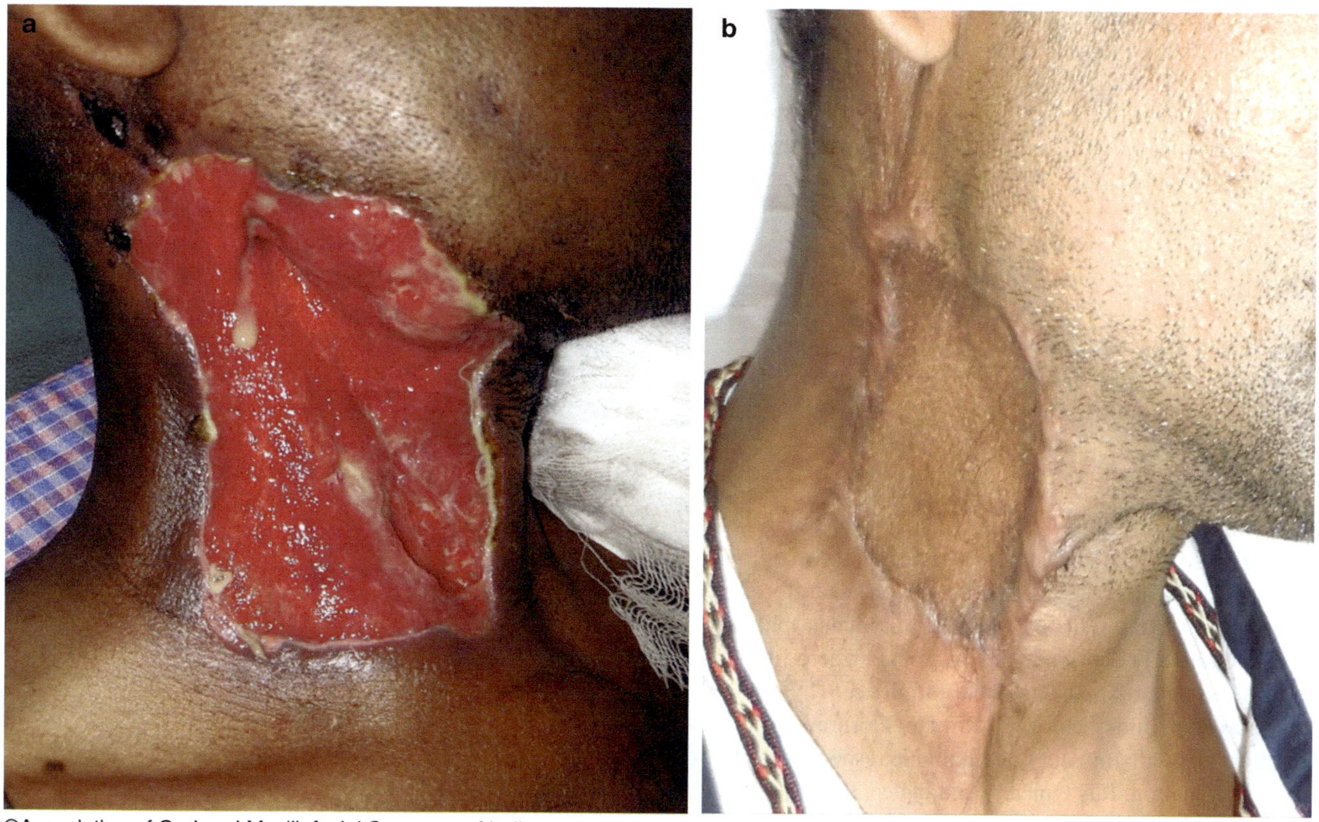

Fig. 49.12 Depicting a case of necrotizing fasciitis of the right side of the neck due to infection from right mandibular third molar. The patient was promptly and aggressively managed by sequential debridement followed by anterolateral thigh skin graft

Table 49.2 Phases of wound healing

Phases of wound healing	Time period	Mechanism of healing
Inflammatory phase	Immediate till 5th day	• Immediate vascular response • Cellular infiltration—Polymorphonuclear leukocytes initially, followed by monocytes within 24 h, which become dominant by the 5th day and actively engaged in phagocytosis • Formation of new blood vessels at the edges of wound (neovascularization) • Synthesis of granulation tissue
Proliferative phase	Established by 5th day	• Cellular proliferation—Macrophages are preponderant • With time, the number of fibroblasts increases that are active in synthesis of extracellular collagen and proteoglycans (collagen synthesis) • The fibroblasts in the wound are closely followed by the endothelial buds of capillaries. The wound is filled with vascular granulation tissue containing new capillaries, fibroblasts, macrophages, and mast cells • An intrinsic increase in the mechanical strength of the wound at the end of this phase
Maturation phase		• Extensive remodeling as a result of a decrease in the numbers of fibroblasts and macrophages concurrent with a decrease in vascularity • Increase in wound strength • Formation of scar tissue

49.10 Principles of Soft Tissue Healing

The three phases of repair in soft tissue wounds are overlapping and include

- The inflammatory phase
- The proliferative phase
- The maturation phase (Table 49.2)

Any alteration in the local environment of the wounds or the systemic status of the patients can influence the normal process of wound healing.

49.11 Types of Wound Healing

The various types of wound healing include:

1. Primary intention
2. Delayed primary closure
3. Secondary intention

1. **Primary intention**—occurs when full-thickness wound edges are approximated shortly after the primary wound has been created. This type of closure is generally avoided in grossly contaminated wounds, in wounds that cannot be completely debrided, and in wounds where further tissue loss is anticipated as in blast injuries.
2. **Delayed primary closure**—Primary closure is delayed to allow host inflammatory and immune responses to control contamination. It is typically completed 3–4 days after the initial injury but depends on the particular characteristics of the wound. Serial debridements may be performed until the full extent of tissue devitalization is determined.

Table 49.3 Factors that negatively influence wound healing

Local factors	Systemic factors
Presence of foreign bodies	Smoking
Venous insufficiency	Comorbidities like diabetes
Ischemia/ hypoxia to tissues	Systemic condition—malnutrition, chronic illness, deficiency of vitamins
Radiation	Prolonged drug use—corticosteroids, cytotoxic chemotherapy
Salivary contamination	
Scarring	
Hematoma	

3. **Secondary intention**—healing is by natural biologic processes without surgical intervention, and it usually occurs in large wounds associated with soft tissue loss or avulsion. It involves epithelialization and collagen deposition for wound healing. Contraction is the most important phenomenon in the spontaneous closure of large open wounds.

49.12 Complications in Wound Healing

Complications in the normal process of wound healing may occur due to presence of various local and systemic factors which exert a negative impact (Table 49.3).

One of the frequently observed complications is "abnormal wound healing" which presents in different forms such as keloids and hypertrophic scars. These are proliferative scars characterized by excessive net collagen deposition. Keloids and hypertrophic scars (Fig. 49.13) differ histologically from normal scars. The clinical appearance of the two types of scar is described in Table 49.4.

Keloids and hypertrophic scars contain collagen bundles aligned in the same plane as the epidermis. Tension

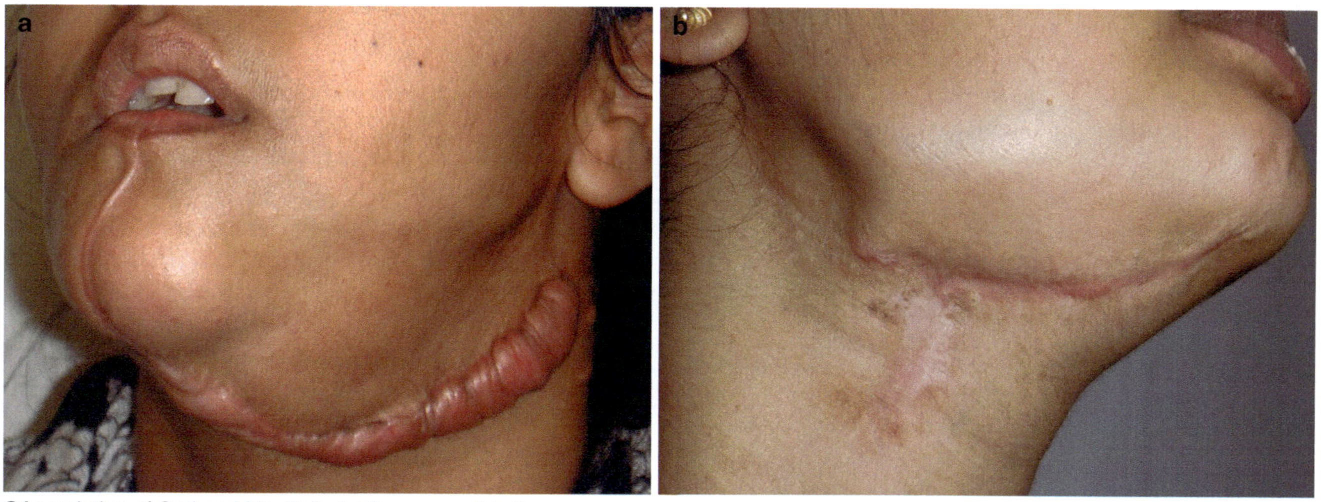

Fig. 49.13 Showing. (**a**) keloid type of scar and (**b**) hypertrophic scar healing

Table 49.4 Difference between keloids and hypertrophic scar

Keloids	Hypertrophic scar
Contain disorganized type I and type III collagen bundles	Primarily contain well-organized type III collagen fibers
The collagen bundles are thicker and form a nodelike structure in the deep layer of skin	Contain islands of aggregates of fibroblasts, small vessels, and collagen fibers throughout the dermis
Cannot be prevented and are often refractory to medical and surgical intervention	Often preventable
Occur above the clavicles, on the trunk, on the upper extremities, and on the face	Prolonged inflammation and insufficient resurfacing (e.g., burn wounds) promote hypertrophic scarring
Grow beyond the borders of the original wounds and rarely regress with time	Raised scars within the confines of the original wound and frequently regress spontaneously
Appear to be genetically predisposed	Represent a reversible hyperproliferative scar phenotype that regresses when the original stimulus (skin tension, stimulatory growth factors) are removed
First-line treatments include pressure therapy and intralesional corticosteroid injections. Intralesional 5-fluorouracil, bleomycin, and verapamil used according to the established treatment protocols. Refractory cases after 12 months of therapy should be considered for surgical excision in combination with adjuvant therapy. Excision alone results in a high recurrence rate of 50–100% and enlargement of the keloid. Immediate postoperative electron beam irradiation or brachytherapy with iridium-192 reduces recurrence rates.	Pressure and silicone therapy combined with selective localized corticosteroid injections in resistant areas. Bleomycin, 5-fluorouracil, and verapamil can be used as adjuncts to corticosteroid therapy. Laser therapy to reduce scar thickness, resurface scar texture, and treat residual redness, telangiectasias, or hyperpigmentation. Early surgery is indicated if the scar causes functional impairment. Scar contracture release procedures in the neck and axilla are best performed with flaps to improve functional and cosmetic outcomes. Widespread large hypertrophic scars may require serial excision or tissue expansion.

over the edges of the wound signals the formation of activated fibroblasts resulting in excessive collagen deposition.

Scars perpendicular to the underlying muscle fibers tend to be flatter and narrower, with less collagen formation than when they are parallel to the underlying muscle fibers. As muscle fibers contract, the wound edges become reapproximated when they are perpendicular to the underlying muscle and tend to gape if placed parallel to it, leading to greater wound tension and scar formation.

49.12.1 Prevention of Hypertrophic or Keloid Scars

The four strategies that reduce adverse scarring immediately after wound closure are:

- Layer-wise closure as to avoid gaping within the layers of the wound
- Closure without tension
- Hydration of the wound with clean dressing
- Use of pressure garments

Postsurgical taping of the wound for 3 months can reduce scarring. Moisturizing lotions and moisture-retentive dressings (silicone sheets and gels) can reduce the thickness, discomfort, and itching and improve the appearance of the scar.

49.13 Recent Advances in Soft Tissue Management

1. Use of **growth factors**—intimate role in the regulation of all phases of wound healing, i.e., chemotaxis, proliferation, matrix synthesis, inflammation, and angiogenesis. The enhancement of soft tissue wound healing can be done by various methods. Topical application of growth factors in a vehicle or by direct seeding of cells topically on the wound can enhance healing. Placement of growth factors or cells can also be done with a fibrin sealant or glue. Use of platelet-rich plasma (PRP) by degranulation of platelets with the secretion of its contents of growth factors into the surrounding fibrin matrix or, more recently, use of tissue-engineered equivalents of skin or mucosa can provide a scaffold that enhances healing.
2. **Gene and stem cell therapy**—in which the gene encoding for the therapeutic growth factor or protein is directly transfected into host cells. This is a promising approach for the treatment of acute and chronic wounds.
3. **Tissue engineering**—In 1987, the National Science Foundation bioengineering panel defined tissue engineering as "the application of the principles and methods of engineering and the life sciences toward the development of biologic substitutes to restore, maintain, or improve function."
   They include—*Bioengineered Skin substitutes vis* [15]

   (a) *Epidermal substitutes*—These are autografts taken from split-thickness skin grafting or from cell line bioreactor expansion and grown in laboratory until enough tissue is produced to be transferred to the wound later.
   (b) *Dermal substitutes*—When the wound is deep and the dermis is destroyed, epidermal substitutes are not enough to ensure wound healing. The dermis is replaced by the one manufactured in the laboratory from the patient-specific cells. This dermis is essential to maintain mechanical resistance and occlude the surface of the wound.
   (c) *Bilayer substitutes*—Integra, developed in 1981, was the first acellular bilayer and has been used successfully to treat burns and chronic wound patients.

49.14 Conclusion

Proper assessment and classification of soft tissue injuries is the primary step in management. Early intervention and closure of soft tissue injuries is associated with optimal functional and esthetic outcomes as well as decreases the risk of complications. The basic principles of management of soft tissue injuries include the control of bleeding, copious irrigation of the wound, debridement of devitalized tissue, and removal of foreign bodies before closure. Administration of antibiotics and tetanus prophylaxis play a vital role in management of contaminated wounds. Wound dressings are mandatory to protect wounds postoperatively and facilitate ideal healing. Soft tissue injuries resulting in loss of tissue must be reconstructed using flaps which may be local, regional, distant, or free microvascular flaps, depending on the type, location, and extent of the injury. Innovative options such as growth factors, stem cell therapy, and bioengineered skin substitutes may be considered.

49.15 Case Scenarios

Case Scenario 1

A 23-year-old male patient met with a road traffic accident and suffered from a perforating injury over the nose, extending to right infra-orbital region. After initial resuscitating of the patient and ruling out the head injury component, the patient was taken up for the management of soft tissue and hard tissue injuries under general anesthesia. Through the existing lacerated wound, open reduction and internal fixation was done within 48 h of the trauma. Simultaneously, the soft tissue closure was performed layer-wise. Closure of the muscle layer was performed followed by the subcutaneous tissue and finally the skin (Fig. 49.14a–e).

Case Scenario 2

A case scenario of a 67-year-old male patient who reported to the department of Oral and Maxillofacial Surgery. He was a victim of ballistic injury while he was working in a marketplace. The penetrating pathway of the bullet could be traced

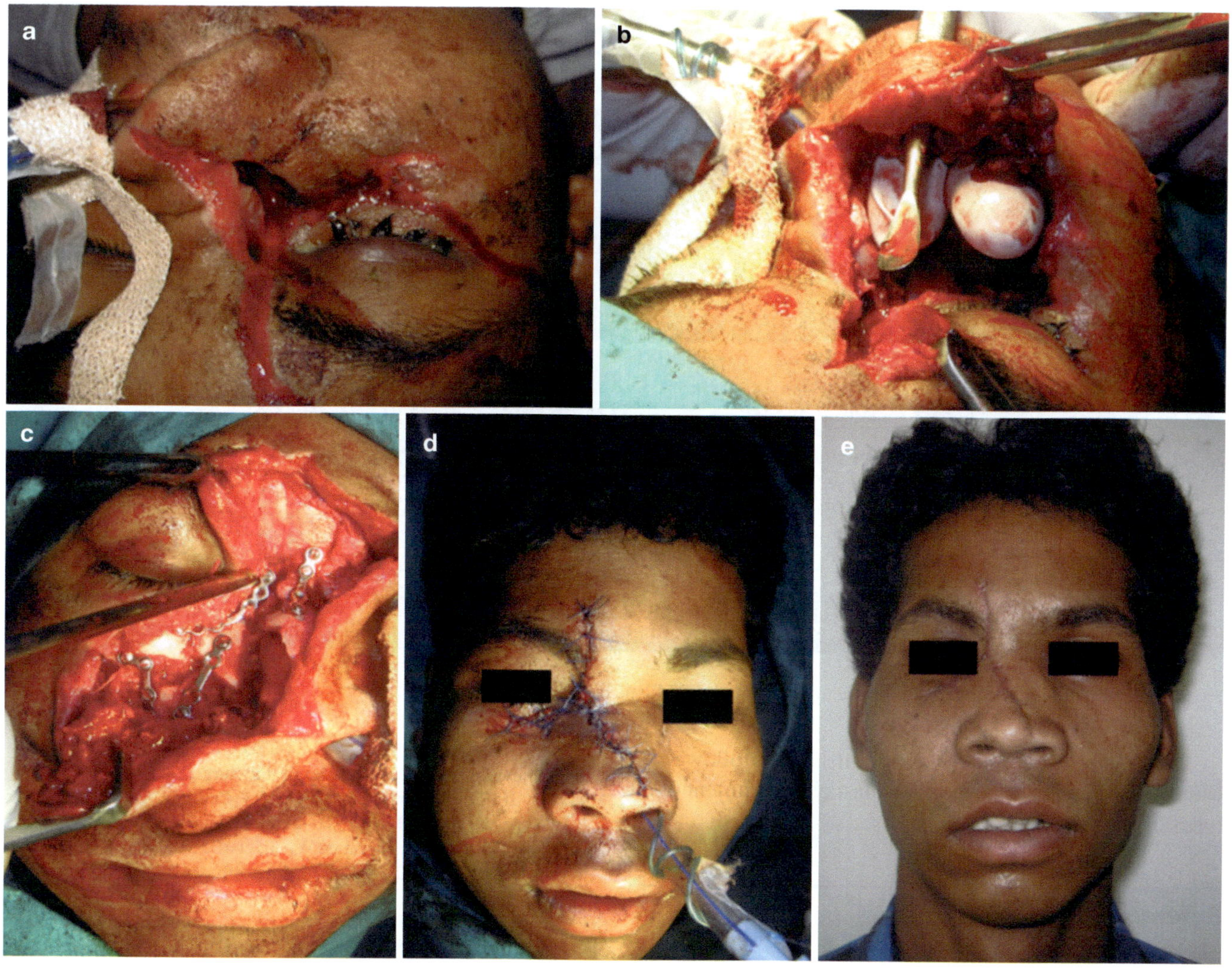

Fig. 49.14 Case scenario 1(a–e): Soft tissue management of a road traffic accident victim

having an entry site over left cheek. An extensive and careful exploration was performed in the OT under general anesthesia after the sections of 3D CT face were obtained (Fig. 49.15a–g). The comminuted fracture of the mandible was reconstructed using reconstruction plate. The bullet was found to be lodged in the carotid triangle just above the bifurcation of the common carotid artery.

Soft tissue management in such type of ballistic injuries becomes very critical. Since the bullet is a foreign material, it has to be removed from the soft tissues. The approach could either be through the entry wound but due to deep seating of the bullet into the neck and proximity of vital structures, one should always think of an extensive approach. The neck dissection was carried out in this case to remove the bullet from the bifurcation of common carotid artery in as atraumatic manner as possible. Bidigital palpation is a crucial step to locate the foreign body in this region. One interesting fact about such injuries is that though they are extensive with crushed and comminuted fractures and they are sterile due to the heat generated by the velocity of the bullet along its path. Such injuries are less prone to infection.

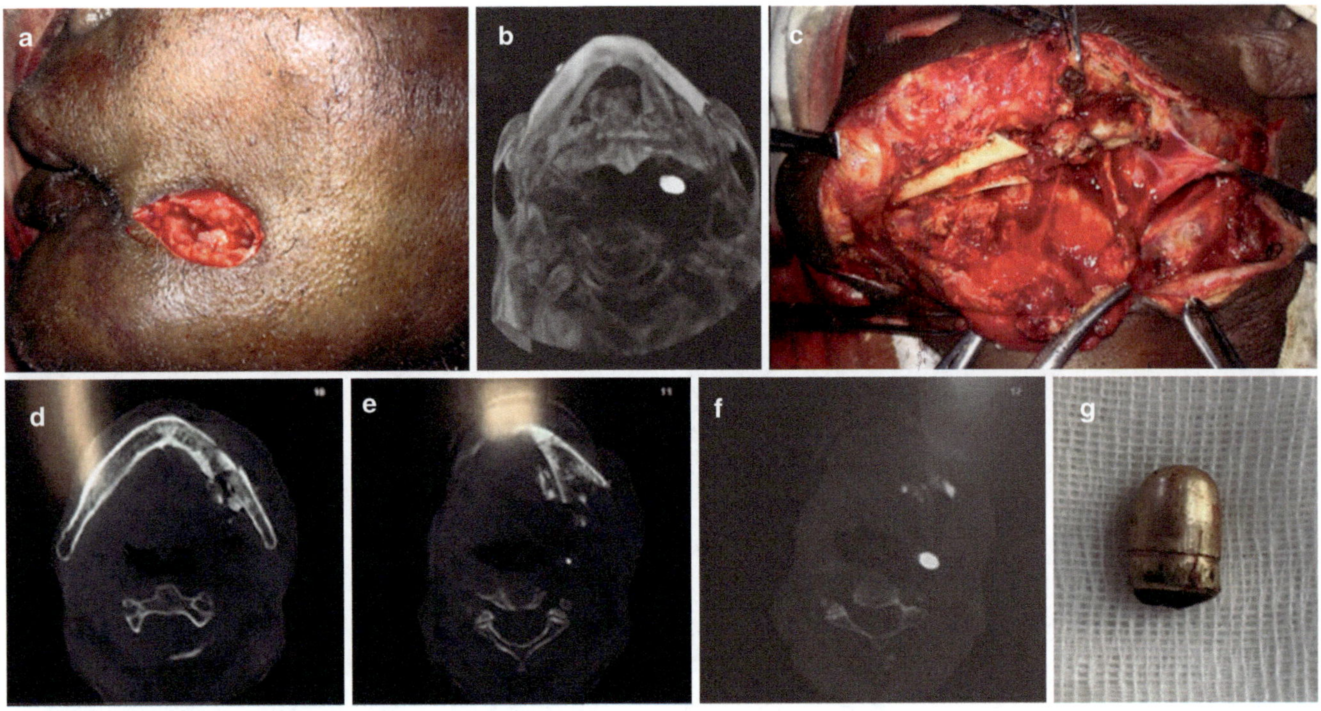

Fig. 49.15 (a–g) Case Scenario 2: Soft tissue management in a ballistic injury

Proper surgical toilet with wound irrigation followed by careful debridement remains the mainstay of treatment of all types of soft tissue injuries.

References

1. Hussain K, Wijetunge DB, Grubnic S, et al. A comprehensive analysis of craniofacial trauma. J Trauma. 1994;36:34.
2. Key SJ, Thomas DW, Shepherd JP. The management of soft tissue facial wounds. Br J Oral Maxillofac Surg. 1995;33(2):76–85.
3. Karlson TA. The incidence of hospital-treated facial injuries from vehicles. J Trauma. 1982;22:303.
4. Fattahi TT. An overview of facial aesthetic units. J Oral Maxillofac Surg. 2003;61(10):1207–11.
5. Seddon HJ, Medawar PB, Smith H. Rate of regeneration of peripheral nerves in man. J Physiol. 1943;102:191–215.
6. Sunderland S. A classification of peripheral nerve injuries producing loss of function. Brain. 1951;74:491–516.
7. Rank BK, Wakefield AR. Surgery of repair as applied to hand injuries. London: Livingstone; 1960.
8. Stefanopoulos PK, Tarantzopoulou AD. Facial bite wounds: management update. Int J Oral Maxillofac Surg. 2005;34(5):464–72.
9. Janis JE. Essentials of plastic surgery. 2nd edn. Boca Raton, FL: Quality Medical; 2014. p. 316–21, 382–5, 390, 480.
10. Frodel JL, Holt GR, Larrabee WF Jr, et al. Facial plastic and reconstructive surgery. In: Papel ID, editor. 4th edn. New York: Thieme; 2016. p. 754–65.
11. Pitt D, Aubin JM. Joseph Lister: father of modern surgery. Can J Surg. 2012;55(5):E8.
12. Morin RJ, Tomaselli NL. Interactive dressings and topical agents. Clin Plast Surg. 2007;34(4):643–58.
13. Lionelli GT, Lawrence WT. Wound dressings. Surg Clin. 2003;83(3):617–38.
14. Argenta LC, Morykwas MJ. Vacuum-assisted closure: a new method for wound control and treatment: clinical experience. Ann Plast Surg. 1997;38:563–77.
15. Greaves NS, Iqbal SA, Baguneid M, Bayat A. The role of skin substitutes in the management of chronic cutaneous wounds. Wound Repair Regen. 2013;21(2):194–210.

Dentoalveolar Injuries and Wiring Techniques

50

Omkar Anand Shetye

50.1 Definition

Dentoalveolar fracture is defined as a fracture in the bone surrounding the teeth without any extension to the basal bones of the maxilla or mandible [1, 2].

50.2 Incidence

Dentoalveolar injuries commonly occur in the age group of 8–12 years. They generally involve teeth, soft tissues, and/or associated bone. Traumatic dental injuries account for a total of 92% of maxillofacial injuries of which 92% involves only the soft tissues and 8% involve the maxillofacial bones [2].

50.3 Introduction

Trauma is the foremost etiological factor that leads to a loss of significant number of teeth annually. The recent advancements in the field of preventive dentistry as well as the development of myriad evidence-based techniques to restore the lost form and function of teeth have made it possible for the dental surgeon to successfully facilitate the improvement in the quality of life of trauma-afflicted patients. Time elapsed post-trauma plays a major factor in determining the outcome of the intervention. Apart from reestablishing the premorbid position of the traumatized tooth in its socket, the goal of the treatment is directed toward achieving the pre-traumatic occlusion and intra-arch contour [3].

Electronic Supplementary Material The online version of this chapter (https://doi.org/10.1007/978-981-15-1346-6_50) contains supplementary material, which is available to authorized users.

O. A. Shetye (✉)
Department of Oral and Maxillofacial Surgery, Goa Dental College and Hospital, Bambolim, Goa, India

50.4 Diagnosis and Treatment Planning

The foundation of diagnosis and management of traumatic dental injuries solely lies on the pillars of a detailed patient history and a clinical examination. **When, Where, and How** forms the "Trauma Triad" of history taking in traumatic dental injuries [4].

When—Time interval between injury and treatment may significantly affect the prognosis for cases of pulp exposure, displacement, and avulsion type of injuries.

Where—The place of injury. The chances of the injury getting infected on a playground compared to an injury that has occurred at home in relatively cleaner surroundings. The place of injury has medico-legal repercussions if the assault or accident has occurred at the place of work. Depending on the cleanliness of the wound, the clinician can also consider protection against tetanus.

How—This may give an indication of concomitant injuries like soft tissue injuries secondary to the trauma [5].

History of immediate local measures employed to reduce the severity of injury helps in eliciting information regarding the original condition of the injured area [6].

History of any systemic disorders that may interfere with treatment or post-operative healing including a history of tetanus vaccination has to be obtained before starting the treatment [7].

"Outside-in" examination (examining the facial structure in three concentric rings paying more attention to the innermost ring) helps in achieving the desired management protocol. Level of consciousness should be assessed prior to the clinical examination [6].

The potential for aspiration, airway compromise, and neurosensory deficit warrants the need for a thorough evaluation of all maxillofacial injuries before managing dental injuries [3].

K. Bonanthaya et al. (eds.), *Oral and Maxillofacial Surgery for the Clinician*, https://doi.org/10.1007/978-981-15-1346-6_50

In a patient with missing tooth fragment or prosthesis, a chest radiograph and abdominal radiograph may be helpful in locating the missing structures and their management. Owing to its anatomic position, the right bronchus is often the site of foreign body dislodgement [3, 6].

50.5 Clinical Examination

Clinical examination of the patient has to be divided into the following subsets [8]:

- Extra-oral soft tissue
- Intra-oral soft tissue
- Jaws and alveolar bone
- Teeth (displacement and mobility)
- Percussion and pulp testing [3]

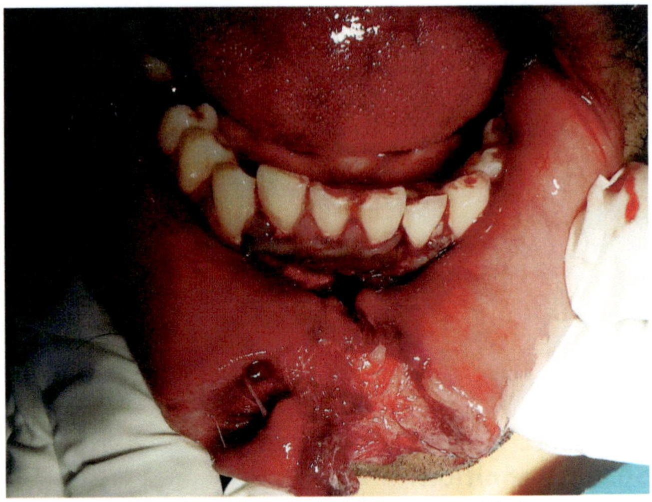

Fig. 50.1 Mandibular anterior lingually displaced dentoalveolar fracture with degloving vestibular wound and ragged lip lacerations

50.5.1 Extra-oral

Asymmetry of the face following trauma could be due to injury to the facial skeleton or swelling. Areas of ecchymosis and hematoma may indicate fracture of the underlying osseous structure. Laceration, contusion, and abrasion of the overlying skin are common with dentoalveolar injuries (Figs. 50.1, 50.2, and 50.3). Mild antiseptic soap should be used to clean the extra-oral abrasions or a saline wash can be used while being careful to not inoculate injury site further with debris or foreign body [4, 8].

50.5.2 Intra-oral

Buccal mucosa lacerations should raise suspicion for a Stensen's duct injury. The lips, floor of the mouth, and tongue are areas which are at a risk of being penetrated or sites for secondary injuries [3].

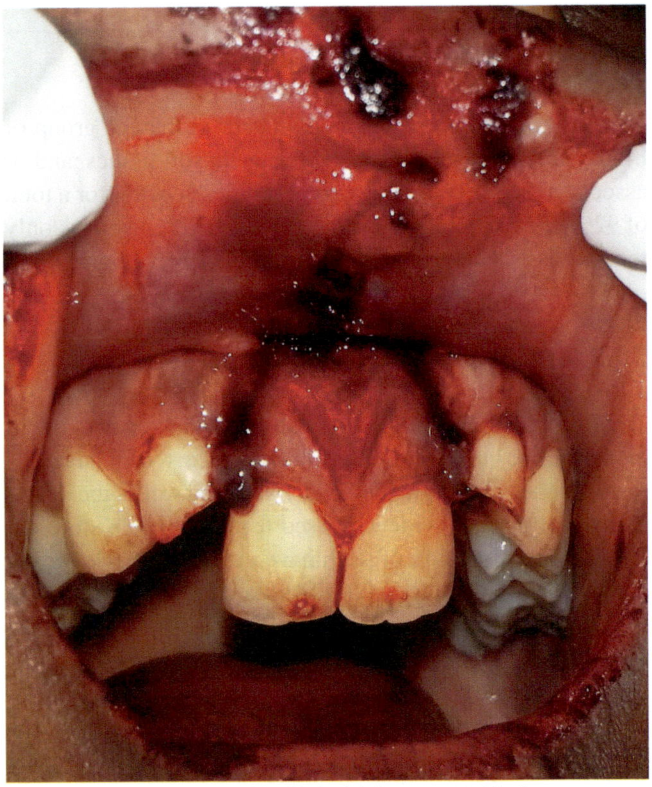

Fig. 50.2 Maxillary anterior palatally displaced and extruded dentoalveolar fracture with associated upper lip injury. Note incisal fractures of the upper lateral incisors (see also Fig. 50.8)

50.5.3 Jaws and Alveolar Bone

Bimanual palpation of the maxillary and mandibular dentition and evaluation of occlusion should reveal areas of discrepancy or mobility. The direction of dislocation of the apex of primary tooth should be diagnosed since these teeth are in close approximation to the succedaneous teeth. Palpating from the vestibular approach makes this diagnosis easier. Sublingual ecchymosis/hematoma (Coleman's sign) at the floor of the mouth is suggestive of underlying mandibular fractures. Step deformity, crepitation, malocclusion, and gingival lacerations raise suspicion for possible bone defects [7, 9].

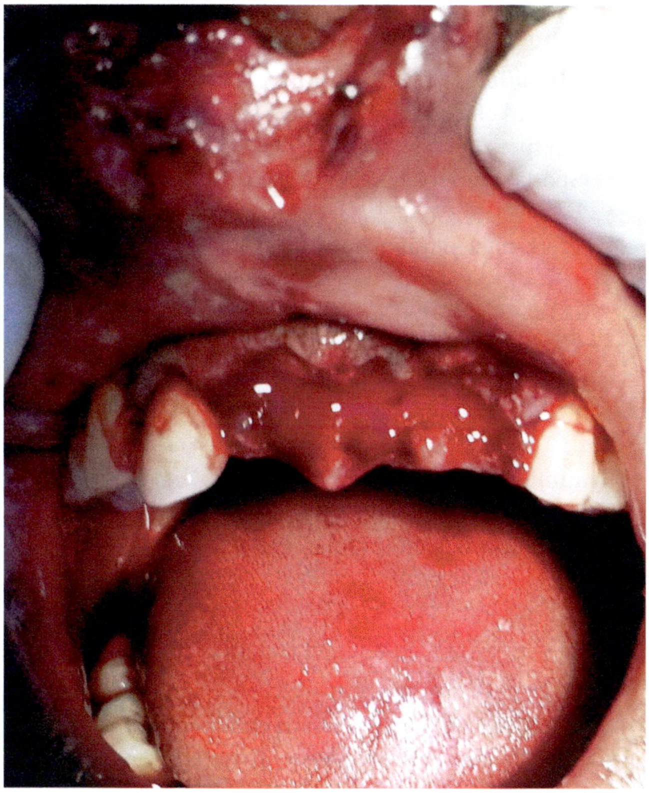

Fig. 50.3 Maxillary anterior teeth complete avulsion with associated upper lip injury

50.5.4 Percussion and Pulp Testing

Percussion test is performed with the end of the handle of an examination mirror. Pain to percussion of a tooth is indicative of damage to the periodontal ligament. Dullness to percussion in one or several adjacent teeth can be indicative of partially luxated teeth or en bloc fracture of tooth or alveolar bone. The percussion test should be started on a non-injured tooth to ensure a reliable response through visual analogue scale [6, 8].

To evaluate the tooth injury thoroughly, pulp vitality is a must. A positive response indicates that the pulp is alive, whereas a negative response indicates that the pulp is dead. Following injury, the tooth may be in a state of shock and may give a false response. Hence pulp testing should also be performed during the subsequent visits to acknowledge the change in response [5].

Electric vitality testing depends on a number of factors including the stage of eruption of tooth, the presence of a restoration or decay, and the ability to isolate the tooth and keep the area clear of blood and saliva [8].

Laser Doppler flowmetry (LDF) is a relatively new pulp testing apparatus. It employs a laser beam directed at the coronal-labial aspect of the pulp which is scattered by pulp blood cells that in turn produce a Doppler frequency shift. The fraction of light scattered back is detected and processed to elicit a signal. The basic theory is that the pulp revascularization process can be monitored. Studies have shown that in cases in which electrometric tests were negative and LDF displayed vascular perfusion, the LDF accuracy of pulp vitality reached 100% [3].

All the teeth should be tested for abnormal mobility both horizontally and vertically. It should be remembered that primary teeth undergoing physiologic root resorption and therefore always exhibit a certain degree of mobility. The typical sign of an alveolar fracture is the movement of adjacent teeth when the mobility of a single tooth is tested [6].

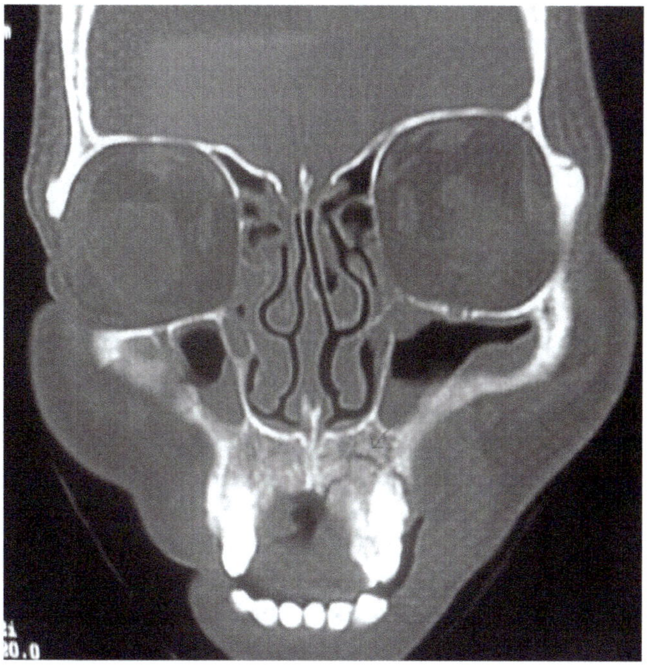

Fig. 50.4 Coronal CT image showing left maxillary high dentoalveolar fracture

50.6 Radiographic Examination

Radiographic techniques are available to evaluate dentoalveolar trauma.

Radiographic examination is essential to determine damage to underlying structures and should include intraoral periapical (IOPA), occlusal, panoramic radiographs (OPG), and cone-beam computed tomography (CBCT) imaging [3, 4].

If conventional CT imaging is done as part of the trauma series, fine axial and coronal cuts will also show the dentoalveolar injuries (Fig. 50.4)

IOPA radiograph provides vital information about root fracture and dislocation of teeth. At times it is difficult to adequately evaluate a fracture on an IOPA radiograph, due to variations in tube-tooth-film geometry. Post-treatment radiographs can confirm the proper repositioning of avulsed or luxated tooth into alveolar bone.

Occlusal radiographs provide a larger field of view, and a steep occlusal exposure is of special value in the diagnosis of root fracture and lateral luxations with displacement of crown [8].

OPG is a useful screening tool and can demonstrate fractures of the mandible and maxilla as well as fractures of alveolar ridges and teeth.

Radiographic evaluation of foreign bodies within soft tissues of the lips and cheeks is done by taking radiographs with the film placed labial to the alveolus. A reduced radiographic exposure time (approximately 1/3rd of the normal) is used.

CBCT scanning is extremely useful in diagnosis of maxillofacial, alveolar bone, and teeth fractures with the advantage of high-resolution three-dimensional images with low radiation.

The etiology of pediatric and adult dentoalveolar injuries were shown in Box 50.1 and Box 50.2 respectively. Box 50.3 and Box 50.4 represents the classification of alveolar bone fracture and classification of alveolar bone fracture based on location and displacement respectively.

Box 50.1: Etiology of Pediatric Dentoalveolar Injuries

Pediatric patients [9]

- Bicycle injuries
- Falls
- Sports injuries
- Car crashes
- Child abuse
- Iatrogenic injuries(dental extractions, endoscopy, oral intubation)
- Industrial accidents

Box 50.2: Etiology of Adult Dentoalveolar Injuries

Adult patients

- Motor vehicular accidents
- Interpersonal violence
- Sports injuries(contact injuries)
- Falls
- Work-related trauma

Box 50.3: Classification of Alveolar Bone Fracture:

Traumatic alveolar bone [9]

Type I: Areas surrounding a single tooth

Type II: Entire dentoalveolar segment dislocation

Box 50.4 Alveolar fracture can be classified by their specific location and movement of displacement [10]

Class I: Edentulous segment fracture

Class II: Little or any displacement of fractured dentulous segment

Class III: Moderate to severe displacement of fractured dentulous segment

Class IV: Multiple fracture lines with combination of fracture of the dentulous segment

Box 50.5: Classification of Dental Injuries and Surrounding Structure

Classification based on level of involvement [11]

1. Fracture involving enamel
2. Fracture involving enamel and dentin
3. Fracture involving enamel, dentin and pulp
4. Fracture involving enamel, dentin, cementum
5. Crown/ root fracture
6. Luxation of tooth
7. Intrusion and extrusion (Fig. 50.5a,b) (Box 50.6)
8. Avulsion (Fig. 50.5c) (Boxes 50.7 and 50.8)

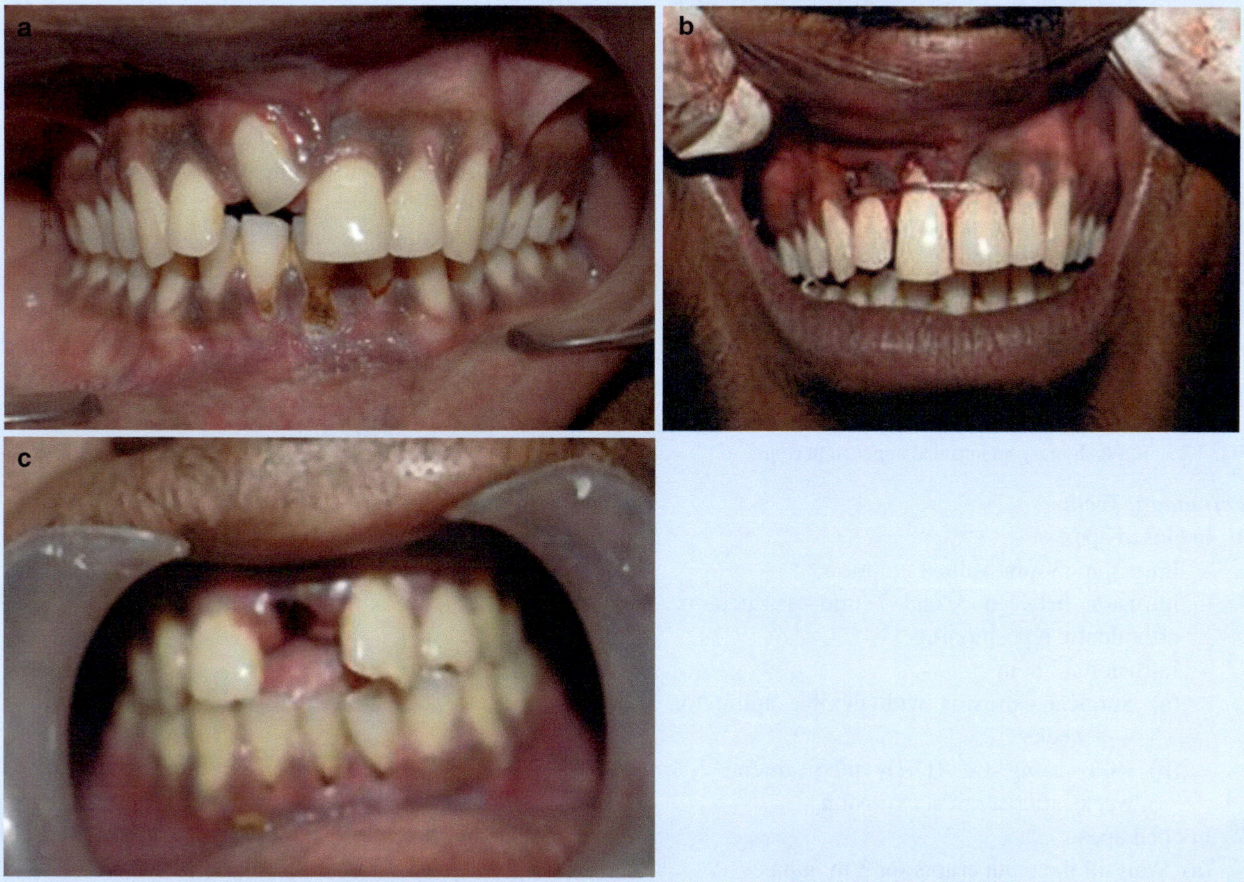

Fig. 50.5 (**a–c**) Clinical images showing tooth (a) intrusion, (b) extrusion, and (c) avulsion

Box 50.6: Management of Intruded Tooth (Fig. 50.6)

Diangelis et al. [12, 13]

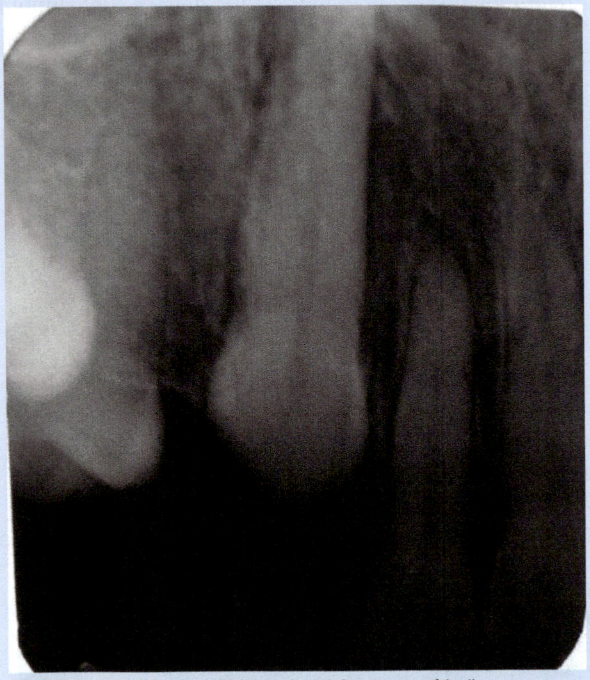

©Association of Oral and Maxillofacial Surgeons of India

Fig. 50.6 IOPA showing an intruded upper right canine

Permanent Teeth

1. In closed apex
   - Intrusion <3 mm—allow eruption
   - Intrusion between 3 and 7 mm—surgical or orthodontic repositioning
   - Intrusion >7 m m
     (a) Surgical extrusion with flexible splint for 4–8 weeks
     (b) RCT using Ca $(OH)_2$ medicament 2–3 weeks after surgical extrusion
2. In open apex
   (a) Wait till the tooth erupts for 3 months
   (b) Place an orthodontic extruding appliance

Primary Teeth

Treatment is debatable

Immediate extraction of the involved tooth

or

More conservative approach

50.6.1 Storage and Transportation Media

If the tooth cannot be reimplanted within 5 min, it should be stored in a medium that will maintain its vitality and periodontal ligament fibers [14–16].

Box 50.7: Principle of Avulsion

- Primary should not be replanted
- Permanent teeth should be replanted as soon as possible and stabilized for 7–10 days up to 2 weeks [14, 15].

Box 50.8: Primary Management of Avulsion by the Patient

What the patient can do:

- To hold the tooth by its crown and not to touch the root surface.
- To rinse the tooth immediately with saliva, tap water or saline solution and reimplant the tooth.
- If the patient cannot replace the tooth, it should be held in the buccal vestibule (only if patient is fully conscious).
- Gentle irrigation with saline or gauze soaked with saline may be employed to remove blood clots or foreign objects from the surface of the root.

What the patient should not do:

- No effort should be made to mechanically cleanse the root of the tooth because this would damage the remaining periodontal ligament.

Transportation media for avulsed teeth include

1. Viaspan: a specialized tissue storage media used when transporting liver for transplantation.
2. Hanks balanced salt solution: both hanks solution and viaspan are physiologic with compatible pH and osmolality. The relative availability and cost-effective hanks solution makes it medium of choice in storage of avulsed teeth.

Commercial products are designed especially for storing avulsed teeth. It has shelf life of 2 years without refrigeration (Box 50.9).

3. Milk: is a readily available medium. It is the medium of choice in the absence of hanks balanced salt solution or viaspan. Milk will only prevent further cellular demise and is used specifically when the teeth has been outside the oral cavity for less than 20 min.

Box 50.9: HBSS Contents

Contents of Hanks balanced salt solution [19]
- Sodium chloride
- Glucose
- Potassium chloride
- Sodium bicarbonate
- Sodium phosphate
- Calcium chloride
- Magnesium chloride
- Magnesium sulfate

Box 50.10: Reagent for Root Surface Therapy

Agents used for root surface treatment to prevent resorption
- Citric acid
- Doxycycline
- Tetracycline
- Fluorides
- Enamel matrix derivative (emdogain)
- Diphosphonates

4. Saliva: is an excellent transport medium and is as effective as saline. It does not matter if the tooth is stored in another person's saliva.
5. Tap water: has been commonly recommended storage solution but due its hypotonicity, it leads to rapid cell lysis and increased inflammation on replantation.
6. Contact lens solution: a compilation of information from a study Blomlof et al. [17] indicates that Hanks buffered saline, isotonic saline, and pasteurized bovine milk may be the most favorable known storage media. If none of these are available, human saliva or contact lens solution is acceptable short-term substitute storage liquid.
7. Culture mediums like minimum essential eagles medium and Dulbecco's storage media [18] have been used as they contain amino acids, vitamins, and bicarbonates that help to maintain the vitality of cells.
8. Propolis: a beehive product which has an excellent anti-inflammatory and anti-bacterial effect has been used as a storage medium.
9. Green Tea: its polyphenol derivative have antioxidative, anti-carcinogenic, anti-mutagenic, anti-inflammatory, antimicrobial, and antiviral effect.
10. Patients own serum have shown to maintain the vitality of periodontal ligament cells up to 1 h.
    Morus rubra (red mulberry), egg white, coconut water, rehydrating solution like Gatorade and ricetral, lens solution, probiotic solutions, saliva officinalis, honey milk, and ascorbic acid have been used as a transportation medium for avulsed tooth.

50.7 Treatment at the Clinic

Traumatically avulsed teeth when out of the mouth for a short period should be reimplanted as soon as possible. After normal reattachment, survival is prolonged. Avulsed teeth which remain out of the mouth for more than 2–3 h generally resorb rapidly and should not be reimplanted indiscriminately.

The outcome of replantation depends on the stage of root development and extra-oral time. If the avulsed tooth has a closed apex and extra-oral time is less than 60 min (early replantation), the reimplanted tooth will have the best prognosis. The ideal time to begin root canal treatment is within 10–14 days post-replantation and before splint removal.

There is a statistically significant association between extirpation within 14 days and an increased likelihood of successful periodontal healing and prevention of external inflammatory root resorption.

It is generally agreed that Ca $(OH)_2$ has a beneficial effect in the outcome because of its antibacterial properties, ability to dissolve necrotic tissue, and its ability to prevent or control inflammatory resorption. The anti-inflammatory and antibacterial action may decrease root resorption by directly inhibiting resorptive cells (Box 50.10).

50.7.1 Delayed Replantation (more than 60 min)

Delayed replantation of avulsed tooth with closed apex has a poor long-term prognosis. The periodontal ligament gets necrotic and healing is delayed. The goal of delayed replantation is to promote alveolar bone growth so as to encapsulate the reimplanted tooth. The eventual outcome is ankylosis.

In children below age of 15 years, if ankylosis occurs and when the infra position of the tooth crown is more than 1 mm, decoronation is recommended to preserve the contour of the alveolar bone.

Root canal treatment (RCT) can be carried out on a tooth prior to reimplantation or it can be carried out within 14 days of reimplantation. The tooth is immersed in 2% sodium fluoride solution for a minimum of 5 min up to 20 min.

Avulsed teeth having open apices and extra-oral time less than 60 min are also reimplanted and stabilized for 7–10 days and up to 2 weeks. The goal of reimplanting developing (immature) teeth in children is to allow for possible revascularization of the tooth pulp.

If there is evidence of the pulpal infection or inflammatory response, the pulp should be removed and Ca $(OH)_2$ placed immediately, aiming to stimulate apexification and halt the inflammatory process.

It is believed that delayed replantation of avulsed teeth with open apices have a poor long-term prognosis. The periodontal ligament gets necrotic and is not expected to heal. Osseous replacement, resorption, or ankylosis will occur. Therefore some authors have concluded that such teeth should not be reimplanted.

The recent guidelines recommend replantation to maintain alveolar ridge contour as ankylosed roots get transformed to bone during the remodeling process. RCT can be performed on the tooth prior to replantation through an open apex (Fig. 50.7a–c).

50.7.2 Stabilization

Stabilization of an avulsed tooth can be achieved using a variety of materials like wires, arch bar wired to the teeth,

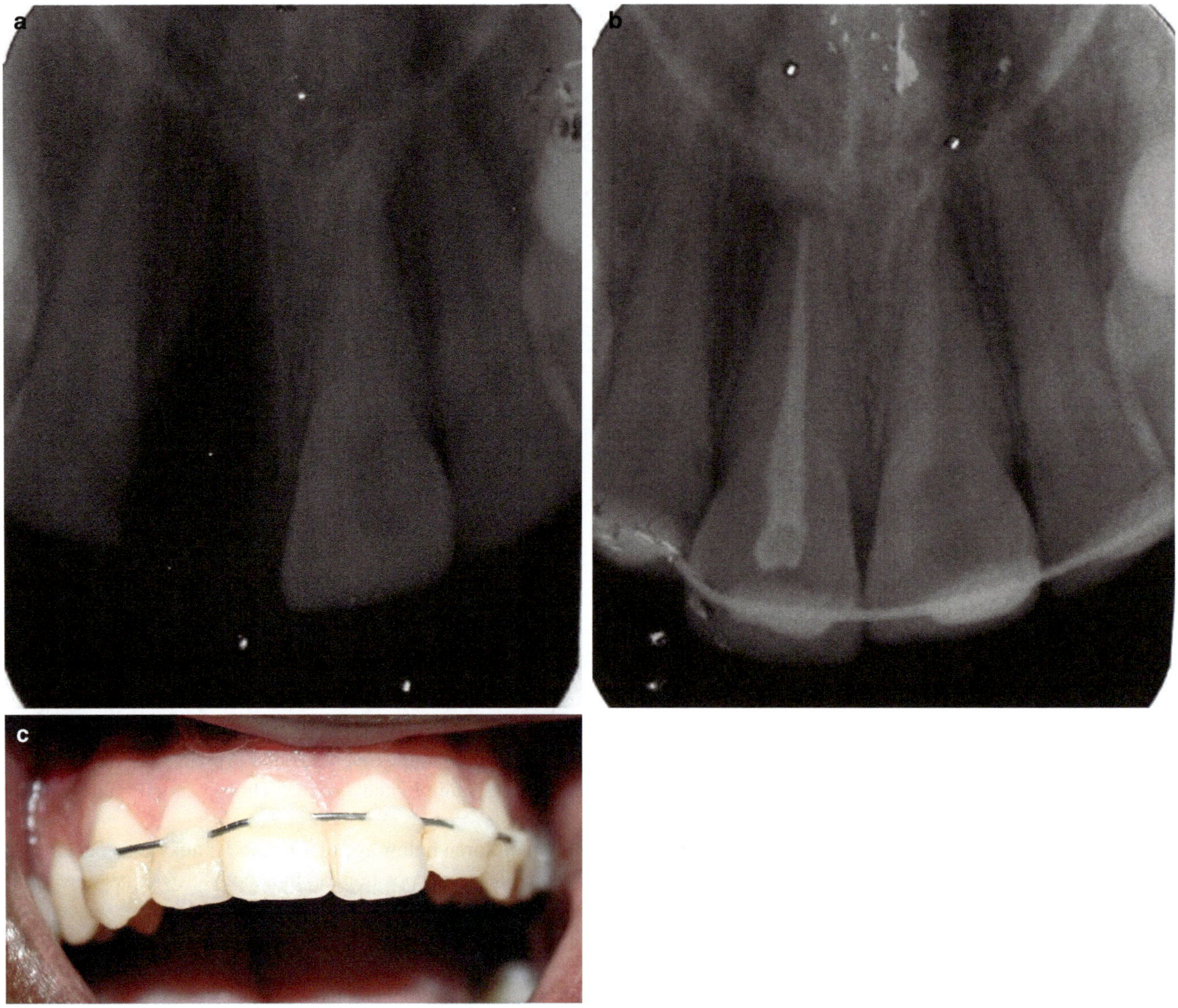

Fig. 50.7 (**a**–**c**) Shows a case of avulsed upper right central incisor in a 24-year-old man, which presented after few hours of avulsion. The tooth was transported in milk by the relatives. A RCT was carried out and the tooth reimplanted and stabilized with wire and composite splint (**a**, IOPA showing avulsed incisor; **b**, IOPA with tooth reimplanted; **c**, shows the clinical image after splinting)

orthodontic band and brackets attached by acid etch technique, combined with orthodontic band and acrylic appliance, or periodontal pack.

They are generally maintained for 7–10 days after replantation to allow gingival reattachment.

Studies by Andreason [20] (1985) have shown that prolonged splinting may be inadvisable because it enhances ankylosis.

The socket should be left undisturbed before replantation. If the alveolar bone has collapsed, a blunt instrument should be inserted carefully into the socket in an attempt to reposition the wall. It should be lightly aspirated if a blood clot is present.

In general, stabilization for reimplanted teeth is required for 7–14 days. The periodontal ligament fibers should have healed sufficiently after the first week to remove the splint. However, the patient should be advised not to bite directly on the reimplanted tooth for 3–4 weeks after injury.

50.7.3 Technique

50.7.3.1 Wire Acid Etch Composite Splint

A wire of moderate stiffness (round 0.030 in. stainless steel) is adapted to the facial surface at least one or more stable teeth on either side of the reimplanted teeth.

The physiologic movement imparted to the reimplanted tooth during function is increased when fewer teeth are included in stabilization of the avulsed tooth.

The facial surface of the avulsed and adjacent teeth is acid etched, and wire is cemented to them with composite.

The wire is generally curved along the middle third of the labial surface of the teeth. 90° terminal bends toward the gingiva are made at the labiodistal angles of the most posterior teeth to be splinted in order to avoid sharp edges and stability. The terminal ends should be about **2 mm** long to reduce the possibility of lateral displacement of the wire [21, 22].

Splinting periods for traumatic dental injuries [6]

Traumatic dental injuries	Splinting period
Subluxation	2 weeks
Extrusive luxation	2 weeks
Avulsion	2 weeks
Lateral luxation	4 weeks
Intrusion(if surgically repositioned)	4–8 weeks
Root fracture(middle third)	4 weeks
Root fracture(cervical third)	4 months

50.7.4 Complications

1. Pulp necrosis
2. Pulp chamber or root canal obliteration
3. Internal resorption
4. External resorption—three types:
   (a) Surface replacement
   (b) Replacement resorption (ankylosis)
   (c) Soft tissue replacement [23]

50.8 Alveolar Process Fracture

Fracture of the alveolar process usually involves the teeth.

↓

Place the segment into position (closed reduction) (Fig. 50.8)

↓

Open reduction/ raise the flap if reduction not possible (Fig. 50.9 a, b)

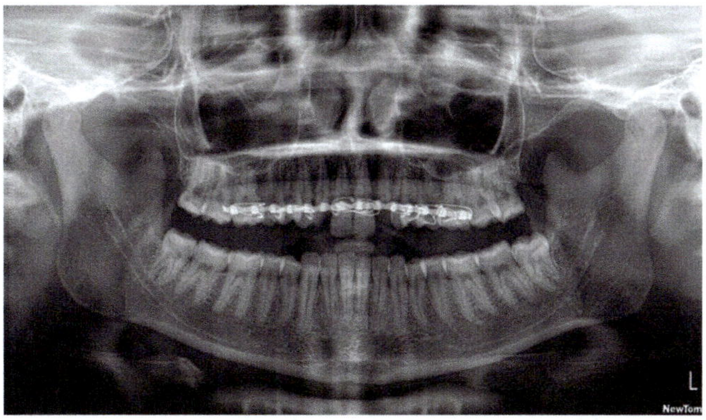

Fig. 50.8 Shows the case in Fig. 50.2, which has undergone closed reduction and fixation by arch bar. Full intrusion and reduction was not achieved. The occlusal discrepancy was planned to be corrected later by RCT and necessary prosthetic work

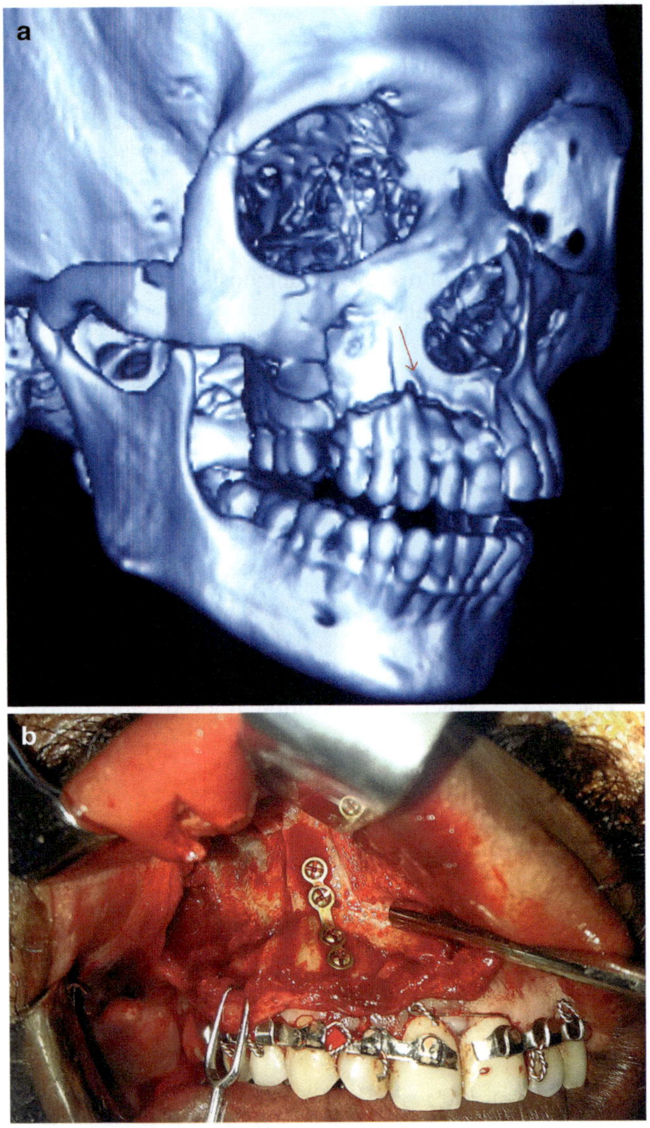

Fig. 50.9 (**a**, **b**) Shows a case of high alveolar process fracture segment in the maxillary right side with associated split between central incisors. Under GA, the extruded displaced alveolar segment was repositioned after placement of split arch bars and bridle wiring between the central incisors. The segment was fixed with mini plate and screws, taking care not to injure the tooth roots. Due to root anatomy, only a single plate was fixed after reduction. Post-operative IMF was given for 2 weeks, for additional stability and to help the healing process

50.9 Management of Dentoalveolar Fracture

The goals of treatment should be:

(a) Anatomic reduction
(b) Re establishment of premorbid occlusion
(c) Early return of function
(d) Preservation of premorbid arch form and facial contour [24]

50.9.1 Treatment Options

1. Arch bars (Fig. 50.8)
2. Loop wiring
3. Orthodontic bands
4. Acrylic/metallic splints
5. Acid etch composite

Model surgery on the plaster models is performed to recreate the normal anatomic relationship of the fractured segment and allow fabrication of accurate splint [9].

50.9.2 Specific Treatment Options

Class I fractures that involve a non-displaced, edentulous alveolar segment often do not require treatment other than a soft diet and observation. If there is concern about the stability of the fracture during the healing process, stabilization may be used.

Class II fractures that involve a displaced dentulous segment and need reduction may require a great deal of force to realign the fractured segment. Posterior fragments are always displaced to the lingual area. Large forceps may be helpful to apply a force suitable to reduce the bony fragment. Reduced fragments are held in place by MMF or splints.

Class III fractures of a moderately or severely displaced dentulous segment may be too difficult to reduce adequately. There may be scant room into which the irregular, displaced segment needs to be replaced. It may be necessary to burr or rasp down the displaced segment or the opening in the remaining bone to successfully reduce the fracture. This is usually accomplished by use of a power drill with a suitable size bur or a fine rhinoplasty rasp. The amount of tissue that is removed should be limited so that the sufficient bone to bone contact remains for bony union as the fracture heals. Maintenance of class III fractures in a reduced fashion may be accomplished with arch bars, MMF, and/or variety of splints.

Class IV fractures that extend into one or more non alveolar fracture lines are usually less challenging than class III fractures because (1) the bone segments are larger, (2) the treatment of the associated fractures gives excellent exposure, and (3) usually no barrier exists to reduction. Plates, screws, arch bars, MMF, and/or variety of splints may be used [7].

50.9.3 Wiring Techniques

In MMF, wires are passed interdentally between teeth in both the jaws followed by tightening of these wires together in a cross arch fashion which serves to stabilize the fracture segments.

Over the period of last century, MMF techniques have evolved dramatically, and more recently, many more easier and effective methods have been introduced like MMF screws, eyelet wiring, and Erich arch bars to name a few. Although it is a quick and efficient way of securing MMF, yet, this technique is criticized for extended periods the patient needs to be closed mouth, difficulty in maintaining oral hygiene, lack or deficient nutritional support via oral route and inability to use this treatment modality in medically compromised patients like epileptics or in immediate post-operative period due to increased risk of aspiration.

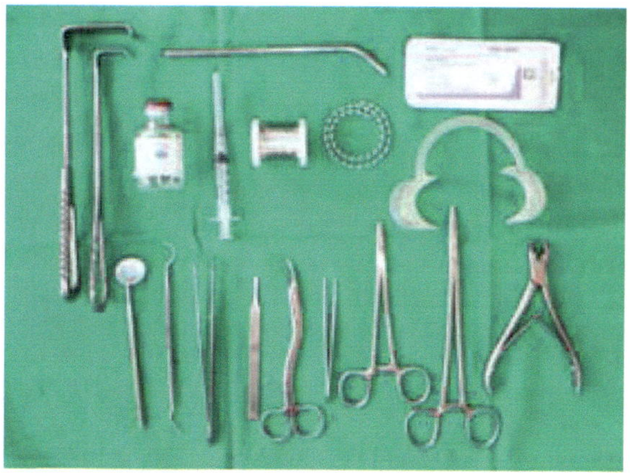

Fig. 50.10 Armamentarium for wiring

50.9.4 Armamentarium and Principles (Fig. 50.10)

A soft stainless steel wire of 0.35–0.5 mm diameter is utilized and pre-stretched to 10% of its original length to prevent loosening of wire once tightened. Overstretching beyond this point should be avoided as this will make the wire brittle and susceptible to breakage.

50.9.5 Principles

Basic principles to be followed are [25]:

1. Continuous tension on the wire while twisting and tightening.
2. Force should be apically directed while tightening.
3. Utilizing a clock wise direction for all tightening/twisting.
4. Only half a turn to be given at a time at the end.
5. Once the tail is cut, it is turned and placed into the inter-proximal embrasures.
6. Once all the wires are in place, move the finger around the arch bar/wire to check for any sharp edge/margin/ wire ending.

50.9.6 Technique

50.9.6.1 Bridle Wire [26, 27]

First advocated by Hippocrates, bridle wire remains one of the oldest yet a conventional method of treating mandibular fractures. This technique represents a temporary way of stabilizing the fractured segments, preventing them from flaying apart.

Advantages include stabilization of the two fractured segments preventing further damage to the adjacent soft tissues, maintenance of the airway patency (especially advantageous for the fractures of the anterior mandible), decrease pain, and reducing damage to the neurovascular bundle from immobilizing the fractured fragments, thereby preventing gross movements and also decreasing muscle cramping.

Technique

Following administration of local anesthesia , a 24–26 gauge wire is passed around the neck of the teeth adjacent to the fracture site on either side (Fig. 50.11a). With both ends being secured in the wire holder (Fig. 50.11b), the fractured segments are manually reduced anatomically, and the wire is tightened in a clockwise fashion till further reduction is achieved (Fig. 50.11c), and the fracture is stabilized

50.9.6.2 Gilmer's Direct Interdental Wiring [26, 27]

This technique represents an easy and fastest method of immobilization.

Technique

A 15 cm pre-stretched wire is passed through the interdental embrasure of the tooth on one side from buccal to lingual. This wire will pass around the tooth and emerge out buccally through the interdental embrasure from the other side. Both ends are held together and twisted to achieve a 3 cm tail (Fig. 50.12a–c). Multiple teeth (at least 5–6) in either jaw are utilized. Following manual fracture reduction and placement of teeth with premorbid occlusion, the tails from opposite arch are twisted together in a cross arch or zigzag fashion to achieve immobilization (Fig. 50.12d). The cut ends of the tail are secured into the interdental spaces. Once all the wires/tails are twisted, complete immobilization is achieved.

The only drawback of this technique is that, in cases of broken /loose wire, all the cross arch wires will have to be removed and redone post placement of twisted wire.

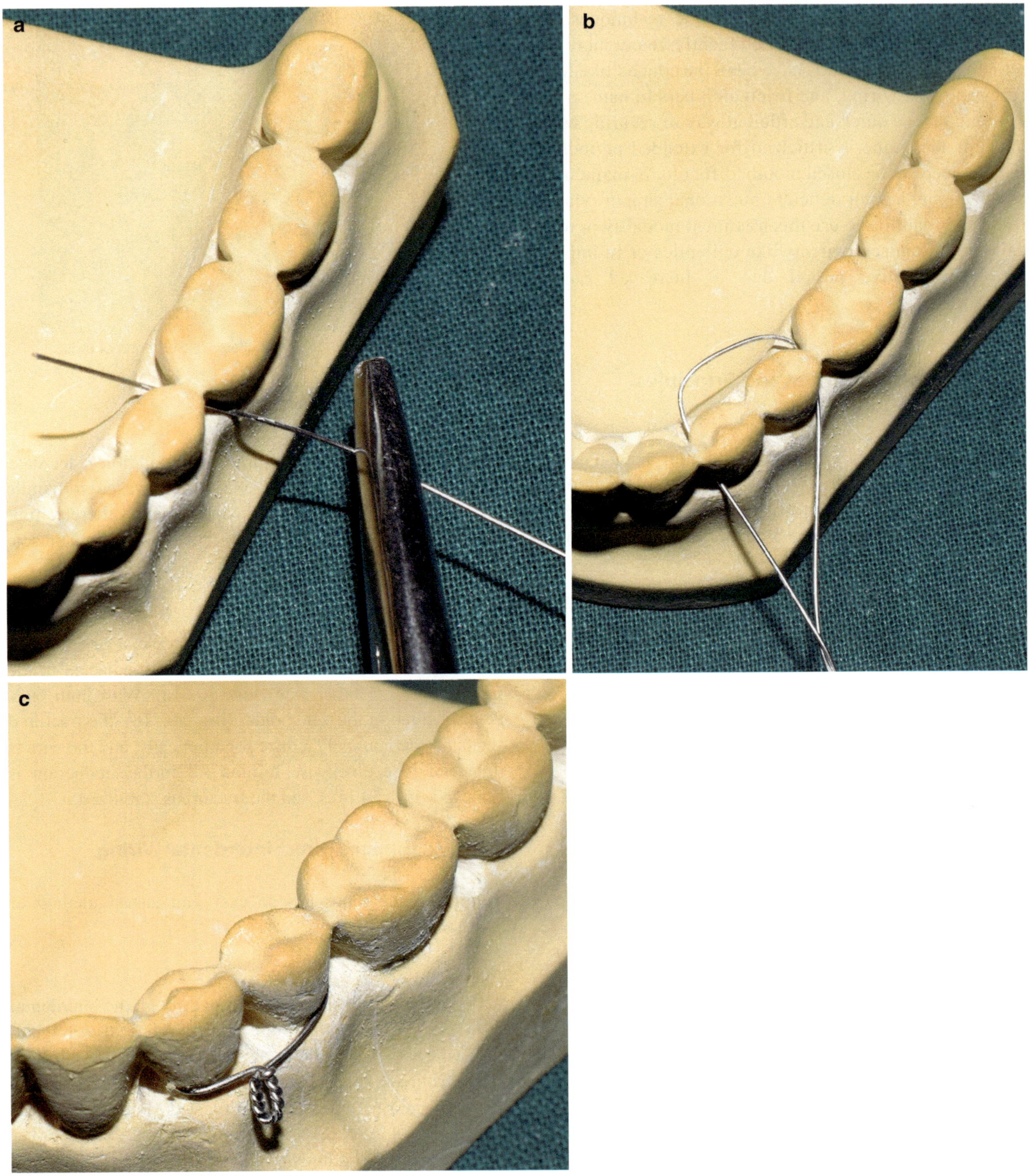

Fig. 50.11 Shows sequential steps bridel wiring. (**a**) Passing of the wire through the tooth embrasure. (**b**) Formation of the wire loop assuming the fracture line is between the two premolars. (**c**) Twisting of both the ends to stabilize the fracture

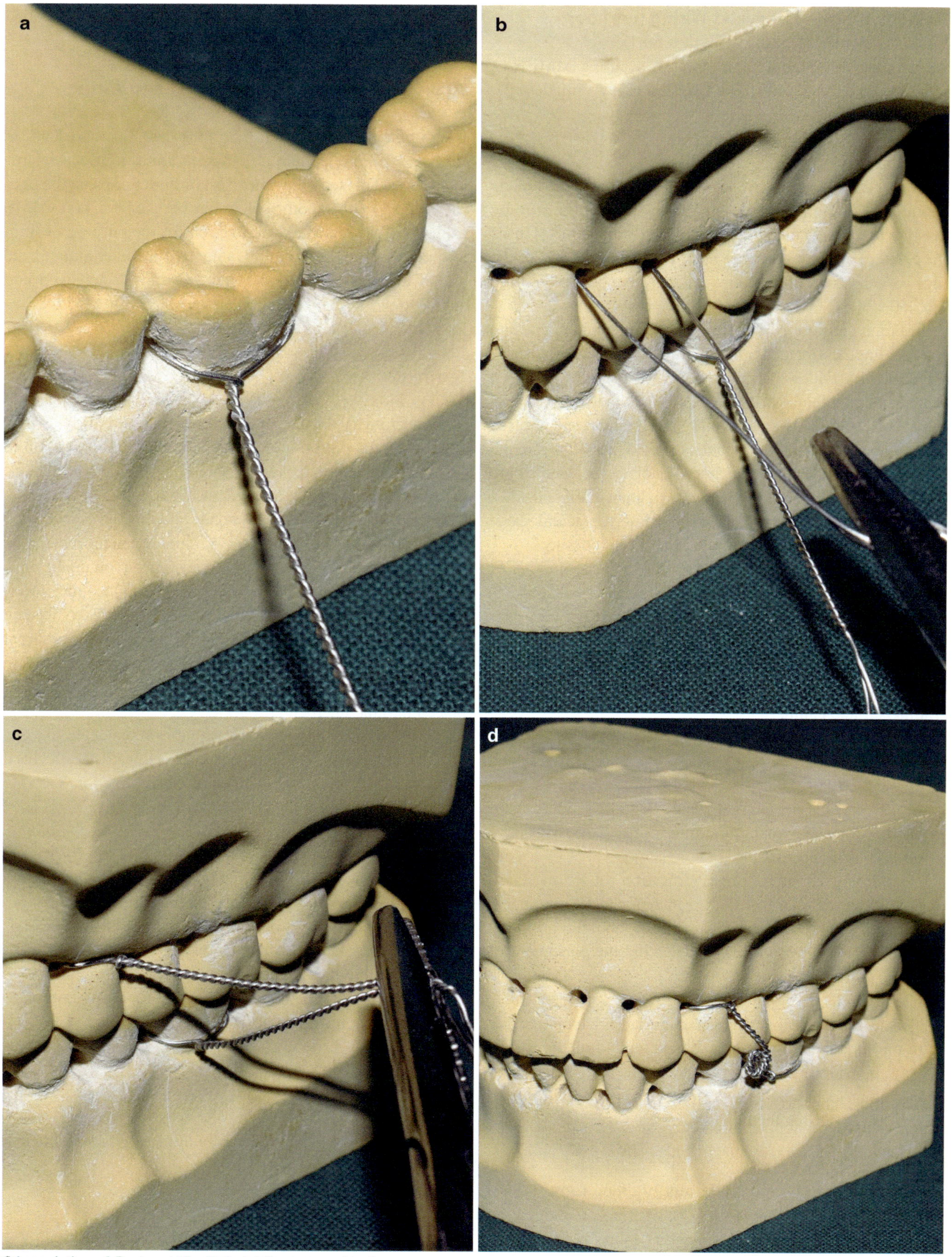

Fig. 50.12 (**a**–**d**) Shows technique of direct Gilmer wiring. Formation of the loop around the tooth in the lower and upper arch followed by twisting both the wires together in order to achieve MMF

50.9.6.3 Interdental Eyelet Wiring (Ivy Loop Method) [26, 27] (Video 50.1)

Yet another easy and quick method of securing MMF was advocated and popularized by Dr. Robert H.Ivy, Philadelphia, USA.

Technique

A pre-stretched 26 gauge/0.35 mm diameter wire was made into an Ivy loop utilizing the middle segment of the wire by twisting it around a metallic rod of 3 mm diameter. 3–4 turns are given to achieve adequate stability to the loop. Both the ends of the wire are then cut in an oblique fashion (Fig. 50.13a).

Both the ends are passed through the interdental space to emerge lingually/palatally so that the loop lies buccally (Fig. 50.13b). Following this, one end of the wire is passed from distal interdental space of the same tooth to emerge buccally. This same wire is passed through the loop and secured to the other end of the wire which is passed mesially from the lingual/palatal side to the buccal side of the adjacent tooth side (Fig. 50.13c,d) . Both the ends are tightened (Fig. 50.13e), and the tail end cut short and secured into the dental space mesially to prevent damage to the adjacent soft tissues.

Stability of the MMF is based on the adequate number of Ivy loops placed in both the arches and secured.

In the maxillary arch, loops can be placed between two molars, two premolars, or between lateral incisor and canine or two central incisors. In the mandibular arch, loops are best placed between two molars, two premolars, or between lateral incisor and canine.

Modifications

1. In 1975, Hallam modified the Ivy loop by addition of another loop proximal to the first for the purpose of ligature/tie wire (Fig. 50.14)

   Although an interesting modification yet the disadvantage observed was that due to increase in length and in patients with short vertical dimension, both the proximal loops would meet one another making the placement of MMF extremely difficult.
2. **Clove hitch**

   This technique helps in placement of an Ivy loop in cases of missing teeth or a single isolated tooth. It is the easiest way to secure MMF where placement of an arch bar or any other technique of securing MMF is difficult due to lack of supporting teeth.

Technique of Clove Hitch

The one end of the wire that has an Ivy loop forms a loop around the lone-standing tooth (Fig. 50.15a) . Continue the wire around the tooth forming another loop for the second time (Fig. 50.15b) . The end of the wire is under the first loop (Fig. 50.15c), and both the ends of the wire are pulled together and tightened (Fig. 50.15d).

50.9.6.4 Continuous or Multiple Loop Wiring [26, 27]

It was first described by Col. Stout in 1943. It represents an easy and simple technique which requires minimal instrumentation. This technique utilizes multiple loops on the buccal surface of the tooth which can be used for both MMF using wire as well as elastic traction for the purpose of fracture reduction. One major advantage of this technique is the use of differential traction force that can be achieved and applied for fracture reduction before securing it with wires for MMF.

Technique

A 30 cm-long pre-stretched wire is placed on the buccal side of the teeth with the anterior end placed as anteriorly as possible while the posterior end extending up to the last tooth to be used. The wire is passed through the interdental space of the posterior most teeth and emerged through its mesial side. The wire is then passed over the buccal wire and passed back into the same interdental space. A 3 mm diameter rod can be used parallel to the buccal wire for adequate loop diameter as well as uniformity of the loop (Fig. 50.16a). Once the wire is passed back through the same interdental space, it then emerges out from the mesial interdental space of adjacent tooth (Fig. 50.16b). This continues till the anterior most teeth where both the ends of the wire are twisted together, cut, and placed into the interdental space (Fig. 50.16c,d). Each loop is then twisted, and loops are made of uniform diameter. In cases of securing MMF, the loops are turned toward the occlusal surfaces of the teeth, but in cases of elastic traction, they are turned in the opposite direction toward the gingiva [27].

Modification

This technique needs modification when some teeth are missing. Herein, once the loop at the mesial end of the tooth adjacent to the missing tooth is formed, both of the free ends of the wires are held together and twisted till the distal end of the next tooth. Once the desired length is achieved, the loop is again formed at the distal end, and the looping continues till the anterior most teeth.

50.9.6.5 Risdon's Wiring [26, 27]

Indications

It is an alternative to an arch bar for a fractured mandible that needs fixation.

Technique

A 25 cm-long wire is passed through the posterior most tooth in the quadrant to emerge bucally, followed by twist-

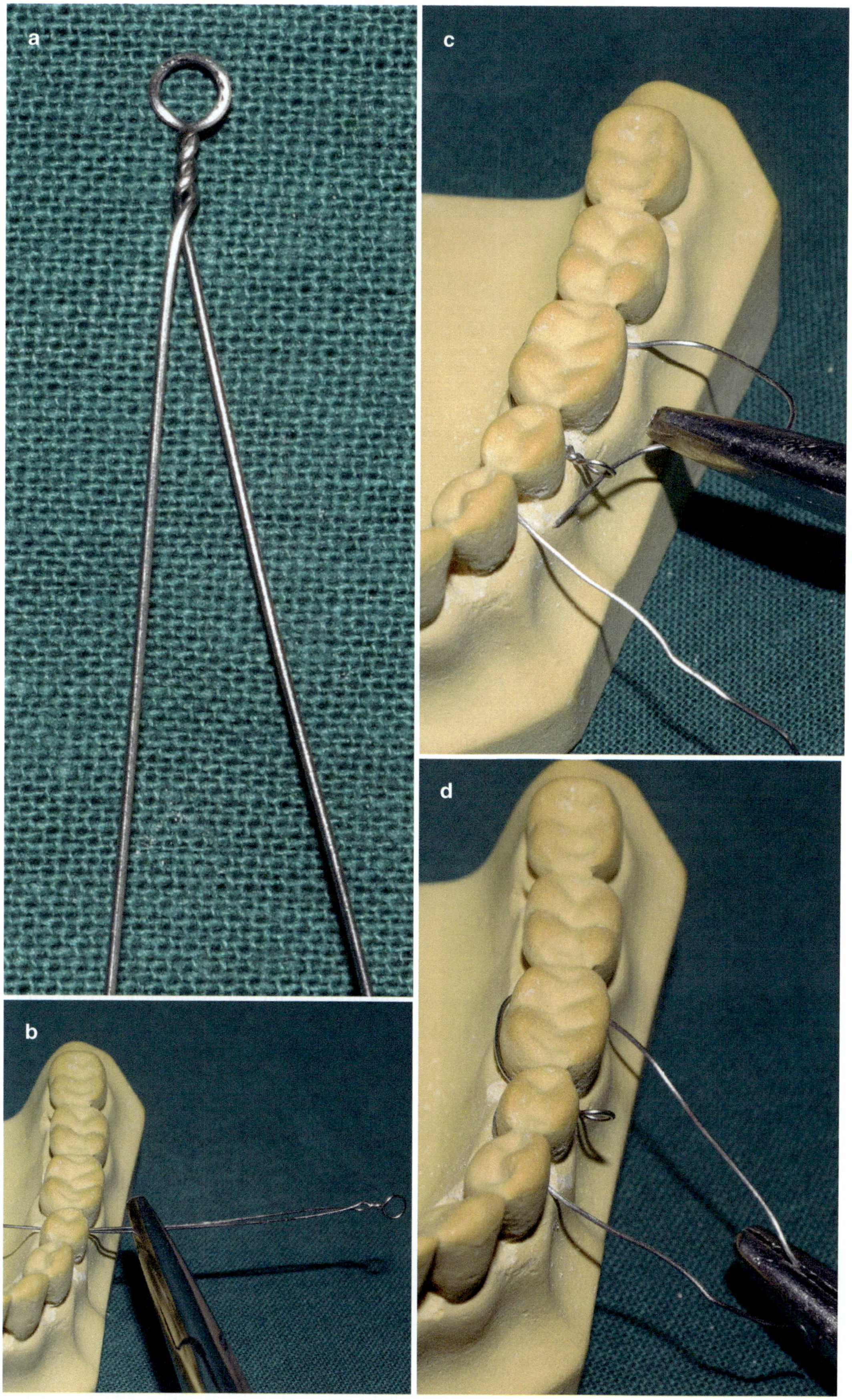

Fig. 50.13 Shows steps in Ivy loop technique. (**a**) Photograph of an Ivy loop. (**b**) Both the ends are held together an passed through the tooth embrasure of the premolar and molar. (**c**) One end passed is passed through the mesial of premolar and other through the distal of molar to emerge buccally. (**d**) Distal end is passed through the loop on the buccal side to emerge mesially. (**e**) Both the ends of the wire are held together and twisted

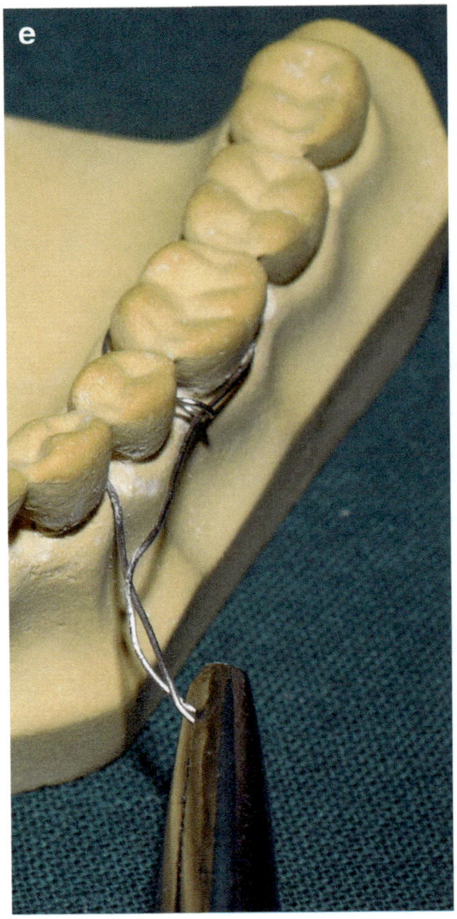

©Association of Oral and Maxillofacial Surgeons of India

Fig. 50.13 (continued)

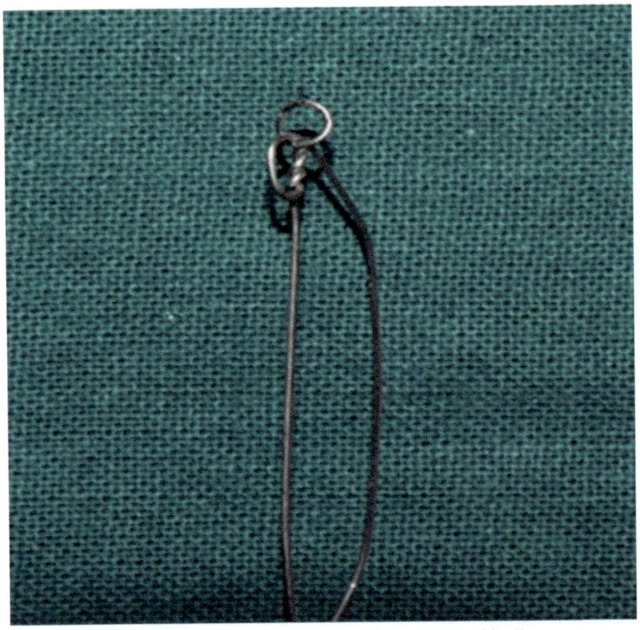

©Association of Oral and Maxillofacial Surgeons of India

Fig. 50.14 Shows a modification of Ivy loop

ing the wire up to its full length till the midline (Fig. 50.17a). Another wire is passed from the opposite quadrant of the same arch and twisted in a similar manner. Both the ends of this twisted wire are tightened at the midline after reducing the fracture segments (Fig. 50.17b,c). Once anatomic reduction is achieved, additional wires are used to stabilize this long wires by passing around the embrasures of the teeth and looping around the wire segment (Fig. 50.17d) [26, 27].

50.9.6.6 Obwegeser Wiring [26, 27]

Technique

This technique utilizes a 30 cm-long wire that is bent into a continuous "W" arcade form as depicted in Fig. 50.18a. The elevated portion of the arcade acts to form the loop, whereas the depressed portion adapts to the contour of the teeth palatally or lingually. The distal end of the wire arcade is kept long enough so that it will follow the buccal contour of the arch, when it is passed through the interdental space of the most posterior tooth from lingual/palatal to buccal side. The elevated ends of the

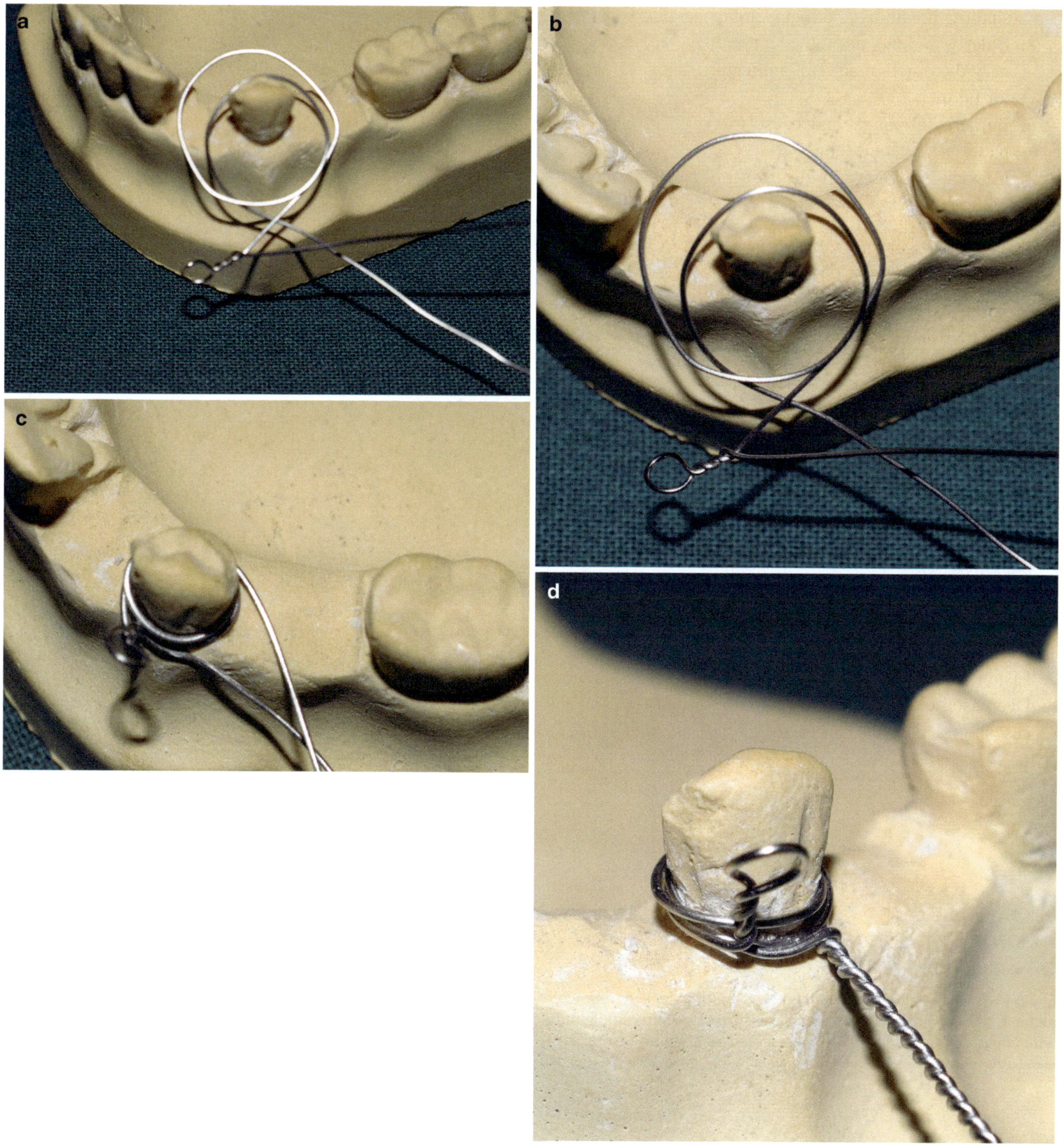

Fig. 50.15 Showing clove hitch technique. (**a–c**) Single loop is passed around the lone-standing tooth followed by second loop under the first one, pulling both the ends together. (**d**) Showing clove hitch wiring technique

arcade have a ligature wire attached to it (Fig. 50.18b), which only suffices the arcade to be pulled through to the interdental space to emerge buccally (Fig. 50.18c,d). The long wire is then passed through this loop (Fig. 50.18e), and a modified hemostat is used to twist this wire to form uniform loops. At the mesial end, both the ends of the wire are held together and twisted (Fig. 50.18f). The loops can be used for both elastic traction and wires for securing MMF.

The disadvantage of this technique is that it is very cumbersome and adequate expertise is needed to carry out this technique.

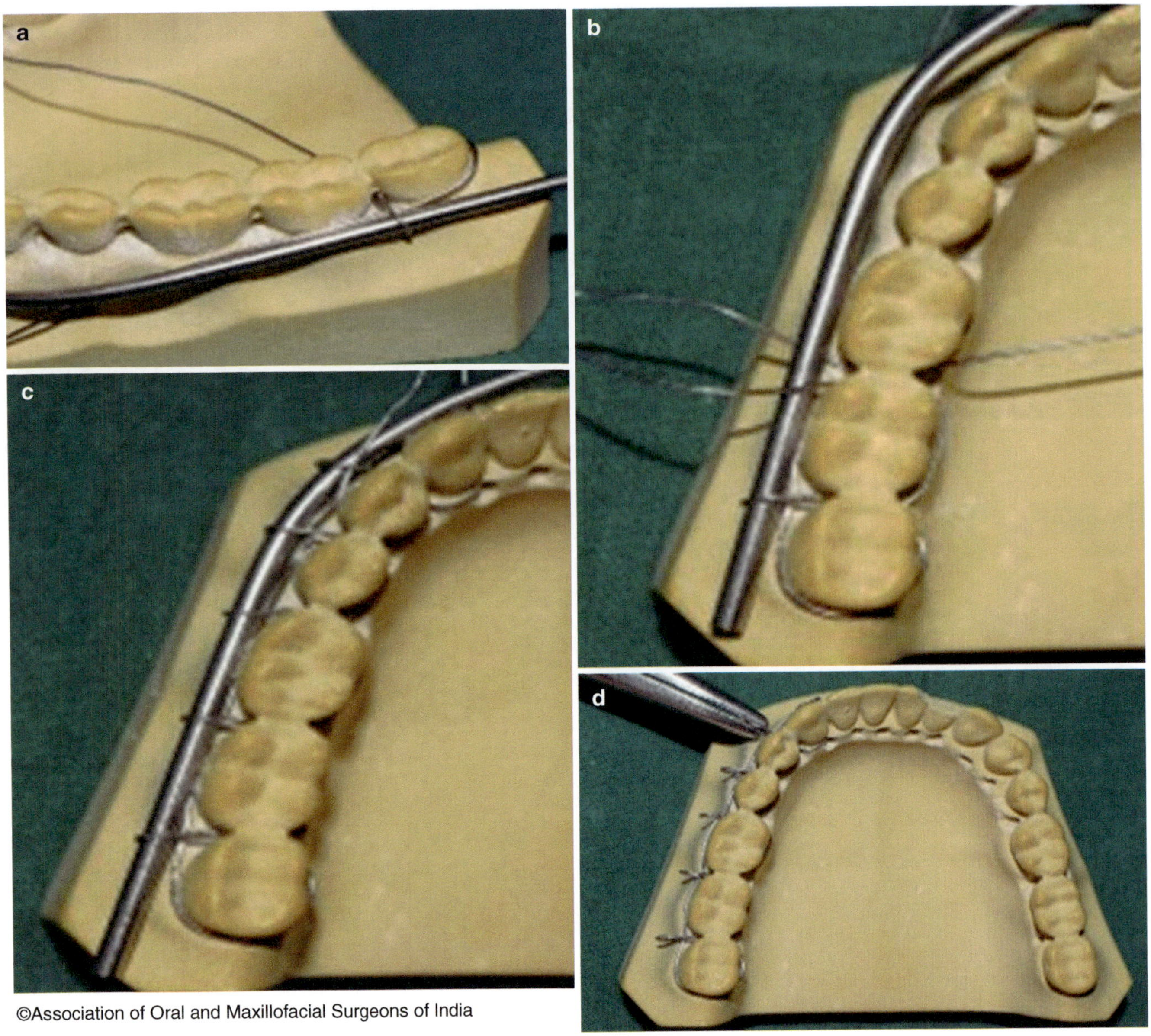

Fig. 50.16 (**a**, **b**) Showing continuous or multiple loop wiring technique, a rod is held parallel to the buccal surface of the teeth, and the wire is passed through the distal most tooth embrasure to emerge buccally and looping around the rod. (**c**, **d**) Continuous loops till the midline are made followed by pulling the buccal rod out to achieve loops

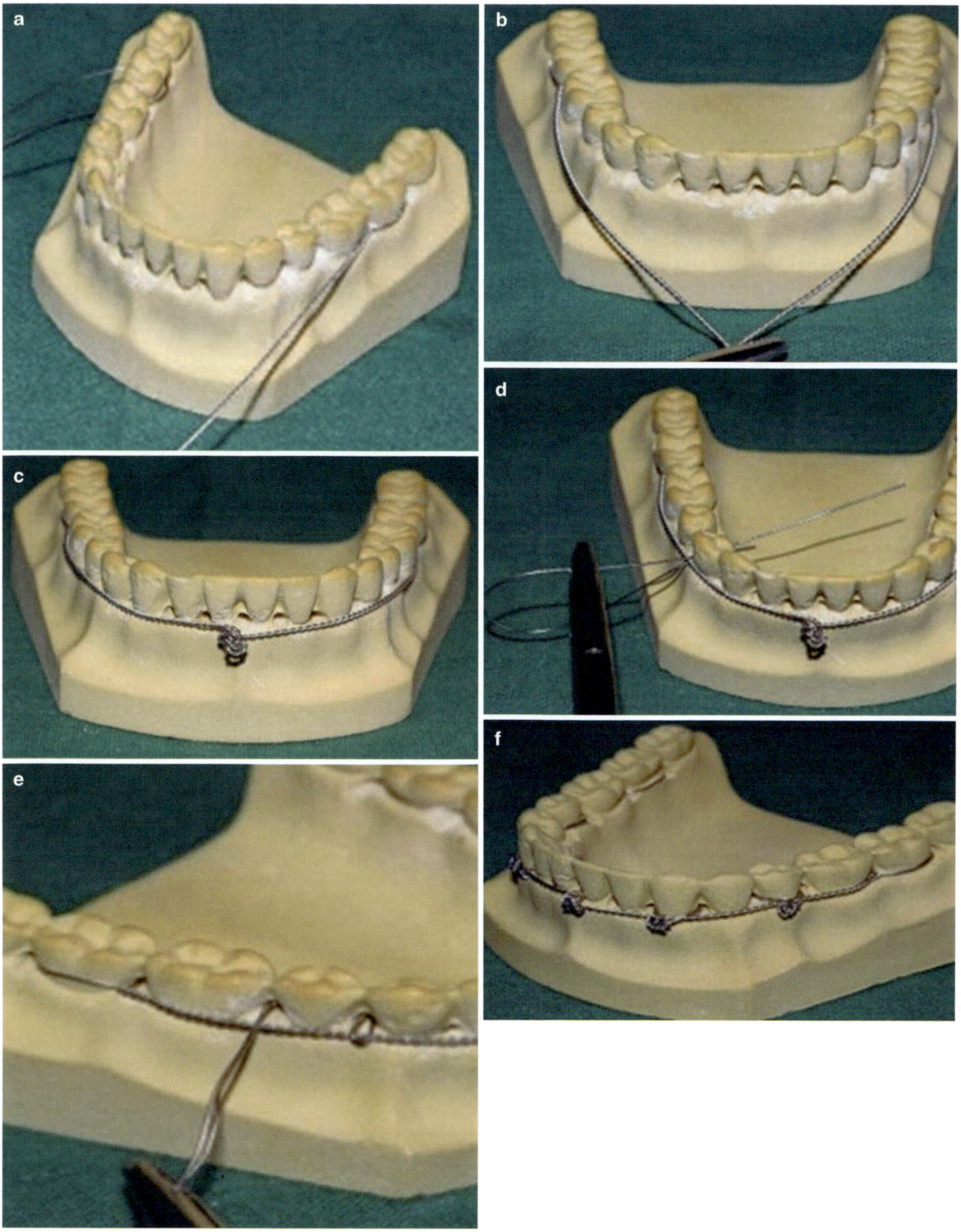

Fig. 50.17 (**a**, **b**) Showing steps in fabrication of Risdon wiring. Distal most tooth is used to loop the wire and twist it. (17c) Showing twisted wire in the midline. (**d**, **e**) Showing wires passed through teeth embrasure to loop around the main wire. (**f**) Alternate method of securing the long wire

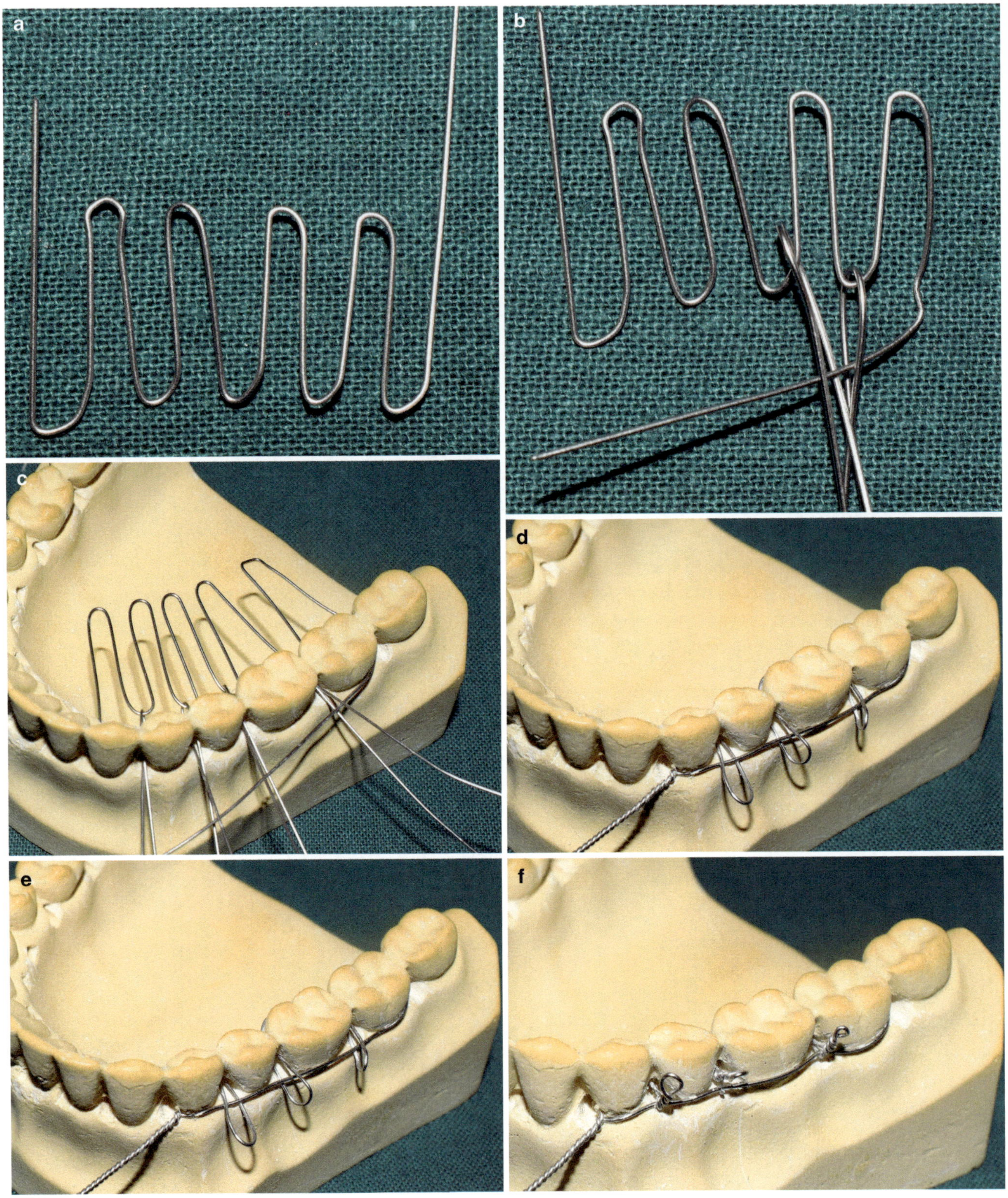

Fig. 50.18 (**a**, **b**) Showing fabricated W arcade used in Obwegeser technique. (**c**) Showing ligature wire pulled from the palatal/lingual side to buccal side. (**d**–**f**) Showing wire from the distal most end passing though the loops to be twisted at the most medial end of the arcade

50.9.6.7 Arch Bar [26, 27] (Video 50.2)

Commercially available arch bars are usually customized or prefabricated. In most clinical scenarios, prefabricated arch bars like Erich's, Jelenko, Winter's, or Schuchardt's suffice the need for placement.

Indications

1. Partially edentulous patients where placement of eyelets is not an option due to insufficient number of teeth.
2. The teeth present are far apart making MMF impossible.
3. For alignment of avulsed teeth/displaced dentoalveolar fracture into proper arch form.
4. Reduction and immobilization of dentoalveolar component/ fracture.
5. As a part of integrated treatment for suspension for treatment of maxillofacial fractures.

Technique

Ideal placement is as close to the interdental spaces, which are then secured with 26 gauge wire. This close placement helps to reduce the arch bar to tooth contact and allows for better adaptability of the arch bar to the arch contour, thereby reducing loosening of arch bar.

In most cases, arch bars are placed from distal of first molar, in one quadrant to the other, maintaining a minimum of two teeth on either side of the fracture line in a dentate patient.

The wire is passed from one interdental space and moved around the tooth to emerge buccally from the other side (Fig. 50.19a). Placement of arch bar by securing it with wire begins (Fig. 50.19b) usually at the midline and proceeds posteriorly or from one end (molar) to another (Fig. 50.19c,d) in order to avoid excess in the center and to achieve uniformity throughout the length of the arch bar. The wires are usually twisted in between the cleats and placed into the interdental space to avoid damage to surrounding soft tissues.

The cleats of the arch bar always face gingivally. MMF is usually secured using 24 gauze wires in box pattern.

Figure 50.19e is showing a model with upper and lower arch bar placement secured with wires, while Fig. 50.19f is showing a clinical photograph of arch bar placement.

Advantages

- Easier to manipulate and maintain the intra-arch form.
- Acts as a tension band, resisting forces acting at the alveolar level of the fractured component.
- Multiple vectors can be provided by using elastics and VW cross bracing in reducing the fracture displacement to achieve premorbid occlusion.

Disadvantages

- One of the major drawbacks is the lack of vertical stop in the anterior region when an arch bar is used. In the posterior region, the opposing teeth act as a vertical stop for occluding teeth which isn't the case with anterior region as the anterior upper teeth may slide over the lower when elastics are stretched between the maxillary and mandibular teeth resulting in extrusion of anterior teeth. This problem can be circumvented, by drilling a hole using a bur in the gingival area apical to the mucogingival junction through the buccal and lingual cortices.

An additional 24 gauze wire is passed from the buccal side of this hole to emerge lingually. The lingual end of the wire is then passed through the interdental space of the tooth to emerge buccally. Both the ends of the wire are then twisted to prevent extrusion.

In the anterior maxilla, anterior nasal spine can be used for additional suspension of the arch bar to prevent downward pull exerted by the elastics.

- Increased operating time.
- High probability of penetrating injuries to the operator.
- Compromised oral hygiene and periodontal tissue damage.
- Post-treatment removal is a traumatic experience.

Complications

Post reduction of the dentoalveolar fracture, the incisal edges of the fractured teeth bearing segment will remain above the normal occlusal plane. This discrepancy can be corrected by application of apical pressure to this segment through MMF, circummandibular wiring, suspension from ANS, lateral piriform, buttress, or using the eye of the maxillomandibular fixation screw.

50.10 Maxillomandibular Fixation (MMF) Screws [28] (Video 50.3)

50.10.1 Introduction

A self-drilling or tapping maxillomandibular fixation screws by Arthur et al. [29] in 1989 reduced the intra and postoperative problem associated with the arch bars.

50.10.2 First Generation

Screws were modified monocortical self-tapping screws that were kept at 4–5 mm above the mucosa for subsequent wire

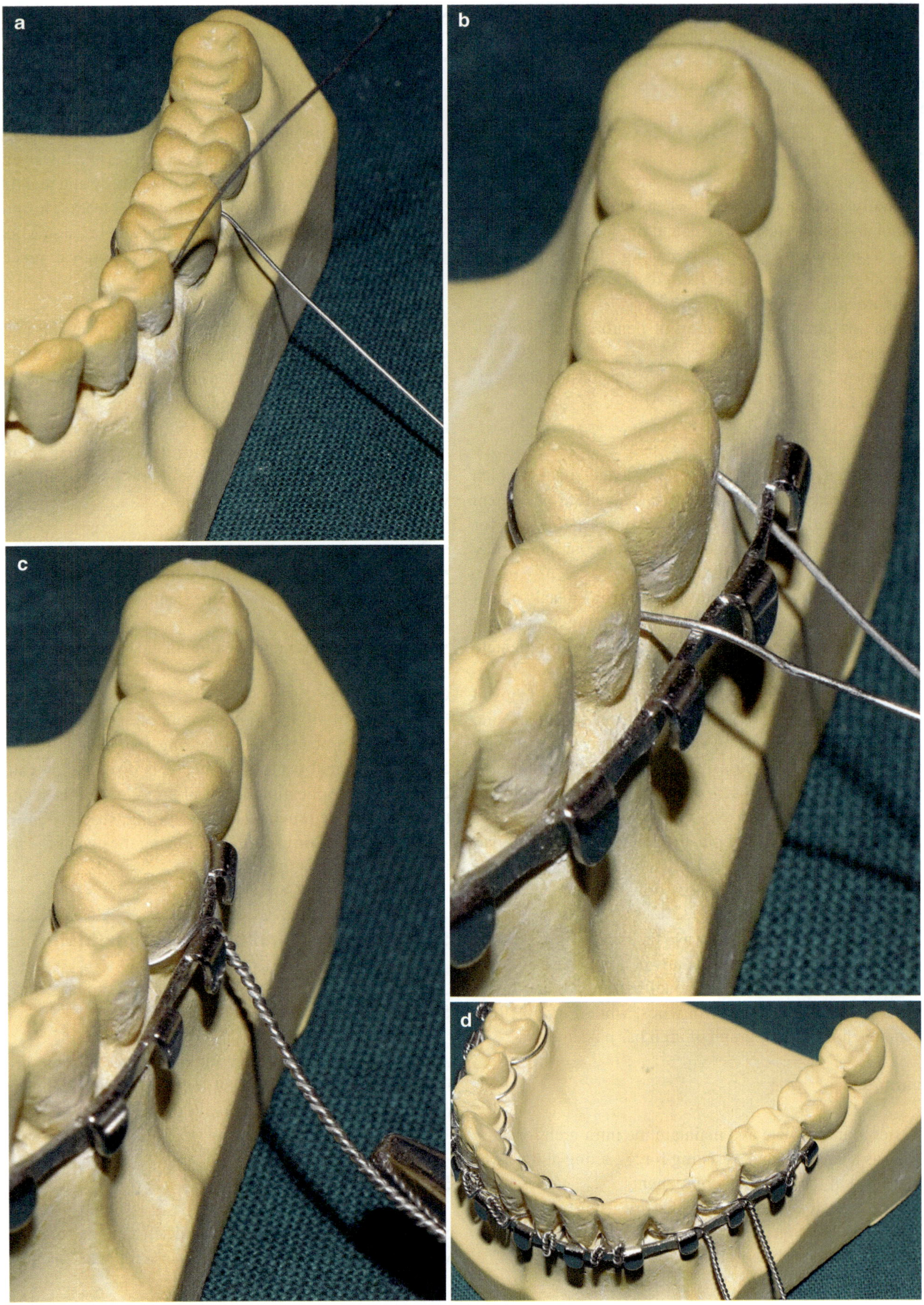

Fig. 50.19 (**a–d**) Showing technique of arch bar placement. The wire is passed through the embrasure or emerge buccally. The wire on the mesial side of the tooth is passed above the arch bar, where as the distal end wire is passed below the arch bar to secure it by twisting. (**e**) Showing a model with upper and lower arch bar placement secured with wires. (**f**) representing a clinical photograph of arch bar placement

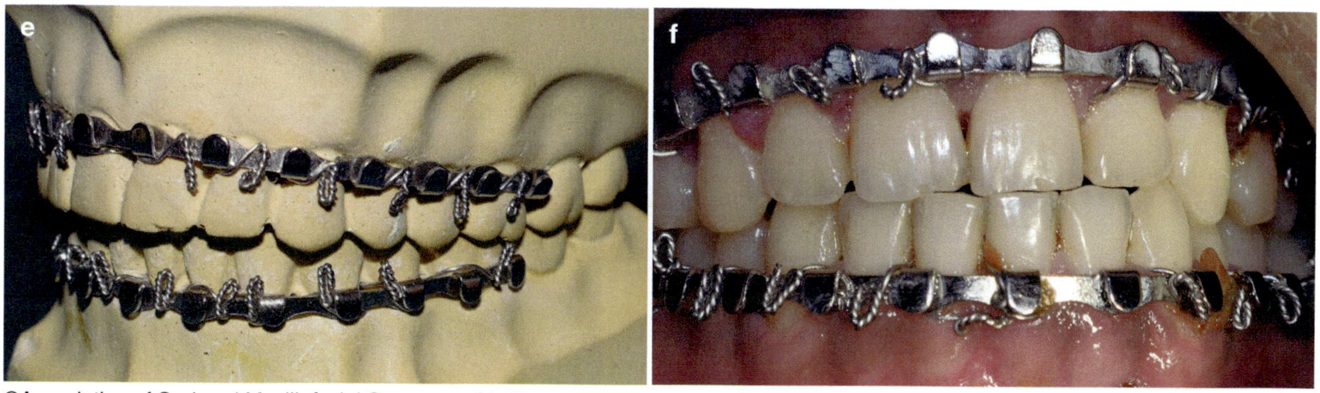

Fig. 50.19 (continued)

splinting. Surgical preparation of the site needed prior to insertion. They were usually wider in diameter with grooves/flutes.

50.10.3 Second Generation

Screws were self-drilling or self-tapping screws which were spool shaped. The central part of the screw head is perforated with one of two channels perpendicular to its axis aiding in the passage of ligature wires. The top of the screw heads is smoothly finished at the contact zone with overlying mucosa.

Clinician should consider fracture location, dentition, surgical exposure, and the quantity of bone for placement of these IMF screws.

Ideal radiographic images obtained are orthopantomogram and CT axial scan to analyze and plan placement of these screws.

Sites include anterior vestibule and anterolateral (canine and premolar regions) as they provide sufficient bone depth, clearance from adjacent tooth, and easy accessibility. Screws should be placed above the root apices as subapical placement leads to mucosal overgrowth (Fig. 50.20a–d).

Ideally one screw should be placed on either side of the fracture line. However, in severely displaced cases, it is advisable to use multiple screws on either side to achieve vectors in different directions.

50.10.4 Advantages

1. Cost-effective
2. Easy placement
3. Lesser operating time
4. Less incidences of penetrating injuries
5. Lesser appliances inside the oral cavity
6. Minimum damage to periodontium
7. Easy maintenance of oral hygiene

50.10.5 Disadvantages

1. Iatrogenic damage to tooth roots
2. Root fracture
3. Ingested hardware
4. Screw loosening resulting in malocclusion [30]
5. Pulpal necrosis
6. Root resorption
7. Tooth loss
8. Soft tissue growth over the screw head [31]

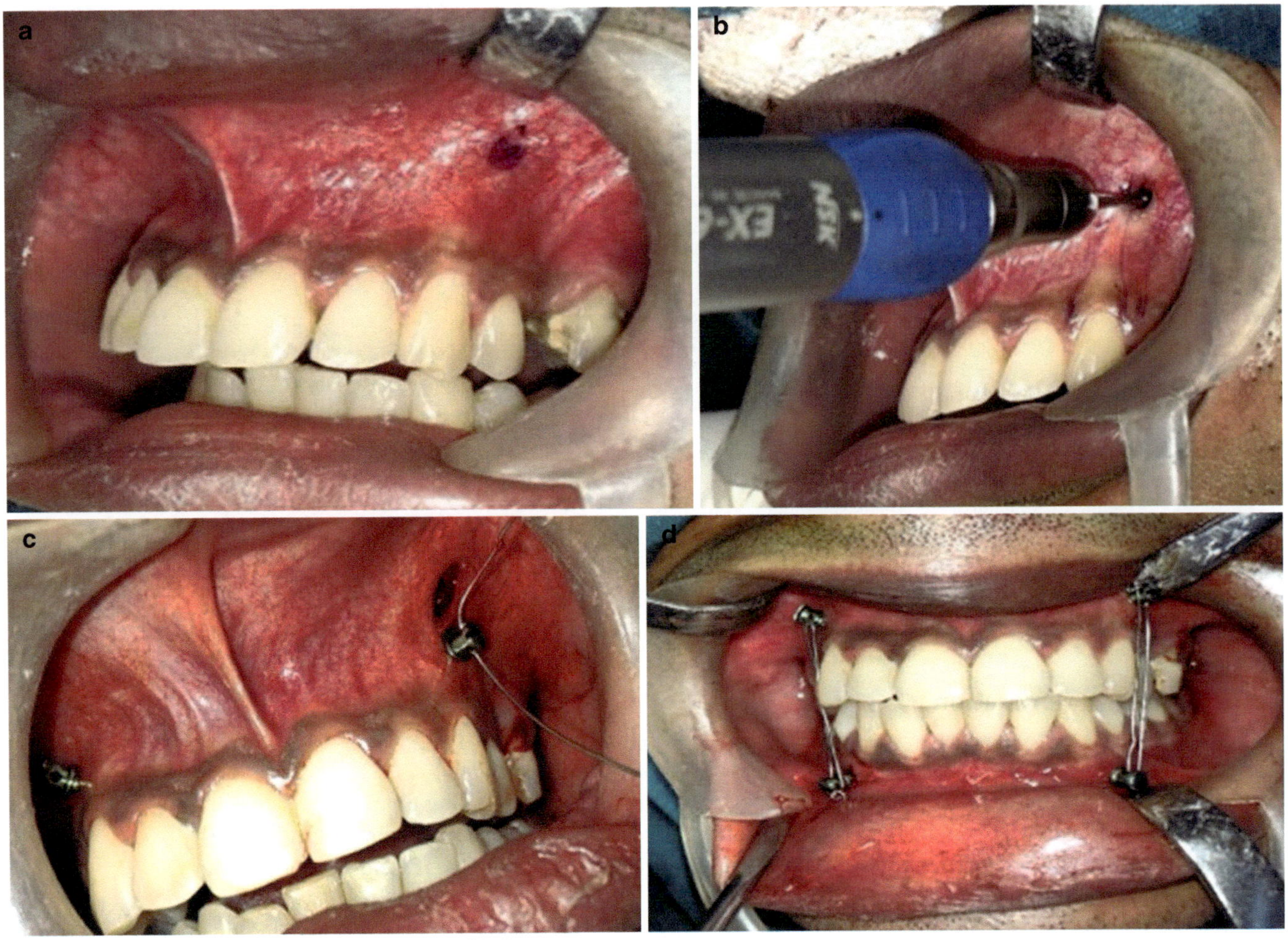

Fig. 50.20 (**a–d**) Showing clinical steps in placement of MMF screw. Technique for placement of MMF screws. Marking is done between the root apices followed by drilling and placement of MMF screw, one in each quadrant. The wire is passed through the eye of the opposing arch and secured to achieve intermaxillary fixation

50.11 Conclusion

Dentoalveolar fracture mostly involves teeth, soft tissues, and associated bones. With the recent advancements in the field of dentistry, the oral and maxillofacial surgeon can restore the lost form and function of teeth to facilitate the improvement in quality of life in trauma-afflicted patients.

Acknowledgments For Figs. 50.1, 50.2, 50.3, 50.4, 50.6, 50.7, 50.8 and 50.9 to Suvy Manuel.

References

1. Nyardady Z, Orsi E, Nagy K, Olasz L, Nyarady J. Transgingival lag screw osteosynthesis of alveolar process fracture. Int J Oral Maxillofac Surg. 2010;39:779–82.
2. Hale ML. Traumatic injuries of the teeth and alveolar process. In: Kruger textbook of oral and maxillofacial surgery. 6th edn. Jaypee; 1968. p. 357–63.
3. Leathers RD, Gowans RE. Management of alveolar and dental fractures. In: Peterson's principles of oral and maxillofacial surgery. Vol 1, 3rd edn. New York: McGraw Hill; 2004. p. 383–405.
4. Ellis E III, Assael LA. Soft tissue and dentoalveolar injuries. In Contemporary oral and maxillofacial surgery. 2nd edn. Elsevier p. 557–86.

5. Sivakumar, Muthu MS. Traumatic injuries of teeth and supporting structures. In Pediatric dentistry principles and practice. 2nd edn. Elsevier. p. 305–26.
6. Pogrel MA, Kahnberg K-E, Andersson L. Traumatic dental injuries. In: Essentials of oral and maxillofacial surgery. 1st edn. Wiley Blackwell; 2014. p. 257–87.
7. Taub PJ, Patel PK, Buchman SR, Cohen MN. Ferraro's fundamentals of maxillofacial surgery. 2nd edn. Springer; 2015. p. 169–73.
8. Margarone JE, Hall R. Management of alveolar and dental fractures. In: Principles of oral and maxillofacial surgery. Vol 1. Philadelphia, PA: J.B. Lippincott; 1992. p. 381–405.
9. Gutmacher Z, Peled E, Norman D, Lin S. Alveolar bone fracture: pathognomonic sign for clinical diagnosis. Open Dent J. 2017;11:8–14.
10. Costello BJ, Martin B. Dentoalveolar trauma. In: Operative oral and maxillofacial surgery. 2nd edn. 2010; p. 475–8.
11. Pagadala S, Tadikonda DC. An overview of classification of dental trauma. IAIM. 2015;2(9):157–64.
12. Faus-Matoses V, Martinez-Vinarta M, Alegre-Domingo T, Faus-Matoses I, Faus-Liacer VJ. Treatment of multiple traumatized anterior teeth associated with an alveolar bone fracture in a 20 year old patient: a 3 year follow up. J Clin Exp Dent. 2014;6(4):e425–9.
13. Diangelis AJ, Andreasen JO, Ebelesder KA, Kenny DJ, Trope M, et al. Guidelines for the management of traumatic dental injuries: fractures and luxations of permanent teeth. Dent Traumatol. 2012;28:2–12.
14. Shulman LE. Transplantation and replantation of teeth. In: Oral and maxillofacial surgery. Vol. 2. St Louis, MO: C V Mosby; 1985. p. 118–42.
15. Turkistani J, Hanno A. Recent trends in the management of dentoalveolar traumatic injuries to primary and young permanent teeth. Dent Traumatol. 2011;27:46–54.
16. Camp JH. Replantation of teeth following trauma. In: McDonalds RE et al., editors. Current therapy in dentistry. Vol 7. St Louis, MO: Mosby; 1980.
17. Blomlof L, et al. Effect of storage in media with different ion strength and osmolaties in human periodontal ligament cells. Scand J Dent Res. 1981;89:180–7.
18. Bag I, Yildirim S. Effect of avulsion storage media on periodontal ligament fibroblast differentiation. Dent Traumatol. 2017;33(6):458–64.
19. William Cornell R. Management of the avulsed tooth. In: Clinical transplantation in dental specialities. 2nd edn. St Louis, MO: C V Mosby; 1980. p. 89–106.
20. Andreasen JO. Periodontal healing after replantation of avulsed human teeth. Assessment by mobility testing and radiography. Acta Odontol Scand 1975;35:325–35.
21. Abu Samra FM. Dentoalveolar injuries classification—management—biological consequences. J Dent Health Oral Disord Ther. 2014;1(4):00025.
22. De Rossi M, De Rossi A, De Queiroz AM, Nelson-Filho P. Management of a complex dentoalveolar trauma: a case report. Braz Dent J. 2009;20(3):259–62.
23. Yamashita D, Cho N. Techniques for maxillomandibular fixation. In: Atlas of oral and maxillofacial surgery. Vol 1. 2nd edn. Elsevier; 2016. p. 638–44.
24. McDonald RE, Avery DR, Dean JA, Jones JE. Management of trauma to the teeth and supporting tissues. In: McDonald and Avery's dentistry for the child and adolescent. 9th edn. 2010. p. 403–42.
25. Coletti DP. Contemporary maxillofacial fixation technique. In: Operative oral and maxillofacial surgery. 2nd edn. Medical; 2010. p. 453–61.
26. Williams JL, Rowe NL. Mandibular fractures: closed reduction. In: Rowe and Williams maxillofacial injuries. Vol. 2. 2nd edn. Churchill Livington; 1995. p. 234–66.
27. Marunick MT. Closed reduction and Immobilization of condylar fractures with intermaxillary fixation alternative techniques of Ivy Loops and Molar wafers. In: Atlas of craniofacial trauma. Lippincott Williams and Wilkins; 2012. p. 36–43.
28. Manjrekar S, Joshi A. Use of mandibulo-maxillary fixation screws for the treatment of maxillofacial fractures. Dentistry. 2017;7(12):467.
29. Arthur G, Berardo N. A simplified technique of maxillomandibular fixation. J Oral Maxillofac Surg. 1989;47(11):1234.
30. Rai A et al. Are maxillomandibular fixation screws a better option than Erich arch bars in achieving maxillomandibular fixation? A randomized clinical study. J Oral Maxillofac Surg 2011;69:3015–3018.
31. Rai A et al.Customised screw for intermaxillary fixation of maxillofacial injuries. Br J Oral Maxillofac Surg. 2009;47: 325–26.

Principles of Internal Fixation in Maxillofacial Surgery

51

Abhilasha Yadav

51.1 Introduction

Road traffic accidents (RTA) are one of the primary etiologies of craniomaxillofacial fractures. Open reduction and internal fixation (ORIF) is the most important treatment modality to restore the compromised form and function. Adequate reduction and fixation with miniplate osteosynthesis is the essential component of management.

51.1.1 Association of Osteosynthesis (AO Principles)

The following are guidelines for internal fixation based on the four basic principles formulated by AO in 1958.

(A) **Anatomic reduction:** Fracture reduction and fixation to restore normal anatomy
(B) **Stable fixation:** Fracture fixation with relative or absolute stability, as required by the patients injury and type of fracture
(C) **Preservation of blood supply:** By gentle reduction and careful handling along with preservation of vascularity of soft tissues and the bone
(D) **Early and active mobilization:** Rehabilitation of the injured part and the patient as a whole with early and safe mobilization

A. Yadav (✉)
Department of Oral & Maxillofacial Surgery, Awadh Dental College & Hospital, Jamshedpur, Jharkhand, India

51.2 History

1. Plating of fractures can be traced back to 1895 when a metal plate was first introduced by Lane for internal fixation. It was abandoned due to its drawback of corrosion [1].
2. Subsequently Lambotte in 1909 and Sheman in 1912 introduced plates for fixation, but due to insufficient strength, their designs were abandoned [1].
3. Eggers in 1948 developed a plate which was structurally weak resulting in instability of fixation [1].
4. In maxillofacial surgery, the interest in rigid fixation began with the treatment of fractures of edentulous mandible, as the fractures located in edentulous mandibular segments were easier to manage.
5. Keys to fast and economic bone healing are optimal reduction of fracture ends and maximum stabilization of fracture area. Simplest way to achieve these goals is to apply the principles of axial compression of fracture ends. This principle was first advocated by Belgian Surgeon Davis in 1994 and later adopted by ASIF (association for the study of internal fixation).

   According to him, there was a need for compression between the fragments of fractures. He used a plate called coaptens to achieve this goal, which increased stability and suppressed interfragmentary motion. The mode of healing initiated by this is called soudure autogene (autogenous welding) now known as primary bone healing.
6. In 1967, mandibular compression screw (MCS) was used in oral and maxillofacial surgery (OMFS) in edentulous fractured mandible while performing first compression osteosynthesis. Self-tightening/automatic MCS plate was developed by Luhr in 1968. Later, dynamic plates were advocated for surgery of long bones with subsequent application in mandibular fractures.

K. Bonanthaya et al. (eds.), *Oral and Maxillofacial Surgery for the Clinician*, https://doi.org/10.1007/978-981-15-1346-6_51

Table 51.1 History of development of fracture management modalities

1881	Glimer	On either sides of the fracture, two heavy rods
1886	Hansmann	Retrievable bone plates
1945	Christiansen	In mandibular fracture-tantalum plates
1956	Bagby	First compression plate
1960	Luhr and Mittlmeir	Improved mandibular compression plates
1969	AO/ASIF	Dynamic compression plates (DCP)
1970s	Brons and Boeriing	Lag screws
1973	Schmoker and Spiessel	(EDCP) eccentric dynamic compression plates
1973	Michelete	Miniplates
1975	Champy	Monocortical screws principal for fixation
1977	Luhr	Compression plates for the first time in management of fracture mandible
1977	Spiessel	For mandible fracture advocated AO/ASIF principle
1989	Bos	Resorbable plates and screws
1994		Dynamic compression plate with locking compression plate
2011		Development of locking compression plate with combination holes

51.2.1 Evolution of Fixation Methods

History of development of fracture management modalities [2–4] (Table 51.1)

51.3 Concept of Bone Healing

51.3.1 Secondary Bone Healing (Fig. 51.1)

51.3.1.1 Stage I: Inflammation Induction

Immediately after fracture, hematoma formation occurs; hematoma plays a vital role in the angiogenesis of the healing fracture. Subsequently, inflammatory cells, stem cells, and fibroblasts initiate inflammatory response and enhance angiogenesis. Cytokines which helps in bone repair are released in this phase and hematoma is removed. Within 3 days, thin layer of fibrous tissue covers the periosteal surface of fractured bone. The cortical bone adjacent to fracture site becomes necrotic which later gets remolded by multinucleated osteoclast.

51.3.1.2 Stage II: Fibrocartilaginous (Soft) Callus Formation

Dense fibrous tissue, cartilage, and fibrocartilage formation occurs due to organization of subperiosteal hematoma; soft callus is composed of internal (endosteum of marrow cavity and lining of Haversian canal) and external components (periosteum and organizing hematoma) and continued proliferation of osteoblasts; fibrocartilaginous tissue begin to calcify as the periosteal and endosteal circulation develops. The conversion of chondrocytes to osteocytes occur and the entire callus is converted to immature woven bone.

51.3.1.3 Stage III: Hard Callus Formation

After 3–4 weeks of fracture, the hard callus begins to form and osseous union of the fractured cortical bone starts.

51.3.1.4 Stage IV: Remodeling

The trabeculae orient themselves in the direction of functional pressures after bone formation.

51.3.2 Primary Bone Healing (Contact and Gap Healing)

Healing without callus formation is called as primary bone healing. When there is direct apposition of cortical bone surfaces, contact healing occurs. Osteoclasts widen the Haversian canals on either side of the fracture and move toward each other. The cortical bridging occurs in 8 weeks and is usually completed in 16 weeks. In gap healing also primary bone healing occurs; gap as wide as 100 μm can be filled with mature lamellar bone (Fig 51.2).

51.4 Biomechanics of Facial Skeleton [5]

51.4.1 Mandible Fractures

The mandible is a class III lever with:

- Condyle as fulcrum.
- Bite load as a resistance force.
- Masticatory muscles as applied force.

Simple beam mechanics described the traditional biomechanical properties of mandible, which represents compression at inferior border and tensile forces on the superior border with an applied anterior load (Fig. 51.3). The "neutral axis" is the line of zero stress where the tensile forces become compressive, and it is approximately at the level of the inferior alveolar canal. Compression and tension will be produced in symphysis region due to torsional forces.

The muscles inserting on the mandible and forces exerted by these muscles during function, determine the tension and compression zone in cases of fracture mandible.

The direction of the muscular forces acting on the mandible by temporalis, lateral pterygoid, pterygomasseteric sling, and suprahyoid musculature is shown by arrows in Fig. 51.4. For successful treatment of facial fractures in the form of rigid fixation, the understanding of biomechanics of facial injury is very important.

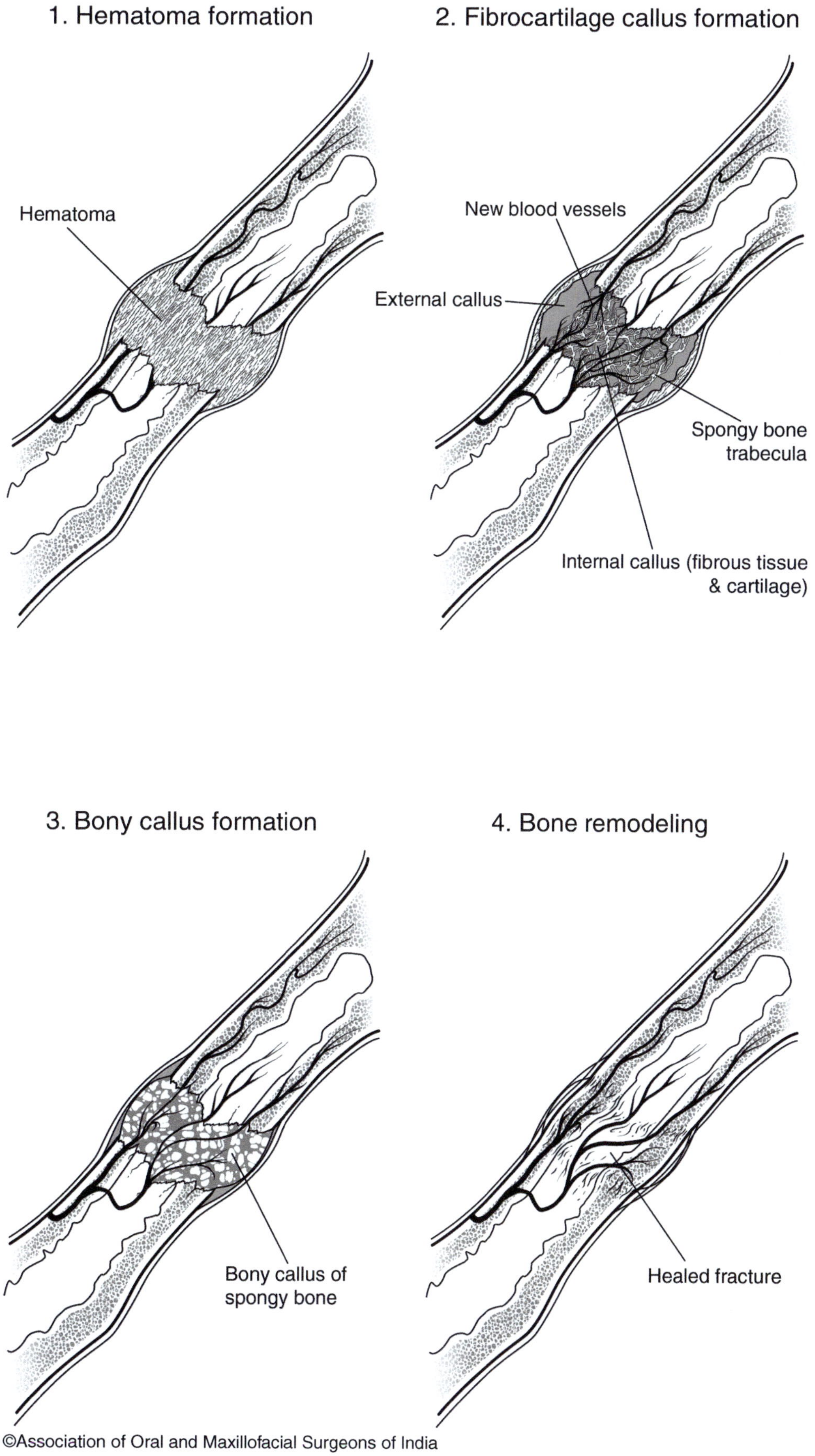

Fig. 51.1 Fracture healing

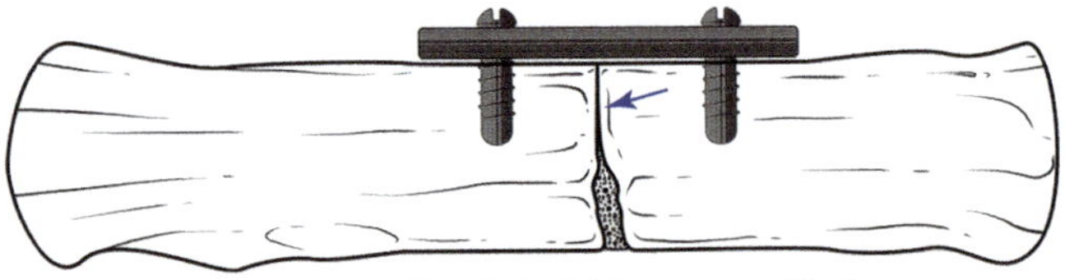

Fig. 51.2 Contact and gap healing (arrow denotes contact healing)

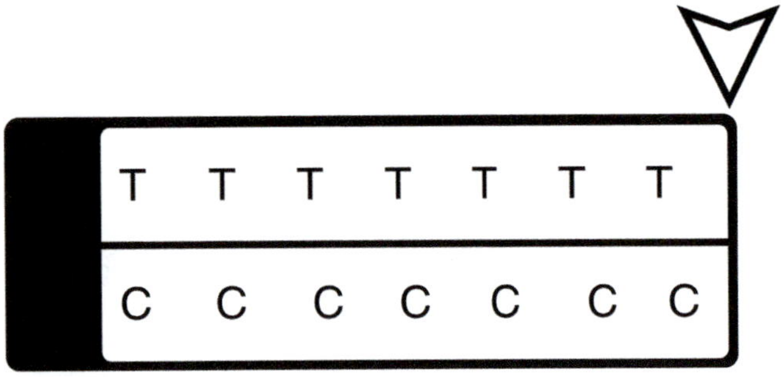

Fig. 51.3 Tensile and compressive force mechanism

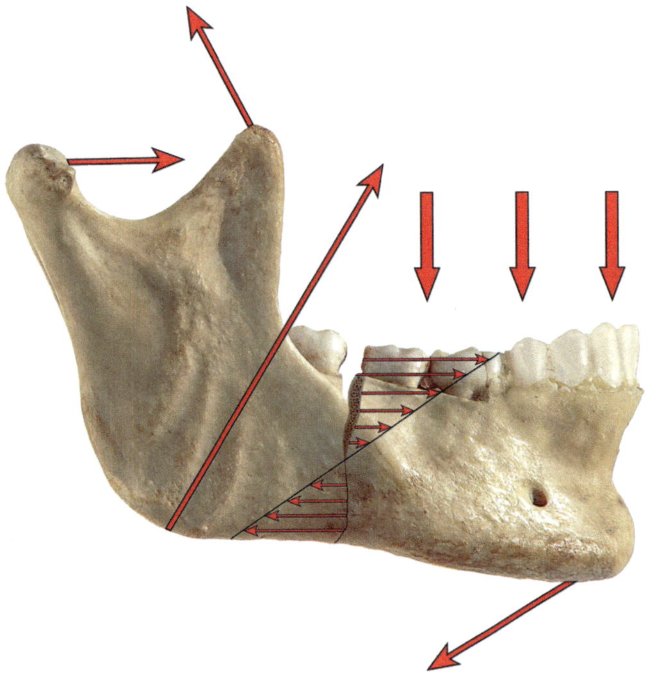

Fig. 51.4 Direction of muscular forces

51.4.2 Midface Fractures

Midface generally does not show muscle forces acting on them except for zygomatic bone, on which masseter exerts the primary force which can create notable bony displacement causing inferior and medial displacement especially in the presence of temporalis fascia disruption (Table 51.2).

Table 51.2 The four articulations of zygoma with their functions in management of fracture

Frontozygomatic suture	Received greatest tensile forces and is the important site for fixation
Infraorbital rim	Thin bone, least important site for fixation
Zygomaticomaxillary buttress	Best site for fixation to counter the force of masseter muscle
Zygomaticotemporal suture	Least important site for plating

51.5 Functions of Plates

51.5.1 Compression

Compressing together the main fragments of a single plane fracture can result in absolute stability, i.e., the complete abolition of interfragmentary movement. Interfragmentary compression in single plane, as in diaphyseal fractures, can be achieved by exploiting the eccentric loading capabilities of the dynamic compression family of plates.

The screw is inserted in a neutral mode, and plate was fixed to the right-hand fragment. In an eccentric (load) mode, a screw is then inserted into the left-hand fragment. As the load screw is fully inserted, it engages and slides down the sloping surface of the plate hole, and the screw and bone move toward the fracture, compressing it.

If the plate that exerts axial compression is exactly contoured to the anatomically reduced fracture surface, there will be some gapping of the opposite cortex when the plate is tensioned by tightening the load screw. This is due to the compression being maximal immediately beneath the plate and not evenly distributed over the whole area of the fracture plane. The solution to this problem is to "overbend" the plate so that its center stands off 1–2 mm from the anatomically reduced fracture surface. Slight gaping of the cortex will occur directly underneath the plate when the neutral side plate is applied to the bone. The tightening of load screw causes tension in the plate and compresses the fracture evenly across the full diameter of the bone.

51.5.2 Neutralization

A primary lag screw fixation, exerting interfragmentary compression, can be vulnerable to disruption by physiological bending and/or rotational forces. Such a primary fixation is usually protected by the use of a plate, spanning from one main fragment to the other—this "neutralizes" the disruptive forces. All such forces are then transmitted via the plate and bypass the primary lag screw fixation.

51.5.3 Tension Band

If a body with a fracture is loaded at each end, over a bending point (fulcrum), tension (distraction) forces are generated, maximal on the side opposite the fulcrum, and angulation occurs. However, if an inelastic band, such as a plate, is anchored to the tension side of the body, same load will generate compression across the fracture interface. This is known as the tension band principle.

51.6 Fixation Methods and Devices [6] (Table 51.3)

Commonly used devices used for fixation are wires, staples, pins, and screws [6].

51.6.1 Material

Most commonly used materials are titanium (Ti-6Al-4V) and stainless steel (316L). Stainless steel has been used because of its greater biocompatibility and corrosion resistance. Since 1980 titanium was used in maxillofacial surgery.

51.6.2 Rigid Fixation

The internal fixation is defined as the placement of wires, plates, screws, rods, pins, and other hardware to stabilize the fracture fragments.

51.6.2.1 Rigid Internal Fixation (RIF)

RIF is defined as "bone fixation of any form in which biomechanical forces are either countered or used to stabilize the fragments of fracture and permits loading of bone to permit active action" [7].

51.6.2.2 Examples of RIF

Examples of RIF are the use of bone plates and screws, two lag screws, and use of reconstruction plate with three screws on each side of the fracture fragment. Use of long compression plate is also included in the rigid internal fixation examples.

Table 51.3 Fixation methods and devices

Fixation methods			
Wires	Staples	Pin	Screws
	Pneumatically driven staples	Kirschner wires	Cancellous screw
	Prebent staple legs		Cortical screw

Healing: In the rigid internal fixation, no callus formation is formed during bone healing. The fracture bones heal by a process of Haversian remodeling. This primary or direct bone union requires immaculate immobilization between osseous fragments, i.e., minimum gap between the rigid fixation. Examples of rigid fixation for fracture mandible are shown in Fig. 51.5a,b.

51.6.3 Nonrigid Internal Fixation

It is a kind of fixation that is not strong enough to prevent interfragmentary motion completely. Thus interfragmentary motion is the differentiating factor between rigid and nonrigid fixation. Any mobility between fragments stabilized through internal fixation on active usage of skeletal structure signifies nonrigid fixation.

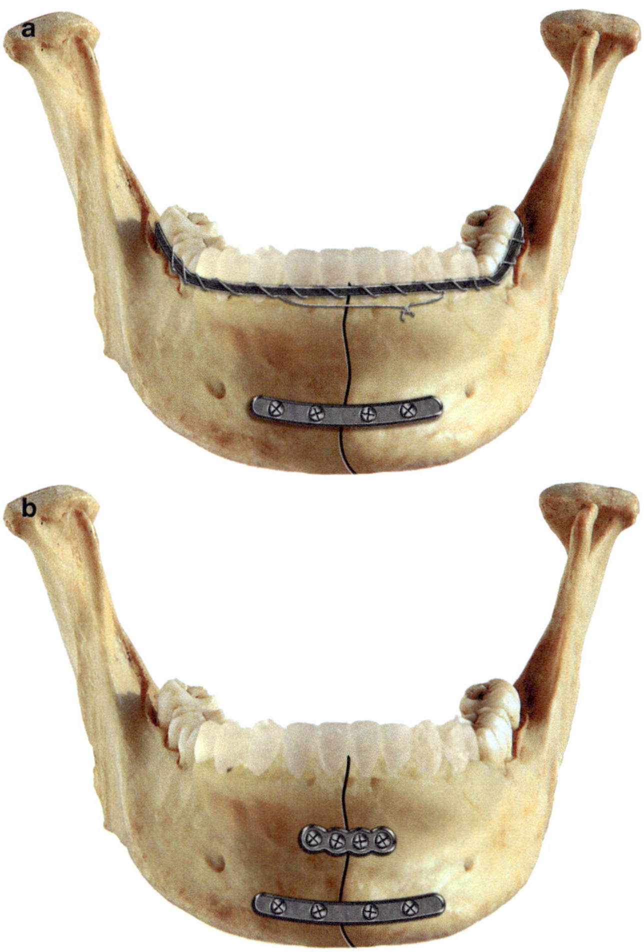

Fig. 51.5 (**a**, **b**) Techniques of rigid fixation for mandibular fracture. (**a**) Fixation with single miniplate and tension band; (**b**) fixation with two miniplates

Transosseous wiring across a fractured mandible is a good example of nonrigid fixation. The wire is unable to neutralize torsion/or shear forces and requires other fixation methods like MMF (maxillomandibular fixation).

Healing: The bone healing that occurs under the condition of mild mobility between fragments is called as secondary bone healing. There is deposition of periosteal callus in such circumstances, followed by resorption of fragment peripheries and tissue differentiation through various stages from fibrous to osseous healing.

51.6.4 Semirigid Fixation

Semirigid fixation is based on load-sharing osteosynthesis. Semirigid fixations include the use of:

- Lag screw
- Miniplates and microplate
- Locking plates
- Resorbable plates
- Three-dimensional plates

51.6.5 Load-Bearing Versus Load-Sharing Fixation (Table 51.4)

Table 51.4 Load-bearing versus load-sharing fixation

	Load-sharing fixation	Load-bearing fixation
Definition/ explanation	Internal fixation of inadequate stability to withstand the functional loads across the fracture	Fixation that is capable of withstand the entire load applied during the functional activities to the mandible
Indication	1. Simple linear fractures 2. Mandibular fractures	1. Mandibular comminuted fractures 2. Loss of segment of mandible due to injury 3. Fracture with very less boney interface because of atrophy
Material used	Stainless steel, titanium 2.0 mm miniplating systems	Stainless steel, titanium 2.3 mm, 2.4 mm, 2.7 mm diameters, mandibular reconstruction bone plate
Complications	Due to inadequate bone stock adjacent to comminuted fractures, load-sharing plates should be avoided	Failure by either screw loosening or plate fracture

51.7 Classification of Plating System [8]

(A) Luhr vitallium maxillofacial systems
  (I) Mandibular compression screw system
  (II) Mini system
  (III) Micro system
  (IV) Mandibular reconstruction system
(B) Champy's system
(C) AO/ASIF maxillofacial implant system
  (I) DCP, EDCP
  (II) Reconstruction plates
(D) The W*ü*rzburg titanium system for rigid fixation

51.7.1 Locking Plate-Screw Systems

In the late 1950s, AO group put forth the tenets which are followed in traditional plates and screws. This included exposure of fracture with anatomic reduction and internal fixation of fracture fragments with the desired result of anatomic bone union [9]. The stability of these plates is achieved by locking the plates by the screws.

Conventional screw – bone plates system requires plate to adapt precisely. In the absence of this contact, the tightening of screw will draw the segments of the bone toward the plate which results in change of the occlusion and bony segments.

On the other hand, the locking plate-screw system does not require the intimate contact of plate to the underlying bone in all the areas. The screw tightening locks the plate and thus stabilizes the bone segments without compressing the bone to the plate. Alteration in reduction is impossible after screw insertion.

According to Herford and Ellis [10], the locking plate and screw system are simple to use. Like compression plate it does not require plate to be compressed to the bone.

Klotch et al. [11] also concluded that the locking plates require less time due to less bending and faster application with good results.

Locking plate and screw come in two designs, i.e.:

- Threaded locking plate and screw (Conventional)
- Tapered locking screw and plate (New generation)

The threaded locking plate - screw system features corresponding machined threads incorporated in both the screw and plate. Whereas, the tapered locking screw - plate system has a screw head which is tapered in shape with machined threads, with the plate either having no machined threads or a single machined thread incorporated into its design. This facilitates a more flexible locking mechanism which allows for screw angulation of upto 10 degrees, in comparison to the threaded locking system which needs absolute perpendicular screw placement [12].

51.7.2 Reconstruction Plates

The rigid plates with 2.7 mm bicortical screws were introduced by AO/ASIF in 1972 [13].

The main advantage attributed to the non-locking reconstruction plate, is its "load bearing" principle. Scolozzi and Richter [14], used the 2.4 mm AO Titanium plates for the management of mandible fractures, with good outcomes and very less complications.

They are available in different shapes for specific areas like angle reconstruction plate (Fig. 51.6), condylar reconstruction plate (Fig. 51.7), and straight reconstruction plate with different lengths.

Indications

1. Large defect of mandible after massive trauma
2. After mandible resection due to tumors or osteoradionecrosis
3. Commonly used in comminuted fractures of mandible, sometimes in combination with miniplates
4. To support the bone grafts in mandibular reconstruction

The advantages of rigid fixation with grafting include immediate jaw function and excellent stabilization of graft. The main disadvantage at the graft site is disuse osteoporosis or "stress shielding." This phenomenon occurs when rigid plates absorb the mandibles functional stress. To protect the long bones from stress, the plate's modulus of elasticity will have to exceed in comparison with the bone to which it is attached. Osteoporosis and reduction in bone strength are the result of protection from stress or shielding in long bones [15].

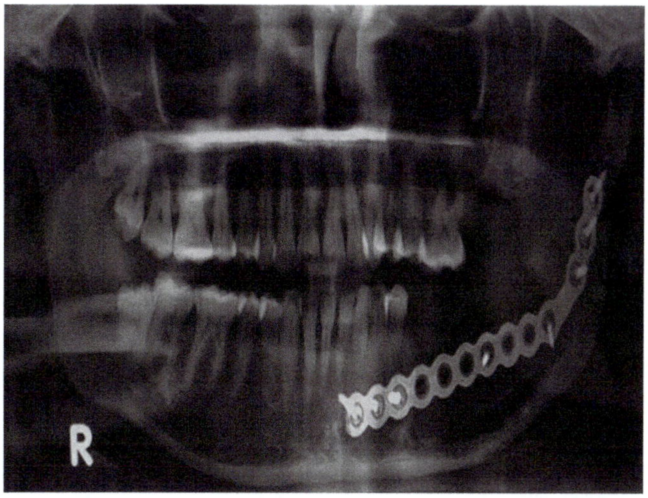

Fig. 51.6 Angle reconstruction plate

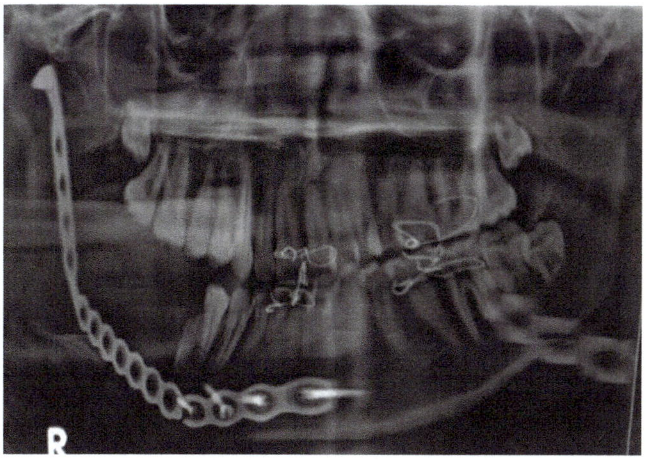

Fig. 51.7 Condylar reconstruction plate

51.7.3 Lag Screw Fixation

In oral and maxillofacial surgery, Brons and Boeriing introduced lag screw fixation for the first time in 1970. According to them two lag screws prevent rotational movements of the fracture fragments in oblique mandibular fractures [16].

51.7.3.1 The Principle of Lag Screw

The lag screw principle is used whenever two wide contact surfaces of the bone should be pressed together (for mandibular oblique sagittal fractures or onlay graft fixation).

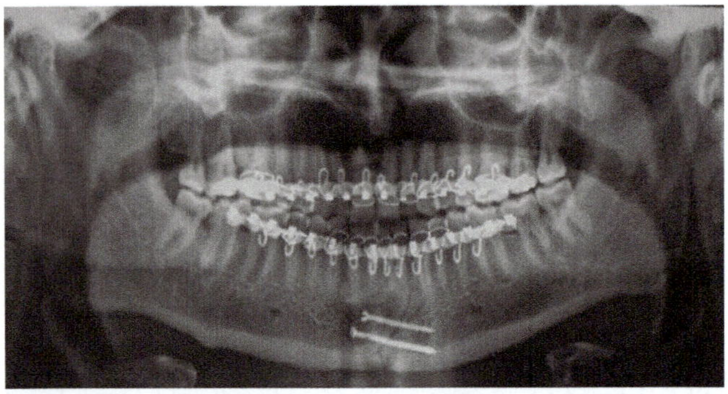

Fig. 51.8 Orthopantomogram showing fixation with lag screws

Through the outer cortex or onlay graft, the drilling of the hole was carried out of the identical diameter to that of screw so that the screw slips through the outer cortex. The lag screw drill, which is of the same diameter as the screw, will simultaneously create a conical countersink to provide an optimal fitting of the screw head. The inner cortex is then perforated with the normal surgical drill, and the screw is inserted. It grips the inner cortex and, when tightened, exerts great force to pull the outer segment into close contact with the inner one. This principle can be used in oblique sagittal mandibular fractures, with the placement of at least three screws, or in combination with the plate, lagging only one or two of the total minimum number of screws (Fig. 51.8).

51.7.3.2 Absolute Rigid Fixation Provided by Lag Screw

Lag screw should be selected in patients having sufficient bone available for placement of two screws; dissolution of the bone around the screws results in cases of micromotion. The lag screw should be placed in the direction perpendicular to the line of fracture to avoid displacement or overriding during tightening of the screws.

Advantages of lag screws over bone plates:

1. Lag screws require less hardware hence cost-effective.
2. Absolute rigid fixation.
3. Quick and easy to use.
4. Accurate reduction.

Disadvantages

As the lag screw fixation relies on compression of bone fragments and if intervening bone is unstable due to comminution or missing, there will be segment overriding or fracture gap shortening, resulting in malocclusion.

51.7.4 Comparison of Lag Screw Fixation Methods with Different Methods of Fixations [17–19]

1. Single lag screw with arch bar, without MMF is sufficient enough in the treatment of anterior mandible indirectly reducing the cost and requiring less hardware and time of healing [17].
2. Lag screw fixation and plating showed excellent outcome in anterior mandible fracture; lag screws technique is difficult but associated with less postoperative complications [18].
3. In mandibular angle fracture, the lag screw demonstrates smaller inter-fragmentary gap in comparison with miniplate fixation [19].
4. Lag screw osteosynthesis is more advantageous for ramus height restoration in comparison with miniplates and Kirschner wires, in patients with condylar process fractures [20].

51.7.5 Champy's System [21]

Different treatment principles using monocortical miniplates without axial compression for treatment of mandibular and midface fractures were introduced, namely, by Michelet et al. in the late 1960s, which they published in 1973.

Michelet's work has been elaborated by Champy et al. for the management of mandibular angle fracture by the use of intraoral monocortical miniplates. The ideal line of osteosynthesis has been followed by Champy for plates fixation (Fig. 51.9).

It is based on the principle of neutralizing unfavorable traction strains while at the same time allowing transmission of favorable compression forces. The biomechanical validity of Michelet principles was confirmed in a series of multidisciplinary experiments performed in Strasbourg, France, between 1971 and 1974 [21].

Advantages

1. Smaller incision required
2. Less soft tissue dissection
3. Less palpable
4. Decrease stress shielding effect
5. Less chance of dental injury because of monocortical screws
6. Less chances of infection

With this type of fixation, there is adequate stability to allow direct bony union and is called as functionally stable fixation. There are many fixation techniques used in oral and maxillofacial surgery (OMFS) which are not rigid fixation truly but classified as functionally stable fixation.

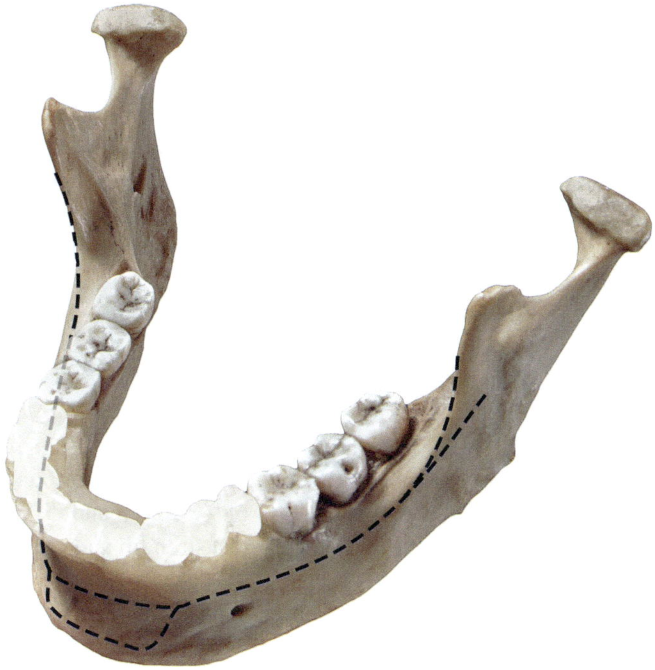

Fig. 51.9 Champy's ideal line of osteosynthesis

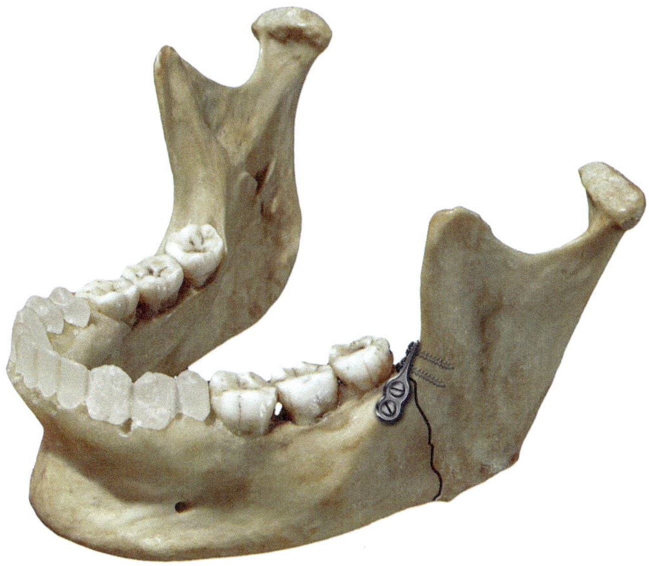

Fig. 51.10 Champy's miniplate

51.7.5.1 Materials

Plates and screws are made up of pure titanium. The miniplates are 2 cm long, 0.9 mm thick, and 6 mm wide. They had an elastic limit of flexibility between 70 and 80 per square millimeter, and their rupture point lies between 95 and 110 decanewton (daN) per square millimeter (Fig. 51.10).

51.7.5.2 Miniplates (Fig. 51.11)

- The miniplates vary in length from 2 to 9 cm with a thickness of 0.9 mm. They come in different lengths such as 2 holes with gap , 3 holes, 4 holes, 6 holes, and 8 holes to 16 holes with gap or continuous plates.
- The four-hole and six-hole plates are available with intermediate spacing.
- A wide variety of pre-shaped plates like L, X, Y, T, and K, delta shaped, and 3D- and H-shaped plates are also available. 2.1 mm is the minimum diameter of the hole in the plate and has a bevel of 30°.

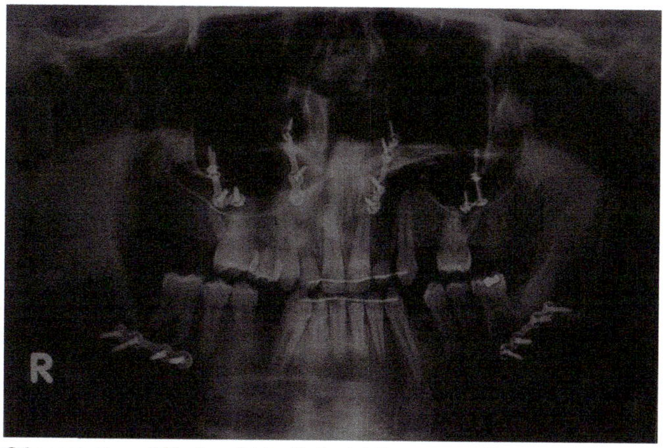

Fig. 51.11 OPG showing fixation with the help of miniplates after Leefort I and bilateral sagittal split osteotomy

51.7.5.3 Screw

- All screws are cortical and self-tapping and have cruciform head.
- Available in lengths of 5, 6, 7, 9, 11, 13, and 15 mm.
- 2 mm is the diameter of the screw with 1.6 core diameter of thread.
- The screw thread is 10/10, so that one turn of the screw corresponds to 1 mm penetration into the bone.
- 2.8 mm is the screw head diameter, and it is designed such that it allows insertion at 30-degree angle with respect to the plate surface.

The drill has the same diameter as the core of the screws—1.6 mm. This ensures firm anchorage of the self-tapping screws.

51.7.5.4 Biomechanical Properties of Screw (Fig. 51.12) [22]

- The external or the outer diameter ranges from 0.8 to 2.0 mm. Core diameter of the screw is its internal diameter. The surgical bone screws act by clamping the bone plate and bone together.

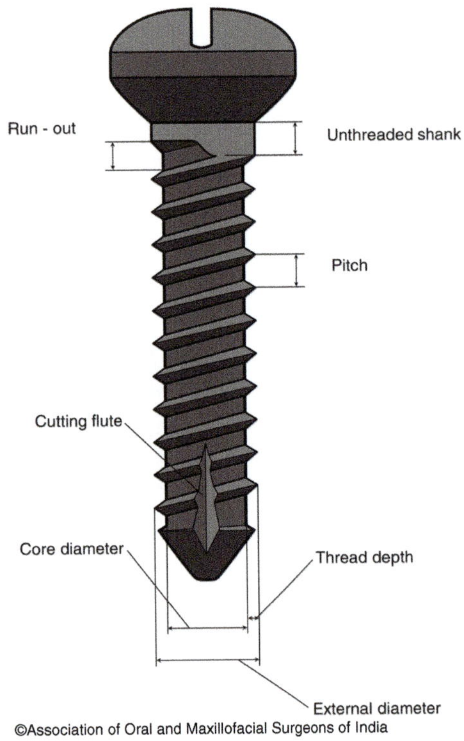

Fig. 51.12 Biomechanical properties of screw

- The pitch of the screw is calculated parallel to the screw axis from a point on one thread to corresponding point on the adjacent thread.
- The difference between core and external diameter is the thread depth.
- The distance between screw runout and screw head is the length of the unthreaded shank.
- The distance between screw runout and plate is the length of the unthreaded shank with plate.

51.7.5.5 Self-Tapping and Drilling Screws [23, 24, 25]

Self-tapping screw: The screw which is inserted into a predrilled hole without tapping a screw head is the self-tapping screw.

Self-drilling screw has a drilled-shaped point to cut and does not require predrilling. Self-drilling screws have several advantages over the self-tapping such as it does not require drilling the hole and prevents thermal damage leading to infection, screw loosening, osteomyelitis, and nonunion. It also prevents damage to tooth roots and nerves by the use of drills and also avoids the complications associated with drill bit fracture.

51.7.5.6 Monocortical vs. Bicortical Screws

The monocortical screws are generally used for fixation of mandibular fractures and after sagittal split osteotomy. Chug H-IJ et al. [26] also concluded that monocortical screws provide stable fixation. Also chances of damage to the vital structure like inferior alveolar and lingual nerve are less with monocortical screws. Bicortical screws are usually used at the lower border of the mandible for fixation.

51.7.6 Microplates

The microplate fixation concept was introduced by Luhr in 1988. They are composed of cobalt, vitallium alloy, and molybdenum in the percentage of 68%, 27%, and 5 %, respectively. It has got excellent physical strength and corrosion resistance.

The thickness of plate is 0.5 mm, and the diameter of the screws is 0.8 mm. In all the three dimensions, they can be contoured and maintained an excellent degree of rigidity for osseous segment stabilization. They are used in:

1. Nasoethmoidal fractures
2. Fractures of infraorbital area
3. Fracture of frontal sinus wall
4. Reconstruction of the skull
5. Infant craniofacial surgery

51.7.6.1 Micromesh

Inspite of its reduced thickness (0.3 mm), micromesh is remarkably strong. It is available in sizes of 40 by 60 and 60 by 100 mm. Template made of a soft, malleable tin alloy comes in various sizes. The template is cut to the shape and size required in the individual case, and then it is contoured to the bone surface. The actual titanium micromesh is then cut out with a wire cutter and contoured on the instrument table reduplicating the individual shape of the template.

51.7.7 AO/ASIF System [27]

The association of osteosynthesis/association for the study of internal fixation (AO/ASIF) were founded by a group of 15 Swiss surgeons in 1958. The group was led by Maurice E. Muller; AO/ASIF investigators have documented the biologic basis for the concepts on which rigid fixation techniques are based.

Spiessl applied AO/ASIF concepts of long bone healing and modified AO/ASIF instrumentations for use in mandible in the late 1960s and early 1970s.

Compression can be achieved through static or dynamic means. The two devices that produce static compression are the self-compression plate and lag screw.

1. The self-compression plate designed by Perren for the ASIF has been called the dynamic compression plate (DCP). It generates interfragmentary compression by spherical guiding principle. The DCP principle causes the movement of screw in both vertical and horizontal direction which compresses the fracture segments.
2. Lag screw principle—when the screw is tightened, it compresses the surface when the screw glides through the cortex of one fragment and engages the cortex of the opposite fragment.

The EDCP (eccentric dynamic compression plate) has outer hole which is oblique causing compression on alveolar side and longitudinal inner holes creating basal side interfragmental compression. EDCPs eccentric action eliminates the need for tension band. This plate has most utility for simple fracture of the posterior region where there are no teeth available for splinting.

The reconstruction plate is a load-bearing plate and absorbs the entire functional load. They are designed for use without the tension band. It is large and reinforced version of basal stabilization plate. They can be adapted to local bony contours and are malleable. Depending on the placement of drill hole, it has two-way DC holes that enable compression to be applied in either longitudinal direction.

51.7.7.1 Plates

(I) Linear system (compression plates)
  (a) DCP plates
  (b) EDCP plates
(II) Universal systems (reconstruction plates)

51.7.7.2 Dynamic Compression Plate (DCP)

These are designed to withstand tensile loading force in the mandible. In mandibular angle, body, and symphysis regions, they can be used comfortably. It can be applied intraorally or through an extraoral incision. It is used with a tension band. The dynamic compression plate was developed in 1969.

The DCP has a self-compressing hole design. The holes are oblong, and the portion of each hole distant from the fracture has a sloping form or "shoulder."

Experimental work showed that the flat undersurface of the DCP interfered with the vascular supply of the underlying cortex onto which it was compressed by the screws. The concept of "footprint" is the area of undersurface of the plate in contact with the underlying bone cortex.

Principles of DCP—The sloping shoulder of the DCP hole has the form of part of an angled cylinder. If a screw is inserted eccentrically, so that its head on final tightening slides down the sloping profile of the hole, the screw/bone unit will be shifted toward the fracture, and the fracture plane will thereby be compressed. Such a screw is often referred to as a load screw.

51.7.7.3 Eccentric Dynamic Compression Plate (EDCP) [27]

It produces a compressive force via arrangement of eccentric and centric (axial) plate holes. EDCP are 8 mm wide and come in four-hole (36 mm long) and six-hole (42 mm long) lengths. The stainless steel plates are 2 mm thick, and the titanium plate is 2.2 mm thick. At the fractures alveolar side, the compression has been provided by the 75° angulation. It is important to place the sloped edge of the angled hole at the mandibular lower border (if the plate is placed upside down, it will tend to distract bone edges at the alveolar border). First central screws are inserted in EDCPs (longitudinal hole eccentrically away from the fracture) than at the lower border; screws are placed in the 75-degree oblique holes eccentrically and in the last rest of the screws inserted in a neutral position. When the plates and tension band splint cannot be used, in those situations EDCP plates are used. The reduction forceps with pressure splinting are useful initially to reduce and compress the fragments when applying the EDCP plate.

51.7.8 Bioresorbable Fixation Systems

Use of titanium plates and screws is time-tested for their use in management of craniofacial fractures. However, it has many drawbacks including infection, hardware palpation and visibility, hypersensitivity to temperature changes, and stress shielding effect. They also interfere with radiographic examination. Sometimes, metal ions leach out into soft tissues. In view of these complications, bioresorbable implants were developed hoping to reduce hardware-associated complications as well as the necessity for hardware removal.

The use of bioresorbable fixation devices must be limited as their mechanical strength is inferior as compared to the titanium hardware. They can be effectively used in low load-bearing areas of maxillofacial skeleton like maxilla, zygoma, and upper regions of face. The bioresorbable system may not be strong enough to provide adequate stability in mandible fractures which are comminuted, as it is a load-bearing bone. It can be used in simple mandibular fractures.

Bioresorbable fixation systems stabilize fracture segments long enough for fracture healing and union to occur then dissolve, thereby reducing complications frequently encountered with metallic hardware such as palpability, visibility, cold sensitivity, and need for removal. Most commonly polylactic acid (PLA) is used in bioresorbable plates.

Complications [28]

1. For allowing the polymer chains to bend without breaking, a heat source is required. Also, the working time is limited to 8–10 s.
2. Screw insertion requires pretapping the screw.
3. Increased operative time.
4. More expensive.
5. PLA decreases stress shielding compared to LD-DC plates.

51.8 Recent Developments

To reduce the stress shielding, reduction in modulus is the answer to correct the disadvantages of internal fixation. To improve the healing of the fracture under the plates, the only solution is to allow micromotion through the fracture site; the design should be made in such a way that it resists torsional, bending, and shear movements.

51.8.1 Three-Dimensional (3D) Plates (Fig. 51.13)

The two miniplates are connected by interconnecting crossbars which are used as 3D plates. Technically, they are not three-dimensional structures, but their closed quadrilateral shape provides stability in all three dimensions.

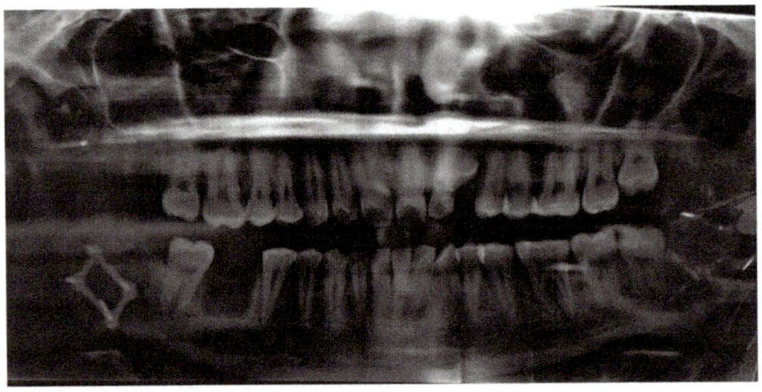

Fig. 51.13 Orthopantomogram showing fixation with three-dimensional plate

51.8.2 Virtual Surgical Planning, Computer-Assisted Design, and 3D Modelling

The management of the facial fracture is very challenging due to its unique three-dimensional contours and nonlinearity of facial skeleton. The recent development in the software technology and 3D modeling has revolutionized the treatment. They can be used as an adjunct to the standard preoperative preparation.

To reduce the operating time in the operation theater, the 3D models can serve as a template on which pre contouring of the fixation plates can be done. Custom-designed titanium implants can be made with the help of 3D printers to get the accurate fit. They can be preferred over the conventional implants and reduce the surgical time. The model design and virtual surgical planning help in constructing the guides which can be used perioperatively, can design the optimal approach preoperatively, and can compare the actual outcome to the virtual design. To reconstruct the multitude of craniomaxillofacial defects of mandible, zygoma, midface, and orbit, these technologies are very helpful. 3D modeling and computer-assisted surgical planning have been very helpful in managing the complications associated with these injuries.

51.8.3 Intraoperative Imaging [29]

Intraoperative imaging is very important in assessing the reduction and fixation of all maxillofacial fractures, and according to its feedback, the surgeons can immediately make corrections of any error that occur during reduction and fixation, which indirectly reduces the complications and avoids potential resurgeries. Computed tomography (CT) is commonly used for the same purpose.

51.9 Conclusion

For the treatment of maxillofacial fractures, many fixation methods have been used with great success. To reestablish the pre-injury esthetics, the normal masticatory function and the proper occlusion in cases of such fractures are the main objectives of the treatment. Maxillomandibular fixation can be done for the conservative management of such fractures which can be carried out with the help of arch bars, wiring, and cap splints and in edentulous patients by gunning splints. The open reduction and internal fixation can be carried out with the help of miniplates, microplates, 3D plates, and reconstruction plates. Different plating systems and wiring techniques make the management of these maxillofacial fractures predictable with high success rate.

Acknowledgment Author wishes to thank Dr. Anshul Rai for providing Figs. 51.6, 51.7, 51.11, and 51.13.

References

1. Uhtoff HK, Poitras P, Backman DS. Internal plate fixation of fracture: short history and recent developments. J Orthop Sci. 2006;11:118–26.
2. Fonseca RJ, Walker RV, Barber HD, Powers M, Frost DE. Oral and maxillofacial trauma. China: Saunders; 2013.
3. Ehrenfeld M, Manson PN, Prein J, AOCMF. Principles of internal fixations of craniomaxillofacial skeleton, trauma, & orthognathic surgery. Basel: Thieme; 2012.
4. Rowe NL, William JL. Maxillofacial injuries. 1st edn. New York: Churchill Livingstone. ISBN: 978-81-312-1840-2.
5. Rudderrnan RH, Mullen RL. Biomechanics of the facial skeleton. Clin Plast Surg. 1992;19:11.
6. Greenberg AM, Prein J. Craniomaxillofacial reconstructive and corrective bone surgery. Principles of internal fixation using the AO/ASIF technique. New York: Springer. p. 101–3.
7. Allgöwer M, Spiegel PG. Internal fixation of fractures: evolution of concepts. Clin Orthop. 1979;138:26–9.
8. Uhthoff HK, Poitras P, Backman DS. Internal plate fixation of fractures:short history and recent developments. J Orthop Sci. 2006;11:118–26.
9. Egol KA, Kubiak EN, Fulkerson E, Kummer FJ, Koval KJ. Biomechanics of locked plates and screws. J Orthop Trauma 2004;18:488–93.
10. Herford AS, Ellis E. Use of a locking reconstruction bone plate/screw system for mandibular surgery. J Oral Maxillofac Surg. 1998;56:1261.
11. Klotch DW, Gal TJ, Gal RL. Assessment of plate use for mandibular reconstruction: Has changing technology made a difference? Otolaryngol Head Neck Surg. 1999;121:388.
12. Coletti DP, et al. Comparative analysis of the threaded and tapered locking reconstruction plates. J Oral Maxillofac Surg. 2007;65:2587–93.
13. Spiessl B. Rigid internal fixation of fractures of lower jaw. Reconstr Surg Traumatol. 1972;13:124–40.
14. Scolozzi P, Richter M. Treatment of severe mandibular fractures using AO reconstruction plates. J Oral Maxillofac Surg. 2003;61:458–61.
15. Waris P. Torsional strength of cortical and cancellous bone grafts after rigid plate fixation. Acta Orthop Scand. 1981;52:249.
16. Bansal P, Kumar S, Mishra V, Jaiswal Y, Das G. Evaluation of titanium lag screw osteosynthesis in the management of mandibular fractures. World J Dent. 2017;8(4):315–20.
17. Emam HA, Stevens MR. Can an arch bar replace a second lag screw in management of anterior mandibular fractures? J Oral Maxillofac Surg. 2012;70(2):378–83.
18. Ellis E. Is lag screw fixation superior to plate fixation to treat fracture of mandibular symphysis? 3rd J Oral Maxillofac Surg. 2012;70(4):875–82.
19. Schaaf H, et al. Comparison of miniplate versus lag screw osteosynthesis for fractures of mandibular angle. Oral Surg Oral Med Oral Pathol Oral Radiol Endod. 2011;111(1):34–40.
20. Sugiura T, et al. A comparative evaluation of osteosynthesis with lag screws, miniplates, or Kirschner wires for mandibular condylar process fractures. J Oral Maxillofac Surg. 2001;59(10):1161–8, 1169–70.
21. Michelet FX, Deymes J, Dessus B. Osteosynthesis with miniaturized screwed plates in maxillo-facial surgery. J Maxillofac Surg. 1973;1(2):79–84.
22. You Z-H, et al. Biomechanical properties of small bone screws. J Oral Maxillofac Surg. 1994;52:1293–302.
23. Champy M, Lodde JP, Schmitt R, et al. Mandibular osteosynthesis by miniature screwed plates via the buccal approach. J Maxillofac Surg. 1978;6:14.
24. Baumgart FW, Cordey J, Morikawa K, et al. AO/ASIF self-tapping screws (STS). Injury. 24 (suppl 1):S1.
25. Heidemann W, Gerlach KL, Gröbel KH, et al. Drill free screws: A new form of osteosynthesis screw. J Craniomaxillofac Surg. 1998;26:163.
26. Chung H-IJ, et al. Postoperative stability after sagittal split ramus osteotomies for a mandibular setback with monocortical plate fixation or bicortical screw fixation. J Oral Maxillofac Surg. 2008;66:446–52.
27. Yaramchuk MJ, Gruss JS, Manson PN. Rigid fixation of the craniomaxillofacial skeleton: Part II: Implant system for rigid fixation of craniomaxillofacial skeleton.
28. Cutright DE, Hunsuck EG. The repair of fractures of orbital floor using biodegradable polylactic acid. Oral Surg. 1972;33:28–34.
29. Meaike JD, Hollier LH. Updates in facial fracture management. J Trauma Treat. 2015;4:4

Fractures of the Mandible

52

Anshul Rai

52.1 Definition

A fracture is defined as "A breach in the continuity of bone."

52.2 Introduction

The mandible which is the only mobile bone of the maxillofacial region forms the lower third of the face. Owing to the prominence of the symphysis of the mandible, it is most vulnerable site to be traumatized during the road traffic accidents and, at the same time, most tempting site to be hit during the assault. Thus, the fractures of the mandible are one of the most common in maxillofacial area. It also affects the social life of the patients (Box 52.1).

The word "mandible" derives from the Latin word mandere "to chew" and -bula (instrument) which literally translates to mandibulaie "instrument used for chewing."

The bone is formed in the fetus from a fusion of the left and right mandibular prominences and the point where these sides join, the mandibular symphysis. Like other symphysis in the body, this is a midline articulation where the bones are joined by fibrocartilage, but this articulation fuses together in early childhood.

Box 52.1: General Effect of Mandible Fracture on Social Life [1]

1. Absence from work.
2. Hospital and ICU stay results in separation from family members and friends.
3. Financial loss.
4. Difficulty in feeding.
5. Weight loss (average 5% of total body weight).
6. Increased mental stress.
7. Delayed recovery in medically compromised and mentally challenged patients.

52.3 Surgical Anatomy

The mandible is a horseshoe-shaped only mobile bone of the facial skeleton. It is the strongest bone with thick cortices. Symphysis is the most prominent part of mandible, and the condyles articulate with glenoid fossa of temporal bone. The inferior alveolar neurovascular bundle passes through the bone, and in the case of fracture, it may get traumatized and can lead to hematoma and neurological deficit.

52.3.1 Angle of the Mandible

By definition, there are three types of angle as described below:

1. **Clinical angle:** It is the junction between the alveolar bone and ramus at the origin of internal oblique ridge.
2. **Surgical angle:** It is the junction between body of the mandible and ramus at the origin of the external oblique ridge.
3. **Anatomical angle or (gonion):** It is the junction where the lower border meets the posterior border of ramus.

Electronic Supplementary Material The online version of this chapter (https://doi.org/10.1007/978-981-15-1346-6_52) contains supplementary material, which is available to authorized users.

A. Rai (✉)
Department of Dentistry, All India Institute of Medical Sciences, Bhopal, Madhya Pradesh, India
e-mail: anshul.dentalsurgery@aiimsbhopal.edu.in

K. Bonanthaya et al. (eds.), *Oral and Maxillofacial Surgery for the Clinician*, https://doi.org/10.1007/978-981-15-1346-6_52

Anatomically, mandibular angle is a weaker structure compared to other anatomic subsites.

- The ramus of the mandible is thin as compared to the body. Whenever a thick portion of the bone unites with the thin portion, it constitutes a line of weakness.
- Further the third molars are located in the angle region, and when they are impacted, they occupy lot of space in the bone and undermine it.
- In the case of mesio-angular impaction, the impacted third molar tooth acts as a wedge and predisposes the fracture of angle of mandible, if the direction of force is perpendicular to it.
- The bone grains which are oriented vertically in the ramus change their course at the angle of mandible as they enter the body of mandible. This abrupt change in the course of the bone grains also makes the bone weak. All these factors make the mandible vulnerable for fracture at this site.

52.3.2 Canine Region of the Mandible

In the canine area, also the mandible is weaker as the canine has the longest and the strongest root, and it occupies lot of space in the bone and undermines and weakens it. Thus, the mandible has a tendency to fracture at this site.

52.3.3 Symphysis and Parasymphysis of Mandible

- The symphyseal area is most prominent and most vulnerable to trauma. There is a compression of the outer cortex and expansion of the inner cortex, and the fracture will result when the forces are beyond the limits of the capacity of the bone to withstand them.
- There is a pair of genial tubercles on the lingual cortical plate in the midline, situated supero-inferiorly, which give origin to the genioglossus and geniohyoid muscles, respectively. Whenever there is a bilateral fracture at the parasymphysis area, the tongue tends to lose its anchorage on the bone, and the patient loses control and the tongue tends to fall back. It is especially true for the unconscious patient, where the tongue fall blocks the airway, and it could be fatal if not prevented.

52.4 Classification

The general classification of fractures of bone is described in Table 52.1.

Table 52.1 General classification of fracture of bone

Simple fracture	This type of fracture is not exposed to the external environment as the overlying soft tissue cover is intact
Compound fracture	In such type of fractures, the fracture line is exposed to the external environment. All dentate fractures are compound fracture as they communicate with the oral cavity
Comminuted fracture	Comminuted fractures have multiple fracture lines and more than two bony fragments
Simple comminuted fracture	It is a comminuted fracture not exposed to the external environment
Compound comminuted fracture	This type of fracture is a comminuted one which is exposed to the external environment
Complicated fracture	This fracture involves vital structures like adjacent nerves, vessels, or joint, directly or indirectly
Impacted fracture	The fractured fragments inter-digitate to an extent that there is no appreciable clinical movement. Such a fracture is unusual in the mandible and is commonly seen in the maxilla
Greenstick fracture	It is an incomplete fracture presenting as cortical bending rather than breaking. It is commonly seen in children as their bones are more elastic in nature. This elasticity allows the bone to bend. This type of fracture is commonly seen in long bones and mandibular condyle of children
Pathological fracture	This fracture occurs readily with minimal trauma or sometimes even during normal physiological function as the bone is significantly weak due to existing undermining pathology

52.4.1 Classification of Mandibular Fracture According to Site (Fig. 52.1)

Figure 52.1 highlights the mandibular fracture according to site of fracture with its incidence [2].

52.4.2 Classification of Mandibular Fracture According to the Impact

According to the impact on bone, fracture can be classified as direct fracture and indirect fracture.

During an impact, the force on the cortex results in compression, and the other cortex undergoes tension. If the force of the impact is more than the compressive and tensile strength of the bone, the bone fractures.

In a similar fashion, when there is an impact, the point of application of force gets compressed, and the resultant vector travels along the bone and applies tensor force on the point intersected by this vector. The fracture at the site of impact is called **direct fracture**, and the fracture at the site of intersection with the vector is **indirect fracture**.

For instance, the force applied to the symphysis menti results in a direct fracture at the symphysis. The vector travels to the condylar necks bilaterally and induce indirect fractures

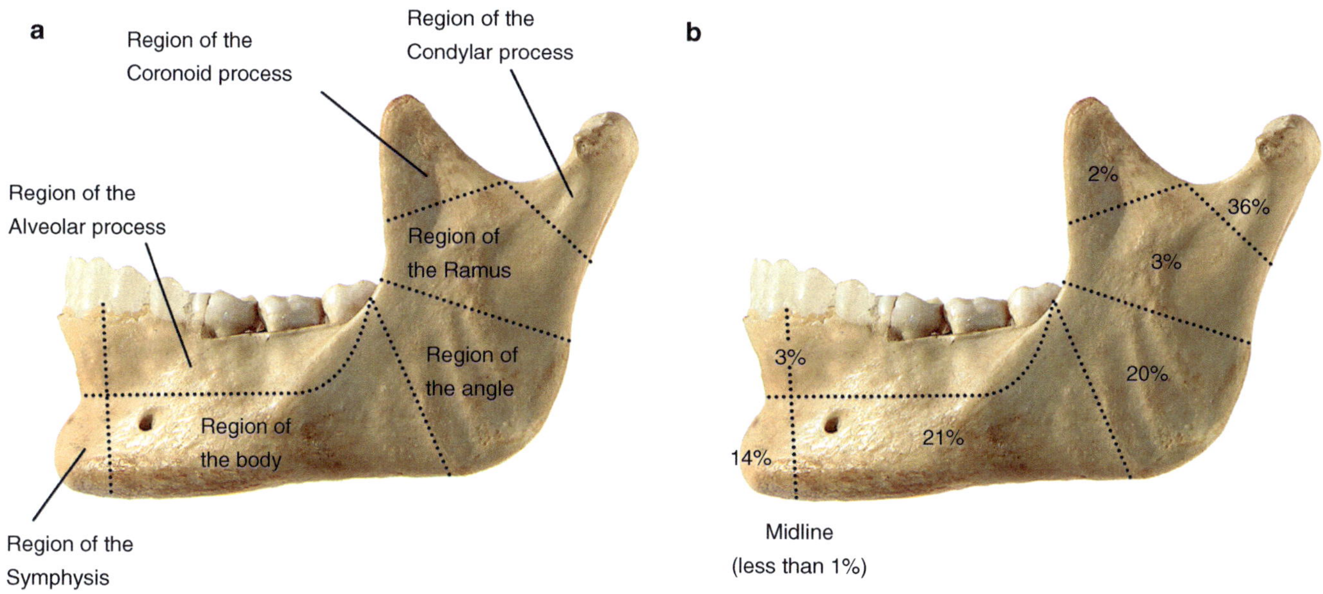

©Association of Oral and Maxillofacial Surgeons of India

Fig. 52.1 (**a**, **b**) Highlights the mandibular fracture according to site of fracture with its incidence

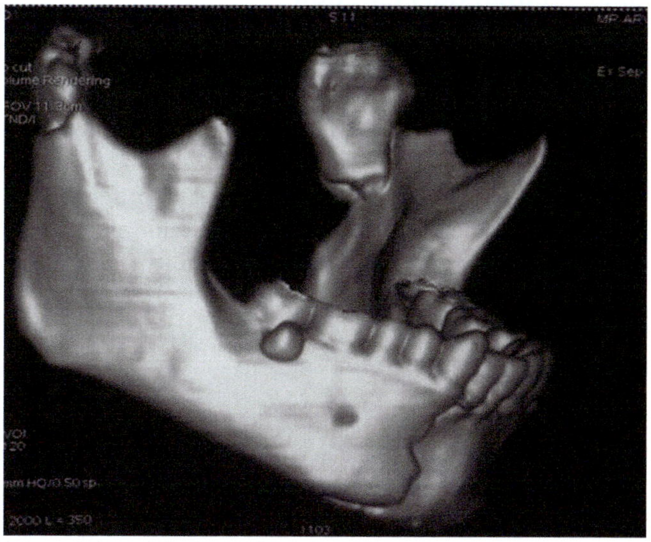

©Association of Oral and Maxillofacial Surgeons of India

Fig. 52.2 3D CT showing parasymphysis and bilateral condyle fracture

Table 52.2 Combination of mandibular fractures

Direct fracture	Indirect fracture
Symphysis fracture	Bilateral subcondylar fracture
Parasymphysis fracture	Contralateral subcondylar fracture
Body fracture	Contralateral angle fracture

of subcondylar areas bilaterally, as the condylar necks are weak. This is called a "tripod fracture" (as the fracture is at 3 points) or "parade ground fracture" or "guardsman's fracture." The later terms are used because these fractures are commonly seen among soldiers who stand upright on the parade ground for a long time. When they faint, they fall on their chin resulting in symphysis and bilateral condylar neck fractures.

52.4.3 Combination of Fracture

The most common mandible fracture seen in the developed countries is angle fracture combined with contralateral body or symphysis of the mandible [3]. Table 52.2 and Figs. 52.2, 52.3, and 52.4 highlight various combinations of direct and indirect fractures in the mandible.

52.4.4 Classification of Mandibular Fracture According to Displacement

The fracture fragments are liable to displacement according to unfavorable muscle pull leading to difficulty in the management of these displaced fractures. Table 52.3 highlights various muscles attached to the mandible with their actions.

According to the displacement of fracture fragments due to muscle pull, the fracture can be classified as:

When viewed from superior aspect:

1. Vertically favorable: When the fracture line is passing from buccal cortical plate to the lingual cortical plate with the buccal end lying mesially and the lingual end of the line lying distally. In such situation the distal fragment will be drawn closer to the proximal fragment due to the pull of the medial pterygoid muscle, and the fracture segments will come closer rather than getting separated in buccolingual plane, and thus the fracture is called as vertically favorable (Fig. 52.5a).
2. Vertically unfavorable: In this case, the fracture line passes buccolingually with the buccal end lying mesially. The distal fragment in this case will be easily viewed from superior border. The distal fragment in this case will easily get drifted

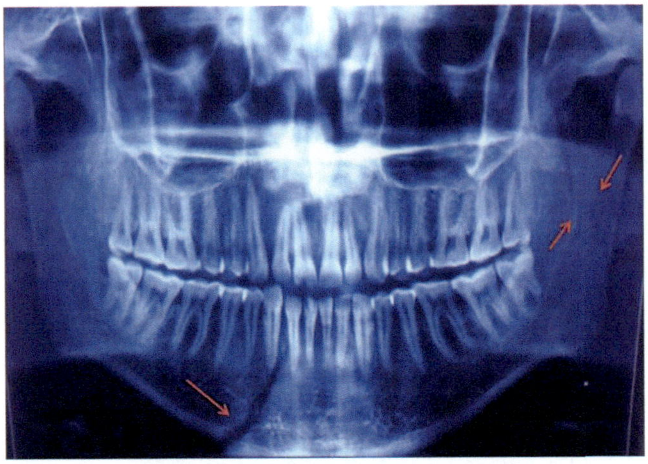

Fig. 52.3 Showing right parasymphysis and left condyle fracture

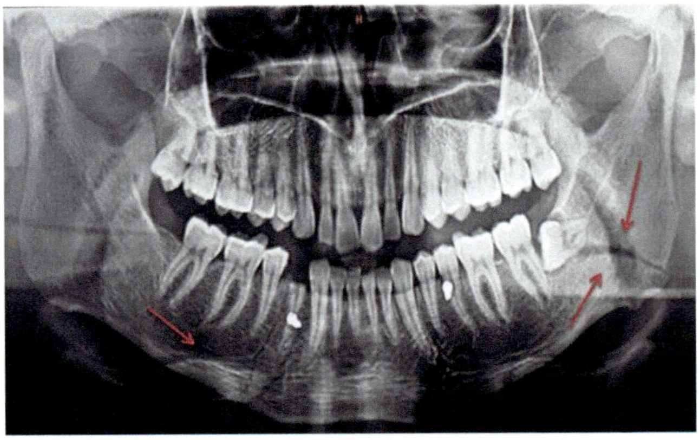

Fig. 52.4 Showing right body and left angle fracture

lingually due to the pull of the medial pterygoid muscle; thus there will be separation of the fragments in the bucco-lingual plane due to the unfavorable muscle pull, and the fracture is said to be vertically unfavorable (Fig. 52.5b).

When viewed from buccal aspect:

1. Horizontally favorable: The fracture line runs supero-inferiorly with its superior end lying posteriorly than its inferior end. In this situation, the muscle pulls from the temporalis, masseter muscle will pull the distal segment superiorly, and the suprahyoid muscles will put the proximal segment inferiorly, thus drawing both the segments closer to each other. This type of fracture is called as horizontally favorable fracture (Fig. 52.6a).
2. Horizontally unfavorable: The fracture line runs supero-inferiorly with its superior end lying anteriorly and the inferior end lying posteriorly; thus, the muscle pull becomes unfavorable and drifts the proximal and distal fracture segments apart. This is described as a horizontally unfavorable fracture (Fig. 52.6b).

Table 52.3 Muscle attachments over the mandible with their actions

Muscle	Action	Attachment
Masseter-medial pterygoid	Elevators of the mandible	Ramus of the mandible
Temporalis	Elevators of the mandible	Coronoid process of mandible
Lateral pterygoid	Depressors of the mandible, lateral movements	Ptreygoid fovea
Suprahyoid muscles (digastricus, geniohyoid, mylohyoid)	Depressors of the mandible	Body and the genial tubercles

52.5 Clinical Features

The clinical features of the fractures are described in Table 52.4 (Figs. 52.7, 52.8, 52.9, 52.10, 52.11, 52.12, 52.13, and 52.14).

52.6 Clinical Examination

52.6.1 Bimanual Palpation

The abnormal mobility at the fracture site can be elicited by the bimanual palpation. The mandible is grasped on either side of the suspected fracture line in such a way that the index finger is on the occlusal surface of the teeth and the thumbs are on the inferior border. The proximal and distal segments are moved in supero-inferior and antero-posterior direction, to elicit abnormal mobility (Fig. 52.15).

52.6.2 Compression Test

When there is a hairline, undisplaced fracture of the mandible especially at the symphysis or angle or in the subcondylar areas and it is not conspicuous clinically and radiologically, a compression of the mandible at the symphysis area and both the sides over the body, using both the palms by the operator, elicits tenderness which may suggest the fracture (Fig. 52.16a, b).

52.7 Radiographic Examination

As a rule, in orthopedics, the X-ray must be taken in two planes perpendicular to each other, i.e., in the anteroposterior and mediolateral. The most common radiographs to detect fracture of the mandible are:

1. Orthopantomogram (OPG) (Fig. 52.17)
2. Posterio-anterior view of the mandible (PA mandible) (Fig. 52.18)
3. Lateral oblique view is taken for body, angle, ramus, and subcondylar fractures.

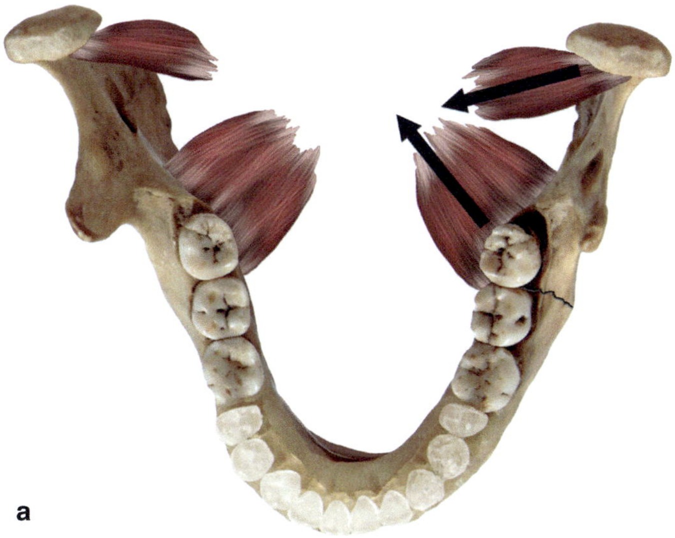

Fig. 52.5 (**a**) Vertically favorable. (**b**) Vertically unfavorable

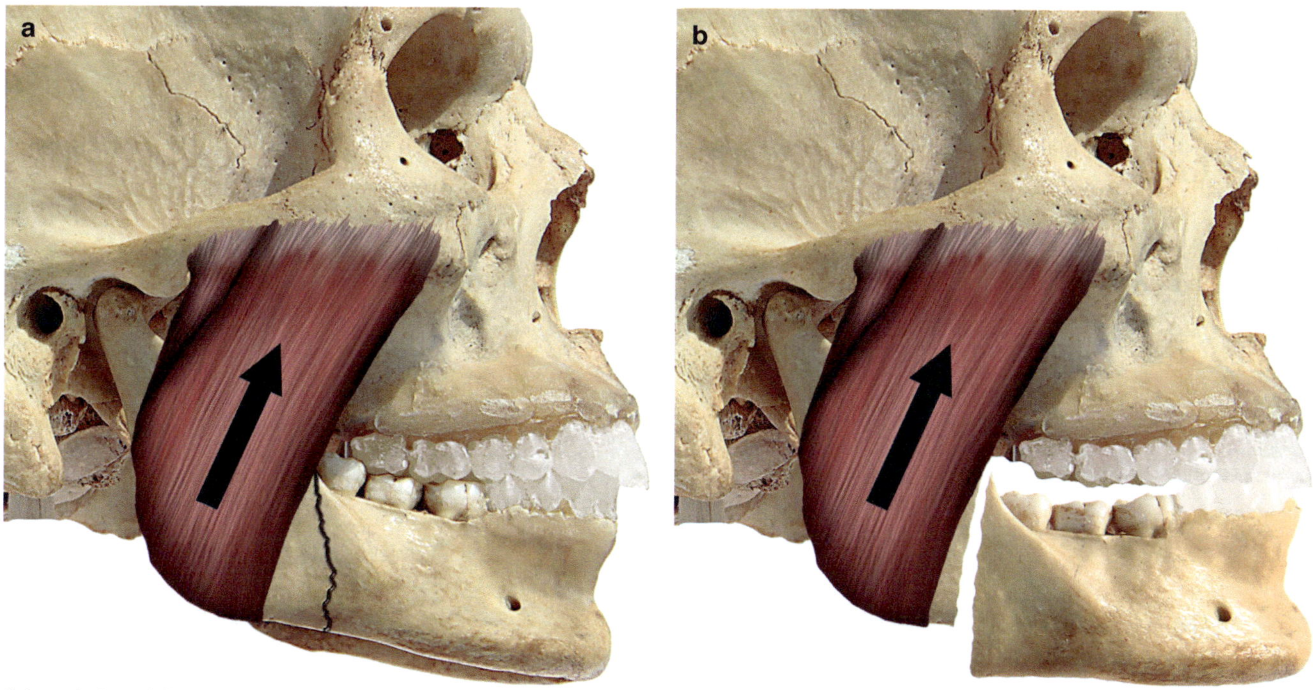

Fig. 52.6 (**a**) Horizontally favorable. (**b**) Horizontally unfavorable

4. Computed tomography (CT) scan (Fig. 52.19)
5. Digital visual tomography (DVT) (Fig. 52.20)
6. Cone beam computed tomography (CBCT) (Fig. 52.21)

- CT, DVT, and CBCT are the most commonly performed radiographs for the accurate diagnosis of mandibular fracture.
- Radiographs should not be advised unnecessary, and they should always be performed after clinical examination and after making provisional clinical diagnosis.
- Surgeons should not depend on the radiologist's report for their diagnosis; radiographs should help in confirming the clinical diagnosis and for the medicolegal record-keeping purpose as much as possible.

Table 52.4 Clinical feature of mandibular fracture

General symptoms	Signs on inspection	Signs on palpation
Pain	Presence of hematoma (Fig. 52.9)	Crepitus over fracture site
Swelling (Fig. 52.7)	Facial asymmetry	Abnormal mobility across fracture site
Difficulty in opening mouth (Fig. 52.8)	Presence of abrasion, contusion, or laceration (Fig. 52.10)	Fracture/mobility/extrusion/intrusion/avulsion of teeth
Tenderness over fracture site	Discoloration of the skin/echymosis (Fig. 52.11)	Tenderness over fracture site
Inability to chew	Trismus due to protective myo-spasm	Intersegmental mobility on bimanual palpation
Inability to swallow	Limited excursive movements of mandible	Positive compression test
Bleeding from the ear/mouth	Visible step deformity in cases with displacement of fractured segments (Fig. 52.12)	
	Malocclusion (Fig. 52.13)	
	Sublingual hematoma (Fig. 52.14) Coleman's sign	
	Tongue fall back in bilateral anterior mandible fracture	

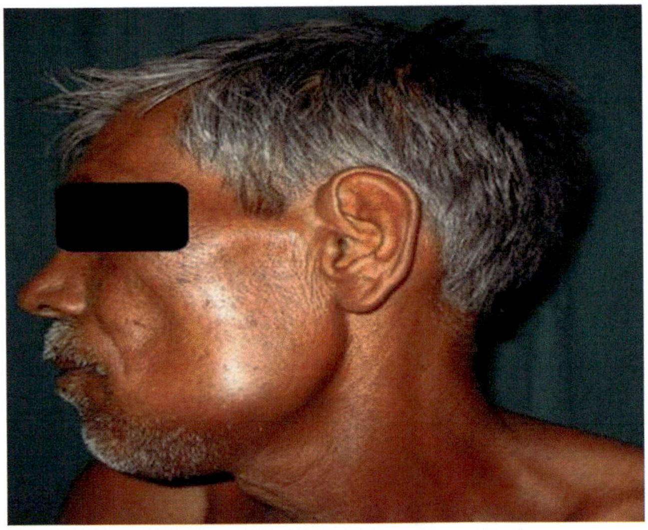

Fig. 52.7 Swelling in angle region after fracture

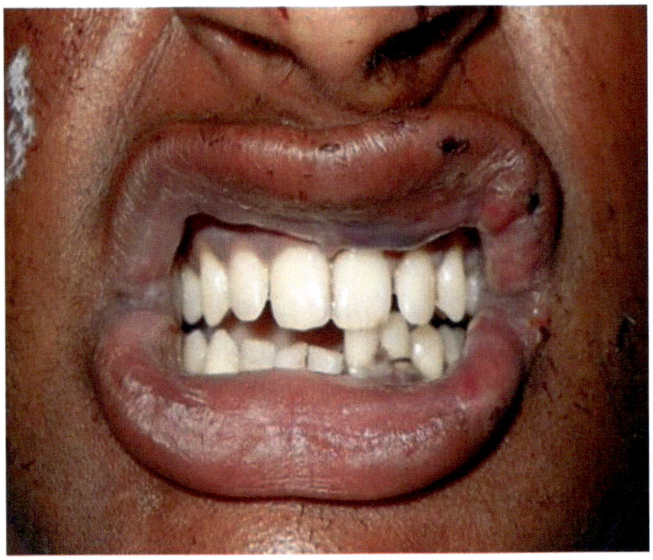

Fig. 52.8 Difficulty in mouth opening due to displacement and deviation of fracture

52.7.1 Are Postoperative Radiographs Necessary?

The answer is no. The reasons behind this is:

1. More than 100–250 deaths occur worldwide from cancer due to unnecessary radiation from diagnostic radiology as suggested by Royal College of Radiologists [4]
2. If somehow retreatment is required for the patient, it generally depends most commonly on the clinical findings rather than radiographic

However, the postoperative radiographs are required in few cases of:

- Mandibular fracture treated with closed reduction
- In medicolegal cases to prevent judicial complications [5]
- Patients who enrolled in the research activities

Bergh van den et al. [6] also suggested that postoperative radiography is not necessary. The advantages of avoiding postoperative radiographs are:

1. Exposure reduction of patients to ionizing radiation
2. Reduced cost
3. More efficient discharge

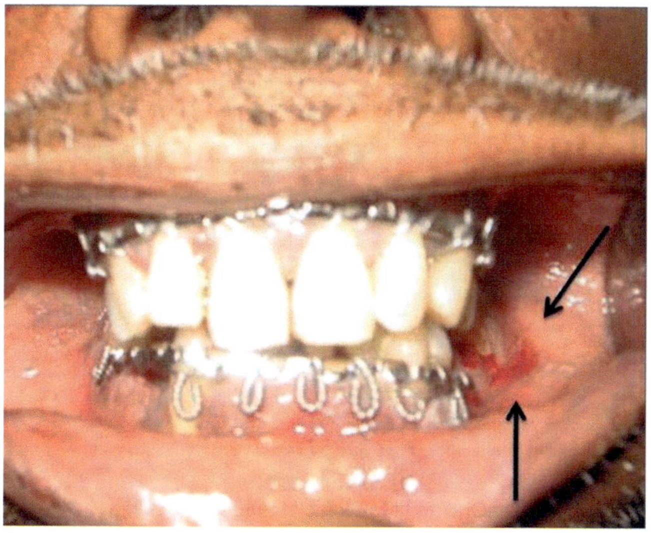

©Association of Oral and Maxillofacial Surgeons of India

Fig. 52.9 Hematoma in the angle region

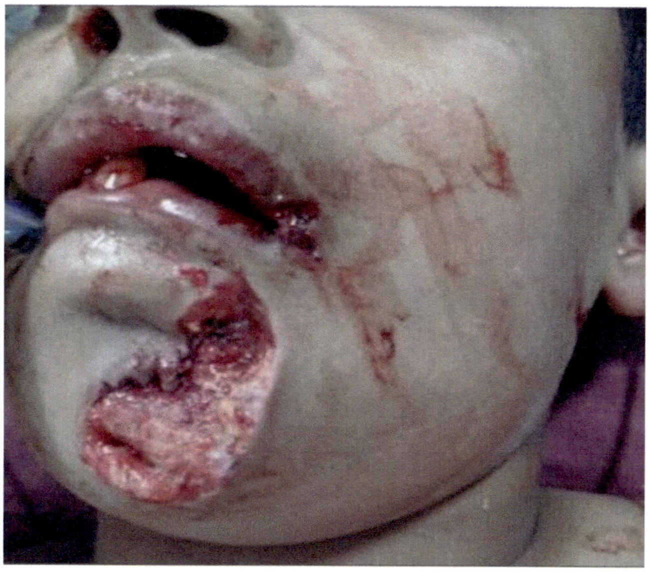

©Association of Oral and Maxillofacial Surgeons of India

Fig. 52.10 Presence of abrasion, contusion, or laceration

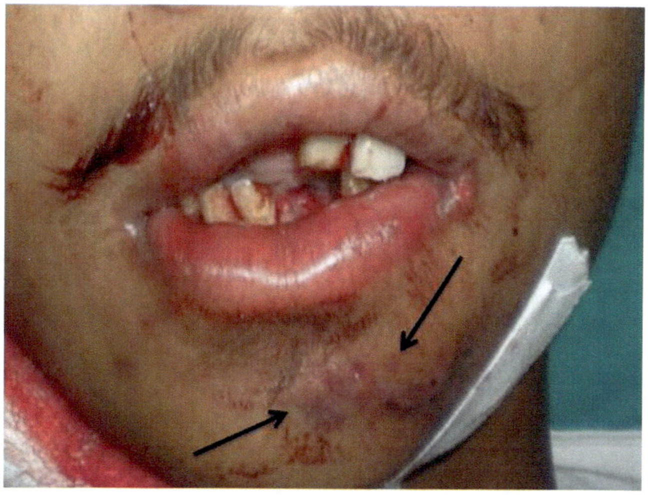

©Association of Oral and Maxillofacial Surgeons of India

Fig. 52.11 Discoloration of skin

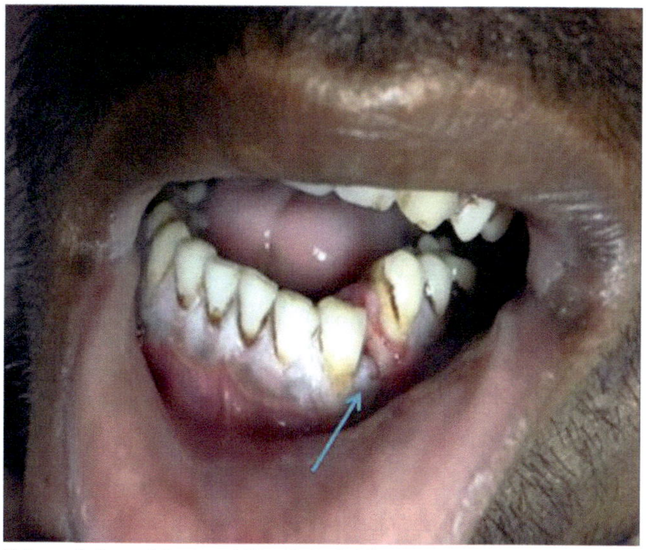

©Association of Oral and Maxillofacial Surgeons of India

Fig. 52.12 Visible step deformity in cases with displacement of fractured segments

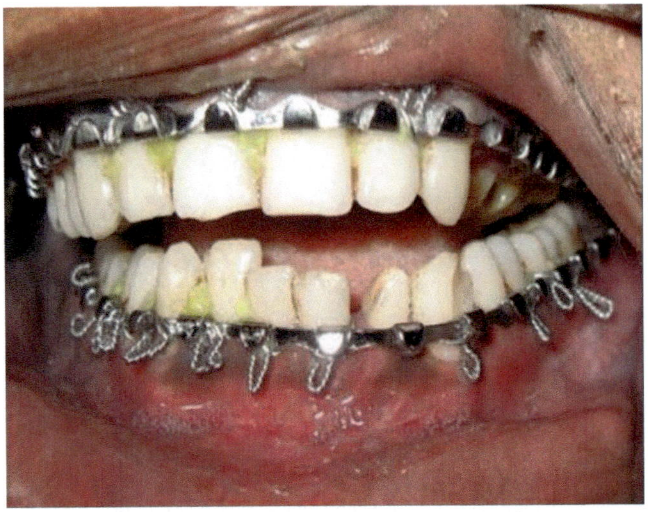

Fig. 52.13 Malocclusion

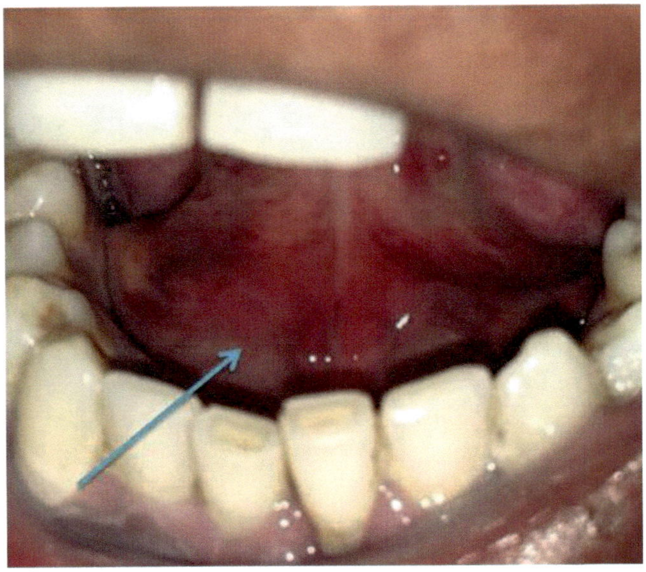

Fig. 52.14 Sublingual hematoma (Coleman's sign)

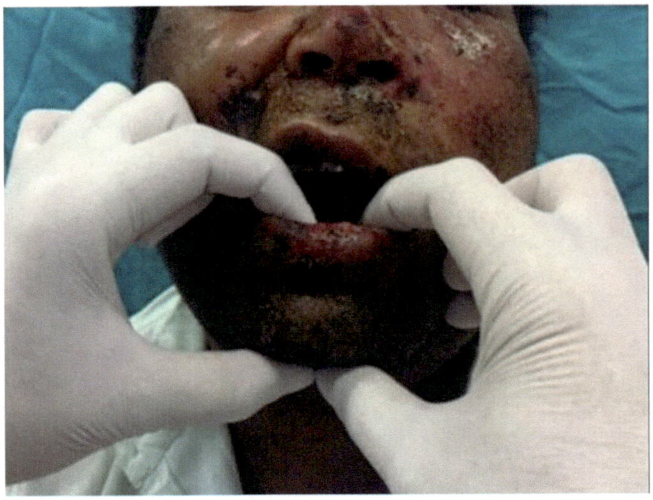

Fig. 52.15 Bimanual palpation

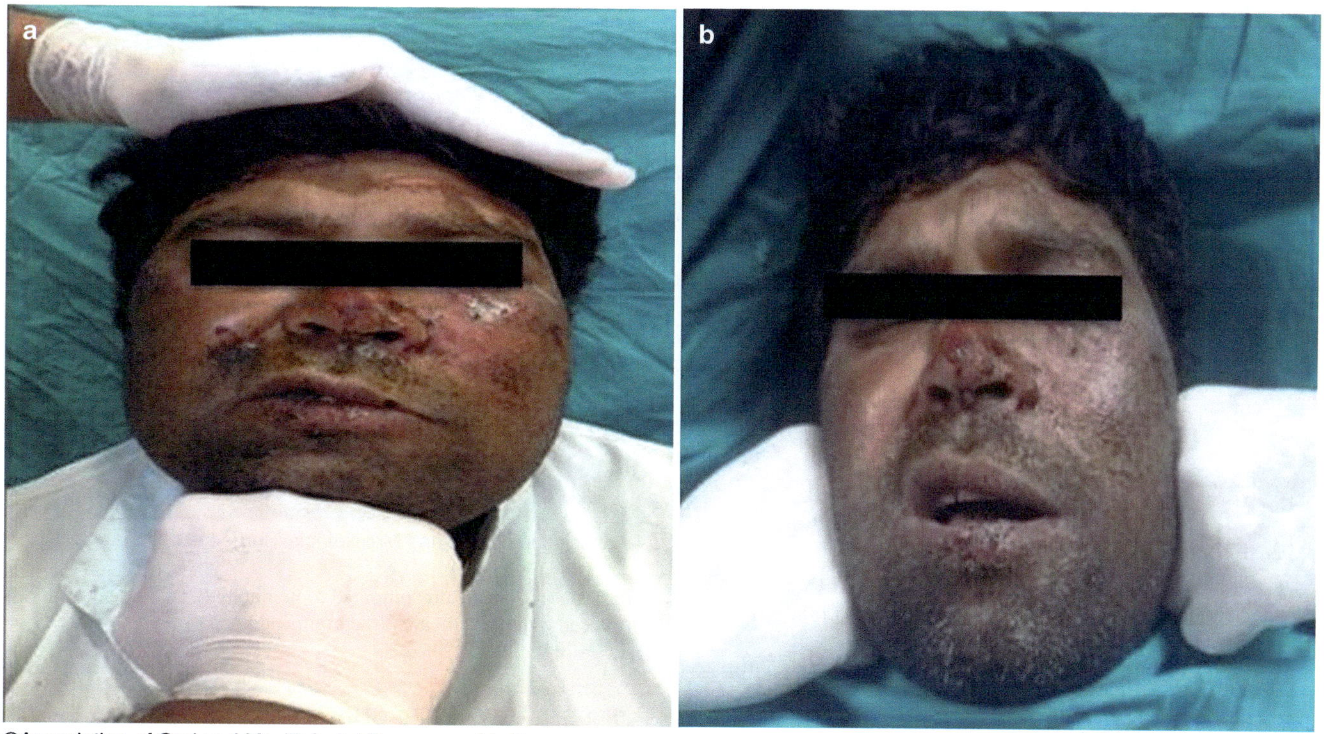

Fig. 52.16 (**a**, **b**) Vertical and horizontal compression test

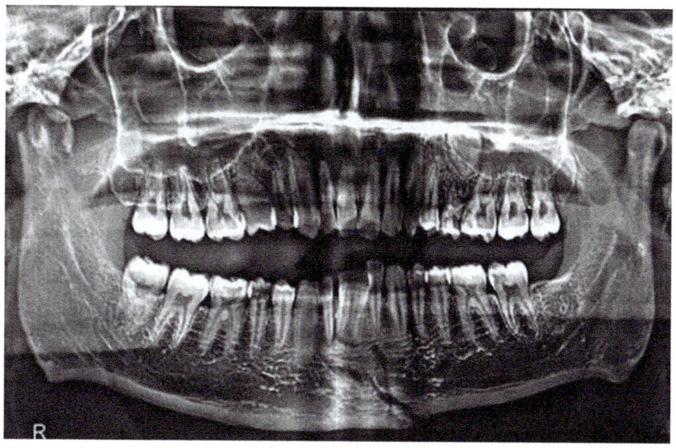

Fig. 52.17 OPG demonstrating parasymphysis and contralateral condylar fracture

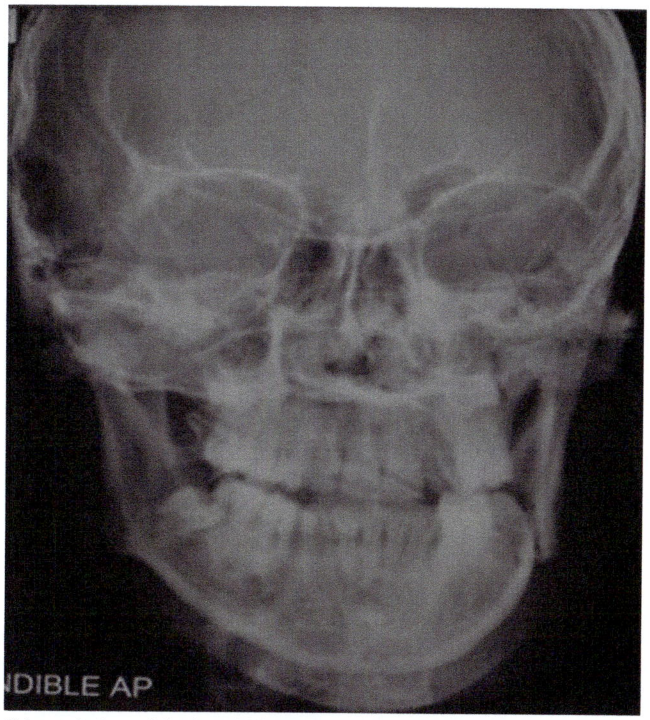

Fig. 52.18 PA view mandible showing left mandibular angle fracture

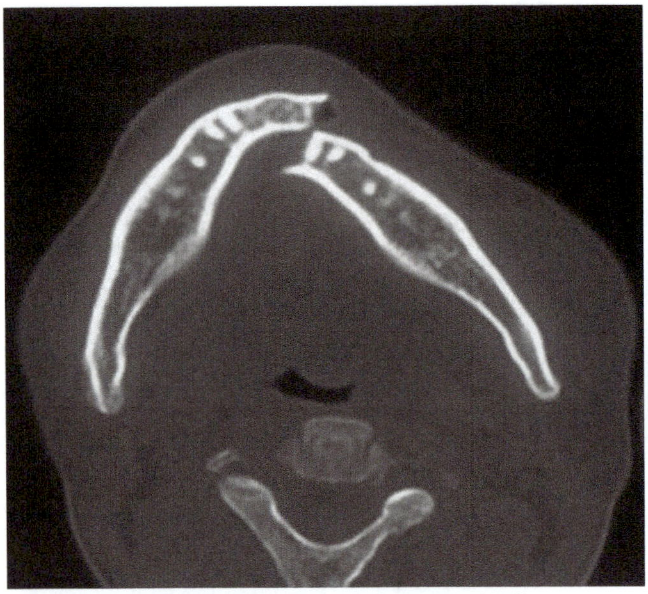

Fig. 52.19 Computed tomography (CT) scan demonstrating displaced left para median fracture

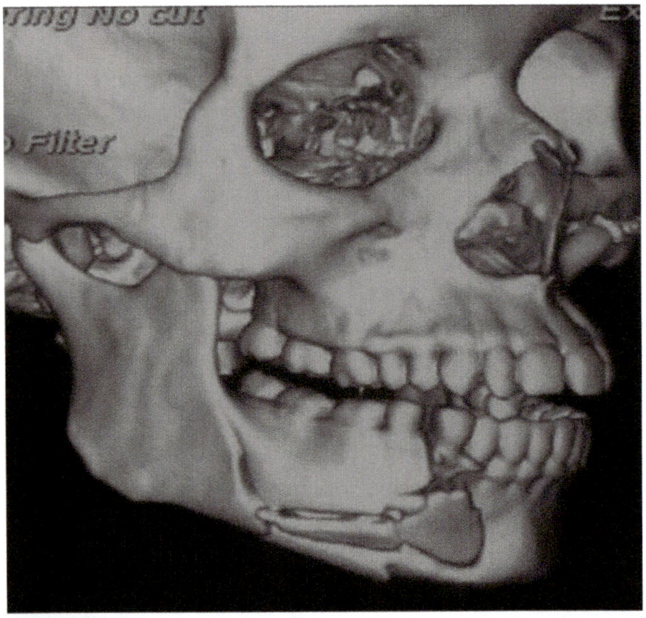

Fig. 52.20 Digital visual tomography (DVT) demonstrating comminuted right body fracture

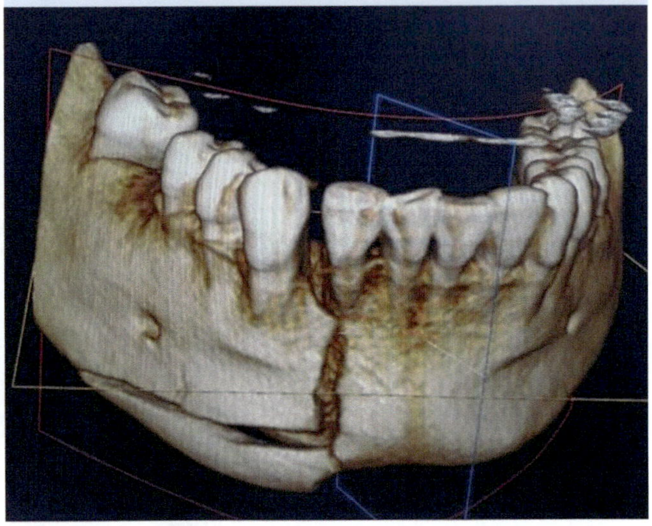

Fig. 52.21 Cone beam computed tomography (CBCT) demonstrating displaced right para median fracture mandible

52.8 Emergency Management (refer Chap. 48 of this book)

Once the basic Airway, breathing, circulation (ABC) in the emergency management has been secured, the suturing of the extra-/intraoral wounds and initial stabilization and immobilization of the fracture fragments are important. Box 52.2 shows advantages of immobilization of fracture fragments.

Initial stabilization and immobilization is done by:

1. **Bridle wiring (refer Chap. 50 of this book)**

   It is a type of temporary stabilization and reduction of the fracture fragments of the dentate segment with the help of 24- or 26-gauge wires under local anesthesia.

   The wire should be wrapped around two healthy teeth adjacent to the fracture line; if the tooth adjacent to the fracture are mobile, the wire should be wrapped around the second tooth adjacent to the fracture (Fig. 52.22a, b).
2. **Supportive bandage**

   These bandages are commonly used to temporarily stabilize the fracture of the lower jaw. Small crepe bandages can be used for mandible fracture.

   (a) Barrel bandage (Fig. 52.23)

   (b) Four-tailed bandage (Fig. 52.24)

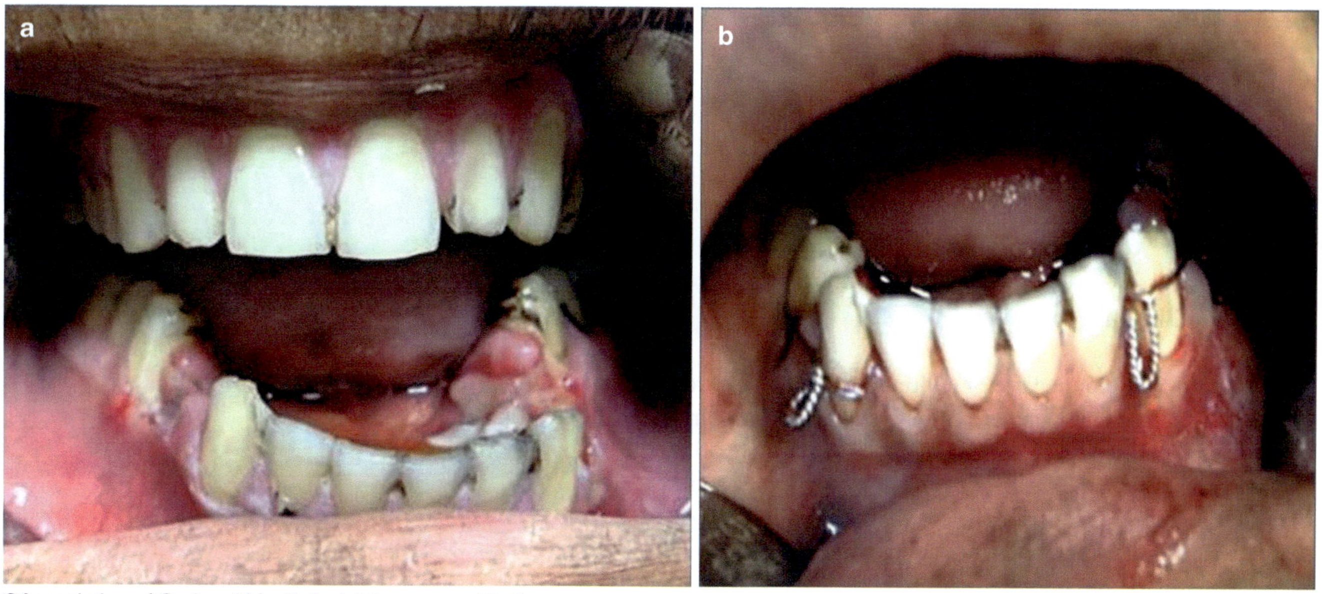

Fig. 52.22 (**a**, **b**) Temporary stabilization of a grossly displaced bilateral body fracture by bridle wiring

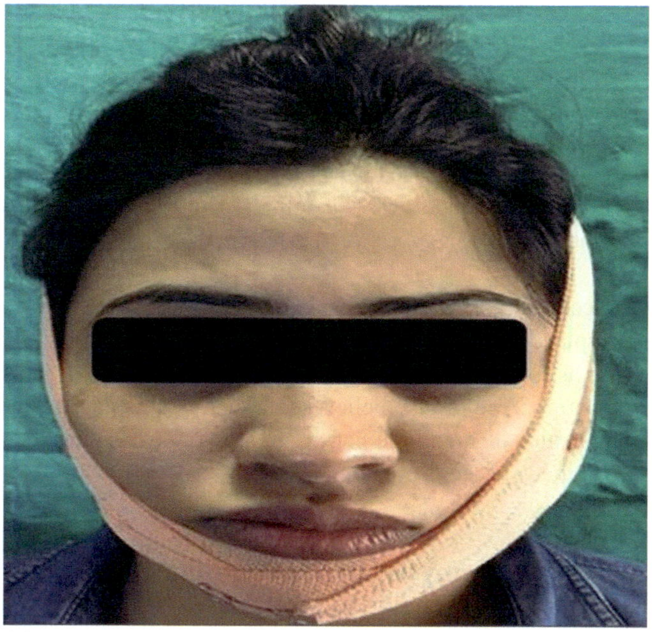

Fig. 52.23 Barrel bandage

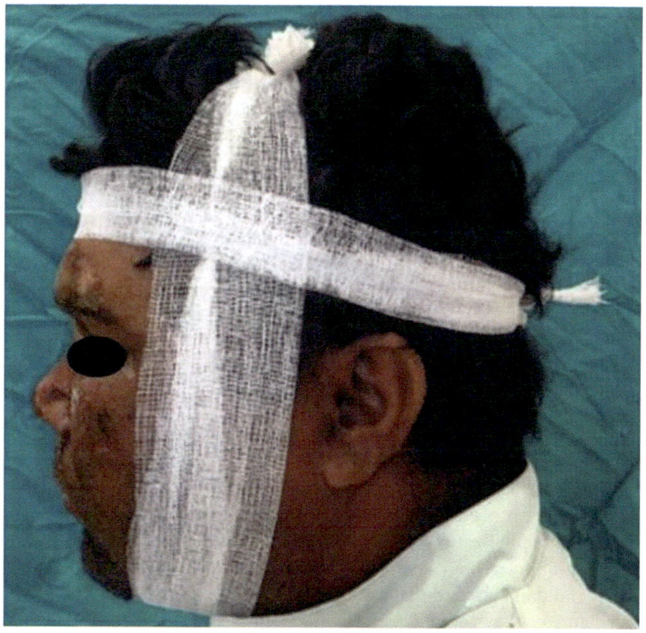

Fig. 52.24 Four-tailed bandage

52.9 Goals of Treatment of Mandibular Fracture (Table 52.5)

52.10 Treatment Options for Different Sites

52.10.1 Closed Reduction (Table 52.6)

52.10.2 Clinical Tip

Wiring techniques required use of multiple wires. These wires cause inadvertent finger puncture to the operator's fingers and increases the risk of spread of blood-borne diseases like HIV and hepatitis. To avoid such complication, Rai [7] recommended the use of dynaplast adhesive tape over all fingertips before wearing sterile gloves while doing Maxillomandibular Fixation (MMF) (Fig. 52.25).

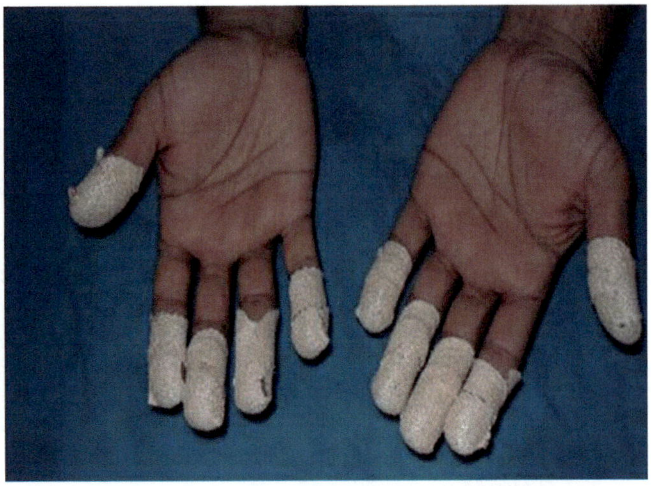

Fig. 52.25 Finger protection before wiring

52.10.3 Open Reduction (Table 52.7)

52.10.4 Steps in Open Reduction Internal Fixation (ORIF) of Mandible Fracture

1. Incision (extra-/intraoral) (Fig. 52.26a, b).
2. Exposure of the fracture site (Fig. 52.27).
3. Curettage to remove the granulation tissues and irrigation with normal saline.
4. Reduction of the fracture (with the help of bone-holding forceps) (Fig. 52.28a–c). Chin retractor is also helpful in reduction of fracture fragments (Fig. 52.29a, b).
5. Immobilization with MMF.
6. Fixation with plates and screws.
7. Closure of the incised site.
8. Pressure bandage over the surgical site to avoid postoperative hematoma formation in required cases (Fig. 52.30).

Table 52.5 Treatment goals for mandibular fracture

1.	Anatomical restitution
2.	Immobilization
3.	Prevention of postoperative complications
4.	Rehabilitation of Functions

Table 52.6 Advantages and disadvantages of closed reduction

Advantages	Disadvantages
1. Day-care procedure, not require hospitalization 2. Cost-effective and safe 3. Avoid damage to the vital structures	1. Restriction of mouth opening for minimum of 4 weeks 2. Patients can take only liquid diet 3. Difficult to maintain oral hygiene 4. Challenging in partially edentulous patients 5. Weight loss 6. Partial trismus for few weeks 7. Contraindicated in asthmatic, in parkinsonism, mentally challenged patients

Table 52.7 Advantages and disadvantages of open reduction

Advantages	Disadvantages
1. Early return to function 2. Exact anatomic reduction under direct visualization 3. No need of MMF in most of the cases 4. Less chances of postoperative complications	1. Requires hospitalization 2. Risk of general anesthesia 3. Extra oral scarring 4. Risk of injuries to the vital structures 5. Expensive to patients when compared to closed reduction

According to Dimitroulis [8] MMF is unnecessary in undisplaced angle fracture if there is a skilled assistant present to assist and help manually reduce the fracture fragments for plating. Author also believes that many undisplaced, single fracture of mandible can be fixed without MMF when two skilled surgeons operate the case.

52.10.5 Symphysis and Parasymphysis Fracture (Video 52.1)

Various internal fixation techniques were mentioned in the literature for both symphysis and parasymphysis fractures [9]. They are enumerated in Table 52.8.

Note: Readers has to refer Chap. 51 on plating systems to know the principles of osteosynthesis, tension banding, zone of compression/tension, etc.

Fixation with two miniplates is widely used for the fixation of symphysis and parasymphysis fractures (Fig. 52.31). Some authors preferred use of two lag screws (Fig. 52.32a, b) for the fixation of symphysis fractures, but their uses are less in comparison to two miniplates because they are technique sensitive. Three-dimensional plates require less manipulation and adaptation which indirectly reduce the operating time

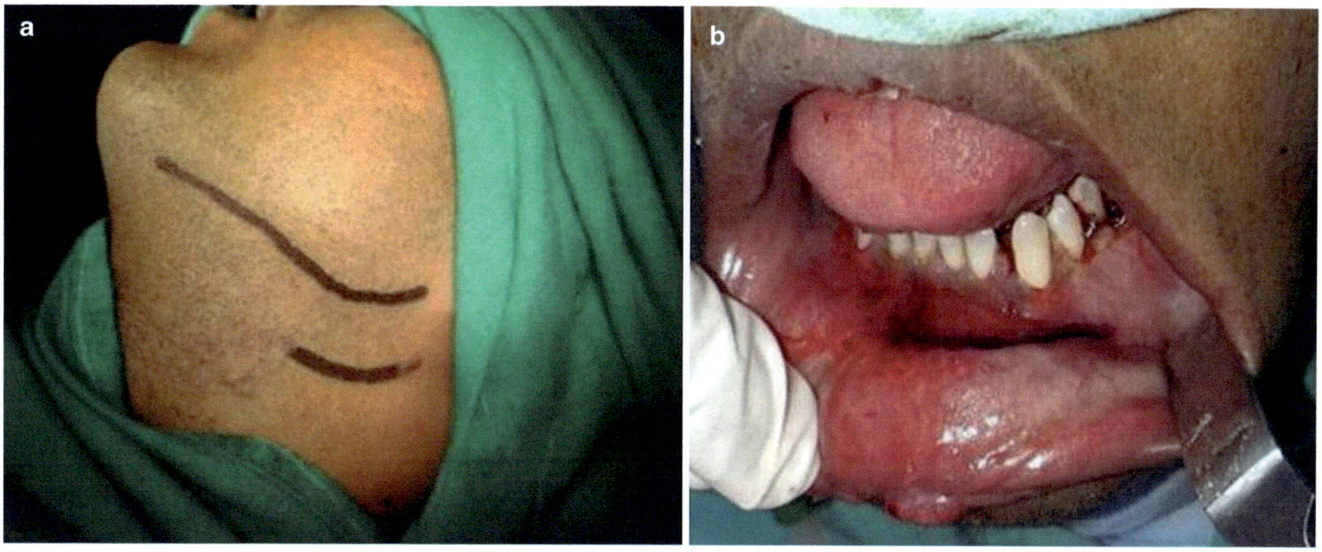

Fig. 52.26 (**a**, **b**) Extraoral sub mandibular incision and intraoral vestibular incision

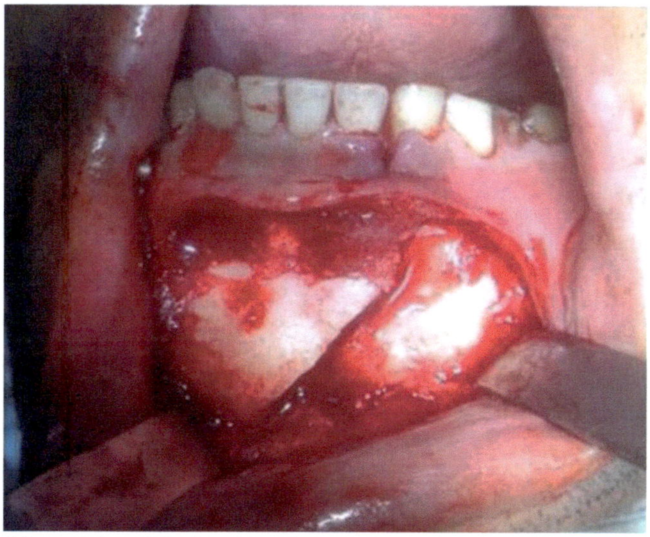

Fig. 52.27 Exposure of the fracture site (left paramedian mandible via vestibular incision)

(Fig. 52.33), but use of it is questionable when fracture fragments are multiple even in isolated symphysis fractures.

Usually, an intraoral approach is preferred for management of symphysis and parasymphysis fractures. However, if an existing laceration or scar is present, it should be utilized for exposure of fractured segments and subsequent management (Fig. 52.34).

52.10.6 Parasymphysis Fracture

1. Mental nerve: The anatomic challenge in ORIF.
2. Plating should be done after the blunt dissection and retraction of the neurovascular bundle.
3. One miniplate above and another below the mental nerve used for fixation of parasymphysis fracture (Fig. 52.35).

52.10.7 Mandibular Angle

The prevalence of angle fractures ranges from 16.5 to 37 % in the literature. Presence of third molar (3M) increases the chance of angle fracture by 3.27 times, and class II-B positions of 3M are the most favorable for angle fracture, while class I-A act as protective factors [10].

52.10.7.1 Impact of Presence or Absence of Impacted Mandibular Third Molar (IM3M) on Angle and Condylar Fracture

- Presence of IM3M generates a weak area in the mandibular angle and predisposes the angle region to fracture after injury; on the other hand, IM3M can decrease the occurrence of condylar fracture which is supposed to be the weakest area of mandible [11].
- Angle fracture is seen most commonly in patients having superficially impacted (vs deeply impacted) third molars (M3s) [12]. The reason behind this is that the mandibular strength is derived from maintenance of cortical and not the medullary bone integrity; this cortical integrity of the external ridge is disrupted by the presence of superficial impacted M3s which produce the point of weakness in the mandible and make it more prone to fractures [13].

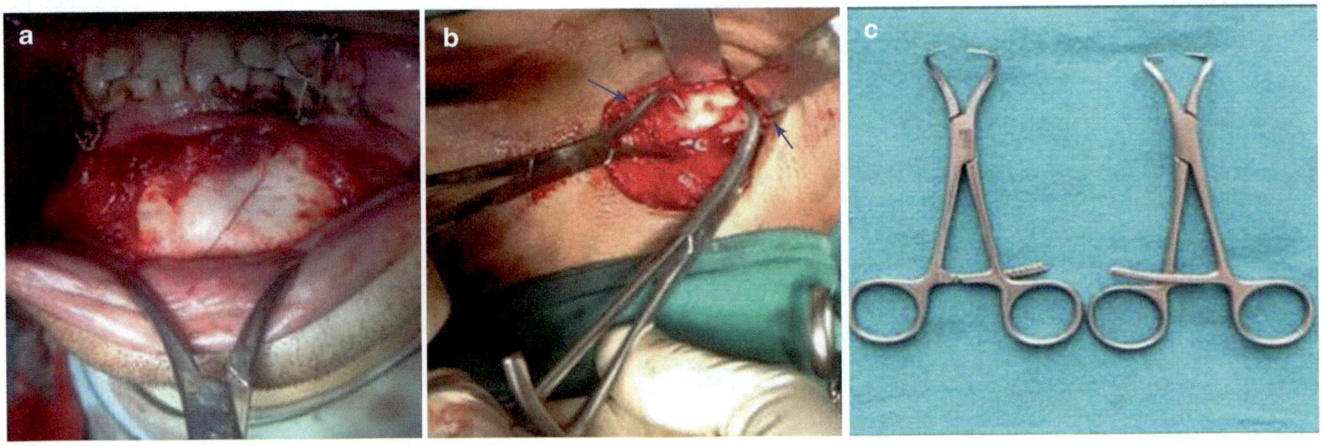

Fig. 52.28 (**a**–**c**) Reduction of the fracture (with the help of bone holding forceps)

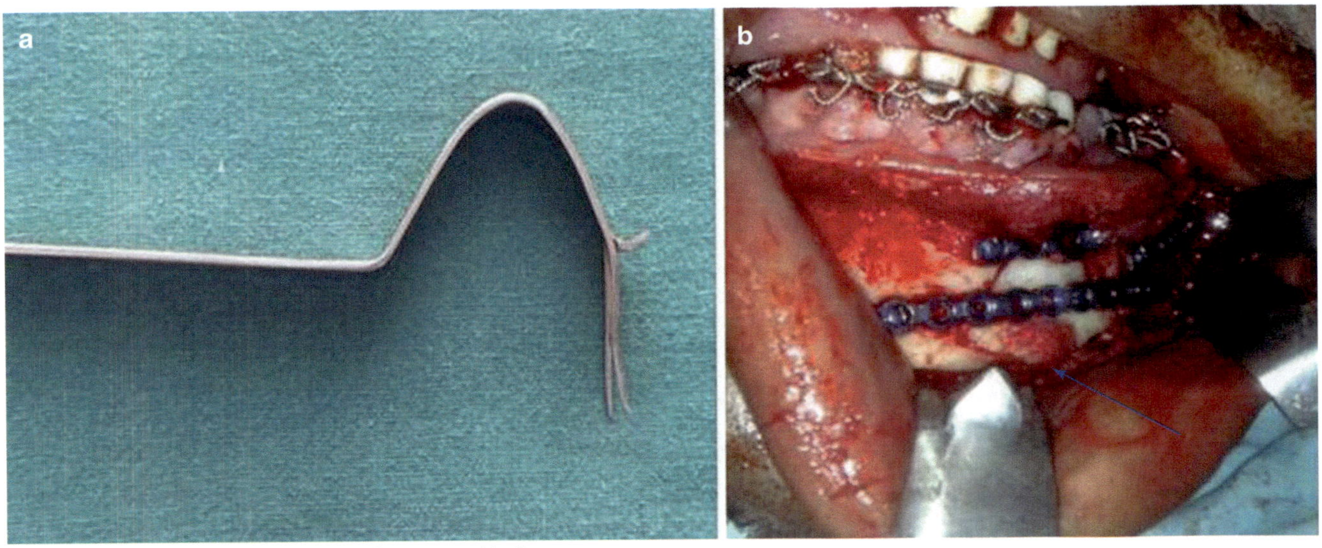

Fig. 52.29 (**a**, **b**) Use of chin retractor in reduction of fracture fragments

52.10.7.2 Open vs. Closed Reduction

Closed reduction is advisable for patients who are medically unfit for surgery (due to any reasons) or those who did not give consent for open reduction internal fixation (ORIF).

52.10.7.3 Approaches for ORIF

1. Intraoral (Fig. 52.36)
2. Extraoral (Fig. 52.26a)
3. Transbuccal (Fig. 52.37)

Intraoral incision is advocated for ORIF with single miniplate, but higher infection rate of 13% was reported in comparison with 2% when extraoral incision was used for plating. Marginal mandibular nerve showed weakness in 8% of cases, and it sometimes has prominent extraoral scarring in patients treated with extraoral approach [14] .

Sugar [15] concluded that the combined use of transbuccal and intraoral approach is safe and effective than the intraoral approach alone for ORIF. Author too prefers the same approach.

52.10.7.4 Advantages of Transbuccal Approach [16]

1. Less operative time
2. Minimal scar formation
3. At the time of plating, direct visualization of the occlusion
4. Low risk of injury to facial nerve

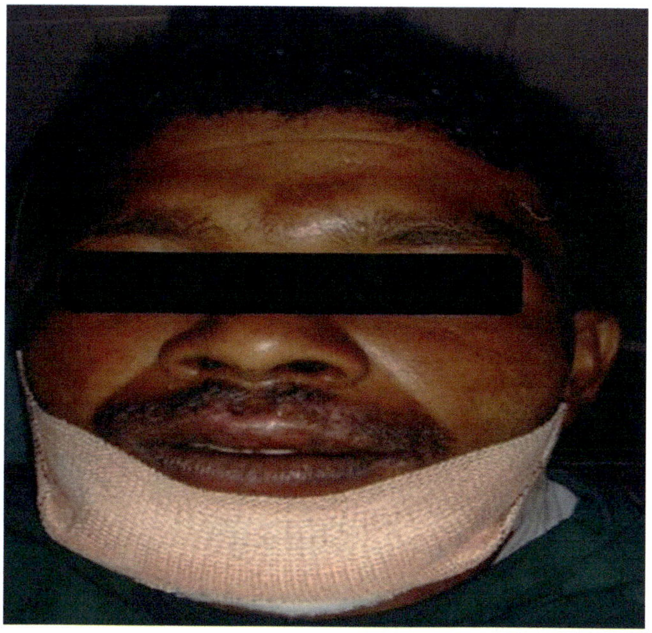

Fig. 52.30 Application of pressure bandage

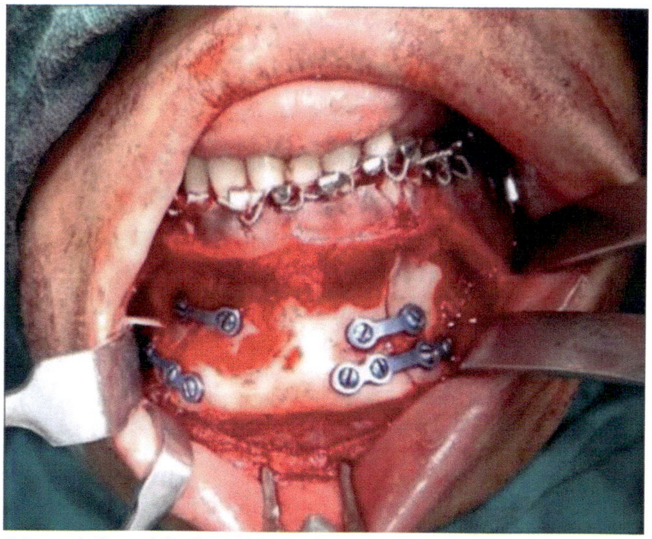

Fig. 52.31 Fixation bilateral paramedian fracture mandible with 2 miniplates each on either side

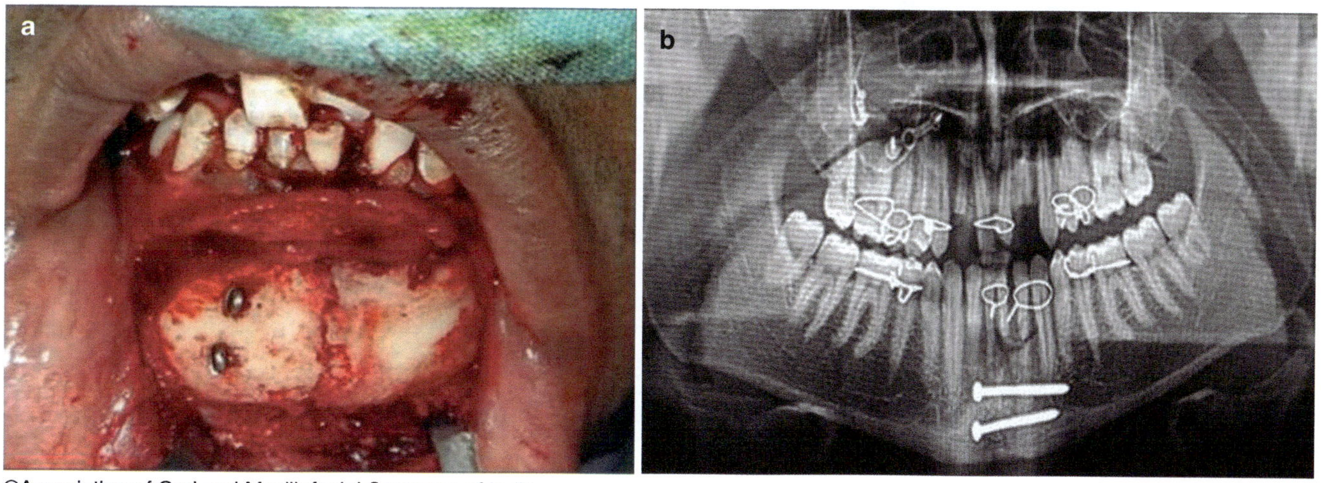

Fig. 52.32 (**a**, **b**) Fixation left para median fracture mandible with lag screws

Position of Trocar Placement [17] (Fig. 52.37)

Gulses et al. described a safe zone to place the trocar in the form of a triangle created by drawing three lines on the face.

Line 1: At the lower border of mandible (mandibular line)
Line 2: Gonial-canthal line which ran from the gonion to the outer canthus of the eye
Line 3: Trago-basal line which ran from tragus to the groove over the body of the mandible at infero-anterior angle of the masseter (at the point of entry of the facial artery over the body of the mandible)

Table 52.8 Various fixation techniques for anterior mandibular fracture

1.	Reconstruction bone plates
2.	Single strong nonreconstruction bone plate
3.	Double miniplates
4.	Two lag screws
5.	Three-dimensional (3D) plate
6.	Segmental arch bar with single large and stronger bone plate

Through a small stab incision, a blunt dissection is performed with dissecting scissors till the mandibular periosteum is torn and the trocar is placed through the dissected channel.

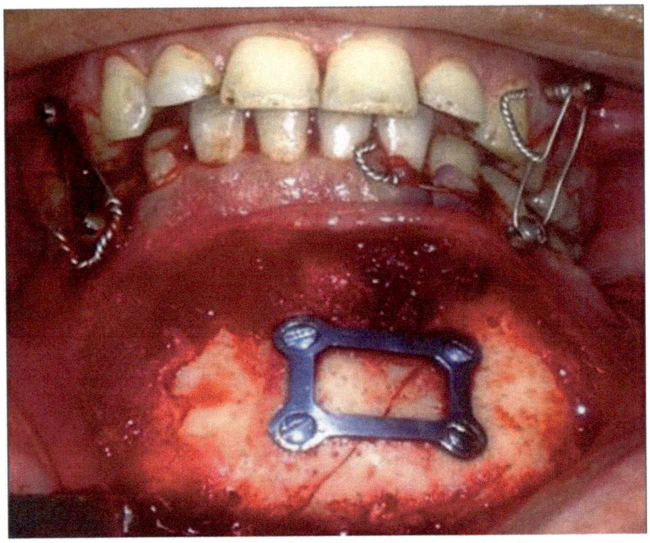

Fig. 52.33 Fixation of anterior mandible with three-dimensional plate

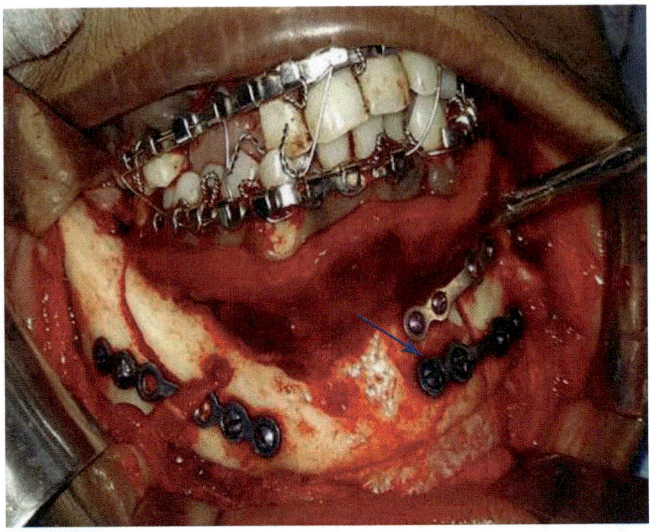

Fig. 52.35 One miniplate above and another below the mental nerve used for fixation of parasymphysis fracture

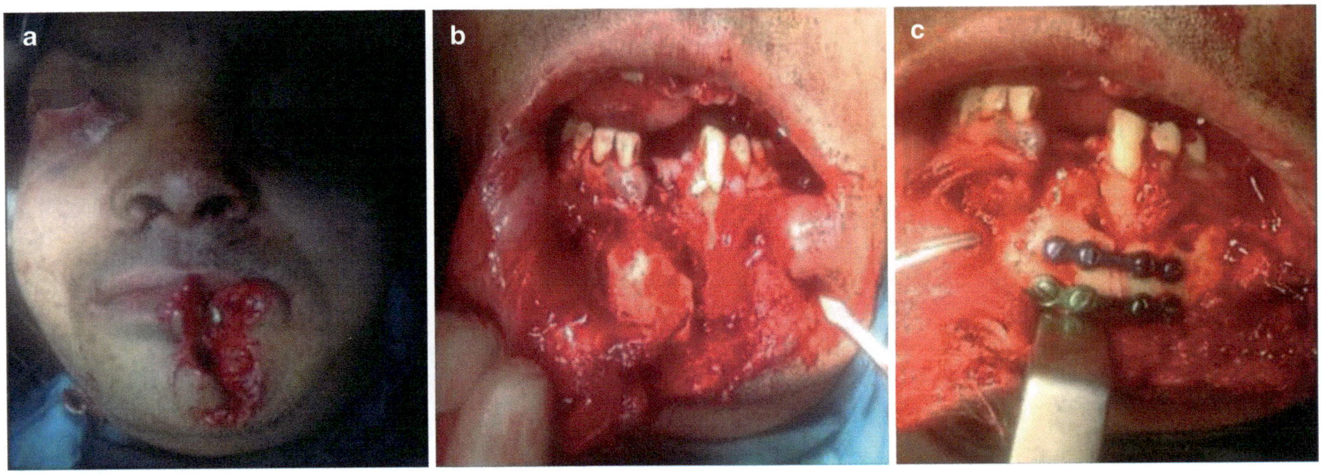

Fig. 52.34 (**a–c**) Existing laceration has been used as access for fixation of the anterior mandible fracture

Various techniques are mentioned in the literature for internal fixation of angle fracture (Box 52.3) [18]:

Box 52.3: Fixation Techniques for Angle Fracture

1. Wire osteosynthesis (obsolete)
2. Single miniplate on the superior border (Fig. 52.38)
3. Single plate on inferior border
4. Two plates, one at superior and another on inferior border (Fig. 52.39a, b)
5. Lag screws
6. Three-dimensional plates (Fig. 52.40)

52.10.7.5 Single vs. Two Plates vs. 3D Plates

Al Moraissi [19] in a meta-analysis showed that the incidence of wound infection, dehiscence, hardware failure, and overall complications were less in patients treated with one miniplate on external oblique ridge in comparison to two.

Ellis III [20] also advocated use of single miniplate on superior border because:

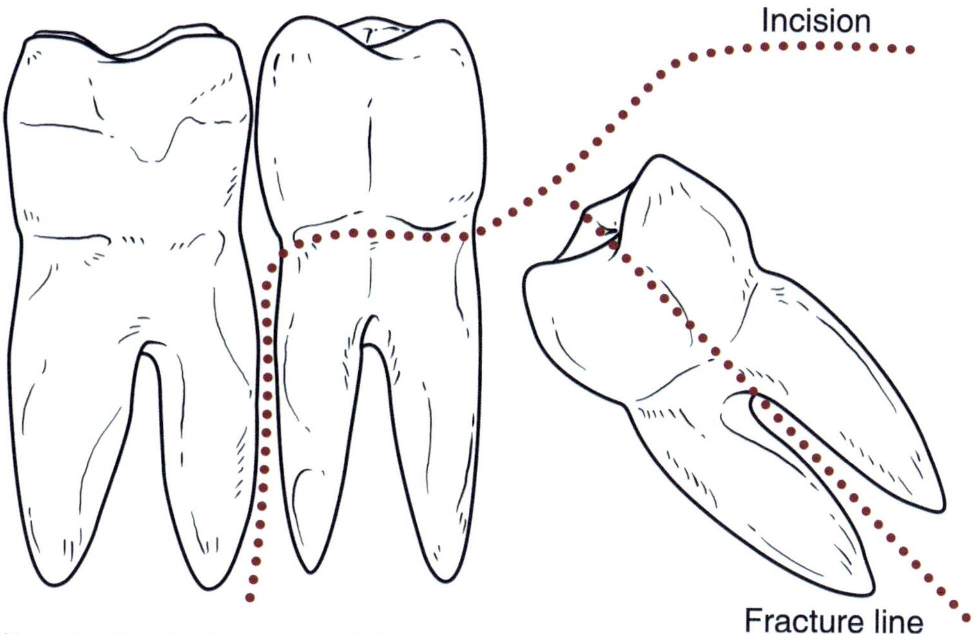

Fig. 52.36 Intraoral incision for exposure

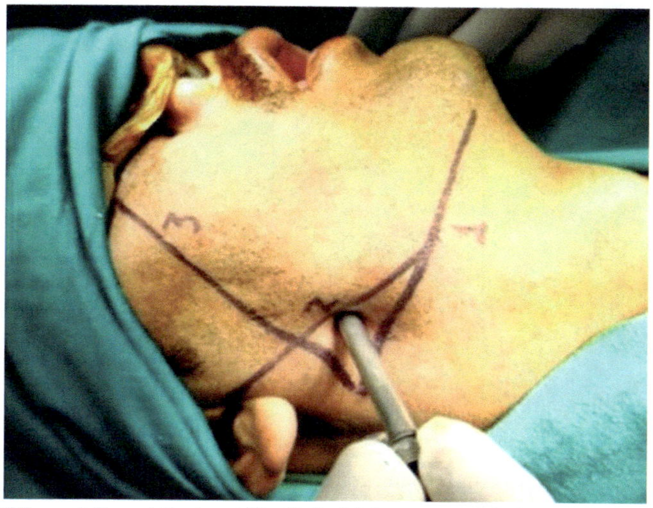

Fig. 52.37 Transbuccal approach used for fixation of angle fractures

- High rate of sequestrectomy, infection, and subsequent second surgery was more in two-plate technique.
- Fixation with two plates took more time, i.e., average 37 min in comparison to an average of 23.5 min in single miniplate fixation from incision to suturing.
- Second plate fixation at inferior border is more difficult and requires more experience.

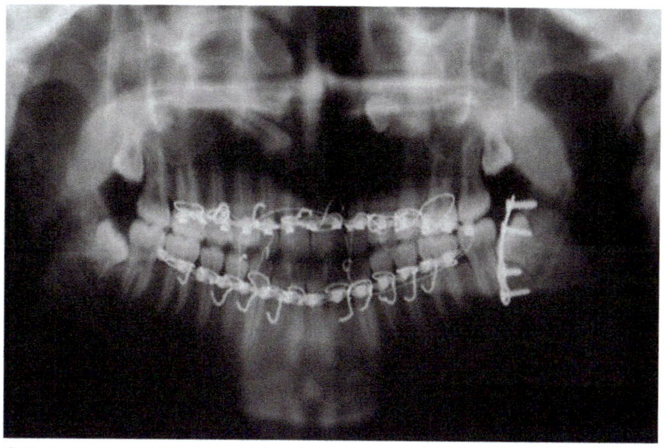

Fig. 52.38 Fixation of mandibular angle fracture using single miniplate

- If infection occurs, retrieval of single miniplate can be done under local anesthesia in a clinic, but two plates commonly required general anesthesia which indirectly increases the cost and prolonged the hospital stay.

Rai et al. [21] also conclude better results with two-plate fixation. Second miniplate is supposed to increase stability and protects the fracture site against torsion and bending.

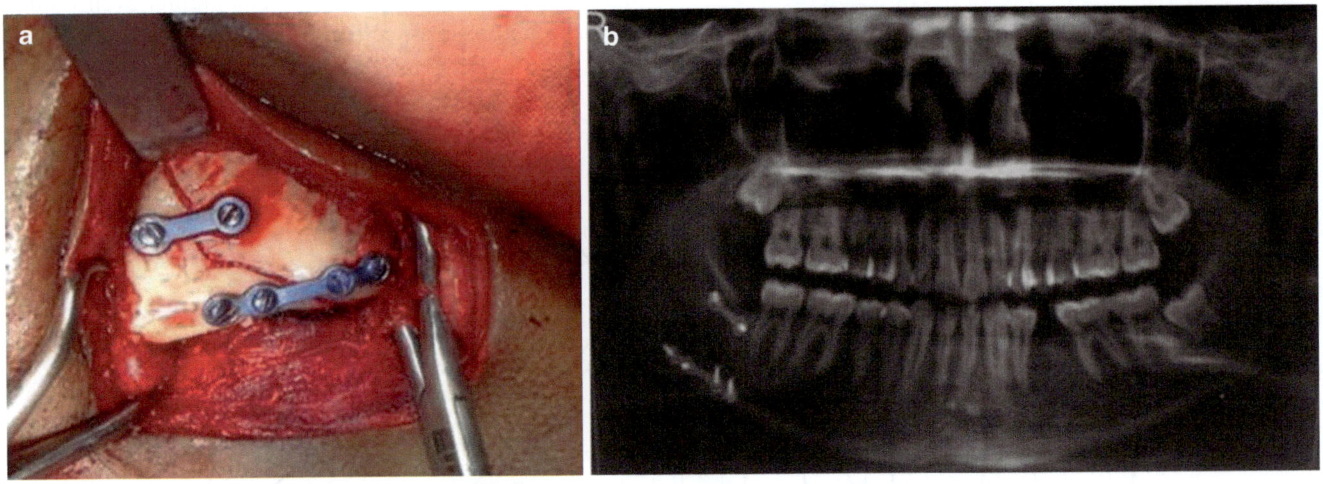

Fig. 52.39 Fixation of mandibular angle fracture using two miniplates. (**a**) Clinical picture, (**b**) orthopantamogram

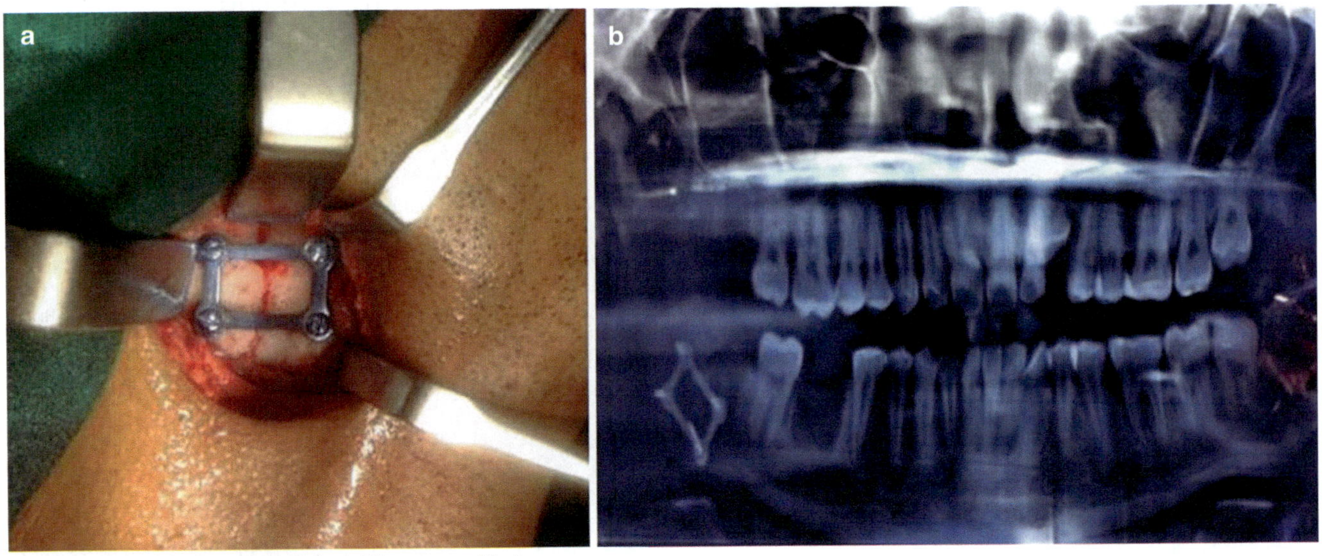

Fig. 52.40 Fixation of mandibular angle fracture using 3D plate. (**a**) Clinical picture, (**b**) orthopantamogram

Theoretically second plate establishes a second line of osteosynthesis.

Levy et al. [22]advocated two-plate fixation superior for ORIF of angle fracture. According to them two miniplates provide better stabilization and have reported lowest complication rate in comparison to any other plating technique.

Wusiman et al. [23] demonstrate that three-dimensional (3D) miniplates provide better fixation than standard miniplates. It also provides simultaneous stabilization of tension and compression zones with lower incidence of postoperative complications and good results. According to Zix et al. [24] 1-mm-thick 3D plate is as stable as 2 mm miniplates, and it offers better bending stability and more resistant to out of plane movement or torque.

Ellis III and Ghali [25] used lag screws for treating mandibular angle fractures but reported very high incidence of postoperative infection and bone exposure. Also the fixation of angle with lag screws is technique sensitive and requires expertise.

Kang and Zide used seven-hole angle plate when Champy technique is ineffective and more rigid or semirigid fixation is required [26]. According to them seven-hole angle plate is fixed through transfacial trocar and stabilized intraorally. On the other hand, Champy plate required bending, lacks rigidity, difficulty in screw hole drilling, inaccurate centric placement of screws.

52.10.7.6 Extraction vs. Retention of IM3M in Angle Fracture

The use of postoperative MMF and extraction versus retention of teeth in the line of fracture did not influence any of the outcomes [27]. Increase rate of infection by extraction of a tooth was found in the study by Ellis and Walker in 1994 [28]. However, in another study published in 2002, Ellis [29] reported an increased incidence of infection if teeth were left in the line of fracture. Author advocates extraction of 3Ms at the time of ORIF for better results.

52.10.8 Body Fracture

A single four hole with gap miniplate (Fig. 52.41) below the root apex and the inferior alveolar canal is sufficient for fixation of body fracture of mandible through the intraoral approach most of the times, except when a patient is having extraoral soft tissue injury/scar or having severely comminuted fracture fragments.

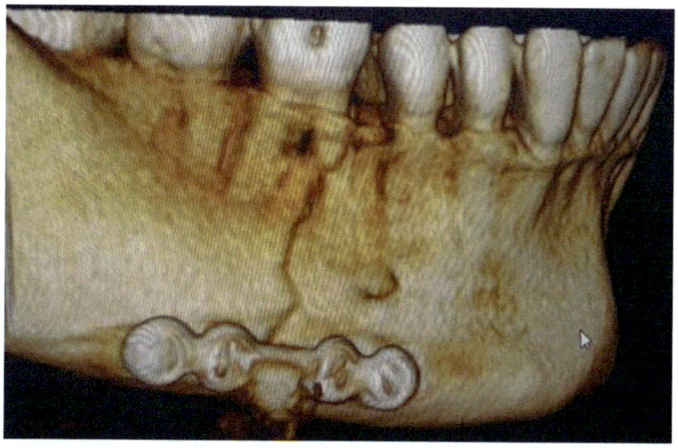

Fig. 52.41 Fixation of body fracture with single miniplate

52.10.9 Ramus Fracture

Mandibular ramus (MR) fracture occurs rarely and ranked third least common fracture after alveolar and coronoid fracture [30]. MR fractures are very rare in isolation. It can be horizontal or vertical. Its incidence ranges from 0.9 to 5.5% [31]. Isolated ramus fracture can be managed by closed reduction, but ORIF is the treatment of choice when it is associated with other maxillofacial fractures. To correct the facial height when midface is also fractured, the vertical rami become the only determinant, and re-establishment of these buttresses is very important before repositioning the crushed midfacial bones [32] (Fig. 52.42a–c).

52.10.9.1 Management of Triangular Fragments (TF) at the Lower Border

Heslop et al. [33] advocated repositioning of TF if they are attached to the muscle or periosteum and remove them if they are very small or detached from the periosteum.

According to Blinder et al. [34] to prevent infection and preserve vascularization, TF should be unexposed and unreduced. TF should be sandwiched between the two fracture lines by rigid fixation without exposure, and preserving vascularization may be the treatment of choice

TF of bone at the angle region were more often shown to get infected in comparison to body, symphysis, or parasymphysis because thick, better vascularized, and more cancellous bone presents in these areas as compared to angle region. It's better to remove small fragments in the angle region to avoid postoperative discomfort.

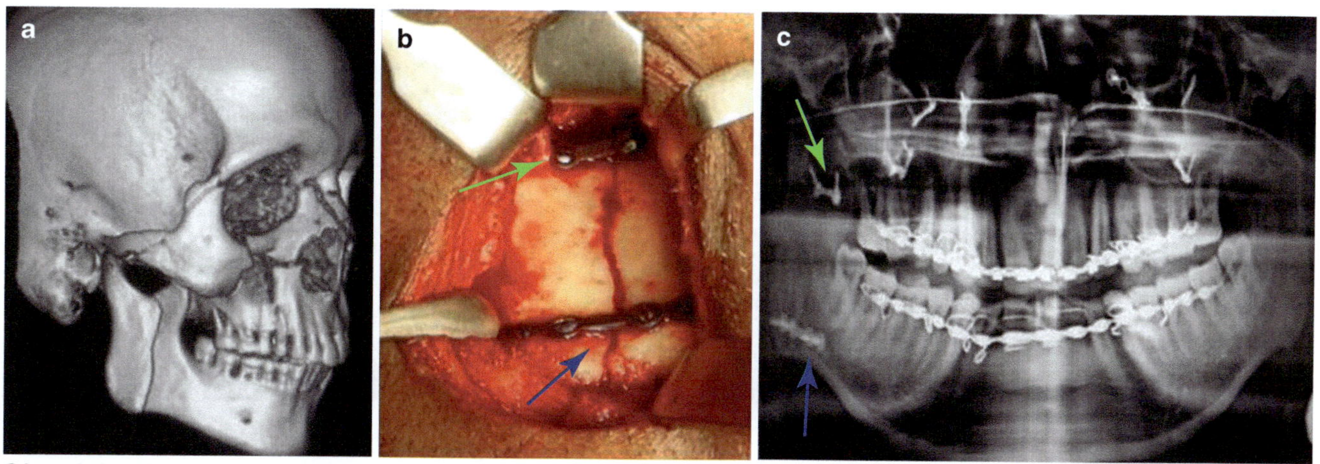

Fig. 52.42 Management of mandibular ramus fracture. (**a**) DVT showing mandibular ramus fracture, (**b**) fixation using two miniplates, (**c**) postoperative orthopantamogram showing fixation of mandibular ramus and midface fractures (blue arrows point to lower border plates and green arrows point to upper border plates)

52.10.10 Coronoid Fracture

It generally occurs in combination with other fracture of the mandible (Fig. 52.43a), and with zygomatic complex fracture (commonly with arch) (Fig. 52.43b), rarely does it occur in isolation. It can be treated by extraoral or intraoral approaches. Later, having low incidence of facial nerve injury and no facial scar. Coronoid fracture ranges from 0.6 to 4.7% of all facial fractures and 1–2.9% of all mandibular fractures [35].

It manifests as [36, 37]:

- Swelling below the zygomatic arch
- Ecchymosis in the retromolar trigone area
- Restricted mouth opening, malocclusion, and facial collapse when occurs in association with other facial fractures

52.10.10.1 Indications for Conservative or Open Reduction of Coronoid Fractures (Table 52.9)

Conservative management in the form of soft diet and mouth opening exercises to avoid bony adhesions to the surrounding structures [38]. If patients are treated with MMF and trismus occurs, it can be managed by removal of the coronoid process [39].

52.10.11 Bilateral Fracture of Mandible

Over half of the mandibular fractures are bilateral; in the case of angle fracture, most of the times, it occurs in combination of contralateral mandibular body and symphysis [40]. ORIF is the treatment of choice most of the times.

Clinical Tip: An MMF screw can be effectively used for reduction of a bilateral mandibular fracture by placing the screw in the symphysis region. A wire is passed through the screw, and the fracture segment can be manipulated for reduction (Fig. 52.44).

Table 52.9 Indications of closed and open reduction for coronoid fractures

Conservative	ORIF
Minimal displacement	Significant fracture displacement and
	Limited mouth opening
	Associated with zygoma, zygomatic arch, mandibular ramus
	Patients who are bad candidates for MMF

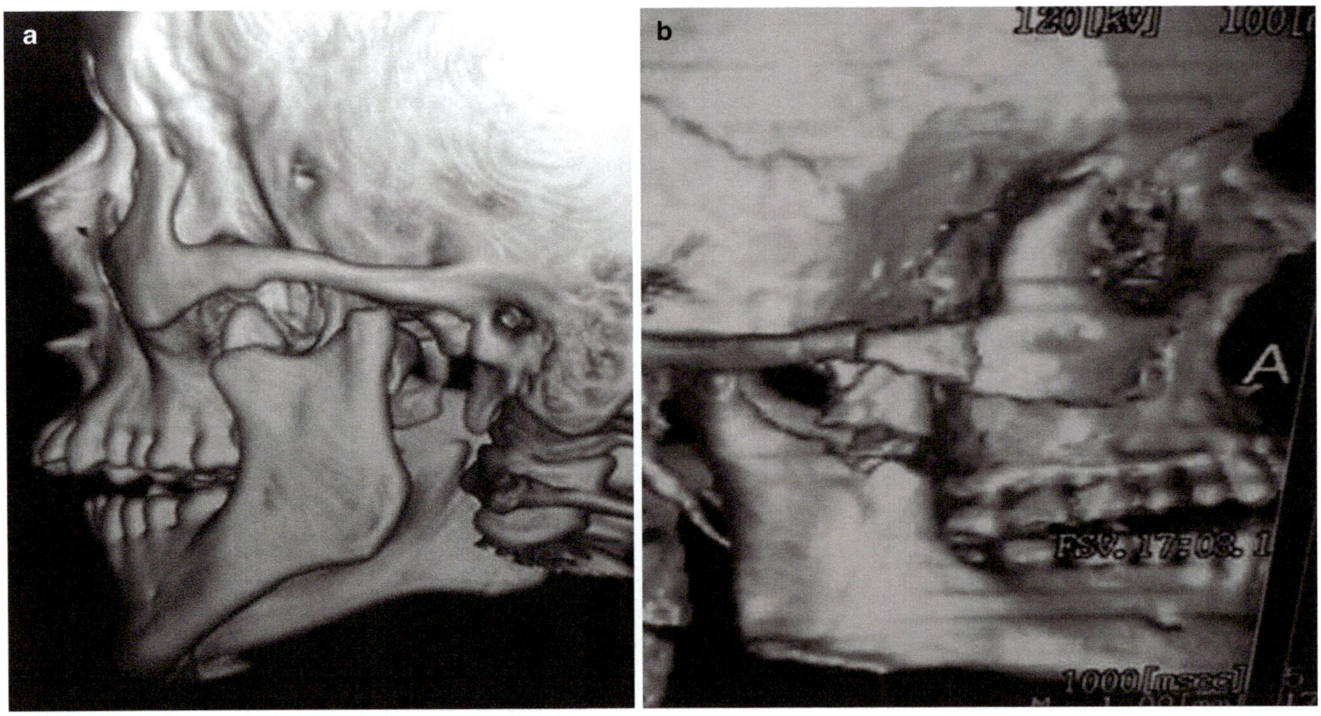

Fig. 52.43 Coronoid fracture (**a**) associated with condylar fracture, (**b**) associated with zygomatic arch

52.10.12 Comminuted Mandible Fractures

Comminution is defined as presence of multiple fracture lines in many small pieces within the same area of mandibular angle, body, ramus, and symphysis [41]. This type of fracture rarely occurs in the condyle region. In a comminuted fracture, bone is "crushed, broken, splintered" into number of pieces, creating multiple small fragments (at least two free segments of bone) (Fig. 52.45a, b).

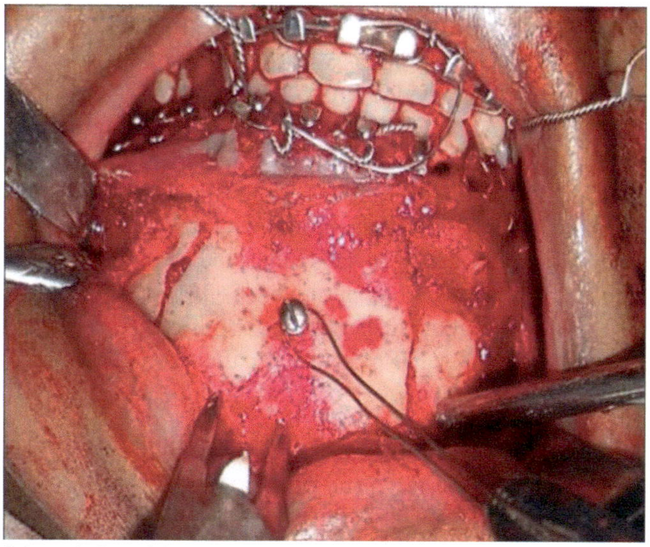

Fig. 52.44 Use of MMF screw in reduction of bilateral parasymphysis fracture

To fix small fragments, multiple options are mentioned in the literature like miniplate, microplate, screws, steel wires, and absorbable sutures. A fragment larger than 1 cm should be conserved, reduced, and fixed [42].

Ellis et al. [43] advocated that more complications are associated with multiple fragment fractures in comparison to fractures having few segments. Therefore, comminuted fractures need load-bearing fixation.

The bone fragments will not provide buttressing to help stabilize the fracture; therefore surgeons operating comminuted mandibular fractures having two or more free bone fragments and/or requiring bone fragment removal should opt for reconstruction plates. Miniplates can be used when comminuted mandibular fractures have only one free bone fragment. Combination of reconstruction and miniplates can be used when multiple small fragments are there in comminuted mandible fracture (Fig. 52.46). Implants used for fixation of comminuted fractures are mentioned in Box 52.4.

Use of reconstruction plates required expertise and it is time-consuming. Sometimes contour is also not favorable

Box 52.4: Implants Used for Fixation of Comminuted Fractures

1. Multiple miniplates
2. Reconstruction plates
3. Combination of mini- and reconstruction plates
4. Titanium Mesh

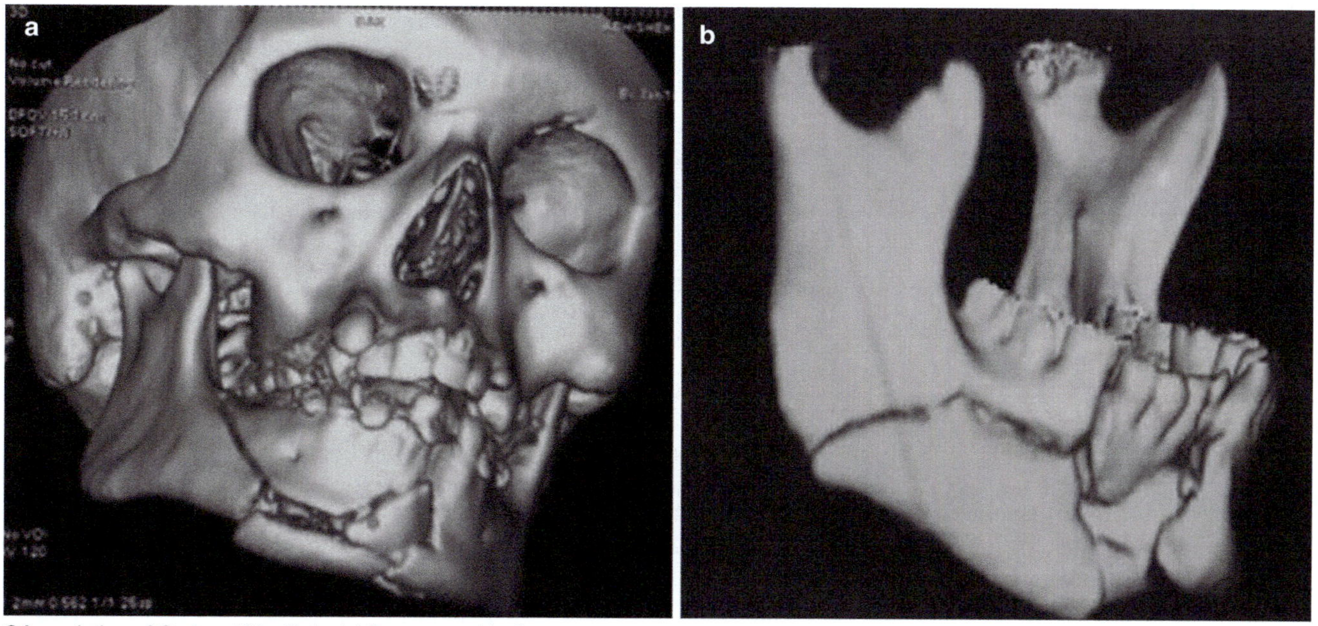

Fig. 52.45 (**a**, **b**) Comminuted fractures

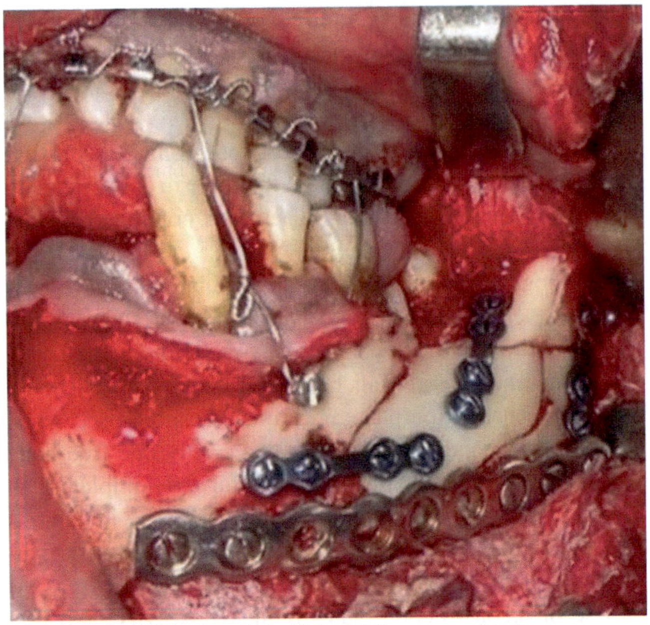

Fig. 52.46 Combination of reconstruction and miniplates in management of comminuted fractures

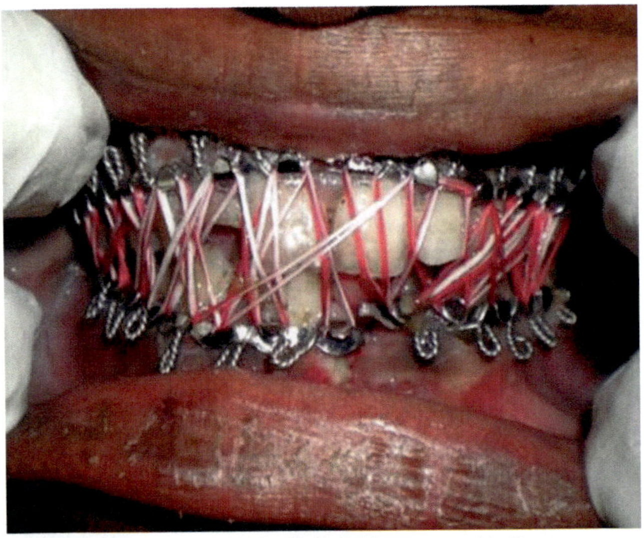

Fig. 52.47 Postoperative elastics for correction of minor occlusal discrepancies (Inter maxillary elastics- IME)

which can create slight malocclusion but can be managed by postoperative elastics and selective occlusal adjustments (Fig. 52.47).

Dia et al. [44] used titanium mesh for the treatment of comminuted mandible fracture with successful results. According to them mesh required little soft tissue exposure, had low infection rate, and provides favorable mandibular morphology.

52.11 Inferior Alveolar Nerve (IAN) Injury in Mandible Fracture

According to the literature, the incidence of IAN injury was [45]:

1. 5.4–81.4% before treatment
2. 0.4–91.3% after intervention
3. 0–46.6% after 1 year

The neurosensory testing was done both before and after the treatment of mandibular fracture in which nerve injury is suspected. Two-point discrimination and pinprick testing can be used to assess the level of IAN injury. Preoperative knowledge of the patient's IAN position (based on CT/CBCT) is very important in decision-making regarding fixation position of the fracture fragments with miniplates. Plating should be done above or below the course of IAN. ORIF in the area of IAN takes longer duration to normalization of sensation, and it ranges from 1 week to 12 months. Postoperative CT/CBCT is mandatory if operating surgeon suspected the impingement of screw on the IAN or no relief of sensation after 6 weeks of ORIF for further management. Surgeons should not hesitate to redo the surgery in cases of IAN injury by miniplates and screws.

52.12 Geriatric Mandibular Fracture

With old age, the incidence rate of maxillofacial fracture increases, with mandibular fracture appearing with a greater frequency. As the age advances, the weakening of the mandible occurs due to:

- Loss of teeth
- Reduced vascularity or decreased blood flow in elderly
- Loss of bone mass

The most common mechanisms of injury in geriatric patients are [46]:

1. Fall
2. Assaults
3. Motor vehicle accidents

Fractures of the edentulous mandible pose unique challenges. Old age itself is a risk factor for poor outcomes following trauma. There are associated comorbidities like hypertension, diabetes mellitus, dementia, or stroke which limit the functional capacity of the patient to bear the stress of surgery and postoperative recovery. Also, the atrophic mandible has compromised blood supply with little osteogenic potential resulting in delayed bone healing. Bilateral mandibular fracture (bucket handle fracture) occurs most commonly in elderly (Fig. 52.48).

52.12.1 Management

Controversy exists in the treatment of edentulous mandibular fracture. One school of thought advocated closed reduction, and another school is in favor of open reduction and internal fixation. According to Bradley [47] the major blood supply to the mandible is "sub periosteal Plexus," and reflection of periosteum in ORIF may seriously impair vascular supply to the bone resulting in non-union.

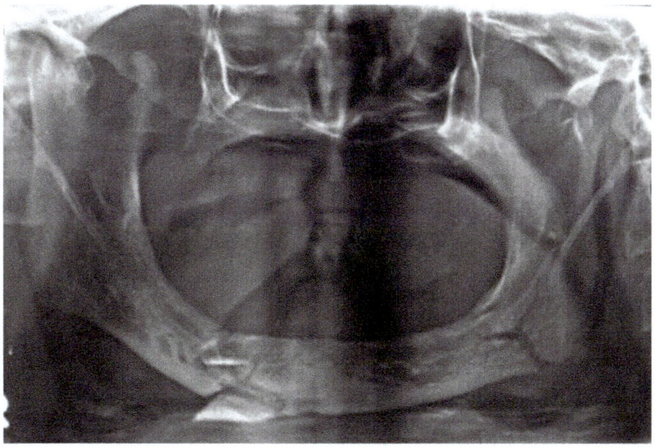

Fig. 52.48 Bilateral mandibular fracture (bucket handle fracture) in edentulous patients

Controversy again exists in the use of bone grafts in edentulous mandible. Are bone grafts necessary? Answer is not always. Reconstruction plates (load-bearing plates) can be used for comminuted fractures and with large defects. Bone morphogenic proteins and tricalcium phosphate can be used as alternative to autogenous grafts in patients whom multiple comorbidities may influence local or systemic outcomes [48].

Few authors advocated extramucosal intraoral plating for the ORIF of the edentulous mandibular fracture. It preserves the blood supply to the mucosa and bone, at the same time provides adequate stability [49, 50].

The techniques of edentulous atrophic mandible fracture management are:

1. Closed reduction (CR)

   This technique is opted when the patient's systemic condition does not allow for an open surgery. CR can be accomplished if the mandibular height is at least 30 mm. It is difficult to achieve CR if the mandibular height is <10 mm. CR can be accomplished using a preexisting denture. If there is no denture, gunning splint can be prepared. The denture/splint is used for immobilization and fixed to the mandible with circum-mandibular wiring (Fig. 52.49a, b).

   Advantages: Periosteal supply to the bone is maintained.

   Disadvantages: Chances of infection and pulmonary issues
2. Open reduction and internal fixation (ORIF)

   This involves use of plates and screws for fixation of fractures. Options for ORIF include use of miniplates or larger reconstruction plates. Miniplates are small and

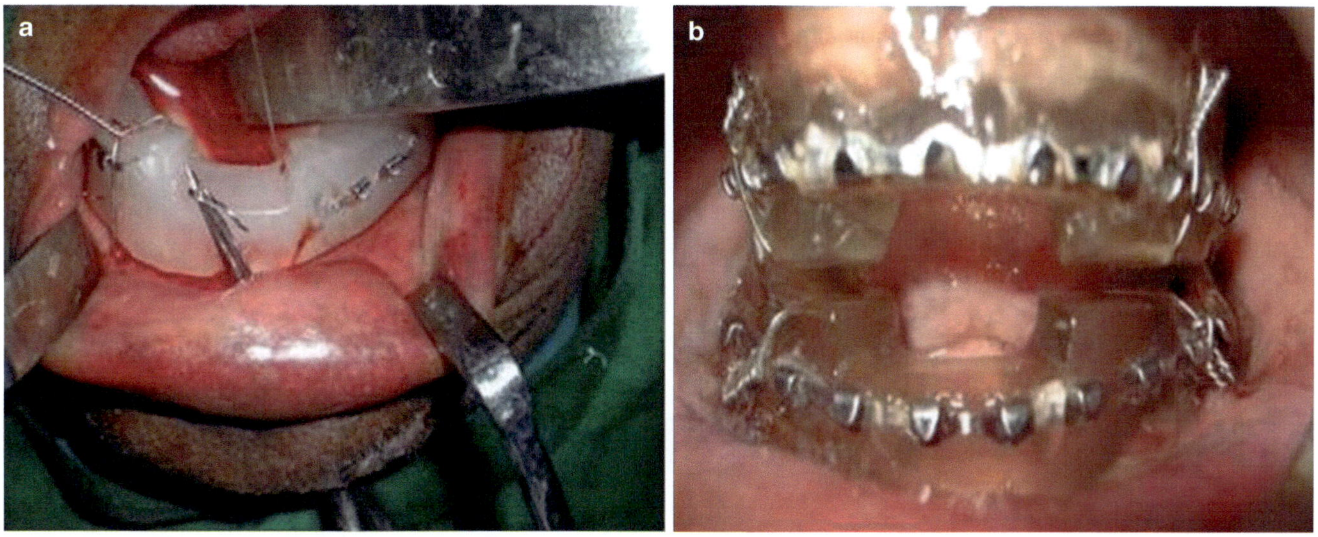

Fig. 52.49 (**a**) Securing gunning splint by circum-mandibular wiring, (**b**) MMF with gunning splint in situ

hence require smaller incision. Screws of miniplates are also small which can easily involve thin fragments. However, in cases of larger fractures, a load-bearing reconstruction plate is preferred.

Advantages: Adequate fixation with no/minimum MMF

Disadvantages: Delayed healing with periosteal blood supply loss

52.13 Pediatric Mandibular Fractures

Among all the maxillofacial fractures, the incidence of pediatric facial fracture is 1–15%. After nasal bone fracture, the second most common fractures in children are mandibular fracture with an incidence of 5–50% [51]. In mandible, the condyle is the commonest site of fracture in pediatric patients followed by symphysis and parasymphysis. The most common mechanisms of injury in children are [52]:

1. Fall from height
2. Bicycle falls
3. Automobile and sports accidents
4. Violence

In children, the developing tooth buds of canine approximate the lower border of mandible. This creates a stress point making the mandible susceptible to fracture in this location. Once the canine erupts, this weak point is reinforced with the bone and is not weaker than any other regions of the mandible. This is the reason probably why parasymphysis fracture is more common in children than adolescents.

With increasing age, the skull-to-face ratio decreases. The larger cranium shields the smaller middle and lower thirds of the face from injuries. This prevents mandibular fracture in small children; however, with increasing age the mandible becomes more prominent resulting in more injuries to this region.

52.13.1 Management

The management of pediatric mandibular fractures is different in comparison to adults due to [53]:

1. Relatively small size of maxillofacial bones
2. Presence of tooth germs
3. Soft bone with good elasticity
4. Instability of deciduous or mixed dentition
5. Rapid repair process
6. Difficulties in cooperation and acceptance

Pediatric mandibular fractures are treated in the following ways:

1. Undisplaced fractures: Managed conservatively with close observation, soft diet, analgesics, and activity prevention
2. Fractures with minor malocclusions: A short period of MMF with the help of bondable buttons and wires for 7–14 days
3. Malocclusion with displacement of segments: Closed reduction using cap splint secured to mandible by circum-mandibular wiring (Fig. 52.50a–c)
4. Malocclusion with severe displacement requiring three-dimensional stabilizations: open reduction and internal fixation

However the absence of teeth due to exfoliation and poor retention of wires on the deciduous teeth crowns makes the ligature wire and traditional use of arch bars difficult or sometimes impossible [54]. In such cases splinting with acrylic splint retained with circum-mandibular wires remains a viable option in treatment of pediatric mandibular fractures.

Cap splints are secured to mandible by circum-mandibular wiring. Kelsey Fry bone awl is used for this purpose. A wide-bore needle can also be used for the same (Fig. 52.51a, b). Intravenous cannula stillete (IVCS) is also mentioned in the literature for performing circum-mandibular wiring. The 16-gauge IVCS was used instead of conventional awl [55].

However, management of pediatric mandibular fracture with ORIF is controversial as the fixation of plates may hamper the growth and development of jaw. Titanium miniplates have been successfully used for ORIF, but the implants are to be removed within 3- to 12-month period [56].

Yerit et al. [57] proposed use of biodegradable plates for ORIF. These plates should be mechanically strong and must undergo resorption within a predictable time frame.

The advantages of biodegradable plates (polyglycolic and poly-L-lactic acid plating system) in comparison to titanium plates are [58]:

1. Does not require second operation for removal, indirectly becoming cost-effective and requiring less hospital visit.
2. Does not cause growth disturbances.
3. Monocortical plates and screws do not cause damage to the tooth buds.

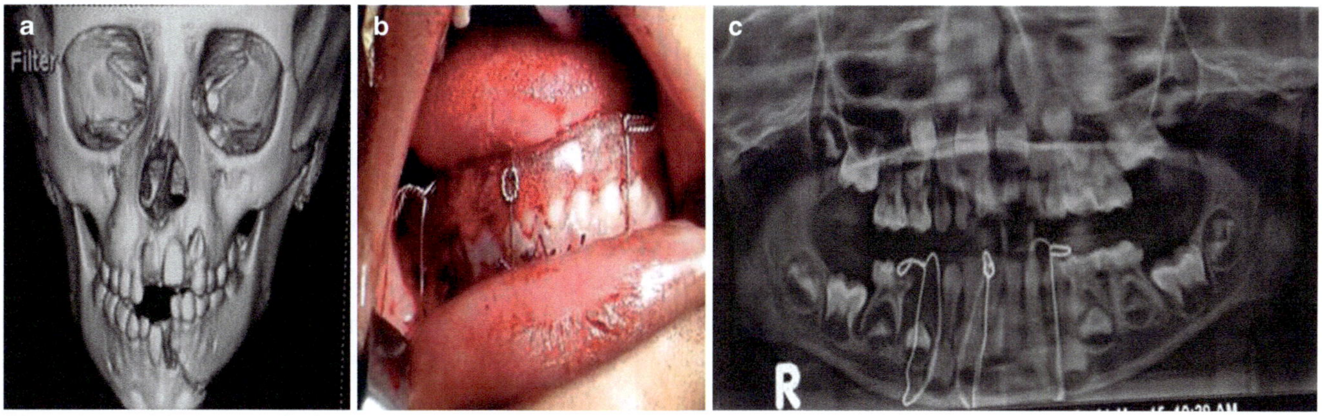

Fig. 52.50 (**a**) Pediatric mandibular fracture, (**b**) cap splint secured using circum-mandibular wiring, (**c**) postoperative orthopantamogram

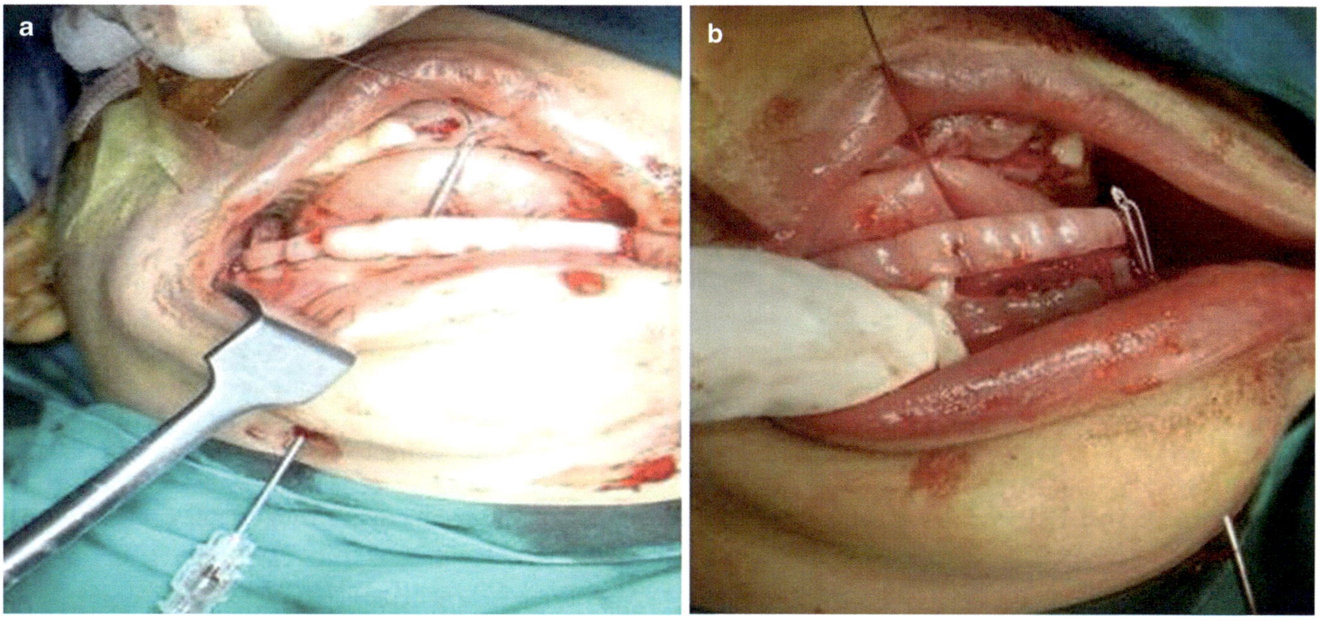

Fig. 52.51 (**a**, **b**) Securing cap splint by circum-mandibular wiring using wide-bore needle

52.14 Use of Bone Grafts in Mandible Fracture Treatment

Anterior iliac crest (cancellous or cortico-cancellous) and fibula (free microvascular reconstruction) are the most commonly used sites from where the bone grafts are used for mandibular reconstruction. All the cases required bone grafting in cases of mandibular fracture treated with ORIF should be kept in MMF of 4 weeks postoperatively.

Bone grafts are indicated in some cases of:

1. Severely comminuted fractures
2. Gunshot wounds
3. In non-union
4. Atrophic mandibular fractures

Rachmiel et al. [59] advocated two-stage reconstruction of mandibular bone defect after trauma by bone grafting followed by alveolar distraction osteogenesis (ADO). This modality helps in correction of intermaxillary vertical relationship and provides sufficient amount of bone for the placement of dental implants and prosthesis.

52.15 Postoperative Care

- Pressure dressing over the site to avoid postoperative hematoma in required cases.
- Elastic traction for correction of minor discrepancies in occlusion (Fig. 52.47).
- Soft and liquid diet.
- Maintenance of oral hygiene by oral rinses.
- Recall visit for review.
- Follow-up appointments and if results are not satisfactory frequent follow-up required.
- If patient is not satisfied, plan for retreatment.

52.16 Complications of Mandible Fracture

Immediate

- Pain
- Swelling

Delayed

- **Infection:** Found to be the most common complication (Fig. 52.52)
- Predisposing factors:
  1. Preoperative oral sepsis
  2. Tooth in the line of fracture
  3. Improper reduction and fixation (Fig. 52.53)
  4. Alcoholic or metabolic disturbances
  5. Prolonged time before treatment
  6. Poor patient compliance
- **Malunion**
  - It indicates that a fracture has healed but in less than an optimal position.
  - It may result when bone is shorter than normal, rotated or twisted in a bad position, or bent.
  - It may cause pain, joint degeneration, posttraumatic arthritis, or catching episodes resulting from instability.
- **Non-union**
  - It is a type of uncommon complication of mandibular fracture, with reported incidence of 2.8–3.9% [60].
  - It is failure of fracture hematoma to become transformed into an osteogenic matrix so that it is converted into non-osteogenic fibrous tissue.
  - Non-union identified by mobility in all planes after interval of minimum 10 weeks.
  - Histologically there is absence of identifiable osteogenic tissue.
  - Radiographically no evidence of progressive decrease in radiolucency at the fracture site and rounding off of the bones' end in the later stages. It can be treated by ORIF by rigid fixation (load-bearing reconstruction plate and sometimes in combination with bone graft) (Fig. 52.54a, b).

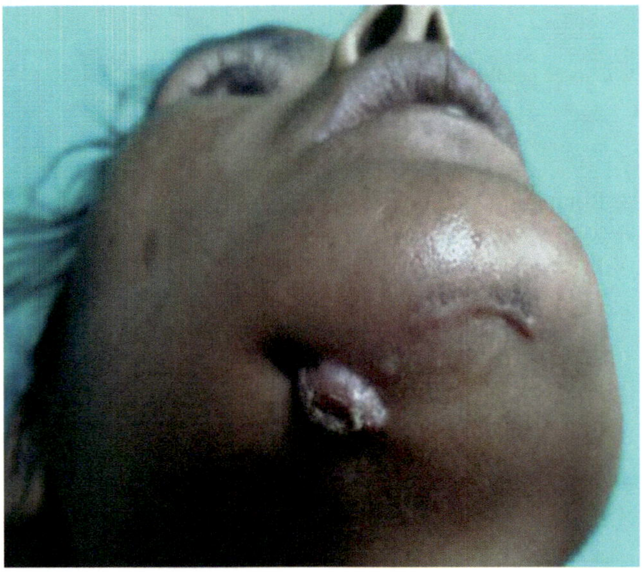

Fig. 52.52 Postoperative infection

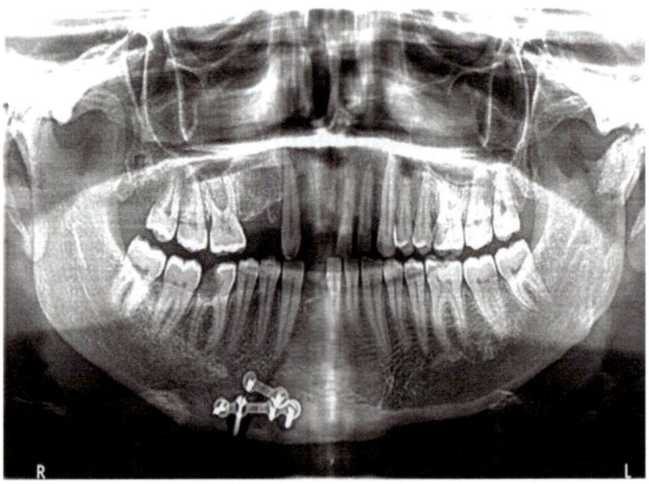

Fig. 52.53 Postoperative infection due to improper reduction and fixation

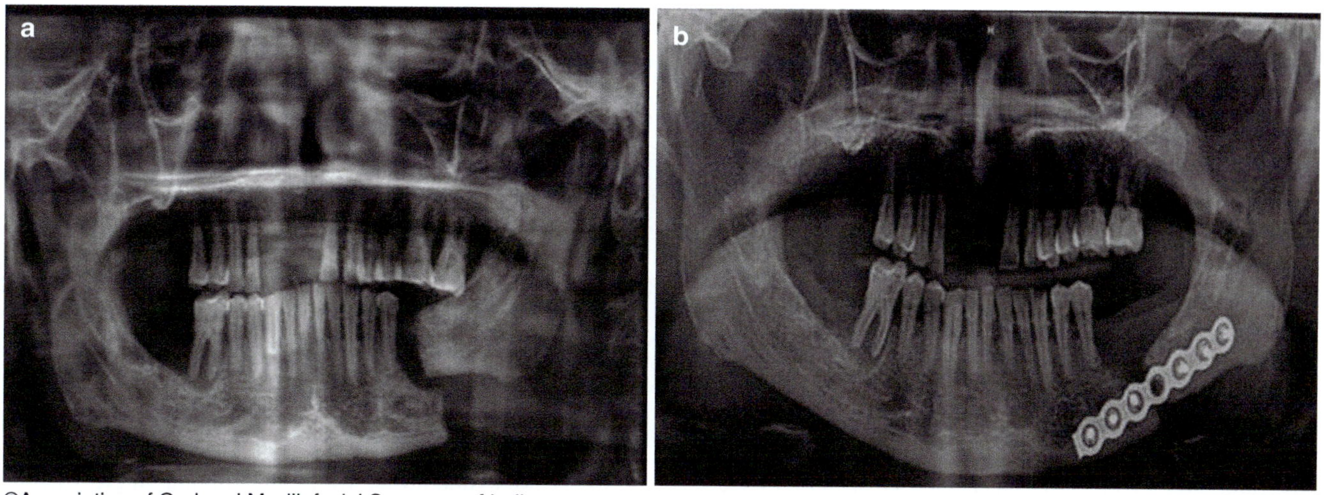

Fig. 52.54 (**a**) Non-union due to closed reduction, (**b**) management of fracture non-union by load-bearing reconstruction plate

Table 52.10 Management of mandibular non-union

If the defect is <1 cm	Defect size: 1–6 cm		Defect > 6 cm
Rigid internal fixation in single stage	***If adequate soft tissue present*** Reconstruction with bone graft in single stage	***If adequate soft tissue absent*** Reconstruction with bone graft at a later stage Reconstruction with vascularized Bone flap in single stage	Reconstruction with vascularized bone flap in single stage

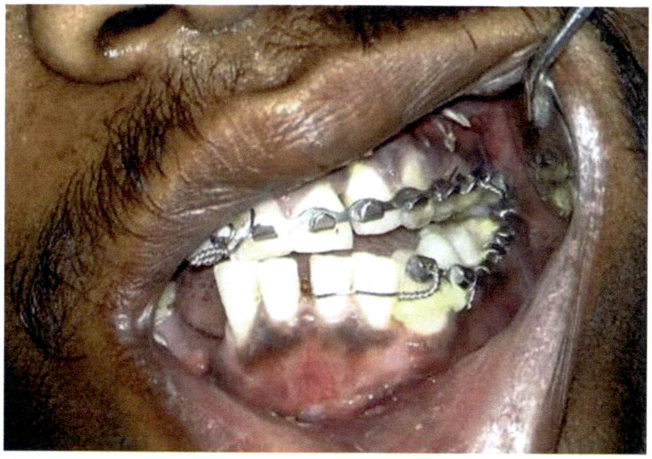

Fig. 52.55 Showing malocclusion

52.16.1 Management of Mandibular Non-union Depending upon the Size of the Defect (Table 52.10) [61]

- Malocclusion (Fig. 52.55)
- Facial asymmetry (Fig. 52.56)

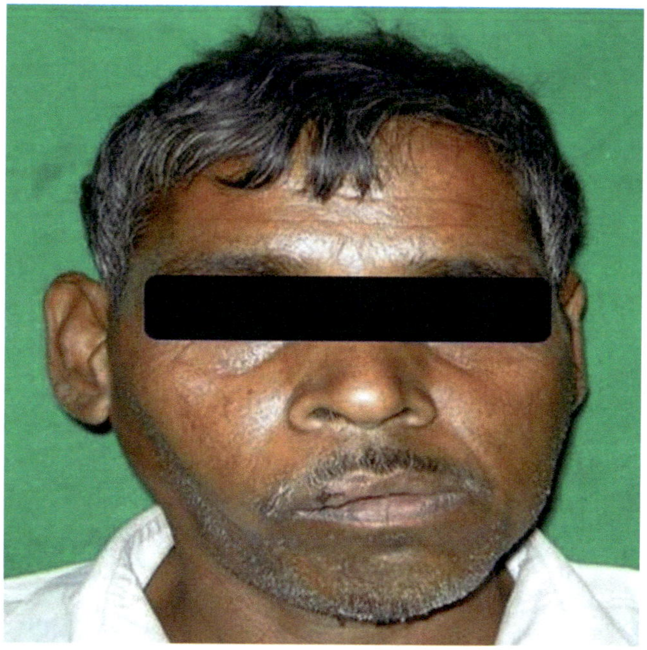

Fig. 52.56 Facial asymmetry

- Mandibular growth disturbances
- Disruption of permanent teeth
- TMJ dysfunction

52.17 Recent Advances

Kokosis et al. [62] advocated use of virtual surgical planning (VSP) with subsequent computer-aided design and manufacturing in management of acute mandibular trauma patients.

The advantages of the use of custom titanium plate in mandibular trauma are:

1. Avoid need for in situ bending.
2. Serving as a guide and confirming accurate reduction.
3. Customized titanium plates are much stronger than conventional plates.
4. Less palpable.

Computer-assisted surgery (CAS) including computer-aided design and manufacturing, surgical navigation techniques, and rapid prototyping (RP) has been used with lot of success in mandibular reconstruction (refer Chap. 41 of this book). CAS helps in [63]:

1. Preoperative planning
2. Preparation of stereolithographic (STL) models or accurate implantation material
3. Implementation of complex design through intraoperative navigation

Some Important Facts from Review of Literature Regarding Mandible Fracture [64, 65]

1. Injuries caused by assaults were more prone to develop postoperative infection, nerve damage, and malocclusion.
2. 11.8-fold more likely to have poor radiographic outcome in patients with comminuted fracture.
3. Dehiscence, nerve injury, and malocclusion occur more commonly in surgeries taking longer duration.
4. Patients with three or more fractures were 13.8-fold more likely to develop postoperative trismus in comparison to single fracture.
5. Chances of complications are more in patients who took discharge against medical advice.
6. Treatment of isolated mandible fracture can be safely delayed to allow for more improved resource distribution and prioritization of more time-dependent interventions.

52.18 Case Scenarios

Case Scenario 1

A male patient reported with a gunshot injury over right side of face. Patient's Glassgow coma scale (GCS) was 15/15 with stable vital signs, but the patient has difficulty in breathing. On maxillofacial examination, a gunshot wound was present over right side of face at the right mandibular angle region. Deviation of mandible was present on right side with cross bite on right side and open bite on left side. Tenderness was present over right mandibular angle region. On palpation, intersegmental mobility was present over right angle region.

Provisional diagnosis: Right mandibular angle fracture following gunshot

Investigation: Apart from blood investigation, a CT scan was performed, and a final diagnosis of comminuted right mandibular ramus and angle fracture with bullet in situ was made (Fig. 52.57a).

Management: Patient was subjected to emergency surgery under general anesthesia with a treatment plan of bullet retrieval, debridement, and open reduction and internal fixation of fracture. After the anesthesia was induced, patient preparation was done; the fracture site was exposed through an extraoral approach. Thorough debridement was done, and bullet was retrieved in multiple pieces (Fig. 52.57b). The bone segments which were detached were removed, and the fracture segments were fixed using a reconstruction plate following achieving occlusion (Fig. 52.57c). The use of bone graft was eliminated considering the risk of postoperative infection due to scattering of bullet particles. Moreover, the fracture site was a nondentate site; hence bone grafting was not mandatorily indicated for postoperative dental rehabilitation. Figure 52.57d shows postoperative OPG and fixation of fracture with reconstruction plate (refer Chap. 59 on Gun shot injuries).

Case Scenario 2

A female patient reported with the chief complaint of difficulty in chewing following operation to treat mandibular fracture. Patient gave a history of fall from height following which she was operated for ORIF elsewhere. The general condition of patient was good. On maxillofacial examination, mandible was deviated on right side with cross bite on right

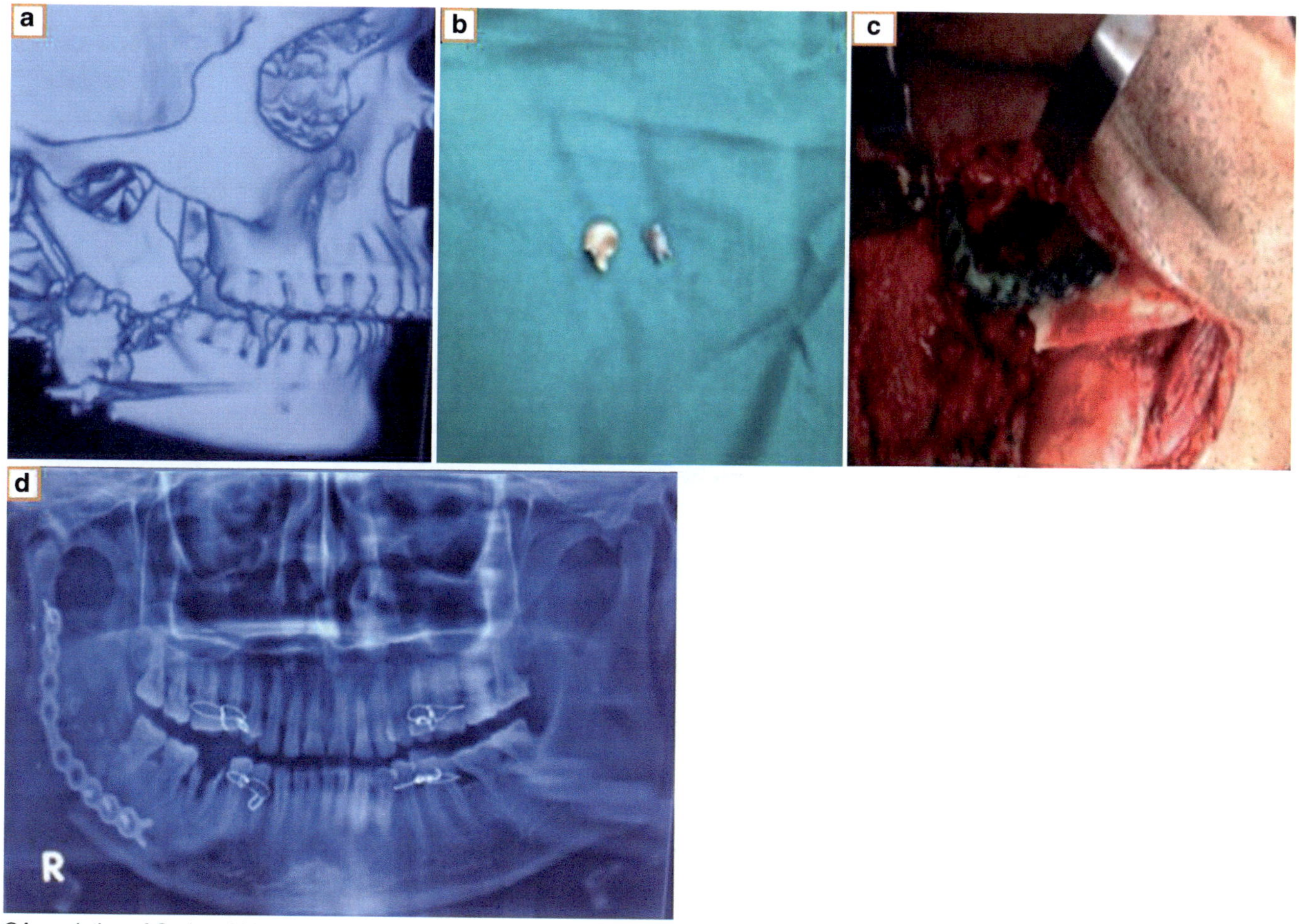

Fig. 52.57 Case Scenario 1 (**a**) DVT showing comminuted right mandibular angle and ramus fracture with bullet in situ; (**b**) retrieved bullet; (**c**) bullet retrieval, debridement, and fixation of fracture with reconstruction plate; (**d**) postoperative OPG showing fixation of fracture with reconstruction plate

side and open bite with lingualized occlusion on left side (Fig. 52.58a). Patient provided us with a pretreatment OPG which revealed right subcondylar with left side mandibular comminuted body and angle fracture (Fig. 52.58b). We subjected the patient to another OPG which revealed improper fixation of left mandibular body fracture and no fixation of left angle and right subcondylar fracture (Fig. 52.58c).

Diagnosis: Malunited left mandibular body, left angle fracture, and right subcondylar fracture

Management: Patient was subjected to general anesthesia. Once the anesthesia was induced, patient preparation was done, and fracture site was exposed through extraoral incision for all the fractures. Existing implants were removed which resulted in removal of few small bone fragments. The fractured and carious teeth were extracted and reduction was done by MMF. Occlusion was achieved (Fig. 52.58d), and fixation was performed using two miniplates at subcondylar site and load-bearing reconstruction plate at the body-angle unit. A postoperative OPG was done (Fig. 52.58e). Patient was discharged in stable condition. After 6 months, dental rehabilitation was performed for missing teeth by delivering dental bridge (Fig. 52.58f).

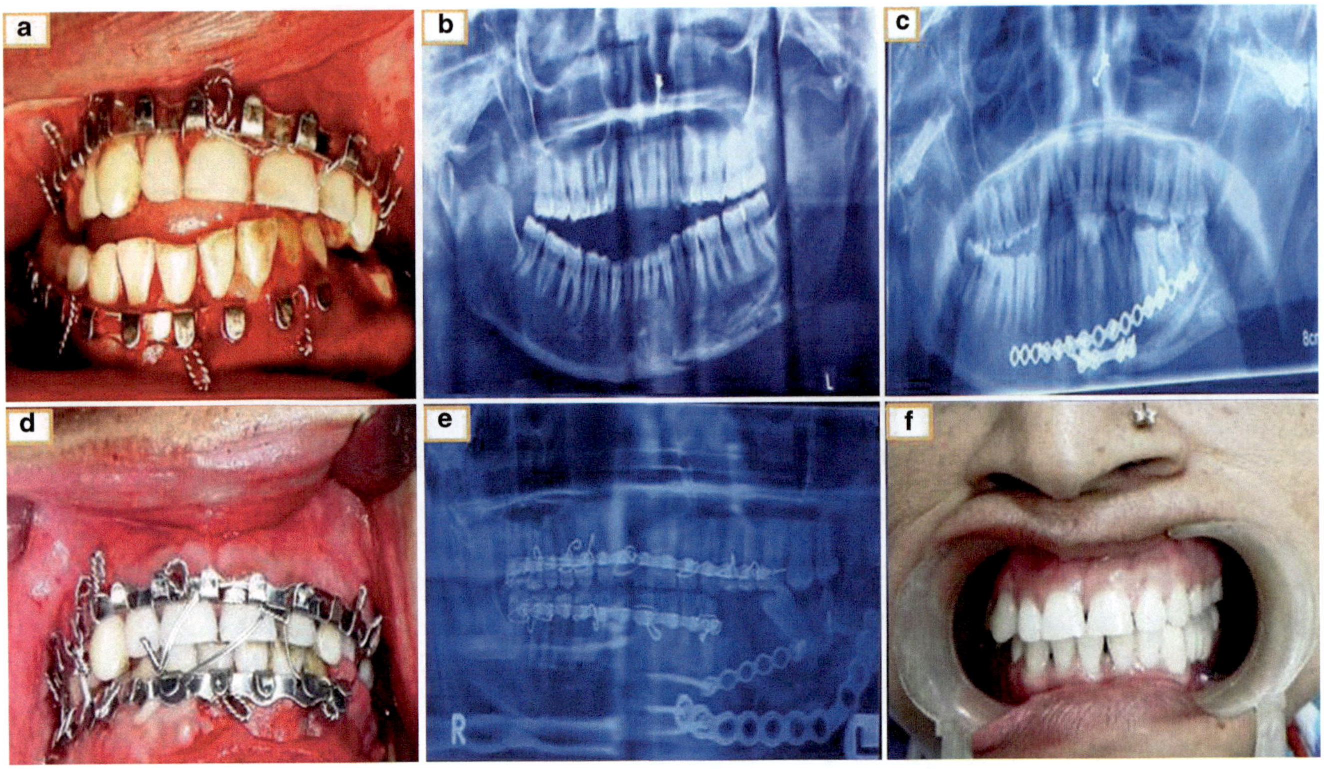

Fig. 52.58 Case scenario 2 (**a**) Deranged occlusion when patient reported to us, (**b**) pretreatment OPG, (**c**) improper fixation of left mandibular body fracture and no fixation of left angle and right subcondylar fracture at other centre, (**d**) intraoperative occlusion achieved, (**e**) postoperative OPG, (**f**) postoperative accurate occlusion

References

1. Christensen BJ, et al. How much weight loss can be expected after treating mandibular fractures? J Oral Maxillofac Surg. 2019;77:777–82.
2. Dingman RO, Natvig P. Surgery of facial fractures. Philadelphia, PA: Saunders; 1964. p. 193.
3. Ellis III E. Open reduction and internal fixation of combined angle and body/symphysis fractures of the mandible: how much fixation is enough? J Oral Maxillofac Surg. 2013;71:726–33.
4. National Radiologic Protection Board. Patient dose reduction in diagnostic radiology. London: National Radiologic Protection Board; 1990.
5. Durham JA, Paterson AW, Pierse D, Adams JR, Clark M, Hierons R, Edwards K. Postoperative radiographs after open reduction and internal fixation of the mandible: are they useful? Br J Oral Maxillofac Surg. 2006;44:279–82.
6. Bergh van den B. Postoperative radiographs after maxillofacial trauma: sense or nonsense? Int J Oral Maxillofac Surg. 2011;40:1373–6.
7. Rai A. A simple method of preventing needle stick type injury to the operator's finger while performing intermaxillary fixation. J Maxillofac Oral Surg. 2014;13(2):215–6.
8. Dimitroulis G. Management of fractured mandibles without the use of intermaxillary wire fixation. J Oral Maxillofac Surg 2002;60:1435–8.
9. Meram AT, Olate S, Palmieri CF Jr. Is the three-dimensional strut plate an adequate fixation technique for mandibular symphysis fractures? J Oral Maxillofac Surg. 2018;76:140–5.
10. Armond ACV, et al. Influence of third molars in mandibular fractures. Part 1: mandibular angle—a meta analysis. Int J Oral Maxillofac Surg. 2017;46:716–29.
11. Mah D-H, et al. Relationship between mandibular condyle and angle fractures and the presence of mandibular third molars. J Korean Assoc Oral Maxillofac Surg. 2015;41:3.
12. Samieirad S, et al. Correlation between lower third molar impaction types and mandibular angle and condylar fractures: a retrospective study. J Oral Maxillofac Surg. 2019;77:556–64.
13. Meisami T, et al. Impacted third molars and risk of angle fracture. Int J Oral Maxillofac Surg. 2002;31:140.
14. Kuriakose M, et al. A comparative review of 266 mandibular fractures with internal fixation using rigid (AO) plates or miniplates. Br J Oral Maxillofac Surg. 1996;34:315–21.
15. Sugar AW, et al. A randomised controlled trial comparing fixation of mandibular angle fractures with a single miniplate placed either transbuccally and intra-orally, or intra-orally alone. Int J Oral Maxillofac Surg. 2009;38:241–5.
16. Kale TP, Baliga SD, Ahuja N, Kotrashetti SM. A comparative study between transbuccal and extra-oral approaches in treatment of mandibular fractures. J Maxillofac Oral Surg. 2010;9:9–12.
17. Gulses et al. Determination of a safety zone for transbuccal trocar placement: an anatomical study. Int J Oral Maxillofac Surg 2012;41:930–3.

18. Braasch DC, Abubaker AO. Management of mandibular angle fracture. Oral Maxillofac Surg Clin North Am. 2013;25:591–600.
19. Al Moraissi EA. One miniplate compared with two in the fixation of isolated fractures of the mandibular angle. Br J Oral Maxillofac Surg. 2015;53:690–8.
20. Ellis E III. A prospective study of 3 treatment methods for isolated fractures of the mandibular angle. J Oral Maxillofac Surg. 2010;68:2743.
21. Rai A, Jain A, Datarkar A. Comparison of single versus two noncompression miniplates in the management of unfavourable angle fracture of the mandible: a prospective randomized clinical study. Oral Maxillofac Surg. 2018;22:157–61.
22. Levy FE, Smith RW, Odland RM, Marentette LJ. Monocortical miniplate fixation of mandibular angle fractures. Arch Otolaryngol Head Neck Surg. 1991;117:149–54.
23. Wusiman P, et al. Management of mandibular angle fractures using 3-dimensional or standard miniplates: A systematic review and meta-analysis. J Cranio Maxillofac Surg. 2019;47:622–8.
24. Zix J, Lieger O, Iizuka T. Use of straight and curved 3-dimensional titanium miniplates for fracture fixation at the mandibular angle. J Oral Maxillofac Surg. 2007;65:1758–63.
25. Ellis E III, Ghali GE. Lag screw fixation of mandibular angle fractures. J Oral Maxillofac Surg. 1991;49:234–43.
26. Kang DR, Zide M. Treatment of mandibular angle fractures using one non compression miniplates. J Oral Maxillofac Surg. 2013;71:327–34.
27. Patel N, Kim B, Zaid W. Analysis of mandibular angle fractures: epidemiology, patterns, treatments, and outcomes. J Oral Maxillofac Surg. 2016;74:1792–9.
28. Ellis E, Walker LR. Treatment of mandibular angle fractures using two non-compression miniplates. J Oral Maxillofac Surg. 1994;52:1032.
29. Ellis E. Outcomes of patients with teeth in the line of mandibular angle fractures treated with stable internal fixation. J Oral Maxillofac Surg. 2002;60:863–6.
30. Subhashraj K, Nandakumar N, Ravindran C. Review of maxillofacial injuries in Chennai, India: a study of 2748 cases. Br J Oral Maxillofac Surg. 2007;8:637–9.
31. Barde D, Madan R, Mudhol A. Prevalence and pattern of mandibular fracture. Central India. Natl J Maxillofac Surg. 2014;5:153.
32. Shaaban I, Gowen GF, Looby JP. Vertical fracture of the ascending ramus of the mandible. Oral Surg Oral Med Oral Pathol. 1967;24:594–97.
33. Heslop IH, Clarke PB, Becker R, et al. Mandibular fractures: treatment by open reduction and direct skeletal fixation. In: Rowe NL, Williams JL, editors. Maxillofacial injuries. London: Churchill Livingstone; 1985. p. 305.
34. Blinder D et al. Management of triangular fragments of the inferior border of the mandible. Oral Surg Oral Med Oral Pathol Oral Radiol Endod 1995;80:398–400.
35. Delantoni A, Antoniades I. The iatrogenic fracture of the coronoid process of the mandible. A review of the literature and case presentation. Cranio. 2010;28:200–4.
36. Philip M, Sivarajasingam V, Shepherd J. Bilateral reflex fracture of the coronoid process of the mandible. A case report. Int J Oral Maxillofac Surg. 1999;28:195–6.
37. Johnson RL. Unusual (coronoid) fracture of the mandible: report of a case. J Oral Surg. 1958;16:73.
38. Rankow RM, Mignogna FV. Ankylosis of the temporalis–coronoid complex of the mandible. Ann Plast Surg. 1978;1:280–5.
39. Shen L, et al. Mandibular coronoid fractures: Treatment options. Int J Oral Maxillofac Surg. 2013;42:721–6.
40. Ellis E 3rd, Walker LR. Treatment of mandibular angle fractures using one noncompression miniplate. J Oral Maxillofac Surg. 1996;54:864–6.
41. Finn RA. Treatment of comminuted mandibular fractures by closed reduction. J Oral Maxillofac Surg. 1996;54:320–7.
42. Li Z, Li Z-B. Clinical characteristics and treatment of multiple site comminuted mandible fractures. J Cranio Maxillofac Surg. 2011;39:296–9.
43. Ellis E, Muniz O, Anand K. Treatment considerations for comminuted mandibular fractures. J Oral Maxillofac Surg. 2003;61:861–70.
44. Dai J, et al. Titanium mesh shaping and fixation for the treatment of comminuted mandibular fractures. J Oral Maxillofac Surg. 2016;74:337–40.
45. Tay Guan AB, et al. Inferior alveolar nerve injury in trauma-induced mandible fractures. J Oral Maxillofac Surg. 2015;73:1328–40.
46. Cillo JE and Holmes TM. Interpersonal violence is associated with increased severity of geriatric facial trauma. J Oral Maxillofac Surg. 2016;74:1023.e1–7.
47. Bradley JC. A radiological investigation into the age changes of the inferior dental artery. Br J Oral Surg. 1975;13:82.
48. Nunez JC, et al. Atrophic mandible fractures: are bone grafts necessary? An update. J Oral Maxillofac Surg. 2017;75:2391–8.
49. Benech A, et al. Intraoral extra-mucosal fixation of fractures in the atrophic edentulous mandible. Int J Oral Maxillofac Surg. 2013;42:460–3.
50. Wood GA, et al. Transmucosal fixation of the fractured edentulous mandible. Int J Oral Maxillofac Surg. 2011;40:549–52.
51. Iatrou I, Theologie-Lygidakis N, Tzermpos F. Surgical protocols and outcome for the treatment of maxillofacial fractures in children: 9 years' experience. J Craniomaxillofac Surg. 2010;38:511–6.
52. Smith DM, Bykowski MR, Cray JJ, Naran S, Rottgers SA, Shakir S, et al. 215 mandible fractures in 120 children: demographics, treatment, outcomes, and early growth data. Plast Reconstr Surg. 2013;131:1348–58.
53. Iatrou I, Theologie-Lygidakis N, Tzermpos F. Surgical protocols and outcome for the treatment of maxillofacial fractures in children: 9 years' experience. J Craniomaxillofac Surg. 2010;38:511–6.
54. Kocabay C, Ataç MS, Oner B, Güngör N. The conservative treatment of paediatric mandibular fracture with prefabricated surgical splint: a case report. Dent Traumatol. 2007;23:247–50.
55. Thomas S, Yuvaraj V. Atraumatic placement of circummandibular wires: A technical note. Int J Oral Maxillofac Surg. 2010;39:83–5.
56. Iatrou I, Theologie-Lygidakis N, Tzermpos F, Kamperos G. Internal fixation of mandibular angle fractures using one miniplate in Greek children: a 5-year retrospective study. J Craniomaxillofac Surg. 2015;43:53–6.
57. Yerit KC, Hainich S, Enislidis G, Turhani D, Klug C, Wittwer G, et al. Biodegradable fixation of mandibular fractures in children: stability and early results. Oral Surg Oral Med Oral Pathol Oral Radiol Endod. 2005;100:17–24.
58. Stanton DC, Liu F, Yu JW, Mistretta MC. Use of bioresorbable plating systems in paediatric mandible fractures. J Craniomaxillofac Surg. 2014;42:1305–9.
59. Rachmiel A, et al. Two-stage reconstruction of the severely deficient alveolar ridge: bone graft followed by alveolar distraction osteogenesis. Int J Oral Maxillofac Surg. 2018;47:117–24.
60. Mathog RH, Toma V, Clayman L, et al. Nonunion of the mandible: An analysis of contributing factors. J Oral Maxillofac Surg. 2000;58:746.

61. Ostrander BT, et al. Contemporary management of mandibular fracture nonunion—a retrospective review and treatment algorithm. J Oral Maxillofac Surg 2018;76:1479–93.
62. Kokosis G, et al. The use of computer-aided design and manufacturing in acute mandibular trauma reconstruction. J Oral Maxillofac Surg. 2018;76:1036–43.
63. Bell RB. Computer planning and intraoperative navigation in cranio-maxillofacial surgery. Oral Maxillofac Surg Clin North Am. 2010;22:135.
64. Hurrell MJ, Batstone MD. The effect of treatment timing on the management of facial fractures: a systematic review. Int J Oral Maxillofac Surg. 2014;43:944–50.
65. Hurrell MJL. A prospective study examining the effects of treatment timing in the management of mandible fractures. Int J Oral Maxillofac Surg. 2018;47:1126–31.

53 Fracture of the Mandibular Condyle

Vikas Dhupar

53.1 Introduction

Maxillofacial surgeons commonly come across a high incidence of condylar fractures in their practice. A French surgeon [1] in the eighteenth century described a high propensity for a narrow portion in the subcondylar region to fracture, which is a common occurrence even today. In spite of a common occurrence, the management has been controversial as there is no established consensus in the treatment of condylar fractures. Traditionally closed reduction has been the treatment of choice for condylar fractures and have been treated by various forms of intermaxillary fixation. With the improvement in radiographic imaging and biomaterials used in the fixation, surgical management has gradually found acceptance as it restores early function.

53.2 Surgical Anatomy

The mandibular condyle forms a part of the temporomandibular joint which is unique (Box 53.1), and it is made of the following structures:

- Condyle of the mandible
- Squamous portion of the temporal bone
- Articular disc (contained within the TMJ)
- Ligaments

Box 53.1. TMJ—Unique Characteristics

- It is a ginglymoarthrodial joint, having both a hinge and a gliding action
- It has an end point closure
- It has a fibrocartilage disc

53.2.1 Condyle

The condyle is one of the two processes of the mandible present on the superior portion of the ramus. The condylar head is ovoid in shape measuring approximately 15–20 mm mediolaterally and 8–10 mm anteroposteriorly in dimension [2]. The mandibular condyle articulates with the glenoid fossa present in the squamous portion of the temporal bone to form the temporomandibular joint (Fig. 53.1). Squamous portion of the temporal bone is as thin as 2 mm as a result; the condylar processes maybe driven into the middle cranial fossa following trauma.

53.2.2 Articular Disc

The squamous portion of the temporal bone and the condyle is separated by a dense fibrous connective tissue called the articular disc. The disc is firmly anchored to the condyle by the medial and lateral collateral ligaments, and it merges with the capsule in the periphery. The joint space is divided into superior and inferior compartments by the disc.

53.2.3 Capsule and Ligaments

The capsule surrounds the TMJ and is reinforced by the medial and lateral ligaments which connect the mandible to the temporal bone. The synovial membrane lines the capsule.

Electronic Supplementary Material The online version of this chapter (https://doi.org/10.1007/978-981-15-1346-6_53) contains supplementary material, which is available to authorized users.

V. Dhupar (✉)
Department of Oral & Maxillofacial Surgery,
Goa Dental College & Hospital, Bambolim, Goa, India

K. Bonanthaya et al. (eds.), *Oral and Maxillofacial Surgery for the Clinician*, https://doi.org/10.1007/978-981-15-1346-6_53

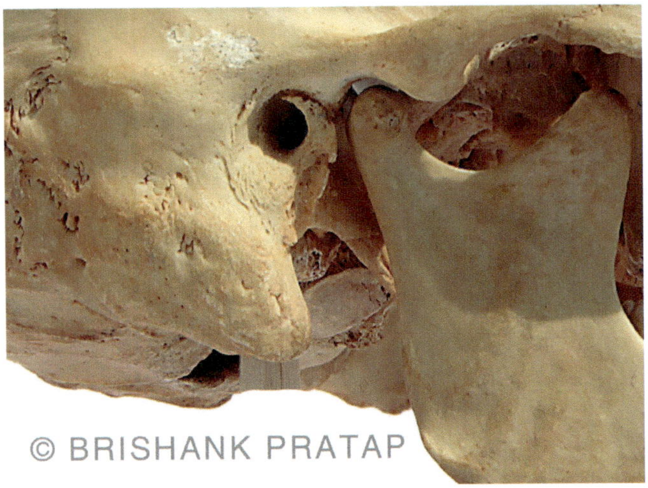

Fig. 53.1 Bony structures of TMJ

This membrane produces synovial fluid which aids in the lubrication and nourishment of the joint. The lateral ligament also known as temporomandibular ligament has a horizontal and an oblique component which stabilizes the joint. The strength of the lateral ligament may be partly responsible for the fracture at the neck of condyle just below the insertion of the ligament [3]. The medial and lateral discal ligaments which are present inside the capsule are also called collateral ligaments. These ligaments connect the disc to the poles of the condyle. In addition to these ligaments, there are two non-capsular ligaments, namely, sphenomandibular and stylomandibular which may have a limited function.

53.2.4 Muscles of Mastication

There are four muscles of mastication, namely, the medial and lateral pterygoid, masseter, and the temporalis. Lateral pterygoid is attached to the pterygoid fovea at the condylar neck and is responsible for the displacement of the condylar fractures. Change in the direction of resultant forces post fracture will alter the function of the mandible during various excursion movements.

53.2.5 Vascularisation

The arterial blood supply to the TMJ is derived from the two terminal branches of the external carotid artery, namely:

- Superficial temporal artery
- Maxillary artery

It may be noted that the condyle receives blood supply from three sources

1. Medullary bone supplied by inferior alveolar artery
2. Overlying periosteum of the condyle
3. Attachment of lateral pterygoid muscle

This may explain the reason for the fractured condyle to remains viable even after stripping of the periosteum during the surgical procedure as the lateral pterygoid muscle remains attached to the fractured fragment [4]. The venous drainage starts in the retrodiscal plexus which drains into the superficial temporal and maxillary veins that join to form the retromandibular vein, which in turn drains into the external jugular vein.

53.2.6 Innervation

It is imperative to understand the innervation of the joint so as to minimize the complications following fracture of the mandible and its management. Both the sensory and motor innervation is encountered while approaching the joint. The sensory nerves are auriculotemporal, masseteric, and posterior deep temporal. Auriculotemporal nerve crosses the condyle medial to it and lies in contact with the condylar neck and capsule [5]. It is encountered in the preauricular incision and may result in postoperative complications.

53.2.7 Facial Nerve

It is the key nerve that transverses the face, and it is liable for the motor function of the muscles of facial expression. This nerve transverses the temporoparietal fascia and finally divides into five terminal branches in the parotid gland (Fig. 53.2). Hence all the extraoral approaches for the condylar fractures are designed keeping the facial nerve in mind. Al-Kayat and Bramley [6] found the nerve was at an average distance of 20 mm with a range of 8–35 mm from the anterior margin of the auditory canal. This is the reason the preauricular incision is given in the skin crease near the tragus or placed endurally. The neck of the condyle can be exposed via the transparotid approach. In this approach the condyle is reached through the space between the temporozygomatic and buccocervical trunks of the nerve. This results in a direct and safe approach to the neck of the condyle. The marginal mandibular nerve is encountered in the submandibular or periangular approach. This branch may further subdivide into two or more branches [7]. As a rule, the submandibular incision is given 2 cm below the lower border of the mandible to prevent paresis of the lower lip.

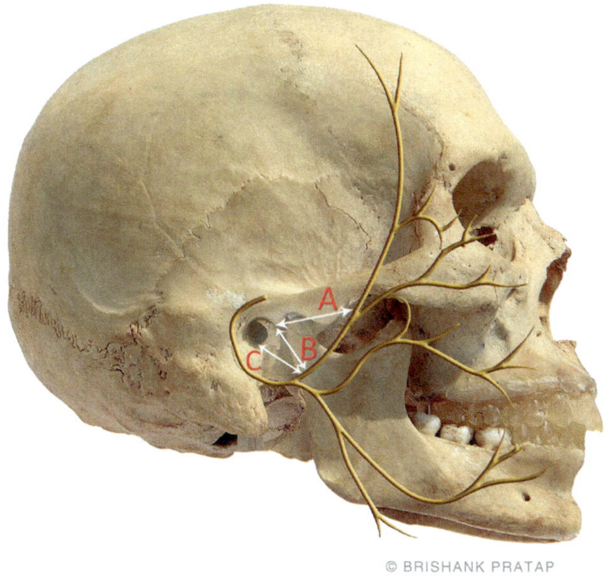

Fig. 53.2 Terminal branches of facial nerve with Al Kayat and Bramely's [6] measurements for trunk of facial nerve. (A) .8–3.5 cm, (B) 2.4–3.5 cm, (C) 1.3 cm

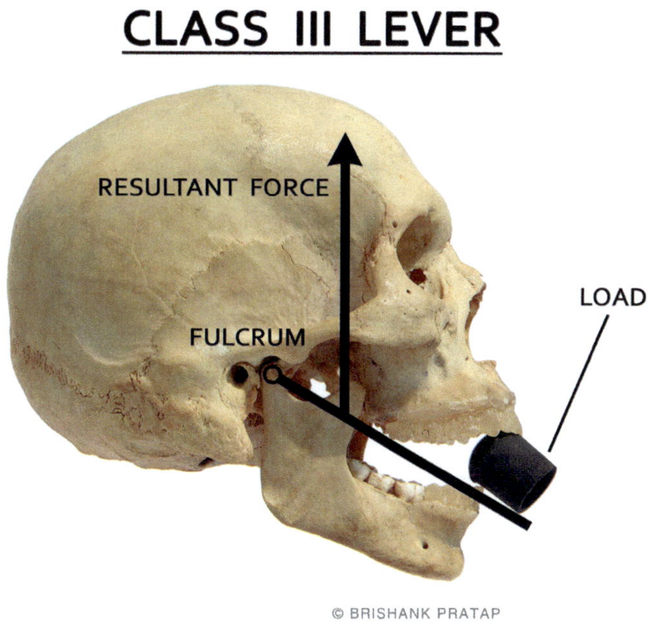

Fig. 53.3 Function of mandible as class III lever

53.3 Biomechanics of Condylar Fracture

U-shaped mandible supports the condyles on either side. There are two major movements while opening the mouth, rotational, and translational which occur in the inferior and superior compartments, respectively. Mandibular function is characterised as a class III lever with the joint being the fulcrum [8]. The musculature applies the force between the joint and the masticatory load (Fig. 53.3).

53.3.1 Mechanism of Injury

Trauma causing condylar fracture was explained by Lindahl [9]. It is important to understand the pattern as it gives the type of injury sustained (Fig. 53.4).

1. Kinetic energy derived from the momentum created by the subject falling on a static object. This is an axial force which is transmitted to the condyle from the lower border of the mandible. Fracture can occur at the site of injury and at the condyles at a higher level. Occluding teeth cannot reduce the force. May also result in fracture of teeth.
2. Kinetic energy derived from the momentum created by a moving object against a static subject. Generally noted in assaults or sport injuries. More or less horizontal forces will result in a fracture both at the site of impact and at the condyle on the opposite side. Fracture is usually at the base of the condyle.
3. Combination of the above two is seen in a road traffic accident and may result in more severe injuries.

An external force applied generally gets distributed over the entire mandible. However these forces result in the fracture of the subcondylar region which is weak and are subject to tensile stresses. A counter-coup injury is often noted in the condylar region. This prevents displacement of the condyles into the middle cranial fossa especially in bilateral fractures resulting from injuries over the chin.

53.3.2 Effect of Condylar Fracture

The signs and symptoms seen following trauma are due to the functional loss resulting from the disruption of the local anatomy. Following trauma a protective mechanism is triggered. It is generally expected that due to premature contact on the fractured side, excessive forces would be generated during loading of the non-fractured site on mastication. However, it is noted there is a shift of mean force vector towards the non-fractured site which results in protecting the fractured site during biting [10]. This results in neuromuscular adaptation. An increase in the muscle activity on the non-fractured side and a decrease of active force on the opposite

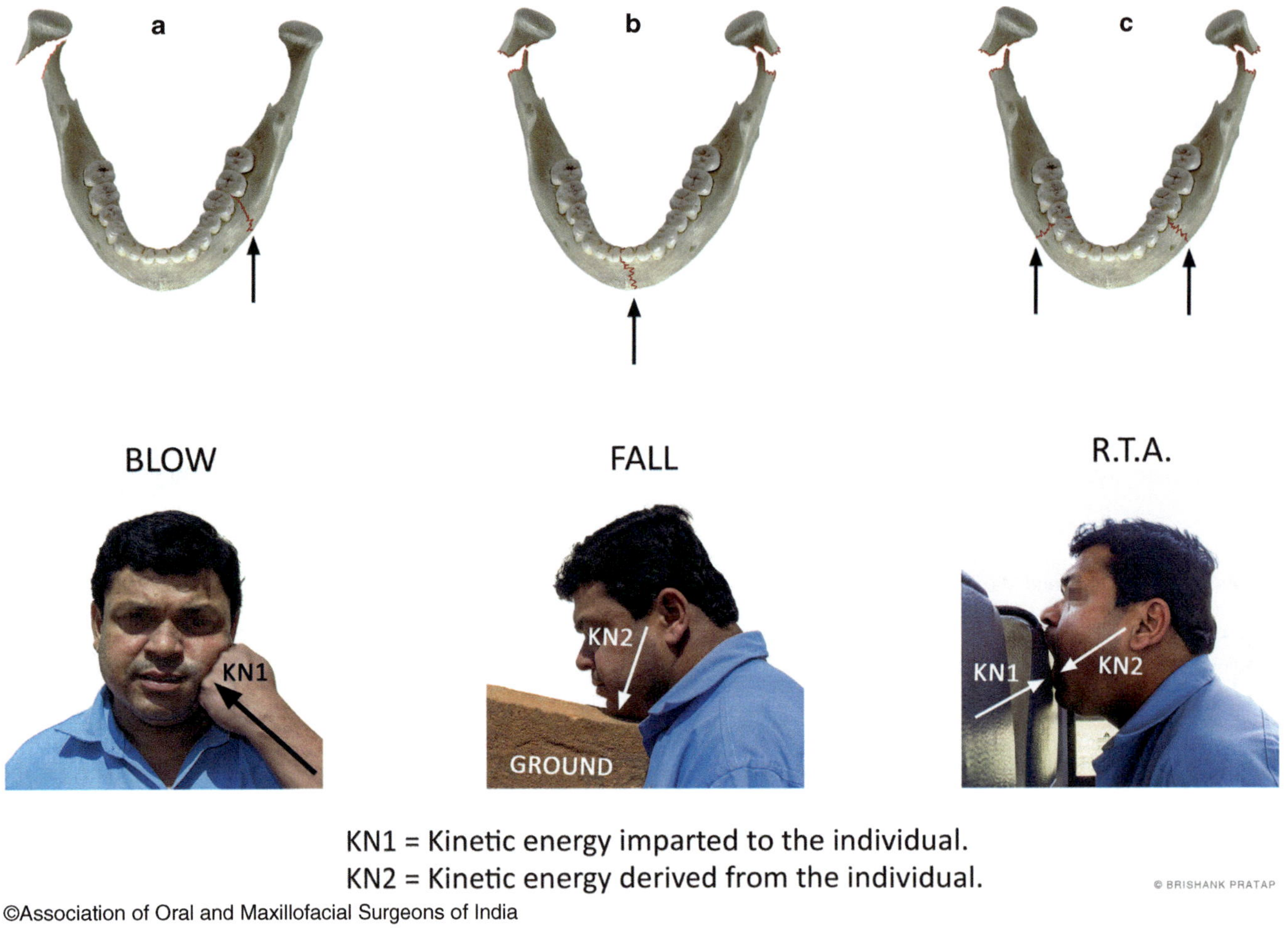

Fig. 53.4 Mechanism of fracture of condyle

side results in this process. Hence most of the masticatory forces are directed towards the non-fractured site and resulting in less neuromuscular adaptation on the fractured site. Refer to the article by Ellis et al. [8] for a comprehensive understanding of the biological considerations of fractures of mandibular condyle.

53.3.3 Adaptation to Fracture

Following condylar fracture of the mandible, patients adapt to the injury by compensation mechanism which is divided as follows:

- Skeletal
- Neuromuscular
- Dental

Intervention by the surgeons either by open or closed reduction minimizes the dental compensation. It is noted that there is a decreased masseter activity on the fractured site transferring load to a non-fractured site. This results in neuromuscular adaptation which may also be a protective phenomenon [8]. In case of an open reduction, there is minimum amount of neuromuscular adaptation. Usually a closed reduction results in an articulation which is inferior and anterior to the articular eminence which may limit the transitional movement. This can be avoided by open reduction and fixation. Minimum complications have been reported in the studies evaluating closed reduction in treatment of condylar fractures as pain and mouth opening were the only criteria which were evaluated. A statistically significant reduction in the incidence of malocclusion and lateral deviation on opening, along with an improved protrusive and laterotrusive movements, were noted in patients treated with surgical therapy vis-á-vis closed therapy in a recent meta-analysis report [10]. Compared to closed reduction where skeletal and neuromuscular adaptation is seen, in open reduction only neuromuscular adaption will take place following treatment.

53.4 Classification of Condylar Process Fractures

Condylar fractures can be described as a fracture line above the mandibular foramen that runs from the posterior border of the ramus to sigmoid notch or the condylar head (Fig. 53.5). Literature mentions numerous classifications of condylar fractures. Most classifications described the fracture based on the anatomical site, displacement, and fracture level, inclined towards close reduction. With the advancement of imaging modalities and better understanding of open reduction procedures, classifications which are relevant are discussed.

Various terms describing the condylar fractures have appeared in the English literature (Fig. 53.6):

- No displacement—Fracture maintains anatomic position
- Deviation—Fragments are in primary contact
- Displacement—There is no contact of the fracture fragments
- Dislocation—Extra articulation of the joints

In 1927 **Wassumund** [11] differentiated between the head and neck fractures of the condyle. Early classification only described anatomical position but had no relevance in treatment as it did not document the angulation of displacement or dislocation. Condylar fractures were classified as:

- Base fracture
- Neck fracture
- Head fracture (diacapitular)

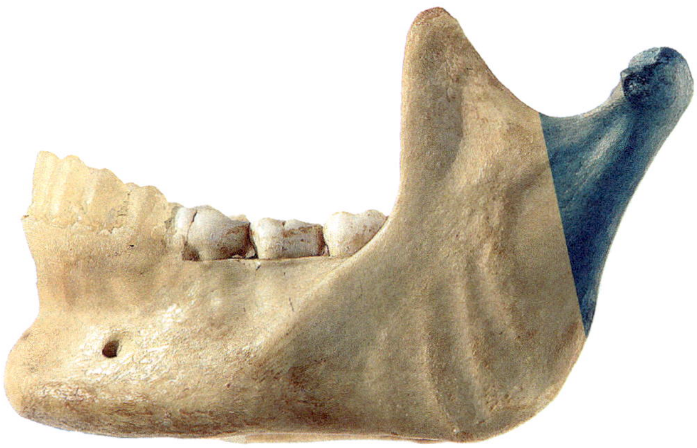

©Association of Oral and Maxillofacial Surgeons of India

Fig. 53.5 Area of condylar fracture

MacLennan [12] was the first to differentiate between simple bending, displacement, and dislocation fractures of the condylar process.

Class I: no deviation (bending)
Class II: deviation (bending) at the fracture level
Class III: displacement (condylar head remains within fossa)
Class IV: dislocation (condylar head outside of fossa)

Spiessl and Schroll [13]. A classification well accepted in the European literature, which differentiated between fractures of the base and neck of the condyle, it also noted the range of angulation with deviation, displacement, or dislocation (Fig. 53.7).

- Type I: condylar neck fracture with no associated deviation/displacement
- Type II: low condylar neck fracture with deviation/displacement
- Type III: high condylar neck fracture with deviation/displacement
  - IIIa: ventral
  - IIIb: medial
  - IIIc: lateral
  - IIId: dorsal
- Type IV: low condylar neck fracture with dislocation
- Type V: high condylar neck fracture with dislocation
- Type VI: intracapsular fracture of the condylar head

There are numerous modifications of Spiessl and Scholl classifications and were given over a period of time as a result subtypes has evolved especially in type V and VI fractures. Modifications included Rasse [14], Neff et al. [15], Hlawitschka and Eckelt [16], and Loukota et al. [17].

- Type A: There is a continuous bony contact within the glenoid fossa, with a component of the remaining condylar head and the fracture supported with no loss of ramal height (Fig. 53.8a).
- Type B: Loss of support within the articulating fossa and with the loss of mandibular ramal height (Fig. 53.8b).
- Type C: The highest portion of the fracture is below the level of the lateral ligament, as a result there in a loss of ramal height (Fig. 53.8c).

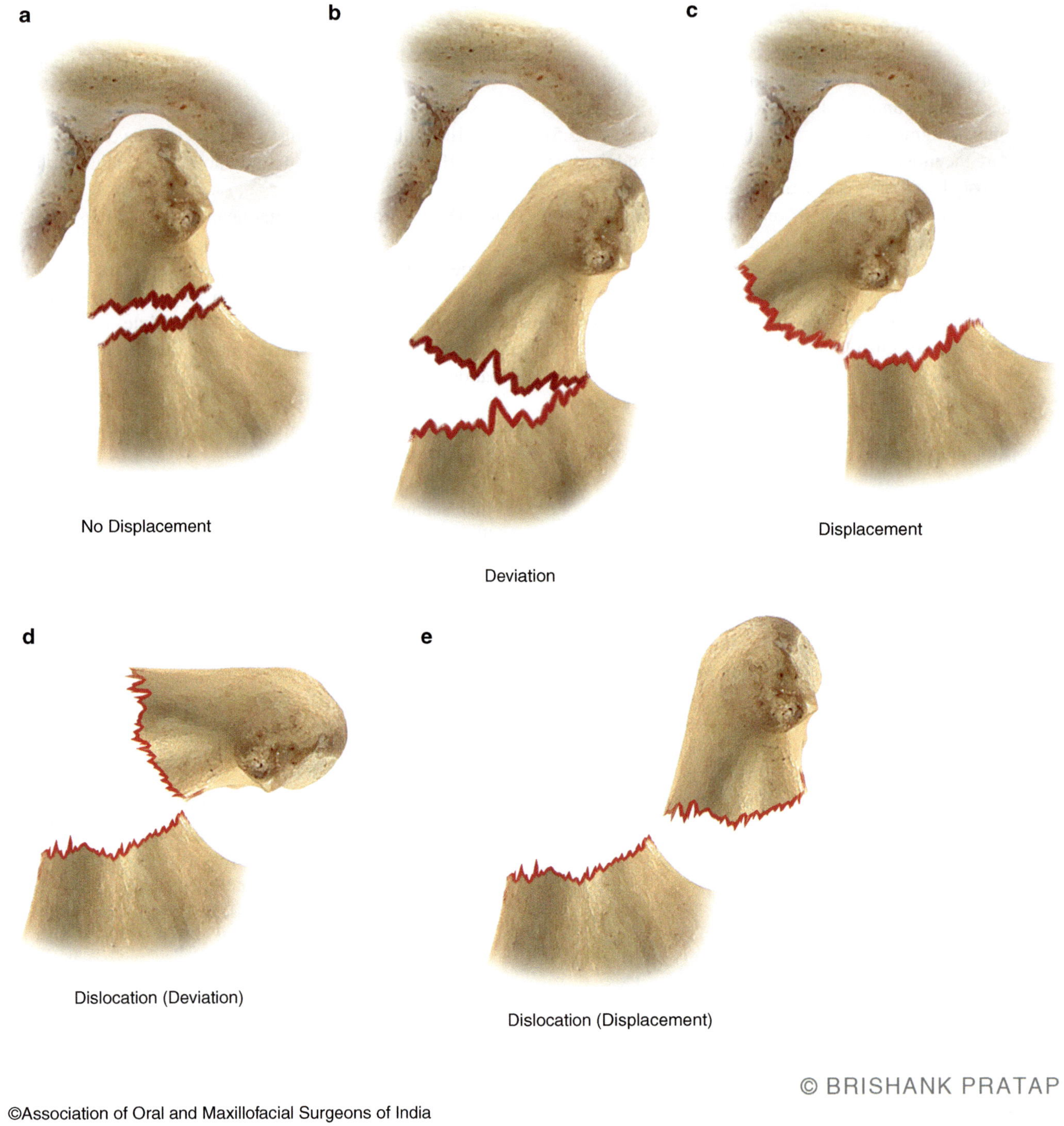

Fig. 53.6 (**a**) No displacement. (**b**) Deviation. (**c**) Displacement. (**d**) Dislocation (deviation). (**e**) Dislocation (displacement)

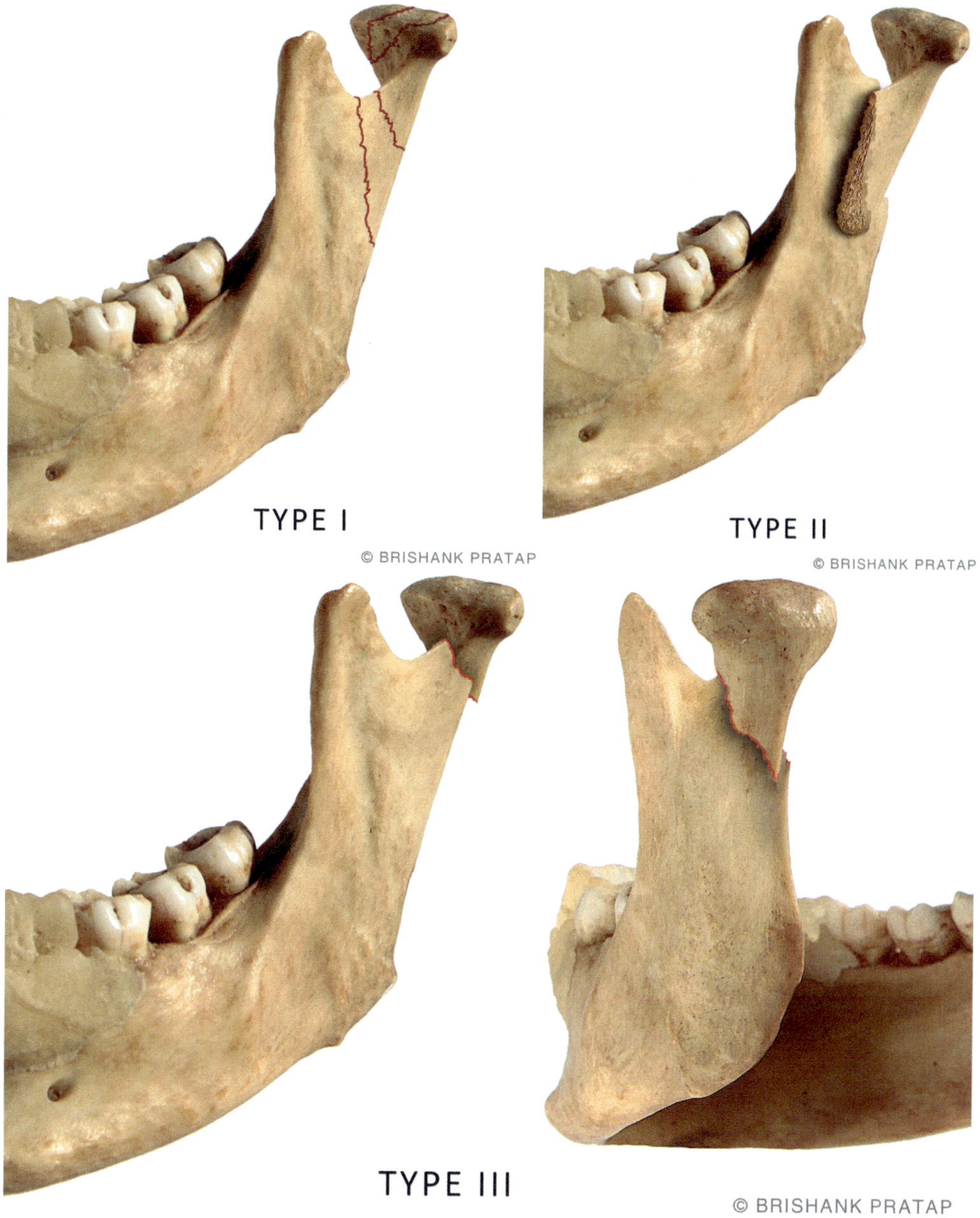

Fig. 53.7 Types I–VI: Spiessl and Schroll classification

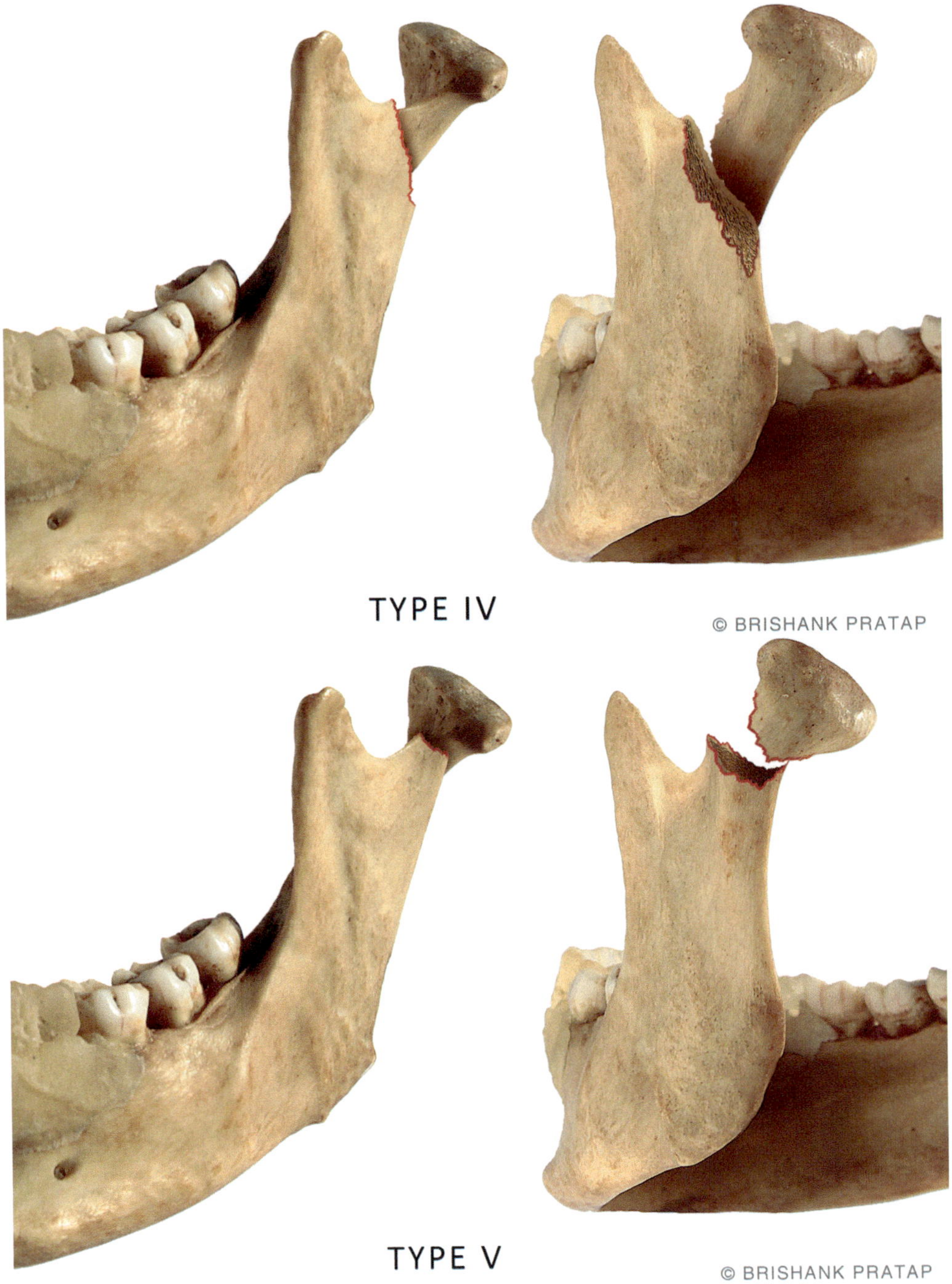

Fig. 53.7 (continued)

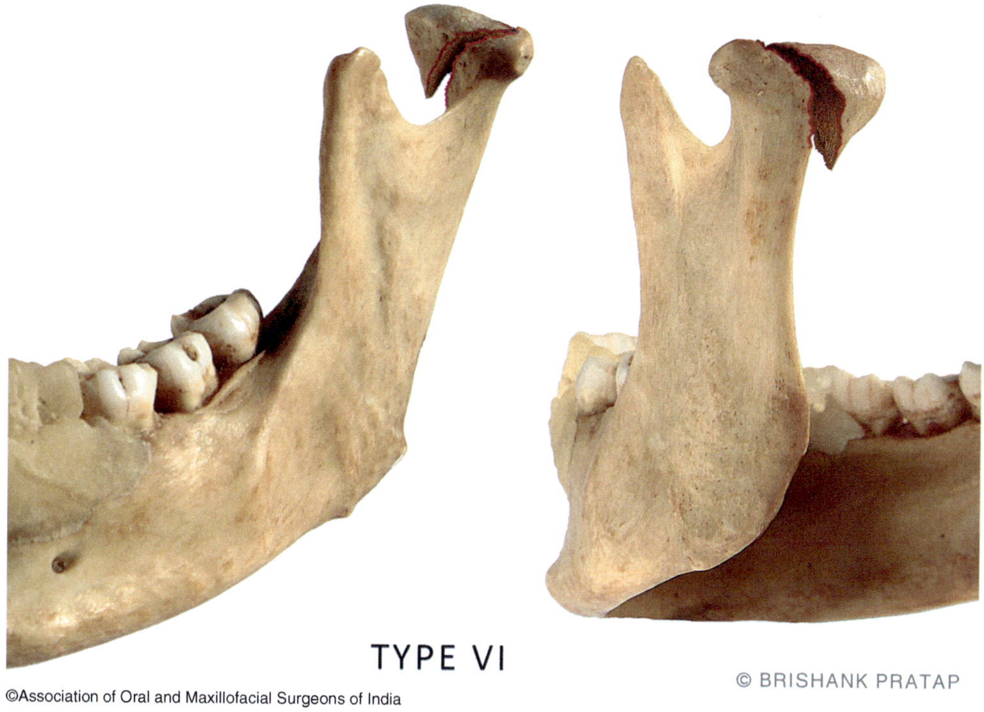

Fig. 53.7 (continued)

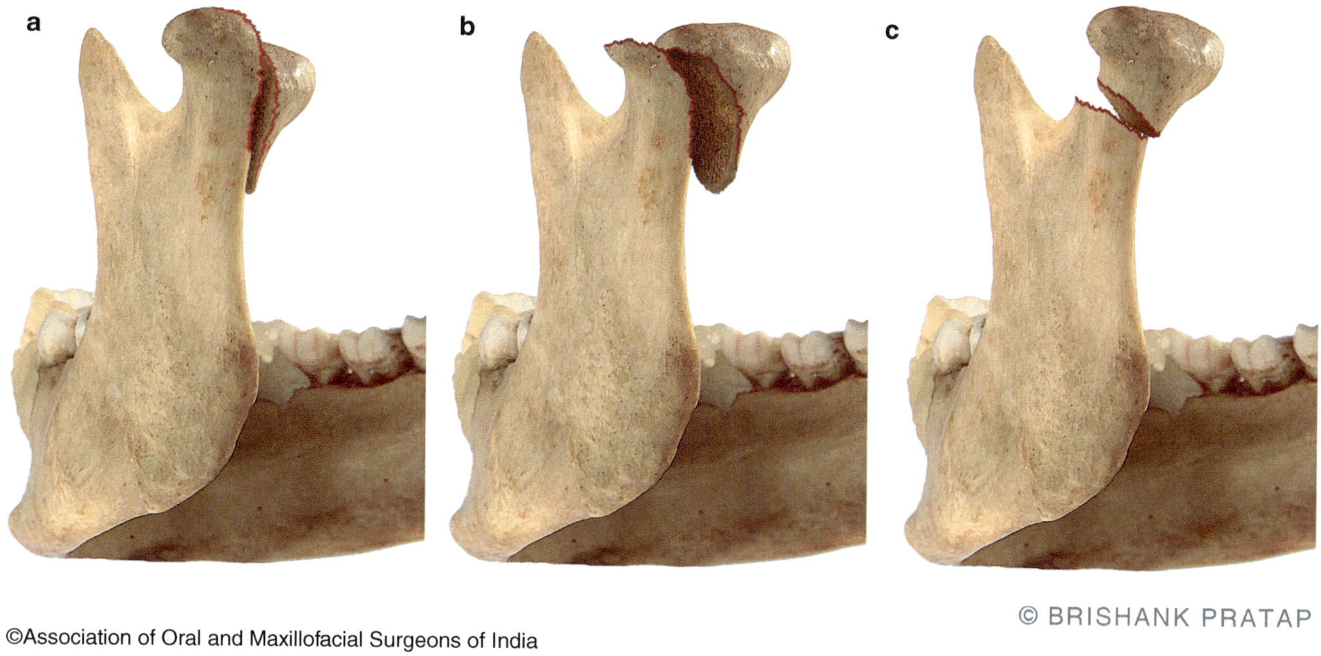

Fig. 53.8 Modified classification Type A, B, C

Lindahl [9] gave the most comprehensive classification. Although descriptive, it is a complicated classification [9].

1. Fracture level
   (a) Condylar head
   (b) Condylar neck
   (c) Subcondylar/condylar base
2. Deviation and displacement
   (a) Bending/deviation with medial overlapping segments
   (b) Bending/deviation with lateral overlapping segments
   (c) Bending/displacement without overlapping
   (d) Nondisplaced fracture without deviation
3. Relation between condylar head and fossa
   (a) No dislocation
   (b) Slight dislocation
   (c) Moderate dislocation
   (d) Severe and/or complete dislocation
4. Condylar head fracture
   (a) Horizontal
   (b) Vertical
   (c) Compression fracture

Lindahl's Definition

- **Subcondylar fracture:** The fracture line starts at the sigmoid notch and extends to the posterior border of the mandible.
- **Condylar neck fracture:** It is located at the condylar process which is below the level of the condylar head.
- **Condylar head fracture:** The majority of the fracture components or the whole fracture is contained within the TMJ capsule.

A most common classification of diacapitular fractures was given by He et al. [18]. The types of fractures that can be recognized are (Fig. 53.9):

- Type A—Lateral third portion of the condylar head has the fracture line, and there is reduction of the ramus height.
- Type B—Central third portion of the condylar head has the fracture line, and there is no reduction of the ramus height.
- Type C—Medial third portion of the condylar head has the fracture line, and there is no reduction of the ramus height.
- Type M—It is a fracture which is comminuted with multiple fragments, usually more than three, of the condylar head.

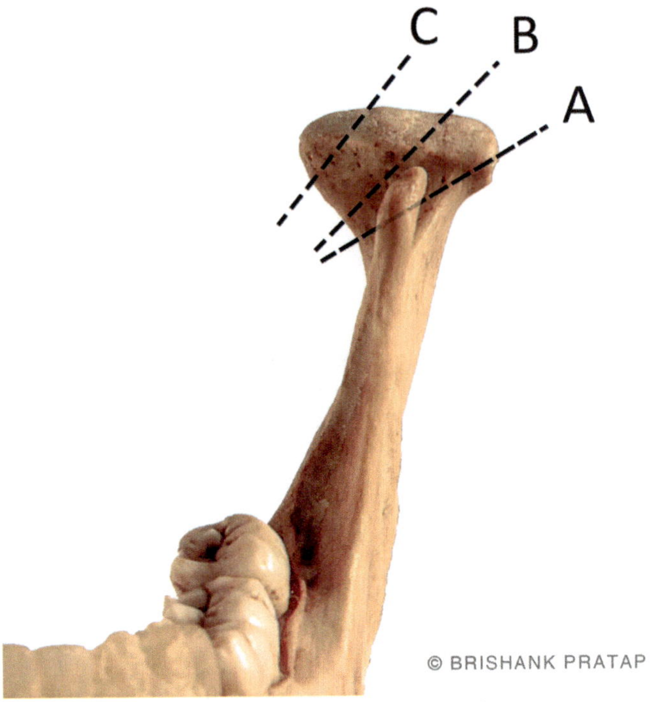

Fig. 53.9 Classification of diacapitular fractures (Type M not shown in figure)

Loukota et al. [19] proposed a system of classification for condylar processes fractures of the mandible. This classification was adopted by SOR group which is based on a line A drawn perpendicular from the lowest portion of the sigmoid notch to the posterior border of the mandible. This helps in identifying the anatomy of the mandibular ramus even in cases following severe trauma. A clarification is also given on the condylar head fracture, and it clearly defined the term minimal displacement.

Diacapitular fracture: Starting in the articular surface the fracture line may extend outside the TMJ capsule (Fig. 53.10a).

Condylar neck: Major portion of the fracture line which starts above the line A remains above it (Fig. 53.10b).

Condylar base: Major portion of the fracture line remains below the line A, and it extends behind the mandibular foramen (Fig. 53.10c).

Minimal displacement: Less than 10^0 displacement or 2 mm overlap of the bone edges or both.

AO Foundation in 2010 expanded on Ellis [20] classification with the determination of "high-neck" and "low-neck" fractures in the online AO Surgery Reference, which pro-

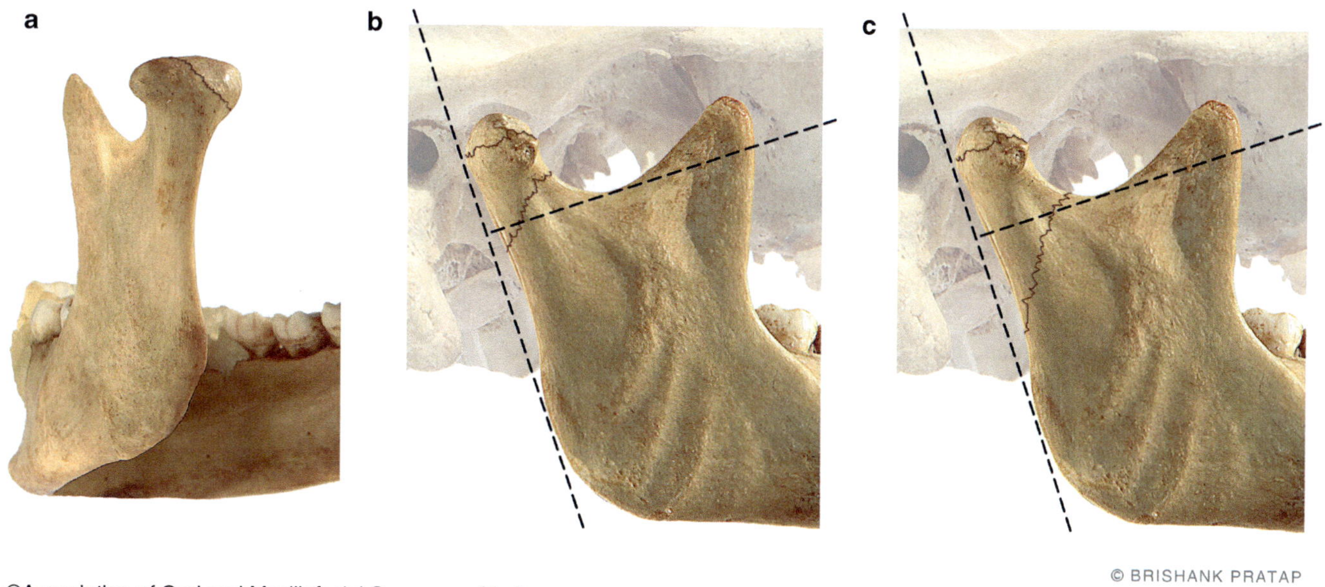

Fig. 53.10 (**a**) Dicapitular fracture. (**b**) Condylar neck. (**c**) Condylar base

vided a great detail to the location of "high and low" fractures as explained by Loukota:

- **Line 1** runs parallels the posterior border of the mandible line .
- **Line 2** as called the sigmoid notch line runs perpendicular to line 1 at the deepest portion the sigmoid notch.
- **Line 3** is perpendicular to the first line and is below the lateral pole of condylar head.
- A line is also drawn half way between the line 2 and line 3 which differentiates between high- and low-neck fractures (Fig. 53.11).

Neff et al. [21] published the Comprehensive AOCMF Classification System: Condylar Process Fractures. It is a system that highlights fracture location, identification, displacement, comminution, and dislocation. Location of the condylar fracture is clearly identified:

- *Condylar head*: the condylar head reference line runs perpendicular to the posterior ramus below the lateral pole of the condylar head.
- *Condylar neck*: the sigmoid notch line running through the deepest point of the sigmoid notch perpendicular to the ramus line extending superiorly to the condylar head.
- *Base of the condylar process*: the sigmoid notch line running through the deepest point of the sigmoid notch perpendicular to the ramus line extending inferiorly.

In the early days classification systems for the condylar fractures were entirely focused in locating the fracture. This was followed by systems which added the relation of the condyle with the adjacent structure. Loukota [19] gave a

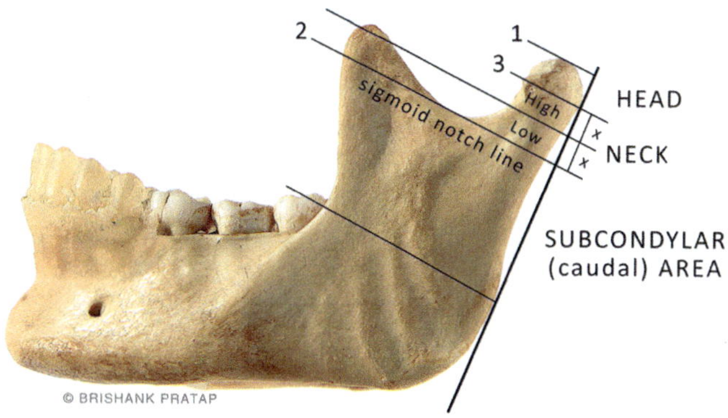

Fig. 53.11 AO foundation classification

classification which accurately locates the fracture with reference to treatment which is a simple classification to follow.

The aim of classifying the condylar fractures of the mandible is to locate the type and nature of the fracture which in turn will give a clear understanding of the nature of injury. This in turn will help the surgeon make a decision on the modality of treatment which may be open or closed.

53.5 Incidence and Pattern

In the facial skeletal, one of the most common bones to fracture is the mandible. Analysis of the fracture of different anatomical sites of the mandible revealed that there was a 10–40% incidence of condylar fractures [22–24]. Ellis et al. [25] published a study that showed condyle fractures represented 29.3% of all mandibular fractures. Zachariades et al. [26] stated that 72% of the condylar fractures were associated with other mandibular fractures. Isolated condylar fractures were rare, and occurrence of malocclusion was more dependent on the site of fracture. Incidence of fractures of condylar base were 57%, neck 31%, and head 12% as reported by Maclennan [27]. Incidence of condylar head was the least with the majority fractures at the condylar base. Frequency of unilateral fractures is higher than the bilateral fractures.

The highest incidence of mandibular fractures in males was 20–30 years and females 30–40 years [25] with the male-to-female ratio 3:1 [26]. Condylar fracture can result from direct or indirect trauma. The degree, direction, magnitude, and point of application of force determine the severity of displacement [27]. Personal violence [28] followed by fall [29–31] is the most common aetiology of condylar fractures.

53.6 Clinical Features

The patient may show mild to severe signs and symptoms following a condylar fracture. These are entirely dependent on the amount of displacement of the fractured fragments. Condylar fractures infrequently occurred in isolation and are generally associated with fractures of other sites of the facial bones. Surgeons may overlook subtle clinical features.

Signs and symptoms:

- Pain and swelling over the preauricular region
- Ecchymosis over the mastoid region
- CSF otorrhea
- Hollowness over the condylar region
- Restricted incisal opening
- Locked mandible

53.6.1 Condylar Fractures: Unilateral

- Premature occlusion on the ipsilateral side (Fig. 53.12a).
- Open bite due to the loss of vertical height on the contralateral side.
- Affected side deviates on opening and is common because of the interruption of the action of the lateral pterygoid muscle.
- Limited laterotrusive movements away from the fractured side but may be maintained towards the fracture.

53.6.2 Condylar Fractures: Bilateral

- Bilateral loss of vertical height results in anterior open bite with posterior gagging (Fig. 53.12b).
- Restricted mouth opening
- May be associated with other fractures

53.6.3 Radiographic Assessment

Condylar fractures can be evaluated by a number of conventional views. A set of two radiographs are usually taken perpendicular to each other for optimum evaluation. However the assessment has become more descriptive with availability of specialized radiographs. Various views which can be taken to evaluate the condylar fracture are as follows (Fig. 53.13):

- Towne's view
- AP mandible coronal position
- Panorex
- CT scan
- MRI

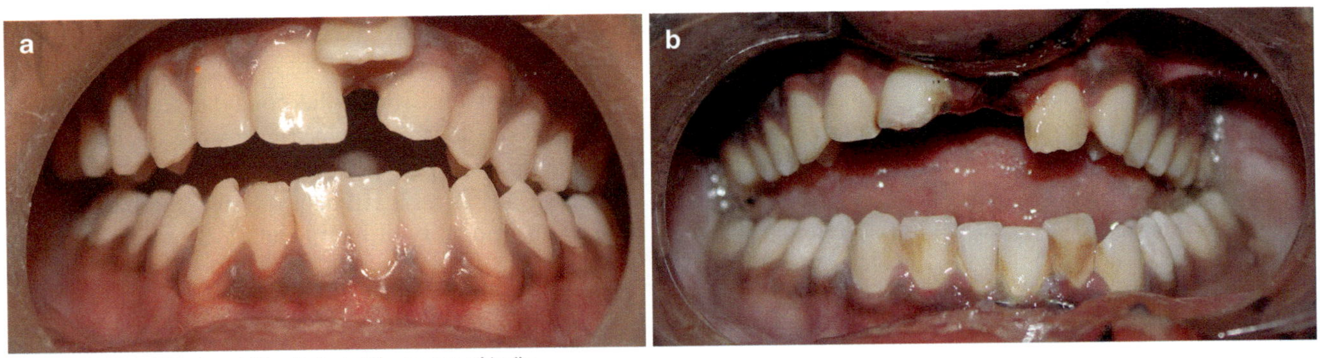

Fig. 53.12 Occlusion post condylar fracture. (**a**) Unilateral condylar fracture of the left. (**b**) Bilateral condylar fracture

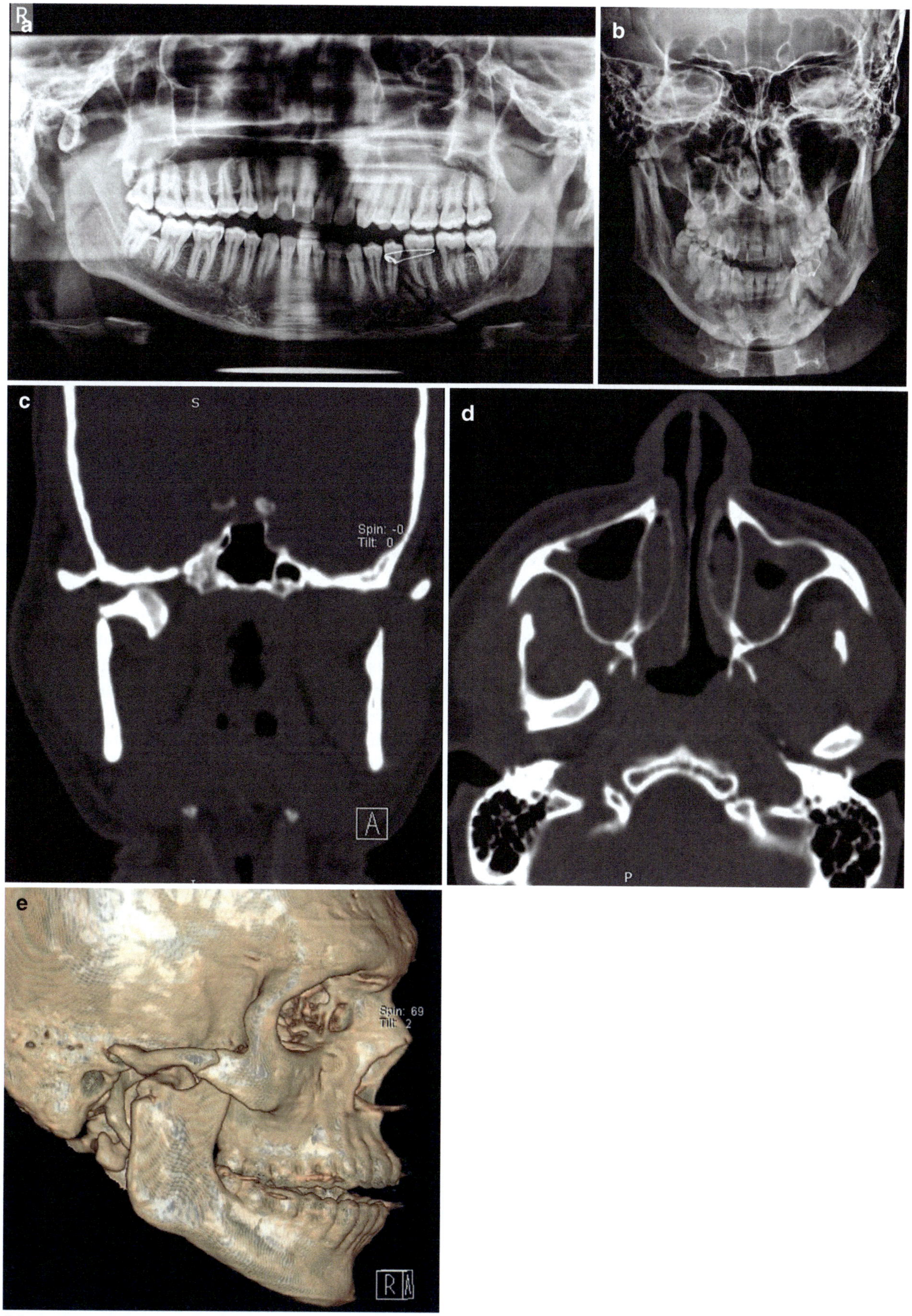

Fig. 53.13 A case of unilateral fracture of the right side of condyle with a left body of mandible. (**a**) OPG. (**b**) PA mandible. (**c**) Coronal view. (**d**) Axial view. (**e**) 3D view of the CT scan

However it may be noted that with conventional radiography, very limited information is available. CT scans in the three plains, namely, coronal, axial, and sagittal, with volumetric studies can reveal the true picture of the fracture both for the terms of evaluation and treatment planning. MRI are essential to evaluate the disc injuries specially in dislocation and intracapsular condylar fractures; however MRI are not taken as a routine practise

53.7 Management

Historically there has been no clear agreement among the surgeons on the line of management of the fractures of the condyle. The goals of treatment which were enumerated by Walker [32] (Box 53.2) are well accepted.

Box 53.2. Treatment Goals [32]

- No pain and minimum interincisal distance of 40 mm on opening the mouth.
- On excursions movements are good.
- Restore pre-injury occlusion.
- Good stable temporomandibular joints.
- Good symmetry of face and jaw.
- Good facial and jaw symmetry

Box 53.3. Indications for Open Reduction
Zide and Kent's [33]

Absolute

- Condyle displaced into middle cranial fossa
- Not possible to obtain adequate occlusion by closed reduction
- Lateral capsular displacement of condyle
- Presence of foreign body

Relative

- Bilateral condylar fracture in an edentulous patient without splint
- Comminuted midface fracture, prognathic or retrognathic jaws having associated bilateral condylar fractures
- Generalized periodontal conditions
- Jaws—totally or partially edentulous
- Unilateral condylar fractures with lack of base

Box 53.4. American Association of Oral and Maxillofacial Surgeons [34]

- Evidence of fracture—clinical
- Evidence of fracture—radiographic
- Malocclusion associated with fractures
- Mandibular dysfunction
- Abnormal maxillo-mandibular relationship
- Foreign body invasion
- Lacerations and/or haemorrhage in external auditory canal
- Cases having hemotympanum, CSF otorrhea, effusion, or hemartorisis

Literature has indicated that closed reduction has been the treatment of choice. This may be due to the complexities involved with open reduction. Surgical approach is technically demanding and associated with complications in inexperienced hands. As a result, some centres have exclusively treated condylar fractures by closed reduction. However as opposed to closed reduction, a few centres follow a protocol for management where open reduction is treatment of choice. Patients managed by surgical treatment have a superior outcome in term of post-treatment malocclusion, protrusion, laterotrusion, and lateral deviation during mouth opening. However, there was a higher infection rate as compared to non-surgical treatment. However, there is no statistical difference in post-treatment pain and maximum mouth opening in the two modalities of management [10]. Management can be divided as non-operative and operative (Box 53.6).

53.7.1 Non-operative

Some patients can be managed by observations provided they have a minimal nondisplaced fracture, dentate with a stable occlusion and having minimum pain. An important factor is that the patient must be complaint. At the onset of the treatment, patient must be explained about the possibility of additional treatment in the form of closed reduction which may be required.

Protocol followed is as follows:

1. Diet: There is no restriction on the diet; generally a patient would be restricted to a soft diet in order to avoid pain.
2. Rehabilitation: Patient is instructed to perform exercises of the jaw such that all the excursion movements are carried out. Goals of rehabilitation are mentioned in the (Box 53.8).

Box 53.5. Indication for Open and Closed Reduction
Fonseca [35] adapted from references [36–43]

Absolute
- Condyle displaced into middle cranial fossa
- Presence of foreign body
- Extracapsular displacement of condyle laterally
- Malocclusion not amenable to closed reduction (e.g., functional reduction of ramus height)

Strong evidence for open reduction
- Bilaterally fractured condyles
- Condyle displacement grossly >45° (severely displaced)
- Anatomic reduction of ramus height ≥ 2 mm
- Condylar fractures with an unstable base (associated midface fractures)
- Unstable occlusion generally seen in periodontal disease, less than three teeth per quadrant
- Condylar fractures for which adequate physiotherapy is impossible

Mixed evidence for open reduction
- Moderate condylar displacement, 10–45°

When to treat with closed reduction
- Nondisplaced or incomplete fractures
- Isolated intracapsular fractures
- Condylar fractures in children (except for absolute indications)
- Reproducible occlusion without dropback or with dropback that returns to midline on release of posterior force
- Medical illness or injury that inhibits ability to receive extended general anaesthesia

Box 53.6. Management of Condylar Fractures

Non-operative:
- Observation, physiotherapy, etc.

Operative:
- Closed procedures:
- MMF (arch bars or screws—elastic or wire)
- Open reduction and internal fixation (ORIF)
  - Approach is determined by:
    - (i) Surgeon preference
    - (ii) Fracture location
    - (iii) Type of fixation

Box 53.7. Factors Taken into Consideration for Treatment
- Location of the fracture
- Amount of vertical reduction in height of the ramus
- Degree of angulation
- Relation of condylar head to the glenoid fossa
- Fragmentation pattern (simple versus complex)
- Association with other mandibular injuries
- Dental occlusion/status of dentition
- Association with other facial bone injuries
- Association with systemic injuries
- Association with the condition of the patient (comorbidity factors)
- Foreign body in temporomandibular joint (TMJ)

Box 53.8. Closed Reduction

Advantages
- Relatively safe procedure
- No injuries to vital structures
- Hospitalization may not be required

Disadvantage
- Long period of intermaxillary fixation
- Growth disturbances can occur in children
- Success depends on patients cooperation
- Long-term follow
- Contraindicated in medically compromised
- Challenge in partially or totally edentulous patients

3. Follow-up: Recall visit is scheduled after 1 week. At this visit progress is recorded. Next visit is scheduled after 2 weeks if the patient is compliant. In case the progress is not satisfactory frequent follow-up would be required or a change in treatment plan.

53.7.2 Closed Reduction

Closed reduction is a misnomer. It is never possible to achieve anatomic reduction as seen in management of other fractures. Closed reduction relies on the functional adaptation where a stable occlusion is achieved. Advantage of this technique is that it is minimally invasive and may not require hospitalization. It is entirely possible to carry out the procedure under local anaesthesia. However adaptation is never complete in adults as opposed to children. It may be possible to treat all types of condylar process fractures by this technique, but the surgeon must exercise his judgement based on the case and patient requirements. Closed reduction may involve the following:

1. Maxillomandibular fixation (MMF): Some surgeons prefer period of MMF which may range over 2–6 weeks. MMF can be obtained by using arch bars, Ivy loops, IMF screws or any other method a surgeon is comfortable; however method used will depend on the use of elastics or wires, and MMF may entirely be based on the level of fracture. The reader is advised to refer Chap. 50 of this book for details on various wiring and IMF techniques The lower the fracture, the longer the period of immobilization. In children immobilization may range from 7 to 10 days as there are high chances of developing ankylosis. This is followed by functional treatment.
2. Functional treatment: At times only, functional treatment may be followed. This treatment relies on guiding elastics and active movements. Elastics are given to achieve repeatable occlusion. Initially heavy elastics are placed and then slowly shifted to light elastics. During the meals elastics are removed. After an initial period of 2–4 weeks, elastics are placed only during the night. Minimum elastics must be used as the aim is to permit maximum mobility of the jaw. Functional treatment can be supported by myofunctional orthodontic treatment employing activator therapy. Myofunctional therapy should be started as soon as the mouth opening enables taking dental impressions.

53.7.3 Open Reduction and Fixation

This modality is technically challenging due to the complexities in terms of anatomy, approach, and fixation. It has been observed that by achieving anatomical reduction irrespective of the type of fixation used, it will result in restoring back the skeletal architecture. This in turn would require only neuromuscular adaptation for full recovery of the patient. According to the reports, this may be the reason for open management to be superior to the closed [36].

Surgical approaches to the condylar fracture are entirely dependent on the following factors (Fig. 53.14):

1. Location of the injury
2. Type of osteosynthesis

Incisions used to approach the fractures are divided as

1. Intraoral
2. Retromandibular
3. Submandibular/ periangular
4. Preauricular/ retroauricular

Box 53.9. Open Reduction and Fixation

Advantages
- Anatomic reduction of fractures
- Short or no intermaxillary fixation
- Early function

Disadvantage
- Complications such as scar and injuries to neurovascular structures
- Infections
- Hospitalization required
- High cost of treatment
- Steep learning curve for surgeon

53.7.3.1 Submandibular/Periangular (Fig. 53.15a, b) (Video 53.1)

This is an approach most maxillofacial surgeons are familiar with in their practise popularly known as Risdon approach. It exposes the base along with the neck of the condyle. Incision can either be parallel to the lower border or placed in a skin crease for maximum cosmetic results. For the condylar, fracture's incision is extended backward and upward to give a maximum exposure hence also referred to as periangular incision. The marginal mandibular nerve is protected by marking the incision 2–3 cm below the lower border of the mandible. Incision transverses through the skin, subcutaneous fat, and platysma. A superior platysmal dissection will expose the marginal mandibular nerve; however this may not be necessary. After dissection of the platysma, superficial layer of deep cervical fascia is transected; this may expose the facial artery and vein. These may be required to be ligated and reflected superiorly. This will protect the marginal mandibular nerve. Then pterygomasseteric sling is divided and periosteum reflected to expose the lower border of the mandible. This gives an adequate exposure for osteosynthesis.

A modification of the submandibular/periangular approach known as the high submandibular approach or the high cervical transmassetric anteroparotid approach provides good aesthetics and reduces the chances of damage to the facial nerve [44]. A curved incision measuring three to five cm in length is placed about 1 cm from the angle of mandible [45]. This is followed by layered dissection. An avascular pouch is created superiorly, and the pterygomasseteric sling is identified. Stripping the masseter muscles of its attachments will lead to the exposure of the fracture [46] (Video 53.2).

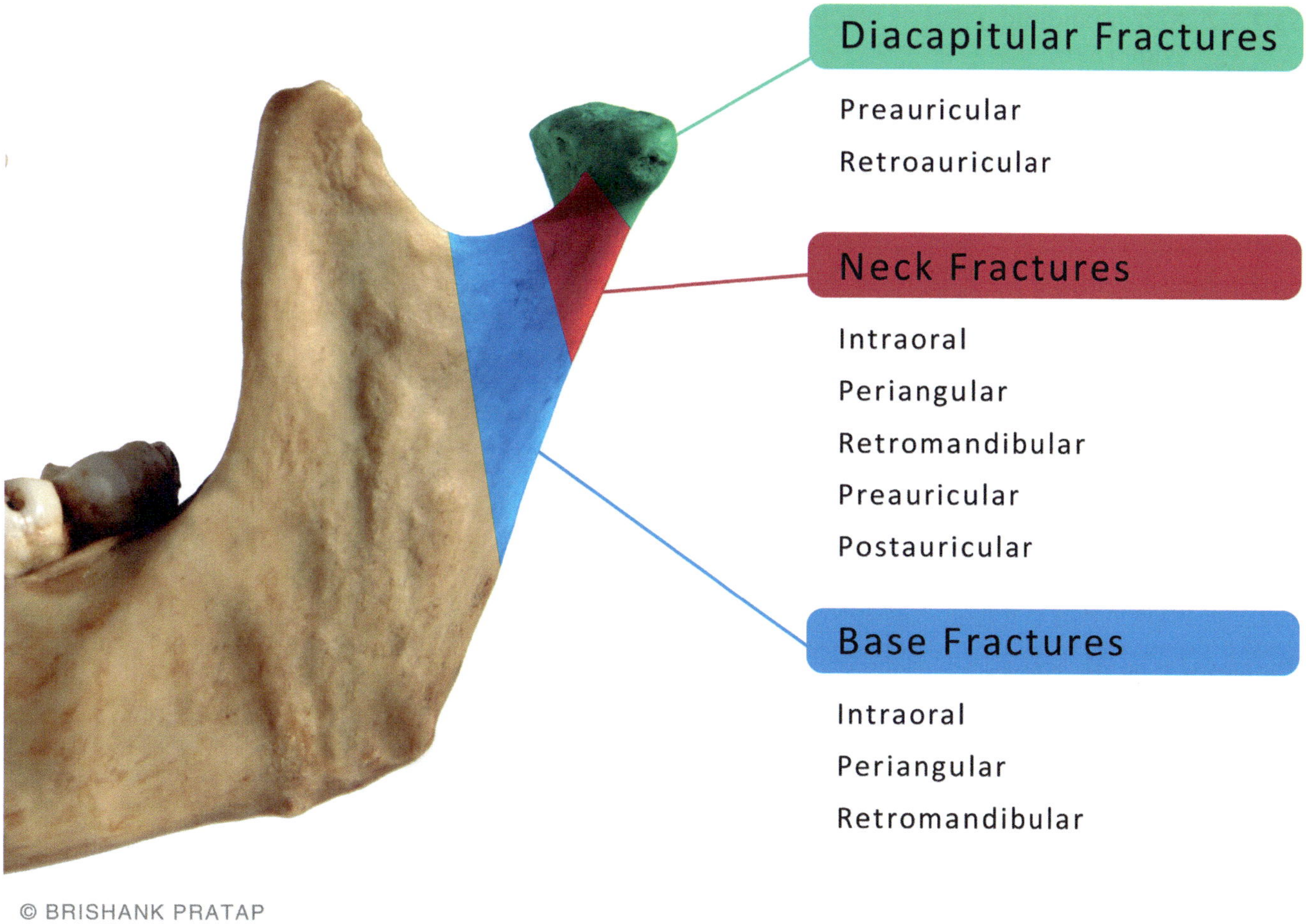

Fig. 53.14 Various incisions possible for condylar fractures based on location

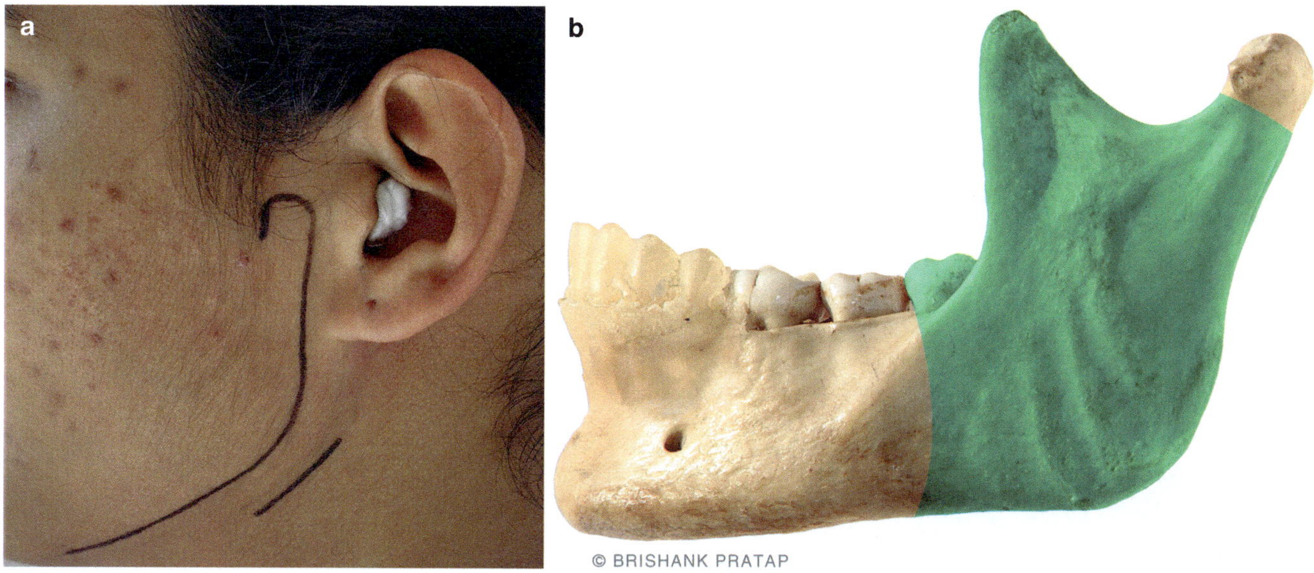

Fig. 53.15 (**a**) Incision for submandibular/periangular approach. (**b**) Area exposed marked green in the mandible

53.7.3.2 Retromandibular (Fig. 53.16a, b) (Video 53.3)

Entire posterior border can be exposed via the retromandibular approach [47]; hence this approach is useful in treating fracture of the condylar neck and the base. The anatomic structures encountered in this approach are the main trunk of the facial nerve and retromandibular vein. It has two main variations transparotid and retroparotid. In both the variation marking of the incision is 5–10 mm below the lobule of the ear, parallel to the posterior border usually 3–4 cm long.

Transparotid Approach

In this approach incision is extends from the skin to the subcutaneous tissue, and it is undermined to reach the parotid capsule which is divided horizontally between the path of the buccal and zygomatic branches of the facial nerve. Dissection is carried out parallel to the direction of the facial nerve branches, and it is not important to locate the branches. Pterygomasseteric sling is sectioned, and periosteal flap elevated to expose the posterior border of the mandible.

Retroparotid Approach

In this approach parotid gland is lifted rather than transected to approach the posterior border of the mandible. Incision in this approach is placed more posterior as compared to transparotid approach as a result exposure is also restricted. After the parotid fascia is identified, dissection is carried out behind the gland. The gland is lifted to expose the posterior border; from here the dissection carried out is the same as the transparotid approach.

The wound is closed in layers to avoid dead space. Also, the parotid fascia should be sutured tightly to prevent sialocele or parotid fistula. Drains can also be placed.

53.7.3.3 Preauricular Approach (Fig. 53.17a, b) (Video 53.4)

This incision is most commonly used by the surgeons in the TM joint surgeries. Diacapitular fractures are approached via this approach [48]. Branches of facial nerve are involved in this approach along with the superficial temporal artery and vein. Incision is placed along the crease of the skin following the tragus and helix of the ear which can be extended in the temple region. This extension on the temple minimizes traction and prevents weakness of facial nerve. Incision is carried from the skin to the subcutaneous tissue till the white glistening temporal fascia is reached. Root of the zygoma is palpated, and an oblique incision is given parallel to the frontal branch of facial nerve. Superficial temporal fascia is incised, and a periosteal elevator is inserted below the fascia to strip the periosteum of the zygomatic arch. This will expose the capsule of the temporomandibular joint. Capsule is incised in an open method to expose the head of the condyle. The neck is exposed by doing a subperiosteal dissection. Closure is done in layers first being the capsule followed by temporalis fascia, subcutaneous tissue, and the skin. The main disadvantage of this approach is an unaesthetic scar. This can be overcome by placing the incision endurally. The scar hides behind the tragus, but it can cause perichondritis.

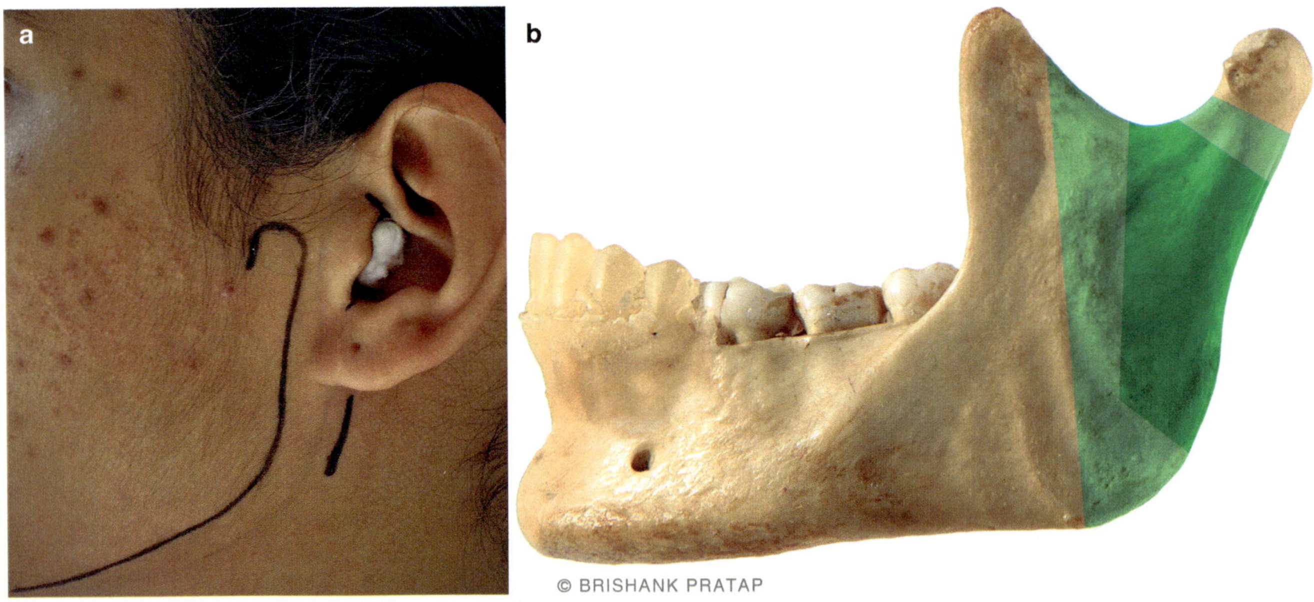

Fig. 53.16 (a) Incision for retromandibular approach. (b) Area exposed marked in mandible (dark green, retro parotid exposure; light green, transparotid exposure)

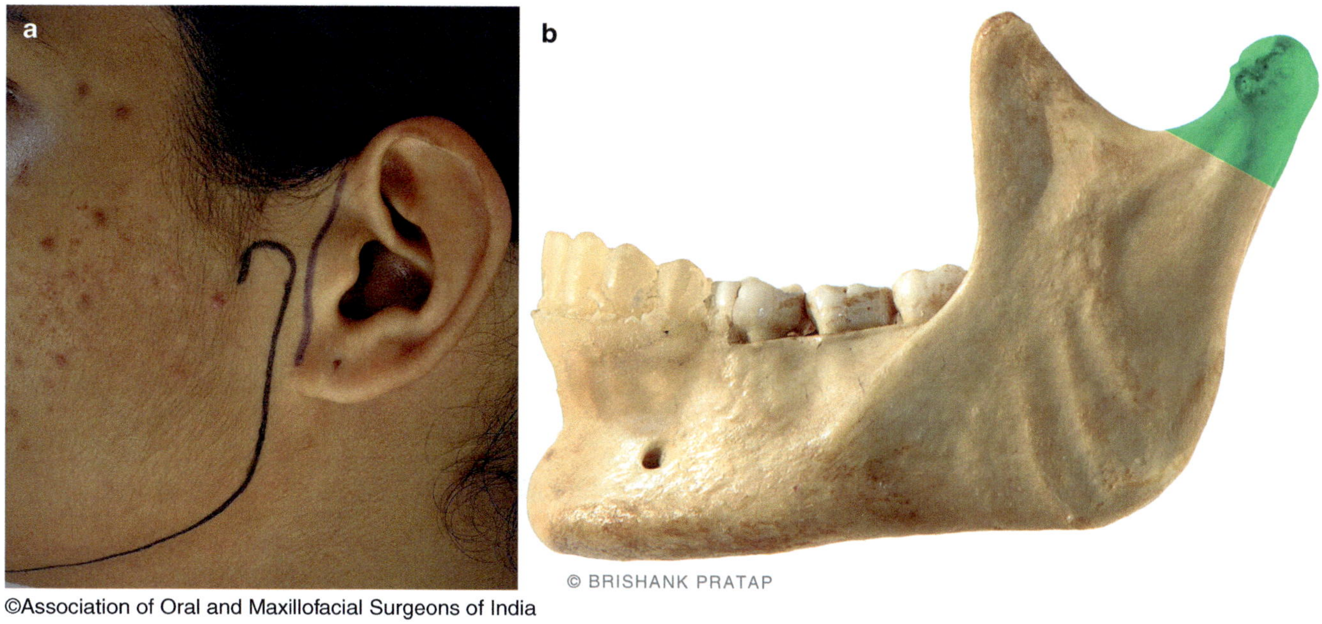

Fig. 53.17 (**a**) Preauricular approach incision. (**b**) Area exposed marked in the mandible

53.7.3.4 Retroauricular Approach

This is an approach which will provide best cosmetic results. However major disadvantage is that it can result in stenosis of the external auditory canal. Also, the closure takes a longer time. Incision runs parallel to postauricular flexure approximately 3 mm behind it. Skin followed by postauricular muscles and fascia overlying mastoid are incised. External auditory canal is identified and completely transected at bony cartilaginous junction. Temporalis fascia is identified, and from here dissection followed is similar to preauricular approach to expose the condylar head. Closure is done in layers with a special attention given to the external auditory canal.

53.7.4 Reduction

After the adequate exposure of the fractured fragments reduction is achieved under direct vision. If the distal fragment is placed laterally, reduction tends to be easy. However, in most of the cases, the fragments tend to be displaced medially resulting from the pull of lateral pterygoid muscle. A medially displaced fragment must be lateralized before an attempt is made to reduce the fracture. For easy manipulation, a plate with a single screw is fixed on the distal fragment. This will help in easy lateralization of the distal fragment and prevent the fragment from slipping back as the lower end of the plate acts as a rest on the proximal segment. Before an attempt is made to reduce the fracture, manual traction is applied to the mandible so that the vertical height of the posterior mandible is restored. This can be achieved as follows (Fig. 53.18a–d):

1. Manual digital traction: Thumb is placed on the lower teeth and fingers support the lower border. Mandible is pulled in inferior and anterior direction.
2. Bite block: A bite block is placed on the same side of the condylar fracture in the molar region. This will result in inferior distraction of the mandible with rotation.
3. Transosseous wire: A transosseous wire can be passed along the posteroinferior border of the mandible. A traction is applied on this wire in an inferior and anterior direction.

Once the fracture is reduced with the help of a clamp in the lowermost hole of the plate, pressure is applied to keep the fractured end in place. Figure 53.19a–d shows the reduction and fixation of a medially displaced condyle fracture.

In a case where two plates are planned for fixation, the smaller plate along the anterior border of the condyle is fixed first with a screw. Once the anterior plate is fixed on the distal segment, similar steps are followed as mentioned earlier for single plate for reduction and fixation.

Sequencing the case of multiple fractures is as follows:

1. Fractures with contralateral condylar fractures—Fractures in the tooth bearing anterior segment are fixed before the condyle is fixed.

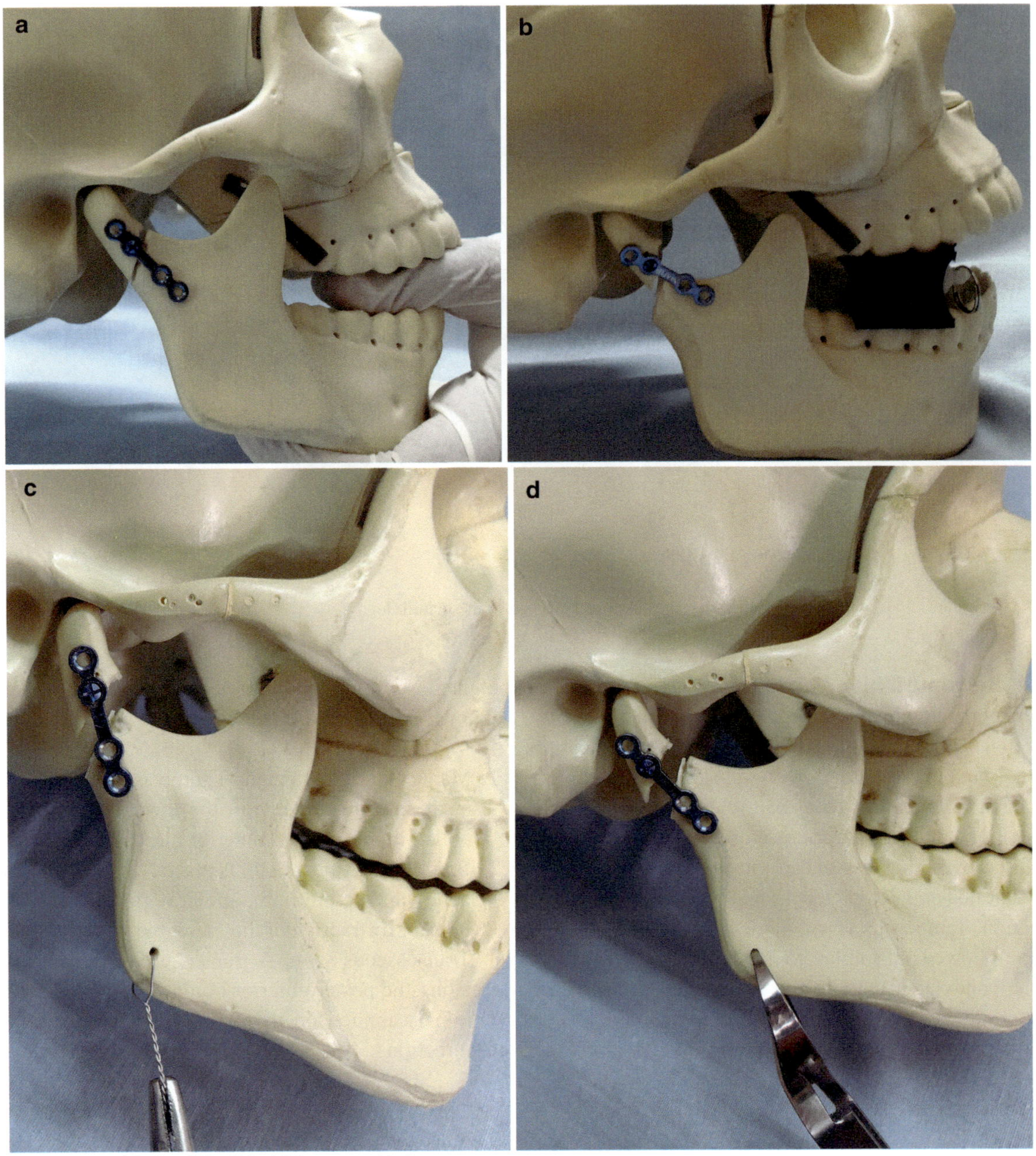

Fig. 53.18 (**a**) Manual digital reduction. (**b**) Traction using bite block. (**c**) Transosseous wiring. (**d**) Towel clip

2. Bilateral condylar fracture with anterior mandible—In these cases there can be flaying of the mandible resulting in increase of transverse dimension of mandible. Anterior fractures are reduced and fixed taking into consideration into the lingual reduction. Anterior fractures are fixed before the posterior.
3. Panfacial trauma—Principal remains the same, mandible is fixed as mentioned above before the midface fractures are reduced and fixed. This may change depending on the sequence followed for fixation of panfacial fractures

53.7.5 Fixation Techniques (Fig. 53.20a–d), (Case 1: Fig. 53.21a–b), (Case 2: Fig. 53.22), (Case 3: Fig. 53.23a–e), (Case 4: Fig 53.24a–d)

The most significant advances that have taken place in the management of fracture of condylar process include the osteosynthesis material and the technique. Fixation with titanium plates and screws has given optimal results when adequate bone, proper site selection with proper techniques

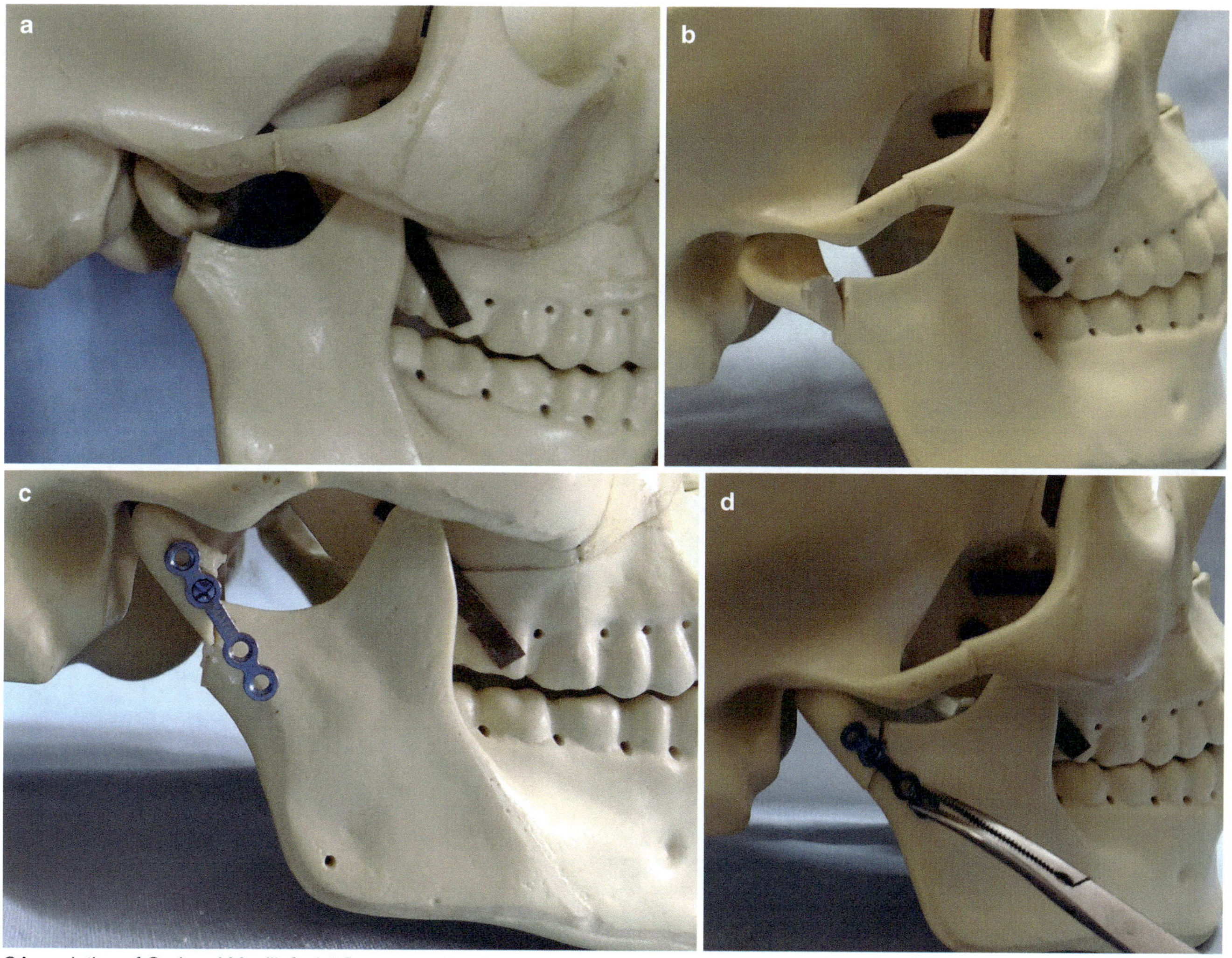

Fig. 53.19 (**a**) Medially displaced condylar fracture. (**b**) Fracture lateralized. (**c**) Distal segment secured with a plate. (**d**) Fracture reduced

followed [49]. At the time of surgery fixation, technique is selected based on the following parameters:

1. Fracture morphology
2. Amount of bone available
3. Surgeon preference

Fixation can be in the form of one plate, two plates, hybrid plates, lag screws, or restorable plates. Studies have shown that use of two plates is superior to one plate [40, 50]. Two plates must be used for lower level fractures to overcome tension and stress in the neck region by placing plates along the anterior and posterior border in a triangular fashion (Fig. 53.20a–d). In cases where there is limited bone, available fixation can be done with heavier single plate. Single plate is fixed along the long axis of the condyle. There are many types of hybrid plates available. These are designed to incorporate the principle of two plates in a single plate. However, this makes the plates bulky as a result it may be at times difficult to fix them especially when there is limited bone available. Irrespective of the type of plate used, there should be at least two screws on either side of fracture.

Fixation of condylar head is a challenge because of the limited space available and the fractures are intracapsular. In addition, there could be multiple small fragments and associated injury to the disc and the capsule which may be required to be repaired. Several osteosynthesis techniques are available for fixation like the mini plates, stainless steel wire, standard lag screws, resorbable screws, resorbable pins, and cannulated lag screws (Fig. 53.25). Reduction and fixation of the condylar head is technically challenging as the small fragments can easily necrose if stripping of the muscle is done. Use of two lag screws would be idle as it will prevent the reduced fragments from displacement during function, but times it may not be possible to fix two screws due to limited space Table 53.1 [51].

Intraoral endosocpic approach for treatment of condylar fractures is given in detail in Chap. 54 of this book.

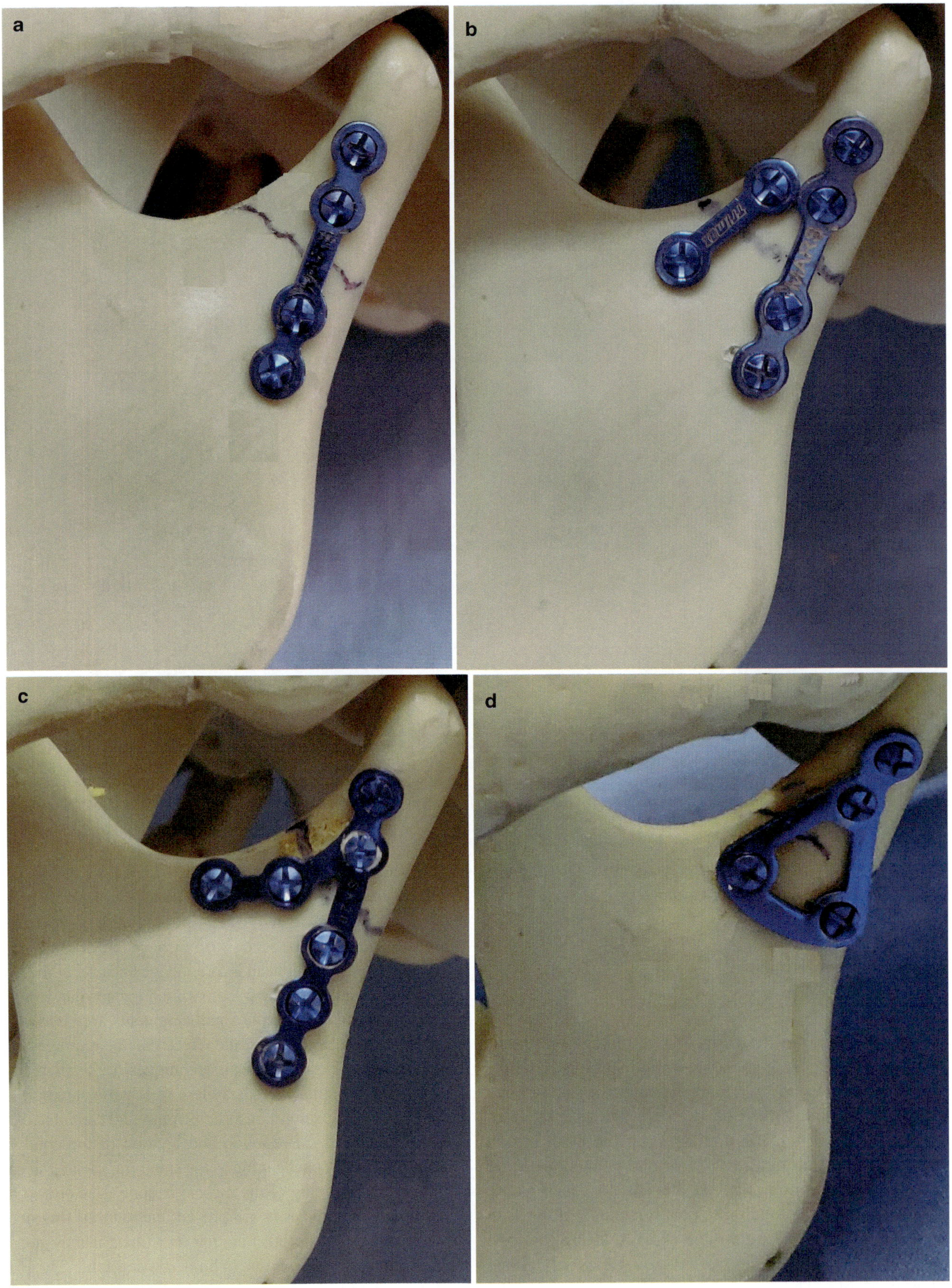

Fig. 53.20 (**a**) Single plate. (**b**) Two plates. (**c**) Lambda plate. (**d**) Delta plate

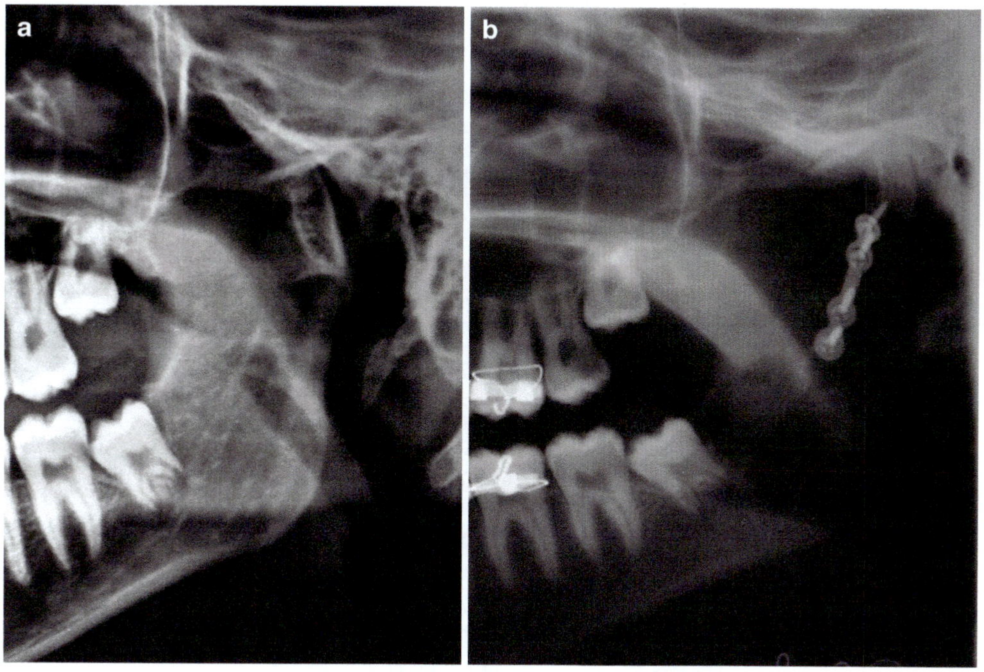

Case 1: Fig. 53.21 (**a**) OPG view showing left condyle fracture (**b**) Post operative OPG showing single plate fixed via retromandibular transparotid approach

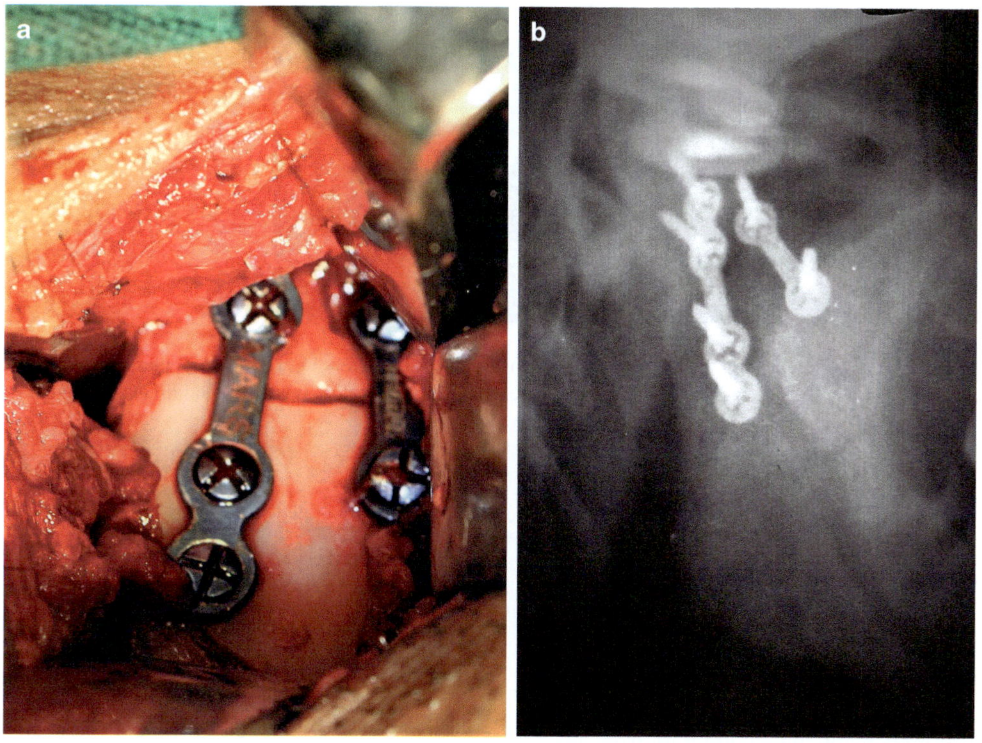

Case 2: Fig. 53.22 (**a**) Intra operative view showing two plates fixed for condyle fracture via retromandibular transparotid approach. (**b**) Post operative radiograph of showing fixation with two plates

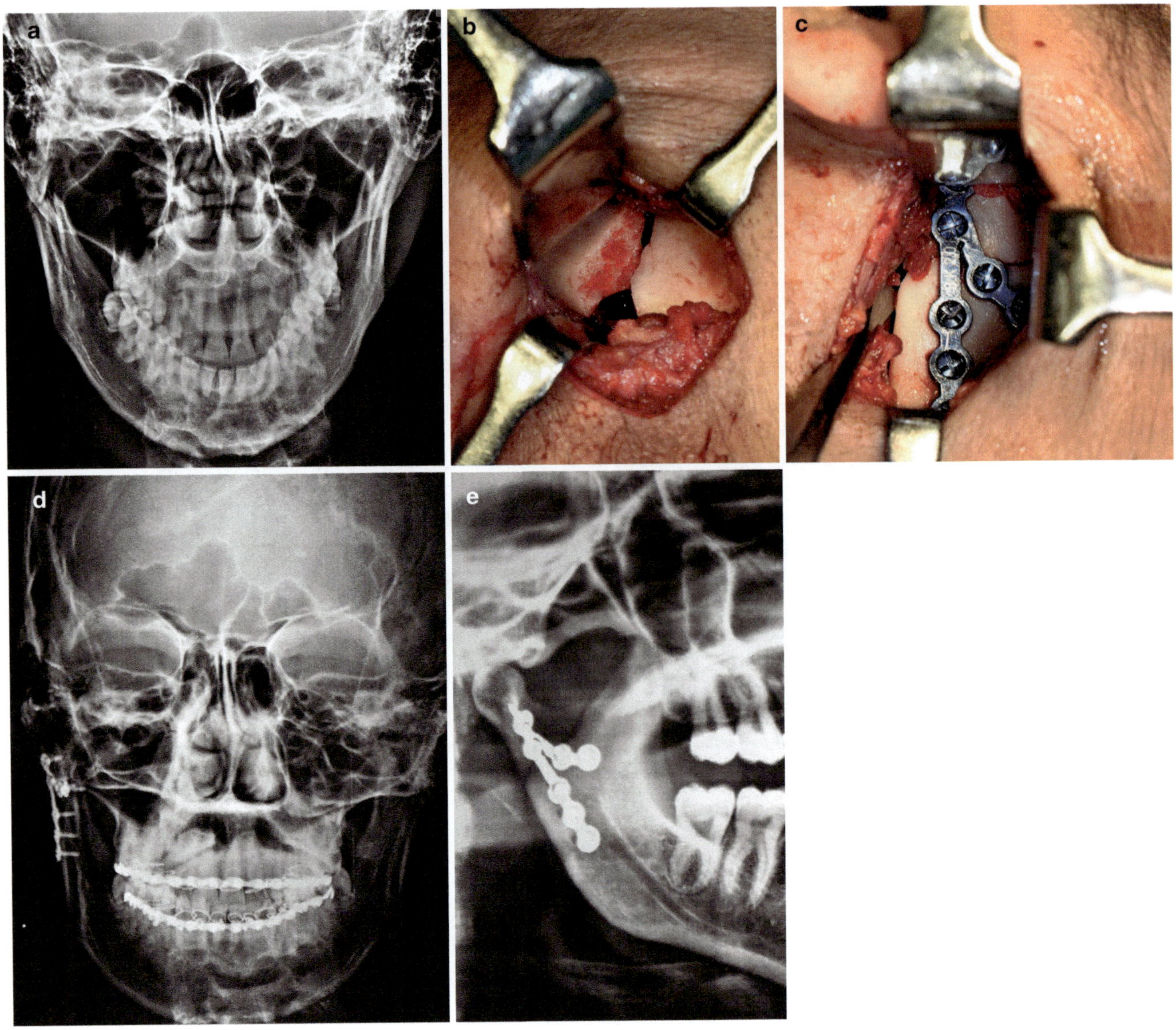

Case 3: Fig. 53.23 (**a**) PA view showing right condyle fracture. (**b**) Intraoperative view via retromandibular transparotid approach shows the displaced condyle. (**c**) Reduction and fixation done with Lambda plate. (**d**, **e**) Post operative PA view and OPG showing the fixed Lambda plates

Box 53.10. Functional Exercise: Rehabilitation Targets [52]

1. Maximal mouth opening > 40 mm
2. Lateral excursive movement > 10 mm
3. Protrusive movement > 10 mm
4. Full range of movements which are pain free
5. Close supervision by the surgeon

53.8 Condylar Fractures in Children

The most common fracture seen in the maxillofacial region in children is fracture of the condylar process [53]. Condyle is unique in children as there is a very thin cortical bone surrounding a highly vascular cancellous bone. This can result in a comminuted type of fracture also called mushrooming. Condylar fractures can result in definitive deformities, both in terms of function as well as

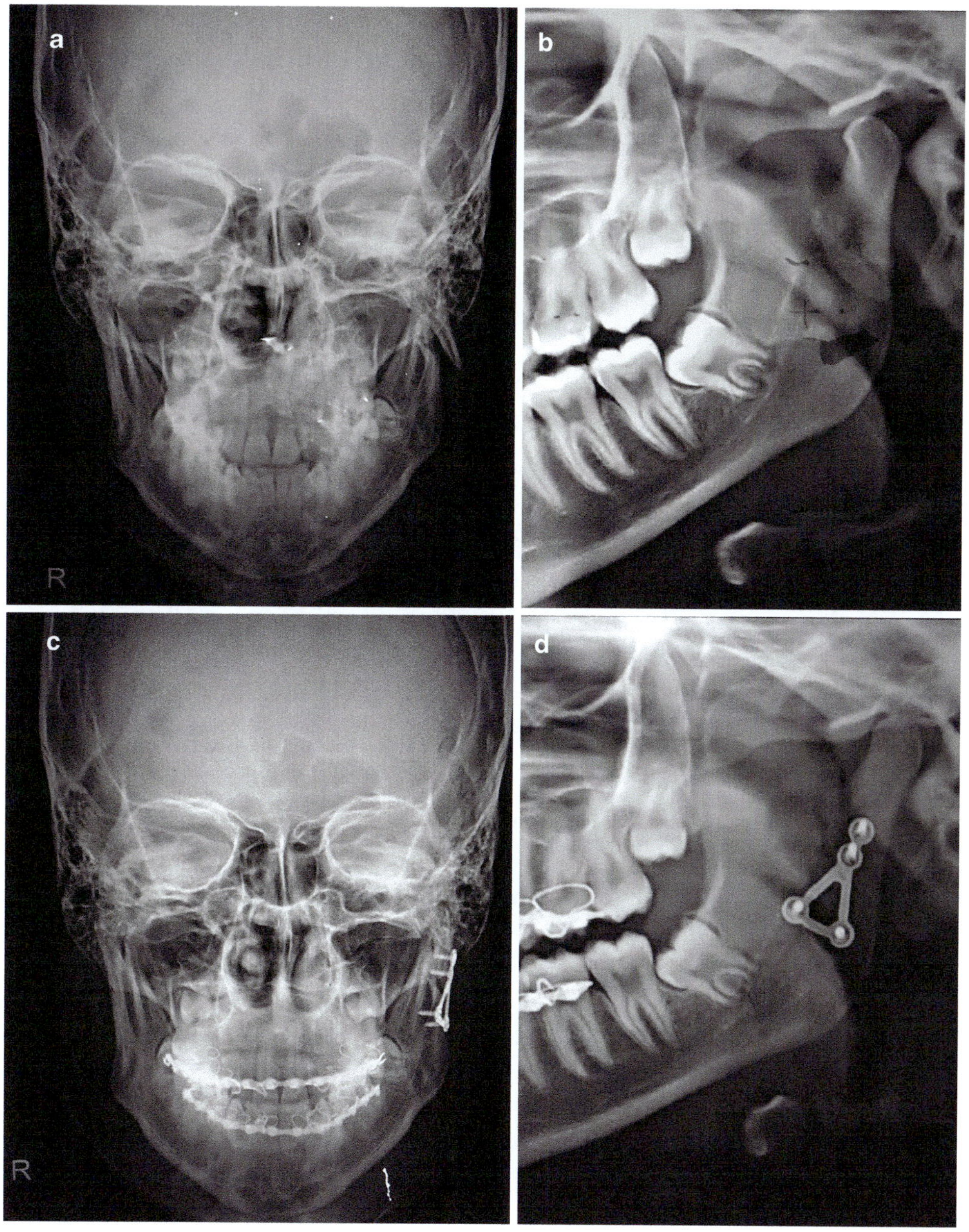

Case 4: Fig. 53.24 (**a**, **b**) Pre operative PA view and OPG showing fracture left condyle. (**c**, **d**) Post operative PA view and OPG showing the fixed Delta plate via Periangular approach

a facial asymmetry in cases of inappropriate treatment. Intracapsular fractures can result in retardation of growth [54, 55] or in excessive growth on the fractured site [56]. Remodelling of the condyle is inversely proportional to age [9, 25, 26]. Children have a better adaptation than the adults. Adaption in children is skeletal, neuromuscular, as well as function. In adults only functional adaptation is seen. For this reason, literature has supported conservative management of fracture of the condylar process. It is paramount to rehabilitate the patient with the restoration of minimum mouth opening, lateral excursion movement with stable occlusion. However, a long-term follow-up showed 50–53% of patients had complaints even though minor in nature irrespective of the type of treatment carried out [57]. Early mobilization is recommended in children below 15 years. Patients are encouraged to be on soft diet to avoid pain. In cases where an open bite is present, guiding elastics will help in restoring the occlusion. There is no concrete evidence of prolonged period of maxillo-mandibular fixation.

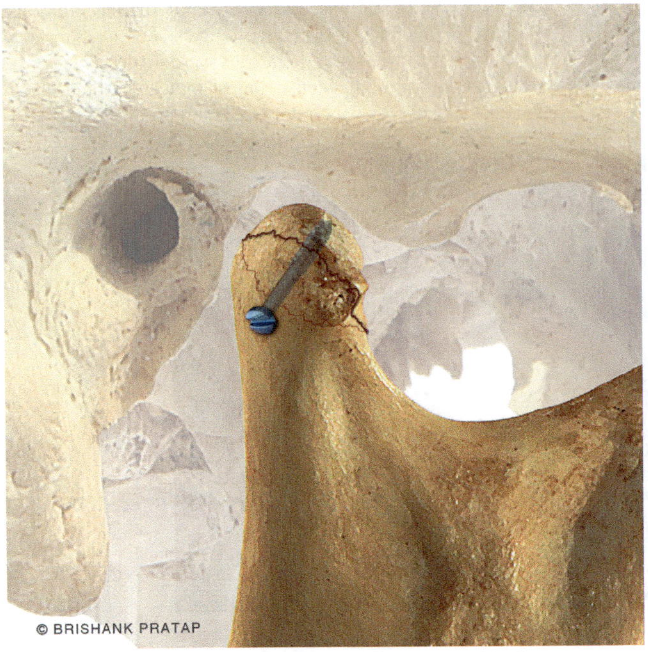

©Association of Oral and Maxillofacial Surgeons of India

Fig. 53.25 Fixation of the condylar head fracture with lag screw

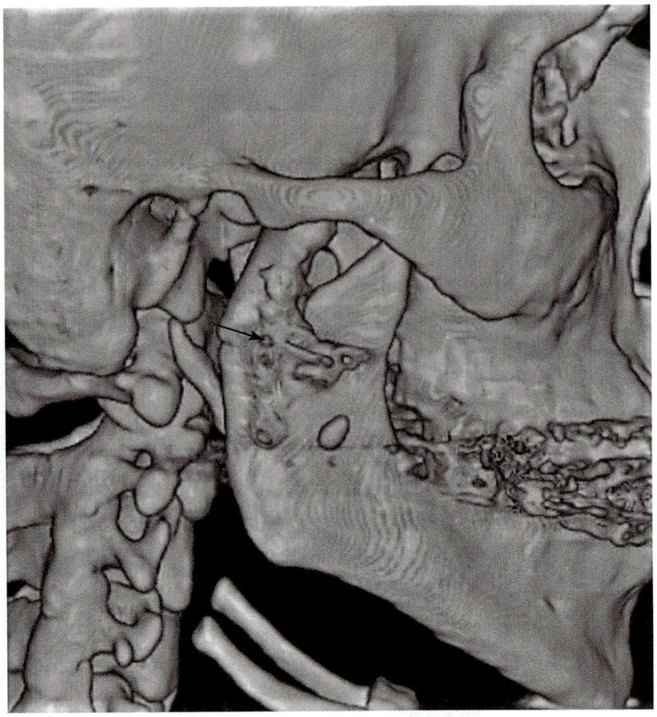

Case 5: Fig. 53.26 Shows improperly reduced fracture condyle which has been fixed in a dislocated position of the condyle-arrow points towards the plate fixed in wrong position

Table 53.1 Comparison of different fixation methods used for fractures of the mandibular condyle

Type of plate used for fixation	Advantage	Disadvantage
Single plate	• Easy to adapt and fix as placed along the long axis of the condyle.	• Does not neutralize the forces acting on the fracture ends. • Relatively heavier plate needed.
Two plates	• Neutralizes the tension and stress along the fracture. • Easy to triangulate. • Aids in reduction of fracture. • Suitable with multiple fractured fragments.	• May be difficult to fix two plates in a narrow neck of the condyle.
Lambda plate	• Single plate neutralizes the tension and stress as the two lower limb follow the anterior and posterior border of the condyle. • Suitable in narrow neck of the condyle.	• Wider exposure is needed. • Junction of two lower and upper limb area of weakness prone for fracture. • Difficult to adapt as the stock plates may not be suited for all types of fractures.
Delta plate	• Single 3D plate neutralizes the tension and stress as two vertical struts follow the anterior and posterior border of the condyle. • Plates don't have an area of weakness.	• Wider exposure is needed. • Difficult to adapt. • At times upper horizontal strut may be wider than the bone available.

53.9 Complications of Condylar Fractures (Case 5: Fig. 53.26) (Case 6: Fig. 53.27a–c)

1. Malocclusion—Quite common with closed reduction if improperly treated. Also seen in patients with prolonged hospitalization [58].
2. Mandibular hypomobility—Prolonged immobilization and delayed physiotherapy, more common in children [59].
3. Ankylosis—seen more commonly in children due to meniscal disruption and lack of physiotherapy. This may be seen in comminuted fractures or disruption of articular disc.
4. Asymmetry—In children due to growth disturbances may result in facial asymmetry, occlusal cants, and reduced ramal height [60]. In adults asymmetry is due to deviation on opening of the mouth.
5. Dysfunctional degeneration—All injured joints can turn arthritic. Factors affecting these are age, long period of immobilization, capsular, or meniscal injury [61].
6. Condylar resorption—Occurs if the condyle becomes devoid of blood supply, but it is extremely rare.
7. Hardware failure—Such as fracture of plates can occur.
8. Infection—Postoperative infection.
9. Chronic pain seen in closed reduction.
10. Neurosensory disturbances—Seen following trauma or inappropriate surgical incisions.

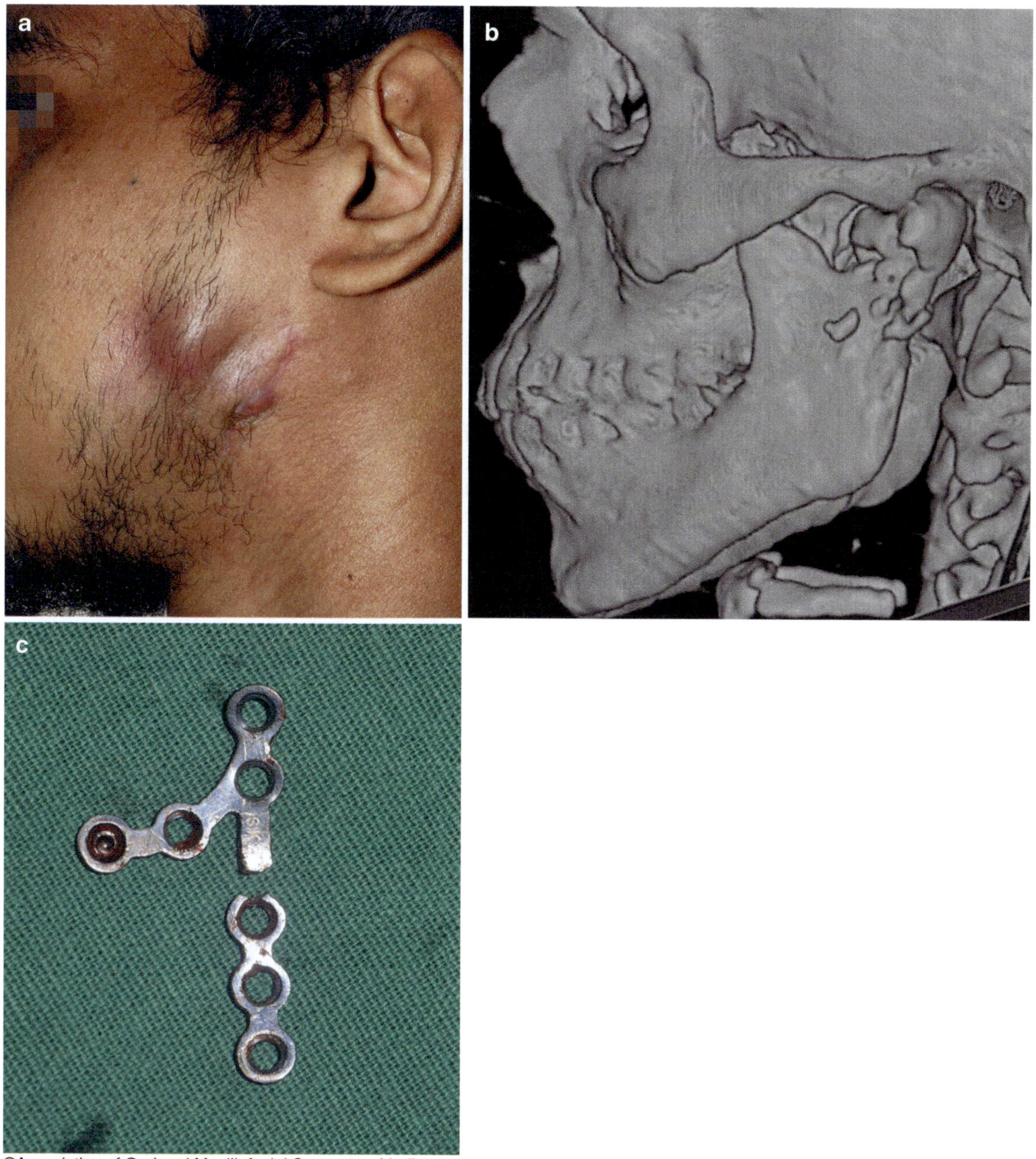

Case 6: Fig. 53.27 (**a**) Chronic infection left side condyle region following reduction and fixation, (**b**) CT scan showed osteomyelitis like changes at left condyle (**c**) the fractured infected plate removed

Box 53.11. Recent Advances [49]

- Improvements in imaging (CT scan/MRI) have resulted in better visualization of fracture site and understanding of soft tissue injuries along with the fracture.
- Surgical approaches better understood, and their application is based on the site of condylar fracture.
- Importance of anatomic reduction which leads to early full range of function.
- Improvement in open or assisted internal fixation techniques.
- Ability to approach and manage intracapsular fractures.
- Need to manage soft tissue injury as and when need.
- There is an improvements and wide choice of fixation materials including resorbable materials.
- Early and effective postoperative rehabilitation.

53.10 Conclusion

There have been numerous controversies in management of condylar fractures. They have ranged from which classification to use, surgical approach, type of fixation, and outcome of the treatment. But till date even with all the advances available to us, we still cannot agree on the two schools of thought for management of condylar fracture that is closed or open. Danda et al. [38] concluded in their study that there was no difference in treatment outcome in both the groups. This can be debated as it is not possible to compare the two modalities of treatment in absolute terms. Although it is pointed out that there are better results in function with open reduction and fixation, there are inherent complications that are only seen in cases treated by open reduction [62] such as nerve injuries and scars.

In an alternative interpretation of evidence, Leon A Assael [63] opined that both open and closed reduction have a critical role in management of condylar fractures. Treatment outcome such as full pain free range of movement and good aesthetics is seen in both the groups. Malocclusion, functional deficit, and internal derangement are seen irrespective of line of treatment. Over the years, complications noted in open reduction have reduced with the better understanding and improvement of technique, but it can be burden on the patient. These complications can only be weighed against the functional advantage patient gets in open reduction and fixation. Treatment of a condylar fracture will entirely be dependent on multiple factors.

To conclude it can be safely stated that management of condylar fractures should be patient centric not entirely based on absolute indications mentioned by various authors. Generally, in children and dentulous adult patients, closed reduction is the choice of treatment, whereas open reduction and fixation would be the choice of treatment for the patients with multiple fractures of mandible, panfacial trauma, partially or totally edentulous jaws, and underlying medical conditions preventing maxillomandibular fixation. Finally, function should be considered as an important parameter while formulating a treatment plan along with the resources available and skill of the surgeon.

References

1. Desault BX. Memoire sur la fracture des condyles de la machoire inferieure. Paris: Euvres Chirurgicales; 1813.
2. Fletcher MC, Piecuch JF, Lieblich SE. Anatomy and pathophysiology of the temporomandibular joint. In: Milora M, Ghali GE, Larsen P, et al., editors. Peterson's principles of oral and maxillofacial surgery. 3rd edn. Shelton, CT: People's Medical Publishing House; 2012. p. 1033–47.
3. Rayne J. Functional anatomy of the temporomandibular joint. Br J Oral Maxillofac Surg. 1987;25:92–9.
4. Walker CJ, Stephen PR. MacLeod: anatomy and biomechanics of condylar fractures. Atlas Oral Maxillofacial Surg Clin N Am. 2017;25:11–6.
5. Schmidt BL, Pogrel MA. The distribution of the auriculotemporal nerve around the temporomandibular joint. Oral Surg Oral Med Oral Pathol Oral Radiol Endod. 1998;86:165–58.
6. Al-Kayat A, Bramley P. A modified pre auricular approach to the temporomandibular joint and malar arch. Br J Oral Surg. 1979;17:91–103.
7. Dingmann RO, Grabb WC. Surgical anatomy of the mandibular ramus of the facial nerve based on the dissection of 100 facial halves. Plast Reconstr Surg Transplant Bull. 1962;29:266–72.
8. Ellis E, Throckmorton GS. Treatment of mandibular condylar process fractures: biological considerations. J Oral Maxillofac Surg. 2005;63:115–34.
9. Lindahl L. Condylar fractures of the mandible. I: classification and relation to age, occlusion and concomitant injuries of the teeth and teeth-supporting structures and fractures of the mandibular body. Int J Oral Surg. 1977;6(1):12–21.
10. Chrcanovic BR. Surgical versus non-surgical treatment of mandibular condylar fractures: a meta-analysis. Int J Oral Maxillofac Surg. 2015;44(2):158–79.
11. Wassmund M. Frakturen und luxationen des gesichtsschädels unter berücksichtigung der komplikationen des hirnschädels. Ihre klinik, und therapie. Berlin: Meusser; 1927.
12. MacLennan WD. Consideration of 180 cases of typical fractures of the mandibular condylar process. Br J Plast Surg. 1952;5(2):122–8.
13. Spiessl, B., Schroll K. Spezielle Frakturen- und Luxationslehre. Ein kurzesHandbuch in fünf Bänden. Band I/1 Gesichtsschädel. Stuttgart: Georg Thieme; 1972. p. 317.
14. Rasse M. Diakapituläre frakturen der mandibula. Eine neue operationsmethode und erste ergebnisse. Stomatolgie. 1993;90:413–28.
15. Neff A, Kolk A, Deppe H, et al. Neue aspekte zur indikation der operativen versorgung intraartikulärer und hoher kiefergelenkluxationsfrakturen [New aspects for indications of surgical management of intra-articular and high temporomandibular dislocation fractures]. Mund Kiefer Gesichtschir. 1999;3(1):24–9. [in German]

16. Hlawitschka M, Eckelt U. Assessment of patients treated for intracapsular fractures of the mandibular condyle by closed techniques. J Oral Maxillofac Surg. 2002;60(7):784–91.
17. Loukota R, Neff A, Rasse M. Nomenclature/classification of fractures of the mandibular condylar head. Br J Oral Maxillofac Surg. 2010;48(6):477–8.
18. He D, Yang C, Chen M, Jiang B, Wang B. Intracapsular condylar fracture of the mandible: our classification and open treatment experience. J Oral Maxillofac Surg. 2009;67(8):1672–9.
19. Loukota RA, Eckelt U, De Bont L, et al. Subclassification of fractures of the condylar process of the mandible. Br J Oral Maxillofac Surg. 2005;43:72–3.
20. Ellis E 3rd, Palmieri C, Throckmorton GS. Further displacement of condylar process fractures after closed treatment. J Oral Maxillofac Surg. 1999;59(2):120–9.
21. Neff A, Cornelius CP, Rasse M, et al. The comprehensive AOCMF classification system: condylar process fractures: level 3 tutorial. Craniomaxillofac Trauma Reconstr. 2014;7(Suppl 1):S44–58.
22. Brasileiro BF, Passeri LA. Epidemiological analysis of maxillofacial fractures in Brazil: A five-year prospective study. Oral Surg Oral Med Oral Pathol Oral Radiol Endod. 2006;102:28–34.
23. Chrcanovic BR, Freire-Maia B, Souza LN, et al. Facial fractures: A 1 year retrospective study in a hospital in Belo Horizonte. Braz Oral Res. 2004;18(1):322–8.
24. Kumar GBA, Dhupar V, Akkara F, Kumar SP. Patterns of maxillofacial fractures in Goa. J Maxillofac Oral Surg. 2013;14(2):138–14.
25. Ellis E, Moos KF, el-Attar A. Ten years of mandibular fractures: An analysis of 2,137 cases. Oral Surg Oral Med Oral Pathol. 1985;59(2):120–9.
26. Zachariades N, Mezitis M, Mourouzis C, et al. Fractures of the mandibular condyle: A review of 466 cases. Literature review, reflections on treatment and proposals. J Craniomaxillofac Surg. 2006;18:151–3.
27. MacLennan WD. Fractures of the mandibular condylar process. Br J Oral Surg. 1969;7:31–9.
28. Sawazaki R, Lima Júnior SM, Asprino L, Moreira RWF, de Moraes M. Incidence and patterns of mandibular condyle fractures. J Oral Maxillofac Surg. 2010;68:1252–9.
29. Silvennoinen U, Iizuka T, Lindqvist C, et al. Different patterns of condylar fractures: An analysis of 382 patients in a 3-year period. J Oral Maxillofac Surg. 1992;50(10):1032–7.
30. Zachariades N, Koumoura F, Konsolaki-Agouridaki E. Facial trauma in women resulting from violence by men. J Oral Maxillofac Surg. 1990;48(12):1250–3.
31. Zachariades N, Papavassiliou D, Koumoura F. Fractures of the facial skeleton in children. J Cranio-Maxillofacial Surg. 1990;18(4):151–3.
32. Robert V. Walker: condylar fractures nonsurgical management. J Oral Maxillofac Surg. 1994;52:1185–8.
33. Zide MF, Kent JN. Indications for open reduction of mandibular condylar fractures. J Oral Maxillofac Surg. 1983;41(2):89–98.
34. AAOMS—special committee on parameter of care indications for open reduction of condylar fractures. https://www.researchgate.net/figure/AAOMS-special-committee-on-parameters-of-care-indications-for-open-reduction-2003_tbl3_230633313. Accessed 1 Feb 2019.
35. Yates DM, Zuniga JR, Zide MF. Traumatic injuries to the mandibular condyle. In: Fonseca RJ, Walker RV, Dexter Barber H, Powers MP, Frost DE, editors. Oral & maxillofacial trauma, 4th ed. 2012. p. 331–53.
36. Schneider M, Erasmus F, Gerlach KL, et al. Open reduction and internal fixation versus closed treatment and mandibulomaxillary fixation of fractures of the mandibular condylar process: A randomized prospective, multicenter study with special evaluation of fracture level. J Oral Maxillofac Surg. 2008;66:2537–44.
37. Eckelt U, Schneider M, Erasmus F, et al. Open versus closed treatment of fractures of the mandibular condylar process—a prospective randomized multi-centre study. J Craniomaxillofac Surg. 2006;34:306–14.
38. Danda AK, Muthuskhar MR, Narayanan V, et al. Open versus closed treatment of unilateral subcondylar and condylar neck fractures: A prospective, randomized clinical study. J Oral Maxillofac Surg. 2010;68:1238–41.
39. Ellis E. Method to determine when open treatment of condylar process fractures is not necessary. J Oral Maxillofac Surg. 2009;67:1685–90.
40. Haug RH, Assael LA. Outcomes of open versus closed treatment of mandibular subcondylar fractures. J Oral Maxillofac Surg. 2001;59:370–5.
41. Silvennoinen U, Iizuka T, Oikarinen K, Lindqvist C. Analysis of possible factors leading to problems after nonsurgical treatment of condylar fractures. J Oral Maxillofac Surg. 1994;52:793–9.
42. Kent JN, Neary JP, Silvia C. Open reduction of mandibular condyle fractures. Oral Maxillofac Clin North Am. 1990;2:69–72.
43. Raveh J, Vuillenium T, Lädrach K. Open reduction of the dislocated, fractured condylar process: Indications and surgical procedures. J Oral Maxillofac Surg. 1989;47:120–6.
44. Pau M, Navisany K, Reinbacher K, et al. Use of a modified high submandibular approach to treat condylar base fractures: Experience with 44 consecutive cases treated in a single institution. J Craniomaxillofac Surg. 2016;44(10):164–45.
45. Trost O, Abu El-Naaj I, Trouilloud P, et al. High cervical transmasseteric anteroparotid approach for open reduction and internal fixation in condylar fracture. J Oral Maxillofac Surg. 2008;66:201.
46. Narayanan V, Ramadorai A, Ravi P, Nirvikalpa N. Transmasseteric anteriorparotid approach for condylar fractures: experience of 129 cases. Br J Oral Maxillofac Surg. 2012;50(5):420–4.
47. Ellis EE, Zide MF. Retromandibular approach. In: Ellis EE, Zide MF, editors. Surgical approaches to the facial skeleton. Baltimore, MD: Williams & Wilkins; 1995. p. 139–53.
48. Cienfuegos R, Cornelius C-P, Ellis E III, Kushner G. Mandible-approaches. In: Figari M, Sánchez Aniceto G, editors. Buchbinder D (general editor) AO surgery reference. https://www2.aofoundation.org/wps/portal/surgery?bone=CMF&segment=Mandible&showPage=approach. Assessed 1 Feb 2019.
49. Kisnisci R. Management of fractures of the condyle condylar neck, and coronoid process. Oral Maxillofacial Surg Clin N Am. 2013;25:573–90.
50. Devlin MF, Hislop WS, Carton AT. Open reduction and internal fixation of fractured mandibular condyles by a retro-mandibular approach: surgical morbidity and informed consent. Br J Oral Maxillofac Surg. 2002;40:23–5.
51. Vesnaver A. Open reduction and internal fixation of intra-articular fractures of the mandibular condyle: our first experiences. J Oral Maxillofac Surg. 2008;66(10):2123–9.
52. Palmieri C, Ellis E, Throckmorton G. Mandibular motion after closed and open treatment of unilateral mandibular condylar process fractures. J Oral Maxillofac Surg. 1999;57:764–75.
53. Lee CYS, McCullon C, Blaustein D, Mahammadi H. Sequelae of unrecognized, untreated mandibular condylar fractures in the pediatric patient. Ann Dent. 1993;52:5–8.
54. Posnick JC, Wells M, Pron GE. Pediatric facial fractures: Evolving patterns of treatment. J Oral Maxillofac Surg. 1993;51:836–4.
55. MacLennan WD, Simpson W. Treatment of fractured mandibular condylar process in children. Br J Plast Surg. 1965;18:423–7.
56. Lund K. Mandibular growth and remodelling processes after condylar fracture: A longitudinal roentgen cephalometric study. Acta Odont Scand. 1974;32:3–117.

57. Levin SC, Frydendall E, Gao D, Chan KH. Temporomandibular joint dysfunction after mandibular fracture in children: A 10-year review. Arch Otolaryngol Head Neck Surg. 2011;137:10–4.
58. Ellis E 3rd. Complications of mandibular condyle fractures. Int J Oral Maxillofac Surg. 1998;27:255–7.
59. De Amaratunga NA. Mouth opening after release of maxillomandibular fixation in fracture patients. J Oral Maxillofac Surg. 1987;45:383–5.
60. Proffit WR, Vig KWL, Turvey TA. Early fracture of the mandibular condyles: Frequently an unsuspected cause of growth disturbances. Am J Orthod. 1980;78:1–24.
61. Palmieri C, Ellis E, Throckmorton G. Mandibular motion after closed and open treatment of unilateral mandibular condylar process fractures. J Oral Maxillofac Surg. 1999;57:764–75.
62. Brandt MT, Haug RH. Open versus closed reduction of adult mandibular condyle fractures: a review of the literature regarding the evolution of current thoughts on management. J Oral Maxillofac Surg. 2003;61:1324–32.
63. Assael LA. Open versus closed reduction of adult mandibular condyle fractures: an alternative interpretation of the evidence. J Oral Maxillofac Surg. 2003;61:1333–9.

Intraoral Endoscopic Approach for Treatment of Condylar Fractures of the Mandible

54

Frank Wilde

54.1 Introduction

The literature is replete with techniques regarding the open reduction and fixation of the condylar fractures of the mandible. The extraoral approach is preferred by the majority of surgeons in comparison to the intraoral approach. Nevertheless, open reduction and internal fixation by an extraoral approach has the evident risk to cause transient or even permanent facial nerve injury [1–4], leads inevitably to a facial scar [1, 5], and can course salivary fistulas, sialoceles [1, 6], Frey syndrome, or disturbance of the great auricular nerve [1]. In contrast, an intraoral approach is minimizing these abovementioned risks and facial scars can be avoided in general [7, 8].

Silverman in 1925 was the first person to mention about the intraoral approach to condylar fractures [9]. However, at that time, the surgeons were facing several difficulties treating those fractures due to a lack of adequate instruments. Fritzemeier and Bechthold developed the 90-degree angular screwdriver, and it served as a milestone in the intraoral management of condylar neck fractures. In their study, there were 32 fractures of which 2 cases showed early failures. Other cases during follow-up showed minor deviation from axis, but there were no evident problems in the temporomandibular joint function [10].

Based thereupon, several authors were reporting about the use of an intraoral approach treating condylar fractures surgically. Forty-eight cases of displaced and shortened mandibular condyle fractures were treated by an intraoral approach and studied by Mokros and Erle in 1996. In 2/3 of the treated fractures, the reduction was successful, and no significant complications were noted in the intraoperative or postoperative period.

TMJ function was good in 90% of the patients, 43% were free of symptoms, and 47% had minor dysfunction. The authors came to the result that proper reduction of the bone fragments is most important for therapeutic success [11].

Schön et al. [8] compared in a study an intraoral endoscopy-assisted approach with an extraoral approach for the treatment of condylar fractures. A reduced risk of facial nerve damage and no visible scars were the major conclusion of the study, and they also opined that intraoral endoscopic approach is a reliable technique for treating condylar fractures [8]. Veras et al. [12] were looking in their study on 25 patients with condylar fractures which were treated surgically by an intraoral approach. The mean mouth opening postoperatively was 4.8 cm. Patients postoperatively did not have clicking of the joint, facial nerve weakness, or pain of the muscles or the joint. They opined that intraoral reduction allowed the anatomic ramus height to be restored and that the functional results were acceptable [12].

Other authors like Jensen et al. [13] or Schneider et al. [14] were not so enthusiastic about the outcome of surgical-treated condylar fractures employing an intraoral approach [13, 14]. Jensen et al. in 2006 stressed on the fact that intraoral approach for the condylar fractures is very technically demanding and there is a chance of getting postoperative complications [13]. Schneider et al. [14] compared in a retrospective study 21 fractures which were treated with an intraoral approach with 24 fractures which were reduced by an extraoral perimandibular approach. In their study, the cases treated by intraoral approach showed suboptimal radiologic findings, and the patients' subjective feelings pointed to less favorable clinical results. They put forward the suggestion that fractures which do not require extensive manipulation and fractures which can be reduced exactly under a limited view only should be approached intraorally. For all other fractures, they recommend extraoral approaches [14].

F. Wilde (✉)
Department of Oral and Plastic Maxillofacial Surgery, Armed Forces Hospital, Ulm, Germany

Department of Oral and Maxillofacial Surgery, University Hospital, Ulm, Germany
e-mail: frank.wilde@uni-ulm.de

K. Bonanthaya et al. (eds.), *Oral and Maxillofacial Surgery for the Clinician*, https://doi.org/10.1007/978-981-15-1346-6_54

54.2 Surgical Technique

From the authors' experience, fractures of the condylar base and the low and medial part of the condylar process can be addressed typically by the following described technique. Treating high condylar neck fractures is demanding and requires experience in using such an approach. Fractures of the condylar head or the transition zone between the neck and head cannot be reached with this approach, and extraoral incisions are still required when this kind of fractures is getting treated surgically.

For the below-described technique, a team of three surgeons (one leading surgeon and two assistant surgeons) are highly recommended.

54.2.1 Special Surgical Instruments and Devices

To facilitate open reduction and internal fixation of condylar fractures via an intraoral approach with predictable results, special equipment is mandatory.

The most important instruments are a 90° angled screwdriver and drill (Fig. 54.1a). The screwdriver should have necessarily a sliding screw-holder which facilitates to hold the screw and plate together (Fig. 54.1b), because positioning a plate with one hand and fixing the screw with the other hand is not appropriate and will lead to unsuccessful procedures. Self-retaining screwdriver-bits or even self-tapping screws should be avoided as well. The authors recommend a straight 90° angled screwdriver with the aforementioned sliding screw-holder and centric-positioned screwdriver-bits. Screwdrivers with eccentric-positioned screwdriver-bits show a lower height indeed. However, they will lead to tilting of the screwdriver during the activation of the device, which results in an inadequate transfer of the force and a frequent loosening of the screws from the bit.

Besides the 90° angled screwdriver and drill, extra-long instruments in the form of raspatories and reposition hooks have to be recommended insistently (Fig. 54.2). They simplify the manipulation and reduction of the fractured condyle with a good direct view into the operation site. Using standard configurated instruments results in less vision due to obstructing the view by the operator's hands.

An appropriate light-intensive headlight is necessary for proper illumination of the operation site (Fig. 54.3).

A 4 mm caliber 30° angled endoscope has to be recommended as well. In combination with a special retractor in which the endoscope can be inserted, a good visualization, especially of the posterior border of the ramus, can be achieved (Fig. 54.4).

In addition, a special retractor with a fiber-optic light guide which can be positioned buccally to the posterior border of the ramus enables good illumination of the surgical site (Fig. 54.5). Nevertheless, having an appropriate headlight, this instrument seems to be dispensable.

It can be further useful to fix the patient during surgery in a Mayfield head clamp as it is commonly used by the neurosurgeons. This allows traction with the retractors without any movement of the head.

Besides the described instruments, there are several special instruments and devices available on the market to facilitate open reduction and internal fixation using an intraoral approach. However, from the authors' experience, the aforementioned instruments and devices are the most helpful in treating condylar fractures by an intraoral approach.

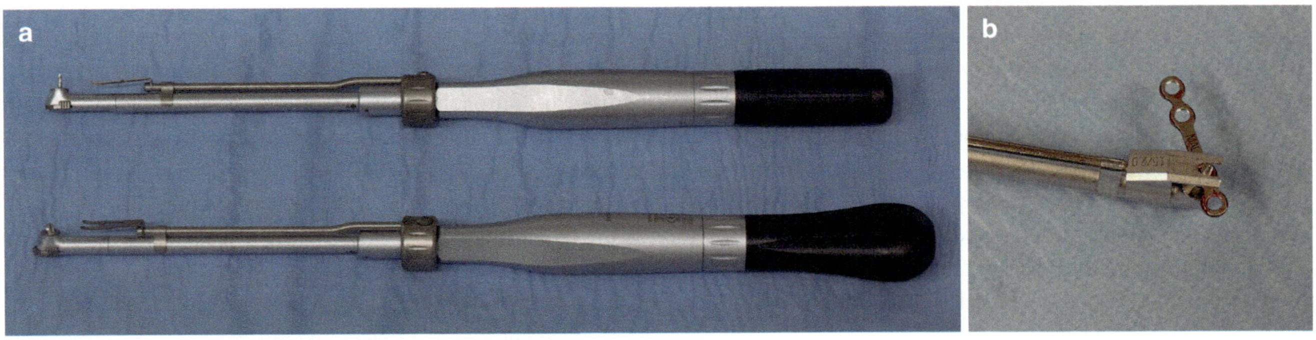

Fig. 54.1 (**a**) 90° angled screwdriver and drill. (**b**) Sliding screw-holder which facilitates to hold the screw and plate together (Medartis, Basel, Switzerland)

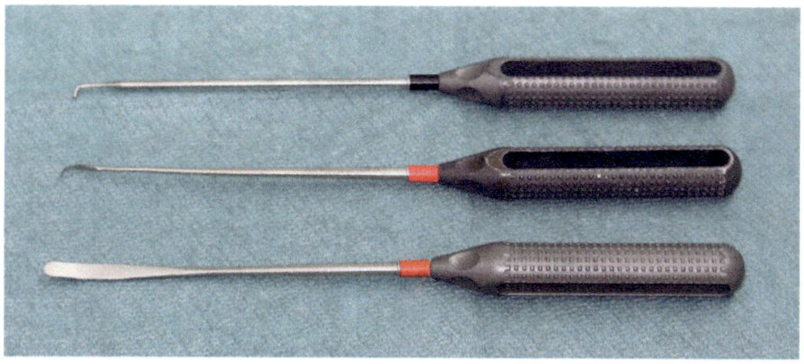

Fig. 54.2 Extra-long instruments in the form of raspatories and reposition hooks (Karl Storz, Tuttlingen, Germany)

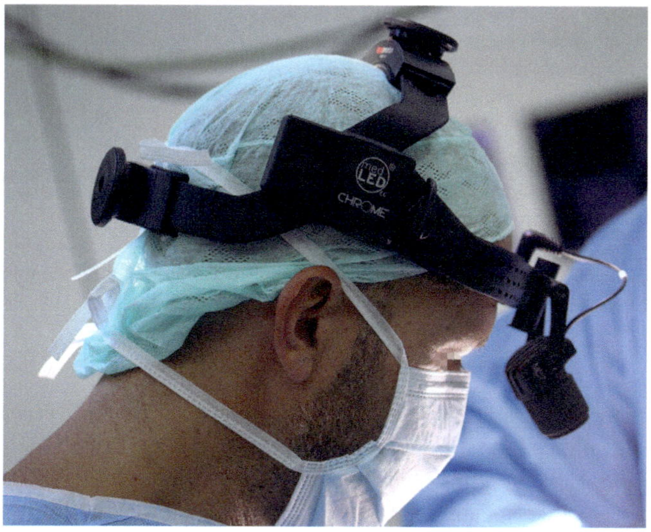

Fig. 54.3 LED headlight (KLS Martin, Tuttlingen, Germany)

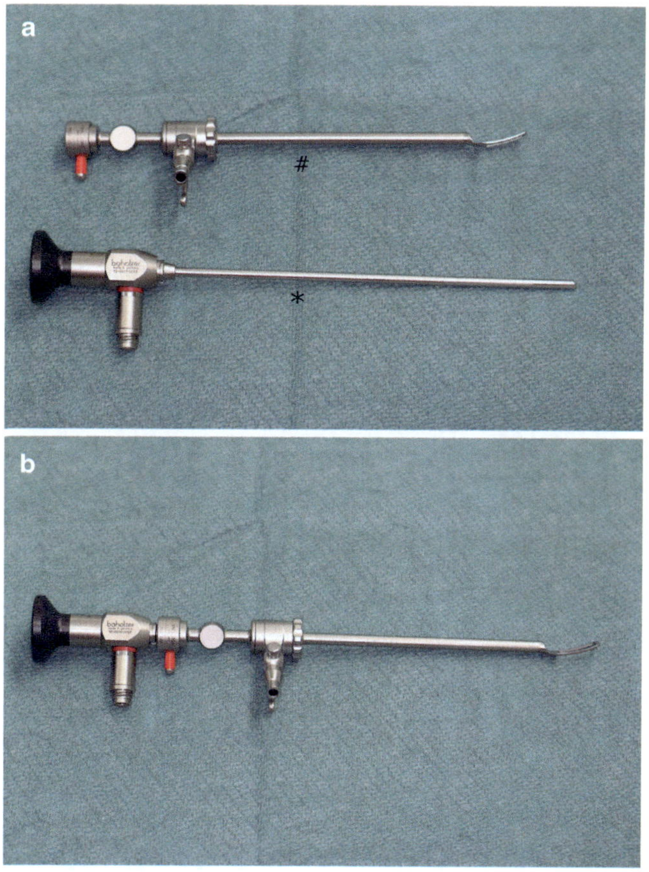

Fig. 54.4 (**a**) 4 mm caliber 30° angled endoscope (asterisk) and retractor in which the endoscope can be inserted (hash symbol). (**b**) Retractor with inserted endoscope (Karl Storz, Tuttlingen, Germany)

54.2.2 Surgical Access

By extending the standard vestibular incision in a superior direction along the ascending ramus, the ramus and the condyle region can be exposed intraorally (Fig. 54.6). The approach is following Obwegeser's principles of avoiding visible scars by extending his approach to the mandibular ramus for sagittal split osteotomy. During the incision of the oral mucosa, the anatomical course of the buccal nerve has to be taken into account. The dissection of the mucoperiosteal flap starts from the mandibular corpus in the region of the first molar to mandibular angle and far up to the condyle until the facture line can be explored. To get an appropriate

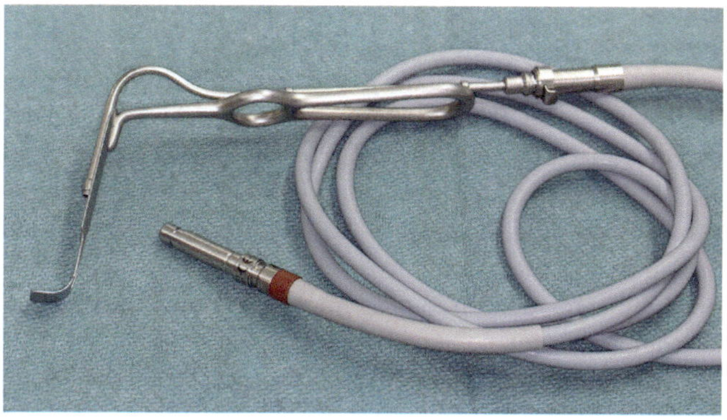

Fig. 54.5 Retractor with a fiber-optic light guide (Karl Storz, Tuttlingen, Germany)

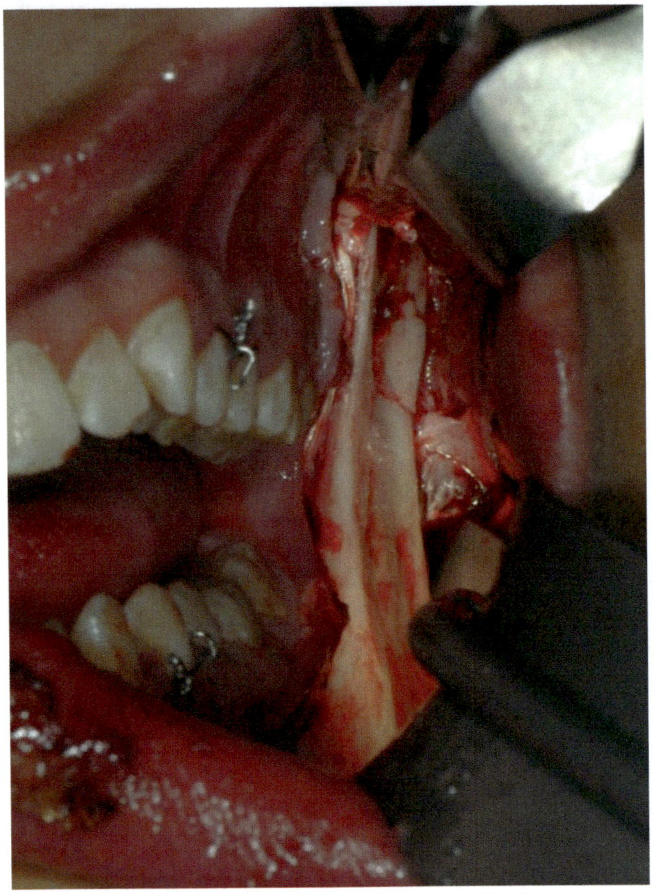

©Association of Oral and Maxillofacial Surgeons of India

Fig. 54.6 Intraoral approach to the condyle region by extending the standard vestibular incision in a superior direction up the ascending ramus

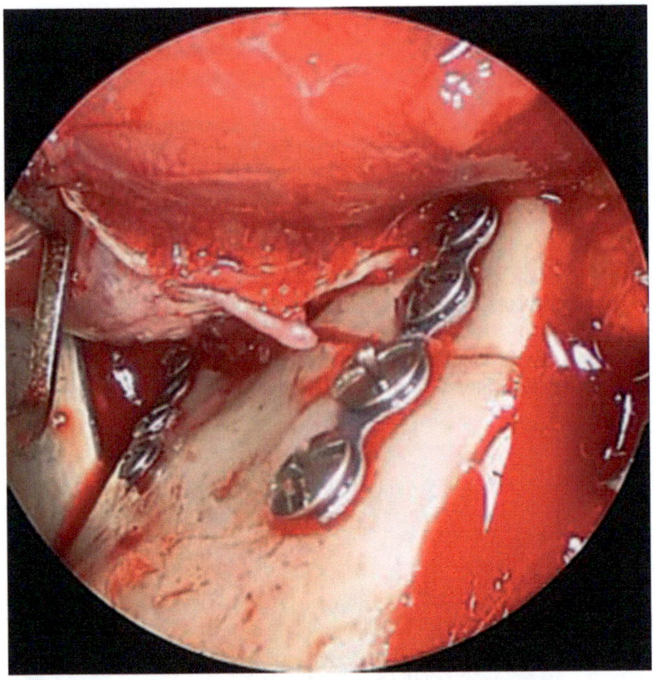

©Association of Oral and Maxillofacial Surgeons of India

Fig. 54.7 After temporary osteotomy and re-fixation of the coronoid process to get better access for repositioning of medial displaced condyle

visualization of the condylar neck region, the mucosa including the fibers of the temporal muscle had to striped from the coronoid process up to or even higher than the mandibular notch. During dissecting the posterior border of the mandibular ramus, the retromandibular vein has to be taken under consideration. Coagulation in this region has to be done carefully, due to the anatomical proximity to the facial nerve which is running laterally in the parotid gland. This is the region where the facial nerve may be damaged during the procedure. In addition to coagulation, vigorous traction can damage the facial nerve in this location as well.

54.2.3 Surgical Procedure

After dissection to get sufficient access to the condylar neck region, the displaced condyle has to be identified. The best instrument for this is the extra-long raspatorium depicted in Fig. 54.2. During this procedure, the ramus has to be distracted. This can be performed by pulling the mandible caudally by hand. Another option is to fix one mini-screw in the mandibular angle to twist a wire around, which is diverted out of the skin in the mandibular angle region by a stab incision. However, this leads to a small extraoral scar.

For this maneuver, a full relaxation of the patient by the anesthesiologist is recommended. Due to the very low risk for facial nerve damage employing this approach, this can be done without increasing this risk.

For medial displaced condyles in high condylar neck fractures, it is sometimes helpful to perform a temporary osteotomy of the coronoid process to get better access for repositioning. A later re-fixation of the osteomized coronoid process by a miniplate is in theory not needed but recommended by the authors (Fig. 54.7).

Once the dislocated fragment is identified, it has to be repositioned anatomically. MMF cannot be recommended in all cases. In some cases, it can be helpful to get a stable reduction during osteosynthesis; however, in most cases, MMF is not very helpful. This decision has to be made individually case by case.

In most cases, the reposition of the proximal fragment is not stable from the beginning (Fig. 54.8). Therefore, the authors recommend to drill the first screw hole in the condyle fragment close to the fracture line in the region of the sigmoid notch. A four- or five-hole 1.0 mm up to 1.2-mm-thick miniplate is fixed in this hole with a 5- to 6-mm-long screw with a diameter of 2.0 mm. The screw should not be tightened completely. Then the reduction of condyle fragment

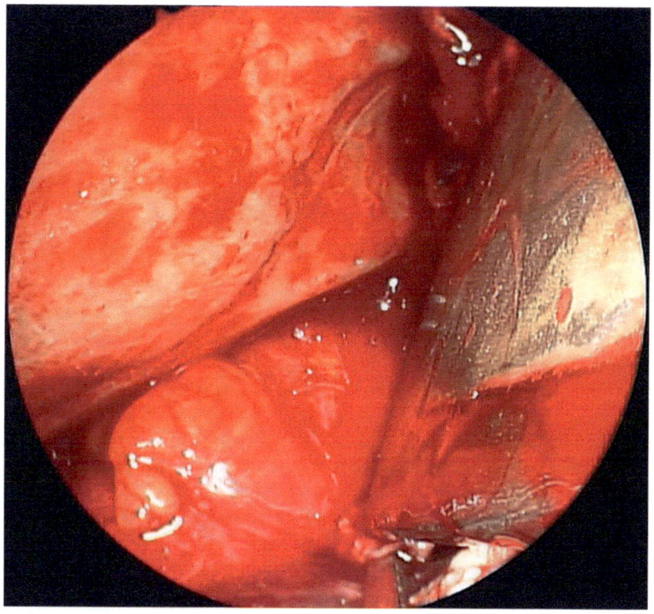

Fig. 54.8 Endoscopic view after repositioning of a condylar neck fracture

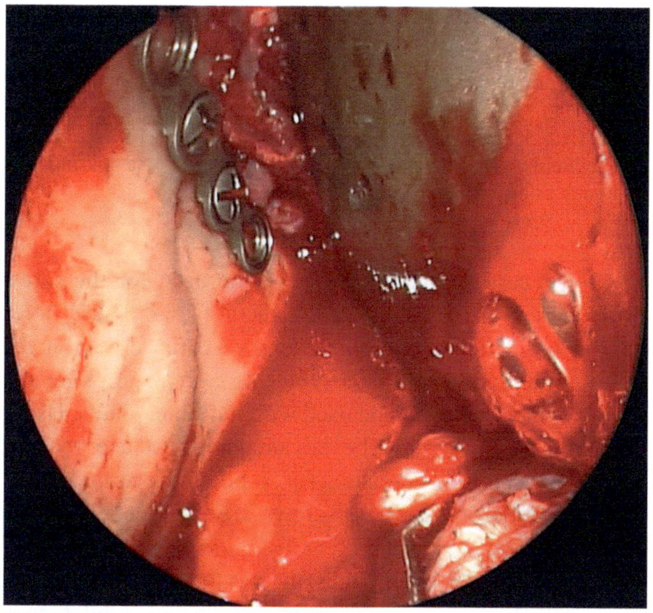

Fig. 54.9 Endoscopic view after fixation of a four-hole miniplate close to the sigmoid notch with two screws adjacent to the fracture line

can be achieved by pulling on the miniplate with one of the extra-long reposition hooks. By visual control of the repositioned fragment, the miniplate should now be fixed in the ramus part of the fracture close to the sigmoid notch by eccentric drilling of the screw hole for fracture line compression during screw insertion. After fixing the second screw, the first screw has to be tightened completely (Fig. 54.9).

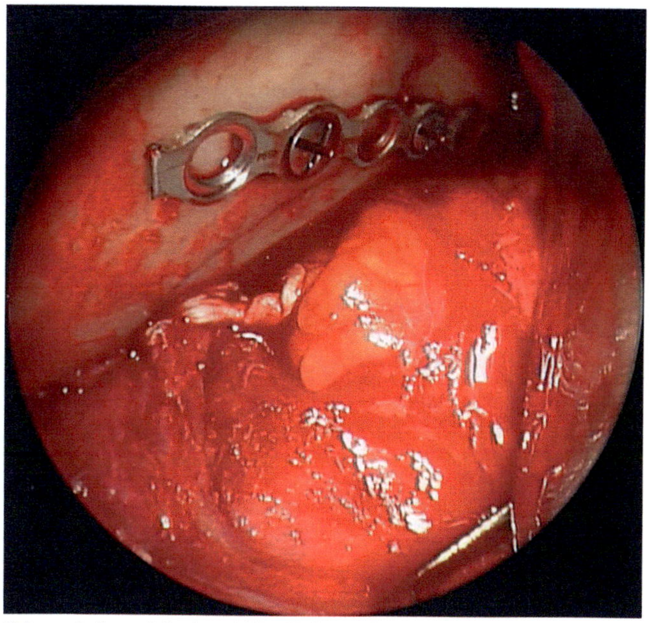

Fig. 54.10 Endoscopic view after fixation of a five-hole miniplate at posterior border with two screws adjacent to the fracture line

Once this is facilitated, often a small gap and flaring can be identified at the posterior border of the condylar neck. To close this gap, a second four- to five-hole miniplate has to be fixed at the posterior border of the condylar neck. Here also the hole has to be drilled in the condyle fragment close to the fracture line. First, the plate has to be fixed in this hole and should be aligned along the posterior border of the condylar neck respectively the ramus. Again, the screw should not be tightened completely at this stage. After exact anatomical reposition of the condyle, the next screw is now drilled for compression osteosynthesis in the ramus part of the ramus close the fracture line and immediately fixed with the fourth screw (Fig. 54.10). The third screw is then tightened completely to stabilize the fracture. After attaining control of the anatomical correct reposition with the endoscope or in low condylar neck fractures even with a simple dental mirror, the other screw holes in both plates are drilled and fixed, starting with the plate at the posterior border and ending with plate close to the sigmoid notch. Figure 54.11 shows the final endoscopic view with the two plates fixed. Figure 54.12 is illustrating the recommended sequencing of plate and screw positioning to facilitate open reduction and internal fixation via an intraoral approach using two miniplates.

In addition, the authors recommend intraoperative imaging with a 3D C-arm device at the end of the procedure when available (Fig. 54.13). This allows the intraoperative radiologic control and documentation of the reduced fracture and of the position of the plates in a multiplanar view and enables an immediate intraoperative correction when the result of the

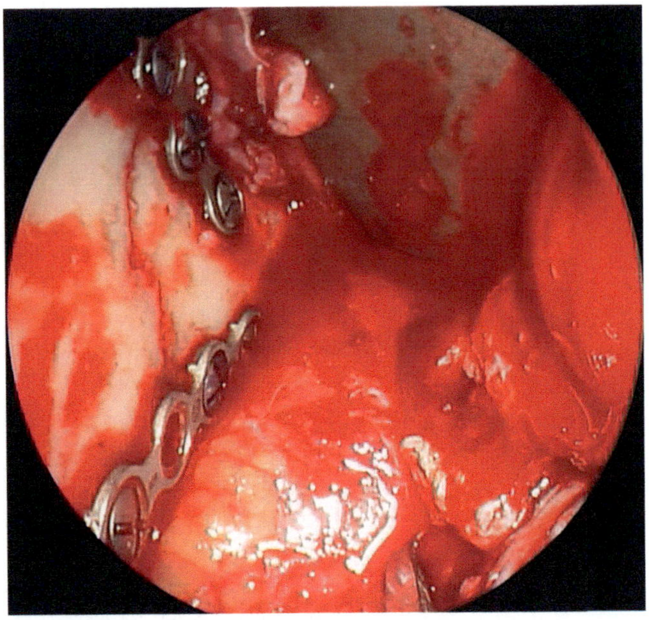

Fig. 54.11 Endoscopic view after complete fixation of a condylar neck fracture with two miniplates. One four-hole plate in the region of the sigmoid notch and a second five-hole miniplate at posterior border

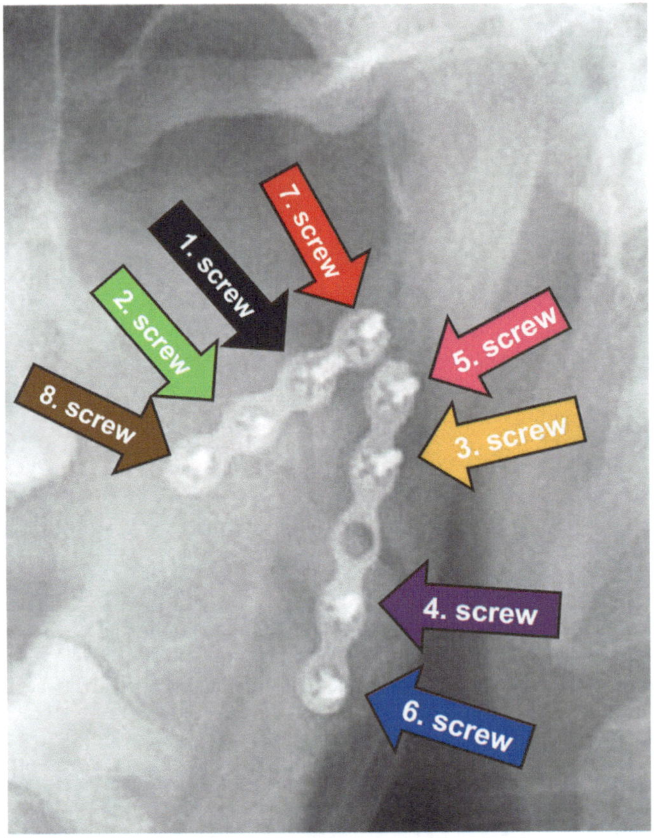

Fig. 54.12 Recommended sequencing of plate and screw positioning to facilitate open reduction and internal fixation via an intraoral approach using two miniplates

procedure is not satisfactory. This reduces the risk for revision surgeries considerably [15, 16].

When the result is satisfactory, the intraoral mucosa has to be closed in the standard way like every intraoral incision. Even when the fracture is reduced and stabilized with success, the authors still recommend a light MMF with elastics strained over two or four MMF screws or arch bars for approximately 1 week for slight immobilization and guidance into the proper occlusion. In case of a postoperative insufficient occlusion, a prolonged functional treatment as in nonsurgical treated condylar fractures with elastics or an orthodontic device like an activator or bionator has to be recommended.

54.2.4 Osteosynthesis Material

As mentioned before, the author is recommending the usage of two miniplates. The plate at the posterior border is responsible for the stability primarily, whereas the plate in the region of the sigmoid notch prevents flaring of the distal fragment during function additionally.

For osteosynthesis, 1.0-mm up to 1.2-mm-thick miniplates can be recommended (Fig. 54.14). It can be favorable to use 1.2-mm-thick miniplates at the posterior border due to stability reasons. The screws should be usually 5–6 mm long with a diameter of 2.0 mm. Locking screws are not necessary and should never be used for the screw holes which are adjacent to the facture line. These holes should be drilled eccentric to achieve compression at the facture line. In modern osteosynthesis systems, locking and non-locking screws can be used with the same plates. Using such a system, it may be advantageous to use locking screws for the fracture-distant screw holes. Nevertheless, as mentioned before, locking screws are not needed in this technique.

Besides standard miniplates, there is the option for the use of so-called 3D plates or special designed condylar neck plates (Fig. 54.15). However, from the authors' experience, plating with two miniplates enables the aforementioned successive repositioning and fixation of the facture most easily and leads to sufficient stability.

There are new developments of anatomically preformed 3D condylar neck plates with integrated reposition wings for the posterior border and the sigmoid notch (Fig. 54.16). Whether these kinds of plates are beneficial or not has to be investigated in the future.

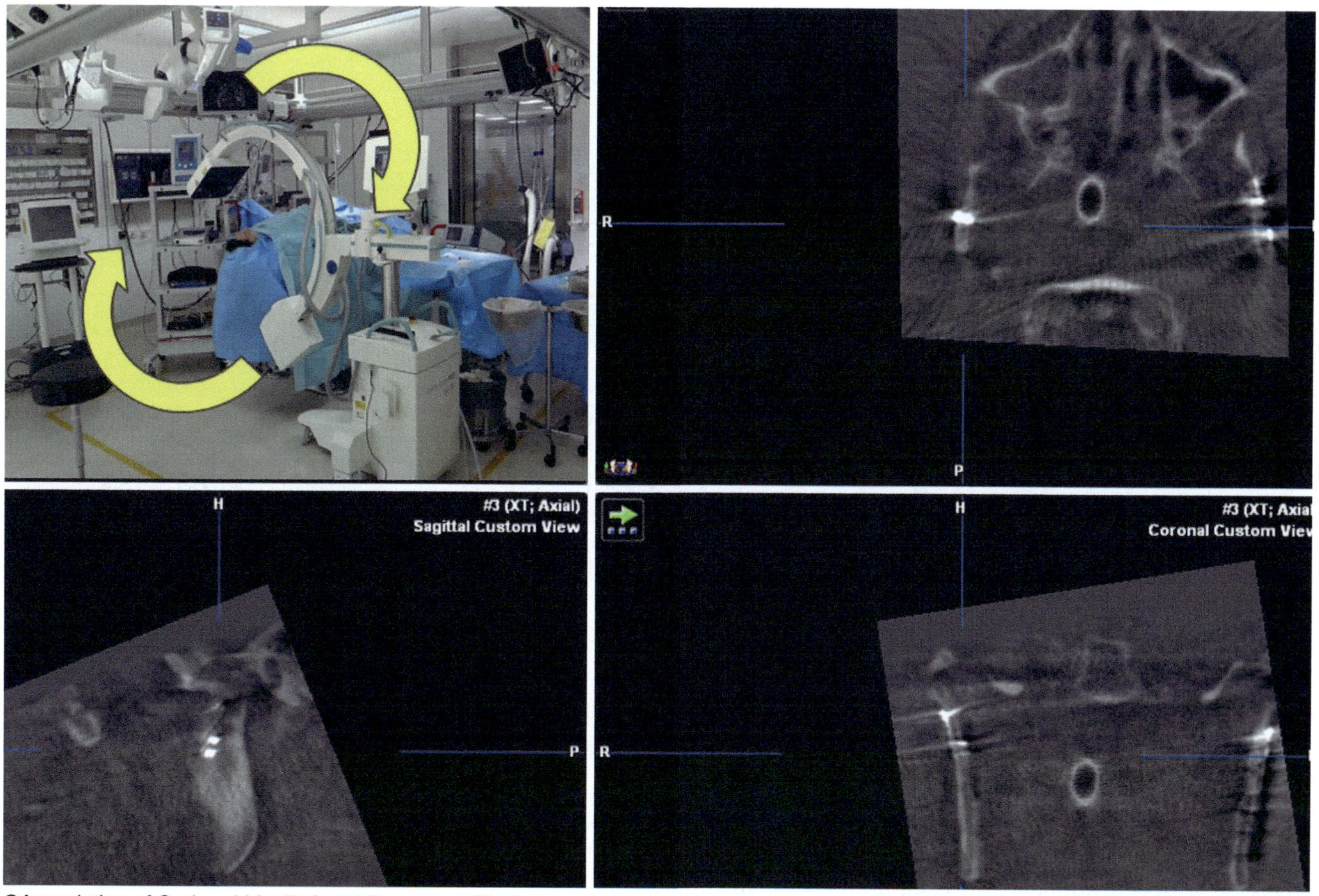

Fig. 54.13 Intraoperative imaging with a 3D C-arm device (Ziehm, Erlangen, Germany) at the end of the procedure and multiplanar view of the surgical result

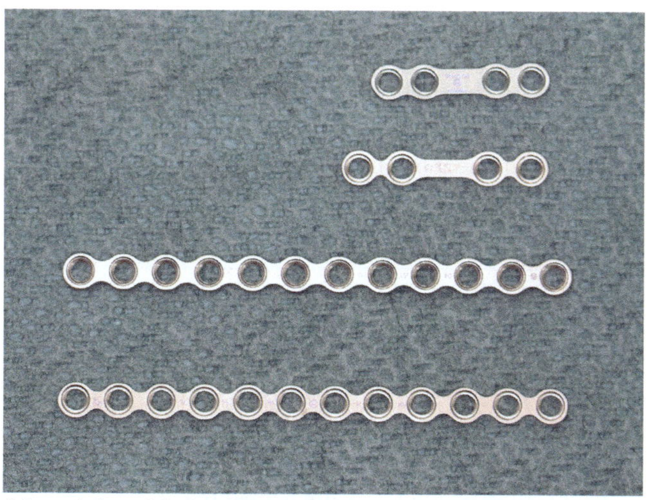

Fig. 54.14 1.0-mm and 1.2-mm-thick standard miniplates (DePuySynthes, Zuchwil, Switzerland)

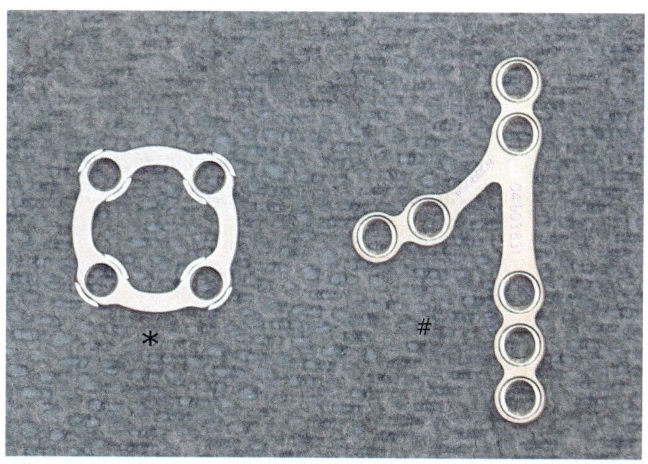

Fig. 54.15 3D miniplate (asterisk) and special condylar neck plate (hash symbol) (DePuySynthes, Zuchwil, Switzerland)

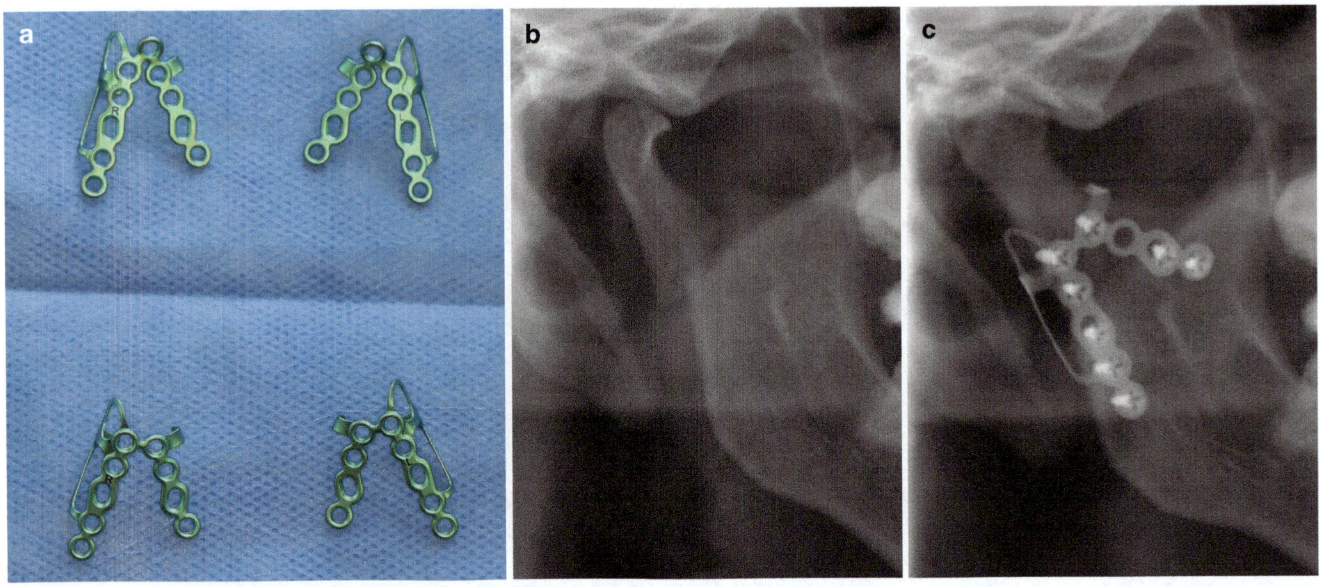

Fig. 54.16 (**a**) Anatomically preformed 3D condylar neck plates with integrated reposition wings for the posterior border and the sigmoid notch (KLS Martin, Tuttlingen, Germany). (**b**) Displaced right condylar neck fracture. (**c**) Condylar neck fracture after repositioning and fixation employing an intraoral approach

54.3 Complications

There is no much difference in complications by treating condylar factures via an intraoral approach in comparison to all other treatment options. Postoperative infection is the most common complication followed by malocclusion. Dysfunctional degeneration of the injured joint can lead to joint clicking, pain, reduced mouth opening, and mandibular deviation during opening and closing. Even severe arthritis or condylar resorption can occur up to the total destruction or loss of the joint. Hardware failure in form of plate fractures or loosening of screws can be seen occasionally as well.

In addition to the avoidance of any visible extraoral scar, the biggest advantage in comparison to all extraoral approaches for surgical treatment of condylar fractures is the very low complication rate concerning facial nerve injuries, salivary fistulas, sialoceles, Frey syndrome, or disturbance of the great auricular nerve.

54.4 Conclusion

The described intraoral approach for the treatment of condylar fractures is favorable for fractures of the condylar base and the condylar process. The biggest benefit and advantage in comparison to all extraoral approaches is the very low complication rate concerning facial nerve injuries and the avoidance of extraoral scars. A disadvantage is the need for special equipment to facilitate this technically demanding procedure with regular success (Table 54.1).

Table 54.1 Advantages and disadvantages of an intraoral approach for the treatment of condylar fractures

Advantages
• No visible scars
• Very low risk for facial nerve damaging
• Very low risk for salivary fistulas, sialoceles or Frey syndrome
• No risk for disturbance of the great auricular nerve
Disadvantages
• Need for special equipment
• Technically demanding
• Not suitable for condylar head fractures

54.5 Case Scenario

History: A 24-year-old female with history of a bicycle accident.

Clinical features: Malocclusion with lateral open bite left. Limited and painful mouth opening. Mobile mandible paramedian region left. Chin hematoma.

Diagnosis: Medial displaced condylar process fracture right and slightly displaced paramedian fracture left (Fig. 54.17a–b).

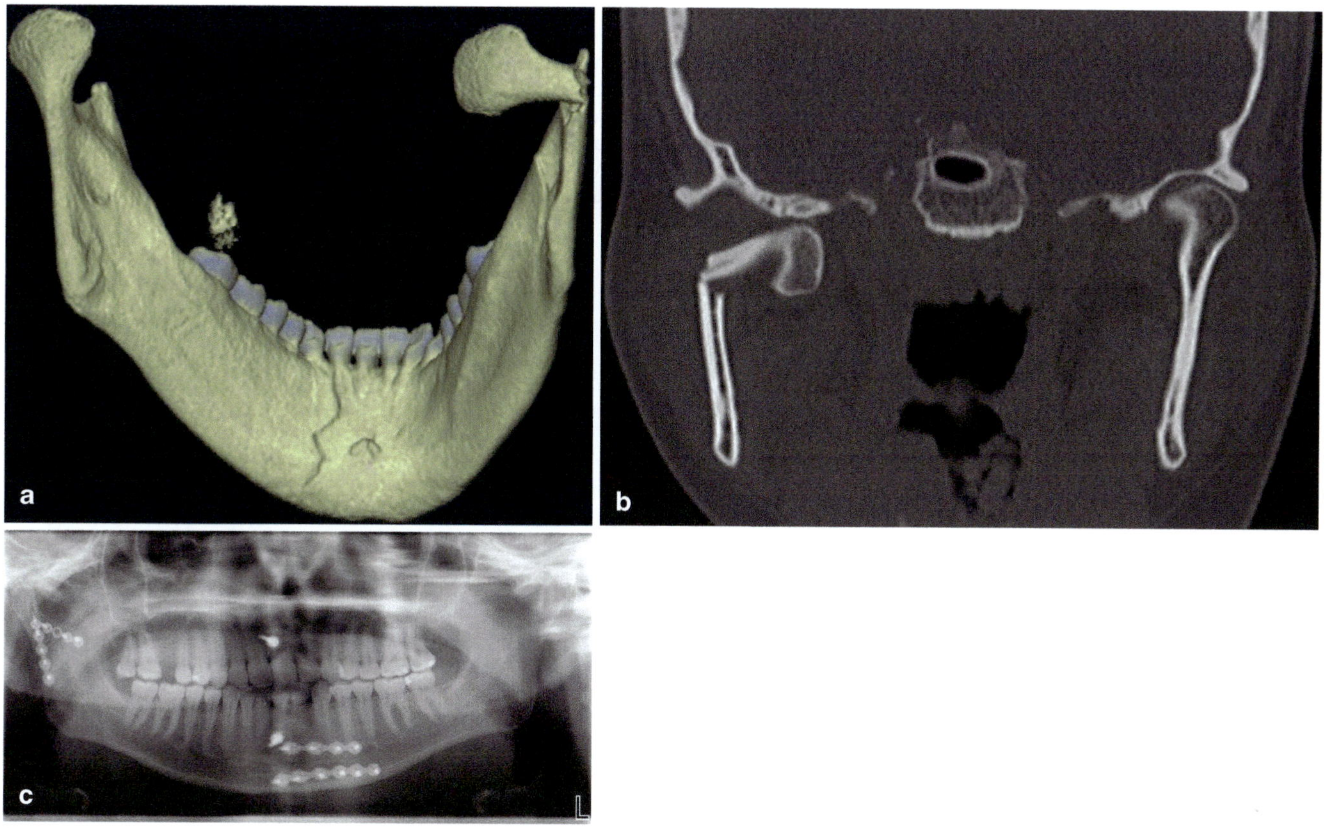

Fig. 54.17 (**a**) 3D reconstruction of the preoperative CT scan showing the medial displaced condylar process fracture right and slightly displaced paramedian fracture left. (**b**) Coronal view of the preoperative CT scan showing the medial out of the fossa displaced condylar process fracture right. (**c**) Postoperative panoramic X-ray showing well-sufficient reduced and with miniplates stabilized fractures paramedian left and at the condylar process right

Surgical plan: Open reduction and internal fixation of both fractures employing an intraoral approach. The paramedian fracture should be fixed first with two miniplates. A gap of the lingual cortex should be prevented by compression of the mandible in the posterior region and overbending the plates. The condylar neck fracture should be fixed second with two miniplates as well.

Postoperative findings: Sufficient reduced and stabilized fractures at the condylar process right and paramedian left (Fig. 54.17c). Proper occlusion and regular mouth opening 4 weeks after surgery without any deviation during function.

References

1. Rozeboom AVJ, Dubois L, Bos RRM, Spijker R, de Lange J. Open treatment of condylar fractures via extraoral approaches: A review of complications. J Craniomaxillofac Surg. 2018;46(8):1232–40.
2. Vural E. Treatment of adult subcondylar mandibular fractures: closed vs open vs endoscopic approach. Arch Otolaryngol Head Neck Surg. 2004;130(10):1228–30.
3. Hall MB. Condylar fractures: surgical management. J Oral Maxillofac Surg. 1994;52(11):1189–92.
4. Ellis E 3rd, Dean J. Rigid fixation of mandibular condyle fractures. Oral Surg Oral Med Oral Pathol. 1993;76(1):6–15.
5. Haug RH, Assael LA. Outcomes of open versus closed treatment of mandibular subcondylar fractures. J Oral Maxillofac Surg. 2001;59(4):370–5. Discussion 375–6
6. Vogt A, Roser M, Weingart D. Transparotidean approach to surgical management of condylar neck fractures. A prospective study. Mund Kiefer Gesichtschir. 2005;9(4):246–50 [Article in German].
7. Patil RS, Gudi SS. Management of subcondylar fracture through intraoral approach with rigid internal fixation. J Maxillofac Oral Surg. 2011;10(3):209–15.
8. Schön R, Gutwald R, Schramm A, Gellrich NC, Schmelzeisen R. Endoscopy-assisted open treatment of condylar fractures of the mandible: extraoral vs intraoral approach. Int J Oral Maxillofac Surg. 2002;31(3):237–43.
9. Silverman SL. A new operation for displaced fractures at the neck of the mandibular condyle. Dental Cosmos. 1925;67:876.
10. Fritzemeier C, Bechthold H. Die Osteosynthese von Unter kiefergelenkfortsatzfrakturen mit alleinigen Zugang von intraoral. Dtsch Z Mund Kiefer Gesichtschir. 1993;17:66–8.

11. Mokros S, Erle A. Transoral miniplate osteosynthesis of mandibular condyle fractures—optimizing the surgical method. Fortschr Kiefer Gesichtschir. 1996;41:136–8.
12. Veras RB, Kriwalsky MS, Eckert AW, Schubert J, Maurer P. Long-term outcomes after treatment of condylar fracture by intraoral access: a functional and radiologic assessment. J Oral Maxillofac Surg. 2007;65:1470–6.
13. Jensen T, Jensen J, Nørholt SE, Dahl M, Lenk-Hansen L, Svensson P. Open reduction and rigid internal fixation of mandibular condylar fractures by an intraoral approach: a longterm follow-up study of 15 patients. J Oral Maxillofac Surg. 2006;64:1771–9.
14. Schneider M, Lauer G, Eckelt U. Surgical treatment of fractures of the mandibular condyle: a comparison of long-term results following different approaches—functional, axiographical, and radiological findings. J Craniomaxillofac Surg. 2007;35:151–60.
15. Schramm A, Wilde F. Computer-assisted reconstruction of the facial skeleton. HNO. 2011;59(8):800–6.
16. Wilde F, Schramm A. Intraoperative imaging in orbital and midface reconstruction. Facial Plast Surg. 2014;30(5):545–53.

55 Maxillary Fractures

Oommen Aju Jacob and Akhilesh Prathap

55.1 Introduction

Complex midface trauma has challenged the diagnostic and operative skills of surgeons through the decades. Robert Marciani in his fifty year review article dated 1993, vividly described the challenges faced by early surgeons regarding the clinical and radiological diagnosis of mid face fractures and the compromised surgical results that may ensue [1].

Table 55.1 Milestones of maxillary fractures

Date	Author	Key finding
1822	Charles Fredrick Reiche	First treatise on maxillary fractures
1823	Carl van Graefe	Use of a head frame to treat a maxillary fracture
1901	René Le Fort	Paper on midfacial fracture patterns
1943	Crawford	Used a Halo frame which was secured directly to the skull using pins

55.1.1 History (Table 55.1)

In an area so anatomically complicated as the midface, the lines of fracture produced in the middle third are classified based upon the experimental studies of René Le Fort in 1901 [2]. The earliest known writings of maxillofacial fractures were recorded in the Edwin Smith papyrus in 1650 BC. Hippocrates who is often portrayed as the "Father of Medicine" described a myriad of facial injuries around 400 BC and his insight provided the basis for bandages and single jaw interdental wiring as methods of fixation and stabilization of facial fractures. Over the subsequent centuries, there appeared many techniques which in essence were variations of what Hippocrates had described. In the nineteenth century, Charles Fredrick Reiche provided the first detailed treatise on maxillary fractures [3]. It was also in the same century that Garretson and Blair advocated mandibular-maxillary fixation with the aid of splints to primarily treat maxillary fractures.

In 1901, a French surgeon René Le Fort published his classic paper on midfacial fracture patterns. He inflicted blunt facial trauma on cadavers, then subsequently removed the soft tissue and examined fracture patterns of the facial skeleton. This study has ever since been the basis for the description of maxillary fractures.

O. A. Jacob (✉)
Department of Oral and Maxillofacial Surgery, Ananthapuri Hospitals and Research Institute, Trivandrum, Kerala, India

Kerala Institute of Medical Sciences, Trivandrum, Kerala, India

A. Prathap
Pushpagiri College of Dental Sciences, Thiruvalla, Kerala, India

K. Bonanthaya et al. (eds.), *Oral and Maxillofacial Surgery for the Clinician*, https://doi.org/10.1007/978-981-15-1346-6_55

55.1.2 Surgical Anatomy/Osteology

The middle third of the facial skeleton is made up of the following bones (Fig. 55.1)

1. Two maxillae
2. Two zygomatic bones
3. Two zygomatic processes of the temporal bones
4. Two palatine bones
5. Two nasal bones
6. Two lacrimal bones
7. The vomer
8. The ethmoid and its attached conchae
9. Two inferior conchae
10. The pterygoid plates of the sphenoid

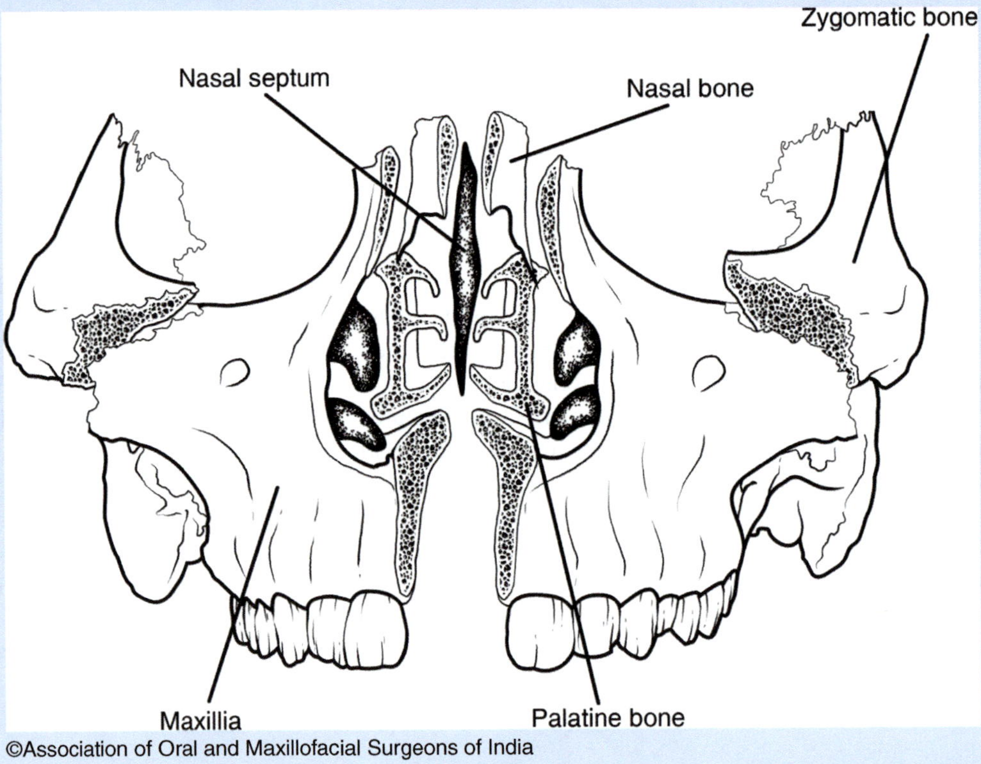

Fig. 55.1 Bones of the midface

The middle third of the face is made up of a number of bones which rarely fractures in isolation. The complex nature of the midface is such that it will withstand the forces of mastication from below and provide protection in certain areas for vital structures. The middle third of the facial skeleton consists of a series of bone struts (buttresses) passing upwards from the upper teeth to the bones of the skull [4] (Fig. 55.2).

The relative fragility of the midface skeleton makes it act as a cushion for trauma directed towards the cranium from an anterior or anterolateral direction. The facial skeleton can be designated by this famous figure, where the skull is similar to a helmet, the midface is similar to a matchbox (crumble zone) and the mandible is similar to a hockey stick (Fig. 55.3). The most common causes of facial fractures in the adult population are assaults and motor vehicle accidents [5].

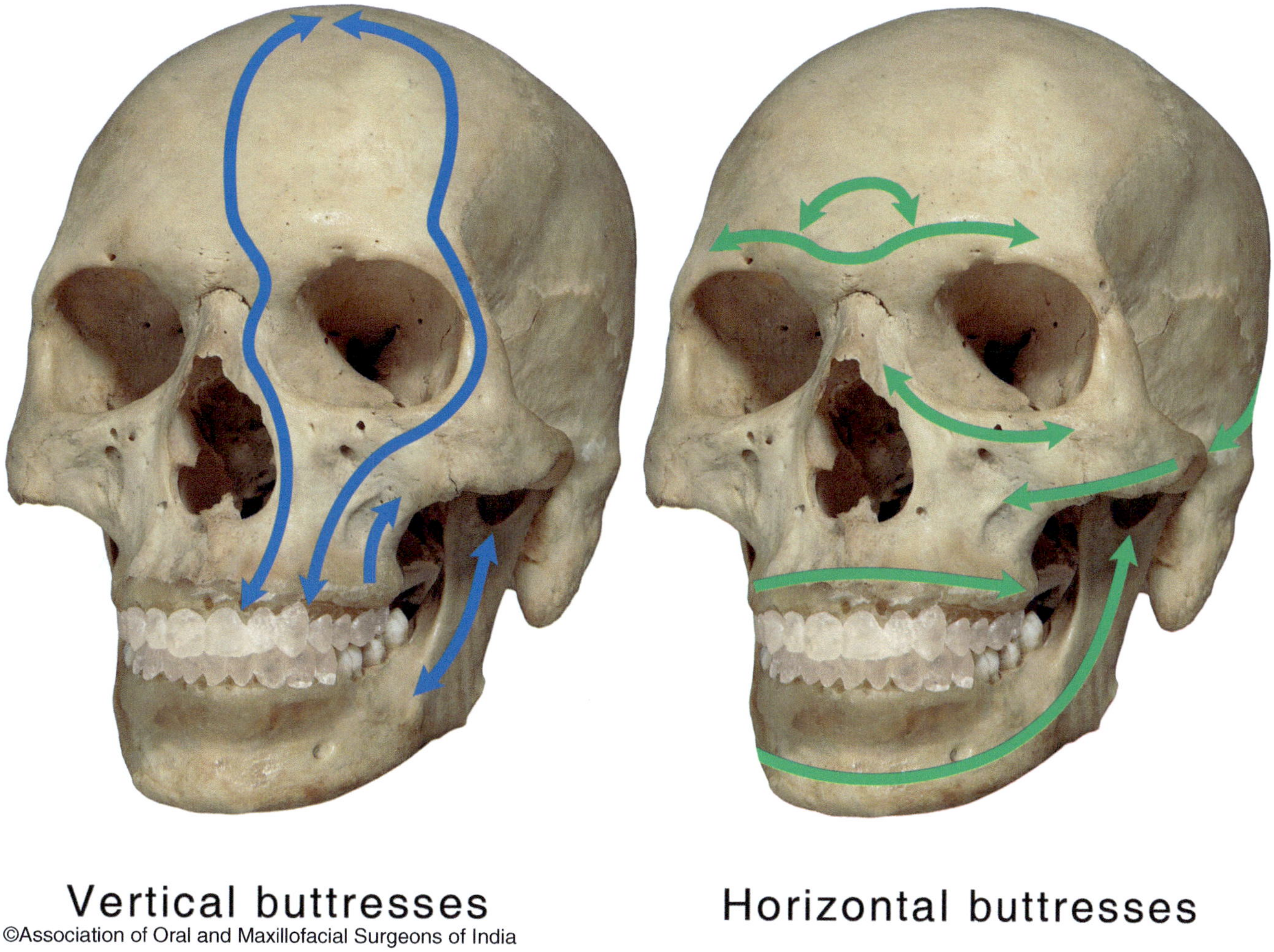

Fig. 55.2 Vertical and horizontal buttresses of the facial skeleton (Also refer Fig. 60.9 and Table 60.2)

55.1.3 Applied Anatomy of the Midfacial Bones

The midface is composed of the nasal, zygoma, maxilla, ethmoid and its conchae, palatine, inferior concha and vomer which are collectively referred to as the middle third of the facial skeleton. The facial bones in isolation are comparatively fragile but gain strength and support as they articulate with each other. It is this strength that has often been described as the facial buttresses which Manson alluded to when describing the vertical and horizontal struts that support the facial skeleton [6]. The horizontal pillars are formed by the frontal bar (composed of the supraorbital rims and nasal process of the frontal bone), the zygomatic arch, the infraorbital rims and the nasal bridge and finally the alveolar process of the maxilla. The vertical pillars are the medial pillar formed by the piriform rims which continues superiorly as the frontal process of the maxilla. The zygomatic buttresses which continue superiorly with the lateral orbital rims form the lateral pillars, and the most caudal pillars are the pterygoid plates.

55.1.3.1 Maxilla

The maxilla consists of a central body and four processes, namely, the frontal, zygomatic, alveolar and palatine process. The body is hollowed out and contains the maxillary sinus. It is pyramidal shaped with the base being the medial surface facing the nasal cavity and the apex being elongated into the zygomatic process. It has an orbital or superior surface which forms the floor and rim of the orbit, a malar or anterolateral surface which forms part of the cheek and a posterolateral or infratemporal surface which contributes to the infratemporal fossa. The base is rimmed inferiorly by the alveolar process. The alveolar process houses the dental arch with the sockets varying in size according to the teeth. The palatine process is a horizontal process from the body to the alveolar process and medially articulates with the palatine process of the opposite maxilla, while posteriorly it articu-

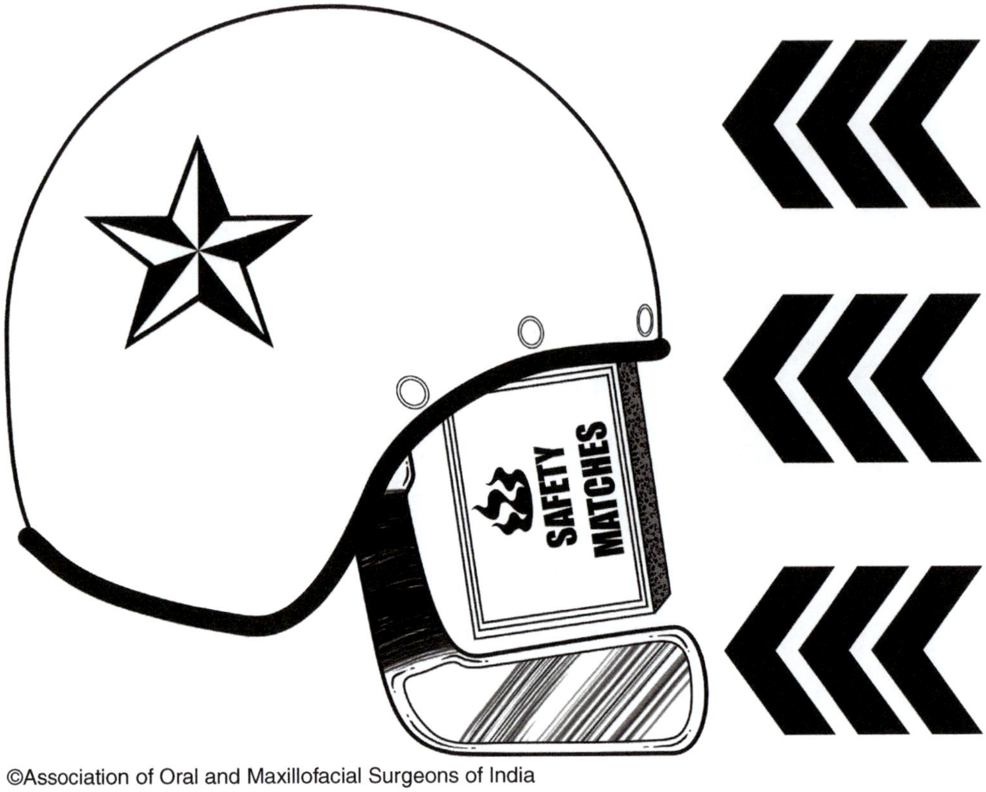

Fig. 55.3 Helmet, matchbox and hockey stick to illustrate relative bone strength (the matchbox is the crumble zone)

lates with the horizontal plate of the palatine bone. The zygomatic process is an extension of the anterolateral surface of the body which contributes to the zygomaticomaxillary suture. The frontal process projects upwards to articulate with the maxillary process of the frontal bone as well as the nasal bone anteriorly and the lacrimal bone posteriorly.

55.1.3.2 Vascular Supply and Innervation

The blood supply to the maxilla and the palatine bones is through the periosteum, the incisive artery and the greater and lesser palatine arteries. The internal maxillary artery lies posterior to the maxillae and the palatine bones and anterior to the pterygoid plates of sphenoid.

The maxillary nerve enters the caudal maxilla ventral to the orbit via the maxillary foramen and runs through the maxilla in the infraorbital canal giving off branches to supply the maxillary cheek and teeth. The nerve then exits the maxilla at the infraorbital foramen.

55.2 Classification

55.2.1 René Le Fort1901 [2]

Maxillary fractures were classified by René Le Fort based on his experiments on cadavers with low velocity unidirectional frontal trauma. Although the present-day maxillary fractures are caused due to high velocity multi directional trauma, the Le Fort classification is still widely followed due to its simplicity and the levels of anatomic differentiation it offers. Other authors have attempted classifications based on the anatomical sites and based on the involvement of the occlusion. Marciani modified the basic Le Fort classification by adding frontal bone and zygomatic fractures.

55.2.1.1 Le Fort I

Low Level Fracture/Guerin Fracture

The fracture line extends backwards from the lateral margin of the anterior nasal aperture below the zygomatic buttress to cross the lower third of the pterygoid laminae. The fracture also passes along the lateral wall of the nose and the lower third of the septum to join the lateral fracture behind the tuberosity (Fig. 55.4a–c).

55.2.1.2 Le Fort II

Pyramidal or Sub-zygomatic Fracture

This fracture runs from the thin middle area of the nasal bones down either side, crossing the frontal processes of maxillae into the medial wall of each orbit; the fracture line crosses the lacrimal bone behind the lacrimal sac before turning forwards to cross the infraorbital margins slightly medial to or through the infraorbital foramen. The fracture now extends downwards and backwards across the lateral wall of the antrum below the zygomaticomaxillary suture and divides the pterygoid laminae about half way up.

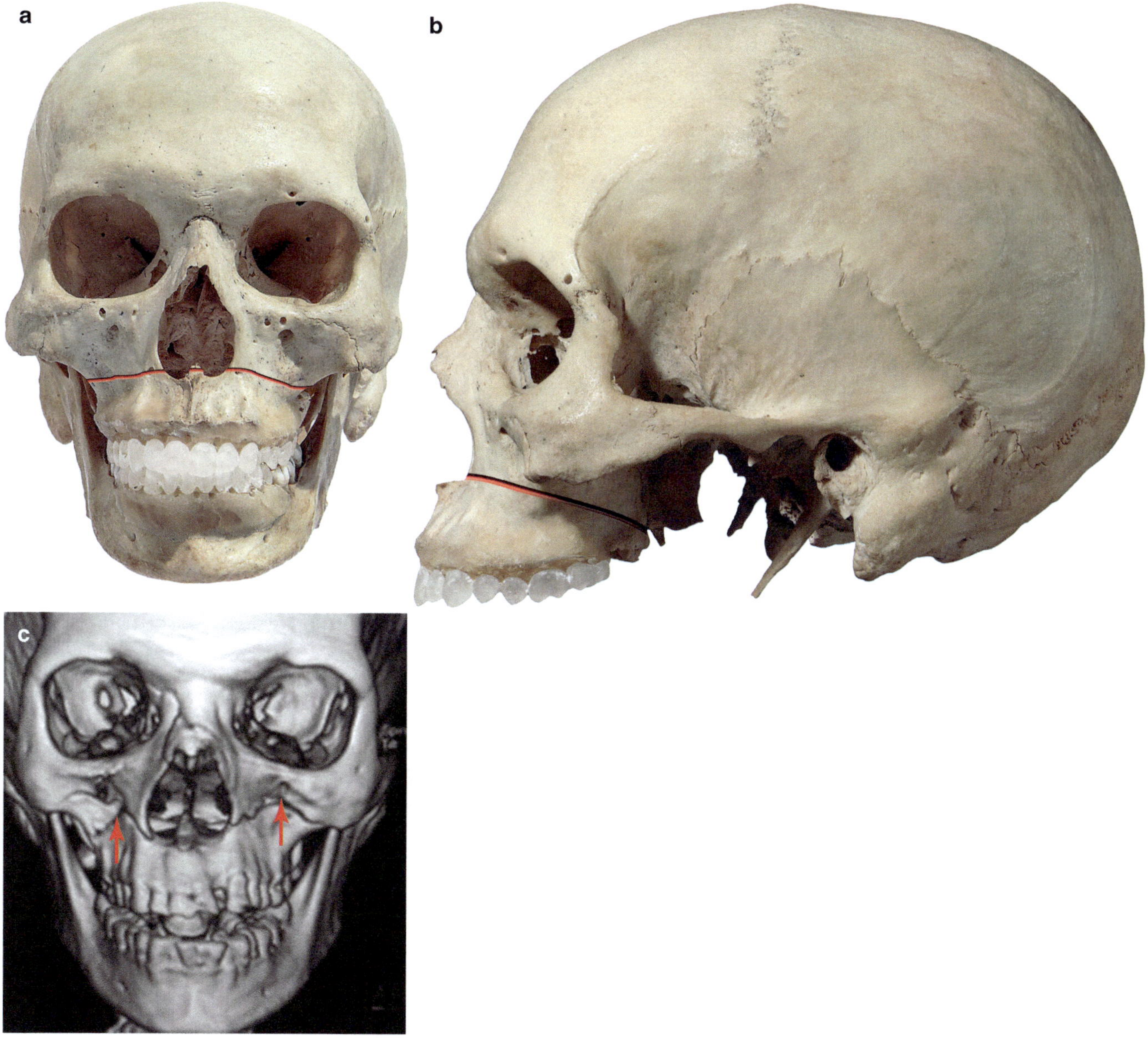

Fig. 55.4 (**a**, **b**) Le Fort I fracture lines. (**c**) CT of Le Fort I fracture

Separation of the block from the base of the skull is completed via the nasal septum and may involve the floor of the anterior cranial fossa (Fig. 55.5a–d).

55.2.1.3 Le Fort III

Transverse or Supra-zygomatic Fracture

The fracture runs from near the frontonasal suture transversely backwards and parallel with the base of the skull and involves the full depth of the ethmoid bone including the cribriform plate. Within the orbit the fracture passes below the optic foramen into the posterior limit of the inferior orbital fissure. From the base of the inferior orbital fissure, the fracture line extends in two directions: backwards across the pterygomaxillary fissure to fracture the roots of the pterygoid laminae and laterally across the lateral wall of the orbit separating the zygomatic bone from the frontal bone. In this way the entire middle third of the facial skeleton gets separated from the cranial base (Fig. 55.6a–c).

Le Fort classification does not take into consideration:

- Dentoalveolar fractures
- Palatal fractures
- Bone loss

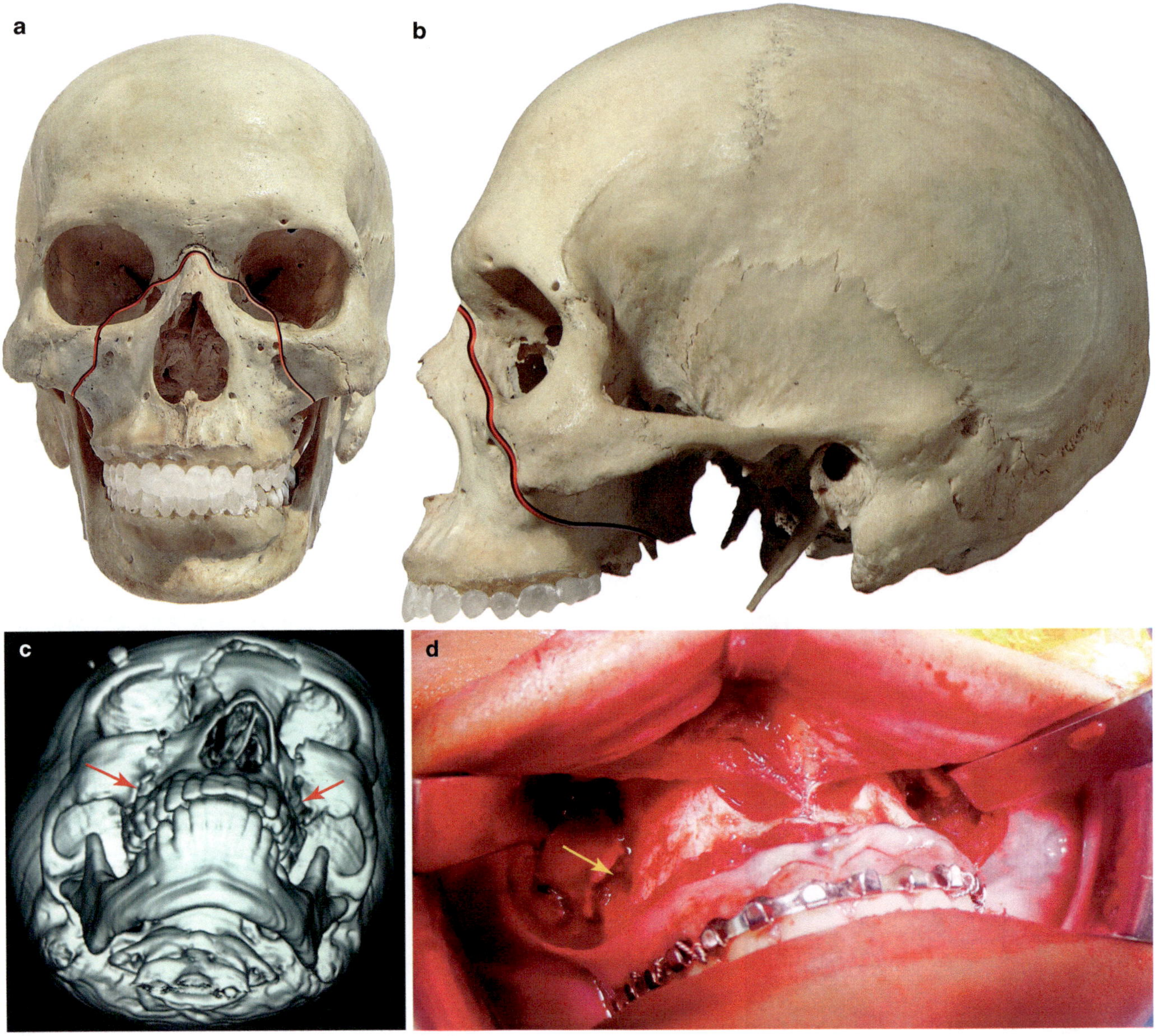

Fig. 55.5 (**a**, **b**) Le Fort II fracture lines. (**c**) CT of Le Fort II fracture showing the midface segment impacted (red arrows). (**d**) Clinical image of case in **c**, showing the impacted area right side Le Fort II (yellow arrow)

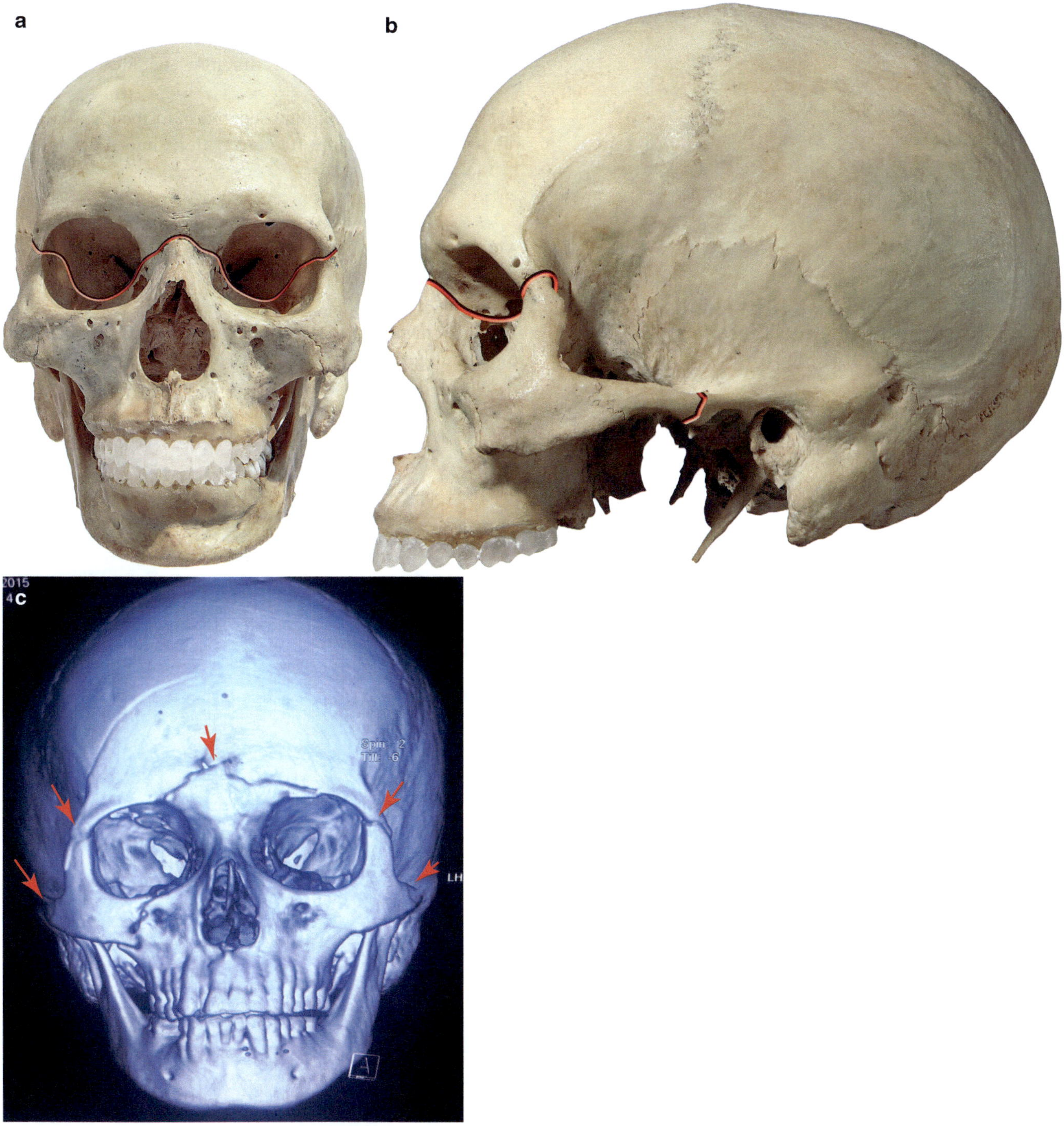

©Association of Oral and Maxillofacial Surgeons of India

Fig. 55.6 (**a**, **b**) Le Fort III fracture. (**c**) CT of Le Fort III fracture (the fracture lines shown with red arrows)

55.2.2 Killey's Classification (1965) [2] (Table 55.2)

Table 55.2 Killey's classification

1. Dentoalveolar fractures
2. Zygomatic complex fractures
3. Nasal complex fractures
4. Le Fort I
5. Le Fort II
6. Le Fort III
7. Extended Le Fort fractures

55.2.3 Rowe and Williams's Classification (1985) [2] (Table 55.3)

Addenda

(i) These fractures may occur unilaterally or be associated independently with a fracture of the zygomatic complex.

(ii) There may be a midline separation of the maxillae and/or extension of the fracture pattern into the frontal or temporal bones.

55.2.4 Marciani (1993: Modification of Le Fort Fractures) [1]

Fractures involving the cranial base and other midface fracture configurations, including severely comminuted segments of the facial skeleton, were not classifiable by the

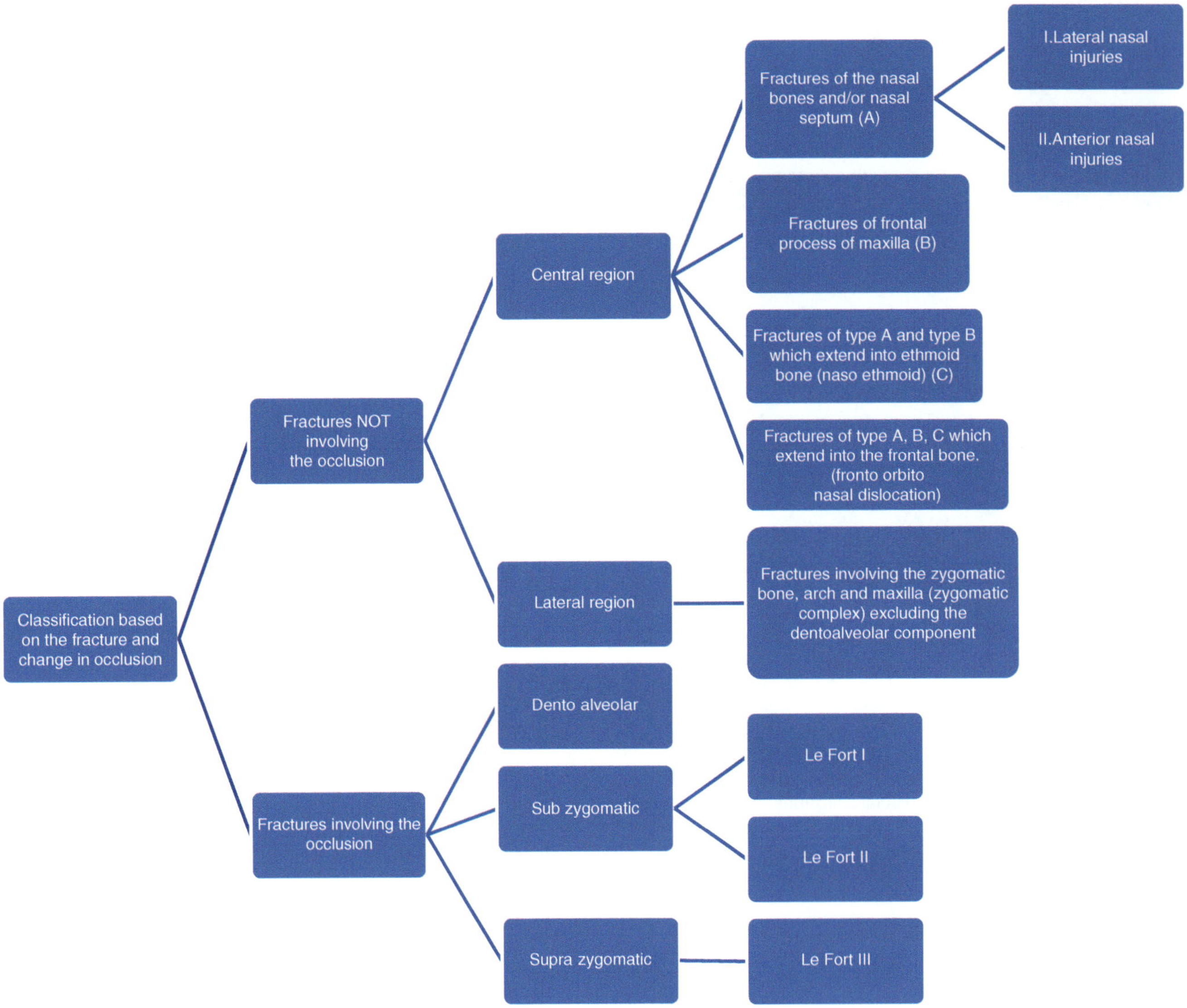

Table 55.3 Rowe and Williams's classification

traditional Le Fort scheme. Hence Marciani proposed a more precise system of describing fracture patterns to define the fracture configuration, establish an accurate diagnosis and to determine potential surgical approaches (Table 55.4).

55.2.5 Palatal Fractures Classification: Hendrickson's Classification (1998) [7] (Figs. 55.7, 55.8, and 55.9; Table 55.5)

Table 55.4 Marciani's modification of Le Fort fracture classification

Marciani (1993-modification of Le Fort fractures)	Le Fort I—Low maxillary fracture	Ia—Low maxillary fracture/ multiple segments
	Le Fort II—Pyramidal fractures	IIa—Pyramidal and nasal fracture
		IIb—Pyramidal and NOE fracture
	Le Fort III—Craniofacial dysjunction	III a—craniofacial dysjunction and nasal fracture
		III b—craniofacial dysjunction and NOE
	Lefort IV—Le Fort II or III and cranial base fracture	IV a—supraorbital rim fracture
		IV b—anterior cranial fossa and supraorbital rim fracture
		IV c—anterior cranial fossa and orbital wall fracture

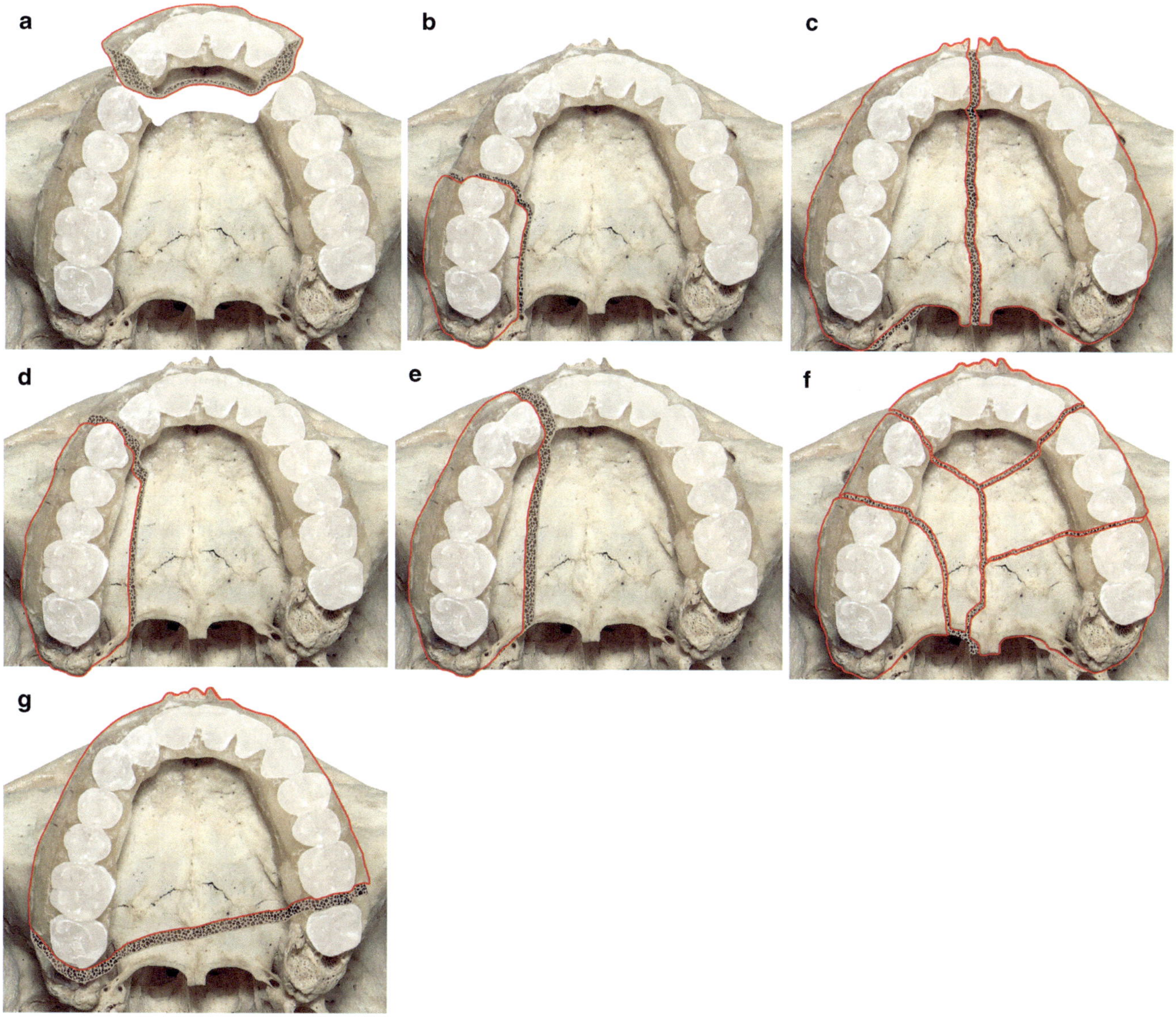

Fig. 55.7 Hendrickson's classification of palatal fractures. (**a**) Type Ia, (**b**) Type Ib, (**c**) Type II, (**d**) Type III ,(**e**) Type IV, (**f**) Type V, (**g**) Type VI

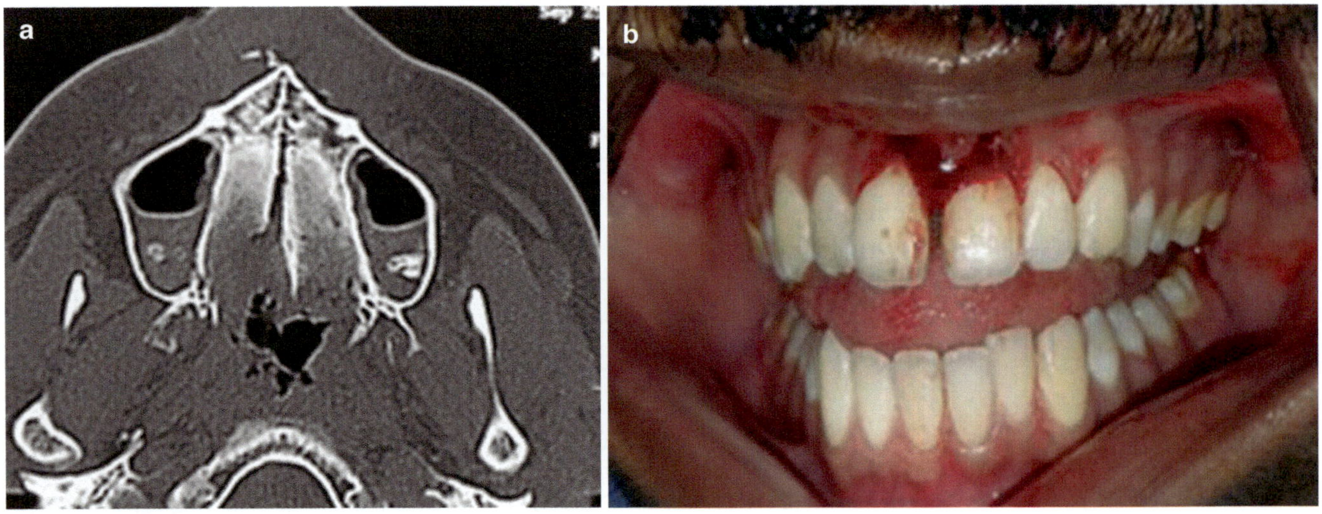

Fig. 55.8 (**a**) CT of Hendrickson's type C fracture. (**b**) Clinical image of case of **a**, showing the midline diastema

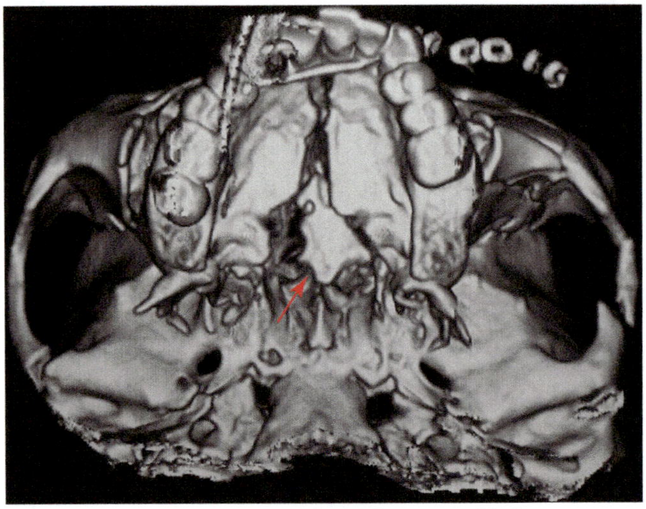

Fig. 55.9 CT of midline palatal fracture with splayed segments, note the posterior displaced fragment, temporary bridle wire has been placed between upper central incisors

55.3 Clinical Features (Box 55.1)

55.3.1 Le Fort I Fractures

Gross facial swelling or facial disfigurement is generally not a feature of Le Fort I fractures, but oedema around the upper lip may occur. Soft tissue injury along the upper lip along with tearing of gingivae may occur due to the causative impact. There can be mobility of the upper dento-alveolus when digital pressure is applied. Mobility of the maxilla at the Le Fort I level must be differentiated from extended maxillary dentoalveolar fracture. Malocclusion may occur if the fracture is displaced or impacted. Dorsal and caudal pull of the medial pterygoid muscles can contribute to the posterior displacement of the maxilla and the resultant anterior open bite (Fig. 55.10a, b). Bilateral epistaxis is rare although emphysema may occur if the patient blows his nose. Ecchymosis in the upper buccal sulcus is a frequent finding. Percussion of the maxillary teeth produces a dull cracked cup sound. In case of inferiorly displaced Le Fort I fractures, the patient may have to keep the mouth open to accommodate the increased vertical dimension. Due to the extreme downward displacement of the maxilla, the nasal base is lost, leading to stretching of the soft tissues of that area, which makes it possible to see directly into the nares.

The posteriorly impacted Le Fort I fracture may result in an anterior open bite and in these cases the maxilla may be immobile. Usually the impacted maxilla can be mobilized by grasping the maxillary teeth and applying a firm anterior pull. A grate may be felt due to the movement between the fractured segments. In posteriorly impacted fractures, there may be damage to the cusps of maxillary teeth usually in the premolar region, caused by the upward impact of the mandibular teeth at the time of the trauma. The complete Le Fort I fracture may be associated with a split along the median palatal suture. Sometimes more than one fracture line may be present in the palate, so that either one or both fragments may be mobile (Fig. 55.11a–c).

55.3.2 Le Fort II Fractures

Marked facial disfigurement resulting from circumorbital ecchymosis and gross oedema can be a feature of Le Fort II fractures. Frequently the patient will not be able to open

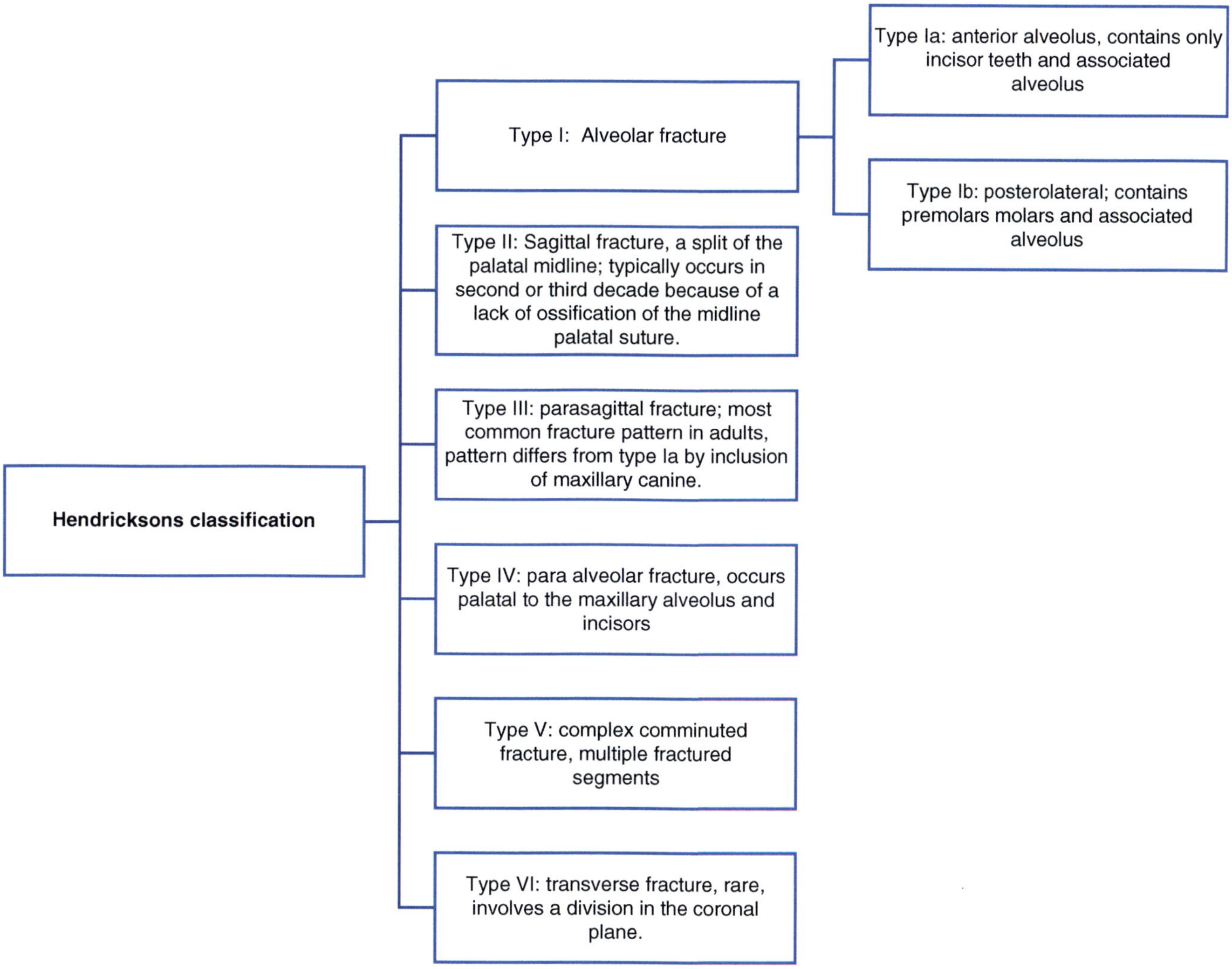

Table 55.5 Hendrickson's classification: of Palate fractures

Box 55.1 Clinical features of Le Fort fractures

Clinical features	Le Fort I	Le Fort II	Le Fort III
Intraoral	• Floating maxilla • Impacted or telescopic fracture • Anterior open bite • Deranged occlusion • Guerin's sign • Palatal fracture in some cases	• Deranged occlusion • Posterior gagging of occlusion • Possible airway obstruction	• Deranged occlusion • Posterior gagging of occlusion • Possible airway obstruction
Extraoral	• Mild swelling and oedema of midface and upper lip • Epistaxis in some cases • Increased visibility of anterior nares	• Moon face appearance • Peri-orbital oedema • Circumorbital ecchymosis • Subconjunctival haemorrhage • Infraorbital step deformity • Altered sensation of cheek • CSF rhinorrhea • Diplopia	• Separation at FZ suture • CSF rhinorrhea • Hooding of eyes • Anti-mongoloid slant • Dish face deformity

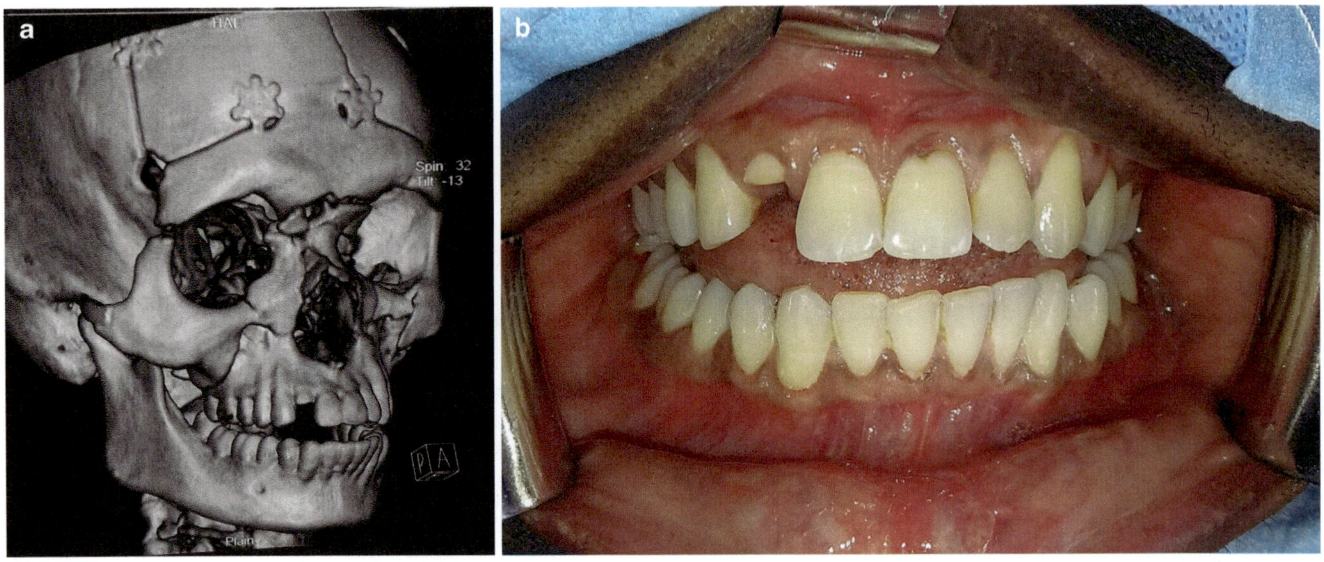

Fig. 55.10 (**a**, **b**) A posteriorly telescoped Le Fort I fracture maxilla clinically manifesting as anterior open bite

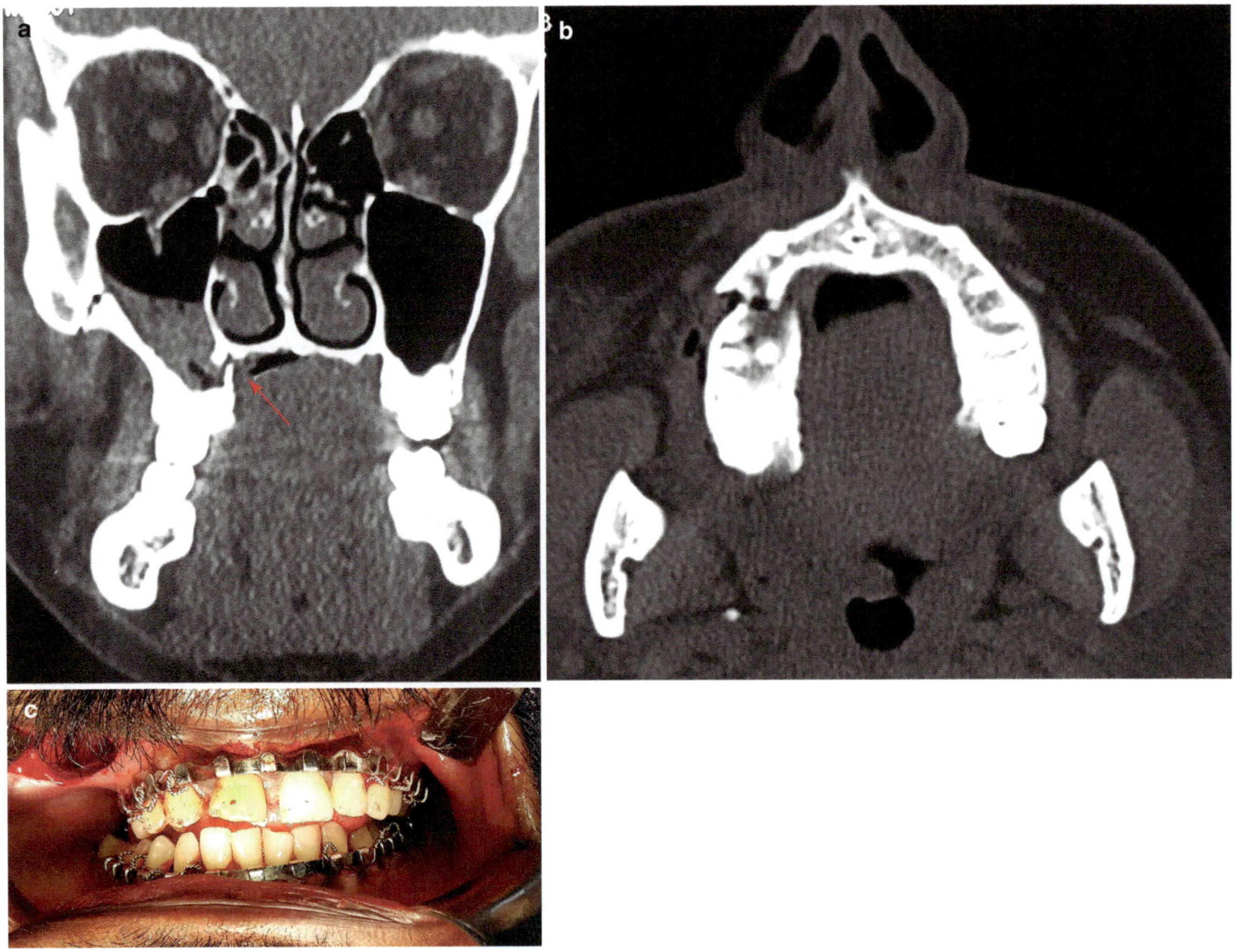

Fig. 55.11 CT images (**a**, **b**) showing a right zygomatic complex fracture associated with a Hendrickson's type B fracture where the right posterior alveolar and palatal segment was displaced palatally and extruded, causing the occlusal discrepancy (crossbite) as seen in **c**

his eyelids to allow an ocular examination. Subconjunctival haemorrhage may be present, the posterior limit of which cannot be identified. Bilateral peri-orbital oedema and circumorbital ecchymosis (described as circumorbital as it follows the shape of the orbicularis oculi muscle) are described as racoon eyes or panda facies. There can be severe oedema of the face which is sometimes described as moon facies. Enophthalmos in case of orbital floor fractures may go undetected due to oedema. Considerable lengthening of face with posterior gagging of teeth can also occur. Bilateral epistaxis is common, and CSF leak may be present. The loss of maxillary prominence may result in a dish face appearance. If the fracture line passes through the infraorbital canal there can be associated paresthesia in the infraorbital nerve region. While clinically mobilizing the maxilla in a Le Fort II fracture, transmitted mobility may be felt at the infraorbital rim and the frontonasal suture. Figure 55.12 shows a CT image where Le Fort II and III lines are seen

55.3.3 Le Fort III Fractures (Also see Fig. 49.5)

This fracture is clinically similar to the Le Fort II fracture but can demonstrate a more serious condition. Bilateral ecchymosis with circumorbital oedema may close the eyes completely. As in Le Fort II, the posterior limit of the subconjunctival haemorrhage cannot be seen. The lengthening of the face occurs due to the loss of bony fixation to the base of the skull. The flattening of the face from the disrupted zygomatic bones is usually masked by the gross oedema. The fracture passes above the Whitnall's tubercle and so the support by Lockwoods, suspensory ligament is lost. This results in hooding of upper eyelid which becomes obvious when the oedema subsides. Gagging of occlusion and shift of the maxillary midline may occur. Gross posterior displacement of the maxilla can result in the soft palate touching the posterior part of the tongue causing airway and speech impairment. As with other maxillary fractures, percussion of teeth might produce a cracked cup sound. .

The clinical differentiation between Le Fort II and Le Fort III fractures can be assessed by palpating for step deformity in the infraorbital rim in the former.

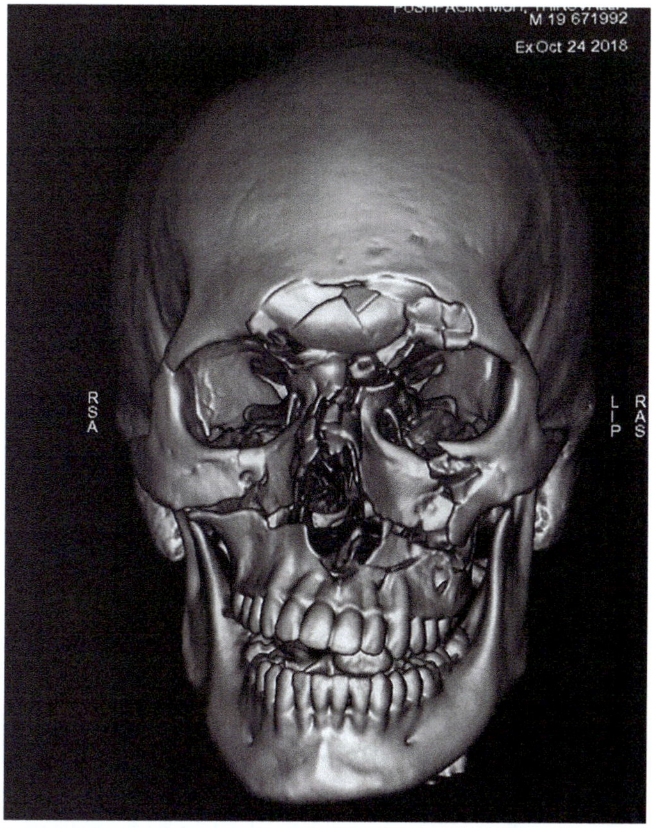

Fig. 55.12 CT image showing Le Fort I and II fractures. Note that maxilla is rotated to the right side with canting on the left side.

55.3.4 Unusual Fracture Patterns

The Le Fort fractures may manifest without the classic fracture patterns as described above. An unilateral fracture at Le Fort I level may occur (identified through imaging) which warrants no intervention unless accompanied by a palatal fracture causing occlusal derangement and/or mobility. Such a unilateral fracture pattern can cause unilateral gagging causing open bite on the contralateral side

The clinician must be aware of the two types of Le Fort I fractures, the mobile and impacted variants; lack of mobility should not be presumed as absence of fracture.

55.4 Radiographic Examination

It is difficult to diagnose fractures of the middle third of the face with plain films and CT scans have now largely replaced radiographs.

The commonly used radiographs for identifying maxillary fractures are occipitomental view (OMV) 10° and 30° and paranasal sinus view 37° (PNS -Waters view).

While assessing maxillary fractures with these radiographs, Mcgregor-Campbell and Trapnell's lines and Dolan's lines (elephant of Rogers) may be kept in mind [8].

McGregor-Campbell's lines:

These lines were described by McGregor and Campbell for ease of searching on an occipitomental view 10-degree frontal projection.

1. First line across the zygomaticofrontal, the superior margin of the orbit and the frontal sinus
2. Second line across the zygomatic arch, zygomatic body, inferior orbital margin and nasal bone

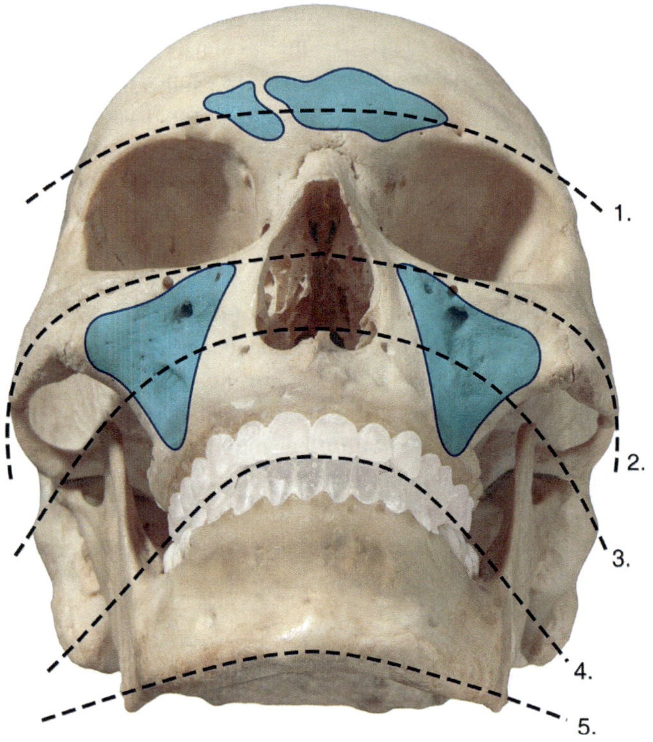

Fig. 55.13 McGregor-Campbell and Trapnell's lines

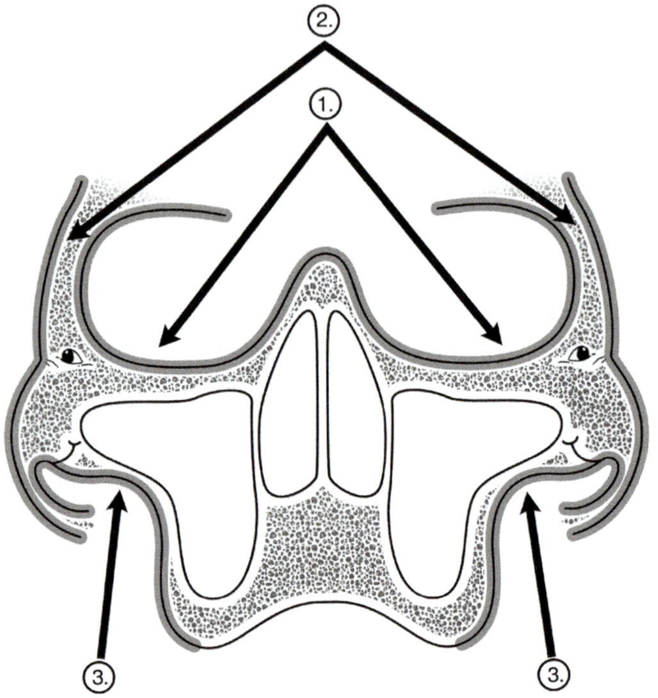

Fig. 55.14 Dolan's lines (also see Fig. 56.22)

3. Third line across the condyles, coronoid process and the maxillary sinus / Zygomatic buttress region
4. Fourth line across the mandibular ramus, occlusal plane
5. Fifth line (Trapnell's line, added later) across the inferior border of the mandible from angle to angle (Fig. 55.13)

The **four S's described by Delbalso, Hall and Margarone** [8]

In PNS view, the following four features are to be verified/compared with the unaffected side

1. Symmetry
2. Sharpness
3. Sinus
4. Soft tissues

Dolan's Lines [8] (Fig. 55.14)

Dolan's lines are the collective name given to three lines described by Dolan and Jacoby that aid in evaluating for maxillofacial fractures on an occipitomental skull radiograph. They are usually used as an adjunct to McGregor-Campbell lines.

- **Orbital line (line 1)** traces the inner margins of the lateral, inferior and medial orbital walls and the nasal arch.
- **Zygomatic line (line 2)** traces the superior margin of the zygomatic arch and body extending along the frontal process of the zygoma to the zygomaticofrontal suture.
- **Maxillary line** (line 3) traces the inferior margin of the zygomatic arch, body, and buttress and the lateral wall of the maxillary sinus.

Elephant of Rogers [8]

Lee Rogers pointed out that the second and third lines of Dolan give the outline of the head of an elephant.

55.4.1 CT Scans

CT scans are now the gold standard for a definitive diagnosis in fractures of the maxilla. A CT scan in all three planes (axial, sagittal and coronal) along with a 3D reconstruction will aid the surgeon in accurate assessment of fracture patterns and also will aid in preoperative planning. The surgeon must never rely on the 3D CT alone but should correlate the images with those obtained in axial sagittal and coronal planes, as there could be reconstruction-related errors which appear as fracture lines or bone defects. CT scan-based fracture patterns may be classified as low, middle or high energy, defined solely by the pattern of segmentation and displacement in the CT scan [9].

55.5 Treatment of Maxillary fractures

The primary aim of treatment of maxillary fractures is to re-establish the dental occlusion and masticatory efficiency. The contribution of the maxilla to the projection and contour of the midface has also to be considered in the management of maxillary fractures and requires a clear understanding of the facial buttress system, subunit anatomy and inter-relationships of the various bones [10]. This aesthetic aspect is often compromised by associated injuries of the zygomatic complex, nose and orbits.

The basic principles of the treatment of maxillary fractures are:

1. Direct exposure and manual reduction of the fractures
2. Reconstitution of the bony buttresses of the mid-face so as to prevent elongation of the face and/or antero-posterior collapse of the maxilla
3. Re-enforcement of the paranasal and zygomatic buttresses with mini-plates
4. Replacement of missing/grossly comminuted bone at the buttresses with autogenous bone grafts [5]

Factors that influence improved treatment outcome in maxillary fractures are:

1. Early definitive treatment
2. Anatomic and functional repair of naso-orbito-ethmoidal injuries
3. Wide exposure of fracture segments
4. Anatomic repositioning and stable fixation of fracture segments in all planes of space [11]

55.5.1 General Considerations in Treatment of Maxillary Fractures

Proper reduction of maxillary fractures is the key to achieving good dental occlusion and needs proper clinical examination of the fracture pattern after all the accessible fracture sites are exposed. A repeat study of the CT scans (axial, coronal and 3D) and correlation with the exposed maxilla will aid the surgeon in planning adequate reduction and rigid fixation. It should be kept in mind that the fractured maxilla is usually displaced backwards and downwards and hence the reduction should in the forward and upward direction. To obtain reproducibly good results, even with the most extensive facial dislocations, the surgeon should restore the facial architecture at the Le Fort I Level [12]. In rare occasions, lateral en bloc displacement of the maxilla is seen, and this requires transverse reduction to achieve the correct dental occlusion. A depressed zygomatic fracture can physically prevent reduction of the maxilla. Hence the fractured zygomatic bone should be reduced prior to manipulating the maxilla.

The most useful instruments for reduction of the maxilla are the Rowe's disimpaction forceps. Even in cases where the fractured maxilla appears to be minimally displaced, it is prudent to mobilize the bone with the disimpaction forceps so as to overcome any bony interferences and thus freeing the maxilla completely. When using this paired forceps, care should be taken to avoid injury to the anterior teeth and also to the palatal mucosa. Mobile, extruded and proclined anterior teeth are at particular risk, and an assistant should closely observe the anterior teeth, while the surgeon is manipulating the fractured maxilla. It would also be advisable to obtain informed consent regarding mobility or loss of these teeth. Trauma to the nasal floor is inevitable when mobilizing the maxilla using the reducing forceps, and some nasal bleeding is usually observed, but this rarely requires a nasal pack.

Adequate reduction of the fractured maxilla is confirmed by:

1. Good dental occlusion
2. Alignment of the paranasal, zygomatic and fronto-zygomatic bony buttresses
3. Adequate reduction of all the observable fracture lines

Problems arise when the patient has few or no teeth and when there is gross comminution of maxilla. In these situations the surgeon has to make do with whatever landmarks are available, and in such cases compromised functional and cosmetic results are not uncommon.

Direct manipulation at the fracture lines is sometimes required especially when the fractured maxilla is telescoped into the superior normal bone. Care must be taken to prevent additional fractures at the bony margins during direct manipulation as this would make fixation more demanding. Using tie wires at the zygomatic buttresses, around the second maxillary premolars/first molars bilaterally and through anterior nasal spine is often useful to physically disimpact and pull the maxilla forwards and upwards thus ensuring good reduction.

When the maxilla is fractured in multiple levels (e.g. Le Fort I and III levels), reduction using the disimpaction forceps alone may not be adequate. The dental occlusion can be achieved, but the midface projection may be compromised. Here also a combination of reduction with disimpaction forceps, direct manipulation at the fracture site and the use of the above mentioned tie wires is often indicated.

Once adequate reduction of the fractured maxilla is obtained, it is mandatory that rigid maxillomandibular fixation (MMF) is applied. In almost all cases, well-adapted maxillary and mandibular arch bars are required as this ensures multiple points for the MMF. Failure to obtain rigid MMF or manually maintaining the dental occlusion during fixation can result in post-operative occlusal discrepancies. If surgical reduction and fixation of the maxilla has to be delayed, elastic traction will be helpful in obtaining a functional occlusion. The use of MMF screws definitely saves operating time but can be problematic if elastic traction is required later.

If the mandibular condylar fracture exists, this should be reduced and fixed prior to the MMF. Failure to do so may result in an open bite due to loss of posterior mandibular height.

55.5.2 Suspension Wiring

Internal wire suspension involves sandwiching the fractured portion of the maxilla between the mandible and the superior part of the facial skeleton/skull that is not fractured. The use of internal suspension wires is more or less obsolete unless there is severe comminution which precludes rigid internal fixation. Suspension wiring may also be the surgeon's choice when there is presence of severe infection at the site of surgery (Fig. 55.15).

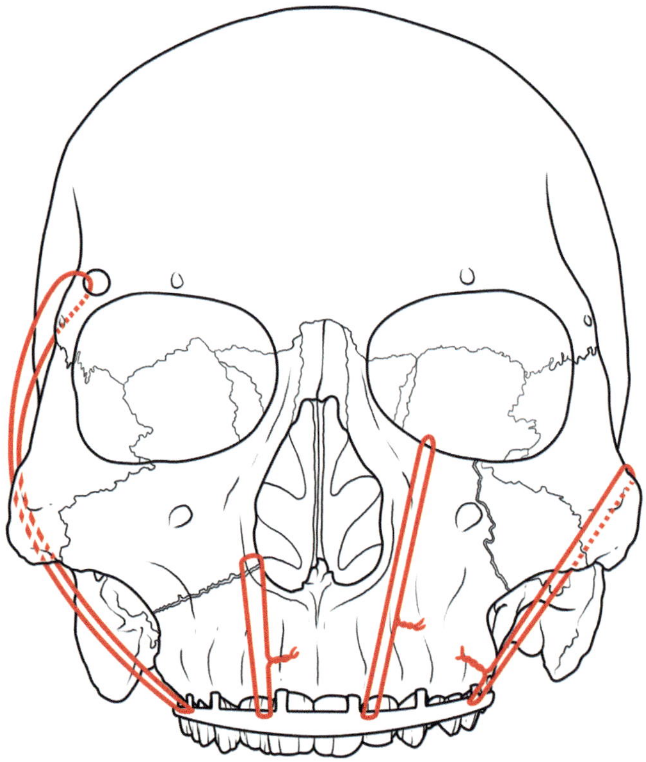

Fig. 55.15 Various types of suspension wiring employed for midface fractures

55.5.3 Rigid Internal Fixation

Although many wiring techniques were practised in the past, rigid internal fixation with titanium bone plates and screws of sufficient rigidity is now the standard of care. For internal fixation of the maxilla, titanium bone plates and screws of sufficient rigidity are used. For providing rigidity, screws with an outer diameter of 1.5 mm is commonly used.

55.5.4 Approaches to the Maxilla

When treating a very high Le Fort I fracture and in Le Fort II and III fractures, it may be necessary to use one or more of the following incisions, which are described in chapter 56 and 57 of this book:

1. Skin incisions for exposure of the infraorbital rim. Extension of this incision medially ensures access to the lateral nasal area, while a lateral extension would give access to the upper portion of the zygomatic body.
2. Upper eyelid or lateral eyebrow incision (blepharoplasty) to expose the fronto-zygomatic suture.
3. An existing laceration with or without conservative extension for increased surgical access.

55.5.4.1 Maxillary Vestibular Approach

The maxilla can be approached through a variety of incisions, the most common being the maxillary vestibular approach. In addition to providing access to the lower part of the entire midfacial skeleton, this approach results in a hidden intraoral scar. This approach may result in disruption of the attachments of the facial muscles of the nasolabial region; hence careful repositioning during closure is recommended to avoid unaesthetic changes to the face. The muscles of importance are the nasalis group, the levator labii superioris alaeque nasi, the levator labii superioris, the levator anguli oris and the orbicularis oris. The vestibular incision and subsequent dissection causes stripping of origin/insertion of most muscles originating in the maxilla. These muscles tend to get reattached in a shortened manner due to the action of the zygomaticus muscle. Deepening of the alar groove and splaying of the alar bases, nostrils and nasal tip may occur following lateral displacement of the nasal modiolus. Soft tissue fullness loss in the naso-alveolar region may result in thinning and retraction of upper lip, reduced vermillion exposure and a obtuse nasolabial angle. Detachment of the levators of the upper lip may cause down turning of the corner of the mouth (Fig. 55.16).

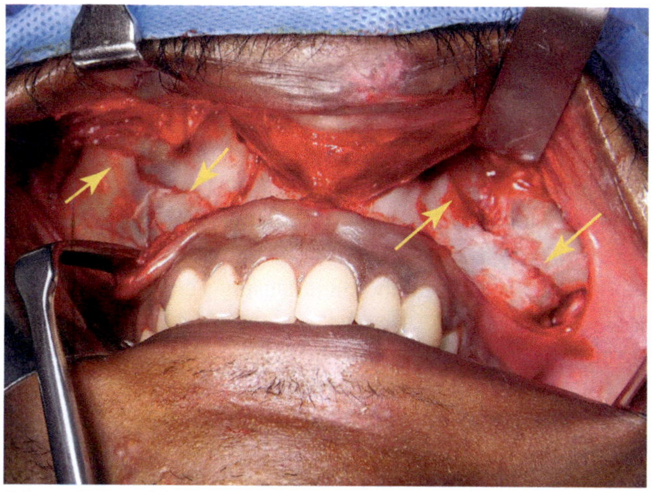

Fig. 55.16 Maxillary vestibular incision with adequate gingival cuff. Yellow arrows denoted the Le Fort I fracture lines

Clinical Tips for approaching the Le Fort fracture via maxillary vestibular incision

- The use of liquid paraffin will minimize trauma to the lips and corners of the mouth especially in patients with a small oral aperture.
- It is important to place a high vestibular incision to ensure a wide gingival cuff of tissue which will aid in closure of the incision.
- "Counter" elevation of the gingival cuff would aid in closure and also expose the root prominences, and this would be helpful during adaptation of the mini-plates and the subsequent screw fixation.
- It is also recommended that the opening of the Stenson's duct be identified so that injury to this structure is avoided when the buccal sulcus is stretched while making the incision.
- Some surgeons mark the midline to ensure proper reapproximation of the tissues during closure. This is important in cases where one is forced to use an oral endotracheal tube exiting from one corner of the mouth which may distort the oral tissues.
- Extension of the posterior end of the incision beyond the first molars may cause buccal fat herniation into the surgical site. This is of minimal concern but can be annoying to the surgeon during plate fixation.
- Sharp elevation of the superior flap will ensure a subperiosteal plane of dissection, but this may not always be possible due to adherent tissue at the fracture sites and the presence of bony fragments in comminuted fractures. As far as possible, sizable fragments of loose bone with soft tissue attachments should be retained to avoid large gaps at the fracture site which might delay healing. Even completely denuded bone can be replaced as free autogenous grafts and fixed in place with tissue glue or fine stainless steel wires.
- As the superior dissection proceeds, care should be taken to identify and protect the infraorbital nerve which may be involved in the fracture. It is also prudent to palpate the infraorbital margin to ensure that inadvertent entry into the orbit is avoided especially when comminution of the infraorbital rim and floor is present.
- Once the flap has been adequately raised, long Langenbeck retractors placed superiorly and cheek retractors at the corners of the mouth will ensure good surgical exposure and adequate lighting and thus aid in reduction and fixation of the fracture (Fig. 55.17).
- A variation which can be done is giving two separate vestibular incisions bilaterally without incising the midline frenal attachment. This variation will not disturb the mid line lip anatomy in cases where exposure of the anterior nasal spine region is not required.

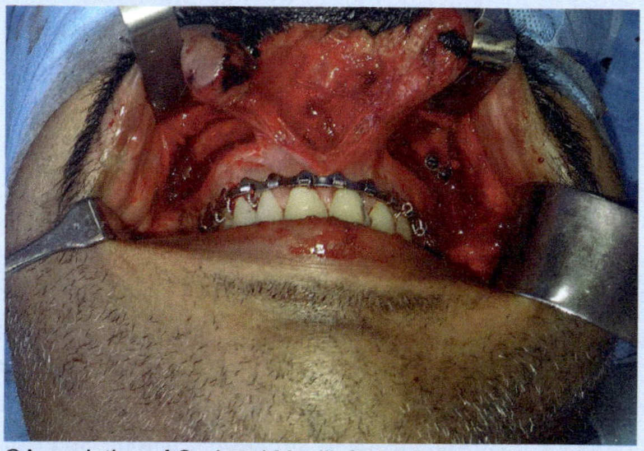

Fig. 55.17 A clinical situation where the separate vestibular maxillary incisions were given to approach anterior maxilla, due to deep through and through lip laceration upper lip extending down to the frenum region

Early intervention (7–10 days) with open reduction and fixation is the treatment of choice for maxillary Le Fort I fractures. Restoration of normal facial contour and occlusion is considered as optimal outcome of treatment. Bone reconstruction should be completed as early as possible to minimize shrinkage, stiffness and scarring of soft tissues [12].

In complex panfacial fracture management, many authors have stressed the importance of managing the Le-Fort fracture while reconstituting the facial architecture [13, 14].

55.5.5 Fixation of Le Fort I

Adequate fixation of the fractured bone depends on two factors, namely, the rigidity of the plate and the friction between the bone fragments (buttressing of the bony segments). When a gap exists between the bone ends, the latter factor is missing. In these cases, non/fibrous union can result if the masticatory forces are greater than the rigidity of the plate. As a general principle, the paranasal and zygomatic buttresses must be rigidly fixed. The plates should be well adapted especially where the bone stock is poor. At least two screws must be present on either side of the fracture and more the number of screws, better the, load sharing, between the plate and the subjacent bone. Opposed to this is when there is no bone buttressing and the plate has to be 'load bearing'. Also a minimum of two threads of the screw should engage the cortical bone. This may be a problem in thin areas as the anterior wall of the maxillary sinus and the alveolus where roots are present. In the edentulous maxilla, the bone quality is often compromised, and the lower end of the plate may need to be placed on the alveolus. This may necessitate removal of the plate prior to prosthodontic rehabilitation.

Obtaining rigid fixation becomes difficult when the buttresses are comminuted. If only one buttress is amenable for plating the reduction at this fracture interface along with reconstitution of the occlusion must be used as the template for repositioning the maxilla. When all the buttresses are comminuted, the surgeon has to "eye ball" the maxilla into the reduced position. In these situations, a long-span plate extending from the body of the zygomatic bone to the relatively thick bone in the area of the anterior nasal spine with or without a bone graft is often the only option available to maintain the vertical position of the floating maxilla. It has been stated that the lip-tooth relationship is helpful in deciding the position of the reduced maxilla, but in practice this is of limited use.

Loss of bone at the buttresses may require the use of primary bone grafts [10]. Though it has been suggested that a gap of more than 5 mm at the buttresses requires a graft, rigid plate fixation followed by MMF is often enough to ensure bony healing.

In essence the decision to graft will depend on:

1. The extend of the bony gap
2. The quality of the bone available for plate fixation
3. The rigidity of the fixation
4. Use of post-operative MMF
5. Loss of a large part of the anterior wall of the maxillary sinus (Fig. 55.18) (causing the overlying soft tissue to fall into the sinus causing a contour defect)

Primary bone grafting can be done using iliac bone (Fig. 55.26), split calvarium or split ribs. The calvarium is the preferred source because of the following reasons:

1. Large amount of graft available
2. Proximity to the operative field
3. Minimal donor site morbidity

The disadvantage is that these grafts are brittle and cannot be contoured. The bone graft has to be mortised to fit the defect and must be fixed rigidly to the plate or lag screwed.

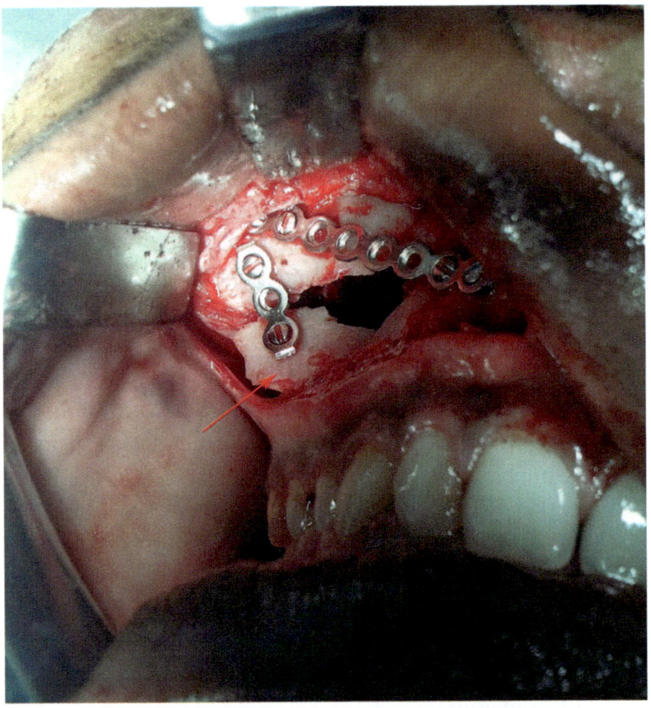

Fig. 55.18 A clinical situation where the defect in the anterior wall maxilla due to comminution of the wall was partly covered by fixing the free segment (red arrow). The long-span plate from the buttress to the anterior maxilla region can also be seen

Incisions for open reduction can be placed from first molar to first molar regions through a vestibular approach for wide exposure of the fracture sites. Rowe's disimpaction forceps and/or Hayton-Williams forceps can be used for mobilizing and reducing the fracture into position. The impacted type of Le Fort I fracture manipulation has to be done by grasping the maxilla with two pairs of Rowe's disimpaction forceps. Osteotomizing the maxilla should be considered if there is significant interval between the time of trauma and surgery. Whenever possible a passive reduction of the maxilla with condyles firmly seated in their correct position should be ensured to avoid post-operative anterior open bite (Figs. 55.19, 55.20, and 55.21).

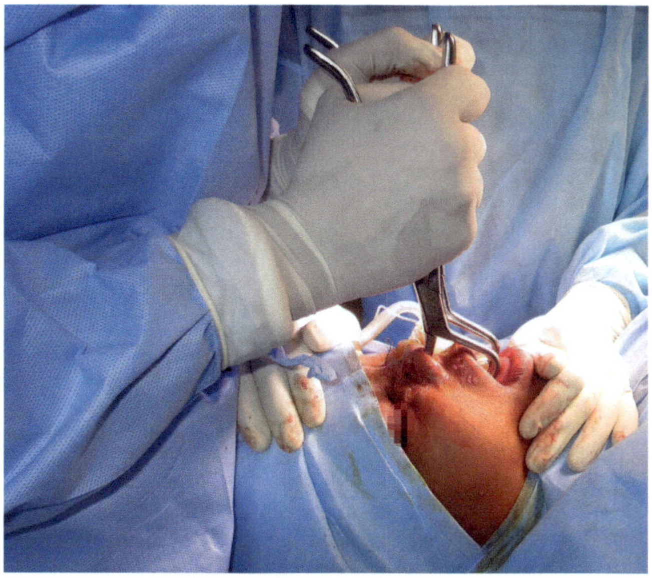

Fig. 55.19 The surgeon stands behind the patient and applies the disimpaction force, while the head is stabilized by the assistant surgeon

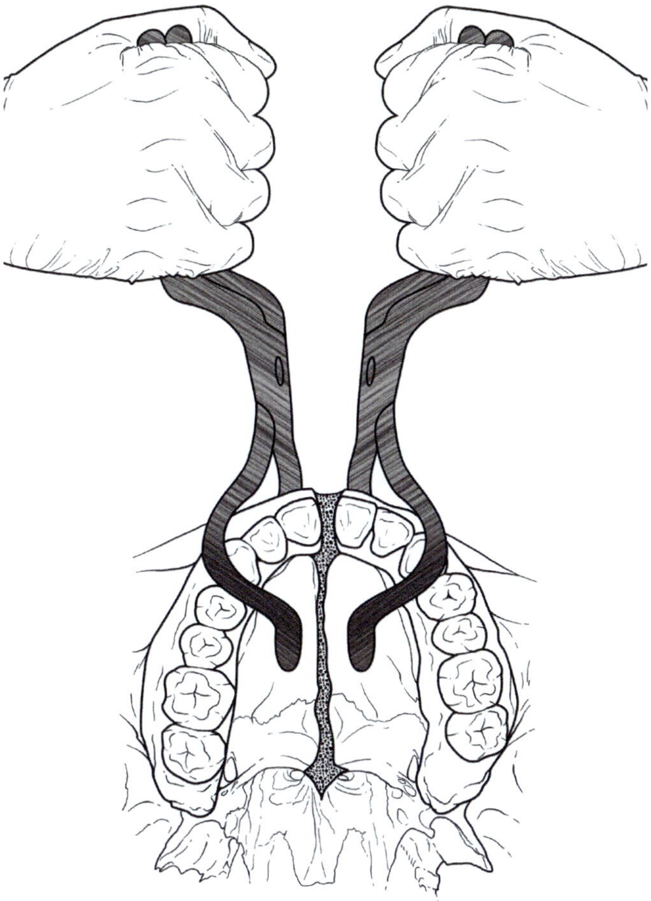

Fig. 55.20 Use of Rowe's disimpaction forceps

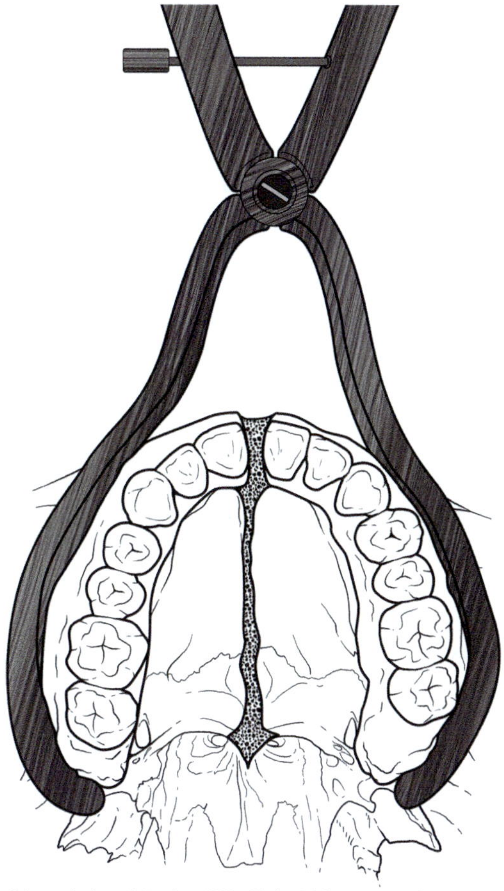

Fig. 55.21 Use of Hayton-Williams forceps

Use of Rowe's disimpaction forceps	Rowe's disimpaction forceps are available as paired (right and left) instruments
	Each instrument has two blades, one for engaging the palate (to be padded before use to avoid injury to the palatal mucosa) and one to be inserted through the nostril
	The instrument has an outward bend at the handle which aids in the use of two forceps simultaneously
	After engaging the forceps, the maxilla has to be moved in all planes to ensure adequate mobilisation

Use of Hayton-Williams forceps	The Hayton-Williams forceps is used to hold the fractured maxilla together
	The instrument is inserted after vestibular incision and is engaged at the pterygoid region
	This is the instrument of choice especially in cases with palatal bone fracture

After reduction the maxilla should be placed into maxillomandibular fixation. The fixation of the fracture sites (four-point fixation) is done at the vertical pillars of nasomaxillary and zygomaticomaxillary (lateral piriform rim and zygomatic buttress regions) for which the preferred plates and screws used are 1.5-mm thickness with 6-mm long screws. In the zygomatic buttress regions, 2.0-mm profile plates also can be used. The mini-plates are fixed as close as possible to the lateral pyriform rim as the bone is thickest there. Usually stabilization of the fracture is achievable even if any three of the four buttresses are fixed. Apparently, gross communition at one of the buttress regions will not cause a significant risk of inadequate stabilization. The associated anterior wall of the maxillary sinuses is generally not fixed due to the relative thin nature of bone in this region. The larger free bone fragments can be repositioned and immobilized using wires or be used for reconstruction of orbital floor defects. The circumvestibular incision is closed with running resorbable sutures after ensuring that the midline of upper lip coincides with the facial midline (Fig. 55.22).

Maxillomandibular fixation of up to 6 weeks also can be considered as alternative for treatment though the results may be less satisfactory with added morbidity to the recovering patient. The readers are advised to refer chapter 50 to read about closed reduction / wiring and intermaxillary fixation techniques.

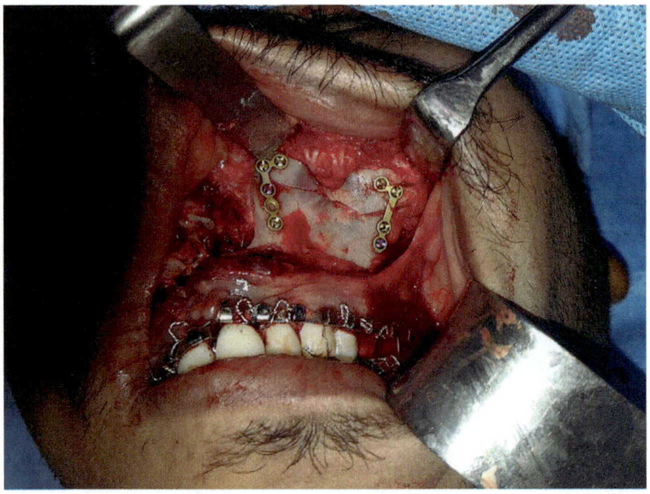

Fig. 55.22 The zygomatic buttress and paranasal buttress fixed in a classical Le Fort I fracture maxilla

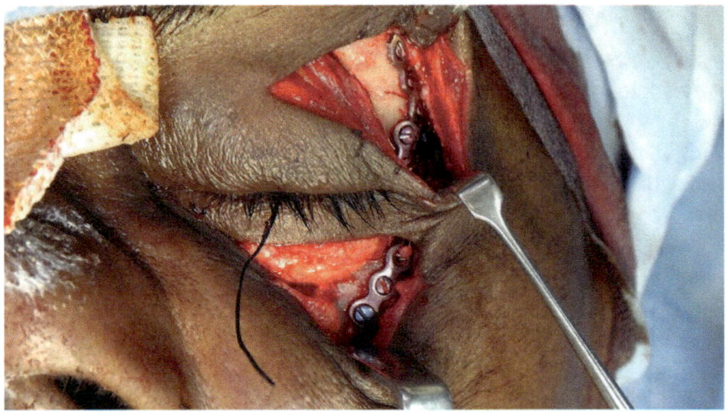

Fig. 55.23 Le Fort II fracture lines at the infraorbital rim area may have to be accessed directly, if required, especially with associated zygomatic/orbit fractures. In this case the lateral orbital rim reconstruction is done via combined access from left sub ciliary incision and left supra tarsal incision

55.5.6 Fixation of Le Fort II Fractures

The pyramidal fracture has the apex of the fracture located at the nasofrontal suture region or at the midnasal bone level. The Le Fort II fractures are ideally fixed at the frontonasal suture region, bilateral infraorbital rims and also both zygomaticomaxillary buttresses. However in majority of the clinical situations fixation at the infra orbital rims and the zygomatic buttress regions gives reasonably good results. Most Nasal bone fractures associated with Le Fort II fractures can be adequately managed by closed reduction techniques. This may require the anaesthetist to change nasal intubation to oral intubation. A submental intubation may also be considered at the beginning of the procedure. If the nasofrontal segment is unstable, fixation of the area can be done through various approaches (existing laceration, Gull wing approach, etc.). A maxillary vestibular incision can frequently provide access to infraorbital fracture alignment and fixation in some cases. The lower eyelid approaches are not always mandatory for fixation unless simultaneous exploration and reconstruction of orbital floors are also planned.

In Le Fort II fractures that are complicated by an associated palatal fracture, surgical splints may be helpful in obtaining adequate reduction. Placement of maxilla mandibular fixation will ensure accurate alignment of midface structures (Fig. 55.23).

55.5.7 Fixation of Le Fort III Fractures

These are complex fractures which rarely occur in isolation and results in a dysjunction of the facial skeleton from the base of the cranium. The ideal repair time should be within 10–14 days following the injury but may get delayed due to neurosurgical issues and other comorbidities.

Incision design for Le Fort III fractures should facilitate adequate access for reduction as well as fixation of the naso-frontal, frontozygomatc and in some cases the zygomatic arches. Using existing lacerations for access avoids need of a coronal incision, as this allows for complete visualization, reduction and fixation of the frontal area and zygomatic arches. A lateral brow or upper blepharoplasty (supra-tarsal fold) incision may be used to approach the lateral orbital rims. Also in such cases, a thicker plate (2.0) placement at the lateral orbital rim may be beneficial. A coronal approach may have to be considered if bilateral fronto-zygomatic and nasofrontal fracture fixation is planned.

The occlusion is a reliable indicator of adequate reduction in cases where direct visualization of the fractured segment is not possible.

In Le Fort III fractures associated with other fractures (open facial/condyle fractures), various surgical sequences can be followed, which is discussed in chapter 60 on Panfacial fractures.

Rarely, Le Fort fractures may present without mobility, but show occlusal disturbances like crossbite, open bite or loss of intercuspation. These can be managed by using traction elastics but at times warrant mobilization and subsequent rigid fixation [15].

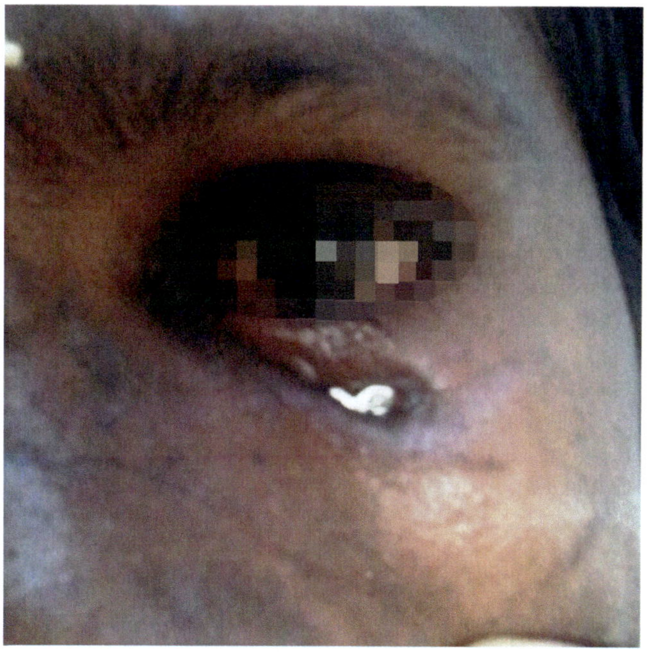

Fig. 55.24 Infraorbital plate exposure

55.6 Complications of Le Fort Fractures (Table 55.6)

General	Le Fort I	Le Fort II	Le Fort III
• Bleeding • Enopthalmous • Infection • Altered vision • Non-union • Mal-union • malocclusion • Epiphora (due to obstruction of nasolacrimal duct) • Scarring • Sinusitis • Exposed hardware (Fig. 55.24) • Foreign body reactions	Maxillry hypoperfusion • Wound dehiscence Necrotic teeth	• CSF leak (rhinorrhea and /or otorrhea) • Palatal fistula • Nasal Septal deviation • Infra orbital paraesthesia	• CSF leak (rhinorrhea and /or otorrhea) • Facial Nerve paralysis • Trigemminal nerve injury

Table 55.6 Complications of Le Fort fractures

55.7 Palatal Fractures

Unlike many other areas of the midface, the palatal bone is relatively thick, and hence palatal fractures are not common. A palatal split makes reduction and fixation of maxillary fractures more difficult mainly due to the transverse instability which can cause medial collapse or outward splaying of the maxilla. The use of the Hayton-Williams forceps along with the disimpaction forceps will control outward splaying of the maxilla but at the risk of medially displacement of the dentate segment of the maxilla. Moreover, the use of all the three forceps effectively requires some amount of surgical expertise.

Moss et al. [16] have proposed a classification for palatal fractures. There is no consensus regarding the management of palatal fractures, but various options have been suggested.

1. Transpalatal wires in the first molar region.
2. Direct exposure of the fracture through an existing palatal laceration or an incision and rigid plate fixation.
3. External fixation by fixing a screw on either side of the fracture and immobilization with a wire connecting the screws. Alternatively a palatal splint can be fabricated after sectioning a plaster model of the palate.
4. Plating the labial fracture line.
5. Plating the nasal floor.

Transpalatal wires are simple to apply and do not have the problems of soft tissue dehiscence and infection seen in the more invasive methods [17]. However, the reduction of the palatal fracture cannot be ensured, and the wires can be cumbersome to the patient as it affects speech and swallowing. If the palatal wires are passed through an infant feeding tube or a small gauge urinary catheter, injury to the dorsum of the tongue can be minimized. It is also noticed that palatal wires tend to become slack after a few days, and then their value in reduction and fixation of the fracture is questionable. Moreover, these wires are not an option in the edentulous maxilla.

Direct exposure and plate fixation are surgically demanding, but the fracture can be reduced and fixed under direct vision. Ceinfuegos et al. have described the technique of fixing the plate over the palatal mucosa, but this plate would have to be removed at a later date [18]. An alternative would be to use a resorbable plate and screws.

Ma et al. has documented the use of self-drilling screws on either side of the palatal fracture with wires to fix the fracture [19].

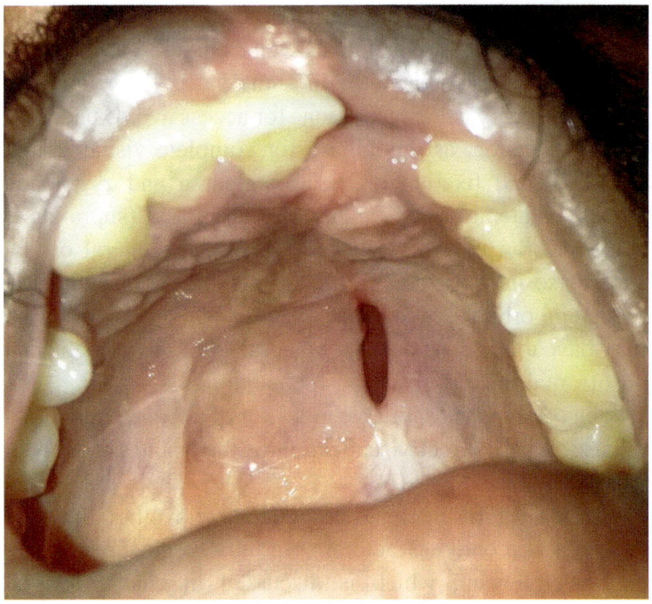

Fig. 55.25 Oronasal fistula in a patient who had sustained palate fracture

Palatal fractures of the sagittal or parasagittal variety can be stabilized by placing a mini-plate across the fracture line on the labial side. Occasionally the prominence of the anterior nasal spine has to be reduced to facilitate mini-plate placement.

The transpalatal reduction should be supplemented by fixation at the zygomaticomaxillary and nasomaxillary buttresses and the use of an arch bar [20].

Palatal fractures accompanied by soft tissue lacerations often cause a serious challenge to the surgeon regarding its management. The healing of the palatal soft tissue laceration is dependent on the exact reduction of the palatal vault and stabilization. Overzealous attempts at closure of the laceration without accurate reduction may compromise wound healing. A tension-free closure of the palatal mucosa is imperative for wound healing. In some cases, the ensuing oronasal communication will have to addressed secondarily (Fig. 55.25).

55.7.1 Surgical Splints

Concomitant fractures of the palate present additional challenges to the treatment of Le Fort fractures. They complicate the re-establishment of proper width and height of the maxilla. Depending on the fracture type, patient comorbidities and associated injuries, either closed reduction and wiring or rigid fixation may have to be performed. Dental impressions can be obtained and occlusion assessed prior to surgery.

Fabrication of an acrylic splint may help in re-establishing the transverse width of the palate.

In cases of gross comminution with partial dentition, palatal splints are helpful. Splints are fabricated on casts on which model surgery has been performed. They are designed such that they cover the occlusal surfaces and heights of contour, and care should be taken as to not disturb the soft tissues. Holes placed in the occlusal surfaces in the splint aid in separately ligating it to the arch bar [21]. In case of edentulous patients, Gunning splints are usually used.

55.8 Special Considerations

55.8.1 Maxillary Fractures in Geriatric Patients

Advanced age and compromised medical fitness may increase the morbidity associated with surgical management of maxillary fractures. Loss of teeth leading to reduced alveolar bone, reduced vascularity of maxilla and greater pneumatisation of the maxillary sinuses, should be taken into consideration before attempting an open reduction and internal fixation. Modification of existing dentures or Gunning splints are viable options in this population.

55.8.2 Maxillary Fractures in Children

The long-term effects of maxillary fractures on skeletal growth are inconclusive at present. Mobile-displaced maxillary fractures in paediatric patients warrant open reduction and fixation. Removal of hardware in growing patients may be considered to overcome complications of plate translocation (shifting of the position of metal plate due to appositional bone growth), extrusion and possible growth restriction. Resorbable plating systems may offer a solution to overcome such complications.

55.8.3 Haemorrhage Control in Maxillary Fractures

Branches of the internal maxillary artery provide much of the vascular supply to the midface. In patients with epistaxis or bleeding, ligation of this artery may be necessary. Due to anastomoses from other branches of the internal and external carotid circulation, vascular insufficiency of the maxilla is unlikely even after ligature of maxillary artery. In certain conditions of intractable bleeding not amenable to control by normal packing methods, embolization methods have been used effectively.

55.9 Recent Advances

The use of pre-surgical stereolithographic models helps in plate contouring and precise positioning of fractured segments. Facilitation of the intraoperative three-dimensional bone positioning is possible due to development of sophisticated computed tomography, computer graphics hardware and image processing software capable of reproducing anatomic templates. Automated preoperative "mirroring" of the contralateral uninjured orbito-zygomaticomaxillary complex to the affected side can result in improved results. The use of intraoperative surgical navigation systems along with mobile cone beam CT improves intraoperative quality control. Endoscopic midface fracture management facilitates smaller incisions, reduced recovery time and minimal post-operative complications. These developments are discussed in the Chap. 41.

55.10 Conclusion

Maxillary fractures can sometimes occur with significant cosmetic and functional implications. Accurate diagnosis and early surgical intervention is essential for successful management of these fractures. The surgeon should keep in mind that the surgical management of maxillary fractures primarily aims at restoration of the vertical and horizontal support buttresses.

55.11 Case Scenario - A case of maxillary Lefort I fracture where bone grafting was done (Fig. 55.26a–g)

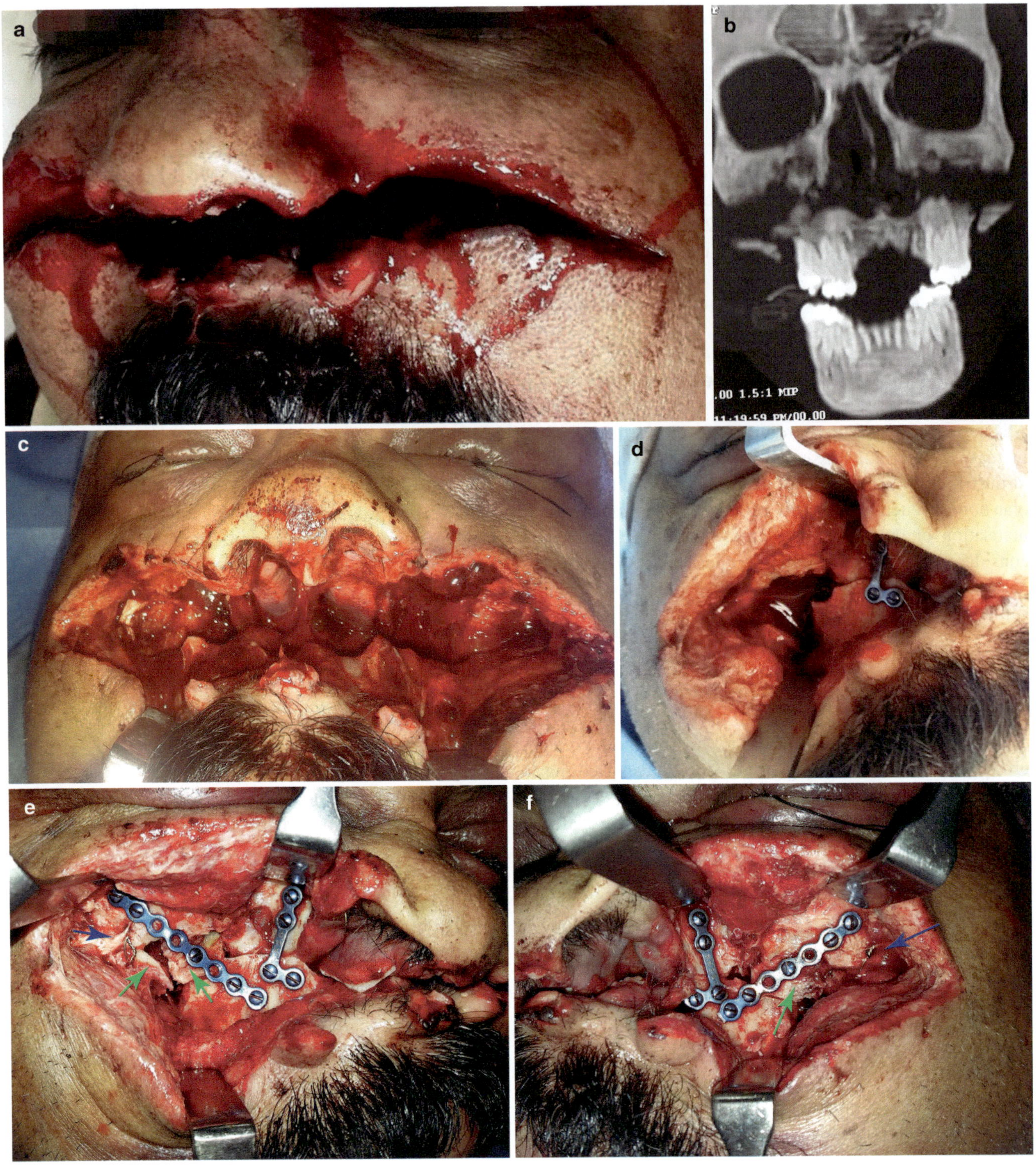

Fig. 55.26 Case scenario (fracture maxilla fixation done with grafting in the anterior maxillary sinus wall). (**a**) 43-year-old man sustained bone deep laceration on face causing Le Fort I like fracture pattern. In the emergency department, oral intubation was required due to heavy bleeding. Nasal packs were placed, and the wound was primarily tacked as adjunct measures. (**b**) MIP view of CT scan showing the maxillary segment displaced downwards will loss of anterior maxillary wall height. (**c**) Intraoperative view showing the severely displaced maxillary segment. Access for the fixation was via the existing laceration. A maxillary vestibular incision was not placed. (**d**) The paranasal buttress was maintained, but loss of bone structure seen at the anterior wall sinus region. To attain primary healing and to avoid malunion, iliac crest bone grafts were procured and split into separate pieces. (**e**) (Right side maxilla) the green arrows point to the graft segments. Initially the graft segment was fixed with wire (blue arrow) and was attached to the titanium plate with screws (the plate was spanned from the zygomatic body to the displaced main fracture segment). (**f**) Similar technique done on left side. (**g**) Immediate post-operative view after closure of the laceration. Patient had arch bars fixed and underwent a period of intermaxillary fixation to help in primary union. Post-operative review showed good stability for maxilla and the occlusion was maintained

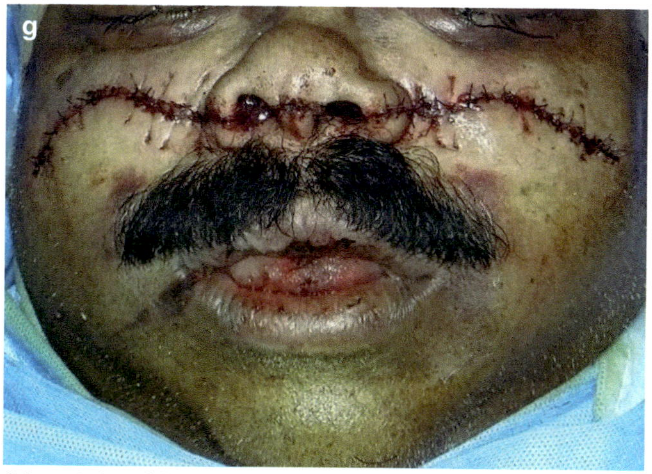

©Association of Oral and Maxillofacial Surgeons of India

Fig. 55.26 (continued)

References

1. Marciani RD. Management of midface fractures: fifty years later. J Oral Maxillofac Surg. 1993;51(9):960–8. Review
2. Rowe and Williams' maxillofacial injuries (ed 2): Williams JL (ed), with 51 contributors, New York: Churchill Livingstone; 1994, 1067 pages (2 volumes), illustrated. J Oral Maxillofac Surg. 1996;54(3):378.
3. Cunningham LL, Haug RH. Management of maxillary fractures. In: Miloro M, Ghali GE, Larson P, Waite P, editors. Peterson's principles of oral and maxillofacial surgery. BC Decker; 2004. chapter 23.1, p. 434–8.
4. Gruss JS, Mackinnon SE. Complex maxillary fractures: role of buttress reconstruction and immediate bone grafts. Plast Reconstr Surg. 1986;78(1):9–22.
5. Louis M, Agrawal N, Kaufman M, Truong TA. Midface fractures I. Semin Plast Surg. 2017;31(2):85–93.
6. Manson PN, Hoopes JE, Su CT. Structural pillars of the facial skeleton: an approach to the management of Le Fort fractures. Plast Reconstr Surg. 1980;66:54–62.
7. Hendrickson M, Clark N, Manson PN, Yaremchuk M, Robertson B, Slezak S, Crawley W, Vander KC. Palatal fractures: classification, patterns, and treatment with rigid internal fixation. Plast Reconstr Surg. 1998;101(2):319–32.
8. Bowley NB, Brown J. Radiology for maxillofacial trauma. In Booth PW, Schendel SA, Hausamen J-E, editors. Maxillofacial surgery. Churchill Livingstone Elsevier; 2007. p. 278–9.
9. Manson PN, Markowitz B, Mirvis S, Dunham M, Yaremchuk M. Toward CT-based facial fracture treatment. Plast Reconstr Surg. 1990;85(2):202–12. Discussion 213–4
10. Gruss JS, Mackinnon SE. Complex maxillary fractures: role of buttress reconstruction and immediate bone grafts. Plast Reconstr Surg. 1986;78(1):9–22.
11. Nastri AL, Gurney B. Current concepts in midface fracture management. Curr Opin Otolaryngol Head Neck Surg. 2016;24(4):368–75.
12. Marciani RD, Gonty AA. Principles of management of complex craniofacial trauma. J Oral Maxillofac Surg. 1993;51(5):535–42.
13. Kelly KJ, Manson PN, Vander Kolk CA, Markowitz BL, Dunham CM, Rumley TO, Crawley WA. Sequencing Le Fort fracture treatment (Organization of treatment for a panfacial fracture). J Craniofac Surg. 1990;1(4):168–78.
14. Markowitz BL, Manson PN. Panfacial fractures: organization of treatment. Clin Plast Surg. 1989;16(1):105–14.
15. Romano JJ, Manson PN, Mirvis SE, Dunham M, Crawley W. Le Fort fractures without mobility. Plast Reconstr Surg. 1990;85(3):355–62.
16. Moss WJ, Kedarisetty S, Jafari A, Schaerer DE, Husseman JW. A review of hard palate fracture repair techniques. J Oral Maxillofac Surg. 2016;74(2):328–36. Review
17. Chen CH, Wang TY, Tsay PK, Lai JB, Chen CT, Liao HT, Lin CH, Chen YR. A 162-case review of palatal fracture: management strategy from a 10-year experience. Plast Reconstr Surg. 2008;121(6):2065–73.
18. Cienfuegos R, Sierra E, Ortiz B, Fernández G. Treatment of palatal fractures by osteosynthesis with 2.0-mm locking plates as external fixator. Craniomaxillofac Trauma Reconstr. 2010;3(4):223–30.
19. Ma D, Guo X, Yao H, Chen J. Transpalatal screw traction: a simple technique for the management of sagittal fractures of the maxilla and palate. Int J Oral Maxillofac Surg. 2014;43(12):1465–7.
20. Manson PN, Glassman D, Vanderkolk C, Petty P, Crawley WA. Rigid stabilization of sagittal fractures of the maxilla and palate. Plast Reconstr Surg. 1990;85(5):711–7.
21. Cohen SR, Leonard DK, Markowitz BL, Manson PN. Acrylic splints for dental alignment in complex facial injuries. Ann Plast Surg. 1993;31(5):406–12.

Fractures of the Zygomaticomaxillary Complex

56

Elavenil Panneerselvam, Poornima Ravi, and B. Sasikala

56.1 Introduction

The zygomaticomaxillary complex (ZMC) refers to the skeletal unit [1] formed by the zygomatic bone and maxilla (Fig. 56.1). These two bones are referred to as a complex, because of the structural and functional relationship between them; they articulate with each other over a wider area, and any traumatic impact on one bone generally influences the other. This duo complex also constitutes a major part of the orbit, spanning the infra-orbital rim, lateral wall, and floor. Hence the ZMC is also termed *orbitozygomaticomaxillary complex* [2]. Because of its multiple articulations, various names are commonly used to describe ZMC fractures such as "tripod, tetrapod, or pentapod" [3, 4] fractures.

Fractures of the ZMC commonly result in severe cosmetic and functional deficits because of the prominent anatomical position of the zygoma and its proximity to adjacent vital structures such as the globe. Precise reduction and fixation of these fractures is challenging due to their complex anatomic form, multiple articulations, and deformation in multiple planes. The scope of this chapter encompasses the biodynamics of ZMC fractures, clinical implications, and guidelines for successful management.

Disclosure: Authors have no financial conflicts to disclose.

Electronic Supplementary Material The online version of this chapter (https://doi.org/10.1007/978-981-15-1346-6_56) contains supplementary material, which is available to authorized users.

E. Panneerselvam (✉)
Department of Oral and Maxillofacial Surgery, SRM Dental College, Ramapuram, Chennai, Tamil Nadu, India

Department of Orbit and Oculoplasty, Aravind Eye Hospital, Chennai, Tamil Nadu, India

P. Ravi · B. Sasikala
Department of Oral and Maxillofacial Surgery, SRM Dental College, Ramapuram, Chennai, Tamil Nadu, India

56.2 Surgical Anatomy

The term zygoma denotes a "yoke or bar," in Greek. Quite aptly, the zygoma extends as a prominent, sturdy bar across the face, contributing to its transverse width and anteroposterior projection. The clinical significance of this bony complex is attributed to its role in defining facial esthetics and globe function.

56.2.1 Articulations

The zygoma articulates with four bones [5]; superiorly frontal, medially maxilla, laterally temporal bone, and posteriorly sphenoid, through five processes [4] (Fig. 56.1), namely, the zygomaticotemporal (ZT), zygomaticomaxillary (ZM), infra-orbital (IOR), fronto-zygomatic (FZ), and sphenozygomatic (SZ) or zygomaticosphenoid (ZS). These processes are clinically significant in establishing the three-dimensional structural integrity of the upper lateral face.

Fractures of the ZMC have been traditionally called the "tripod or trimalar fractures" because it involved separation at the three processes of the zygoma—the FZ, IOR, and the ZM processes (Fig. 56.2a). The terminology was later modified to "quadripod or quadramalar fracture" to include separation at the fourth point of articulation, the ZT process (Fig. 56.2b). However, the importance of SZ articulation along the lateral wall of the orbit has been recognized lately, and, hence, ZMC fracture is currently called a pentapod fracture (Fig. 56.2c), to emphasize the necessity of restoring the five articulations during fracture management.

56.2.2 Relations

- Zygoma and orbit: ZMC forms the lateral and inferior part of the orbit, protecting as well as supporting the globe and associated soft tissues. The Whitnall's tubercle present on the zygoma (inferior to the FZ suture) provides

K. Bonanthaya et al. (eds.), *Oral and Maxillofacial Surgery for the Clinician*, https://doi.org/10.1007/978-981-15-1346-6_56

attachment to the suspensory ligament of Lockwood that maintains the horizontal axis of the globe [6] (Fig. 56.3a). A fracture line located above the Whitnall's tubercle leads to inferior displacement of zygoma as well as the lateral attachment of Lockwood ligament resulting in anti-mongoloid slant to the eye (Fig. 56.3b). Thus ZMC fractures greatly influence the structure and function of the orbit. Further, the contents of the orbit including the globe, extraocular muscles, and orbital fat are intimately related to the zygoma and may be affected in fractures of the ZMC or its surgical manipulation.

- Zygoma and mandible: The zygoma and zygomatic arch are anatomically close to the coronoid process of the mandible. Therefore, a fractured zygoma or arch, when retro/medially positioned, may impede mandibular movements [7]. A displaced and untreated fracture of zygoma/arch which is in close proximity to the coronoid process can result in extra-articular ankylosis [8].
- Zygoma and maxillary sinus: Fractures of the ZMC (except the isolated zygomatic arch fractures) involve the maxillary sinus and show features of hemosinus [4] or sinusitis [3].

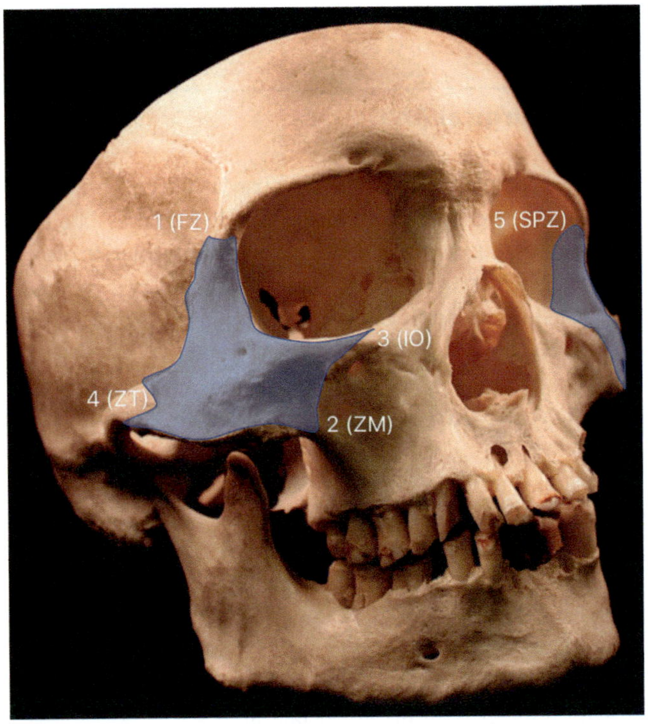

Fig. 56.1 ZMC skeletal unit. Articulations of zygoma with facial skeleton and articulating processes

56.2.3 Muscle and Fascia Attachments

The muscles attached to ZMC are the zygomaticus major, zygomaticus minor, orbicularis oculi, and masseter [9]. Masseter is attached to the zygomatic arch on the lateral and inferior aspect as well as the zygomatic tuberosity (Fig. 56.4a). The downward displacing forces of the masseter have been considered by many as the principal cause of post-reduction instability [10].

The temporal fascia attached to the arch superiorly plays a major role in resisting the downward displacement of fractured ZMC or arch due to the inferior pull of the masseter (Fig. 56.4b) [1].

56.2.4 Zygomatic Arch

The arch is the key parameter for re-establishing the sagittal projection as well as transverse width of the face [11]. An arch which is bent outward or inward gets shortened [4]. This leads to retrodisplacement of zygoma resulting in altered facial width (Fig. 56.5b). It is important to remember

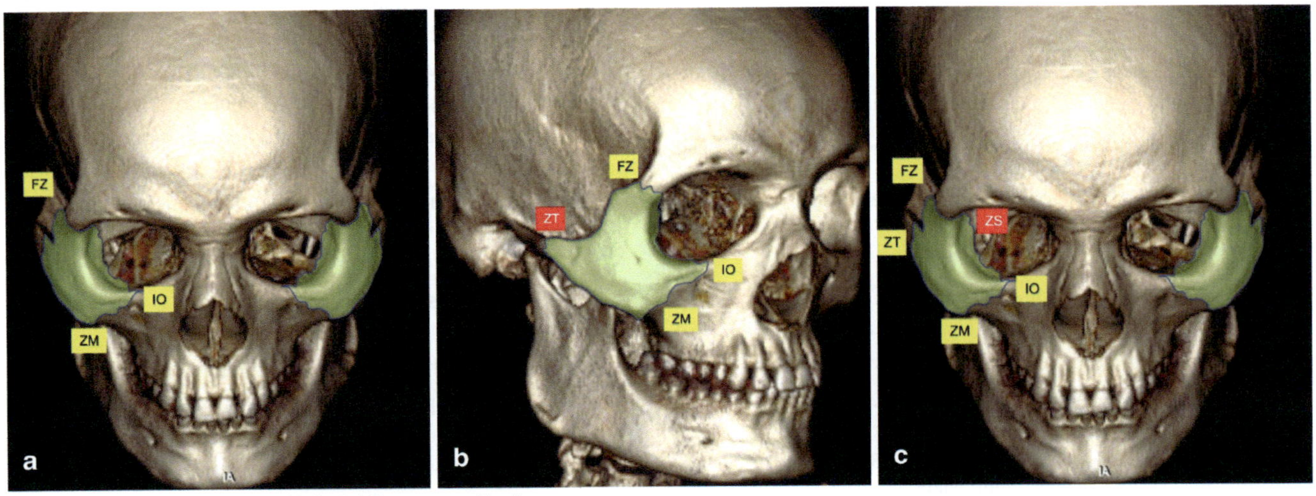

Fig. 56.2 Types of ZMC fractures. (**a**) Tripod fracture. (**b**) Tetrapod fracture. (**c**) Pentapod fracture

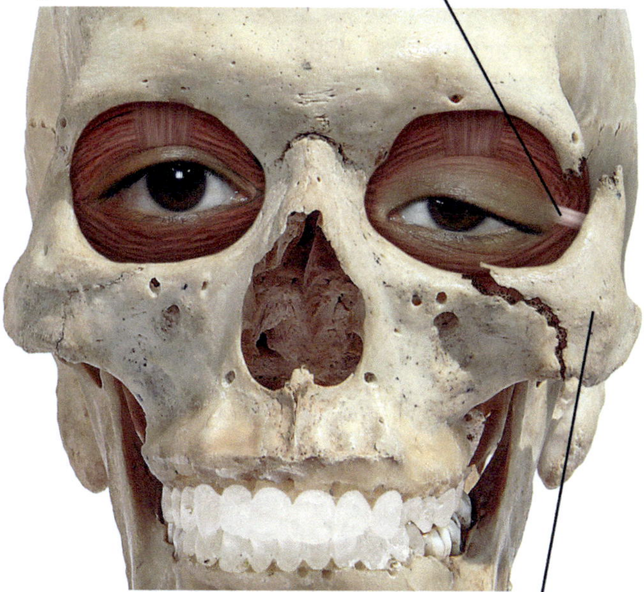

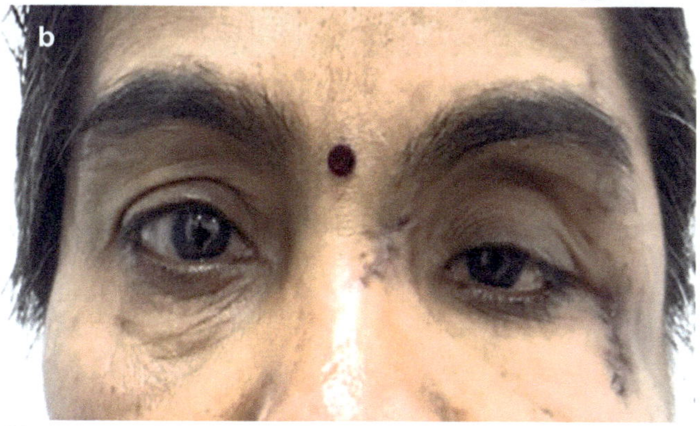

Fig. 56.3 Relation of suspensory ligament to zygoma. (**a**) Displacement of suspensory ligament of Lockwood leading to anti-mongoloid slant. (**b**) Clinical appearance of anti-mongoloid slant

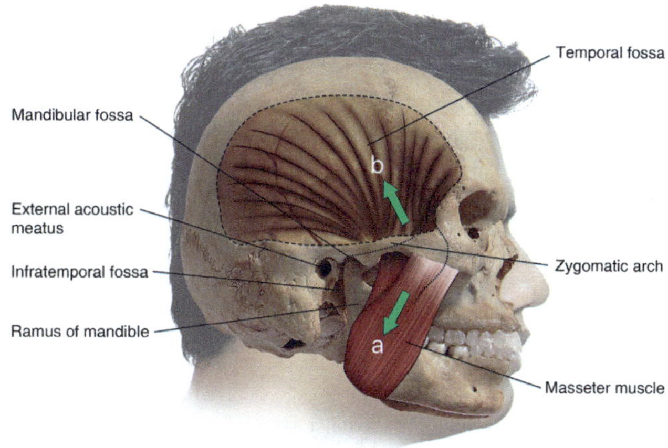

Fig. 56.4 Displacing forces acting on the zygoma and arch. (**a**) Masseter exerting downward force. (**b**) Temporalis with a superior vector

that in spite of being referred to as an arch, it does not have an exaggerated curvature. Therefore, overzealous contouring during reduction of zygomatic arch fractures can result in compromised esthetics. The arch is encased by a thick periosteal and fascial envelope which counteracts the displacing forces of the masseter [1]. However, when the periosteal envelope is damaged due to high-velocity injuries, the fracture segments show more displacement.

56.2.5 Nerves and Blood Vessels

The nerves in close proximity to the ZMC are (1) infraorbital nerve and (2) zygomatic nerve [12] (Fig. 56.6a). The infra-orbital nerve runs along the ION groove and enters the ION canal giving off the superior dental plexus of nerves before exiting through the ION foramen onto the face. Here it innervates the lower eyelid, lateral aspect of the nose, and upper lip of the ipsilateral side. The zygomatic nerve which enters the orbit through the inferior orbital fissure divides into two branches, the zygomatico-facial and zygomatico-temporal which emerge onto the face through their respective foramina. The zygomaticofacial nerve innervates the skin over the malar area, while the zygomaticotemporal nerve supplies the skin over the anterior temporal region. These nerves may be injured due to trauma or during surgery. The severity of paresthesia which arises is generally proportional to the degree of displacement of a fractured zygoma [13]. The other nerves whose function may be affected in ZMC fractures are the optic nerve [14] and facial nerve [15]. Blood vessels of importance related to the ZMC are infra-orbital artery and vein [16] (Fig. 56.6b) which accompany the infra-orbital nerve. Uncontrolled forces delivered during elevation of zygoma may injure these vessels resulting in severe intra-op bleeding.

56.3 Classification

56.3.1 Classification of ZMC Fractures

Numerous classifications have been proposed for ZMC fractures; this chapter would discuss the most practical ones which help in understanding the biodynamics of fracture as well as facilitate quick decision-making regarding the treatment.

- The classification proposed by Rowe and Williams [1] (Fig. 56.7) is based on the axis of rotation of ZMC and the

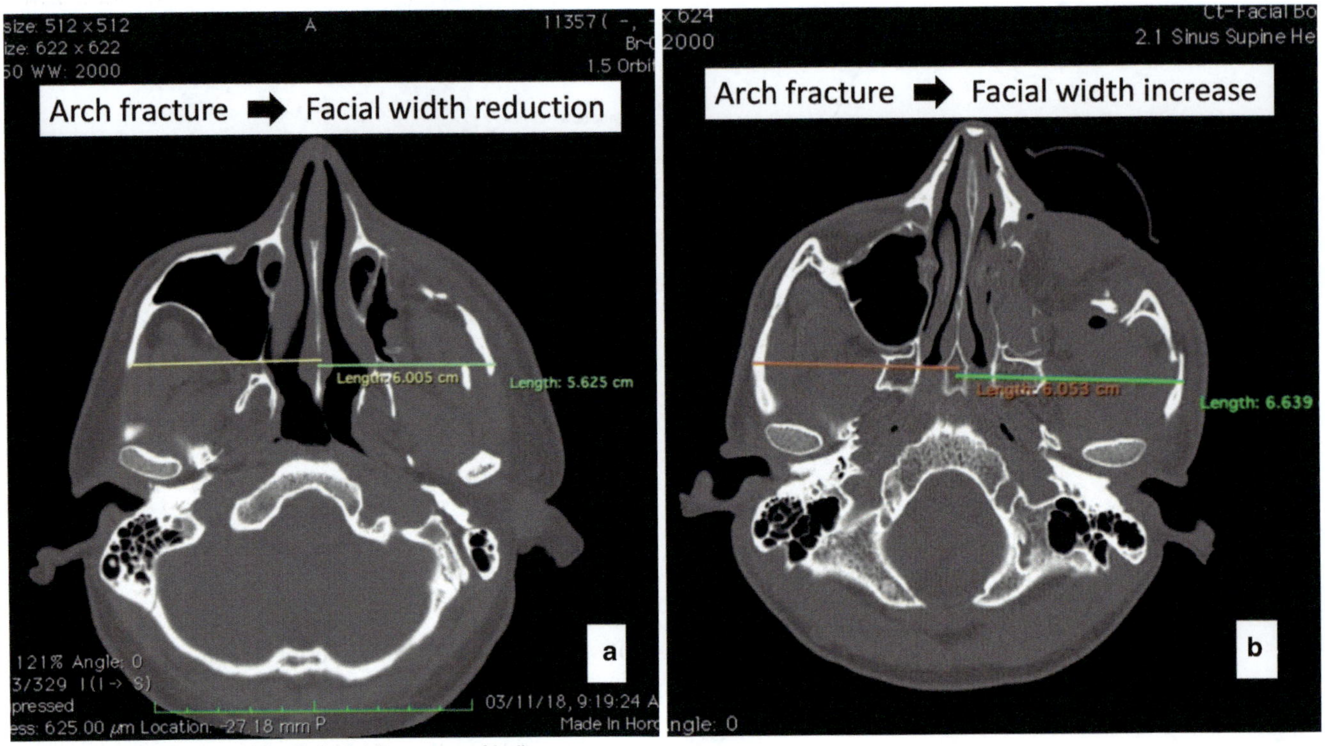

Fig. 56.5 Change in facial dimension in zygomatic arch fractures. (**a**) Inward bowing of arch. (**b**) Outward bowing of arch

stability after reduction. Following trauma, the zygoma may undergo rotation along two axes: vertical axis extending through the FZ suture and first molar and horizontal axis running across the infra-orbital foramen and zygomatic arch. According to this classification, fractures were considered as *stable after elevation* when they demonstrated (1) arch only fracture with medial displacement and (2) rotation around vertical axis (medially/laterally), while fractures were categorized as *unstable after reduction* when the following features were observed: (1) arch only fracture with inferior displacement (Fig. 56.8), (2) ZMC fracture rotated around horizontal axis (Fig. 56.7), (3) dislocated en bloc (inferiorly/laterally/medially) (Fig. 56.9a), and (4) comminuted (Fig. 56.9b).

This classification provides clinical guidance regarding the stability of fracture after reduction and the necessity for fixation.

- ZMC fractures have also been classified on the basis of "severity of traumatic impact" [4] into low-, medium-, and high-energy patterns, as demonstrated on CT; low-energy type is associated with non-displaced/minimally displaced "en bloc" fractures, medium-energy type is displaced fractures with or without fragmentation, and high-energy type is associated with fractures with massive displacement, comminution, or fragmentation.
- Zing et al.'s [17] classification (Fig. 56.10a–e) is a simple but practically useful method based on the anatomic site involved; type A1 refers to isolated zygomatic arch fracture, and types A2 and A3 are separation at the FZ suture and IOR, respectively. Type B is a complete monofragment type with separation at all five sites of articulation and type C which is multifragmented.

A special and rare variant of zygoma injuries includes ***avulsion*** of zygoma [18] (Fig. 56.11). These injuries result from tangentially directed forces with high velocity or greater energy. The fractured zygomatic fragment characteristically becomes a non-vascularized-free graft whose management is complex.

56.3.2 Classification of Arch Fractures

The fractures involving the zygomatic arch constitute a separate entity.

The various patterns of zygomatic arch fractures have been described by **Ozyazgan et al.** [19] (Fig. 56.12) based on the number of fracture lines and displacement of fracture fragments:

- Type 1 constitutes the isolated zygomatic arch fractures which are subdivided into (1) dual fracture (type I A) and (2) more than two fractures (type I B). This is further classified into V-shaped (type I B-V) and displaced fracture (type I B-D).
- Combined zygomatic arch fractures are referred to as type II, which can present as two variants: single (type II A)

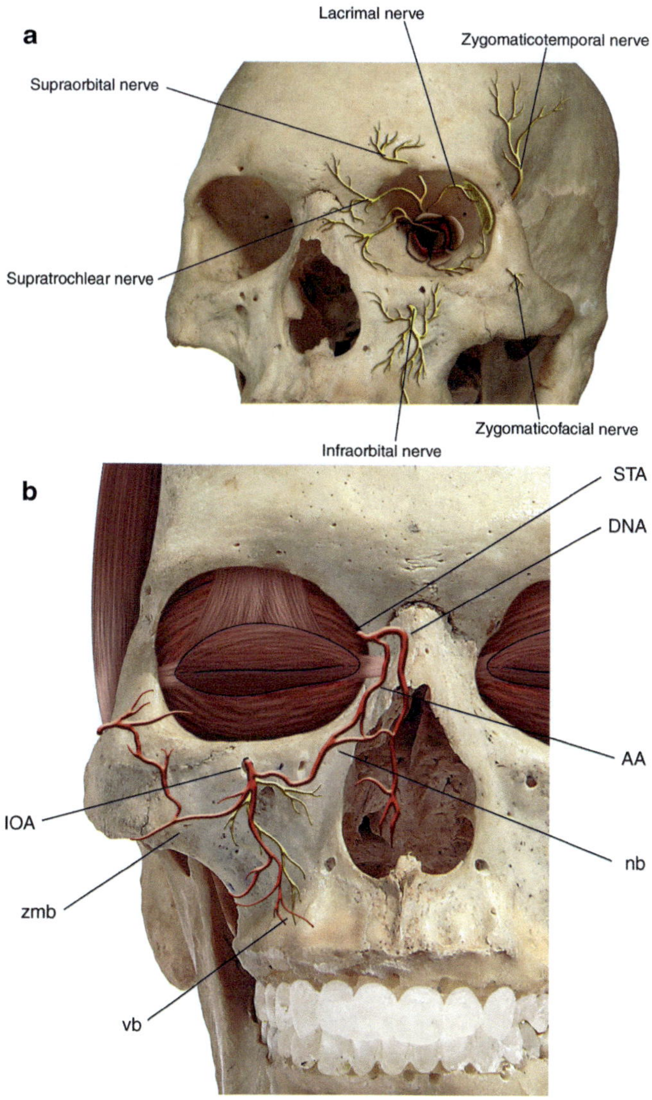

Fig. 56.6 **a**, **b** Neurovascular structures related to ZMC fractures. OA, ophthalmic artery; nb, nasal branch; zmb, zygomatico-malar branch; vb, vestibular branch

and plural fracture (type II B). Plural fractures are termed type II B-R when they are approximated or reduced and type II B-D, when displaced.

Yamamoto et al. classification [20] (Fig. 56.13) differentiates fractures based on displacement: type I, no displacement; type II, displacement with bone contact at all fracture lines; type III, displacement without bone contact at one fracture line; type IV, displacement without bone contact at two fracture lines; and type V, comminution or displacement without bone contact at three or more fracture lines. **Honig Merten et al**. [21] (H-M classification) (Fig. 56.14) classified zygomatic arch fractures based on CT findings as class I which indicated isolated tripod fracture, class II as an isolated stick fracture of the arch, and class III a combined fracture of the malar bone and the zygomatic arch.

56.4 Clinical Assessment

The clinical assessment of ZMC fractures is performed by a thorough examination of the face and the eye. As the zygoma forms an integral part of the orbit (floor and lateral wall), any trauma to the ZMC may have profound impact on the integrity of the globe and vision [2, 22]. This mandates a primary ophthalmic examination prior to facial examination.

56.4.1 Examination of the Eye

The globe is meticulously assessed for its form, position, and function. This is performed by a comprehensive examination protocol called "8-point eye exam" [23] provided by the American Academy of Ophthalmology (refer to Chap. 57).

56.4.2 Examination of the Face

The facial examination should focus on assessment of (1) facial symmetry and morphology and (2) functions such as mouth opening, vision, sensory perception, and occlusion.

The clinical characteristics of ZMC fractures [1, 4, 5] may be divided based on their cosmetic and functional implications (Box 56.1) .

Box 56.1: Clinical Features of ZMC Fractures

Cosmetic deficits	Functional deficits
• *Facial asymmetry due to* – Periorbital edema – Hematoma – Emphysema	• *Vision* – Diplopia – Loss of vision (partial/ total)
• *Facial asymmetry due to malpositioned zygoma* – Depression of malar prominence – Transverse facial widening – Changes in AP projection – Orbital dystopia	• *Restricted mouth opening* • *Malocclusion* • *Neurological deficit* – Paresthesia (i) Infra-orbital nerve (ii) Zygomaticofacial nerve (iii) Zygomaticotemporal nerve
• *Discoloration* – Subconjunctival hemorrhage – Periorbital ecchymosis	– Paresis/palsy (i) Facial nerve
• *Altered morphology/position of eye* – Anti-mongoloid slant – Increased scleral show – Hypoglobus/hyperglobus – Enophthalmos/ exophthalmos	• *Epistaxis/nasal congestion* • *Compartment syndromes* – SOF syndrome – Orbital apex syndrome

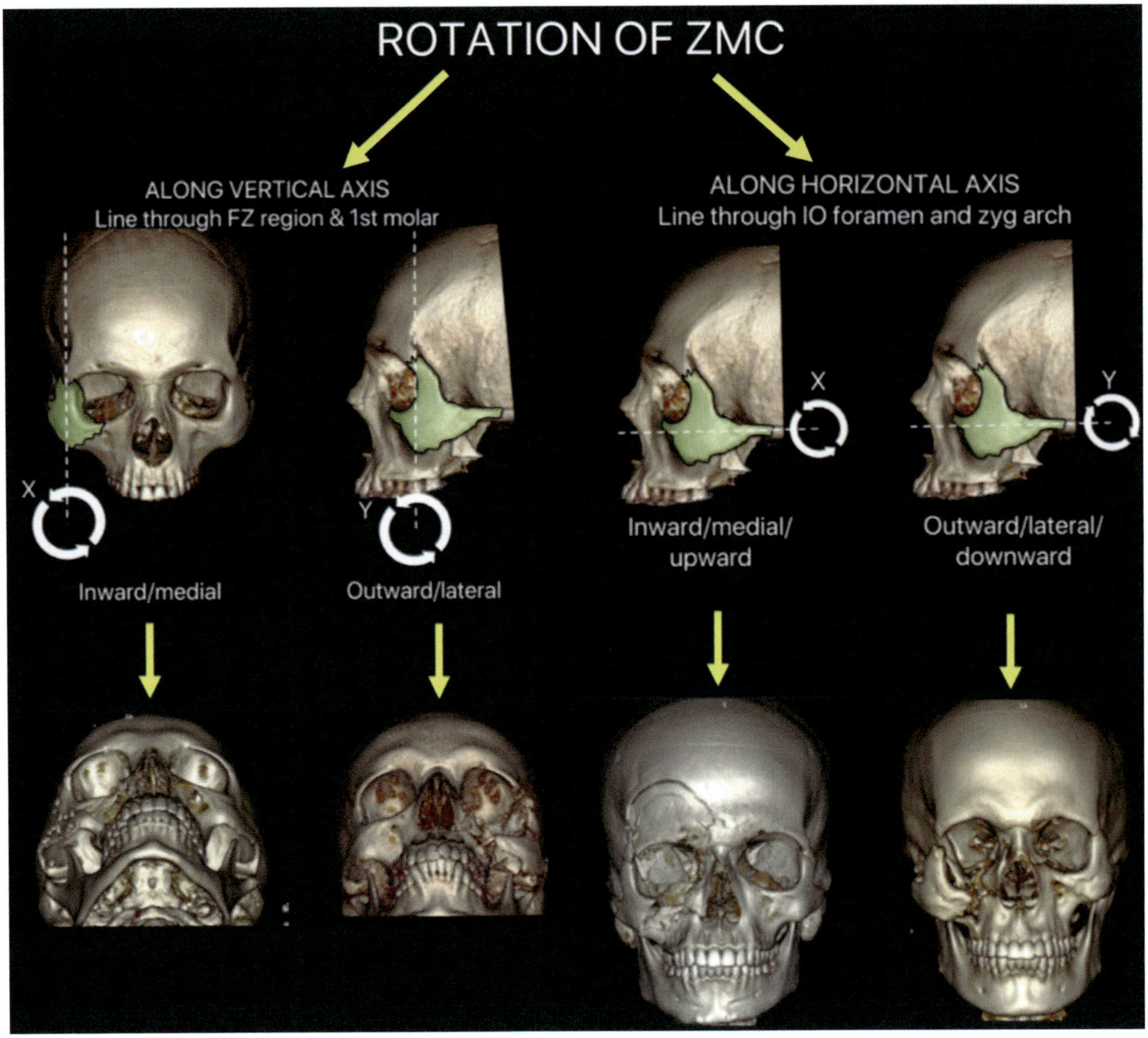

Fig. 56.7 Axes of rotation of ZMC fractures

A description of clinical features with their associated pathophysiology is provided below.

- *Periorbital edema and ecchymosis:* The edema and ecchymosis in ZMC fractures are more dramatic due to the loose connective tissue in the periorbital region. Ecchymosis is commonly seen in the circumorbital region and maxillary buccal sulcus (Fig. 56.15).
- *Subconjunctival hemorrhage (SCH):* Subconjunctival hemorrhage or hyposphagma (Fig. 56.15) often occurs in ZMC fractures due to collection of the blood into the subconjunctival space, secondary to hemorrhage from the surrounding periosteum. Characteristically, SCH in ZMC fractures does not have a posterior limit in contrast to SCH due to globe injuries [24]. It is important to note that SCH without a posterior limit is also seen in skull base fractures [25].Chemosis and hyphema are also seen in some cases.
- *Epistaxis:* Occasional epistaxis may be observed due to escape of pooled blood from the maxillary sinus following ZMC fracture. This is typically ipsilateral. Resultant nasal congestion is a common clinical finding.
- *Loss of facial prominence:* Displacement of zygoma due to trauma leads to the characteristic flattening of malar prominence (Fig. 56.16). This is well observed in bird's eye and worm's view. Examination by palpation is done

from behind the patient to detect malar depression. However, the flattening cannot be appreciated in the presence of moderate or severe edema.

- *Eye signs:* The eye signs are a very striking feature of zygomatic injury especially when rotated and inferiorly displaced. Inferior displacement of zygoma results in hypoglobus and an anti-mongoloid slant to the eye (Fig. 56.3b). Inferior or posterior displacement of the infra-orbital rim also causes lowering of the lower eyelid leading to increased scleral show (Fig. 56.17).

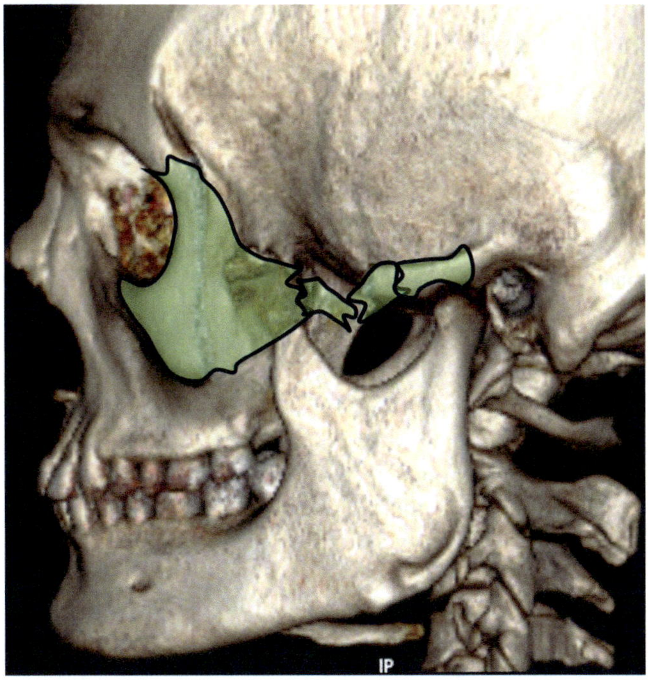

Fig. 56.8 Inferior displacement of zygomatic arch

The commonly observed variations in globe position are exophthalmos in posteriorly/medially displaced zygoma (Fig. 56.18a–c) and enophthalmos in laterally and inferiorly displaced zygoma (Fig. 56.19). En/exophthalmos resulting from ZMC fractures must be differentiated from enophthalmos arising from blow-out fractures involving the orbital floor. The clinical implications of the above are explained under "preoperative planning." Also, it is important to remember that the traditional assessment of en/exophthalmos by Hertel's exophthalmometer does not reflect the true position of the globe in displaced ZMC fractures because it uses the orbital rim as a point of reference. Naugle's which utilizes supraorbital rim as a reference is ideal in such cases [26]. However CT evaluation is the most preferred modality [27] (refer Chap. 57 on orbital fractures).

- *Tenderness* and *step deformity:* When edema is severe and inspectory findings are not conclusive, palpation gives more details. Tenderness on digital palpation, step deformity at the fronto-zygomatic, zygomatic buttress, and IOR are good indicators of fracture.
- *Air emphysema:* Palpation also helps to elicit air emphysema in the form of subcutaneous crackling. This occurs when there is a fracture through a sinus wall which allows air escape into the facial soft tissues. It usually disappears spontaneously, in 2–4 days [28]. However, this can be a potential cause of infection [29].
- *Reduced mouth opening:* Restriction in mouth opening can arise because of two reasons [30]: (1) mechanical obstruction to movement of the mandible by a retrodisplaced zygoma or a fractured zygomatic arch (Fig. 56.20a, b) and (2) a fractured arch impinging on the temporalis muscle causing reflex spasm/trismus. Likewise, injury to the masseter also can lead to trismus.

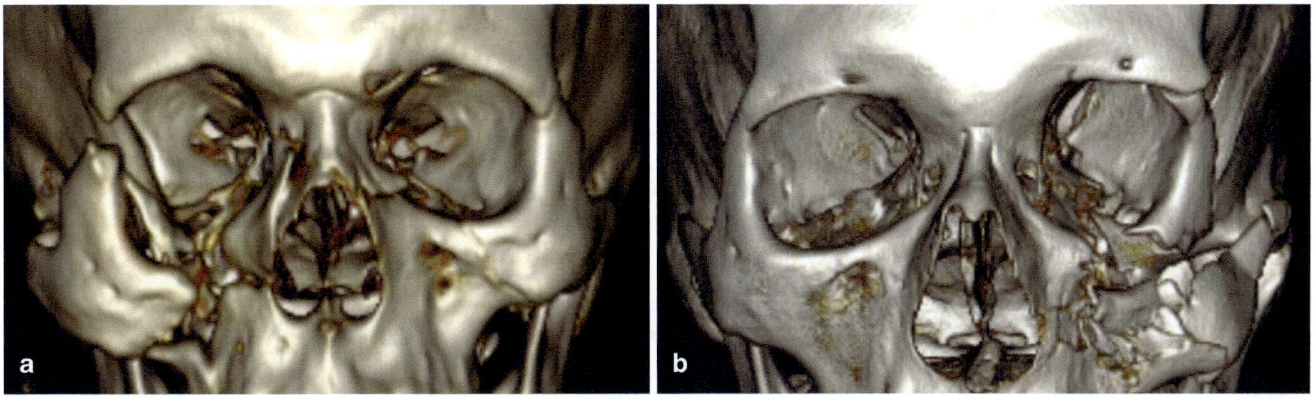

Fig. 56.9 En bloc and comminuted ZMC fractures. (**a**) En bloc displacement of the right ZMC. (**b**) Comminuted ZMC of left side

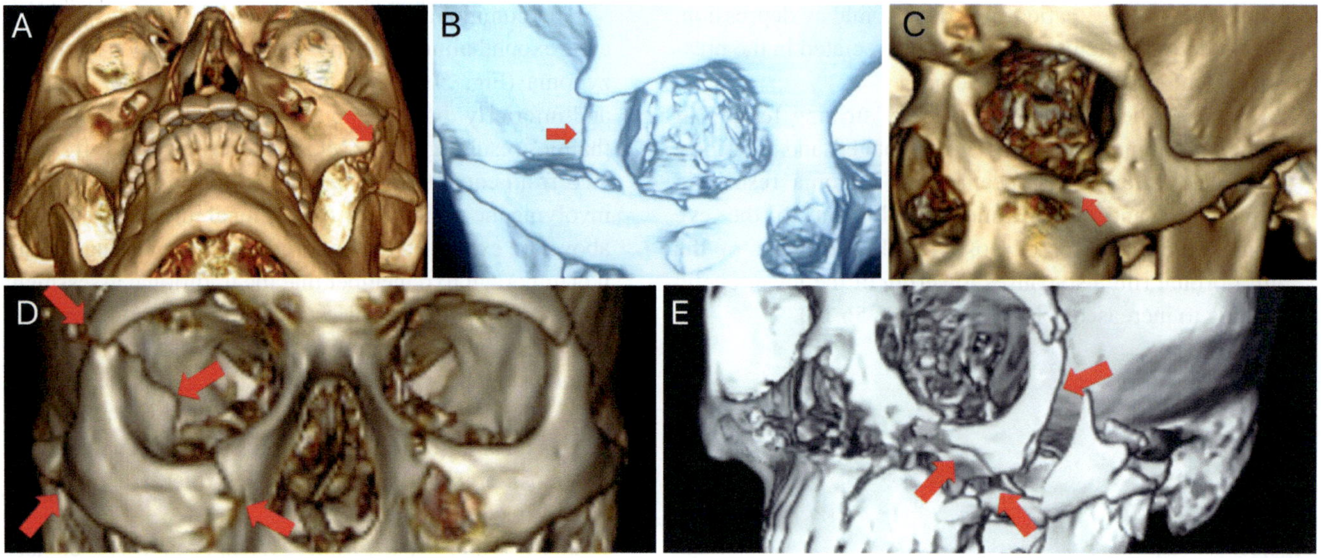

©Association of Oral and Maxillofacial Surgeons of India

Fig. 56.10 Zing's classification of ZMC fractures. (**a**) arch only (Type A1), (**b**) separation at fronto-zygomatic suture (Type A2), (**c**) separation at infra-orbital rim (Type A3), (**d**) complete mono-fragment (Type B) and (**e**) multi-fragment (Type C)

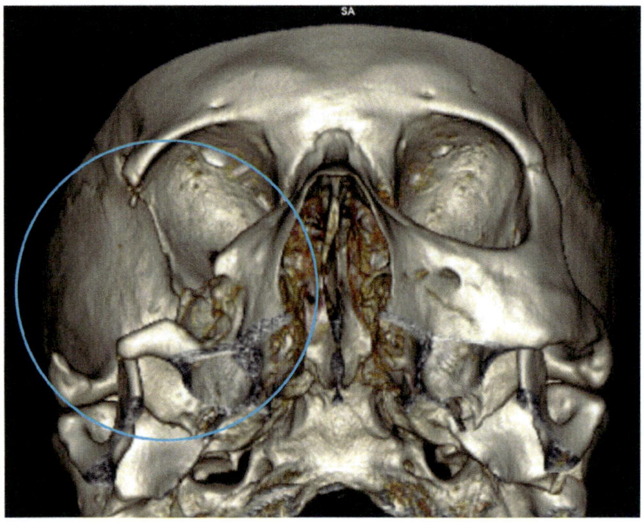

©Association of Oral and Maxillofacial Surgeons of India

Fig. 56.11 Avulsion of zygoma

- *Paresthesia:* Infra-orbital nerve being closely related to the zygoma gets compressed or pulled in displaced or comminuted ZMC fractures leading to paresthesia along the lower eyelid, upper lip, and lateral aspect of the nose. Occasionally, a patient may also have altered sensation involving the maxillary teeth leading to a perception of altered dental occlusion [5]. The other theory put forward for altered occlusion is the flexing of the ipsilateral maxillary alveolus leading to premature molar contact [31]. Paresthesia involving the zygomaticofacial and zygomaticotemporal nerves may be present. In rare occurrences, injury to the facial nerve leading to paresis has been observed in severely displaced or high-velocity injuries of the zygoma [15].
- *Altered/loss of vision:* Binocular diplopia is a common finding. The diplopia that develops following trauma can be the result of soft tissue (muscle or periorbital) entrapment, neuromuscular injury, intra-orbital or intramuscular hematoma/edema, or a change in orbital shape, with displacement of the globe [32]. A forced duction test (FDT) (Fig. 56.21) would confirm any physical impediment to ocular motility [4]. Diplopia due to edema/hematoma resolves in a few days, while that due to muscle entrapment does not, necessitating surgical correction.

Another rare but serious sequel to ZMC fractures is traumatic optic neuropathy which may present as total or partial loss of vision [33].

56.5 Imaging for ZMC Fractures

Radiological assessment is essential for accurate diagnosis and assessment of severity of the fracture.

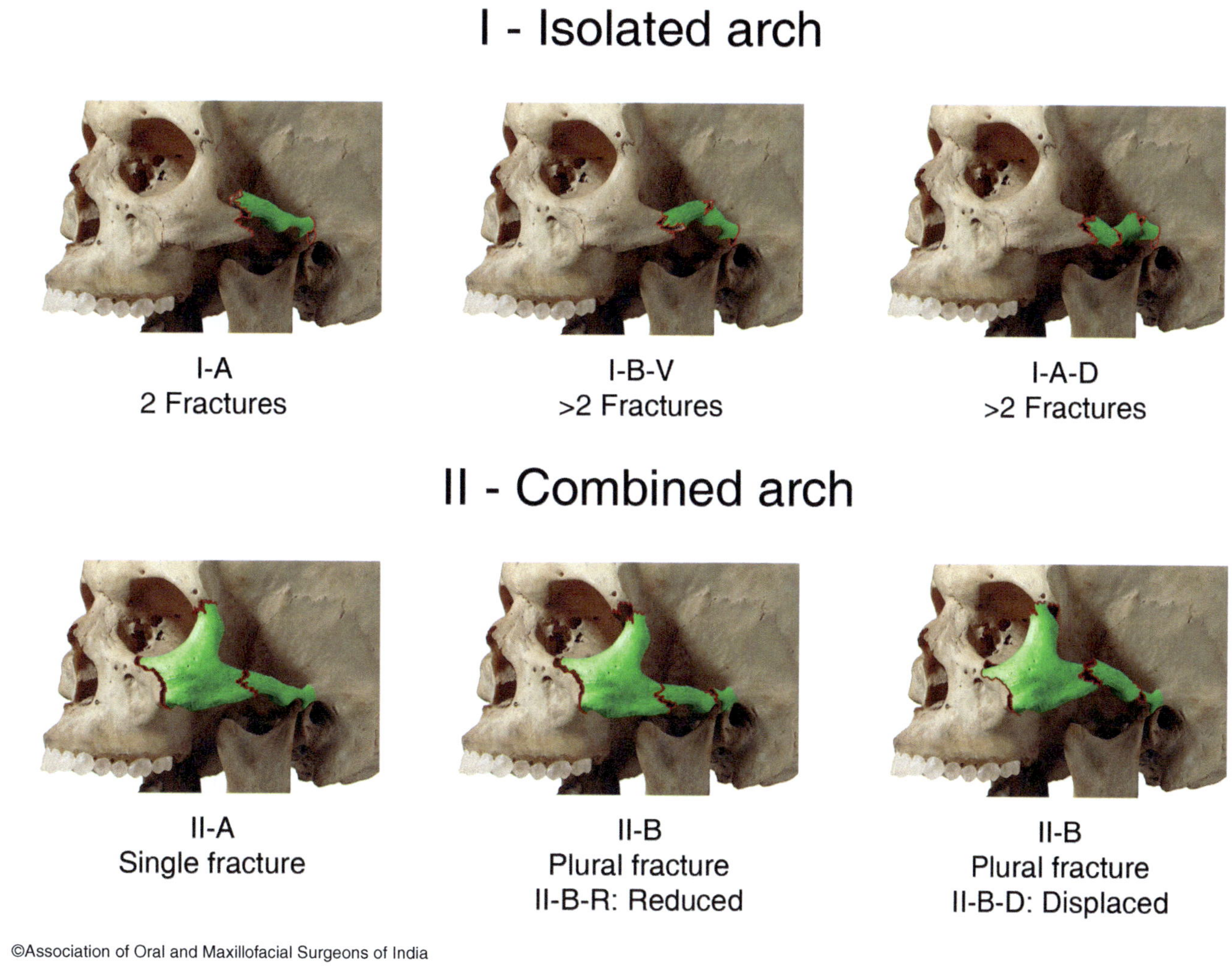

Fig. 56.12 Ozyazgan et al. classification of zygomatic arch fractures

- *Plain radiographs* [31]*:* Conventional radiographs continue to remain the mainstay of imaging at some centers. Conventional radiographs may also be useful in the post-operative phase, to assess fracture reduction. However conventional radiographs are limited by superimposition of structures.

  The commonly used views include the waters view (37° occipitomental) (Fig. 56.22) which provides good visualization of the fractured zygoma and helps in comparing with the contralateral side. Tracing the McGrigor-Campbell lines [34] (refer Chap. 55) or the Dolan's lines [35] are useful in identification of fractures on the Water's view (Box 56.2).

Box 56.2 (Fig. 56.22): Radiographic Appearance in ZMC Fracture

- Disruption of the Dolan's lines
  - Orbital line
  - Zygomatic line
  - Maxillary line
- Loss of elephant trunk appearance

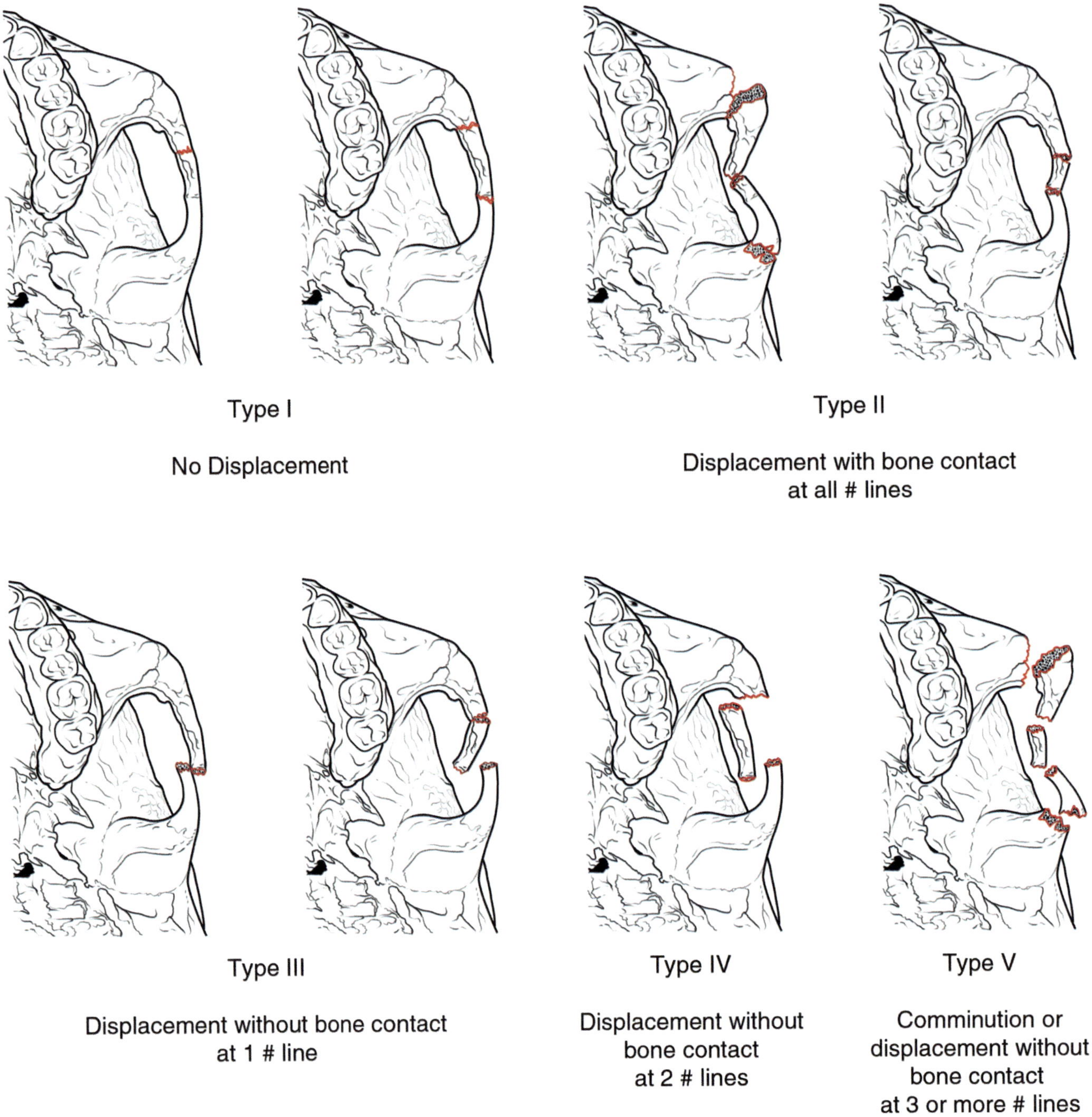

Fig. 56.13 Yamamoto et al. classification of zygomatic arch fractures

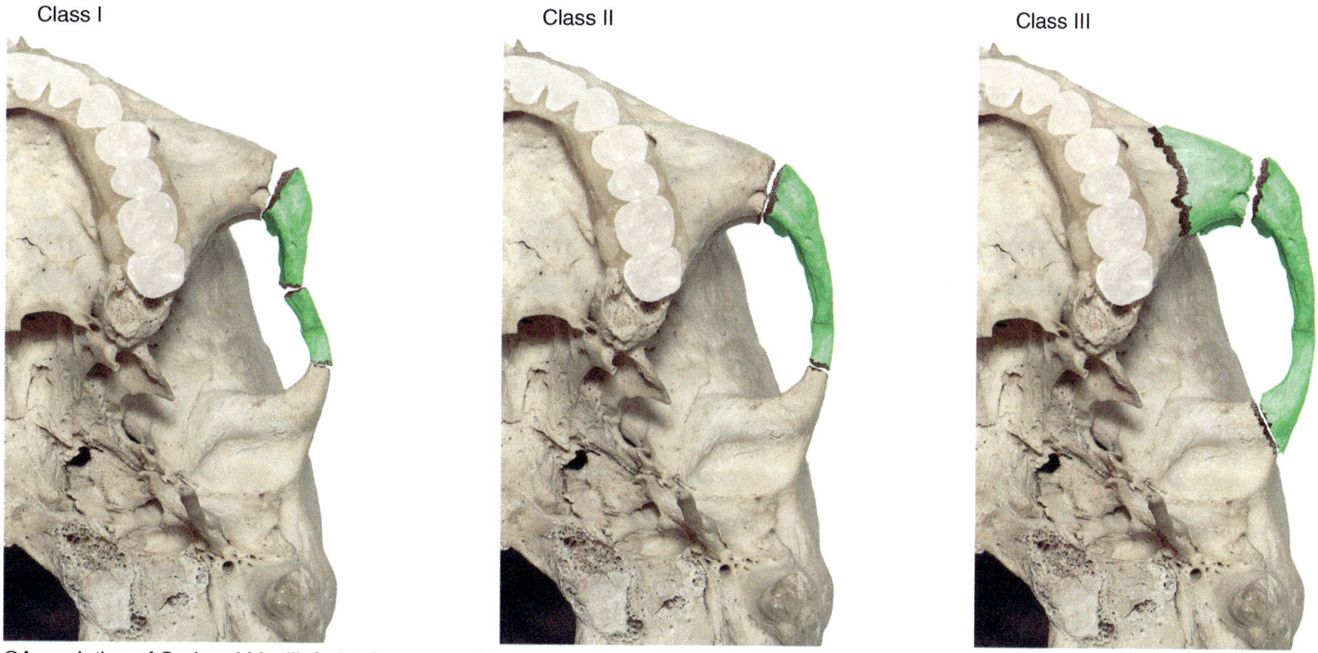

Fig. 56.14 Hönig Merten (HM) et al. classification of zygomatic arch fractures

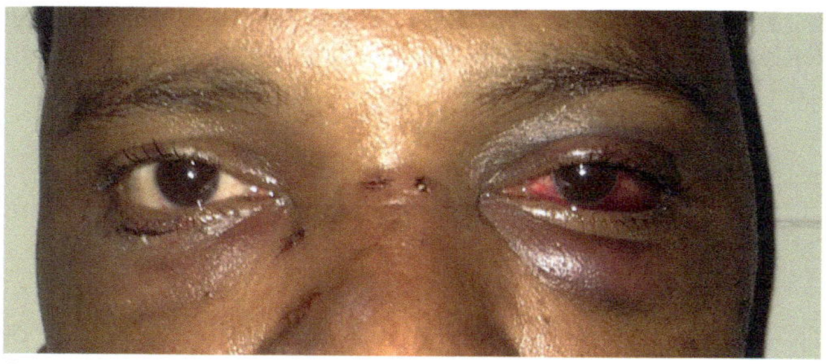

Fig. 56.15 Periorbital edema, ecchymosis, and subconjunctival hemorrhage

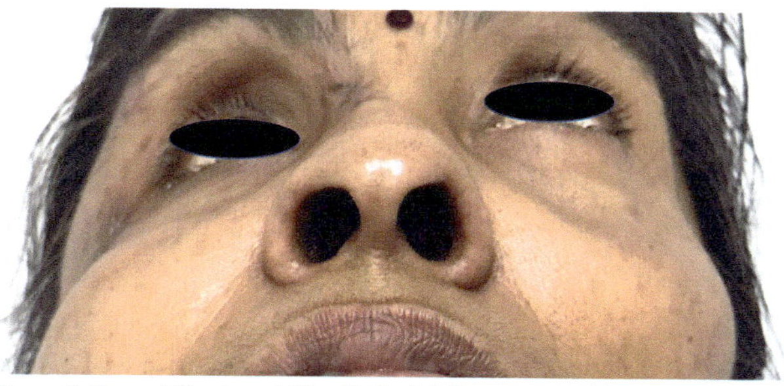

Fig. 56.16 Loss of facial prominence in right malar region

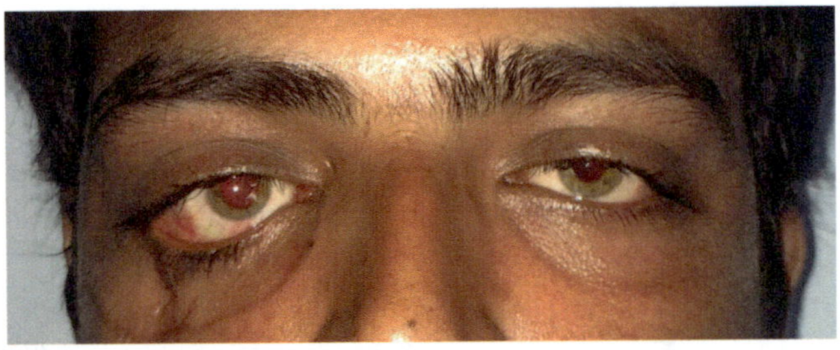

Fig. 56.17 Increased scleral show on right side

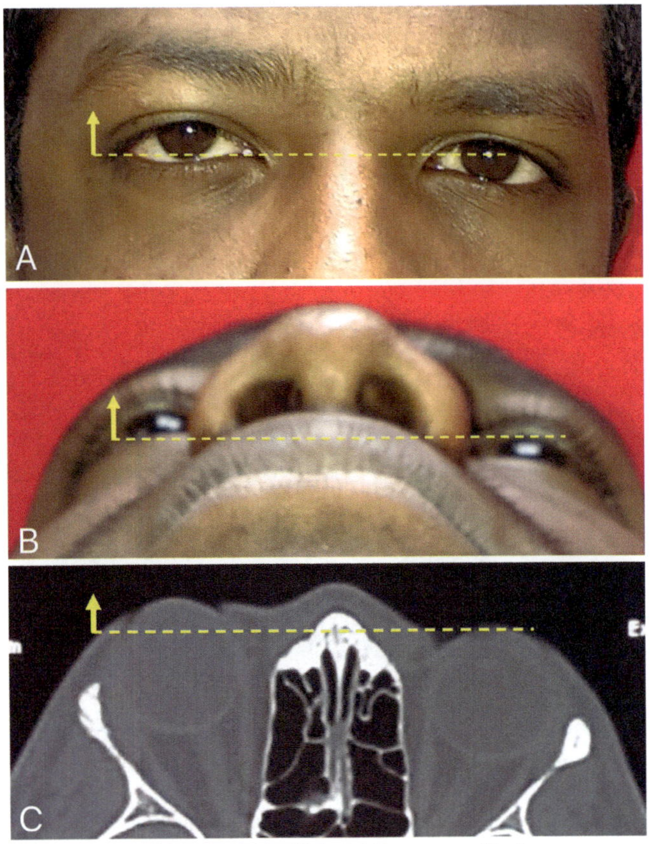

Fig. 56.18 Exophthalmos. (**a**) Frontal view demonstrating exophthalmos and hyperglobus on right side. (**b**) Basal view of the same patient showing exophthalmos on right side. (**c**) Axial CT section demonstrating exophthalmos of the right eye

- The submentovertex/jug handle view [31] (Fig. 56.23) offers the best representation of fractures of the arch. Loss of elephant trunk appearance which is indicative of arch fracture is well appreciated in this view.

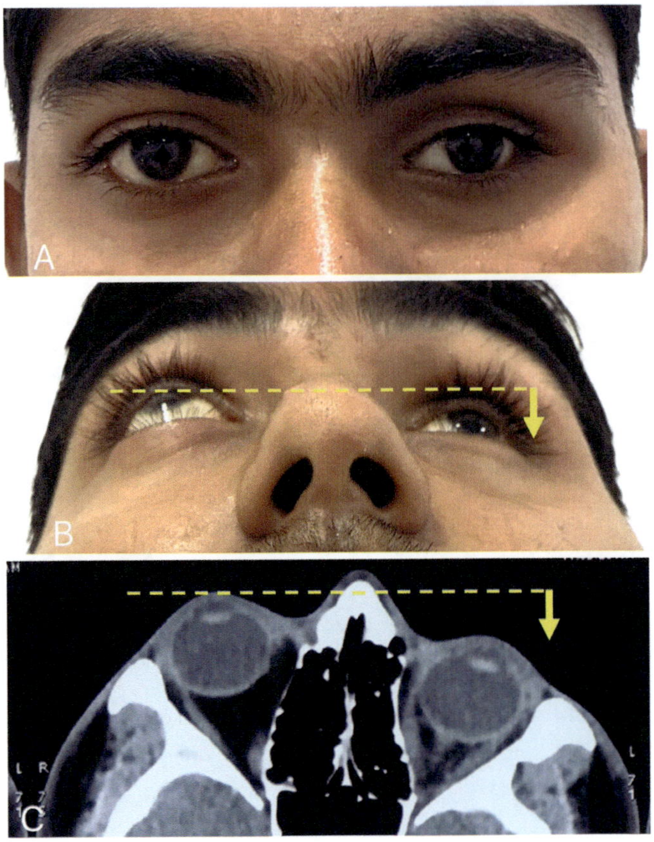

Fig. 56.19 Enophthalmos. (**a**) Frontal view showing enophthalmos on left side. (**b**) Basal view of the same patient showing enophthalmos on left side. (**c**) Axial CT section demonstrating enophthalmos of the left eye

- *Computed tomograms:* CT remains the gold standard [31]. It enables a three-dimensional assessment of the fracture along with demonstration of soft tissue entrapment between the fracture fragments. Identification of sphenozygomatic diastasis is best appreciated on CT scans. They also aid in volumetric analysis of the orbital cavity and deficits of the orbital floor. The features demonstrated in different CT sections are highlighted (Fig. 56.24a–d). Figure 56.25 demonstrates CT scan image with volume rendering, which is useful in assessing the spatial orientation of fractured ZMC.
- *USG* is a useful tool for diagnosis of ZMC fractures with high degree of sensitivity for fractures of the arch and infra-orbital rim with the significant advantage of “zero” radiation exposure [36].

The role of intra-operative imaging is discussed in the later segments of the chapter.

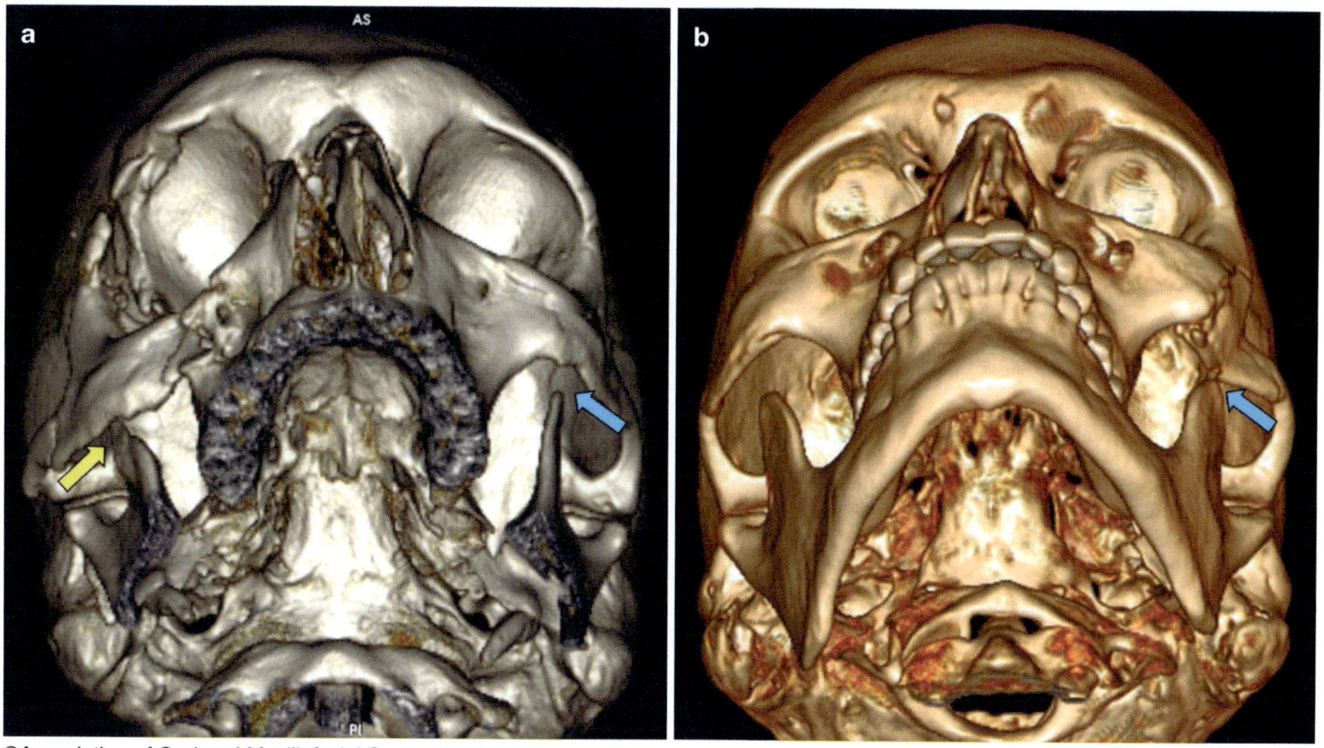

Fig. 56.20 Restricted mouth opening in ZMC fractures. (**a**) Retrodisplaced zygoma impinging on the coronoid. Yellow arrow demonstrating restriction of space between the body of zygoma and coronoid. Process, blue arrow demonstrating normal space. (**b**) Fractured arch impinging on the coronoid (Here, blue arrow demonstrates reduced space)

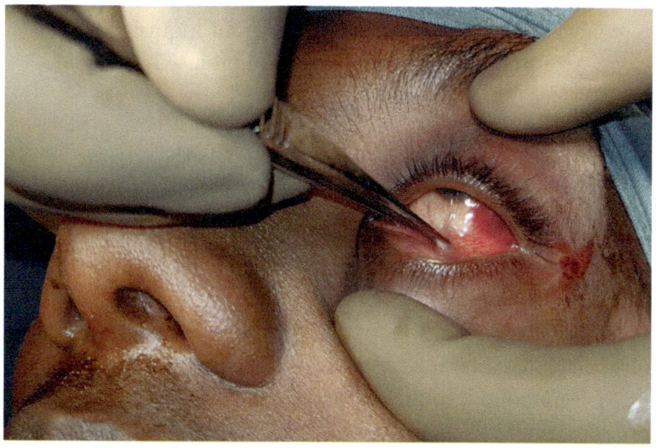

Fig. 56.21 Forced duction test

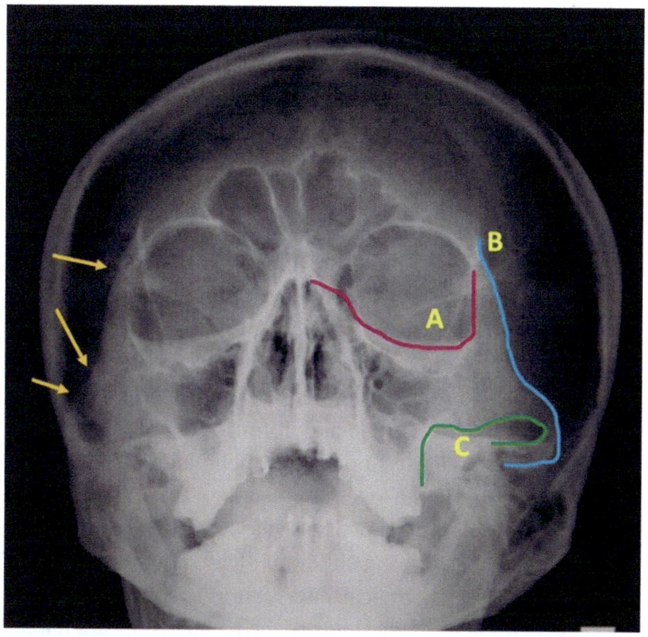

Fig. 56.22 Waters view with Dolan's lines. (**A**) Orbital line, (**B**) Zygomatic line and (**C**) Maxillary line. The yellow arrows indicate fracture separations noted on the right ZMC

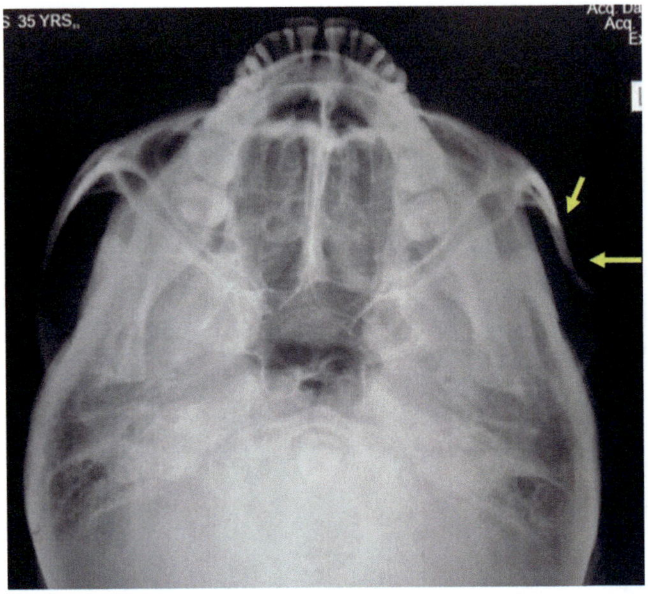

Fig. 56.23 Submentovertex view demonstrating fractured arch on left side

56.6 Principles of Management

56.6.1 Indications and Contraindications for Intervention [5, 37]

Surgical outcome of ZMC fractures is greatly influenced by two important factors: (1) choosing the right indications for intervention and (2) ideal time for surgery. Not all fractures of the ZMC require surgical intervention. The decision to intervene should be based on signs and symptoms and presence of functional impairment (Fig. 56.26).

1. It is not necessary to intervene surgically if the fracture is incomplete, undisplaced, or minimally displaced with no compromise in esthetics or function. But such patients must be advised to follow soft, non-chewy diet for 2–6 weeks and monitored to identify displacement [38].
2. Indications for surgery include (1) presence of cosmetic defects in the form of facial deformity, loss of lower eyelid support, or ocular dystopia; (2) functional deficits such as limitation of mouth opening, sensory nerve deficit, and impaired ocular movements; and (3) ZMC fracture associated with OCR reflex in children (please refer to Chap. 57).
3. Postponement of surgical intervention is considered when the general neurologic status of the patient is questionable.
4. Surgical intervention is relatively contraindicated when the involved side has the only seeing eye. In a patient willing for surgery, "potential loss of vision" has to be included in the informed consent.

56.6.2 Timing of Intervention [39]

ZMC fractures are not emergencies, and treatment can be delayed, if necessary.

- When the decision is "no immediate intervention," surgery may be postponed for up to 2 weeks, following which a reassessment may be made.
- When the indications are questionable, for example, presence of severe edema or fractures with minimal displacement, it is advisable to wait for the edema to subside so that the deformity may be assessed better.
- When the indications are definite, immediate intervention provides better outcomes due to minimal soft tissue scarring and easier reduction of fractures.

56.6.3 Surgical Objectives

Management of ZMC fractures is aimed at achieving the surgical objectives highlighted in Box 56.3 [37].

Box 56.3: Surgical Objectives in ZMC Fracture
- Restoration of facial esthetics
- Restoration of premorbid ocular function
- Correction or prevention of enophthalmos/exophthalmos
- Restoration of premorbid antral function
- Restoration of mandibular range of motion
  Mouth opening of 40 mm, excursion – 4–6 mm

56.6.4 Need for Prophylactic Antibiotics

ZMC fractures may be categorized into three classes based on their propensity to develop postsurgical infection: clean fractures (isolated arch fractures), clean-contaminated (ZMC fractures compound into the antrum), and dirty (fracture which is open to exterior). While type three fractures require regular antibiotic prophylaxis, types 1 and 2 show minimal rates of infection and may either need "no" antibiotic prophylaxis [40] or a modified single-day postsurgical regimen [41].

56.7 Preoperative Planning [42]

ZMC fractures show high propensity for over or under reductions due to lack of objective intra-operative measures to assess reduction. This may be overcome with accurate pre-

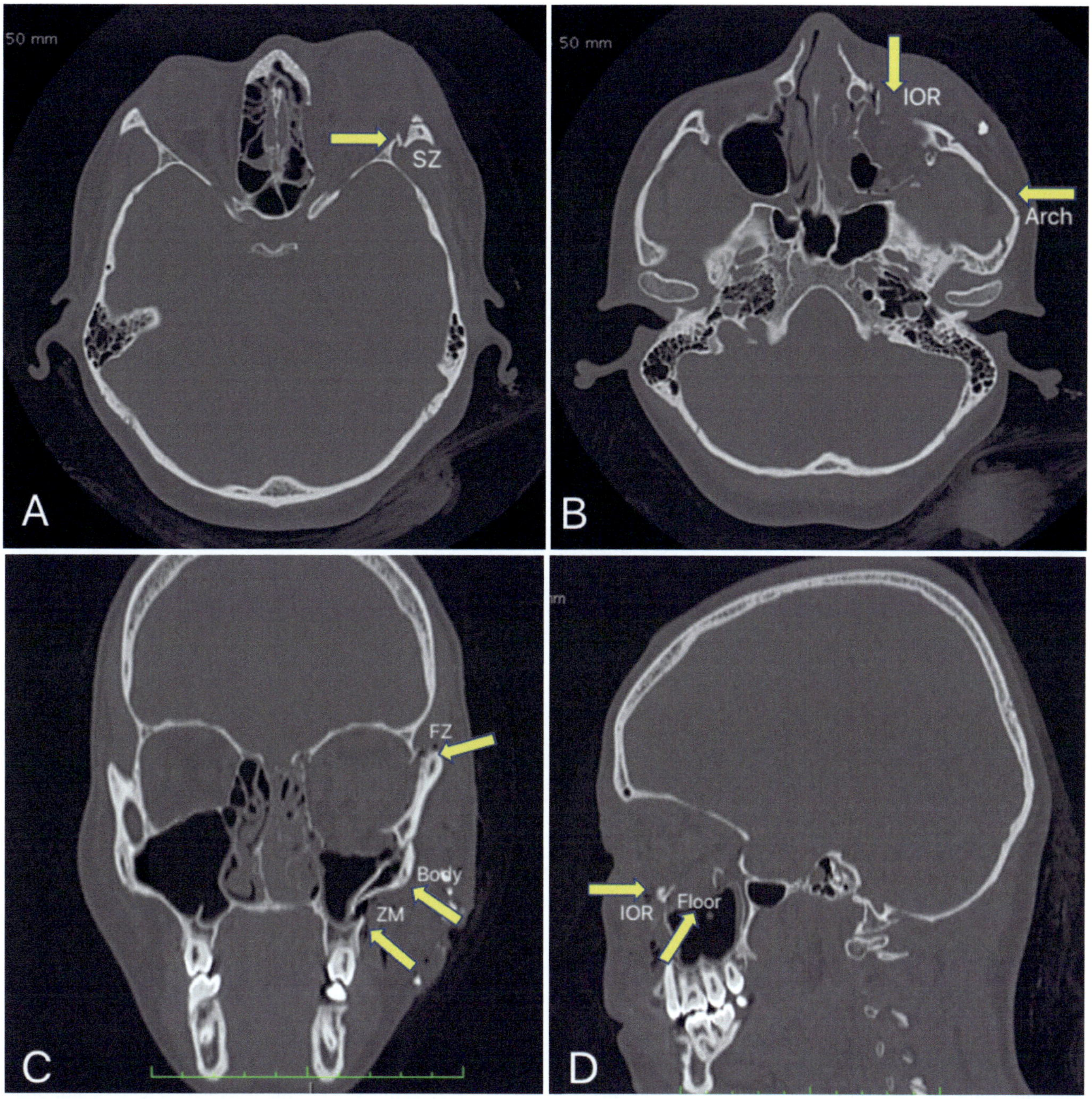

Fig. 56.24 CT scan of patient with left ZMC fracture. (**a**) Axial view demonstrating overriding of fracture fragments at SZ suture. (**b**) Axial section demonstrating fracture at the IOR and buckling of arch. (**c**) Coronal section showing separation at the FZ and ZM sutures with medial displacement of the body of zygoma. (**d**) Sagittal section demonstrating posterior displacement of IOR and large blow-out fracture of orbital floor

operative planning which helps in realizing surgical objectives in a predictable manner.

Preoperative planning includes three vital steps:

(i) CT evaluation
(ii) Model surgery
(iii) Soft tissue analysis

56.7.1 CT Evaluation

Proper CT evaluation is absolutely essential for choosing the ideal treatment; CT plays a very important role in differentiating en/exophthalmos due to ZMC fractures from those due to orbital fractures. This helps in arriving at a decision regarding internal orbit reconstruction (Box 56.4).

Box 56.4: Relative vs. Absolute En/Exophthalmos

	Enophthalmos in ZMC **Relative**	Enophthalmos in ZMC +orbit fracture **Absolute**
Etiology	Change in globe position due to displaced zygoma	Change in globe position due to fracture of orbital floor
Surgical management	Restoration of orbital rims by reduction and fixation of ZMC fracture alone	Restoration of orbital rims by reduction of ZMC fracture as well as reconstruction of orbital floor

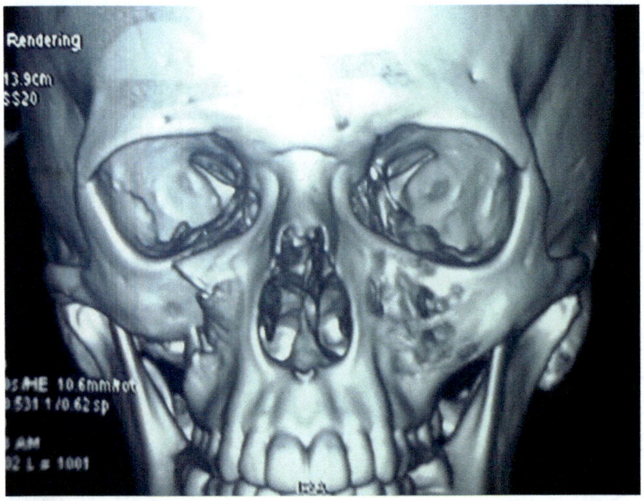

Fig. 56.25 CT with 3D volume rendering demonstrating medially rotated right ZMC fracture

56.7.2 Model Surgery

The process begins with obtaining CT scans of the patient with minimum slice thickness of 0.6 mm. This is followed by two different sequences of workflow (Fig. 56.27) which are described below.

(A) **Planning Using Physical Models**

The first step involves generation of a physical stereolithographic model (STL) from the CT scan of the patient. There are two methods by which this can be done.

1. **STL model with the actual deformity:** This model presents the post-traumatic deformity, as observed clinically. A routine model surgery is then performed, by which the displaced fragments are cut and repositioned to obtain optimal anatomical form.

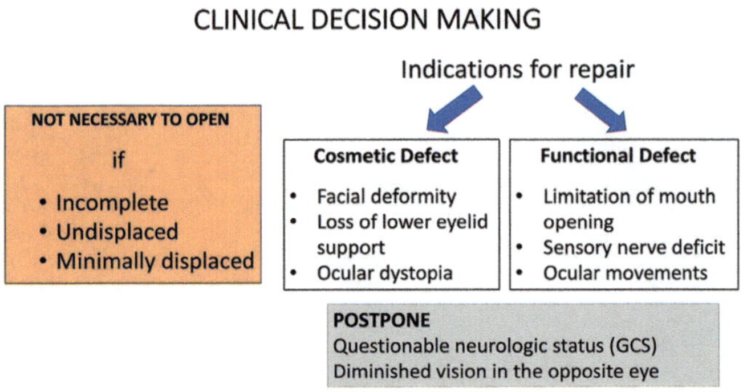

Fig. 56.26 Indications and contraindications for intervention

The repositioned fragments are stabilized temporarily with wax. The fixation devices (miniplates) are then pre-contoured over the model. Such pre-contoured implants are used to guide intra-operative fracture reduction as well as fixation. Figure 56.28a–d demonstrates the sequence described.

2. **STL model after mirroring:** CT scan is used to generate a virtual model wherein the normal side is mirrored onto the fractured side. The virtual model is used to print a physical model which demonstrates the skull which is bilaterally symmetrical, mimicking ideal reduction status. Similar to the earlier method, implants for fixation are pre-contoured over this model to help achieve optimal results intra-operatively. Figure 56.29a–d demonstrates a similar clinical scenario.

(B) **Planning Using Virtual Models**

This method utilizes the complete spectrum of computer-assisted surgical planning. A CT scan is obtained to create a virtual model on which the entire surgical sequence of reduction is performed and on which the stents for intra-operative guidance are designed. Intra-operative stents are printed from these virtual designs. There is no physical "handheld" model here (Refer Chap. 41).

- In the case of a unilateral ZMC fracture, the normal side is mirrored to the fractured side to obtain bilateral symmetry. CAS technology is then utilized to design "guidance stents" on the mirrored side. These stents can be utilized intra-operatively to (1) verify ideal reduction position in primary trauma or (2) design the osteotomy and repositioning, in secondary corrections. Another important advancement in recent years is the design and printing of "patient-specific implants" (PSI) using virtual planning. These customized fixation devices double up as guidance stents also (Refer Fig. 57.54).
- In bilateral ZMC fractures [43], mirroring is not an option, and the ideal sequencing for such cases is discussed in Sect. 56.14, of this chapter.

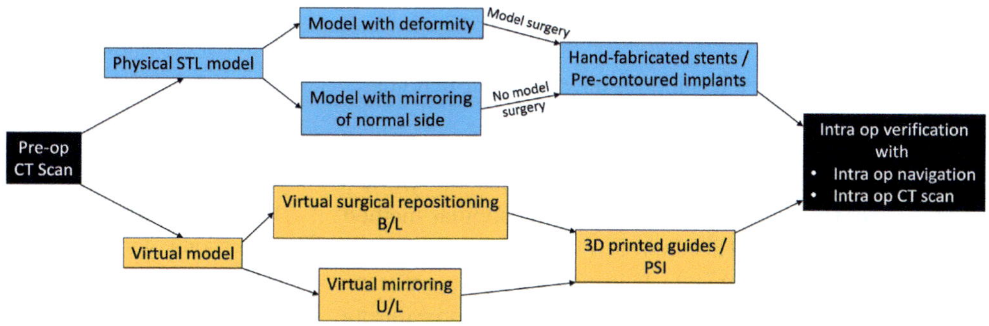

Fig. 56.27 Flow chart for preoperative planning in ZMC fractures

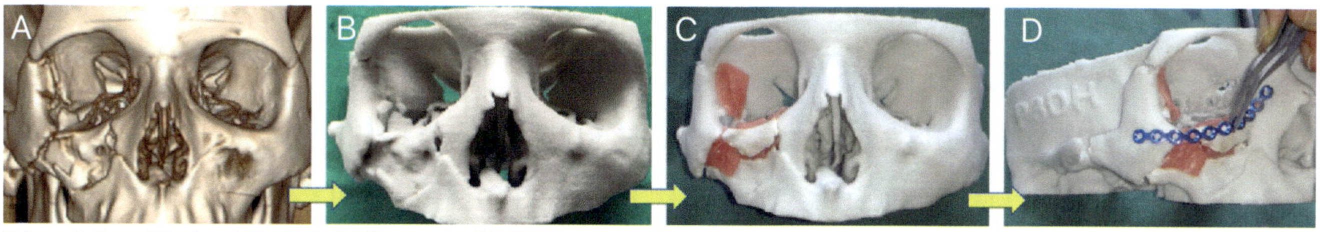

Fig. 56.28 Model surgery for pre-contouring of implants. (**a**) CT image demonstrating fractured ZMC of right side. (**b**) STL model demonstrating deformity. (**c**) Repositioning of fracture fragments to anatomical position. (**d**) Pre-contouring of implants

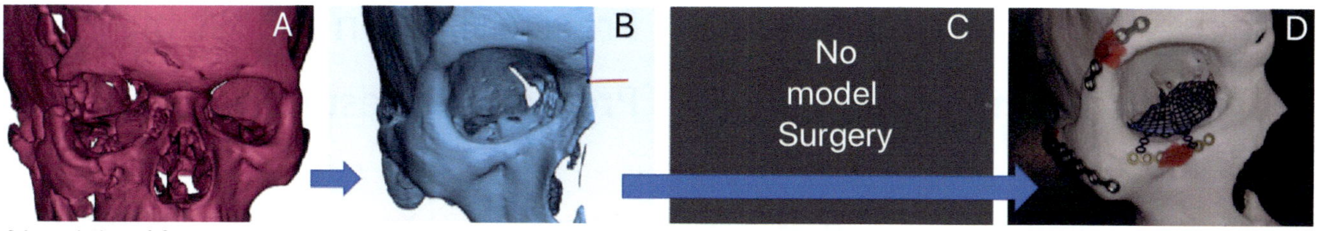

Fig. 56.29 Use of mirrored models for pre-contouring of implants. (**a**) 3D CT image of fracture. (**b**) Mirroring of zygoma of normal side to fractured side. (**d**) Generation of mirrored STL model and pre-contouring of implants

56.7.3 Soft Tissue Analysis

Li et al. [44] have described a technique for 3D simulation and prediction of soft tissue—outcome analysis in ZMC fractures. This process enables prediction of postoperative soft tissue changes in patients with ZMC fractures who are indicated for primary/secondary surgical interventions. The planning involves utilization of CT data and 3D stereophotography for the analysis. The technique may also be utilized for evaluation of postsurgical results.

56.8 Reduction of ZMC Fractures

Reduction of zygoma is unique in two aspects:

1. Unlike the other facial bones, "reduction alone" may be the sole treatment in many cases of ZMC fractures.
2. The surgical approach for reduction may be different from that for fixation.

Fracture reduction may be done either by direct or indirect method, and the approaches may be extraoral or intraoral [1].

56.8.1 Direct vs. Indirect Method

The indirect method is a blind technique where fracture is reduced without exposure of the fracture site (e.g., Gillies reduction), while direct method involves reduction of the fracture under direct visualization (e.g., coronal approach to reduce arch fracture). The differences between the two methods are shown in Fig. 56.30. However, indirect method is more commonly practiced. Open method is resorted to when the ZMC fracture is (1) severely displaced, (2) complex or comminuted, (3) when stable reduction is doubtful, and (4) there is a need for internal orbit reconstruction. However, no "single technique" is superior, and sometimes, a combination of techniques is more effective.

56.8.2 Extraoral Techniques

The extraoral reduction techniques may be either percutaneous, temporal, or endoscopic [1, 45].

- ***Temporal approach*** [46], commonly called the Gillie's (Figs. 56.31a–f and 56.32a), is the most popular method of ZMC reduction. This approach is favored because the incision is placed within the hairline which does not leave a visible scar. It also offers a very predictable force during reduction and may be used for reduction of both the arch as well as the zygoma. The technique is based on the anatomical basis that the plane between the temporalis fascia and the temporalis muscle offers direct access to the zygomatic arch and zygoma. The only contraindication to this approach is the presence of concomitant temporal bone fracture. The incision is placed at a level 2 cm above the helix of the ear, paralleling the anterior branch of the superficial temporal artery, well within the hairline (Fig. 56.33). Dissection is carried down through the skin, subcutaneous tissue, and galea aponeurotica (temporoparietal fascia—TPF) to reach the temporalis fascia.

INDIRECT / CLOSED	DIRECT / OPEN
# site is not visualized Incision & Instrumentation away from # site	# site is visualized Instrumentation at # site
Difficult to assess reduction	Can assess reduction
Precise fixation is not possible	Precise fixation is possible
Surgical outcome- not predictable	Predictable results

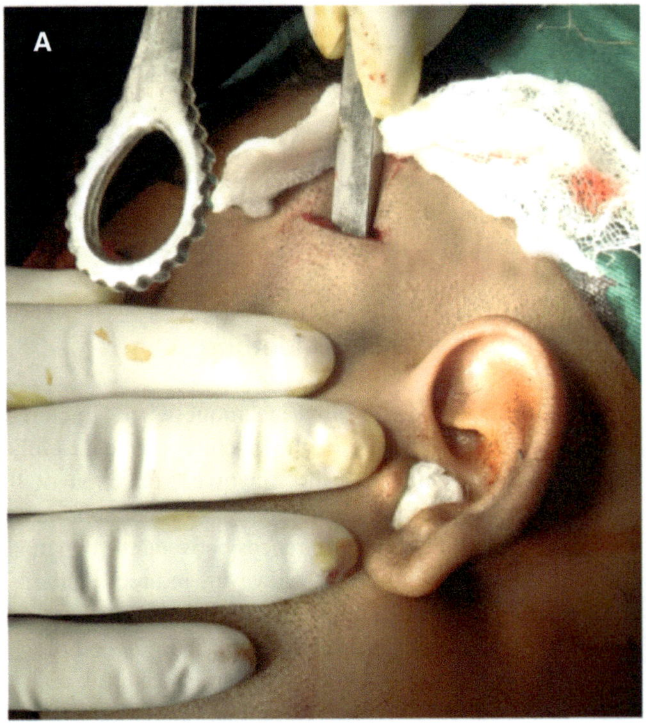

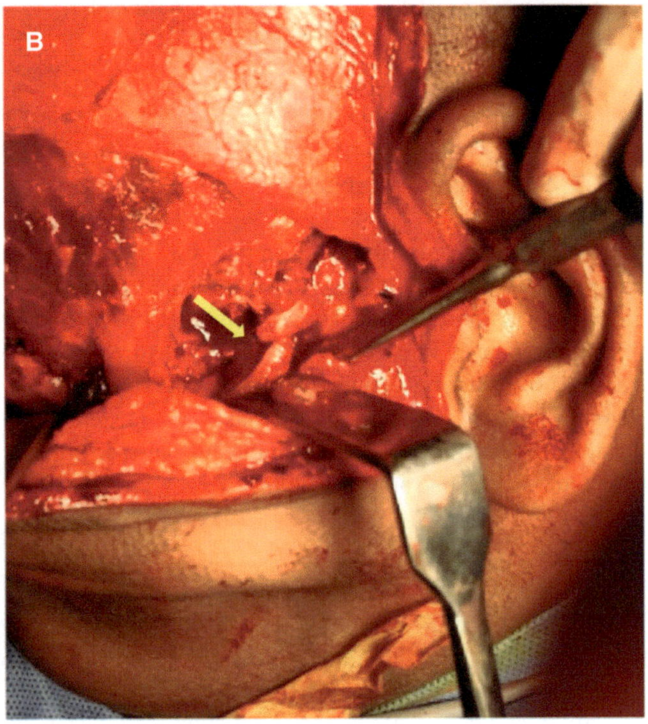

Fig. 56.30 (**A**) Indirect vs (**B**) direct reduction

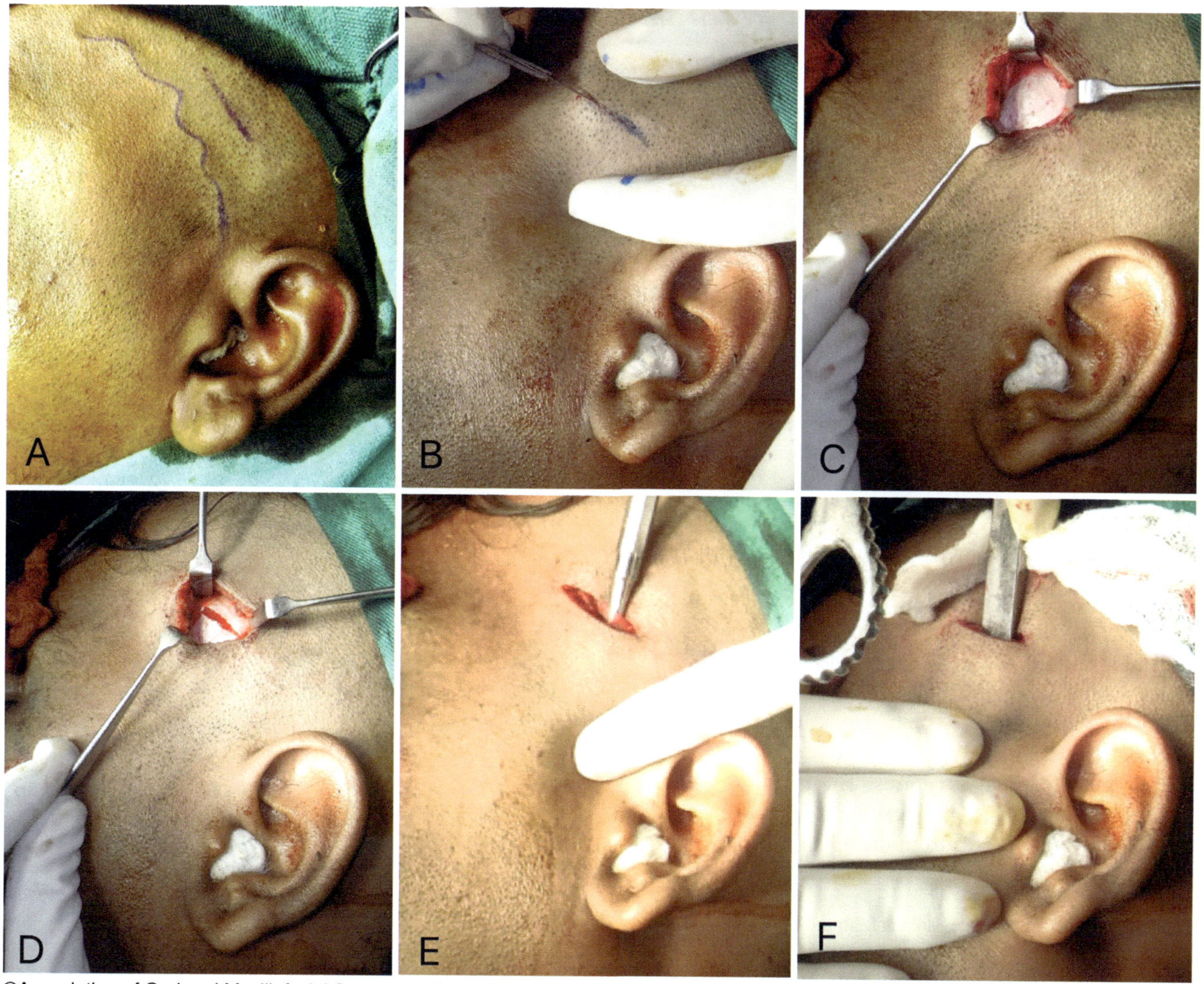

Fig. 56.31 Gillies temporal approach. (**a**) Marking of incision parallel to frontal branch of superficial temporal artery. (**b**) Placement of incision. (**c**) Exposure of deep temporal fascia. (**d**) Incision through deep temporal fascia exposing temporalis muscle. (**e**) Developing plane of elevation with periosteal elevator. (**f**) Placement of Rowe's zygomatic elevator for elevation

An incision is made through the temporalis fascia to reveal the underlying temporalis muscle. A Howarth's elevator is inserted between the temporalis fascia and the muscle, to create a plane for the zygomatic elevator. Two types of zygomatic elevators, namely, the Bristow's and Rowe's (Fig. 56.34a), are commonly used; the Bristow' s has a single flat and elongated working tip attached to a handle and is used like a spatula for elevation, while the Rowe's elevator has an additional arm attached to the working tip which serves two purposes: (1) to provide the necessary countertraction during elevation so that it relieves the fulcrum off the temporal bone and (2) to evaluate the approximate depth of insertion of the working tip when inserted into the tissue. The zygomatic elevator is positioned in the plane created, directed inferiorly to reach the deeper surface of the zygoma and carefully elevated, while an ironing motion is used to smoothen the collapsed arch form. Care is taken not to lever the elevator against the skull (Video 56.1).

Clinical Tip

1. It is good practice to keep a roll of gauze under the zygomatic elevator to prevent injury to the temporal bone.
2. Instead of extensive shaving of the temporal hair for a Gille's approach, a small patch (1cm by 3cm) of shaving/close trimming of hair can be done for better cosmesis.

- **Percutaneous methods** make use of a minimal facial skin incision, usually right over the zygoma or the lateral brow (Dingman's method) through which instruments may be inserted to manipulate and elevate the displaced zygoma.

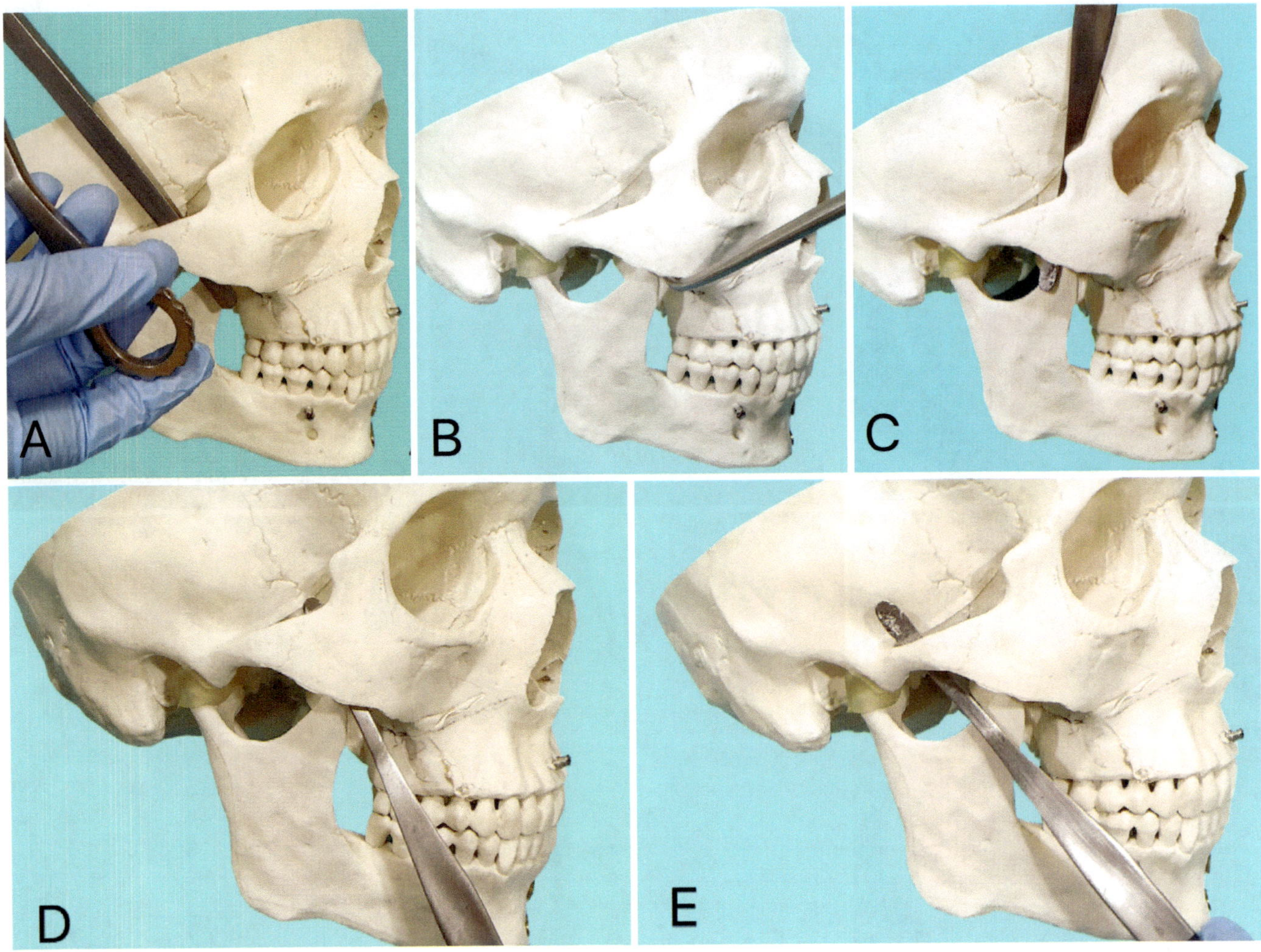

Fig. 56.32 Different approaches for reduction of fractured ZMC. (**a**) Gillie's. (**b**) Poswillo. (**c**) Dingman. (**d**) Balasubramaniam. (**e**) Quinn

- *Poswillo's* approach. This involves a stab incision made at the point of intersection of two imaginary lines—a horizontal from the base of the nose and a vertical from lateral canthus (Fig. 56.35a, b). The incision is oriented along the skin crease, just enough for a Poswillo hook [47] to be engaged underneath the body of the zygoma (Fig. 56.32b and Fig. 56.34b). And the impacted zygoma is pulled upward or outward. Skin incision is closed with a single suture. Reduction through a zygoma approach may also be performed by using a Carroll-Girard screw [48]/universal bone reduction screw (Fig. 56.34c).
- *Dingman's lateral brow approach* [49] (1964) (Fig. 56.32c)

  This technique is performed through a standard lateral brow approach where the fracture is visualized by a direct approach to the bone after incising through the skin, subcutaneous tissue, and periosteum. An elevator is then passed laterally and posterior to the orbital rim into the temporal fossa. The temporal aponeurosis (attachment of the deep temporal fascia to the lateral orbital rim) is incised, and the elevator is passed beneath it to lift the arch or the body of the zygoma in an upward, forward, and outward fashion. The original description by Dingman utilized trans-osseous wiring for stabilization of the front-zygomatic suture. However current methods incorporate the use of miniplate osteosynthesis through this approach.

56.8.3 Intraoral Techniques

The greatest advantage of intraoral techniques is "no skin incision." Commonly followed methods are:

- *Balasubramaniam's/Keen's approach* (upper buccal sulcus approach) [50] (Fig. 56.32d)

  This approach uses a vestibular incision behind the zygomatic buttress. A Howarth's periosteal elevator is inserted in a supraperiosteal plane to engage the infratemporal surface of the zygoma. Reduction is achieved with an upward, forward, and outwardly directed force. When greater force is needed to elevate as in impacted zygomas

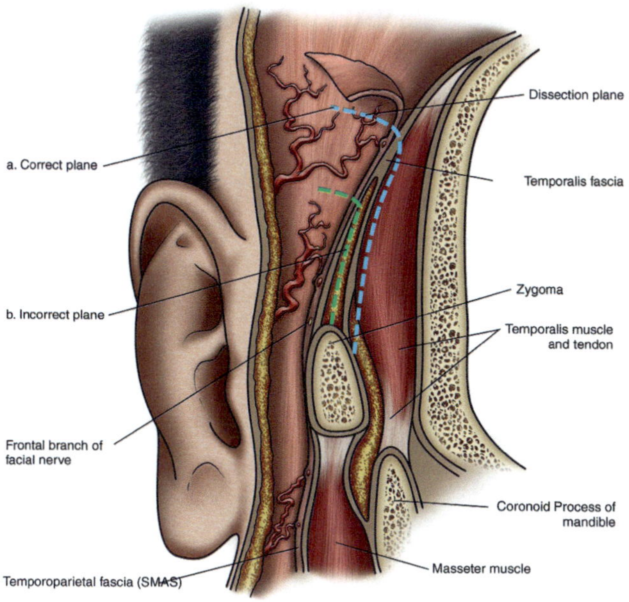

Fig. 56.33 Gillie's correct plane for elevation. It is important to understand that the deep temporal fascia divides into two, to enclose the zygomatic arch and the fat above, approximately 2 cm above the arch. An incision placed too low may mislead the young surgeon into the fat plane (b, lateral to the arch) rather than the subfascial plane (a, medial to the arch) (Also refer Fig. 85.1a)

or delayed presentation, a Bristow's/Rowe's zygomatic elevator (Fig. 56.36) or the arm of an upper anterior forceps may be used. The technique offers more mechanical advantage than the extraoral method; less force is needed to elevate, because the force is directed entirely at the center of the zygomatic body, which is considered more effective.

- *Quinn's procedure* (lateral coronoid approach) [51] (Fig. 56.32e) employs an incision over the anterior border of the ramus. An elevator is inserted in a supraperiosteal plane, lateral to the coronoid process and paralleling the temporalis tendon to reach the medial surface of the zygomatic arch. Elevation of the arch may be done in an ironing fashion.

Both the abovementioned intraoral techniques are supraperiosteal methods.

56.8.4 Reduction of Zygomatic Arch

Elevation of the depressed arch is usually performed in an indirect manner, using the Gillie's technique. However numerous techniques have been advocated in literature. These include the "roller-coaster" lateral brow technique [52] and methods using percutaneous towel clip [53], traction suture [54], Foley's catheter [55], K wire [56], and Dingman elevator [57] to restitute the arch anatomy.

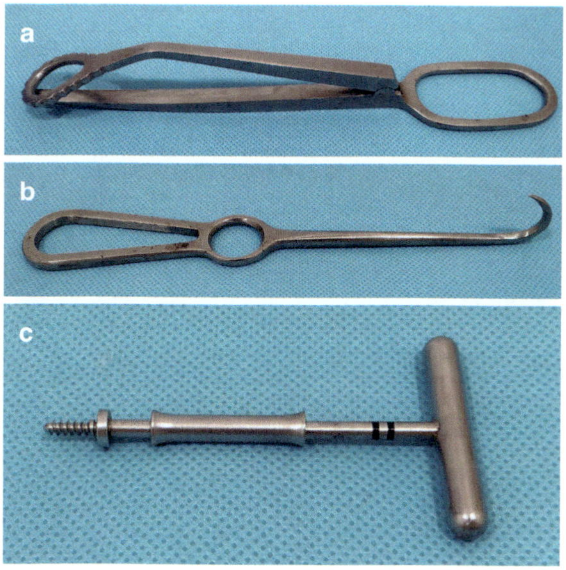

Fig. 56.34 Instruments for reduction. (**a**) Rowe's . (**b**) Poswillo hook. (**c**) Universal bone reduction screw

56.8.5 Intra-operative Assessment of Reduction

The intra-operative assessment of reduction is a critical step in zygoma management, especially in closed reduction. The methods commonly used are (1) clinical assessment, (2) imaging, and (3) use of prefabricated guides/stents.

1. ***Clinical assessment*** is usually done by eyeballing, comparing with the normal side or palpation of the rims for steps. However, the adequacy of reduction may be difficult to assess intra-operatively because of edema as well as patient position. Audible click during manipulation is also indicative of reduction [58]. Surgical exposure of multiple suture sites is the other method to confirm reduction [59] but is less favored because of surgical morbidity. However, exposure at all sites of articulation is not required; two sites are considered perfect indicators of accurate reduction [5] (Box 56.5).
2. ***Intra-operative imaging*** [58] such as C-arm [60] (Fig. 56.37a, b), CT [59], O arm [61], or endoscopes [45] are valuable guides in confirming reduction of ZMC fractures. However, use of intra-op imaging other than endoscopes mandates use of lead aprons by operating room personnel to prevent radiation exposure.
3. ***Prefabricated guides/ stents*** [62] are valid tools which ensure accuracy of reduction, intra-operatively.

Box 56.5: Indicators of Accurate Reduction of ZMC #

Reduction along the vertical axis—SZ suture
Reduction along the horizontal axis—ZM suture

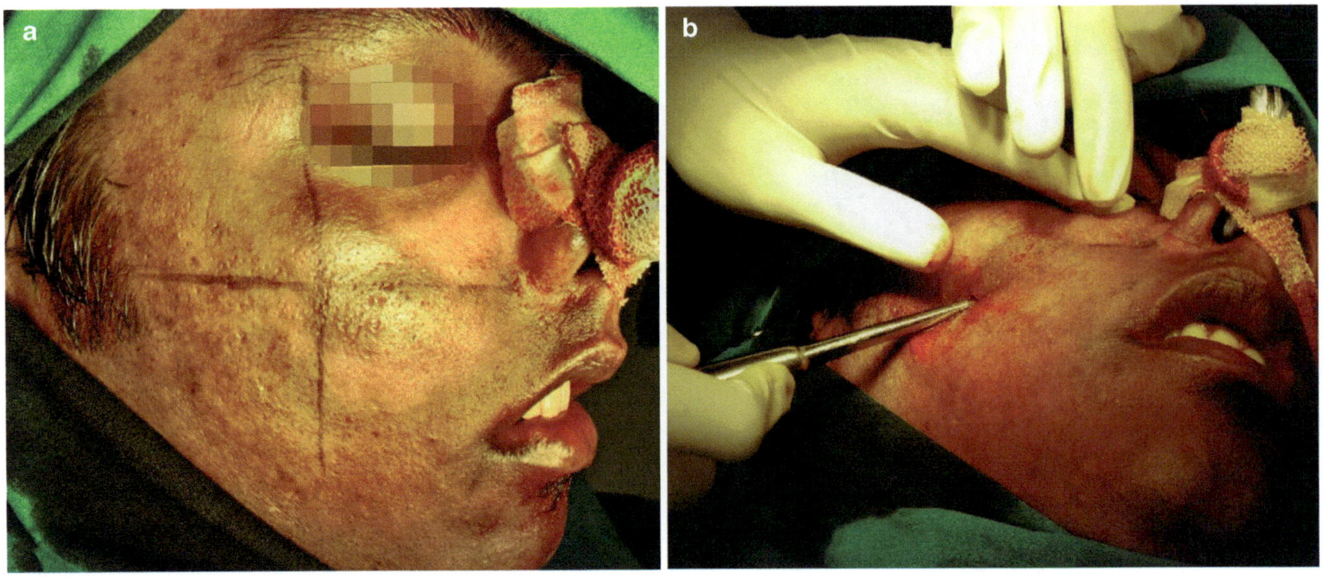

Fig. 56.35 Percutaneous reduction with Poswillo's technique. (**a**) Marking on skin. (**b**) Percutaneous insertion of bone hook

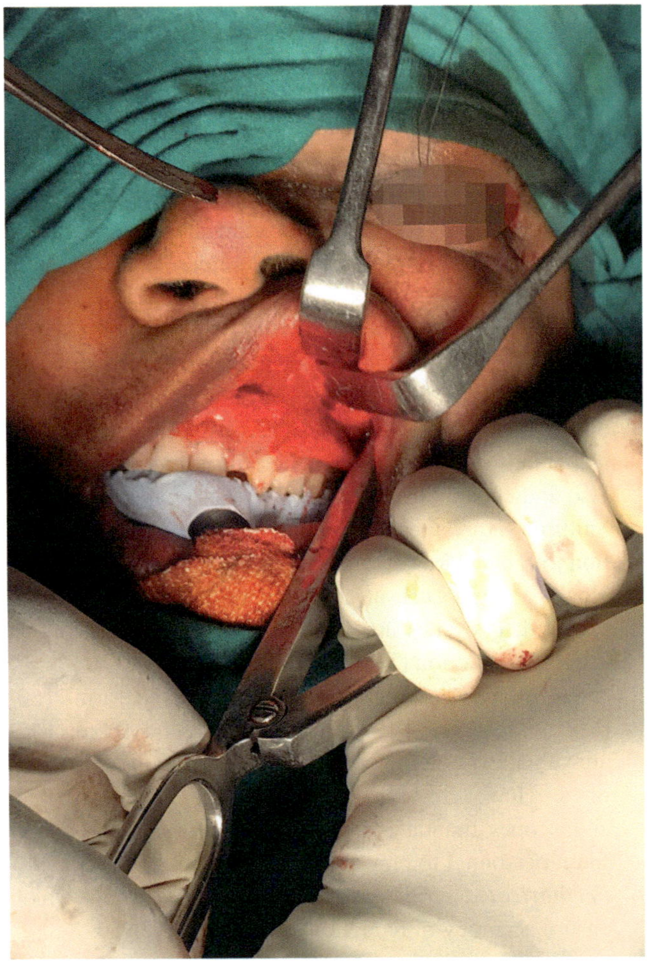

Fig. 56.36 Balasubramaniam's technique

56.8.6 Precautions During and After Reduction

Manipulation of zygoma during reduction has been known to cause certain complications such as bleeding from infra-orbital vessels [16]. Use of controlled force during indirect reduction greatly reduces such complications. It is prudent to watch out for stimulation of Oculocardiac reflex (OCR) [63] as described later in the text. OCR may also be prevented by administering regional blocks before elevation [64].

Once the reduction is completed and found satisfactory, the fracture fragments need to be maintained in the reduced state. A Zimmer splint [65] (preformed aluminum splint with foam on the undersurface) may be adapted to the reduced arch and secured with sutures. It is maintained in situ for 2–3 weeks.

Finally, it is mandatory to do a force duction test (FDT) after elevation of zygoma [5] (Box 56.6).

Box 56.6: FDT Is Mandatory After Reduction of ZMC Fractures (Fig. 56.21)

During reduction of ZMC fractures, as the fractured bones get realigned to normal anatomical position, entrapment of surrounding soft tissue or muscles may occur between the fragments

This may lead to port-surgical diplopia, necessitating a surgical revisit.

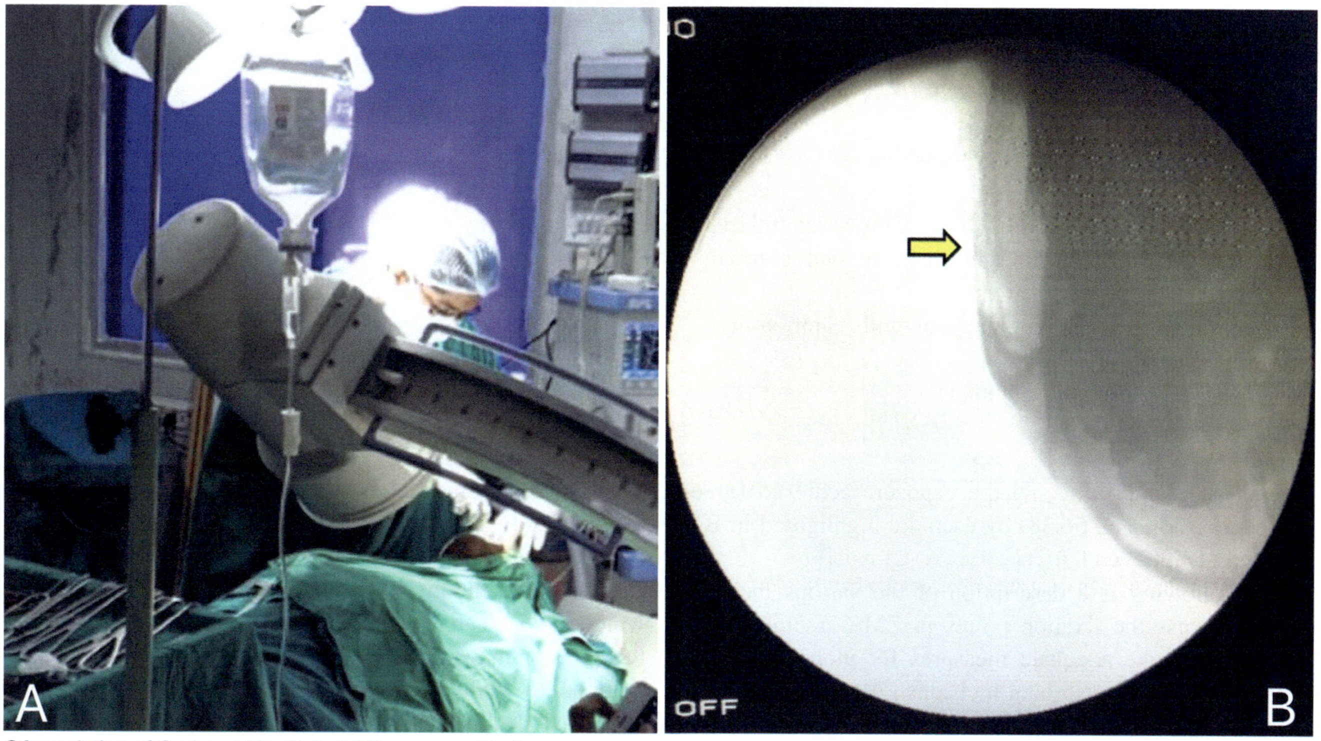

Fig. 56.37 Intra-operative assessment of reduction using C-arm. (**a**) Intra-operative positioning of C-arm. (**b**) Image demonstrating zygomatic arch after reduction

56.9 Fixation and Stabilization of ZMC Fractures

56.9.1 Need for Fixation

Fixation needs of ZMC fractures depend on the post-reduction stability. Classification of fracture patterns by Rowe and Williams [1] provides guidance on assessment of fracture stability after reduction. Any fracture classified as stable after reduction does not require fixation, while those considered unstable, mandate fixation. However, a practical method would be to apply moderate digital pressure on the malar eminence after reduction. Displacement secondary to this maneuver, requires fixation [59]. The algorithm proposed by Rodrigo and Belini et al. is also a practical guide to manage ZMC fractures which are not associated with orbital component [3]. For ZMC fractures with orbital involvement, Ellis and Perez advocate guidelines for orbital reconstruction based on CT evaluation. Most of the studies indicate increase of fixation points from 1 to 2, 3, and 4 points based on the status of intra-operative stability after reduction. Involvement of orbit leading to changes in intra-orbital volume requires orbital reconstruction [59].

Box 56.7: Ideal Sequence of Fixation

1. Vertical buttress—to restore facial height
2. Zygomatic arch—to restore anteroposterior projection

56.9.2 Fixation Principles

The current dictum is "any zygoma which when fractured and displaced must be fixed" [37]. The objectives are to achieve a 3D reconstruction (transverse width, vertical height, and anteroposterior projection) and establish the buttresses. Attention needs to be given to the order of restoration [66, 67]. The results of various biomechanical experiments indicate that the vertical buttress needs to be fixed first, to restore the facial height. Then, the anteroposterior projection may be achieved by restoring the arch (Box 56.7).

56.9.3 Surgical Access to Fixation

Surgical approaches for ZMC fixation are chosen based on the fracture pattern and fixation needs. A single or multiple incision may be used for the surgical exposure of ZMC fractures [30, 68, 69].

The incisions may be broadly classified as:

- Cutaneous (upper eyelid, lateral brow, subciliary, subtarsal, infra-orbital, preauricular, and coronal incisions)
- Conjunctival (transconjunctival with canthotomy/ transcaruncular)
- Mucosal (intraoral vestibular)

The list of incisions and the exposure achieved (green shaded areas on Fig. 56.38) by each are highlighted in Box 56.8 (Fig. 56.38)

The following is a description of the various incisions used to access the fixation points in ZMC fractures. It is important to take adequate measures for globe protection while placing any periorbital incisions [70]. The commonly followed methods include either a temporary tarsorrhaphy (Fig. 56.39) or a corneal shield (Fig. 56.40). The tarsorrhaphy also offers the additional advantage of being used as a retraction suture during surgery.

Box 56.8: Approaches to ZMC Fractures

Intraoral vestibular incision	ZM, IOR
Lower eyelid cutaneous incisions (Subtarsal, subciliary, infraorbital)	IOR, orbital floor
Transconjunctival	SZ, FZ, IOR, floor
Lateral brow	FZ, SZ
Upper eyelid	SZ, FZ
Coronal	SZ, FZ, arch
Preauricular	Arch

56.9.3.1 Supraorbital/Lateral Brow Incision (Fig. 56.38)

The lateral brow incision is otherwise called as "in the brow" incision and offers a fast and direct access to the fronto-zygomatic suture and lateral part of the supraorbital rim. The extensions for the incision must be well within the eyebrow which provides an ideal camouflage (Fig. 56.41a). However, this incision may not be ideal in people who are cosmetically inclined to maintain a higher eyebrow. Absence of any important neurovascular structures in this area makes this incision easy to perform, even by beginners.

After infiltration of LA solution containing vasoconstrictor, a 2 cm long incision is placed along the curve of the

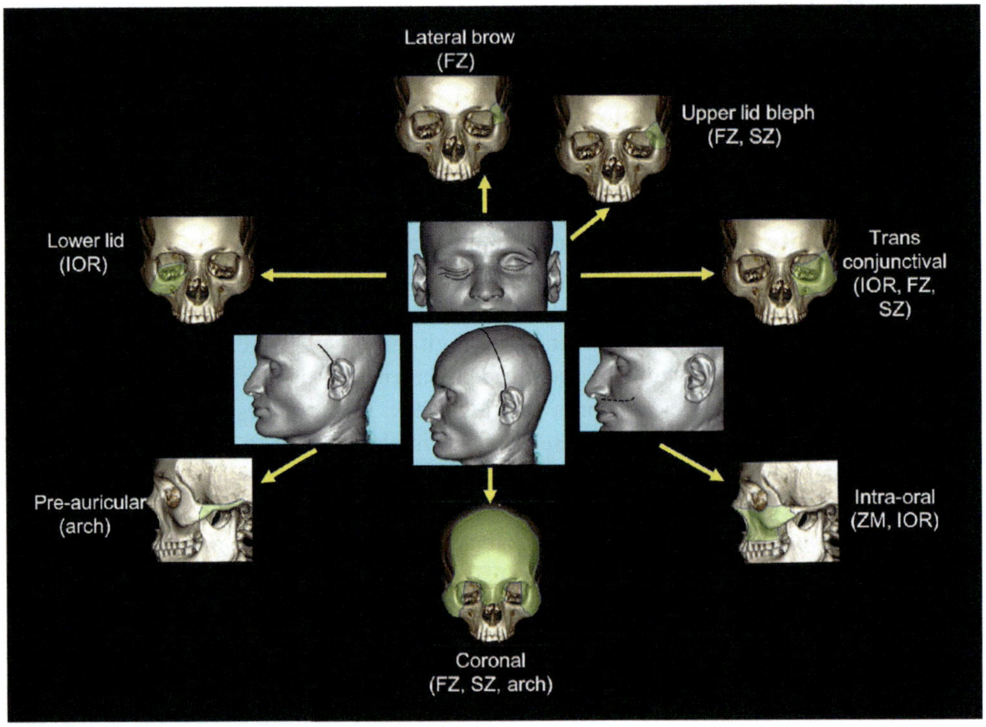

Fig. 56.38 Incisions to access ZMC fractures

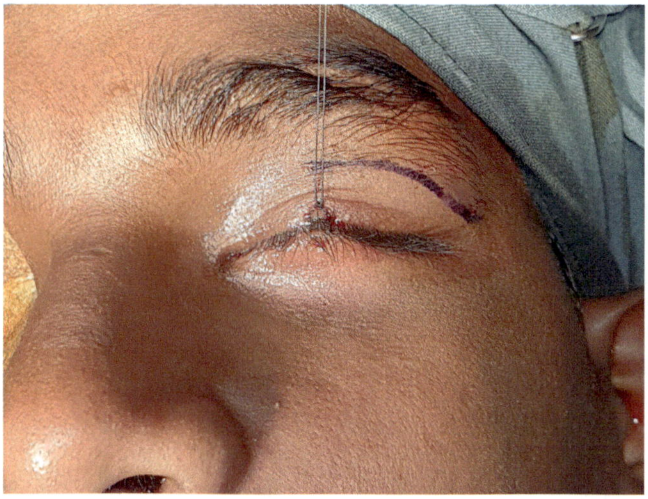

Fig. 56.39 Tarsorrhaphy

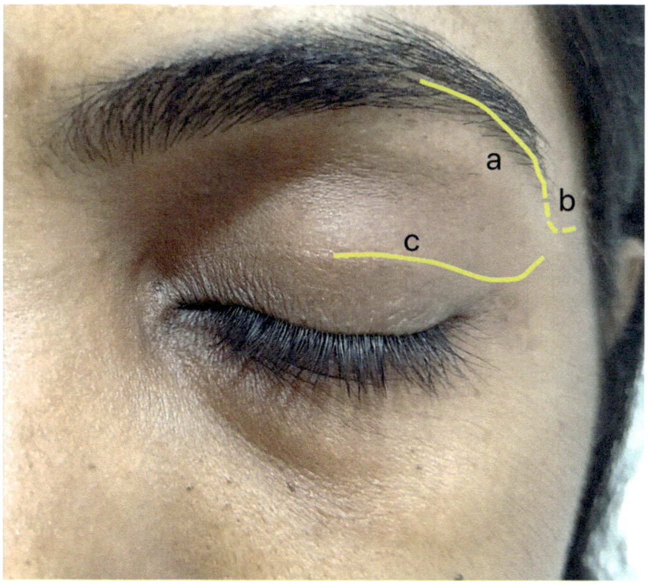

Fig. 56.41 Periorbital incisions for FZ suture. (a) Lateral brow incision. (b) Lateral brow extension (shown in dotted lines). (c) Upper lid blepharoplasty

superolateral part of the orbital rim. Care is taken to incline the blade parallel to the hair so that the shafts are not transected. Failure to do so may cause linear alopecia along the incision line, which may be unaesthetic. Incision is carried through the skin, subcutaneous tissue, and the orbicularis oculi muscle. The flap is undermined in the supraperiosteal plane to permit ease of retraction. A periosteal incision is then placed above the fronto-zygomatic suture for reduction and fixation (Fig. 56.42a, b).

When additional exposure is needed on the medial aspect, the incision is extended up to the supraorbital nerve. For additional inferior extension, a gradual 90° turn into the

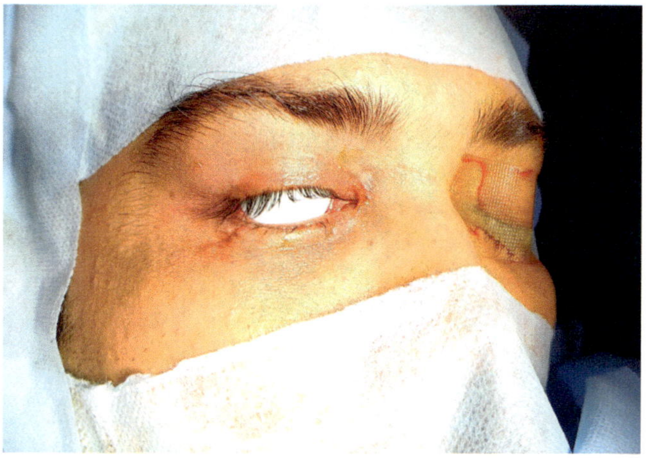

Fig. 56.40 Corneal shield

crow's feet wrinkle which is restricted to the skin only, is utilized to provide a much wider access [70] (Fig. 56.41b). This extension must remain 6 mm superior to the lateral canthus. Inferior limit of the incision along the lateral orbital rim should not cross the RSTL (resting skin tension lines) to avoid unaesthetic scars.

Closure is performed in layers with approximation of the periosteum and subcutaneous tissues (Video 56.2).

56.9.3.2 Upper Eyelid Blepharoplasty Incision (Fig. 56.38)

The upper lid blepharoplasty incision is otherwise called as the ***supratarsal fold*** or ***upper eyelid crease*** incision. It offers the most esthetically favorable approach to the fronto-zygomatic suture region. The incision is made along the eyelid crease, 10 mm above the free margin of the eyelid (Fig. 56.41c). As the incision extends laterally, it should be at least 6 mm above the lateral canthus. When eyelid anatomy is distorted with edema or hematoma, the contralateral lid crease measurements are used to mark the incision.

The incision is placed through the skin and muscle and is raised as a skin-muscle flap for good viability of the overlying skin. The plane of dissection is below the orbicularis oculi in a superior and lateral fashion to reach the periosteum (Fig. 56.43a, b). The periosteum is sharply incised to expose the bone underneath. Further dissection along the bony margins is strictly subperiosteal; any violation of the periosteum may cause herniation of the lacrimal gland which is present in the superolateral concavity of the orbit. Closure of the incision is done in layers, starting with periosteum, followed by the orbicularis oculi, and the skin.

An important advantage of the upper lid blepharoplasty incision is the extensive access it offers to the entire superolateral aspect of the orbit. It also permits good visualization and access to the spheno-zygomatic suture which is the most important indicator of reduction of ZMC fractures.

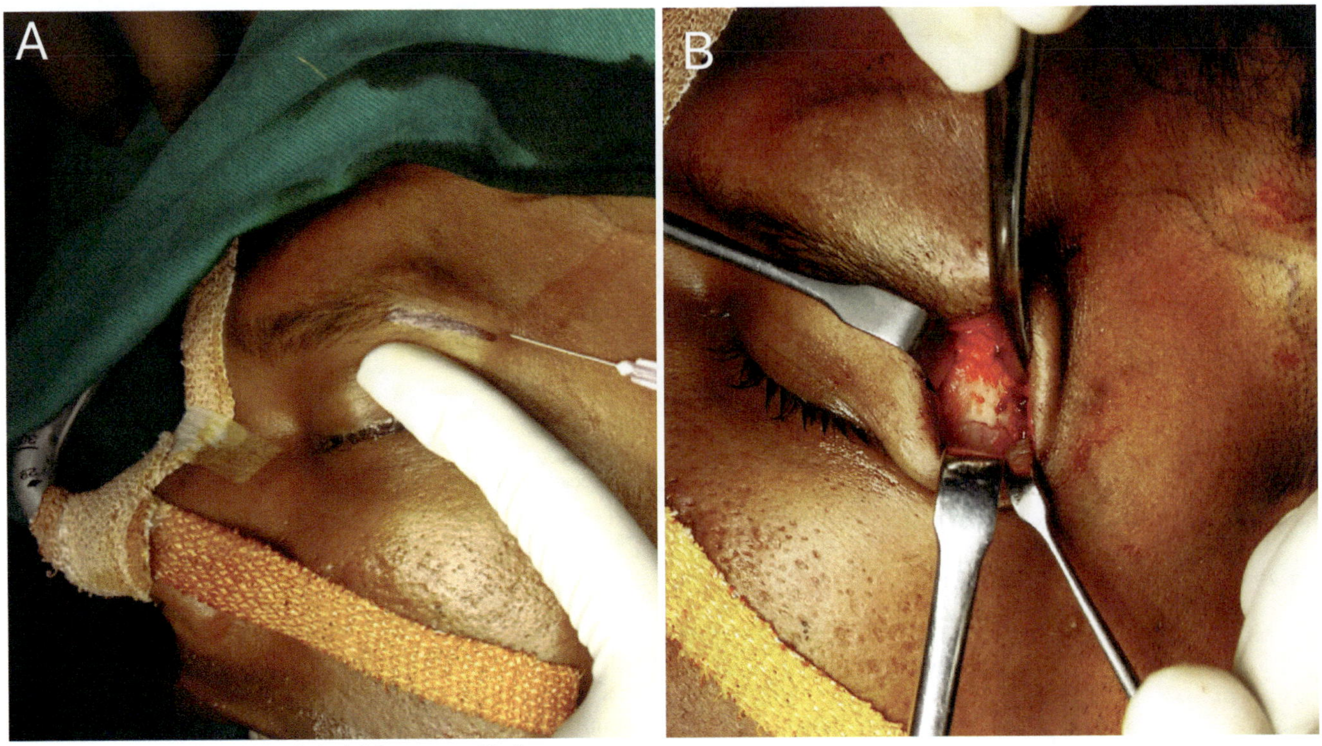

Fig. 56.42 Lateral brow incision—intra-operative. (**a**) Marking. (**b**) Exposure

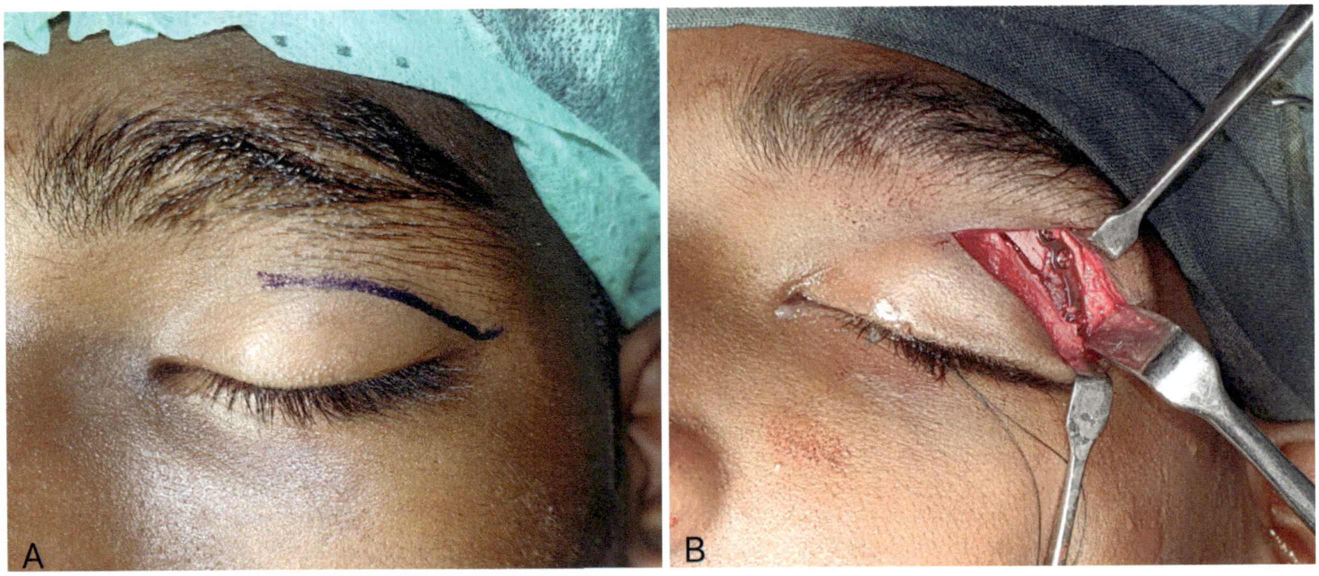

Fig. 56.43 Upper lid blepharoplasty intra-operative. (**a**) Marking. (**b**) Exposure demonstrating ORIF

56.9.3.3 Subciliary Incision [71, 72] (Figs. 56.38, 56.44a and 56.45a, b)

The subciliary incision is a commonly used transcutaneous approach which offers good exposure of the infra-orbital rim along with the entire orbital floor. This may be a very useful approach in the management of ZMC fractures which involve the orbital floor also.

The skin incision is placed along the entire length of the lower eyelid, 2 mm below the level of the eye lashes to conceal the future scar.

The incision must not be extended more than 2 cm lateral to the lateral canthal ligament. This prevents any inadvertent damage to the temporal branch of the facial nerve which is present about 3 cm lateral to the lateral canthal ligament.

Once the skin is incised, the dissection may proceed in three different ways [30, 70] (Fig. 56.45b) (Box 56.9):

(i) ***"Skin-alone" flap technique*** where the plane of dissection is along the *subcutaneous plane between the skin of the eyelid and the orbicularis oculi.* On reaching the facial surface of the infra-orbital rim, the orbicularis muscle along with the periosteum is incised to reach the rim. The periosteal incision is generally placed at least 3–4 mm below the level of the infra-orbital rim (Fig. 56.45a and 56.45b1).

(ii) ***"Skin-muscle" technique:*** the incision is carried down from the skin into the pre-tarsal fibers of the orbicularis oculi, and the flap is dissected along the *plane deep to the muscle but superficial to the tarsal plate*. The dissection is then carried out superficial to the orbital septum till the rim is reached. Exposure of the rim is performed after sharp dissection of the periosteum just below the level of the rim (Fig. 56.45b2).

(iii) ***"Step" approach*** is performed in two different levels and is considered the best approach as it prevents most of the complications which are associated with the two former approaches. The incision is first placed through the skin, and the plane of dissection is carried in the *subcutaneous plane, maintaining the pre-tarsal fibers of the orbicularis oculi.* As the lower end of the tarsal plate is reached, the orbicularis oculi muscle is divided, and the plane is changed to include the muscle along with the skin as a "skin-muscle" flap (Fig. 56.45b3).

The development of a skin-alone flap at the marginal level and a "skin-muscle" flap at the subtarsal level creates a ***step*** in the plane of dissection. The dissection then proceeds caudally toward the infra-orbital rim in a submuscular plane superficial to the orbital septum. On reaching the rim, the periosteum is incised sharply about 3–4 mm below the level of the rim on the facial aspect.

Box 56.9: Comparison of Variants of Subciliary Incisions

	Skin flap	Skin-muscle flap	Stepped skin-muscle flap
Skin incision	2 mm below the cilia	2 mm below the cilia	2 mm below the cilia
Muscle incision	Just below the infra-orbital rim	Same level as skin incision	2–3 mm below the skin incision
Periosteum incision	Just below the infra-orbital rim	Just below the infra-orbital rim	Just below the infra-orbital rim
Plane of dissection	Between skin and orbicularis muscle	Between orbicularis muscle and septum	• Stepped • Between skin and orbicularis muscle in pre-tarsal region • Between orbicularis muscle and septum—inferior to the tarsal region
Preservation of pre- tarsal fibers of orbicularis oculi	Preserved	Incised	Preserved
Complications	Skin buttonholing, discoloration	Septal perforation Ectropion Lid shortening Scleral show	Lesser incidence of complications

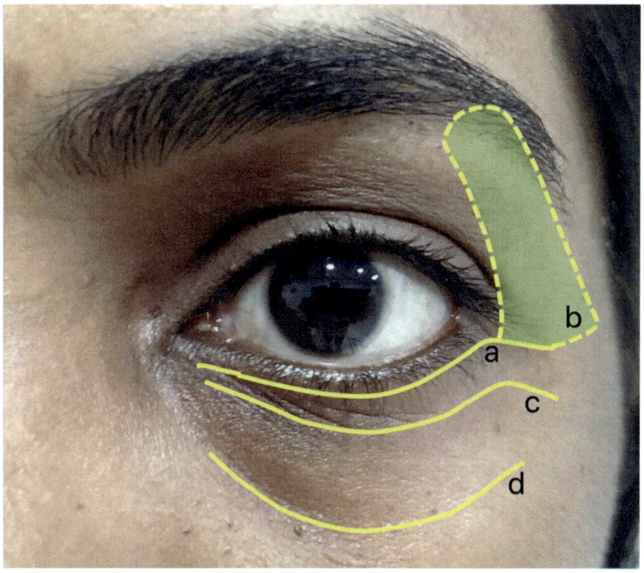

Fig. 56.44 Lower eyelid incisions. (a) Subciliary. (b) Extended subciliary showing area of exposure shaded. (c) Subtarsal incision. (d) Infra orbital

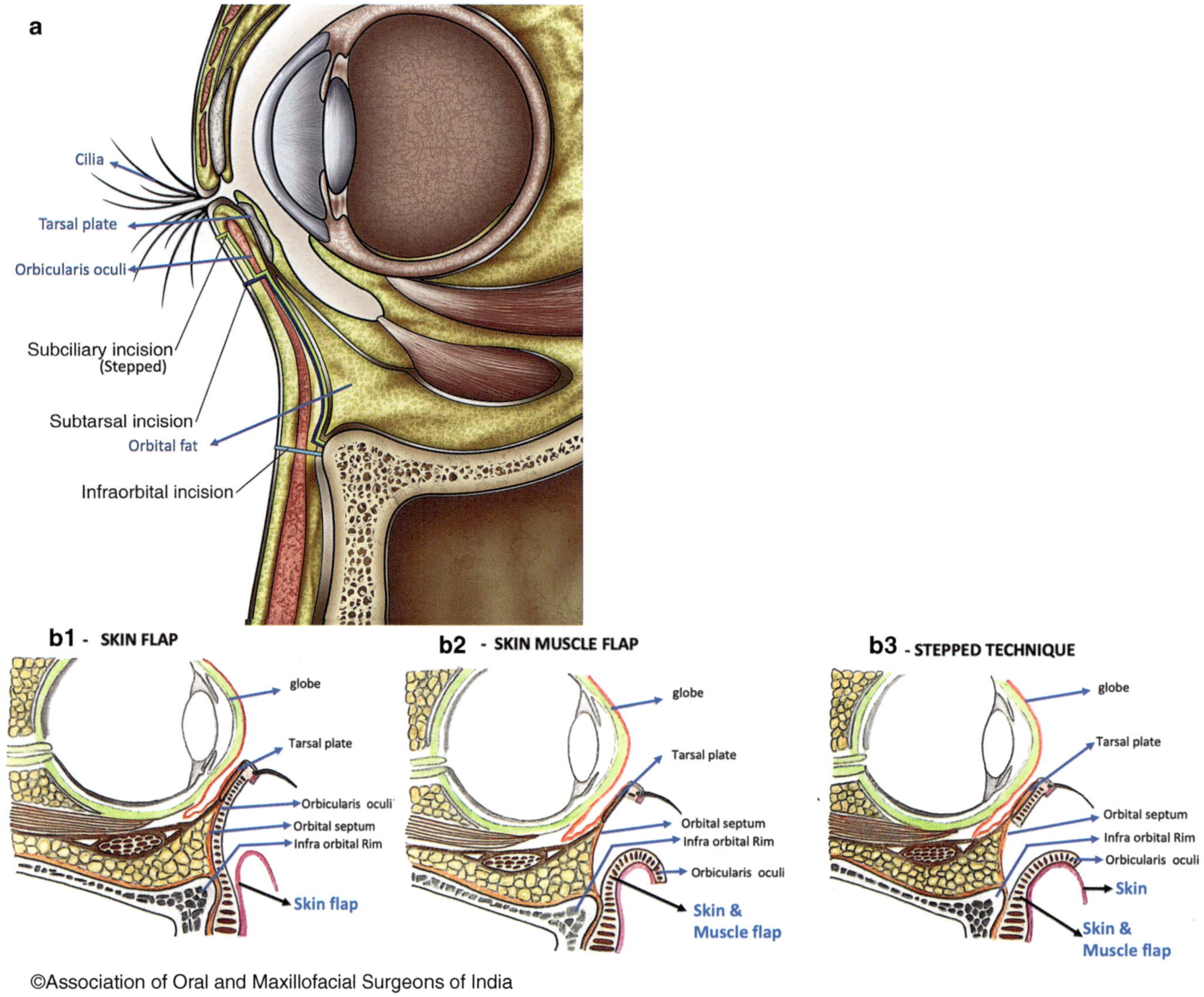

Fig. 56.45 Lower eyelid incisions—sagittal view. (a) Subciliary, sub tarsal and infra-orbital (b) Variants of sub-ciliary incision

The incision of the periosteum at this level not only helps preserve the attachment of the orbital septum along the rim margin but also lies above the level of the infra-orbital foramen which is seen about 7–8 mm below the level of the rim. Dissection of the periosteum can be performed along the entire length of the infra-orbital rim, anterior maxilla, and the zygoma to provide excellent exposure.

> Advantages of the stepped approach include (1) minimal chances of buttonholing or darkening of the skin due to vascular compromise (2) lesser incidence of ectropion and entropion (3) reduced scarring at the eyelid margins due to preservation of the pre-tarsal orbicularis oculi fibers.

The differences between the three variants of subciliary incision are highlighted in Box 56.9 (Figs. 56.45b).

56.9.3.4 Extended Lateral Exposure with the Subciliary Approach Fig. 56.46 [70]

After placing a standard subciliary incision, supraperiosteal dissection is performed along the lateral orbital rim in the cephalic direction till the FZ suture or a few millimeters beyond (Figs. 56.44b and 56.46). This releases the skin flap and makes it amenable to easy retraction to reach the FZ region. The periosteum is then divided in the center of the lateral orbital rim along its length. In most cases the lateral canthal ligament may be stripped in a subperiosteal fashion to facilitate comfortable access to the FZ suture. This approach may be used to avoid an additional incision for exposure of the FZ suture.

56.9.3.5 Subtarsal Approach [73] (Figs. 56.38, 56.44c and 56.47)

Subtarsal or ***mid-lid incision*** was also described by Converse. The incision is marked 5–7 mm below the inferior lid margin corresponding to the lower border of the tarsal plate, along

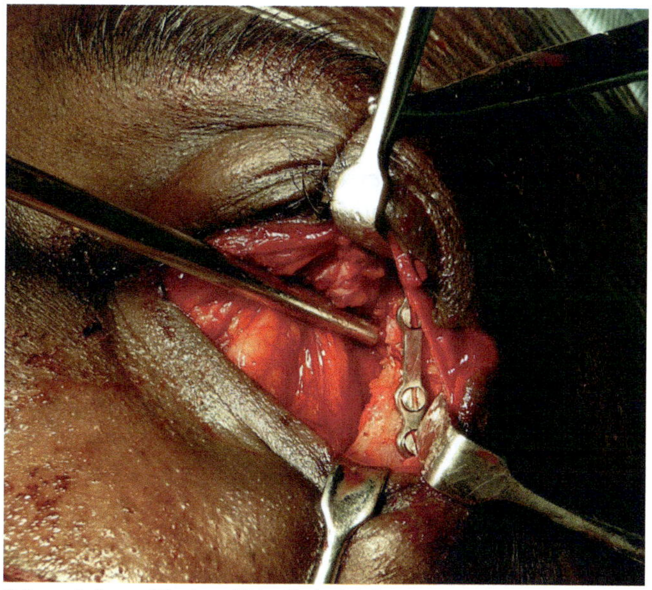

Fig. 56.46 Subciliary with lateral extension demonstrating exposure of the FZ suture after ORIF

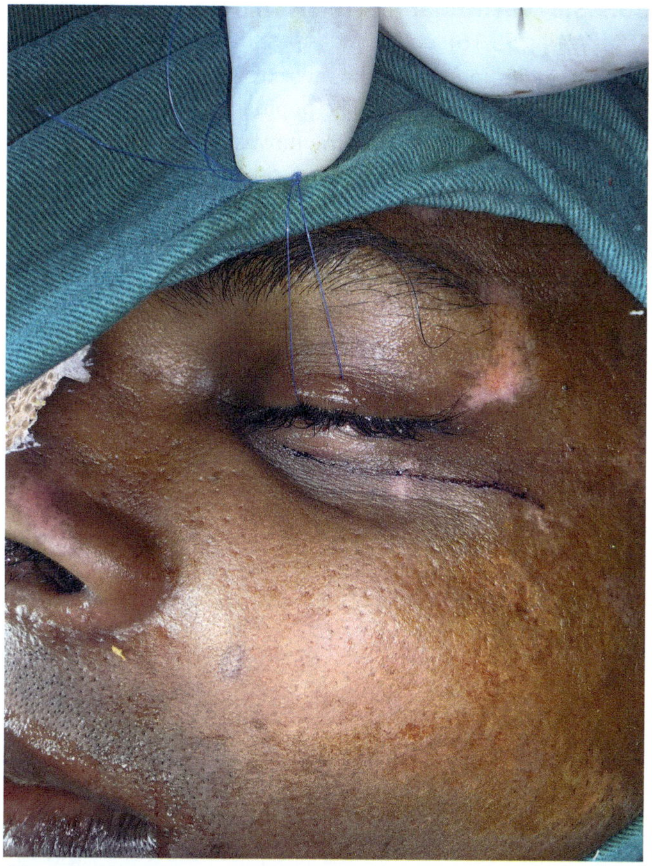

Fig. 56.47 Subtarsal marking intra-operative

the subtarsal crease (Fig. 56.47). The lateral extension of the incision may be extended up to 2 cm beyond the lateral canthal ligament similar to the subciliary incision, along one of the resting skin tension lines. The incision is made through the skin and subcutaneous tissue. The *pre-septal fibers of the orbicularis oculi are also divided at the same level*, and the plane of dissection is maintained superficial to the orbital septum. The dissection is carried out caudally to reach the infraorbital rim, and the periosteum is divided below the level of the rim on the anterior surface of the maxilla and zygoma.

The subtarsal approach is favored more than the subciliary [73] due to its easier technique and lesser incidence of complications (Box 56.10).

Box 56.10: Subtarsal vs. Subciliary Incision

	Subtarsal	Subciliary
Ease of technique	Easy	Technically demanding due to • Stepped dissection and closure • Interference of lashes in the surgical field
Time taken for the approach	Quick	Takes almost twice the amount of time
Incidence of scleral show or ectropion	2.7–7.7%	17–42%
Cutaneous scar	More visible	Less visible

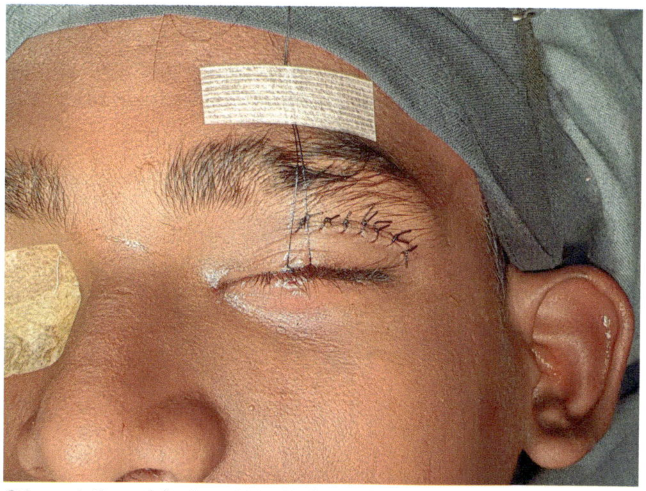

Fig. 56.48 Figure demonstrates use of frost suture for ZMC fracture approached by transconjunctival and upper lid blepharoplasty incision. *Technique for frost suture. A 4-0/5-0 nonabsorbable suture on a 3/8th circle needle is passed to engage the inferior tarsal plate, at the middle of the lower eyelid margin. The suture is taken either through the gray line or through the pre-tarsal skin to include the skin, orbicularis, and the tarsus. Appropriate tension is applied in superior direction by the anchoring the suture ends, to the supraorbital skin, 5 mm above the eyebrow using adhesive tapes*

An important consideration following lower eyelid approaches is the application of the "frost suture" [74] (temporary lower eyelid suspension suture) (Fig. 56.48), to prevent postoperative ectropion. Frost suture also permits visualization of the globe in the postoperative phase, when required (Refer Fig 11.13).

Nevertheless, lower rim incisions are often associated with postoperative ectropion and scleral show. While scleral show/lid traction refers to abnormal exposure of sclera (1 mm or more) with contact between bulbar conjunctiva and the lid, ectropion refers to eyelid eversion with no contact between bulbar conjunctiva and lid [75]. Ectropion requires correction for cosmetic reasons as well as functional problems arising from keratinization of exposed conjunctiva. Treatment varies from conservative modalities to surgical procedures [76, 77] (Box 56.11).

Box 56.11: Measures to Correct Ectropion and Scleral Show

- *Conservative measures*
  Corneal protection measures; artificial tears, ointment, temporary tarsorrhaphy
- *Surgical procedures*
  Release of cicatrization, sutures, skin/mucosal grafts, cartilage grafts, rotation flaps

56.9.3.6 **Infra-orbital Incision** (Figs. 56.38 and 56.44d)

This is performed as an incision which simultaneously divides the skin, orbicularis muscle, and periosteum, along infra-orbital rim. Though the infra-orbital incision offers the most direct approach to the infra-orbital rim and orbital floor, it is seldom preferred in contemporary surgery due to the unsightly postoperative scar and prolonged edema of the lower lid region due to disruption of lymphatic drainage.

56.9.3.7 **Transconjunctival Incision** [78, 79] (Figs. 56.38 and 56.49)

Transconjunctival incision has gained popularity because it completely negates the unesthetic scarring associated with skin incisions. This incision offers good access to the infra-orbital rim and SZ regions with either a pre-septal or retro-septal approach. Refer to the Chap. 57 for a detailed description of the approach. The modified transconjunctival incision with a cutaneous Y extension when combined with lateral canthotomy offers excellent exposure to the IOR, SZ, as well as the FZ region [80–82]. The complications of transconjunctival incisions include entropion [82], in-curling of lashes (trichiasis) [83], or growth of the eyelashes in two layers (distichiasis) [84]. Malposed lateral canthus has also been observed following improper repositioning of the lateral canthus after canthotomy [82].

56.9.3.8 **Vestibular** [85] **Incision** (Figs. 56.50 and 55.16)

The vestibular incision is the most frequently used approach to access the ZM buttress. The popularity is due to its application for reduction of ZMC fracture as well as fixation at the ZM buttress. Refer to the Chap. 55 for description of the technique. The author of this chapter (EP) uses the vestibular approach to also fix the zygomatic arch fractures which override at the zygomaticotemporal suture, with transbuccal instrumentation (transoral arch fixation technique) (Refer to recent trends section 56.16).

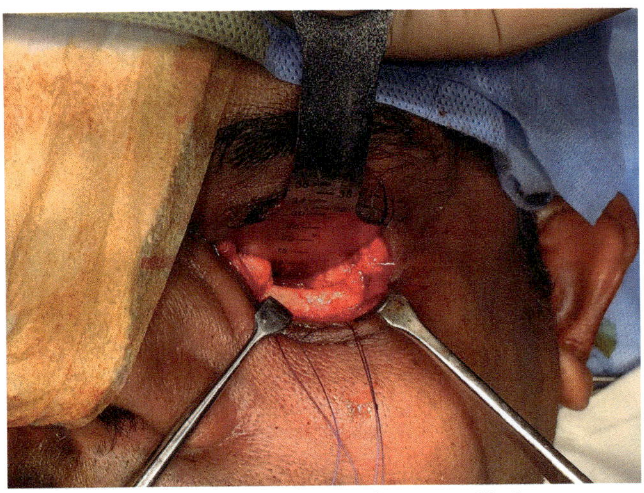

Fig. 56.49 Transconjunctival intra-operative

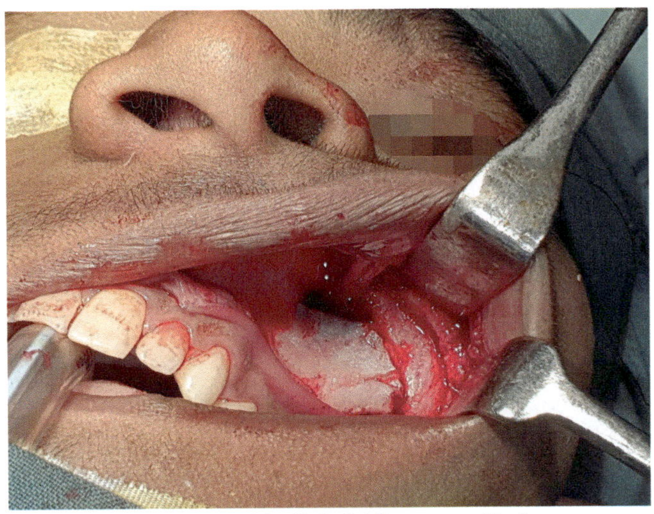

Fig. 56.50 Vestibular incision demonstrating fracture at ZM buttress

56.9.3.9 Preauricular [86] (Figs. 56.38, 56.51, 53.17a, b and 65.6) (Refer Video on pre auricular approach in Chap. 53)

Preauricular incision is useful for open reduction and fixation of arch fractures. After the routine skin incision, adopting the deep subfascial approach provides better protection to the facial nerve as compared to the other commonly used approaches, namely, the subfascial and suprafascial procedures [87]. Figure 56.51 demonstrates the use of preauricular incision with deep subfascial dissection to expose a malunited zygomatic arch fracture.

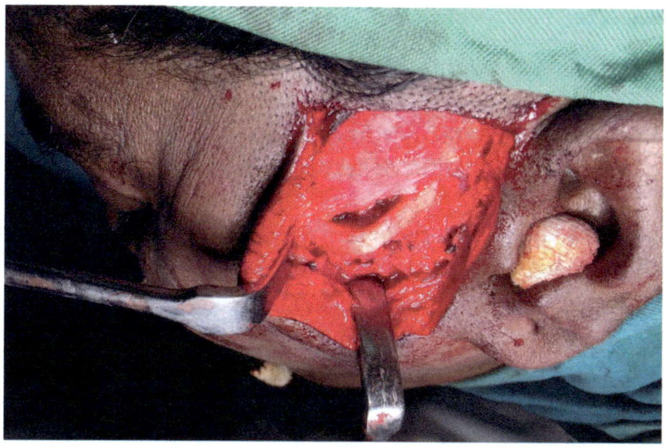

Fig. 56.51 Preauricular approach demonstrating exposure of malunited zygomatic arch fracture

56.9.3.10 Coronal Incision [88] (Figs. 56.38, 56.52a, b and 85.1)

Tessier introduced the use of coronal incision to access the superior and lateral orbits bilaterally along with naso-orbito-ethmoid complex in congenital facial reconstruction. The approach can be extended with a preauricular incision to include the exposure of the zygomatic body and the arches bilaterally. This incision also facilitates the temporal approach to the SZ suture [82]. Disadvantages of the approach include the extensive length of incision, dissection, temporal hollowing, scar alopecia, risk of injury to the supra-orbital nerve, and temporal branch of the facial nerve.

56.9.4 Fixation Methods

Fixation methods for ZMC fractures have evolved through the ages.

Three basic fixation methods are available for ZMC fractures [1] (Table 56.1):

1. Temporary support
2. Indirect fixation and
3. Direct fixation

The trend has gradually shifted from nonrigid fixation methods such as trans-osseous wiring, external pin fixation, and K wires to functionally rigid fixation methods including

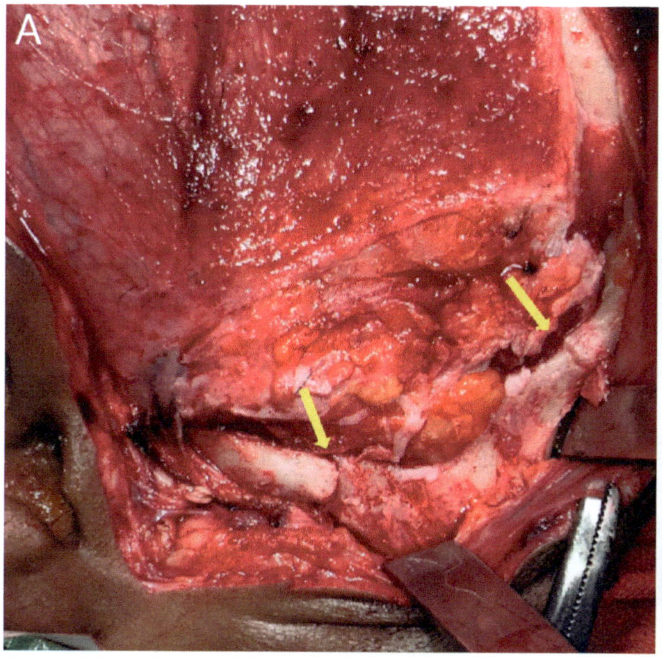

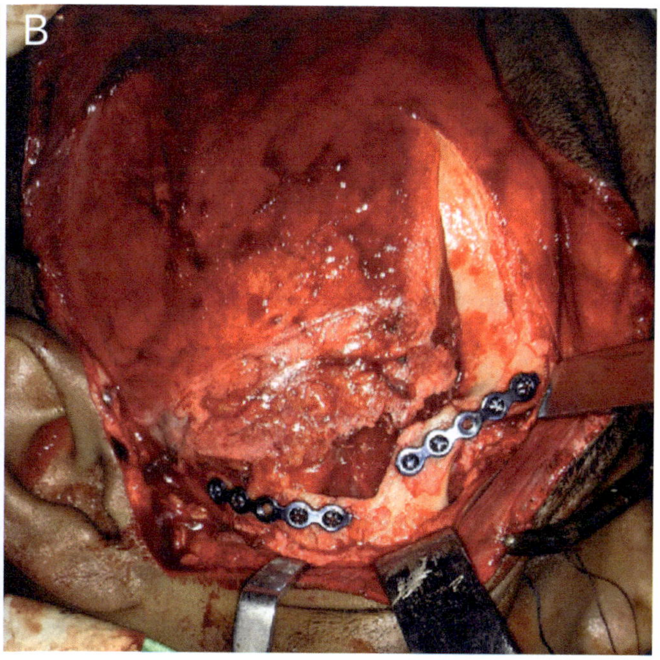

Fig. 56.52 Coronal approach, intra-operative. (**a**) Exposure of arch demonstrating fractured zygomatic arch and FZ region (yellow arrows). (**b**) Arch after reduction and fixation at ZT and FZ region

Table 56.1 Fixation methods for ZMC fractures

	Temporary support	Indirect fixation	Direct fixation
Access to fracture	Fracture is not visualized	Fracture is not visualized	Fracture is visualized by surgical exposure
Fixation technique	Provide support to reduced fragments	Indirectly fixed using anchorage from a distant site	Directly fixed
Modalities	• Antral pack • Antral balloon • Silicone wedge • Percutaneous wire with splint (arch)	• Trans-osseous pins (K wire, Steinmann pins) • External fixatorsCranio-zygomaticFronto-zygomatic	• Trans-osseous wiring • Miniplates and screws • Microcompressive screws
Advantages	Less surgical morbidity	Less hardware Less invasive	• Functionally stable/semi rigid/rigid (lag screw) • Anatomic reduction possible
Limitations	• Nonrigid • Not precise • Chances of infection • Poor patient compliance	• Poor patient compliance • Non-precise • Chances of pin track infection • Requires second intervention for removal	• Wiring is nonrigid • Surgical morbidity
Indications	When the surgery must be delayed (eg. compromised systemic status)	• Comminuted fractures • Inability to visualise fracture site (Please add bullets for both these points)	For most fractures, unless contraindicated

miniplates and compressive screws. However, some of the nonrigid fixation modalities are still applicable in certain clinical situations. A brief description of all fixation methods is provided below along with their indications and limitations.

- ***Trans-osseous wiring*** using stainless steel wires is rarely used in current practice due to its nonrigid mode of fixation that compromises post-reduction stability. However, it still remains a useful technique for fracture reduction by traction, especially at the FZ and IOR. The advantages include minimal periosteal stripping and lesser hardware as compared to use of miniplates and screws.
- **Antral packing** [89] with gauze or balloon/Foley's catheter is used in special scenarios where the ZMC is comminuted. But it is an inaccurate technique with high relapse potential and increased possibility of infection.

  Antral packing may be done either with a roller gauze pack or balloon. The technique followed for both is similar. The anterolateral wall of the maxilla is exposed by a Caldwell-Luc incision in the vestibule through which the fracture is inspected and manipulated to achieve reduction of the fragments. A trans-nasal antrostomy port is created in the inferior meatus. (refer Sect. 24.10, Fig. 24.24)

  – The *medicated ribbon gauze* pack is introduced into the antrum through trans-nasal antrostomy, and one end of the gauze is packed tight in the antrum under direct visualization through the vestibular incision. The oral layer is closed, once the desired level of packing is achieved. The other end which is free is pulled out through the nostril and taped to the cheek. This is later used to retrieve the pack once the healing phase is complete.

  – The *inflatable balloon* is positioned within the sinus cavity in a similar manner and verified through the vestibular approach. The balloon is then inflated with about 20cc of saline till adequate support is obtained for the reduced fragments. The vestibular approach is then closed meticulously without damaging the balloon. The balloon is left in situ for the fracture to heal. Removal is accomplished by deflating the balloon and pulling it out through the antrostomy port.
- **Kirchner or K wires and Steinmann pins** [1, 90] (Fig. 56.53a–c) are still popular in some units as they serve as tools of reduction as well as fixation. But these techniques are associated with cutaneous scars and poor patience compliance due to the transcutaneous presence of pins. The noteworthy advantages of external pin fixation are the reduced cost and the possibility of adjusting the fixation in the immediate postoperative period.
- K wires and Steinmann pins constitute an indirect method of fixation whereby the fractured zygomatic bone is fixed in a secure fashion to another stable point in the craniofacial skeleton. Such indirect anchorage may be obtained by using pins (1) to secure the fractured fragment to other stable bones or (2) to provide anchorage for connectors of an external fixator. The different techniques of indirect fixation that have been advocated for management of ZMC fractures include (Fig. 56.54):

  (A) ***Trans-zygomatic***—by this technique, the zygoma is first reduced through an intraoral approach to

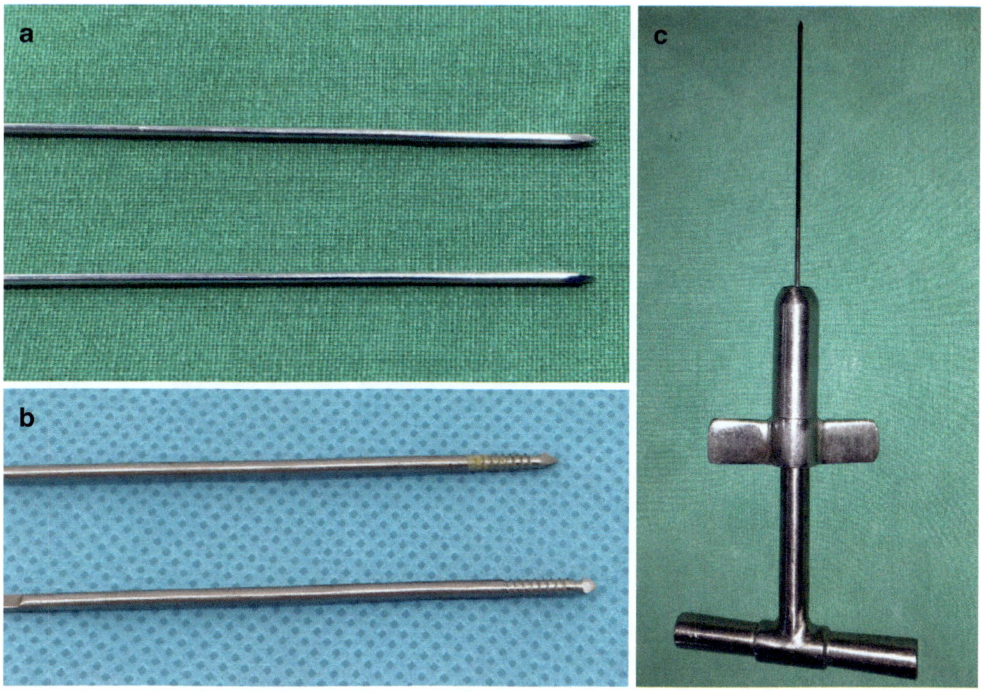

Fig. 56.53 Armamentarium for indirect fixation. (**a**) K wire. (**b**) Steinmann pin. (**c**) Manual K-wire driver

enable adequate visualization of the entry of K wire/pin thorough the vestibular incision. The reduced ZMC is then stabilized by transfixing it to the contralateral zygoma using a K wire. The K wire is passed from the body of the reduced zygoma in a trans-facial fashion to engage the stable cortex of the contralateral zygoma by the use of a K-wire driver.

(B) ***Naso-zygomatic***—this method involves the use of a K wire to stabilize the reduced ZMC to the frontal process of the maxilla on the contralateral side. The wire is driven from the frontal process of the maxilla in a forward and downward direction to engage the antral surface of the zygomatic body. This must be done with care to prevent any inadvertent damage to the nasolacrimal duct which lies adjacent to the path of pin.

(C) ***Zygomatico-palatal***—this procedure involves fixation of the reduced ZMC to the palatal surface of the contralateral maxilla, by passing a K wire through the reduced ZMC in a downward and oblique direction.

Indirect fixation may also be performed by the use of external fixators or a halo frame that can be attached to pins for anchorage. This may include the techniques described below.

(D) ***Fronto-zygomatic fixation***: This technique involves the use of a Steinmann pin for anchorage onto the reduced ZMC fragment. The pin is then anchored to another pin which is fixed on the stable orbital process of the frontal bone by the use of an external fixator device.

(E) ***Cranio-zygomatic fixation:*** This method is performed in the same fashion as the fronto-zygomatic method, except that the stable component for anchorage is from a halo frame that is cranially anchored, rather than a single pin on the frontal bone.

- **Lag screws** [91] have been found to be an effective alternative at the FZ region because of the additional stability offered by interfragmentary compression. But this technique requires adequate bone stock for fixation.
- **Micro screws** [92]: Micro screws are 2 mm screws which are used to fix sagittal zygomatic fractures by using the lag screw technique. These screws also reduce hardware (Fig. 56.55a–c).
- **Miniplates** [3, 4]: The principal method of fixation is miniplate osteosynthesis. Miniplates are chosen based on

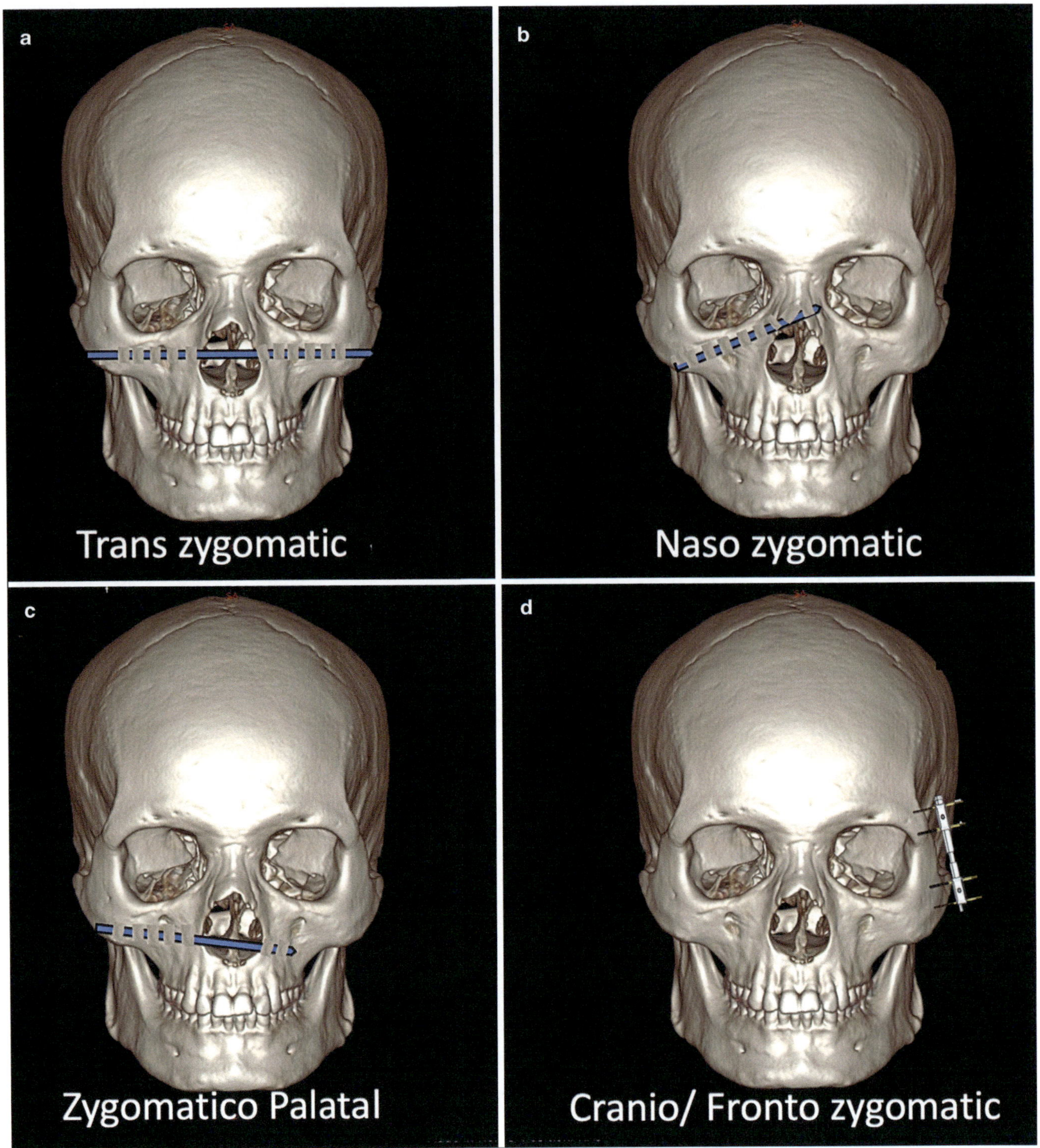

Fig. 56.54 Techniques for indirect fixation

rigidity requirements, anatomical site involved, presence of bone deficits, and biological considerations pertaining to protection of adjacent vital structures.

Shape of plates: The plates are chosen according to the contour of the bone that needs to be fixed; L plate for the ZM suture and a curved plate for the IOR.

Presence of bone loss: Comminuted fractures or bone loss may result in sagging of overlying soft tissues, especially in the ZM buttress region. This may be negated by using a broad mesh that bridges defects.

Biological considerations: Care must be taken to protect the roots, infra-orbital nerve and eye during fixation. In regions where the skin is thin, low-profile plates are preferred, 2 mm system for the ZM buttresses and 1.5 mm at the FZ, IOR, arch, and SZ suture [72].

Stability requirements: For ideal stability, screws of 6 mm length with a minimum of two screws on either side of fracture are essential. The only exception being the SZ suture where one screw on either side of the fracture line is adequate.

- *Fixation points:* The number of fixation points is directly proportional to the requirements of stability. Five different possibilities exist (Fig. 56.56a–f):
  - One-point fixation [92] refers to fixation at either the FZ or ZM suture. This has been found to be adequate in resisting post-reduction in-stability in simple tripod fractures while reducing hardware and surgical exposure.

    Comparative studies have shown that one-point fixation at the ZM buttress has been found to more advantageous due to many reasons: (1) absence of external scarring; (2) ease of surgical access; (3) unlike the FZ region, adequate soft tissue cover is present; and there are no issues of plate palpability; (4) easier to remove the plate, when needed; and most importantly (5) ZM buttress is a better indicator of zygoma alignment than the FZ region due to the wider area of articulation. However, FZ may be used in fractures with comminuted ZM buttress.
  - Two-point fixation indicates fixation at ZM and FZ/IOR [93, 94].
  - Three-point fixation/tripoding includes fixation at the FZ, IOR, and the ZM. A recent meta-analysis indicates that three-point fixation is the most effective in ensuring absolute clinical stability against displacing forces after reduction [94].
  - Four-point fixation/tetrapoding [95] involves fixation at the FZ, IOR, arch, and the ZM. This may be indicated in panfacial fractures requiring fixation of the arch to restore the anteroposterior projection of the face (case scenarios 1 and 2).
  - Five-point fixation/pentapoding [4] is used to manage severely comminuted or dislocated ZMC fractures wherein the SZ suture is also fixed, in addition to the other four sites of fixation. The SZ fixation may be performed either through a temporal or an intra-orbital approach

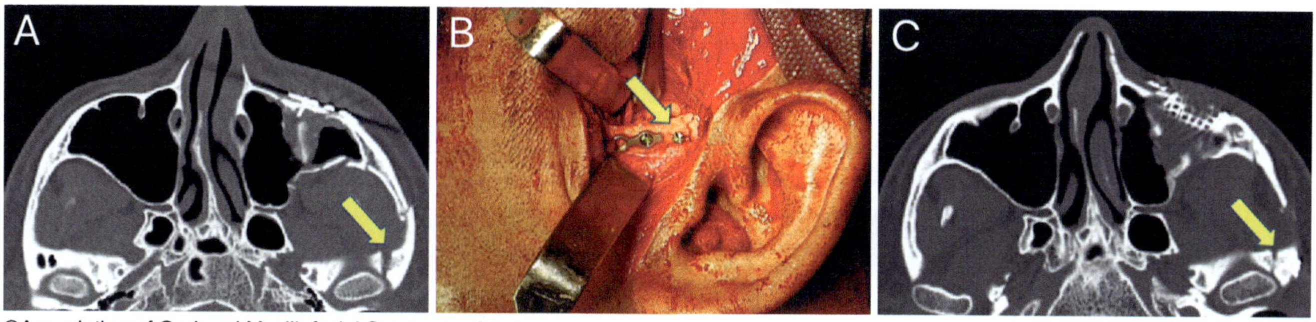

Fig. 56.55 Fixation of zygomatic arch fracture with microcompressive screws a, b, and c. (**a**) Preoperative CT showing diastasis at the zygomatic root. (**b**) Intra-operative picture showing arch fixation with screw. (**c**) Postoperative CT showing adequate fracture reduction and screw fixation

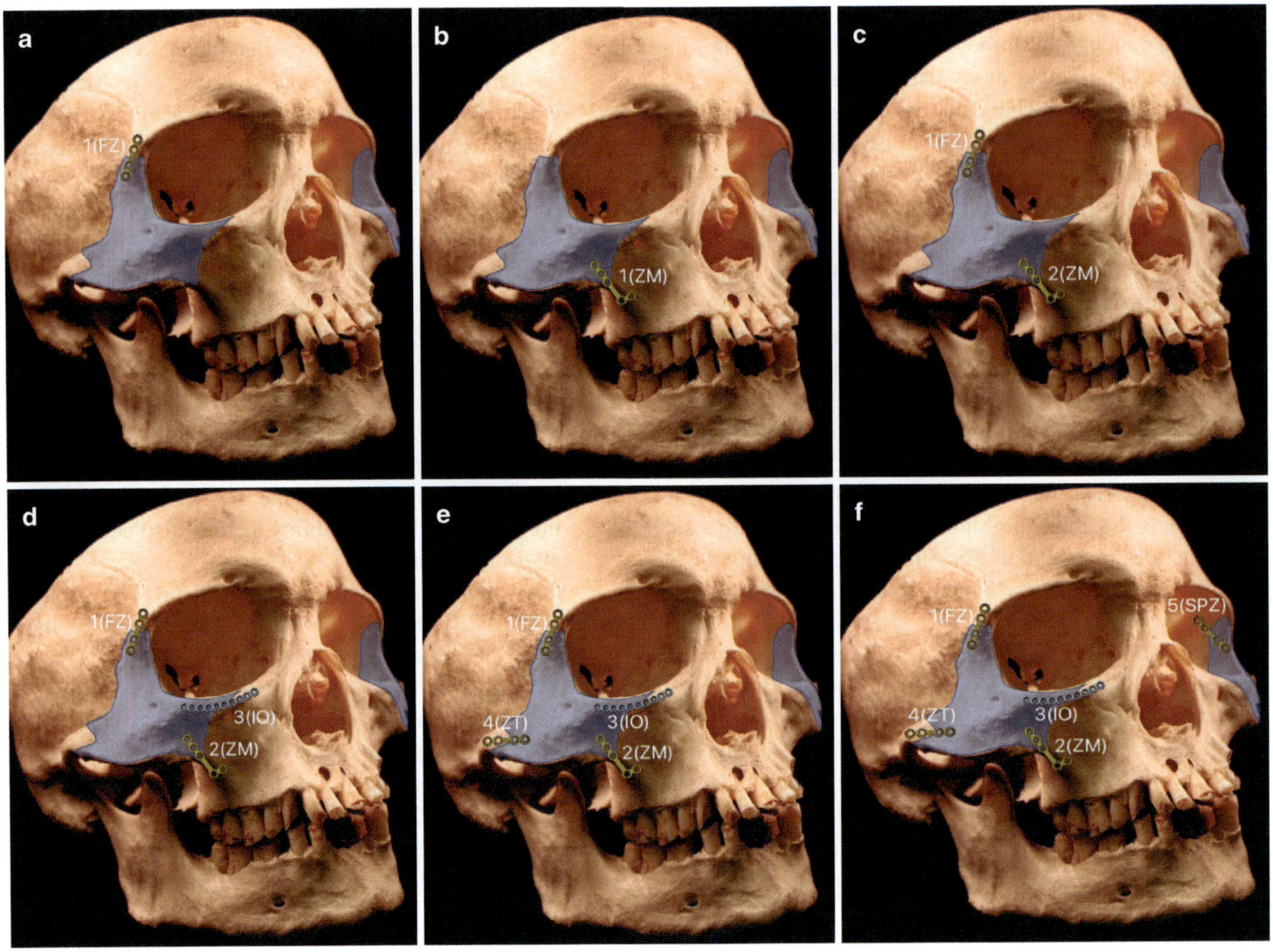

Fig. 56.56 Types of fixation using miniplates. (**a**) One-point fixation at FZ suture; (**b**) one-point fixation at ZM buttress; (**c**) two-point fixation; (**d**) three-point fixation; (**e**) four-point fixation; and (**f**) five-point fixation (the 5th articulation (SPZ) of the right is unseen and hence is depicted on the contralateral side for better understanding)

– ZMC fractures requiring orbital reconstruction [59]: irrespective of the type of fixation, when ZMC fracture is associated with orbit, the orbital rims are fixed first. This is important because it is safer and easier to gauge the depth of orbital dissection from the restored infraorbital rim and also to facilitate floor reconstruction [66] (case scenario 2). Also, the size of the orbital defect is better assessed when the rims are aligned.

- **Bio-resorbable plates** [96, 97]

  Though titanium miniplates are more commonly used to fix ZMC fractures, substantial clinical success has been obtained with use of bio-resorbable plates. They offer comparable post-reduction stability along with the added advantages of preventing thermal sensitivity and avoiding the need for second surgery to remove plates. Limitations associated with bio-resorbable plates are its technique sensitivity and increased operating time.

56.9.5 Fixation of Zygomatic Arch

The ORIF of arch fracture is indicated when the fragments are unstable after closed reduction and in cases where re-establishment of sagittal projection of face is needed. Fixation may be performed by one of the three methods, based on the fracture pattern (Fig. 56.57a, b, c): (1) a miniplate for an arch demonstrating a single fracture line (Fig. 56.52b), (2) a spanning adaptation plate (Fig. 56.62b) when the arch is multi-fragmented [98], and (3) a micro screw for an outfractured root or sagittal fracture of the arch [99] (Fig. 56.55). Kim et al. proposed plating on the superior surface of the upper border as an alternate line of arch fixation which negated the drawbacks associated with the conventional fixation [100] (Fig. 56.57).

56.10 Soft Tissue Resuspension [101, 102]

Accurate reduction and fixation of ZMC fractures frequently necessitates the use of multiple incisions on the midface which deglove the entire periosteum-muscle-fat complex of the midface and zygoma. Failure to re-approximate the dissected tissues may lead to undesirable changes in the soft tissue projection and form.

> The various changes that may be a sequel to wide subperiosteal dissection of the midface include (1) cheek ptosis, (2) descent of the lower eyelid skin and infraorbital hollowness, (3) loss of malar prominence due to inferior displacement of the malar fat pad, and (4) exaggeration of the nasolabial fold [101].

Over the years many authors have documented these undesirable changes and proposed soft tissue resuspension methods to minimize them. This can be achieved by various methods (Fig. 56.58a): (1) re-approximating the incised periosteum using absorbable sutures, (2) by suspending the periosteum using heavy absorbable or nonabsorbable sutures to a drill hole placed in a superiorly positioned bony landmark

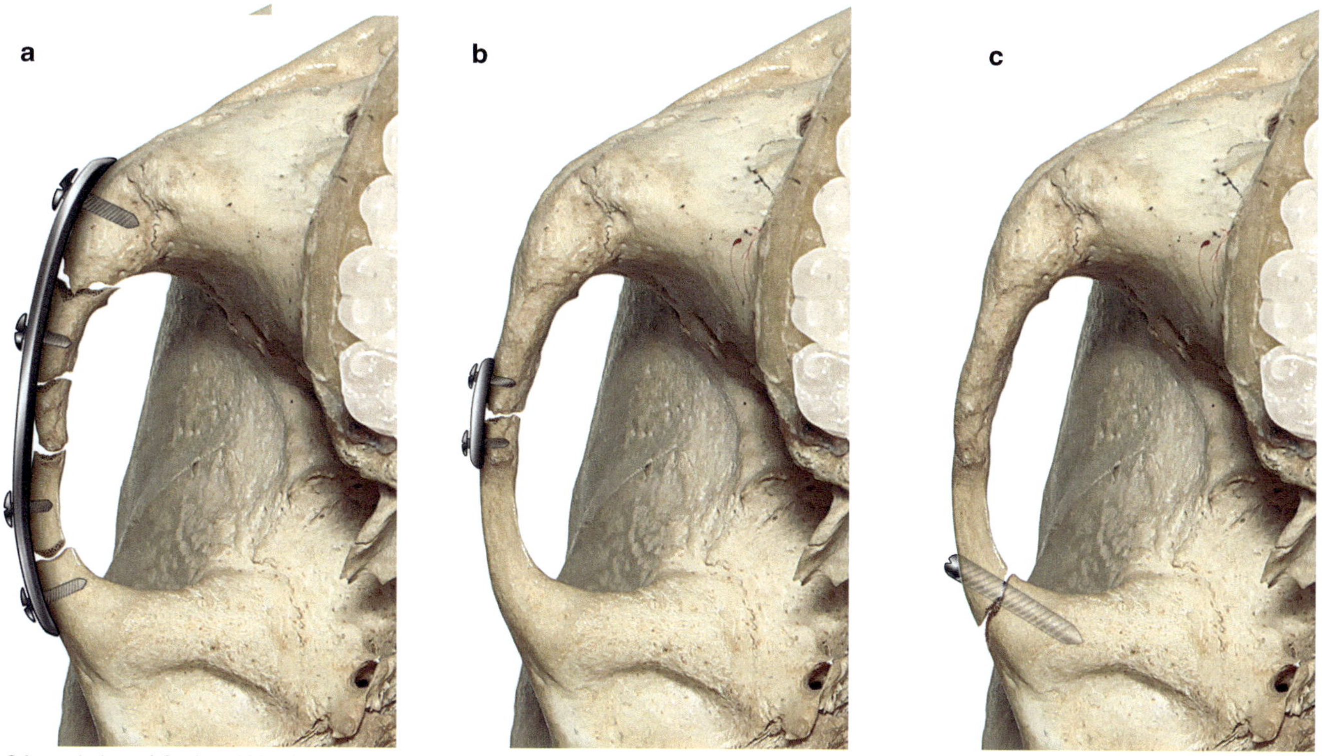

Fig. 56.57 Different fixation options for zygomatic arch fractures. (**a**) Adaptation plate. (**b**) Miniplate. (**c**) Compressive screw

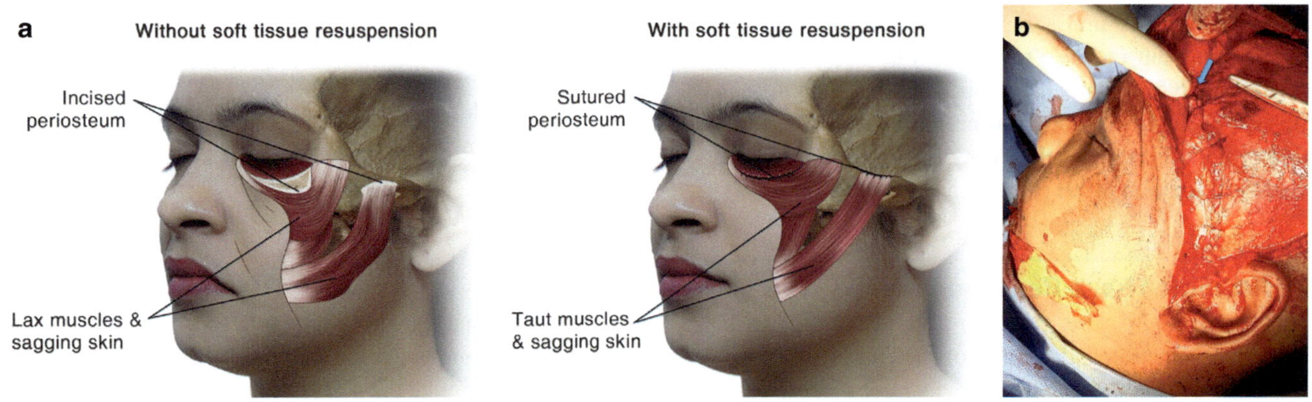

Fig. 56.58 Soft tissue resuspension. (**a**) Graphical representation. (**b**) Resuspension of temporal soft tissues to deep temporal fascia (blue arrow)

such as the orbital rim [103], (3) resuspension of lateral facial and temporal soft tissues to the deep temporal fascia in the temporal region [104] (Fig. 56.58b), and (4) prophylactic endoscopic midface lift [101].

56.11 Postoperative Care

Following reduction of ZMC fractures, with or without fixation, the following measures are taken to maintain post-surgical stability and prevent soft tissue complications (Box 56.12):

Box 56.12: Postsurgical Care

- Soft diet
- Protection of surgical site and eye
- Frost suture
- Post-op sinus regimen
- Periodic assessment of vision
- Anti-edema measures
- Anti-emphysema measures
- Physiotherapy (eye and mouth opening)

- Soft diet: Patients managed with conservative methods are advised soft diet for a period of 2 weeks.
- Protection of surgical site: The reduced zygoma or the arch must be protected with a tape labelled "do not touch" to provide cognitive input to the patient and people around.
- Frost suture: This temporary suspension suture is maintained for 3–5 days in any patient undergoing an inferior eyelid approach for the prevention of ectropion.
- Post-op sinus regimen [105]: A sinus regimen including prophylactic antibiotics for sinus coverage and decongestants is advocated by some authors.
- Periodic assessment of vision [66]: Periodic ophthalmic examination for the first 2 postoperative weeks is mandatory, in an awake patient. In an unconscious patient, it is achieved by swinging flashlight test or VEP (visual evoked potential).
- Anti-edema measures: Head end elevation must be maintained to prevent facial edema.
- Anti-emphysema measures, such as avoiding nose blowing [106].
- Protection of eye with ophthalmic ointments.
- Physiotherapy to prevent postoperative trismus: Postoperative trismus is a common phenomenon following ORIF of ZMC fractures due to hematoma, reflex muscle spasms, and fibrosis. Measures such as physiotherapy, forced mouth opening using gag [107], and kinesiologic tapes [108] may be used to improve mouth opening.
- Eye movement exercises are encouraged to facilitate resolution of edema and expedite restitution of movements [66].

56.12 Pediatric Considerations

56.12.1 Nonsurgical vs. Surgical Intervention [109]

The incidence of ZMC fractures is high in pediatric population due to its prominence [109]. In children, most authors favor a "nonsurgical" management or "reduction without fixation" of ZMC fractures due to concerns regarding "surgery/implant-induced" growth disturbances of facial skeleton and injury to teeth. However, literature supports ORIF of zygoma fractures which are grossly displaced or unstable after reduction. This is very important in pediatric population to (1) correct the facial asymmetry which may cause psychological impact, (2) restitute normal mouth opening to permit mastication, and (3) restitute globe position and function to enable normal vision and prevent development of phthisical eye or hypoplasia of zygoma, in the future.

56.12.2 Approaches and Fixation Principles

The preferred approaches include vestibular and lateral brow with minimal soft tissue dissection. Literature suggests one-point fixation at FZ region as adequate for pediatric ZMC fractures because of the short lever arm forces between the FZ and IOR [110]. But current studies have demonstrated that two-point fixations provide adequate stability and are associated with the least complication rates when compared with one and three-point fixations. Similarly, fixation at the zygomaticomaxillary buttress had the least complications when compared against the fronto-zygomatic and infra-orbital fixations [111]. In contrast, Defazio et al. proposed that plating at the FZ and IOR may be done conveniently in children below 6 years without any risk of damage to tooth buds [112].

56.12.3 Osteosynthesis Methods

Fixation techniques prior to year 2000 advocated titanium miniplates for pediatric midface. However they must be removed after 2 months to prevent any growth disturbances, plate migration, or burying of plate due to bone apposition. Microplates and self-drilling screws are also reported to give adequate stability and fixation in this age group without compromising vital structures [110]. Alternatively, bio-resorbable plates may be used which became popular after year 2004 to negate the need for re-surgery for plate removal [113]. Figure 56.59a–f shows a case of displaced zygoma fracture in a 5-year-old boy managed by ORIF. The plates were removed after 2 months.

56.13 Malunited ZMC Fractures [114]

Malunion of the zygoma may be a sequel to two clinical scenarios, (1) a neglected ZMC fracture which was never treated and (2) an improperly treated fracture. The protocol for the management of the malunited zygoma is based on the type of deformity which may be either cosmetic or functional. The protocol followed by the author is demonstrated in Fig. 56.60.

Deformities producing aesthetic concerns may again be subdivided into those demonstrating facial asymmetry or those showing altered globe positions.

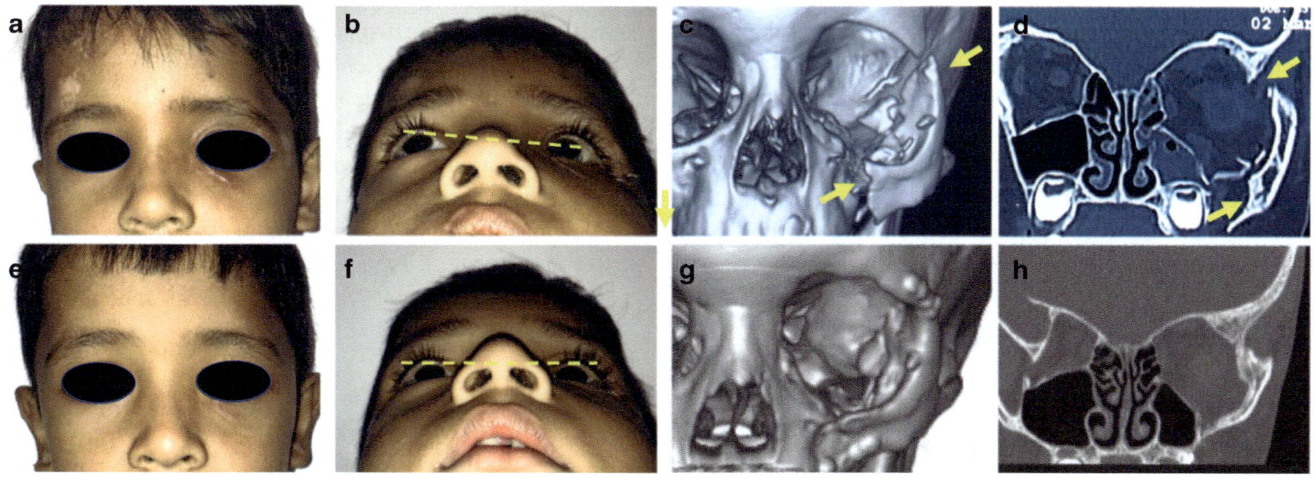

Fig. 56.59 ZMC fracture management in a pediatric patient. (**a**) Frontal view of patient with left-sided ZMC fracture. (**b**) Basal view demonstrating loss of facial projection and enophthalmos of left side. (**c**) Preoperative 3D CT image demonstrating en bloc displacement of ZMC. (**d**) Preoperative coronal section demonstrating separation at FZ suture and lateral displacement of the body of zygoma. (**e**) Postoperative frontal view. (**f**) Postoperative basal view demonstrating restoration of facial projection and enophthalmos correction. (**g**) Postoperative 3D CT. (**h**) Post-operative coronal section

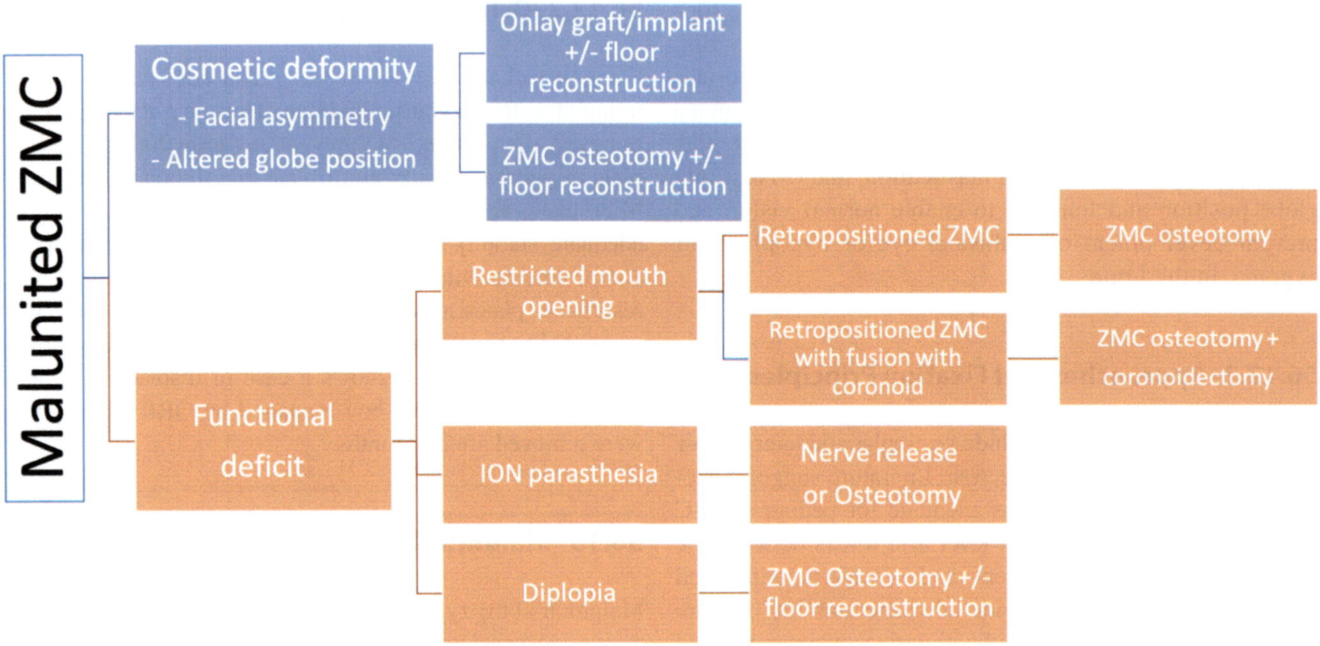

Fig. 56.60 Management of malunited ZMC fracture—algorithm

- The patients with asymmetries involving only the malar or infra-orbital regions with no functional deficits can be treated with onlay grafts which may either be autogenous in nature (rib, iliac crest, calvarium) or alloplastic (Medpore, PEEK (polyether ether ketone), etc.) (Fig. 56.61).
- Patients demonstrating gross facial asymmetry along with orbital dystopia and/or anti-mongoloid slant of the palpebral fissure may not be amenable to treatment with onlay augmentations. In such cases, a conventional osteotomy (re-fracture) and repositioning of the zygomatic complex is advocated (case scenario 2).
- When either of the deformities are associated with large floor defects, they require concomitant orbital floor reconstructions.

Functional deficits secondary to malunited ZMC fractures essentially fall into three categories; Restricted mouth opening, parasthesia and diplopia.

- Restricted mouth opening due to retropositioned zygoma/arch which either (1) forms a mechanical obstacle to mandibular translation or (2) fuses to the coronoid process of the mandible (extra-articular ankylosis) (Fig. 56.62a, b). The choice of treatment in these patients is dictated by the presence or absence of fusion (bony/fibrous); ZMC osteotomy, and repositioning alone are indicated in the absence of fusion, while presence of fusion mandates additional coronoidectomy [8, 115].
- Paresthesia over the infra-orbital nerve (ION) distribution: The entrapment of the ION or constriction of the infra-orbital foramen is not an uncommon finding. The first line of management in these patients is to perform a nerve release by an ostectomy around the infra-orbital foramen or by repositioning of the ZMC when it is compressing the nerve.
- Diplopia: The major cause for diplopia in ZMC fractures may either be gross displacement of the ZMC or mechanical restriction due to entrapment of orbital soft tissues (muscle, orbital septum, or fat) with resultant fibrosis or adhesions. Correction in these instances is achieved only by an osteotomy along with release of the entrapped tissues. These patients may also require orbital floor reconstructions if they present with floor defects that are large (>2 cm^2 in area). Non-resolving diplopia may be subjected to management with prism glasses and/or strabismus surgery.

56.14 Bilateral ZMC Fractures

Bilateral fractures of the ZMC are a rare occurrence and present more difficulty in achieving adequate reduction. In contrast to unilateral fractures where the normal side is used as a guide to achieve symmetry on the fractured side, bilateral ZMC fractures are complex in management. Two options exist: (1) reducing the less displaced or comminuted side first and using it as a reference for the more displaced side [116]. This may however result in compromised results, if three- or four-point fixation is not achieved, and (2) meticulous preoperative planning [43] by virtual surgical procedure to achieve the ideal facial width and projection. This involves a sequence of segmenting and virtually repositioning the fracture fragments to the "best possible fit" position. Once this is completed, the stents for intra-operative guidance can be generated.

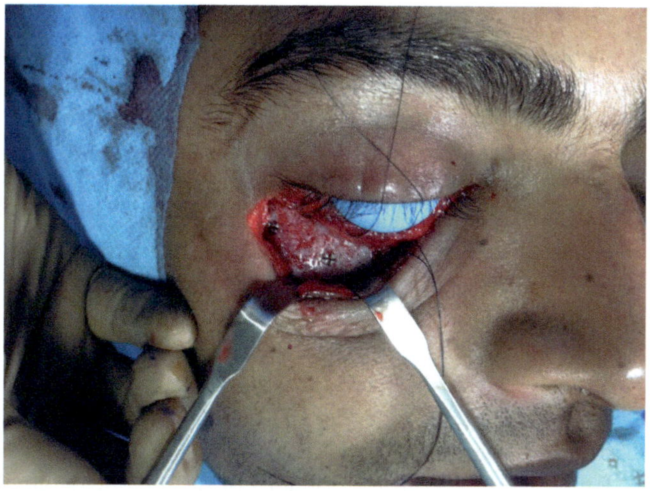

Fig. 56.61 Use of Medpore onlay for malunited fracture

56.15 Complications of ZMC Fractures [3–5]

The incidence of postoperative complications increases with certain risk factors such as severe displacement, presence of sinus infection, and compound/comminuted ZMC fractures [37].

The various complications specific to surgeries of the ZMC may be categorized as intra-operative, immediate post-operative, and delayed postoperative complications.

- ***Intra-operative complications***: Commonly encountered intra-operative complications are bradycardia and bleeding. *Bradycardia due to oculocardiac/trigemino-cardiac* reflex occurs typically during elevation of the ZMC [117]. Manipulation of zygoma stimulates the trigeminal nerve which subsequently stimulates the vagus nerve, due to the neuronal interconnections between them. Vagal stimulation is cardioinhibitory and hence results in bradycardia of varying degrees. This complication can be prevented by identifying risk factors and administering prophylactic vagolytic agents or minimizing nerve stimulation by administering regional blocks. However, management of bradycardia after its onset involves temporary cessation of manipulation and or medical management with atropine or epinephrine [64].

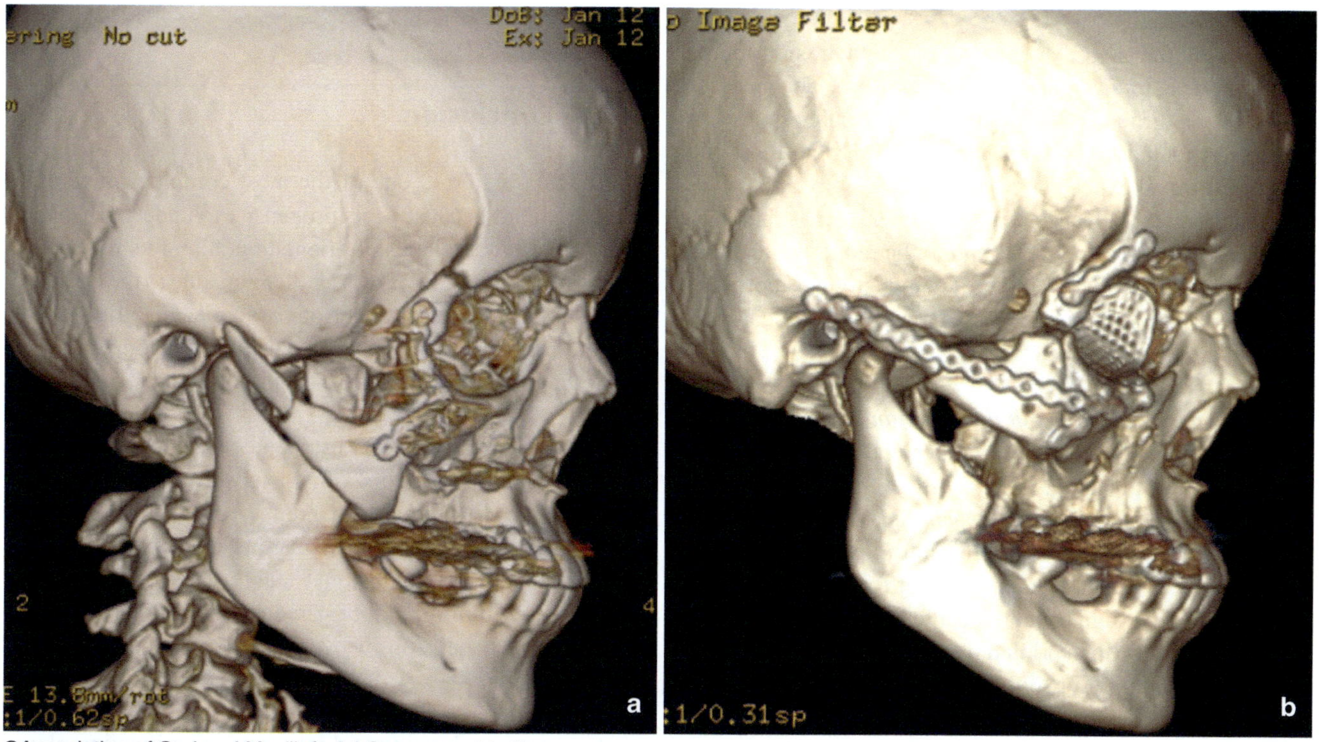

Fig. 56.62 Coronoidectomy for malunited ZMC fracture. (**a**) Pre-operative scan showing malunion of the right ZMC with fusion of the body of zygoma and coronoid process, and (**b**) post-operative scan demonstrating reduction and fixation of the right zmc with ipsilateral coronoidectomy.

Brisk intra-op bleeding can occur due to the sudden rupture of vessels (mainly infra-orbital artery) during reduction.

- **Immediate postoperative complications:** In the immediate postoperative phase, the adverse effects range from maxillary sinusitis, meteorosensitivity [3] (discomfort arising due to change in weather conditions) to infra-orbital nerve paresthesia, diplopia, blindness, and SOF syndrome. The incidence of postoperative infra-orbital nerve paresthesia is higher with ZMC fractures which demonstrate more rotation, displacement, and comminution [118]. Interestingly, recovery from post-trauma ION paresthesia shows better prognosis with reduction and fixation due to de-compression on the nerve. Blindness following surgery may arise either due to direct injury to optic nerve by impingement of fracture fragments or hemorrhage into the optic sheath/retro-bulbar hemorrhage (Refer Fig. 56.16) producing nerve compression [119].
- **Delayed post-op complications** commonly witnessed include enophthalmos and hypophthalmos due to inadequate reduction or inadequate fixation. Oroantral fistula [120], TMJ dysfunction [121], and ankylosis of zygoma to coronoid process, referred to as Jacob's disease [1, 122], are also recorded in literature.

56.16 Recent Trends

Fractures of the ZMC are notorious for their sub-optimal outcomes due to over or under reductions. This may be attributed to difficulty in simultaneous visualization of its multiple articulations without increasing surgical morbidity due to additional exposures.

Technological advancements in the recent years have added ease as well as predictability to the reduction and fixation of these fractures while minimizing surgical morbidity. The most popular methods in contemporary surgical management are discussed below.

1. ***Intra-operative reduction and fixation templates*** [123]
   This has been discussed earlier under the section for preoperative planning.
2. ***Computer-assisted patient-specific implants (PSI)*** [42]: Another method for improving intra-operative accuracy is the use of virtual surgery to plan for reduction of the fracture and design patient-specific implants (PSI). These PSI designs are then printed using a 3D printer which can double up as intra-operative reduction guides also. Refer to section 57.13.2 in Chap. 57 for additional information
3. ***Intra-operative navigation*** [124]: Intra-operative navigation is an excellent method for obtaining intra-operative guidance for precise reduction. Refer to Chap. 41. "Computer-assisted navigation surgery in oral and maxillofacial surgery" for additional information. The margin of error with use of intra-operative navigation is less than 1.2 mm with accurate restoration of facial symmetry. A case of deformity secondary to ZMC fracture treated using intra-operative navigation is illustrated in Fig. 56.63.
4. ***Intra-operative imaging***: Intra-operative imaging greatly improves the accuracy of intra-operative fracture reduction. The various imaging modalities that are available include ultrasound, conventional C-arm (videofluoroscopy), and intra-operative CT. The quality of imaging with videofluoroscopy is not accurate in reflecting the complex anatomy of the cranio-facial skeleton. This makes intra-operative CT a more accurate and reliable tool. However, the associated radiation doses may be a concern. This has been surmounted with the advent of the intra-operative CBCT devices [125]. This device has the significant advantages of portability, ease of use, increased accuracy, and reduced radiation exposure.
5. **Transbuccal Arch Fixation:** A technique involving intra oral reduction of zygomatic arch and its fixation by trans-buccal instrumentation has been described by Panneerselvam et al for fractures of the zygomatic arch which are displaced at the zygomatico temporal articulation. This technique minimises the potential morbidity associated with the coronal approach which is commonly used for ORIF of zygomatic arch [126].

56.17 Conclusion

The ZMC fracture is one of the most complex fractures to reduce and fix, because of its propensity to undergo displacements in all three planes of orientation, along its five articulations. Accurate reduction is challenging due to the difficulty in intra-operative assessment of reduction, inability to predict the rotation of the zygoma during reduction, and complexity involved in concomitant orbital fractures.

> The surgical objectives must include (1) choice of incisions which provide maximal exposure with minimal morbidity, (2) increase in number of fixation points with increase in severity of fracture displacement, (3) achieving three-dimensional stability of ZMC complex and minimizing post-reduction complications, and (4) resuspension of overlying soft tissues to prevent sagging.

Preoperative planning and intra-operative imaging play a great role in improving accuracy of fracture reduction while minimizing surgical exposure and post-reduction complications.

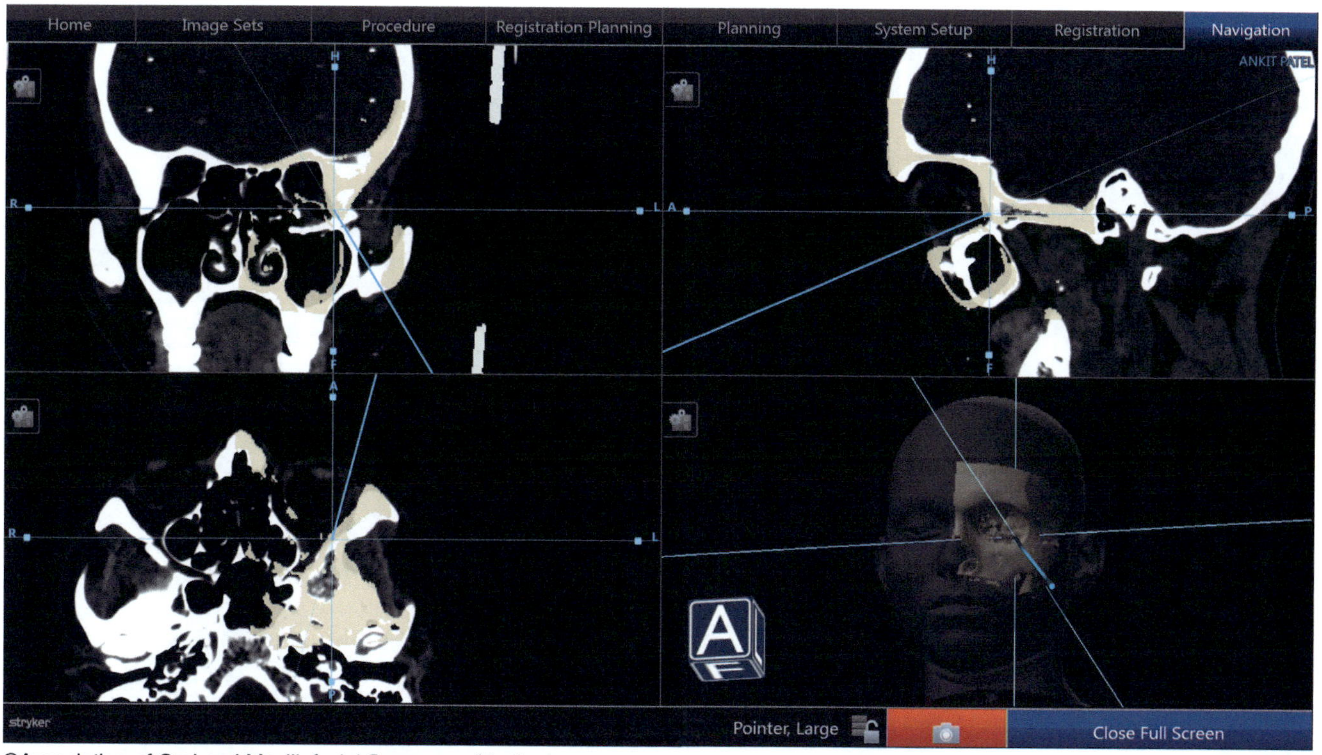

Fig. 56.63 Intra-operative navigation for ZMC fracture. Multiplanar sections demonstrating superimposition of patient CT (white) and surgical. Plan (pink) with use of intra-operative navigation to verify position during surgery (blue pointer)

Acknowledgment The authors would like to acknowledge the efforts of the postgraduate trainees Dr. Vijitha and Dr. Logitha Sri towards the illustrations.

56.18 Case Scenarios

Case Scenario 1: Fracture of right ZMC (Fig. 56.64)

Patient: 21-Year-Old Male, with History of RTA

Preoperative CT (Fig. 56.64a, c) showing right-sided fracture of the ZMC and arch with undisplaced frontal bone.

The sections demonstrate:

- Medial displacement with reduction of the transverse dimension of the face
- Diastasis at the FZ and ZM sutures
- Overriding of fragments at the IOR and SZ suture
- Medial displacement of the right zygomatic arch

Surgical plan: Reduction of ZMC fracture with four-point fixation

Surgical procedure:

- The exposure of fracture sites was done by:
  1. Trans-conjunctival incision with extended lateral approach
  2. Intraoral buccal sulcus approach
- Reduction of ZMC fracture and arch fracture by Balasubramaniam's approach
- Four-point fixation of fracture was performed at FZ, IOR, ZM, and SZ (Fig. 56.64f) regions with miniplates

Postoperative CT (Fig. 56.64b, d, e):

CT demonstrating optimal reduction of fractured ZMC and arch. The successful surgical outcome may be appreciated by the approximation and fixation at the SZ suture, which is the most reliable indicator of accurate ZMC reduction.

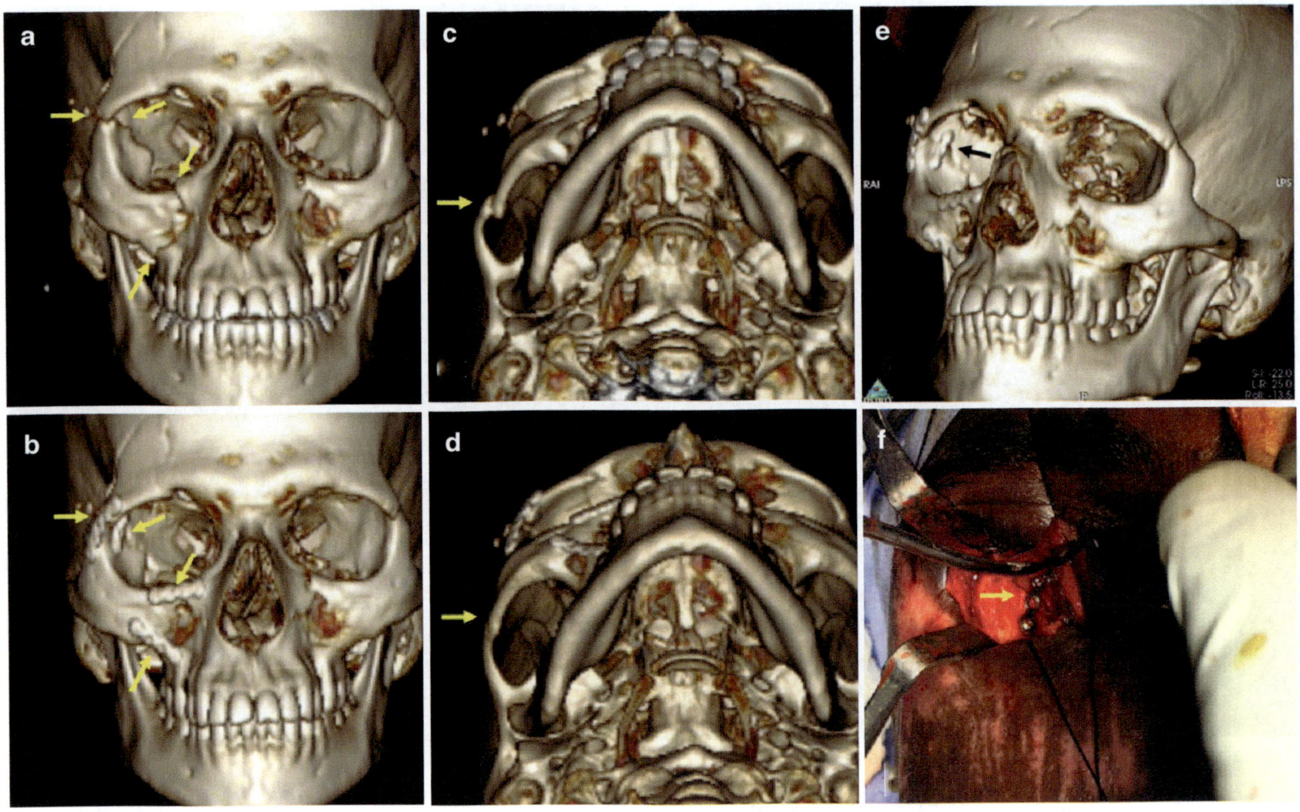

Fig. 56.64 Case scenario 1. (**a**) Preoperative 3D CT-frontal view demonstrating fractures. (**b**) Postoperative 3D CT-frontal view demonstrating fixation. (**c**) Preoperative 3D CT-basal view demonstrating arch fracture. (**d**) Postoperative 3D CT-basal view demonstrating arch reduction. (**e**) Postoperative 3D CT demonstrating fixation at SZ suture. (**f**) Intra-operative fixation at SZ suture

Case Scenario 2: Fracture of left ZMC and orbital floor (Fig. 56.65 a–h)

Patient: 27-Year-Old Male with History of RTA and delayed presentation after 2 months

Preoperative CT findings (Fig. 56.65a, b):

- En bloc fracture of the left ZMC with diastasis at the left infra-orbital rim, zygomatic arch, and FZ and SZ sutures.
- The fracture shows posterior, inferior, and lateral displacement and comminution at the infra-orbital rim, zygomaticomaxillary buttress, and the arch.
- The CT also demonstrates a concomitant left orbital floor fracture with resultant enophthalmos and hypo-ophthalmos (Fig. 56.65g).

Surgical plan: ZMC osteotomy, repositioning, and internal fixation

Surgical procedure:

- Virtual surgical planning to generate a mirrored STL model for pre-contouring of implants (Fig. 56.65c, d)
- Surgical exposure of the fracture through a transconjunctival (infra-orbital rim and floor), upper lid blepharoplasty (FZ and SZ sutures), vestibular for the ZM buttress, and preauricular approaches for the zygomatic arch.
- Mobilization of the malunited ZMC after osteotomy and ORIF with pre-contoured implants
- Fixation of the fracture performed at the FZ, infra-orbital rim, and the zygomatic arch regions
- Orbital exploration and reconstruction with pre-contoured left-sided anatomical titanium orbital implant

Postoperative features (Fig. 56.65e, f and h):

The postoperative CT demonstrates optimal reduction and fixation of the left ZMC with reconstruction of the left orbital floor defect with titanium implant.

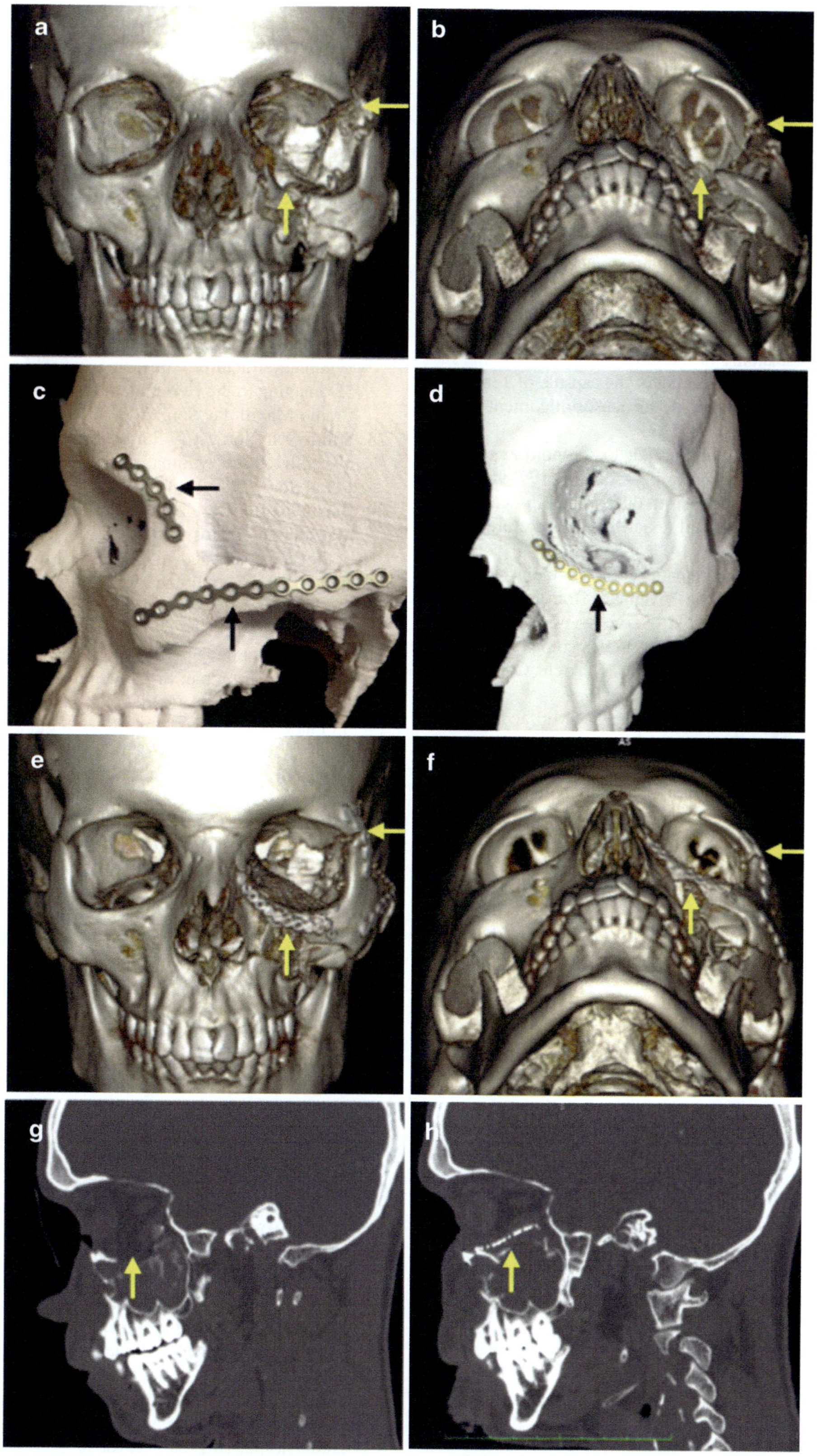

Fig. 56.65 Case scenario 2. (**a**) Preoperative 3D CT-frontal view demonstrating fractures. (**b**) Preoperative 3D CT-basal view. (**c**) STL model surgery with pre-contoured plate. (**d**) STL model demonstrating mirroring of normal side and plate adaptation. (**e**) Postoperative 3D CT-frontal view demonstrating fixation. (**f**) Postoperative 3D CT-basal view demonstrating fixation. (**g**) Preoperative CT-sagittal view demonstrating floor fracture. (**h**) Postoperative CT-sagittal view demonstrating reconstruction of floor with orbital mesh

References

1. Rowe NL, Williams JL. Maxillofacial injuries, Vol 1. Edinburgh: Churchill Livingstone; 1985. p. 435–537.
2. Maturo S, Lopez MA. Zygomatico-orbito-maxillary complex fractures. Oper Tech Otolaryngol. 2008;19:86–9.
3. Marinho RO, Freire-Maia B. Management of fractures of the zygomaticomaxillary complex. Oral Maxillofac Surg Clin North Am. 2013;25:617–36.
4. Ehrenfeld M, Manson PN, Prein J. Principles of internal fixation of the craniomaxillofacial skeleton trauma and orthognathic surgery. AO Foundation. p. 205–22.
5. Fonseca RJ, Walker RV. Oral and maxillofacial trauma, vol. 1. Philadelphia: Saunders; 1991.
6. Lockwood CB. The anatomy of the muscles, ligaments, and fasciae of the orbit, including an account of the capsule of Tenon, the check ligaments of the recti, and the suspensory ligaments of the eye. J Anat Physiol. 1885;20:i2–i25.
7. Brusati R. Mouth opening limitations due to coronoid-zygomatic-malar interference. Minerva Stomatol. 1975;24(4):177–98.
8. Lee SM, Baek JA, Kim Y. Ankylosis of the coronoid process to the zygomatic bone: a case report and review of the literature. J Oral Maxillofac Surg. 2019;77:1230.e1–11.
9. Cohen AJ, Narayanan D. Zygomatic complex facial fractures. 2017 (Cited September 17, 2018) Available from https://emedicine.medscape.com/article/1284142-overview.
10. Karlan MS, Cassisi NJ. Fractures of the zygoma. A geometric, biomechanical, and surgical analysis. Arch Otolaryngol. 1979;105:320–7.
11. Louis M, Agrawal N, Kaufman M, Truong TA. Midface fractures I. Semin Plast Surg. 2017; 31(2): 85–93.
12. Buehler JA, Tannyhill RJ 3rd. Complications in the treatment of midfacial fractures. Oral Maxillofac Surg Clin North Am. 2003;15:195–212.
13. Zachariades N, Papavassiliou D, Papademetriou I. The alterations in sensitivity of the infraorbital nerve following fractures of the zygomaticomaxillary complex. J Craniomaxillofac Surg. 1990;18:315–8.
14. Jamal BT, Pfahler SM, Lane KA, Bilyk JR, Pribitkin EA, Diecidue RJ, Taub DI. Ophthalmic injuries in patients with zygomaticomaxillary complex fractures requiring surgical repair. J Oral Maxillofac Surg. 2009;67:986–9.
15. Cavalcante JR, Junior JR, Peixoto TS, de Albuquerque TT, Cavalcanti AL. Reduction and fixation of unstable fractures of the zygomatic arch: report of a series of cases. J Surg Tech Case Rep. 2015;7:29–31.
16. Susarla SM, Bojovic B. Acute intraorbital hemorrhage following reduction of a displaced orbitozygomaticomaxillary complex fracture. Craniomaxillofac Trauma Reconstr. 2015;8:221–7.
17. Zingg M, Laedrach K, Chen J, et al. Classification and treatment of zygomatic fractures: a review of 1,025 cases. J Oral Maxillofac Surg. 1992;50:778–90.
18. Colin-Durand J, Czerwinski M, Parker WL, Crepeau RJ. Repair of an avulsed zygoma: defining optimal management. J Oral Maxillofac Surg. 2008;66:2615–6.
19. Ozyazgan I, Günay GK, Eskitaşçioglu T, Ozköse M, Coruh A. A new proposal of classification of zygomatic arch fractures. J Oral Maxillofac Surg. 2007;65:462–9.
20. Yamamoto K, Murakami K, Sugiura T, Fujimoto M, Inoue M, Kawakami M, Ohgi K, Kirita T. Clinical analysis of isolated zygomatic arch fractures. J Oral Maxillofac Surg. 2007;65:457–61.
21. Hönig JF, Merten HA. Classification system and treatment of zygomatic arch fractures in the clinical setting. J Craniofac Surg. 2004;15(6):986–9.
22. Ellis E, El-Attar A, Moos KF. An analysis of 2,067 cases of zygomatico-orbital fracture. J Oral Maxillofac Surg. 1985;43:417–28.
23. Rupp J. The 8-Point Eye Exam [Internet]. American Academy of Ophthalmology. 2019 [cited 21 May 2019].
24. Qayyum Z, Khan A, Khitab U. Characteristics and etiology of zygomatic complex fractures. Pak Oral Dent J. 2007;27(1):93–6.
25. King AB, Walsh FB. Trauma to the head with particular reference to the ocular signs: Part I. Injuries involving the cranial nerves. Am J Ophthalmol. 1949; 32(2):191–206.
26. Jeon HB, Kang DH, Oh SA, Gu JH. Comparative study of Naugle and Hertel exophthalmometry in orbitozygomatic fracture. J Craniofac Surg. 2016;27(1):142–4.
27. Nkenke E, Benz M, Maier T, Wiltfang J, Holbach LM, Kramer M, Häusler G, Neukam FW. Relative en-and exophthalmometry in zygomatic fractures comparing optical non-contact, non-ionizing 3D imaging to the Hertel instrument and computed tomography. J Cranio Maxillofac Surg. 2003; 31(6):362–8.
28. Smith SN, Nortjé CJ. Surgical emphysema following an undisplaced fractured zygoma: an unusual radiographic appearance. Br J Oral Surg. 1980;18(3):202–4.
29. Brasileiro BF, Cortez AL, Asprino L, Passeri LA, de Moraes M, Mazzonetto R, Moreira RW. Traumatic subcutaneous emphysema of the face associated with paranasal sinus fractures: a prospective study. J Oral Maxillofac Surg. 2005;63(8):1080–7.
30. Markiewicz MR, Gelesko S, Bell RB. Zygoma reconstruction. Oral Maxillofac Surg Clin North Am. 2013;25(2):167–201.
31. Perry M, Holmes S. Atlas of operative maxillofacial trauma surgery—primary repair of facial injuries. London: Springer; 2014.
32. Roth FS, Koshy JC, Goldberg JS, Soparkar CN. Pearls of orbital trauma management. Semin Plast Surg. 2010;24(4):398–410.
33. Bossert RP, Girotto JA. Blindness following facial fracture: treatment modalities and outcomes. Craniomaxillofac Trauma Reconstr. 2009;2:117–24.
34. McGrigor B, Campbell W. The radiology of war injuries. IV. Wounds of the face and jaw. Br J Radiol. 1950;23(276):685–96.
35. Dolan KD, Jacoby CG. Facial fractures. Semin Roentgenol. 1978;13(1):37–51.
36. Ogunmuyiwa SA, Fatusi OA, Ugboko VI, Ayoola OO, Maaji SM. The validity of ultrasonography in the diagnosis of zygomaticomaxillary complex fractures. Int J Oral Maxillofac Surg. 2012;41(4):500–5.
37. Ochs M, Chung W, Powers D. Trauma surgery. J Oral Maxillofac Surg. 2017;75(8):e151–94.
38. Ellstrom CL, Evans GR. Evidence-based medicine: zygoma fractures. Plast Reconstr Surg. 2013;132(6):1649–57.
39. Hurrell M, David M, Batstone M. A multi-outcome analysis of the effects of treatment timing in the management of zygomatic fractures. Int J Oral Maxillofac Surg. 2015;44:e83.
40. Knepil GJ, Loukota RA. Outcomes of prophylactic antibiotics following surgery for zygomatic bone fractures. J Craniomaxillofac Surg. 2010;38(2):131–3.
41. Soong PL, Schaller B, Zix J, Iizuka T, Mottini M, Lieger O. The role of postoperative prophylactic antibiotics in the treatment of facial fractures: a randomised, double-blind, placebo-controlled pilot clinical study. Part 3: Le Fort and zygomatic fractures in 94 patients. Br J Oral Maxillofac Surg. 2014; 52(4):329–33.
42. Zhang X, Han CY, Dai MJ, Chen JL, Zheng XH, Long J, Tang W, Tian WD, Liu L. Application of computer-assisted surgery techniques in the management of zygomatic complex fractures. Chin J Traumatol. 2018;21(5):281–6.
43. Xia JJ, Gateno J, Teichgraeber JF. A new paradigm for complex midface reconstruction: a reversed approach. J Oral Maxillofac Surg. 2009;67(3):693–703.

44. Li P, Zhou ZW, Ren JY, Zhang Y, Tian WD, Tang W. Accuracy of three-dimensional facial soft tissue simulation in post-traumatic zygoma reconstruction. Int J Oral Maxillofac Surg. 2016;45(12):1665–70.
45. Krimmel M, Cornelius CP, Reinert S. Endoscopically assisted zygomatic fracture reduction and osteosynthesis revisited. Int J Oral Maxillofac Surg. 2002;31(5):485–8.
46. Gillies HD, Kilner TP, Stone D. Fractures of the Malar-zygomatic compound: With a description of a new X-ray position. Br J Surg. 1927;14(56):651–6.
47. Poswillo D. Reduction of the fractured malar by a traction hook. Br J Oral Surg. 1976;14(1):76–9.
48. Lee EI, Mohan K, Koshy JC, Hollier LH. Optimizing the surgical management of zygomaticomaxillary complex fractures. Semin Plast Surg. 2010;24(4):389–97.
49. Dingman RO, Natvig P. Surgery of facial fractures. Philadelphia: WB Saunders; 1964. p. 212–3.
50. Balasubramaniam S. Intra-oral approach for reduction of malar fractures. Br J Oral Surg. 1966;4:189–91.
51. Quinn JH. Lateral coronoid approach for intraoral reduction of fractures of the zygomatic arch. J Oral Surg. 1977;35(4):321–2.
52. Pilanci O, Basaran K, Datli A, Kuvat SV. "Roller coaster maneuver via lateral orbital approach" for reduction of isolated zygomatic arch fractures. J Craniofac Surg. 2013;24(6):2082–4.
53. Carter TG, Bagheri S, Dierks EJ. Towel clip reduction of the depressed zygomatic arch fracture. J Oral Maxillofac Surg. 2005;63(8):1244–6.
54. Ahn HC, Youn DH, Choi MSS, Chang JW, Lee JH. Wire or hook traction for reducing zygomatic fracture. Arch Craniofac Surg. 2015;16(3):131–5.
55. Bazani PL, Bonardi JP, Magro-Filho O. The use of foley catheter for treatment of unstable fracture zygomatic arch. J Craniofac Surg. 2016;27(4):1012.
56. Camilleri AC, Gilhooly M, Cooke ME. Stabilisation of the unstable fractured zygomatic arch with a Kirschner wire. Br J Oral Maxillofac Surg. 2005;43(2):183–4. PubMed PMID: 15749224
57. Yoon H, Kim J, Chung S, Chung YK. Effectiveness of dual-maneuver using K-wire and dingman elevator for the reduction of unstable zygomatic arch fracture. Arch Craniofac Surg. 2014;15(2):59–62.
58. van Hout WM, van Cann EM, Muradin MS, Frank MH, Koole R. Intraoperative imaging for the repair of zygomaticomaxillary complex fractures: a comprehensive review of the literature. J Craniomaxillofac Surg. 2014;42(8):1918–23.
59. Ellis E 3rd, Perez D. An algorithm for the treatment of isolated zygomatico-orbital fractures. J Oral Maxillofac Surg. 2014;72(10):1975–83.
60. Menon A, Karikal A, Shetty V. Does C-arm guidance improve reduction of zygomatic arch fractures? A randomized controlled trial. J Oral Maxillofac Surg. 2018;76(11):2376–86.
61. Cannizzaro D, Revay M, Mancarella C, Colletti G, Costa F, Cardia A, Fornari M. Intraoperative imaging O-Arm™ in secondary surgical correction of post-traumatic orbital fractures. Oral Maxillofac Surg Cases. 2017;3(3):56–60.
62. Bujtar P, Steele P, Holland I, Halsned M. Buttress guide: direct positioning splint to align a complex fracture of the zygoma. Br J Oral Maxillofac Surg. 2017;55(1):97–9.
63. Lubbers HT, Zweifel D, Gratz KW, Kruse A. Classification of potential risk factors for trigeminocardiac reflex in craniomaxillofacial surgery. J Oral Maxillofac Surg. 2010;68:1317–21.
64. Shearer ES, Wenstone R. Bradycardia during elevation of zygomatic fractures. A variation of the oculocardiac reflex. Anaesthesia. 1987;42:1207–8.
65. Padaki P, Graham R, Markose G. Modified Zimmer finger splint revisited. Br J Oral Maxillofac Surg. 2017;55(10):e141.
66. Cornelius C, Gellrich N, Hillerup S, Kusumoto K, Schubert W. Midface - indication - zygoma, zygomatic complex fracture—AO Surgery Reference [Internet]. www2.aofoundation.org. 2019 [cited 18 June 2019]. Available from:. https://www2.aofoundation.org/wps/portal/surgery?bone=CMF&segment=Midface&classification=92-Zygoma,%20Zygomatic%20complex%20fracture&showPage=indication
67. Gruss JS, Van LW, Phillips JH, Antonyshyn O. The importance of the zygomatic arch in complex midfacial fracture repair and correction of posttraumatic orbitozygomatic deformities. Plast Reconstr Surg. 1990;85(6):878–90.
68. Humphrey CD, Kriet JD. Surgical approaches to the orbit. Oper Tech Otolaryngol Head Neck Surg. 2008;19(2):132–9.
69. Farber SJ, Nguyen DC, Skolnick GB, Woo AS, Patel KB. Current management of zygomaticomaxillary complex fractures: A multidisciplinary survey and literature review. Craniomaxillofac Trauma Reconstr. 2016;9(04):313–22.
70. Ellis E, Zide MF, editors. Surgical approaches to the facial skeleton. Lippincott Williams & Wilkins; 2006.
71. Al-Moraissi EA, Thaller SR, Ellis E. Subciliary vs. transconjunctival approach for the management of orbital floor and periorbital fractures: A systematic review and meta-analysis. J Cranio Maxillofac Surg. 2017;45(10):1647–54.
72. Cornelius C, Gellrich N, Hillerup S, Kusumoto K, Schubert W. Midface - indication - zygoma, zygomatic complex fracture—AO Surgery Reference [Internet]. www2.aofoundation.org. 2019 [cited 18 June 2019]. Available from:. https://www2.aofoundation.org/wps/portal/surgery?contentUrl=/srg/92/04-Approaches/A30_2-lower-eyelid-transcutan.jsp. Accessed 12 June 2019.
73. Wilson S, Ellis E. Surgical approaches to the infraorbital rim and orbital floor: the case for the subtarsal approach. J Oral Maxillofac Surg. 2006;64(1):104–7.
74. Connolly KL, Albertini JG, Miller CJ, Ozog DM. The suspension (Frost) suture: experience and applications. Dermatol Surg. 2015;41(3):406–10.
75. Al-Moraissi EA, Elsharkawy AT, Al-Tairi NH, Farhan AH, Abotaleb BM, Al-Sharaee YA, Olufunmilayo OF, Alzubaidi A. What surgical approach has the lowest risk of the lower lid complications in the treatment of orbital floor and periorbital fractures? A frequentist network meta-analysis. J Craniomaxillofac Surg. 2018;46:2164–75.
76. Sebastiani AM, Trento GS, Antonini F, Kluppel LE, Scariot R, Costa DJ, Rebellato NL. Cicatricial ectropion correction in the inferior eyelid with cartilaginous tissue graft: Case report. Int J Med Surg Sci. 2014;1(3):217–2.
77. Pascali M, Avantaggiato A, Brinci L, Cervelli V, Carinci F. Tarsal sling: an essential stitch to prevent scleral show in lower blepharoplasty. Aesthet Surg J. 2015;35(1):11–9.
78. Kushner GM. Surgical approaches to the infraorbital rim and orbital floor: the case for the transconjunctival approach. J Oral Maxillofac Surg. 2006;64(1):108–10.
79. Elsheikh E, Hussein AM, Tantawy AA, Abdelbaki YM. Transconjunctival versus subciliary approach to the infraorbital margin for open reduction of zygomaticomaxillary complex fractures: a randomized feasibility study. Oral Maxillofac Surg. 2017;21(2):187–92.
80. Ishida K. Evolution of the surgical approach to the orbitozygomatic fracture: From a subciliary to a transconjunctival and to a novel extended transconjunctival approach without skin incisions. J Plast Reconstr Aesthet Surg. 2016;69(4):497–505.
81. Martinez AY, Bradrick JP. Y modification of the transconjunctival approach for management of zygomaticomaxillary complex fractures: a technical note. J Oral Maxillofac Surg. 2012;70(1):97–101.

82. Sharma R, Singh S, Patrikar S. Retroseptal transconjunctival approach for fractures of the zygomaticomaxillary complex: a retrospective study. Br J Oral Maxillofac Surg. 2018;56(1):29–33.
83. Yoon SH, Lee JH. The reliability of the transconjunctival approach for orbital exposure: measurement of positional changes in the lower eyelid. Arch Craniofac Surg. 2017;18(4):249.
84. Salhi S, Cordoba C. Distichiasis following transconjunctival approach to the inferior orbital rim and orbital floor. JPRAS Open. 2015;5:29–33.
85. Courtney DJ. Upper buccal sulcus approach to management of fractures of the zygomatic complex: a retrospective study of 50 cases. Br J Oral Maxillofac Surg. 1999;37(6):464–6.
86. Choi KY, Ryu DW, Yang JD, Chung HY, Cho BC. Feasibility of 4-point fixation using the preauricular approach in a zygomaticomaxillary complex fracture. J Craniofac Surg. 2013;24(2):557–62.
87. Massimo P, Corrado T, Roberto C, Fabia C, Massimo R. The deep subfascial approach to the temporomandibular joint. J Oral Maxillofac Surg. 2004;62:1097–102.
88. Zhang QB, Dong YJ, Li ZB, Zhao JH. Coronal incision for treating zygomatic complex fractures. J Craniomaxillofac Surg. 2006;34(3):182–5. Epub 2006 Mar 14.
89. Erich JB. Treatment of fractures of the zygoma and floor of the orbit. Am J Surg. 1966;112(3):432–5.
90. Park BY, Song SY, Yun IS, Lee DW, Rah DK, Lee WJ. First percutaneous reduction and next external suspension with Steinmann pin and Kirschner wire of isolated zygomatic fractures. J Craniofac Surg. 2010;21(4):1060–5.
91. Chotkowski G, Eggleston TI, Buchbinder D. Lag screw fixation of a nonstable zygomatic complex fracture: case report. J Oral Maxillofac Surg. 1997;55(2):183–5.
92. Stevens MR, Menis MA. Microscrew fixation of zygomatic arch fractures. J Oral Maxillofac Surg. 1993;51(10):1158–9.
93. Kim ST, Go DH, Jung JH, Cha HE, Woo JH, Kang IG. Comparison of 1-point fixation with 2-point fixation in treating tripod fractures of the zygoma. J Oral Maxillofac Surg. 2011;69(11):2848–52.
94. Jazayeri HE, Khavanin N, Jason WY, Lopez J, Shamliyan T, Peacock ZS, Dorafshar AH. Fixation points in the treatment of traumatic zygomaticomaxillary complex fractures: a systematic review and meta-analysis. J Oral Maxillofac Surg. 2019.
95. Sharma R, Muralidharan CG, Roy ID, Jain NK, Patrikar S. Radiological evaluation of sphenozygomatic suture fixation for restoration of orbital volume: a retrospective study. J Craniomaxillofac Surg. 2016;44(12):1903–8.
96. Wu CM, Chen YA, Liao HT, Chen CH, Pan CH, Chen CT. Surgical treatment of isolated zygomatic fracture: outcome comparison between titanium plate and bioabsorbable plate. Asian J Surg. 2018;41(4):370–6.
97. Chu SG, Lee JS, Lee JW, Yang JD, Chung HY, Cho BC, Choi KY. Comparisons among four types of absorbable plates used for internal fixation of zygomaticomaxillary complex fractures. J Craniomaxillofac Surg. 2019;47(3):383–8.
98. Xie L, Shao Y, Hu Y, Li H, Gao L, Hu H. Modification of surgical technique in isolated zygomatic arch fracture repair: seven case studies. Int J Oral Maxillofac Surg. 2009;38(10):1096–100.
99. Ribeiro AL, de Souza Rodrigues TM, de Melo A-JS, Pinheiro JD. Interfragmentary screw fixation of the zygomatic arch in complex midface and zygomaticomaxillary fractures. J Oral Maxillofac Surg. 2015;73(3):494–8.
100. Kim H, Yoon J, Lee BI. Radiological morphometric analysis of the zygomatic arch: Application of osteosynthesis on the upper arch border for rigid fixation. J Plast Reconstr Aesthet Surg. 2019;72(5):831–41.
101. Brown R, Lozada K, Kadakia S, Gordin E, Ducic Y. Prophylactic midface lift in midfacial trauma. Facial Plast Surg. 2017;33:347–51.
102. Gruss JS, Whelan MF, Rand RP, Ellenbogen RG. Lessons learnt from the management of 1500 complex facial fractures. Ann Acad Med Singapore. 1999;28:677–86.
103. Phillips JH, Gruss JS, Wells MD, Chollet A. Periosteal suspension of the lower eyelid and cheek following subciliary exposure of facial fractures. Plast Reconstr Surg. 1991;88:145–8.
104. Frodel JL Jr, Rudderman R. Facial soft tissue resuspension following upper facial skeletal reconstruction. J Craniomaxillofac Trauma. 1996;2:24–30.
105. Susarla SM, Peacock ZS. Zygomaticomaxillary complex fracture. Eplasty. 2014;14.
106. Mahmood S, Keith DJ, Lello GE. When can patients blow their nose and fly after treatment for fractures of zygomatic complex: the need for a consensus. Injury. 2003;34(12):908–11.
107. Chang CM, Ko EC, Kao CC, Chang PY, Chen MY. Incidence and clinical significance of zygomaticomaxillary complex fracture involving the temporomandibular joint with emphasis on trismus. Kaohsiung J Med Sci. 2012;28(6):336–40.
108. Ristow O, Pautke C, Kehl V, Koerdt S, Schwärzler K, Hahnefeld L, Hohlweg-Majert B. Influence of kinesiologic tape on postoperative swelling, pain and trismus after zygomatico-orbital fractures. J Craniomaxillofac Surg. 2014;42(5):469–76.
109. Ferreira P, Marques M, Pinho C, Rodrigues J, Reis J, Amarante J. Midfacial fractures in children and adolescents: a review of 492 cases. Br J Oral Maxillofac Surg. 2004;42:501–5.
110. Zimmermann CE, Troulis MJ, Kaban LB. Pediatric facial fractures: recent advances in prevention, diagnosis and management. Int J Oral Maxillofac Surg. 2006;35:2–13.
111. Luck JD, Lopez J, Faateh M, Macmillan A, Yang R, Davidson EH, Nam AJ, Grant MP, Tufaro AP, Redett RJ, Manson PN, Dorafshar AH. Pediatric zygomaticomaxillary complex fracture repair: location and number of fixation sites in growing children. Plast Reconstr Surg. 2018;142:51e–60e.
112. DeFazio MV, Fan KL, Avashia YJ, Danton GH, Thaller SR. Fractures of the pediatric zygoma: a review of the clinical trends, management strategies, and outcomes associated with zygomatic fractures in children. J Craniofac Surg. 2013;24:1891–7.
113. Iatrou I, Theologie-Lygidakis N, Tzerbos F. Surgical protocols and outcome for the treatment of maxillofacial fractures in children: 9 years' experience. J Craniomaxillofac Surg. 2010;38:511–6.
114. Perino KE, Zide MF, Kinnebrew MC. Late treatment of malunited malar fractures. J Oral Maxillofac Surg. 1984;42(1):20–34.
115. Rikalainen R, Lamberg MA, Tasanen A. Extra-articular fibrous ankylosis of the mandible after zygomatic fracture. J Maxillofac Surg. 1981;9:132–6.
116. Ramanathan M, Cherian MP. Isolated bilateral zygomatic complex and arch fracture: a rare case report. Craniomaxillofac Trauma Reconstr. 2010;3(04):185–8.
117. Loewinger J, Cohen M, Levi E. Bradycardia during elevation of a zygomatic arch fracture. J Oral Maxillofac Surg. 1987;45:710–1.
118. Benoliel R, Birenboim R, Regev E, Eliav E. Neurosensory changes in the infraorbital nerve following zygomatic fractures. Oral Surg Oral Med Oral Pathol Oral Radiol Endod. 2005;99:657–65.
119. Buckley SB, McAnear JT, Dolwick MF, Aragon SB. Monocular blindness developing 7 days after repair of zygomaticomaxillary complex fracture: A clinical report. Oral Surg Oral Med Oral Pathol. 1985;60(1):25–8.
120. Dym H, Wolf JC. Oroantral communication. Oral Maxillofac Surg Clin North Am. 2012;24:239–47.
121. Rajantie H, Snäll J, Thorén H. Postoperative temporomandibular dysfunction in patients with fractures of the zygomatic complex: a prospective follow-up study. Br J Oral Maxillofac Surg. 2018;56(7):573–7.

122. i de la Torre ÒE, Klok EV, i Roig AM, Mommaerts MY, i Ayats JP. Jacob's disease: report of two cases and review of the literature. J Craniomaxillofac Surg. 2001;29(6):372–6.
123. Liu XZ, Shu DL, Ran W, Guo B, Liao X. Digital surgical templates for managing high-energy zygomaticomaxillary complex injuries associated with orbital volume change: a quantitative assessment. J Oral Maxillofac Surg. 2013;71:1712–23.
124. Gong X, He Y, An J, Yang Y, Huang X, Liu M, Zhao Y, Zhang Y. Application of a computer-assisted navigation system (CANS) in the delayed treatment of zygomatic fractures: a randomized controlled trial. J Oral Maxillofac Surg. 2017;75:1450–63.
125. Pohlenz P, Blake F, Blessmann M, Smeets R, Habermann C, Begemann P, Schmelzle R, Heiland M. Intraoperative cone-beam computed tomography in oral and maxillofacial surgery using a C-arm prototype: first clinical experiences after treatment of zygomaticomaxillary complex fractures. J Oral Maxillofac Surg. 2009;67:515–21.
126. Panneerselvam E, Balasubramanian S, Kempraj J, Babu VR, Raja VBKK. Management of Zygomatic Arch Fractures by Intraoral Open Reduction and Transbuccal Fixation: A Technical Note. Craniomaxillofacial Trauma & Reconstruction. 2020 Jun;13(2):130-132. DOI: 10.1177/1943387520911866.

57 Orbital Fractures

Ananthanarayanan Parameswaran, Madhulaxmi Marimuthu, Shreya Panwar, and Beat Hammer

57.1 Introduction

Orbital fractures are unique among cranio-maxillofacial (CMF) fractures. They have functional, cosmetic, and psychological implications. Most importantly they are among the few true emergencies in the realm of CMF trauma. Management of orbital fractures poses a challenge to every surgeon because of its complex anatomy, relationship to vital structures such as the globe and the brain, and its direct influence on the most precious of senses, *Vision.*

The orbit is a small bony cone filled with numerous vital and delicate structures, which require absolute precaution while handling and immense precision in its reconstruction. The principles of managing orbital trauma differ significantly from rest of the CMF fractures, which mandate a thorough understanding of its morphology and biodynamics. Choosing the appropriate indication for intervention and management protocol is critical in achieving the desired surgical outcome. This chapter aims to answer the questions of the *When*, *Why*, and *How* of managing orbital trauma.

57.2 Surgical Anatomy of the Orbit

The orbits are bilateral bony cavities which house the globes. Each orbit is made up of seven bones: the maxilla, frontal bone, zygomatic, sphenoid, ethmoid, lacrimal, and the palatine bones (Fig. 57.1). The orbital cavity is a pyramidal structure with a quadrilateral base anteriorly, forming the orbital aperture, and the apex posteriorly which ends at the optic foramen. The apex is superomedially placed, while the base is directed anterior and lateral. The orbit encases two fissures: (1) the inferior orbital fissure also called the sphenozygomatic fissure and (2) the superior orbital fissure otherwise called as the inter-sphenoidal fissure (Fig. 57.2). The major structures within the orbit are provided in Box 57.1.

Electronic Supplementary Material The online version of this chapter (https://doi.org/10.1007/978-981-15-1346-6_57) contains supplementary material, which is available to authorized users.

A. Parameswaran (✉)
Department of Oral and Maxillofacial Surgery, Meenakshiammal Dental College and Hospital, Chennai, India

Department of Orbit, Oculoplasty, Reconstructive and Aesthetic Surgery, Shankara Nethralaya, Chennai, India

Department of Orbit and Oculoplasty, Aravind Eye Hospitals, Chennai, India

M. Marimuthu
Department of Oral and Maxillofacial Surgery, Saveetha Dental College and Hospital, Chennai, India

S. Panwar
Department of Oral and Maxillofacial Surgery, Meenakshiammal Dental College and Hospital, Chennai, India

B. Hammer
CFC Hirslanden Kopf Zentrum, Aarau, Switzerland
e-mail: Beat.Hammer@hirslanden.ch

K. Bonanthaya et al. (eds.), *Oral and Maxillofacial Surgery for the Clinician*, https://doi.org/10.1007/978-981-15-1346-6_57

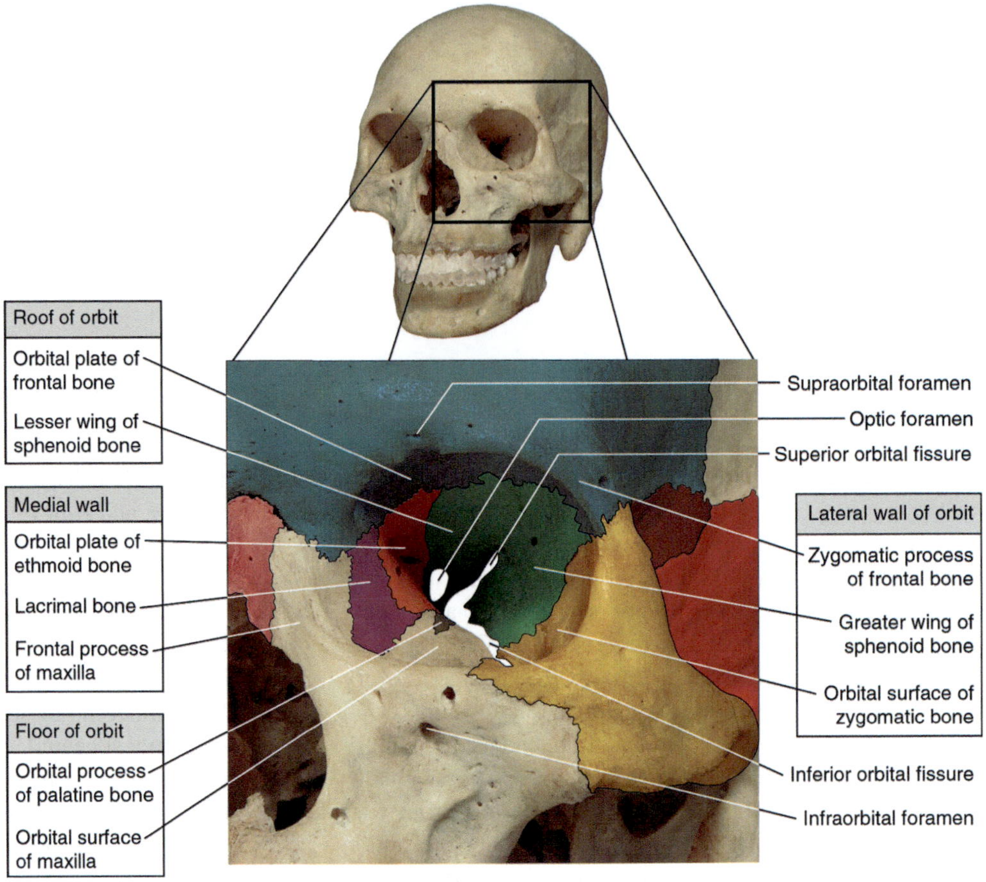

Fig. 57.1 Bones forming the orbit

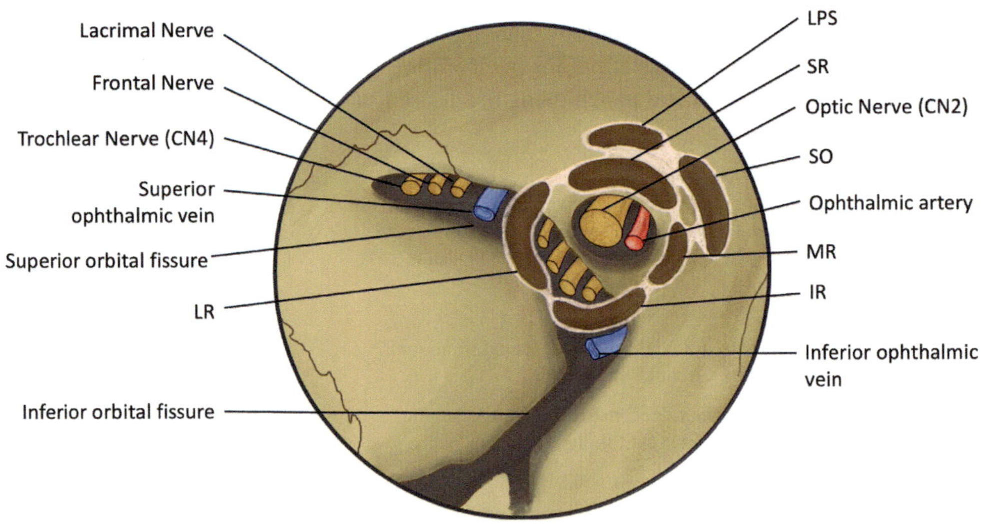

Fig. 57.2 Structures passing through the superior and inferior orbital fissures

Box 57.1 The Major Structures that Occupy the Orbit

- Eye/globe
- Orbital fat
- Extraocular muscles
- Ciliary parasympathetic ganglion
- Nasolacrimal apparatus
- Optic nerve
- Oculomotor
- Trochlear
- Abducent nerves
- V1 and V2 of trigeminal nerve
- Ophthalmic vessels

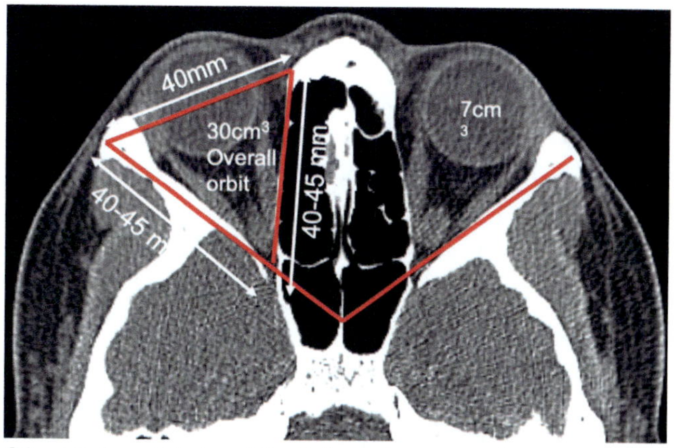

Fig. 57.3 Diagrammatic representation of the various measurements of the orbit and the globe

The orbits have an average height of 35 mm and a medio-lateral width of 40 mm [1–3]. The intra-orbital volume of an adult is approximately 30 cc, while the volume of the globe is 7 cc [4]. Generally, the orbital and globe volumes are bilaterally symmetrical at any stage of growth. The medial walls are parallel to each other and around 45–50 mm in length, while the lateral walls are around 90° to each other and 40–45 mm long (Fig. 57.3).

The orbital skeleton may essentially be divided into walls and rims. These include the orbital roof, floor, and medial and lateral walls. The rims include the inferior, superior, medial, and lateral orbital rims. A brief description of the structure of the orbital cavity is provided below.

57.2.1 Orbital Walls

The roof (Fig. 57.4a) is formed by a concave broad plate of the frontal bone which delineates the orbital contents from the cranial cavity. The posterior portion of the roof has a small contribution from the lesser wing of the sphenoid. The anterolateral portion has a shallow depression called the lacrimal fossa, while 5 mm behind the medial aspect of the supraorbital rim is the trochlear fossa which has the cartilaginous pulley of the superior oblique muscle. The roof is triangular in shape and ends in optic foramen, which is the entry of the optic nerve into the orbit.

In older patients there may be spots of resorption in the orbital roof which may cause the dura to adhere to the periorbita of the roof. The junction of the medial wall and the roof has a suture line which lies in close proximity to the cribriform of the ethmoid and is prone for fragmentation. This may be a major concern for CSF leak into the orbits or the nose or at times both.

The roof is separated from the lateral orbital wall by the superior orbital fissure which serves as a passage of entry for the cranial nerves III, IV, V1, and VI into the orbit. The other structure coursing through the fissure is the ophthalmic vein. On the anterior aspect of the roof, at the junction between the medial 1/3rd and the lateral 2/3rd of the supraorbital rim is the supraorbital foramen which transmits the supraorbital neurovascular bundle [1–3, 5].

The medial wall (Fig. 57.4c) is quadrangular in shape and is constituted by the ethmoid bone in the center. The antero-superior aspect is formed by the frontal bone, while the antero-inferior part is formed by the lacrimal bone. The sphenoid bone forms the posterior part of the medial wall. The infra-orbital rim continues along the anterior aspect of the medial wall forming the anterior lacrimal crest which is a part of the frontal process of the maxilla, while the superomedial aspect of the supraorbital rim continues inferiorly as the posterior lacrimal crest which is formed by the lacrimal bone. Between these crests lie the fossa which houses the lacrimal sac. This is of importance during access planning for surgery of the medial wall and the anteromedial aspect of the infra-orbital rim.

The anterior and posterior ethmoidal foramen are located along the fronto-ethmoidal suture which signifies the height of the cribriform plate. The anterior ethmoidal foramen which transmits the anterior ethmoidal artery and nerve lies approximately 22–25 mm behind the medial orbital rim while the posterior ethmoidal foramen which transmits the posterior ethmoidal artery and the spheno-ethmoidal nerve is present about 12 mm posterior [6]. The optic foramen is in continuation of the medial wall and is approximately placed 45–50 mm behind the medial rim. The safe distances the sur-

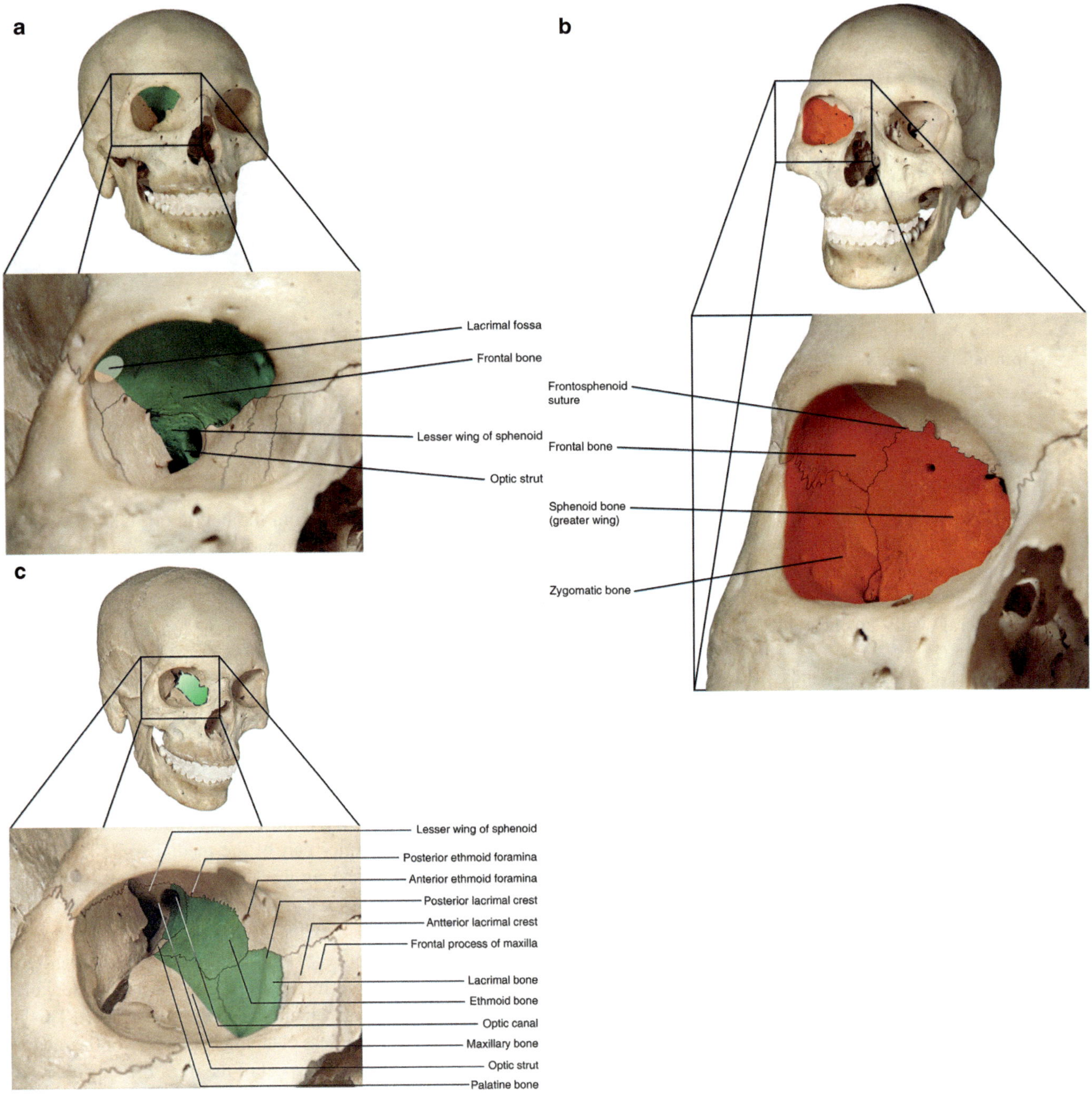

Fig. 57.4 (**a**) Roof, (**b**) lateral wall, and (**c**) medial wall of the orbit

geon needs to remember are 24 mm for the anterior ethmoidal artery, with an additional 12 mm for the posterior ethmoidal vessel and a further 6 mm as the limit to stay away from the optic foramen making it *24-12-6*, an easy formula to remember. One important structure which may be involved in medial wall trauma is the medial rectus muscle which can get entrapped causing ocular motility disturbances.

The lateral wall (Fig. 57.4b) is the thickest wall and is made primarily by the orbital surface of the zygomatic bone and the greater wing of the sphenoid. A small bony projection seen on the lateral wall is the Whitnall's tubercle which lies 11 mm below the fronto-zygomatic suture and 4 mm behind the rim (Fig. 57.7).

This tubercle forms the attachment of the 4L's:

1. The suspensory ligament of Lockwood
2. The lateral horn of the levator aponeurosis
3. The ligaments of the lateral rectus muscle
4. The lateral palpebral ligament

A small groove may be seen at the anterior end of the inferior orbital fissure which transmits the zygomatico-facial and zygomatico-temporal vessels. These course through the zygoma and exit through independent foramina to supply the face and the temporal regions.

The floor (Fig. 57.5a, b) follows a gentle slope from its medial to lateral side. The highest point lies in the posteromedial aspect of the floor forming a bulge called the "Hammer's key area" [7] (Fig. 57.5a), which influences the position of the globe in the anteroposterior axis. In the sagittal view, the floor follows a "lazy S" shape with the anterior part concave and the posterior convex. The reconstruction of this convexity is important to maintain the anterior position of the globe (Fig. 57.5b). The floor is separated from the lateral wall by the inferior orbital fissure. The fissure communicates with the pterygopalatine fossa extra-orbitally. The maxillary division of the V nerve and its branches, the infraorbital artery, and branches of the sphenopalatine ganglion are transmitted through the posteromedial aspect of the fissure, while the inferior ophthalmic veins pass through the lateral aspect to communicate with the pterygoid plexus. The floor is formed by the zygomatic bone and the maxilla with a small contribution from the orbital process of the palatine bone in the posteromedial aspect. A rough area at the anteromedial angle of the floor behind the infra orbital rim forms the attachment of the inferior oblique muscle. The infraorbital groove originates from the inferior orbital fissure and transmits the infra-orbital neurovascular bundle.

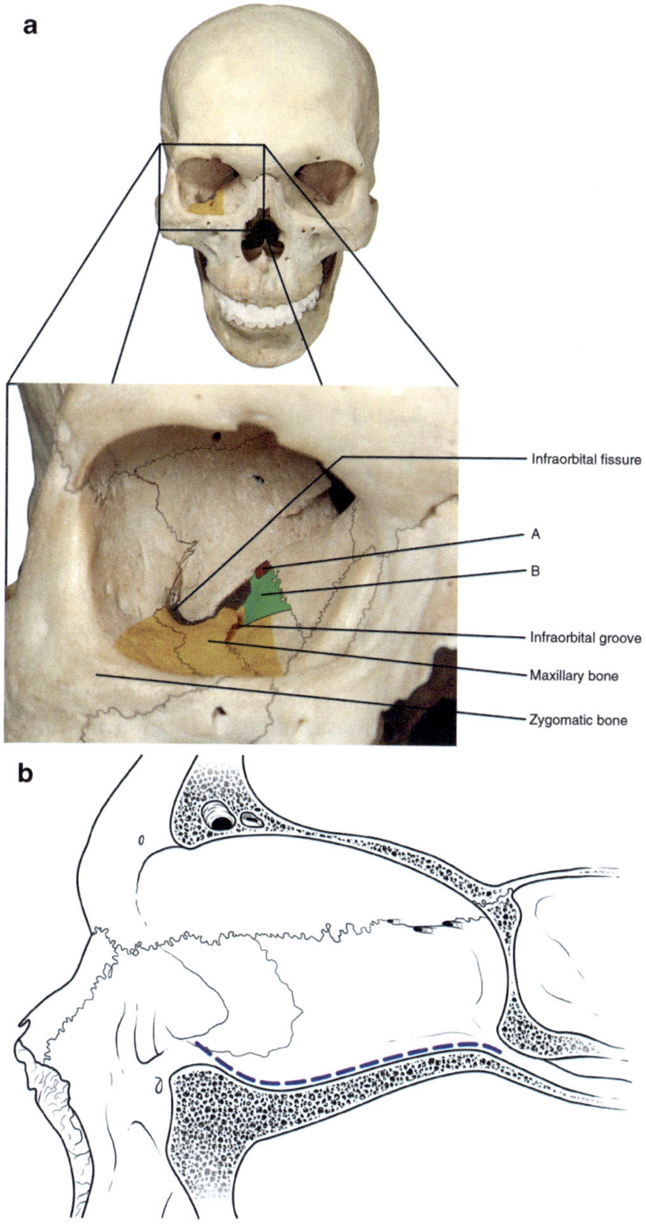

Fig. 57.5 The orbital floor in (**a**) frontal view demonstrating the (A) orbital process of palatine bone and (B) "Hammer's key area." (**b**) Sagittal view of the floor with the "lazy S" form

Orbital Rims:
The rims are superior, inferior, medial, and lateral. Three major bones—the maxilla, zygomatic bone, and frontal bone—make up the rims of the orbit. The width of the rims is greater than its height making it into a rectangular form. The presence of the maxillary sinus and the insertion of the inferior oblique muscle make the infra-orbital rim more prone for fracture and comminution.

57.2.2 Muscles of the Orbit (Fig. 57.6a)

Muscles in relation to the orbit can be divided into

- the muscles associated with the lids
- and the muscles associated with the globe.

The muscles of the lid are:

1. The orbicularis oculi which has a palpebral portion (upper and lower eyelids), the intervening orbital septum, and the inner layer connecting the tarsus
2. The levator palpebrae superioris which is the elevator of the upper eyelid
   The levator palpebrae superioris along with the four recti, and the two obliques form the seven extraocular muscles of the human eye.

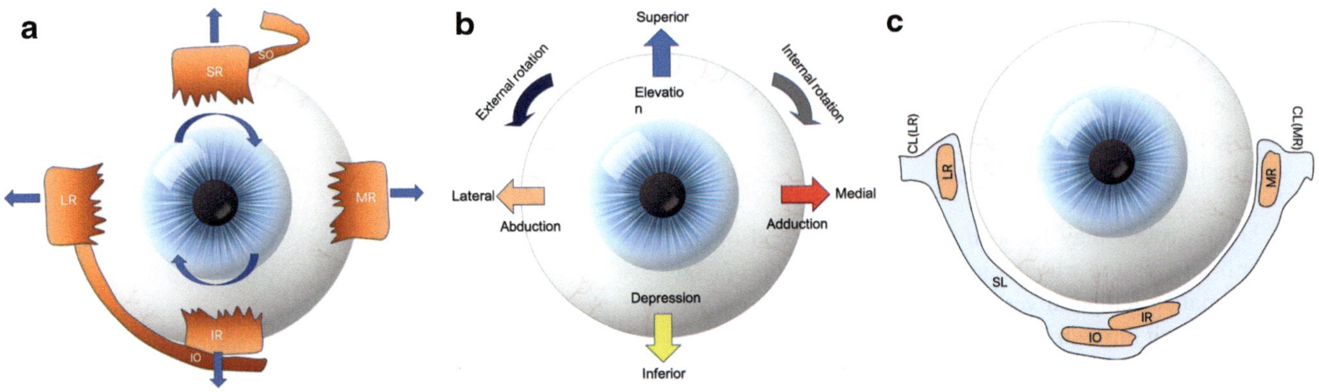

Fig. 57.6 Diagram of right eye demonstrating (**a**) the extraocular muscles and (**b**) the movements they cause. (**c**) The fascial sheath. (*SR* - Superior Rectus, *IR* - Inferior Rectus, *MR* - Medial Rectus, *LR* - Lateral Rectus, *SO* - Superior Oblique, *IO* - Inferior Oblique, *CL(MR)* - Check Ligament of Medial Rectus, *CL(LR)* - Check Ligament of Lateral Rectus, *SL* - Suspensory Ligament

The origin of the superior rectus is from the common tendinous ring superolateral to the optic canal, and its insertion is into the upper part of the sclera. Its function is to produce elevation of the eye and to move the cornea upward and medially helping in adduction and medial rotation.

The origin of the medial rectus is from the medial aspect of the tendinous ring and inserts into the medial surface of the sclera. The medial rectus helps in moving the eye medially (adduction), and bilateral action of the medial rectus helps in medial convergence of both the corneas. A suspensory attachment to the lacrimal crest is also seen on the medial orbital wall where it blends with the medial canthus and the check ligament (Fig. 57.6c) [2, 3, 6, 8]. The origin of the lateral rectus is from the lateral part of the common tendinous ring, and it inserts into the lateral surface of the sclera. Its primary function is to move the eye laterally (abduction).The inferior rectus arises from the common tendinous ring, below the optic canal, and inserts into sclera below the cornea. It is responsible for depression and lateral rotation of the eye.

The inferior rectus followed by the medial rectus are the most common muscles to be entrapped secondary to orbital trauma and may need to be explored and released surgically as indicated. Delayed release of the recti may cause significant necrosis and fibrosis of the muscles hampering return to normal function.

The superior oblique arises superomedial to the optic canal. It has a pulley action at the trochlea on the anteromedial aspect of the orbital roof and inserts into the sclera behind the equator of the globe. The contraction of the muscle produces depression of the cornea and movement of the eye laterally with medial rotation (intorsion).

The inferior oblique muscle arises from the orbital surface of the maxilla lateral to the nasolacrimal groove and inserts into the lateral part of the sclera behind the equator between the inferior and lateral recti muscle. It produces elevation of the cornea and helps in moving the eye laterally with lateral rotation (extorsion).

57.2.3 Movements of the Eye and Their Innervation

Box 57.2 The Movements of the Eye

- Elevation
- Depression
- Adduction
- Abduction
- Intorsion
- Extorsion (Fig. 57.6b)

The different movements of the eye are enumerated in Box 57.2. These are facilitated by the extraocular muscles described above and are contained by the check ligaments. The inferior oblique and inferior rectus muscles which course the floor of the orbit serve as the inferior check ligaments. The fascia of the levator palpebrae superioris, which is anchored to the Whitnall's tubercle laterally and the trochlea medially, acts as the superior check ligament [8].

The contraction of the orbicularis oculi innervated by the facial nerve dictates the closure of the upper eyelid. The movements of the globe within the orbit are however dictated by the synchronous movements of the extraocular muscles of the orbit. The oculomotor nerve innervates all the extraocular muscles other than the lateral rectus which is supplied by the abducent nerve and the superior oblique supplied by the trochlear nerve. Reflex closure of the eyelids occurs via the sympathetic pathways traveling to the smooth muscles of the upper and lower eyelids.

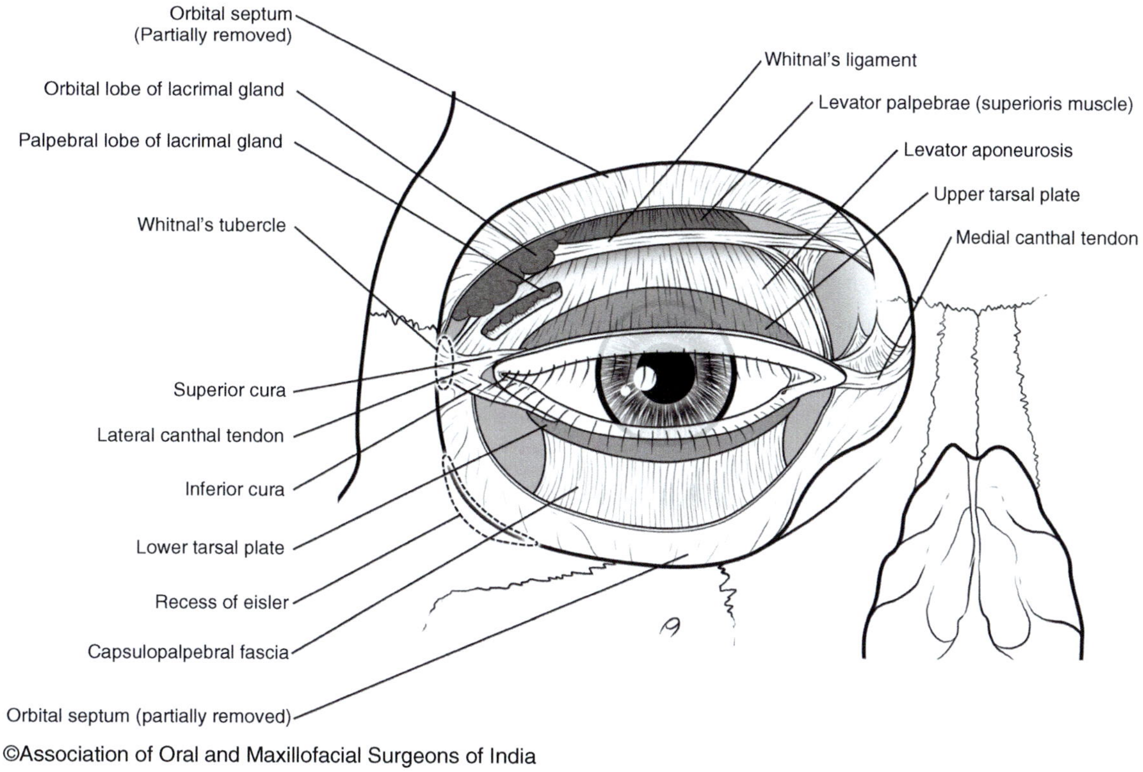

Fig. 57.7 The tarsal apparatus and the orbital septum

57.2.4 Orbital Septum and Tarsal Plates (Fig. 57.7)

The supporting framework for the eyelid is formed by a dense fibrous tissue called the orbital septum which condenses at the lids as the tarsal plates. The orbital septum which separates the orbital and lid contents attaches to the bone and becomes the periorbita inside the orbit and periosteum outside the orbit. The septum of the lower eyelid attaches to the orbital rims, while the septum of the upper eyelid is attached intra-orbitally behind the equator of the globe. The tarsal plates add rigidity to the lids and also serve attachments of multiple muscles and membranes [1, 3].

57.2.5 Conjunctiva

The conjunctiva is the transparent mucous membrane that covers the front surface of the globe and the inner surface of the eyelids.

This has two segments:

1. The bulbar conjunctiva that covers the anterior part of the sclera (the "white" of the eye)
2. The palpebral conjunctiva otherwise known as tarsal conjunctiva which covers the inner aspect of the eyelids

57.2.6 Fascial Sheath of the Eyeball (Fig. 57.6c)

The fascial sheath of the eyeball is called the Tenon's capsule [8]. It extends from the optic foramen to the sclerocorneal junction enveloping the eyeball on the inferior aspect. It attaches to the sclera on the anterior and posterior surfaces of the eyeball and becomes continuous with the fascia of the muscles posteriorly and around the inferior oblique muscle. The fascial sheath of all muscles blend together and form a continuous fascial band called the suspensory ligament of the eye that provides support for the eyeball [8, 9].

57.2.7 Orbital Fat

The orbital fat is present both intra- and extra-conally. They cushion the globe and muscles of the orbit. The extra-conal fat determines and influences the position of the globe. This may be altered either due to herniation or atrophy secondary to fractures of the orbit resulting in enophthalmos.

57.3 Classification System

Manson [10] and colleagues classified the fractures based on the energy of impact, the degree, and extent of comminution and displacement observed on CT:

(a) Trap door fractures—low-velocity injuries
(b) Medial blowout fractures—intermediate-velocity injuries
(c) Lateral blowout fractures—high-velocity fractures

Converse and Smith [11] termed them "pure" or "impure" based on the involvement of orbital rims (Fig. 57.8):

(a) Pure (blow-in or blowout fractures)—fracture of the internal walls with intact rims
(b) Impure (complex with involvement of one or more rims)—associated fractures of the rims

Hammer [7] described four classes of orbital fractures based on their occurrence with other fractures of the face (Fig. 57.9):

(a) *Type I*: Orbito-zygomatic fractures—These involve the fractures of the walls of the orbit along with the zygomatic complex.
(b) *Type II*: Internal orbital fractures—These involve isolated fractures of any of the walls, roof, and floor.
(c) *Type III*: Naso-orbito-ethmoid-type fractures—These involve fractures of the naso-orbito-ethmoid complex which involve the orbit.
(d) *Type IV*: Complex fractures of the face—This type involve fractures of the orbit with concomitant fractures of the face other than the ones mentioned above [7].

57.4 Blowout and Blow-In Fractures

Smith and Converse in 1960 recognized the phenomenon of blowout fractures (Fig. 57.10a). These fractures may involve entrapment or herniation of periorbital tissues resulting in restricted eye movements and/or enophthalmos due to reduction in the volume of intra-orbital contents [3, 11].

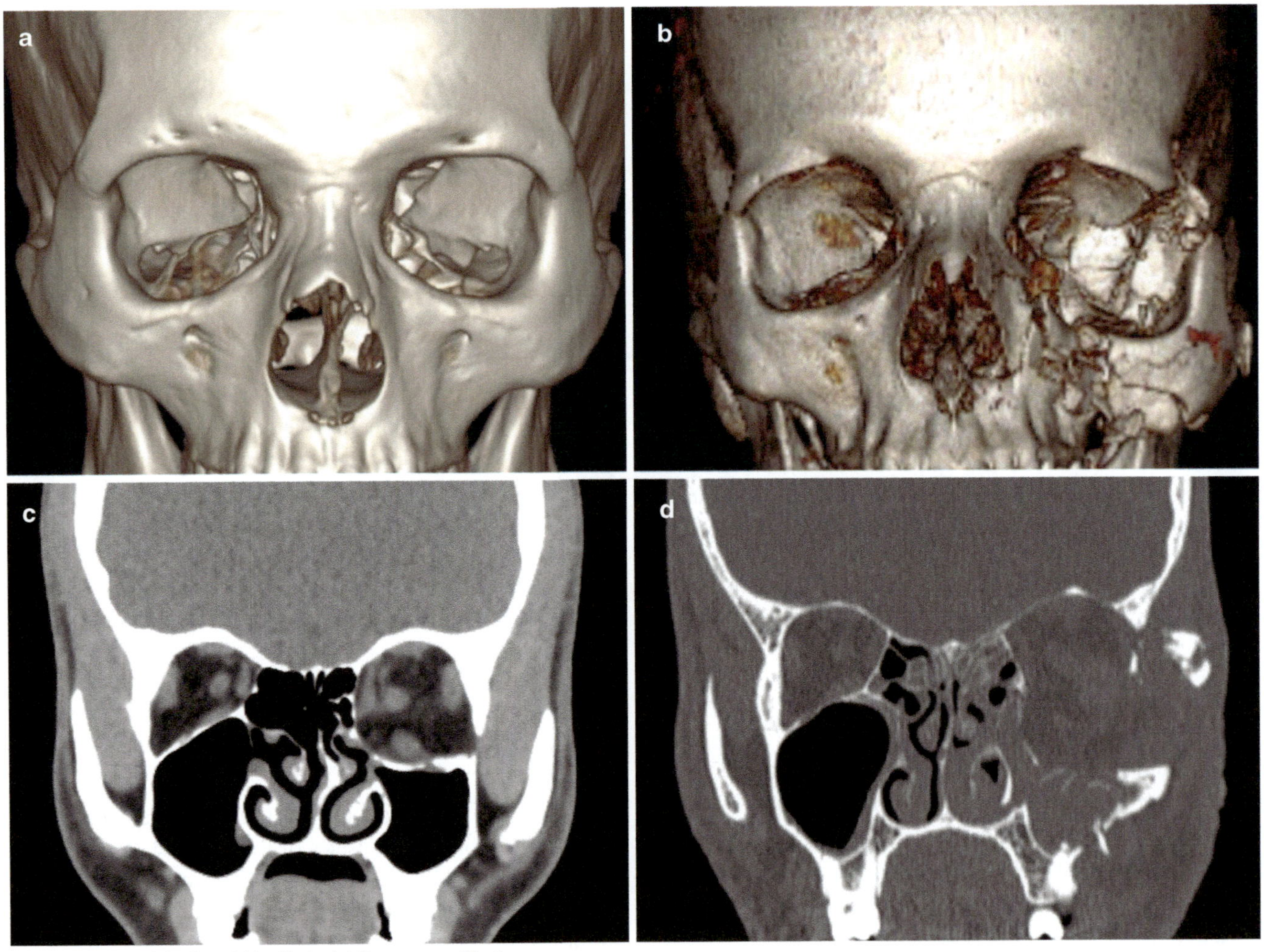

Fig. 57.8 CT scans showing Pure (**a** and **c**) and impure (**b** and **d**) blowout fractures of the orbit

"Blow-in" type of orbital fractures was described by Dingman and Natvig [3, 12] in 1964 wherein the intra-orbital space is reduced by an internally displaced bony fragment (Fig. 57.10b). Such types of fractures are usually accompanied with proptosis on the affected side [13].

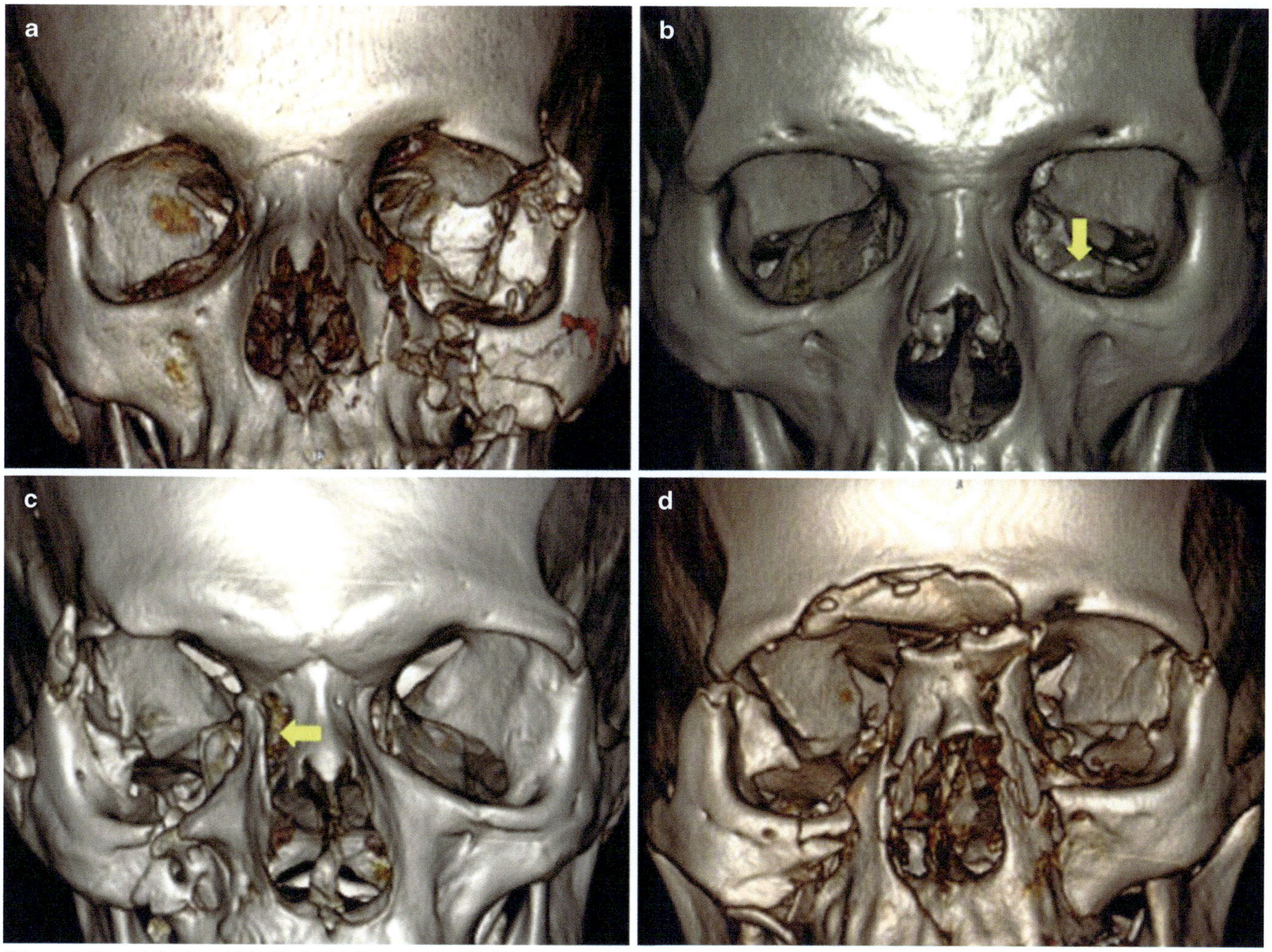

Fig. 57.9 CT scan images showing types of orbital fractures: (**a**) orbito-zygomatic, (**b**) internal orbital, (**c**) naso-orbito-ethmoid type, and (**d**) orbit with complex facial fractures

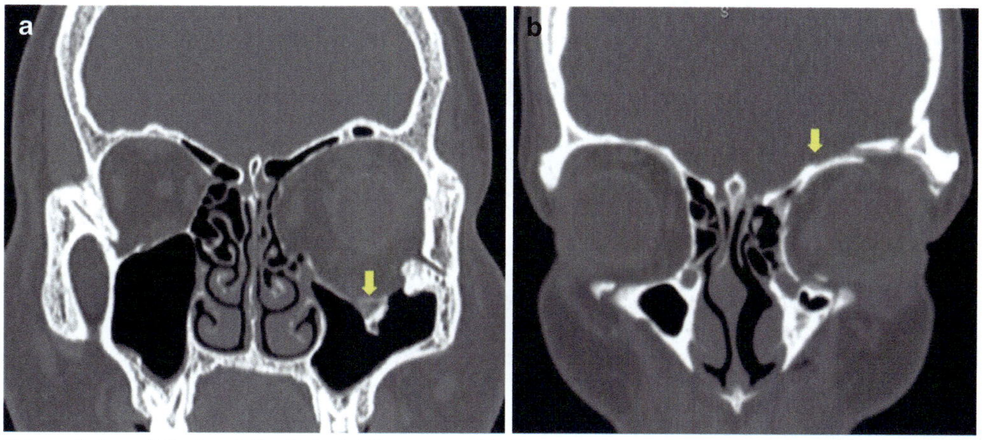

Fig. 57.10 CT scans demonstrating a blowout of the medial orbital wall and floor (**a**) and a blow-in fracture of the orbital roof (**b**)

57.5 Biomechanics of Injury

One of the first mechanisms of orbital wall fractures was suggested by Pfeiffer [14] in 1943, called *globe-to-wall theory or hydraulic theory* (Fig. 57.11a), wherein posterior displacement of the globe after sustaining a direct hit was propounded to transmit force along the walls resulting in fracture of the thinner walls. There are two more widely accepted mechanisms of orbital wall fractures, namely, the:

(i) *Retropulsion theory* (Fig. 57.11b)
(ii) *Buckling mechanism* [15] (Fig. 57.11c)

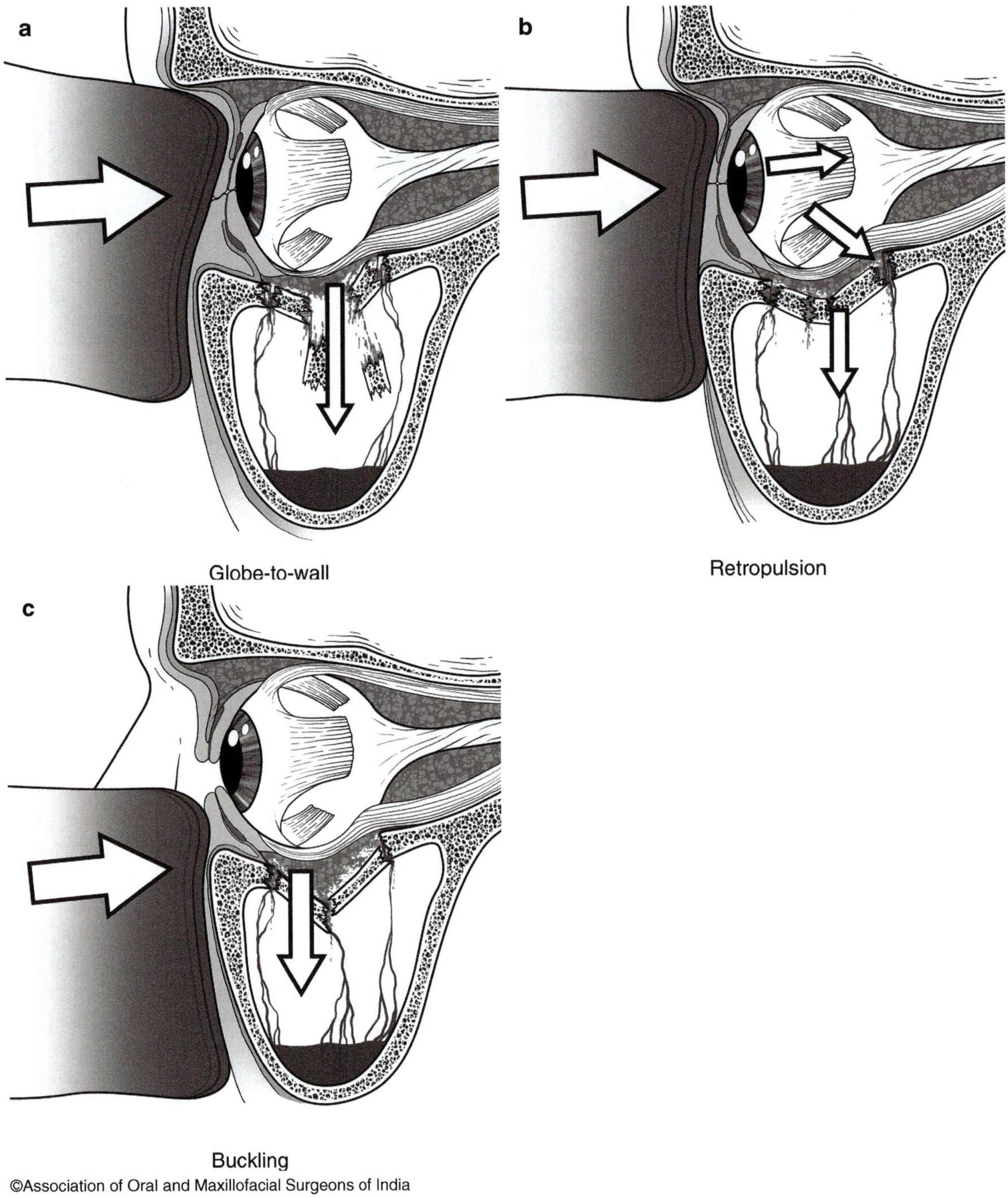

Fig. 57.11 Diagrammatic representation of (**a**) hydraulic theory, (**b**) retropulsion theory, and (**c**) buckling mechanism

First proposed by King [16] in 1944, retropulsion theory suggests that sudden increase in intra-orbital pressure caused by direct hit from a large object creates stresses along the orbital walls resulting in fractures at the areas of least thickness. The buckling theory or transmission theory explains the injury through a ripple effect created in the floor. The ripple thus created causes compression in an anteroposterior direction and resultant fracture at the posteromedial part of the orbital floor commonly [17, 18].

57.6 Initial Assessment

After initial stabilization of the patient, a thorough facial examination is performed in a way similar to any facial fracture. Special consideration is given to a detailed ophthalmic evaluation followed by eliciting signs and symptoms significant for periorbital trauma which are discussed below. The frontal area and supraorbital rim are examined first, with a logical progression downward, including the lateral and infra-orbital rims, although extensive edema in this area may obscure any steps making the palpatory examination difficult [3, 7, 19–22].

57.6.1 Ophthalmologic Examination

The American Association of Ophthalmology [23] advocates an 8-point ophthalmological examination which includes the following (Box 57.3):

1. *Visual acuity*: Visual acuity test for each eye is recorded using a Snellen chart (Fig. 57.12a) and includes ability to read letters, count fingers, perceive hand movements, and light perception. If visual acuity is extremely poor and recording of a chart test fails, the patient is subjected to a finger counting test or at times even assessed for primary light perception alone.
2. *Pupillary examination*: Pupillary examination is done to note the
   (a) size,
   (b) shape,
   (c) symmetry,
   (d) and direct/indirect reflex to light.
   Glaucoma, previous history of surgery, and/or injury to ocular system may also account for anisocoria or irregular pupils. Peaked or irregular pupils may also be indicative of perforation of the globe. The swinging flashlight test is performed for relative afferent pupillary defect (RAPD) (Fig. 57.12b).
3. *Extraocular motility and alignment*: The patient is first screened for all the six cardinal gazes (Fig. 57.12c). First checked binocularly for versions of both sides and then checked monocular for ductions. A thorough heterotropia check is also performed. Diplopia and restrictions in gazes are noted. Clinically, a forced duction test under topical anesthesia is done to elicit mechanical impediment to movement of the globe. This may also be performed under general anesthesia intraoperatively (Figs. 56.21, 57.13). A Hess chart examination is a part of the orthoptic assessment protocol for evaluation of ocular motility.
4. *Intraocular pressure*: Tonometry should be performed to evaluate intraocular pressure either in a clinic setting using a Goldmann applanation method or outside using a mobile/portable device. This examination is skipped if there is a suspicion of ruptured globe. The normal IOC

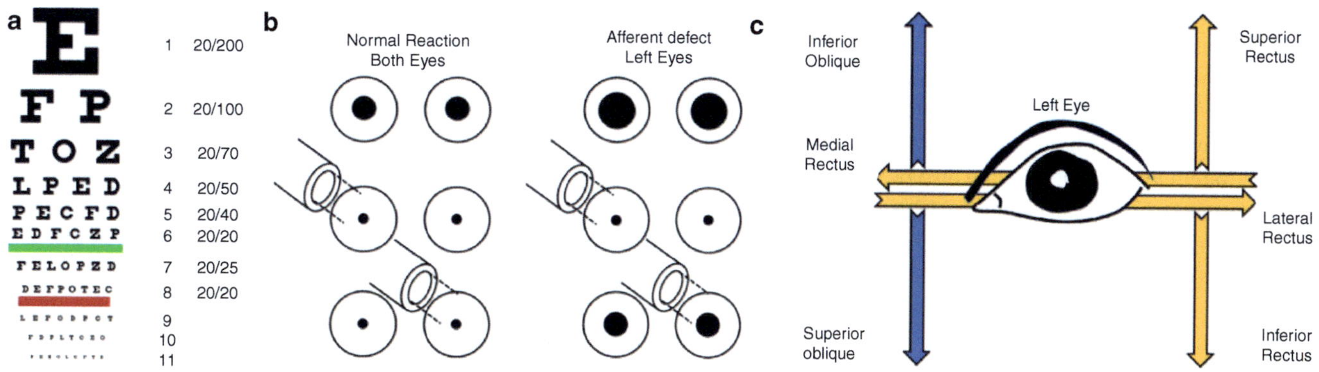

Fig. 57.12 Picture showing (**a**) the Snellen chart, (**b**) swinging flash light test, and (**c**) the six cardinal signs of gazes

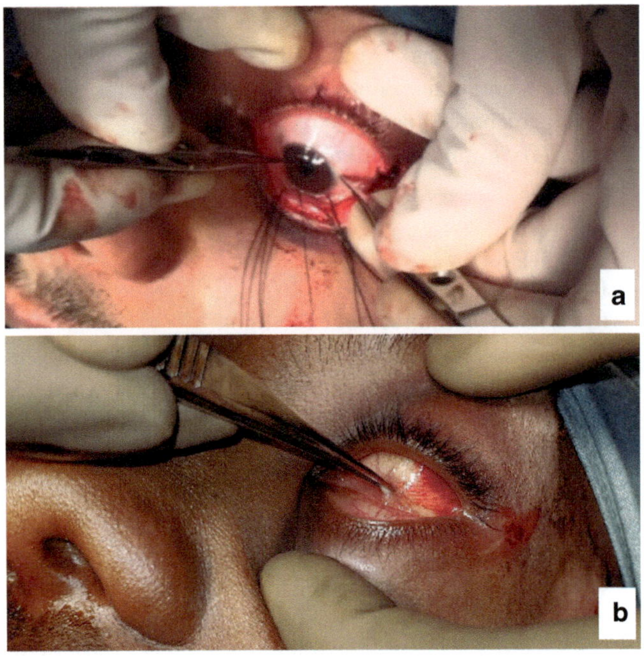

Fig. 57.13 Demonstration of the method of performing intraoperative forced duction test (**a**) by grasping the limbus (sclero-corneal junction) and (**b**) by grasping the inferior rectus muslce

is a range between 10 and 21 mmHg with the mean being around 15 mmHg. Low IOP may be suggestive of a ruptured globe or detached retina, while increased IOP may indicate hyphema, glaucoma, or an orbital compartment syndrome like "retrobulbar hemorrhage." A pressure of more than 30 mmHg is an ophthalmological emergency.

5. *Visual fields*: Visual fields for each eye are checked by asking the patient to determine movements at the periphery of the examiner's own visual field, while at a distance of about 2 ft from each other. Loss of field may be suggestive of compressive or ischemic injuries to the optic nerve with or without damage to the visual pathway. Goldmann visual field test can also be employed to objectively chart binocular visual field loss wherein patient is asked to look at a center of the chart and is required to track a point source of light.
6. *External examination/periorbital screening*: A thorough clinical evaluation is performed to note down all clinical features detailed below. Orbital trauma is generally associated with possible adnexal injuries which also need to be assessed for intervention and management.
7. *Slit-lamp examination*: A formal slit lamp test is performed if it may be allowed. This provides information about the lids, lashes, lacrimal system, conjunctiva, sclera, anterior chamber, iris, the lens, and the anterior vitreous.
8. *Fundoscopic examination*: A fundoscopic examination is performed to assess the retina, optic nerve head, and the vessels. This is done by the use of an ophthalmoscope. It also provides information about presence of intraocular hemorrhages and foreign bodies.
9. *Globe position*: An important feature in examination of orbital trauma from a cranio-maxillofacial perspective includes the examination of globe positions. This is performed both clinically and by using an exophthalmometer. The Hertel's exophthalmometer is used in common settings for the evaluation of proptosis or enophthalmos. In case of injuries involving the lateral face, like a fracture of the ZMC, the Naugle's exophthalmometer is used.

Box 57.3 "8-Point" Ophthalmic Examination Advocated by the American Association of Ophthalmology [23]

1.	Visual acuity and visual fields
2.	Pupillary examination
3.	Extraocular motility and alignment
4.	Intraocular pressure
5.	External examination/periorbital screening
6.	Slit-lamp examination
7.	Fundoscopic examination
8.	Globe position

57.6.2 Clinical Features

A good evaluation of the skeletal and soft tissue components of the orbit as well its associated adnexa (eyelids, lacrimal apparatus, etc.) is mandated. The common clinical features that are presented with in orbital trauma are provided in Box 57.4.

Box 57.4 Common Clinical Features in Orbital Trauma Are Enumerated Below

- Periorbital edema (Fig. 57.14a)
- Periorbital ecchymosis and subconjunctival hemorrhage (Fig. 57.14b)
- Contusions and hematomas
- Subcutaneous emphysema with crepitus
- Lacerations involving the eyelids (Fig. 57.14c)
- Injuries to the canthal apparatus (medial and lateral)
- Neurological deficits of the infra-orbital and facial nerves

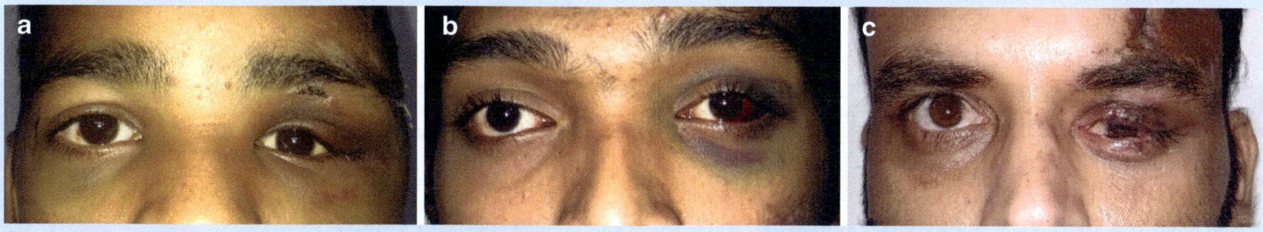

Fig. 57.14 Clinical pictures demonstrating (**a**) edema of the left periorbital region, (**b**) left-sided periorbital ecchymosis and subconjunctival hemorrhage, and (**c**) soft tissue injury of the left eyelid and supraorbital region

Clinical signs and symptoms that are more exclusive to orbital trauma are discussed further in more detail.

57.6.2.1 Enophthalmos/Hypophthalmos (Fig. 57.15a, b)

Any change in the orbital volume directly impacts the position of the globe and its anteroposterior projection and supero-inferior position [24]. Clinically enophthalmos can be detected by an exaggerated suprapalpebral fold and reduced projection on viewing from an inferior view or worm's view. Hertel's or Naugle's exophthalmometer can also be used to quantify and measure the discrepancy. Other causes of enophthalmos implicated are traumatic atrophy of intra-orbital fat, infections causing cicatricial contraction of retrobulbar tissues, and dislocation of trochlear attachment of superior oblique muscle due to trauma [25, 26]. Hypophthalmos is noted as a change in the horizontal pupillary levels.

57.6.2.2 Retrobulbar Hemorrhage (Fig. 57.16)

Retrobulbar hemorrhage is a vision threatening emergency which occurs due to accumulation of blood in the retrobulbar space. This causes increased intra-orbital pressure resulting in compression or stretching of the optic nerve and reduced perfusion to the eye. Orbital trauma especially blunt injury may be associated with retrobulbar hemorrhage which warrants immediate attention. However this may also occur as a complication following surgery to the orbit or pathologies like an aneurysm. Acute post-septal hemorrhage limited anteriorly by the orbital septum and posteriorly by bone may cause permanent loss of vision by creating a compartment syndrome [27]. It presents as reduced ocular motility, elevated intraocular pressure, proptosis, and diminishing vision. In unconscious patients, pupillary assessment, increased pressure, and presence of relative afferent pupillary defect or RAPD are usually diagnostic.

57.6.2.3 Lacrimal System Injuries

Due to its close topographical location to the orbital complex, nasolacrimal system especially the duct may be involved in traumatic injuries to the orbit. Injury to the canaliculi or the nasolacrimal ducts in naso-orbito-ethmoidal injuries may present as epiphora [28]. Patency of

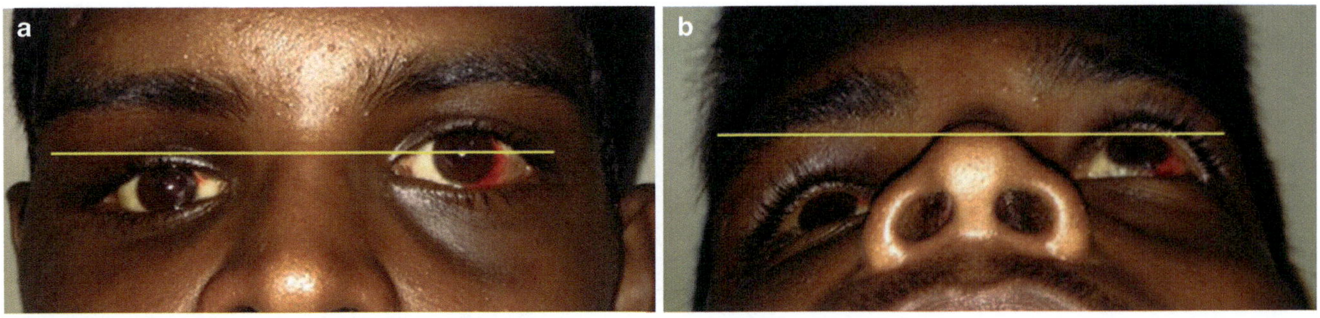

Fig. 57.15 Clinical photograph of a patient with both (**a**) hypophthalmos and (**b**) enophthalmos of the right globe

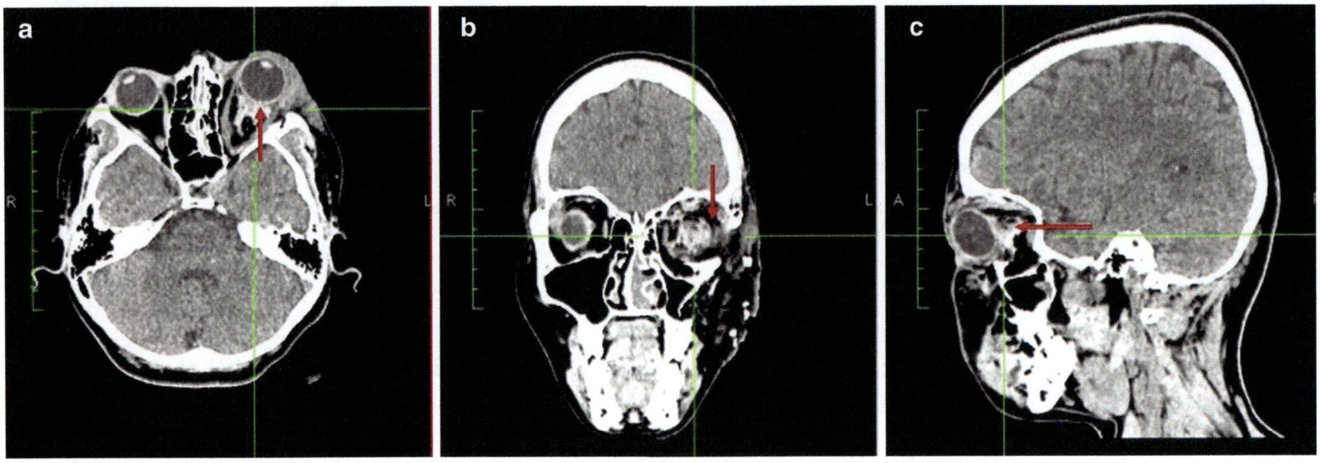

Fig. 57.16 (**a**) Axial, (**b**) coronal, and (**c**) sagittal section CT scan images demonstrating left-sided retrobulbar hemorrhage

the naso-lacrimal duct and sac can be verified by the Jones tests 1 and 2 or by a simple lacrimal probing test with insertion of a Crawford silicone intubation tubes though the canaliculi and visualization of the same at the distal end of the disruption. ROPLAS test or regurgitation on pressure over lacrimal sac may be performed clinically to elicit post-traumatic blockage of the nasolacrimal duct (Fig. 57.17c). Confirmation however is obtained with a CT dacryocystogram or CT-DCG (Fig. 57.17a, b). Reconstruction of the lacrimal drainage system is achieved by simple intubations or a formal dacryocystorhinostomy as indicated by the clinical scenario.

57.6.2.4 Oculocardiac Reflex (Trigeminocardiac Reflex)

First described by Dagnini and Aschner in 1908, oculocardiac reflex is bradycardia on manual compression of the eyes. The most common traumatic etiology is the incarceration of inferior rectus muscle in trap-door fractures of the orbital floor [29, 30]. Other causes that may present with oculocardiac reflex are retrobulbar hemorrhage, white-eyed blowout fractures and orbital surgery.

57.6.2.5 Superior Orbital Fissure Syndrome (Box 57.5)

Post-traumatic superior orbital fissure syndrome may be attributed to pressure exerted on the contents of the superior orbital fissure due to hemorrhage or impingement by fractured fragments.

Superior orbital fissure syndrome was first described by Hirschfield in 1858 [31, 32] and symptoms include:

(i) Ophthalmoplegia due to involvement of III, IV, and VI cranial nerves.
(ii) Paresthesia over the forehead due to involvement frontal nerve of first division of trigeminal nerve.
(iii) Ptosis due to impeded action of levator palpebrae superioris and Muller's muscle.
(iv) Pupillary dilatation due to paresis of circular sphincter muscle and unrestricted action of dilator pupillae.
(v) Impairment of direct pupillary reflex due to blocked ipsilateral efferent arc, whereas consensual reflex is preserved due to intact ipsilateral efferent and contralateral efferent arcs.

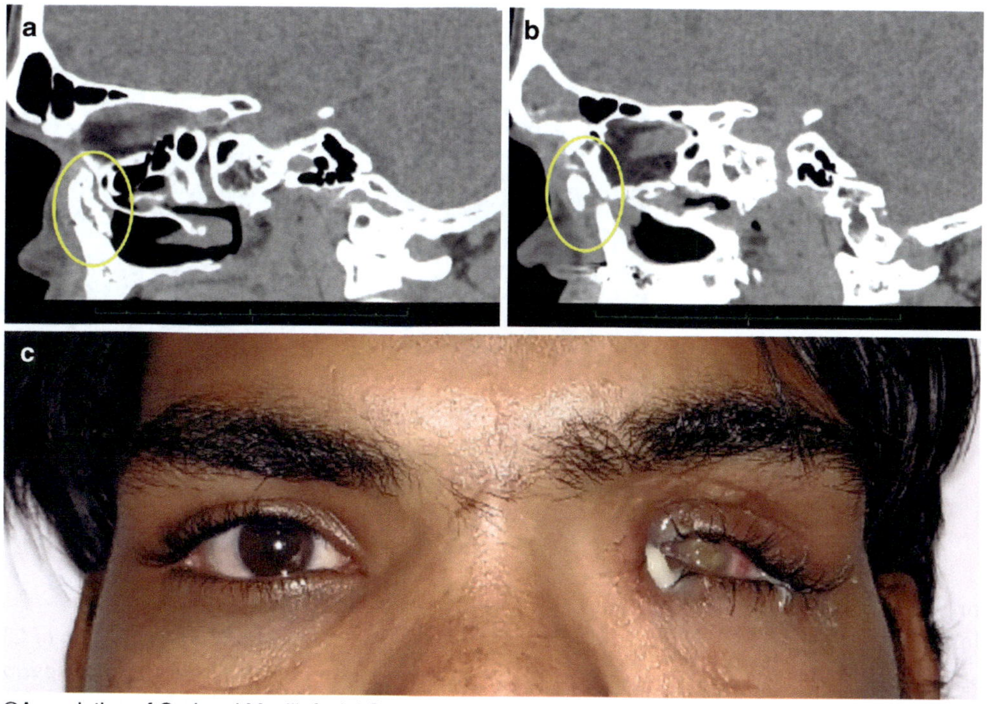

Fig. 57.17 (**a**) Sagittal section CT DCG demonstrating patent NLD with draining dye and (**b**) blocked NLD with no drainage of the dye. (**c**) Clinical photograph of patient with left-sided NOE fracture demonstrating regurgitation of contents due to blocked left naso-lacrimal duct ROPLAS positive

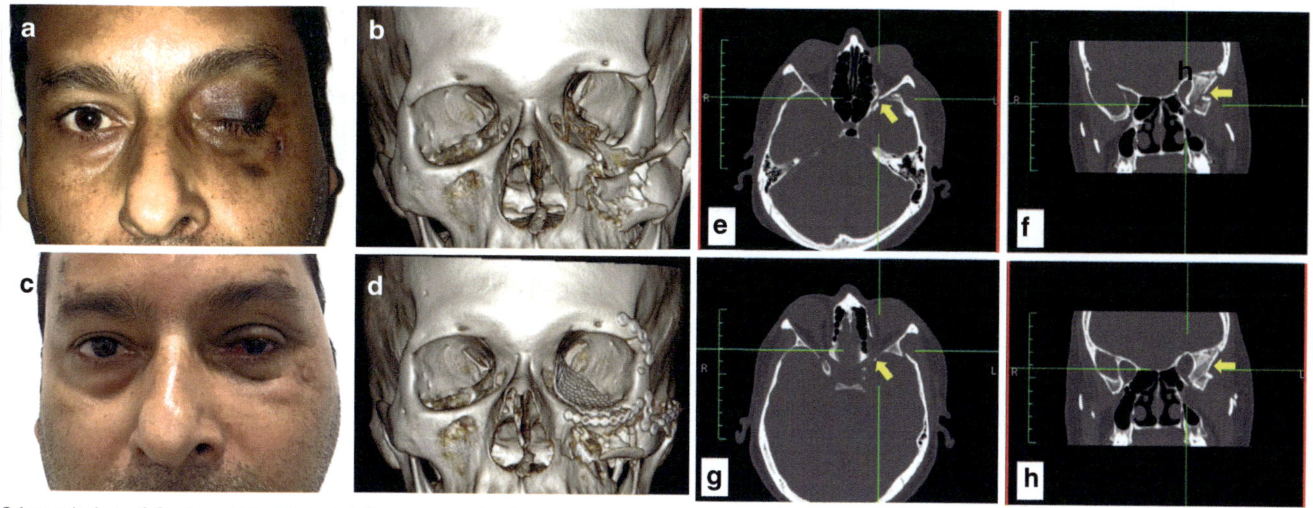

Fig. 57.18 Clinical pictures and CT scans of patient with orbital apex syndrome. (**a**) Clinical picture demonstrating left-sided orbito-zygomatic trauma with clinically evident ptosis, (**b**) 3D CT demonstrating comminuted zygomatico-orbital fracture with medial displacement of the greater wing of sphenoid, (**c**) clinical picture of patient 2 weeks post-surgery with resolution of ptosis, (**d**) post-operative 3D CT showing ORIF, (**e**) pre-operative axial CT demonstrating total compression of the left optic canal (yellow arrow), (**f**) pre-operative coronal CT demonstrating compression of the left superior orbital fissure (yellow arrow), (**g**) post-operative CT showing decompressed left optic canal (yellow arrow) and (**h**) post-operative coronal CT showing decompresison of the left superior orbital fissure (yellow arrow)

(vi) Impaired accommodation is because of impaired parasympathetic pathway to the ciliary ganglion.
(vii) Loss of corneal reflex due to lack of transmission via the nasociliary branch of ophthalmic nerve.
(viii) Proptosis either due to presence of hemorrhage or paresis and laxity of extraocular muscles which normally aid in globe retraction.

Management may be conservative or exploratory surgery of the orbit including surgical decompression [33].

57.6.2.6 Orbital Apex Syndrome (Fig. 57.18) (Box 57.5)

In severe orbital trauma, optic nerve may also be implicated due its close proximity to the superior orbital fissure [31, 34]. The term orbital apex syndrome was first coined by Kjaer in 1945 [35], and the symptoms include all features

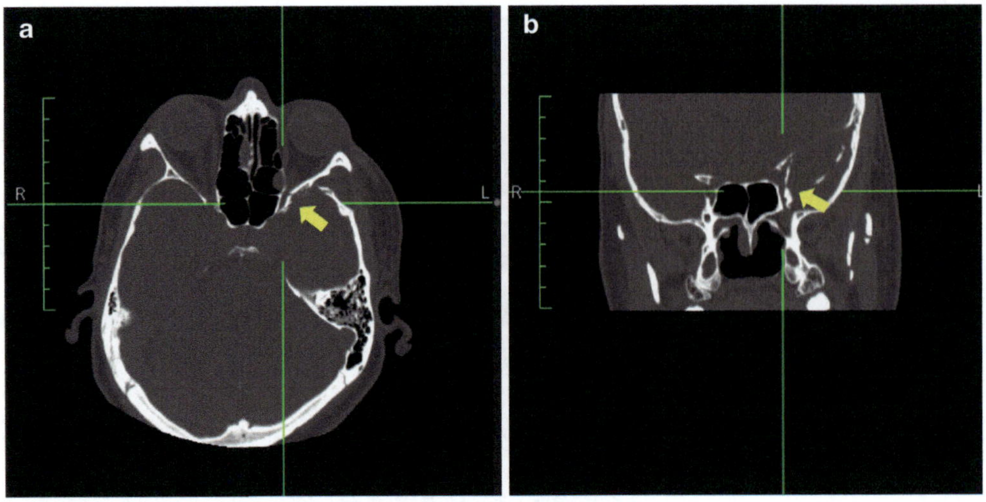

Fig. 57.19 (**a**, **b**) Axial CT scan of patient with direct traumatic optic neuropathy demonstrating a skull base fracture and bony spicule at the entry of the optic nerve into the canal

of superior orbital fissure syndrome along with partial or loss of vision.

57.6.2.7 Traumatic Optic Neuropathy (TON) (Box 57.5)

TON may be defined as an acute injury to the optic nerve with impairment of visual function. It may occur as a result of:

(i) Direct trauma to the optic nerve (Fig. 57.19) (physical damage or nerve sheath compression due to compartment syndromes)
(ii) An indirect insult due to diffuse axonal damage secondary to conduction of forces from blunt head trauma

The occurrence may be unilateral or bilateral.

Clinical features of TON include:

(i) Afferent pupillary defect
(ii) Diminished visual acuity
(iii) Diminished color perception
(iv) Varying reduction in visual fields

Management of TON is handled under the section of orbital emergencies.

Box 57.5 Comparison of Clinical Features of Traumatic Optic Neuropathy, Superior Orbital Fissure, and Orbital Apex Syndromes

Traumatic optic neuropathy (TON)	Superior orbital fissure syndrome	Orbital apex syndrome
Unilateral or bilateral	Ophthalmoplegia with involvement of cranial nerves III, IV, & VI	All features of superior orbital fissure syndrome
Relative afferent pupillary defect (RAPD) except in symmetrical bilateral cases	Forehead paresthesia	Partial or total loss of vison
Variable loss of visual acuity (from normal to no vision)	Ptosis	
Impaired color vision	Dilated pupil	
Variable visual field defects	Impaired direct but preserved consensual pupillary reflex. Impaired accommodation	
	Loss of corneal reflex	
	Proptosis	

57.6.3 Investigations

Conventional radiographs have a minimal role in the diagnosis and planning of orbital fractures. CT scans (Fig. 57.20a–c) have long been considered the "gold standard" in orbital trauma. The scans are usually ordered in fine cuts of 0.5 mm and taken in all the three planes. The coronal and the sagittal scans are important in the diagnosis

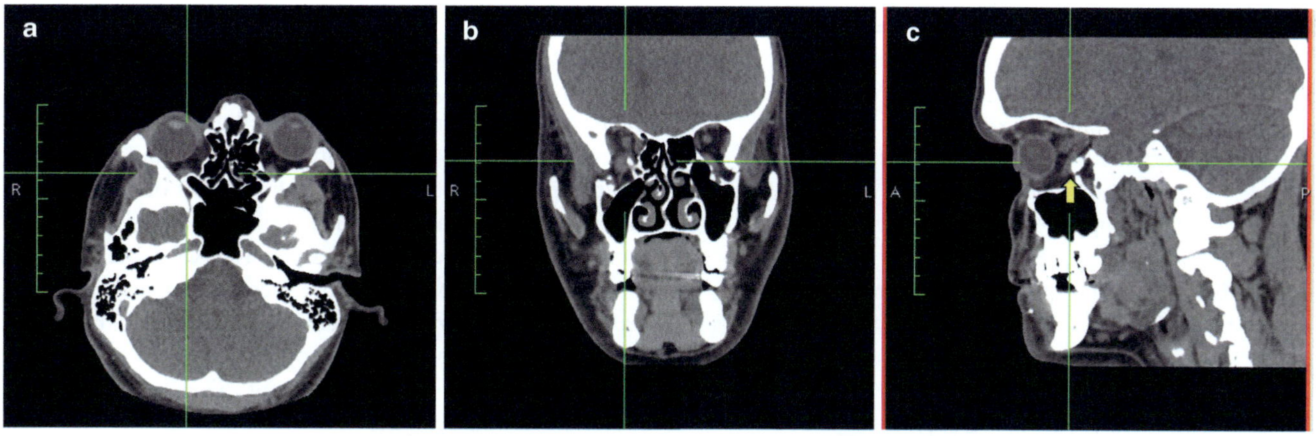

Fig. 57.20 CT scans showing (**a**) axial section with fracture of the medial wall of the right orbit, (**b**) coronal section showing fractures of the medial wall and floor, and (**c**) sagittal section showing fracture of the floor with fibrosis of the inferior rectus to the posterior ledge (yellow arrow)

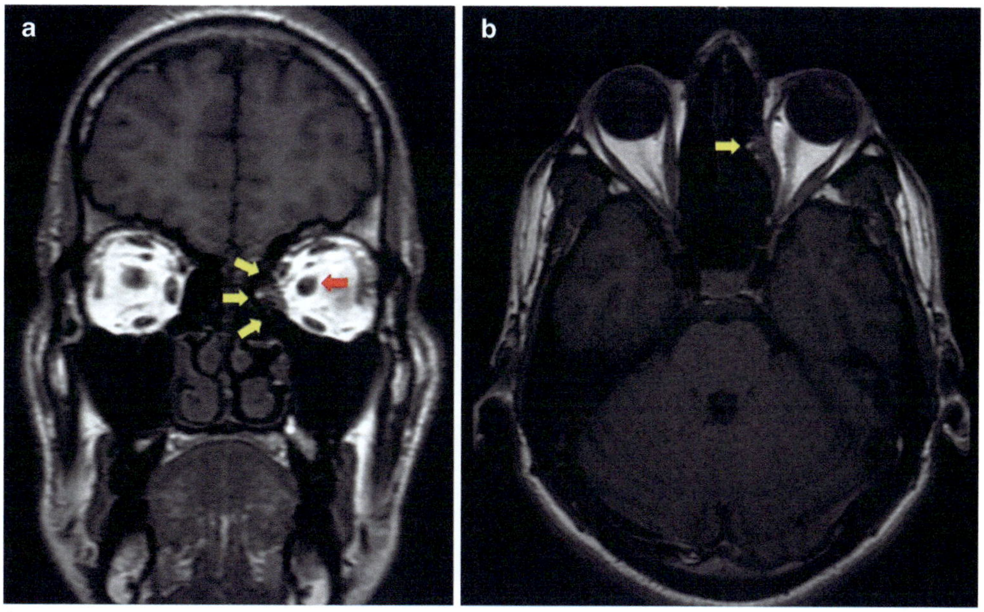

Fig. 57.21 MRI (**a**) coronal and (**b**) sagittal sections, demonstrating entrapment of the medial rectus (yellow arrows) and medial displacement of the optic nerve (left orbit)

of fractures of the floor and the roof, while the axial scans provide better information regarding the fractures of the medial and lateral walls. Axial sections are also important to study the optic canal integrity.

Indications for an MRI (Fig. 57.21a, b) scan are limited to determining soft tissue injuries and entrapment of muscles and to assessing damage to the optic nerve. It is also used to identify intra-orbital herniation of brain in the case of blow-in fractures.

57.7 Approaches to the Orbit

Box 57.6 Surgical Approaches to the Orbit

- Transcutaneous-medial and lateral
- Trans-caruncular
- Transconjunctival

57.7.1 Transcutaneous Approaches

1. Lynch
2. Extended glabellar approach
   (a). Lateral transcutaneous approaches
      (i) Lateral brow incision
      (ii) The upper lid blepharoplasty and the sub brow approaches
   (b). Lower eyelid approaches (Also refer Figs. 56.44, 56.45)
      (i) Sub-ciliary
      (ii) Sub-tarsal
      (iii) Infra-orbital (Video 57.1)

57.7.1.1 Lynch

This incision described by Lynch [36] in 1921 is a semilunar-shaped incision (Fig. 57.22a) placed between the nasal dorsum and the medial canthal ligament that provides direct access to the canthal apparatus and the medial orbital rim and wall. The major drawbacks of this particular incision are chances of developing a web and hence an unsightly scar. There may also be risk of damage to the medial canthal tendon and the lacrimal apparatus that is present infero-laterally. Recent modifications of the Lynch incision have accommodated options to reduce the scarring by the use of "Z" plasties (Fig. 57.22b, c) and other esthetic incision designs.

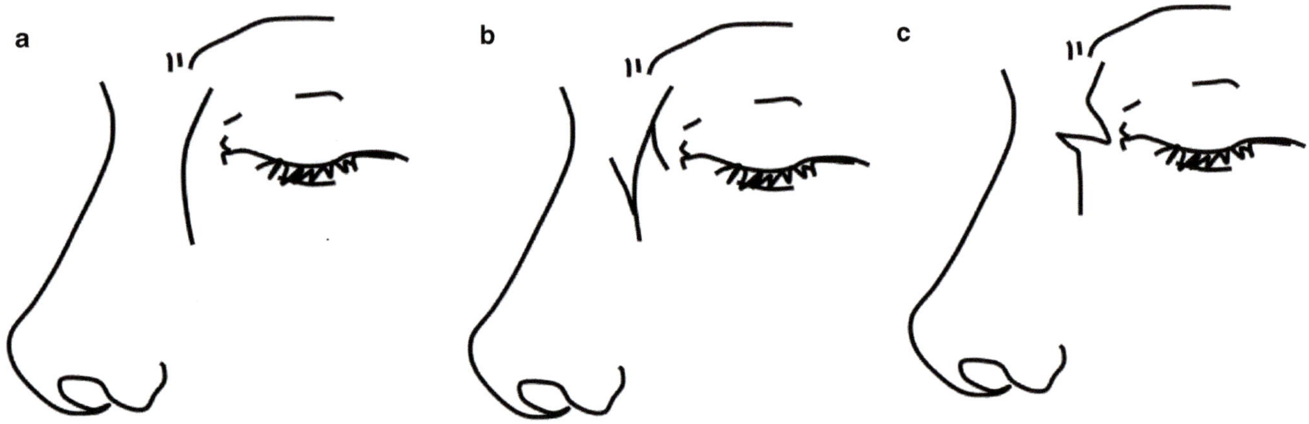

Fig. 57.22 Diagrammatic representation of the (**a**) classical Lynch incision and (**b, c**) modification with "Z" plasty

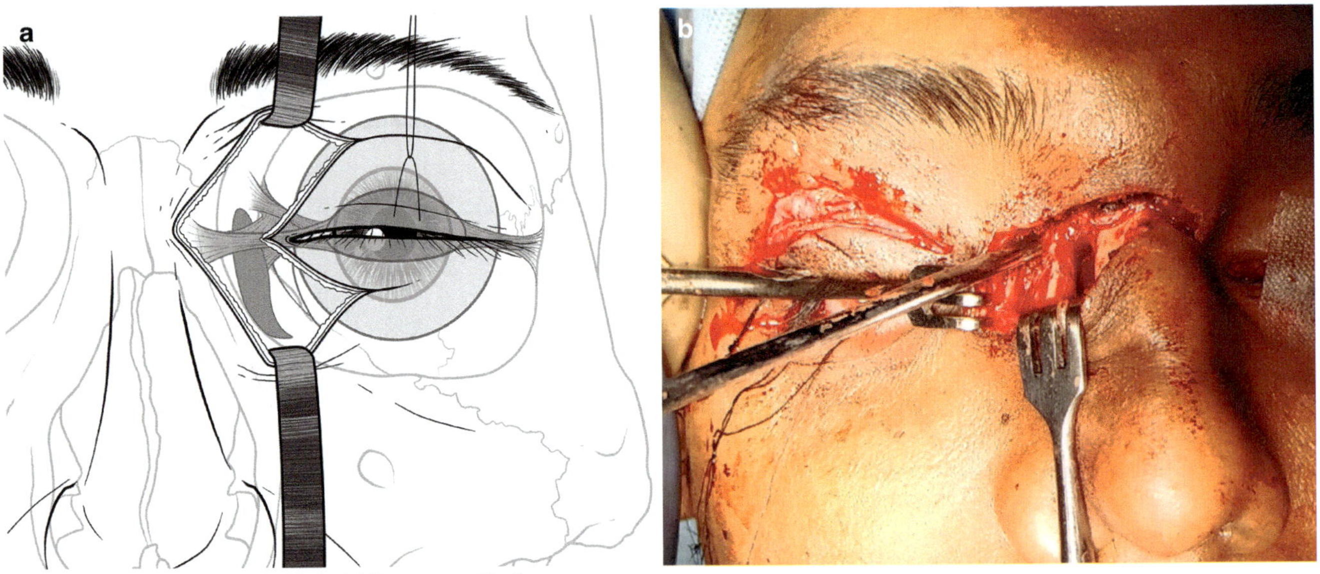

Fig. 57.23 Diagram and intraoperative picture showing extended glabellar approach to the medial orbit

57.7.1.2 Extended Glabellar Approach (Fig. 57.23)

The extended glabellar incision or a horizontal "Y" approach involves a small Y-shaped incision with the fork extending over the upper and lower lid crease with the long arm across the nasal dorsum over the glabellar region. This approach provides excellent access to the medial canthal tendon apparatus and also provides enough room for medial orbital wall exploration cephalad to the tendon.

57.7.2 Trans-caruncular Approach

The trans-caruncular route provides excellent exposure to the medial orbit without causing any esthetic concern. The caruncle is a papular structure seen medial to the plica semilunaris which is a fold of conjunctiva in medial canthal region. An avascular plane is located deep to the caruncle between the medial orbital septum and the Horner's muscle which on dissection exposes the medial wall of the orbit (Fig. 57.24a) [37].

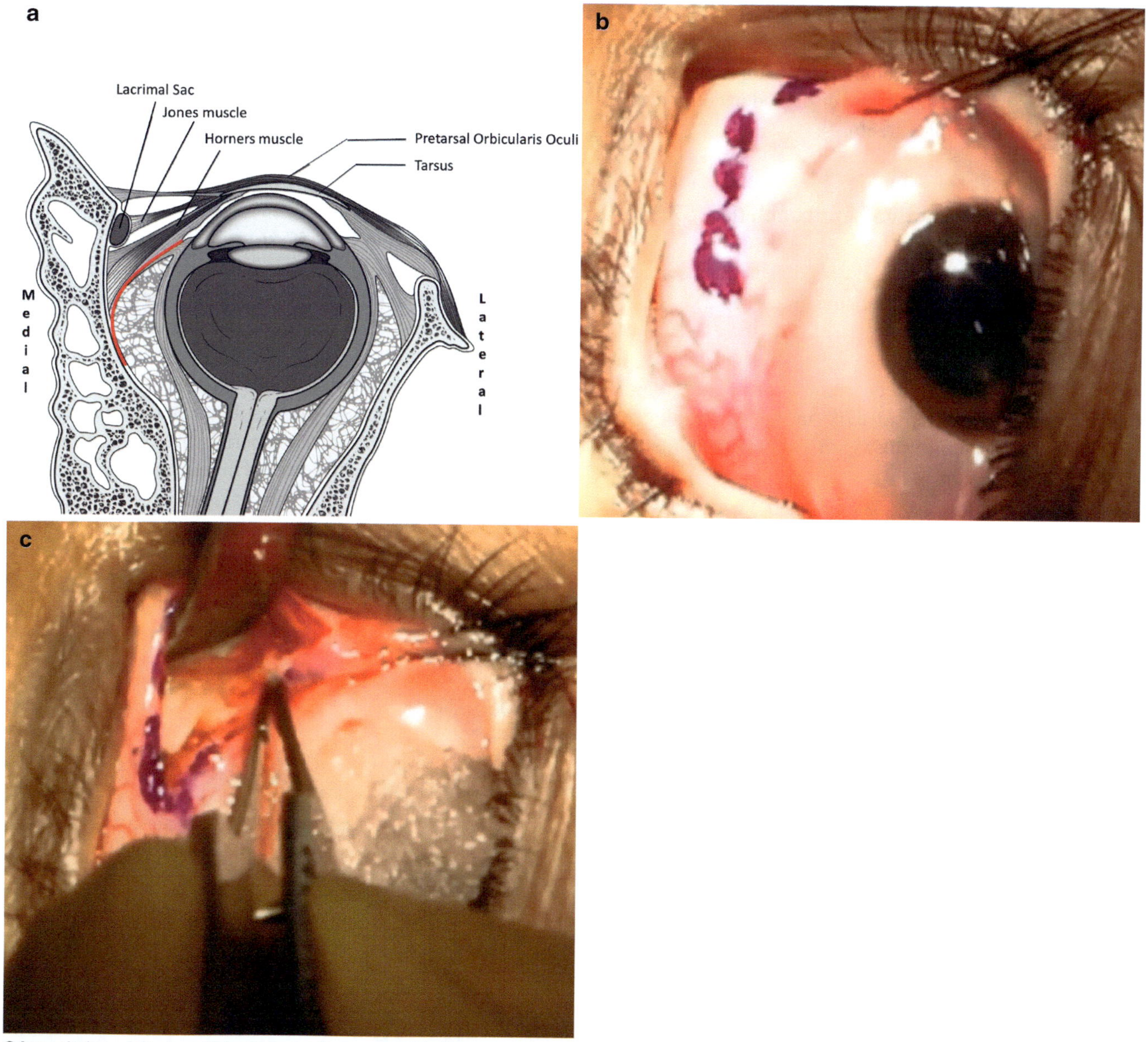

Fig. 57.24 (**a**) Diagram and (**b**) intraoperative pictures showing marking for trans-caruncular approach to the medial orbit and (**c**) exposure of the medial orbital wall. (Courtesy: Dept of Orbit & Oculoplasty, Shankara Nethralaya, Chennai)

After placing retraction sutures on upper and lower eyelids, gentle medial traction is applied over the skin of the nasal dorsum, and incision is placed lateral to the caruncle, while avoiding injury to the lacrimal puncta or canaliculi (Fig. 57.24b). The length of the incision is between 1.5 and 2.5 cm. Dissection through the fibers of the Muller's muscle exposes the medial wall just posterior to the posterior lacrimal crest (Fig. 57.24c). For additional exposure of associated orbital floor fractures, a C-shaped approach can be used including a transconjunctival incision with or without lateral canthotomy and inferior cantholysis in conjunction with the trans-caruncular approach.

As the lateral transcutaneous and lower lid approaches also find use in the management of fractures of the zygomatic complex fractures, they are discussed in detail in chapter on zygomatic complex fractures.

A historical perspective of the description of the transconjunctival approach and its evolution into the most favored approach for access to the floor and medial wall of the orbit along with the infra-orbital rim is provided in Box 57.7.

Box 57.7 Evolution and Modifications of the Transconjunctival Approach

Author	Year	Description
Bourget J	1924	Conjunctival approach for blepharoplasty
Tenzel & Miller	1971	Post-septal approach
Tessier P	1973	Pre-septal approach
McCord & Moses	1979	"Swinging eyelid" with lateral canthotomy
Garcia GH	1998	Trans-caruncular approach

57.7.3 Transconjunctival Approach (Fig. 57.25)

The infra-orbital rim and orbital floor defects can be accessed through a transconjunctival incision (Video 57.2).

Its advantages include:

(i) Excellent cosmesis
(ii) Minimal incidence of ectropion
(iii) Extensive access up to 270° including the floor and medial and lateral walls, with the modifications to the conventional approach

Pre-septal Approach (Fig. 57.26)

The incision is marked 2–3 mm posterior to the tarsal plate along the mediolateral length of the lower palpebral conjunctiva. Dissection is performed along the subconjunctival plane and is carried down toward the inferior orbital rim. This maintains the plane anterior to the orbital septum. Retraction sutures may be placed on the vestibular portion of the conjunctival flap with traction in superior direction, to provide additional protection to the globe. On reaching the facial surface of the infra-orbital rim, the periosteum is incised about

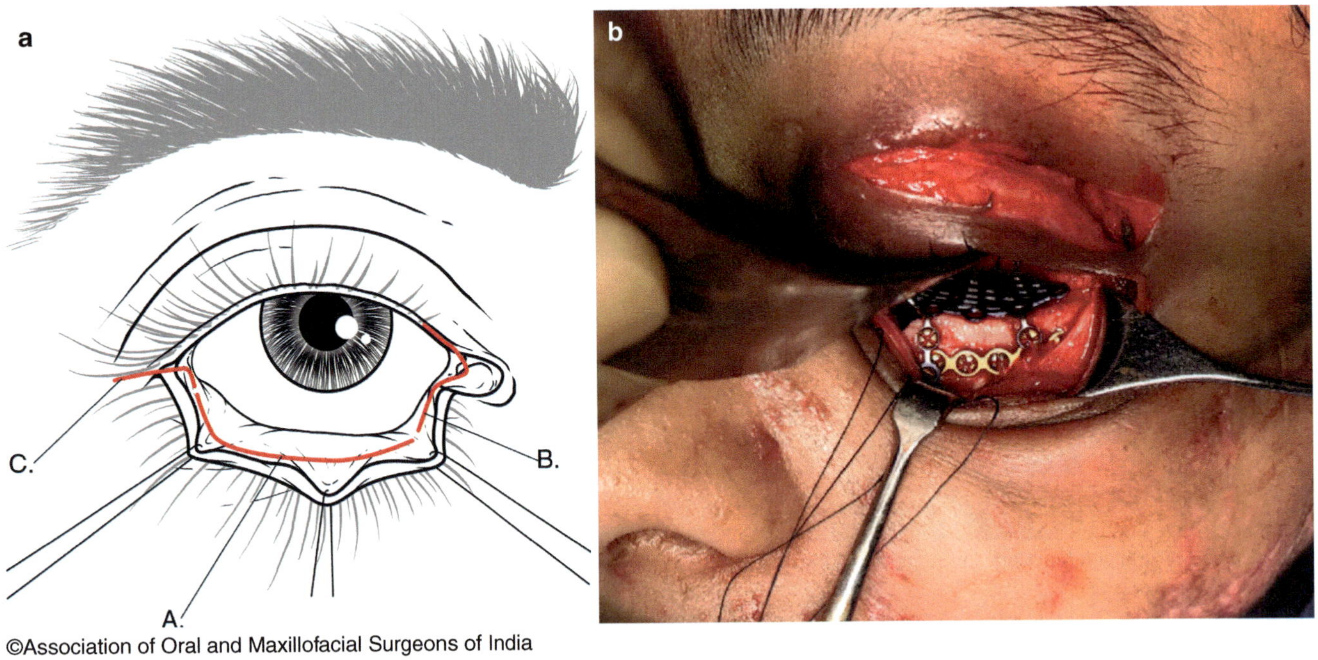

Fig. 57.25 (**a**) Diagram showing trans-conjunctival approach and its modifications - A. Transconjunctival, B. Trans-caruncular & C. Lateral canthotomy. (**b**) Intra-operative picture of trans-conjunctival with the lateral canthotomy modification. The picture also shows an upper lid blepharoplasty incision used to access the fronto-zygomatic suture

2 mm inferior to the rim. This is followed by subperiosteal dissection and exploration of the orbital floor by retracting the globe and orbital contents superiorly. Approximately 2–3 mm distance must be maintained from the lower end of the tarsal plates while making the initial conjunctival incision failing which there is vertical shortening of the lower eyelid and entropion post-operatively.

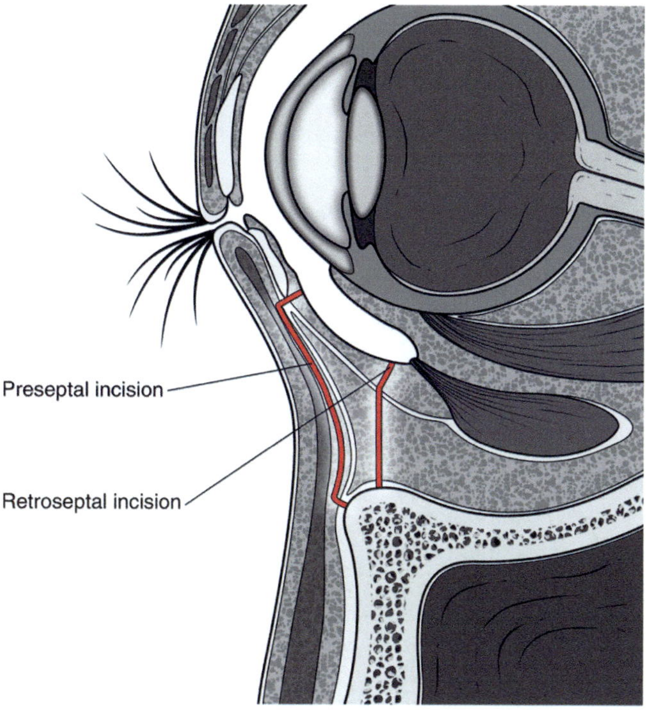

Fig. 57.26 Diagrammatic representation of the pre-septal and retroseptal modifications of the transconjunctival approach

Retroseptal Approach (Fig. 57.26)
In the retroseptal type, the conjunctival incision is made near the fornix spanning mediolaterally just short of the caruncle. Dissection is posterior to the orbital septum providing a fast and direct access to the floor when compared to the preseptal type [38]. However, orbital fat is encountered before approaching the orbital floor, which may prove bothersome for dissection and manipulation. The periorbita is incised immediately posterior to the rim after superior retraction of the fat and globe with a malleable retractor. This is followed by subperiosteal dissection and exploration of the floor defect. Excessive manipulation of the orbital fat during orbital reconstruction increases the risk of enophthalmos due to fat disintegration [39, 40]. Placement of the incision too low into the fornix may damage the inferior oblique muscle and retractors of the lower eyelid, compromising esthetics post-operatively due to lower lid entropion.

57.7.4 Trans-antral Endoscopic-Assisted Approach (Fig. 57.27a, b)

The trans-antral approach was attempted by Converse and Smith [41] as early as the 1960s. Entry to the antrum is gained through a transoral Caldwell Luc procedure and a 0° or 30° endoscope may be used to visualize the orbital floor.

57.7.5 Coronal Approach

The coronal approach offers the most extensive exposure of the entire upper and middle third of the face including the orbit. A detailed description of the same is provided in Chap. 85 on access osteotomies.

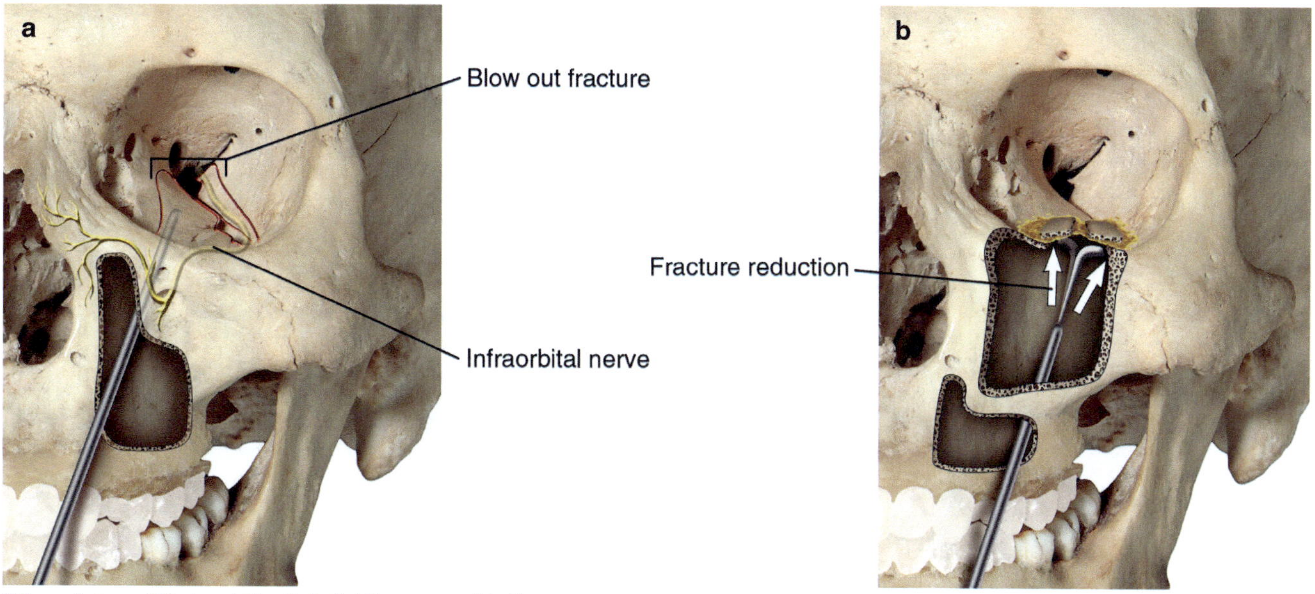

Fig. 57.27 (**a**, **b**) Diagram of the trans-antral endoscopy assisted approach to the orbital floor

57.8 A Clinical Sequence for Treatment Planning and Management of Orbital Fractures

A clear understanding of the various patterns of orbital fractures and their clinical implications is absolutely necessary to design and formulate a plan for their reconstruction. The basic management guidelines for the common variations in orbital fractures are detailed below (see Hammer [7] classification, Fig. 57.9).

57.8.1 Type I (Orbito-Zygomatic)

Concomitant fractures of the zygomatic complex and the orbit mandate ORIF of the zygomatic complex first, followed by internal orbital reconstruction. This sequence is favored because the orbital rims provide the most accurate guidance for restoration of the internal orbital architecture.

Box 57.8 The Surgical Objectives for Type I Fractures

- Restoration of transverse dimension of the face, malar prominence, and the arch anatomy
- Restoration of rim architecture
- Correction of orbital dystopia
- Correction of the axis of the palpebral fissure and
- Reconstruction of the internal orbit

Figures 57.28a–d and 57.29a–d demonstrate a type I fracture managed using the above principles.

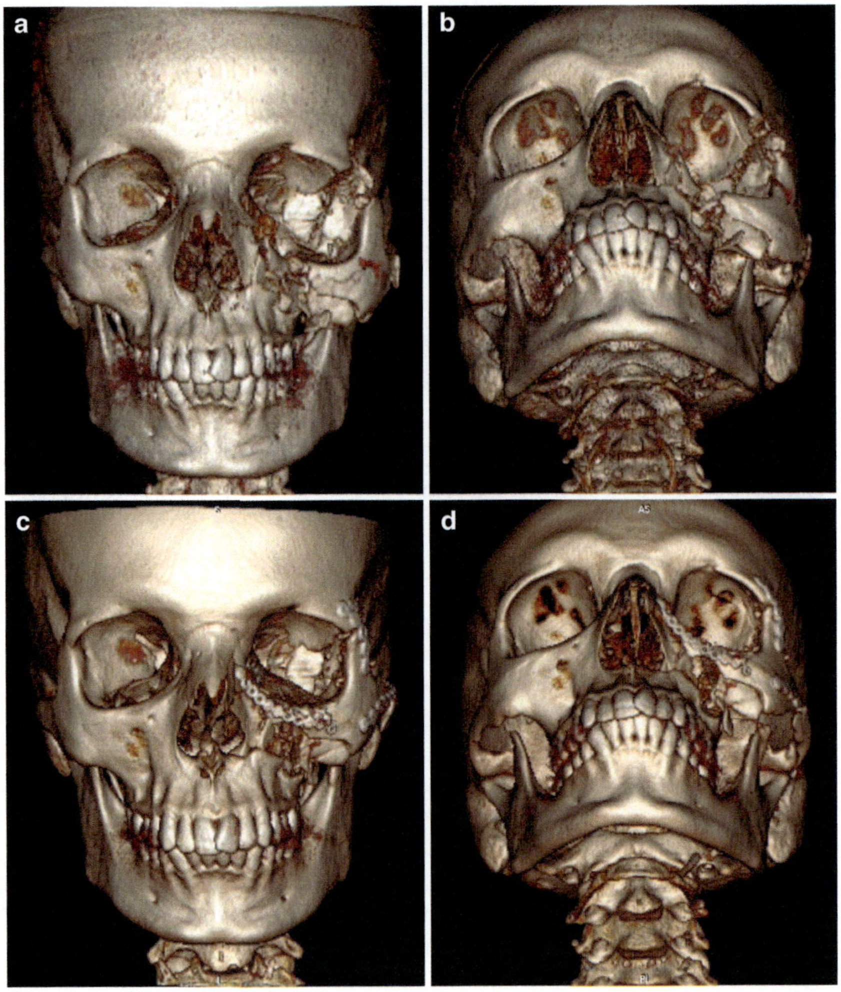

Fig. 57.28 3D CT scans of patient with orbito-zygomatic fracture. (**a** and **b**) Preoperative frontal and basal views demonstrating the fracture, (**c** and **d**) post-operative frontal and basal views demonstrating fixation of fractures

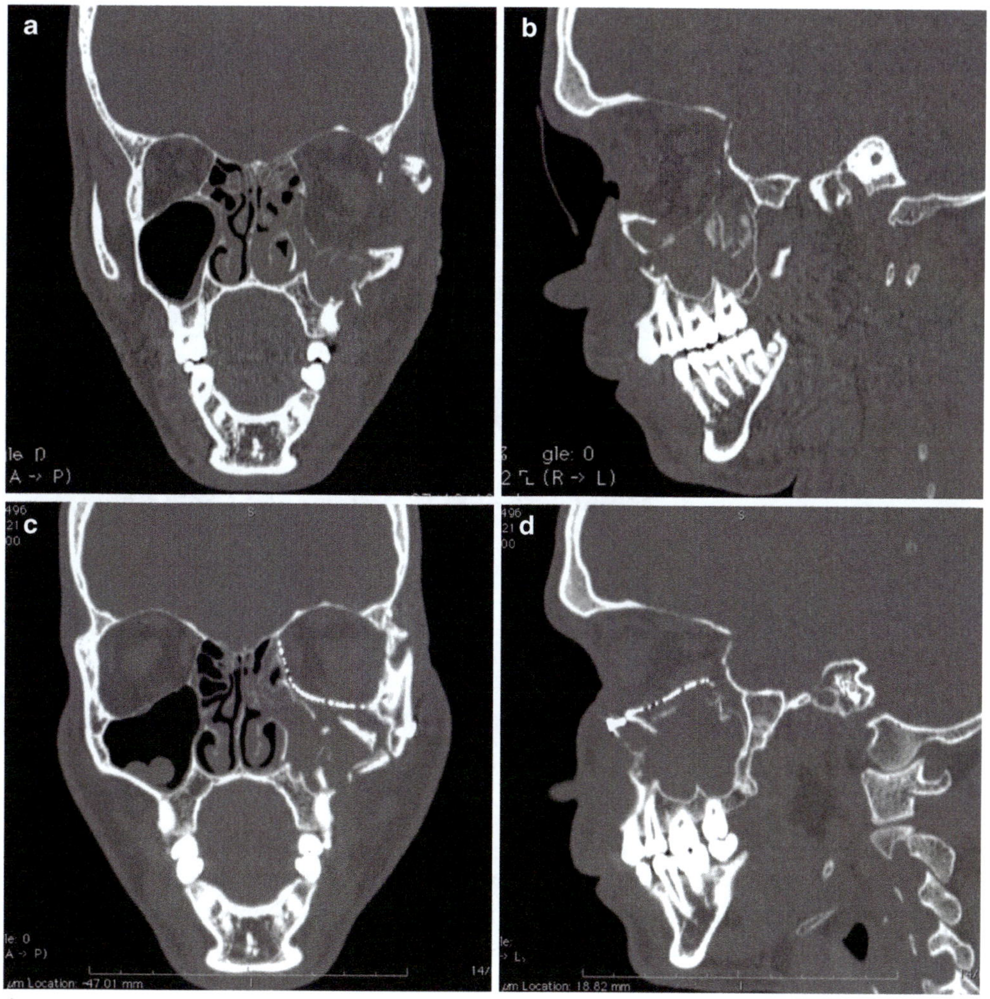

Fig. 57.29 Axial and sagittal scans of the patient in Fig 57.28, with orbito-zygomatic fracture. (**a** and **b**) Sections demonstrating fracture of the left zygomatic complex with a large defect of the orbital floor. (**c** and **d**) Post-operative sections revealing optimal reduction of the fracture and floor reconstruction with anatomical orbital floor implant

57.8.2 Type II (Internal Orbital)

Management of type II orbital fractures, which are essentially the internal fractures (both blow-in and blowout) of the orbit including (1) the roof, (2) the floor, and (3) the medial and (4) lateral walls are detailed below.

> **Box 57.9 The Management of All Internal Orbital Fractures Can Be Handled Essentially by Answering the Following Basic Questions** *(Clinical Tip)*
>
> (i) Is there a need for intervention?
> (ii) When is the best time to intervene?
> (iii) Is there a need for reconstruction?
> (iv) What to use for reconstruction?

57.8.2.1 Fractures of the Orbital Roof

Isolated fractures of the orbital roof are extremely rare. They usually occur as a part of fronto-basilar fractures, fractures of the frontal sinus, or may occur concomitant with fractures of the supraorbital rim. Orbital roof fractures are present in approximately 5% of all orbital and cranial fractures, while incidence of isolated orbital roof fractures may be as low as 0.7% of all orbital and cranial fractures. The most common etiological factors include motor vehicle accidents, assaults, or falls.

Orbital roof fractures may be associated with more severe neurological symptoms including dural tears, CSF leak, tension pneumocephalus, diffuse cerebral edema, and contusions of the frontal lobe [42]. It is imperative for a neurological and ophthalmological consult prior to management.

In general, orbital roof fractures may be categorized into four types (Fig. 57.30).

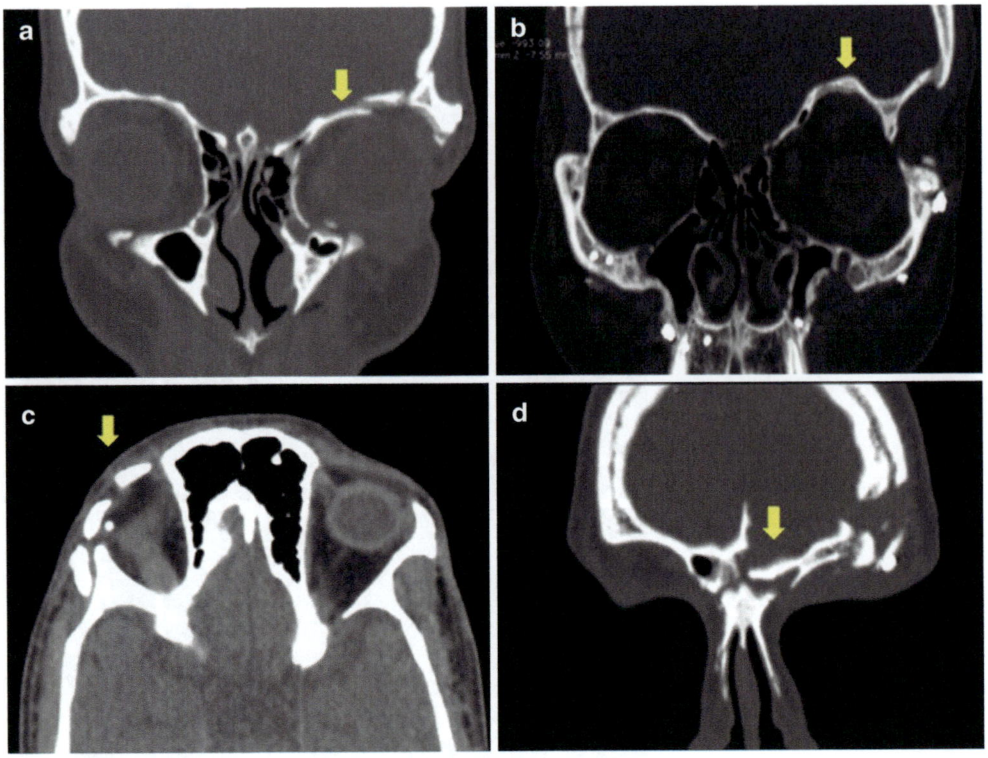

Fig. 57.30 CT scan images showing types of roof fractures (**a**) blow-in fracture, (**b**) blowout fracture, (**c**) fracture of the supraorbital rim, and (**d**) fronto-basilar fracture

- I—Blow-in fractures of the orbital roof where there is caudal displacement of the orbital roof with or without herniation of the brain. These may be undisplaced or displaced fractures. Comminuted fractures may leave fragments within the orbital cavity and may produce functional deficits with ophthalmic signs including restriction of extraocular muscle movement, diplopia, ptosis, and even blindness. These are generally caused due to increase in the intra-cranial pressure secondary to injuries.
- II—Blowout fractures of the orbital roof where there is cephalad displacement of the orbital roof into the cranial cavity due to increased intra-orbital pressure pushing the roof above. These injuries may be associated with neurological symptoms.
- III—Fractures involving the supraorbital rim. These may be seen as impure fractures of the orbital roof with an associated fracture of either a blow-in or a blowout nature.
- IV—Fractures involving the frontal sinus and the fronto-basilar complex. These fractures are more severe in nature and may often be associated with severe neurological implications.

Less than 10% of orbital roof fractures may need any form of surgical intervention [42]. Most are amenable to conservative management with observation and follow-up of neurological and ophthalmic status.

The need for management of fractures of the orbital roof may depend on:

(i) The presence of CSF leak which may need to be addressed
(ii) The necessity to retrieve displaced intra cranial fragments
(iii) Ophthalmic signs with compromise on vision
(iv) Large displacement of fragments which may act as mechanical impediments or significantly alter intra-orbital volume producing enophthalmos or exophthalmos.

Interventions may be indicated immediately or late primary depending on the indications mentioned above. Reconstruction of the roof of the orbit is not a procedure routinely indicated. However in cases where there is an absolute necessity for reconstruction like prevention of brain herniation or restoration of intra orbital volume which has been significantly altered, the choice may vary between the use of titanium meshes (Fig. 57.31) or porous polyethylene implants fixed with micro-screws to split calvarial grafts.

Figure 57.32a–f demonstrates the management of a malunited fronto-basilar fracture along with a blow-in fracture of the orbital roof compressing the eyeball producing restriction of movement.

57.8.2.2 Fractures of the Lateral Orbital Wall

Lateral orbital walls are the strongest of all the orbital walls [43]. The lateral wall generally shows diastasis and displacement in the case of fractures involving the zygomatico-orbital complex and is restored to its normal anatomy when the reduction of the zygomatic complex is achieved [44]. However this wall gets comminuted in high-velocity injuries [45] necessitating reconstruction in the primary intervention.

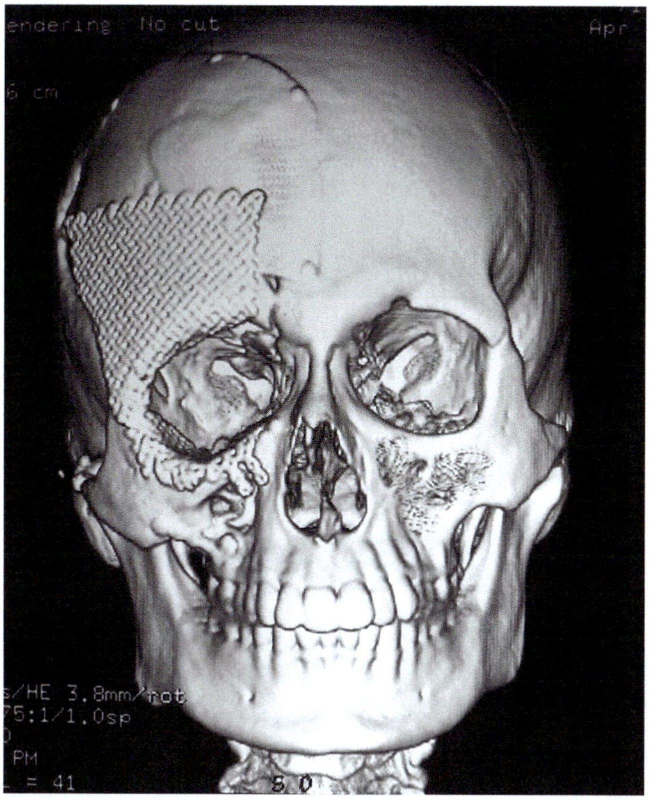

Fig. 57.31 Reconstruction of complex defect of the frontal bone, orbital roof, and supraorbital rim with a titanium mesh

The anatomy of the lateral wall plays an important role in the internal orbital volume as demonstrated by development of enophthalmos in unrestored lateral wall fractures [46]. Restoration of the architecture or augmentation of the same ensures correction of enophthalmos.

> Reconstruction of the lateral orbital walls is usually accomplished with the use of:
> (i) Alloplasts including titanium meshes, porous polyethylene sheets, and custom-made polyether ether ketone (PEEK) implants
> (ii) Bone grafts which may be harvested from either the calvarium or ilium

Figure 57.33a, b demonstrates the management of fracture of the lateral walls of the orbit in a patient with concomitant fracture of the zygomatic complex.

57.8.2.3 Medial Wall Fractures

The medial wall and the floor are the thinnest walls of the orbit and have the propensity to fracture the most [47, 48]. Though the incidence of concomitant fractures of the medial wall with that of the orbital floor have been reported over a wide range of 5–71%, its occurrence in isolation is very rare. Most fractures of the medial wall are incidental findings when CT scans are obtained to study other cranial, facial, or orbital fractures.

The most common type of clinical presentation would either involve a combination of the medial wall and floor (36%) or medial wall, floor, and zygomatic complex (28%) [49–51].

Fractures of the medial wall were managed conservatively in the past, but current literature proposes clear indications [49–51] for the exploration and reconstruction of the medial wall fractures and defects, which include:

1. Restriction of ocular motility
2. Diplopia
3. Clinically significant enophthalmos

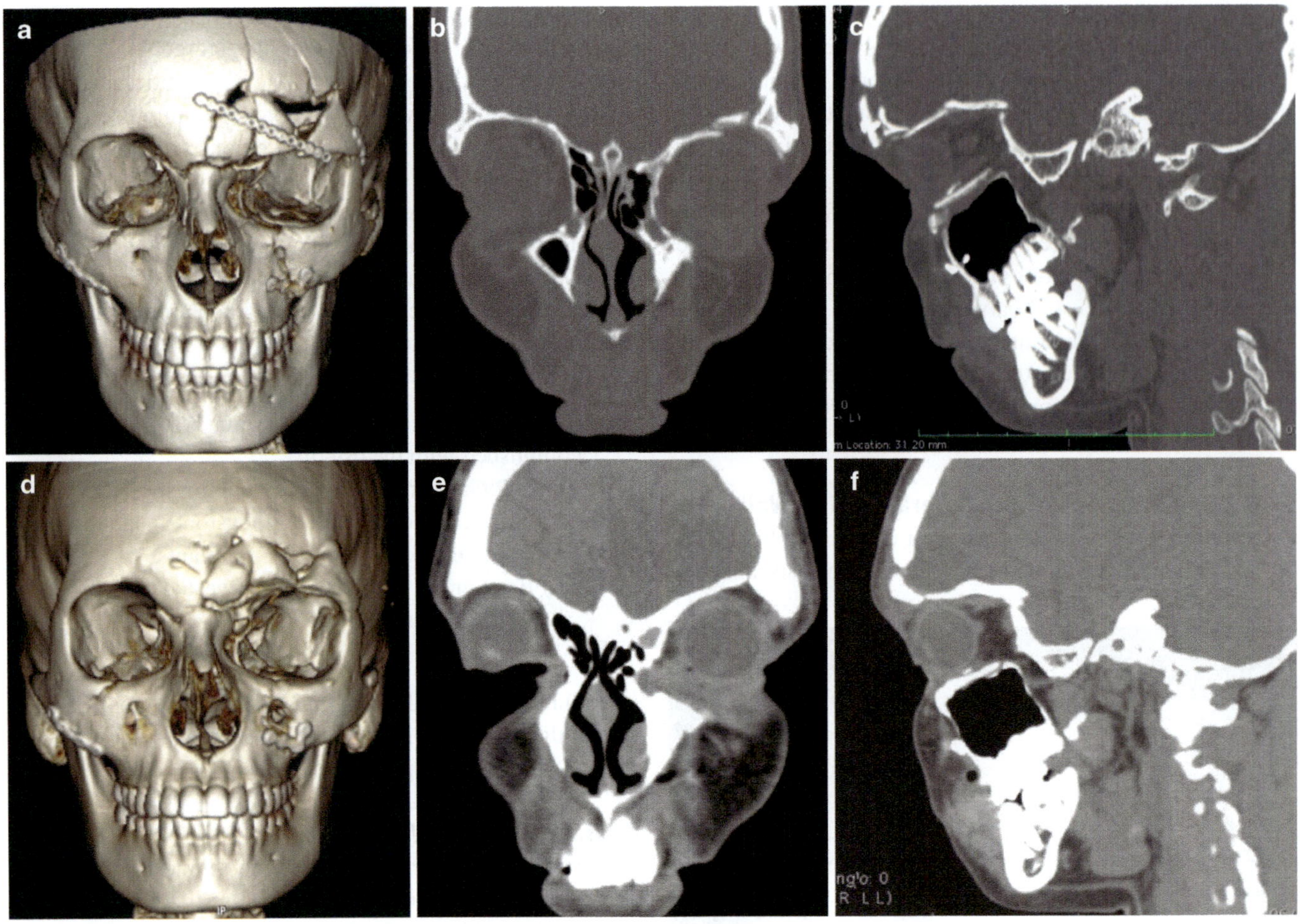

Fig. 57.32 CT images of patient with malunited fractures of the orbital roof. (**a–c**) Pre-operative images demonstrating malunited fracture of the frontal bone and orbital roof of the left side with decrease in intra-orbital volume and compression on the globe. (**d–f**) Post-operative images showing recontouring of the supraorbital rim and roof using ultrasonic aspirator system, with resultant expansion of the intra-orbital volume

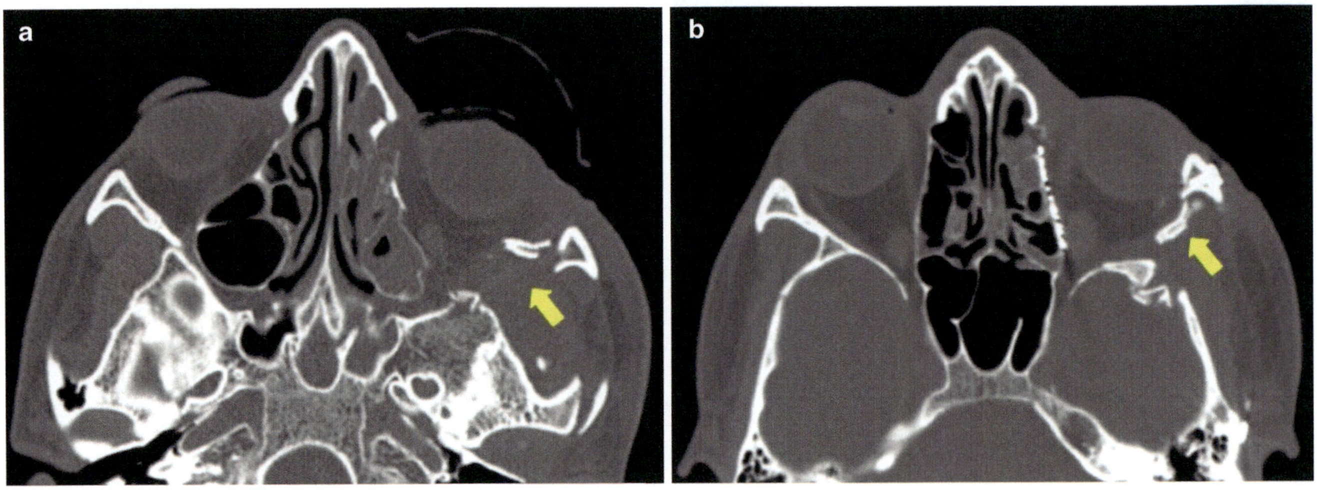

Fig. 57.33 CT scan images of lateral orbital wall with concomitant fracture of the zygomatic complex. (**a**) Pre-operative image showing fracture and displacement of the lateral wall and (**b**) post-operative image showing reduction of the lateral wall and re-establishment of the sphenozygomatic suture continuity

Box 57.10 A Clinically Useful Classification of Medial Wall Fractures Has Been Described by Nolasco et al. [47] **in 1995 Based on CT Scan Findings**

They describe four patterns of presentations (Fig. 57.34)

- Type I: Isolated medial wall fractures
- Type II: Fracture involving the medial wall and the orbital floor
- Type III: Fractures involving the medial wall, floor, and the zygomatic complex
- Type IV: Medial wall plus complex fractures of the face (maxillary, NOE, etc.)

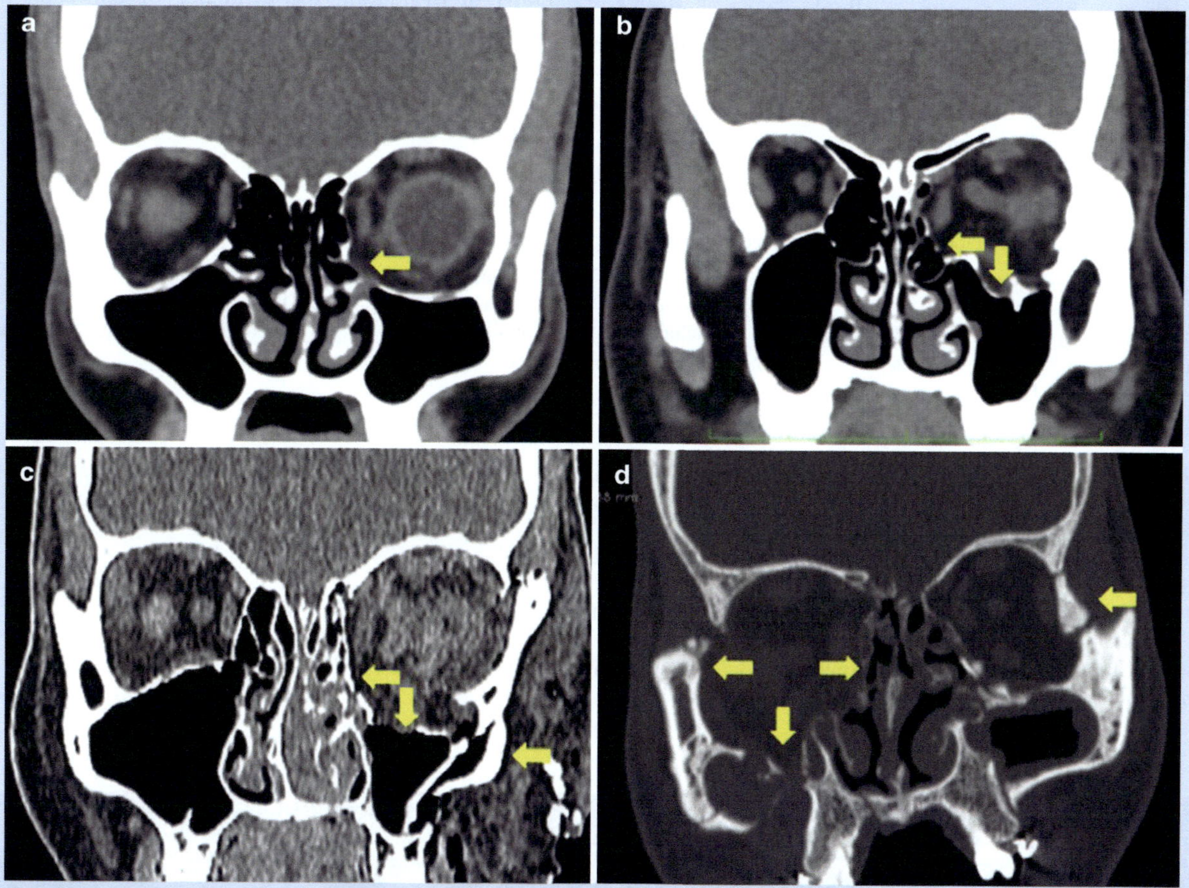

Fig. 57.34 CT scans showing types of medial wall fractures. (**a**) Isolated medial wall fracture; (**b**) fracture of medial wall with floor; (**c**) fracture involving medial wall, floor and zygomatic complex; and (**d**) concomitant fractures of the medial wall, floor, and midface at LeFort 3 level

Contrary to earlier belief the loss of medial wall integrity also significantly contributes to development of enophthalmos [49]—with any defect involving an area of more than 1.9 cm^2 or volume expansion of excess of 0.9 ml [50, 51] producing clinically significant enophthalmos (2 mm or more).

Approaches to the medial wall have already been described in detail earlier. The most favored being the transcaruncular/retro-caruncular approaches which give excellent exposure and access to the medial wall for both exploration and reconstruction [37, 52].

Options for reconstruction include a multitude of materials which may be autogenous or alloplastic as shown in Table 57.1. Bioactive resorbable sheets are also found to produce good outcomes [53].

Figure 57.35a, b demonstrates reconstruction of a medial wall fracture with a Titanium mesh.

57.8.2.4 Orbital Floor Fractures

The fractures involving the orbital floor are the most common fractures of the internal orbit either in isolation or concomitant with other facial fractures. A comprehensive classification of floor fractures with clinical guidelines for management is described by Jaquiery [54] et al. which lays emphasis on the morphology of the defect and the role of the infero-medial strut of the inferior orbital fissure.

> The internal orbit is divided into three zones which helps in evaluating the difficulty of approach and exposure:
> (i) Anterior third
> (ii) Middle third
> (iii) Dorsal third

Table 57.1 Commonly used biomaterials for orbital reconstructions

Material	Stability / fixation (S/F)	Contouring	Biological behavior	Permeability for inflammatory exudate	Donor site morbidity	Radio-opacity	Availability
Titanium	S+++ F++	++	++ (allows tissue in-growth)	+	+	+	+
Bone graft	S++ F+	-	+++	-	-	+	+/−
Porous polyethylene	S+/− F+/− (when thin)	+	++ (allows tissue in-growth)	−	+	-	+
Composite porous polyethylene/Ti	S++ F++	+	++ (allows tissue in-growth)	−	+	+	+
Resorbable (PLLA)	S+/− F+/−	+	+ (inflammatory response)	(non-perforated)	+	−	+
Pre-formed anatomical implant	S+++ F++	+++ (minimal contouring needed)	++ (allows tissue in-growth)	+	+	−	+

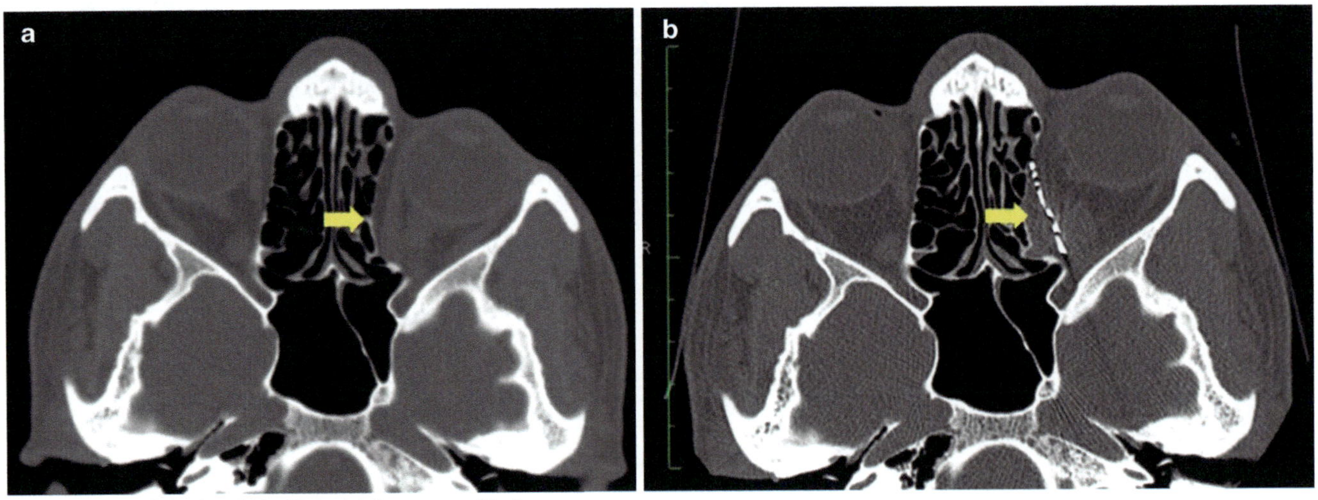

Fig. 57.35 CT images of patient with medial wall fracture. (**a**) Fracture of the medial orbital wall of the left orbit showing displaced medial rectus. (**b**) Post-operative image demonstrating medial orbital reconstruction with titanium mesh

Table 57.2 The classification of orbital wall defects (Jaquiery et al. modified by Dubois et al.) [53–55]

Category of fracture	Complexity of reconstruction	Defect description	Clinical finding
I	Low	Isolated defect of floor or medial wall, 10–20 mm² within zone 1 or 2	
II	Moderate	Defect of floor and/or medial wall >20 mm² within zone 1 and 2	Bony infero-medial strut of the inferior orbital fissure present
III	High	Defect of floor and/or medial wall >20 mm² within zone 1 and 2	Infero-medial strut of inferior orbital fissure absent
IV	High	Defect of the entire orbital floor with medial wall involving zone 3	Infero-medial strut of inferior orbital fissure absent. The posterior ledge of the floor also may be absent

The fractures themselves are then classified into four categories of defects (Table 57.2; Fig. 57.36a–d).

Which Fractures of the Orbital Floor Need Intervention?

Indications and contraindications for floor exploration and repair are well defined.

Absolute Indications

1. Acute injury to the orbit showing evidence of immediate clinical enophthalmos and/or hypophthalmos [55] (Fig. 57.15), necessitating a primary surgical intervention. Post-surgical outcome may get compromised with delay due to progressive atrophy of intra-orbital fat.
2. Severe restriction of ocular motility with CT or MRI evidenced muscle entrapment or incarceration of periorbital soft tissue.

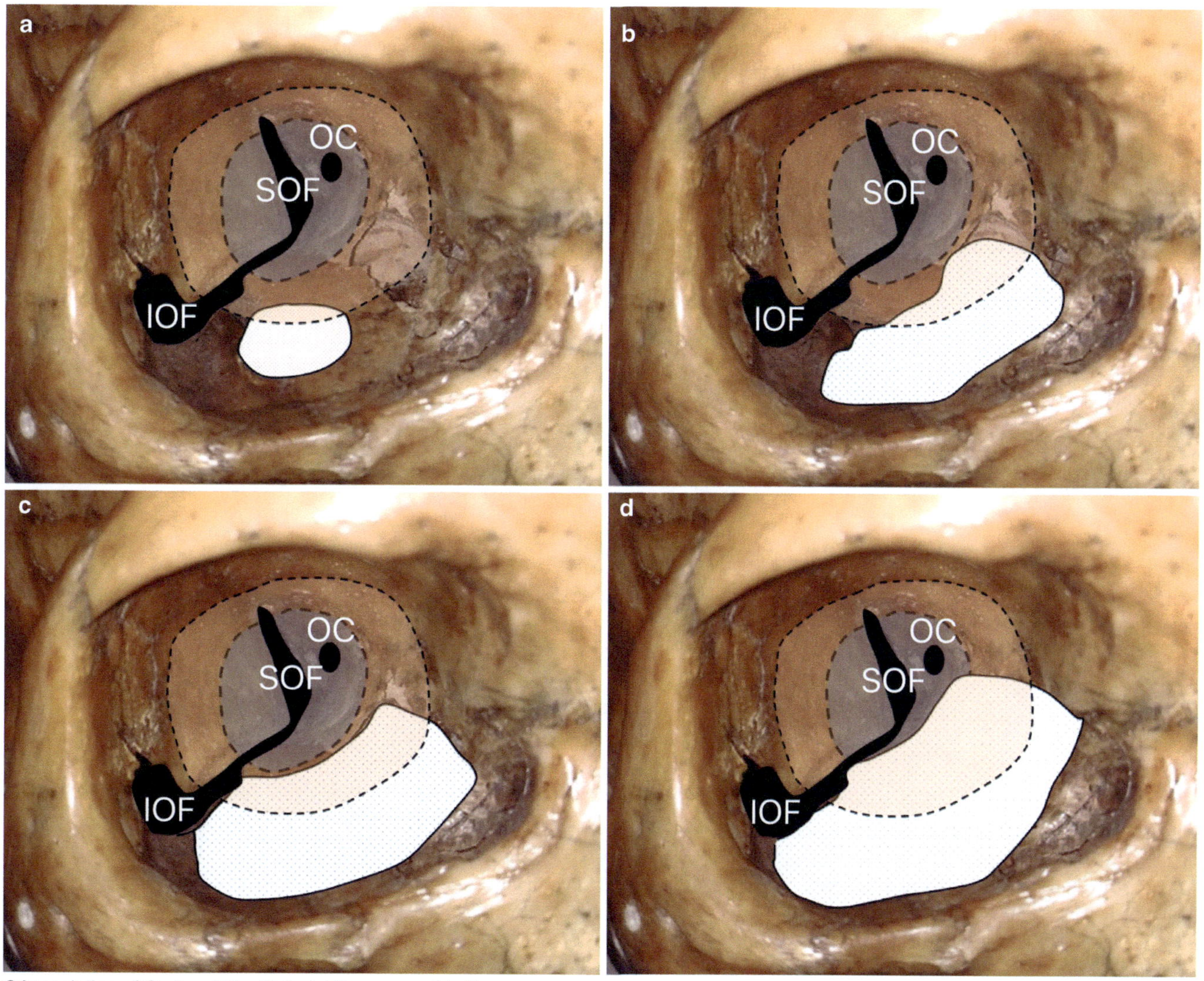

Fig. 57.36 Diagrammatic representation of the different types of defects of the orbital floor which indicate the grades of difficulty to reconstruct. (**a**) Type I, (**b**) Type II, (**c**) Type III and (**d**) Type IV

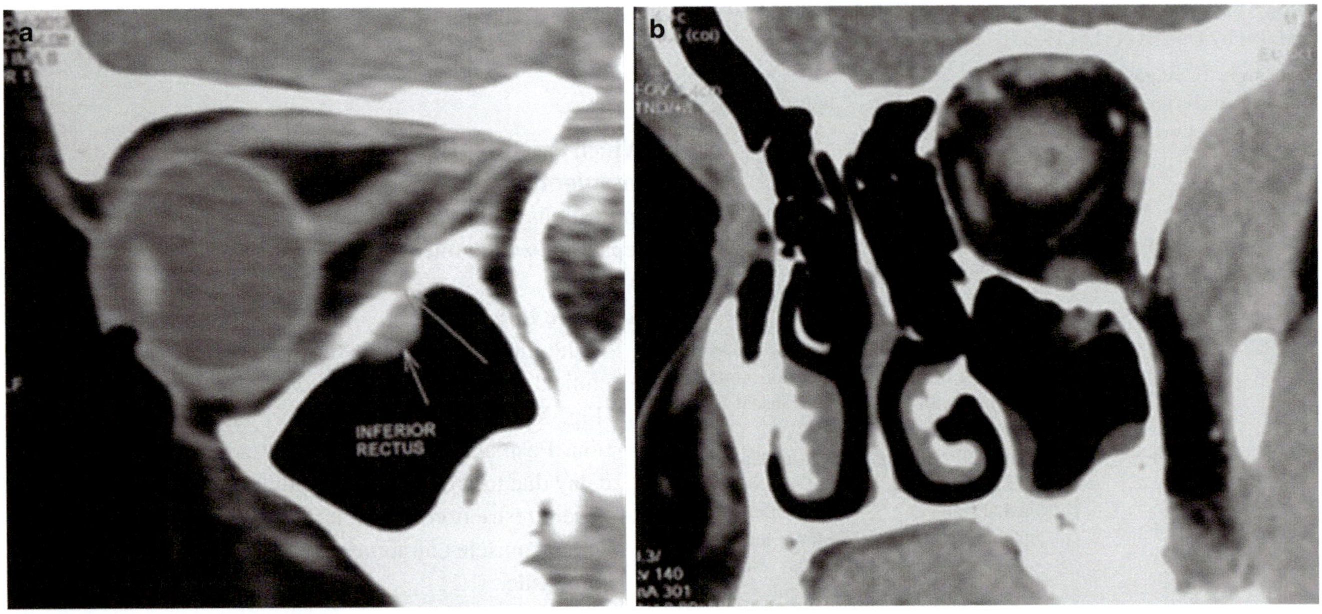

Fig. 57.37 CT scan images of a young boy with history of orbital trauma. (**a**) Sagittal and (**b**) coronal sections demonstrating a "springing trapdoor" fracture of the orbital floor on the left side with entrapped inferior rectus muscle. (Courtesy: Dept of Orbit & Oculoplasty, Shankara Nethralaya, Chennai)

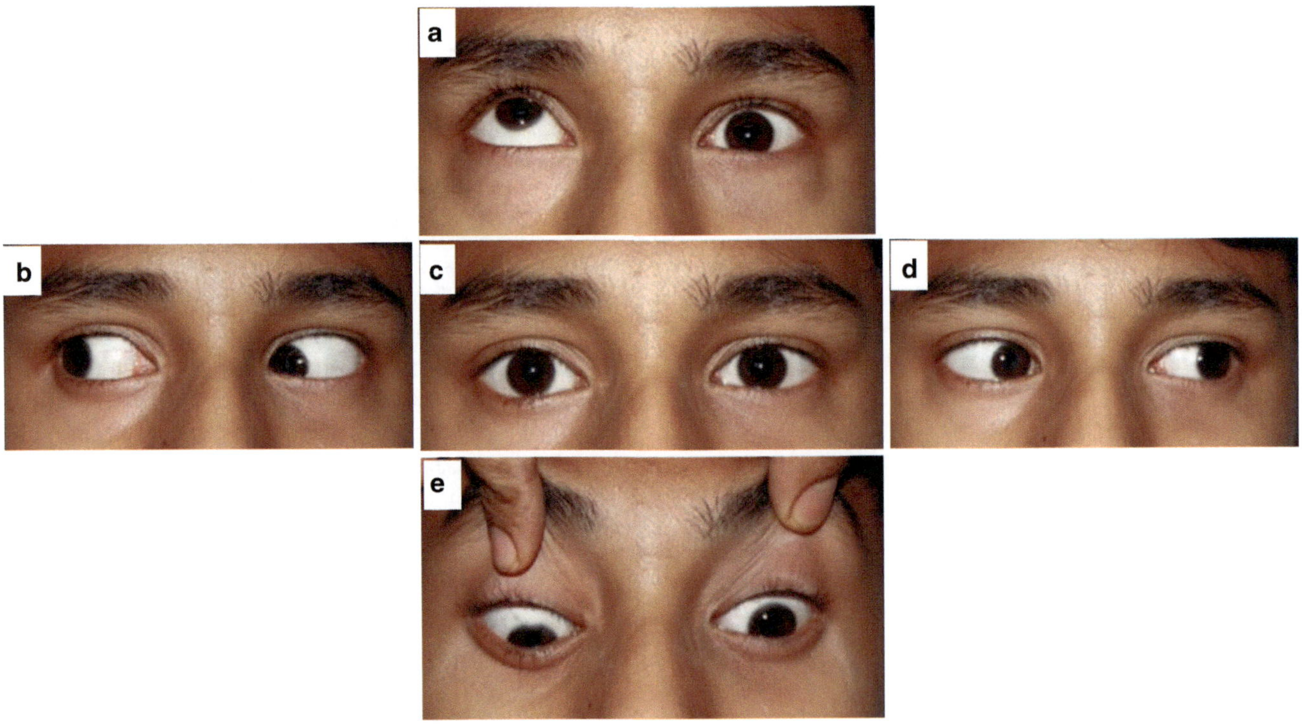

Fig. 57.38 Clinical photographs of a boy with "White eye blowout" fracture, showing restriction of ocular motility in the left eye in the superior (**a**) and inferior (**e**) gazes. The other gazes (**b**, **c** and **d**) show no abnormalities. (Courtesy: Dept of Orbit & Oculoplasty, Shankara Nethralaya, Chennai)

3. "White eye blowout" fracture in a child or young adult with severe restriction of ocular motility (Figs. 57.37a, b and 57.38) and vagal symptoms.

Relative Indications

1. Defects of the orbital floor often larger than 50% of the orbital floor area or greater than 20 × 20 mm of defect size especially in the zone between the floor and the medial wall (Fig. 57.39a).
2. Diplopia which is non-resolving and persistent for more than 2 weeks due to entrapment or fibrosis of orbital soft tissue (Fig. 57.39b) [56, 57].

Relative Contraindications

1. Associated ophthalmic injuries like retinal tears, hyphema, displacement of lens, ruptured globe, avulsion injuries of the globe, etc.
2. Loss of vision in one eye with the only seeing eye involved in a fracture

Figure 57.40a–f demonstrates the delayed management of a patient with an isolated fracture of the floor and medial walls. The CT scan shows fibrosis and adhesion of the inferior rectus muscle to the residual posterior ledge producing diplopia and restriction in superior gaze.

Surgery for Special Indications in Orbital Floor Fractures

Enophthalmos

Enophthalmos is the displacement of the eyeball in a posterior direction and is attributed to increase in the intra-orbital volume. Numerous studies have shown that there is a correlation between increase in intra-orbital volume and the presenting enophthalmos. It is proved that an increase in intra-orbital volume by 0.5–1 cc would produce posterior displacement of the globe by 1 mm. Enophthalmos of 2 mm or more may be clinically perceivable and warrant surgical intervention [58, 59]. An important aspect of orbital reconstruction lies in the fact that it is the only fracture in CMF region where the onus is not in recreating the anatomical form but rather in the restitution of the intra-orbital volume. Care should be taken to reconstruct the posteromedial aspect of the orbit (Hammer's key area) to achieve anterior projection of the globe. It is imperative to understand that reconstruction of the floor posterior to the equator of the globe influences anterior projection of the globe, while reconstruction of the equatorial region of the floor influences only the supero-inferior position of the globe (Fig. 57.41).

Figure 57.42a–d shows a case of delayed correction of enophthalmos in a patient with an orbital floor fracture.

Hypophthalmos

This is otherwise called hypoglobus and signifies the downward displacement of the globe due to the interruption in the anatomical integrity of the orbital floor. The clinical presence of hypoglobus needs to be differentiated from orbital dystopia which essentially means that the entire bony orbit with its contents is displaced caudally, unlike hypophthalmos, where only the globe is displaced caudally.

However decision-making for surgical intervention based on both enophthalmos and hypophthalmos is challenging as they may or may not present immediately following trauma. (Refer to clinical scenario 1. Figs. 57.57, 57.58 and 57.59).

Diplopia

Clinically demonstrable double vision is termed diplopia. Generally post-traumatic diplopia due to edema and hemorrhage is self-limiting and shows spontaneous resolution.

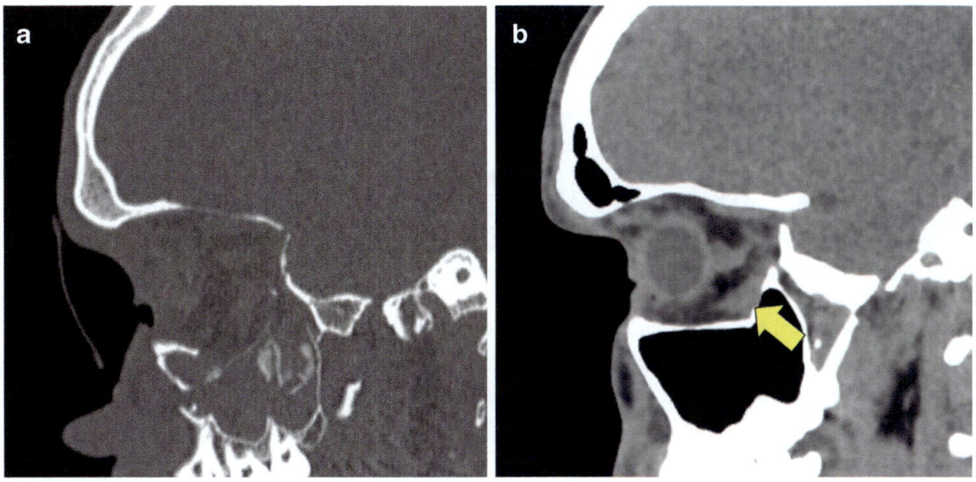

Fig. 57.39 (**a**) Sagittal section CT demonstrating large defect of the orbital floor. (**b**) Sagittal section CT demonstrating fibrosis and adhesion of the inferior rectus (yellow arrow) to the posterior ledge of the orbital defect

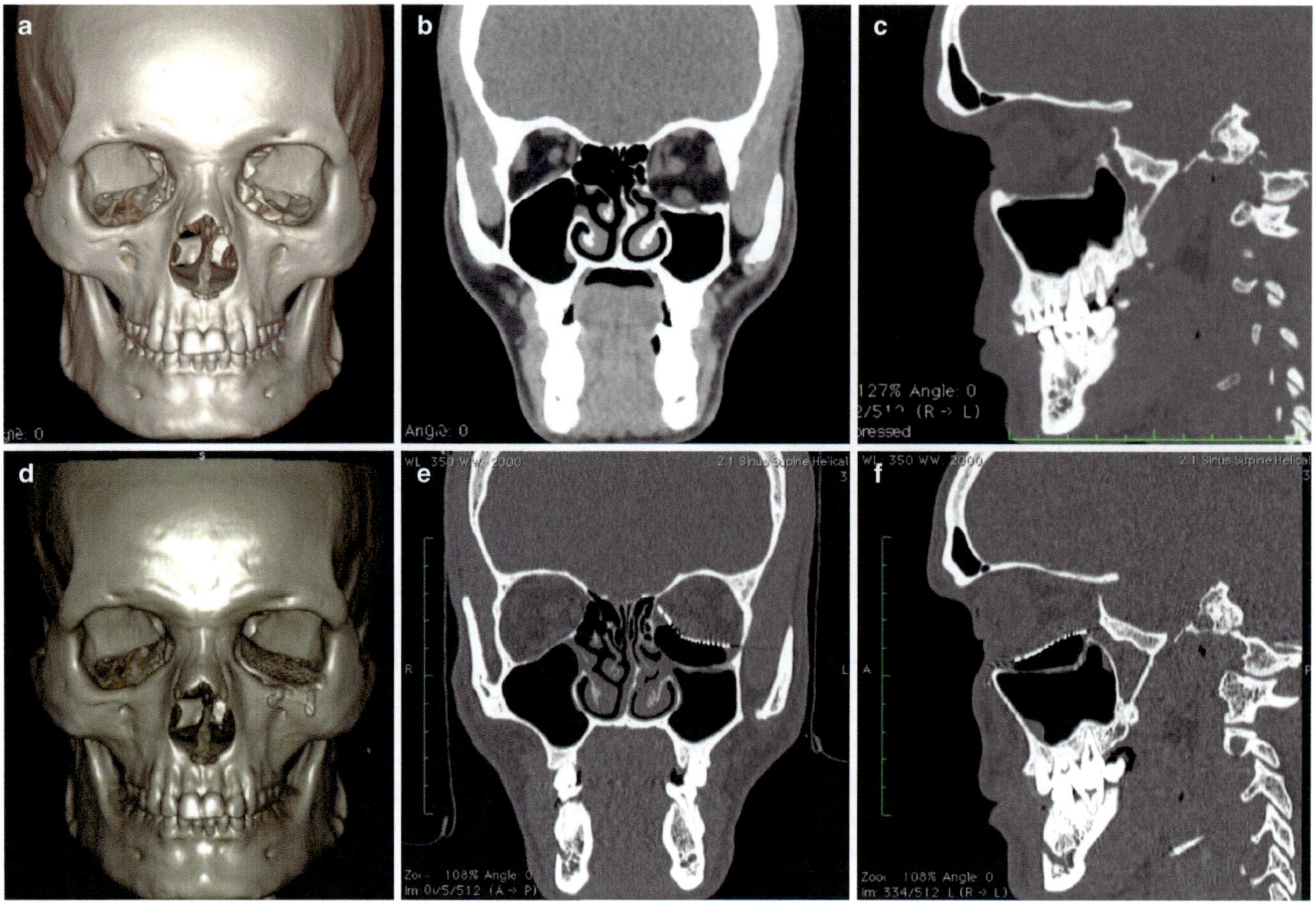

Fig. 57.40 CT scan images of patient with internal orbital fracture. (**a–c**) 3D, coronal, and sagittal images demonstrating isolated fracture of the left orbital floor and medial wall. (**d–f**) post-operative images demonstrating reconstruction of the defect with anatomical orbital implant

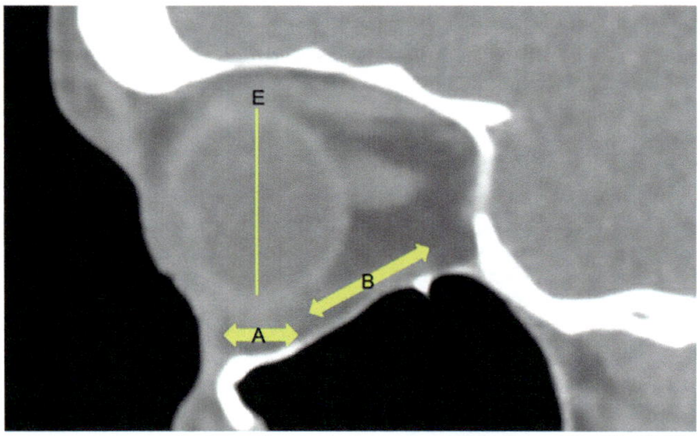

Fig. 57.41 Graphical representation of the equator of the globe (E) and the associated equatorial (A) and post-equatorial (B) zones of the floor

Diplopia can manifest in two forms:

(i) Monocular (diplopia present when seeing through one eye with the other eye closed) which is of more concern where the pathology is generally due to an ophthalmic problem (corneal, retinal, etc.) or neurological where the problem may be due to the optic nerve or the optic disk being injured.

(ii) Binocular diplopia (diplopia present only when seeing with both eyes, while absent on seeing with one eye) with CT proven muscle entrapment is seen as an indication for immediate intervention. However, it may also be attributed to other reasons including (a) intra-orbital edema or hemorrhage, physical bony spicules or fragments acting as impediments following trauma, (b) entrapment of the periorbita, and in rare cases (c) large changes in intra-orbital volume including massive

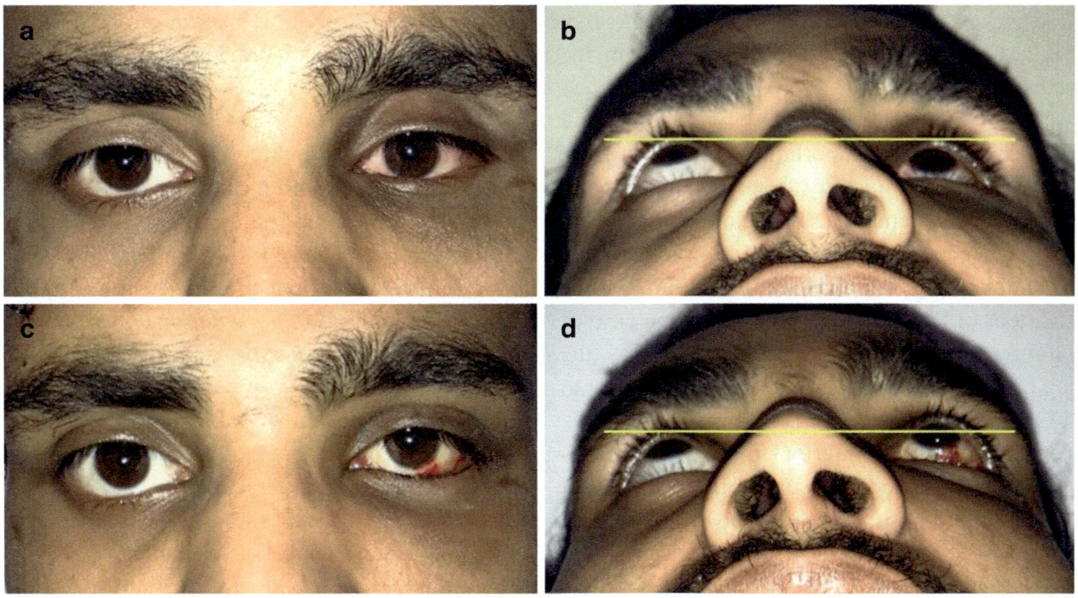

Fig. 57.42 Clinical photographs of patient with enophthalmos. (**a** and **b**) Pre-operative pictures demonstrating significant enophthalmos of the left globe. (**c** and **d**) Post-operative pictures demonstrating good surgical outcome

herniations or atrophy of periorbital fat, which do not mandate immediate intervention. Refer to clinical scenario 2.

When Is the Right Time to Intervene?

The timing for intervention for fractures of the orbital floor can be divided into three categories—immediate, early, and late. The indication for all three categories are well discussed in literature [57] and are listed in Fig. 57.43.

Indications for immediate repair are of an urgent nature and may require priority as surgical emergencies, generally less than 6 h following trauma.

What to Use for Reconstruction of the Orbital Defect?

A plethora of material both autogenous and alloplastic have been used and documented. A table is provided with the list of the most commonly used materials and their relative merits (Table 57.1). However, contemporary literature favors the use of stock titanium meshes and custom patient specific implants which provide optimal corrections (Fig. 57.44a, b).

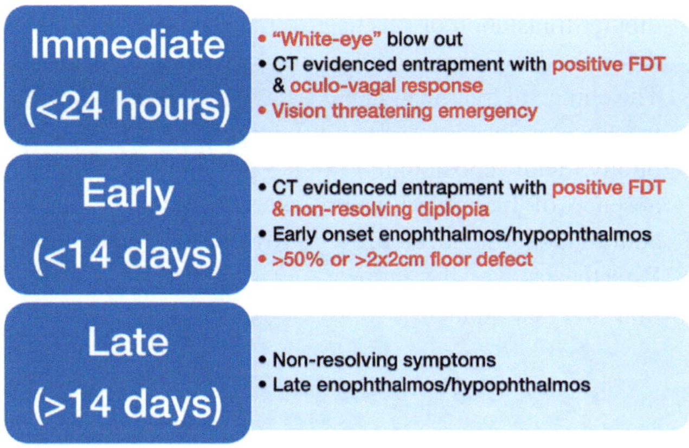

Fig. 57.43 Chart showing timing for intervention for orbital reconstruction

Guidelines for Deep Orbital Dissection

The dissection of the deep orbit is always a challenge for the surgeon due to the high concentration of vital structures within a limited space [60]. A few anatomical landmarks that have been suggested for guidance while dissecting in the deep orbit include:

(a) *Infra-orbital nerve*: the course of the infra-orbital nerve within the orbit is a very important landmark in floor dissection. The point of its entry from the pterygopalatine fossa at the genu/bend where inferior orbital fissure takes a turn and ascends laterally to continue as the superior orbital fissure signifies the safe limit for the posterior extent of floor dissection. Even in the case of badly comminuted fractures or delayed corrections, the nerve may be identifiable and provides a reliable clue to the end of the pre confluence area.

(b) *Inferior orbital fissure*: the inferior orbital fissure forms a pathway for an extended exposure of the lateral orbit as the contents of the fissure can be safely divided using bipolar cautery dissection. This facilitates easy navigation into the deep orbit behind the fissure and trace the greater wing of sphenoid. It may be of clinical relevance to note that the structures of the lateral orbit are much stronger and less prone to comminution when compared to the medial orbital structures. This makes the lateral approach to the deep orbit more predictable. Furthermore, the medial strut of the inferior orbital fissure is an important entity to identify and utilize for reconstruction of the internal orbit.

(c) *The greater wing of the sphenoid*: this is a thick and strong bony structure which forms the majority of the lateral orbit and bridges the inferior and superior orbital fissures. Its robust nature makes it less prone for comminution and hence forms a predictable landmark to find even in severe trauma.

(d) *Orbital process of the palatine bone*: the Orbital process of the palatine bone forms the highest point of the posterior-medial bulge of the orbital floor. This is an integral part of the posterior orbit that needs to be reconstructed to get adequate positioning of the globe in the anteroposterior and vertical directions.

(e) *Orbital confluence*: the orbital confluence (Fig. 57.45a, b) is formed by the convergence of two bony shelves forming the genu of the internal orbital fissures. This signifies the safe limits of the dissection of the orbital floor. The confluence is formed by the perpendicular plate of the palatine bone on the medial aspect and the bony inferior margin of the greater wing of the sphenoid laterally.

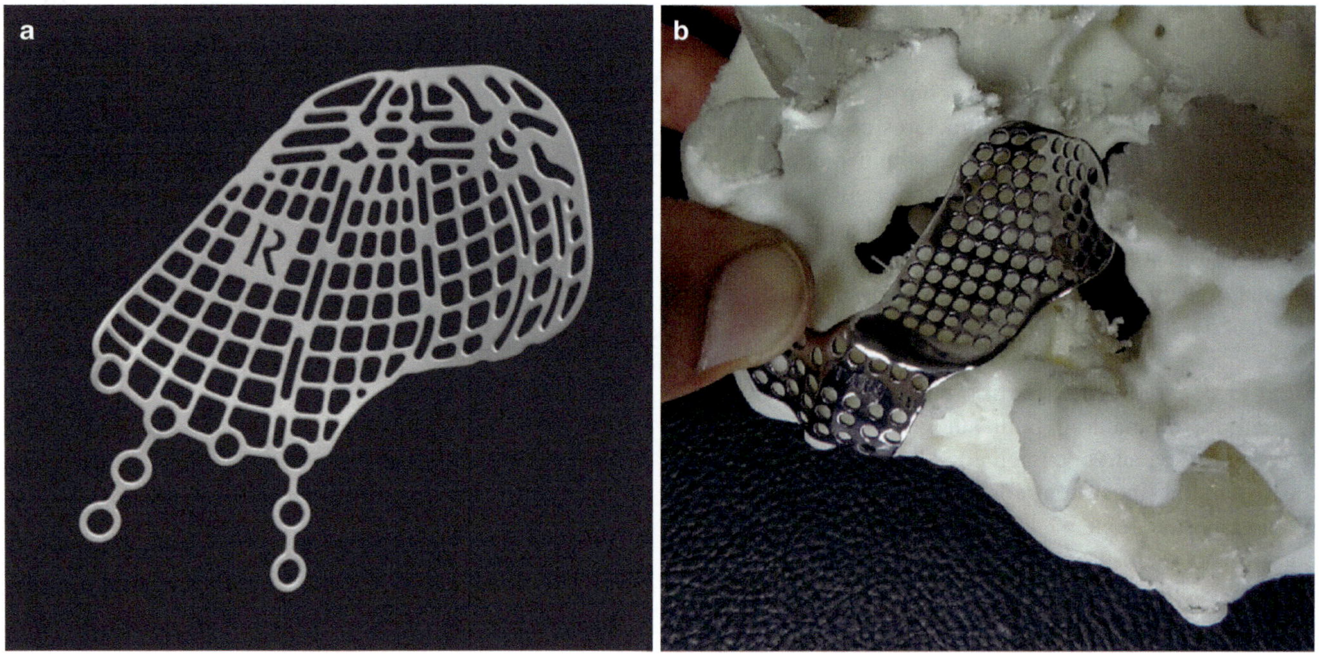

Fig. 57.44 Photographs of (**a**) Stryker^{R} preformed anatomical orbital floor implant and (**b**) titanium "patient-specific implant" (PSI)

(f) *Safe distances within the orbit*: an important formula to remember safe distances within the orbit is 24-12-6, where 24 is the distance in mm of the anterior ethmoidal foramen from the medial orbital rim; an additional 12 mm deeper (36 mm) would indicate the posterior ethmoidal foramen followed by another 6 mm deep for the optic nerve (42 mm) [6].

(g) *Globe protection*: protection of the globe is of vital importance in orbital surgery. Adequate care should also be exercised for the protection of other vital structures like nerves and vessels also. Use of protection devices like specific retractors (Fig. 57.46a, b, c) and corneal shields is mandatory.

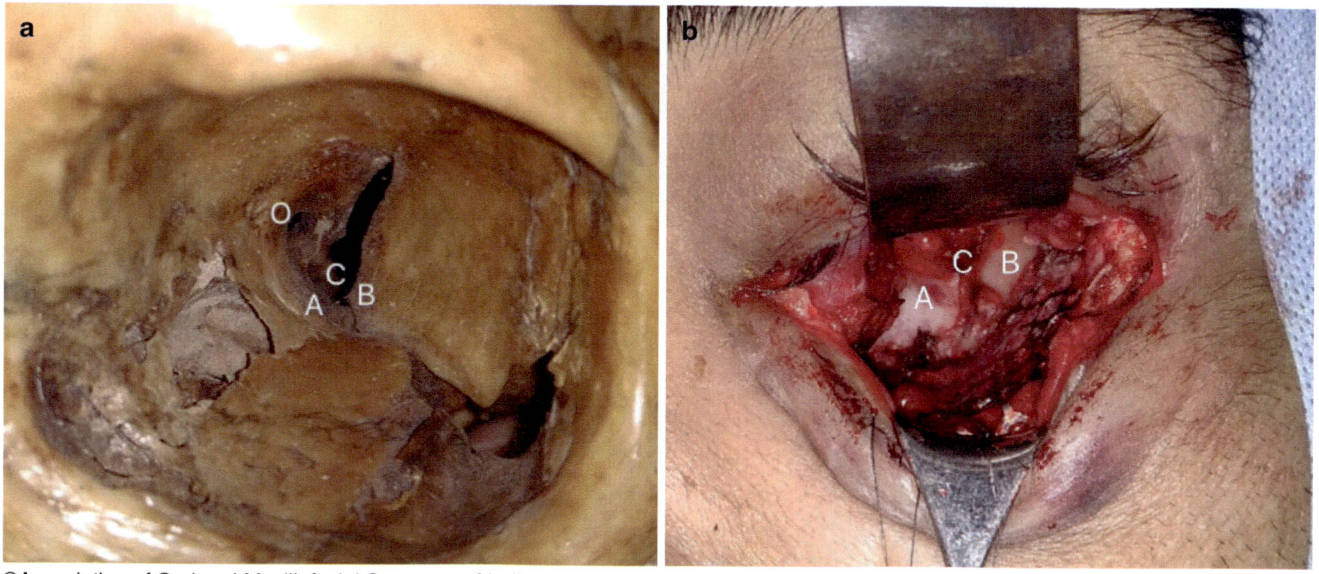

Fig. 57.45 (**a**) Demonstration of landmarks on dry skull. (A) Perpendicular plate of the palatine bone. (B) Medial lip of the greater wing of the sphenoid. (C) Orbital confluence and (O) Optic foramen. (**b**) Intraoperative photograph demonstrating the structures of the deep orbit in a patient undergoing secondary surgery for floor reconstruction with implant replacement

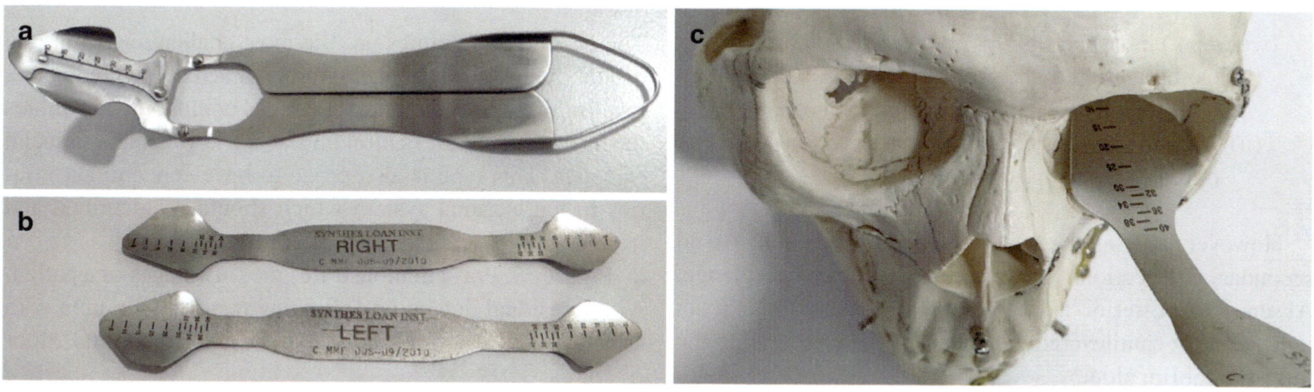

Fig. 57.46 Photographs showing globe protection devices. (**a**) Stryker^R globe retractor, (**b**) Synthes^R globe retractor and (**c**) Synthes^R retractor in anatomical position demonstrating the use of calibration to aid intraoperatively

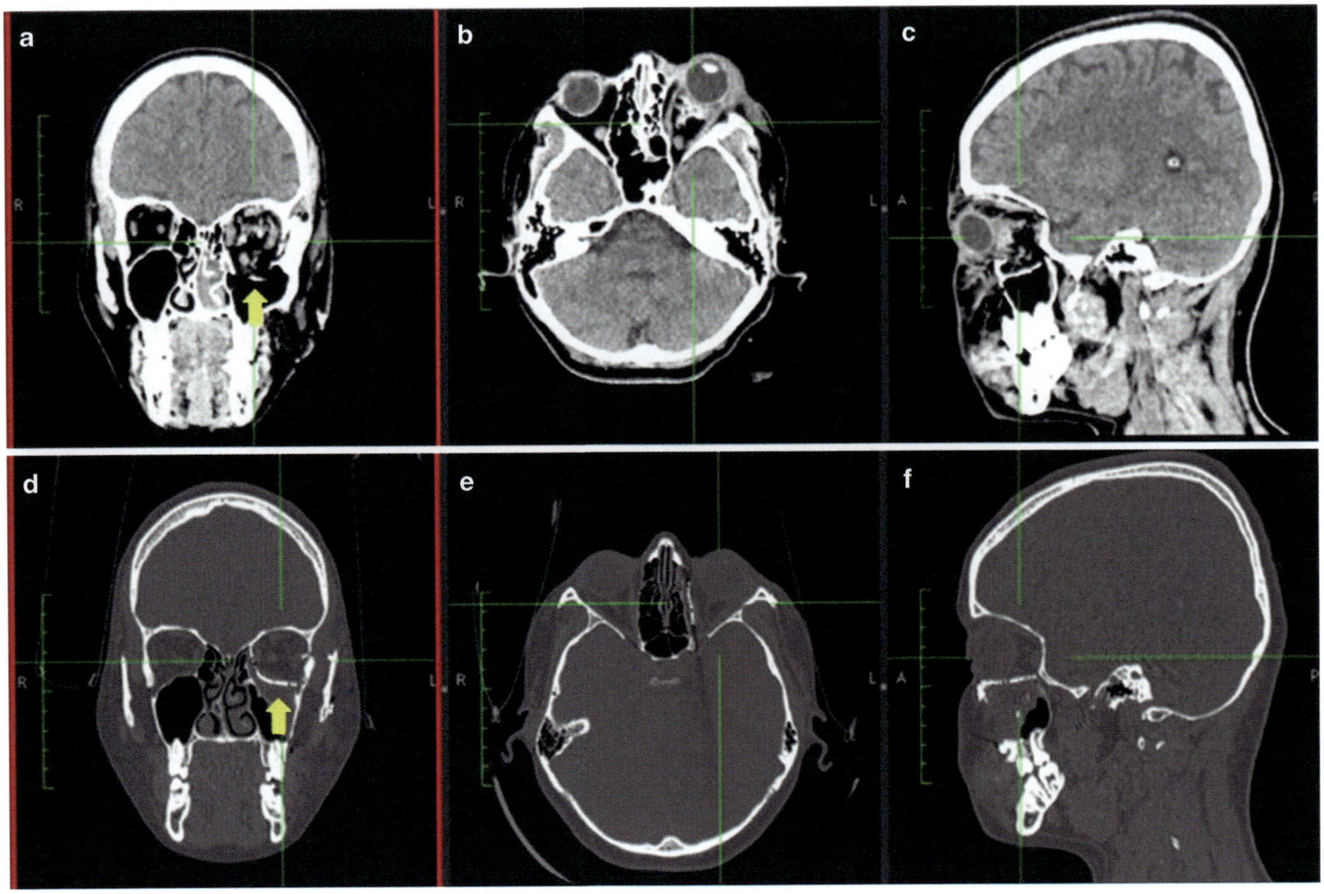

Fig. 57.47 CT scans images demonstrating optimal de-herniation of orbital contents and restoration of intra-orbital volume. (**a**–**c**) Pre-operative, (**d**–**f**) post-operative

De-herniation of the Orbital Contents and Locating the Posterior Ledge

> Two important aspects of floor reconstruction are:
> (i) De-herniation of the orbital (Fig. 57.47a–f) contents to *restore* the internal orbital volume
> (ii) Locating the posterior ledge (Fig. 57.48a–d) for optimal implant positioning

However, locating the posterior ledge in large defects and secondary corrections may be a significant challenge. Absence of posterior ledge in severe orbital trauma is an indication for cantilevered implants which are secured to the infra-orbital rim alone.

57.8.3 Type III (Naso-Orbito-Ethmoid Type) (Refer Chap. 58)

The NOE-type fractures are the most challenging of all the orbital fractures to manage in terms of achieving predictable results. The management of the NOE complex reconstitutes the facial form of the central midface: a key element in facial esthetics. This type is also prone to have concomitant injuries to the lacrimal system which should be identified and treated.

Figure 57.49a–f demonstrates the CT images of a patient with a residual deformity following pan-facial trauma with a right-sided type I NOE and neglected orbital floor fractures.

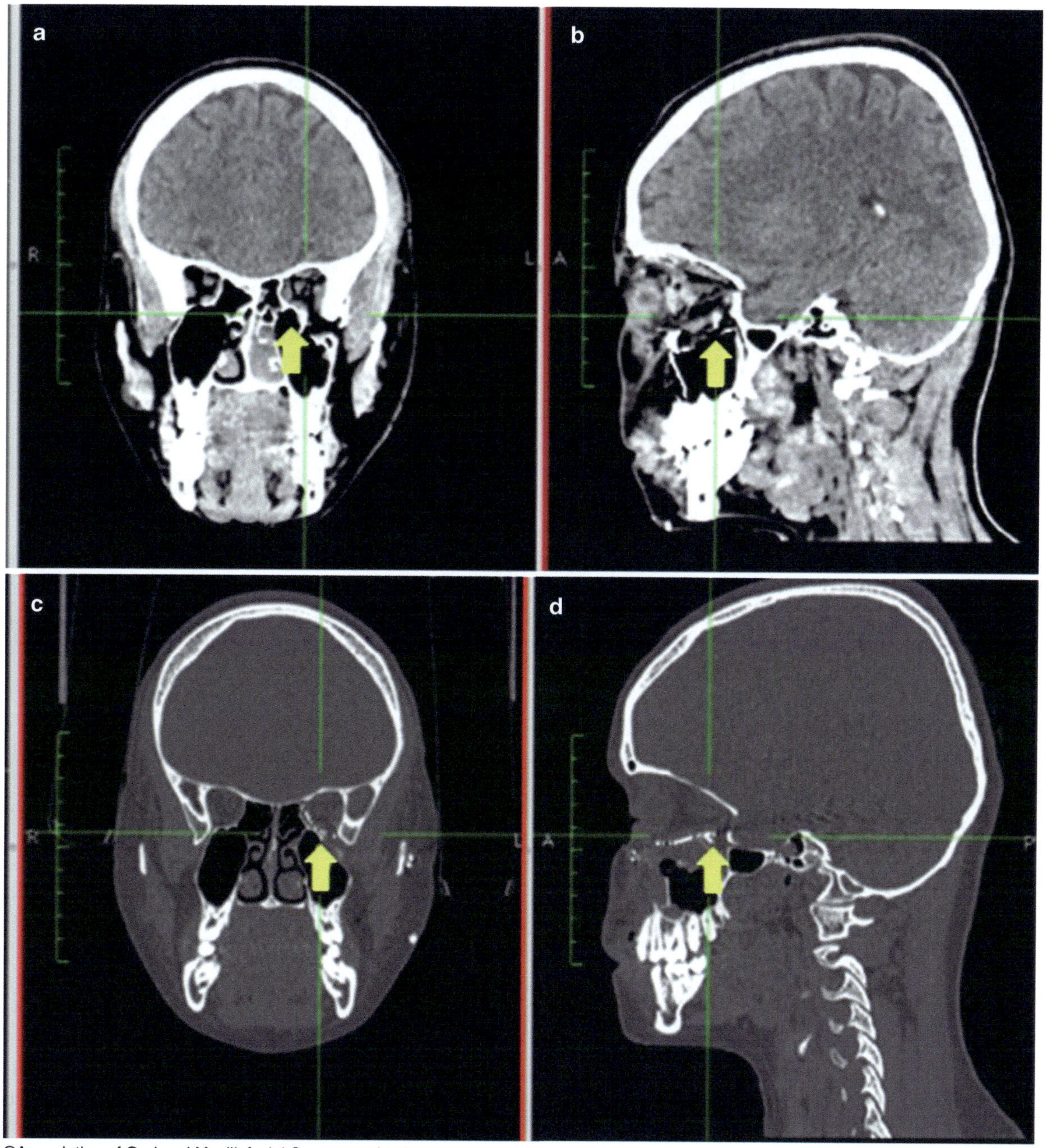

Fig. 57.48 (**a** and **b**) Pre-operative coronal and sagittal section CT images demonstrating the location of the posterior ledge of the floor defect. (**c** and **d**) Post-operative images showing the placement of the anatomical orbital floor implant in the appropriate position to bridge the defect

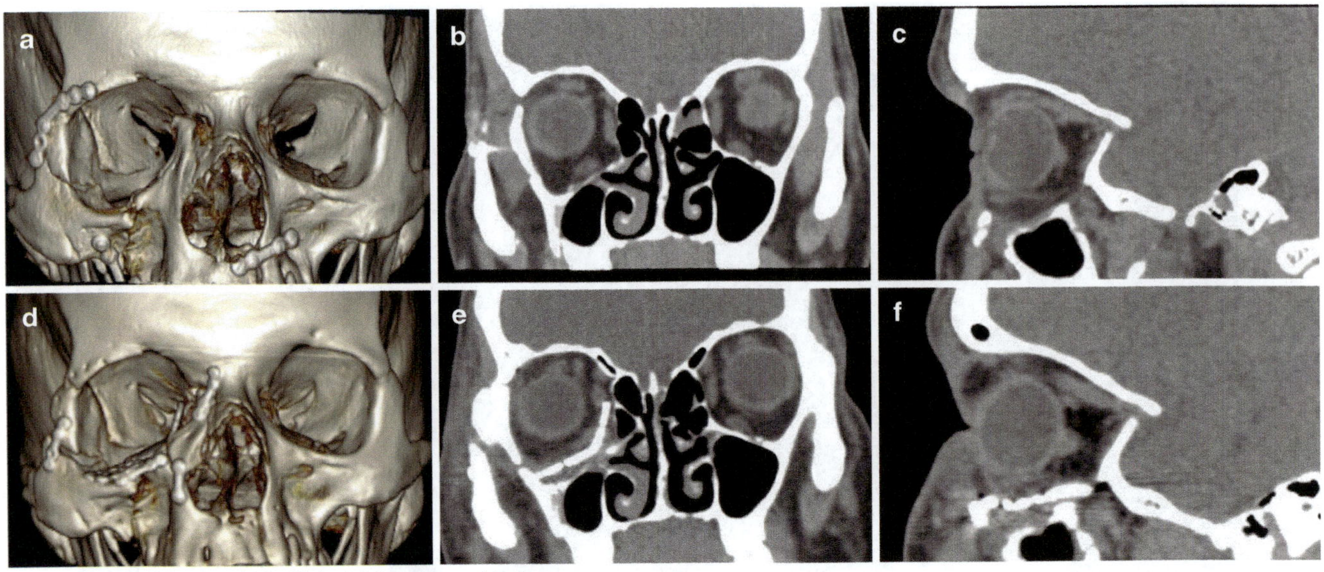

Fig. 57.49 CT scan images of patient with type I NOE fracture, plus orbito-zygomatic complex on the right side. (**a–c**) 3D, coronal and sagittal images demonstrating the fractures and the floor defect. (**d–f**) Post-operative images demonstrating ORIF of the right NOE fracture, redo of the orbito-zygomatic complex and floor reconstruction with anatomical orbital implant

Box 57.11 The *Key Elements* for Managing Type III Fractures

- Management of the medial canthal tendon (MCT) as indicated: this can be performed according to the description of Markowitz et al. [61] with the focus being the attachment or avulsion of the medial canthal tendon (MCT) to the fracture fragment
- Management of the soft tissue drape after reposition of the MCT
- Restoration of the nasal dorsum projection, which is of paramount importance
- Evaluation of injuries to the lacrimal system: canaliculi, sac and the nasolacrimal duct (NLD), and its management

57.8.4 Type IV (Complex Fractures of the Face with Orbital Fractures)

This type includes all the combinations of the fractures of the face which do not fall into the types described above. Sequencing of fractures (refer Chap. 60) such as these including pan-facial fractures requires a thorough understanding of the principles to obtain optimal outcomes. It is to be borne that sequencing and fixation of all facial fractures need to be completed prior to the reconstruction of the internal orbit.

Figures 57.50a–d and 57.51a–d demonstrate a patient with residual facial deformity following RTA. Patient had sub-optimally treated pan-facial and orbital fractures and a malunited mandible fracture. He was operated for a revision surgery addressing his midface and dental occlusion.

57.9 Management of Orbital Emergencies

(a) *Retrobulbar hemorrhage*: investigations with a CT scan or an MRI as the clinical situation mandates help us with a diagnosis of retrobulbar hemorrhage. 20% mannitol 2 g/kg body weight or 500 mg acetazolamide is administered to reduce the intraocular pressure in conjunction with 100 mg hydrocortisone for management of edema. Hourly examinations of pupils, visual acuity, and IOP are of great significance as stable ophthalmic status with diminishing signs of vision can be managed medically. Deterioration of vision or changes in visual fields may be considered an emergency [62]. Inferior cantholysis is the most commonly employed procedure for decompression of the retrobulbar space [63–65].

(b) *Traumatic optic neuropathy*: the management of traumatic optic neuropathy includes observation, use of steroids, and surgical decompression [66]. However, the use of corticosteroids in acute brain trauma is now debatable, and the general consensus is non-use of steroids in patients having concomitant brain trauma [67]. Many clinicians now restrict the use of steroids (bolus

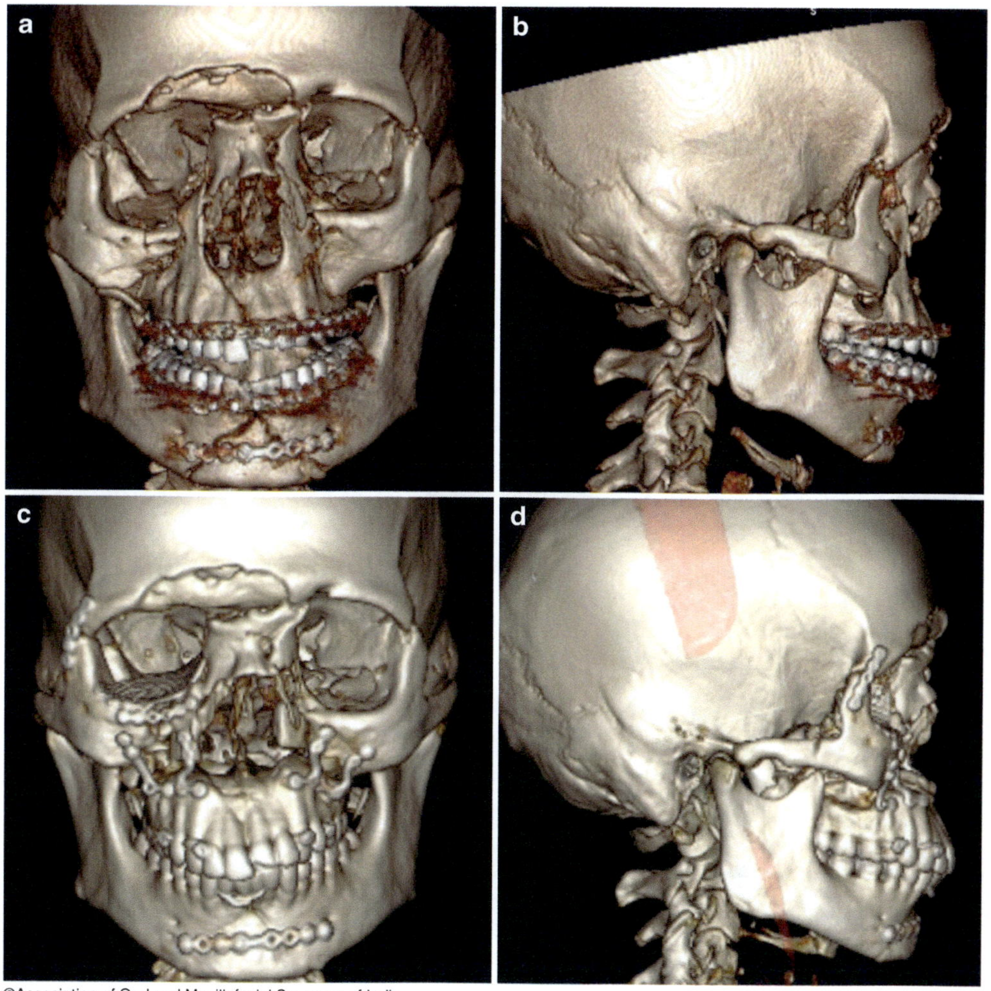

Fig. 57.50 3D CT images of patient with neglected pan facial injury and associated orbital fracture. (**a** and **b**) Images demonstrating frontal and lateral views showing malunited pan-facial fracture with facial deformity and significant dental malocclusion. (**c** and **d**) Post-operative images demonstrating ORIF of the right orbito-zygomatic complex and a Lefort I osteotomy with restoration of skeletal form, midface projection, and restoration of functional occlusion

dose of 30 mg/Kg body weight of methyl prednisolone followed by 3 mg/Kg/h for 24 h) within the first 8 h of injury, in cases of severe primary vision loss or progressive vision loss.

(c) *Compartment syndromes*: this includes both superior orbital fissure and orbital apex syndromes. The current protocols indicate early surgical decompression where indicated. The role of steroids is debatable as indicated above.

57.10 Pediatric Considerations (Figs. 57.52a–d and 57.53a, b)

Pediatric consideration in orbital trauma necessitates the discussion of four important aspects which clearly delineate the management principles from adults.

(a) *Ratio of cranium to facial fractures in children*
The face to cranium ratio of an infant is 1:8, while that of a child who is between 4 and 6 is about 1:4. This clearly establishes the fact that the cranium in an infant or a child is much larger than the face and is more exposed to potential trauma. The incidence of orbital roof fractures is much more common in children who are younger than 5 years, while beyond the age of 7, the floor fracture is more commonly seen.

(b) *Pediatric orbital roof fractures*
Roof fractures in children occur in the growing age [68] and cause an entity called the "growing skull fracture," where the fracture fragments continue to separate due to growth, causing "leptomeningeal" herniation which involves herniation of the meninges and part of the frontal lobe into the orbital cavity. Management of these need to be planned in conjunction with neurosurgical support.

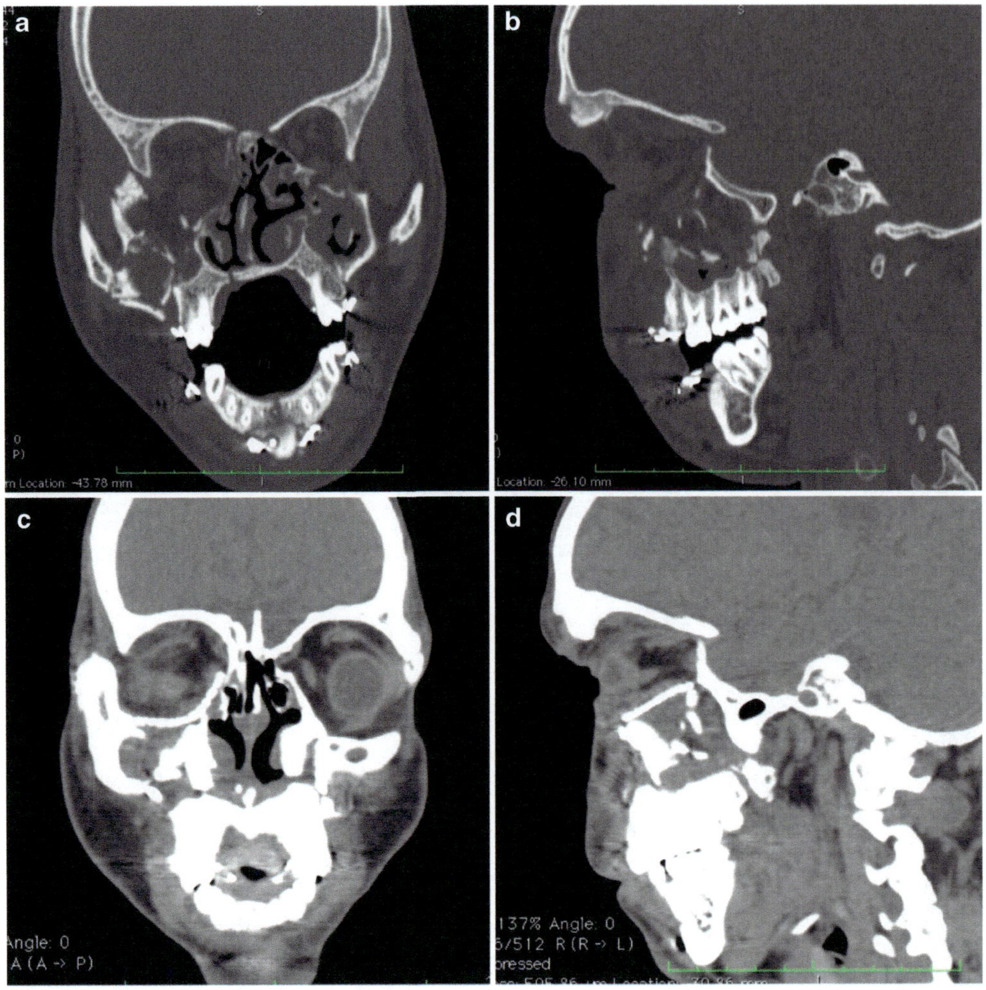

Fig. 57.51 Coronal and axial CT images of the patient in Fig 57.50. (**a** and **b**) Images demonstrating comminuted fractures of the midface and orbit. (**c** and **d**) Post-operative images showing optimal restoration of form of the face and orbit

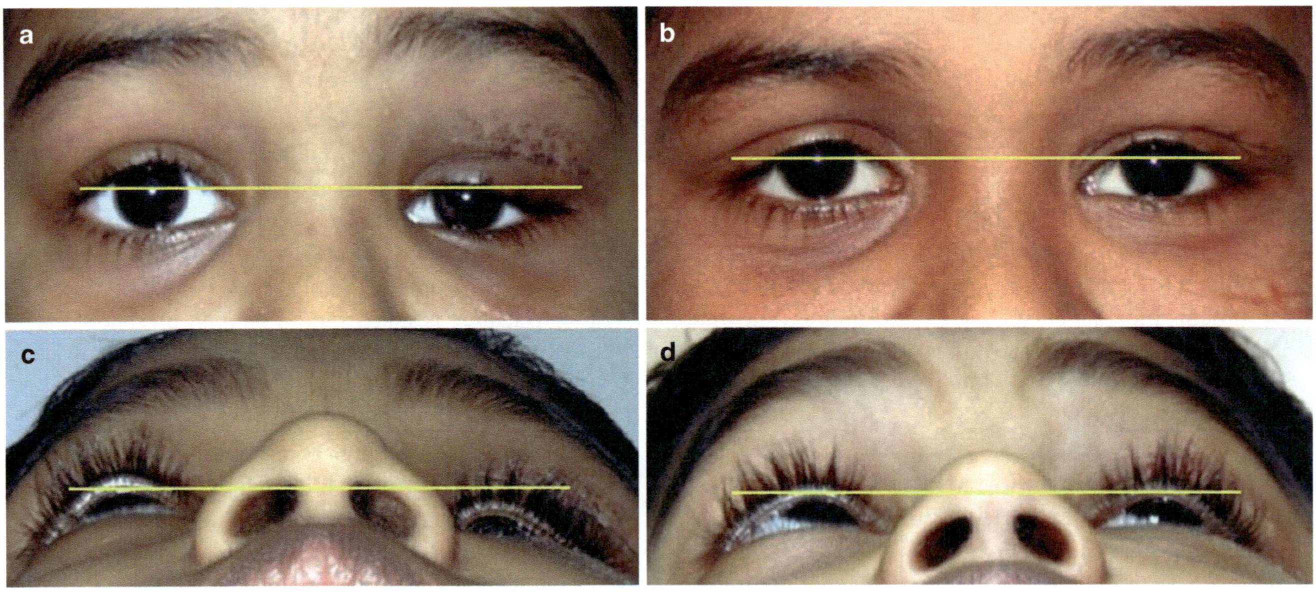

Fig. 57.52 Clinical photographs of a 6-year-old child with left sided orbital trauma (**a** and **c**) frontal and basal views demonstrating immediate-onset enophthalmos and hypophthalmos. (**b** and **d**) post-operative photographs showing optimal post-surgical outcome. (Courtesy: Dept of Orbit & Oculoplasty, Shankara Nethralaya, Chennai)

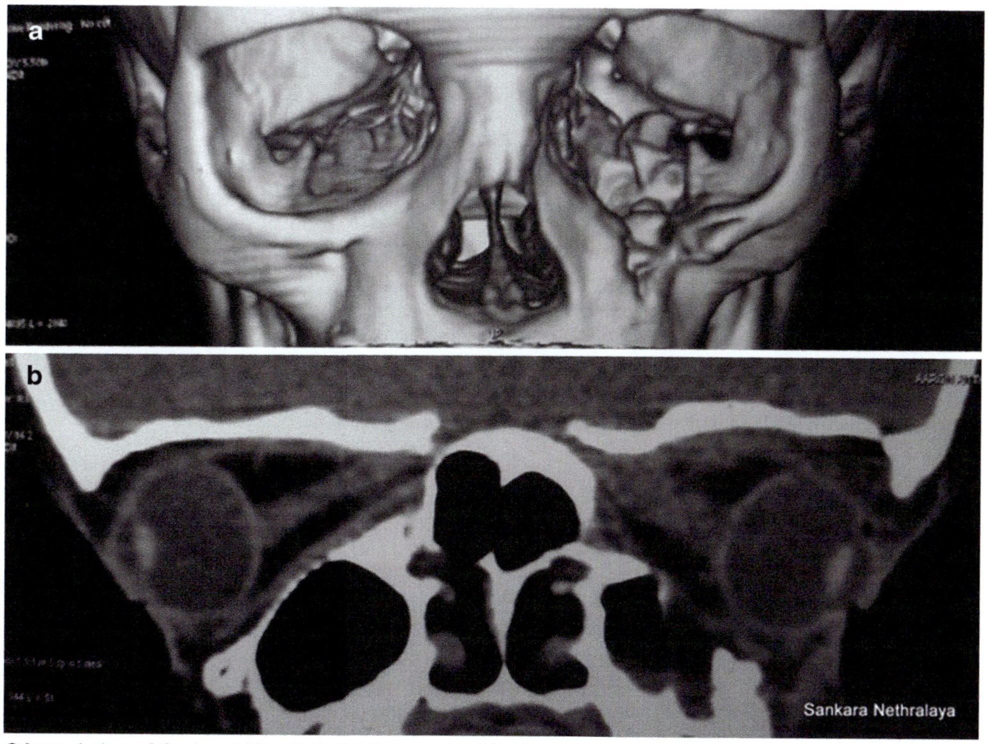

Fig. 57.53 CT scan images (**a**) 3D image demonstrating fracture involving the left infra-orbital rim and orbital floor in a 6 year-old child, (**b**) sagittal sections of both orbits showing left sided floor fracture. (Courtesy: Dept of Orbit & Oculoplasty, Shankara Nethralaya, Chennai)

(c) *White eye blowout*
The presence of floor fractures with restriction in superior gaze, with or without oculo-vagal responses and devoid of any physical signs of hemorrhage or ecchymosis in the eye or periorbital region [69–71]. This is a feature which may be seen in children and young adults as a result of a "self-reducing trapdoor" fracture which entraps the inferior rectus. The white eye blowout is considered a surgical emergency and necessitates immediate intervention.

(d) *Role of resorbable implants*
The cranium and upper face exhibit rapid growth in the early years. The orbit completes almost 80% of its growth within the first 2 years of life and another 10% within the next 2–3 years. Choice of implants in the growing orbit is to be taken into consideration by the surgeon who has to plan for the residual growth of the orbit and possible chances of migration of implants.

57.11 Secondary Correction of Orbital Deformities

Secondary corrections of the internal orbit demand great degrees of skill and are technically demanding even for the trained surgeon due to the nature of fibrosis and contracture that is already set in and the distortion of bony landmarks within the orbit. This may necessitate more extensive dissection and mobilization of the orbital contents and yet yield sub-optimal outcomes.

57.12 Complications

Complications associated with management of orbital fractures may be categorized into immediate and delayed complications.

Box 57.12 Indications for Secondary Deformity Correction of the Internal Orbit Generally Are

(a) Restricted ocular movement, which may be either due to muscle entrapments or adhesions of intra orbital and/or periorbita
(b) Diplopia due to physical impediments like bony interferences and/or soft tissue adhesion/entrapment
(c) Enophthalmos and/or hypophthalmos

57.12.1 Immediate Complications

The most common immediate complications that are secondary to orbital surgery include:

- edema,
- infection,
- would dehiscence,
- aberrant implant position,
- extrusion of implants.

Hemorrhage may be an infrequent complication which may happen during the surgery or in the immediate post-operative period.

Complications associated with specific ophthalmic implications like injuries to the cornea, extraocular muscles, lacrimal apparatus, or the optic nerve also may occur.

Blindness is a rare but grievous complication which has to be borne in mind.

The last group includes neurosensory disturbances like paresthesia or dysesthesia associated with the infra-orbital nerve and carrying grades of facial nerve palsy or weakness [72, 73].

57.12.2 Delayed Complications

Delayed complication may present in the form of:

- Persistent enophthalmos/hypophthalmos
- Persistent or worsened diplopia with altered vision
- Restricted ocular movement due to fibrosis and adhesion

Other adverse outcomes include:

- Entropion
- Ectropion
- Hypertrophic scars/keloids
- Change in the axis of the palpebral fissure

57.13 Recent Advances in Management of Orbital Fractures

Orbital reconstruction still remains one of the most challenging and enigmatic areas in the management of cranio-facial trauma and most certainly attracts the latest in terms of technology and developments to refine and improve outcomes. Significant advances in the field of orbital reconstruction include:

1. Computer-assisted surgery
2. Intraoperative imaging and navigation (refer Chap. 41)
3. Patient-specific implants for reconstruction

57.13.1 Navigation and CAS for Orbital Fractures and Reconstruction

Computer-assisted surgery allows virtual pre-operative planning of the desired reconstruction using pre-operative CT scans (Fig. 57.54a–d) [74]. This virtual plan gives real-time guidance during surgery. Navigation helps visualize the actual surgical outcome during surgery in relation to the pre-operative plan (Fig. 57.55). With this technique, sub-optimal reduction of fractures and positioning of implants can be identified and corrected during surgery, thereby reducing the need for secondary procedures [75–77].

57.13.2 Patient-Specific Implants (Fig. 57.56a–c)

Custom implants for the reconstruction of complex defects and deformities have become vogue now. They offer the advantages of accurate planning and infallible positioning intraoperatively which enormously improve post-surgical

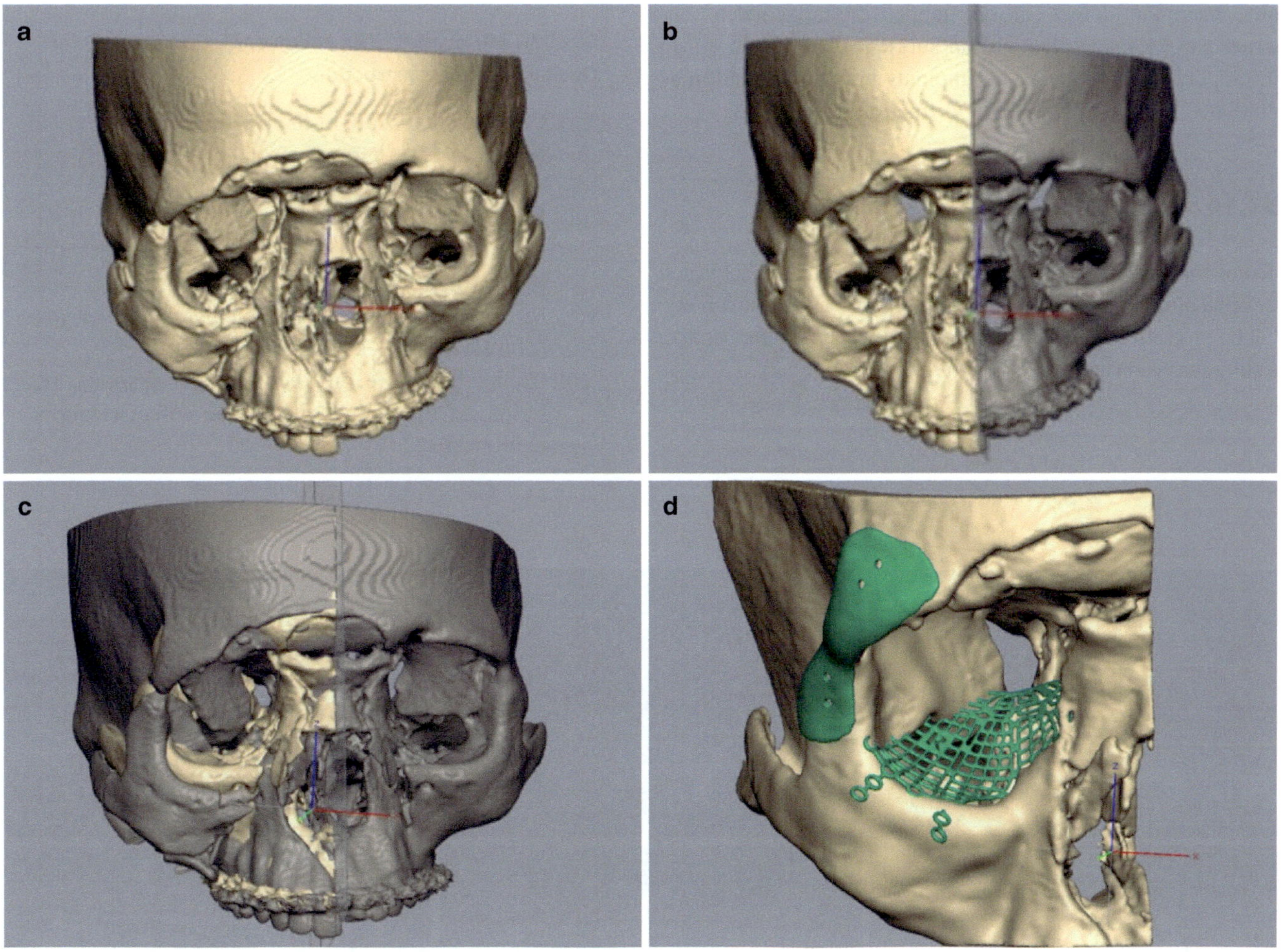

Fig. 57.54 Photographs depicting stages in computer-assisted surgery for orbito-facial reconstruction. (**a**) Generation of virtual 3D model; (**b**) segmentation and mirroring of normal side; (**c**) superimposition of the mirrored object on the affected side, enabling a better understanding of the deformity; and (**d**) creation of patient specific implant design for the fronto-zygomatic region and importing the virtual model of the anatomical orbital implant for floor reconstruction

outcomes. The defect can be mapped digitally and a construct can be made after virtual surgical planning to aid in intraoperative guidance. The implants may also function as guidance stents and double up as fixation devices too.

57.14 Conclusion

To conclude, all patients with orbital trauma need to be subjected to ophthalmological examinations both pre- and post-surgery. Globe protection, gentle retraction of tissues, and intraoperative testing for vision are mandatory during orbital surgery.

Box 57.13 Principles to Be Followed During Surgery for Orbital Floor Reconstruction

(i) Complete exposure of the fracture and defect
(ii) Meticulous de-herniation of the orbital soft tissues with restitution of intra-orbital volume
(iii) Identification of the posterior ledge in floor defects which is the posterior limit for reconstruction
(iv) Restoration of the posteromedial bulge of the orbit (Hammer's key area) [7]
(v) Choice for the reconstruction material should be based on the complexity of the defect (Dubois et al.) [55]

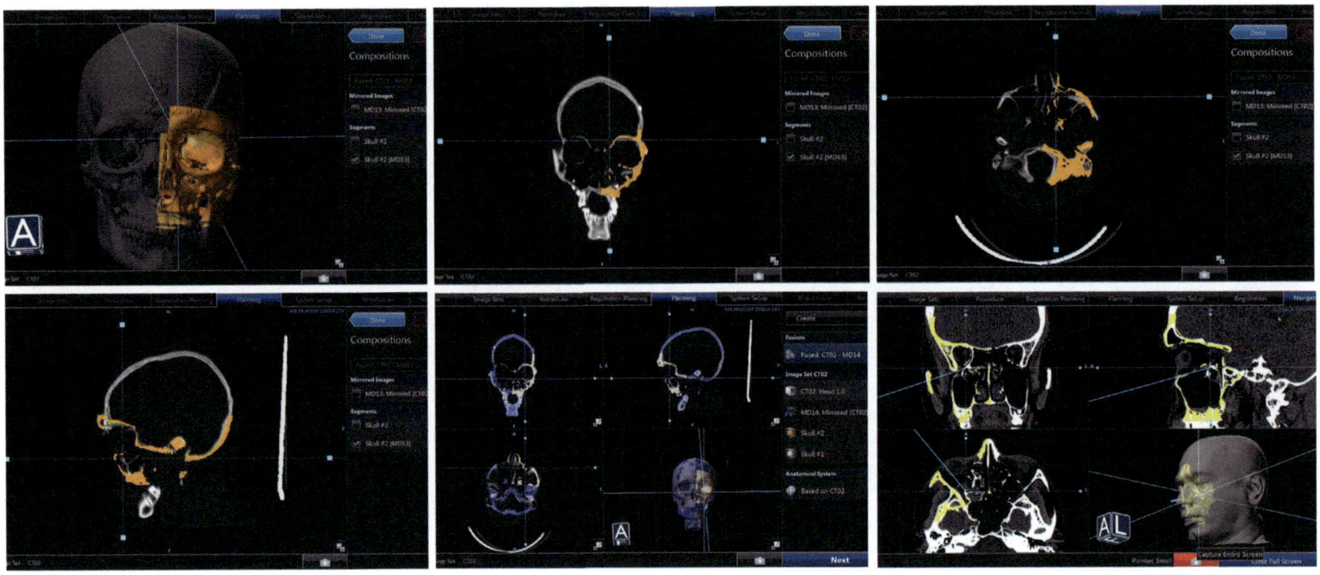

Fig. 57.55 Screenshot images of a left-sided orbital floor with an anatomical orbital floor implant that is virtually planned and executed with the help of intraoperative navigation

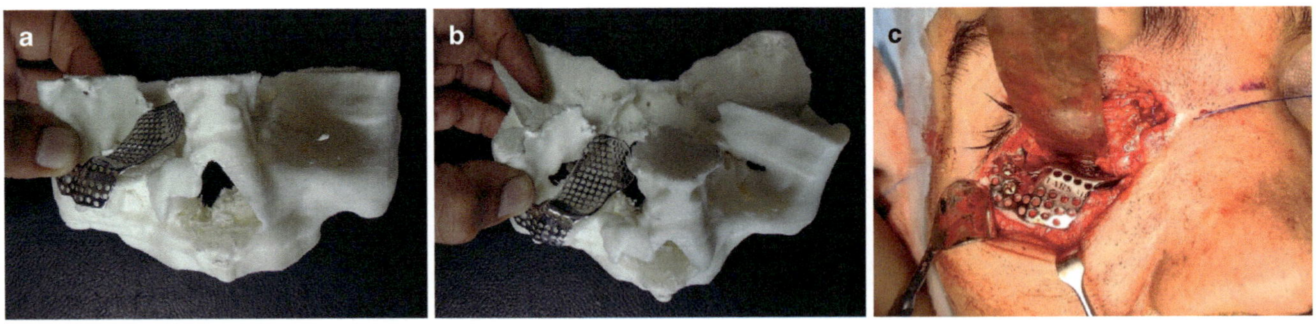

Fig. 57.56 PSI designed for reconstruction of a large floor and medial wall defect in the right orbit. (**a**) Frontal view of PSI on an STL model of the patient, (**b**) superior view, and (**c**) intraoperative photograph showing placement of the PSI "in situ"

57.15 Case Scenarios

Case 1

Patient with a history of facial trauma 8 months back presented with complaints of change in the position of his eyeballs. He had a history of surgical intervention for management of his pan-facial fractures immediately following the trauma. No intervention was performed for the orbital fractures primarily. Subsequent clinical evaluation performed 8 months later revealed enophthamos, hypophtalmos and restriction in superior gaze in the right eye. CT scans revealed a large orbital floor defect on the right side with fibrosis and adhesion of the inferior rectus to the posterior ledge of the floor defect. The patient was subjected to secondary surgery for correction of the above mentioned complaints. An orbital exploration was performed on the right side to release the inferior rectus, the infra-orbtial rim was augmented with a ramal graft and the floor defect was reconstructed with a "Stryker" anatomical orbital implant. Post-surgical evaluation revealed optimal corrections of the enophthalmos, hypophthalmos and good repositioning of the inferior rectus muscle (Figs. 57.57a–d, 57.58a, b and 57.59a–f).

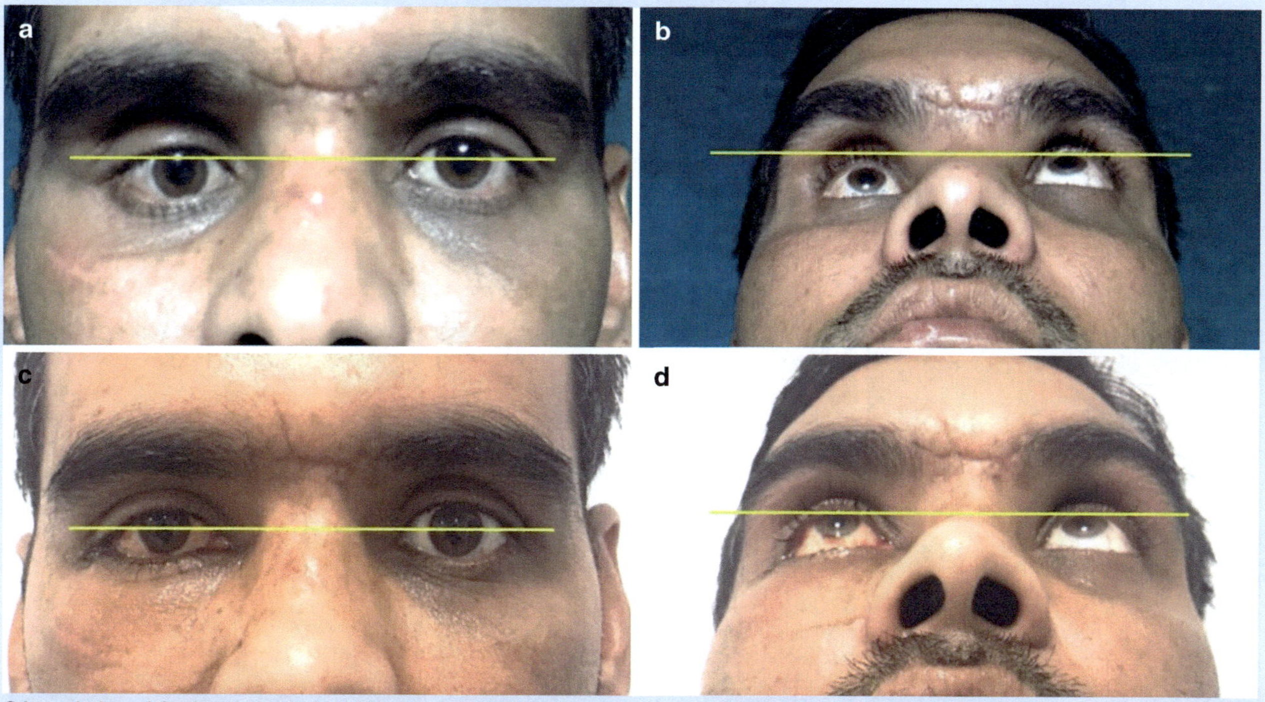

Fig. 57.57 (**a** and **b**) Pre-operative clinical photographs of patient demonstrating right sided enophthalmos and hypophthalmos. (**c** and **d**) Post-operative clinical photographs showing optimal surgical outcomes

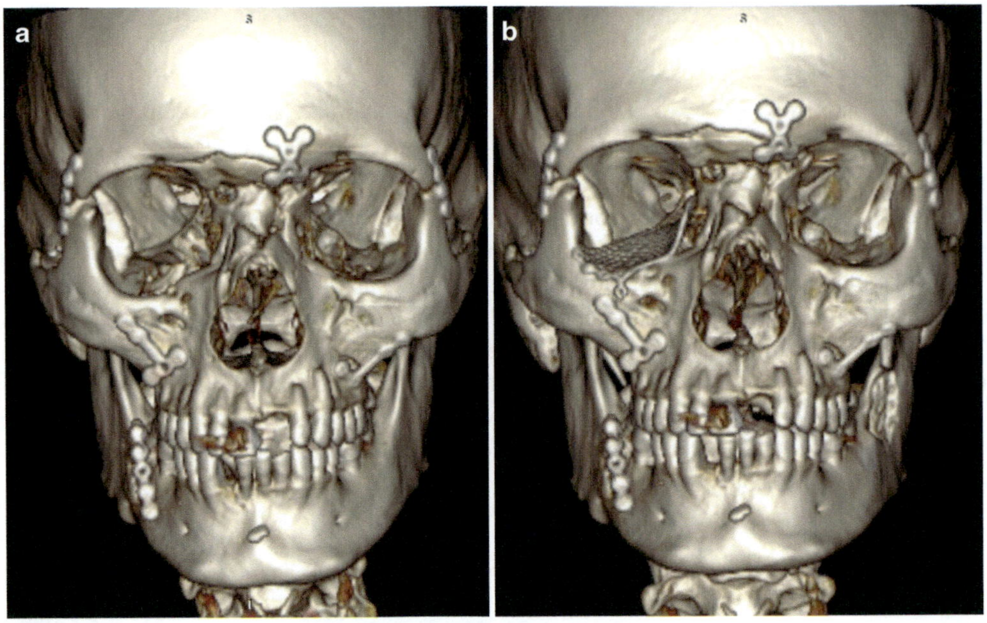

Fig. 57.58 3D CT reconstructions of patient in Fig 57.57 demonstrating (**a**) right-sided malunited zygomatic complex fracture with orbital floor defect and (**b**) post-surgical scan image showing reconstruction of the right orbital floor defect with an anatomical orbital implant after augmentation of the infra-orbital rim with a mandibular ramus bone graft

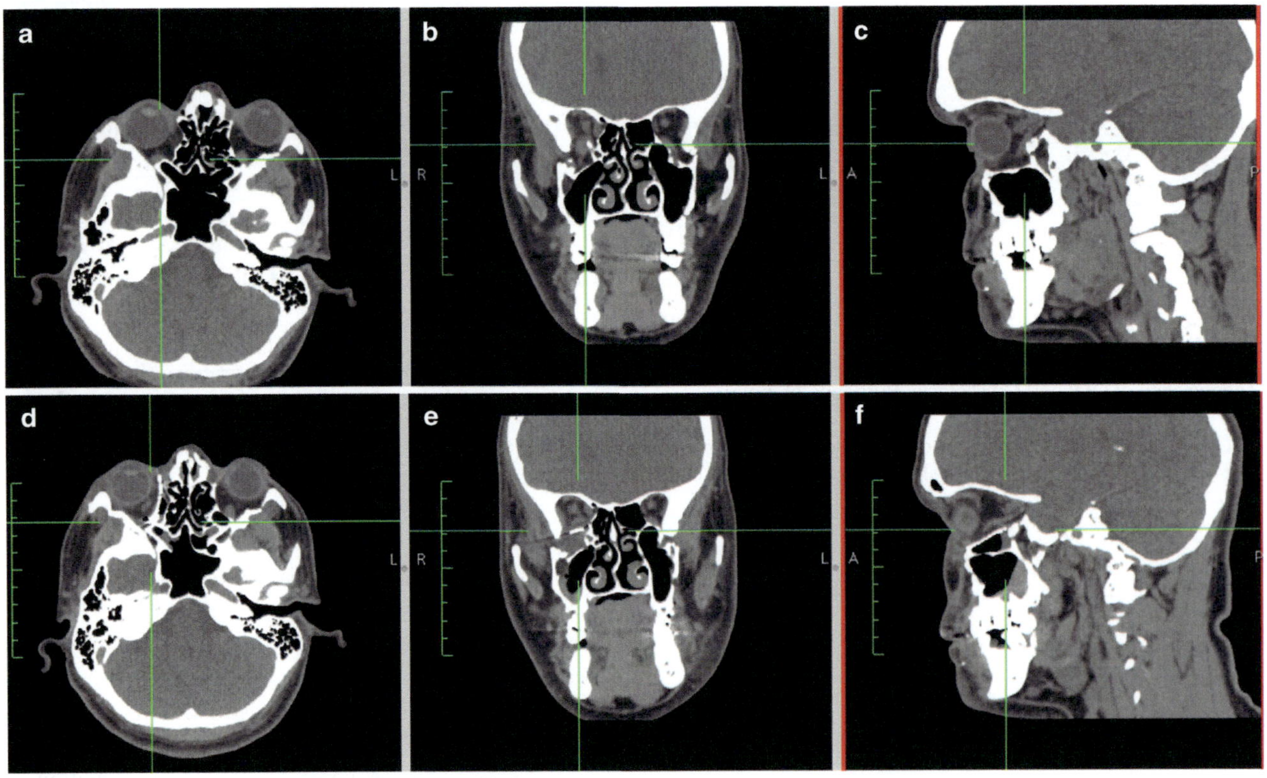

Fig. 57.59 (**a–c**) Pre-operative axial, coronal, and sagittal scans of patient in Fig 57.57 with large defect of the right orbital floor. (**d–f**) Post-operative sections demonstrating the correction of the floor defect with an anatomical orbital implant

Case 2

A 12 year old girl presented to the surgical OPD with history of blunt injury to the left eye. On examination she had no external signs of injury but revealed restriction in superior gaze in the left eye. CT scan revealed a springing trapdoor fracture of the left orbital floor with entrapment of the inferior rectus muscle. A diplopia charting was performed which revealed moderate to severe restriction of the left eye in the superior gaze. The patient was taken up for immediate surgery for orbital exploration and release of the entrapped muscle with/without floor reconstruction. The exploration was successful and the patient required no reconstruction of the floor. Post operatively the patient demonstrated complete resolution of the symptoms with the full range of ocular movements restored. (Figs. 57.60, 57.61, 57.62a, b) (Courtesy: Dept of Orbit & Oculoplasty, Shankara Nethralaya, Chennai)

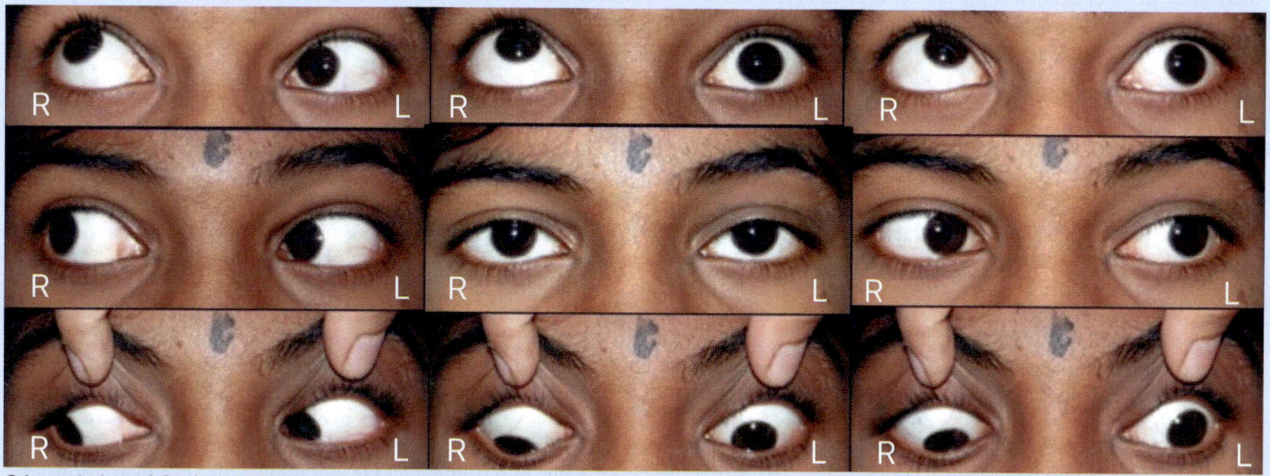

Fig. 57.60 Pre-operative photograph demonstrating the nine gazes of a young girl with a "White eye blowout" fracture of the left orbital floor with entrapment of the inferior rectus. (Courtesy: Dept of Orbit & Oculoplasty, Shankara Nethralaya, Chennai)

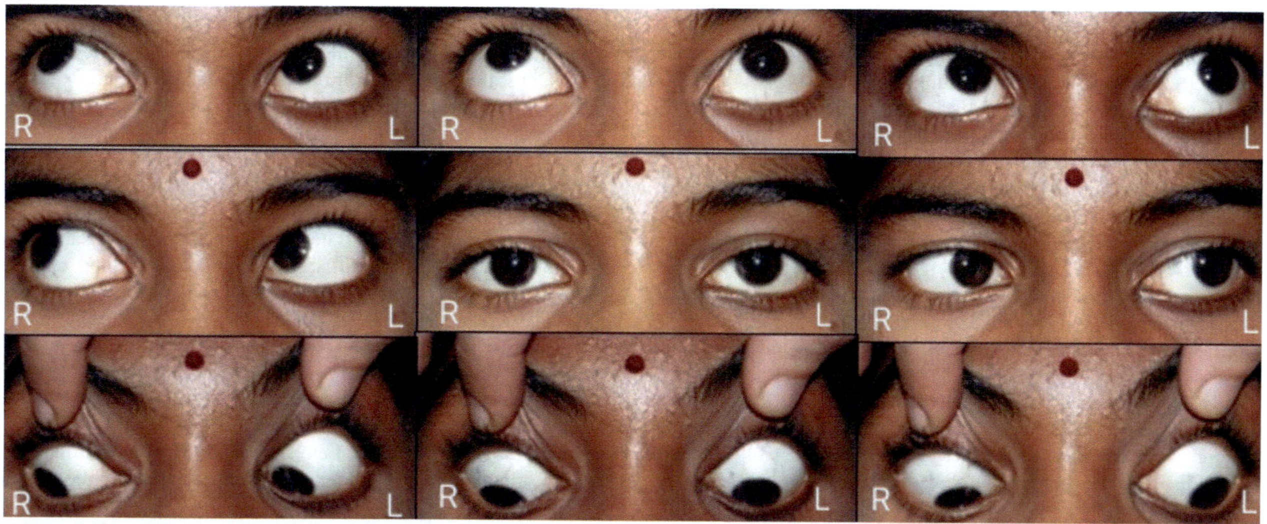

Fig. 57.61 Post-operative photograph demonstrating resolution of symptoms after 3 weeks of surgery (Courtesy: Dept of Orbit & Oculoplasty, Shankara Nethralaya, Chennai)

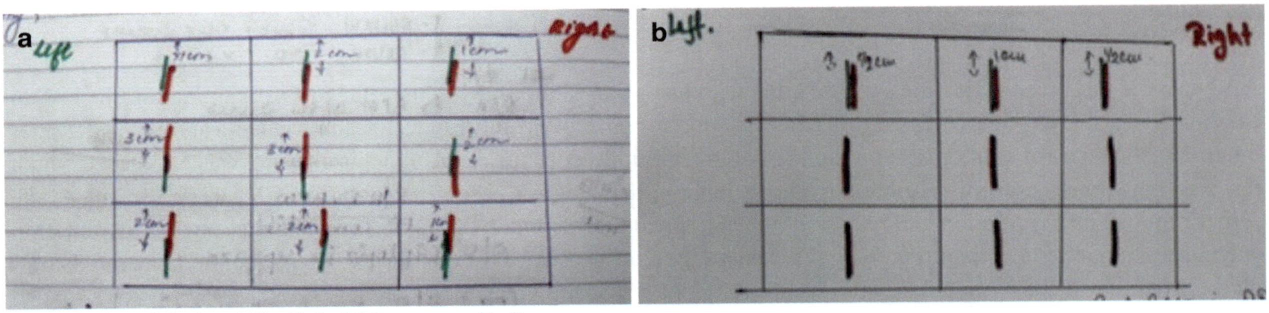

Fig. 57.62 Photograph of documentation of diplopia by charting with two colors (green for left and red for right eyes). The left and right sides are marked in the orientation that the patient sees an object in front of him/her. (**a**) Pre-operative and (**b**) post-operative (Courtesy: Dept of Orbit & Oculoplasty, Shankara Nethralaya, Chennai)

References

1. Turvey TA, Golden BA. Orbital anatomy for the surgeon. Oral Maxillofac Surg Clin North Am. 2012;24(4):525–36.
2. Ochs MW, Buckley MJ. Anatomy of the orbit. Oral Maxillofac Surg Clin North Am. 1993;5:419–29.
3. Rowe NL, Williams JL. Maxillofacial injuries. Edinburgh: Churchill Livingstone; 1985.
4. Furuta M. Measurement of orbital volume by computed tomography: especially on the growth of the orbit. Jpn J Ophthalmol. 2001;45(6):600–6.
5. Bron AJ, Tripathi RC. Wolff's anatomy of the eye and orbit. London: Chapman and Hall Medical; 1997.
6. Zide BM, editor. Surgical anatomy around the orbit: the system of zones. Philadelphia: Lippincott Williams & Wilkins; 2006.
7. Hammer B. Orbital fractures: diagnosis, operative treatment, secondary corrections. Toronto: Hogrefe & Huber; 1995.
8. Manson PN, Clifford CM, Su CT, Iliff NT, Morgan R. Mechanisms of global support and posttraumatic enophthalmos: I. The anatomy of the ligament sling and its relation to intramuscular cone orbital fat. Plast Reconstr Surg. 1986;77(2):193–202.
9. Martins C, Costa e Silva IE, Campero A, Yasuda A, Aguiar LR, Tatagiba M, Rhoton A. Microsurgical anatomy of the orbit: the rule of seven. Anat Res Int. 2011;2011:468727.
10. Manson PN, Markowitz B, Mirvis S, Dunham M, Yaremchuk M. Toward CT-based facial fracture treatment. Plast Reconstr Surg. 1990 Feb;85(2):202–12.
11. Converse JM, Smith B. Blowout fracture of the floor of the orbit. Trans Am Acad Ophthalmol Otolaryngol. 1960;64:676–88.
12. Dingman RO, Natvig P. Surgery of facial fractures. London: Saunders; 1964.
13. Fujino T. Experimental "blowout" fracture of the orbit. Plast Reconstr Surg. 1974;54(1):81–2.
14. Pfeiffer RL. Traumatic enophthalmos. Trans Am Ophthalmol Soc. 1943;41:293–306.
15. Brady SM, Mcmann MA, Mazzoli RA, Bushley DM, Ainbinder DJ, Carroll RB. The diagnosis and management of orbital blowout fractures: update 2001. Am J Emerg Med. 2001;19(2):147–54.
16. King EF, Samuel E. Fractures of the orbit. Trans Ophthalmol Soc U K. 1944;64:134–53.
17. Ahmad F, Kirkpatrick NA, Lyne J, Urdang M, Waterhouse N. Buckling and hydraulic mechanisms in orbital blowout fractures: fact or fiction? J Craniofac Surg. 2006;17(3):438–41.
18. Nagasao T, Miyamoto J, Shimizu Y, Jiang H, Nakajima T. What happens between pure hydraulic and buckling mechanisms of blowout fractures? J Cranio-Maxillofac Surg. 2010;38(4):306–13.
19. Al-Qurainy IA, Dutton GN, Titterington DM, Stassen LF, Moos KF, El-Attar A. Midfacial fractures and the eye: the development of a system for detecting patients at risk of eye injury. Br J Oral Maxillofac Surg. 1991;29(6):363–7.
20. Soparkar CN, Patrinely JR. The eye examination in facial trauma for the plastic surgeon. Plast Reconstr Surg. 2007;120(7):49S–56S.
21. Al-Qrainy IA, Dutton GN, Stassen LF, Moos KF, El-Attar A. The characteristics of midfacial fractures and the association with ocular injury: a prospective study. Br J Oral Maxillofac Surg. 1991;29(5):291–301.
22. Ochs MW. Orbital and ocular trauma. In: Peterson's principles of oral and maxillofacial surgery. 2nd ed. Hamilton: London; 2004. p. 463–90.
23. American Academy of Ophthalmology. 8-point eye exam. Adopted May 24, 2016 (Cited May 21, 2019). Available from https://www.aao.org/young-ophthalmologists/yo-info/article/how-to-conduct-eight-point-ophthalmology-exam
24. Al-Qurainy IA, Dutton GN, Stassen LF, Moos KF, El-Attar A. Diplopia following midfacial fractures. Br J Oral Maxillofac Surg. 1991;29(5):302–7.
25. Tahernia A, Erdmann D, Follmar K, Mukundan S, Grimes J, Marcus JR. Clinical implications of orbital volume change in the management of isolated and zygomaticomaxillary complex–associated orbital floor injuries. Plast Reconstr Surg. 2009;123(3):968–75.
26. He D, Li Z, Shi W, Sun Y, Zhu H, Lin M, Shen G, Fan X. Orbitozygomatic fractures with enophthalmos: analysis of 64 cases treated late. J Oral Maxillofac Surg. 2012;70(3):562–76.
27. Goodall KL, Brahma A, Bates A, Leatherbarrow B. Lateral canthotomy and inferior cantholysis: an effective method of urgent orbital decompression for sight threatening acute retrobulbar haemorrhage. Injury. 1999;30(7):485–90.
28. Gruss JS, Hurwitz JJ, Nik NA, Kassel EE. The pattern and incidence of nasolacrimal injury in naso-orbital-ethmoid fractures: the role of delayed assessment and dacryocystorhinostomy. Br J Plast Surg. 1985;38(1):116–21.
29. Woernley TC, Wright TL, Lam DN, Jundt JS. Oculocardiac reflex in an orbital fracture without entrapment. J Oral Maxillofac Surg. 2017;75(8):1716–21.
30. Schaller B. Trigeminocardiac reflex. J Neurol. 2004;251(6):658–65.
31. Fonseca RJ, Marciani RD, Turvey TA. Oral and maxillofacial surgery. Missouri: Saunders Elsevier; 2009.

32. Chen CT, Chen YR. Traumatic superior orbital fissure syndrome: current management. Craniomaxillofac Trauma Reconstr. 2010 Mar;3(01):009–16.
33. Zachariades N. The superior orbital fissure syndrome: Review of the literature and report of a case. Oral Surg Oral Med Oral Pathol. 1982;53(3):237–40.
34. Warburton RE, Brookes CC, Golden BA, Turvey TA. Orbital apex disorders: a case series. Int J Oral Maxillofac Surg. 2016;45(4):497–506.
35. Antonyshyn O, Gruss JS, Kassel EE. Blow-in fractures of the orbit. Plast Reconstr Surg. 1989;84(1):10–20.
36. Lynch RC. The technique of a radical frontal sinus operation which has given me the best results.(original communications are received with the understanding) that they are contributed exclusively to the laryngoscope. Laryngoscope. 1921;31(1):1–5.
37. Ellis E, Zide MF, editors. Surgical approaches to the facial skeleton. Philadelphia: Lippincott Williams & Wilkins; 2006.
38. Perry M, Holmes S. Manual of operative maxillofacial trauma surgery. London: Springer; 2014.
39. Cline RA, Rootman J. Enophthalmos: a clinical review. Ophthalmology. 1984;91(3):229–37.
40. Athanasiov PA, Prabhakaran VC, Selva D. Non-traumatic enophthalmos: a review. Acta Ophthalmol. 2008;86(4):356–64.
41. Converse JM, Smith B, Obear MF, Wood-Smith D. Orbital blowout fractures: a ten-year survey. Plast Reconstr Surg. 1967;39(1):20–36.
42. Cossman JP, Morrison CS, Taylor HO, Salter AB, Klinge PM, Sullivan SR. Traumatic orbital roof fractures: interdisciplinary evaluation and management. Plast Reconstr Surg. 2014;133(3):335e–43e.
43. Alsuhaibani AH. Orbital fracture: significance of lateral wall. Saudi J Ophthalmol. 2010;24(2):49–55.
44. Stanley JR, Sires BS, Funk GF, Nerad JA. Management of displaced lateral orbital wall fractures associated with visual and ocular motility disturbances. Plast Reconstr Surg. 1998;102(4):972–9.
45. Manolidis S, Weeks BH, Kirby M, Scarlett M, Hollier L. Classification and surgical management of orbital fractures: experience with 111 orbital reconstructions. J Craniofac Surg. 2002;13(6):726–37.
46. McNichols CH, Hatef DA, Thornton JF, Cole PD, de Mitchell CA, Hollier LH Jr. A paradigm shift in correcting medial orbital fracture–related enophthalmos: volumetric augmentation through a lateral approach. J Craniofac Surg. 2012;23(3):762–6.
47. Nolasco FP, Mathog RH. Medial orbital wall fractures: classification and clinical profile. Otolaryngol Head Neck Surg. 1995 Apr;112(4):549–56.
48. Burm JS, Chung CH, Oh SJ. Pure orbital blowout fracture: new concepts and importance of medial orbital blowout fracture. Plast Reconstr Surg. 1999;103(7):1839–49.
49. Lee WT, Kim HK, Chung SM. Relationship between small-size medial orbital wall fracture and late enophthalmos. J Craniofac Surg. 2009;20(1):75–80.
50. Jin HR, Shin SO, Choo MJ, Choi YS. Relationship between the extent of fracture and the degree of enophthalmos in isolated blowout fractures of the medial orbital wall. J Oral Maxillofac Surg. 2000;58(6):617–20.
51. Saiepour D, Messo E, Hedlund AJ, Nowinski DJ. Radiologic and long-term clinical outcome from treatment of isolated medial orbital wall blowout fractures. J Craniofac Surg. 2012;23(5):1252–5.
52. Lee CS, Yoon JS, Lee SY. Combined transconjunctival and transcaruncular approach for repair of large medial orbital wall fractures. Arch Ophthalmol. 2009;127(3):291–6.
53. Dubois L, Steenen SA, Gooris PJ, Bos RR, Becking AG. Controversies in orbital reconstruction—III. Biomaterials for orbital reconstruction: a review with clinical recommendations. Int J Oral Maxillofac Surg. 2016;45(1):41–50.
54. Jaquiéry C, Aeppli C, Cornelius P, Palmowsky A, Kunz C, Hammer B. Reconstruction of orbital wall defects: critical review of 72 patients. Int J Oral Maxillofac Surg. 2007;36(3):193–9.
55. Dubois L, Steenen SA, Gooris PJ, Mourits MP, Becking AG. Controversies in orbital reconstruction—I. Defect-driven orbital reconstruction: a systematic review. Int J Oral Maxillofac Surg. 2015;44(3):308–15.
56. Palmieri CF, Ghali GE. Late correction of orbital deformities. Oral Maxillofac Surg Clin North Am. 2012;24(4):649–63.
57. Dubois L, Steenen SA, Gooris PJ, Mourits MP, Becking AG. Controversies in orbital reconstruction—II. Timing of post-traumatic orbital reconstruction: a systematic review. Int J Oral Maxillofac Surg. 2015;44(4):433–40.
58. Koo L, Hatton MP, Rubin PA. When is enophthalmos "significant"? Ophthalmic Plast Reconstr Surg. 2006;22(4):274–7.
59. Sung YS, Chung CM, Hong IP. The correlation between the degree of enophthalmos and the extent of fracture in medial orbital wall fracture left untreated for over six months: a retrospective analysis of 81 cases at a single institution. Arch Plast Surg. 2013;40(4):335.
60. Gooris PJ, Muller BS, Dubois L, Bergsma JE, Mensink G, van den Ham MF, Becking AG, Seubring K. Finding the ledge: sagittal analysis of bony landmarks of the orbit. J Oral Maxillofac Surg. 2017;75(12):2613–27.
61. Markowitz BL, Manson PN, Sargent L, Vander CAK, Yaremchuk M, Glassman D, et al. Management of the medial canthal tendon in nasoethmoid orbital fractures: the importance of the central fragment in classification and treatment. Plast Reconstr Surg. 1991;87(5):843–53.
62. Hayreh SS, Weingeist TA. Experimental occlusion of the central artery of the retina. IV: Retinal tolerance time to acute ischaemia. Br J Ophthalmol. 1980;64(11):818–25.
63. Vassallo S, Hartstein M, Howard D, Stetz J. Traumatic retrobulbar hemorrhage: emergent decompression by lateral canthotomy and cantholysis. J Emerg Med. 2002;22(3):251–6.
64. Gerbino G, Ramieri GA, Nasi A. Diagnosis and treatment of retrobulbar haematomas following blunt orbital trauma: a description of eight cases. Int J Oral Maxillofac Surg. 2005;34(2):127–31.
65. Amrith S, Saw SM, Lim TC, Lee TK. Ophthalmic involvement in cranio-facial trauma. J Cranio-Maxillofac Surg. 2000;28(3):140–7.
66. Levin LA, Beck RW, Joseph MP, Seiff S, Kraker R, International Optic Nerve Trauma Study Group. The treatment of traumatic optic neuropathy: the International Optic Nerve Trauma Study. Ophthalmology. 1999;106(7):1268–77.
67. Steinsapir KD, Goldberg RA. Traumatic optic neuropathy. Surv Ophthalmol. 1994;38(6):487–518.
68. Hoffmeister B. Pediatric maxillofacial trauma. In: Maxillofacial surgery. London: Churchill Livingstone; 2017. p. 193–9.
69. Sugamata A, Yoshizawa N. A case of blowout fracture of the orbital floor in early childhood. Int Med Case Rep J. 2015;8:155–8.
70. Tiwana PS, Vickers A. Pediatric cranio-maxillofacial trauma: mandibular fractures. In: Current therapy in oral and maxillofacial surgery. Philadelphia: WB Saunders; 2012. p. 841–50.
71. Yew CC, Shaari R, Rahman SA, Alam MK. White-eyed blowout fracture: diagnostic pitfalls and review of literature. Injury. 2015;46(9):1856–9.
72. Benoliel R, Birenboim R, Regev E, Eliav E. Neurosensory changes in the infraorbital nerve following zygomatic fractures. Oral Surg Oral Med Oral Pathol Oral Radiol Endod. 2005;99(6):657–65.

73. Kumar P, Godhi S, Lall AB, Ram CS. Evaluation of neurosensory changes in the infraorbital nerve following zygomatic fractures. J Maxillofac Oral Surg. 2012;11(4):394–9.
74. Bell RB, Markiewicz MR. Computer-assisted planning, stereolithographic modeling, and intraoperative navigation for complex orbital reconstruction: a descriptive study in a preliminary cohort. J Oral Maxillofac Surg. 2009;67(12):2559–70.
75. Lauer G, Pradel W, Schneider M, Eckelt U. Efficacy of computer-assisted surgery in secondary orbital reconstruction. J Cranio-Maxillofac Surg. 2006;34(5):299–305.
76. Wilde F, Lorenz K, Ebner AK, Krauss O, Mascha F, Schramm A. Intraoperative imaging with a 3D C-arm system after zygomatico-orbital complex fracture reduction. J Oral Maxillofac Surg. 2013;71(5):894–910.
77. Wilde F, Schramm A. Intraoperative imaging in orbital and midface reconstruction. Facial Plast Surg. 2014;30(05):545–53.

Additional Reading

Bater MC, Ramchandani PL, Brennan PA. Post-traumatic eye observations. Br J Oral Maxillofac Surg. 2005;43(5):410–6.

58 Frontal and Naso-Orbito-Ethmoid Complex Fractures

Kannan Balaraman

58.1 Introduction

Naso-orbito-ethmoid (NOE) region is a confluence of critical structures of the face including the nose, orbit and skull base. Hence injuries to the region have a major impact on the function of these regions as well as aesthetics. A deformity of the NOE region tends to catch the eye much more than a deformity elsewhere in the face and hence affecting the individual. The injuries to this area are about 5% of maxillofacial injuries in adults and about 15% in children [1, 2] and mostly occur as a result of road traffic accidents (RTA) [1] especially in the Indian subcontinent. This is especially so due to two-wheeler injuries. Considering the proximity of the region to the brain and globe, these injuries may need multidisciplinary evaluation before embarking on a definitive treatment plan.

58.2 Applied Surgical Anatomy

The NOE complex is a part of the medial vertical buttress system of the face abutting the cranium. It is made of the nasal bones, the ethmoid bones encompassing the sinuses which also form the medial wall of the orbit articulating above with the frontal bone at the anterior skull base. This ethmoid labyrinth which separates both the orbits acts like a shock absorber during trauma thus minimizing force dissipation into critical structures like the orbital and cranial cavities. Extensive injury or comminution can result in associated anterior cranial base fractures causing cerebrospinal fluid (CSF) leak as well. The frontal process of maxilla and the lacrimal bone also is an integral part of the complex owing to their proximity and involvement in the fracture pattern occurring in the region.

K. Balaraman (✉)
Department of Oral and Maxillofacial Surgery, Ganga Medical Centre and Hospitals, Coimbatore, Tamil Nadu, India

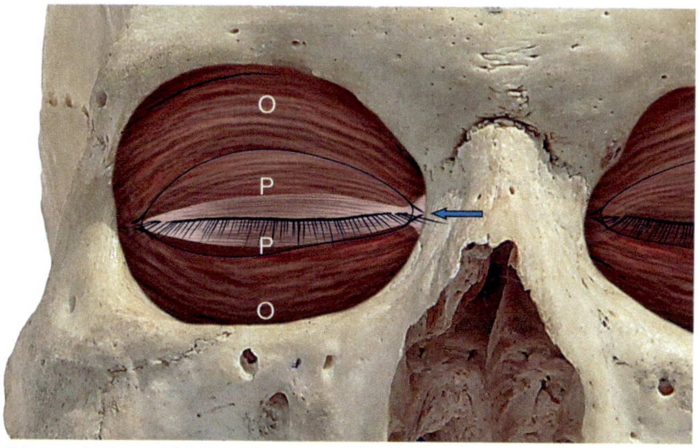

Fig. 58.1 MCL anchoring eyelids (O-occular, P-palpebral)

Apart from the bony parts, the medial canthal ligament (MCL) is an important soft tissue of the complex (Fig. 58.1). The ligament not only anchors the upper and lower eyelids to the nasal complex but also encompasses the lacrimal sac at its anterior, posterior and superior aspect [3]. Certain authors have found that the posterior limb is not always present or clearly defined in certain instances [4]. The ligament being attached to the edges of the lacrimal fossa in the lacrimal bone in these areas helps in emptying of the lacrimal sac during blinking thus effecting drainage of the lacrimal sac. Hence injuries to the region affecting the attachment of the medial canthal ligament can impact the medial eyelid attachment and/or draining off tears from lacrimal sac. The skin and soft tissues drape over the complex like a cloth over a framework, and when the region crumples following an injury, the soft tissue envelope collapses as well causing distinct deformity which if not treated well can result in persistent deformity of the region. The collapsed soft tissue heals/scars over the deformed bony complex and secondary correction at a later date do not help achieve the pre-injury status. Hence optimal primary realignment and repair offer the best chance of achieving optimal results [5].

K. Bonanthaya et al. (eds.), *Oral and Maxillofacial Surgery for the Clinician*, https://doi.org/10.1007/978-981-15-1346-6_58

58.3 Historical Perspective and Classification [6]

The treatment of NOE complex injuries has evolved from the previous century. Though nasal bone fractures have been recognized for a long time, the fracture of ethmoids was highlighted by Dawson and Fordyce in 1953. Converse and Smith in 1963 identified the involvement of medial orbital wall and termed it as naso-orbital. Stranc was the first to in modern English literature to adopt the terminology naso-ethmoid. Epker recognized the present-day terminology of naso-orbito-ethmoid in 1973, whilst Gruss in 1985 preferred the term naso-ethmoid-orbital [6].

58.3.1 Classification

Rowe and Williams [7] in their classic text highlighted the complexity of the area and stressed the need for primary management. Their classification was quite simple, depending on side involved and association with other fractures.

- Unilateral or bilateral
- Isolated or associated with other facial fractures

Markowitz and Manson (1991) [8] identified the importance of canthal ligament, and their classification reflected the need for getting the position of the canthal ligament either by manipulating the fragment or anchoring the canthus directly. Their classification was as follows (Box 58.1):

Box 58.1 Markowitz and Manson Classification

Type I	Simple fracture with canthal ligament attachment intact
Type II	Comminuted fracture with intact canthal attachment in the large fragment (positioning this fragment helps in securing the canthus in the right place)
Type III	Gross comminution with the canthal attachment in a small fragment or detached canthus both necessitating canthopexy

58.3.2 Paediatric NOE Fractures (Fig. 58.2) Classification: Burstein et al.'s [9] (Box 58.2)

Box 58.2 Paediatric NOE Fracture Classification

Paediatric NOE fractures classification types are:

- *Burstein type I fracture*—localized to the upper NOE complex and frontal bone, medial to superior orbital foramen
- *Burstein type II fracture*—involves half of the superior orbital wall, although it does not involve the NOE
- *Burstein type III fracture*—is bilateral and involves the superior orbital walls, upper NOE and bilateral frontal bones

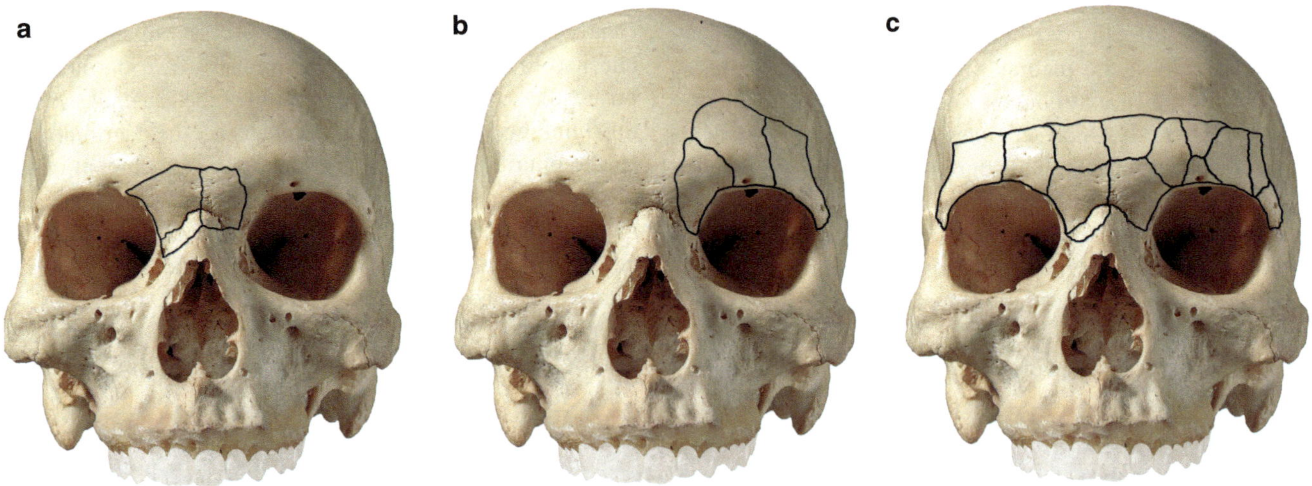

Fig. 58.2 Paediatric NOE fractures classification

Markowitz classification of adult NOE fractures does not take into account the differences in paediatric population such as:

- Midface-skull proportions
- Frontal sinus pneumatization

58.4 Aetiology, Clinical Features and Diagnosis

The most common aetiology of the fracture of NOE complex is trauma be it road accidents in unprotected individuals, assaults or fall from height [10].

Initial presentation can be disconcerting for the individual and bystanders due to profuse nasal bleeding and gross oedema around the midfacial skeleton. The signs and symptoms are given in Box 58.3 (symptoms) and Box 58.4 (signs).

Box 58.3 Symptoms of NOE Fracture

Periorbital swelling
Pain and discomfort
Epistaxis
Nasal blockade
– Widening of NOE area

Box 58.4 Signs of NOE Fracture

Nasal deformity with crepitus
Epistaxis—blood or mixed with CSF
Depressed nasal bridge
Upturned nasal tip
Rounded medial canthus
Altered palpebral fissure shape
Blockage of nasolacrimal duct
– Accentuation of the nasojugal skin fold
– Formation of obtuse angle at the base of columela with tension on upper lip
– Lip separation caused due to ruptured tip of nose
Telecanthus
(a) lose of almond shape of palpebral fissure
(b) Transverse shortening of the palpebral aperture
(c) Eyelids become lax
(d) Epicanthal fold become more prominent
(e) Flattening of the bottom of naso-orbital valley
(f) Obliteration of the caruncle
(g) Diminished tension of canthal ligament

From the point of view of the examining clinician, Advanced Trauma Life Support (ATLS) protocols take precedence however gross the presenting scenario is (Refer Chap. 48 of this book). Once primary survey is completed and the patient cleared for secondary survey, definitive clinical examination starts. It is also imperative to rule out underlying injuries to the head/brain, ophthalmologic or associated structures prior to comprehensive maxillofacial assessment.

The main indicators suggesting an underlying NOE fractures include:

- Depressed nasal bridge (with or without upturned nasal tip) is a result of the loss of bony morphology (Fig. 58.3a, b). When the medial canthal ligament attachment is lost, the manifestations include loss of contour of palpebral fissure with rounded medial canthal region. The almond shape of the palpebral fissure is lost and becomes larger, and Bowstring test becomes positive (Fig. 58.4).
- Traumatic telecanthus is a direct indicator of the MCL disruption or widening of the fragments. When there is an intercanthal distance of 35 mm or more, then it may be an indication of the fragment with MCL being displaced. Direct physical examination is useful in identifying the collapsed complex.

Measurement of Intercanthal Distance (ICD):

Normal values are 32–33 mm for females and 33–34 mm for males. The rule of thirds can be applied whilst evaluating NOE fractures. Normally ICD equals the palpebral fissure width. However, in NOE fractures, increased ICD is found, called telecanthus (Fig. 58.5).

Telecanthus deformity is characteristic; the lateral displacement of MCT leads to rounding of the medial palpebral fissure, widening of the NOE region and transverse shortening of the palpebral aperture.

- Care should be taken to rule out CSF leak and also damage to the nasolacrimal duct. However the latter is difficult to assess primarily in some of the cases and may become apparent much later. Clear discharge from the nose or watery bloody discharge should arouse a high index of suspicion necessitating further biochemical investigations to differentiate CSF from nasal discharge. Glucose content is more in CSF, but assessment of Tau protein (beta 2 Transferrin) is the confirmatory diagnostic factor. Thorough neurologic and ophthalmologic assessment is also essential. In the acute setting, clinical examination is challenging due to the discomfort and

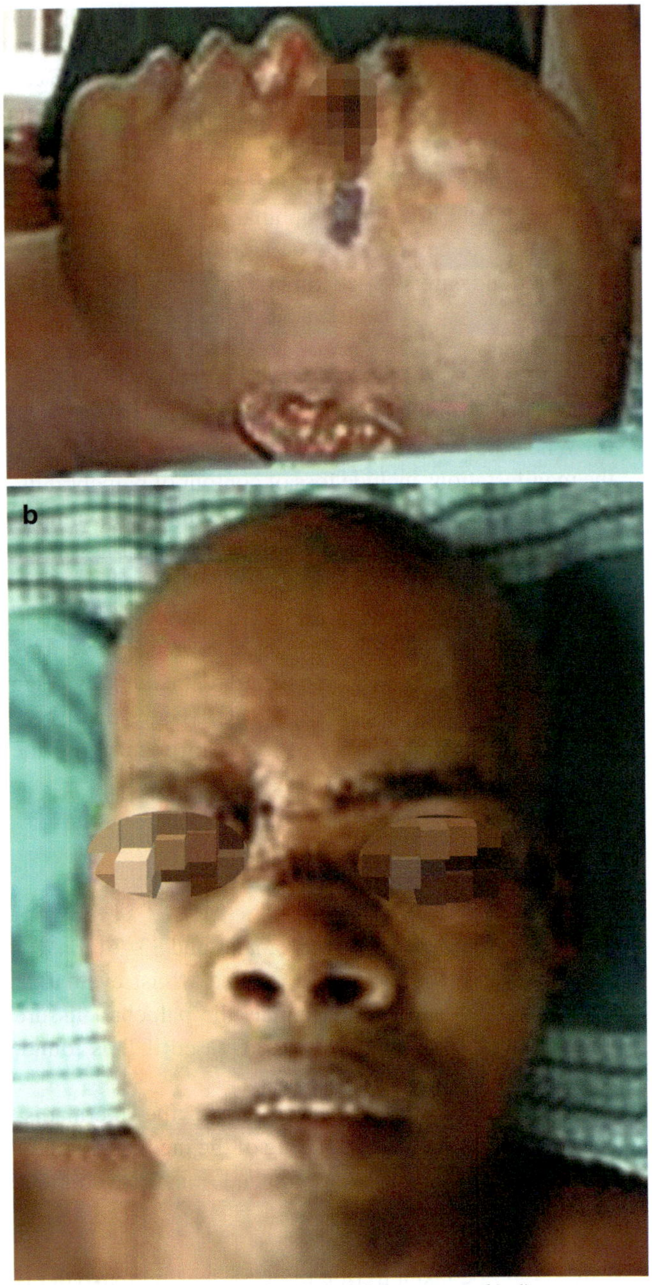

Fig. 58.3 (**a**, **b**) Depressed, widened nasal complex with upturned tip of the nose

always may be inadequate [11, 12], and hence radiological investigations are mandatory. The diagnosis and understanding of the fractures has evolved over the last century with the advent of CT imaging. CT scan imaging in all planes is the norm in these fractures and helps in ruling injuries to the adjacent structures as well as assess-

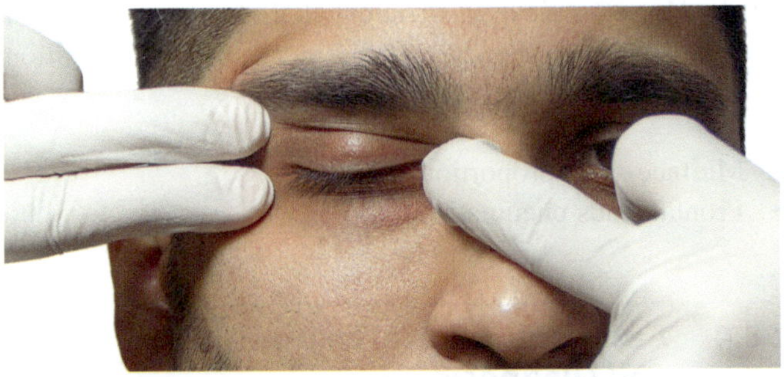

Fig. 58.4 Bowstring test for assessment of MCL attachment patency

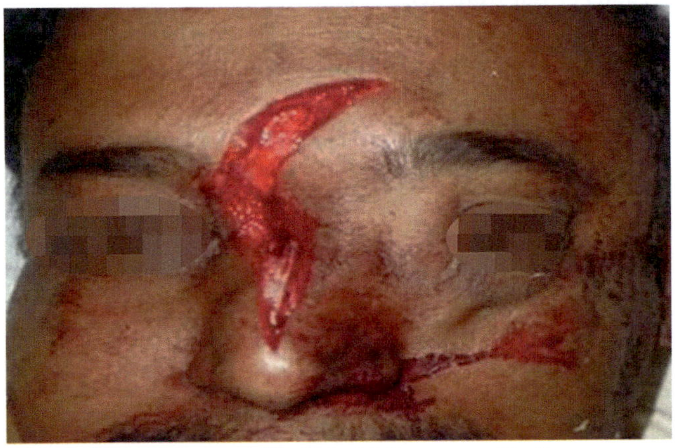

Fig. 58.5 Traumatic telecanthus

ing the extent and nature of displacement of NOE complex injuries.

- High-resolution CT scan images in all planes (axial, coronal (Fig. 58.6a–d)) help to identify and assess the fracture pattern accurately. Thin sections (0.6 mm) not only help in better evaluation but also facilitate surgical planning or fabrication of models if required. The CT scans will be mandatory anyway to assess the head injury status in such cases, and these images can be a part of the head injury screening imaging. Communicating with the radiology department of the importance of such images will ensure that the required sections being done at the same instance of head injury assessment scans thus avoiding repeat scans. The axial sections show if there is disruption of the nasal complex or there is splaying of the ethmoid complex. The coronal sections depicts the displacement in the mediolateral aspect (thus the status of the fragment with the MCL), whilst the sagittal sections

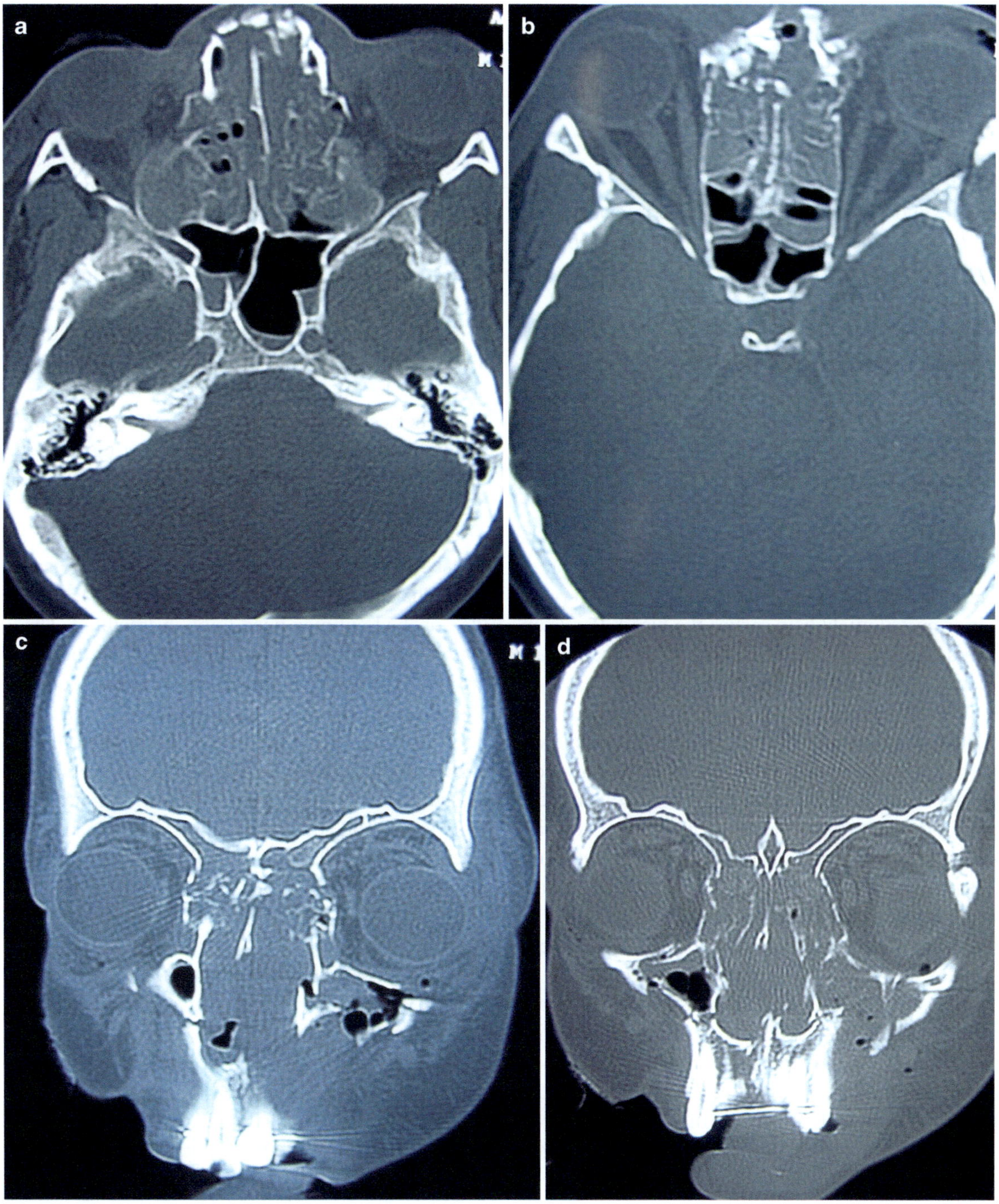

Fig. 58.6 (**a–d**) Axial and coronal CT scan images of NOE fracture

depict the displacement in the anteroposterior (AP) aspect (depression).

- 3D reconstructed images show the gross morphologic status and are as accurate as the thinness of the sections. Such images are good to plan the surgical management, discuss with the assistants the treatment goals and also explain to the patient the nature of the injury and proposed treatment plan as part of informed consent.

Test to Assess Integrity of MCT

NOE fracture is positive if mobility of the medial canthal tendon is appreciated.

It is revealed by a Bowstring or a bimanual test.

- Bowstring Test:
  When the eyelid is pulled laterally, a lack of resistance or detection of movement of the underlying bone at the tendon area is indicative of a fracture.
- Bimanual Test:
  An instrument is placed in the nose and pushed laterally. Instability and crepitation felt at the tendon area suggests NOE fracture.

58.5 Management

The initial presentation of such patients occasionally may be dramatic due to profuse epistaxis which may exacerbate in someone lying down. Keeping patients sitting up with packs in the anterior nostril might help reduce the bleed. Persistent profuse bleed may necessitate intubation to secure the airway and packs in both anterior and posterior nasal passages to help prevent aspiration.

The patient once stabilized, and fit to undergo surgery will need a discussion with the anaesthesiologist about options of intubation. Fractures not involving occlusion can be managed by oral intubation, whilst if involving occlusion then options like submental intubation or even tracheostomy of the patient requires prolonged ventilation or due to have further surgical procedures (as in poly trauma patients).

The presence of CSF leak might pose a tricky problem. Instances of CSF leak are higher whenever there is pneumocephalus. Hence in such instances, an approach combined with neurosurgical team may be mandatory, whilst involvement of an ophthalmologist is mandatory when there is involvement of lacrimal drainage system or lid adnexa. The treatment goals of NOE are shown in Box 58.5.

Box 58.5 Treatment Goals of NOE Fracture

Treatment goals
Restoring the nasal projection
Restoring nasal dorsal height with adequate nasofrontal angle
Re-establishing the MCL attachment
Restoring the latency of nasolacrimal duct

Conventionally the nasal complex was treated with closed reduction till Adam et al. [6] reported on the importance of nasal wiring. The importance of involving the medial canthal region in the treatment plan was initiated by Converse and Smith in 1963 [6]. They emphasized the importance of manipulating the segment with the MCL, forward positioning the fragment and trans nasal wiring over a perforated plate.

The case for open reduction and internal fixation (ORIF) was highlighted by Dingman and Natvig [13]. They reported superior results have been achieved in the more serious injuries (with minimum of effort and with the greatest degree of comfort to the patient) by open reduction with direct fixation. The need and feasibility of identifying MCL and anchoring it across to the other side was described by Mustarde in 1964 [14]. The need for primarily bone grafting when there is severe comminution of the nasal dorsum rendering primary reduction incomplete and also help achieve single-stage reconstruction was highlighted by Cruse [15] and Gruss [16].

Reduction of the nasal complex may be done with Walsham's forceps to realign the deviated/displaced complex. The collapsed complex may be out-fractured, and complex opened out may need to be in-fractured. The depressed complex may be elevated into position by the septal forceps (Ash's). However in displaced or comminuted scenarios, closed reduction isn't optimal. Hence trans nasal wiring may be needed to keep the splayed segments well reduced and minimize telecanthus. In the absence of gross comminution, closed reduction and trans nasal wiring has been proved quite useful and adequate to achieve optimal results as advocated by some authors especially in patients with associated maxillary fractures [17].

58.5.1 Surgical Access for NOE

1. Existing laceration (Fig. 58.7)
2. Glabella approach—a horizontal skin incision over the glabella region (Fig. 58.8)
3. Bicoronal approach (Fig. 58.9)
4. Butterfly incision (combination of Gullwing and open sky incision) (Fig. 58.10)
5. Vertical incision (Fig. 58.11)
6. H-shaped incision (Fig. 58.12)

Ed Ellis et al. [11] reported on having a sequential plan to proceed with the surgical sequence. They emphasized on adequate exposure for identification of the bone fragment with the MCL tendon, realigning the medial rim and canthopexy if required. The nasal dorsum reconstruction is planned at the end.

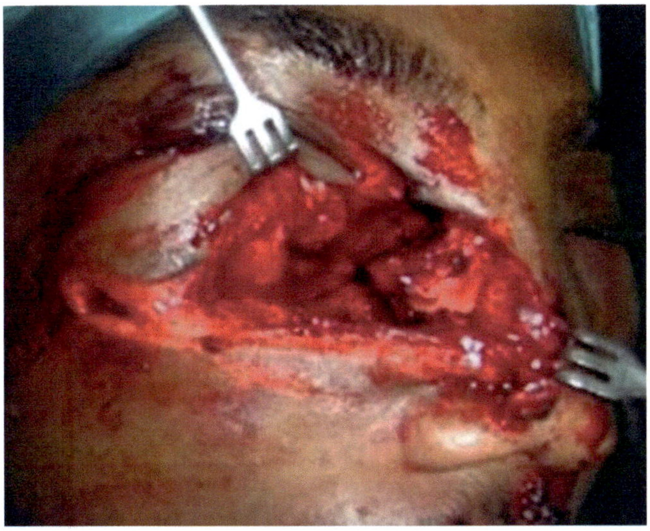

Fig. 58.7 Existing laceration used as an approach

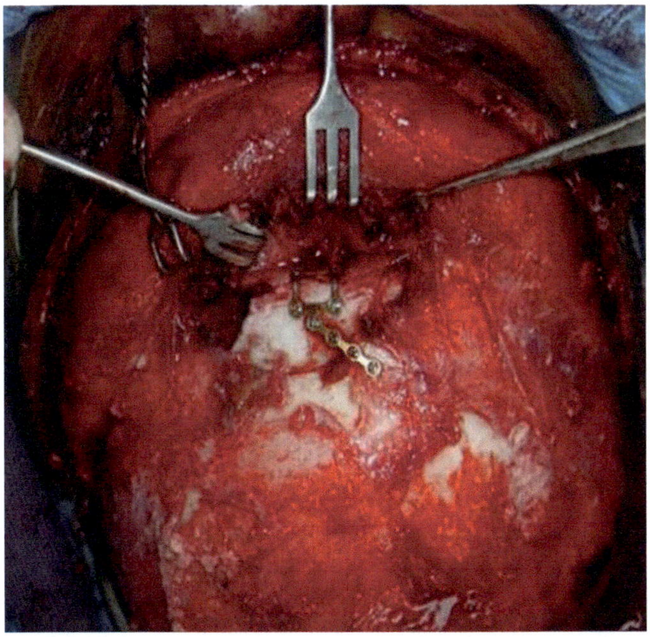

Fig. 58.9 Bicoronal approach

According to them pre-treatment photographs are very important in getting good results, and deformity should be overtreated than undertreated because secondary deformity which occurs is difficult to treat.

Trans nasal wiring:

Closed reduction in established fractures with telecanthus rarely helps achieve adequate reduction and MCL repositioning and hence may need trans nasal wiring as well to help with MCL positioning [6, 13]. Using a K wire driver or an awl will help pass a trans nasal wire across the nasal complex and help narrow the area by bringing the sides together. To help achieve adequate narrowing and restore

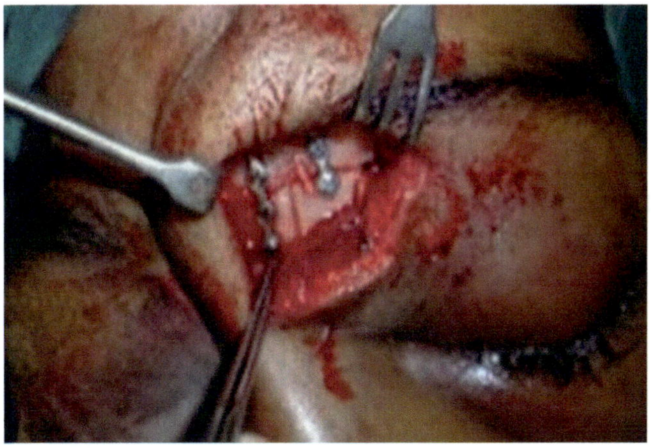

Fig. 58.8 Glabella approach

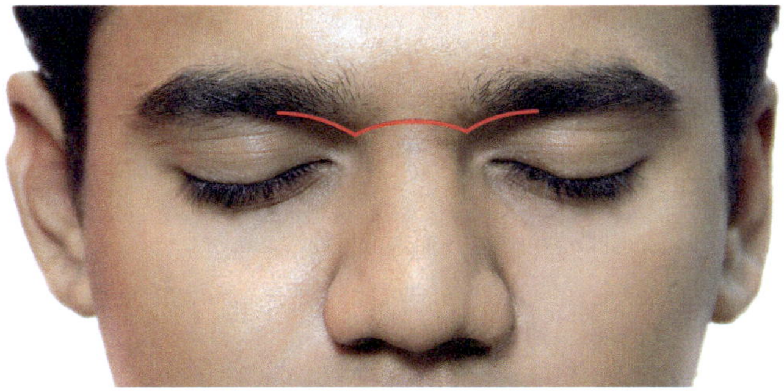

Fig. 58.10 Butterfly incision (combination of Gullwing and open sky incision)

Steps in Management

- Step1: Good exposure
- Step 2: Identify the medial canthal tendon/tendon-bearing bone
- Step 3: Reduce and reconstruct medial orbital rim
- Step 4: Reconstruction of medial orbital wall
- Step 5: Trans nasal canthopexy
- Step 6: Reduce septal fracture/displacement
- Step 7: Nasal dorsum reconstruction/augmentation with bone graft
- Step 8: Soft tissue readaptation (nasal splint, trans nasal bolsters, silicone sheeting)

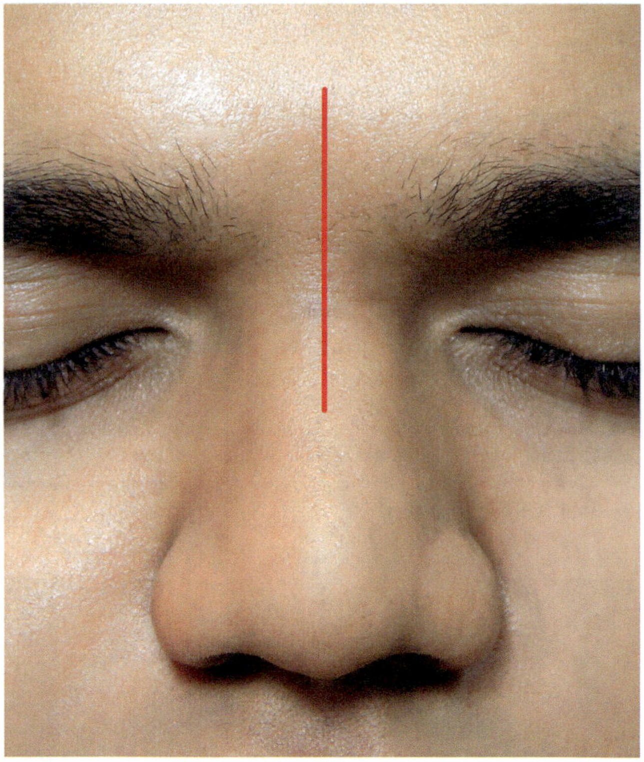

Fig 58.11 Vertical incision

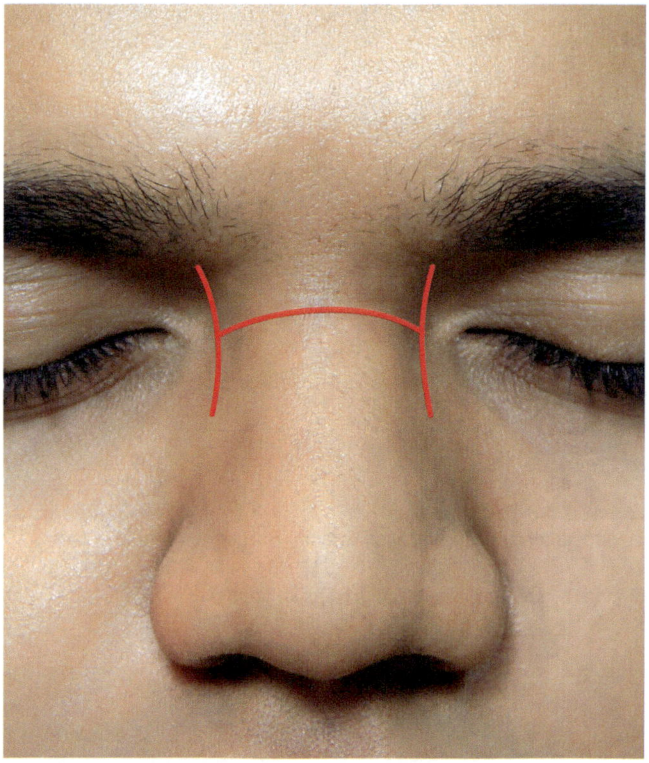

Fig. 58.12 H shaped incision

the canthal distance, the entry area on the affected site should be just superior and posterior to the posterior lacrimal crest to which the posterior limb of the ligament is attached. The wire entry point anterior to the area can result in widening of the telecanthus as the posterior aspect flares laterally.

As long as a large fragment with MCL attachment is identifiable, open reduction and fixation of the fragment can help in achieving our objectives. Using very low profile titanium plates (1.1–1.3 mm depending on the system used) helps achieve adequate fixation. Rigid fixation needs exposure of a stable area to help achieve the same and may necessitate exposing the glabella or frontal bone superior to it for adequate results. Realignment of the fragments and fixation will help in achieving better results in cases of fracture having multiple fragments and reconstruction with bone graft wherever required (Fig. 58.13 a, b).

MCL disruption or a tiny bony fragment with MCL might necessitate a canthopexy.

58.5.2 Trans Nasal Canthopexy

The objectives of trans nasal canthopexy are:

- To medialize the central fragment
- To position the tendon posterior and superior to posterior lacrimal crest that would give an ideal vector.

The commonly used methods are the trans nasal wiring (Fig. 58.14) or using a canthal barb. The identified ligament edges are either anchored with a suture (size 2–0 prolene) or a wire (26 gauge) and guided to the opposite side. The entry point is posterior and superior to lacrimal crest to ensure adequate positioning. One way to help achieve this is to adapt a plate in medial aspect extending from lateral nose onto the medial wall extending just beyond the lacrimal crest (Fig. 58.15).

The wire or suture anchoring the MCL is passed through a hole of the plate just beyond the lacrimal crest brought to

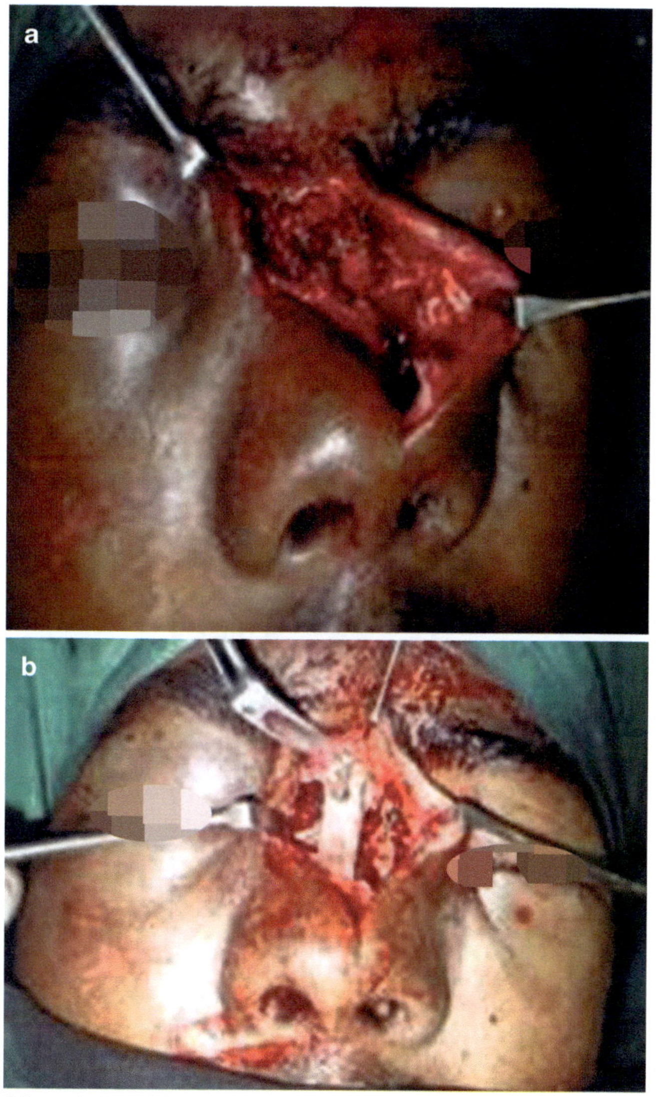

Fig. 58.13 (**a**) Alignment and fixation of stable fragments. (**b**) Bone grafting of the dorsum of nose

the opposite side and secured around a screw in the forehead adjacent to the midline or a plate to prevent the wire cutting through the bone. Special barbed wires have been advocated by certain authors to engage the MCL and anchor it to help with medial canthopexy with small incisions around the medial canthus. These help especially when there is medial canthal disruption without bony disruption [18, 19].

Figure 58.16 shows a clinical case where the MCL has be anchored to the holes of the plate on either sides (arrows) with SS wires.

Paediatric injuries of the naso-maxillary complex are generally under treated, but they need similar management protocols like that of an adult to achieve optimal results [20]. The use of resorbable implants will be of prudence in the paediatric patients [3].

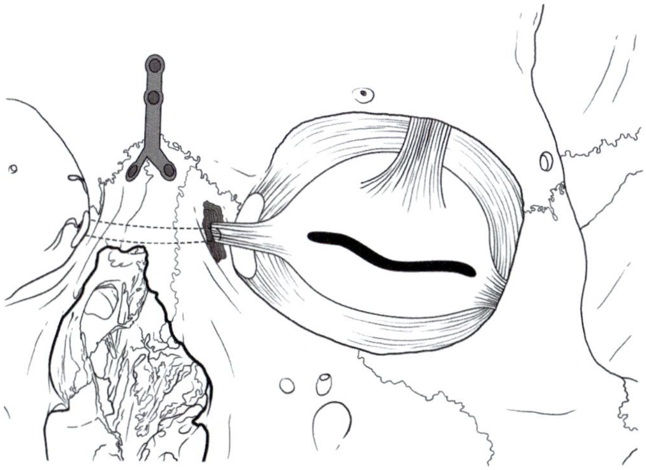

Fig. 58.14 Canthopexy with SS wire (note the wire shown as dotted lines)

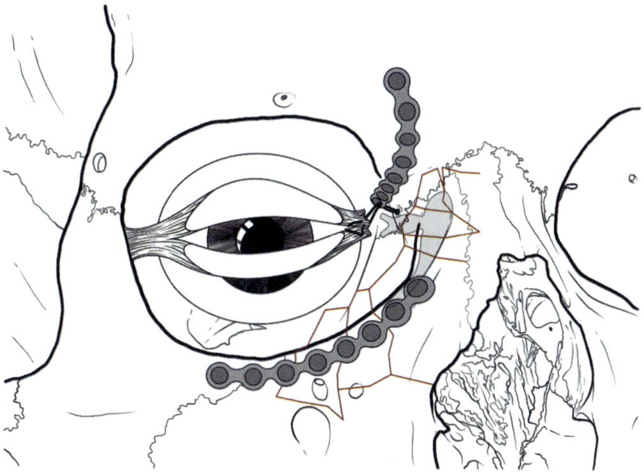

Fig. 58.15 Use of plate to guide MCL reattachment (note the MCL fixed to plate with a wire, the red lines denote the fractured bones)

Post-operative aesthetic assessments of outcomes done for the management options comparing the canthal position and nasofrontal angle measurements have indicated that bone grafting may result in obtunded nasofrontal angle as compared to ORIF. Closed reduction of the complex has resulted in under projection of the nasal bridge region [20].

58.5.3 Soft Tissue Readaptation

A post-operative nasal bolster splint is very important after ORIF or NOE fractures. It plays the following functions:

- It reduces post-operative swelling due to oedema and haematoma.

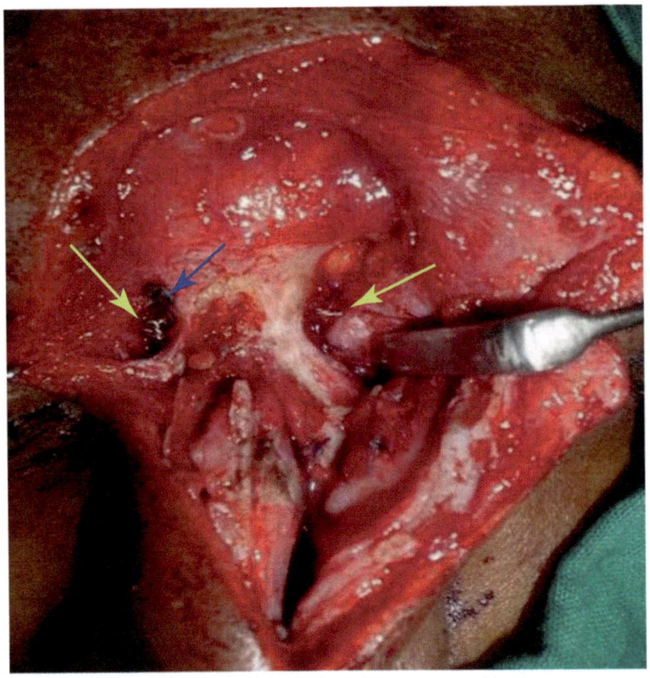

Fig. 58.16 shows a clinical case where the MCL has been anchored to the holes of the plate (blue arrow) on either sides with SS wires (yellow arrow)

Redrapes soft tissues to underlying skeletal framework and prevents *pseudo telecanthus* (increase in intercanthal distance, in spite of accurate reduction and fixation of facture fragments. This occurs due to non-adaptation of soft tissues to the underlying NOE complex, with resultant fibrosis of tissues). *Bolster splints may cause skin necrosis if used inappropriately*. After reduction and fixation of NOE, nasal packing has been done with ribbon gauge soaked in paraffin/flavine emulsion or bismuth iodoform paraffin paste (BIPP). Over packing should be avoided. Sometimes it obstructs the airway and a potential source of infection and required removal after 72 h postsurgery.

58.5.4 Post-operative Evaluation [20]

It includes evaluation of:

- Nasofrontal angle
- Nasal prominence and
- Intercanthal width

The average distance between the medial canthus should be approximately 1/3rd (33%) of the distance between lateral canthus. The distance from the lateral canthus of the eye to cornea and cornea to nasofrontal junction will be compared, and they should be in 1:1 relationship. The ideal naso-orbital angle is approximately 115–130°. All the three parameters should be checked post-operatively to assess the surgical results (Figs. 58.17, 58.18, and 58.19).

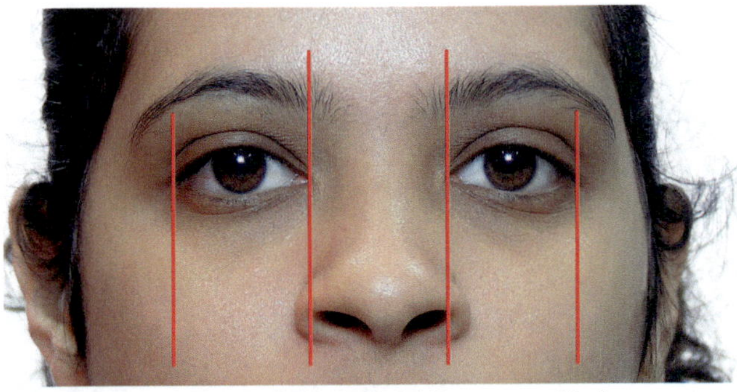

Fig. 58.17 Ideal intercanthal distance

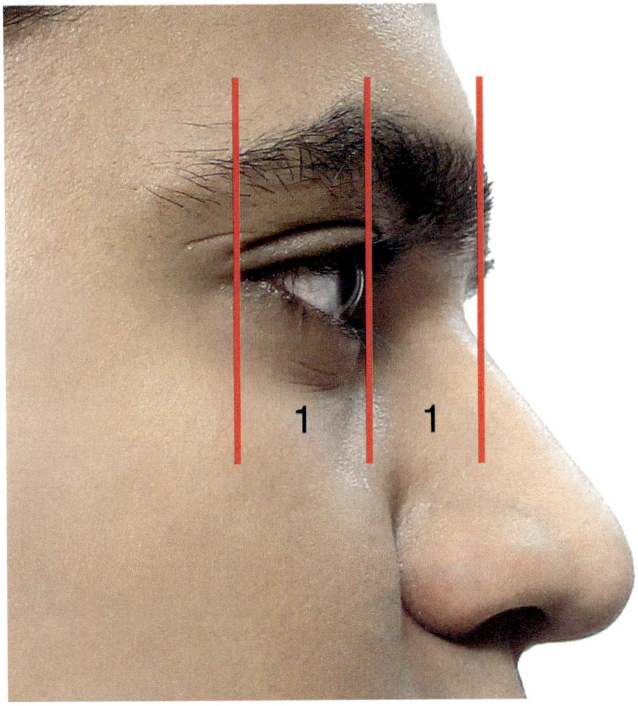

Fig. 58.18 Ideal nasal projection (1:1)

58.6 Complications

Inadequate assessment and treatment planning may result in incomplete management of the NOE complex resulting in secondary deformity which can aesthetically inadequate. Deformities of the NOE are quite easily noticeable compared to those in other regions, and hence appropriate management helps achieve good results. The aesthetic issues like persistent telecanthus or depressed nasal bridge are difficult to correct secondarily with suboptimal results. Hence the first time is the best time to address the central nasal component [21,

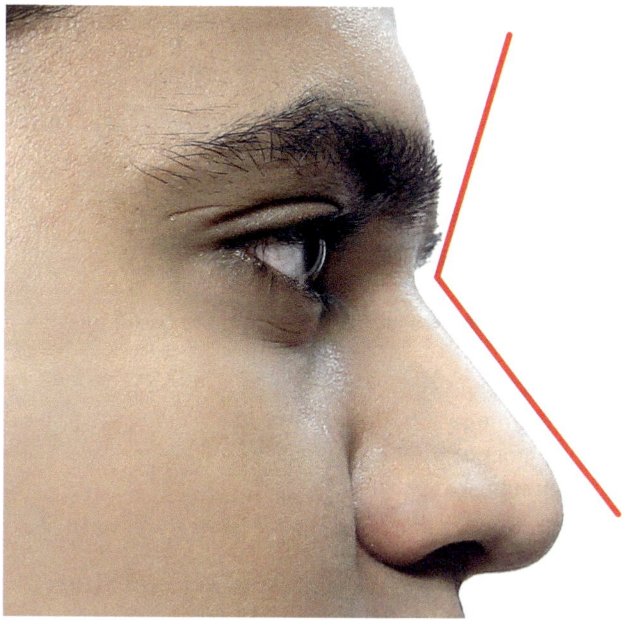

Fig. 58.19 Ideal frontonasal angle

22]. Apart from aesthetic complications, functional issues like epiphora due to nasolacrimal duct injury or obstruction may manifest which may need stenting [23] or dacryocystorhinostomy (creating a osteum in the lateral nasal wall adjacent to the lacrimal sac along with stenting) to establish patency. Involvement of the medial wall may result in diplopia [24] which if not addressed adequately may persist. Another important issue overlooked is anosmia, but if it should occur, recovery is unpredictable, and prior discussion with patients is better. In cases with concomitant brain injuries or CSF leak, risk of associated sequelae is present, and a multidisciplinary approach helps. Though improperly placed trans nasal wires may occlude/impede the lacrimal drainage apparatus, it remains a popular modality to help treat these fractures [25, 26].

58.7 Frontal Sinus Fracture

58.7.1 Introduction

Fractures of the frontal sinus are frequently associated with orbital, NOE, nasal and anterior cranial fossa injury. Frontal sinus is most frequently damaged as a result of high velocity motor vehicle accidents. 70% of frontal sinus fractures were due to automobile accidents and 20% due to assaults. Proximity of sinus to the brain makes untreated disease in this area potentially fatal. Inappropriate treatment of frontal sinus fracture can lead to mucocele formation, recurrent sinusitis, osteomyelitis of frontal bone, brain abscess or thrombosis of cavernous sinus, encephalitis, etc. [27].

58.7.2 Applied Anatomy of Frontal Sinus

Frontal sinuses are two asymmetric sinuses separated by a thin bony septal plate. The average dimensions of frontal sinus are as follows [28]:

- Height: 32 mm
- Width: 26 mm
- Depth: 17 mm
- Surface Area: 720 mm^2

The frontal sinus is an air-filled cavity lined by pseudostratified ciliated columnar epithelium encased in bone. It becomes visible radiographically at the age of 6 years. The posterior table is thinner than the anterior table. The posterior table separates the sinus from dura of frontal lobe. Anterior table is covered by a soft tissue layer of frontalis muscle, orbicularis oculi muscle, supraorbital and supratrochlear nerves, vessels and skin. Posteriorly, the floor of the frontal sinus consists of orbital plate of frontal bone. Anteriorly, the floor of the sinus overlies the anterior ethmoidal sinus and nasal cavity. The frontonasal drainage area of the sinus originates from the posteromedial part of sinus floor. The frontal sinus drains through the frontonasal ducts into the middle meatus of the nasal cavity or directly through the ostia into the nasal cavity.

58.7.3 Functions of Frontal Sinus

Following are the various functions of the frontal sinus:

1. Production and storage of mucus
2. Resonator for voice
3. Humidification and warming of inhaled air
4. Accessory area of olfaction
5. Conservation of heat from the nasal fossae
6. Definition of facial contours
7. "Surge Tank" to dampen the pressure differential that develops during inspiration

The diagnosis of the frontal sinus fracture based on the proper history and physical examination of the patient which includes inspection and palpation of the affected area.

The detailed history includes the following points:

1. Information about events
2. Visual difficulties
3. Numbness
4. Pain
5. Rhinorrhea
6. Sense of smell
7. Previous history of nasal or sinus disease surgery

58.7.4 Clinical Features [29]

1. Forehead laceration (58%)
2. Forehead pain (82%)
3. Swelling
4. Frontal bone depression (25%)
5. Periorbital ecchymosis
6. CSF rhinorrhea (1/3rd patients)

58.7.5 Radiographic Features

For an accurate diagnosis of frontal sinus fracture, a CT scan (Fig. 58.20a, b) in different views must be examined [30].

1. Axial view: It reveals location, severity and degree of comminution of anterior and posterior table fractures.

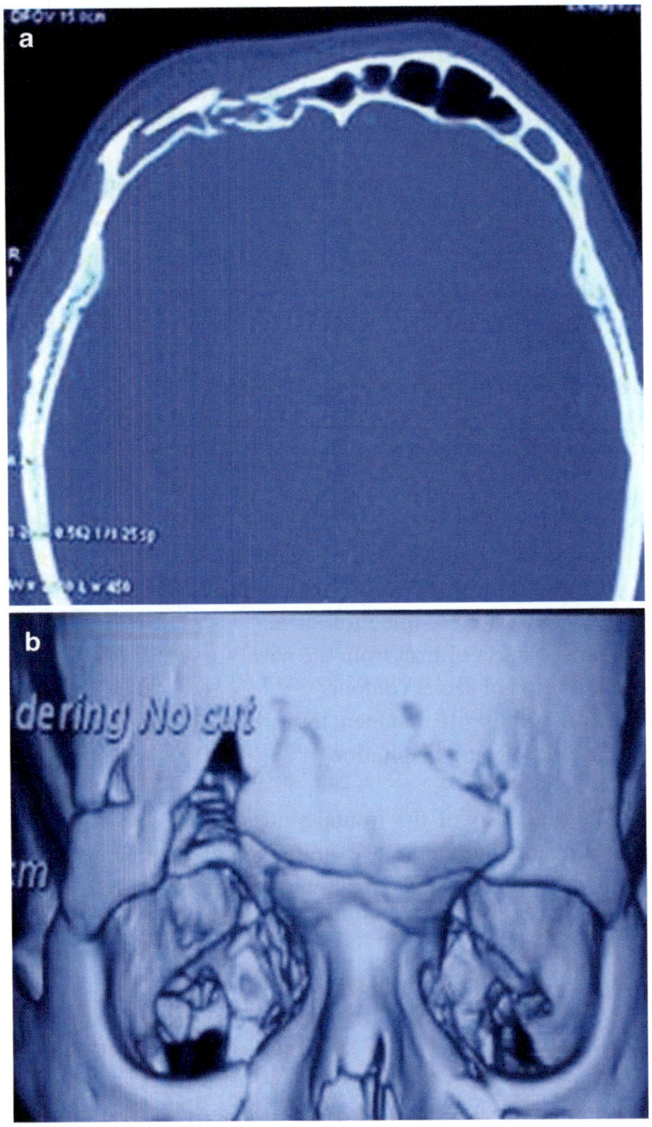

Fig. 58.20 (**a**, **b**) 3D CT and axial CT image with frontal sinus fracture

2. Coronal view: It reveals frontal sinus floor and orbital roof fractures.
3. Sagittal view: It assesses frontonasal duct.
4. Submentovertex view and lateral view: It visualizes anterior and posterior tables.

58.7.6 Classifications

Frontal sinus fractures are usually classified based on:

- Location
- Extent of injury
- Involvement of frontonasal duct
- Current injury to the dura

58.7.7 Stanley's Classification of Frontal Sinus Fracture [31]

- *Type I: Anterior Table Fracture*
  - Isolated to anterior table
  - Accompanied by supraorbital rim fracture
  - Accompanied by naso-ethmoid complex fracture
- *Type II: Anterior and Posterior Table Fractures*
  - It is a linear fracture either on transverse direction or in vertical direction
- *Type III: Comminuted Fractures*
  - Isolated to both tables
  - Accompanied by naso-ethmoid complex fracture

58.7.8 Gonty Et al. Classification of Frontal Sinus Fracture [32]

- *Type I: Anterior Table Fracture*
  - Isolated to anterior table
  - Accompanied by supraorbital rim fracture
  - Accompanied by naso-ethmoid complex fracture
- *Type II: Anterior and Posterior Table Fractures*
  - A linear fracture either on transverse direction or in vertical direction
  - Comminuted fracture either isolated to both tables or accompanied by naso-ethmoid complex fracture
- *Type III: Posterior Table Fracture*
- *Type IV: Through and Through Frontal Sinus Fracture*

58.7.9 Management (Box 58.6) [33]

Surgical Access:

1. Through existing laceration
2. Butterfly incision (Fig. 58.10)
3. Gullwing or eyeglass incision (Fig. 58.21)

Box 58.6 Guiding Principles for Frontal Sinus Management

- To separate nasal cavity from sinus
- To eliminate dead space
- To separate the frontonasal duct from frontal sinus by obstructing the duct
- To eliminate a functional sinus, sinus mucosa is removed, and sinus is obliterated

4. Bicoronal approach (Fig. 58.9): Khan et al. in 2018 [34] suggests sterile surgical glove tourniquet intraoperatively to get the haemorrhage control and blood less surgical field in elevation of bicoronal flap for the surgical management of frontal sinus fracture.

58.7.10 Indications of Surgery in Frontal Sinus Fractures [35]

1. To avoid immediate complications such as CSF leak, meningitis
2. To avoid long-term complications such as frontal sinusitis, meningitis and brain abscess formation
3. To provide aesthetic contour to the forehead
4. To provide exposure for anatomic reduction of NOE fractures

58.7.11 Management of Anterior Table Fracture [36–38]

Decision-Making:

- Simple greenstick or undisplaced fracture does not require surgical intervention.
- In depressed anterior wall fracture, frontal sinus explored, careful irrigation carried out, fragments reduced and stabilize by internal fixation. In posterior wall fracture without CSF leak or pneumoencephalus, reconstruction of only anterior wall is done.

Other than surgical intervention, antibiotics, sinus decongestants and analgesics are prescribed to keep the frontonasal duct patent and to prevent infection.

Rai et al. [39] suggested bone mapping/sketching in management of anterior table frontal sinus fracture with great success. To get good post-operative contour, each fracture fragment is to be placed at the original position after debridement of the sinus. For the same purpose, numbers have to be given to the fracture fragments on a plane paper (sterile glove covering paper) or green sheet (Fig. 58.22a–c).

Yoo MH et al. suggested endoscopic trans nasal reduction of anterior table fracture [40]. To support the reduced fragments, they advocated use of custom made latex glove balloon to be inserted into the frontal sinus then expanded and maintained for 3 weeks. It avoid use of coronal incision is the advantage of endoscopic reduction. It should be avoided in severe comminuted fractures, displaced posterior table fracture with evidence of dura tear, associated orbital roof blow in fracture and extensive skull bone fractures.

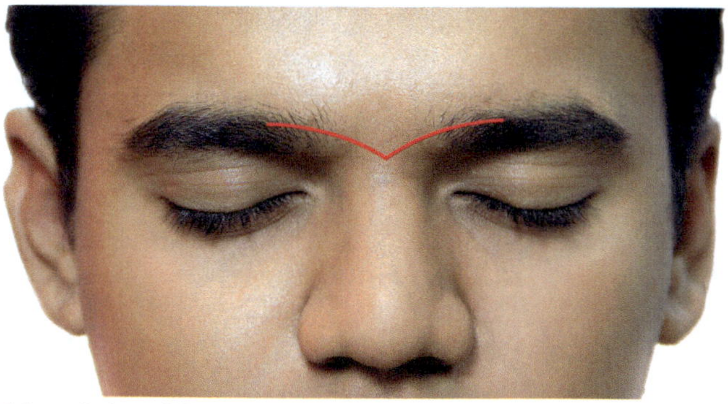

Fig. 58.21 Gullwing or eyeglass incision

58.7.12 Treatment of Posterior Table Fracture [41]

Patients with displaced and comminuted posterior wall combined with or without anterior wall require the support of a neurosurgeon because of dural and intracranial lesions. To get the good exposure, bifrontal craniotomy is indicated to eliminate the posterior wall.

To widen the neurosurgical access to the anterior floor of the cranium, the supraorbital bandeau will be temporarily removed. The sinus mucosa carefully removed with bur, and sinus is cranialized, and then repair of the dura will be carried out. Calvarial bone graft used to obliterate the nasofrontal duct and bone powder can be used to cover the remaining dead space. Anterior table can be stabilized with bone plates and screws. Bone defect will be treated with calvarial bone graft or titanium mesh. With patent duct and no concurrent dural tears or brain injury exist, any amount of posterior table displacement is inconsequential and managed by observation.

58.7.13 Methods of Treatment of Damaged Frontonasal Duct [42]

The damage to the nasofrontal duct and frontal sinus obstruction increases the risk of mucocele formation and inflammatory complications post-operatively. Obliteration of the duct is indicated in such situation. The muscle, temporalis fascia, bone chips, etc. are the materials used commonly to obstruct the duct.

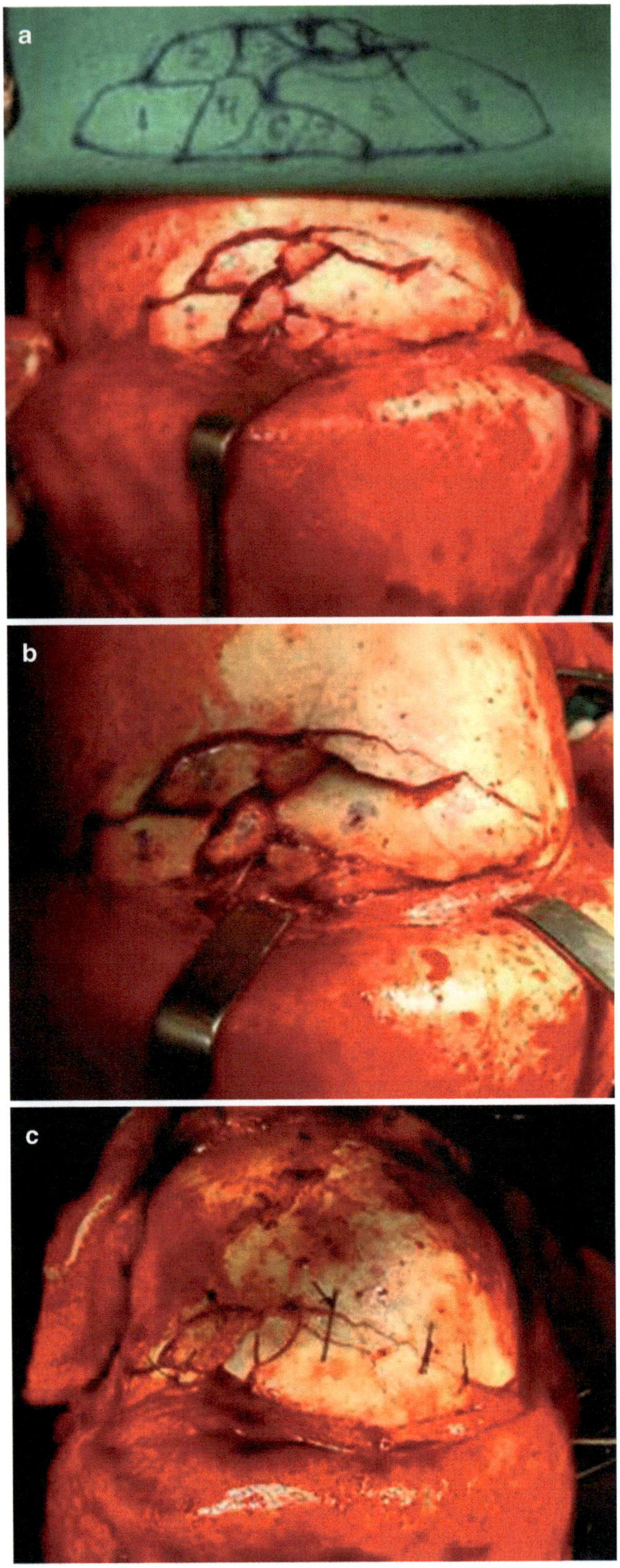

Fig. 58.22 (**a**–**c**) Bone mapping/sketching in management of anterior table frontal sinus fracture

Box 58.7 Complications of Frontal Sinus Fractures [46]

Immediate complications	Late complications
1. Wound infection	1. Mucocele
2. CSF leak	2. Mucopyocele
3. Paresthesia of supraorbital nerve	3. Late frontal sinusitis
4. Frontal sinusitis	4. Brain abscess
5. Meningitis	5. Osteomyelitis of frontal bone
6. Neurological injuries secondary to penetrating trauma or displacement of frontal bone into neurocranium	

58.7.13.1 Material Used for Sinus Obliteration [43]

1. Hydroxyapatite
2. Glass wool
3. Bone
4. Cartilage
5. Muscle
6. Absorbable gelatin sponge
7. Temporalis fascia
8. Oxidized segmented cellulose
9. Acrylic or methyl methacrylate
10. Fat (commonly used)

58.7.14 Cranialization [44, 45]

It is another technique to minimize the dead space in sinus. It involves removing posterior table thus permitting brain to expand into frontal sinus resulting in confluence between sinus cavity and anterior cranial fossa. It is done in cases with CSF leak and neurological injury due to displaced posterior table fracture. To isolate the splanchnocranium from the frontal sinus, a pericranial flap is used.

58.7.15 Key Points

- Actual or suspected fractures involving the frontonasal duct are an indication to remove the outer table, so the duct can be inspected.
- If outer table is comminuted and a bony segment over 1.5 cm in missing, a bone graft should be harvested to restore the outer table contour.
- The most common treatment for outer table fracture with injury to duct without inner table fracture is obliteration of frontal sinus to seal the frontonasal duct to prevent nasal infection.
- Adipose tissue from abdomen is used to fill the dead space of frontal sinus because of its resistance to infec-

tion, slow resorption rate, and it is gradually replaced by the fibrous tissue.

Complications of frontal sinus fractures is given in Box 58.7.

58.8 Conclusion

The management of NOE and frontal sinus fracture is always a challenging task .The proper handling of MCL and naso-frontal duct is mandatory to get good post-operative results. Proper treatment planning in the form of incision selection, method of fixation and use of bone graft should be done to avoid unaesthetic results.

References

1. Milad Etemadi SH, Shahnaseri S, Soltani P, Motamedi MRK. Management of naso-orbito-ethmoid fractures: a 10-year review. Trauma Mon. 2017;22:292–30.
2. Brasileiro BF, Passeri LA. Epidemiological analysis of maxillofacial fractures in Brazil: a 5-year prospective study. Oral Surg Oral Med Oral Pathol Oral Radiol Endod. 2006;102(1):28–34.
3. Rosenberger E, Kriet JD, Humphrey C. Management of naso-ethmoid fractures. Curr Opin Otolaryngol Head Neck Surg. 2013;21:410–6. (Anatomy of MCL, physical examination of the complex and displacement)
4. Poh E, Kakizaki H, Selva D, Leibovitch I. Anatomy of medial canthal tendon in Caucasians. Clin Exp Ophthalmol. 2012;40:170–3.
5. Merkx MA, Freihofer HP, Borstlap WA, van't Hoff MA. Effectiveness of primary correction of traumatic telecanthus. Int J Oral Maxillofac Surg. 1995;24:344–7.
6. Heine D, Catone GA, Bavitz B, Grenadier MR. Naso-orbital-ethmoid injury: report of a case and review of the literature. Oral Surg Oral Med Oral Path. 2005;69(5):542–9.
7. Rowe NL. Rowe and Williams' maxillofacial injuries, vol. 2. 2nd ed. Edinburgh: Churchill Livinstone; 1994.
8. Markowitz BL, Manson PN, Sargent L, et al. Management of the medial canthal tendon in nasoethmoid orbital fractures: the importance of the central fragment in classification and treatment. Plast Reconstr Surg. 1991;87:843–853.
9. Burstein F, Cohen S, Hudgins R, Boydston W. Frontal basilar trauma: classification and treatment. Plast Reconstr Surg. 1997;99(5):1314–21.
10. Balaraman K, Ramani V, Bharathi R, Venkataramani H, Sabapathy SR. Outcome assessment of Nasoethmoid fractures. Int J Oral Maxillofac Surg. 2013;42(10):1220.
11. Ellis E III. Sequencing treatment for naso-orbito-ethmoid fractures. J Oral Maxillofac Surg. 1993;51:543–558.
12. Nguyen M, Koshy JC, Hollier LH Jr. Pearls of nasoorbitoethmoid trauma management. Semin Plast Surg. 2010;24:383–8.
13. Dingman RO, Grabb WC, Oneal RM. Management of injuries of the naso-orbital complex. Arch Surg. 1969;98:566–71.
14. Mustarde JC. Epicanthus and telecanthus. Int Opthalmol Clin. 1964;4:359.
15. Cruse C, Blevins PK, Luce EA. Naso-ethmoid-orbital fractures. J Trauma. 1980;20:551.
16. Gruss JS. Naso-ethmoid-orbital fractures: classification and role of primary bone grafting. Plast Reconstr Surg. 1985;75:303.
17. Baliga S, Urolagin SB. Transnasal fixation of NOE fracture: minimally invasive approach. J Maxillofac Oral Surg. 2012;11(1):34–7.
18. Timoney PJ, Sokol JA, Hauck MJ, Lee HB, Nunery WR. Transcutaneous medial canthal tendon incision to the medial orbit. Ophthal Plast Reconstr Surg. 2012;28:140–4.
19. Goldenberg DC, Bastos EO, Alonso N, Friedhofer H, Ferreira MC. The role of micro-anchor devices in medial canthopexy. Ann Plast Surg. 2008;61:47–51.
20. Pawar SS, Rhee JS. Frontal sinus and naso-orbital-ethmoid fractures. JAMA Facial Plast Surg. 2014;16:284–9.
21. Herford AS, Ying T, Brown B. Outcomes of severely comminuted (type III) nasoorbitoethmoid fractures. J Oral Maxillofac Surg. 2005;63:1266–77.
22. Potter JK, Muzaffar AR, Ellis E, Rohrich RJ, Hackney FL. Aesthetic management of the nasal component of naso-orbital ethmoid fractures. Plast Reconstr Surg. 2006;117(1):10e–8e.
23. Vora NM, Fedok FG. Management of the central nasal support complex in naso-orbital ethmoid fractures. Facial Plast Surg. 2000;16(2):181–91.
24. Becelli R, Renzi G, Mannino G, Cerulli G, Iannetti G. Posttraumatic obstruction of lacrimal pathways: a retrospective analysis of 58 consecutive naso-orbitoethmoid fractures. J Craniofac Surg. 2004;15:29–33.
25. Wei J-J, Tang Z-L, Liu L, Liao X-J, Yu Y-B, Jing W. The management of naso-orbital-ethmoid (NOE) fractures. Chinese J Traumatol. 2015;18:296–301.
26. Bell RB, Dierks EJ, Homer L, Potter BE. Management of cerebrospinal fluid leak associated with craniomaxillofacial trauma. J Oral Maxillofac Surg. 2004;62:676–84.
27. Gerbino G, Roccia F, Benech A, Caldarelli C. Analysis of 158 frontal sinus fractures: current surgical management and complications. J Craniomaxillofac Surg. 2000;28:133–139.
28. Haug RH, Cunningham LL. Management of fractures of the frontal bone and frontal sinus, selected Readings. Oral and Maxillofacial Surgery. 2002;10(6):1–32.
29. Wallis A, Donald PJ. Frontal sinus fractures: a review of 72 cases. Laryngoscope. 1988;98:593.
30. Finkle DR, Ringler SL, Luttenton CR, Beernink JH, Peterson NT, Dean RE. Comparison of the diagnostic methods used in maxillofacial trauma. Plast Reconstr Surg. 1985;75(1):32–41.
31. Stanley RB Jr. Fractures of the frontal sinus. Clin Plast Surg. 1989;16(1):115–23.
32. Gonty AA, Marciani RD, Adornato DC. Management of frontal sinus fractures: a review of 33 cases. J Oral Maxillofac Surg. 1999;57:372–9.
33. Rohrich RJ, Hollier LH. Management of frontal sinus fractures. Changing concepts. Clin Plast Surg. 1992;19:219–32.
34. Khan M, Rai A, Jain A. A simple and effective scalp tourniquet for controlling scalp hemorrhage. J Maxillofac Oral Surg. 2018;17(2):264–5.
35. Manolidis S. Frontal sinus injuries: associated injuries and surgical management of 93 patients. J Oral Maxillofac Surg. 2004;62:882–91.
36. Fattahi T, Salman S. An aesthetic approach in the repair of anterior frontal sinus fractures. Int J Oral Maxillofac Surg. 2016;45(9):1104–7.
37. Cole P, Kaufman Y, Momoh A, et al. Techniques in frontal sinus fracture repair. Plast Reconstr Surg. 2009;123(5):1578–9.
38. Weathers WM, Wolfswinkel EM, Hatef DA, Lee EI, Brown RH, Hollier LH Jr. Frontal sinus fractures: a conservative shift. Craniomaxillofac Trauma Reconstr. 2013;6(3):155–60.

39. Rai A, et al. “Bone mapping/sketching” in management of anterior table frontal sinus fracture. J Maxillofac Oral Surg. 2017;16(1):127–30.
40. Yoo MH, et al. Endoscopic transnasal reduction of an anterior table frontal sinus fracture: technical note. Int Journal Oral Maxfac Surg. 2008;37:573–5.
41. Freeman JL, Winston KR. Breach of posterior wall of frontal sinus: management with preservation of the sinus. World Neurosurg. 2015;83(6):1080–9.
42. Rohrich RJ, Hollier L. The role of the nasofrontal duct in frontal sinus fracture management. J Craniomaxillofac Trauma. 1996;2:31–40.
43. Mickel TJ, Rohrich RJ, Robinson JB Jr. Frontal sinus obliteration: a comparison of fat, muscle, bone, and spontaneous osteoneogenesis in the cat model. Plast Reconstr Surg. 1995;95(3): 586–92.
44. Scholsem M, Scholtes F, Collignon F, et al. Surgical management of anterior cranial base fractures with cerebrospinal fluid fistulae: a single institution experience. Neurosurgery. 2008;62: 463–71.
45. Pollock R, Hill J, Davenport D, et al. Cranialization in a cohort of 154 consecutive patients with frontal sinus fractures (1987–2007): review and update of a compel- ling procedure in the selected patient. Ann Plast Surg. 2013;71(1):54–9.
46. Guy WM, Brissett AE. Contemporary management of traumatic fractures of the frontal sinus. Otolaryngol Clin North Am. 2013;46(5):733–48.

Gunshot Injuries of the Maxillofacial Region

59

Lt Col Rohit Sharma and Maj Anson Jose

59.1 Introduction

Gunshot injuries to the maxillofacial region in particular present a challenging situation for the facial reconstructive surgeon. These injuries are relatively rare and hence the true incidence is unknown [1]. Feature common to most maxillofacial gunshot injuries is extensive tissue destruction. The degree of tissue loss, depth of the injury, associated necrosis, and concomitant central nervous system (CNS) injuries may not be apparent at initial presentation [2]. Comprehensive management of such wounds is often challenging because of its heterogeneous nature, composite 3D tissue destruction, and complex structural and functional anatomy of the face.

In contrast to blunt facial trauma, the literature on the management of ballistic facial injury is relatively scarce [1]. The management strategies for patients with facial gunshot wounds are almost as diverse as the case presentation itself. While there has been a gradual shift from conservative delayed operative repair to an early aggressive one-stage management approach, the controversies surrounding the timing and extent of intervention have not yet ceased to exist. Such an ongoing debate is largely due to the fact that the majority of treatment outcomes of gunshot facial injuries continue to be unsatisfactory regardless of treatment methodology adopted. On the other hand, new principles have evolved including the early definitive repair of hard tissues with precise anatomic rigid fixation using bone grafts and definitive soft tissue management with local or vascular flaps allowing for early rehabilitation of patients to their pretraumatic appearance. This paradigm shift away from delayed to a more immediate definitive reconstruction has been predominantly due to the widespread use of free tissue transfer, diagnostic computed tomography (CT) scan, and deeper understanding about zone of injury in such cases [3].

Presently the management of gunshot injuries comprises the following steps:

1. Conservative debridement followed by fracture stabilization and primary closure
2. Early reconstruction of missing hard and soft tissues
3. Antibiotics and prevention of infection
4. Postoperative physiotherapy and psychiatric assistance
5. Residual deformity correction and oral rehabilitation [3–6]

This review describes the current management strategies, damage control surgery, and basic protocols employed in the management of high-velocity ballistic injuries to the face.

59.2 Pathologic Anatomy and Classification

Traditionally gunshot injuries have been classified as penetrating, perforated, or avulsive [7]. As the gamut of injuries continues to evolve, the severity and magnitude of facial ballistic wounds demand an expanded classification and can be appropriately classified based on the wounding effects and terminal location of projectile as:

- Penetrating
- Perforating
- Avulsive
- Blast
- "Chop off" injuries

Lt Col R. Sharma (✉)
Department of Oral and Maxillofacial Surgery, 11 Corps Dental Unit, Jalandhar Cantt, India

Maj A. Jose
Department of Oral and Maxillofacial Surgery, ADC R&R, New Delhi, India

K. Bonanthaya et al. (eds.), *Oral and Maxillofacial Surgery for the Clinician*, https://doi.org/10.1007/978-981-15-1346-6_59

Penetrating injuries are caused when a low-velocity projectile pierces the tissues without making an exit wound (Fig. 59.1).

On the other hand, perforating injuries are distinguished by the presence of a definite exit wound in addition to the entry wound (Figs. 59.2 and 59.3). The exit wounds are often larger with ragged or stellate margins. Avulsive injuries are basically penetrating injuries, characterized by an acute loss and destruction of tissue as a consequence of the passage of the projectile within and out of the body (Fig. 59.4). Blast

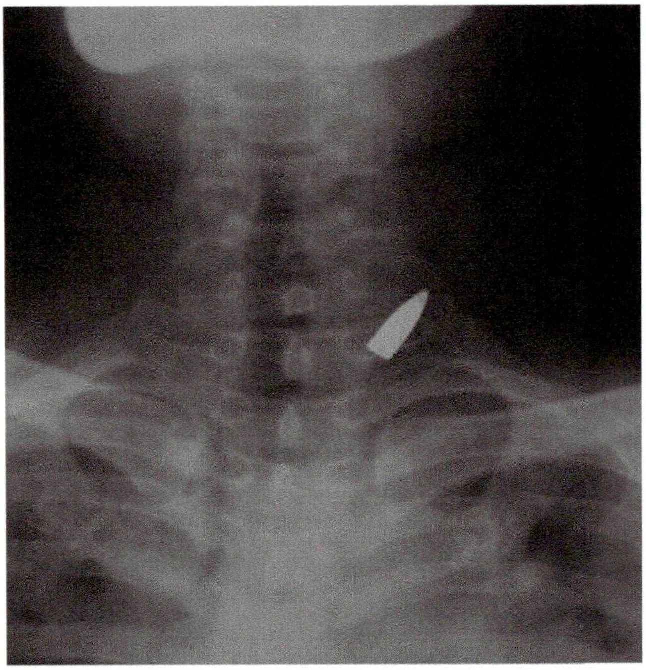

©Association of Oral and Maxillofacial Surgeons of India

Fig. 59.1 Penetrating injury with bullet lodged inside the neck

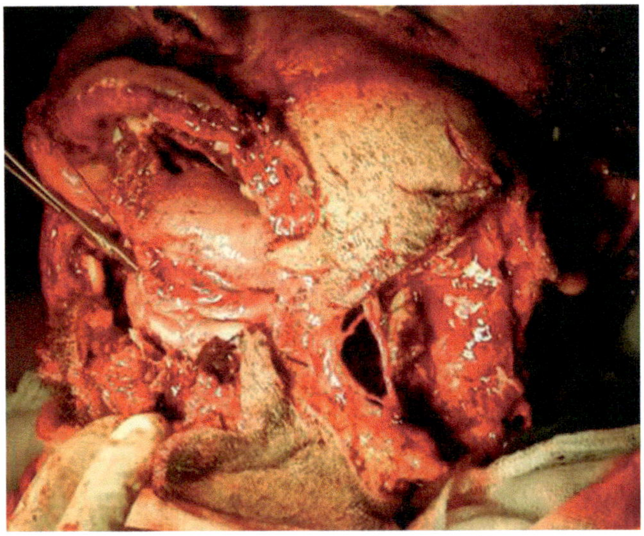

©Association of Oral and Maxillofacial Surgeons of India

Fig. 59.2 Perforating injury caused by 7.62 × 39 mm AK-47 rifle. Note the effects of high-energy bullet impact and explosive effects of cavitation on soft tissues resulting in stellate wound margins at the exit

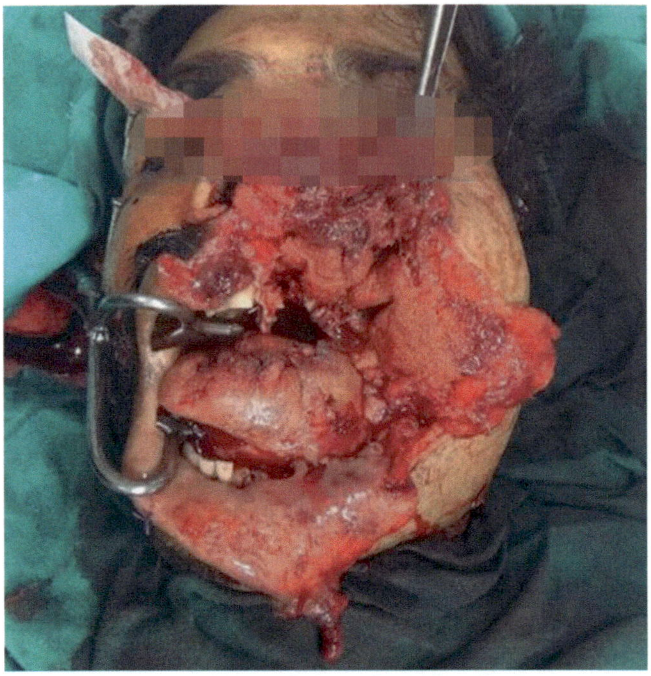

©Association of Oral and Maxillofacial Surgeons of India

Fig. 59.3 Avulsive injury of midface caused by a short-range high-velocity impact. The hallmark of high-velocity injuries are comminuted fractures of the facial skeleton with avulsion of soft tissues

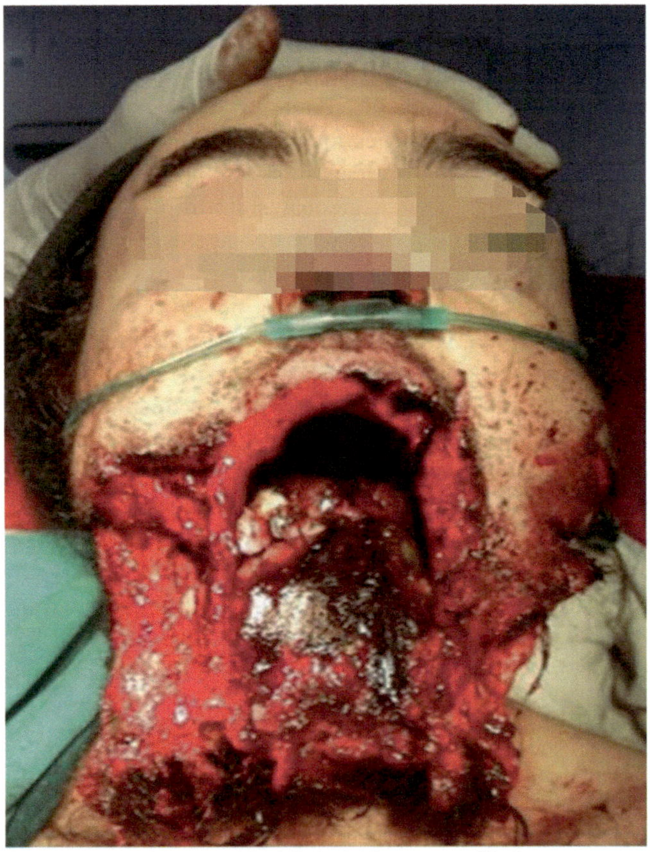

©Association of Oral and Maxillofacial Surgeons of India

Fig. 59.4 “Chop off” injury with complete avulsion of the mandible and associated soft tissue caused by velocity projectile from a military assault rifle injuries are the result of direct or indirect exposure to an explosion caused by military weapons or explosive devises (Fig. 59.5). "Chop off" injuries represent wounds with extensive hard and soft tissue loss as a consequence of high-velocity close-range gunshots [8]. In all these varieties of injuries, the tissue damage is directly proportional to the kinetic energy transferred by the bullet, time taken for the energy transfer, and area over which the energy is transferred. Hence, the type and variant of injury have significant implications in management.

Apart from this conventional nomenclature, various other classifications have been used for categorizing penetrating

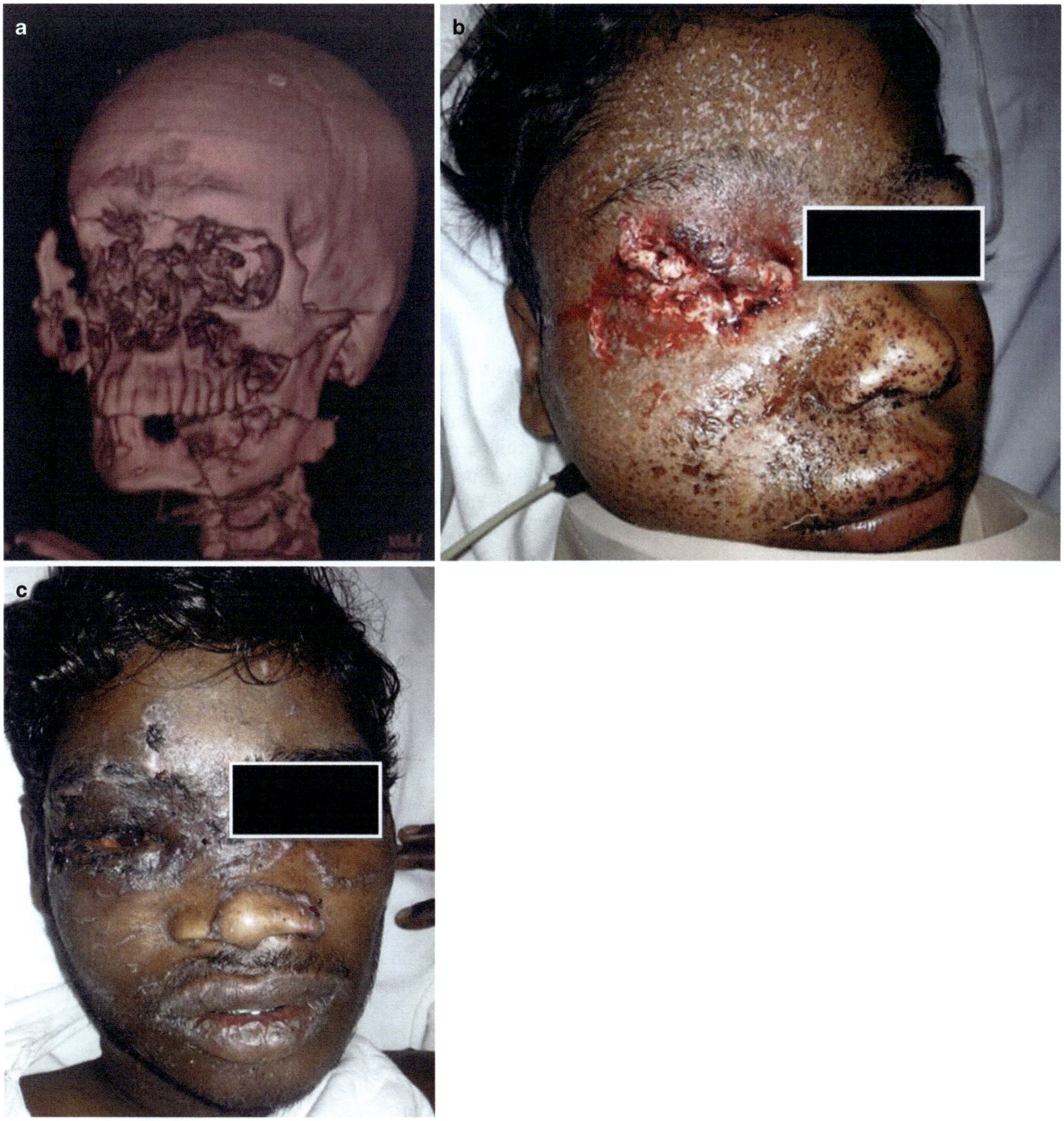

Fig. 59.5 (**a**, **b**, **c**) Blast injury caused by propagation of shock waves from the projectile. Soft tissue injury is minimal in such cases with severe comminution of the underlying skeleton

facial injuries; however, its application in clinical scenario is debatable. Similarly, many authors have developed an algorithm for the workup of ballistic wound based on the location of entry wound. Despite having limited application, no significant correlation has been found between site of entrance wound and therapeutic outcome of gunshot wounds [9].

A pragmatic approach to the management of such injuries involves:

1. Establishing an airway
2. Control of hemorrhage
3. Damage control surgery and identifying concomitant injuries
4. Early definitive repair of hard and soft tissues
5. Aesthetic refinements and rehabilitation

59.3 Initial Evaluation, Triage, and Damage Control Surgery

Initial management of gunshot wounds is based on the advanced trauma and life support protocols (also refer Chap. 48 of this book). Gibbons and Breeze [10] have elaborated the modified military protocols pertaining specifically to combat-related ballistic facial injuries. These include emergency management procedures that followed the CABC (catastrophic hemorrhage, airway, breathing, circulation) protocol proposed by Hodgetts et al. [11] which focused the need to control catastrophic bleeding as a priority over airway complications in a polytrauma patient. In a parallel manner, initial evaluation and damage control maxillofacial surgery should commence within the golden hour for effective patient management. Damage control surgery may be perceived as an immediate assessment of life-threatening injuries and addressing them promptly by means of early life-saving resuscitation and surgeries [12]. It is not regarded as a separate entity; it is seen as an essential, initial component in the management of any severely injured patient. In order to clear confusion clouding this highly debated area, a proposed set of damage control procedures that can be applied to ballistic maxillofacial injuries involving the maxillofacial region is given (Table 59.1).

Fortunately, the mortality rate directly attributable to maxillofacial firearms injuries is as low as 2–3% and predominantly due to a compromised airway [10]. Airway compromise is a serious consequence of all gunshot injuries to the face, and it can be due to a direct or an indirect injury to the airway. Injury to tissues and resultant edema in the vicinity of the air passages invariably handicaps the airway indirectly. Additionally, loss of muscle attachments and fractures of the anterior mandible significantly debilitates the airways. Manual repositioning of the fractured segments of mandible and base of tongue are the fundamental measures to be executed to prevent posterior airway collapse. While nasopharyngeal and oropharyngeal airways afford interim relief, endotracheal intubation is the established approach in emergency condition. This however presents a challenge on account of the edema, bleeding, and avulsed soft tissues that may possibly block the airway [13].

In the author's experience, a vast majority of maxillofacial gunshot wounds require surgical tracheostomy. The probability of concomitant intracranial injuries with low Glasgow Coma Scale (GCS) is also high in such patients [14]. Since most patients in this category require prolonged intubation and most gunshot wounds to the face require multi-phased surgical approach, the authors view surgical tracheostomy as having distinct advantage over other methods. Management of hemorrhage and its allied complications are well known in maxillofacial injuries as emphasized by previous writers on war surgery, yet it needs a descriptive analysis owing to the fatality it can cause. Hemorrhage is an inevitable consequence of all gunshot injuries to the face. Management of bleeding is an important aspect of damage control surgery, and adequate hemodynamic resuscitation is essential for the early physiological recovery of the victim [15].

Bleeding from high-energy ballistic injuries is practically impossible to control by external pressure tamponade due to the presence of bony structures and the inherently vulnerable condition of fragile anatomic structures like the eyes, brain, and airway seen in such injuries. In open injury scenario, hemorrhage can be easily managed by meticulous examination to recognize all the bleeding vessels followed by their ligation. Closed injuries necessitate balloon tamponade with Foley catheter (Fig. 59.5) to control bleeding. If bleeding is not controlled by the usual techniques, external carotid ligation or selective embolization method is used, which is by far the most predictable method to control bleeding from external carotid artery and its tributaries [13, 16].

Table 59.1 Algorithm in the treatment of Gun Shot Wounds (GSW)

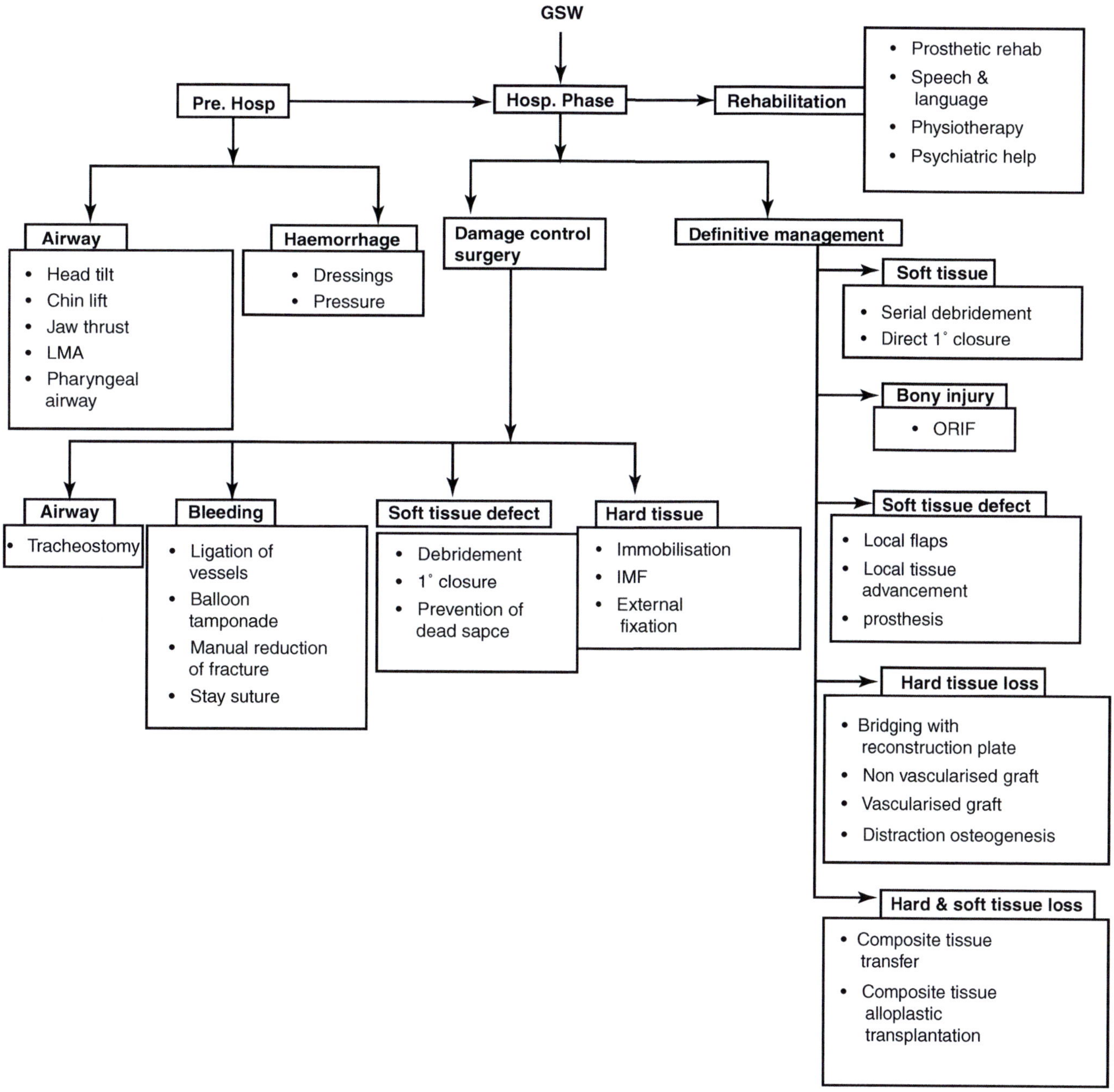

59.4 Diagnostic Imaging

Once airway is secured and bleeding is controlled, attention should be directed toward radiological assessment of the injury. Depending on the severity of injury a plain X-ray, CT scan and CT angiography can be requested [15]. The extent of injury, degree of hard tissue fragmentation, location of metallic splinters, damage to C-spine, and any occult brain injuries can be easily delineated with the help of a CT scan. Similarly, involvement of great vessels, any concealed bleeding, and flow dynamics of vessels suitable for microvascular reconstruction can be studied using CT angiogram. Apart from the damage characteristics of the wound, another crucial factor which needs to be assessed during radiological examination is the status of C-spine.

Any injury of such magnitude enough to fracture the facial skeleton can invariably cause an occult C-spine injury. The incidence of C-spine injuries varies from 8 to 11% in all maxillofacial traumas [17]. Hence, potential cervical spine injury should be always considered unless proven otherwise clinically or radiologically. It is pertinent to immobilize the cervical spine to prevent further damage especially in unconscious patient (Fig. 59.6). However, substantial evidence is still lacking about the safety and efficacy of cervical collars

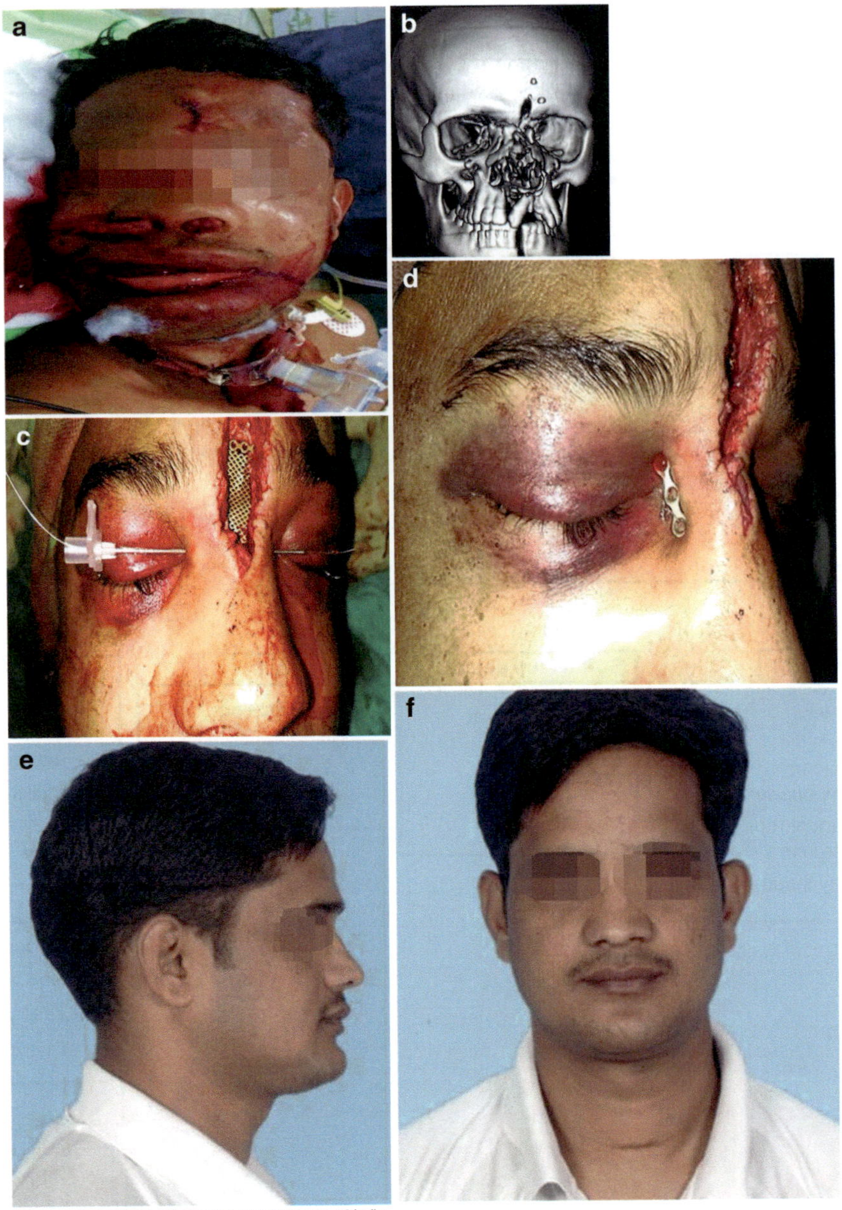

Fig. 59.6 (**a**–**e**) Low-velocity close-range handgun injury—3D CT showing comminution of maxilla and NOE complex. The case was treated by ORIF mandible, maxilla, frontal bone, and cathopexy using iv cannula and wire. Three years post-surgery—adequate restoration of width and projection of midface

used in such injuries. Moreover, placement of rigid collars interferes during airway management, central line placement, and definitive repair of facial injuries [13].

59.5 Definitive Management of Facial Gunshot Wounds

The prime goal in the management of facial gunshot wounds is to rehabilitate the patient to pre-injury function and aesthetics. However, it is not always easy to get a flawless postoperative outcome with one particular treatment modality or a particular surgical technique. Hence, the treatment should be timed and tailored depending upon the type and severity of the injury, amount of tissue loss, general health status of the patient, surgeon's expertise, and availability of resources. Before initiating any treatment procedures, a thorough assessment of the wound by a multidisciplinary team is imperative as gunshot injury cases are seldom comparable. A comprehensive evaluation and discussion by a diverse panel gives the surgeon valuable perspectives which in turn has a positive impact on the final outcome.

59.6 Debridement

Modern high-velocity firearms transfer heavy cavitation energy inside tissues causing physiological and morphological alterations resulting in hemorrhage, thrombosis, and necrosis [18]. The tissue response toward the high-velocity projectile varies with the type of tissues and elastic deformation it can sustain. The dermis is viscoelastic, and injuries will result in abrasion, traumatic tattooing, and contusion particularly in close-range shots. Muscle tissues can withstand elastic deformation up to four times the size of the projectile, but at a cellular level, it may undergo significant necrosis, devitalization, and denaturation rendering the microenvironment favorable for bacterial multiplication [19]. The injuries to neurovascular bundles behave similar to muscles, thereby causing tearing, shearing, and rupture of blood vessels. At microscopic level, all the three layers of blood vessels get affected resulting in the formation of thrombus, inflammation, and persistent spasm [20]. Cortical bone on the other hand is crystalline in consistency; therefore, penetrating injury causes fragmentation of bone with formation of multiple secondary projectiles. Conventional management of firearm injuries involves initial wound debridement, wound toilet, adequate soft tissue closure, and administration of antibiotics followed by delayed repair of deformities [4]. However, with the advent of vascular flaps and new reconstruction methods, there has been a colossal shift in the management of such injuries to a more definitive early single-stage repair [21].

The management commences with meticulous debridement of wounds to the point of active surgical bleeding. This strategy is particularly important in case of crushed and contaminated wounds wherein the active surgical bleeding encourages the formation of a healthy granulation tissue [18]. Furthermore, it also improves adequate microcirculation at wound margins, thereby promoting rapid healing and tissue resistance to infection. A serial debridement with judicious excision of the necrotic and non-contractile muscle tissues is done to achieve a wound with non-contaminated healthy margins [22].

After generous tissue excision, debridement should be assisted with soft scrubbing brushes and copious irrigation. Removal of deeply embedded splinters or metallic foreign bodies is controversial regarding any particular clinical benefits it offers [10]. The wound debridement should be prompt, and any delay (6–12 h) further complicates the wound management by progressive tissue necrosis. The development of progressive necrosis is a salient feature of gunshot wounds, and contrary to the popular belief, the tissue necrosis is not directly related to energy transfer but rather to the depth of tissues destroyed by the movement of the projectile. Animal studies have shown that beyond that critical time period, identification of necrotic margins will be difficult and hence it complicates the debridement and surgical control of the wound [23].

There are two main areas of conflicts pertaining to debridement in gunshot wounds. Many authors recommend immediate careful conservative soft tissue excision followed by secondary debridement of all tissues with questionable viability at a later stage [24, 25]. These researchers are of the view that it is practically impossible to distinguish between vital and non-vital tissues at initial intervention. On the contrary, a few other professionals believe in single-stage radical debridement on initial intervention [26].

Experimental evidences have shown that the extent of tissue necrosis after gunshot injury is 2 mm and 8 mm from the wound margins in skin and muscle tissues, respectively. In bony skeleton, it may extend up to 5 mm from the fracture line [27]. Thus, there is no convincing evidence to preserve fragmented bone of 1 cm or less during debridement even if it is attached to soft tissues. Similarly, a serial debridement of such wound is often required to deal with the evolving pattern of tissue necrosis over a period of 24–36 h. This allows for early identification of the demarcation zone between vital and non-vital tissues before reconstructive procedures are planned. The consensus of radical wound debridement at initial intervention aims to remove foreign bodies, necrotic tissues, and microbial contamination as early as possible. It also minimizes inflammation, prevents infections, and helps in achieving favorable wound healing. Any late wound management in our opinion eventually increases the chances of infection, operating time, toxemia, and subsequent surgical intervention.

Concomitant injuries to salivary gland ducts and facial nerve are often encountered during initial debridement. The ducts and facial nerve are usually tagged with Prolene sutures for future repair. Most of the ductal injuries can be managed by cannulation and primary repair or by rerouting it into oral cavity. Non-salvageable glands should be removed without hesitation to prevent sialocele, salivary fistula, and complicated wound healing. Damage to facial nerve is mainly by thermal, avulsion, and stretch injury caused by the cavitation. Preferably the nerve should be repaired within 72 h for predictable results. Lacerated nerve is repaired primarily by coaptation or using nerve grafts harvested from greater auricular nerve. The nerve damage caused by cavitation may extend as far as 1.8 cm from the bullet track, and that should be considered during nerve grafting procedure [19]. Any facial nerve injury anterior to a line connecting mental foramen and lateral canthus is generally not repaired as spontaneous recovery is very likely in such cases.

59.7 Infection and Role of Antibiotics

Ballistic facial injuries are often compound and contaminated with high propensity for infection (class IV wounds). Contrary to the popular belief, all ballistic injuries are inherently contaminated, and the infection is primarily by the inoculation of microorganisms carried by the bullet and secondarily as a result of wound contamination in transit or in hospital environment. The actual incidence of infection rates remains elusive and ranges from 7 to 100% of all military facial injuries [28]. However, a general consensus is lacking in the timing, choice, and duration of antimicrobial therapy in combat injuries. Nonetheless the usage of broad-spectrum antibiotics for 10–14 days which provides cover against staphylococci, *Clostridium perfringens*, and *Acinetobacter baumannii* is commonly used [14, 29]. The critical level of bacteria required for initiating an infection reaches peak at 6 h of injury (10^5 bacteria/gm. of tissue), and studies have shown that early administration of antibiotics is paramount and any delay of greater than 6 h renders the treatment ineffective [30]. The accepted guidelines for combat-related injuries recommend administration of short-course, broad-spectrum antibiotics preferably within 3 h of injury [31]. The use of antibiotics is an adjunct to scrupulous debridement for the prevention of infection and should always be considered in the initial management of ballistic injuries.

59.8 Soft Tissue Reconstruction

Gunshot wounds result in composite 3D defects with involvement of the skin, musculature, facial skeleton, and mucosa. The various reconstruction methods for wounds of these natures are prosthetic obturation, non-vascularized grafts with local tissue advancement, loco-regional flaps, and free flaps for large composite defects (Also refer Chaps. 86 and 88 of this book). Before initiating the reconstructive procedure, it should be kept in mind that the management of such wounds is often complicated by the ambiguity in prognosis caused by tissue loss, progressive necrosis, and infection. Therefore most critical facet while handling avulsive wounds lays in achieving and maintaining a favorable intraoral wound closure to minimize the chances of wound infection and wound dehiscence due to oral contamination [32]. It is always crucial to close the wound primarily because of the high propensity toward scarring and functional debility of wounds that heal secondarily. Most gunshot wounds can be closed primarily, and delayed wound closure in maxillofacial region is rarely necessary. However, two exceptions to this are (1) wounds which are not possible to debride completely at initial operation and (2) wounds with questionable vitality of tissues.

Sequencing of primary reconstruction of oro-facial region should follow an inside-out principle [33]. The injuries of the oropharynx are first addressed by repairing the musculature and mucosa. This is followed by repair of oral mucosa, floor of the mouth, and the tongue. The reconstruction of lips, cheeks, and other extra-oral tissues is performed later after oral cavity has been reconstructed. Nonetheless if an acceptable intraoral closure is difficult to achieve, a maxillomandibular fixation is done, and it is prudent to leave the wound to heal secondarily. While selecting a reconstructive option, it is important to consider a treatment plan which reduces the treatment time, patient morbidity, number of surgical intervention, and hospital stay [34]. The best possible function and aesthetics are achieved when debridement and reconstruction of hard and soft tissues are done at an early stage and the residual soft tissue deformities are addressed at a later stage with revision surgeries and local flaps [2]. Extra-oral wounds that cannot be closed primarily due to excessive tissue loss are best managed by employing local, regional pedicled flaps and microvascular flaps.

Use of local flaps and regional flaps at the initial operation appears to be most favorable as far as aesthetics and function are concerned (Fig. 59.6a). Motamedi [2] advised early use of local flaps in patients with gunshot wounds of the face. He reviewed 30 GSW patients and reported excellent cosmetic and functional outcomes. However, the disadvantages of local flaps are that composite defects cannot be addressed and its availability, limited bulk, and pedicle length. Local tissue rearrangements and local flaps with nonvascular grafts like iliac crest, rib, or cranium can be used for small defects. But large 3D defects and poorly vascularized surrounding tissues caused by cavitation often preclude the use of bone grafts with local tissue rearrangements unlike in tumor reconstruction.

Major avulsive and chop off injuries demand vascularized bone grafts with skin paddle for their reconstruction. Composite free tissue transfer is predictable, provides adequate bulk of well-vascularized tissue to fill the dead space, rehabilitates the buttresses, and reinstates the soft tissue envelope in a limited period of time [15]. The variables affecting the selection of flap depend on the type and amount of tissue loss, location, length of pedicle, donor site injury, and, certainly, surgeon's preference. The most commonly used flaps for facial reconstruction are anterolateral thigh flap, radial forearm, and fibula with skin paddle [5]. It is obligatory to reconstruct both bone and soft tissues in composite defects, and without osseous support, soft tissue-only reconstruction tends to droop over time. After primary healing, the flap is contoured, subsequently unaesthetic skin paddle is excised, and local tissue can be re-advanced for better aesthetic outcomes. Similarly, if adequate vascularized tissue is not used for reconstruction, complications like scar contracture, bone graft resorption, fistula formation, and ultimately collapse of facial envelope will result.

It is clear that reconstruction of avulsive facial defects with free flap should be addressed as early as possible to prevent soft tissue contracture. Nonetheless, how much grace period is required before initiating a free flap reconstruction for optimizing the reconstructive outcomes is still not clear. High-energy cavitation in soft tissue may temporarily damage the local vasculature and hemodynamics at a distance from the margin of permanent wound. While planning a treatment based on microvascular reconstruction, it is imperative to have a conception of the zone of injury in its actual extent. Animal studies have shown that it is safe to place an anastomosis 3 cm away from the margin of wound track [35]. Furthermore, experimental evidences have shown superior results in integrity and patency of facial vessels anastomosed 3 days after injury than those repaired immediately after the injury [20]. If it is so, a composite free tissue transfer as a part of immediate reconstruction in avulsive ballistic injuries should be delayed till 3–4 days. This time period helps in adequate assessment of the extent of devitalized tissues, formulating a treatment plan based on available resources and optimizing the results by executing the treatment before the onset of soft tissue fibrosis and when the blood vessels are devoid of spasm.

Despite several arguments favoring immediate reconstruction for excellent aesthetic outcomes, it is to be noted that scar contracture is inevitable irrespective of the timing of treatment and reconstruction method adopted, although the frequency is more with delayed treatment [36]. Therefore, a review to determine the need for secondary corrective procedures should be conducted in consultation with the interdisciplinary team. Scar contracture is usually managed later by revision surgeries after the maturation of scar. The total number of revision surgeries required for a free flap is less as compared to local or regional flaps. The outcomes of revision surgery depend on the type of flap used, complexity of the defect, and location of the defect with nasal, orbits, and lips requiring the highest number of aesthetic refinements [5]. Similarly other expected soft tissue complications like trismus, microsomia, and other functional disabilities can be addressed by fat grafting, coronoidectomy, commissuroplasty, and Botox injections [37]. Very often the reconstructive surgeries of aesthetically prominent regions of the face like nose and orbits are always suboptimal, and in such cases, prosthetic rehabilitation can be considered even though not physiological and patient compliance is less.

59.9 Fracture Stabilization and Hard Tissue Reconstruction

The methodology for treatment varies and ranges from:

1. Debridement only
2. Debridement and closed reduction with or without fixation
3. Debridement, open reduction, and plate osteosynthesis

In patients without continuity defect, infection and minimal comminution open reduction and internal fixation (ORIF) is simultaneously done along with debridement at the initial stage.

Once initial stabilization is ensured, fixation is generally accomplished by miniplates or reconstruction plates. However, wounds with limited soft issue coverage require a different strategy as the granulation tissues may fail to cover thickness of plate resulting in subsequent plate exposure. Thus, if adequate soft tissue cover cannot be achieved, debridement, external pins, and maxillomandibular fixation (MMF) are the method of choice [33]. Until the introduction of surgical screws and plates, closed treatment was the preferred mode of treatment. The treatment ideology was directed to treat the whole wound as a "bag of bones" using external fixation or MMF in order to avoid periosteal stripping and devitalization of small fragments of bone. Although this therapeutic concept is advocated by several authors, who have reported significantly lesser rates of infection with this technique when compared with ORIF and plates, the value approach continues to be underestimated [38].

The advantages of external fixation are manifold. It helps to prevent bone devascularization, allows for bone regeneration, and also provides adequate support to the comminuted fracture fragments. Additionally, it also enhances the osteogenic potential of the injury site by helping in spontaneous bone regeneration. This phenomenon is more commonly seen in young patients due to hypoxia and acidosis-induced activation of local bone morphogenic proteins (BMPs). The high-velocity trauma causes extensive damage to adjacent muscles and periosteum. This damage along with the effects of local inflammation, hypoxia, and increased carbon dioxide concentration activates BMPs resulting in spontaneous bone formation. The concept and knowledge regarding facial buttress and its implication in trauma management have added a new dimension in the functional and aesthetic reconstruction of the face. As a result, internal fixation using locking plates has greatly replaced external fixators over a period of time. It is currently the most widely used technique in management of GSWs with bone loss and is used if the fracture fragments are large enough to accept screws.

Additionally, bone defects if any should be grafted with harvested iliac crest, ribs, or cranium depending upon the size of the defect (Fig. 59.7). However, the infection rates associated with internal fixation are comparatively higher as quoted by many authors. The increased rates of infection associated with ORIF are due to loosening of hardware and subsequent micromotion at the fracture site and possibly by contamination by oro-nasal flora. Motammedi [2] reported that it is almost impossible to achieve occlusion without arch bars and MMF in majority of gunshot fractures. Presently ORIF along with arch bars continue to be the mainstay in the management such patients. With the advent of new techniques of reconstruction supplemented by innovative plates and screws, vascular grafts and antibiotics have heralded a paradigm shift in the treatment philosophy. Current principles clearly favor early definitive reconstruction of hard tissues with ORIF using rigid fixation supplemented by MMF and bone grafts whenever required (Fig. 59.8).

59.10 Timing of Definitive Reconstruction

An area of ongoing debate and controversy in the management of gunshot wounds of the face is regarding the timing of definitive reconstruction [6, 39]. Although previous teachings and practices were in favor of delayed reconstruction, the more recent studies demonstrate predictable functional and aesthetic outcomes with immediate definitive reconstruction [40–42]. Scientific studies suggest carrying out definitive reconstruction within a time frame of 48 h would yield the best possible outcome [2].

Advocates of delayed reconstruction believe that the delay in treatment reduces the probability of infection, necrosis, and postoperative wound complications exponentially. Additionally delay in treatment reduces the chances of mortality and morbidity due to infection and progressive tissue necrosis [43, 44]. Any increase in postoperative temperature, raised leukocyte counts, and other local signs of infection may invariably cause a failure in flap due to risk of venous thrombosis. It has also been suggested that the decreased inflammation and edema aid surgeons to have a better assessment of the extent of injury, thereby helping in precise and desired treatment planning which in turn could lead to a better outcome. Therefore in their opinion, it is prudent to wait before applying any principles of primary reconstruction until a healthy tissue bed is achieved. On the other hand, the disadvantages of delayed treatment are increased treatment time, prolonged hospital stay, increased cost of treatment, and patient distress caused by psychosocial impact of disfigurement associated with gunshot injury (Tables 59.2 and 59.3).

Advocates of early primary treatment claim superior functional and aesthetic outcomes, early restoration of facial form, and limited hospital stay with early return to normal

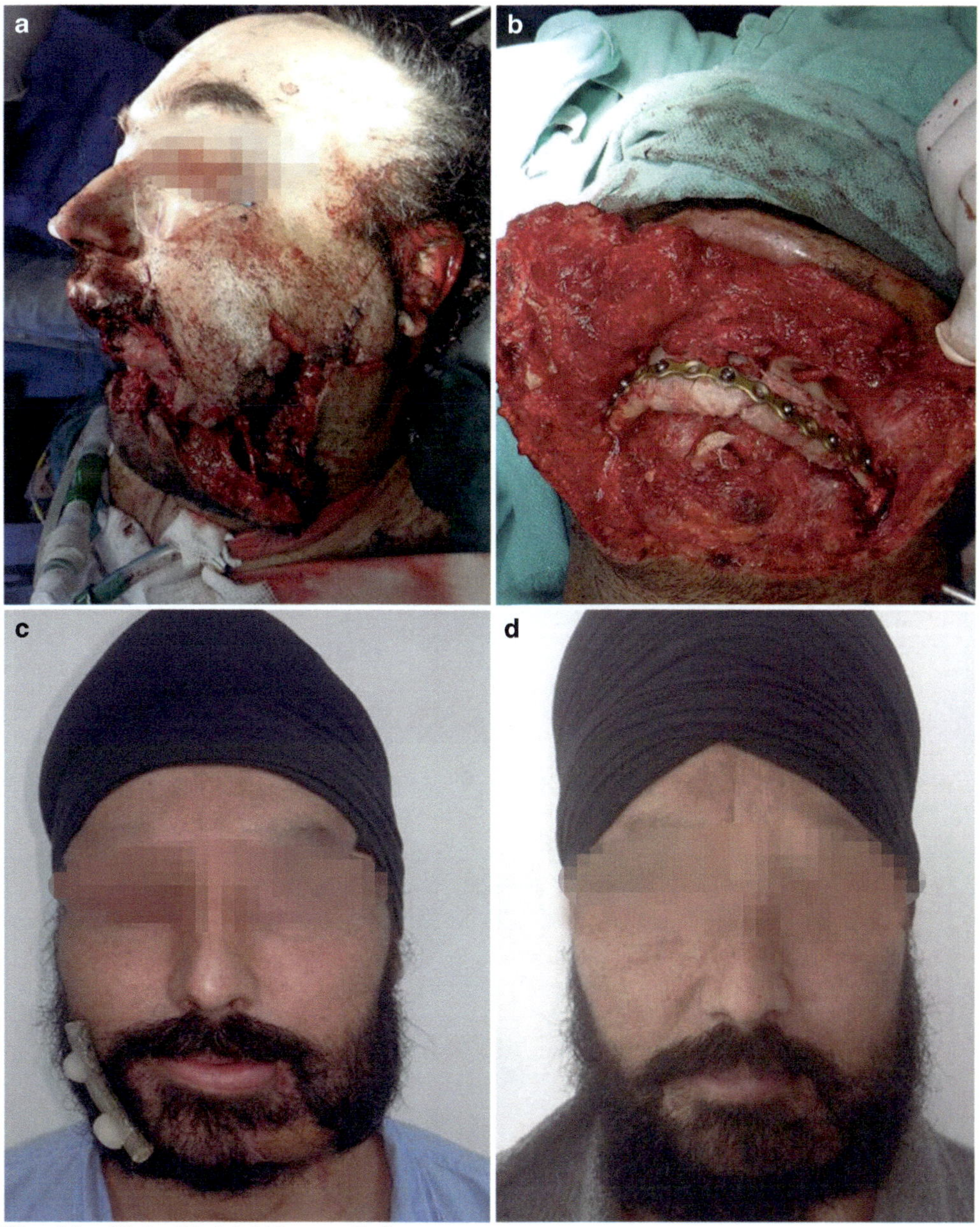

Fig. 59.7 (**a–d**) High-velocity close-range assault rifle injury with comminution of mandible and soft tissue loss. Managed initially by non-vascularized graft and later by free fibula osteocutaneous flap reconstruction. External fixator for stabilizing fibula in place. Follow-up after complete treatment

function [4, 14, 45]. These benefits are predominantly due to the elimination of soft tissue contracture by proper anatomic coverage of soft tissue at an early stage [21]. Vasconez et al. [42] compared the infection rates of gunshot wounds that have been managed by early and late reconstruction in a series of 33 cases. In their observation, they could not found any significant difference in infection rates between the two groups. However, the delayed group showed an apparent increase in the incidence of scar contracture with significant functional and aesthetic complications. Similarly, several other studies have also reported excellent clinical outcomes when immediate reconstruction is carried out [46].

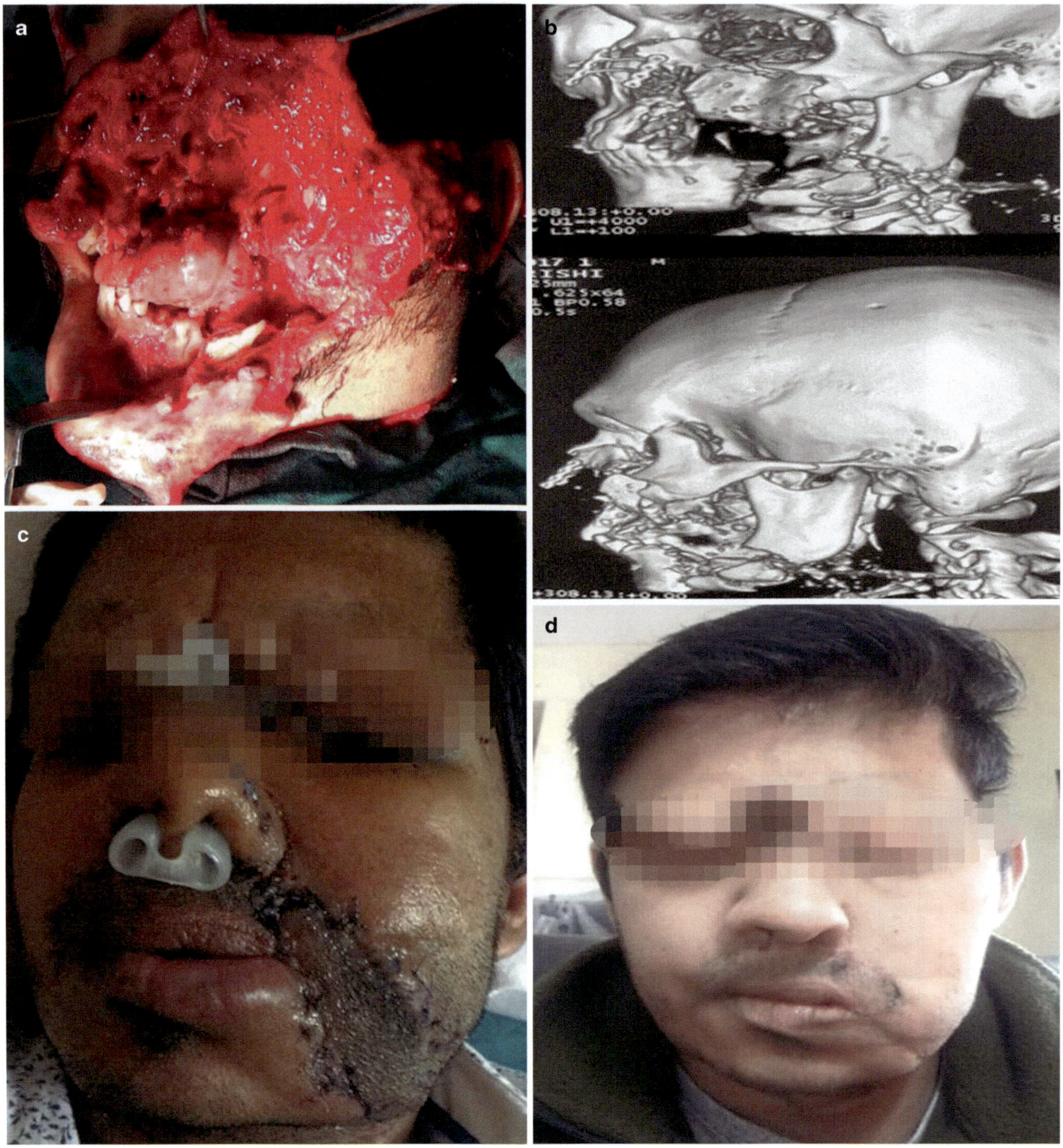

Fig. 59.8 (**a**–**d**) High-velocity assault rifle injury to the face with loss of hemimaxilla and mandible along with partial loss of upper lip was done. Reconstruction of the upper lip by hair-bearing submental island flap. Mandible reconstruction is performed by vascularized fibula

Definitive management of most maxillofacial injuries is not a surgical emergency, and treatment is often delayed in polytrauma patients. A standard consensus for delaying treatment and adopting a staged approach in such cases is due to the inability of a critically injured patient to undergo surgical intervention. However, as soon the patient is deemed to be medically stable, operative intervention targeted toward managing the facial injuries should be initiated. It is imperative to address the bony and soft tissue injuries soon after the resolution of edema and before the initiation of fibrosis of

Table 59.2 Advantages and disadvantages of immediate reconstruction

Advantages of immediate reconstruction	Disadvantages of immediate reconstruction
Less scar contracture, better postoperative function and aesthetics	The margins of devitalized tissues and its extent cannot be appreciated during early repair
Early return to function and less hospital stay	Correction of subtle deformities is difficult and such minor correction always requires second intervention
Less psychological impact on patient because of early recovery	Surgeon's expertise and availability of resources
Proper anatomical coverage of defect so chances of infection are less	Tissue edema immediately following the injury will hamper the judgment of surgeon resulting in suboptimal outcome

Table 59.3 Advantages and disadvantages of delayed reconstruction

Advantages of delayed reconstruction	Disadvantages of delayed reconstruction
Correction of defects after the resolution of edema will give a clear picture of the defect size	Severe scar contracture, less postoperative functional and aesthetic outcome
Correction of minor deformities is possible which may have been missed during immediate reconstruction	Number of hospital stay is increased with more psychological burden to the family and patient due to disfigured face
The necrotic margins can be easily assessed before reconstruction	High chances of infection due to open wound

soft tissues and malunion of fractures. This grace period will allow the surgeon to have an accurate and swift identification of subtle deformities for a major single-stage intervention rather than repeated assault to soft tissues causing fibrosis and decreased vascularity.

The essential difference in the management of routine maxillofacial injury and gunshot wounds of the face is the requirement of a multidisciplinary team for the management of gunshot wounds. Therefore, a short-term delay or temporizing such wounds allows time to procure diagnostic images and study models and lastly for a discussion on inputs from the medical and surgical team. In general, the formulation of treatment plan should be based on the general health status of the patient, availability of resources, surgeon's expertise, and patient's will.

In a vast majority of cases despite the primary management approach, a significant number of gunshot injuries are plagued with residual functional and aesthetic problems. Hence, a good postoperative outcome is multifactorial and is the reflection of all the above factors and not just the early definitive repair. However, a large number of maxillofacial gunshot wounds can be treated definitively at the time of initial intervention if the general condition of the patient and expertise of surgeon permit and the benefits of such an approach are manifold.

> The general physical status of the patient, timing of surgery, extent of composite tissue damage, good surgical techniques, use of appropriate hardwares, antibiotics, and proper rehabilitation are the factors which determine the final outcome and aesthetic result in a penetrating facial injury.

59.11 Recent Advances

Several recent advances have significantly improved the morbidity and survival rates in complex maxillofacial gunshot injuries. More importantly they serve as a support system to the surgeons, enabling them to appreciate and attend to the finer aspects of complex composite injuries. This in turn paves the way to achieve far more superior reconstructive outcomes. Contemporary techniques employ virtual surgical planning, patient-specific stereolithographic models, as well as intraoperative navigation and imaging (Refer Chap. 41 of this book). These modern-day techniques help elevate the surgical experience to one that is more precise, faster, and minimally invasive.

Composite tissue alloplastic transplantation or face transplantation is yet another recent innovation in this field. This treatment is rendered for patients with massive loss of hard and soft tissues of the face or in cases where the final outcome is suboptimal even after multiple surgeries. However, it is not in the mainstay treatment of gunshot wound of the face because of the difficulties in finding an appropriate donor, lack of expertise, requirement of long-term immunosuppressants, absence of long-term follow-up, and associated ethical issues.

59.12 Conclusion

In conclusion, the management strategies of patients with facial gunshot wounds are almost as diverse as the case presentation itself. This chapter ascertains that the blueprint for actions in the management of facial gunshot injuries has undergone significant change over the last decade. A new understanding of the inherent osteogenic potential of the human body in the face of contemporary warfare coupled with the availability of state-of-the-art equipments and facilities favors a brisk early approach. Thus, present guidelines essentially direct surgeons to do as much as possible for the gunshot patient with regard to hard and soft tissue reconstruction of the face and jaws within 48 hours. The treatment in such cases is more comprehensive with intent to simultaneously debride and reconstruct.

References

1. McLean JN, Moore CE, Yellin SA. Gunshot wounds to the face—acute management. Facial Plast Surg. 2005;21:191–8.
2. Motamedi MHK. Primary management of maxillofacial hard and soft tissue gunshot and shrapnel injuries. J Oral Maxillofac Surg. 2003;61:1390–8.
3. Robertson BC, Manson PN. High-energy ballistic and avulsive injuries. A management protocol for the next millennium. Surg Clin North Am. 1999;79:1489–502.
4. Motamedi MH, Behnia H. Experience with regional flaps in the comprehensive treatment of maxillofacial soft-tissue injuries in war victims. J Craniomaxillofac Surg. 1999;27:256–65.
5. Doctor VS, Farwell DG. Gunshot wounds to the head and neck. Curr Opin Otolaryngol Head Neck Surg. 2007;15:213–8.
6. Kummoona R. Management of missiles injuries of the facial skeleton: primary, intermediate, and secondary phases. J Craniofac Surg. 2010;21:976–81.
7. Williams CN. Immediate and long-term management of gunshot wounds to the lower face. Plast Reconstr Surg. 1988;82:433–9.
8. Shuker ST. Emergency treatment strategy and the biodynamic effects of massive, & "chopped off" mandibular tissue and a prolapsed tongue. J Craniomaxillofac Surg. 2013;41:e59–63.
9. Chen AY, Stewart MG, Raup G. Penetrating injuries of the face. Otolaryngol Neck Surg. 1996;115:464–70.
10. Breeze J, Tong D, Gibbons A. Contemporary management of maxillofacial ballistic trauma. Br J Oral Maxillofac Surg. 2017;55:661–5.
11. Hodgetts TJ, Mahoney PF, Kirkman E. Damage control resuscitation. J R Army Med Corps. 2007;153:299–300.
12. Tong DC, Breeze J. Damage control surgery and combat-related maxillofacial and cervical injuries: a systematic review. Br J Oral Maxillofac Surg. 2016;54:8–12.
13. Jose A, Nagori SA, Agarwal B, Bhutia O, Roychoudhury A. Management of maxillofacial trauma in emergency: an update of challenges and controversies. J Emerg Trauma Shock. 2016;9:73–80.
14. Powers DB, Will MJ, Bourgeois SL, Hatt HD. Maxillofacial trauma treatment protocol. Oral Maxillofac Surg Clin North Am. 2005;17:341–55.
15. Futran ND, Farwell DG, Smith RB, Johnson PE, Funk GF. Definitive management of severe facial trauma utilizing free tissue transfer. Otolaryngol Head Neck Surg. 2005;132:75–85.
16. Cole RD, Browne JD, Phipps CD. Gunshot wounds to the mandible and midface: evaluation, treatment, and avoidance of complications. Otolaryngol Head Neck Surg. 1994;111:739–45.
17. DuBose J, Teixeira PGR, Hadjizacharia P, Hannon M, Inaba K, Green DG, et al. The role of routine spinal imaging and immobilisation in asymptomatic patients after gunshot wounds. Injury. 2009;40:860–3.
18. Shvyrkov MB, Yanushevich OO. Facial gunshot wound debridement: debridement of facial soft tissue gunshot wounds. J Craniomaxillofac Surg. 2013;41:e8–16.
19. Cunningham LL, Haug RH, Ford J. Firearm injuries to the maxillofacial region: an overview of current thoughts regarding demographics, pathophysiology, and management. J Oral Maxillofac Surg. 2003;61:932–42.
20. Tan YH, Zhou SX, Liu YQ, Liu BL, Li ZY. Small-vessel pathology and anastomosis following maxillofacial firearm wounds: an experimental study. J Oral Maxillofac Surg. 1991;49:348–52.
21. Clark N, Birely B, Manson PN, Slezak S, Kolk CV, Robertson B, et al. High-energy ballistic and avulsive facial injuries: classification, patterns, and an algorithm for primary reconstruction. Plast Reconstr Surg. 1996;98:583–601.
22. Clasper JC, Hill PF, Watkins PE. Contamination of ballistic fractures: an in vitro model. Injury. 2002;33:157–60.
23. Berlin R, Janzon B, Nordström G, Schantz B. The extent of muscle tissue damage in missile wounds one and six hours after the infliction of trauma studied by the current method of debridement. Acta Chir Scand. 1978;144:213–7.
24. Rich NM. Vietnam missile wounds evaluated in 750 patients. Mil Med. 1968;133:9–22.
25. Reis ND, Zinman C, Besser MI, Shifrin LZ, Rosen H. A philosophy of limb salvage in war: use of the fixateur externe. Mil Med. 1991;156:505–20.
26. Al-Shawi A. Experience in the treatment of missile injuries of the maxillofacial region in Iraq. Br J Oral Maxillofac Surg. 1986;24:244–50.
27. Zhou S, Lei D, Liu Y, Tan Y, Gu X. Experimental study on firearm wound in maxillofacial region. Chin Med J. 1998;111:114–7.
28. Suominen E, Tukiainen E. Close-range shotgun and rifle injuries to the face. Clin Plast Surg. 2001;28:323–37.
29. Petersen K, Hayes DK, Blice JP, Hale RG. Prevention and management of infections associated with combat-related head and neck injuries. J Trauma. 2008;64:S265–76.
30. Mellor SG, Cooper GJ, Bowyer GW. Efficacy of delayed administration of benzylpenicillin in the control of infection in penetrating soft tissue injuries in war. J Trauma. 1996;40:S128–34.
31. Hospenthal DR, Murray CK, Andersen RC, Bell RB, Calhoun JH, Cancio LC, et al. Executive summary: guidelines for the prevention of infections associated with combat-related injuries: 2011 update. J Trauma Inj Infect Crit Care. 2011;71:S202–9.
32. Ray JM. The Treatment of Maxillofacial Trauma in Austere Conditions. Atlas Oral Maxillofac Surg Clin. 2013;21:9–14.
33. Kummoona R, Muna AM. Evaluation of immediate phase of management of missile injuries affecting maxillofacial region in Iraq. J Craniofac Surg. 2006;17:217–23.
34. Xavier SP, de Barros Pontes C, Silva ER, de Santana Santos T, Zatiti SC, de Mello Filho FV. Three-stage mandible reconstruction after firearm injury. J Craniofac Surg. 2013;24:e87–8.
35. Tan Y, Zhou S, Liu Y, Li Z. A gross and microscopic study of cerebral injuries accompanying maxillofacial high-velocity projectile wounding in dogs. J Oral Maxillofac Surg. 1998;56:345–8.
36. Behnia H, Motamedi MH. Reconstruction and rehabilitation of short-range, high-velocity gunshot injury to the lower face: a case report. J Craniomaxillofac Surg. 1997;25:220–7.
37. Gassner HG, Sherris DA, Otley CC. Treatment of facial wounds with botulinum toxin A improves cosmetic outcome in primates. Plast Reconstr Surg. 2000;105:1948–53.
38. Manson PN, Crawley WA, Yaremchuk MJ, Rochman GM, Hoopes JE, French JH. Midface fractures: advantages of immediate extended open reduction and bone grafting. Plast Reconstr Surg. 1985;76:1–12.
39. Kaufman Y, Cole P, Hollier L. Facial gunshot wounds: trends in management. Craniomaxillofac Trauma Reconstr. 2009;2:85–90.
40. Hollier L, Grantcharova EP, Kattash M. Facial gunshot wounds: a 4-year experience. J Oral Maxillofac Surg. 2001;59:277–82.

41. Mladick RA, Georgiade NG, Royer J. Immediate flap reconstruction for massive shotgun wound of face. Case report. Plast Reconstr Surg. 1970;45:186–8.
42. Vásconez HC, Shockley ME, Luce EA. High-energy gunshot wounds to the face. Ann Plast Surg. 1996;36:18–25.
43. Spira M, Hardy SB, Biggs TE, Gerow FJ. Shotgun injuries of the face. Plast Reconstr Surg. 1967;39:449–58.
44. Kassan AH, Lalloo R, Kariem G. A retrospective analysis of gunshot injuries to the maxillofacial region. SADJ. 2000;55:359–63.
45. Finch DR, Dibbell DG. Immediate reconstruction of gunshot injuries to the face. J Trauma. 1979;19:965–8.
46. Gruss JS, Antonyshyn O, Phillips JH. Early definitive bone and soft-tissue reconstruction of major gunshot wounds of the face. Plast Reconstr Surg. 1991;87:436–50.

Panfacial Fractures

60

Kiran S. Gadre, Balasubramanya Kumar, and Divya P. Gadre

60.1 Introduction

Most facial fractures occur in combinations involving various subunits of craniomaxillofacial (CMF) skeleton [1] (Fig. 60.1). Severity of these injuries is determined by multiple factors such as its aetiology, causative factor, force of impact, pre-existing patient factors, etc. High velocity road traffic accidents RTA / assaults are the most common cause of panfacial fractures. With a large number of different patterns these fractures project, it is challenging to have a proper definition of "panfacial fractures". It is well-known that fractures involving multiple bones of the face is known as panfacial fracture. It could be described as "fractures involving upper third, middle third, and lower third of face with at least one condyle, palate and fronto-naso-orbito-ethmoidal complex (FNOE) fracture" (Fig. 60.2). When there is skull base or co-existing neurosurgical involvement, it is termed as craniofacial fracture. Managing these cases is extremely complicated as each of them present with unique pattern of hard and soft tissue injury. This demands a team approach as these injuries are commonly seen in polytrauma with multisystem involvement. Airway compromise, severe haemorrhage, large open wounds, severe ocular/orbital injuries and coincidental surgical procedure being performed are the only indications for immediate definitive surgical intervention. Restoration of form and function at the earliest opportunity should be the goal of maxillofacial surgeons.

K. S. Gadre (✉)
Gadre Clinic, Pune, Maharashtra, India

Department of Oral and Maxillofacial Surgery, Bharati Vidyapeeth Dental College and Hospital, Pune, Maharashtra, India

B. Kumar
Department of Maxillofacial Surgery, St. Marthas's Hospital, Bangalore, Karnataka, India

Bhagwan Mahaveer Jain Hospital, Vikram Hospital, Bangalore, Karnataka, India

D. P. Gadre
Gadre Clinic, Pune, Maharashtra, India

60.2 Epidemiology

Global status report on road safety (2015) indicates that more than 1.25 million deaths, and 15–20 million injuries occur in road traffic accidents (RTA) costing most countries 3% of their GDP [2]. Countries with low and middle income having 54% of vehicles account for 90% of RTA-related fatalities, mostly of subjects aged between 15 and 44 years. RTA is the main cause of mortality in three quarters of males in 15–29 years age group. The true economic and public health impact is not estimated in most developing countries due to lack of infrastructure and resources [3].

Panfacial fractures are caused by high-energy impact, usually generated as a result of RTA or firearm injury directed at CMF skeleton, and it also has a contrecoup component causing associated cranio-cerebral or cervico-spinal injuries with a low Glasgow coma scale. These injuries can also cause associated injuries like rib fracture/pulmonary contusion, pneumothorax or intra-abdominal injuries, limb and pelvic injuries and require immediate treatment.

60.3 Management Philosophy

Restoration of form and function is the ultimate goal in treating panfacial injuries. Proximity to important structures like the brain, eyes, auditory apparatus and spine necessitates a holistic approach to their management involving neurosurgeons, ophthalmic surgeons, ENT surgeons, maxillofacial surgeons and anaesthetists.

It is challenging to follow an established pattern of repair as each case is unique and requires skill and expertise of the surgeon to restore the pre-traumatic anatomy of facial function with aesthetics. Despite all the aggressive treatment, many patients with panfacial trauma may need further correction of residual deformities.

K. Bonanthaya et al. (eds.), *Oral and Maxillofacial Surgery for the Clinician*, https://doi.org/10.1007/978-981-15-1346-6_60

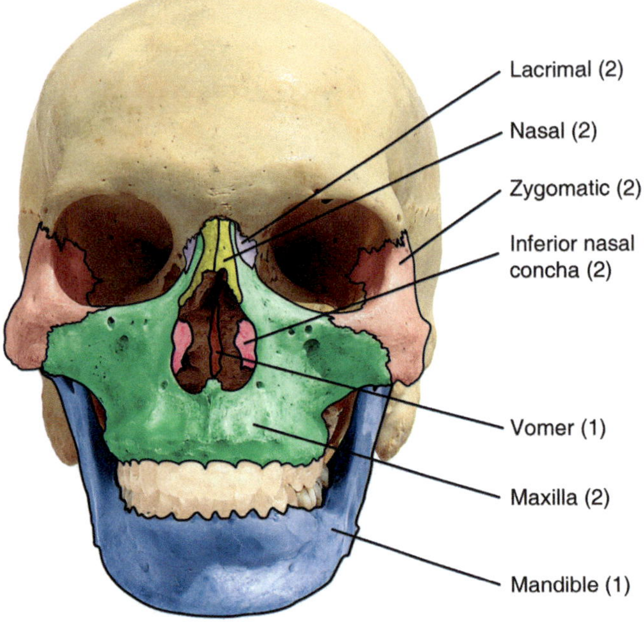

Fig. 60.1 Schematic diagram depicting subunits of facial skeleton

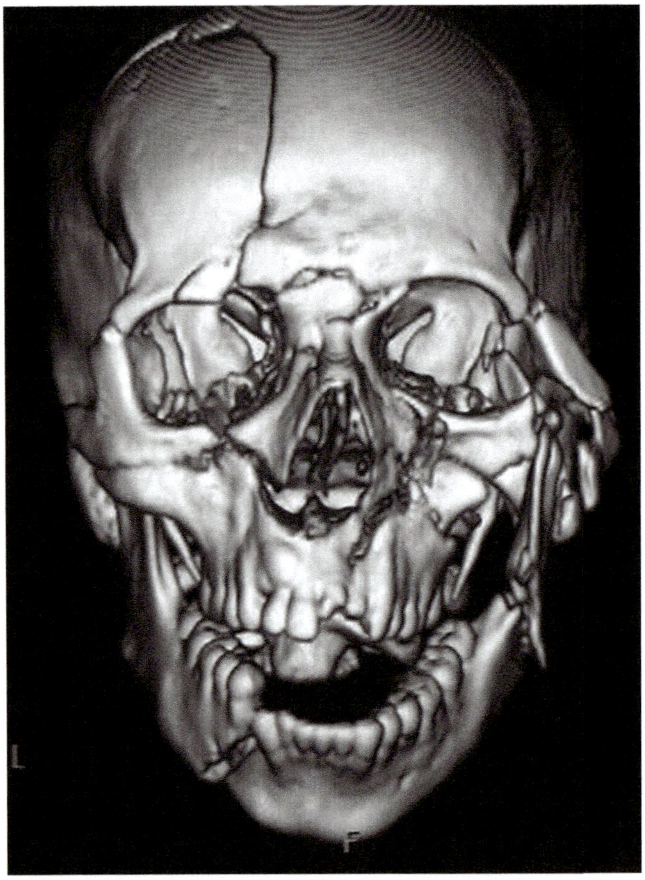

Fig. 60.2 3D CT scan image showing panfacial fracture involving the upper, middle and lower third of face

60.3.1 History of Management

The management of panfacial fractures has changed during past few decades, particularly after the 1990s, when indigenous plating systems were more freely available.

1. Prior to the 1980s, most panfacial fractures were treated with closed reduction using Plaster of Paris (POP) head caps and cranial frames. A variety of trans/interosseous wiring techniques (see Chap. 50 for details on various wiring techniques) and internal suspension methods like cranio-mandibular/maxillary suspension were used (Figs. 60.3a, b and 55.15).
2. The surgeons of the 1990s generation started using combination of plating at key buttresses and internal suspension techniques [4]—the approach which may be attributed to early learning curve of internal fixation (Fig. 60.4).
3. Use of internal fixation has revolutionised the management of panfacial fractures [4] (Fig. 60.5a, b), leading to faster recovery and satisfactory outcome of these injuries. (See Chap. 51 for details on Principles of internal fixation)
   A better understanding of anatomy, pathophysiology, anaesthesia, sterilization and asepsis with advances in intubation techniques (transmylohyoid/submental, bronchoscopic) and instrumentation (fiberoptic and endoscopic) and instrumentation has influenced the management of these complex injuries significantly (Chap. 7 deals with Anesthesia and intubation techniques in maxillofacial surgery). Use of engineering technology like three-dimensional planning, stereolithographic models, endoscopic and navigation techniques has simplified the accurate treatment of these fractures, avoiding injury to other vital structures and saving intra-operative time (Fig. 60.6a–d).

60.3.2 Indications

Panfacial fractures can be disfiguring and cause significant functional problems like difficulty in mastication, deglutition, speech, olfaction and abnormalities of vision. Early fixation of displaced fractures causing the above problems is warranted. Undisplaced/minimally displaced fractures can be left for a few days, buying some time to manage other grievous injuries. It is necessary to understand that sense of urgency for treatment should exist in treating any panfacial fracture (within 15 days, provided other parameters are permitting).

60.3.3 Contraindications

There are no absolute contraindications but relative contraindications which cause delay of treatment, are presented below.

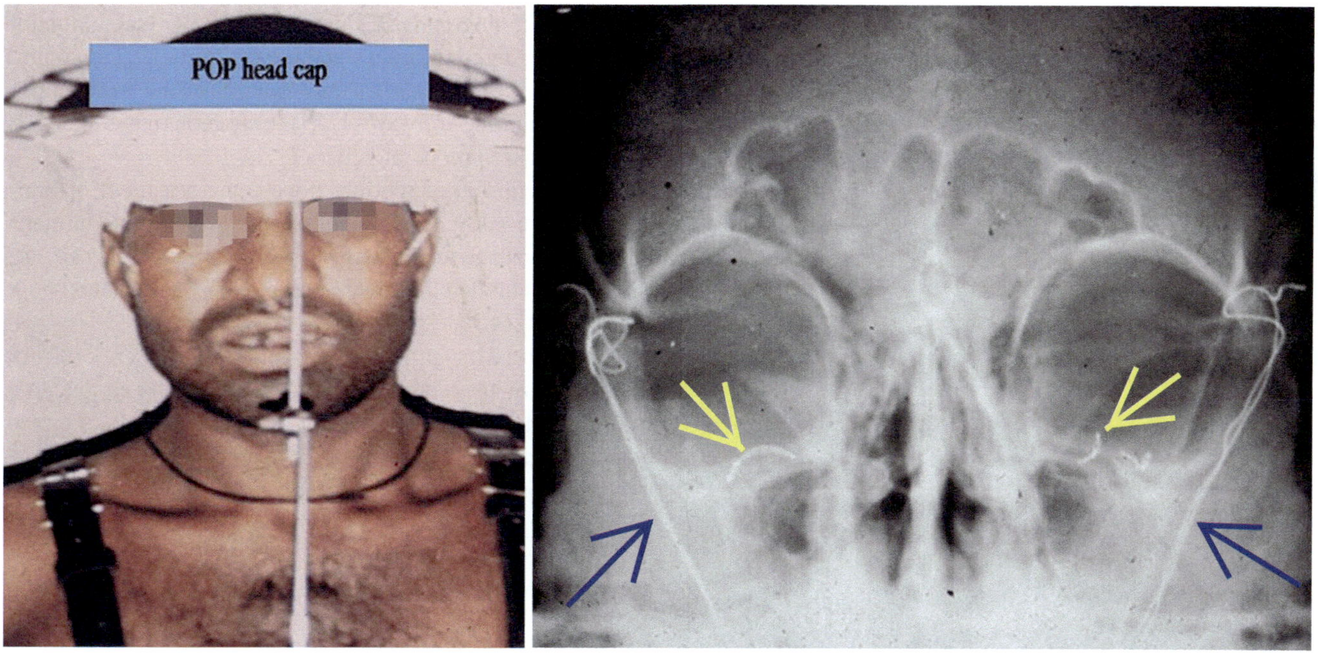

Fig. 60.3 (**a**) POP head cap used in traditional days. (**b**) Interosseous wiring (yellow arrow) with internal suspension (blue arrow)

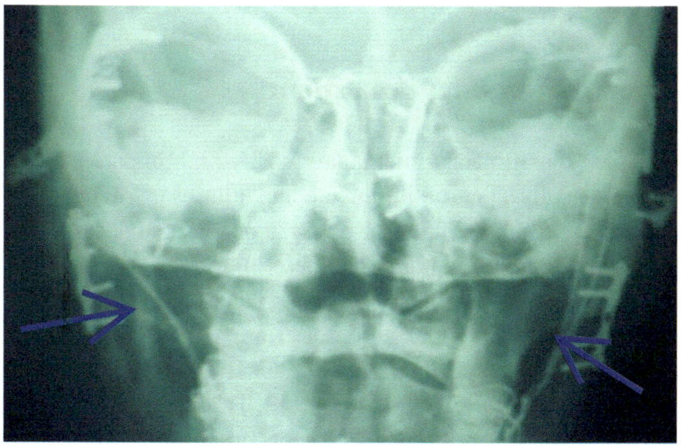

Fig. 60.4 Plating with internal suspension (blue arrows)

1. Definitive treatment of panfacial injuries may be delayed up to 2 weeks in presence of severe, compromising, concomitant systemic or head injury.
2. It is advisable to operate only when patients are neurologically and systemically stable. This period should be used for further surgical assessment and planning.
   Reduction of facial oedema further unmasks the underlying fractures and facial deformity. This gives an opportunity to review the imaging and prepare necessary splints (see Sect. 55.7.1) (Fig. 60.7a, b). These are very essential to establish width, height and anteroposterior projection of the facial skeleton, particularly where large dento-alveolar segments have been lost along with the presence of bilateral condylar fracture.
3. When a combination of avulsive injury (Chap. 49 deals with management of Soft tissue injuries in maxillofacial region) and panfacial fractures is present, golden hour reconstruction should be utilised, if circumstances and conditions permit. This is the best time as patient is in optimal physiologic and physical condition.

60.3.4 Clinical Findings

The clinical findings in panfacial trauma are a combination of signs and symptoms as seen in various subunits of facial fractures with increased severity (readers are advised to refer the respective chapters on maxillofacial trauma for signs and symptoms and management of fractures of mandible in Chap. 52, Fractures of the Condyle in Chaps. 53 and 54, fractures of maxilla in Chap. 55, fractures of the zygomatic complex in Chap. 56, fractures of the orbit in Chap. 57, fractures of the frontal naso orbit ethmoid region in Chap. 58 and Gun shot injuries in Chap. 59).

Facial oedema makes examination and standard radiography difficult. Bilateral raccoon's eyes and elongated dish-shaped face, with presence of orbital dystopia, traumatic telecanthus and deranged occlusion, are commonly seen. There may be elements of severe dento-alveolar trauma and soft tissue injury which may vary from minor contused or lacerated wounds (CLW) to avulsive injuries.

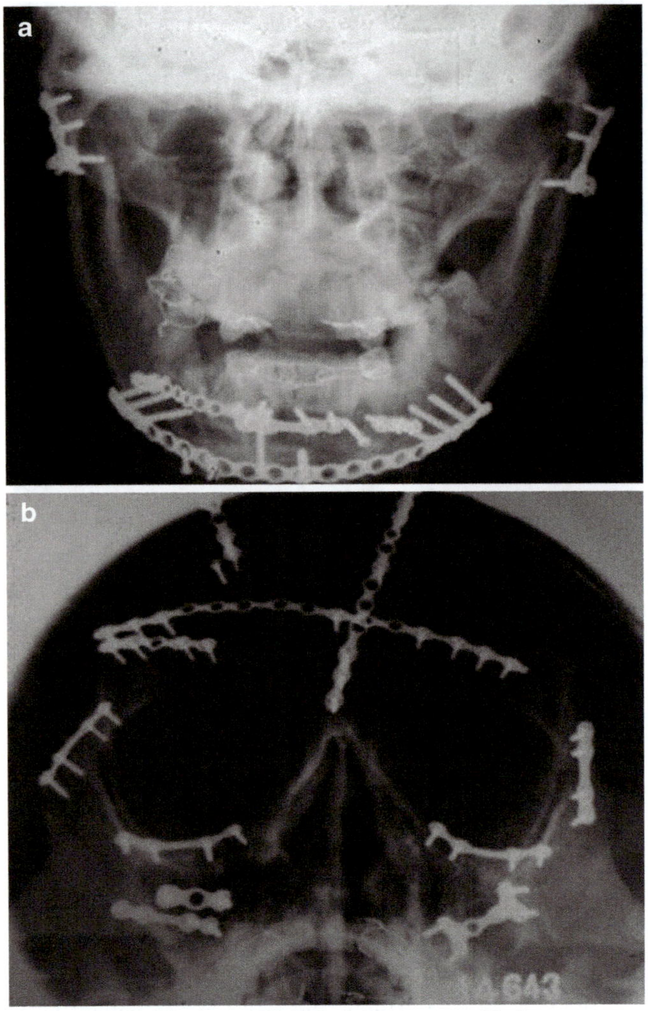

Fig. 60.5 (**a**, **b**) Plating of panfacial fractures as seen on (**a**) posterior-anterior Caldwell view of mandible and (**b**) posterior-anterior Water sinus view radiographs

Presence of cervical, cranial and other concomitant injuries must be assumed till proved contrary. Similarly absence of teeth, dentures in mouth must be assumed to have been swallowed or aspirated until proven otherwise.

60.4 Workup

The pre operative planning consists of two parts: (a) imaging and (b) diagnostic procedures.

Imaging:
Standard radiographs like posterior-anterior (PA) view, Caldwell view of mandible, Water's view, submento-vertex view, cervical spine radiographs have been used as a baseline in any emergency and are easily available in most settings. Computed tomography (CT) images with 3D reconstruction is now considered the gold standard in complex facial trauma patients as it provides a 1:1 information of the fracture pattern. 3D planning softwares help the surgeon in meticulously planning cases preoperatively.

CT imaging is commonly done for assessment of brain and spinal cord in a head injury patient to exclude intracranial haemorrhage and other grievous injuries. Facial skeleton should be included in the same scan in suspected facial bone fractures.

Coronal and sagittal sections of the CT scan could be obscured by the endotracheal tube in intubated patients. Axial and three-dimensional images with computer-generated models can be used for assessing most facial fractures in these cases (Fig. 60.8a, b).

Diagnostic Procedures:
Occlusion of teeth is the key to reduction and fixation of facial bone fractures. Mock surgery using dental models help in repositioning the teeth-bearing segments including dento-alveolar and palatal fractures and aid in fabricating acrylic stents and splints (Fig. 60.7). They are essential in cases where there is gross occlusal disturbance, splaying of basal bone or multiple fractures of dento-alveolar segment.

60.5 Emergency Treatment

Complex maxillofacial trauma are mostly high impact injuries and are usually a part of life-threatening injuries involving other organ systems like central nervous system, chest, abdomen, pelvis or limbs. It is important that these injuries be assessed and managed prior to or simultaneously as facial injuries.

Current standards of care for trauma patients, whether polytrauma or those involving the CMF skeleton, mandate that one must follow the Advanced Trauma Life Support (ATLS) protocol relating to airway, breathing, circulation, disability and exposure in that sequence. Airway and circulation should have the highest priority (Table 60.1). This is followed by an assessment of the patient's neurological, visual and cervical spine status. The details of primary and emergency management of polytrauma patients are dealt in Chap. 48 of this book.

Patients with polytrauma/panfacial fractures can require immediate or late treatment depending on the mechanism and kind of injury. Occasionally, immediate treatment can be the definitive procedure. An immediate intervention may be done merely for initial stabilization of the patient; procedures demanding a more detailed assessment and planning will need to be postponed. Immediate initial treatment in patients with maxillofacial injuries is indicated in following situations.

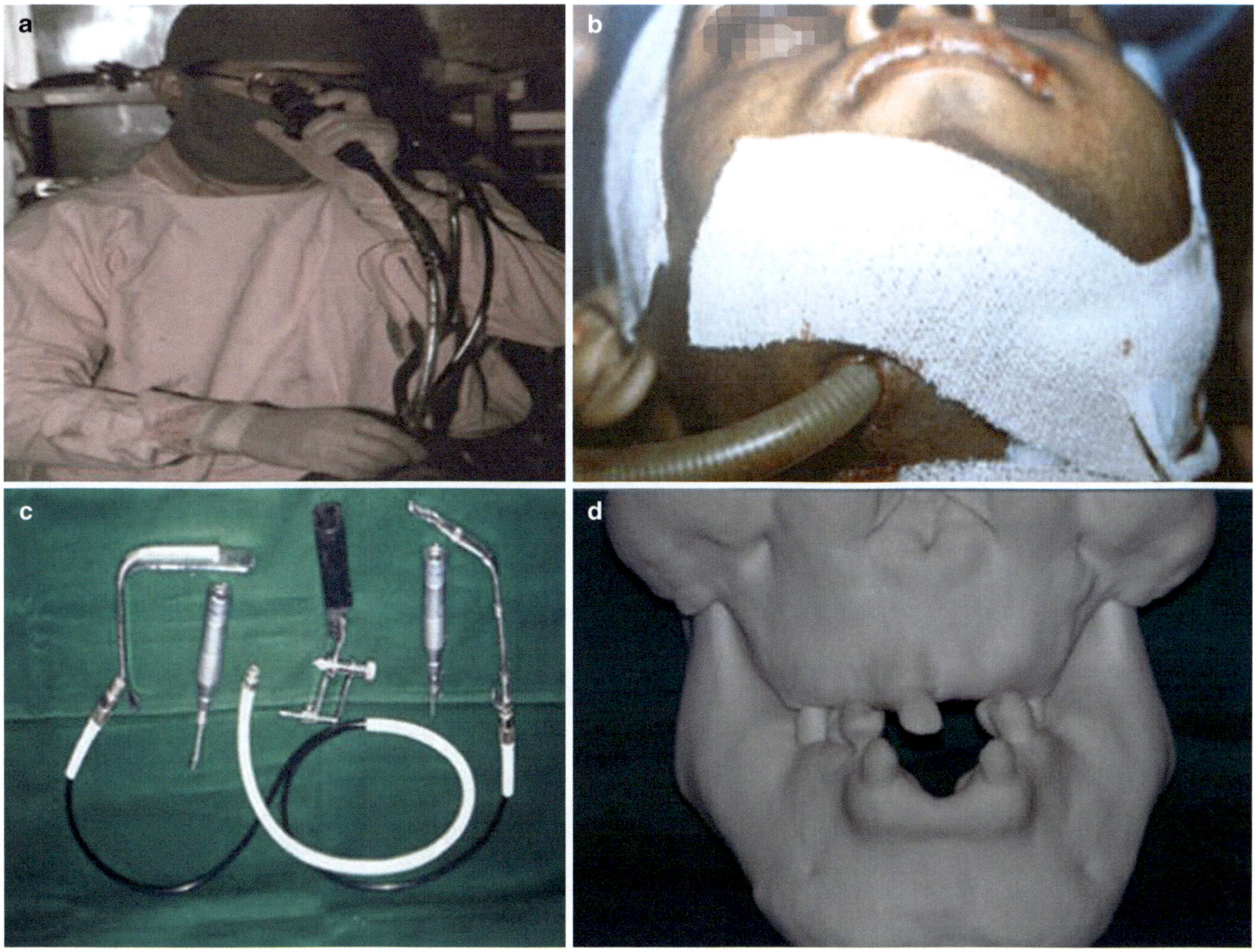

Fig. 60.6 (**a**–**d**) Showing few of advances from various specialities of medicine and engineering contributing to advances in management of panfacial fractures. ((**a**) Bronchoscopic intubation, (**b**) transmylohyoid intubation, (**c**) fibreoptic instruments, surgical saw, (**d**) stereolithographic model)

60.5.1 Airway Compromise

Obstructed airway is an important sequel of panfacial fractures and is managed either by temporarily reducing and stabilizing the fractured facial bones and attached soft tissues or performing a surgical tracheostomy. Patients with C-spine injury can be challenging to intubate due to inability to flex or extend the neck, as is establishment of a surgical airway like tracheostomy.

60.5.2 Severe Haemorrhage

Reduction and stabilization of fractured segments not only helps to correct airway but also controls severe bleeding. Haemorrhage not amenable to the above procedure may necessitate packing, identification of causative bleeder and its cauterisation or ligation. Occasional ECA control may be required, if multiple ipsilateral bleeding areas or unidentified areas of bleeding are seen. In centres where the facility is available, uncontrollable bleeding from facial region (especially after comminuted midface fractures) is controlled with selective embolisation by a interventional radiologist.

60.5.3 Large Open Wounds

These are commonly used to fix the fractures beneath them. In such situations initial washout and primary approximation should be done when possible for haemostasis and maintaining continuity of vascular supply, especially in cartilaginous areas like the ears and nose. This closure is basically a primary tacking of the wound margins. Layered closure is better done under controlled conditions along with fixation of the fractures under anesthesia [1].

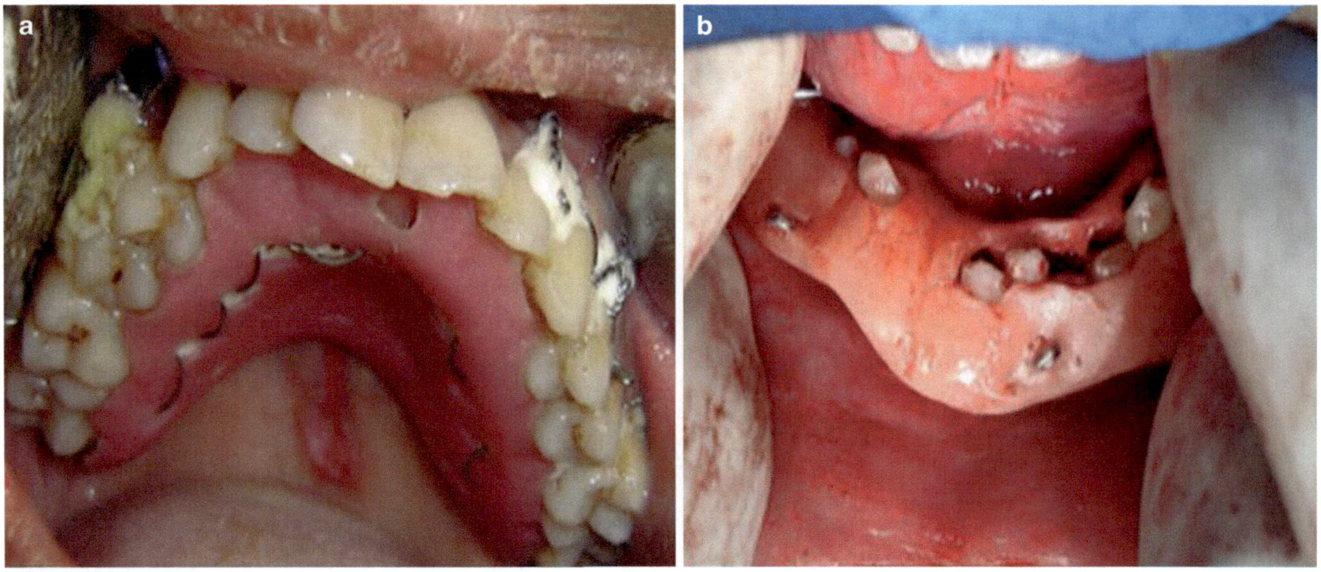

Fig. 60.7 (**a**, **b**) Showing utility and essentiality of splints in management of panfacial fractures

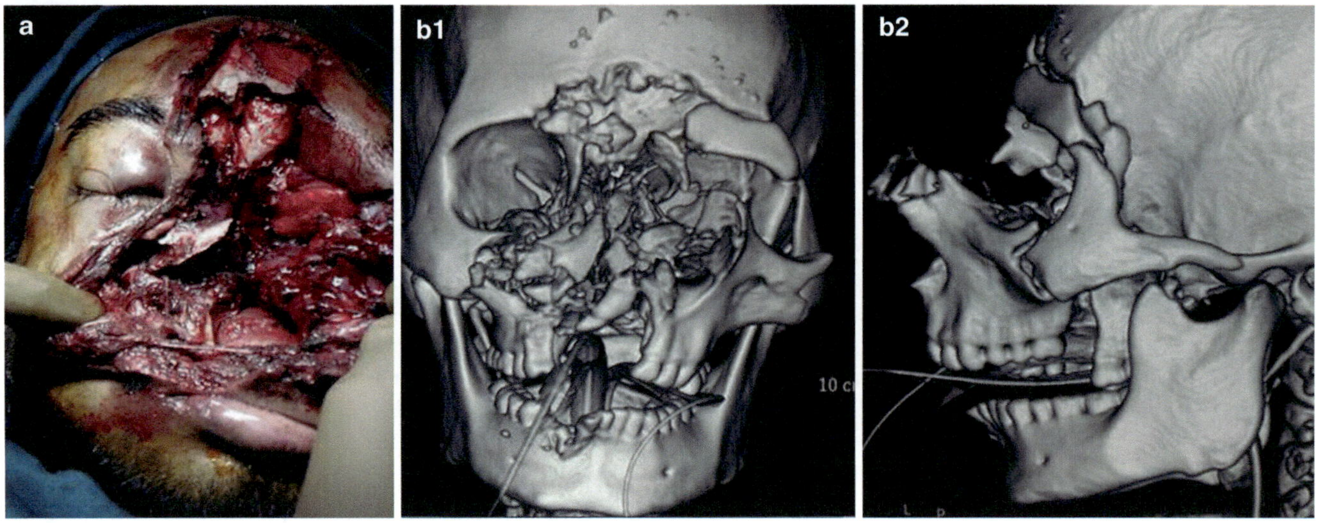

Fig. 60.8 (**a**, **b**) Depicting importance of high-resolution CT scan in an avulsive injury to assess nature and extent of injury and achieve predictable outcomes

60.5.4 Surgery for Associated Life-Threatening Injuries

Occasionally, patients with polytrauma undergo immediate surgery to treat other grievous injuries. This provides an opportunity to perform initial debridement, assessment and stabilisation and make dental impressions for fabrication of a customised splint. Considering the planning and surgical time required for comprehensive management of panfacial fractures, it is usually not advisable or possible to perform fixation during emergency management of other more severe injuries (neurological/abdomen/long bones/chest).

It is always wise to initiate assessment of a head injury or polytrauma patient using the ATLS (Advanced Trauma Life Support) protocol. A detailed record of all maxillofacial injuries should be made. Diagrams and representations of fracture patterns and soft tissue injuries make it easy for the understanding and execution of treatment. It is important to document the whereabouts, mechanism and time of injury accurately, to minimise medico-legal problems at a later date. Photographs are a good medium of educating the patients with their attenders and recording the preoperative soft tissue injuries.

Table 60.1 Immediate management of a polytrauma patient

Management	Option 1	Option 2
Airway	Suction, recovery position, Intubation	Tracheostomy. More so with C spine injury
Hemorrhage	Pressure	Ligation
	Grouping cross-matching	Fluids 1–2 liters in adults and 20ml/kg for children
IV	Peripheral with 16 G intra-cath	Central
Catheterization	Nasogastric tube insertion; caution when FNOE fractures	Foley's catheter for input - output chart
Immunisation	Anti gas gangrene	Tetanus
Laboratory	Routine	ABG
Imaging	CT scan: HFN, Chest, Pelvis	Chest X-ray, USG abdomen
Assessment	Circulatory	Neurological

60.5.5 Definitive Treatment

Paul Manson's quote "you never get a second chance" has to be kept in mind, i.e. the time frame [5] regarded appropriate for primary fracture treatment is limited to 2 weeks. After 2 weeks, the treatment is regarded as delayed and may necessitate secondary post-traumatic reconstruction (see Chap. 60 on residual deformities of the maxillofacial region).

60.6 Preoperative Documentation and Planning

Preoperative treatment planning is essential for successful outcomes. One must gather enough information and documentation to help in formulating an accurate treatment plan.

This can include:
1. The topography and extent of fracture involvement
2. Loss of hard and soft tissues with their residual defects
3. Involvement of teeth and teeth-bearing segments
4. Assessment of important structures like parotid and submandibular glands, nasolacrimal duct, trigeminal nerve, facial nerve, muscles of eye and most importantly vision

A proper evaluation by ophthalmologist, ENT surgeon and Neuro Surgeon is mandatory before proceeding with panfacial fracture fixation, and these allied specialities may be part of the surgical team for comprehensive management of the panfacial injuries.

Large bony defects with loss of soft tissue are best treated immediately or secondarily with local, pedicled non-vascularised or vascularised-free flaps provided the wound is clean and non-infected. Tissue shrinkage should be avoided as much as possible in these special situations by using techniques of maxillomandibular fixation (MMF) and internal or external fixation devices or splints. Immediate reconstruction can be planned in clean wounds. Need for transmylohyoid/submental endotracheal intubation as an alternative to tracheostomy should be explored in discussion with the anaesthesia team [6], especially in panfacial trauma involving nasal bones and skull base fractures needing fixation of maxilla and mandible.

60.7 Intra-operative Details

The essential in treating panfacial fractures is obtaining adequate fixation at key buttresses (Fig. 60.9a, b, Fig 55.2). Its description was first given by Cryer in 1916 [7]. This helps in creating the outer framework for fixation of other fractures.

60.7.1 Buttresses of the Facial Skeleton

These are the regions of thick bones which neutralise the forces applied onto them.

Outcome of maxillofacial reconstruction in terms of restoration of facial height, width and projection in addition to restoring the occlusion depends on proper reduction and fixation of these buttresses [8, 9] (Table 60.2).

They are important to:
1. Maintain projection and protection of airway
2. Anchor suspension of musculo-aponeurotic system
3. Protection of skull base and structures above like brain and eye with their adjoining structures from masticatory forces

60.7.2 Key Contributors to Facial Architecture

- Central facial width: fronto-naso-orbital-ethmoid (FNOE) complex, palate and the mandibular arch
- Lateral facial width: Frontal bar, zygomatic arches, malar eminences and mandibular angles
- Projection: frontal bone, frontonasomaxillary buttresses, zygomatic arches and mandible from angle to symphysis
- Facial height: frontal bone, midface buttresses, mandibular angles and condyles

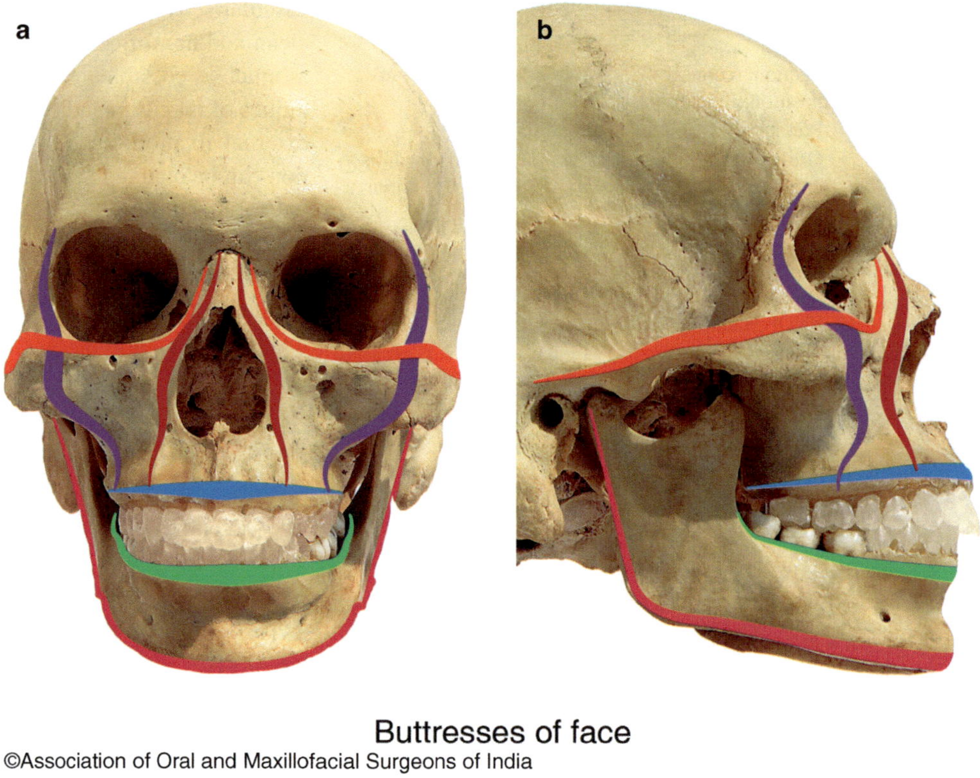

Fig. 60.9 (**a**, **b**) Schematic markings of facial buttresses (Correlate with Table 60.2) (Also see Fig. 55.2)

Table 60.2 Buttress of facial skeleton (colour codes of Fig. 60.9 marked)

Vertical buttresses	Horizontal buttresses
Nasomaxillary (red)	Frontal (orange)
Zygomaticomaxillary (purple)	Zygomatic (orange)
Pterygomaxillary	Maxillary (blue)
Condyle and posterior mandible (pink)	Mandibular (green)

60.7.3 Various Approaches to Facial Skeleton

Approaches to individual facial bones are discussed in the respective sections of the book. They are enumerated here for quick reference and revision.

Facial lacerations overlying fractures should be used for access when possible (Fig. 60.10a–d). In situations without any such lacerations, appropriate incisions for respective fractures should be used as described in other sections of this book.

Subciliary or transconjunctival incisions are commonly used to provide access to infraorbital rim and orbital floor; lateral brow or upper blepharoplasty incisions provide access to frontozygomatic suture and lateral wall of orbit; intraoral vestibular incision provides access to maxilla and zygomatic buttress; and coronal incision provides access to frontal, fronto-naso-ethmoid complex, zygomatic arches and roof of orbit.

Mandible symphysis, parasymphysis, can be approached through intraoral vestibular or crevicular incisions. Mandibular angle is approached intraorally through an extended 3rd molar incision alone or in combination with a transbuccal approach using a trochar and cannula. The condylar head will need to be approached through preauricular or bicoronal incision, whereas the mandibular subcondyle and ramus can be approached through retromandibular or peri-angular incision. Endoscopic approach to the mandibular condyle is been popularised in a few units (see Chap. 54 for details on endoscopic approach to condylar fractures).

Sequencing of fixation in panfacial fractures is a challenging task. The sequencing will alter slightly depending on clinical and radiological evaluation.

60.8 Sequencing Options

There are two options for sequencing:

1. *Bottom to top* [10, 11]: This involves restoring the maxillomandibular unit using occlusion as guide and fixing maxilla and mandible using semi-rigid or rigid fixation techniques. Thereon reduction and fixation proceeds in caudal direction starting from calvarium. The other fractures are then restored in a build-out fashion with maxilla and mandible being a stable base
2. *Top to bottom*: This involves starting with the reduction and fixation at the level of the calvarium. Then the operator proceeds in a caudal direction with reduction and fixation. In this top to bottom sequencing technique, establishing proper occlusion with MMF is no less

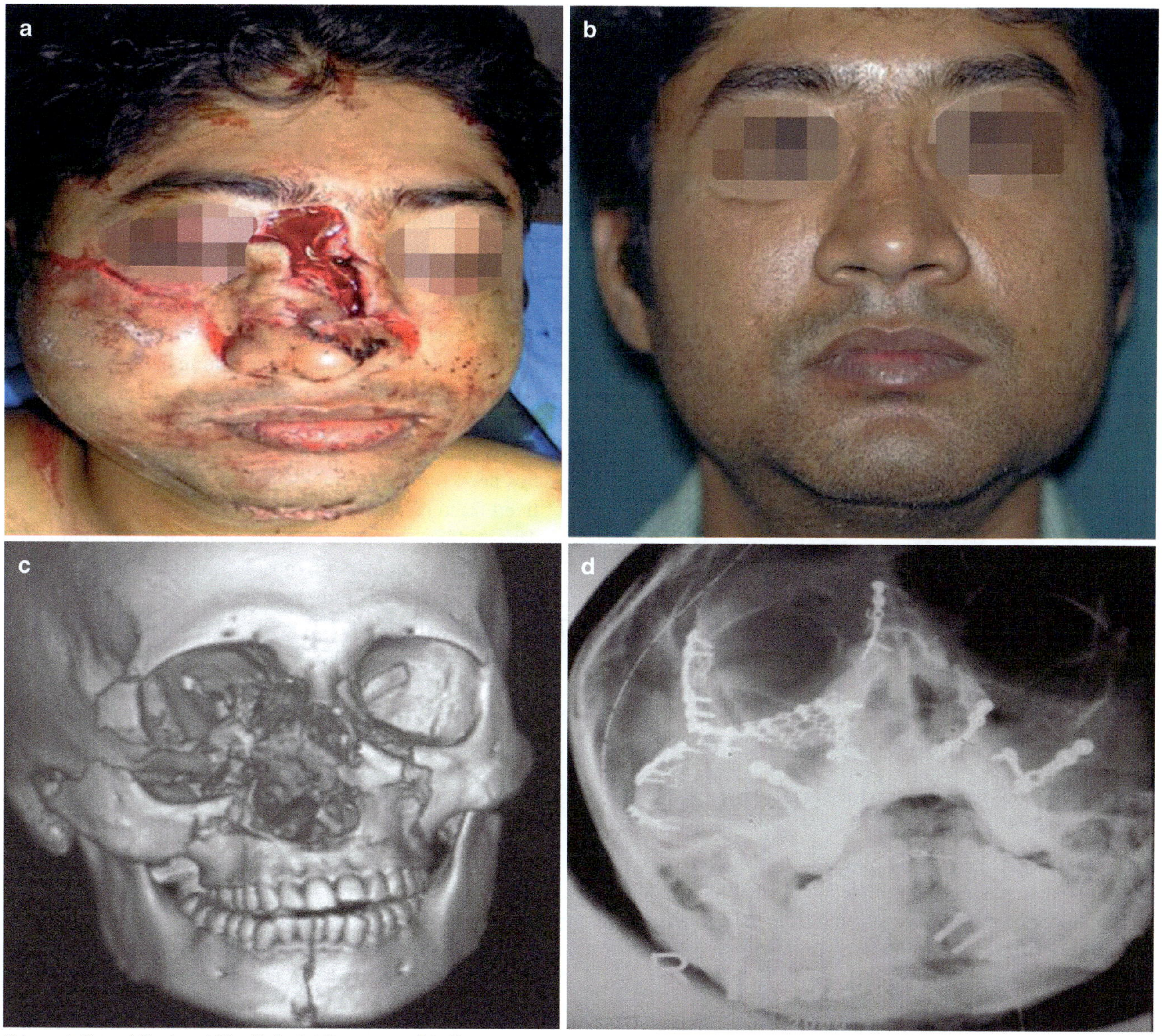

Fig. 60.10 (**a–d**) Use of existing laceration to achieve optimal results

important,and is surely done prior to rigid fixation of Leforte I and mandibular fractures.

Although author's preference is "bottom to top" approach, as establishing functional occlusion is of prime importance, a combination of both the approaches might be necessary in many situations (Fig. 60.11).

60.8.1 Bottom to Top Approach

1. When using this approach one is committed to using the mandible as guide for establishing the height, width and projection of face. Hence after occlusion is established, the mandible is rigidly fixed from one condyle to the other. This makes it necessary to plate minimum one condyle in case bilateral condylar fracture. It is necessary to ensure proper seating of mandibular condyle into the glenoid fossa.
2. Further sequencing will depend on presence or absence of palatal fracture and its nature (comminuted or not). In any case it is very important to establish width of midface correctly so as to achieve optimal functional and aesthetic results.
3. Use of splints made on dental models after model surgery serves an ideal and desirable method to establish correct width of middle and lower face particularly when there is comminution of maxilla and mandible. Use of conventional acrylic splints is the easiest and least time consuming. 3D splint has led to more accurate and predictable results but adds on to the time and cost.

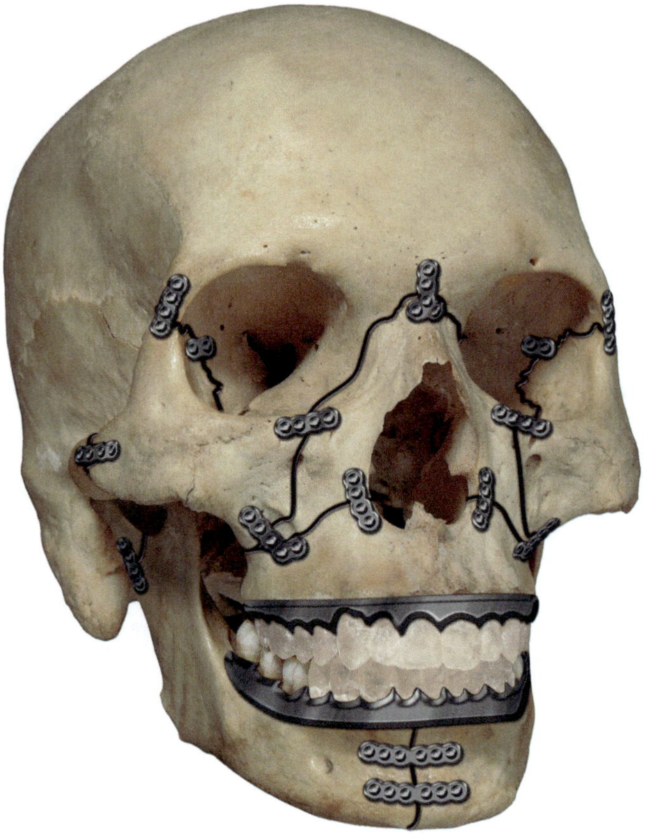

Fig. 60.11 Use of combination techniques to achieve stable fixation schematic diagram

4. The next step is to begin the reduction and fixation of the remainder of the midface starting from the calvarium and working in a caudal direction similar to "top to down" sequencing.

60.8.2 Top to Bottom Approach

1. The reconstruction sequence to re-establish midfacial pillars (buttresses) and dimensions starts with the most reliable and stable point on calvarium and on the side with the least comminution.
2. The calvarial, frontal sinus and orbital roof fractures are addressed first using stable point/region on calvarium as reference point for reconstruction of midface.
3. The zygoma is positioned into its proper three-dimensional position, almost as a flat structure and confirming that lateral wall of orbit is in alignment with the greater wing of sphenoid. This helps proper establishment of width and anterior-posterior projection of face. Approximation of the sphenozygomatic suture in the lateral wall of the orbit should be a guide to reduction in cases of comminuted zygomatic fractures [12]

   Fixing the zygomatic arch increases the accuracy of multidimensional reconstruction (frontozygomatic suture, infraorbital rim, zygomaticomaxillary buttress, zygomatic arch) of fractured and comminuted zygoma [13, 14].
4. The infraorbital rims and NOE complex are properly aligned to complete the reconstruction of the periorbital area.
5. Where reconstruction of the medial canthal tendon is necessary, it can be addressed towards the end of the procedure.
6. The next step in midface reconstruction is fixation across the Le-Fort I and II level. Maxillomandibular fixation may be done at this stage. If everything has been perfectly aligned, these fractures should also align adequately. Splints play a significant role in determining the facial width at Le-fort I level. Malalignment at this level signifies need for reassessment and realignment of previously fixed fractures.

   The midface, because of weak bone structure and comminuted fracture pattern, must be considered a dependent and less stable structure.
7. From an aesthetic standpoint, a minimal malalignment at the Le-Fort I level is not as noticeable as a malalignment of the orbits.
8. Fractures of the inferior orbital rim and orbital floor can be now addressed as the true volume of the orbital defect can be seen once other fractures are aligned.
9. The mandibular fractures are then fixed. Condyle fractures may be addressed with separate incisions or managed conservatively depending on the displacement and influence on the vertical height of the mandible, as discussed previously.

   Tulio etal advocated fixation of condylar fractures as the first step in fixation of pan facial fractures. In their study there was no evidence of dental or skeletal alterations and measurement of the mandibular ramus and radiographic examination show that posterior facial height as well as projection and width of the inferior lower third of the face, was restored. The correct timing of surgical intervention and the use of rigid fixation allows the restoration of the morphological and functional nature of the face after pan facial fractures [15].
10. The occlusion should be rechecked, and rigid or elastic maxillomandibular fixation may be considered as necessary for 4–6 weeks. The occlusal splints may be fixed using wires for the period of MMF as a guide to maintaining the occlusion.

    The sequencing for pan-facial fractures depends more on the clinical situation, than on predefined algorithms as the patterns of clinical presentation may be diverse. However, the general consensus in current literature emphasizes that the the dental units are given priority for providing guidance. The dental arches are first stabilised to form a

Table 60.3 Bottom-up inside-out and top-down outside-in, comparison of sequencing

Bottom-up	Top-down
Maxillomandibular fixation (MMF), splints for palate and mandibular lingual in case of gross comminution	Fix calvarium, frontal sinus and orbital roof fractures sequentially
Fix mandibular fractures (symphysis/body/ramus)	Fix zygomaticomaxillary complex (including arch) fractures, with proper alignment of infraorbital rims
Fix condylar fractures, at least one when fracture is bilateral	Fix naso-orbito-ethmoid complex, and nasal fractures
Fix maxilla at LeFort I level	Maxillomandibular fixation (MMF), splints for palate and mandibular lingual in case of gross comminution
Fix calvarium, frontal sinus and orbital roof fractures sequentially	Fix maxilla at Lefort I level
Fix zygomaticomaxillary complex (including arch) fractures, with proper alignment of infraorbital rims	Fix condylar fractures, at least one when fracture is bilateral
Fix naso-orbito-ethmoid complex, and nasal fractures	Repair of Mandibular fractures

cohesive unit, followed by the mandible in its horizontal and vertical dimensions (10, 19) (also see Manson 2012 in additional reading). The mid face is then managed using a top-down or a bottom-up method depending on the presence or absence of bony defects in the calvarium.

60.8.3 Essentials in Either Approach

1. Soft tissue repair and closure of wounds/incisions of intraoral and pharyngeal areas should be done prior to maxillomandibular fixation. In some cases it might be essential to temporarily release MMF to close lacerations and redo MMF later.
2. Laceration which would be concealed under the splint should be closed prior to fixation of splints.
3. Thoroughly debride perforating wounds before closure.
4. Extraoral incisions and lacerations communicating with the oral cavity should be closed from deep (mucosal) to superficial (skin) in multiple layers.

The sequence of the above approaches are compared in Table 60.3.

Author follows the *"Wire before you plate"* principle.

It is author's preference to use initial wire osteosynthesis stainless steel (SS) for better alignment and anatomical reduction at multiple sites before plating. This technique also does away with the requirement of holding fragments together, and with less of instrumentation in the surgical field, there is an obvious ease of plating more precisely. Wire osteosynthesis should be removed following fixation of the fractures to avoid or prevent reaction between dissimilar metals, namely, SS (stainless steel) and Ti (titanium).

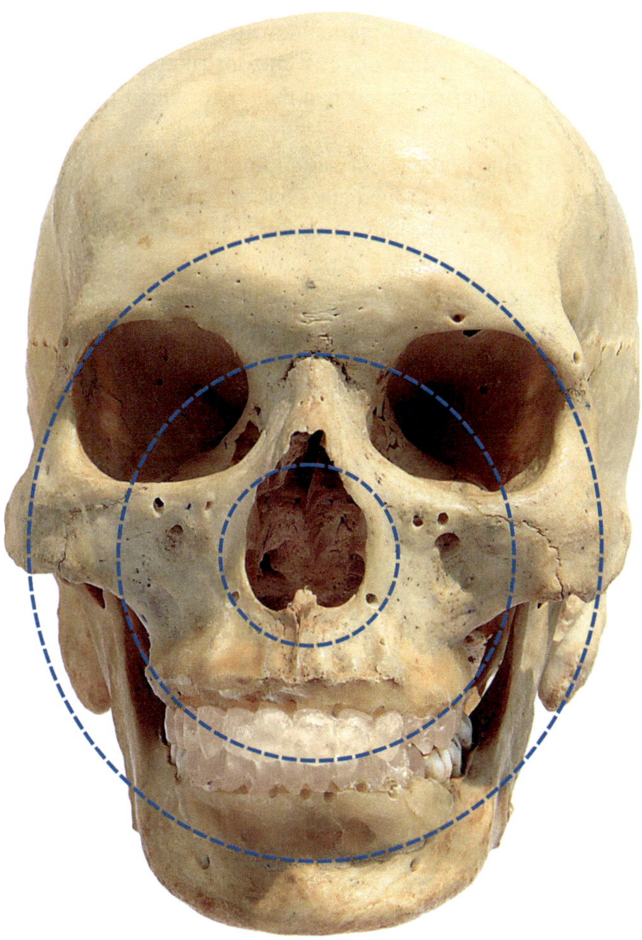

Fig. 60.12 Three concentric circles used as a guide to the reduction of panfacial fractures (Adapted from: H.C Killey. Fractures of Middle-third of facial Skeleton, Issue 3 of Dental Practitioners Handbook, No.3)

There are other sequencing methodologies and philosophies as suggested by other authors.

Manson et al. put forward a highly conceptualised treatment protocol where face is divided into groups, units and sections, and each section is assembled in three dimensions. Soft tissue is considered the "fourth dimension" of facial reconstruction. They advised bone reconstruction to be completed as early as possible to minimise soft tissue shrinkage, stiffness and scarring of soft tissues in non-anatomic position [1, 16].

Killey and Kay demonstrated the fixation of panfacial fractures first in the outer ring followed by the middle ring and lastly the nasal complex in the inner ring (Fig. 60.12).

Inside-out sequence was also found to show good results by Kim et al. [17].

The occlusion first approach, with initial reduction of larger segments, enables effective reconstruction of multiple segments. Smaller segments can then be oriented to fixation of these fractures [18].

Role of bone grafts in very comminuted fractures or missing bone demands immediate bone grafting to produce a stable outcome. Commonly used areas of bone and cartilage grafts are rib, calvarium, iliac crest and conchal cartilage [19]. Recipient site requirements determine the ideal donor site for replacing bone. Revascularisation potential and mechanical needs of the donor site are two factors known to influence this [20].

60.9 Paediatric Panfacial Fractures

They are rare and different as the cranium to face ratio is 8:1, and also differential growth in eyes, brain and face makes a difference in pattern and incidence of fractures. Children should not be treated as small adults as its not only important to restore them to normal form and function, but the growth potential also should be taken into consideration. One must remember that both injury and treatment can lead to growth disturbances, and hence many times conservative management is preferred. Splints are the mainstay in treatment of paediatric fractures (Figs. 52.50 and 52.51). Panfacial fractures are preferably treated with resorbable plates to prevent growth disturbances and damage to tooth buds. This also avoids second surgery for plate removal. Furher, it must be kept in mind that minor occlusal discrepancies are self-corrective during transitional dentition phase or can be treated easily with orthodontics at later date. Major emphasis should be on preventing deformities in central midface. Paediatric patients have to be followed up till growth has completed. In developing countries wire/resorbable suture osteosynthesis can be utilised for economic reasons and availability [21].

60.10 Complications

Complications associated with panfacial injuries include those associated with individual fractures of frontal sinus, nasal and fronto-naso-ethmoid, zygomatic, maxillary and mandibular fractures.

- Motor and sensory deficits of motor and sensory nerves like anaesthesia, paresthesia and weakness
- Reduction in posterior facial height
- Anterior open bite
- Increase in facial width secondary to reduction of anterior-posterior facial projection
- Traumatic telecanthus
- Orbital deformities
- Lacrimal apparatus injuries/dacryocystitis
- Malocclusion
- Nasal obstruction and external nasal deformity
- Cerebrospinal fluid leak
- Anosmia
- Blindness
- Temporomandibular joints dysfunction
- Oro nasal fistula from wide palatal fractures (Fig. 55.25)

60.11 Tips and Tricks

1. Panfacial fractures do not follow specific patterns but occur in variety of combinations involving all facial subunits.
2. Discuss with patients' relatives about realistic outcomes of surgery. Use of patient photographs prior to injury may act as a guide for the surgeon to establish treatment goals. This may be challenging to assess with the oedema and disfigurement following trauma. Making a record of intra-operative and post-operative photographs is a good practice for comparison and documentation.
3. In patients with displaced midface fractures and bilaterally displaced mandibular condyles, it is important to fix at least one condyle anatomically by open method in order to obtain adequate mandibular positioning and posterior facial height.
4. In either approaches to panfacial fractures seating of condyle into glenoid fossa is absolutely mandatory.
5. If prolonged ventilation is anticipated tracheostomy, percutaneous endoscopic gastrostomy (PEG) should be considered.
6. Vertical and horizontal buttresses should be established and fixed (to attain correct facial width and height) before orbital walls and rim correction.
7. Special attention should be paid to soft tissue repair and need for suspension, more particularly to fractures involving FNOE region.
8. Bicoronal exposure allows simultaneous harvesting of calvarial bone graft for bony augmentation and reconstruction like in blow-out orbital fractures.
9. Establish zygomatic arch as linear structure to get perfect facial projection and width.
10. Inadequate and delayed FNOE complex fractures treatment is usually a disaster and at most times is only partially correctable by secondary surgeries.

11. Preoperative arch impressions and splints fabrication have a major role to play in preventing oro-nasal communication and establishing facial width.
12. MMF is mandatory for proper occlusion intra-operatively. Elastics may be needed during follow-up.
13. Most common residual deformity associated with panfacial fractures is lack of projection, increased facial width, malocclusion, enophthalmos and lacrimal dysfunction.
14. Complete removal of all mucosa and blockage/sealing of fronto-nasal duct should be done before cranialisation or obliteration of frontal sinus.
15. Documentation of details of injury is essential of medico-legal reasons, more so of the mechanism and time of injury; these details if necessary can be noted from other observers. Photographs can serve as legal documentation. These should be taken following a valid patient consent.
16. Close soft tissues from deep to superficial and from intraoral to extraoral. Complete intraoral closure prior to securing the MMF. Debride contaminated wounds thoroughly before closure.
17. Forced duction test is essential before and during surgery in fractures involving orbital walls (Fig. 56.21).
18. Caution: removal of throat pack is a joint responsibility of the anaesthetist and surgeon.

60.12 Case Scenario

Case 1:
(Figs. 60.13a–d, 60.14a–f, and 60.15a–c) Shows Management of a Case of Pan Facial Fracture

Figure 60.13 shows the pre operative CT scans, Fig. 60.14 show the various surgical approaches used for internal fixation and Fig. 60.14 shows the post operative radiographs showing the fixation.

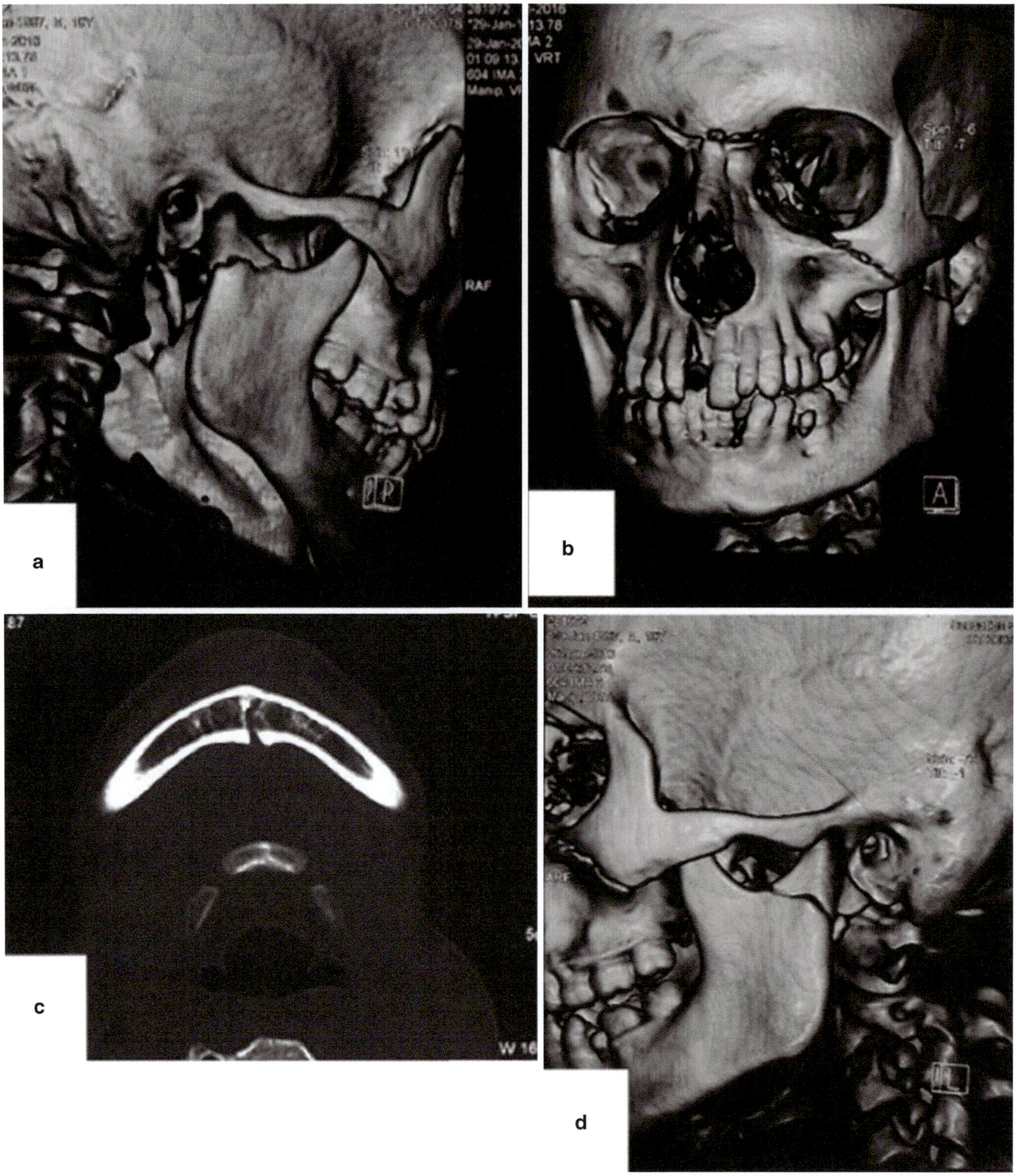

Fig. 60.13 (**a**–**d**) Panfacial trauma preoperative CT scan. (**a**) Right condylar fracture. (**b**) Naso-ethmoid complex fracture, left zygomatic buttress and infraorbital rim fracture. (**c**) Mandibular symphysis fracture. (**d**) Left condylar fracture

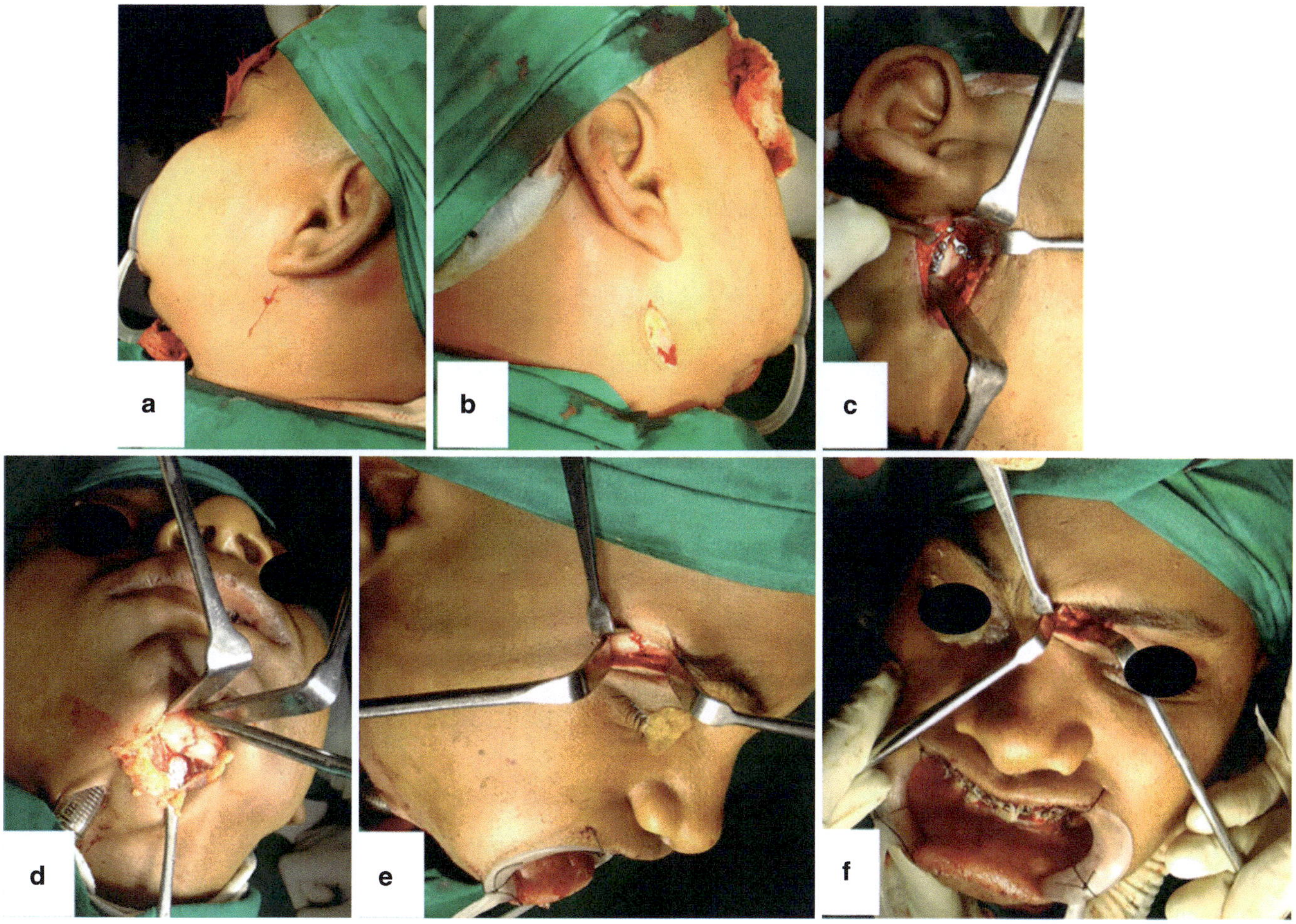

Fig. 60.14 (**a**–**f**) Panfacial trauma intra-operative images of case shown in Fig. 60.14. (**a**) Left retromandibular approach (**b**) Right retromandibular approach. (**c**) Right condyle plating. (**d**) Symphysis exposure. (**e**) Right frontozygomatic fracture. (**f**) Naso-ethmoid fracture exposure

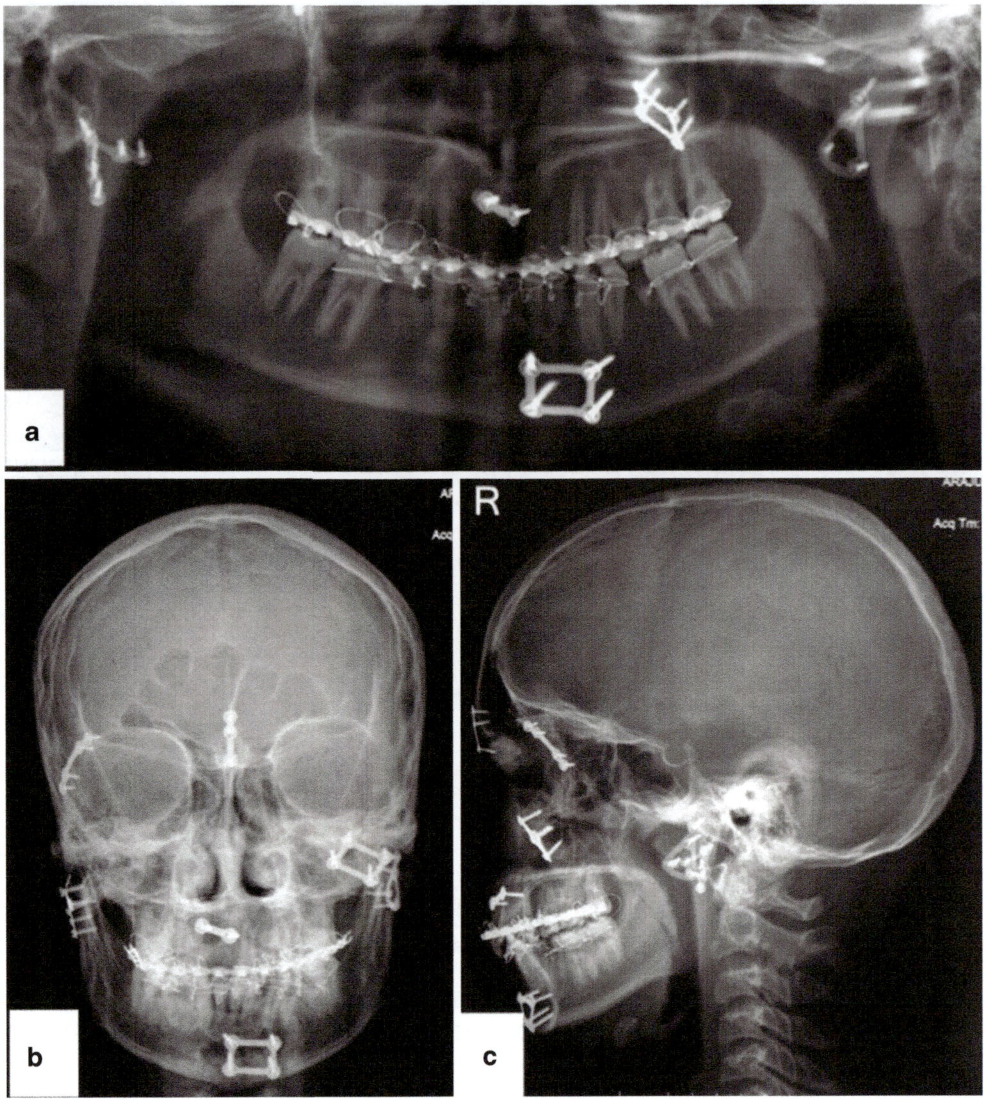

Fig. 60.15 (**a**–**c**) Panfacial trauma post-operative radiographs of case shown in Fig. 60.14. (**a**) OPG. (**b**) PA cephalogram. (**c**) Lateral cephalogram

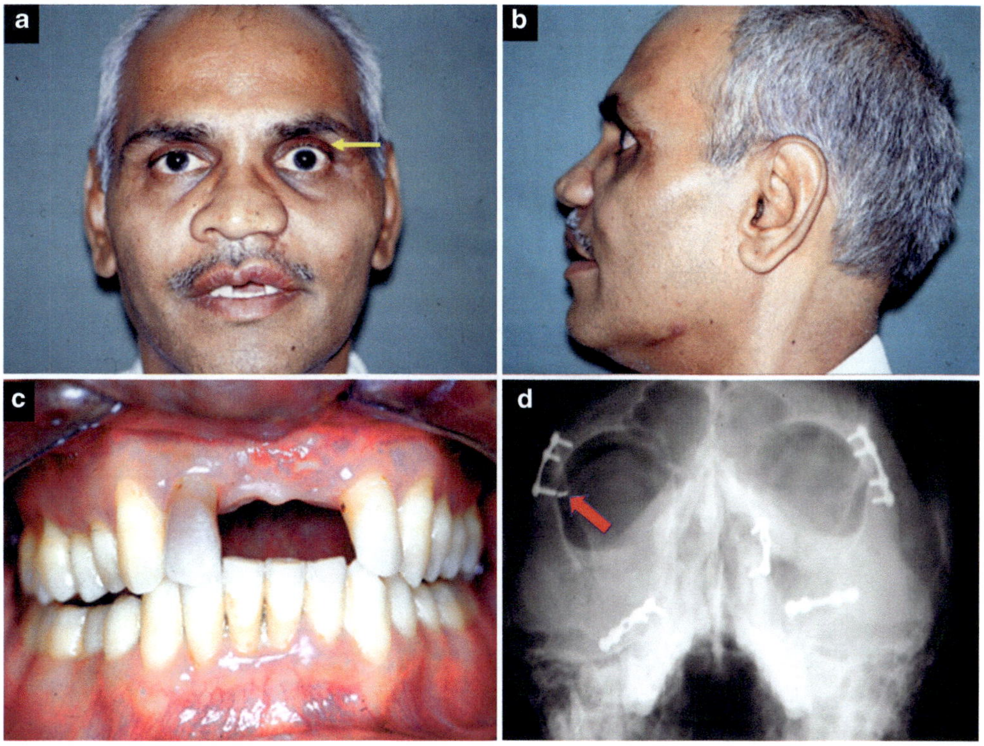

Fig. 60.16 (**a–d**) Pre-operative photographs. (**a**) Frontal view showing asymmetrical face, alar bases, lip and deepened supra tarsal fold (yellow arrow). (**b**) Lateral view showing upturned lip, increased vertical dimension, scar on left body of mandible. (**c**) Malocclusion with anterior open bite. (**d**) Pre-operative P.A. Waters view showing inadequate fixation of midfacial fractures and foreign body within right orbit (Red arrow)

Case 2 (Figs. 60.16a–d, 60.17a–e, and 60.18a–d)

Back ground:

This case was treated in 1997 by the first author, when CT scan was a novelty rather than necessity. Plating system used was stainless steel.

A 43 years male with no comorbidities was referred by dental surgeon for correction of malocclusion and asymmetrical face. Patient had a history of RTA with panfacial fractures, and head injury, cerebral oedema 3 months prior. He was treated conservatively for head injury and had no residual neurological deficit. He was treated by other specialist for panfacial fractures by ORIF and then referred to dentist for prosthetic correction of occlusion. Patient insisted upon simultaneous correction of occlusion and asymmetric face.

Patient reported with complaints of:

Inability to masticate, changed pattern of upper and lower teeth meeting , crooked nose with asymmetric nasal bases, sunken left eyeball, diplopia on superior gaze, and changed facial appearance compared to preinjury status.

Clinical Findings (Fig. 60.16a–d)

1. Significant change in facial appearance as compared to pre-trauma, pre-treatment appearance
2. Elongated face
3. Upturned upper lip and acute nasolabial angle
4. Deviated and depressed nose, with dissimilar alar bases
5. Enophthalmos with increased supratarsal fold left eye. (yellow arrow)
6. Changed pupillary levels, and excessive scleral show of left eye
7. Increased width of face more so on left side
8. Malocclusion, with anterior open bite, increased vertical dimension of face due to posterior and inferior displacement of maxilla with gagging.
9. Scars in Bilateral frontozygomatic, left infraorbital, left mandibular body region.
10. Left mandibular body fracture fixed adequately but patient had left marginal mandibular nerve paresis/ injury.
11. Total mobility of middle third of facial skeleton suggestive of non-union/malunion.

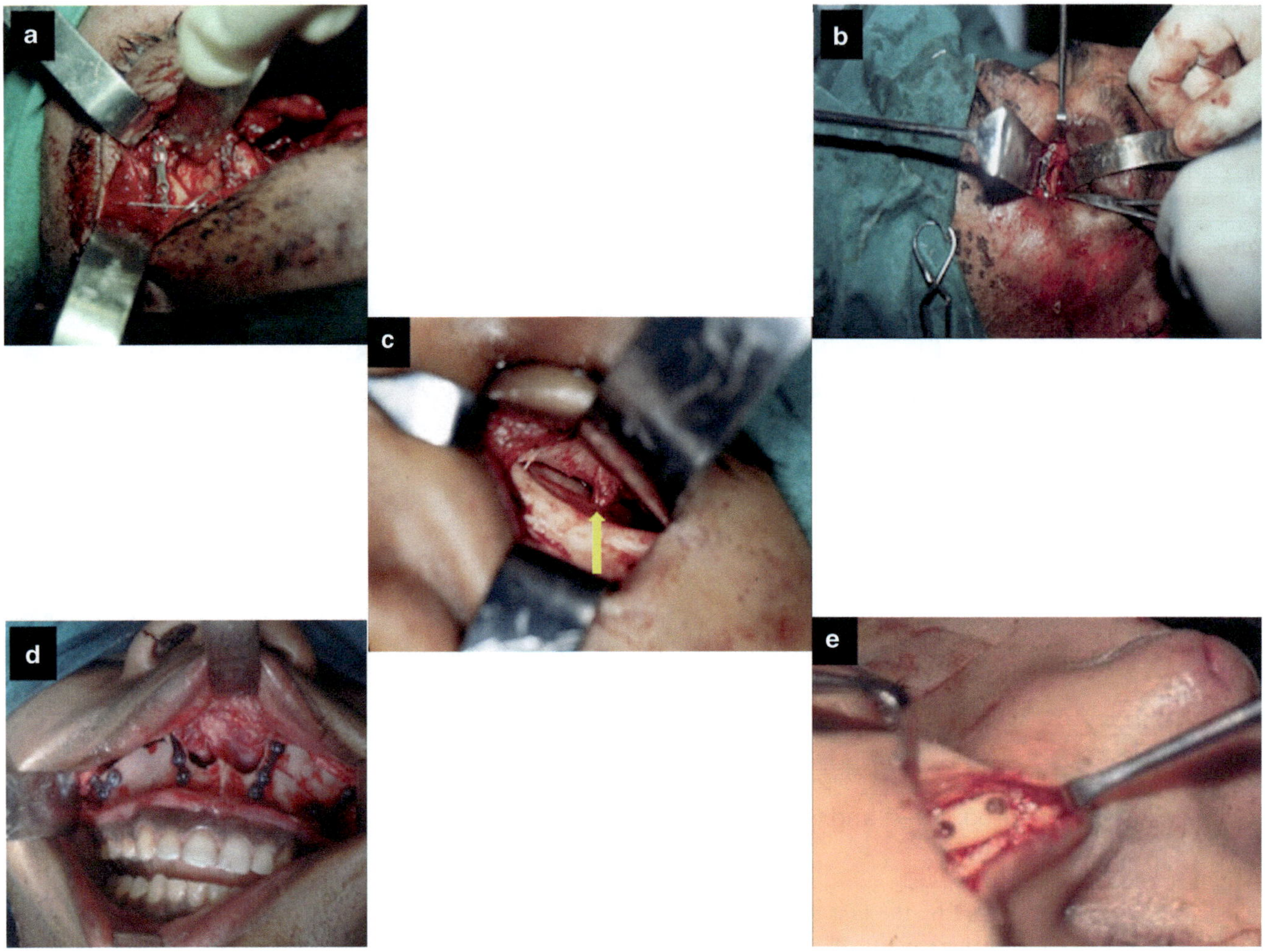

Fig. 60.17 (**a–d**) Intra-operative representative photos. (**a**) Fixation at FZ suture. (**b**) Fixation at inferior orbital rim. (**c**) Entrapment of inferior rectus, left orbital floor (yellow arrow). (**d**) Fixation of LeFort I fracture. (**e**) Fixation of bone graft to augment nasal bridge

Diagnosis:

1. Patient was counselled and asked to undergo X-rays to have 3 dimensional orientation. 1. PA Caldwell.
2. PA Water sinus (full face),
3. Base of skull for zygomatic arches and mandible.
4. Upper and lower occlusal topographic. CT scan of face with 3D reconstruction was not done for financial reasons. Remember CT scans were relatively expensive then.
5. Routine preoperative preparation.

Radiological Findings

Inadequate fixation seen at bilateral Fronto Zygomatic (FZ) suture, LeFort I,II,III level, and FNOE complex. A Foreign body (broken drill) was seen in Right orbit near FZ suture (red arrow). Mandible was fixed adequately both radiologically and clinically.

Plan of action/surgical approach (Fig. 60.17a–e)

1. Transmylohyoid intubation.
2. Mandible fracture being adequately fixed during previous surgery was not addressed
3. Mobilisation/osteotomy of midfacial skeleton to achieve adequate occlusion, projection of midface and reduce mid-facial width.
4. Approach midface fractures through existing scars at FZ suture, and left infraorbital region, subciliary approach to right infraorbital region.
5. Horizontal incision at nasal bridge for alignment of FNOE complex. (Fig 60.17e)
6. Intraoral sub labial approach for LeFort I fracture.
7. Iliac bone grafting at LeFort I level and nasal bridge to achieve prominence and augment the same.
8. Bone graft at left floor of orbit to correct enophthalmos and diplopia.
9. Alar cinch for flared left ala of nose.

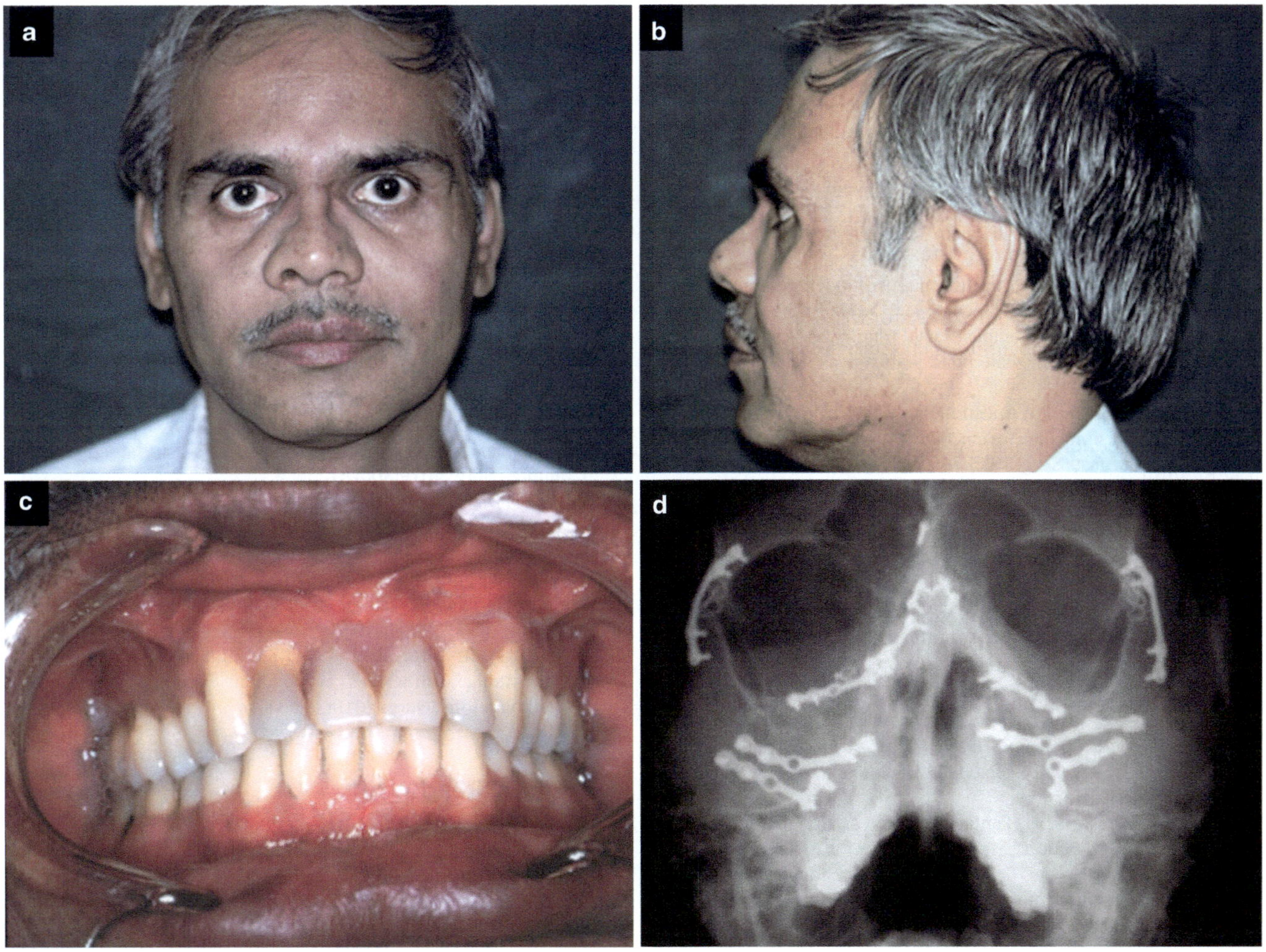

Fig. 60.18 (a–d) Ten years Post-operative photographs. (a) Frontal view showing restored symmetry. (b) Lateral view showing correct lip positioning, corrected vertical dimension, scar on left body of mandible. (c) Corrected occlusion. (d) Post-operative P.A. Waters view (Full face) showing adequate fixation of midfacial fractures at all the struts

10. Avoid MMF. Post-op X-ray (Fig. 60.18d) shows plating with wires, they were not removed as hardware used then was stainless steel so there was no issue of Eddy's current due to dissimilar metals.

60.13 Conclusion

The increasing number of RTA and related CMF injuries suggests the need for immediate attention from the concerned authorities, to enforce strict laws like mandatory use of seat belts and total head and face guard (that suit climatic conditions) rather than the conventional helmets. Restricting the use of mobile phones and head phones while driving may lead to decrease in the incidence of RTA. If RTA is considered an epidemic of modern times, then prevention is its vaccine. Increasing public awareness towards voluntary use of safety measures for their own safety rather than merely obeying the rules can reduce most of the cranio-maxillofacial injuries.

Panfacial trauma can appear complex and challenging to treat but is actually the conglomeration of treating individual fractures that are a common place in maxillofacial injuries (it would be wise to "simplify" the fracture in the minds' eye view and formulating a treatment plan). Adhering to a treatment protocol and treating each fracture as a unit, with adequate fixation, enable the surgeon to obtain good results. Development of a sequential and methodical treatment plan prior to surgery and adherence to the basic principles of maxillofacial trauma is vital in treatment of these patients.

References

1. Kelly KJ, Manson PN, Vander Kolk CA, Markowitz BL, Dunham CM, Rumley TO, Crawley WA. Sequencing LeFort fracture treatment (Organization of treatment for a panfacial fracture). J Craniofac Surg. 1990;1(4):168–78.
2. Gadre KS, et al. Incidence and pattern of cranio-maxillofacial injuries: a 22 year retrospective analysis of cases operated at major trauma hospitals/centres in Pune, India. J Maxillofac Oral Surg. 2013;12(4):372–8.
3. Hazen A, Ehiri JE. Road traffic injuries: hidden epidemic in less developed countries. J Natl Med Assoc. 2006;98:73–82.
4. Gruss JS, Phillips JH. Complex facial trauma: the evolving role of rigid fixation and immediate bone graft reconstruction. Clin Plast Surg. 1989;16:93–104.
5. Manson PN, Crawley WA, Yaremchuk M, et al. Midface fractures: advantages of immediate extended open reduction and bone grafting. Plast Reconstr Surg. 1985;76:1–12.
6. Gadre KS, Waknis PP. Transmylohyoid/submental intubation: review, analysis, and refinements. J Craniofac Surg. 2010;21:516–9.
7. Cryer MH. The maxillae. In: The internal anatomy of the face. Philadelphia, PA: Lea & Febiger; 1916. p. 76–7.
8. Manson PN, Hoopes JE, Su CT. Structural pillars of the facial skeleton: an approach to the management of Le Fort fractures. Plast Reconstr Surg. 1980;66:54–62.
9. Manson PN, Clark N, Robertson B, Slezak S, Wheatly M, Vander Kolk C, Iliff N. Subunit principles in midface fractures: the importance of sagittal buttresses,soft-tissue reductions, and sequencing treatment of segmental fractures. Plast Reconstr Surg. 1999;103(4):1287–306.
10. Curtis W, Horswell BB. Panfacial fractures: an approach to management. Oral Maxillofac Surg Clin North Am. 2013;25(4):649–60.
11. Yang R, Zhang C, Liu Y, Li Z, Li Z. Why should we start from mandibular fractures in the treatment of panfacial fractures? J Oral Maxillofac Surg. 2012;70(6):1386–92.
12. Rohner D, Tay A, Meny CS, et al. The sphenozygomatic suture as a key site for osteosynthesis of the orbitozygomatic complex in panfacial fractures: a biomechanical study in human cadavers based on clinical practice. Plast Reconstr Surg. 2002;110:14630–71.
13. Stanley RB Jr. The zygomatic arch as a guide to reconstruction of comminuted malar fractures. Arch Otolaryngol Head Neck Surg. 1989;1150:1459–62.
14. Gruss JS, Van Wyck L, Phillips JH, Antonyshyn O. The importance of the zygomatic arch in complex midfacial fracture repair and correction of posttraumatic orbitozygomatic deformities. Plast Reconstr Surg. 1990;85(6):878–90.
15. Tullio A, Sesenna E. Role of surgical reduction of condylar fractures in the management of panfacial fractures. Br J Oral Maxillofac Surg. 2000;38(5):472–6.
16. Markowitz BL, Manson PN. Panfacial fractures: organization of treatment. Clin Plast Surg. 1989;16:105–14.
17. Kim J, Choi JH, Chung YK, Kim SW. Panfacial bone fracture and medial to lateral approach. Arch Craniofac Surg. 2016;17(4):181–5.
18. Choi JW, Kim MJ. Treatment of panfacial fractures and three-dimensional outcome analysis: the occlusion first approach. J Craniofac Surg. 2019;30(4):1255–8.
19. Gruss JS, Mackinnon SE, Kassel EE, et al. The role of primary bone grafting in complex craniomaxillofacial trauma. Plast Reconstr Surg. 1985;75:17–24.
20. Phillips JH, Forrest CR, Gruss JS. Current concepts in the use of bone grafts in facial fractures. Basic science considerations. Clin Plast Surg. 1992;19:41–58.
21. Iatrou I, et al. Surgical protocols and outcome for the treatment of maxillofacial fractures in children: 9 years' experience. J Craniomaxillofac Surg. 2010;38:511–6.

Additional Reading

Gruss JS, Bubak PJ, Egbert MA. Craniofacial fractures. An algorithm to optimize results. Clin Plast Surg. 1992 Jan;19(1):195–206.

Manson PN. Panfacial Fractures. In: Ehrenfeld M, Manson PN, Prein J, editors. Principles of Internal Fixation of the Craniomaxillofacial Skeleton, Trauma and Orthognathic Surgery. Thieme; 2012. p 292–305.

Residual Deformities of the Maxillofacial Region

61

Samson Jimson

61.1 Introduction

A maxillofacial surgeon plays a vital role in not only restoring the structural form of the maxillofacial unit but also aims to restore the pre-traumatic functional status of the patient. Diagnosis, clinical evaluation with enhanced treatment planning and restoration of aesthetics and function is the key for any maxillofacial surgery. However, it is not always possible to achieve the most appropriate results in all cases. It is not uncommon to see failure or mediocre outcomes following maxillofacial trauma surgery. The outcome of the primary treatment may depend on factors such as the extent of the injury/defect, delay in diagnosis/management, improper treatment plan, lack of utilizing modern diagnostic/treatment planning utilities, poor execution of treatment plan and inexperience of the surgeon. These may lead to not expecting the eventful deformities and not coordinating with other specialists to yield the most standard and deserving treatment for the patient with restoration of both form and function [1–3].

Residual deformities are seen following primary treatment of trauma due to one more reason mentioned earlier. Correction of such residual deformities may be challenging to the surgeon but very often a life-changing experience for patients. It is the experience of the surgeon that helps to recognise the challenges ahead in restoring the form and function. Residual deformities are often evaluated by the extent of deformities following primary management. Apart from reasons that may pertain to the experience of the operating surgeon, pathobiology of the healing zone may also contribute to the residual deformities. A variety of such reasons contributes to both soft tissue and hard tissue defects in the maxillofacial unit. This chapter aims to discuss in detail the clinical evaluation, diagnosis, protocols, management and post-operative care of hard tissue deformities in oral and maxillofacial surgery with emphasis on current trends and future propositions.

S. Jimson (✉)
Department of Oral and Maxillofacial Surgery, Tagore Dental College and hospital, Chennai, India
e-mail: jimsons@tagoredch.in

61.1.1 Preventive Wound Management [4]

Wound management begins right after the soft tissue injury in the primary or acute stage.

Post-traumatic scarring can be reduced considering the following measures:

- Removal of foreign bodies/debris
- Reduce bacterial carriage by copious irrigation
- Judicious debridement to reduce the persistent scarring
- Management of the adjacent tissue with appropriate closure
- Tension free closure, minimising scar formation
- Wound care management by the use of agents that promote healing
- Prophylactic antibiotics in necessary conditions

Soft tissue injuries/scar revision/soft tissue and hard tissue reconstruction related to management of residual deformities have been dealt in detail in respective chapters of this book (refer Chaps. 36, 49, 86 and 88*). Wound care and management begin with preventive measures.*

61.1.2 Volume Issues in Deformities [3]

This section briefly discusses management of volume defects using tissue expanders. Volume issues are to be considered with all excision techniques. Loss of tissue volume due to trauma or contraction of the scar may lead to depression and

K. Bonanthaya et al. (eds.), *Oral and Maxillofacial Surgery for the Clinician*, https://doi.org/10.1007/978-981-15-1346-6_61

distortions that are more obvious than the original scar. Such loss of tissue may require volume replacement that can be achieved by other techniques. Surgical flaps may be commonly used to fill the tissues. Likewise, biological fillers can also be taken into consideration in managing depressed or irregular areas. Tissue debulking can be done whenever there is an excess of tissue volume.

Two methods of tissue transfer can be opted whenever there is loss of tissue: a free skin graft and a skin flap. A free skin graft of limited thickness involves the complete removal from the donor site and then placement on the recipient site for survival. This type of graft will not survive in avascular recipient sites. A skin flap with underlying subcutaneous tissue will carry its blood supply necessary for the survival of the flap. These skin flaps are further divided into local flaps or distant flaps (from distant sites). Single-stage transfer of flaps may be done with microvascular surgical techniques (Chart 61.1 shows types of soft tissue deformities with relation to the volume defects).

61.1.2.1 Minor Loss of Tissue [3]

- Local flaps should always be considered in case of minor loss of tissue. Facial tissue is naturally the first choice due to the colour and texture for replacement of tissue defects that are not too extensive. In such cases of local flaps, skin bordering the deformity should be raised and rotated into the defect, approximating the scar in a favourable position.
- Small scar defects may not yield a good result with split skin grafts, but full-thickness grafts can potentially give good aesthetic results in the repair of small defects.
- Lower eyelid scarring due to ectropion may be corrected using full-thickness graft (Wolfe's graft) that results in predictable function and aesthetics.

61.1.2.2 Major Loss of Tissue [3]

- Traumatic or gunshot injuries may result in a substantial loss of tissues. Majorly these injuries are associated with loss of soft tissue and skeletal structure.
- The replacement of tissue should involve necessary covering, lining and support to the bone or cartilage.
- Flaps used in all anatomical structures like the antrum, orbit, mouth and nose should have necessary lining epithelium; otherwise it will result in contraction of the tissues and exposure of underlying tissues.
- Complications like nasal airway stenosis, oral stenosis, microsomia and obliterated buccal/labial sulcus may occur.
- A split skin graft may be used in case of nasal or buccal defect.
- Double flap with both inner and outer aspects composed of full-thickness skin or subcutaneous tissue may help to increase the flexibility in case of a cheek flap. In such cases, the extent of fibrosis is decreased and thereby helps in increasing flexibility due to the underlying vascularity.
- *Nasal* lining may be provided by approximating the adjacent in-turned flaps of skin around the surrounding defects. A split skin graft should be preferred whenever such approximation is not possible. Hard tissue nasal deformities are discussed elsewhere.
- *Lip defects* may result in loss of larger tissue. Contraction due to lip re-suture may result in the loss of one-third of the available tissue. Local tissue flaps as full-thickness flaps should be considered ahead of tube pedicle flaps. Whenever permissible, it is better to take a full-thickness flap of the cheek or buccal mucosa, rotate it and form a lip and fill the subsequent secondary defect with tube pedicle.

Chart 61.1 Types of soft tissue residual deformities

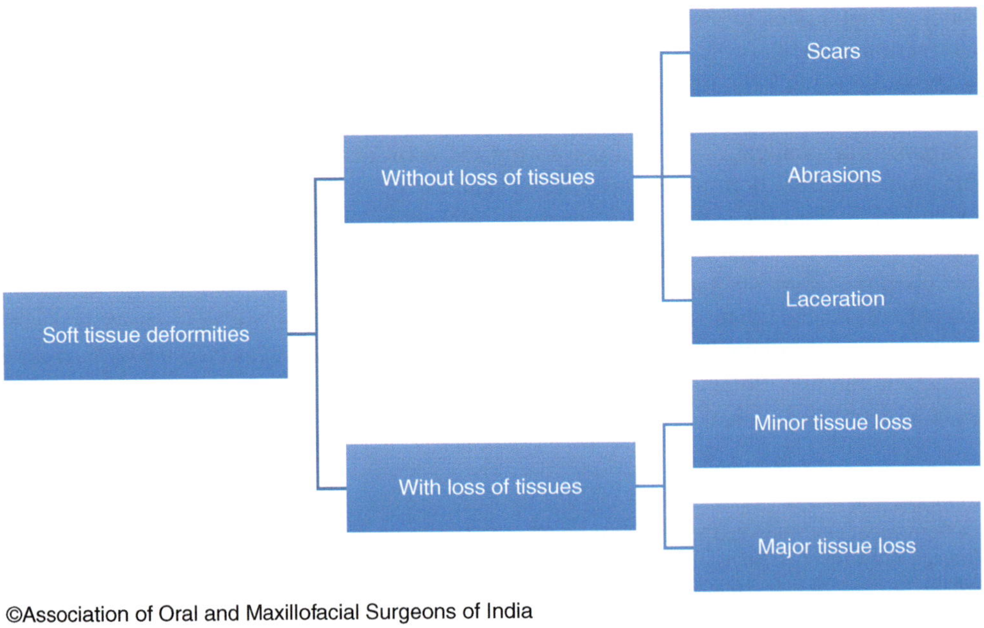

- *Scar adhesions* of the sulcus or obliteration of sulci due to deficient tissues may predispose the difficulty in the construction of a functional and stable prosthesis. The fibrous scar tissue may be excised, or the sulci may be created with dissection followed by insertion of a free split skin graft.
- *Palate*: Substantial loss of tissue may involve the hard palate, soft palate or both areas. Generally, loss of tissue in the hard palate may be closed with an obturator. Scar tissue associated with the hard tissue defect may be managed by dividing the fibrous scar bands and restoring the residual tissues. Rotational flaps may also be used to close the defects. Tissues from additional sources may be used in the closure by using full-thickness flaps. Two-staged full-thickness flaps from the lateral third of the tongue are used, the base of which is divided after 3 weeks. In case of larger defects, myofascial temporalis flaps may be used with downward rotation, and following osteotomy of the zygomatic arch, it may be passed through a mucosal tunnel to reach the oral cavity. Both the flaps provide better results, but the advantage of the latter is being a single-staged technique [3].

61.1.3 Tissue Expanders [4–6]

Tissue expanders are the advised treatment technique when the loss of tissue or the scar surface areas are larger. It is indicated in revision or excision of scar where local or regional flaps may not be feasible to be used in the immediate reconstruction. Although commonly employed for tissue expansion in forehead and scalp, it may be beneficial for any areas with larger defects. Tissue expansion becomes an ideal choice in the scalp due to its inelasticity. It allows replacement of defects with adjacent surrounding tissue which is similar in colour, texture, adnexal structures and innervation (Fig. 61.1)

61.1.3.1 Properties of Tissue Expanders [4, 5, 7–9]

Silastic balloons with self-sealing valves which are used as tissue expanders are implanted beneath the skin.

- These tissue expanders are available in different shapes and sizes and can also be custom-made to fit an irregularly bordered defect.
- It is important to choose an expander of sufficient size to provide the necessary expansive force required for the need in tissue gain for reconstruction.
- The expander has to be 2.5 times that of the scar to be corrected while using a rectangular or crescent-shaped expander. On the other hand, the diameter of the base of the circular expander should be 2.5 times that of the scar to be replaced.
- The expanders must be implanted in a position where ideally a simple advancement, rotation or transposition flaps may be developed later.
- The goal is to have the adjacent healthy tissue expanded and not the scar itself. Hence, the proper placement of the tissue expander is vital.
- Scarred, atrophic areas or sites that have undergone prior radiation therapy are contraindicated.
- Sufficient expander volume must be available.

61.1.3.2 Biomechanical Properties

During the period of tissue expansion, a capsule is formed, and the epidermis is thickened and expanded. Increased mitotic activity is seen evidently using the microscope during the expansion. The dermal thickness, which decreases during the expansion phase, returns to normalcy in 2–3 years. Expanders may also result in decreased adjacent muscle thickness, but without any loss of function. The adipose cells may decrease in number, and subcutaneous thinning may also be seen. Viability of expander is maintained with increased angiogenesis. Bone remodelling may also take place beneath

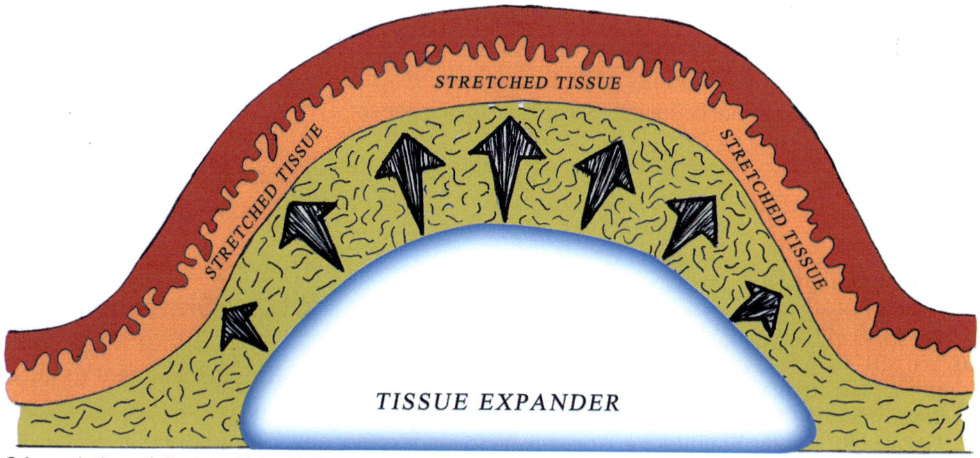

Fig. 61.1 Schematic representation of a tissue expander

the expander. The morphology and number of hair follicles are usually not affected, and hence this is a key in scalp expansion. Treatment duration can be reduced in areas where more than one expander can be placed. The gradual stretching of the tissue over the expanding subcutaneous tissue is called biological creep. Placement of the balloons and allowing a series of inflations and deflations to result in the stretching of the skin are the principles behind tissue expanders. This inherent nature of the skin to expand beyond its natural extensibility is referred to mechanical creep [4, 10].

61.1.3.3 Technique

Expanders are implanted by making incisions at the junction of the scar and the healthy tissue. A pocket is made in an avascular fascial plane. Wound closure is done with layers over the expander. 10% volume of expander may be added at the time of surgery to minimise chances of hematoma formation around the expander. Necrosis of the overlying tissues may occur if any wrinkles are present over the surface of the expanders. If the site allows area for placement for more than one expander, it may reduce the overall treatment duration. Two weeks after placement, the expanders are inflated once or twice in a week. Patient discomfort or blanching over the surface of expander should be observed. Overexpansion of tissue is necessary as there will be a degree of contraction after removal of the expander. Likewise, bony contour changes usually regress without any intervention. The capsule of the expander is released along its margins but is left intact (Fig. 61.2). Generally, a waiting period of 2 weeks should be observed before proceeding to the next stage of the surgery/procedure. This allows the skin tension to reduce before the next stage of the surgery [4, 5].

Advantages

Local usage of tissue by expansion helps in the preservation of the sensation, vascularity and the adnexal structures. This aids well in both aesthetic and functional aspects.

Disadvantages

- Two operative procedures are usually required.
- Frequent inflation of the expanders.
- A temporarily visible deformity when the expander reaches its full inflation may not be socially acceptable by the patient.

Complications

- Pain
- Infection
- Implant failure
- Implant exposure
- Necrosis and tissue breakdown leading to exposure of the expander
- Bony erosion below the implant
- Decreased patient compliance and psychological stress for the patient as the expander increases in size creating a transient compromise in aesthetics

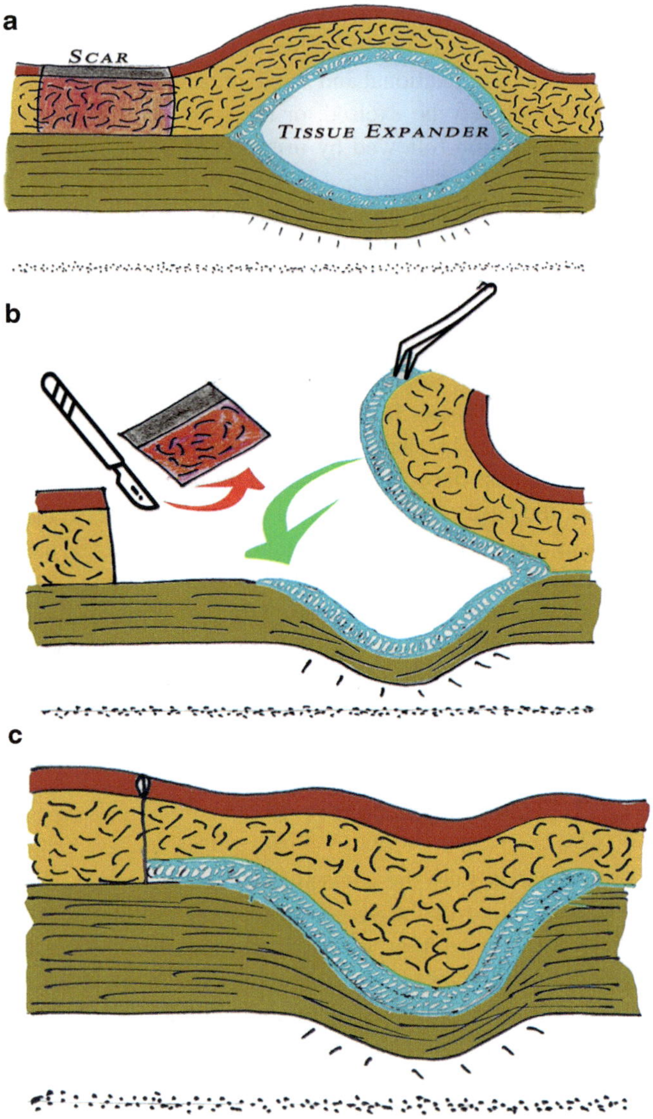

Fig. 61.2 Conventional method of tissue expander in management of scar tissue. (**a**) Expander placed near scar tissue and tissue expansion seen. (**b**) Adjacent scar tissue removed before closure. (**c**) Overexpanded tissue closed with adjacent scar tissue removed and the capsule is left intact with release along its margin

This chapter further discusses the use of grafts in residual deformities, management of hard tissue residual deformities and recent advances.

61.2 Grafts in Residual Deformity

Soft tissue and hard tissue defects are best managed by the use of grafts. Secondary or residual use of grafts and flaps is essential in restoring the hard tissue and soft tissue defects. The scope of this chapter briefly describes grafts used in residual deformities. This section also outlines the

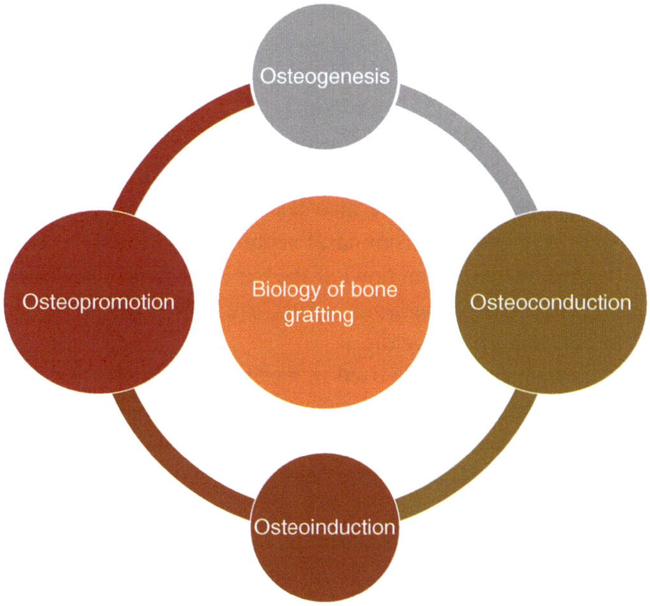

Chart 61.2 Essentials in biology of bone grafting

Table 61.1 Biology of bone grafting

Osteoconduction	Mechanism in which the graft substance serves as a scaffold for new bone growth aided by native bone. Osteoblasts from the source utilize the bone graft as a structural scaffold on which new bone generation takes place. A bone graft should be ideally osteoconductive. Ex: Calcium sulphate, calcium phosphate cements, ceramics, collagen, synthetic polymers
Osteoinduction	Mechanism involves stimulation of osteoprogenitor cells → differentiation into osteoblasts → formation of new bone. Ex: Bone morphogenic proteins. It is ideal to have grafts that are osteoconductive and osteoinductive in nature Ex: DBM (Demineralised Bone Graft), BMPs, growth factors, genetic therapy
Osteopromotion	Enhancing osteoconduction without osteoinductive properties. It promotes action and can't grow bone independently. Ex: Enamel matrix derivative enhances the osteoinductive property of demineralised freeze-dried bone allograft
Osteogenesis	Formation of new bone with the help of osteoblasts originating from the bone graft material. Ex: Bone marrow aspirate (BMA)

biology behind bone grafting and types of bone grafts (Chart 61.2).

61.2.1 Ideal Characteristics of Bone Graft Material [11]

- Biocompatible
- Promotes cell differentiation and proliferation
- Less risk of infection
- Non-toxic
- Non-immunogenic
- Maintains volume over time
- Balance in resorption rate and bone formation
- Ability to replace site with new bone growth

61.2.2 Biology of Bone Grafting

Biology of bone grafting includes the following rationale [12–17] (Table 61.1):

1. Osteoconduction
2. Osteoinduction
3. Osteopromotion
4. Osteogenesis

61.2.2.1 Types and Tissue Sources for Grafting (Table 61.2 and Chart 61.3)

Boyne's Ideal Characteristics of Bone Grafts [18]

- It should be easily and readily available and should not require additional surgical intervention in a second donor site.
- It should not stimulate any immunological response.
- It should stimulate rapid osteogenesis.
- It should enhance re-vascularisation and neo-angiogenesis.
- It should be highly osteoinductive.
- It should be osteoconductive in nature.
- It should not affect or impede bone growth.

Grafts play a major role in primary or secondary/residual management, eventually playing plays a vital role in reconstruction. Bone grafts in residual deformities are ideal to fill volume defects and also aid in reconstruction. Various types and sources of grafts have already been listed (Chart 61.3).

Table 61.2 Types of bone grafts

Type	Highlights
Autografts	• Bone grafting from the same individual • Bone harvesting from nonessential sites • Less risk of graft rejection • Osteoconductive, Osteoinductive and osteogenic • Requires an additional surgical site and risk of infection, pain and complications in the donor site • Gold standard and available in many forms
Allografts	• Bone grafting from another individual (Human donors). Bone is taken from cadavers. Although it can be from living donors, it is more likely to come from dead individuals • Properties may be limited due to preparation and sterilisation • Preparation removes risk of antigenicity • Limited risk of disease transmission • Osteoinductive • Gold standard and available in many forms
Synthetic variants	Artificial bone substitutes. Constitutes mineral to organic matrix ratio close to that of normal human bone. Grafts not taken from living donors
Xenografts	Grafts from species other than humans
Alloplastic grafts	• Strictly a synthetic bone substitute • Osteoconductive in nature • No risk of disease transmission • Unlimited graft options
Growth factors	Produced by recombinant DNA technology. Consists of human growth factors or morphogenic proteins

61.2.3 Bone Grafts in Hard Tissue Residual Deformities

61.2.3.1 Nasal Deformities [19]

- Bone grafts for nasal deformities can be readily obtained from cranial bone or iliac bone crest. Costochondral and tibial bone grafts have also been used earlier. Cartilage may be harvested from nasal septum. It may also be harvested from conchal bowl of the ear in case of septal bone loss. *Osteocartilaginous grafts are discussed in nasal reconstruction in detail.*
- Alloplastic materials used in nasal surgeries are silicone, Mersilene mesh, porous polyethylene, proplast, alloderm, etc. The usage depends on the type and size of defects and can be used alone or along with autogenous grafts.

61.2.3.2 Orbital Deformities [19]

- Autogenous bone grafts were earlier considered to be ideal for treatment of orbital floor deformities, but are currently replaced by alloplastic materials. Silastics are currently not considered due to reports of post-operative infection.

Most commonly used alloplastic materials in orbital reconstruction:

- Titanium mesh.
- High-density porous polyethylene implants (e.g. Medpore).

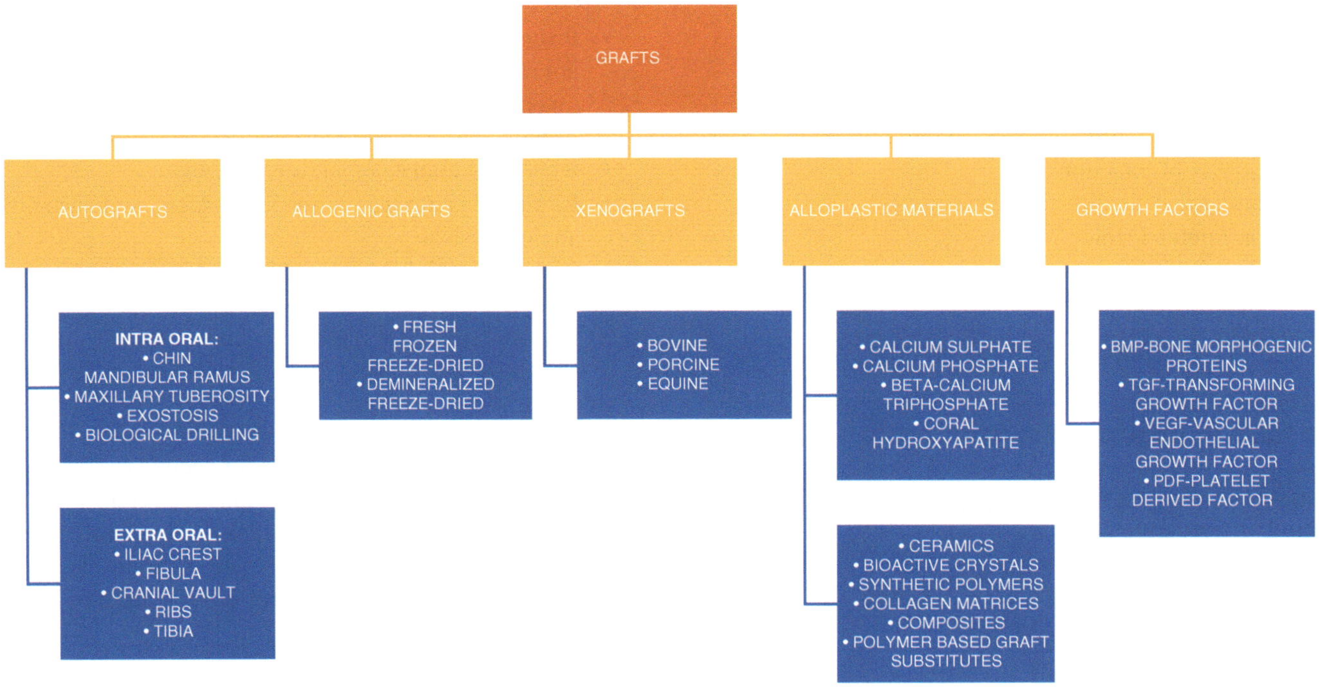

©Association of Oral and Maxillofacial Surgeons of India

Chart 61.3 Sources of bone grafts

- Orbital floor implants are used by manual adaptation of implants according to the contour of the damaged site. However, custom designed implants with computer-guided surgical planning is best utilised in management of late deformities as there is time to assess, plan, design and custom manufacture the precise implants. Orbital titanium implants can also be manufactured by this method.

61.2.4 Alloplastic Materials [19–24]

Alloplastic materials have been used in surgeries since 1930s, and newer materials are available since then. Prime advantages of alloplastic materials are reduced donor site morbidity, easily usable, good patient compliance and shorter working time compared to autogenous grafts. Sources and types of graft materials are listed in Chart 61.3.

Goal of Alloplastic Materials
- *Biocompatible*
- *Resistant to infection*
- *Easy to use*
- *Cost effective*

Their role in maxillofacial reconstruction is still controversial. These porous alloplastic materials are high-density polyethylene implants that are very stable and flexible in nature and also help in new vascular and tissue growth within. This makes alloplasts an essential commodity in management of maxillofacial defects and also in reconstruction.

Alloplastic materials used in the region of defects for reconstruction are available in various forms like titanium mesh, porous polyethylene (Medpor) and PEEK (poly ether ether ketone) which can be customised as needed. *Medpore (stock)* can be manipulated and adapted in situ according to the defect. It is also possible to make *custom-made Medpore, silicone and PEEK* with the computer-aided designing. Even though they are known to produce good clinical outcomes, it may be predisposed to infection. Careful handling, understanding patient's history and surgical placement are essential to avoid any complications or to manage any failures. Medpore along with fat grafting may serve to restore the contour as well as the volume. These custom-made implants are widely used in management of defects and deformities as part of maxillofacial reconstruction. Applications of MEDPORE are chin augmentation procedures, correcting congenital deformities and improving aesthetic outcome in nasal, subnasal, paranasal, malar, orbital, and mandibular (angle and body) areas. It is essentially suited for midfacial contouring in patients treated for cleft. The use of these alloplastic materials ideally helps to establish three-dimensional anatomical harmony in correcting defects. Polyether ether ketone (PEEK) is another valuable alloplastic material that precedes with advantages similar to that of Medpore Custom-made patient-specific PEEK implants have proven to offer excellent facial rehabilitation. The durability and malleable property of PEEK make it a biomaterial of choice for maxillofacial surgeons with which complex maxillofacial defects following trauma or neoplastic can be corrected. Often, the use of alloplastic materials may be an adjunct or combined with prosthesis to further complete the facial rehabilitation process.

61.2.5 Use of Grafts in Associated Residual Structural Damages

Traumatic or iatrogenic reasons causing structural or residual damages are areas of concern during maxillofacial surgery. Important structural damages involving nerve tissues, salivary gland apparatus and nasolacrimal system should be identified and best managed during the primary surgery. If left untreated, secondary or delayed management leads to further complications. It is the skill of the surgeon to carefully carry out the surgery with no or minimal trauma to adjoining structures, and it is experience that will help to predict any relative functional damages and manage it accordingly.

Nerve Injuries: Injuries to the peripheral branches of the trigeminal nerve following maxillofacial trauma or surgery often result in sensory and functional problems. Spontaneous recovery of inferior alveolar nerve and infraorbital nerve after facial fractures depends on a number of factors like age, gender, fracture displacement, site, type of management and time interval between injury and management. Localisation and determination of the pattern of injury of trigeminal nerve are done by careful examination of the neurosensory dysfunction (NSD) of sensory dermatome of trigeminal nerve. It may be very difficult in establishing the exact cause in secondary NSD damages. Such residual defects due to injuries can be from nerve compression due to displaced old fracture segments, laceration due to fracture components, dislocated nerve from a displaced fracture, and compression due to soft tissue oedema or secondary ischemia. Injuries may also be related to crushing, avulsion and partial or total nerve transection [25–28].

Determining the exact aetiology of post-operative residual or secondary NSD damage is difficult, and the best way to manage is assessing the damage during the primary surgery. Accessing and operating the site for correction secondarily may itself cause further damage if not handled properly. Nerve grafts can be used in the management of such damages. It involves microsurgical repair of nerve that requires reconstruction of any continuity defect using an autogenous nerve graft (*donor site—sural or great auricular nerve*). Microsurgical repair helps in improving the clinical outcome in such conditions. Nerve allografts have proven to be successful in improving the neurosensory recovery. Allografts are further beneficial as it alleviates the donor site morbidity. Ichihara et al. suggest the use of alloplastic tubes in short span nerve defects as artificial nerve guides. However, studies need to ascertain their use in long span trigeminal nerve defects. Similar use of autogenous and allogenic grafts is applicable for facial nerve injury as well. The successful outcome of grafts depends on the length/size of the defect and patient factors like age/gender/nutritional status, and it is also important to address factors like previously irradiated sites [29–32].

Salivary Gland/Duct Injuries: Trauma, lacerations, deep injuries and iatrogenic injuries in the parotid region can result in injuries to the important related structures like the buccal branches of facial nerve, Stenson's duct and transverse facial artery and vein. Surgical and non-surgical management of injuries to the salivary gland or its duct is done to improve the clinical outcomes. Non-surgical management includes the use of anti-sialagogues, elastic bandages and reduced oral intake until the defect heals. Microsurgical repair may be done to preserve remaining ductal structures using autologous vein grafts. Reconstruction of the duct is done using autologous vein grafts like saphenous vein, antebrachial vein, facial vein, etc. Alloplastic Gore-Tex has been used, and the outcome was found to be similar to anastomosis in autologous vein grafts in parotid duct reconstruction. Gore-Tex tube carries advantages like decreased graft morbidity and shorter operation time. Timely correction of salivary ducts is important to avoid complications like sialocele, salivary fistula, etc. [33–38].

Nasolacrimal Duct Injury: It is important to reconstruct the nasolacrimal system if damage is seen following orbital or midface trauma. It is similar to other ductal and nerve management. The nasolacrimal duct system can be reconstructed with autogenous and allogenic grafts. Greater saphenous vein can be used as autogenic grafts in such cases. Buccal mucous membrane grafting also shows improved outcomes in removing obstructions in the ducts. Silicone stent intubation is also used in the repair of damaged nasolacrimal duct. Primary management is essential in this condition since delayed management may be difficult to carry out [39–41].

Future of Grafting

Future in grafting promises advances in gene therapy, tissue-engineering, and 3D scaffold. It has created greater perspective with the inclusion of growth factors, stem cells and biological scaffolds that will help in production of laboratory-engineered tissue substitutes in oral and maxillofacial surgery.

> Three-dimensional (3D) computed tomography (CT) has brought major changes to visualisation, planning and treatment of maxillofacial defects ever since its introduction. The scanning and surgical planning software have advanced in such a way that a surgeon can meticulously plan a patient-specific protocol to carry out procedures effectively. Preformed and custom printed alloplastic has more accuracy, reduced operative time and a predictable outcome in management. However, conventional implants require intraoperative adaptations and longer duration of operation. All these have been possible with the advances in reconstructive surgeries with CAD-CAM (computer-aided design-computer-aided modelling) software. Such major advances will lead to further improvement in patient-specific implants (PSI) in the three-dimensional management of defects in reconstructive procedures [23, 24, 42, 43].

61.3 Hard Tissue Deformities

Deformities in the maxillofacial bones are due to a variety of causes like pathology, trauma, infection and congenital disabilities. Residual deformities are such defects that are observed even after the primary surgical management and need further cosmetic and functional intervention for an outcome. The size of the defects in the maxillofacial region may vary from small alveolar clefts and nasal deformities to maxilla-mandibulectomy-type defects. Restoration of the deformities to its closest healthy anatomical structure and their essential functioning are the primary goals of any re-intervention procedure.

Any defect (size, shape, position or amount) of the osseous structure can be replaced by reconstructive surgery. The aim is to replace it with the missing structure, i.e. the bone. Various types of bone grafts may be used for this purpose. Correction of soft tissue defects needs a complete understanding of the wound healing biology. Likewise, in hard tissue deformities, it is essential to know the bone physiology, immunology and surgical principles to make the reconstruction a successful procedure.

61.3.1 Patient Assessment

Although general rule implies to replace or reconstruct the lost osseous defect, it is important to evaluate every patient thoroughly before proceeding with any intervention. Analysis should include evaluation of hard tissue and associated soft tissues. When accompanied by soft tissue deformities, it is important to treat with caution considering the soft tissue changes over time as well [44].

61.3.2 Residual Mandibular Deformities [3, 45–50]

General Assessment Points for Mandibular Defects:
- Careful and complete clinical examination.
- Necessary radiographs to assess the amount of osseous defects.
- Site and size of the defect to be taken into detailed evaluation. Such evaluation is of utmost importance in mandibular osseous defects.

Causes for Post-traumatic Mandibular Deformities:
- Poor diagnosis
- Improper surgical methods—inadequate reduction and/or fixation
- Infection
- Healing disorders

Residual Deformities in Mandible:
- Causes like trauma, gunshot wounds and infection may result in loss of a portion of the mandible.
- Loss of tissues results in functional and aesthetic concerns. Small deformities may often go unnoticed.
- Loss of a portion of the alveolar process leading to loss of teeth is a less serious complication.
- Malunion of mandibular fractures can often result in serious consequences in occlusion among adults and children. More serious changes may affect the mandibular growth in children following condylar fractures.
- Loss of anterior attachment of the tongue due to tissue loss causes an airway hazard that needs to be corrected primarily.
- Loss of bone in mental region or large areas:
  - Difficulty in speech
  - Difficulty in swallowing
  - Drooling of saliva
  - Un-aesthetic appearance

61.3.2.1 Deformity in the Ascending Ramus of the Mandible

No treatment is often required if the occlusion is satisfactory. Complete fusion of the bony segments to the temporomandibular joints may occur following the destruction of the developing mandibular condyle after trauma or secondary infection. In this case, the destruction of the articular disc allows the contact between the bony fragments of ascending ramus and the glenoid fossa, finally resulting in ankylosis. When this occurs in children bilaterally, it shows reduction in lower third dimension resulting in appearance called "Bird Face deformity". This usually results in aesthetic and airway concerns, and psychological disturbances. Airway disturbances should be viewed with greater importance. Ankylosis in adults will result in occlusal abnormalities and difficulty in enunciation of speech and communication. Sometimes pseudo-ankyloses may also be observed.

61.3.2.2 Surgical Options for Post-traumatic Residual Deformities

Post-traumatic deformities include *non-union, malunion/malocclusion and facial asymmetry*, and they may require secondary correction. These deformities can occur alone or in conjunction, sometimes as a sequel to a deformity.

61.3.2.3 Non-union [45–50]

They are fractures with arrested healing that requires further surgical treatment for correction. It is considered to be non-union when a fractured segment is mobile for 4 weeks without treatment or 8 weeks after surgical treatment.

Causes for Non -union	
• Soft tissue infection	• Improper reduction
• Large fracture gaps	• Delayed treatment
• Comminuted fractures	• Teeth in the line of fracture
• Severe atrophic fractures	• Smoking and alcohol abuse
• Osteomyelitis	• Poor treatment planning
• Movements	• Inadequate surgical skills
	• Poor patient compliance

Diagnostic considerations:
Clinical Examination:
- Identify persistent mandibular deformity.
- Tenderness at fracture site.
- Malunion in closed reduction techniques may be identified after release of maxillo-mandibular fixation.

Radiographic Findings:
Irregular radiolucency with mottled fracture ends.

Management:
- Extra-oral approach is the best option as it allows good visualisation. Transoral approaches may be considered in indicated cases.
- It is followed by the debridement for removal of any fibrous tissue, necrotic bone or failed hardware.
- Following this, adequate occlusion and maxillo-mandibular fixation is achieved. The fracture is reduced,

and then reconstruction plates are fixed with the help of screws away from the fracture.

- Considering less mineral (even though appearing normal) content in the site near the fracture, it is recommended to place screws no closer than 7–10mm.
- Autogenous bone grafting may be used to re-establish continuity of mandible in areas where the bone contact is inadequate.
- In younger patients and well-vascularised areas, union of small gaps is successful.

61.3.2.4 Malunion/Malocclusion: [46, 51, 52]

It can occur in any type of mandibular fracture when segments heal in improper alignment. Malunion is often due to inadequately established occlusion, inadequate anatomic reduction and poor adaptation of fixation plate.

Figs. 61.3, 61.4, 61.5, and 61.6 depicts malocclusion related management of deformities.

Diagnostic Considerations:
It is often diagnosed with malocclusion and more associated with rigid internal fixation. Dental models are used to study and plan the occlusion.

Management Considerations:

- Revisit of the surgical site may be necessary to correct the errors due to rigidity.
- Minor occlusal corrections can be done with orthodontic treatment.

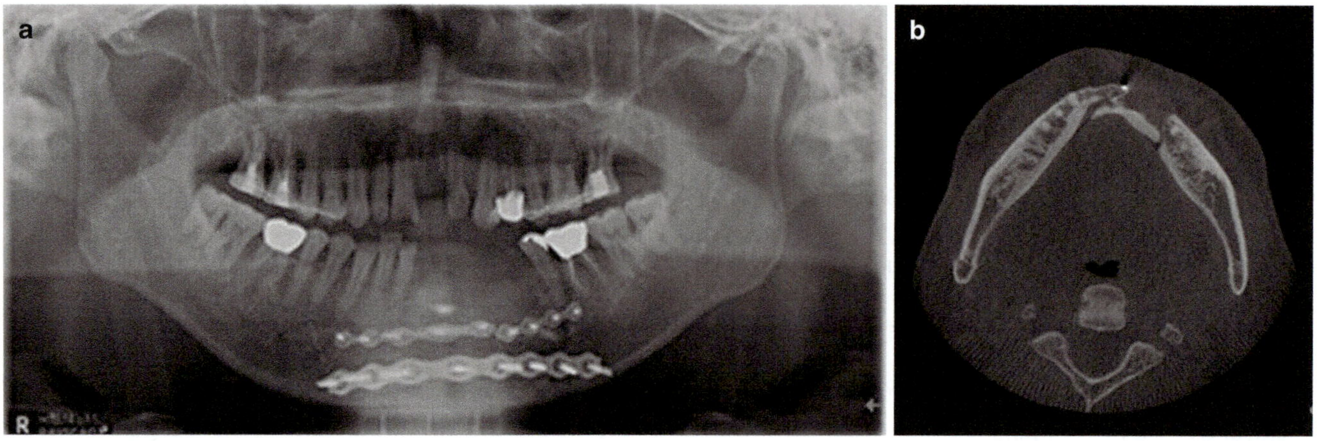

Fig. 61.3 Malocclusion following trauma surgery with multiple loss of teeth in mandible and associated osteonecrosis. Patient managed with iliac grafting of mandibular osteonecrosis site, followed by implant rehabilitation and vestibuloplasty. Preoperative radiograph. (**a**) Panoramic radiograph (**b**) Cone beam computed tomography scan. (Reference for Figs. 61.3, 61.4, 61.5, and 61.6) (http://creativecommons.org/licenses/by/4.0/), Kim SY, Choi YH, Kim YK. *Maxillofac Plast Reconstr Surg*. 2018;40(1):27. Published 2018 Oct 15. doi:10.1186/s40902-018-0167-z (springer open)

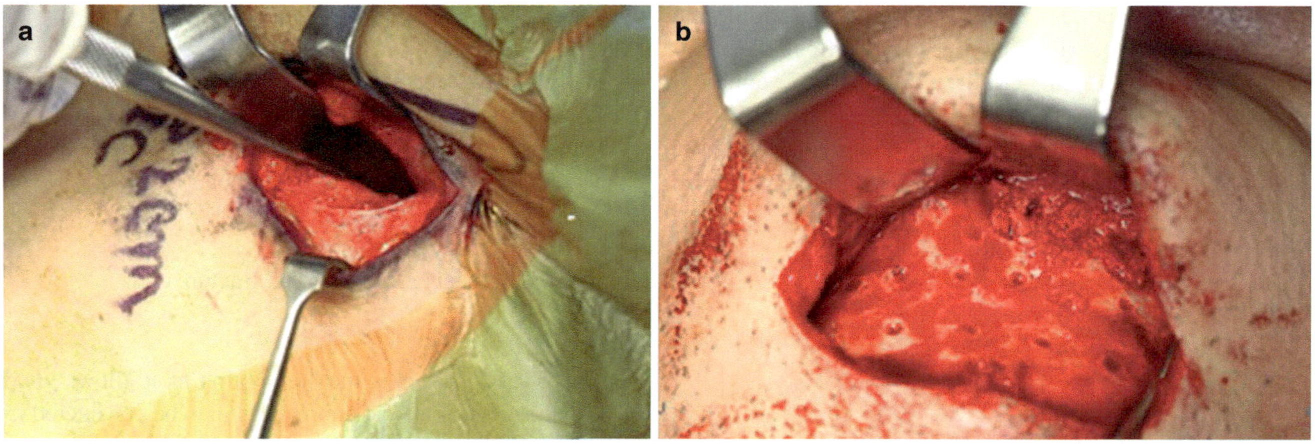

Fig. 61.4 Clinical intra-oral photograph showing. (**a**) Iliac bone harvesting. (**b**) Grafting of the harvest iliac bone into the mandible defect

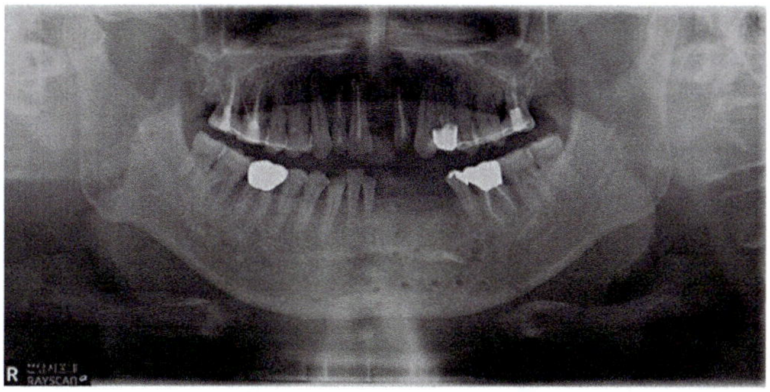

Fig. 61.5 Post-operative OPG

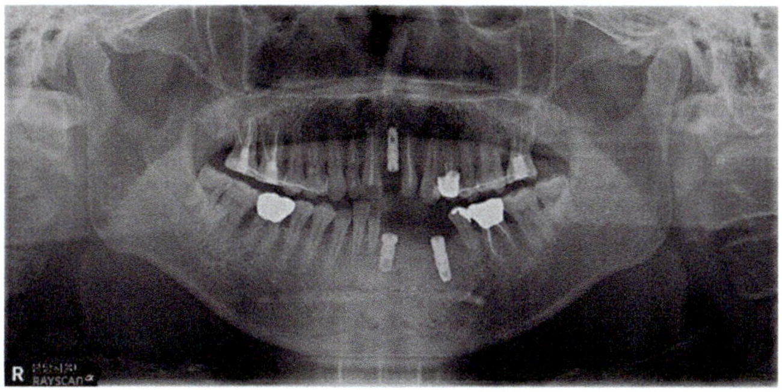

Fig. 61.6 Post-operative OPG after implant placement for dental rehabilitation

61.3.2.5 Early Malunions

- Surgical approach is similar to the primary treatment.
- Old hardware is removed → adequate occlusion achieved → with maxillo-mandibular fixation → fracture reduction if necessary → new fixation is done → new occlusion is verified with release of the fixation.

61.3.2.6 Late Malunions

- Surgical approach is determined based on type of osteotomy.
- Study models are used to study the occlusion and plan a mock surgery.
- Management includes osteotomies for proper establishment of anatomy and occlusion.
- Mandible is re-fractured → occlusion is achieved with the help of a surgical splint → maxillo-mandibular fixation is obtained → new rigid fixation → occlusion is verified after the release of maxillo-mandibular fixation.
- Bone grafts may be used to close gaps whenever necessary.

61.3.2.7 Malunions/Malocclusion and Condylar Fractures [53–56]

- Majority of condylar fractures when treated "closed" may develop malunion. However, condylar malunion may not always cause malocclusion.
- Quality of the functional rehabilitation of the mandible is an more important factor than the type of treatment (closed or open).

Diagnostic Considerations:

- Radiographs and malocclusion are key in examination.
- No treatment or previous unsuccessful treatment is a main reason for malocclusion following condylar fractures.
- Degree of mandibular ramus deformity is essential to determine the necessity for a re-surgery to correct malocclusion following condylar fracture.

Treatment Considerations:

- Unilateral or bilateral fractures.
- Time period between fracture and treatment of malocclusion.
- Availability of remaining stable dentition.

Management Considerations:

- *Minor occlusal discrepancies* may be treated with orthodontics, prosthetic rehabilitation, reconstruction and occlusal adjustments if indicated.
- *TMJ reconstruction* may be indicated—when the remaining ramus is short with multiple fragments and large movements are required to correct occlusion.
- *Orthognathic surgery* may be indicated in long-standing malocclusions.
- *Functional therapy* can be done up to 3 months for management of malocclusion.

61.3.2.8 Facial Asymmetry [46]

- Usually as a sequel to malunion, non-union and inadequate fixation.
- A number of clinical scenarios may present itself to facial asymmetry

Diagnostic Considerations:

- *Early stages*: Difficult to diagnose because of the swelling.
- Antero-posterior cephalometry or CT scans are confirmatory.
- Facial, dental and radiographic analyses are done.

Management Considerations:

- Treatment similar to malunions and malocclusions.
- In cases where the defect is diagnosed early, the mandible can be approached through the initial surgical wound, the hardware may be removed, mal union corrected and new fixation can be placed.
- Orthognathic surgeries in cases of established facial asymmetries. Surgical splints and model surgeries help in

surgical planning. Asymmetry is corrected, and new occlusion is verified with new fixation. The procedure similar to principle treatment. Additional osteotomy may be required depending on the type of original injury.

61.3.2.9 Principles of Mandibular Reconstruction [45, 57]

Reconstruction of larger defects of the mandible is discussed in Chap. 88.

Marx and Saunders listed the goals of mandibular reconstruction in order to consider a grafting procedure successful.

- *Restoration of continuity* is the key since the mandible is a bone with two articulating ends supported by muscles with opposing forces. Deviated mandibular segments need to be realigned not only to improve facial aesthetics but also to restore essential function movements.
- *Restoration of alveolar bone* is another essential aspect to aid in the functional rehabilitation of the patient. The process of mastication and the efficiency to masticate are possible only once the necessary alveolar bone height has been obtained. In patients with osseous defects, this helps in the placement of a prosthesis.
- *Restoration of osseous bulk* is vital to provide the required amount of osseous tissue to withstand forces and perform normal function. Fracture of the graft area may occur when the area is too thin, lacking the bulk to withstand functional forces directed towards the bone.

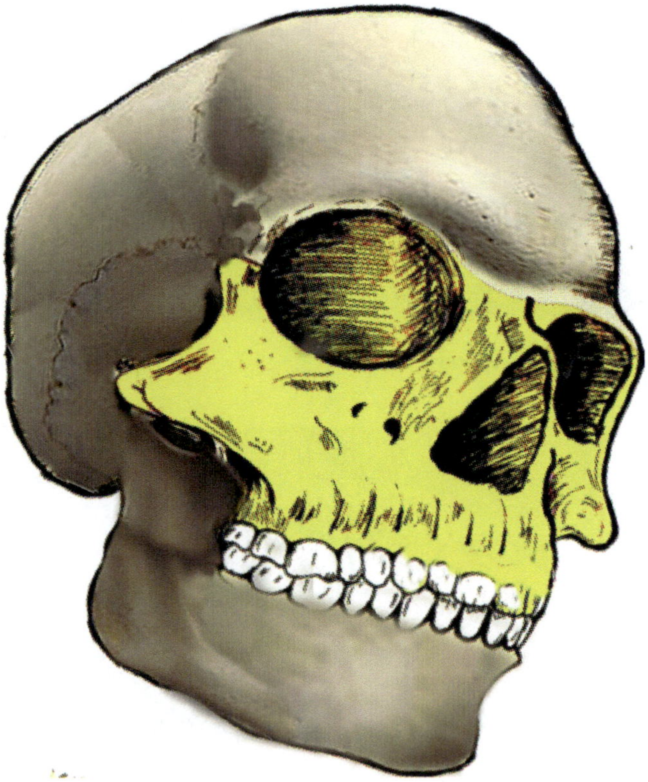

©Association of Oral and Maxillofacial Surgeons of India

Fig. 61.7 Highlighted (yellow) areas represent midface region

61.3.3 Midface Deformities [3, 58]

The midface is a critical zone of the maxillofacial region concerning both aesthetics and function. Midface includes structures like the maxilla, palate, orbit, cheek, upper lips, eyelid and nose. It is often an area that poses a significant challenge to a maxillofacial surgeon for reconstruction. Orbit is usually challenging to reconstruct in secondary setting mainly due to chances of scarring. Due to the difficulty in obtaining good results in primary surgery, the nose and auricle are best considered for correction in a secondary setting. Figure 61.7 shows areas of the midface.

Objectives in Correcting Midface Deformities [58]

- Restoration of midface projection
- Restoration of occlusion
- Providing support for the orbit
- Filling the volume of the orbit
- Restoration of palate competence
- Restoration of functional harmony

Along with the reconstruction of the hard tissue, it is important to correct associated soft tissue defects as well. Failure to correct the primary deformities may result in sequelae of defects of the associated soft tissues and end up in affecting the functional quality of life of the patients.

Indications to Correct Midface Defects [58]

- Untreated/avoided defects during primary reconstruction
- Poor result following primary reconstruction (partial or complete loss of flap, non-union of bone, oro-cutaneous fistula)
- Poor outcome in primary reconstruction due to poor planning
- Post-operative complications that may lead to hematoma and scarring

Diagnostic Workup: [58]

Treatment planning for midface changes requires careful planning and knowledge of previous treatments to achieve the best result.

- Evaluate general status of the patient (age, history of tobacco, alcohol abuse, nutritional status, and presence of co-morbidity)

- Accurate assessment of anatomic defects
- Assessment of quality of tissue involved, surrounding tissues and status of scar
- Availability of healthy surrounding tissue

During the workup, it is necessary to eliminate cases of unresectable conditions like distant metastasis or recurrence in oncology or non-traumatic cases.

Diagnostic Assessment: [58]
Assessment requires evaluation of surface or volume of missing tissues. Assessment should include evaluating defects in the bone, skin, musculature, innervation and mucosa (Chart 61.4).

Treatment Options: [3, 58]
Surgical correction in this region varies from prosthetic replacement to complex microvascular reconstructive surgeries.

Surgical Options:
- Local or regional flaps for small to moderate defects.
- Secondary free flaps: iliac crest flaps, fibula flaps, subscapular free flaps.
- Microvascular surgeries are primarily done in major defects.
- Microvascular flaps provide adequate and necessary amount of well-vascularised bone and/or soft tissue augmentation, thereby enabling a better 3D fitting flap and closure.

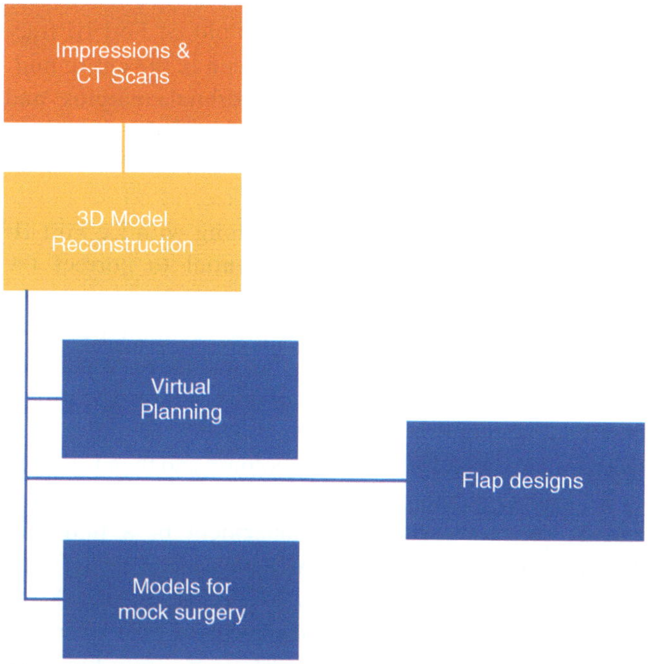

Chart 61.4 Diagnostic assessment

- Critical evaluation is to be done in previously irradiated or operated midfacial defects.

Current methods under development include tissue engineering for ideal regeneration of the tissues in head and neck defects. Facial transplantation has also paved newer paths in this field, but indications are restricted.

Other Non-surgical Options: [58]
Maxillofacial prosthesis:
- Palatal obturators in maxillectomy cases.
- Complex defects affecting structures like the nose, orbit and those which cannot be restored with flap reconstruction may be managed by maxillofacial prosthesis. Recent advancements include supporting the prosthesis with dental implants.

Ancillary Procedures: [3, 58–61]
- Additional supportive techniques may help to improve the outcome of a correction in midface re-operative procedures.
- CT images are useful in designing adequate fronto-orbital facial contours.
- Free bone grafts for facial contouring are indicated for upper midface defects. The bone grafts can be obtained from calvaria and synthetic implants—porous polyethylene, methyl methacrylate and titanium mesh. However, it is contraindicated in a previously irradiated area and in cases of oral cavity communication.
- Combination of titanium mesh and soft tissue may be helpful to provide support for the globe.
- *Liposuction* is an excellent alternative technique to fill certain residual defects following midface reconstruction. Microvascular flaps may help fill residual flattened areas.
- *Distraction osteogenesis*: Mainly indicated in mandibular repair, it is also used in the repair of minor maxillary bone defects which cannot be treated with bone flap reconstruction (refer Chap. 87).

Oral Rehabilitation:
- Implant-supported prosthesis with good osseointegration is often considered as the best option in oral rehabilitation. Peri-implant hygiene and osteointegration are important for the success of dental/zygomatic implants in oral rehabilitation procedures.
- Dental implants are most helpful for oral rehabilitation. Implants may be placed during the primary reconstructive procedure or preferably as a secondary procedure.
- Zygomatic implants may also be used when regular alveolar bone reconstruction is not possible.
- Implant placement in previously irradiated areas may not give the best results, and hence it is a contraindication.

61.3.4 Residual Maxillary Deformities [3, 58]

Goals in Correction of Maxillary Deformities
- Restoration of function
- Restoration of occlusion
- Restoration of original relationship between thirds of the face

Common Maxillary Deformities May Be Due to:
- Malpositioned maxillary fractures
- Undiagnosed fractures—untreated dislocated fractures
- Severely comminuted fractures with associated damages
- Untreated old fractures
- Edentulous displaced maxilla
- Post-traumatic hypertelorism

Essentials for Treatment Planning:
- Preoperative *photographs* (full face, profiles pictures, frontal and lateral views of occlusion, palate, floor of the mouth and other required projections).
- Detailed *clinical assessment* and treatment of other existing carious and inflammatory conditions of the oral cavity.
- *Models and radiographs*—OPG, lateral cephalometric X-rays
- Current imaging and planning techniques: CBCT helps in *3D virtual planning* to design flaps and to create 3D models for planning and mock surgery (61.5).

61.3.4.1 Immediate Repositioning of Maxilla and Midface Complex

Open Surgical Immediate Mobilisation Treatment: This is indicated in conditions where total mobilisation is not possible. These are cases that are treated after 6 weeks or more after trauma, or even years later, usually cases where partial or complete consolidation has already taken place. The principle of surgical treatment is often the same as in the treatment of primary maxillary and midface treatments.

Old Fracture Segments: Old fracture segments in the anterior maxilla can be corrected by techniques described by Wassmund (1935) and Wunderer (1962) in cases of protruded maxilla. It is key to observe any scars in the labial vestibule as that may affect the vasculature to the alveolar process. Wassmund's method should be preferred when a scar is present; otherwise, Wunderer's method may be followed in which maintenance of labial blood supply is essential. In contrast, Schuchardt K suggested a single-stage technique which involved an osteotomy of the lateral alveolar process and relocation to its original alveolar location [62–64].

61.3.4.2 Old Le Fort I and II Fractures [3]

Untreated Le Fort I Fractures: An incision may be made at a point horizontally through lateral and anterior maxillary sinus walls. Osteotomy is done to ensure that the plates are placed on both sides of the stable bone region. Line of osteotomy does not precisely follow the line of fracture.

Old Le Fort II Fractures [3]: If there's no cosmetic significance or less damage to the nasal region—similar procedure may be followed. Le Fort II osteotomy is indicated when the nose has sunken, and the midface is shortened.

In the above scenarios, Le Fort I and II osteotomies may be done when either occlusion needs to be restored or there is an aesthetic concern. Bone grafts may be used in the region of the bridge of the nose below the buttress and also between pterygoids and the maxillary tuberosity if possible (Figs. 61.8 and 61.9).

61.3.4.3 Displaced Edentulous Maxilla [3]

- *Minor displacements* may be corrected with osteotomies, only if the disturbance along the intermaxillary relationship in the sagittal plane is minimal. Otherwise, it is justifiable to treat with a prosthesis.
- *In case of severe displacements* of maxilla which results in the appearance of a skeletal Class III, the maxilla has to be surgically replaced to its original place with the help of bone grafts.

61.3.4.4 Old Le Fort III Fractures (Figs. 61.10 and 61.11)

Le Fort III osteotomy is indicated in old Le Fort III fractures when the deformities may be seen in the entire midface region with dislocations in orbital margins and zygoma. Unilateral osteotomy may be indicated when only one side of the face is affected. Occasionally in cases of comminuted fractures of the midface, a Le Fort I osteotomy may be needed to be done along with Le Fort III osteotomy procedure. This is essential to correct the occlusion in untreated midface fractures. It may be challenging to carry out a re-treatment for comminuted midface fractures. Segments may be stabilised separately considering the complex nature of the fracture. The procedure can be simplified by first mobilising the entire midface complex with Le Fort III osteotomy and then followed by Le Fort I osteotomy (Figs. 61.12, 61.13, 61.14, 61.15, and 61.16 shows surgical management of a mid face deformity by onlay grafting; All images 61.12–61.16 are from the same patient) (Figs. 61.17, 61.18, and 61.19 shows clinical images of management of post operative malocclusion; all images 61.17–61.19 are from the same patient).

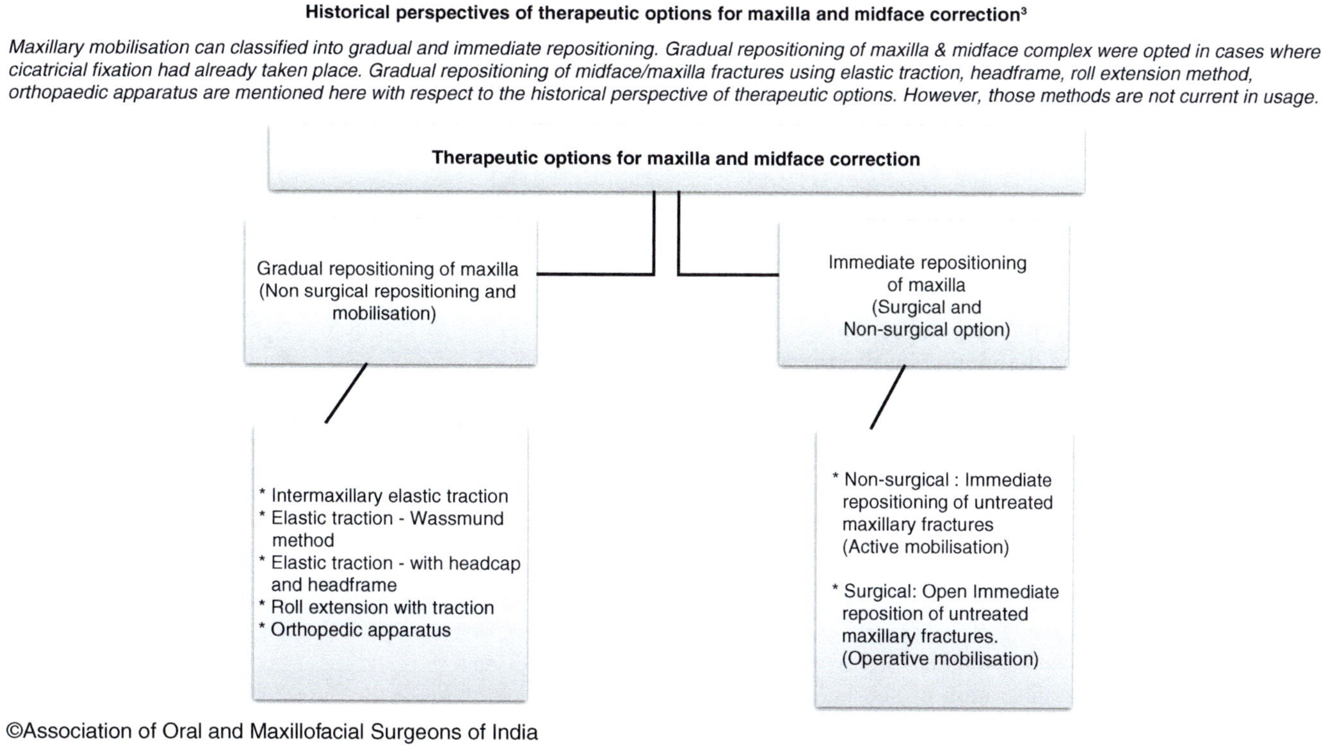

Chart 61.5 Historical perspectives of therapeutic options for maxilla and midface correction [3]

Fig. 61.8 Schematic diagram showing preoperative old untreated midface fractures

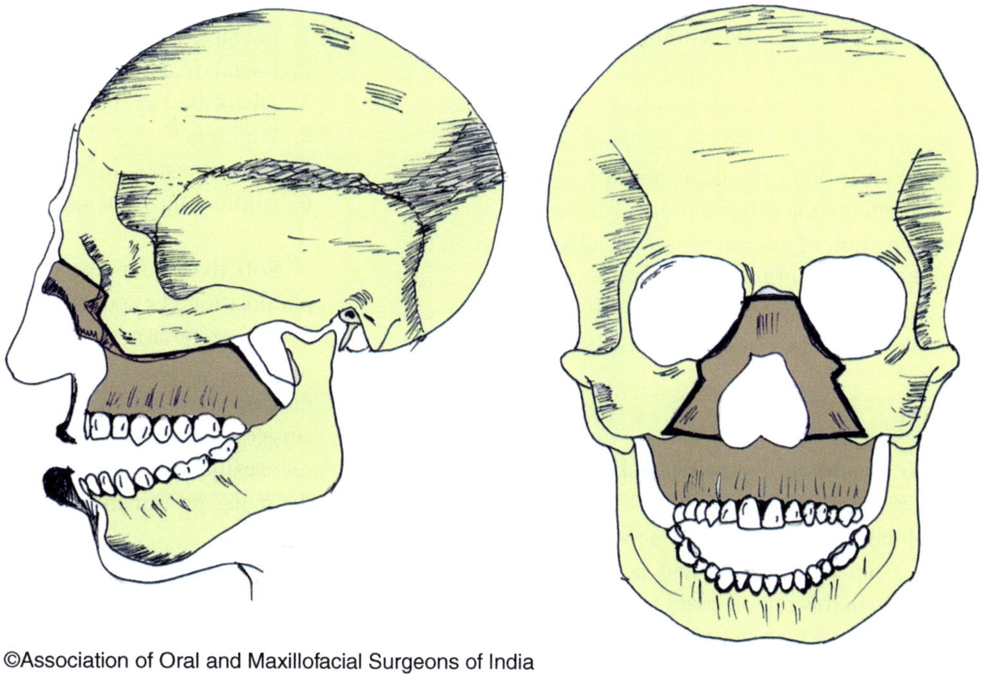

61.3.5 Post-traumatic Hypertelorism [3, 44, 65–71]

It is a complication that may arise in fractures of midface complex when there is a dislocation of one or both orbits. Treatment is similar to congenital hypertelorism, and procedure may follow as suggested by Tessier et al. (1967). Stereolithographic models are best used for treatment planning. Although Tessier developed the extra and intracranial approach to correct the deformity, it was further refined later by Tessier, Converse, Van der Meulen et al., Monasterio

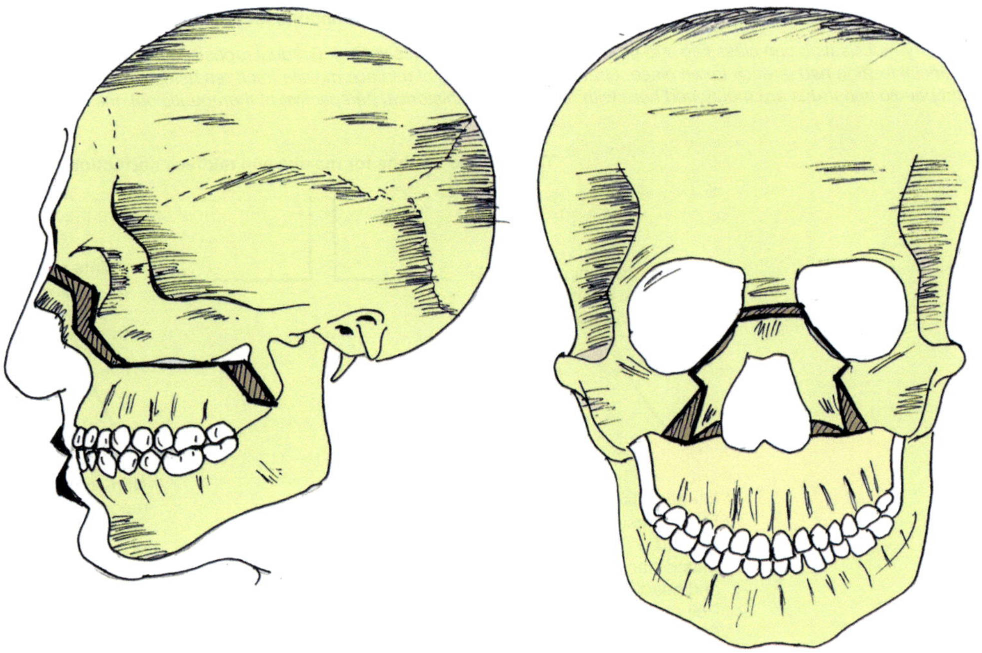

Fig. 61.9 Schematic diagram showing post-operative scenario following combined Le Fort 1 and Le fort II. Defects as a result of repositioning shaded as brown are areas to be filled with bone graft

et al. and Marchac et al. They were able to visualise the bony orbit in two parts with the outer square box containing the globe and the inner cone housing the optic nerve. It was established that if these two parts could be separated, the outer box can be moved without affecting the vision.

Goals of surgery for hypertelorism include:
- Correction of orbital dystopia
- Bringing the orbits closer together
- Creation of normal nose with adequate projection
- Narrowing of the nasal dorsum
- Correction of associated soft tissue defects over the nose, nasal clefts or even displaced eyebrows

61.3.6 Residual Zygomatic Deformities [3, 58]

Periorbital area is often a zone of interest in the midface region from a functional and aesthetic point of view. An imbalance in this region could result in aesthetic concern and altered vision. This can be due to malunion of the fracture of the zygomatic complex. Any untreated fracture for longer than *10 weeks* is considered to be an *old fracture* and results in malunion—a stage at which a procedure needs to be done to correct any deformity.

Clinical Signs and Symptoms
1. Facial asymmetry
2. Facial disharmony
3. Dislocated eyeball
4. Diplopia
5. Paraesthesia—infraorbital nerve
6. Limited movements of the mandible

Soft tissue damage like a torn lateral canthal ligament, malpositioned zygomatic bone, zygomatic arch or fragments of the orbital arm may result in an asymmetry of the lateral midface. Corrective surgeries may be required in case of a destroyed orbital bone as well. More often, patients visit the surgeon for aesthetic reasons. It may be often difficult to correct aesthetics when it involves post-traumatic deformities in the malar prominences (Table 61.3).

61.3.6.1 Associated Defects of the Orbital Zone [3]

- *Dislocated eyeball*: Usually occurs as a sequel to zygomatic fractures, and slight dislocation may be seen after primary treatment. Displaced orbital floor due to enlargement of the socket or the loss of the orbital content due to

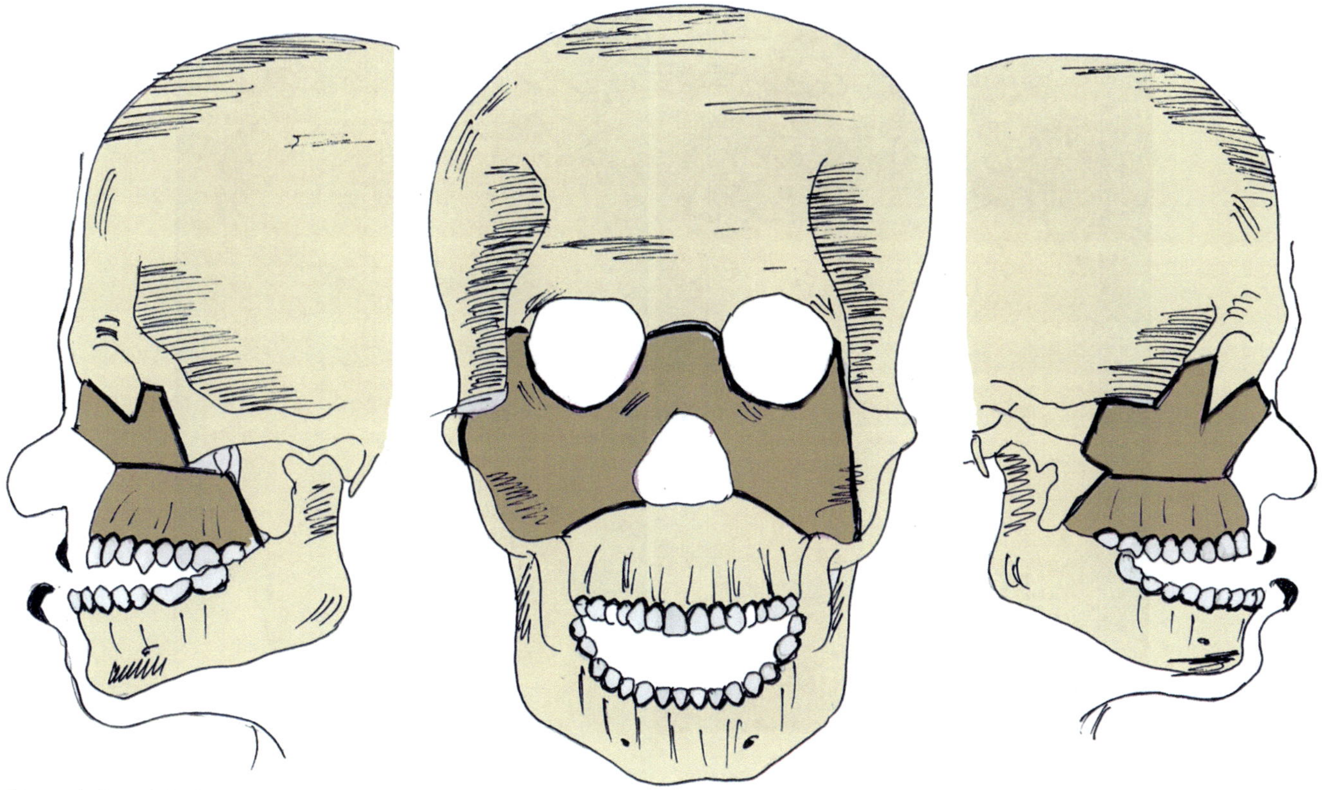

Fig. 61.10 Schematic diagram showing old untreated Le fort III fractures

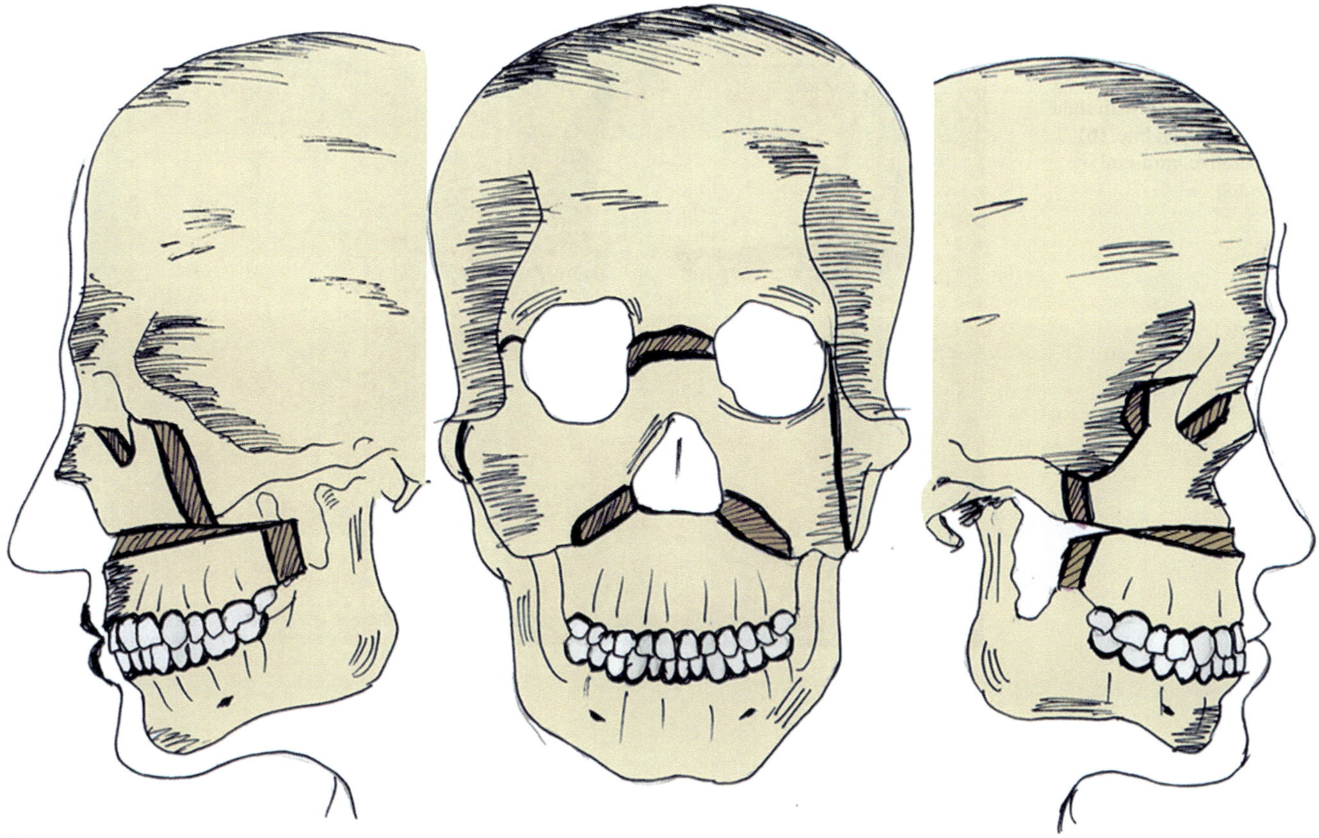

Fig. 61.11 Schematic diagram showing post-operative following combined Le Fort I and Le fort III. Defects as a result of repositioning shaded as brown are area to be filled with bone graft

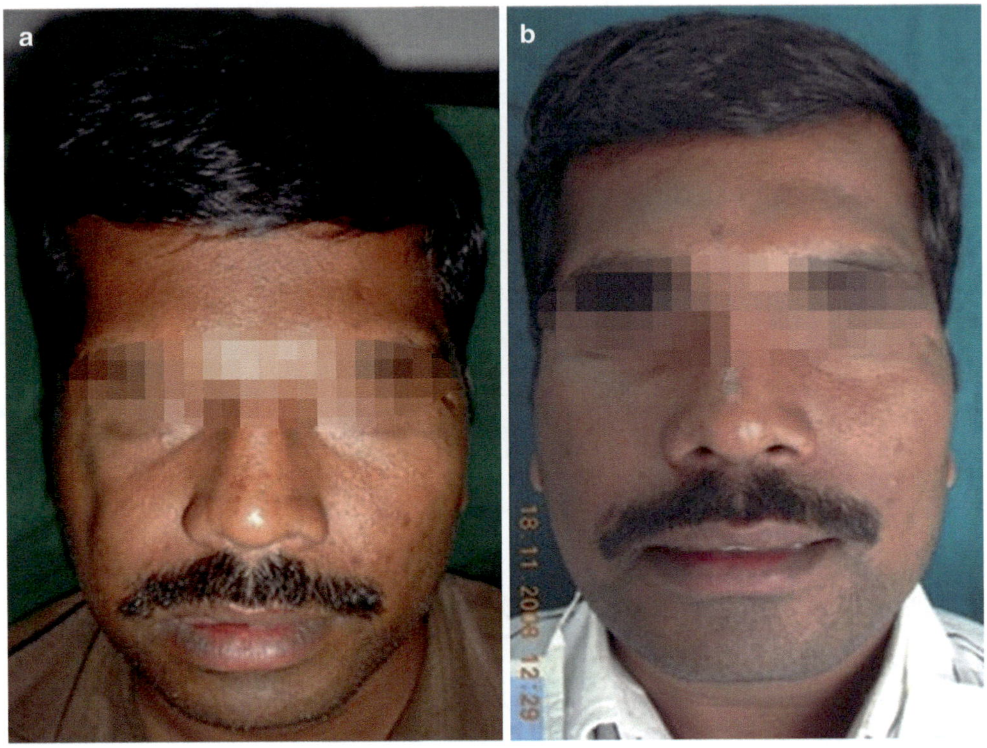

Fig. 61.12 Midface deformities showing residual deformities. (**a**) pre-operative extra-oral photograph showing facial asymmetry, depressed malar prominence (right side), and incompetent lips. (**b**) Post-operative extra-oral photograph. (Reference for Figs. 61.12, 61.13, 61.14, 61.15, and 61.16: Ranganath K, Hemanth Kumar HR. The correction of post-traumatic pan facial residual deformity. *J Maxillofac Oral Surg*. 2011;10(1):20–24. https://doi.org/10.1007/s12663-010-0088-6) *springer publishers*

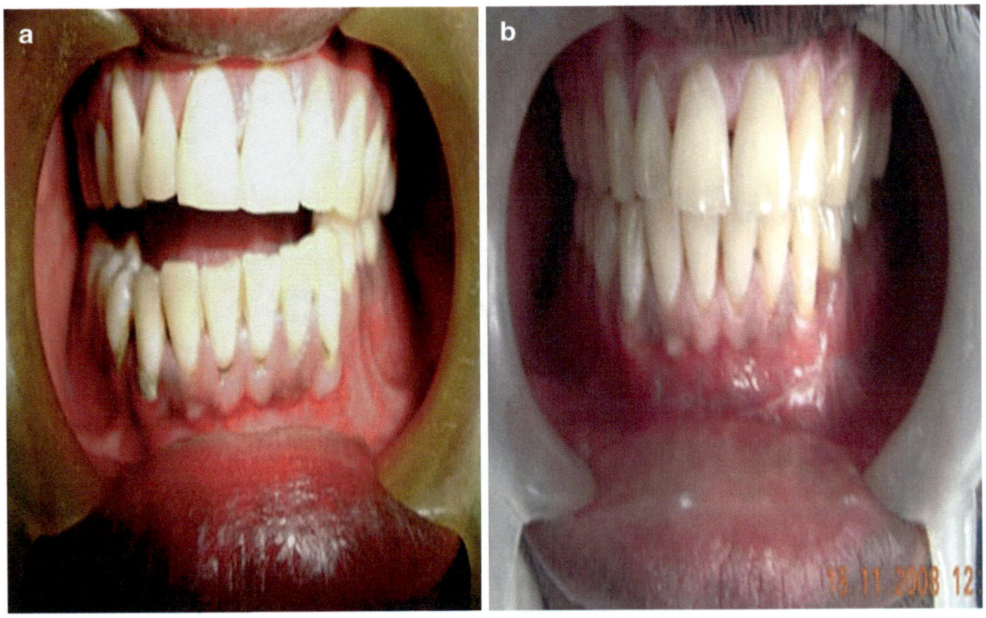

Fig. 61.13 (**a**) Preoperative intra-oral photograph showed deranged occlusion with right anterolateral open bite. (**b**) Post-operative intra-oral photograph

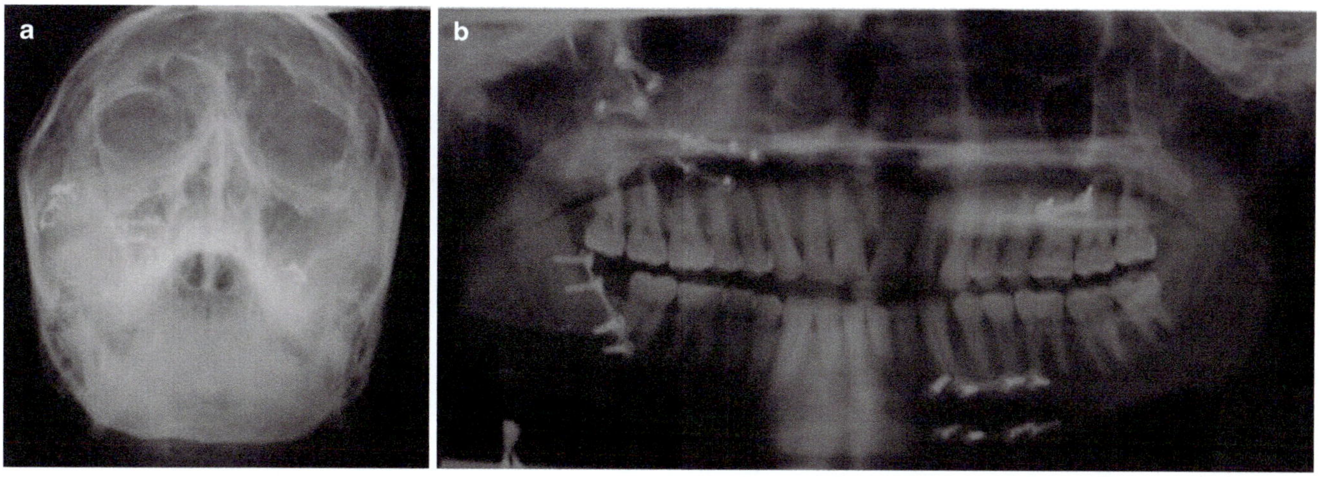

Fig. 61.14 (**a**) Post-operative PNS radiograph. (**b**) Post-operative orthopantomograph

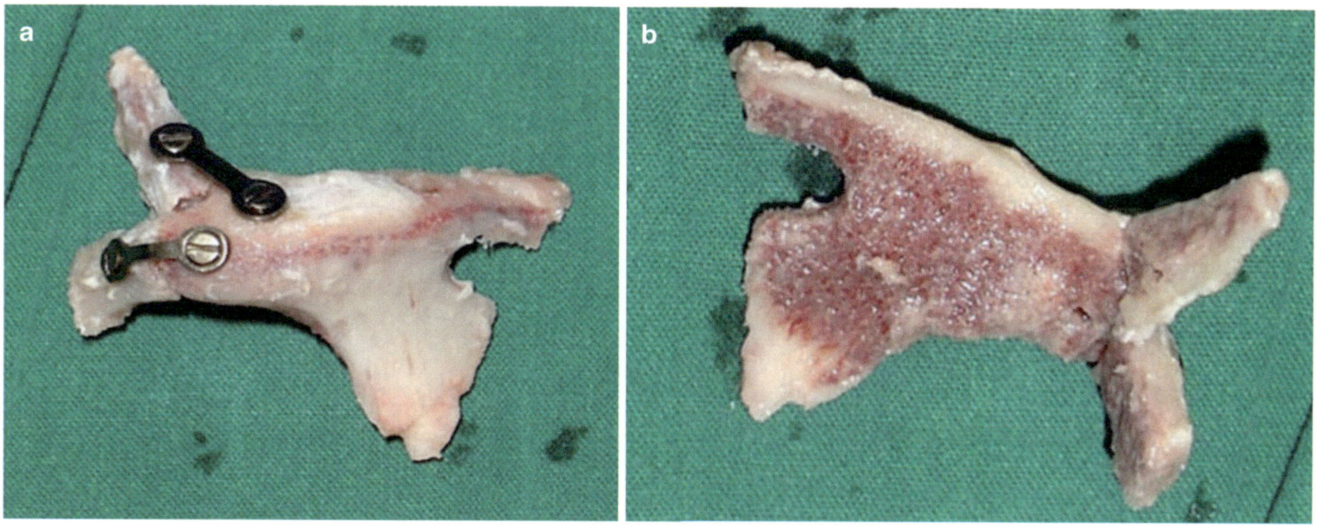

Fig. 61.15 (**a**, **b**) Sculptured iliac bone onlay graft

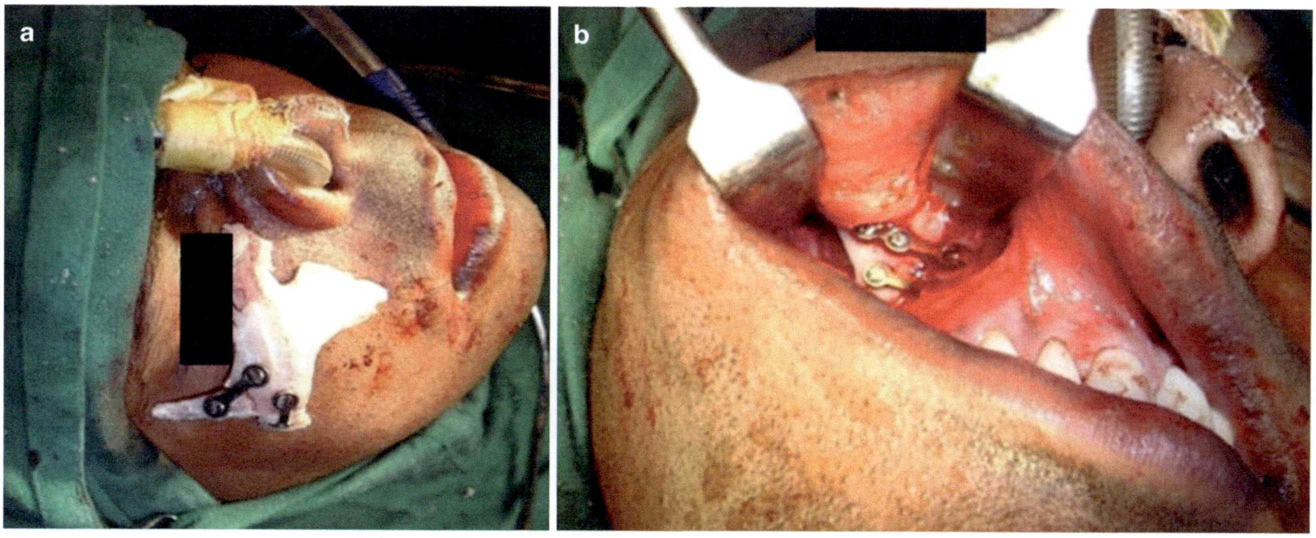

Fig. 61.16 (**a**) Onlay graft positioned on the patient. (**b**) Onlay graft plated to the maxilla

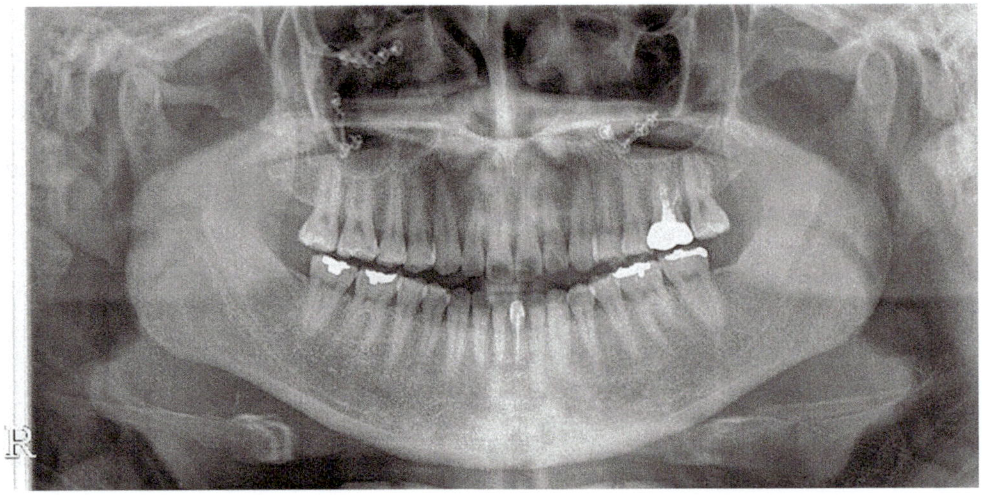

Fig. 61.17 Patient complains of open bite, malocclusion, deviation of maxilla and TMJ tenderness after trauma surgery. Preoperative OPG showing malunion in maxilla and malocclusion. (Reference for Figs. 61.17, 61.18, and 61.19: Kim, Sang-Yun et al. "Post-operative malocclusion after maxillofacial fracture management: a retrospective case study." Maxillofacial plastic and reconstructive surgery vol. 40,1 27. 15 Oct. 2018, https://doi.org/10.1186/s40902-018-0167-z. (http://creativecommons.org/licenses/by/4.0/), springer open

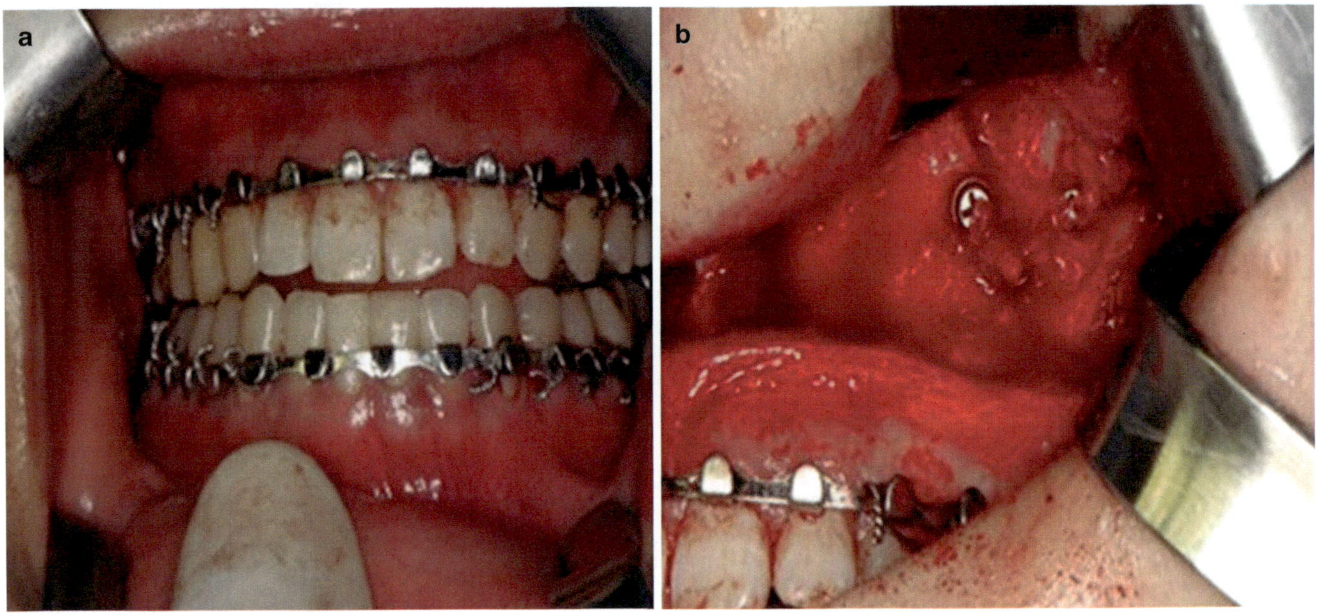

Fig. 61.18 Photograph during the operation. (**a**) Shows severe malocclusion before second operation. Arch bar placed for intermaxillary fixation. (**b**) Fracture site exposed, malunion segments detected

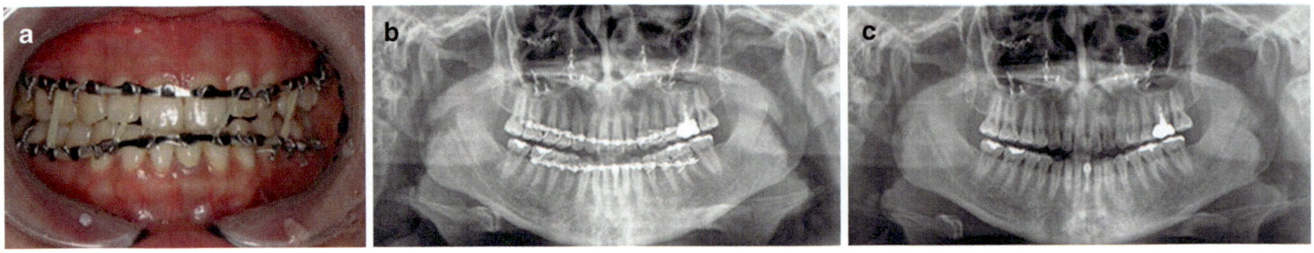

Fig. 61.19 Le fort I osteotomy done under general anaesthesia to resolve malunion and malocclusion. TMJ pain resolved following the treatment. (**a**) Post-operative (1 month) photograph showing resolution of malocclusion. (**b**) OPG after 1 month. (**c**) OPG 1 year after operation

soft tissue displacement or necrosis may result in enophthalmos and/or downward displacement of the globe.
- *Diplopia*: Usually due to severe dislocation of the eyeball, but severe diplopia may more likely occur as a consequence to trauma to the cranial nerves, scarring of the extraocular muscles or prolapse and entrapment of orbital soft tissue. Waiting period before re-treatment of diplopia neural and muscle damage is at least 12 months and 15 months, respectively, to observe if the diplopia subsides. Diplopia is differentiated into heterotropia and heterophoria. While sometimes heterophoria may not even need a correction, in certain cases of severe heterotropia, the patient is advised to maintain a titled head position to avoid any double vision. Sometimes double vision may persist even after the fracture has been corrected.
- *Paraesthesia of the distributing area* due to crushing or tearing of the nerve within the infraorbital canal or foramen. Recovery of the nerve by itself may take at least 1 year.
- *Limited mandibular movements* are caused due to a depressed zygoma impinging on the coronoid process of the mandible, restricting the free excursion of the coronoid process. Patient complains of difficulty to open the mouth, and some cases of difficulty to close the mouth may be due to an open mouth during the blow to the zygomatic complex.
- *Pseudoarthrosis* between the coronoid process and temporal process of the zygomatic bone may occur rarely in old untreated cases [72].

Indications for Surgery: [3]
- Aesthetically *unacceptable asymmetry of the orbital rims*. Pathological difference between the two malar prominences more than 5mm.
- *Diplopia* caused due to downward displacement (*more than 3mm*) of the eyeball due to orbital floor displacement and *not primarily due to neural or muscle damage.*

Table 61.3 Radiographic assessment for detecting malunion at fracture sites

Type of x-ray/ view	Use
Occipito-mental (Waters View)	To examine fronto-zygomatic suture, inferior orbital rim and maxillary sinus
Postero-anterior view	To examine orbital floor and rim
Vertico-submental	"Jug-handle" appearance. To view zygomatic arch
Tomograms	To examine orbital floor, space between coronoid process and zygomatic arch
CBCT	To obtain and study oblique images from the three-dimensional data for fracture detection, displacement evaluation, soft tissue herniation

- *Enophthalmos in combination* with displacement of the orbital floor.
- *Paraesthesia of the orbital nerve* after at least 12 months of post-surgical repositioning of bone fragments.
- *Depression of zygomatic arch* impinging the coronoid process that is radiographically evident in causing limited mandibular movement.

Surgical correction of traumatic zygomatic complex fractures is discussed in Chap. 56.

Treatment options: [3] (Chart 61.6) (Table 61.4)
Surgical approach is decided once the operative procedure has been finalised. Common approaches include [3]:
- Periorbital (Chart 61.7)
- Preauricular (Chart 61.7)
- Oral (Chart 61.8)
- Old facial scar

Complications: [3]
- Failed surgery due to insufficient fixation of the refractured site or failure due to the implanted materials.
- Untreated pre-existing chronic sinusitis may result in an orbital abscess or phlegmon.
- Serious complications that may lead to blindness.
  - Fracture of bone at the optic canal
  - Misplaced implant that may result in compression of nerve
- Retrobulbar haemorrhage

61.3.7 Secondary Orbital Reconstruction [5, 72, 73]

Post-traumatic secondary deformities include:
- Enophthalmos
- Dystopia

Both deformities are difficult to correct.

Factors Responsible for Globe Malposition:
- Displaced or missing periorbital bone
- Orbital fat loss
- Contracture of scar

Factors Responsible for Enophthalmos:
- Pathological increase in bony orbit
- Dislocated zygomatic bone

Rotated and displaced zygomatic bone leads to separation of the structures from its normal articulation with the greater wing of the sphenoid and maxilla. A substantial increase in the volume of the orbital cavity is accompanied by fissures along the floor and lateral wall of the orbit. Also, naso-ethmoidal fractures can result in canthal distortion and mal-

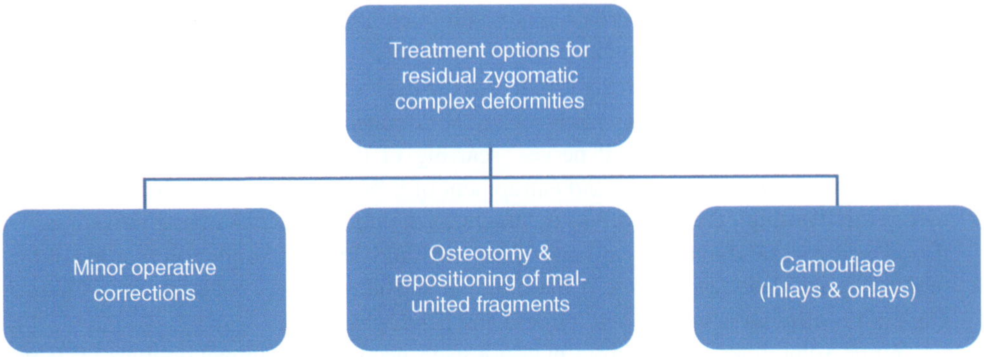

Chart 61.6 Treatment options for residual zygomatic complex deformities

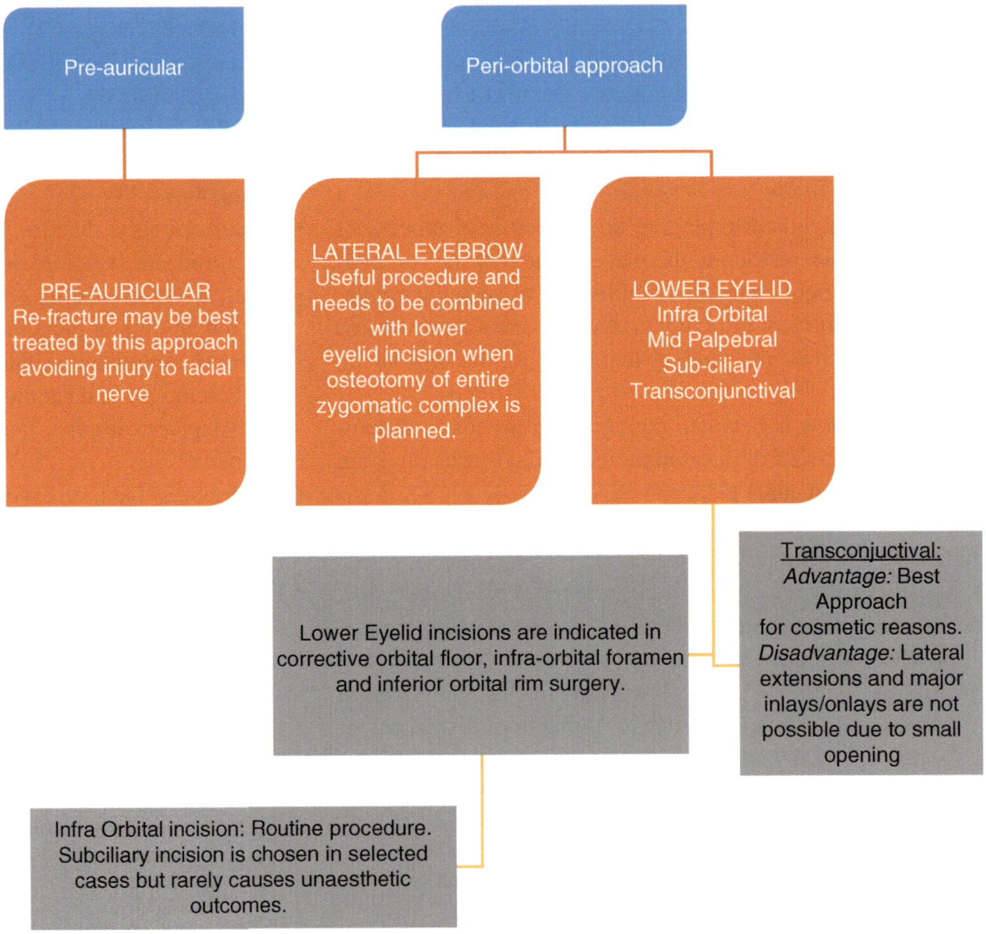

Chart 61.7 Treatment options for residual zygomatic complex deformities—Preauricular and periorbital approach

position. Telecanthus and canthal height distortion can be difficult to correct if there is a significant loss of soft and hard tissue.

Any excess or deficiency in the horizontal position of the globe is called dystopia and is easier to correct. Inferior displacement (horizontal displacement) is managed by augmenting the sub-periosteum of the anterior orbital wall, anterior to the axis of the globe. This technique helps to produce superior movement of the eyeball but does not correct enophthalmos even with the overall decrease in orbital volume [5].

Chart 61.8 Treatment options for residual zygomatic complex deformities–Oral approach

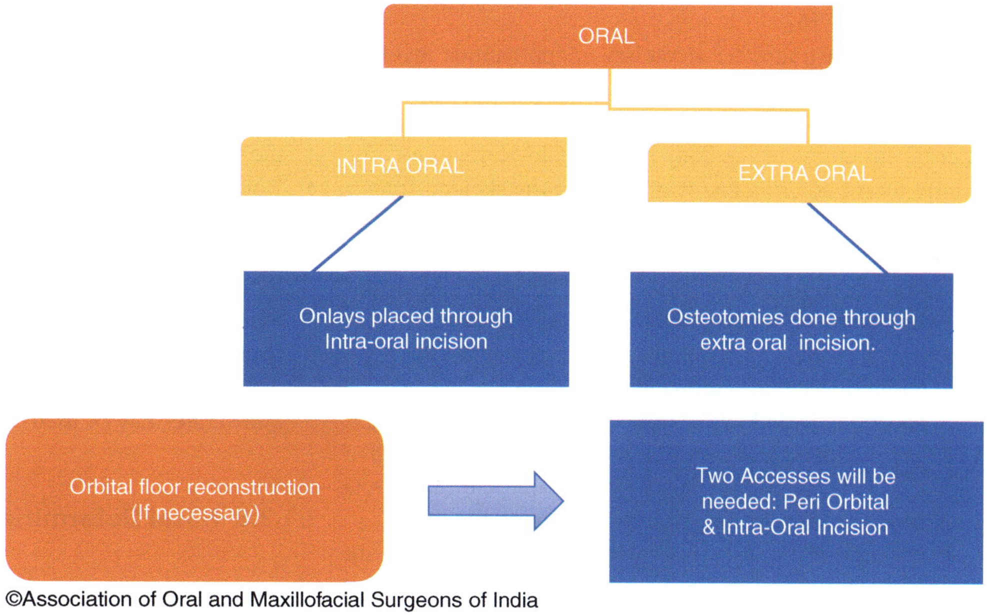

Table 61.4 Surgical options for zygomatic residual fractures [3]

Indications	Clinical presentation	Treatment
Removal or reposition of mal-united fragments	• Sequelae of old, mal-united and consolidated fracture of zygomatic complex	Corrective surgery considered
	• No disturbance to intercuspation and occlusion • No abnormal ophthalmic findings • Good overall symmetry and harmony of the face	No major osteotomy is indicated
	• Visible bony step at the orbital rim	*Surgically removed* through lower eyelid incision. During this, the orbital floor needs to be observed for any adhesions
Paraesthesia	• Persistent paraesthesia is an indication for surgery	*Infra orbital foramen* is widened to free the nerve When only paraesthesia is present—can be accessed through an intra oral approach When additional exploration of the infra orbital canal is required—lower eyelid incision is indicated
Depressed Zygomatic arch	• Hindering the coronoid process' free excursion	*Refracture, reposition and wire fixation* Surgical Approach: Curvilinear, pre-auricular and/or lateral eyebrow incision *Older surgical approach:* Removal of coronoid process
Complete Zygoma Dislocation	• Depressed malar prominence, caudally displaced eyeball and diplopia	• *Treated with osteotomy* • *Camouflage surgery* as a second option • Lateral eyebrow incision and infra-orbital incision to explore the zygomatic complex and detach from the frontozygomatic suture at the inferior orbital margin, inferior and lateral walls of the orbit, and the zygomatic arch (if necessary) • Reposition the segments • Fixation of the fragment is further assured by placing bone graft in the gap in lateral or inferior orbital rim • Orbital Floor is finally covered with lyophilised dura. Procedure is done to ensure good support to the malar bone and orbital floor
	• To prevent post-operative relapse after above surgery	*Over compensate* the pre-operative displacement to a certain extent
	• If downward displacement of globe is not completely resolved after the surgery.	*Free transplant of lyophilized dura could be an option*

Enophthalmos: [5]

Managing post-traumatic secondary enophthalmos involves reducing the volume of orbital cavity posterior to the globe axis. The three-dimensional anatomy of both external and internal structures of the bony orbit should be restored efficiently by refracturing and rearticulating the skeletal framework (including zygomatic bone).

- The zygomatic bone may be accessed by complete exposure using surgical techniques to free the bone and also to establish the correct alignment.
- The zygomaticofrontal suture and the zygomatic arch are exposed through the coronal flap, and facial and muscular connections including the masseter muscle are released.
- Inferior orbital rim and orbital floor are exposed through a lower eyelid incision. Upper lip gingivobuccal incision is done to uncover the zygomatico-maxillary articulation.
- Bony cuts mimicking zygomatic complex fracture are made with a reciprocating bone saw.
- The zygomatic bone is freed and then replaced into the new position with rigid fixation. Necessary bone grafting needs to be done to close the gaps and also to augment the orbital volume.
- The globe should be left slightly exophthalmic (1–2 mm). If an autologous bone is used in augmenting the orbital volume, this exophthalmos is left behind expecting resorption over the next few months. However, this may be difficult to achieve in cases of excessive scarring.
- Placement of the graft plays a very important role as improper placement of grafts, or displacement into the intramuscular cone can result in dysfunction of the extraocular muscles or damage/injure the optic nerve.
- Management of complication: Creating safe pockets for the graft by carefully dissecting off the periorbita from the underlying bone. The grafts may be placed external to the extraocular muscles if the periorbita had been disrupted from previous trauma.
- Enophthalmos and diplopia may worsen further due to scarring or displacement of the implant. However, postoperatively globe position may moderately improve and is often long-lasting [5, 72–74].

Complications in Correction of Enophthalmos: [12, 74]

- Worsening vision.
- Diplopia—may improve to certain degree.
- Dystopia.
- Persistent enophthalmos.
- Graft displacement/retrobulbar hematoma may result in changes in vision.
- Pressure from grafts posterior to the globe may result in retinal folds and ischemia.

Telecanthus: [74]

- Lateral displacement of the medial canthus is called telecanthus.
- Corrected using medial orbital osteotomy by positioning the tendon and the overlying soft tissue medially.
- Bone cuts that are made along the fracture lines (typical as in nasoethmoid complex fractures) help to free bone segment that inserts into the point of the tendon, followed by medially relocating the bone to its normal anatomical location.
- Rigid fixation of the bone is done to the surrounding bone over the maxilla and inferomedial forehead. Autologous bone grafts may be used to replace missing bone segments.

61.3.8 Nasal Deformities [3, 75]

Residual nasal deformities occur as a consequence of the displacement of bony and cartilaginous components of the nasal skeleton. The basic anatomy of the nasal skeleton includes the nasal bone and the cartilaginous part of the nasal septum. The frontal process forms the lateral walls, and the vomer forms the osseous part of the nasal septum. The nose is the most commonly traumatised area due to its prominent central location and its elevation from the frontal facial plane. However, secondary deformities to nasal trauma are not rare [3].

Reasons for secondary nasal deformities [75]	
• Inadequate diagnosis • Improper patient selection • Inadequate surgical skills • Improper surgical planning • Inadequate primary treatment • Delayed primary treatment • Inadequate post-operative stabilisation • Post-operative recurrent trauma	• Unstable bony and cartilaginous structures due to fracture • Poor nasal septal management—aggressive septal management • Poor nasal narrowing • Poor management of nasal tip/base surgery • Improper intranasal incisions (too many or incorrect) • Incorrect dorsal hump reduction

61.3.8.1 Potential Complications Associated with Nasal Deformities [3] (Chart 61.9)

Clinical Evaluation: [3, 75]

The patient needs to be aware and educated on the options for a secondary rhinoplasty to correct the residual nasal deformities as the pathology may concern the functional and cosmetic needs of the patient.

- The intensity of the trauma is relative to the type of deformity that may follow.
- Initial low intensity trauma → nasal tip may become malpositioned. There is an evident inward rotation of the lower portion and an upward-outward rotation of the upper portion. This results in a depressed supra tip and a small cephalic hump.
- Increased force → fracture of the bones, cartilage or the nasal dorsum
- Incomplete fracture → late deviation

Preoperative Examination: [3]
- Identify the aesthetic and functional concerns of the patient
- External examination of the nose and the face as a whole
  - Deformity
  - Symmetry
- Internal examination with endoscope and speculum
- Airway examination
- Radiological examination to aid in diagnosis

Morphological Considerations: [3]
- Profile:
  - Shape/contour
  - Prominence of the nasal bridge
- Symmetrical position: Position and relation with the naso-orbital angles
- Degree of angulation and contour of frontal and the nasal margins at nasofrontal angle
- Evaluation of naso-labial angle

It is important to evaluate the injury as it may be related to [3]
- Exterior framework
- Posterior ethmoidal maxillary bony base
- Superior fronto-ethmoidal complex

Residual deformities may fall in the following groups and are discussed in brief
- Deformities of the nasal bridge or nasomaxillary region.
- Deformities of the naso-orbital angle or naso-ethmoidal region.
- Deformities associated with nasofrontal angle.
- Complex deformities involving the naso-ethmoido-frontal complex.

61.3.8.2 Deformities of the Nasal Bridge or Nasomaxillary Region [3]

Deformities involving the nasal bridge and lateral walls of the nose not extending into the frontal or orbital regions.

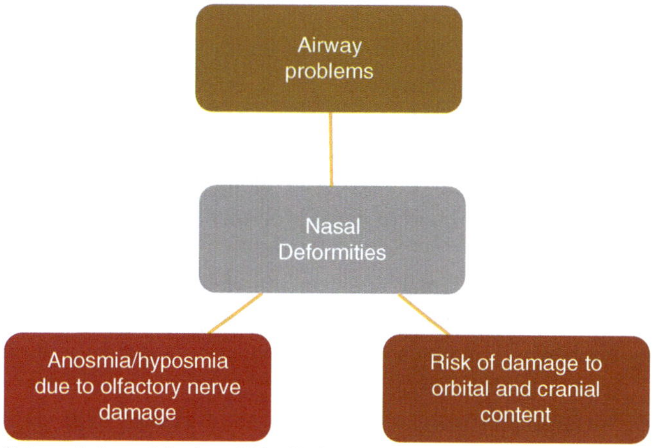

Chart 61.9 Potential complications associated with nasal deformities

Pathogenesis:
- Fractures of → nasal bone, frontal process of the maxilla, septal cartilage → untreated and/or inadequately treated fractures, displaced fragment → resorption associated with fibrous union/malunion with excess callus formation.
- Malunion depends on the direction and point of contact of the blow of the original injury.
- Residual callus and subsequent deformity will be evident following fracture of bony or cartilaginous structures or both tissues.
- Force directed from the lateral aspect → deviation of the bridge and lateral wall to the opposite side.
- Force → antero-posterior plane → depression of the nasal bridge and crushing of associated supporting posterior bony elements.
- Blow from the lateral aspect → displacement or bent/twisted nature of the nasal septum → one surface of the septum is therefore outwardly bent → airway obstruction.
- Impact → antero-posterior or sagittal plane → telescoped or folded septum → reduces nasal patency → obstruction of airway

Clinical Features:
- Obvious external deformity—aesthetic concern for the patient.
- Nose deviated towards one side or crushed inwards or both deformities together.
- Deviation → curvature of the septum.
- When seen from the front, the bridge and the dorsum of the nose may appear to be in a straight line, but the tip and the base of the septum are deviated, also leading to deformation of the nasal orifice.

Nose:

- Convex on one side (*or*) upper half/lower half—convex, another half—concave.
- Tip of nose may often be straight but is angulated when the cartilaginous dorsum is displaced.
- Profile—straight or depressed along the entire length/depression confined to nasal prominence (upper or lower half).
- Malunion of septal component—deformity leading to alteration in patency of the nasal airway.
- Narrowing of patency—Unilateral or bilateral → ultimately leads to obstruction.
- Nasal disturbances—Important to evaluate with age, occupation, pre-existing illness or any pulmonary pathology.
- Nasal airway disturbance → may lead to complications of airway tract and paranasal sinuses.
- Depression of nose—depression along the entire nasal crest or depression involving only the lower half.

Surgical Approach for nasal deviation:

- Intranasal approach for aesthetic rhinoplasty—this avoids any external cutaneous scars.
- Dissection is done by Separating or freeing the external investing tissues → elevation of mucous membrane that lines the nasal fossae.
- Dissection includes separation of underlying soft tissues and separation of mucosa.
- Bony and cartilaginous structures freed from the external and internal harvesting tissues.
- This is followed by chondrotomies and osteotomies.
- Chondrotomies are done to mobilise the septal cartilage.
- Osteotomies are done to reduce the displacement of the nasal bridge and dorsum – lateral and median osteotomy.
- Immobilisation aids in maintaining the fragments in position during the union. Careful immobilisation is done internally and externally.

61.3.8.3 Depression of Nose [3] (Saddle-Shaped Deformity)

Treatment differs based on extent of the deformity along the nasal crest (entire length or lower half).

- This deformity is best treated with placement of a bone graft in the region of depression of the bone.
- Intranasal: Best indicated surgical approach but less nasal exposure is a disadvantage.
- Vertical columella incision: Gives good exposure but may leave scars.
- A combined incision with both internal and external incision gives best exposure and leaves a less obvious transnasal scar in the anterior one-third of columella. This is almost invisible in the upright position due to its presence in a "dead angle".
- Surgical steps involve preparation of bony bed at receptor site and preparation of bone graft for placement.
- Stabilisation of bone graft by firm fixation in median, vertical and sagittal planes. Ensure the maintenance of columnar support.
- Sutures placed with adequate immobilisation.

61.3.8.4 Depression of Lower Half of Nasal Crest [3]

Two types of concepts are followed in treatment of such deformities:

- Reduce false or relative prominence by resection of upper half of the nasal crest. Nasal profile is converted to being straight. This might increase the width of the upper half of the nasal crest for which osteotomy of lateral walls may be essential. This concept is to be applied when adequate nasal bone is available to produce a healthy and aesthetic profile.
- The other concept involves the placement of a cartilaginous graft to cover the depression. Fixation may however be difficult in this scenario.

61.3.8.5 Naso-Orbital Deformities [3]

Deformities not only involving the nasal pyramid but also affecting the ethmoid and maxillary components.

Pathogenesis:

- Severe impact → nasal complex → results in extension of fracture lines and displacement of associated components.
- Deformities may extend into the frontal process of the maxilla and the two orbital plates of ethmoid bone (which support the nasal bones).
- Due to the complex anatomy of this region, various combinations in deformities, fracture pattern, injury and pathology may be seen.

Anatomical Characteristics: [3]

Frontal process of the maxilla—

- Determines the morphology of nasal pyramid.
- Determines the orbito-nasal angle
- Forms the lacrimal fossa (anterior part)
- Serves as a point of insertion for the medial palpebral ligament in the anterior crest

Ethmoid bone—

- Determines the formation of lacrimal canal on lateral aspects.
- Continues posteriorly as the orbital plate which forms the medial wall of the orbit.
- Contributes to the formation of the posterior part of the nasal septum.

Clinical Features:

Nasal crest—

- Deviated or often depressed → consequent lateral displacement or antero-posterior crushing of the nasal bones.
  Orbito-nasal angle—
- Reduced/obliterated/displaced outwards
  Widening of bridge—
- Due to displacement of frontal processes of the maxillae outwards and backwards
- Due to malunion of a comminuted type of fracture.
  Displacement of medial canthus—
- External displacement may produce telecanthus.
- Anterior displacement will further increase in obliteration of the orbito-nasal angle.
- Inferior dystopia—vertical displacement deranges the symmetry of two medial canthi.
- Dystopias are due to the bony fragments impinging on the tissues and causing rupture of the medial canthal ligament, avulsion of the ligament and displacement of frontal process of maxilla which houses the medial canthal ligament.
  Lacrimal passages—
- The lacrimal canal is blocked due to discontinuity in nasolacrimal apparatus. Bony fragments of comminuted fractures may cause tearing of the lacrimal sac. This may result in epiphora.
- Epiphora → watering of eyes — → dacryocystitis.
  Nasal airway patency problems due to —
- Deviation of posterior part of nasal septum.
- Blockage caused by nasal septum may further be accentuated by displacement of anterior cartilaginous part of the nasal septum.

Essentials in Correcting the Deformity:
- Repair the base of the nose.
- Repair the naso-orbital angle.
- Restore the lacrimal passages.
- Nasal reconstruction must be carried out while correcting the above mentioned during the same procedure.

61.3.8.6 Surgical Management

Key Points in Treatment:
- Reconstitution of the nasal base is the basic procedure in reconstruction of the nasal pyramid. It has to be supported by a solid base.
- Base has to be aesthetically appealing, smooth, regular and well proportioned.
- Reconstitution of the naso-orbital angle is essential.
- Symmetrical placement of the two medial canthi is necessary. Any asymmetry can affect the appearance of the nose.
- Approach to the lacrimal passages may be obtained by dividing the medial canthal ligament that can be reattached later.
- Quality of repair is subsequently affected in cases of infected lacrimal passages.
- Any deviation of the nasal septum negatively influences nasal reconstruction.

61.3.8.7 Nasofrontal Deformities [3]

Deformities due to secondary post-traumatic lesions involving not only the nasal pyramid but also the nasal base and area of the frontal bone. Concentration of injuries at the nasofrontal angle is proportionate to the degree of violence encountered, thereby resulting in fractures and displacement of tissues.

Nasofrontal angle profile is affected by
- Frontal region (median)
- Paranasal region (inferior)
- Secondary malunited callus

Pathogenesis:

- Trauma → nasal spine of frontal bone→ displacement of nasal spine involving middle part of the inferior wall or floor of the sinus
- Trauma → anterior wall of sinus → fracture extending into the anterior wall of sinus or posteriorly communicating with the posterior wall
  Lesions on anterior wall—
- When isolated and not involving the other walls → has only aesthetic significance
- Malunited depressed fracture → hollow midline → significant reduction of the nasofrontal angle
  Lesions of inferior wall—
- Depression → hollow midline → reduction in nasofrontal angle → has a cosmetic influence and also affects patency of frontonasal duct →blockage of canal → blockage of outflow tract
- Lateral aspect of lesions → involving medial portion of orbital roof → deformed naso-orbital angle → subsequent risk of spread of the infection
  Lesions of posterior wall—
- Injury in this zone affects the brain and the meninges.
- Fracture → unhealed fissures → spread of infection to the meninges.
- Deformity in the continuity of bone → herniation of the brain and meninges.
- Sharp bony defect → penetrates the meninges → CSF rhinorrhoea.
  Associated lesions—
- When more than one wall is involved → increased deformity of the nasofrontal angle → complications in sinus drainage, brain and meninges
- Resorption of fractured margins → loss of continuity in the anterior or posterior walls → deformed nasofrontal angle

Clinical Features:

- Profile is altered—depression and deviation of nasal bones → unaesthetic profile of the frontonasal angle.
- Greater degree of depression is relative to the retrusion or displacement of middle frontal segment posteriorly, extending above the orbits as far as the bridge of nose.
- Resorption or loss of bony tissue → protrusion of tissue between bony margins → meningocele → increased prominence.

Associated pathological changes—

- Osteitis in fracture zone
- Improper drainage → persistence of infection
- Meningitis
- CSF rhinorrhoea
- Brain abscess

Essentials in Surgical Management:

- Morphological and functional defects should be corrected to avoid any vital injury in the future.
- In case of depression of the nasal crest and deformities involving only the anterior wall of sinus, onlay bone graft is essential to augment the defect.
- Grossly deranged sinus must be treated first and then followed by nasal reconstruction.
- Grafting is not enough when deformities involve the inferior wall/floor and/or posterior wall as it carries the risk of damaging the sinus, brain and meninges.

The principles of the management of nasofrontal deformities in delayed conditions are similar to managing post-traumatic nasofrontal deformities but should be done with caution and must address associated complications seen at the stage of delayed management. In case of nasofrontal deformities, it is important to address post-traumatic dehiscence of frontal sinus wall in delayed management cases. Certain degree of bone loss due to resorption is seen during the post-traumatic phase, and this may increase when the management is delayed. Hence, in such cases it is important to be cautious in resection of minimal tissue of the posterior wall, and it needs to be carefully performed. Reconstruction of the anterior wall with bone grafts may be done, also including the orbital roof and the ethmoidal region if necessary [3].

61.3.8.8 Naso-Fronto-Ethmoidal Deformities [3]

Deformities involving the nasal bony mass are caused due to greater degree of force. The impact may extend as far as the ethmoid bone which forms the upper wall/roof in the posterior part.

Pathogenesis:

- Fractures lines extending from the front, passing behind and across the nasal spine and extending into the cribriform plate
- Displacement due to fracture → affects the passage of olfactory nerve → further lacerates the dura mater → cerebrospinal fluid leakage or CSF rhinorrhoea

Clinical Features:

- Clinically, it may be similar to the deformities involving nasofrontal fractures. A mere extension into the cribriform plate does not increase the severity of the deformity. Features may differ based on the involvement of anterior wall.
- Anosmia—loss of smell sensation.
- If the meningeal tear is not sealed immediately → CSF rhinorrhoea.
- The meningeal tear is always predisposed with long-term risk of leak (even after the leakage has dried) due to lack in quality of scar tissue and increased permeability of the malunited callus.

Essentials in Management of Naso-Fronto-Ethmoidal Deformities:

- Surgery may be carried out by combined neurosurgical and maxillofacial teams.
- Meningeal tear repair can be managed by trans-ethmoidal (low level) approach. However, trans-frontal approach is considered to be safer and effective.
- Sinus-associated lesions should be managed along with nasal reconstruction procedure.
- *The principles of the management of naso-fronto-ethmoidal deformities in delayed conditions are similar to managing post-traumatic naso-fronto-ethmoidal deformities or naso-orbito-ethomoidal complex fractures but should be done with caution, addressing associated complications seen at the stage of delayed management.*

61.3.8.9 Delayed Management of Orbital Hypertelorism and Naso-Orbito-Ethmoidal (NOE) Fractures [73, 75–77]

Acute trauma in the naso-orbito-ethomoidal region could result in chronic orbital and naso-orbital deformities. It is important to be aware of the acute injury to correct the deformity that will be established later. Secondary late corrections in cases of severe orbital hypertelorism may be very difficult to correct. The severity of orbital hypertelorism can be assessed with the help of Tessier score.

Traumatic orbital hypertelorism due to NOE complex fractures
Goals of management:
- Symmetrical restoration of medial canthal anatomy
- Maintenance of physiologic function of the lacrimal system
- Avoid frontal sinus-related complications
- Restoration of globe position and volume

Surgical Management:
- Coronal approach gives the most predictable access and visualisation for the surgeon.
- Frontal sinus should also be evaluated and operated at this stage.
- Reconstruction should be considered in the following order starting first with cranial base, frontal region and outer orbital zone, followed by fixation of the orbital rim and frontonasal buttress. Grafts and plates may be used to restore the nasal dorsum and nasal projection.
- It is then followed by repositioning and fixation of the mini-plate in the medial orbital wall and medial canthal tendon. Mesh and trans-nasal wiring may be used for repositioning the displaced medial canthal tendon.
- It is important to establish a good frontonasal angle and nasal projection to have good aesthetic outcome. Deformity could result in poor aesthetics when there is poor frontonasal angle and poor nasal projection along with orbital hypertelorism.

61.3.8.10 Secondary or Delayed Management of Orbital Hypertelorism Associated with NOE Complex Fractures [75–77]

- Goal is to restore the normal interorbital distance.
- Acute management of chronic long-standing deformities is essential. It is very difficult to correct severe orbital hypertelorism, especially in cases which includes intracranial osteotomies. Such cases are associated with increased post-operative morbidities. Subcranial osteotomies may be opted in milder cases.
- Aesthetic and functional outcomes in late correction may not be satisfying, and hence the best strategy is to repair the deformities as early as possible following the first injury and hence not delay the treatment.

61.3.8.11 Conclusion

- Repair and reconstruction of nasal deformities are often challenging and technique sensitive for the surgical team (maxillofacial and neurosurgical). It is emotionally and psychologically challenging for the patients as well. Hence, it is essential to identify the pitfalls and carefully carry out the surgical treatment plan. Sometimes, further revision may be necessary even with the best planned surgical procedures. Therefore, it is important for the surgeon and the patient to understand the limitations of the available surgical techniques.

61.4 Post-oncological Deformities

Management of Post-oncological Deformities:
Post-oncological deformities here refer to the soft tissue and hard tissue defects that may be encountered following a primary treatment. Unlike a primary cosmetic therapy, predicting the result of an oncological treatment is often more technique sensitive and should be considerate in establishing the overall physical and mental well-being of the patient. Management of deformities should also aim at a comprehensive functional, aesthetic and social well-being of the patient.

Reconstruction of soft tissue and hard tissue structures following trauma or oncological surgical therapy is primarily essential. Correction of the residual deformities should be carried out along with the principles of reconstructive management.

Reconstruction generally includes the following steps in management [78]:
- Healing by secondary intention
- Primary closure
- Grafting—split or full-thickness graft
- Composite grafts
- Local grafts
- Regional pedicle grating
- Free tissue transfer

We have already discussed in detail the use of above methods in management of traumatic residual deformities in this chapter.

Recurrences, untreated tumours and metastasis which are considered to be residual in nature after primary management are not considered under management of post-oncological deformities. It is important for the surgeons to be more accurate with the surgical margins when surgically operating malignancies. Any re-surgical procedure for recurrence or deformities is often challenging due to factors like previously irradiated areas, previously operated surgical field, under nourished status due to the pre-existing malignant condition and also due minimal surgical options for such patients.

Residual deformities associated with post-oncosurgery results in external facial disfigurement/defects, intra-oral defects and also changes that may affect certain functions. These deformities are often relative to structures which were primarily involved and their corresponding functional deformities. Deformities occurring following surgical treatment of head and neck oncology usually require reconstruction procedures as the complete removal of tumours with margins may involve increased loss of soft or hard tissues.

61.4.1 Lip Deformities [79–83]

Post-oncosurgical defects of the lip are often seen with loss of tissues. Management of such defects is usually considered according to the size of the defects. Secondary deformities of the lower lip after reconstruction are described in (Table 61.5), and they need to be treated accordingly with cosmetic surgeries. *Lip reconstruction is discussed in soft Tissue reconstruction chap.* 86.

Table 61.5 Secondary deformities of lower lip following reconstruction

Type of Flap	Deformities	Complications
Abbe	Relative Microsomia Trap Door deformity due to thickened scar	Vermillon notching Lip asymmetry Scarring beyond submental crease
Estlander	Commissure violation and may require commissuroplasty	
Karpandzic	Microstomia Inversion vermillion Flat mentolabial junction	Dysthesia or Anesthesia of lip
Gillies fan	Oral incompetence may result	
Bernard burrow	Adynamic reconstruction	Post-operative drooling

61.4.2 Management of Intra-oral Defects Involving Floor of the Mouth and Alveolar Ridge Tumours

Defects in these regions are relative to the size of tissues lost and may be corrected with augmentation and reconstruction procedures.

- *Correction of small intra-oral defects is best done with* primary closure in the buccal and tongue region, but scar contracture is seen with grafting. Closure by secondary intention can be done in alveolar and hard palate defects where the scar contracture is insignificant [84].
- *Correction of large intra-oral defects using* free flaps is considered ideal in reconstruction procedures [84–86].
- *Advanced large defects* may be seen in cases which require large resection of tissues, as in cases of advanced tumours which may include cortical or segmental mandibulectomy, composite resections, and glossectomy (total/sub-total) procedure. These defects may also involve the lip or skin of the lower third of the face when tumour extends anteriorly [86]. Hemi- or partial loss of mandible may result in severe functional or psychological morbidity for the patients. The loss of anterior mandible results in a defect called as "Andy-Gump" deformity [87]. En bloc resection is best reconstructed with regional free tissue transfer or free flaps. Bony defects are managed with osteocutaneous free flap or with free tissue transfer.

61.4.3 Management of Defects of Oropharynx

Oropharyngeal defects are managed with primary closure, skin grafts, local pedicle flaps and microvascular-free flaps. Current goals in reconstruction include restoration of the function and closure of defects as well.

61.4.3.1 Management of Soft Palate Defects [88]

- Soft palate defects cause *velopharyngeal incompetency* resulting in inability to seal the oropharyngeal and nasopharyngeal cavity during speech and deglutition.
- *Rhinolalia aperta* is caused due to small soft palate defects leading to change in resonance of voice as a result of air escape due to incompetent velum.
- *Smaller defects* are best closed primarily or along with a split-thickness skin graft.
- *Radial forearm flaps* are used in cases following surgical ablation of *soft palate and tonsillar defects.*

- *Large or extensive palatomaxillary defects* are managed with obturator prosthesis or with vascularised osteocutaneous free flaps.

61.4.3.2 Management of Tongue Defects [89, 90]

Tongue defects are usually difficult to treat and reconstruct. Management of tongue defects primarily involves improving the functional outcome.

- *Small defects* are managed with primary closure.
- *Large defects* are treated with myocutaneous flaps (rectus or pectoral major flaps and fasciocutaneous flaps)

61.4.3.3 Management of Posterior Pharyngeal Wall [90]

- Primary closure with/without split thickness skin graft is used for closure of small defects. Free flap reconstruction is necessary for large defects.

61.4.4 Deformities Associated with Intra-oral Disfigurement [91–98]

The primary goal in surgical management of oral tumours is to gain surgical access for assessment and visualisation of margins and anatomic relations for resecting the tumours. Surgical margins are vital in establishing a tumour-free zone. Although it is important to have a follow-up on recurrence of tumours and metastasis, it is the complex nature of the oral cavity and head and neck anatomy that requires careful yet skilful management of the adjacent normal tissues by proper closure and post-operative management.

The goal earlier was to achieve access to the tumours, but now it also involves incisions that will facilitate an aesthetic access to the pathology. Increased incidence of dehiscence and unaesthetic scar formation are common in neck incisions (with trifurcation extensions) that do not lie along the natural skin creases. Irradiated areas may cause worsening of scar appearance, or even superficial necrosis may occur. Inadequate, delayed and infected tracheostomy may also result in an unaesthetic tracheostomy scar formation. Prevention of unaesthetic scars can be done by careful tissue handling. It is also essential to protect the skin from additional trauma due to traction, tension or electrocautery. Flaps with adequate vascularity further help to minimise the chances of unaesthetic scars. Following access through the lip to certain tumours in the oral cavity, the site requires to be exactly oriented and aligned with the vermilion lip border, as well as interdigitating orbicularis oris muscle, re-orienting lip skin and oral mucosa to replicate lip competence, aesthetics and function [92–97].

Even though reconstruction of maxillectomy defects is an option, maxillary defects can also be corrected with prosthetic obturators. Maxillary obturator provides adequate structural support to preserve speech, swallowing and essential mastication. Clinically, a good obturator can be fabricated only by the skills of a good prosthodontist [98].

It is important to evaluate any history that may contribute to poor wound healing and also lead to post-operative wound dehiscence and compromised flap vascularity resulting in improper scarring.

61.4.5 Deformities Associated with Healing Tissues [91, 92, 99, 100]

Surgical procedure involving the upper aerodigestive tract through neck incision may lead to fistula formation as a result of salivary leakage.

The formation of fistulas is contributed majorly due to:

- Incision design
- Tumour type
- Tumour stage
- Improper surgical site management
- History of operative site
- Physical and nutritional status of patient

Biological Factors that Contribute to Fistula Formation:

- Effect of radiation on surgical wound closure: Radiation dose and timing play an important role in delayed wound healing, formation of fistula and dehiscence.
- Low oxygen tension: Proportional to flap vascularity and viability.
- Vascularity: Decreased blood supply affects the wound healing property.

Signs and Symptoms of Fistulas:

- Occurs post-surgery as early as 1 week and somewhere between 3 and 4weeks in late cases of fistula formation. Persistent fistulas are present for more than 1 month.
- Low-grade fever.
- Inflamed and indurated areas of skin that facilitate the drainage.

Management:

- Early assessment of fistula can help to explore the surgical wound and aid in directing saliva from vital structures.
- Site may be explored, irrigated and closed. This is followed by antimicrobial therapy and nutritional support.
- Persistent fistulas are managed with excision of the fistulous tract with closure of oral mucosa and/or skin.

- Hardware failure due to infection can be managed with local debridement, removal/replacement of existing failed hardware and closure with local and regional flaps.
- Management can be combined with anti-cholinergic medications to decrease salivary flow if necessary and only if indicated.

61.4.6 Functional Deformities Associated with Oro-Oncological Surgery

Surgical cancer resection may cause the following functional defects [101]:

- Difficulty in speech, swallowing and chewing
- Difficulty in masticatory function and nutrition
- Neurological complications

61.4.6.1 Spinal Accessory Nerve

Iatrogenic injury may cause "shoulder syndrome", for which physical therapy may help to improve the functional outcome. Pain, weakness of muscles, restrained shoulder movement, deformity of the upper extremity and inability to abduct upper extremity above 90degress occur due to denervation of trapezius muscle [91, 92, 102, 103].

61.4.6.2 Phrenic Nerve

Iatrogenic damage causes paralysis of ipsilateral diaphragm. It may even result in long-term pulmonary complications. Such damage can be prevented by limiting surgical dissection to the layer superficial to pre-vertebral fascia and thereby prevent injury to nerve [92, 101, 104].

61.4.6.3 Hypoglossal Nerve and lingual Nerve [92, 101, 104]

- Iatrogenic damage to both the nerves is possible during head and neck dissection. This is aggravated with damage to lingual nerve during excision of tongue and floor of the mouth. Hypoglossal and lingual nerves are often preserved unless there is extensive neural invasion of the tumour.
- Hypoglossal nerve dysfunction/damage causes deviation of tongue to ipsilateral side of injury, tongue biting, dysarthria and difficulty in mastication and deglutition. Bilateral nerve injury may result in upper airway obstruction when the patient is in supine position. Atrophy of tongue muscles may also be observed.
- Damage to lingual nerve may cause ipsilateral loss of sensation, further impacting mastication, speech and swallowing. Injury to tongue during speech and mastication may also be observed.
- Rehabilitation by physical therapy is often useful for improving the speech and swallowing.

61.4.6.4 Vagus Nerve, Recurrent Laryngeal Nerve and Superior Laryngeal Nerve [91]

- Injury to these nerves may occur during dissection around the carotid sheath.
- Injury to recurrent laryngeal nerve causes unilateral vocal cord paralysis. The damage is usually compensated by the intact contralateral vocal cord. Mild hoarseness is experienced by the patient. Upper airway obstruction is seen with bilateral injury.
- Injury to branches of superior laryngeal nerve occurs due to dissection around the superior thyroid branch of external carotid artery. The following changes may be associated:
- Minor swallowing difficulty
- Decreased sensation in laryngeal inlet
- Decrease in tensor capability of true vocal cord
- Fatigue
- Decreased ability to reach high phonated/pitched sounds

Management usually begins with accurate diagnosis of the neurological origin. It is best to prevent such injuries with careful dissection.

61.4.6.5 Sympathetic Trunk [92, 101, 104]

Damage or disruption to the sympathetic trunk can result in ipsilateral Horner's syndrome. Careful evaluation is necessary to diagnose Horner's syndrome due to damage of nerve fibres, and it involves the following:

- Blepharoptosis (drooping of upper eyelid)
- Miosis or pupillary constriction
- Lack of perspiration of forehead skin
- Enophthalmos
- Vascular dilation (ipsilateral to injury)

61.4.6.6 Marginal Mandibular Branch of Facial Nerve [92, 105]

Injury to This Nerve Causes:

- Altered mobility of corner of the mouth as a result of disruption in innervation to orbicular oris and depressor anguli oris.
- Inability to control lower lip movements during liquid consumption.
- Functional and cosmetic disturbances are seen.

Management:

Careful design and incision considering the anatomic location of the nerve during flap elevation help to prevent iatrogenic injuries and resultant deformities. It may take several months for neurosensory recovery when the neurologic injury is due to traction and not due to severance.

61.5 Recent Advances

61.5.1 Endoscopy in Residual Deformitites [106, 107]

Recent trend in oral surgery includes the use of an endoscope to facilitate oral and maxillofacial procedures. Endoscopy techniques can be used in diagnosis and for treatment with minimal complications in many oral and maxillofacial surgical procedures like TMJ disorders, pathologies of jaw, nasal deformities, trauma and aesthetic procedures. The techniques and applications of endoscopy in oral and maxillofacial surgery are explained in detail elsewhere in this book. The advantages and applications of endoscopy-assisted maxillofacial surgical procedures make its usage a favourite option for maxillofacial surgeons. Minimal complications, good success rates and its efficiency make endoscopy-assisted procedures a viable option.

The following are the best-known applications of endoscopy currently in oral and maxillofacial surgery:

- Trauma
- Orthognathic deformities
- Obstructive salivary gland pathology
- Maxillary sinus surgery
- Trigeminal nerve injury
- Temporomandibular disorders
- Nasal deformities
- Trauma

Endoscopy-assisted minimally invasive technique is used in traumatic deformities like the following:

Orbital Floor Fracture: Requires trans antral approach. Care should be taken to protect the intraorbital contents like musculature, periorbita and optic nerve. Intraoperative conditions may necessitate the need for an additional periorbital approach during the surgery.

Mandibular Angle Fracture: Here, endoscopy can be used to fix the mandible with the superior and inferior plate with the best approximation possible. Endoscopic reduction helps in complete visualisation of the entire fracture line with inclusion of the inferior border. Management with endoscopy-assisted surgery also reduces the risk of facial nerve injury. A single transbuccal trocar technique is used for positioning and fixation of the plates with easy visualisation of the fracture line. Some surgeons prefer a locking cannula for the precise placement of the fixation hardware. Endoscope is then used to confirm proper fixation and reduction, and it is then closed. Endoscope also aids in appropriate documentation of the procedure.

Sub-condylar Fractures: (Refer Chap. 54 on endoscopic approach for treatment of condylar fractures of mandible) Endoscopy can be applied in management of sub-condylar fractures by open technique, reducing risks of scars, fistula formation and facial nerve injury. Extra-oral and transoral approach may also be used. Although the procedure is technique sensitive, it is proposed with advantages of improved visualisation, magnified field of view, less trauma to tissues, less bleeding, better patient compliance, good reduction and decreased post-operative complications.

Frontal Sinus Fractures: Endoscopy in the management of frontal sinus fractures helps to avoid large incisions and its associated complications like alopecia, paraesthesia, scarring, nerve injury, etc. It helps in better visualisation of sinus wall fractures, nasofrontal duct and the posterior wall of sinus.

- The use of *endoscopy in orthognathic surgery* helps to visualise aspects of the osteotomy so as to improve the efficiency of the surgical outcome.
- Best application of endoscopy in salivary gland pathologies is the usage of sialoendoscopy in the diagnosis and treatment of salivary gland/ductal pathologies in a non-invasive manner.
- TMJ arthroscopy is another area that has gained greater attention.
- Endoscopy is also best utilised in removal of foreign bodies from the cranio-maxillofacial region as it allows visualisation of anatomical structures without extensive incisions.

Endoscopy in nasal deformities: is a developing concept, and there has been an increase in its extensive usage in sinus endoscopic surgeries. The use of endoscope in correction of septal deformities like deviation, aids in better visualisation of the target site and reduced time of the procedure. The primary advantages are improved field of view, reduced morbidity, decreased post-operative swelling and more accuracy in surgical procedure. Endoscopy in nasal corrections is very essential in cases that have gone for prior septal cartilage resection, reducing the need for repeated incisions or extent of dissection. Studies also suggest lesser post-operative symptoms in endoscopic-assisted nasal septal corrective surgeries [107].

61.6 Conclusion

Careful planning, eminent skills and excellent knowledge of the clinical anatomy are of utmost importance in carrying out secondary corrective procedures in treating residual deformities following trauma or oncological procedures. It is the skill of the surgeon to predict the functional and aesthetic outcome of the treatment so as to facilitate a proper treatment planning. It is also the role of the surgeon to educate the patient about the condition and options available for the correction, to provide the best possible outcome. It is recommended that surgeons use available imaging techniques (routine X-rays, CT scans, CBCT, etc.) in their treatment plans and also make best usage of the current trends in 3D models and visual planning software in treatment planning. The use of CAD/CAM-designed patient-specific alloplastic (e.g. Medpore, PEEK) implants should be considered in surgical management. Treatment plan should often accommodate recommendations from other specialities that may be a part of the surgical team.

Both soft tissue and hard tissue deformities should be dealt together in a well-planned manner to provide the patient with an acceptable aesthetic outcome and functional rehabilitation. Likewise, mastication and prosthetic rehabilitation can be aided by dental and zygomatic implants. Most often correction of residual deformities may go together with reconstruction of the lost structures. It becomes essential to carry out the entire treatment phase in a well-planned manner to provide the patient with a final, socially and psychologically acceptable outcome with or without post-operative physical therapy. Surgeons are also recommended to be updated about endoscopy-assisted surgeries and transoral robotic surgeries to further enhance the quality of outcome of the treatment.

References

Introduction

1. Ranganath K, Hemanth Kumar HR. The correction of post-traumatic pan facial residual deformity. J Maxillofac Oral Surg. 2011;10(1):20–4.
2. David DJ, Abott JR, Jay M, Nugent MAC. Deformities, textbook of craniomaxillofacial trauma, Chap. 21. New York: Churchill Livingstone; 1995. p. 545–618.
3. Evans AJ, Burwell RG, Merville L, Pfeifer G, Gundlach K, Sailer HF, et al. Residual deformities. In: Rowe NL, Williams JL, editors. Maxillofacial injuries, vol. 2. Edinburgh: Churchill Livingstone; 1985. p. 765–868.
4. Ardeshirpour F, et al. Improving posttraumatic facial scars. Otolaryngol Clin N Am. 2013;46(5):867–81.
5. Dolan R. Facial plastic, reconstructive and trauma surgery (Textbook). 2016 Apr. p. 716–29.
6. Hoffmann JF. Tissue expansion in the head and neck. Facial Plast Surg Clin North Am. 2005;13(2):315–24.
7. Van Rappard JHA, Molenaar J, Van Doorn K, Sonneveld GJ, Borghouts JMHM. Surface are increase in tissue expansion. Plast Reconstr Surg. 1988;82:833–7.
8. Kane WJ, McCaffrey TV, Wang TD, Koval TM. The effects of tissue expansion of previously irradiated skin. Arch Otolaryngol Head Neck Surg. 1992;118:419–26.
9. Kabaker SS, Kridel RWH, Krugman ME. Tissue expansions in the treatment of alopecia. Arch Otolaryngol. 1986;112:720.
10. Gibson T. The physical properties of skin. In: Converse JM, editor. Reconstructive plastic surgery, I. Philadelphia, PA: WB Saunders; 1977. p. 70–7.

Grafts in Residual Deformities

11. Hupp JR, Tucker MR, Ellis E. Contemporary oral and maxillofacial surgery, 6th ed. 2014.
12. Labres XR, Camps AR, Salas EJ, Albuquerque R, Ortega EV, et al. Graft materials in oral surgery: revision. J Biomimetics Biomater Tissue Eng. 2014;19:124.
13. Kumar P, et al. Bone grafts in dentistry. J Pharm Bioallied Sci. 2013;5(Suppl 1):S125–7.
14. Laurencin C, Khan Y, El-Amin SF. Bone graft substitutes. Expert Rev Med Devices. 2006;3:49–57.
15. Giannoudis PV, Dinopoulos H, Tsiridis E. Bone substitutes: an update. Injury. 2005;36(Suppl 3):S20–7.
16. Conrad EU, Gretch DR, Obermeyer KR, Moogk MS, Sayers M, Wilson JJ, et al. Transimission of the hepatitis-C virus by tissue transplantation. J Bone Joint Surg Am. 1995;77:214–24.
17. Centres for disease control and prevention. Septic arthritis following anterior cruciate ligament reconstruction using tendon allografts: Florida and Louisiana, 2000. MMWR Morb Mortal Wkly Rep. 2001;50:1081–3.
18. Boyne PJ, Sands NR. Secondary bone grafting of residual alveolar and palatal clefts. J Oral Surg. 1972 Feb;30(2):87–92.
19. Meara DJ. Acquired defects of the nose and naso-orbitoethmoid (NOE) region. Oral Maxillofac Surg Clin North Am. 2013;25(2):131–49.
20. Rieck KL, Fillmore WJ, Ettinger KS. Late revision or correction of facial trauma-related soft-tissue deformities. Oral Maxillofac Surg Clin North Am. 2013;25(4):697–713.
21. Khorasani M, et al. Maxillofacial reconstruction with Medpor porous polyethylene implant: a case series study. J Korean Assoc Oral Maxillofac Surg. 2018;44(3):128–35.
22. Schwaiger M, Echlin K, Atherton D, Haers P. The use of Medpor implants for midface contouring in cleft patients. Int J Oral Maxillofac Surg. 2019.
23. Scolozzi P. Maxillofacial reconstruction using polyetheretherketone patient-specific implants by "mirroring" computational planning. Aesthet Plast Surg. 2012;36(3):660–5.
24. Kim MM, Boahene KDO, Byrne PJ. Use of customized polyetheretherketone (PEEK) Implants in the reconstruction of complex maxillofacial defects. Arch Facial Plast Surg. 2009;11(1):53–7.
25. Salomon D, Miloro M, Kolokythas A. Outcomes of immediate allograft reconstruction of long span defects of the inferior alveolar nerve. J Oral Maxillofac Surg. 2016.
26. Bagheri SC, Meyer RA, Khan HA, Steed MB. Microsurgical repair of peripheral trigeminal nerve injuries from maxillofacial trauma. J Oral Maxillofac Surg. 2009;67(9):1791–9.

27. Renzi G, Carboni A, Perugini M, et al. Posttraumatic trigeminal nerve impairment: A prospective analysis of recovery patterns in a series of 103 consecutive facial fractures. J Oral Maxillofac Surg. 2004;62:1341.
28. Thurmuller P, Dodson TB, Kaban LB. Nerve injuries associated with facial trauma: Natural history, management, and outcomes of repair. Oral Maxillofac Surg Clin North Am. 2001;13:283.
29. Meyer RA. Nerve harvesting procedures. Atlas Oral Maxillofac Surg Clin North Am. 2001;9:77.
30. Joohee J, et al. Per-oral cross-facial sural nerve graft for facial reanimation. Maxillofac Plast Reconstr Surg. 2018;40(1):22.
31. Lu X, Cai Z, Peng X, Yu G. Reconstruction of peripheral facial nerve injury. Int J Oral Maxillofac Surg. 2009;38(5):511.
32. Ichihara S, Inada Y, Nakamura T. Artificial nerve tubes and their application for repair of peripheral nerve injury: an update of current concepts. Injury. 2008;39(Suppl 4):29–39.
33. Gheisari R, et al. Parotid duct repair by facial vein graft versus gore-tex: a sialographic evaluation. J Dent (Shiraz, Iran). 2013;14(2):53–6.
34. Raveenthiran V. Reconstruction of traumatically avulsed parotid duct using buccal mucosa flap: report of a new technique. J Trauma. 2008;65:732–5.
35. Lewkowicz AA, Hasson O, Nahlieli O. Traumatic injuries to the parotid gland and duct. J Oral Maxillofac Surg. 2002;60:676–80.
36. Parekh D, Glezerson G, Stewart M, Esser J, Lawson HH. Posttraumatic parotid fistulae and sialoceles. A prospective study of conservative management in 51 cases. Ann Surg. 1989;209:105–11.
37. Ananthakrishnan N. Vein graft repair of a chronic parotid duct fistula. J Oral Maxillofac Surg. 1983;41:266–7.
38. Heymans O, Nélissen X, Médot M, Fissette J. Microsurgical repair of Stensen's duct using an interposition vein graft. J Reconstr Microsurg. 1999;15:105–7.
39. Tao JP, Luppens D, McCord CD. Buccal mucous membrane graft-assisted lacrimal drainage surgery. Ophthalmic Plast Reconstr Surg. 2010;26(1):39–41.
40. Balaji SM. Management of nasolacrimal duct injuries in midfacial advancement. Ann Maxillofac Surg. 2015;5(1):93–5.
41. Tao H, Wu H-Y, Hou S-K. Lacrimal duct reconstruction with grafting of great saphenous vein or labial mucosa via endoscopic transnasal dacryocystorhinostomy: a group comparison in 18 cases. J Clin Rehabil Tissue Eng Res. 2009;13(44):8797–800.
42. Terino EO, Edwards MC. Customizing jawlines: the art of alloplastic premandible contouring. Facial Plast Surg Clin North Am. 2008;16:99–122.
43. Scolozzi P, Martinez A, Jaques B. Complex orbitofrontotemporal reconstruction using computer-designed PEEK implant. J Craniofac Surg. 2007;18:224–8.

Hard Tissue Deformities

44. Van der Meulen JC. Medial faciotomy. Br J Plast Surg. 1979;32:339–42.
45. Hupp JR, Tucker MR, Ellis E. Surgical reconstruction of defects of jaw. Contemporary oral and maxillofacial surgery, 7th ed. 2019. p. 628–40.
46. Vega LG. Reoperative mandibular trauma: management of posttraumatic mandibular deformities. Oral Maxillofac Surg Clin North Am. 2011;23(1):47–61, v–vi.
47. Haug RH, Schwimmer A. Fibrous union of the mandible: a review of 27 patients. J Oral Maxillofac Surg. 1994;52(8):832–9.
48. Mathog RH, Toma V, Clayman L, et al. Nonunion of the mandible: an analysis of contributing factors. J Oral Maxillofac Surg. 2000;58(7):746–52.
49. Furr AM, Schweinfurth JM, May WL. Factors associated with long-term complications after repair of mandibular fractures. Laryngoscope. 2006;116(3):427–30.
50. De Souza M, Oeltjen JC, Panthaki ZJ, et al. Posttraumatic mandibular deformities. J Craniofac Surg. 2007;18(4):912–6.
51. Ellis E. Complications of rigid internal fixation for mandibular fractures. J Craniomaxillofac Trauma. 1996;2(2):32–9.
52. Koury M. Complications of mandibular fractures. In: Kaban L, Pogrel A, Perrott D, editors. Complications in oral and maxillofacial surgery. 1st ed. Philadelphia: WB Saunders; 1997. p. 121–45.
53. Ellis E, Walker R. Treatment of malocclusion and TMJ dysfunction secondary to condylar fractures. Craniomaxillofac Trauma Reconstr. 2009;2(1):1–18.
54. Laskin DM. Management of condylar process fractures. Oral Maxillofac Surg Clin North Am. 2009;21(2):193–6.
55. Becking AG, Zijderveld SA, Tuinzing DB. Management of posttraumatic malocclusion caused by condylar process fractures. J Oral Maxillofac Surg. 1998;56(12):1370–4.
56. Ellis E, Throckmorton G. Treatment of mandibular condylar process fractures: biological considerations. J Oral Maxillofac Surg. 2005;63(1):115–34.
57. Marx RE, Saunders TR. Reconstruction and rehabilitation of cancer patients. In: Fonseca RJ, Davis WH, editors. Reconstructive preprosthetic oral and maxillofacial surgery. Philadelphia, PA: WB Saunders; 1986.
58. Acero J, García E. Reoperative midface reconstruction. Oral Maxillofac Surg Clin North Am. 2011;23(1):133–51, vii.
59. Kokemueller H, Tavassol F, Ruecker M, et al. Complex midfacial reconstruction: a combined technique of computer-assisted surgery and microvascular tissue transfer. J Oral Maxillofac Surg. 2008;66:2398–406.
60. Zizelmann C, Gellrich NC, Metzger MC, et al. Computer-assisted reconstruction of orbital floor based on cone beam tomography. Br J Oral Maxillofac Surg. 2007;45(1):79–80.
61. Coleman SR. Facial recontouring with lipostructure. Clin Plast Surg. 1997;24:347–67.
62. Wassmund M. Lehrbuch der praktischen Chirurgie 6es Mundes und der Ki.efer, Bd. I. Meusser, Leipzig 1935
63. Wunderer S. Die Prognathieoperation mittels frontal gestieltem Maxillafragment. Ost Z Stomat. 1962;59:98.
64. Schuchardt K. Formen des offenen Bisses und ihre operativen Behandlungsmöglichkeiten. Fortschr Kiefer Gesichtschir. 1955;1:222–30.
65. Tessier P, Guiot G, Rougerie J, Delbet JP, Pastoriza J. Cranio-naso-orbito-facial osteotomies. Hypertelorism. Ann Chir Plast. 1967;12:103–18.
66. Tessier P. Total facial osteotomy. Crouzon's syndrome, Apert's syndrome: oxycephaly, scaphocephaly, turricephaly. Ann Chir Plast. 1967;12:273–86.
67. Tessier P. Experiences in the treatment of orbital hypertelorism. Plast Reconstr Surg. 1974;53:1–18.
68. Converse JM, Ransohoff J, Mathews ES, Smith B, Molenaar A. Ocular hypertelorism and pseudohypertelorism. Advances in surgical treatment. Plast Reconstr Surg. 1970;45:1–13.
69. Van der Meulen JC, Vaandrager JM. Surgery related to the correction of hypertelorism. Plast Reconstr Surg. 1983;71:6–19.
70. Ortiz-Monasterio F, del Campo AF, Carrillo A. Advancement of the orbits and the midface in onepiece, combined with frontal

repositioning, for the correction of Crouzon's deformities. Plast Reconstr Surg. 1978;61:507–16.
71. Marchac D, Renier D, Arnaud E. Infrafrontal correction of teleorbitism. In: Whitaker L, editor. Proceedings from the seventh meeting of the ISCFS. Santa Fe: Menduzzi; 1997. p. 173–5.
72. Marin PC, Love T, Carpenter R, Iliff NT, Manson PN. Complications of orbital reconstruction: misplacement of bone grafts within the intramuscular cone. Plast Reconstr Surg. 1998;101:1323–7.
73. Wolff J, Sándor GK, Pyysalo M, Miettinen A, Koivumäki AV, Kainulainen VT. Late reconstruction of orbital and naso-orbital deformities. Oral Maxillofac Surg Clin North Am. 2013;25(4):683–95.
74. Cohen SR, Kawamoto HK Jr. Analysis and results of treatment of established posttraumatic facial deformities. Plast Reconstr Surg. 1992;90:574–84.
75. Sandor GK, Clokie CM. Hypertelorism. In: Fonseca RJ, editor. Oral and maxillofacial surgery, vol. 6. Philadelphia: W.B. Saunders Company; 2000. p. 221–38.
76. Tessier P. Anatomical classification of facial, craniofacial, and latero-facial clefts. J Maxillofac Surg. 1976;4:69–89.
77. Lanigan DT, Stoelinga PJ. Fractures of the supraorbital rim. J Oral Surg. 1980;38(10):764–70.

Post Oncological Deformities

78. Hurvitz KA, Kobayashi M, Evans GR. Current options in head and neck reconstruction. Plast Reconstr Surg. 2006;118(5):122e–33e.
79. Renner G. Reconstruction of the lip. In: Baker S, editor. Local flaps in facial reconstruction. 2nd ed. Philadelphia, PA: Mosby; 2007. p. 475–525.
80. Abbe R. A new plastic operation for the relief of deformity due to double harelip. Plast Reconstr Surg. 1968;42(5):481–3.
81. Ong WC, Lim J, Lim TC. A modification of the bilobed and Karapandzic flap used for reconstruction of the lower lip. Plast Reconstr Surg. 2005;115(7):2154–5.
82. Anvar BA, Evans BC, Evans GR. Lip reconstruction. Plast Reconstr Surg. 2007;120(4):57e–64e.
83. Ozdemir R, Ortak T, Kocer U, Celebioglu S, Sensoz O, Tiftikcioglu YO. Total lower lip reconstruction using sensate composite radial forearm flap. J Craniofac Surg. 2003;14(3):393–405.
84. McConnel FM, Pauloski BR, Logemann JA, Rademaker AW, Colangelo L, Shedd D, et al. Functional results of primary closure vs flaps in oropharyngeal reconstruction: a prospective study of speech and swallowing. Arch Otolaryngol Head Neck Surg. 1998;124(6):625–30.
85. Yu P. Characteristics of the anterolateral thigh flap in a Western population and its application in head and neck reconstruction. Head Neck. 2004;26(9):759–69.
86. Vos JD, Burkey BB. Functional outcomes after free flap reconstruction of the upper aerodigestive tract. Curr Opin Otolaryngol Head Neck Surg. 2004;12(4):305–10.
87. Aziz SR. Andy Gump and his deformity. J Oral Maxillofac Surg. 2010 Mar;68(3):651–3.
88. Genden EM, Wallace D, Buchbinder D, Okay D, Urken ML. Iliac crest internal oblique osteomusculocutaneous free flap reconstruction of the postablative palatomaxillary defect. Arch Otolaryngol Head Neck Surg. 2001;127(7):854–61.
89. Rieger JM, Zalmanowitz JG, Li SY, Sytsanko A, Harris J, Williams D, et al. Functional outcomes after surgical reconstruction of the base of tongue using the radial forearm free flap in patients with oropharyngeal carcinoma. Head Neck. 2007;29(11):1024–32.
90. Seikaly H, Rieger J, Wolfaardt J, Moysa G, Harris J, Jha N. Functional outcomes after primary oropharyngeal cancer resection and reconstruction with the radial forearm free flap. Laryngoscope. 2003;113(5):897–904.
91. Kolokythas A. Long-term surgical complications in the oral cancer patient: a comprehensive review. Part II. J Oral Maxillofac Res. 2010;1(3):e2.
92. Kim DD, Ord RA. Complications in the treatment of head and neck cancer. Oral Maxillofac Surg Clin North Am. 2003;15(2):213–27.
93. Friess CC, Fontaine DJ, Kornblut AD. Complications of therapy for oral malignant disease. Otolaryngol Clin N Am. 1979;12(1):175–81.
94. Ramon Y, Hendler S, Oberman M. A stepped technique for splitting of the lower lip. J Oral Maxillofac Surg. 1984;42(10):689–91.
95. Lewis VL Jr, Manson PN, Stalnecker MC. Some ancillary procedures for correction of depressed adherent tracheostomy scars and associated tracheocutaneous fistulae. J Trauma. 1987;27(6):651–5.
96. Waldron J, Padgham ND, Hurley SE. Complications of emergency and elective tracheostomy: a retrospective study of 150 consecutive cases. Ann R Coll Surg Engl. 1990;72(4):218–20.
97. Hayter JP, Vaughan ED, Brown JS. Aesthetic lip splits. Br J Oral Maxillofac Surg. 1996;34(5):432–5.
98. Haug SP. Maxillofacial prosthetic management of the maxillary resection patient. Atlas Oral Maxillofac Surg Clin North Am. 2007;15(1):51–68.
99. Shah JP, Candela FC, Poddar AK. The patterns of cervical lymph node metastases from squamous carcinoma of the oral cavity. Cancer. 1990;66(1):109–13.
100. Kerawala CJ. Complications of head and neck cancer surgery—prevention and management. Oral Oncol. 2010;46(6):433–5.
101. Kolokythas A. Long-term surgical complications in the oral cancer patient: a comprehensive review. Part I. J Oral Maxillofac Res. 2010;1(3):e1.
102. Cappiello J, Piazza C, Nicolai P. The spinal accessory nerve in head and neck surgery. Curr Opin Otolaryngol Head Neck Surg. 2007;15(2):107–11.

103. Saunders JR Jr, Hirata RM, Jaques DA. Considering the spinal accessory nerve in head and neck surgery. Am J Surg. 1985;150(4):491–4.
104. Schauber MD, Fontenelle LJ, Solomon JW, Hanson TL. Cranial/cervical nerve dysfunction after carotid endarterectomy. J Vasc Surg. 1997;25(3):481–7.
105. Dingman RO, Grabb WC. Surgical anatomy of the mandibular ramus of the facial nerve based on the dissection of 100 facial halves. Plast Reconstr Surg Transplant Bull. 1962;29:266–72.

Recent Advances: Endoscopy in Management of Residual Deformities

106. Pedroletti F, Johnson BS, McCain JP. Endoscopic techniques in oral and maxillofacial surgery. Oral Maxillofac Surg Clin North Am. 2010;22(1):169–82.
107. Gupta N. Endoscopic septoplasty. Indian J Otolaryngol Head Neck Surg. 2005;57(3):240–3.

Part XVII

Temporomandibular Joint Disorders

Myofascial Pain Dysfunction Syndrome

62

Mirza Farhatullah Baig and Yashoda Ashok

62.1 Introduction

There is an accepted concept of triple complex involving both joints and intact dentition forming an integrated system which is carefully monitored by an arthrokinetic reflex muscular activity to ensure a controlled and stable pattern of painless mandibular movement. A disturbance in the co-ordinated activity of this musculature arising from malocclusion often accentuated by psychological factors inducing neuromuscular tension forms the basis for majority of problems involving temporomandibular joint (TMJ) dysfunction.

There is a large pool of evidence that clearly shows that mind and body are not independently functioning entities but closely interrelated in all aspects of pain direction, detection and perception. TMJ disorders is an umbrella term referring to a classification of musculoskeletal disorders impacting the masticatory muscles and/or the TMJ and is usually subdivided into three main categories. Box 62.1 enumerates the three categories of musculoskeletal disorders, often clubbed as TMJ disorders.

Box 62.1 Subcategories of TMJ Disorders (TMDs)

1. Myofascial pain disorder
2. TMJ disc interference disorders
3. TMJ degenerative diseases

It has always been a challenging job for the clinician to manage temporomandibular disorder (TMD) as it is a conundrum wrapped in enigma.

Management of TMD is controversial because science takes a back seat. We need scientific studies especially randomised clinical trials to overcome this problem. Matching the diagnosis to the treatment is still the most problematic aspect of TMD practice. The solution lies in making an accurate diagnosis to match an appropriate method of treatment.

62.2 Definitions

The definitions for TMJ pain are not universally used. Three currently accepted definitions of TMJ pain are:

1. Temporomandibular pain and dysfunction syndrome (International Association for the Study of Pain: Merskey and Bogduk [1])
   (a) Aching in the muscles of mastication often associated with restricted jaw movements and popping sounds
2. Oromandibular dysfunction [2] (International Headache Society: Oleson 1988)
   (a) Temporomandibular joint sounds on movement
   (b) Limited or jerky jaw movements
   (c) Pain during jaw function
   (d) Lock jaw on opening
   (e) Gnashing of teeth (bruxism)
   (f) Miscellaneous parafunction (tongue, lips or cheek biting)
3. Facial arthromyalgia [3]
   (a) Chronic or intermittent pain of TMJ and of its associated musculature

M. F. Baig (✉)
Department of Oral and Maxillofacial Surgery, Saveetha Dental College, Chennai, India

Y. Ashok
Department of Oral and Maxillofacial Surgery, Meenakshi Ammal Dental College and Hospitals, Chennai, India

K. Bonanthaya et al. (eds.), *Oral and Maxillofacial Surgery for the Clinician*, https://doi.org/10.1007/978-981-15-1346-6_62

62.2.1 Evolving Terminologies

Over many years, functional disorders of the masticatory system have been referred by many terms contributing to the confusion regarding aetiologic mechanisms and manifestations in this area.

In 1934 James Costen [4], an otolaryngologist, described a set of symptoms focused around the ear and temporomandibular joint (TMJ) leading to the earliest nomenclature of Costen syndrome. Costen believed these symptoms were due to the backward displacement of condyle after overclosure of the bite. Auriculotemporal nerve is found behind the tympanic bone which prevents nerve compression. Hence this theory was rejected.

Schwartz [5] (1959) described myofascial pain dysfunction syndrome (MPDS) characterised by clicking, muscle tenderness, pain in the TMJ region and restricted mouth opening. Following this, much later the term TMJ disturbances became popular, and then, in 1959, Shore [6] introduced the term TMJ dysfunction syndrome. Later Ramfjord and Ash [7] brought forth the term functional TMJ disturbances. To establish a connect with the aetiology, terms such as occluso-mandibular disturbance and myoarthropathy of the TMJ [8] were introduced. When pain and associated muscle involvement became the focus, terminologies such as pain-dysfunction syndrome [9], myofascial pain-dysfunction syndrome [10] and TM pain-dysfunction syndrome [11] arose.

Currently it has been established that these terms attempt to describe conditions with symptoms not always isolated to the TMJ, and for the need of a broader, umbrella term to classify these conditions, some authors believe that the title craniomandibular disorders [12] should be used. Finally, the term which has gained large-scale acceptance was suggested by Bell [13]—"temporomandibular joint disorders".

62.2.2 Current Definition

Myofascial pain dysfunction syndrome (MPDS) is a well-known term that is used in many other branches of medical science [14–16]. But in the last few decades, this term has been employed to describe orofacial chronic pain [17–19] often abbreviated in the literature as MPDS.

Presently, myofascial pain can be defined as "a regional myogenous pain condition characterised by local areas of firm, hypersensitive bands of muscle tissue known as trigger points" [20] alternatively called myofascial trigger point pain. The presence of central excitatory effects is a defining characteristic of this myalgic disorder. The presence of referred pain is common, often resembling a tension-type headache.

62.3 Etiopathogenesis and Proposed Mechanisms

A number of mechanisms have been put forth to explain myofascial pain, even though currently a holistic understanding of aetiologies remains elusive (Fig. 62.1):

1. Continuous source of input leading to deep pain [21, 22]
2. Heightened emotional stress [21, 23]
3. Sleep disturbances [21, 24]

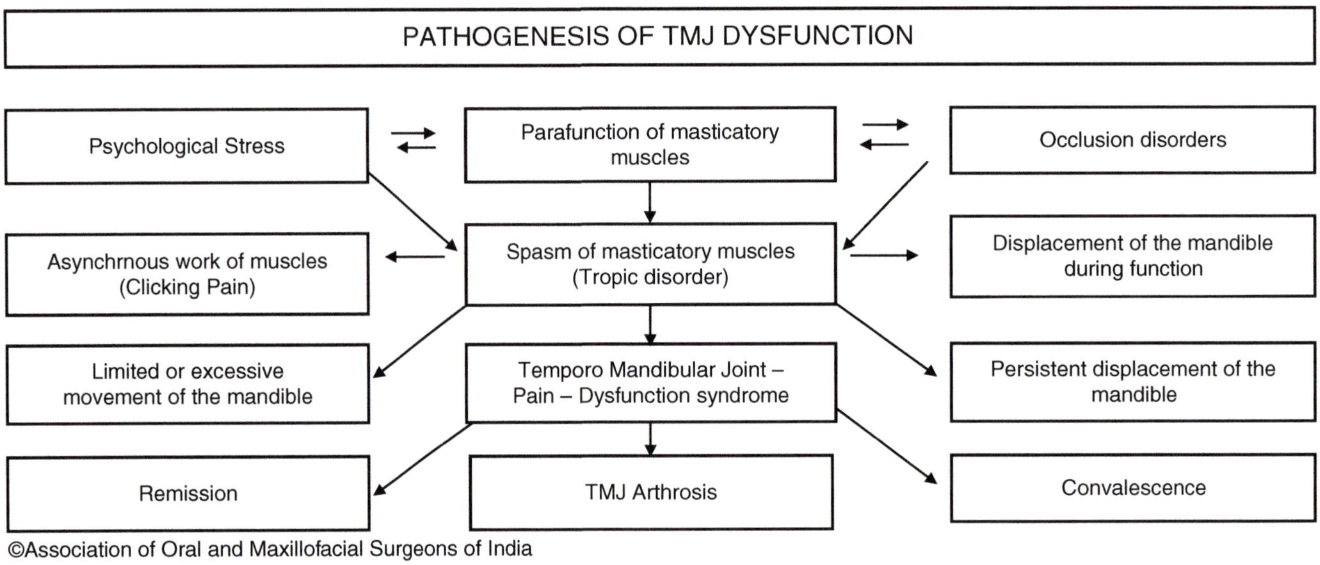

Fig. 62.1 Pathogenesis of TMJ dysfunction

4. Local factors that govern muscle health, namely, habits, posture and muscle strains
5. Systemic factors like nutritional deficiencies [21], poor physical status, chronic fatigue and viral infections [21]

62.4 Patient History and Clinical Characteristics

The patient's main complaint is often directed towards the site of referred pain and rarely the exact source of pain (the trigger points). The clinician may accidentally direct treatment towards the secondary sites of pain resulting in failure to treat the actual cause of the pain, thereby leading to unsuccessful treatment. History taking must specifically include incidences of repetitive muscle trauma, improper postural habits, presence of occlusal parafunction and mental and emotional stress.

On clinical examination, the patient will display decreased range and speed of mandibular movement which usually correlates to the location and intensity of trigger point pain. The pain is commonly described as a dull ache or pressure which can be throbbing and severe. The masticatory muscles are tender on palpation with identifiable trigger points on palpation [25].

Trigger points are described as firm knots within muscles which are more tender on palpation than the surrounding muscle tissue. The pain that is generated is usually within and beyond the muscle and may occasionally elicit referred pain to a distant site and even an autonomic response.

Temporary inactivation can be tried through a trigger point anaesthetic injection, vapocoolant sprays, transcutaneous electrical nerve stimulation (TENS), etc. [26] which are used by certain practitioners to temporarily inactivate trigger points.

From a clinical standpoint, if the muscle is tender to palpation and none of the other masticatory muscle disorders better describe the patient's condition, the suggested diagnosis is myofascial pain.

62.5 Examination

- Questions concerning pain and restricted mandibular movements and TMJ sounds
  - Visual examination of the head and neck.
  - Palpation of the head and neck—This includes palpation of the individual masticatory muscles for tenderness (Figs. 62.2a, b and 62.3).
  - Listening to TMJ sounds and joint palpation (Fig. 62.4).

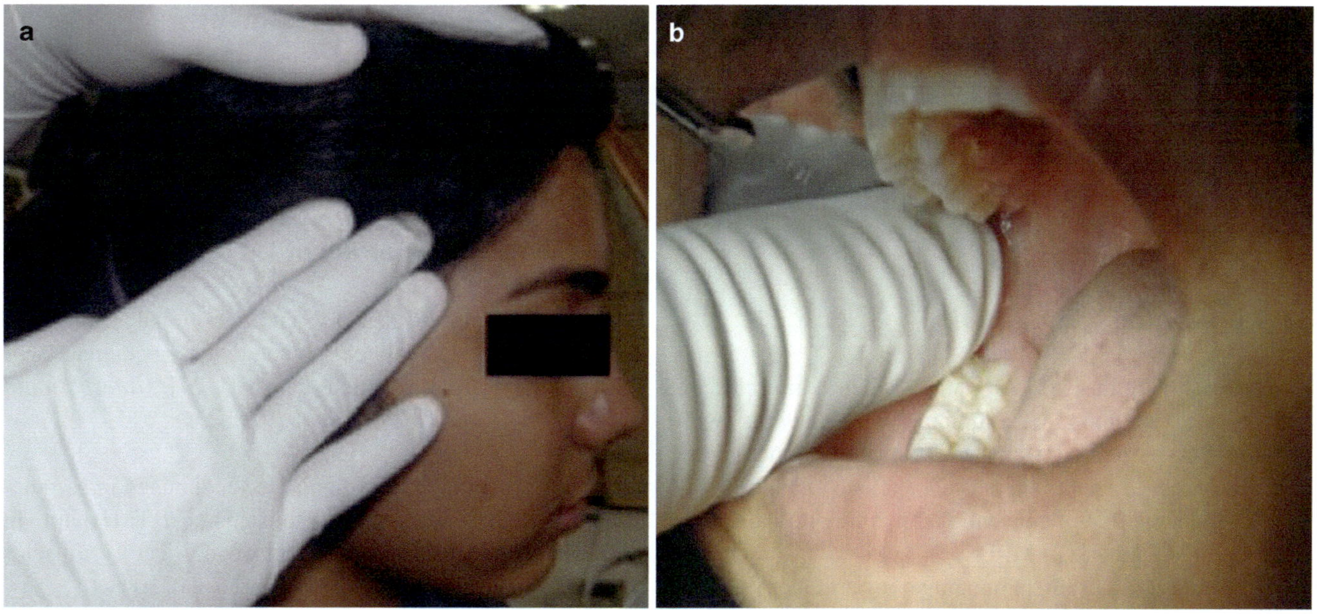

Fig. 62.2 (**a**, **b**) Palpation of temporalis

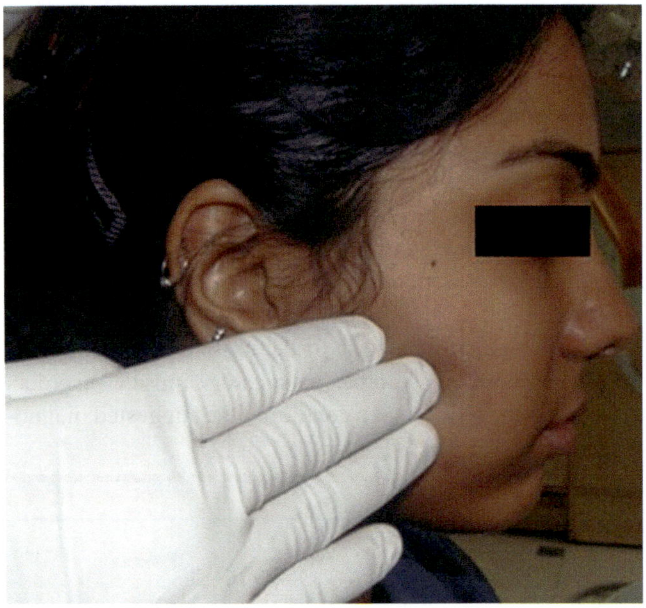

Fig. 62.3 Palpation of masseter

- Mandibular movements—For range of motion and deviation.
- Radiographs and other imaging techniques—An OPG (Fig. 62.5) may be easily available in most clinical set-ups. Dental cone beam CTs (Fig. 62.6) offer the advantage of lowered radiation dose with reasonable hard tissue detailing, articular surface erosions and joint space dimensions. MRIs are useful for imaging soft tissues such as the articular disc and joint ligaments (Fig. 62.7a, b).
- General oral examination.
- Occlusion.

62.5.1 Imaging Techniques

Pain in relation to the TM joint and masticatory muscles are among the commonest complaints of patients with TMD. MPDS is unique in that the contributing factors are neurogenic, psychogenic and musculoskeletal in nature. This greatly limits the role of conventional imaging modalities in clinching the diagnosis of MPDS.

OPG and CT are useful in imaging bony articular surfaces for erosions and changes in the joint spaces. MRI is excellent for imaging the disc, capsule and TM joint ligaments. However the usefulness of these imaging techniques appears restricted to ruling out other contributing factors to the patients' pain such as internal derangement and osteo-degenerative disorders. These features may often overlap with myofascial pain, often adding to confusion in diagnosis.

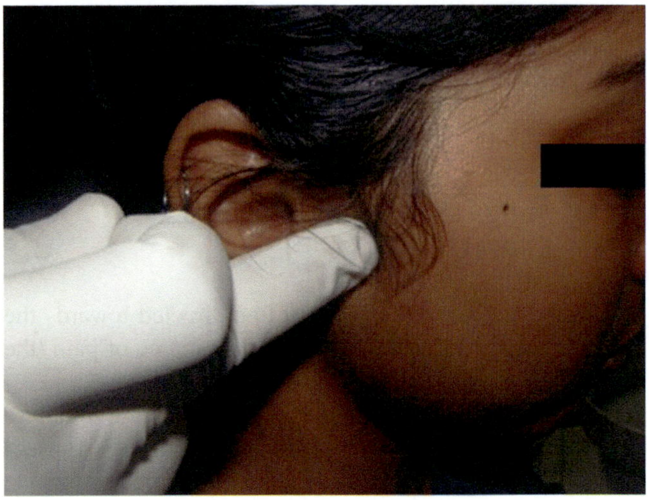

Fig. 62.4 Palpation of temporomandibular joint

A thorough clinical examination is the most reliable way to arrive at a diagnosis of MPDS with imaging investigations assisting in ruling out other causative factors. Figures 62.5, 62.6 and 62.7 demonstrate some of the conventional methods of imaging the TM joint and associated structures with relevant findings.

62.6 Psychological Assessment

It is mandatory to do psychological assessment or screening of the patient for history of anxiety, depression and pain-related disability.

62.7 Pathophysiology of TMJ Pain

Pain An unpleasant sensory and emotional experience associated with actual or potential tissue damage, or described in terms of such damage [27] (*International Association for the Study of Pain 1979*).

Inflammatory Pain Intra-articular tissue damage in association with disc displacement results in local TMJ pain. In addition, it can elicit reflex spasm of masticatory muscles resulting in pain from regions other than TMJ.

Arthrogenous Pain The patient can point to the worst spot with one finger in the TMJ region. The pain is relieved by giving auriculotemporal nerve (ATN) block.

Myogenous Pain Not relieved by block and diffuse in nature over the muscle.

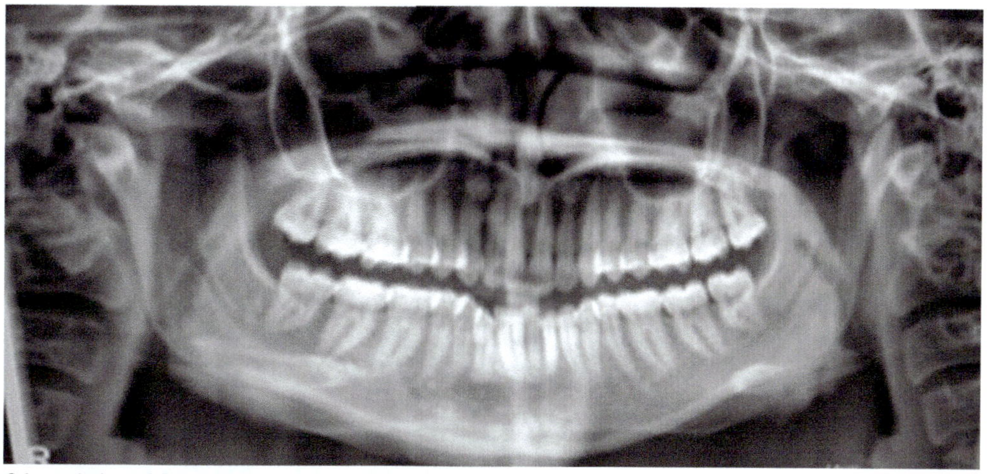

Fig. 62.5 OPG showing bony articular surfaces of TMJ

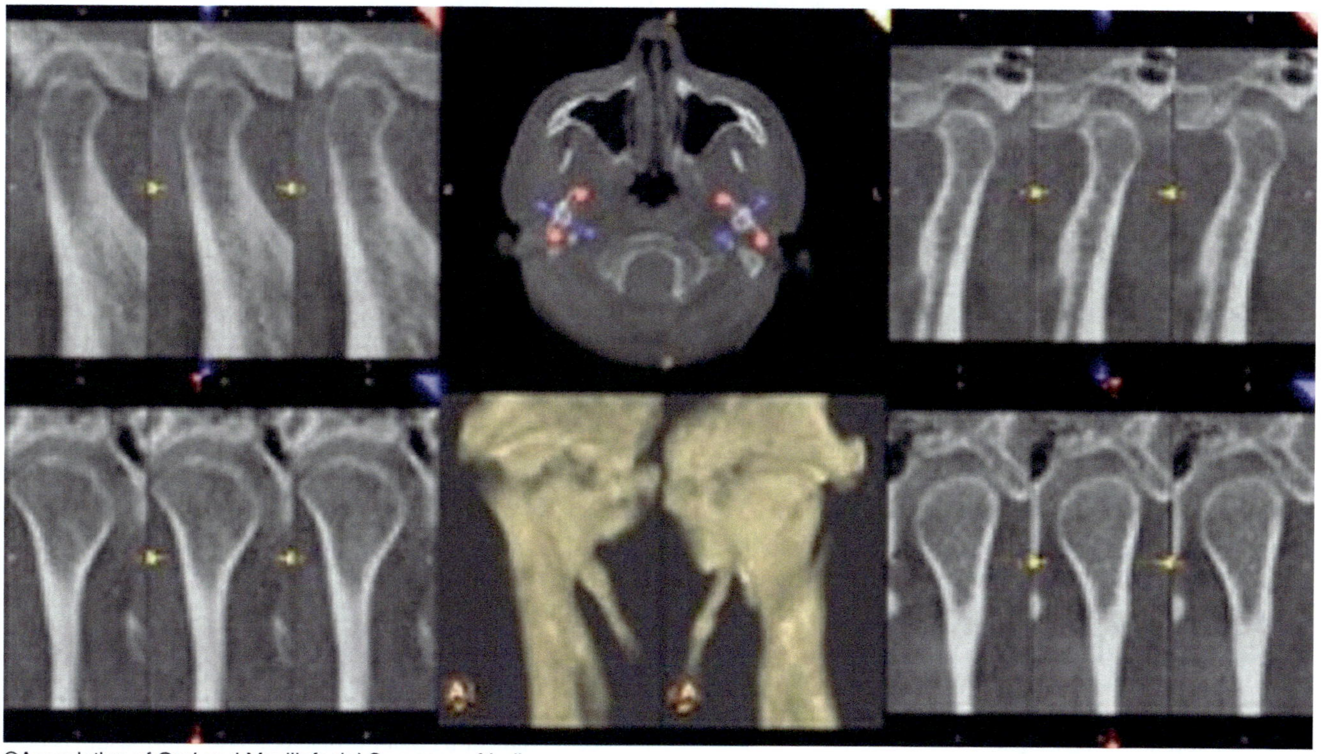

Fig. 62.6 CBCT shows erosions and craters in the head of the condyle and increased joint space

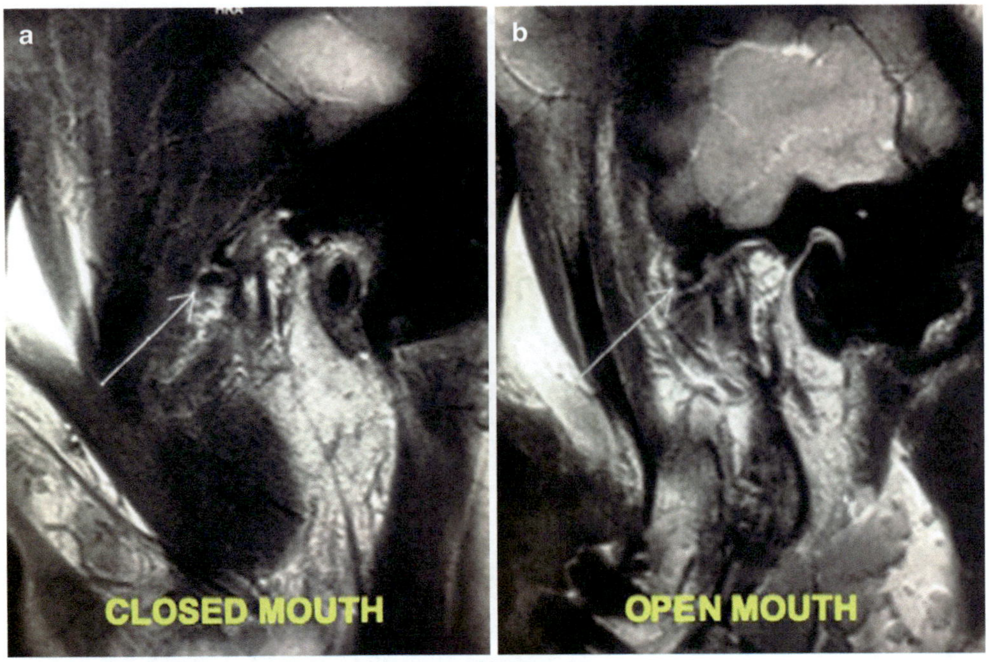

Fig. 62.7 (**a**, **b**) MRI showing disc displacement without reduction in open and closed positions

62.8 Role of Parafunctional Habits

62.8.1 Bruxism

- Bruxism is defined as an oral habit of involuntary rhythmic non-functional gnashing or clenching of teeth outside of masticatory movements of the mandible [28]—"tooth grinding neurosis".
- Associated with REM, commonly seen in patients with high trait anxiety or increased depressive symptoms.
- This sustained muscle contraction leads to non-serous inflammatory reaction in masticatory muscles, subsequent fatigue and pain.
- Signs of bruxism: Fig. 62.8a–c
  - Attrition of teeth
  - Scalloping of the tongue
  - Cheek ridging—linea alba

A complete process of risk evaluation and assessment helps to highlight the problematic causative factors. These may include central and peripheral causes as shown in Table 62.1.

62.9 Clinical Signs of MPDS

- Pain in TMJ region
- Clicking/popping noise
- Restriction of mouth opening
- Deviation of mandibular midline to the affected side on mouth opening before clicking
- Restricted laterotrusive jaw movements to the contralateral side (Fig. 62.9a)
- Unrestricted laterotrusive jaw movements to the affected side (Fig. 62.9b, Table 62.2)

62.9.1 Clinical Test

To diagnose clicking caused by disc displacement with reduction:

- Patient is instructed to occlude the teeth firmly together.
- Patient is instructed to open the mouth until jaw clicking occurs indicating that the disc/condyle relationship is now reduced into normal position.
- No clicking sound is heard after placing the spacer (Fig. 62.10a, b).

62.10 Principles of Management

62.10.1 Role of Evidence-Based Management

The varying manifestation of myofascial pain (MFP) can range from single muscle involvement to complex cases involving multiple sites of pain and numerous contributing

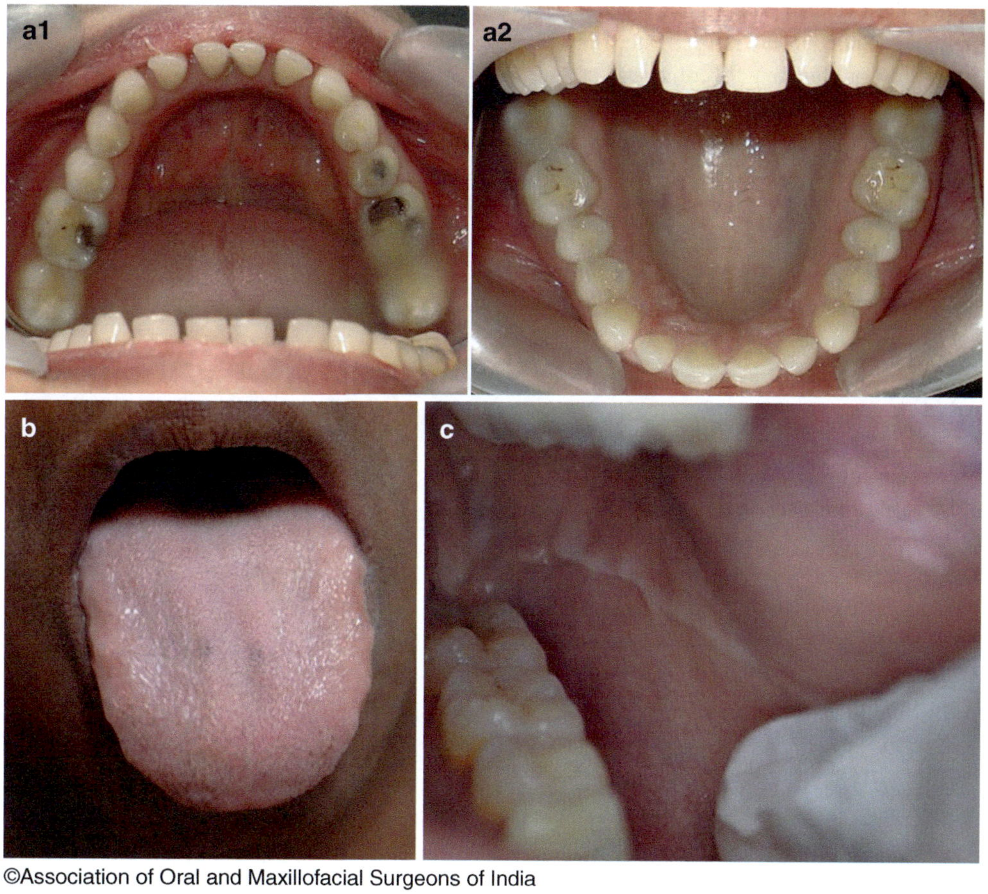

Fig. 62.8 (a) Attrition of teeth from bruxism. (b) Scalloping of tongue margins (c) Linea alba

Table 62.1 Central and peripheral causes of MPDS

Central causes	Peripheral causes
Stress	Adverse postural issues
Anxiety	Repetitive localised strain in the form of occlusal parafunction
Depression	

factors. The challenge in management consists of educating patients about the lifestyle factors that contribute to MFP, the persistence of which tends to result in treatment failure. Studies by Fricton and Aronoff [29, 30] et al. indicate that patients with MFP visit multiple practitioners in their quest for relief and are often treated with multiple modalities in a disorganised manner without experiencing improvement other than on a temporary basis.

62.10.2 Formulating a Comprehensive Problem List

Patient must be encouraged to adopt therapeutic lifestyle changes such as diet modification, exercise, proper sleep habits, social support and coping mechanisms which may contribute to more holistic and long-lasting positive outcomes.

62.10.3 Role of Interdisciplinary Management for the Complex Patient

Patients exhibiting multiple and often overlapping risk factors are best approached via an interdisciplinary involvement that uses a team of specialists to address the varied nuances

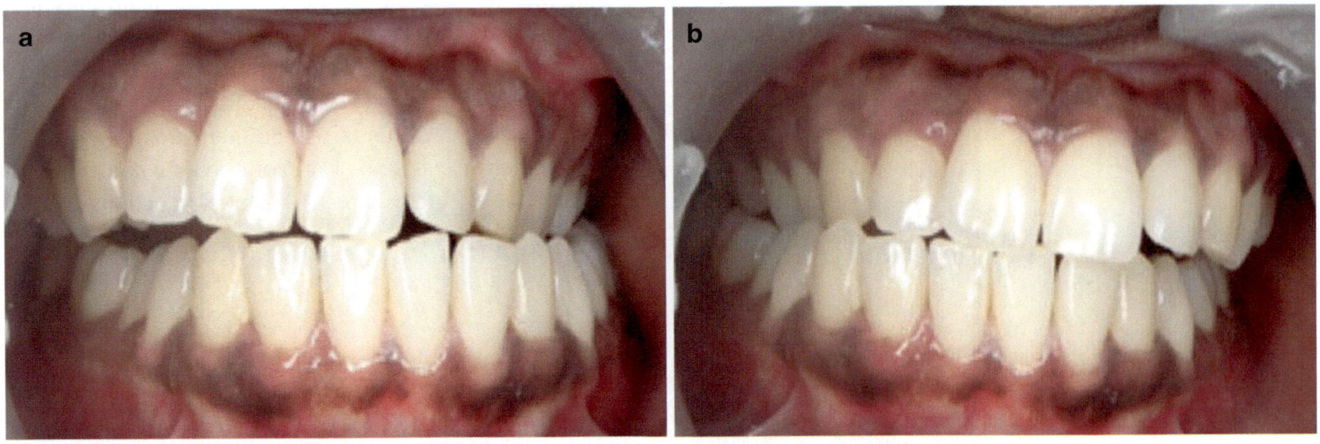

Fig. 62.9 (**a**) Restricted laterotrusive jaw movements—contralateral side (**b**) Unrestricted laterotrusive jaw movements—affected side

Table 62.2 Causes of clicking

Causes of clicking
1. Disc displacement with reduction
2. Hypermobility of the condyle
3. Loose intra-articular bodies like arthroliths, intra-articular fracture fragments of the articular surface [29]
4. Thickening of the soft tissue on the slope of articular eminence

of the problem in an organised manner. In both simple and complex cases, the clinician needs to isolate the individual problem area and arrive at a customised solution best suited to the patient.

62.10.4 The Role of Occlusal Splint: Termination of the Cycle of Habitual Pain

Chronic pain is a learnt pattern that arises from repetition and is generated by the CNS. This habitual pattern must be arrested before attempting to treat MPDS. Treatment of MPDS is dependent on breaking the repetitive pattern generated by the central nervous system. Nociceptive responses are carried from peripheries into the central nervous system (CNS) through myelinated (type A-delta) or unmyelinated (type C) nerve fibres [31]. Dental malocclusion as a causative factor for MPDS has been found in literature since most treatment modalities hint at occlusal alteration one way or another. In a study by Laskin et al. [32], the authors remarked that many aspects of MPDS are yet to be explored; many have agreed that rapid improvement of symptoms is noticed with splint therapy. Splint therapy is an effective method of isolating occlusion as the causative factor as the interposition of a splint can immediately and dramatically break the pain pattern generated by the CNS. It is however necessary that splint therapy be initiated by skilled practitioners.

Soft splints are constructed of polyvinyl worn at night. It may act as a habit breaker.

The anterior bite plane or Lucia Jig is recommended for short-term use and is to be worn at night. Stabilisation splints help to disocclude the jaws, thereby restoring normal joint space with prolonged wear. These are also used to correct disc dislocations in internal derangement. The anterior repositioning splint allows the patient to close the mandible in a forward direction; however, this has not yielded successful results in many circumstances.

The gnathological splint was designed based on Roth's philosophy of correction of centric relation-centric occlusion discrepancies. It is a permissive type of hard splint made of heat cure clear acrylic fabricated using a semi-adjustable articulator (SAM 3, AD2, PANADENT articulators). It is usually worn full time in maxillary or mandibular arch. The splint is designed on the concepts of gnathology to correct the centric relation-centric occlusion (CR-CO) discrepancies, which are a sequence of progressive disc derangements.

A few important factors to be considered prior to splint fabrication include diagnosis and institution of therapy by skilled clinicians, and alteration of occlusion results in

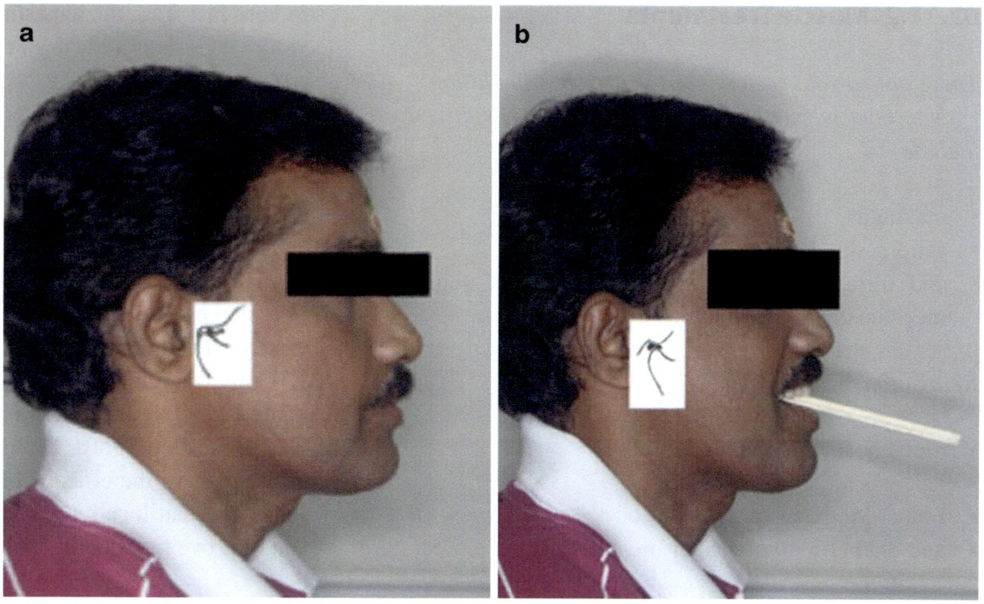

Fig. 62.10 Diagnosis of clicking sound in the TMJ. (**a**) Patient in closed mouth position, with anterior disc displacement (shown by TMJ superimposition) and (**b**) Condyle translating over the displaced disc (TMJ superimposition), to produce clicking sound

changes in masticatory behaviour which in turn alters neuromuscular activity and learnt patterns of pain generation. Regular follow-up is essential after splint usage. This helps to identify any complications as a result of splint therapy which might mandate stoppage of splint therapy altogether [33, 34]. The specific type of splint and duration of treatment must be carefully titrated for individual patients. Overuse of the right splint can also result in worsening of the condition by creating open bites, intrusion of teeth and loss of occlusal contact and worsening of MPDS symptoms [35–37].

62.10.5 Occlusal Adjustments

Wang et al. advocated elimination of premature contacts using occlusal adjustment as one of the most crucial methods for breaking the neuromuscular cycle in MPDS [38]. A thorough occlusal analysis has consistently been an instrumental diagnostic criterion to resolve MPDS symptoms.

62.11 Modalities of Management of MPDS

Because of the prolonged and occasionally varied treatment phases in the management of myofascial pain, the healthcare provider must develop a long-term association with the patient and direct the goals towards fostering a positive attitude towards therapy and commitment to long-term change [39, 40].

62.11.1 Muscle Exercises

Muscle exercises are the most effective for muscle rehabilitation. Active muscle stretching combined with passive exercises diminishes the sensitivity of trigger points. Postural exercises reduce trigger point reactivation, while strengthening exercises serve to enhance circulation and suppleness of the muscles. Determination of the muscular range of motion is the preliminary requirement prior to prescribing physiotherapy.

Postural exercises function to teach the patient to adopt a more neutral and relaxed body position, thereby ameliorating fatigue from undue stress on a set of muscles. Inter-incisal mouth opening is an effective indicator of muscle range of motion, and limited mouth opening is indicative of tender points in the masticatory muscles. Adverse postures such as jaw thrust and forward head position must also be discouraged.

Correctional exercises include:

1. Placement of the tip of the tongue on the roof of the mouth with the teeth parted.
2. Instruction in proper posture for daily activities like sitting, standing and lifting of objects.
3. Encourage sleeping on the side or back. This is effective for patients who complain of muscle stiffness upon awakening.
4. Incorporate a form of aerobic exercise into the daily routine to improve mood, circulation, strength and muscle endurance [41].

62.11.2 Muscle Treatments

There are various techniques for muscle stimulation.

Non-invasive methods of trigger point (TrPs) inactivation include

- massages,
- acupressure therapy
- and ultrasound application which act as non-invasive mechanisms of disruption.

Relaxation measures include

- moist heat applications,
- ice packs,
- Fluori-Methane sprays
- and diathermy which alter muscle and skin temperature.

Electrical current stimulation through

- transcutaneous electrical nerve stimulation (TENS),
- electro-acupuncture
- and direct current application stimulates the muscles and TrPs.

Methods of chemical and mechanical alteration of TrPs are achieved by:

- acupuncture and
- TrP injections with local anaesthetic,
- saline
- and corticosteroids.

Spray and stretch technique: Local muscle vapocoolant spray application alongside passive stretching renders instant pain relief [21, 42]. Failure of this technique has been attributed to:

(a) Inadequate achievement of full muscle dimension due to bone or joint abnormalities, muscular contractures or the patient's inability to voluntarily relax
(b) Incorrect technique of spraying
(c) Failure to attenuate causative factors

62.11.3 Trigger Point (TrP) Injections

Pain reduction, improvement in range of motion, better exercise tolerance and generalised enhancement of circulation in muscles are some of the positive effects of trigger point injections as documented by Cifala et al. [43] and Jaeger and colleagues [44].

Trigger point injections act by physical disruption of the trigger point from needle entry, and the pain relief may be seen to last from the anaesthetic duration to several months. Saline injections and "dry needling" have also been reported with varying degrees of success. Dry needling, frequently known as myofascial trigger point dry needling, is an alternative medicine practice comparable to acupuncture. It is carried out by physical therapists where permissible by state laws. The use of a combination of sub-anaesthetic doses of local anaesthetic agents has also been found to be successful. The results of a double-blind controlled trial by Simons et al. [45] suggested 3% chloroprocaine and 5% procaine (without vasoconstrictors) to be effective.

Corticosteroid in combination with a local anaesthetic administered as a local intramuscular injection was first practised in the early 1950s. Though there haven't been randomised trials to prove the efficacy of the same, Gray and colleagues suggested that locally delivered corticosteroids mitigate pain and improve function in patients with MPDS [46].

62.11.4 Trigger Points

These are areas of taut, inflamed muscle bands that elicit pain on palpation. Pain of this origin is usually referred to other sites in the local region. Figure 62.11a–e demonstrates the various muscles of the head and neck and the related trigger points elicited in MPDS.

62.11.5 Bite Adjustment

Despite many MPDS cases being treated from an occlusion-related standpoint, literature has shown dental occlusion or partial and total edentulism to be weakly correlated as causative or maintenance factors of TMPDS [47, 48].

Therapies ranging from occlusal adjustments on natural teeth to extensive prosthetic dental rehabilitation have been reported. Other treatments include oral appliances and orthodontics. Marbach [49] et al. demonstrated that missing teeth, malocclusion and night-time bruxism in control group patients did not correlate with facial pain and vice versa.

62.12 Intraoral Appliance Therapy *(Refer to suggested reading at the end of the chapter)*

Stabilisation appliances are well accepted, but the clinician must ensure that they are not ill-fitting, bulky, etc., so it is imperative to adjust them for patient comfort and better compliance. Regular reviews and inspection for soft tissue ulceration, dental pain, oral malodours, speech impairment, caries, tooth mobility and occlusal alterations must be carried out.

Splints: Box 62.2 enumerates the broad classification of splints conventionally used in the management of MPDS.

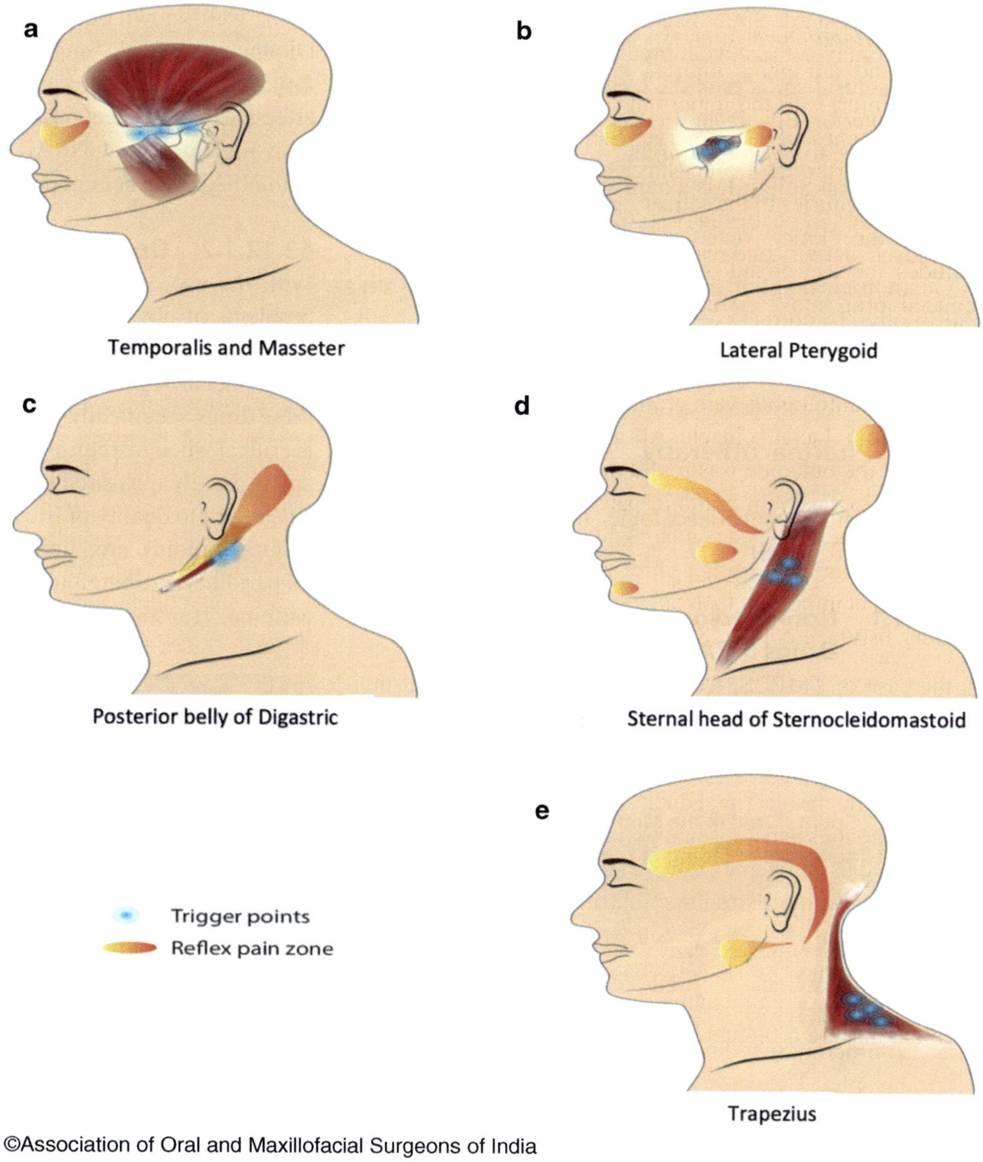

Fig. 62.11 Trigger points (blue) in chewing muscles, neck muscles and reflex pain zone (yellow-orange): (**a**) Masseter and temporalis. (**b**) Lateral pterygoid. (**c**) Posterior belly of digastric. (**d**) Sternocleidomastoid (**e**) Trapezius

Soft Bite Guard: Splint is constructed of polyvinyl worn at night. It may act as a habit breaker and also serves to protect the occlusal surfaces of the teeth (Fig. 62.12).

The Anterior Bite Plane or Lucia Jig (Fig. 62.13): For short-term use to be worn at night.

Stabilisation Splint: It is a hard splint made of acrylic for the restoration of occlusion (Fig. 62.14). It minimises abnormal muscle activity and restores neuromuscular balance.

Gnathological Splint: A specialised splint based on Roth's philosophy: To correct centric occlusal-centric relation discrepancies (Fig. 62.15a, b).

62.12.1 Pharmacotherapy

Multiple different pharmacologic therapies have found application in MPDS.

62.12.1.1 Non-steroidal Anti-inflammatory Drugs (NSAIDs)

In the case of TMPDS, few controlled trials exist that indicate daily use of NSAIDs offers little benefit when compared to the well-known occurrence of side effects as reported by Dionne et al. [50]. Singer and colleagues concluded that a 4-week trial of ibuprofen 1500 mg per day was no more effective than a placebo [51]. Patients report short-term relief with high doses of NSAIDs; however, long-term therapy with NSAIDs is not encouraged.

62.12.1.2 Opioids and Narcotic Analgesics

With the use of opioid and narcotic analgesics comes the problems of physical dependence, addiction and drug tolerance. There is a lack of controlled studies in literature to guide the clinician regarding the same which restricts the use of these drugs specifically to recalcitrant cases. Patient selection is critical when instituting opioid therapy, and success of therapy is usually measured by reports of reduction in pain intensity, return to quality of life and achievement of a stable dose.

Oral opioids are, namely, sustained release morphine, meperidine and butalbital in combination with aspirin and caffeine. Transdermal fentanyl is effective in some cases.

Box 62.2 Splints Used in the Management of MPDS (Refer to suggested reading at the end of the chapter)

Types of splint:
1. Permissive/muscle deprogrammers, e.g. stabilization splints, gnathological splint—Roth philosophy
2. Non-permissive/directive, e.g. anterior repositioning splint

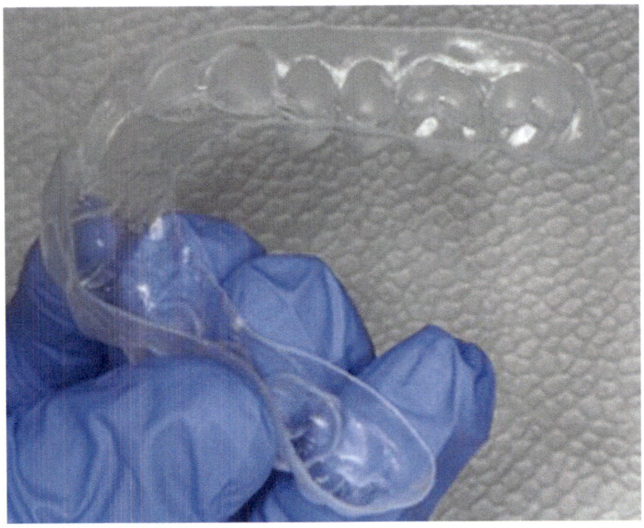

Fig. 62.12 Soft splint

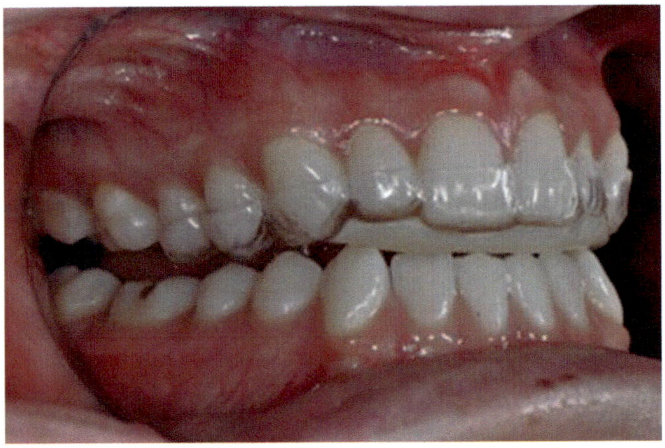

Fig. 62.13 Anterior bite plane or Lucia Jig

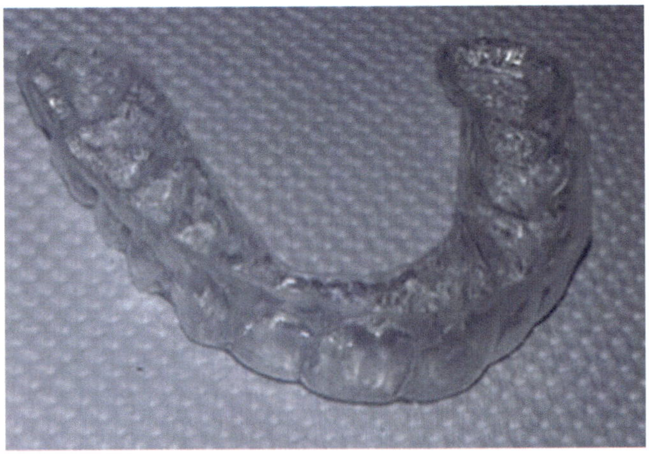

Fig. 62.14 Stabilisation splints (hard split)

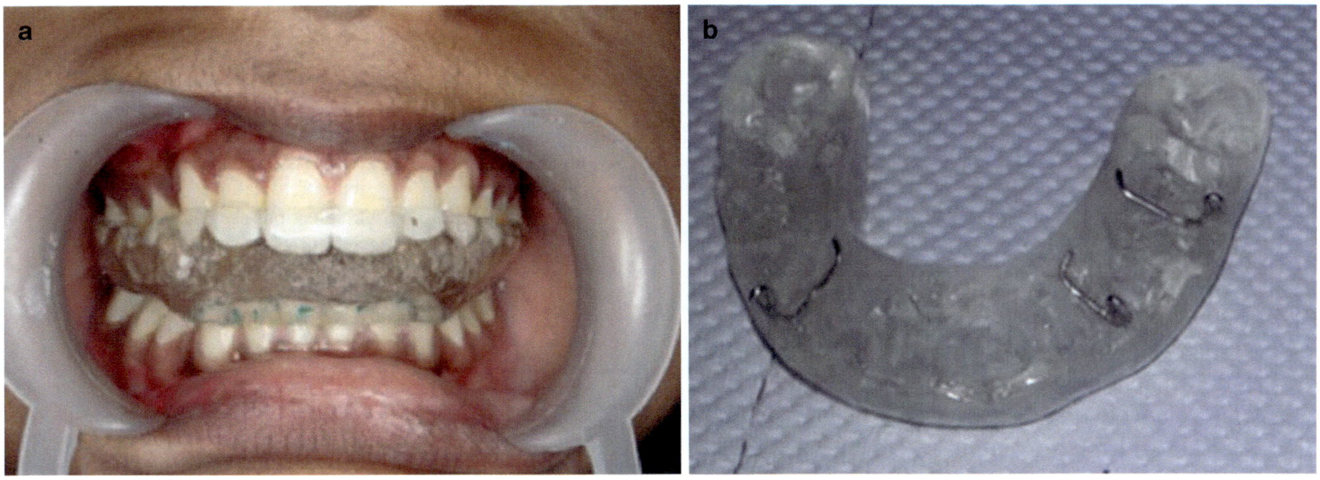

Fig. 62.15 (**a**) Gnathological splint (intraoral) (**b**) Gnathological splint (in vitro)

62.12.1.3 Antidepressants

Antidepressant drugs are frequently used in the management of a number of pain conditions, including MPDS. Studies indicate that these drugs behave independent to their role as antidepressants since they are effective at low doses (on average 23.6 mg for pain relief as opposed to a mean of 129 mg for depression) [52].

Amitriptyline and imipramine have been widely researched for their antidepressant and pain control properties. Dosage is initiated at 10 mg during bedtime and, if needed, is raised in 10 mg increments up to 30–40 mg. Analgesic effects are noted to occur within a few days. Side effects include sedation, constipation and dry mouth. TMPDS case reports have shown anecdotal evidence suggestive of agitation arising from selective serotonin reuptake inhibitors. Citalopram, a Selective Serotonin Reuptake Inhibitor (SSRI), had comparable effects to a placebo in the treatment of fibromyalgia [53]. Earlier sources of literature have also highlighted the efficacy of monoamine oxidase inhibitor drugs (phenelzine, tranylcypromine) in the treatment of orofacial pain conditions [54].

62.12.1.4 Muscle Relaxants

In the short term, diazepam and related muscle relaxants bring about relief from painful muscle spasms but are effective only for a short-term basis.

Benzodiazepines are associated with development of tolerance when used for a long period of time among other side effects. Varying degrees of relief have been reported with relatively low (diazepam, 5 mg bid; clonazepam, 0.5 mg bid or tid) doses, and usually an increase in dosage is not mandated.

62.12.2 Supportive Therapy

62.12.2.1 Ultrasound and Electrogalvanic Stimulation

Painful trigger points have been demonstrated to be managed effectively with therapeutic modalities such as ultrasound application and electrogalvanic stimulation (EG) [55]. Ultrasound causes localised muscle relaxation by producing heat deep within the fibres corresponding to the trigger points [56]. Low-voltage EG stimulation is used to stimulate muscles in a phased and rhythmic manner. This results in muscle relaxation and reduced muscle hyperactivity [57, 58]. These techniques are generally considered conservative and are extremely useful in mild to moderate cases of MPDS.

Box 62.3 outlines the prognosis and some of the important pearls to be borne in mind by the clinician attempting to treat MPDS.

Box 62.3 Clinical Pearls for Successful Outcomes and Prognosis of MPDS

Successful outcomes and prognosis of MPDS are dependent on the following factors:

- Accurate diagnosis—It is essential to isolate MPDS from a host of conditions that may mimic symptoms such as internal derangement, migraines and cluster headaches.
- Appropriate case selection—This necessitates the correct identification of the disease phase and institution of appropriate treatment measures.
- Clinician factors—Experience and patient rapport.
- Patient factors—Compliance, understanding, expectations.
- Multidisciplinary team approach—Effective communication between maxillofacial, orthodontic, orthopaedic and physiotherapy colleagues can ensure holistic management of the patient's condition.

62.13 Treatment Summary

The management of MPDS can be summarised as follows (Table 62.3). (Refer also to Chap. 63 - Internal Derangements of the Temporomandibular Joint)

62.14 Recent Advances

Newer management methods that have emerged in the recent years for treatment of MPDS include botulinum toxin injections as well as cold and soft laser therapy.

62.14.1 Botulinum Toxin Injections

Botulinum toxin injection enhances vascularity by augmenting the blood flow to the affected muscles and releases the taut muscle fibres caused by abnormally contracting muscles [59]. It has also been reported to increase endogenous endorphin secretion by way of needle insertion into trigger points [60, 61]. However, studies reveal that 3–10% of patients develop neutralising antibodies with long-term adverse effects that include muscular atrophy [62].

The injection solution is prepared by dissolving 100 IU of botulinum toxin into 1.0 mL of sterile saline solution (0.9%) at room temperature to be done immediately before injection. An insulin syringe with a hypodermic needle may be used for administering the injection. Small increments of this solution may be injected into trigger points in different muscles. (refer Chap. 33 for more details)

Table 62.3 Summary of MPDS stages and authors' recommendation for management

Phase	Treatment approach
I (Fatigue and spasm causing pain and dysfunction)	• Avoidance of clenching and grinding • Soft diet • NSAIDs and muscle relaxants—ibuprofen, Valium
II (Unsuccessful phase I)	• Medications are continued • Splints (bite appliances) are introduced to prevent muscle overuse, including bruxism • Encourage to wear night and day • Medications discontinued if relief is obtained
III (Unsuccessful phase II)	• Physical therapy of muscles • Ultrasound
IV (Unsuccessful phase III)	• Psychological counselling • Referral to multidisciplinary centres • Surgery for recalcitrant cases

62.14.2 Cold and Soft Lasers

Cold laser therapy or low-level laser therapy (LLLT) has been shown to play a substantial role in the treatment of generalised musculofascial disorders and facial pain relief [63–66]. After a thorough clinical examination of the patient that must reveal clearly the affected muscles, a treatment cycle is formulated which usually consists of low-level laser application like Ga-Al-As (Endolaser) of wavelength 780 mm for 4–6 weeks.

Theories put forth to explain pain reduction via low-level laser therapy include hyperpolarisation of neuronal cell membranes and resultant elevation of pain threshold alongside an increase in the secretion of morphine-like substances such as encephalin and endorphin which have an analgesic and anti-inflammatory effect [11].

Since trigger points are known to be of inflammatory nature [6], it can be concluded that laser application alleviates oedema, inflammation and pain by inhibiting inflammatory components such as prostaglandin (PGE2), prostacyclins, histamine and kinin.

62.15 Summary and Conclusion

It would be appropriate to conclude that successful outcomes and prognosis of MPDS are dependent on accurate diagnosis, appropriate case selection and above all an interdisciplinary involvement that uses a team of specialists to address the various nuances of the problems in an organised manner.

The clinician needs to isolate the individual problem area and arrive at a customised solution best suited for the patient.

The following salient points must be borne in mind by the reader on completion of the chapter on MPDS as shown in Box 62.4.

Box 62.4 Summary of Important Points

- Myofascial pain dysfunction syndrome is mainly a pain disorder related to muscles and fasciae, distinct from TMJ disc interference disorders and temporomandibular degenerative diseases.
- Myofascial pain can be defined as "A myogenous pain condition characterised by Local areas of firm, hypersensitive bands of muscle tissue known as trigger points".
- Bruxism and other parafunctional habits lead to sustained muscle contraction and eventually non-serous inflammatory reaction in masticatory muscles, muscle fatigue and pain.
- Splint therapy as interposition can dramatically break the pain pattern. "Lucia Jig" or anterior bite plane recommended for short-term use helps to disocclude the posterior teeth, thereby relieving muscle fatigue and pain caused by sustained muscle contraction due to clenching.
- Non-invasive method of muscle treatment includes inactivation massage, ice packs and Fluori-Methane sprays.
- Trigger point (TrP) injections with local anaesthetic, saline and steroids mitigate pain and improve function.
- Anti-depressants like amitriptyline in small doses (10 mg) at bedtime along with "Lucia Jig" for short-term use give good pain control results.

62.16 Case Scenarios

Case 1: (Fig. 62.16a–c)

A 29-year-old female patient complained of pain in the head and jaw for the past 2 years and underwent medical treatment for the same with little relief. On examination, muscles of mastication were sore and there was difficulty in manipulation of the jaw, and the patient showed a deep bite (Fig. 62.16a). CBCT showed increased joint space and MRI showed normal imaging. Having diagnosed with MPDS, the patient was advised gnathological splint (Fig. 62.16b) for full-time wear. The symptoms improved over 6–8 months. Post splint therapy, the bite was considerably opened (Fig. 62.16c), relieving pressure on the joint structures, and the patient was forwarded for orthodontic settling.

Case 2: (Fig. 62.17a–c)

A 48-year-old female patient complained of pain in the head and neck for the past 1 year. All the symptoms started with dental procedures which lasted long. On examination there was severe muscle spasm with tenderness in muscles of mastication and difficulty in opening mouth due to muscle spasm, and deviation on mouth opening was also seen. Intraorally, she had a deep anterior bite which was almost closed in relation to 11, 21, 31, 41 (Fig. 62.17a). CBCT and MRI showed normal imaging, and hence she was advised a gnathological splint (Fig. 62.17b) for her myofascial pain and to open the bite. The symptoms improved over 3–5 months of full-time wear, the bite was significantly opened and the patient was referred for orthodontic settling of the bite.

Case 3: (Fig. 62.18a–c)

A 21-year-old female patient who was a dental student reported with clicking sounds and pain on both sides of the lower jaw and severe teeth grinding at night for the past 6

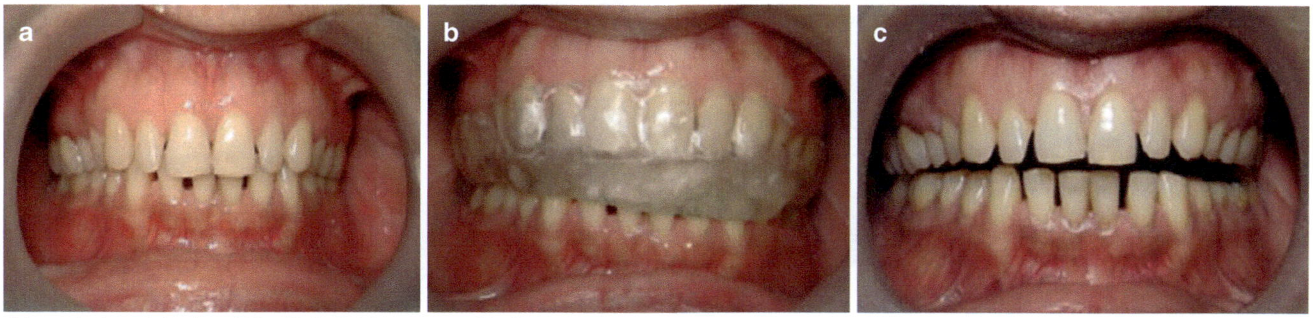

Fig. 62.16 (**a**) Anterior deep bite with spacing in the lower anteriors. (**b**) Gnathological splint in place. (**c**) Post splint therapy correction of deep bite prior to orthodontic settling

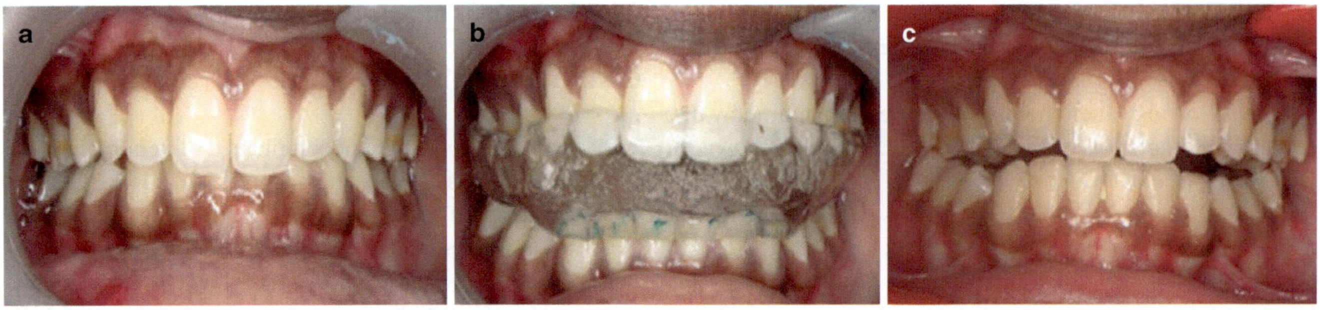

Fig. 62.17 (**a**) Pretreatment occlusion showing anterior deep bite. (**b**) Gnathological splint in place. (**c**) Post splint therapy

Fig. 62.18 (**a**) Palpation of tender points on the temporalis and masseter muscles. (**b**) The Lucia Jig. (**c**) Patient wearing the Lucia Jig

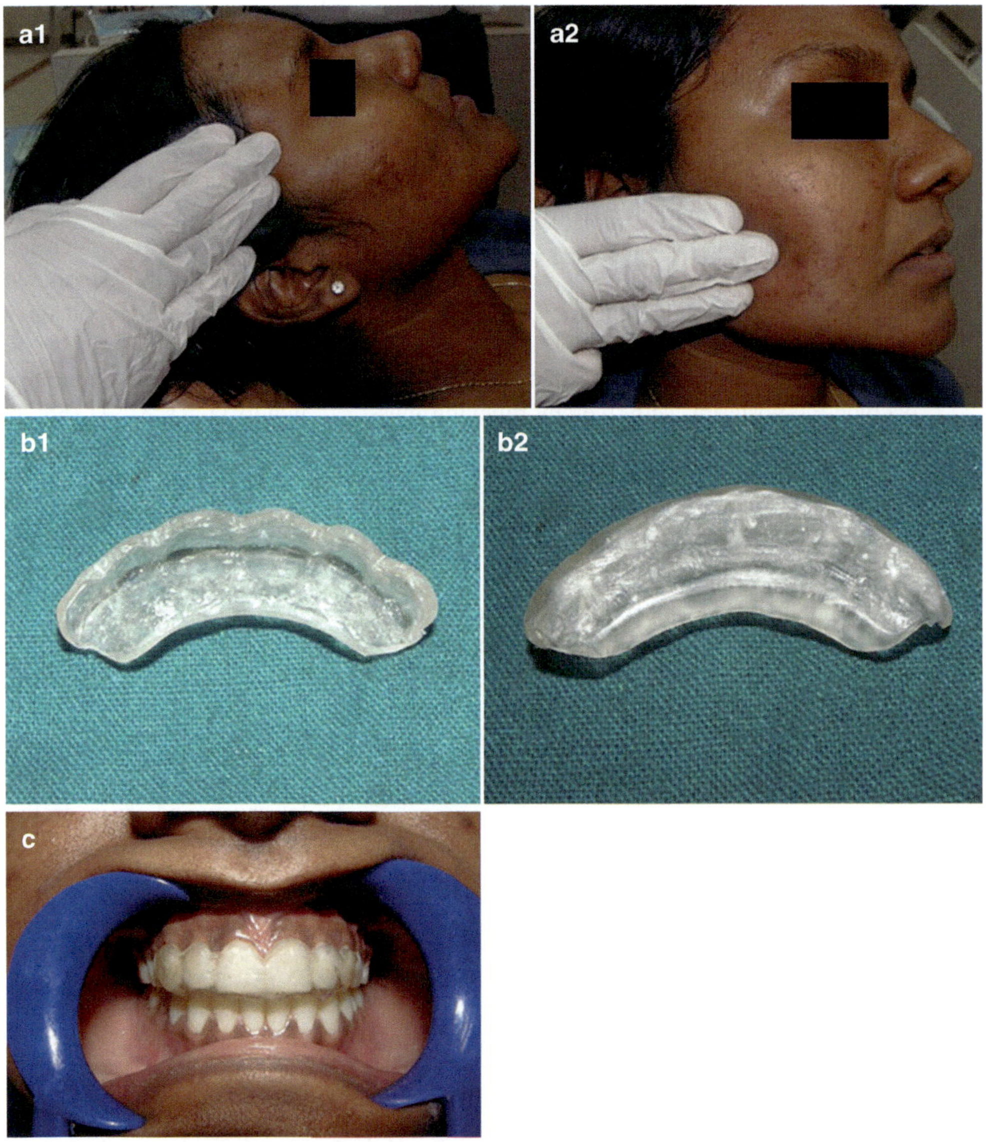

months. The patient was clinically examined, severe tenderness was elicited on palpating the masseters and temporalis bilaterally (Fig. 62.18a), and intraoral signs of enamel wear from attrition were apparent. Imaging of the TMJ via MRI showed a normal study. She was advised to wear a Lucia Jig (Fig. 62.18b, c) for 3 months in order to disocclude the posterior teeth. In addition, she was prescribed amitriptyline (10 mg) once a day at night which she took for the same period. On follow-up after 3 months, she had complete relief from the pain and reported complete cessation of the parafunctional habit.

Acknowledgement The authors would like to acknowledge the invaluable contributions of a few who helped make this chapter a rewarding endeavour. We would like to thank Dr Elavenil P for her tireless efforts towards shaping important nuances of this chapter for the textbook. Dr Faisal Tajir and Dr Arvind Muhthukrishnan are sincerely appreciated for their timely contribution of clinical photographs and case scenarios included herein. The authors would like to extend heartfelt thanks to Dr Vidya Devi for the illustrations in this chapter.

Disclosure Authors have no financial conflicts to disclose.

References

1. Merskey H, Bogduk N. Classification of chronic pain descriptions of chronic pain syndromes and definitions of pain terms. Task force on taxonomy of the International Association for the Study of Pain. 2nd ed. Seattle, WA: IASP Press; 1994.
2. Jensen R, Rasmussen B. Prevalence of oromandibular dysfunction in a general population. J Orofac Pain. 1993, Spring;7(2):175–182, 8p.
3. Feinmann C, Harris M. Psychogenic facial pain. Part 2: management and prognosis. Br Dent J. 1984;156:205–12.
4. Costen JB. Syndrome of ear and sinus symptoms dependent upon functions of the temporomandibular joint. Ann Otol Rhinol Laryngol. 1934;3:1–4.
5. Schwartz RA, Greene CS, Laskin DM. Personality characteristics of patients with myofascial pain-dysfunction (MPD) syndrome unresponsive to conventional therapy. J Dent Res. 1979;58:1435–9.
6. Shore NA. Occlusal equilibration and temporomandibular joint dysfunction. Philadelphia: Lippincott; 1959.
7. Ramfjord SP, Ash MM. Occlusion. Philadelphia: Saunders; 1971.
8. Gerber A. Kiefergelenk und Zahnokklusion. DtschZahnaerztl. 1971;26:119.
9. Graber G. Neurologische und psychosomatische Aspekte der Myoarthropathien des Kauorgans. Zwr, 1971;80:997–1005.
10. Laskin DM. Etiology of the pain-dysfunction syndrome. J Am Dent Assoc. 1969;79(1):147–53.
11. Schwartz L. Disorders of the temporomandibular joint. Philadelphia: Saunders; 1959.
12. McNeill C, Danzig D, Farrar W, et al. Craniomandibular (TMJ) disorders—state of the art. J Prosthet Dent. 1980;44:434–7.
13. Bell WE. Clinical management of temporomandibular disorders. Chicago: Year Book; 1982.
14. Bennett R. Myofascial pain syndromes and their evaluation. Best Pract Res Clin Rheumatol. 2007;21(3):427–45.
15. Palla S. Trigger points as a cause of Orofacial pain. J Musculoskelet Pain. 2004;12(3–4):29–36.
16. Ge HY, Monterde S, Graven-Nielsen T, Arendt-Nielsen L. Latent myofascial trigger points are associated with an increased intramuscular electromyographic activity during synergistic muscle activation. J Pain. 2014;15(2):181–7.
17. Svensson P. Pain mechanisms in myogenous temporomandibular disorders. Pain Forum. 1997;6(3):158–65.
18. Kerstein RB. Disclusion time-reduction therapy with immediate complete anterior guidance development to treat chronic myofascial pain-dysfunction syndrome. Quintessence Int. 1992;23(11):735–47.
19. Kerstein RB. Treatment of myofascial pain dysfunction syndrome with occlusal therapy to reduce lengthy disclusion time—a recall evaluation. Cranio. 1995;13(2):105–15.
20. Nilner M. Prevalence of functional disturbances and diseases of the stomatognathic system in 15–18 year olds. Swed Dent J. 1981;5(5-6):189–97.
21. Simons DG, Travell JG, Simons LS. Travell & Simons' myofascial pain and dysfunction: the trigger point manual, chapter 4. 2nd ed. Baltimore: Williams & Wilkins; 1999. p. 220–7.
22. Sarlani E, Grace EG, Reynolds MA, Greenspan JD. Evidence for up-regulated central nociceptive processing in patients with masticatory. Myofascial pain. J Orofac Pain. 2004;18(1):41–55.
23. Younger JW, Shen YF, Goddard G, Mackey SC. Chronic myofascial temporomandibular pain is associated with neural abnormalities in the trigeminal and limbic systems. Pain. 2010 May;149(2):222–8.
24. Moldofsky H, Scarisbrick P. Induction of neurasthenic musculoskeletal pain syndrome by selective sleep stage deprivation. Psychosom Med. 1976;38(1):35–44.
25. Sciotti VM, Mittak VL, DiMarco L, Ford LM, Plezbert J, Santipadri E, Wigglesworth J, Ball K. Clinical precision of myofascial trigger point location in the trapezius muscle. Pain. 2001;93(3):259–66.
26. American Academy of Orofacial Pain. In: Okeson JP, editor. Orofacial pain: guidelines for assessment, diagnosis and management. Chicago: Quintessence; 1996. p. 127–41.
27. IASP Subcommittee on Taxonomy. The need of a taxonomy. Pain. 1979;6:249–52.
28. The glossary of prosthodontic terms. J Prosthet Dent. 2005;94(1):10–92
29. Fricton JR, Velly A, Ouyang W, et al. Does exercise therapy improve headache? A systematic review with meta-analysis. Curr Pain Headache Rep. 2009;13(6):413–9.
30. Aronoff GM, Evans WO, Enders PL. A review of follow-up studies of multidisciplinary pain units. Pain. 1983;16(1):1–11.
31. Greene SA. Chronic pain: pathophysiology and treatment implications. Top Companion Anim Med. 2010;25(1):5–9.
32. Greene CS, Laskin DM. Splint therapy for the myofascial pain-dysfunction (MPD) syndrome: a comparative study. J Am Dent Assoc. 1972;84(3):624–8.
33. Harden RN, Bruehl SP, Gass S, Niemiec C, Barbick B. Signs and symptoms of the myofascial pain syndrome: a national survey of pain management providers. Clin J Pain. 2000;16(1):64–72.
34. Donovan TE, Anderson M, Becker W, Cagna DR, Hilton TJ, JR MK. Annual review of selected scientific literature: report of the committee on scientific investigation of the American Academy of Restorative Dentistry. J Prosthet Dent. 2012;108(1):15–50.
35. Conti PCR, De Alencar EN, Da MotaCorrêa AS, Lauris JRP, Porporatti AL, Costa YM. Behavioural changes and occlusal splints are effective in the management of masticatory myofascial pain: a short-term evaluation. J Oral Rehabil. 2012;39(10):754–60.
36. Gozler S, Vanlioglu B, Evren B, Gozneli R, Yildiz C, Ozkan YK. The effect of temporary hydrostatic splint on occlusion with computerized occlusal analysis system. Indian J Dental Res. 2012;23:617–22.
37. Aldemir K, Üstüner E, Erdem E, Demiralp AS, Oztuna D. Ultrasound evaluation of masseter muscle changes in stabilization splint treat-

ment of myofascial type painful temporomandibular diseases. Oral Surg Oral Med Oral Pathol Oral Radiol. 2013;116(3):377–83.
38. Wang C, Yin X. Occlusal risk factors associated with temporomandibular disorders in young adults with normal occlusions. Oral Surg Oral Med Oral Pathol Oral Radiol. 2012;114(4):419–23.
39. Institute of Medicine. Relieving pain in America: a blueprint for transforming prevention, care, education, and research. Washington, DC: National Academies Press; 2011.
40. US Department of Health and Human Services. National Institutes of Health PA-13-118. Available at: http://grants.nih.gov/grants/guide/pa-files/PA-13-118.html. Accessed 29 Jun 2016
41. Fricton JR. Management of masticatory myofascial pain. Semin Orthod. 1995;1(4):229–43.
42. Halkovich LR, Personius WJ, Clamann HP, et al. Effect of Fluori-Methane spray on passive hip flexion. Phys Ther. 1981;61(2):185–9.
43. Cifala J. Myofascial (trigger point pain) injection: theory and treatment. Int J Osteopath Med. 1979:31–6.
44. Jaeger B, Skootsky SA. Double blind, controlled study of different myofascial trigger point injection techniques. Pain. 1987;4(Suppl):S292.
45. Simons DG. Myofascial pain syndrome: one term but two concepts, a new understanding. J Musculoskeletal Pain. 1995;3:7.
46. Gray RG, Tenenbaum J, Gottlieb NL. Local corticosteroid injection treatment in rheumatic disorders. Semin Arthritis Rheum. 1981;10:231.
47. Pullinger AG, Seligman DA, Gornbein JA. A multiple regression analysis of the risk and relative odds of temporomandibular disorders as a function of common occlusal features. J Dent Res. 1993;72:968.
48. Seligman DA, Pullinger AG. The role of functional occlusal relationships in temporo-mandibular disorders: a review. J Craniomandib Disord Facial Oral Pain. 1991;5:265.
49. Marbach JJ, Raphael KG, Dohrenwend BP, et al. The validity of tooth grinding measures: etiology of pain dysfunction syndrome revisited. J Am Dent Assoc. 1990;120:327.
50. Dionne RA. Pharmacologic treatments for temporomandibular disorders. In: Sessle BJ, Bryant PS, Dionne RA, editors. Temporomandibular disorders and related pain conditions. Seattle: IASP Press; 1995. p. 363.
51. Singer EJ, Sharav Y, Dubner R, et al. The efficacy of diazepam and ibuprofen in the treatment of chronic myofascial orofacial pain. Pain. 1987;30:S83.
52. Sharav Y, Singer E, Schmidt E, et al. The analgesic effect of amitriptyline on chronic facial pain. Pain. 1987;31:199.
53. Norregaard J, Volkmann H. Danneskiold-Samsoe 8: a randomized controlled trial of citalopram in the treatment of fibromyalgia. Pain. 1995;61:445.
54. Lascelles RG. Atypical facial pain and depression. Br J Psychiatry. 1966;112:651.
55. Ay S, Dogan SK, Evcik D, Baser OC. Comparison the efficacy of phonophoresis and ultrasound therapy in myofascial pain syndrome. Rheumatol Int. 2011;31(9):1203–8.
56. Zohn DA, Mennell JM. Musculoskeletal pain: diagnosis and physical treatment. Boston: Little Brown; 1976. p. 126–37.
57. Bonica JJ. Management of myofascial pain syndromes in general practice. J Am Med Assoc. 1957;164(7):732.
58. Kamyszek G, Ketcham R, Garcia R, Radke J. Electromyographic evidence of reduced muscle activity when ULF-TENS is applied to the Vth and VIIth cranial nerves. Cranio. 2001;19(3):162–8.
59. Von Lindern JJ, Niederhagen B, Bergé S, Appel T. Type A botulinum toxin in the treatment of chronic facial pain associated with masticatory hyperactivity. J Oral Maxillofac Surg. 2003;61:774–8.
60. Aoki KR. Evidence for antinociceptive activity of botulinum toxin type A in pain management. Headache. 2003;43(Suppl 1):S9–15.
61. Jabbari B. Botulinum neurotoxins in the treatment of refractory pain. Nat Clin Pract Neurol. 2008;4:676–85.
62. Anderson TJ, Rivest J, Stell R, Steiger MJ, Cohen H, Thompson PD. Botulinum toxin in the treatment of spasmodic torticollis. J R Soc Med. 1992;85:524–9.
63. Gur A, Sarac AJ, Cevik R, Altindag O, Sarac S. Efficacy of 904 nm gallium arsenide low level laser therapy in the management of chronic myofascial pain in the neck: a double-blind and randomize-controlled trial. Lasers Surg Med. 2004;35:229–35.
64. Venanciorde A, Camparis C, Lizarerellirde F. Low intensity laser therapy in the treatment of temporomandibular disorders. J Oral Rehabil. 2005;32:800–7.
65. Nunez SC, Garcez AS, Suzuki SS, Ribeiro MS. Management of mouth opening in patients with temporomandibular disorders. Photomed Laser Surg. 2006;24:45–9.
66. Dundar U, Eucik D, Samli F. The effect of gallium arsenide aluminum laser therapy in the treatment of temporomandibular joint disorders. J Clin Rhematol. 2006;33:229–35.

Suggested reading

Basics of Occlusal Splint Therapy (Internet). Dentistry Today 2002 (Cited October 21, 2020). Available at https://www.dentistrytoday.com/prosthodontics/prosthetics/1716.

Internal Derangements of the Temporomandibular Joint

63

Gary Warburton

63.1 Introduction

The term "internal derangement" has been used for more than a century in surgical and orthopedic literature to describe conditions that interfere with normal joint function [1, 2]. In the knee, the term internal derangement is broadly used to describe a torn, ruptured, or deranged meniscus of the knee, a partial or complete cruciate rupture, with or without injury to the capsular ligament of the knee, resulting in ongoing or intermittent signs and symptoms such as pain, instability, or abnormal mobility. Alterations in the disc, condyle-fossa relationships in the temporomandibular joint (TMJ) were suspected as early as 1887 by Sir Astley Cooper and published by Annandale in the Lancet "on displacement of the inter-articular cartilage of the lower jaw, and its treatment by operation" [3]. The term internal derangement was adopted and used to describe disturbances between the articulating components of the TMJ, alluding to the damage to the internal structures and dysfunction of the joint associated with changes in the position of the disc [4, 5].

In the TMJ literature, the term has evolved to be synonymous with disc displacement. In the 1970s and 1980s, TMJ internal derangement was perceived as a mechanical problem and resulted in attempts to reposition or replace the disc. In 1979, McCarty and Farrar stressed on the relevance of disc displacement as a major disorder of the TMJ [5]. It was believed that a displaced or abnormal disc was a progressive problem that led to degenerative joint disease and as a result importance was given to repositioning the displaced disc. Conservative therapy was done by mandibular manipulations and oral appliances, and surgical repositioning was performed for patients who had persistent symptoms. A commonly performed surgical procedure was repositioning of the disc, and if the disc was perforated or beyond repair, even discectomy was performed. Various materials and tissues were used for disc replacement (cartilage, dermis, muscle fascia, fat, silastic, and Proplast-Teflon). However, the use of Proplast-Teflon resulted in severe destruction of the articular surfaces due to foreign body giant cell reactions [6–8].

Over the past few decades, there has been a conceptual shift from internal derangement and disc displacement being a primary diagnosis toward our current understanding that disc displacement/internal derangement is an endpoint and a manifestation of a process in which there is damage to articular tissues and biomechanical failure from a specific cause that must be identified if treatment is to be successful.

Clinical and basic science research has led us to the conclusion that internal derangement represents a variety of stages of biomechanical failure of the joint tissues, resulting from different causes.Wilkes staging system (Table 63.1) categorizes the extent of joint damage in internal derangement without being specific for the underlying cause that is responsible for the failure of the joint tissues. With this limitation in mind, Wilkes classification [9] is still useful today in communicating severity and guiding treatment.

The realization in the 1990s that arthroplasty with disc repositioning or discectomy often leads to degenerative joint disease and fibrosis, coupled with the fact that the disc repositioning was not reliably maintained, caused a major change in surgical management. Arthroscopic surgery of the TMJ was shown to be an effective alternative to arthroplasty. Arthroscopy was a reliable procedure to reduce the pain and to improve the maximal incisal opening without causing a change in position of the disc [10–15]. The role of disc displacement and disc position in symptomatic patients has been further questioned due to the fact that MRI studies have documented disc displacement in 32–38% of asymptomatic patients and volunteers [16, 17]. We now know that the abnormally positioned disc is not the primary cause on pain and dysfunction for many

Electronic Supplementary Material The online version of this chapter (https://doi.org/10.1007/978-981-15-1346-6_63) contains supplementary material, which is available to authorized users.

G. Warburton (✉)
Department of Oral and Maxillofacial Surgery, University of Maryland School of Dentistry, Baltimore, MD, USA
e-mail: gwarburton@umaryland.edu

K. Bonanthaya et al. (eds.), *Oral and Maxillofacial Surgery for the Clinician*, https://doi.org/10.1007/978-981-15-1346-6_63

Table 63.1 Wilkes classification

Stage I Early	Painless clicking Anterior disc displacement with reduction
Stage II Early intermediate	Clicking with intermittent pain and locking Anterior disc displacement with reduction
Stage III Intermediate	Pain, joint tenderness, frequent and prolonged locking, restricted motion, No degenerative changes Anterior disc displacement with or without reduction
Stage IV Intermediate-late	Chronic pain, restricted motion, no clicking, degenerative bony changes Adhesions Anterior disc displacement without reduction
Stage V Late	Variable pain, painful function, reduced function, crepitus, advanced degenerative bony changes, gross disc deformity and/or perforation Advanced adhesions Anterior disc displacement without reduction

patients as the majority of patients with displaced discs are asymptomatic through the process of adaptation.

Arthrocentesis was subsequently introduced as another effective yet minimally invasive means of treating patients with symptomatic internal derangement [18–22]. Arthroscopy and arthrocentesis allowed sampling synovial fluid and has been of tremendous value in our understanding of the biochemical mediators and cytokines responsible for inflammation, cartilage degeneration, and destruction of joint tissue leading to internal derangement [23–26].

Diagnostic criteria for temporomandibular disorders (TMD) for research and clinical purposes were recently updated in 2014 [27] and include internal derangement or disc displacement which is presented as:

- Disc displacement with reduction
- Disc displacement with reduction with intermittent locking
- Disc displacement without reduction with limited opening
- Disc displacement without reduction without limited opening

Normal disc position, displacement with reduction, and displacement without reduction are depicted in Fig. 63.1.

63.2 Epidemiology

Internal derangement of the TMJ is a relatively common problem. Farrar estimated that up to 25% of the population has TMJ internal derangement [28]. Epidemiologic studies have shown that TMJ clicking is detectable in up to 31% of the population, and crepitus is detectable in up to 40% of the population on auscultation, with a higher prevalence among women.

MRI studies have documented disc displacement in 32–38% of *asymptomatic* patients and volunteers [15, 16]. The mean age for TMJ disorders is 34 with 90% of patients falling within 15–45 years of age range. Agerberg et al. studied 637 people aged 18–65 and found an incidence of 21% clicking in men and 28% in women, while crepitus was noted in 26% of men and 40% of women [29]. Disc displacement occurs most commonly in the anterior or anteromedial direction, which is the most common direction of displacement followed by lateral and rarely posterior displacement accounting for only 0.7% of displacements [30].

63.3 Etiology

Internal derangement is an endpoint and a manifestation of a process in which there is damage to articular tissues and biomechanical failure from a specific cause that must be identified if treatment is to be successful. The broad etiologic categories resulting in internal derangement are:

- Macrotrauma—major impact to jaw, e.g., sports injury, assault
- Microtrauma—parafunctional habits (clenching and bruxism)
- Systemic arthropathy—rheumatoid, SLE, psoriatic arthritis, HLA B27, infective, etc.

An alternative framework regarding etiology is:

- A normal joint subjected to overload (trauma or parafunction)
- An abnormal joint subjected to normal load (rheumatoid, SLE or psoriatic arthritis, osteochondroma, chondromatosis)

The majority of patients fall into the normal joint subjected to overload etiologic category and in particular due to parafunctional habits of clenching or bruxism during the day or at night.

Historically occlusion has been considered a primary etiologic factor, but this has now been refuted in current evidence-based literature [31, 32].

63.4 Anatomy and Function Relevant to Internal Derangement

The TMJ is a hinging and sliding synovial joint (ginglymoarthrodial joint) and forms the articulation between the mandibular condyle and the temporal bone. The articular surfaces

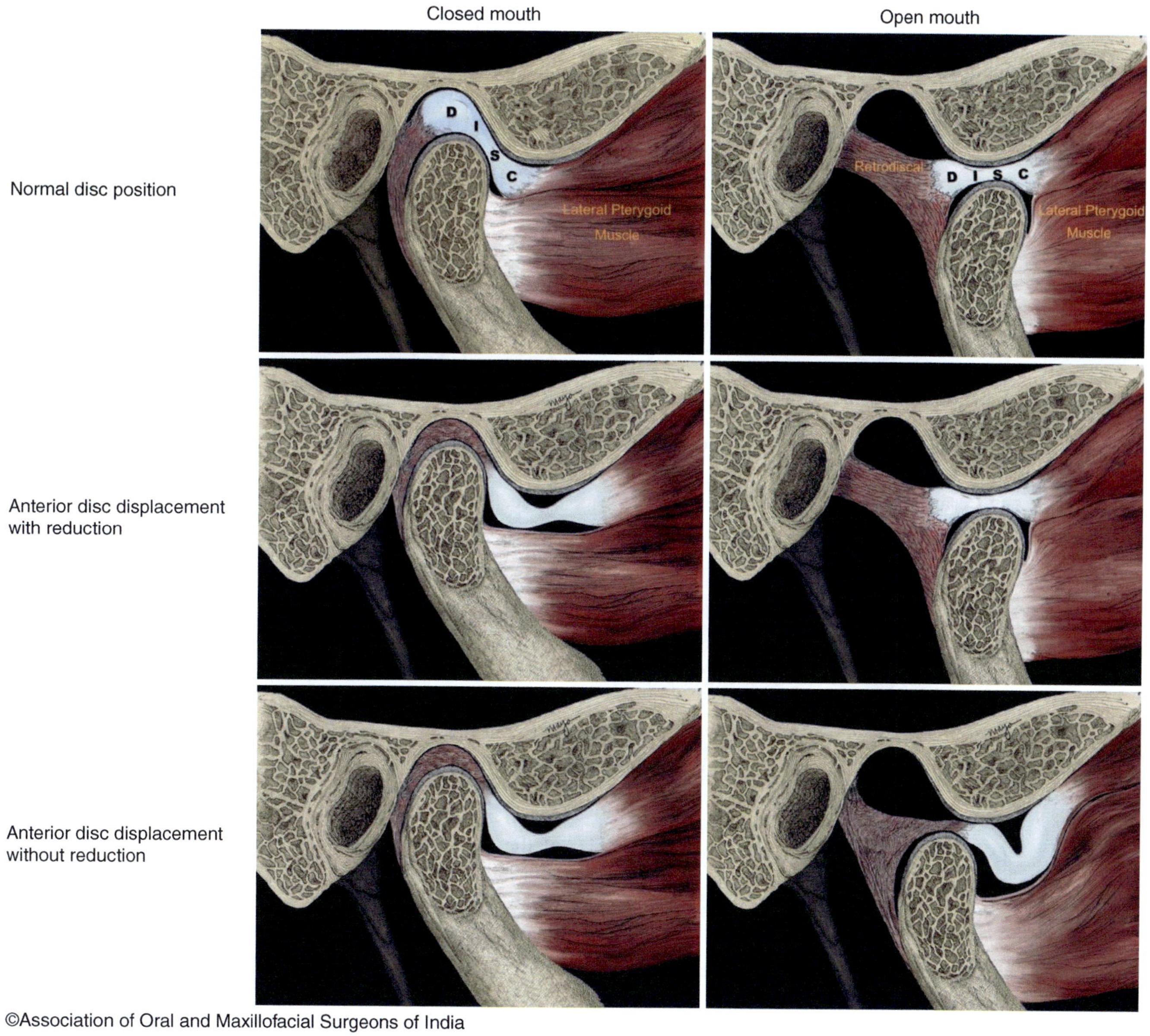

Fig. 63.1 Normal and displaced disc positions, with and without reduction (modified with the permission of Dr. Robert Talley)

are covered with fibrocartilage, while most other synovial joints are composed of hyaline cartilage. Fibrocartilage is composed of fibrochondrocytes, fibroblast-like cells, type I collagen, and proteoglycans. Fibrocartilage is less susceptible to degeneration and also has a greater repair capacity compared to hyaline cartilage [33]. The articular disc or meniscus that is interposed between the mandibular condyle and articular eminence of the temporal bone is also a fibrocartilaginous structure in the shape of a biconcave elliptical disc. It has a thicker posterior and anterior band with a thinner intermediate zone in between (Fig. 63.2). From a lateral viewpoint in the closed mouth position when the condyle is seated in the glenoid fossa, the posterior band is normally positioned at the 12 o'clock position from a point in the center of the condyle. As the condyle rotates and translates forward beneath the disc during mouth opening, the disc comes to lie above the condyle (this has been termed "roofing"). The disc itself is an avascular structure and that has no innervation. The metabolic and nutritional requirements of the avascular disc are provided by the surrounding synovial fluid through a process known as weeping lubrication (whereby a small amount of synovial fluid is forced into and out of the disc during the compressive forces generated by joint function and loading of the disc). The disc is anchored to the medial and lateral poles of the condyle by the collateral (discal) ligaments (Fig. 63.3).

Figure 63.4 shows the attachments of the disc in a sagittal view. The posterior attachment of the disc is the retrodiscal

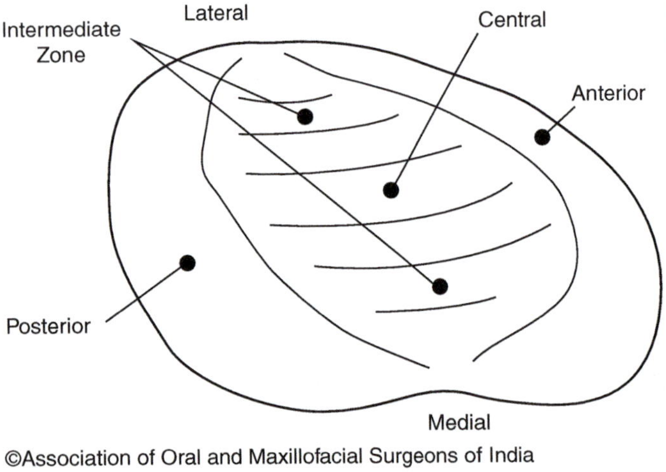

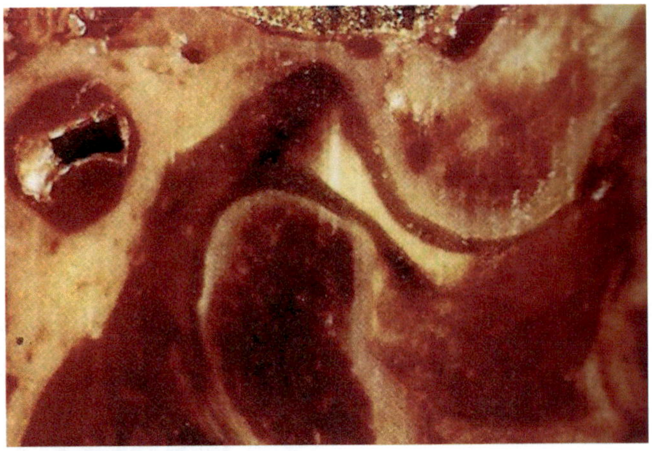

Fig. 63.2 Articular disc or meniscus (normal position) (Also see normal disc position in open mouth and closed position in Fig. 63.1)

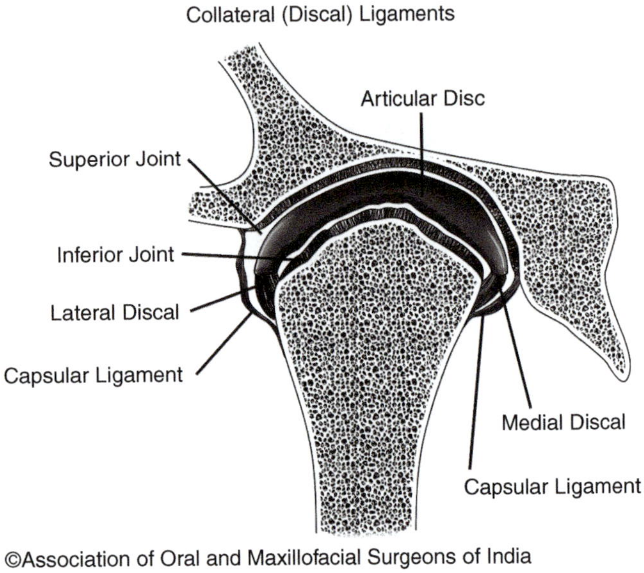

Fig. 63.3 Coronal view of the medial and lateral collateral (discal) ligaments

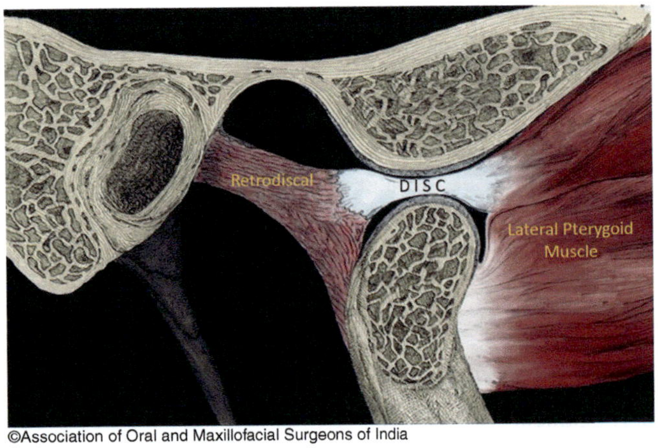

Fig. 63.4 Attachments of the disc in a sagittal view (modified with the permission of Dr. Robert Talley)

tissue. The retrodiscal tissue is a bilaminar structure with a superior lamina, inferior lamina, and intervening loose connective tissue that is very vascular and well-innervated. The retrodiscal attachment connects the disc to the tympanic plate of the temporal bone by the superior lamina, which is composed of connective tissue and elastic fibers. These elastic fibers condense to form a prominence recognized arthroscopically as the posterior oblique protuberance/band. The inferior lamina is composed of collagen fibers and inserts into the condylar neck. The disc and retrodiscal tissue together divide the TMJ into upper and lower joint spaces which are filled with synovial fluid. The anterior attachment of the disc is to the temporal bone, the anterior condylar neck, and the upper head of the lateral pterygoid muscle, while the medial and lateral attachments are to the capsular ligaments as well as the collateral ligaments. All the joint surfaces are covered with synovial lining except the disc itself, glenoid fossa, articular eminence, and condylar head.

It is the collateral (discal) ligaments along with the superior and inferior lamina of the retrodiscal tissue that are disrupted and elongated when the disc is displaced anteriorly in internal derangement.

The glenoid fossa of the temporal bone lies immediately beneath the middle cranial fossa (Fig. 63.5a, b). From both arthroscopic and open surgical standpoints, one must recognize that the bony roof of the fossa is extremely thin. An autopsy study revealed that the glenoid fossa was only 0.2–1.5 mm thick in normal joints and 0.5–2.0 mm thick in joints with disc displacement [34]. Care must be taken not to perforate the thin roof of the fossa during arthroscopic and open TMJ surgical procedures.

The TMJ is innervated by the trigeminal nerve, predominantly through the auriculotemporal branch of the mandibular division which passes behind the condylar neck and penetrates the capsule to enter the joint. However, some innervation also comes from the deep temporal and masseteric branches.

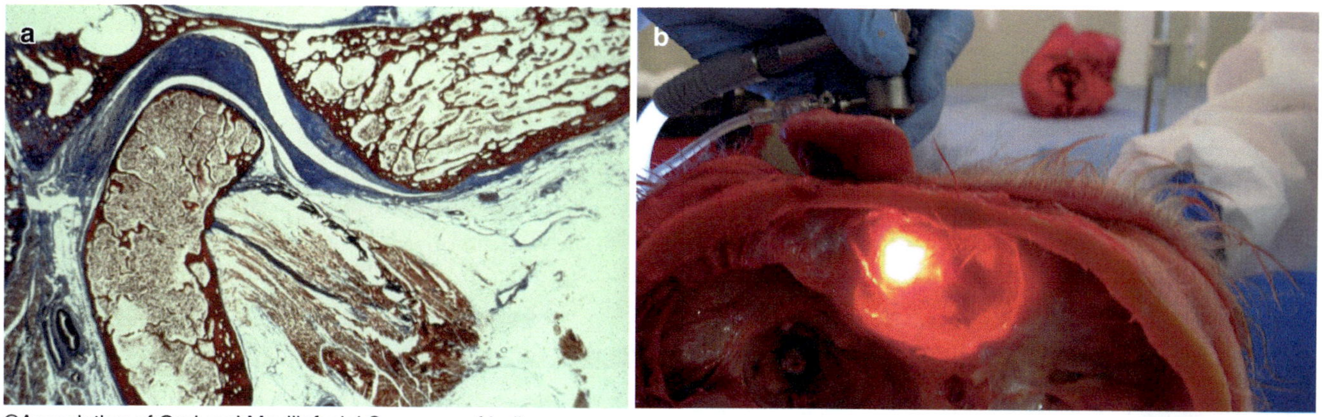

Fig. 63.5 (**a**) Sagittal section through TMJ and glenoid fossa. (**b**) Cadaveric specimen viewed from the middle cranial fossa (brain removed) with an arthroscope in the left TMJ. Both demonstrate the thin roof of the glenoid fossa

63.5 Clinical Features and Diagnosis

The most common presenting complaints in patients with TMJ internal derangement include:

Pain
Joint noises (click or crepitation)
Loss of function
Occasionally a change in occlusion

The loss of function may be due to limited mouth opening (closed lock in anterior disc displacement without reduction), a mechanically obstructive click, or dietary compromise secondary to pain.

63.5.1 Patient History

A good clinical history is essential for accurate diagnosis of any TMJ disorder including internal derangement. Questions including onset and evolution of the problem may reveal a classical story of a clicking or "popping" joint, indicating a disc displacement with reduction, or a story in which a patient with a history of a clicking joint notices that the click suddenly disappears and at the same time develops limited mouth opening and pain indicative of progression to disc displacement without reduction. Questions regarding initiating factors are helpful in identifying the underlying etiology (trauma or parafunction). Patient reports of pain increasing with stress or pain present on waking from sleep are strongly suggestive of parafunctional habits.

Other questions should include details of prior treatment attempts and specific questions regarding pain:

Location
Radiation
Severity
Timing (intermittent or constant)
Duration and frequency of episodes
Exacerbating factors
Relieving factors
Associated symptoms (headache, tinnitus, etc.)

The answers to these pain questions may suggest pain originating from the joint when the pain is localized over the preauricular area, compared to muscular pain when it is more widespread, a critical differentiation in determining appropriate management. Problems with other joints such as pain or laxity may suggest systemic arthritis or even conditions such as Ehlers-Danlos syndrome.

63.5.2 Patient Examination (Fig. 63.6a–c)

Should include examination of the muscles of mastication, TMJ, range of mandibular motion, and intraoral examination to evaluate occlusion and signs of parafunction (buccal mucosal ridging at the level of the occlusal plane, scalloping of the lateral border of the tongue, tooth wear, and fractured teeth or restorations).

When examining each pair of muscles, one should evaluate for tenderness, trigger points, muscle mass, and tone. If the patient reports pain on palpation (indicating myalgia), it is helpful to determine if the pain is localized to the point of palpation (local myalgia), spreading beyond the point of palpation but within the muscle boundary (myofascial pain), or radiates outside the muscle boundary (myofascial pain with referral).

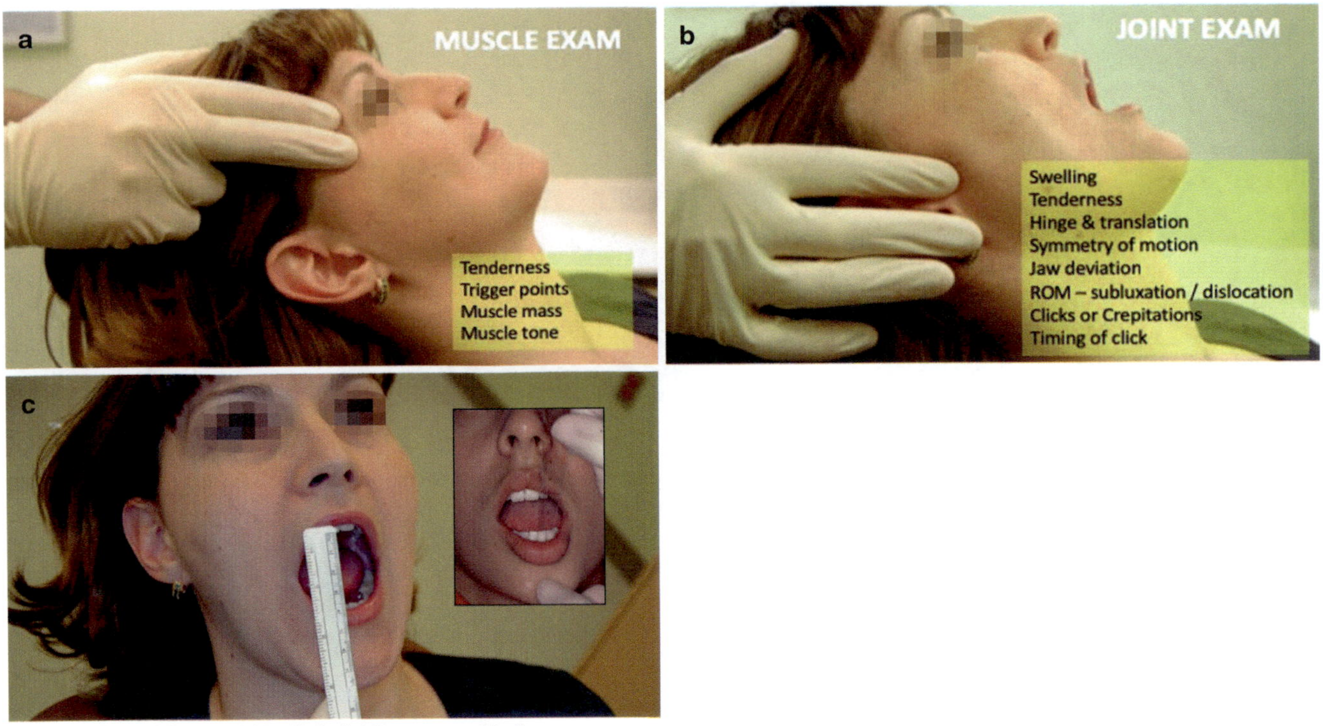

Fig. 63.6 (**a–c**) Examination of muscles, joint, and range of motion

Fig. 63.7 Anterior disc displacement and retrodiscitis (as seen in the inset arthroscopic image) with a positive direct pressure loading test of the right TMJ = biting on tongue blades between left canines loads the right TMJ, and pain is reported in the right TMJ

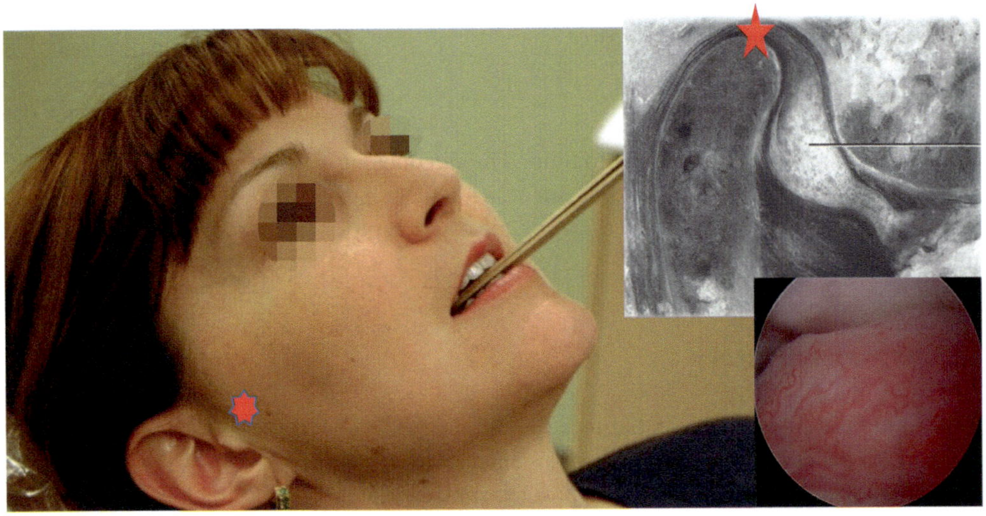

When examining the joint, one should evaluate for tenderness, swelling, range of motion (hinge and translation), symmetry of motion or deviations, subluxation/dislocation, clicks, and crepitation. Joint noises may be audible or palpable, but some may only be detected by auscultation. Timing of any opening click provides clinical information on the extent of disc displacement before reduction. A very early click on condylar translation suggests minimal anterior disc displacement before reduction, while a late click suggests greater anterior displacement of the disc. If the disc is anteriorly displaced, there may be significant retrodiscitis due to the condyle functioning on the retrodiscal tissue rather than the disc itself (Fig. 63.7). If the patient is asked to bite on two wooden tongue blades between the canine teeth and they report pain localized to the contralateral TMJ that is now being loaded, this is pathognomonic for retrodiscitis and is known as a positive direct pressure loading test. Crepitations often indicate perforation, usually in the retrodiscal tissues, and may occur due to long-term function on the retrodiscal tissue or trauma.

63.5.3 Radiographic Evaluation

While plain radiographs and CT scans are useful for evaluating bony changes, MRI scans are best suited for evaluating disc position and displacement and have a diagnostic accuracy of at least 90% [35]. MRI should be ordered with both T1 and T2 images in the open and closed mouth positions (Fig. 63.8a–c); often additional imaging sequences are helpful such as fat suppressed or STIR sequences which help to show edema in tissues that contain fat. This can be helpful in evaluating edema in the cancellous bone of the condylar head. Using MRI, one can assess the bone of the condyle, fossa, and eminence (looking for sclerosis, erosions, flattening, osteophytes, and breaks in cortical continuity), the disc

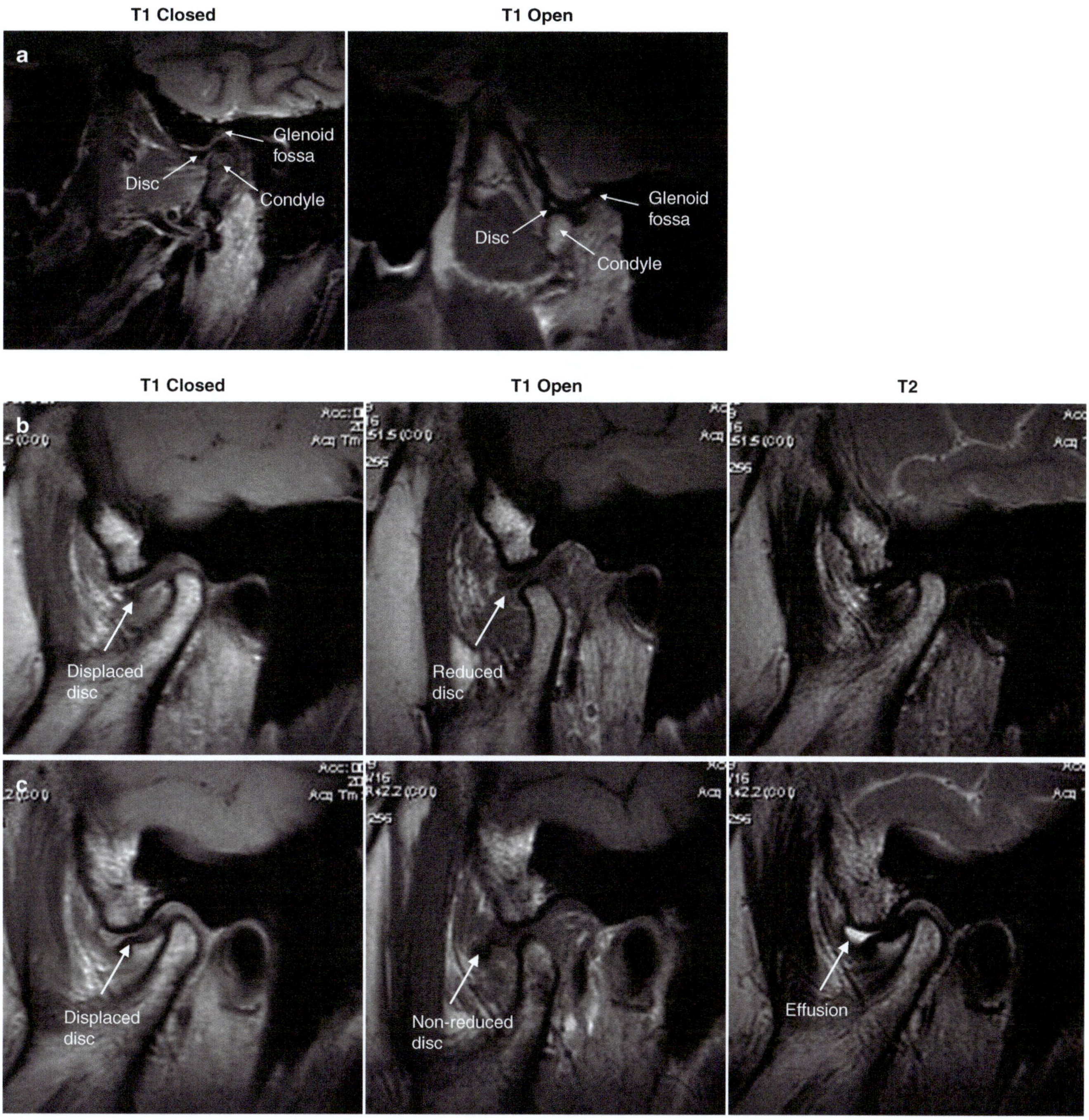

Fig. 63.8 (**a**–**c**) MRI scan—T1 and T2 images in closed and open mouth positions. (**a**) Normal disc position. (**b**) Anterior disc displacement with reduction. (**c**) Anterior disc displacement without reduction and superior joint space effusion

(looking at its position, density, shape, size, and continuity in cases of perforation), effusions which are easily seen on T2 sequences, and finally for collapse of the joint space. The sagittal closed and open mouth images determine if the disc is displaced and whether or not it reduces on opening.

63.5.4 Serology

Is helpful in the diagnosis of primary inflammatory arthritis (Table 63.2). Rheumatoid factors (RFs) occur in 60–80% of patients with rheumatoid arthritis (RA) [36]. While they are sensitive, their diagnostic utility is limited by their relatively poor specificity, since they are also found in 5–10% of healthy individuals, 20–30% of people with SLE, virtually all patients with mixed cryoglobulinemia (usually caused by hepatitis C virus infections), and those with many other inflammatory conditions. Higher titers of RFs (at least three times the upper limit of normal) have somewhat greater specificity for RA. The prevalence of RF positivity in healthy individuals rises with age. More recently, other antibody markers have been utilized. Anti-cyclic citrullinated peptide (anti-CCP) antibodies have a similar sensitivity to RF for RA but have a much higher specificity (95–98%). Anti-CCP antibodies are also present early in the disease, and their presence often correlates with more severe forms of RA, making them better prognostic indicators [37]. HLA-B27 is associated with seronegative spondyloarthropathies, psoriatic and reactive arthritis [38].

Table 63.2 Serology in primary inflammatory arthritis

Serology	• Rheumatoid factor → Rheumatoid arthritis
	• HLA B-27 → Reactive arthritis, ankylosing spondylitis, juvenile reactive arthritis
	• ANA → Autoimmune D/O (e.g. rheumatoid arthritis, systemic lupus erythematosus)
	• Anti-citrullinated protein antibody ACCP → Aid in dx of RA and its prognosis

63.5.5 Diagnostic Local Anesthetic Block

In complex cases where history and examination fail to clearly confirm pain originating from the joint itself, or in cases that have undergone previous surgeries on the TMJ, or in chronic pain patients, an auriculotemporal nerve block and injection of local anesthetic into the superior joint space is very helpful and can demonstrate the amount of pain originating from the joint. The author uses 3% mepivacaine injected using a dental syringe (Fig. 63.9a–c). With the patient in occlusion, the needle is inserted and advanced to contact the posterior condylar neck where half the carpule is injected as an auriculotemporal nerve block. The patient then opens their mouth, and the needle is advanced superiorly to contact the posterior slope of the articular eminence, and the remaining anesthetic is deposited into the superior joint space. The patients pain score before is compared to the pain score 10–15 min after injection. Any portion of pain that has resolved is most likely originating from the joint. This is helpful in determining if surgery is indicated and also in providing realistic postoperative pain expectations for the surgical patient.

63.6 Treatment of Internal Derangement

Treatment for internal derangement can be divided into nonsurgical and surgical options, but the general treatment goals are the same:

Decrease joint overload
Decrease pain
Reduce inflammation
Improvement in the range of motion
Restore function
Causative factors to be identified and controlled

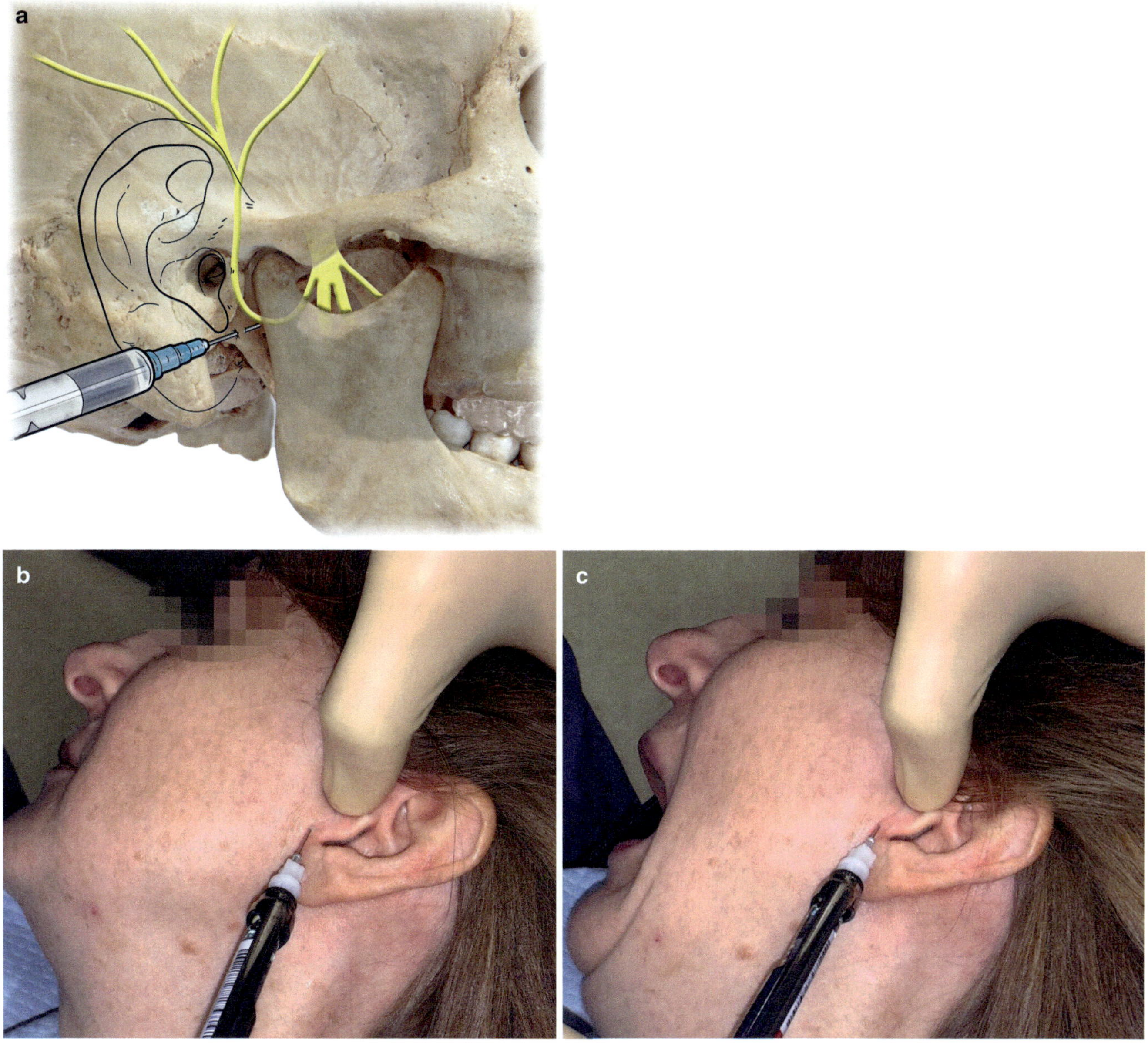

Fig. 63.9 (**a–c**) Diagnostic auriculotemporal nerve block and TMJ injection

Clinical research [39–41] into the natural progression of TMJ internal derangement has shown:

- Without any treatment, improvement is seen in many patients.
- On an average, about 1 year is required for the resolution of symptoms , but this time is variable.
- About 25–33% of patients do not improve.
- Older patients and those with MRI evidence of more advanced disease (osteoarthritis and advanced internal derangement) are at higher risk for not improving spontaneously.

63.6.1 Nonsurgical Treatment

Nonsurgical options include:

Patient education
Soft diet
Occlusal appliance/orthotic devices
Parafunctional habit awareness
Biofeedback
Nonsteroidal anti-inflammatory medication
Muscle relaxants
Botulinum toxin
Physical therapy

Occasionally, psychology referral and counselling are indicated in certain patients.

Patient education is of great value. A simple explanation of the mechanics causing a clicking joint with internal derangement with the information that around 30% of the population have internal derangement can be very reassuring and put a patient's mind at ease. Furthermore, educating the patient in habit awareness to avoid daytime clenching is a key element in the long-term success of any nonsurgical or surgical treatment (Table 63.3).

Orthotic devices or occlusal appliances may help to reduce nighttime parafunctional habits. However, our understanding of orthotic devices has changed significantly over time. In the late 1930s and 1940s, temporomandibular joint disorders (TMD) used to be seen as problems related to occlusal or skeletal disharmony. Costen was an otolaryngologist who in 1934 first suggested the link between occlusion, TMJ disorders, and ear symptoms based on his observations in 11 patients [42]. This evolved into orthotics and occlusal therapies being used for the treatment of TMJ disorders in the 1940s and 1950s. However, a significant paradigm shift has occurred as the classic dental and skeletal etiologic theories have been challenged and refuted by studies conducted around the world, and a biopsychosocial medical model of orthopedics, pain phenomenology, and behavioral factors has gradually replaced them. As a result, the conceptual basis for occlusal appliances/orthotic use has significantly changed over the years. Occlusal appliances/orthotics were initially conceived and used based on these old dental and skeletal etiologies and were thought to produce occlusal disengagement, relax jaw musculature, restore vertical dimension of occlusion, unload the joint(s), or reposition the condyle and or disc. Even today, these are often described as deprogrammers or jaw-repositioning devices that can establish ideal craniomandibular relationships wile relieving pain and restoring function. Until the 1960s, there were no well-controlled, well-designed, systematic studies evaluating the treatment of TMD. Instead, there were a number of anecdotal reports claiming success with various mechano-dental treatments, including various designs of oral appliance or orthotic [43, 44]. As the evidence-based literature has evolved, these reports have been refuted. Lundh [45] divided patients with symptomatic TMJ disc displacement into two treatment groups: one group with no treatment and one group with an occlusal appliance/orthotic and compared outcomes. After 12 months, pain had resolved in around 33% of patients in both groups. 40% of patients reported increased pain in the occlusal appliance/orthotic group compared to 16% in the no treatment group. Truelove [46] evaluated 200 patients with anterior disc displacement with reduction, arthralgia, and myalgia who were randomly assigned into three treatment groups: group 1 had basic nonsurgical treatment (education, self-care, hot/cold packs, and passive stretching), group 2 had hard flat plane occlusal appliance/orthotic, and group 3 had soft splint. Outcomes were evaluated after 3 and 12 months, and there were no significant differences in success among the three groups. Greene [47] and Laskin [48] studied the placebo effect using mock/sham occlusal appliances and sham occlusal adjustments. They found that non-occluding appliances/orthotics helped over 40% of patients and mock/sham occlusal adjustments helped almost two-thirds of patients. Furthermore, the use of occlusal appliances/orthotics may increase the parafunctional habit in some resulting in a patient complaining of increased pain and/or stiffness after use. In addition, partial coverage devices may result in occlusal changes if used for more than a few months due to eruption of teeth. Therefore, our perception of occlusal appliances/orthotics must take into consideration the current evidence-based literature.

Table 63.3 Nonsurgical management

Patient education (explain the condition)
Patient home care instructions
• Soft diet
• Awareness and avoid clenching habits
• Night time bruxism—night guard/orthotic
• Range of motion
• Heat and massage to muscles
Pharmacotherapy
• NSAIDs, muscle relaxants, tricyclics, sedatives, Botox
Occlusal appliance/orthotic
• For nighttime parafunctional habits
Physical therapy
• Posture training
• Mobilization/manipulation/joint distraction
• Massage/muscle conditioning
• Physical agents or modalities
• TENS , ultrasound, iontophoresis, phonophoresis, electrogalvanic stimulation, thermal
Stress reduction
• Psychologist
• Counselor
• Psychiatrist

In review of evidence-based literature on occlusal appliance/orthotics [45–47, 49, 50], we can conclude:

- Symptoms of myalgia and arthralgia may be decreased by occlusal appliances.
- Wear on the dentition caused by parafunctional habits may be reduced.
- Risk is low if they are not worn 24 h a day.
- The disc position is not changed by the appliance.
- Over time, many patients show improvement in signs and symptoms.
- There is no appreciable significant difference between the nontreatment and treatment group.
- Palliative care (NSAIDs, education, diet modification, exercises) seem to be as effective as more expensive appliance therapy.
- All treatments have a powerful placebo effect.

In Klasser's review [50] of occlusal appliances/orthotics, he concludes that rather than trying to establish new horizontal or vertical jaw relationships, occlusal appliance/orthotics today should be viewed as "oromandibular crutches," which are analogous to back braces or ankle support orthotics because they support the joint and provide symptomatic relief while the joints are recovering. Table 63.4 outlines Klasser's conclusions on occlusal appliance use and limitations.

Most often, painful internal derangement causes a reactive muscle response. This muscle response and myalgia can be treated by soft diet, heat, and massage to the affected muscles, limiting the range of motion to within the pain-free range, NSAIDs, muscle relaxants, physical therapy, and even botulinum toxin injections (e.g., Botox).

Table 63.4 Occlusal appliance/orthotic device limitations [50]

Can do	Can't do
• Protect teeth/restorations from fracture due to bruxism/clenching • Reduce/change the loading of the TMJ by reducing intensity, frequency, and duration of bruxism/clenching • Adding a foreign body into the occlusion briefly reduces muscle activity • Reduce headaches related to bruxism/clenching • Reduce internal derangement symptoms related to bruxism/clenching upon awakening • Change the neuromuscular engrams deprogramming	• Unload the disc by pivoting the mandible on the molars and distracting the condyle • Retrain muscle to be less active upon cessation of the appliance • Recapture and reposition discs • Permanently reduce bruxism/clenching • Relieve headaches that are neurovascular or vascular in origin

63.6.2 Surgical Treatment (Fig. 63.10)

The vast majority (approximately 90%) of TMD patients will experience symptom resolution either spontaneously or with nonsurgical treatment [51]. This resolution of symptoms occurs due to the underlying adaptive capacity of the TMJ. Given that internal derangement is a common MRI finding in 32–38% of asymptomatic patients and volunteers [16, 17] and that arthrocentesis or arthroscopy without disc repositioning is so successful, it is evident that the TMJ has the ability to adapt to the disc displacement in the vast majority of patients. Those patients with internal derangement and disc displacement that do not adapt are potential surgical candidates. It is the authors' preference to follow a surgical pyramid algorithm with most patients beginning with arthroscopy unless there are specific indications otherwise (e.g., ankylosis). Since no single surgical procedure carries a 100% success rate, patients who fail one level (phase 1) on the algorithm progress further up the pyramid to a second (phase 2) surgical procedure with phase 2 procedure being determined by the arthroscopic findings of phase 1.

63.6.3 Arthrocentesis

This minimally invasive procedure was introduced after the success of simple arthroscopy was recognized. Arthrocentesis in the TMJ was first described in 1987 by Murakami using a single needle pumping technique to create a hydraulic distention of the upper joint space [52]. Nitzan and Dolwick [18] subsequently modified the technique and used two needles. It provides lysis and lavage of the upper joint space

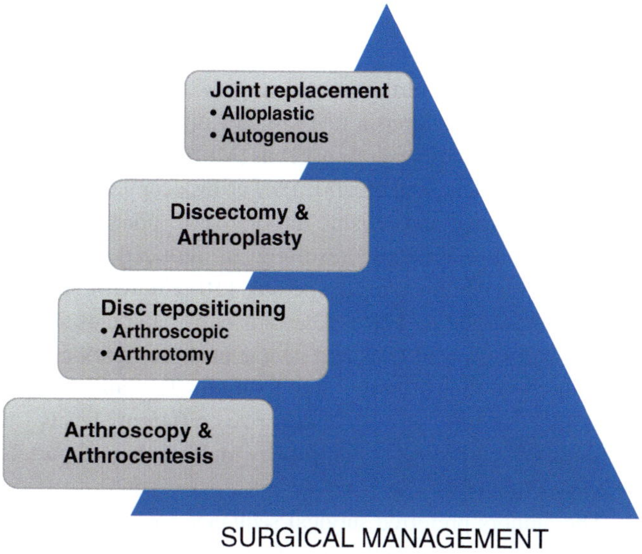

Fig. 63.10 Surgical treatment options

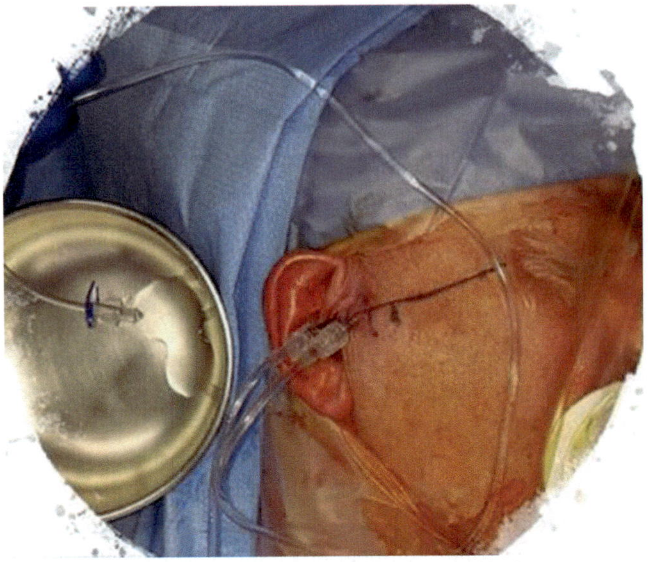

Fig. 63.11 Arthrocentesis—using the Holmlund-Hellsing markings measured along the trago-canthal line (10 mm forward from mid-tragus and 2 mm down correspond to the glenoid fossa entry site)

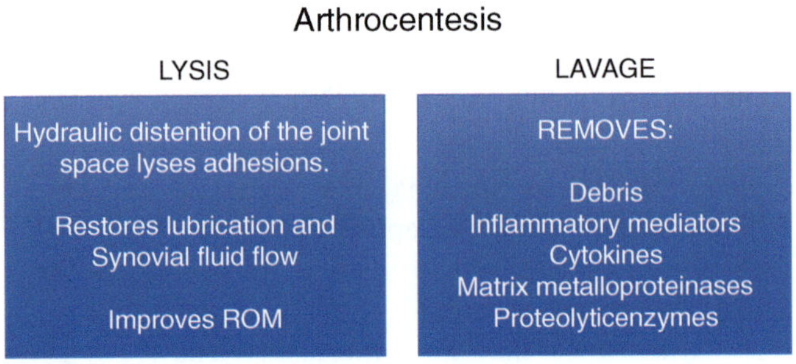

Fig. 63.12 Arthrocentesis—lysis and lavage

using an inflow needle, an outflow needle, and at least 300 ml Lactated Ringer's irrigation solution (Fig. 63.11). The lysis is accomplished by the hydraulic distention of the superior joint space, while the lavage removes inflammatory mediators, cytokines, and debris (Fig. 63.12). It is through the lysis and lavage that the adhesions are separated and the inflammatory mediators and debris are removed. Several authors have since reported success rates of arthrocentesis in the management of internal derangement ranging from 70 to 95% [18–22].

63.6.4 Arthroscopy

Minimally invasive arthroscopic surgery for the TMJ was first performed by Ohnishi in 1974 and subsequently developed in the 1980s by several surgeons (Murakami, Holmlund, McCain, Saunders, and others). TMJ arthroscopy has proven to be an effective and reliable alternative to open joint surgery for many patients, resulting in reduced pain and improved maximum incisal opening [10–15] with success rates as high as 91% [12]. TMJ arthroscopy can be as simple as a visually assisted lysis and lavage or as complex as performing disc repositioning and fixation. The author uses McCain's terminology to categorize different levels of arthroscopy according to complexity and number of portals of entry (Table 63.5).

The authors preferred surgical sequence for performing a level 1 arthroscopy as outlined in Table 63.6 (Video 63.1). All arthroscopy should begin with an examination under anesthesia of the TMJ. The EUA allows the surgeon to anticipate what might be encountered upon entering the joint arthroscopically. The range of condylar translation is noted, and whether translation is onto the peak of the articular eminence stops short of the peak or beyond the peak of the eminence as in subluxation and even dislocation. In addition, if there is very limited translation or just hinging, the surgeon might expect a tight joint space filled with adhesions and a fibrous arthrosis potentially making the arthroscopic puncture, joint access, and visualization difficult. Joint noises (clicking and crepitation) should be noted, and bone-on-bone crepitations are indicative of a perforation in the retrodiscal tissue.

Table 63.5 Levels of TMJ arthroscopy (McCain's terminology)

Level I Arthroscopy
• Single puncture & outflow needle
• Lysis& lavage
• Diagnostic sweep
• Needle/scope adhesiolysis
Level II Arthroscopy
• Double puncture & outflow needle
• Level I
• Instrumentation port (laser, coblation, grasper, probe etc.)
Level III Arthroscopy
• Triple puncture & outflow needle
• Level II
• Discopexy(suture/screw)

Table 63.6 Level 1 arthroscopy sequence

• Examination under anesthesia
• Marking landmarks
• Superior joint space insufflation
• Trocar and cannula puncture
• Backwash
• Insert scope (confirm entry)
• Establish outflow
• Diagnostic sweep
• Medications (Steroid, hyaluronic acid or PRP etc.)
• Manipulation

In addition to the lysis and lavage as in arthrocentesis (Table 63.6), a level 1 arthroscopy provides a diagnosis and identifies intra-articular pathology (Fig. 63.13a–f). A systematic diagnostic sweep through the entire superior joint space is performed to obtain the diagnostic information. Level 1 arthroscopy can be accomplished using a standard operative arthroscope (usually 1.9–2.7 mm) or the more recently available disposable scopes (1.2 mm). While the image quality from a disposable scope is currently not as good as the traditional operative arthroscopes, it does allow for adequate visualization and a diagnosis.

Level 2 arthroscopy includes a second puncture with an operative cannula and allows for additional procedures such as disc mobilization, biopsy, laser ablation, or coblation to be performed. Video 63.2 shows the second cannula being inserted, disc mobilization with a probe, and laser ablation of hyperplastic polypoid synovitis.

Level 3 arthroscopy with multiple cannulas allows for more advanced techniques and disc repositioning with fixation, using sutures, wires, pins, or screws. The author uses a suture technique to anchor the repositioned disc as shown in the Video 63.3. Figure 63.14a, b shows the suture placed through the posterior band of the disc anchoring it into the reduced position. The arthroscopic suture video clearly shows how tightening the suture reduces the anteriorly displaced disc.

Several surgeons have described and published techniques to reposition and fixate the displaced disc [53–59]. Success in the early reports of arthroscopic disc repositioning was not high. Yang reported better success rates with partial and later complete anterior release of the disc from its anterior attachment and suggested that relapse rates without complete anterior release are high [55]. While more recent success rates of disc repositioning as high as 95.3% [60] have been reported, many of these studies have relatively short-term follow-up and/or no MRI confirmation of long-term stability of the disc repositioning.

It is the authors' opinion that level 3 arthroscopy should be performed primarily for functional reasons, e.g., a mechanically obstructive click, closed lock, or subluxation. In McCain's publication on arthroscopic discopexy [59], the

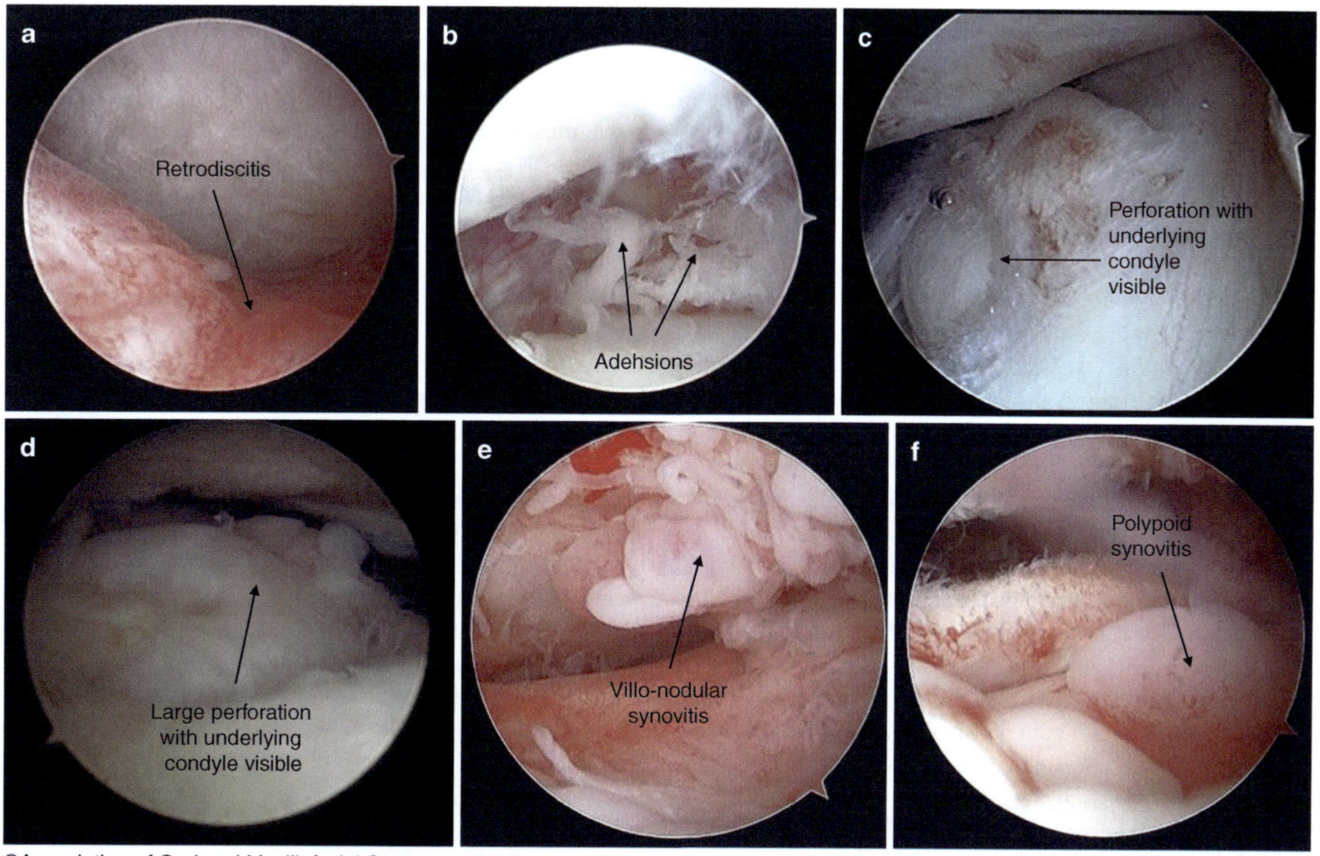

Fig. 63.13 (**a–f**) Arthroscopic pathology. (**a**) Retrodiscitis (**b**) Adhesions (**c**) Small disc tear/perforation (**d**) Large perforation with condyle visible (**e**) Villonodular synovitis (**f**) Polypoid synovitis

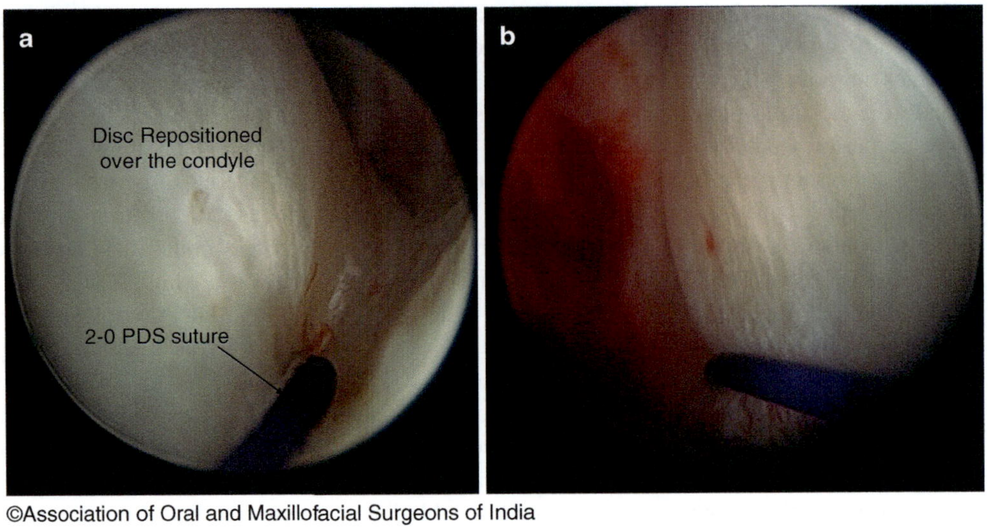

Fig. 63.14 (**a**, **b**) Arthroscopic suture discopexy—suture placed through the posterior band of the disc anchoring it into the correct reduced position

success rate in 42 joints was 86.7% in Wilkes II and III but only 25% in Wilkes IV and V which emphasizes that case selection is a key element to success. For disc repositioning to be indicated and have good outcomes, the disc must be salvageable, and there must be sufficient posterior joint space height in which to reposition the disc. In other words, the disc must be intact, and MRI evaluation must confirm normal disc morphology with adequate posterior joint space height in which to reposition the disc. If the joint space has collapsed as is often the case in longer-standing/chronic disc displacement, the load placed during function on the repositioned disc will be excessive, and the fixation will likely fail, leading to displacement again. Postoperatively, all patients will notice a malocclusion with slight mandibular deviation to the contralateral side. However, the majority of these malocclusions will resolve within 3 weeks. Additional factors to success are the postoperative physical therapy and dietary instructions. The author instructs his patients to perform "limited range of motion" exercises for the first 3 weeks to minimize the risk of the fixation failing or tearing through the disc. This is achieved by instructing the patient to keep the tongue on the roof of the mouth while performing opening exercises. The diet should be soft with minimal chewing and as for all surgical cases and any parafunctional habits should be well controlled. After 3 weeks, the patients gradually increase their mouth opening with daily stretching exercises. Associated myalgias may improve once the joint pain and function improve following arthroscopy, but often concomitant nonsurgical treatment of the muscle disorder is also required.

At the end of the arthroscopic procedure, the surgeon has the option of injecting medications including steroid, hyaluronic acid (HA), and platelet-rich plasma (PRP).

63.6.4.1 Viscosupplementation with Hyaluronic Acid

Hyaluronic acid is a glycosaminoglycan polysaccharide naturally found in synovial fluid. It is produced by the chondrocytes and synoviocytes and plays an important role in joint function and nutrition. HA is the main contributor to the viscosity of synovial fluid and provides protection under joint loading. Inflammatory disorders of the TMJ including internal derangement are associated with reduced quantity and quality of HA through a process of destruction and also the production of HA that is lower in molecular weight [61, 62]. The short half-life of injected HA makes it unlikely that its effectiveness is due to restoration of the viscosity of the synovial fluid [63]. It is suggested that supplementation with injectable HA could have anti-inflammatory and analgesic effects [64]. Altman suggested that injection of HA could lead to repair of the articular cartilage/fibrocartilage and normalize the synthesis of endogenous HA [65].

Viscosupplementation has been described in orthopedic literature for many years, but there are discrepancies in the evidence to support the widespread use of intra-articular hyaluronic acid to treat knee osteoarthritis. However, several recent studies have shown hyaluronic acid to be a viable treatment option showing longer-term improvement in both knee pain and function. Unfortunately, similar uncertainty exists regarding the effectiveness of viscosupplementation using hyaluronic acid in the TMJ [66–68]. Beyond viscosupplementation, there are some additional benefits to using HA in TMJ arthroscopy. If the surgeon is having difficulty maneuvering the scope because of a tight joint space, the lubricant properties of HA may be helpful in minimizing iatrogenic damage to the joint surfaces and disc. It is also helpful at the end of the procedure in reducing the bleeding from a hyperemic joint.

63.6.4.2 Platelet-Rich Plasma

Is a concentration of platelets and growth factors taken from autologous blood. It has reported beneficial effects in joint degeneration and tendinopathy [69–72], and there is both literature supporting its effectiveness in TMJ arthroscopy [73–75] and conflicting literature reporting no benefit [76, 77]. Therefore, the use of PRP after TMJ arthroscopy remains controversial, and further studies are needed [78].

63.6.4.3 Open Joint Surgery and Arthroplasty

The effectiveness of minimally invasive procedures such as arthrocentesis and arthroscopy has significantly reduced the frequency and volume of open joint surgery (disc repositioning or discectomy). However, currently there are very few surgeons trained in the advanced technique of arthroscopic discopexy, and so for patients who fail level 1 or 2 arthroscopy and require disc repositioning surgery, open joint surgery with disc repositioning may be the next surgical step in moving up the surgical pyramid. Annandale first published "On displacement of the inter-articular cartilage of the lower jaw and its treatment by operation" in 1887 [3], but it wasn't until later that surgery for internal derangement became popular. Surgical interest in disc displacement began with reports from McCarty and Farrar [5] claiming disc repositioning success rates of 94% using a wedge resection and suture plication technique. However, other surgeons were not as successful, and the long-term stability of suture plication techniques was low, leading to multiple variations of open surgical disc repositioning and methods of fixation [79–82]. In 2001, Wolford reported a more rigid fixation technique using a Mitek mini-bone anchor to fixate the repositioned disc [83]. In this technique, the anterior and lateral disc attachments are released allowing passive disc repositioning. The disc is separated at its junction with the retrodiscal tissue, and Mitek anchor is inserted into a 2-mm hole drilled into the posterior condyle 8–10mm below articulating surface. Two 0-Ethibond braided sutures are inserted through the posterior band of the disc in a mattress suture fashion fixing the disc to the Mitek anchor (Fig. 63.15a–c). Although radiographs at the longest follow-up showed no condylar resorption and stable position of the metal anchor, the stability of the disc repositioning was not evaluated by MRI. Despite this, Wolford reported that there was a statistically significant reduction in TMJ pain, facial pain, headaches, TMJ noises, and disability and improvement in jaw function and diet.

Alternative fixation and anchoring devices are available on the market today. He et al. use a self-drilling miniscrew and have modified the technique to include a complete anterior release and overcorrection of the disc position for better stability of the repositioning. They report stable short-term (mean 10 months) disc position on MRI in 98.6% of patients [84]. Zhou et al. evaluated the same technique in 149 joints and the long-term stability of the repositioned disc on MRI at a mean longest follow-up of 23.4 months (range 12–84 months) and reported that 95.3% of discs were still in position, whereas 4.7% had relapsed anteriorly [85]. They also reported new condylar bone formation in 74.5% of joints and even greater in young patients (under the age of 20), 90% of whom had new bone formation, suggesting that adolescents may have growth ability after disc repositioning which might reduce facial asymmetry. Mandibular asymmetry in unilateral disc displacement has been reported in the literature. Xie et al. [86] reported mandibular asymmetry in 72% of 165 patients with anterior disc displacement and the severity of the asymmetry correlated with the degree of disc displacement, disc deformity, and condylar shortening. Therefore, disc repositioning may allow for condylar bone formation and reduce mandibular asymmetry that may develop as a result of the displaced disc. The overall clinical outcomes of disc repositioning surgery are good with reduced pain, improved diet, and improved range of motion with 94% of patients reporting improved quality of life [87].

For those patients with discs that are not salvageable, discectomy is the next step in the surgical pyramid. This involves removal of the disc and the area surrounding any perforation in the retrodiscal tissue, and possible replacement of the disc is an option. There are several long-term studies demonstrating greater than 80% success rates following discectomy [88–91] with a few following patients for more than 20 years [92–94] with almost complete resolution of pain and restoration of normal diet. A 5-year follow-up study of discectomy without any disc replacement reported 87% of patients fulfilling the criteria for success with reduced pain on function and increased mouth opening, although pain at rest was unchanged [95]. Following discectomy, radiographs will show altered condylar morphology in the operated joint, and this is thought to be an adaptive process of remodeling because the reduced symptoms do not correlate with the radiographic changes [96, 97]. While the literature demonstrates the long-term success of discectomy without replacement [89, 90], disc replacement options have been explored in attempts to reduce the crepitation these patients experience and also with the intent to reduce the

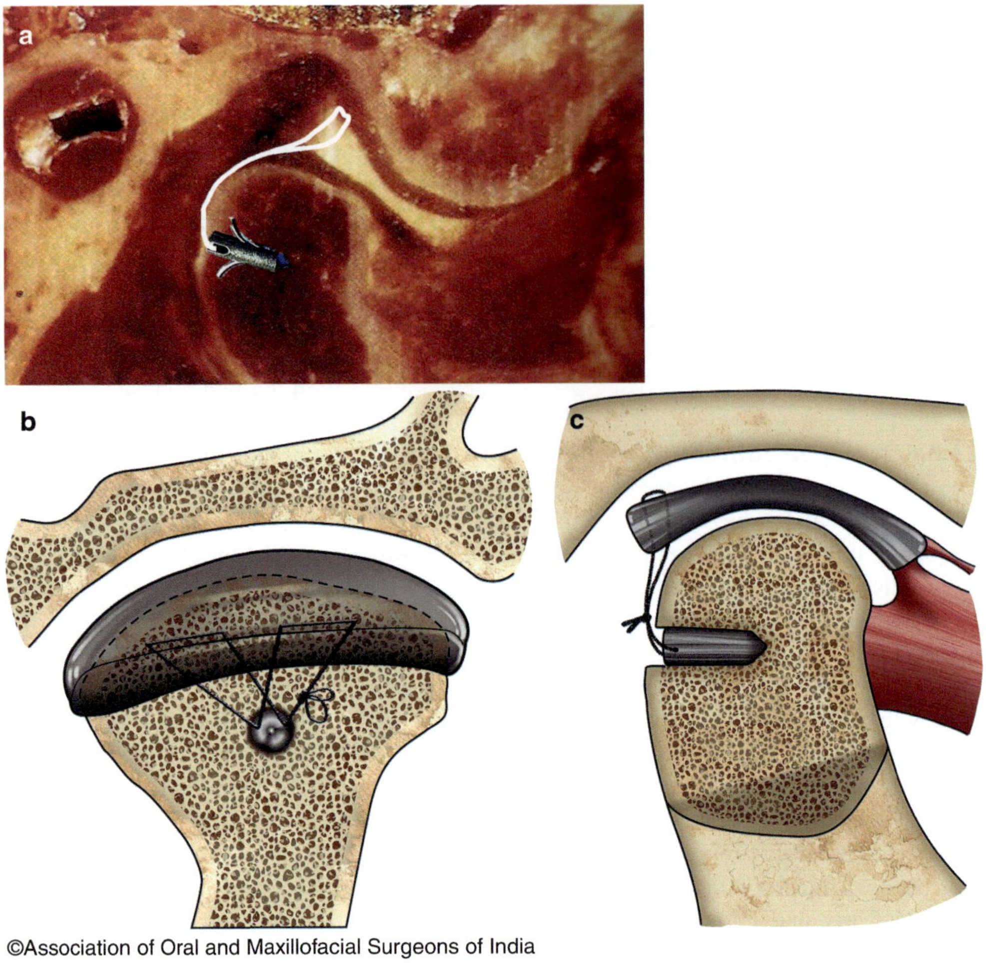

Fig. 63.15 (**a–c**) Use of a Mitek anchor according to Wolford's technique

remodeling. Many autogenous, allogeneic, and alloplastic disc replacements have been tried with varying degrees of success (Table 63.7), and some such as Proplast have caused joint destruction necessitating joint reconstruction and replacement [99]. At the current time, there is a lack of evidence to support the routine use of any disc replacement after discectomy.

Table 63.7 Disc replacement options [98]

Alloplastic	Methyl methacrylate Silastic Proplast-Teflon Fossa prosthesis
Allogenic	Dura (cryopreserved) Cartilage (lyophilized, freeze-dried)
Autogenous	Temporalis muscle/fascia Ear/rib cartilage Dermis skin grafts Abdominal fat
Xenograft	Bovine collagen/cartilage

The use of tissue engineering is emerging as a promising option to repair or potentially replace the diseased tissues of the TMJ and may provide additional treatment options in the future. Progress has already been made toward the development of appropriate tools for TMJ tissue engineering. The goal is to develop an approach to produce new tissues de novo (neotissues) with qualities similar to the native TMJ. This may be accomplished by (1) in situ tissue engineering, which involves an acellular scaffold matrix attracting local cells (cell homing) guiding the process of regeneration, and (2) ex vivo cell seeding on the scaffold, which provides enough competent cells to orchestrate the regenerative process. The second strategy appears better suited for TMJ regeneration because of its limited capacities of self-repair and the rapid regeneration expected [100].

Table 63.9 Algorithm and decision framework

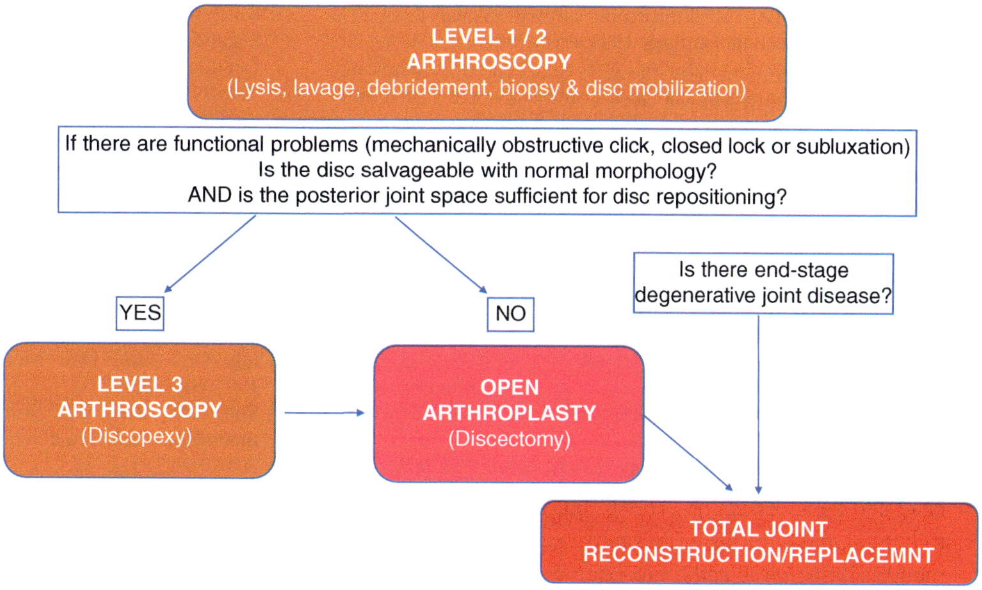

Table 63.8 Failed level 1 or 2 arthroscopy—now what?

• Wilkes II/III/early IV → Discopexy
• Wilkes IV/V → Advanced debridement
• Primary arthritis → Establish diagnosis
• Rheumatology referral
• Joint replacement

63.7 Conclusion

Internal derangement of the TMJ is a common problem resulting in pain and limited function for some patients. While the vast majority of patients adapt to the internal derangement over time or with nonsurgical treatment, surgery may be indicated for those with ongoing problems. There are no surgical procedures for the TMJ that have a 100% success rate; it therefore makes sense to undertake the least invasive procedures first. The surgical pyramid presented in this chapter provides a stepwise progression for TMJ surgical patients. In the authors' clinical practice, most surgical patients begin with a level 1 or 2 arthroscopic surgery and only step up the pyramid if this fails. If the diagnosis after arthroscopy is Wilkes II, III, or early IV, phase 2 procedure would be disc repositioning and discopexy if the disc is intact and has normal morphology and there is sufficient posterior joint space in which to reposition it. In Wilkes IV and V, phase 2 procedure would be joint debridement and discectomy (Table 63.8).

Finally, Table 63.9 presents an algorithm and decision framework that guides the progression through the various surgical procedures discussed in this chapter.

References

1. Steele AB. Internal derangement of the knee joint. BMJ. 1855;3(114):224–5.
2. Annandale T. An address on internal derangements of the knee-joint and their treatment by operation. Br Med J. 1887;1(1363):319–21.
3. Annandale T. On displacement of the inter-articular cartilage of the lower jaw, and its treatment by operation. Lancet. 1887;129(3313):411.
4. Porter RS. In: Porter RS, editor. The Merck manual of diagnosis and therapy, 20th ed. 2018.
5. McCarty WL, Farrar WB. Surgery for internal derangements of the temporomandibular joint. J Prosthet Dent. 1979;42(2):191–6.
6. Kaplan PA, Ruskin JD, Tu HK, Knibbe MA. Erosive arthritis of the temporomandibular joint caused by Teflon-Proplast implants: plain film features. AJR Am J Roentgenol. 1988;151(2):337–9.
7. Smith RM, Goldwasser MS, Sabol SR. Erosion of a Teflon-Proplast implant into the middle cranial fossa. J Oral Maxillofac Surg. 1993;51(11):1268–71.
8. Lypka M, Yamashita D-DR. Exuberant foreign body giant cell reaction to a teflon/proplast temporomandibular joint implant: report of a case. J Oral Maxillofac Surg. 2007;65(9):1680–4.
9. Wilkes CH. Internal derangements of the temporomandibular joint. Pathologic variations. Arch Otolaryngol Head Neck Surg. 1989;115:469–477.
10. Sanders B, Buoncristiani R. Diagnostic and surgical arthroscopy of the temporomandibular joint: clinical experience with 137 procedures over a 2-year period. J Craniomandib Disord. 1987;1(3):202–13.

11. Moses JJ, Poker ID. TMJ arthroscopic surgery: an analysis of 237 patients. J Oral Maxillofac Surg. 1989;47(8):790–4.
12. McCain JP, Sanders B, Koslin MG, Quinn JH, Peters PB, Indresano AT, et al. Temporomandibular joint arthroscopy: a 6-year multicenter retrospective study of 4,831 joints. J Oral Maxillofac Surg. 1992;50(9):926–30.
13. Hoffman DC, Cubillos L. The effect of arthroscopic surgery on mandibular range of motion. Cranio. 1994;12(1):11–8.
14. Dimitroulis G. A review of 56 cases of chronic closed lock treated with temporomandibular joint arthroscopy. J Oral Maxillofac Surg. 2002;60(5):519–24.
15. Dimitroulis G. Outcomes of temporomandibular joint arthroscopy in patients with painful but otherwise normal joints. J Craniomaxillofac Surg. 2015;43(6):940–3.
16. Kircos LT, Ortendahl DA, Mark AS, Arakawa M. Magnetic resonance imaging of the TMJ disc in asymptomatic volunteers. J Oral Maxillofac Surg. 1987;45(10):852–4.
17. Katzberg RW, Westesson PL, Tallents RH, Drake CM. Anatomic disorders of the temporomandibular joint disc in asymptomatic subjects. J Oral Maxillofac Surg. 1996;54(2):147–53.
18. Nitzan DW, Dolwick MF, Martinez GA. Temporomandibular joint arthrocentesis: a simplified treatment for severe, limited mouth opening. J Oral Maxillofac Surg. 1991;49(11):1163–7.
19. Nitzan DW, Samson B, Better H. Long-term outcome of arthrocentesis for sudden-onset, persistent, severe closed lock of the temporomandibular joint. J Oral Maxillofac Surg. 1997;55(2):151–7.
20. Dimitroulis G, Dolwick MF, Martinez A. Temporomandibular joint arthrocentesis and lavage for the treatment of closed lock: a follow-up study. Br J Oral Maxillofac Surg. 1995;33(1):23–6.
21. Hosaka H, Murakami K, Goto K, Iizuka T. Outcome of arthrocentesis for temporomandibular joint with closed lock at 3 years follow-up. Oral Surg Oral Med Oral Pathol Oral Radiol Endod. 1996;82(5):501–4.
22. Sembronio S, Albiero AM, Toro C, Robiony M, Politi M. Is there a role for arthrocentesis in recapturing the displaced disc in patients with closed lock of the temporomandibular joint? Oral Surg Oral Med Oral Pathol Oral Radiol Endod. 2008;105(3):274–80.
23. Quinn JH, Bazan NG. Identification of prostaglandin E2 and leukotriene B4 in the synovial fluid of painful, dysfunctional temporomandibular joints. J Oral Maxillofac Surg. 1990;48(9):968–71.
24. Shafer DM, Assael L, White LB, Rossomando EF. Tumor necrosis factor-alpha as a biochemical marker of pain and outcome in temporomandibular joints with internal derangements. J Oral Maxillofac Surg. 1994;52(8):786–91.
25. Kopp S. Neuroendocrine, immune, and local responses related to temporomandibular disorders. J Orofac Pain. 2001;15(1):9–28.
26. Kubota E, Kubota T, Matsumoto J, Shibata T, Murakami KI. Synovial fluid cytokines and proteinases as markers of temporomandibular joint disease. J Oral Maxillofac Surg. 1998;56(2):192–8.
27. Schiffman E, Ohrbach R, Truelove E, Look J, Anderson G, Goulet J-P, et al. Diagnostic Criteria for Temporomandibular Disorders (DC/TMD) for Clinical and Research Applications: recommendations of the International RDC/TMD Consortium Network and Orofacial Pain Special Interest Group†. J Oral Facial Pain Headache. 2014;28(1):6–27.
28. Farrar WB. Letter: myofascial pain dysfunction syndrome. J Am Dent Assoc. 1975;91(2):205–6.
29. Agerberg G, Inkapööl I. Craniomandibular disorders in an urban Swedish population. J Craniomandib Disord. 1990;4(3):154–64.
30. Santos KCP, Dutra MEP, Warmling LV, Oliveira JX. Correlation among the changes observed in temporomandibular joint internal derangements assessed by magnetic resonance in symptomatic patients. J Oral Maxillofac Surg. 2013;71(9):1504–12.
31. Rinchuse DJ, McMinn JT. Summary of evidence-based systematic reviews of temporomandibular disorders. Am J Orthod Dentofacial Orthop. 2006;130(6):715–20.
32. Türp JC, Schindler H. The dental occlusion as a suspected cause for TMDs: epidemiological and etiological considerations. J Oral Rehabil. 2012;39(7):502–12.
33. Okeson JP. Management of temporomandibular disorders and occlusion. St. Louis: Elsevier Health Sciences; 2007. 1 p.
34. Honda K, Larheim TA, Sano T, Hashimoto K, Shinoda K, Westesson PL. Thickening of the glenoid fossa in osteoarthritis of the temporomandibular joint. An autopsy study. Dentomaxillofac Radiol. 2001 Jan;30(1):10–3.
35. Larheim TA. Current trends in temporomandibular joint imaging. Oral Surg Oral Med Oral Pathol Oral Radiol Endod. 1995;80(5):555–76.
36. Song YW, Kang EH. Autoantibodies in rheumatoid arthritis: rheumatoid factors and anticitrullinated protein antibodies. QJM. 2010;103(3):139–46.
37. Niewold TB, Harrison MJ, Paget SA. Anti-CCP antibody testing as a diagnostic and prognostic tool in rheumatoid arthritis. QJM. 2007;100(4):193–201.
38. García-Kutzbach A, Chacón-Súchite J, García-Ferrer H, Iraheta I. Reactive arthritis: update 2018. Clin Rheumatol. 2018;37(4):869–74.
39. Sato S, Goto S, Nasu F, Motegi K. Natural course of disc displacement with reduction of the temporomandibular joint: changes in clinical signs and symptoms. J Oral Maxillofac Surg. 2003;61(1):32–4.
40. Sato S, Kawamura H, Nagasaka H, Motegi K. The natural course of anterior disc displacement without reduction in the temporomandibular joint: follow-up at 6, 12, and 18 months. J Oral Maxillofac Surg. 1997;55(3):234–8.
41. Kurita K, Westesson PL, Yuasa H, Toyama M, Machida J, Ogi N. Natural course of untreated symptomatic temporomandibular joint disc displacement without reduction. J Dent Res. 1998;77(2):361–5.
42. Costen JB. A syndrome of ear and sinus symptoms dependent upon disturbed function of the temporomandibular joint. 1934. Annal Otol Rhinol Laryngol. 1997;106(10 Pt 1):805–19.
43. Block LS. Diagnosis and treatment of disturbances of the temporomandibular joint especially in relation to vertical dimension. J Am Dent Assoc. 1947;34(4):253–60.
44. Posselt U. The temporomandibular joint syndrome and occlusion. J Prosthet Dent. 1971;25(4):432–8.
45. Lundh H, Westesson PL, Eriksson L, Brooks SL. Temporomandibular joint disk displacement without reduction. Treatment with flat occlusal splint versus no treatment. Oral Surg Oral Med Oral Pathol. 1992;73(6):655–8.
46. Truelove E, Huggins KH, Mancl L, Dworkin SF. The efficacy of traditional, low-cost and nonsplint therapies for temporomandibular disorder: a randomized controlled trial. J Am Dent Assoc. 2006;137(8):1099–107.
47. Greene CS, Goddard G, Macaluso GM, Mauro G. Topical review: placebo responses and therapeutic responses. How are they related? J Orofac Pain. 2009;23(2):93–107.
48. Greene CS, Laskin DM. Splint therapy for the myofascial pain—dysfunction (MPD) syndrome: a comparative study. J Am Dent Assoc. 1972;84(3):624–8.
49. Minakuchi H, Kuboki T, Matsuka Y, Maekawa K, Yatani H, Yamashita A. Randomized controlled evaluation of non-surgical treatments for temporomandibular joint anterior disk displacement without reduction. J Dent Res. 2001;80(3):924–8.
50. Klasser GD, Greene CS. Oral appliances in the management of temporomandibular disorders. Oral Surg Oral Med Oral Pathol Oral Radiol Endod. 2009;107(2):212–3.

51. Randolph CS, Greene CS, Moretti R, Forbes D, Perry HT. Conservative management of temporomandibular disorders: a posttreatment comparison between patients from a university clinic and from private practice. Am J Orthod Dentofacial Orthop. 1990;98(1):77–82.
52. Murakami KI, Iizuka T, Matsuki M, Ono T. Recapturing the persistent anteriorly displaced disk by mandibular manipulation after pumping and hydraulic pressure to the upper joint cavity of the temporomandibular joint. Cranio. 1987;5(1):17–24.
53. McCain JP, Podrasky AE, Zabiegalski NA. Arthroscopic disc repositioning and suturing: a preliminary report. J Oral Maxillofac Surg. 1992;50(6):568–79.
54. Zhang S-Y, Liu X-M, Yang C, Cai X-Y, Chen M-J, Haddad MS, et al. New arthroscopic disc repositioning and suturing technique for treating internal derangement of the temporomandibular joint: part II—magnetic resonance imaging evaluation. J Oral Maxillofac Surg. 2010;68(8):1813–7.
55. Yang C, Cai X-Y, Chen M-J, Zhang S-Y. New arthroscopic disc repositioning and suturing technique for treating an anteriorly displaced disc of the temporomandibular joint: part I—technique introduction. Int J Oral Maxillofac Surg. 2012;41(9):1058–63.
56. Zhu Y, Zheng C, Deng Y, Wang Y. Arthroscopic surgery for treatment of anterior displacement of the disc without reduction of the temporomandibular joint. Br J Oral Maxillofac Surg. 2012;50(2):144–8.
57. Goizueta-Adame CC, Pastor-Zuazaga D, Orts Bañón JE. Arthroscopic disc fixation to the condylar head. Use of resorbable pins for internal derangement of the temporomandibular joint (stage II-IV). Preliminary report of 34 joints. J Craniomaxillofac Surg. 2014;42(4):340–6.
58. Goizueta-Adame CC, Muñoz-Guerra MF. The posterior double pass suture in repositioning of the temporomandibular disc during arthroscopic surgery: a report of 16 cases. J Craniomaxillofac Surg. 2012;40(1):86–91.
59. McCain JP, Hossameldin RH, Srouji S, Maher A. Arthroscopic discopexy is effective in managing temporomandibular joint internal derangement in patients with Wilkes stage II and III. J Oral Maxillofac Surg. 2015;73(3):391–401.
60. Liu X, Zheng J, Cai X, Abdelrehem A, Yang C. Techniques of Yang's arthroscopic discopexy for temporomandibular joint rotational anterior disc displacement. Int J Oral Maxillofac Surg. 2018;48(6):769–78.
61. Nitzan DW. The process of lubrication impairment and its involvement in temporomandibular joint disc displacement: a theoretical concept. J Oral Maxillofac Surg. 2001;59(1):36–45.
62. Sharma A, Rana AS, Jain G, Kalra P, Gupta D, Sharma S. Evaluation of efficacy of arthrocentesis (with normal saline) with or without sodium hyaluronate in treatment of internal derangement of TMJ—a prospective randomized study in 20 patients. J Oral Biol Craniofac Res. 2013;3(3):112–9.
63. Machado RC, Capela S, Rocha FAC. Polysaccharides as viscosupplementation agents: structural molecular characteristics but not rheology appear crucial to the therapeutic response. Front Med (Lausanne). 2017;4:82.
64. Gencer ZK, Özkiriş M, Okur A, Korkmaz M, Saydam L. A comparative study on the impact of intra-articular injections of hyaluronic acid, tenoxicam and betametazon on the relief of temporomandibular joint disorder complaints. J Craniomaxillofac Surg. 2014;42(7):1117–21.
65. Altman RD, Manjoo A, Fierlinger A, Niazi F, Nicholls M. The mechanism of action for hyaluronic acid treatment in the osteoarthritic knee: a systematic review. BMC Musculoskelet Disord. 2015;16(1):321.
66. Ferreira N, Masterson D, Lopes de Lima R, de Souza Moura B, Oliveira AT, Kelly da Silva Fidalgo T, et al. Efficacy of viscosupplementation with hyaluronic acid in temporomandibular disorders: a systematic review. J Craniomaxillofac Surg. 2018;46(11):1943–52.
67. Bouloux GF, Chou J, Krishnan D, Aghaloo T, Kahenasa N, Smith JA, et al. Is hyaluronic acid or corticosteroid superior to lactated ringer solution in the short-term reduction of temporomandibular joint pain after arthrocentesis? Part 1. J Oral Maxillofac Surg. 2017;75(1):52–62.
68. Bouloux GF, Chou J, Krishnan D, Aghaloo T, Kahenasa N, Smith JA, et al. Is hyaluronic acid or corticosteroid superior to lactated ringer solution in the short term for improving function and quality of life after arthrocentesis? Part 2. J Oral Maxillofac Surg. 2017;75(1):63–72.
69. Foster TE, Puskas BL, Mandelbaum BR, Gerhardt MB, Rodeo SA. Platelet-rich plasma: from basic science to clinical applications. Am J Sports Med. 2009;37(11):2259–72.
70. Dai W-L, Zhou A-G, Zhang H, Zhang J. Efficacy of platelet-rich plasma in the treatment of knee osteoarthritis: a meta-analysis of randomized controlled trials. Arthroscopy. 2017;33(3):659–670. e1.
71. Fitzpatrick J, Bulsara MK, O'Donnell J, McCrory PR, Zheng MH. The effectiveness of platelet-rich plasma injections in gluteal tendinopathy: a randomized, double-blind controlled trial comparing a single platelet-rich plasma injection with a single corticosteroid injection. Am J Sports Med. 2018;46(4):933–9.
72. Fitzpatrick J, Bulsara M, Zheng MH. The effectiveness of platelet-rich plasma in the treatment of tendinopathy: a meta-analysis of randomized controlled clinical trials. Am J Sports Med. 2017;45(1):226–33.
73. Bousnaki M, Bakopoulou A, Koidis P. Platelet-rich plasma for the therapeutic management of temporomandibular joint disorders: a systematic review. Int J Oral Maxillofac Surg. 2018;47(2):188–98.
74. Hegab AF, Ali HE, Elmasry M, Khallaf MG. Platelet-rich plasma injection as an effective treatment for temporomandibular joint osteoarthritis. J Oral Maxillofac Surg. 2015;73(9):1706–13.
75. Chung P-Y, Lin M-T, Chang H-P. Effectiveness of platelet-rich plasma injection in patients with temporomandibular joint osteoarthritis: a systematic review and meta-analysis of randomized controlled trials. Oral Surg Oral Med Oral Pathol Oral Radiol. 2019;127(2):106–16.
76. Cömert Kiliç S, Güngörmüş M. Is arthrocentesis plus platelet-rich plasma superior to arthrocentesis plus hyaluronic acid for the treatment of temporomandibular joint osteoarthritis: a randomized clinical trial. Int J Oral Maxillofac Surg. 2016;45(12):1538–44.
77. Fernández Sanromán J, Fernández Ferro M, Costas López A, Arenaz Bua J, López A. Does injection of plasma rich in growth factors after temporomandibular joint arthroscopy improve outcomes in patients with Wilkes stage IV internal derangement? A randomized prospective clinical study. Int J Oral Maxillofac Surg. 2016;45(7):828–35.
78. Haigler MC, Abdulrehman E, Siddappa S, Kishore R, Padilla M, Enciso R. Use of platelet-rich plasma, platelet-rich growth factor with arthrocentesis or arthroscopy to treat temporomandibular joint osteoarthritis: Systematic review with meta-analyses. J Am Dent Assoc. 2018;149(11):940–2.
79. Leopard PJ. Anterior dislocation of the temporomandibular disc. Br J Oral Maxillofac Surg. 1984;22(1):9–17.
80. Walker RV, Kalamchi S. A surgical technique for management of internal derangement of the temporomandibular joint. J Oral Maxillofac Surg. 1987;45(4):299–305.
81. Weinberg S, Cousens G. Meniscocondylar plication: a modified operation for surgical repositioning of the ectopic temporomandibular joint meniscus. Rationale and operative technique. Oral Surg Oral Med Oral Pathol. 1987;63(4):393–402.
82. Zetz MR, Ash DC. Double-layer closure for temporomandibular joint discoplasty. J Oral Maxillofac Surg. 1990;48(4):427–9.

83. Mehra P, Wolford LM. The Mitek mini anchor for TMJ disc repositioning: surgical technique and results. Int J Oral Maxillofac Surg. 2001;30(6):497–503.
84. He D, Yang C, Zhang S, Wilson JJ. Modified temporomandibular joint disc repositioning with miniscrew anchor: part I—surgical technique. J Oral Maxillofac Surg. 2015;73(1):47.e1–9.
85. Zhou Q, Zhu H, He D, Yang C, Song X, Ellis E. Modified temporomandibular joint disc repositioning with mini-screw anchor: part ii-stability evaluation by magnetic resonance imaging. J Oral Maxillofac Surg. 2019;77(2):273–9.
86. Xie Q, Yang C, He D, Cai X, Ma Z. Is mandibular asymmetry more frequent and severe with unilateral disc displacement? J Craniomaxillofac Surg. 2015;43(1):81–6.
87. Abramowicz S, Dolwick MF. 20-year follow-up study of disc repositioning surgery for temporomandibular joint internal derangement. J Oral Maxillofac Surg. 2010;68(2):239–42.
88. Merrill RG. Historical perspectives and comparisons of TMJ surgery for internal disk derangements and arthropathy. Cranio. 1986;4(1):74–85.
89. McKenna SJ. Discectomy for the treatment of internal derangements of the temporomandibular joint. J Oral Maxillofac Surg. 2001;59(9):1051–6.
90. Holmlund AB, Gynther G, Axelsson S. Discectomy in treatment of internal derangement of the temporomandibular joint. Follow-up at 1, 3, and 5 years. Oral Surg Oral Med Oral Pathol. 1993;76(3):266–71.
91. Miloro M, McKnight M, Han MD, Markiewicz MR. Discectomy without replacement improves function in patients with internal derangement of the temporomandibular joint. J Craniomaxillofac Surg. 2017;45(9):1425–31.
92. Silver CM. Long-term results of meniscectomy of the temporomandibular joint. Cranio. 1984;3(1):46–57.
93. Takaku S, Toyoda T. Long-term evaluation of discectomy of the temporomandibular joint. J Oral Maxillofac Surg. 1994;52(7):722–6.
94. Tolvanen M, Oikarinen VJ, Wolf J. A 30-year follow-up study of temporomandibular joint meniscectomies: a report on five patients. Br J Oral Maxillofac Surg. 1988;26(4):311–6.
95. Nyberg J, Adell R, Svensson B. Temporomandibular joint discectomy for treatment of unilateral internal derangements—a 5-year follow-up evaluation. Int J Oral Maxillofac Surg. 2004;33(1):8–12.
96. Agerberg G, Lundberg M. Changes in the temporomandibular joint after surgical treatment. A radiologic follow-up study. Oral Surg Oral Med Oral Pathol. 1971;32(6):865–75.
97. Hansson LG, Hansson T, Petersson A. A comparison between clinical and radiologic findings in 259 temporomandibular joint patients. J Prosthet Dent. 1983;50(1):89–94.
98. Dimitroulis G. A critical review of interpositional grafts following temporomandibular joint discectomy with an overview of the dermis-fat graft. Int J Oral Maxillofac Surg. 2011;40(6):561–8.
99. Henry CH, Wolford LM. Treatment outcomes for temporomandibular joint reconstruction after Proplast-Teflon implant failure. J Oral Maxillofac Surg. 1993;51(4):352–8.
100. Van Bellinghen X, Idoux-Gillet Y, Pugliano M, Strub M, Bornert F, Clauss F, et al. Temporomandibular joint regenerative medicine. Int J Mol Sci. 2018;19(2):446.

Temporomandibular Joint Dislocation

64

V. B. Krishnakumar Raja

64.1 Introduction

Hypermobility disorders of the temporomandibular joint (TMJ) present in two major forms:

1. Dislocation
2. Subluxation [1]

The differences between dislocation and subluxation have been highlighted in Box 64.1.

The condyle may be displaced either anteriorly, posteriorly, medially, or laterally of which anterior dislocation is the most common [1]. The incidence of TMJ dislocation constitutes about 3% of the dislocations occurring in other joints of the body with female predilection. The reported incidence of TMJ dislocation is 7% with a preponderance in people in the second and third decades [2].

Box 64.1 Definition of Dislocation and Subluxation
Dislocation refers the phenomenon in which condyle is displaced out of the glenoid fossa and traverses in front of the articular eminence. In contrast, subluxation is the condition in which the dislocated condyle can be reduced back into the normal position by patient themselves, without any professional assistance.

64.2 Classification (Box 64.2)

Dislocation has been classified by numerous methods. Rowe and Killey [3] based it on the duration of the dislocation episode as:

Box 64.2 Classification of Dislocation
Based on duration of displacement
- Acute dislocation
- Habitual dislocation/subluxation
- Chronic recurrent dislocation
- Long-standing/chronic protracted dislocation

Based on direction of displacement
- Anterior
- Posterior
- Medial
- Lateral
- Superior

Based on side of displacement
- Unilateral
- Bilateral

1. Acute
2. Chronic

Dislocation recurring more than once is termed as chronic recurrent dislocation. The term *chronic protracted dislocation* is used to describe dislocation persisting for more than 1 month, while dislocation present for more than 6 months is called *extra-long-standing dislocation* [4].

Based on the direction of displacement [2], dislocation may be categorized as:

- Anterior
- Posterior
- Lateral
- Superior

Anterior dislocation is the most common type of dislocation due the weakness of the capsule in the anterior region.

V. B. Krishnakumar Raja (✉)
Department of Oral and Maxillofacial Surgery, SRM Dental College and Hospital, Ramapuram, Chennai, Tamil Nadu, India

K. Bonanthaya et al. (eds.), *Oral and Maxillofacial Surgery for the Clinician*, https://doi.org/10.1007/978-981-15-1346-6_64

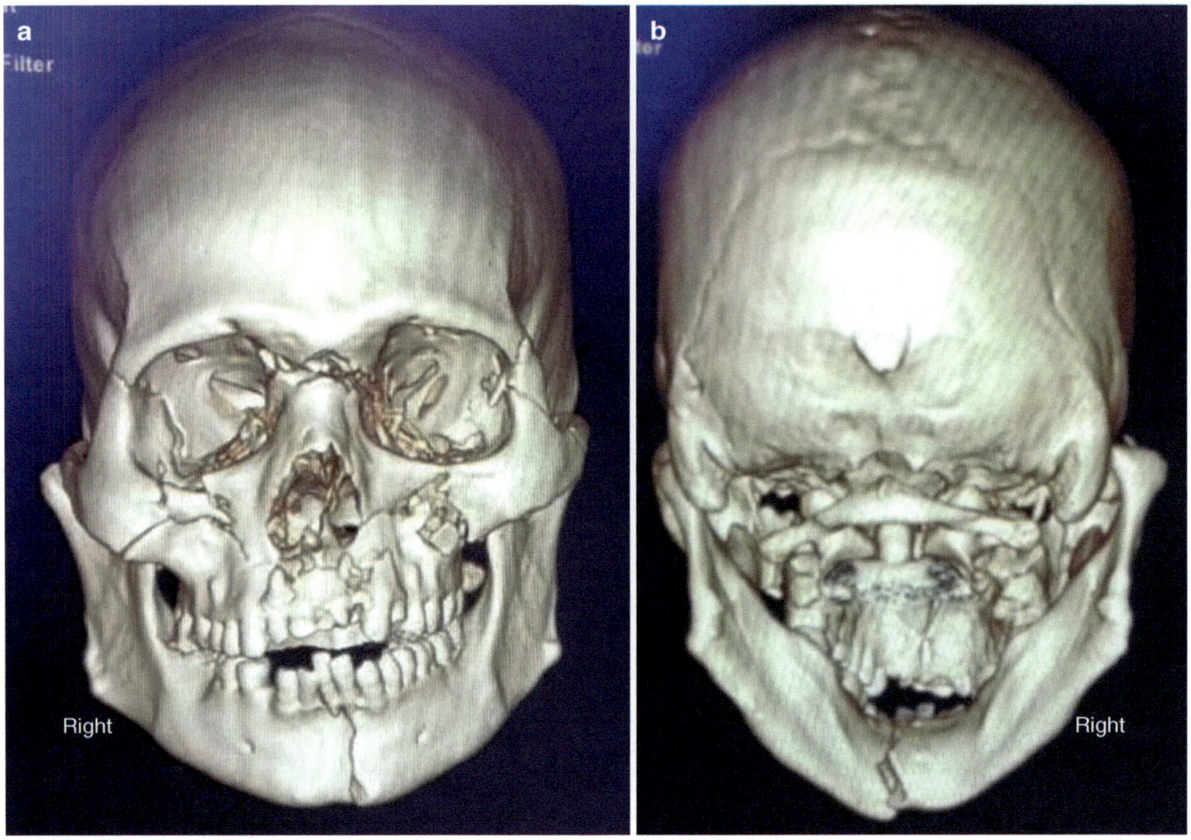

Fig. 64.1 Lateral dislocation of condyle, Post trauma, on the right side. (**a**) Frontal view showing lateral dislocation on right side (**b**) Posterior view showing lateral dislocation on right side

Posterior dislocation occurs following fracture of the external auditory canal and skull base. Allen and Young classified lateral dislocation into Type I and Type II. This type of dislocation occurs in mandibular trauma (Fig. 64.1a, b):

- Type I refers to lateral subluxation.
- Type II indicated lateral and superior dislocation into the temporal fossa [2].

Superior dislocation results when condyle is pushed into the middle cranial fossa accompanied by glenoid fossa fracture. Small and round-shaped condyle is predisposed to this type of dislocation [2].

64.3 Etiopathogenesis (Table 64.1)

A multitude of causes have been described in the etiopathogenesis of TMJ dislocation including congenital, iatrogenic, anatomical aberrations, spontaneous, pharmacological, neurological, neuromuscular, etc. Proper diagnosis of the etiology is important to institute problem-specific treatment.

Table 64.1 Etiology of dislocation

Trauma	
Medical and surgical procedures	Dental procedures which require wide mouth opening for prolonged time Intubation procedures, gastrointestinal endoscopy, laryngoscopy/bronchoscopy ENT procedures
Spontaneous	Laughing Yawning Biting Vomiting Singing Epileptic seizures
Anatomical aberrations	Small condyle Poorly grooved glenoid fossa, shallow/steep articular eminence, laxity of ligaments and capsule for more prone for dislocation
Systemic disorders	Ehlers-Danlos disease Marfan's syndrome Huntington disease Parkinson disease Multiple sclerosis Muscle dystrophies or dystonias
Medications	Antipsychiatric Antiemetic
Occlusal conditions	Edentulous posterior region

Daily activities which involve wide mouth opening such as laughing, yawning, and biting may induce TMJ dislocation. It may also occur spontaneously during epileptic seizures, vomiting, yawning, and singing. Trauma is another cause which might cause posterior, superior, and lateral dislocation in addition to anterior dislocation [5]. Iatrogenic causes include dental procedures which require wide mouth opening for prolonged time, intubation procedures, gastrointestinal endoscopy, and laryngoscopy/bronchoscopy. Anatomical aberrations such as small condyle, underdeveloped glenoid fossa, shallow/steep articular eminence and laxity of ligaments and capsule are more prone for dislocation.

Predisposing risk factors include connective tissue disorders such as Ehlers-Danlos disease and Marfan's syndrome which predispose to laxity of the joint and hypermobility. Muscle spasms occur in neurodegenerative or neurodysfunctional diseases, namely, Huntington disease, Parkinson disease, multiple sclerosis, muscle dystrophies, or dystonias.

Medications which induce dislocation are antipsychiatric (phenothiazines) and antiemetic (metoclopramide) drugs which produce unwanted extrapyramidal reactions which eventually lead to muscular imbalance attributed to dislocation.

Reduced vertical dimension due to loss of posterior teeth in advanced age may also predispose an individual to dislocation [5].

Though various theories of pathogenesis have been described in literature, the most accepted was muscular incoordination during mandibular movements. In the initial stages of mouth closure, elevators are activated prior to the relaxation of depressors mainly lateral pterygoid which pulls the condyle forward. This initial dislocation facilitates the further dislocation [5].

64.4 **Clinical Features** (Mentioned in Box 64.3; Figs. 64.2a, b, 64.3, 64.4a, b, and 64.5a, b)

Box 64.3 Clinical Features of Dislocation

The classical clinical features of dislocation are:

1. Pain in the preauricular and surrounding region.
2. Preauricular depression/hollowing.
3. Protruding chin.
4. Inability to close mouth.
5. Drooling of saliva.
6. Inability to speak, swallow, or masticate.
7. Tense masticatory muscles are also a characteristic feature [6]

Unilateral dislocation is associated with deviation of chin towards contralateral side.

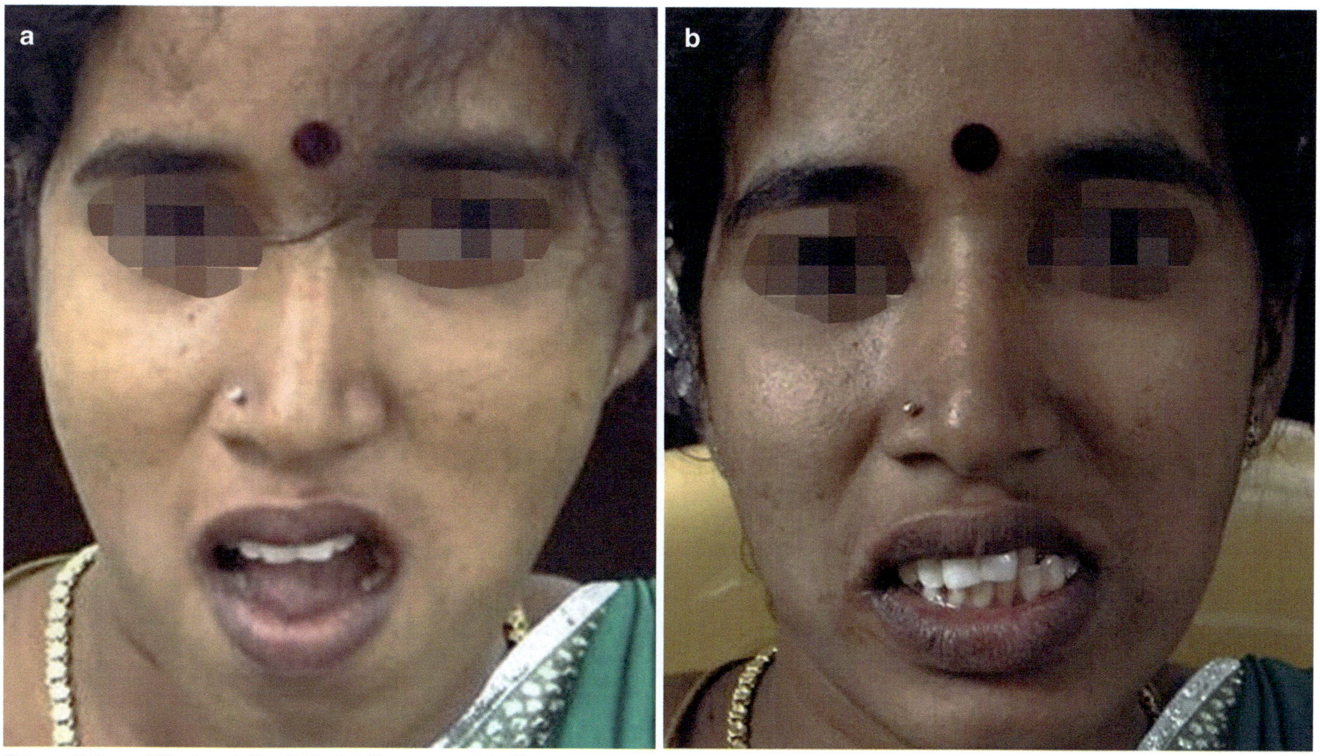

Fig. 64.2 (**a**, **b**) Bilateral TMJ dislocation. (**a**) Before reduction (**b**) After reduction

64.5 Investigations

- *Orthopantomogram* (OPG) (open and closed) (Fig. 64.6)
  This is the commonly used screening modality for the examination of TMJ. Morphology of condyle, articular eminence, and joint space can be evaluated. Open mouth OPG shows the position of the condyle in relation to the articular eminence.

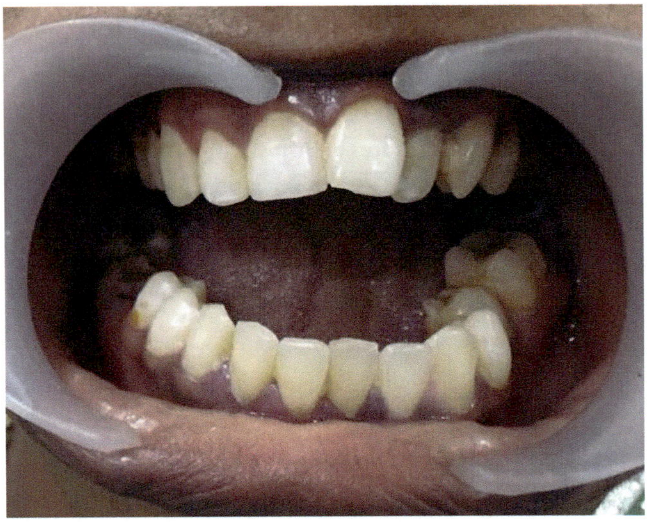

Fig. 64.3 Bilateral TMJ dislocation showing openbite

- *TMJ tomogram*
  Open and closed mouth TMJ images can be obtained in different slices.
- *Computed tomography(CT)*
  Evaluation of the morphology of osseous TMJ components—condyle, articular eminence and the glenoid fossa—are better assessed with CT.
- *Cone beam computed tomography* CBCT
  CBCT facilitates accurate measurement of condylar height, width, and length as well as inclination of articular eminence.
- *Magnetic resonance imaging (MRI)*
  MRI demonstrates the soft tissue morphology, particularly disc shape, displacement, and effusion of the joint frequently associated with dislocation.
- *Electromyography (EMG)*
  EMG evaluates the activity of the muscles which may be hypoactive, normoactive, or hyperactive.
- *Ultrasonography (USG)*
  Thickness and length of the muscles can be evaluated both at rest and clenching by USG.

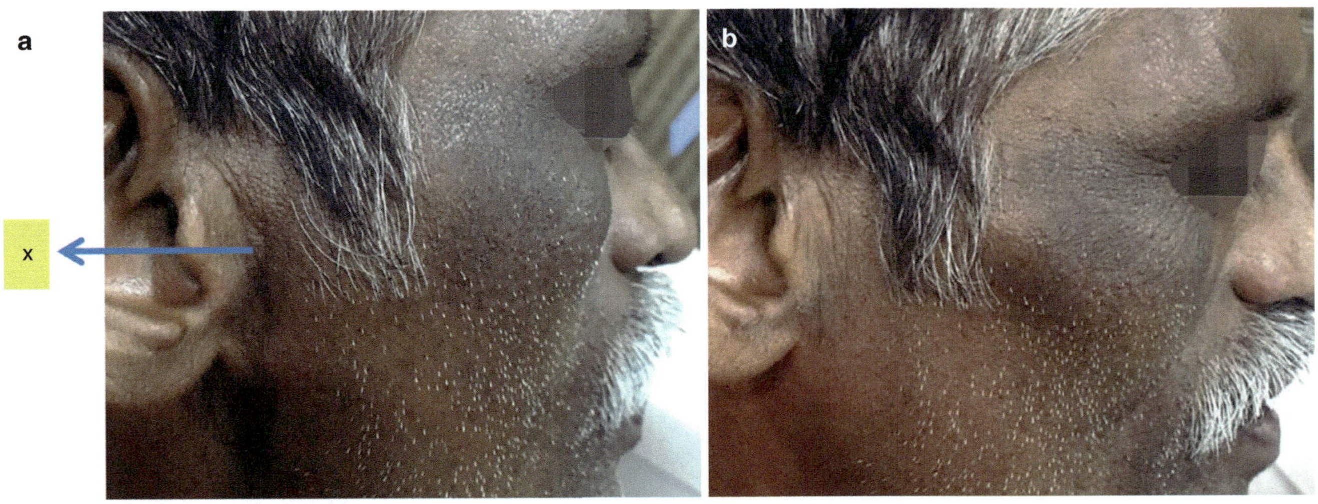

Fig. 64.4 (**a**, **b**) Preauricular depression. (**a**) Before reduction. x—Preauricular depression. (**b**) After reduction

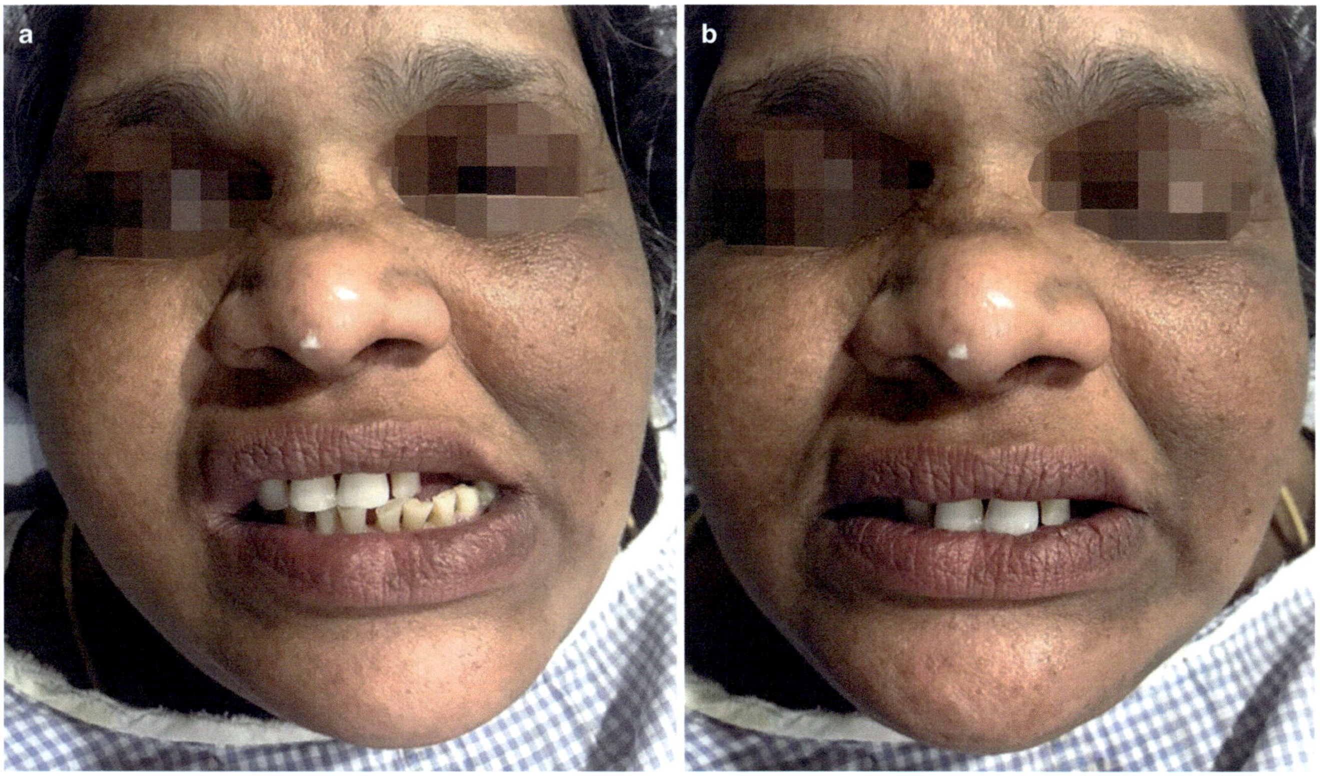

Fig. 64.5 (**a**, **b**) Unilateral TMJ dislocation on the right side. (**a**) Before reduction (**b**) After reduction

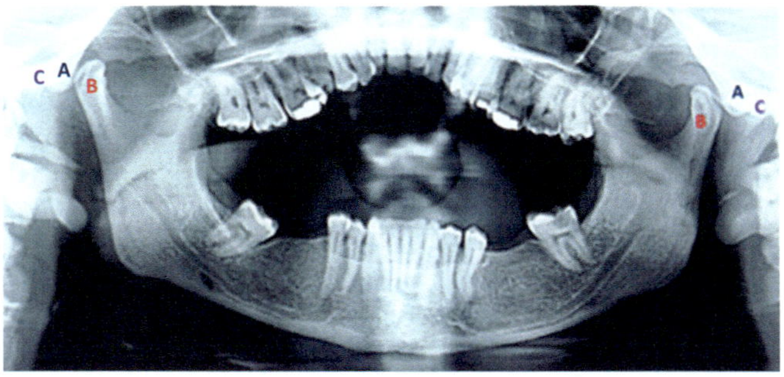

Fig. 64.6 OPG demonstrating dislocation. A: Articular eminence. B: Condyle in front of articular eminence. C: Glenoid fossa

64.6 Management of Dislocation (Box 64.4)

64.6.1 Acute Dislocation

Reducing the dislocated condyle poses a great challenge. Reduction is more complicated with the accompanied muscle spasm persisting for longer duration. In difficult situations, reduction can be facilitated with the help of local anesthesia, conscious sedation, and general anesthesia. Following reduction, a Barton's bandage, chin strap, or intermaxillary fixation is advised for 3–6 weeks to prevent further dislocation. Several reduction techniques have been employed with varying rates of success.

Box 64.4 Management of Acute Dislocation

- Conventional technique—Hippocratic/Nelaton's method
- Wrist pivot technique
- Extraoral technique
- Gag reflex

64.6.1.1 Hippocratic/Nelaton's Technique (Fig. 64.7)

This is the conventional method of reduction of acute dislocation in which physician stands in front of the patient, with the thumb placed either on the external oblique ridge or on the lower molars and other fingers positioned along the lower border of the mandible. A steady downward, backward, and superior force should be given to reduce the dislocated condyle. The thumb should be protected either with a plastic splint or gauze wrapped around it to prevent injury to the thumb while reducing dislocation.

64.6.1.2 Gag Reflex [3]

Gag reflex is induced by probing the soft palate using mouth mirror. In alert individuals, this reflex relaxes the lateral pterygoid muscle through coordinated neuromuscular activities which reduces dislocation in natural way.

64.6.1.3 Wrist Pivot Method [7] (Fig. 64.8)

This method utilizes existing myospasm of the elevators for reduction. The thumb is placed under the chin, while other fingers are placed over the occlusal surfaces of lower teeth.

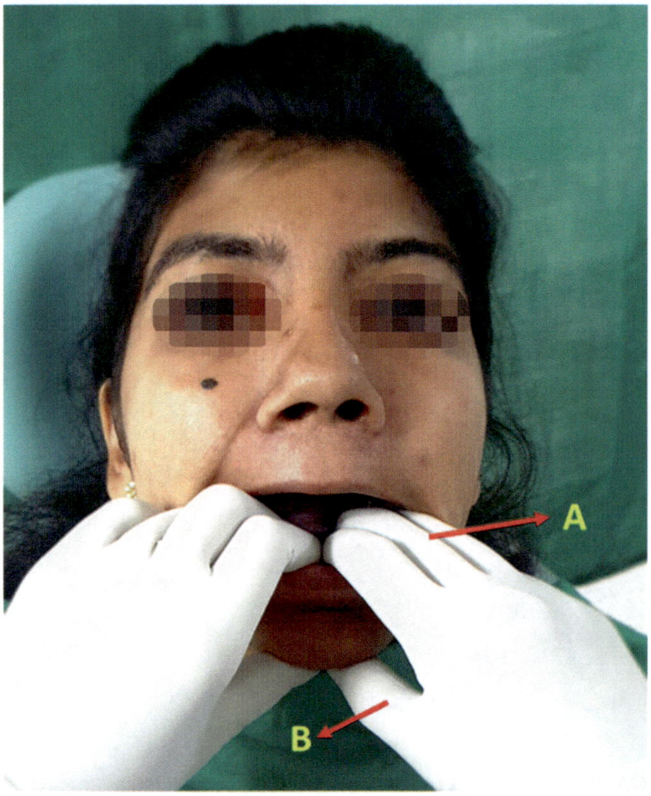

Fig. 64.8 Wrist-pivot method. A: Other fingers intraorally on the occlusal surface lower teeth. B: Thumb on the chin

Then upward movement is applied by the thumb, and concomitant inferior force is given by other fingers with pivoting the wrist. The advantage of this technique is that it utilizes the force created by the muscles of mastication rather than overcoming this force as in Nelaton's technique.

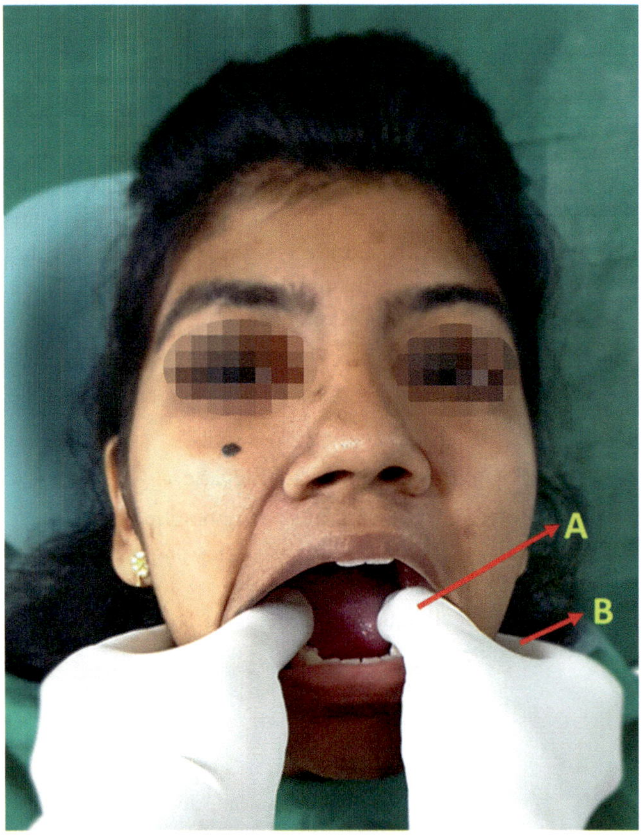

Fig. 64.7 Nelaton's method. A: Thumb intraorally on the occlusal surface lower teeth. B: Other fingers at the inferior border of body and angle of the mandible

64.6.1.4 Extraoral Method [8] (Fig. 64.9a, b)

Intraoral methods described previously have the risk of human bite in which there are chances of infection transmission. To overcome this, extraoral method has been described. In the dislocated mandible, coronoid process comes forward which is easy to palpate. On one side, the thumb is positioned over the coronoid process which pushes the mandible backward, while the other fingers are located over the mastoid process to deliver counteracting force (Fig. 64.9a). On the other side, the mandible is pulled further forward with the thumb on the malar eminence and rest of the fingers on the mandibular angle (Fig. 64.9b). Pulling the mandible on one side with simultaneous pushing of the mandible on the other side reduces the dislocation on one side first and then subsequently on the other side. This technique is applicable in unilateral dislocation as one side is reduced first and then the other is reduced thereafter.

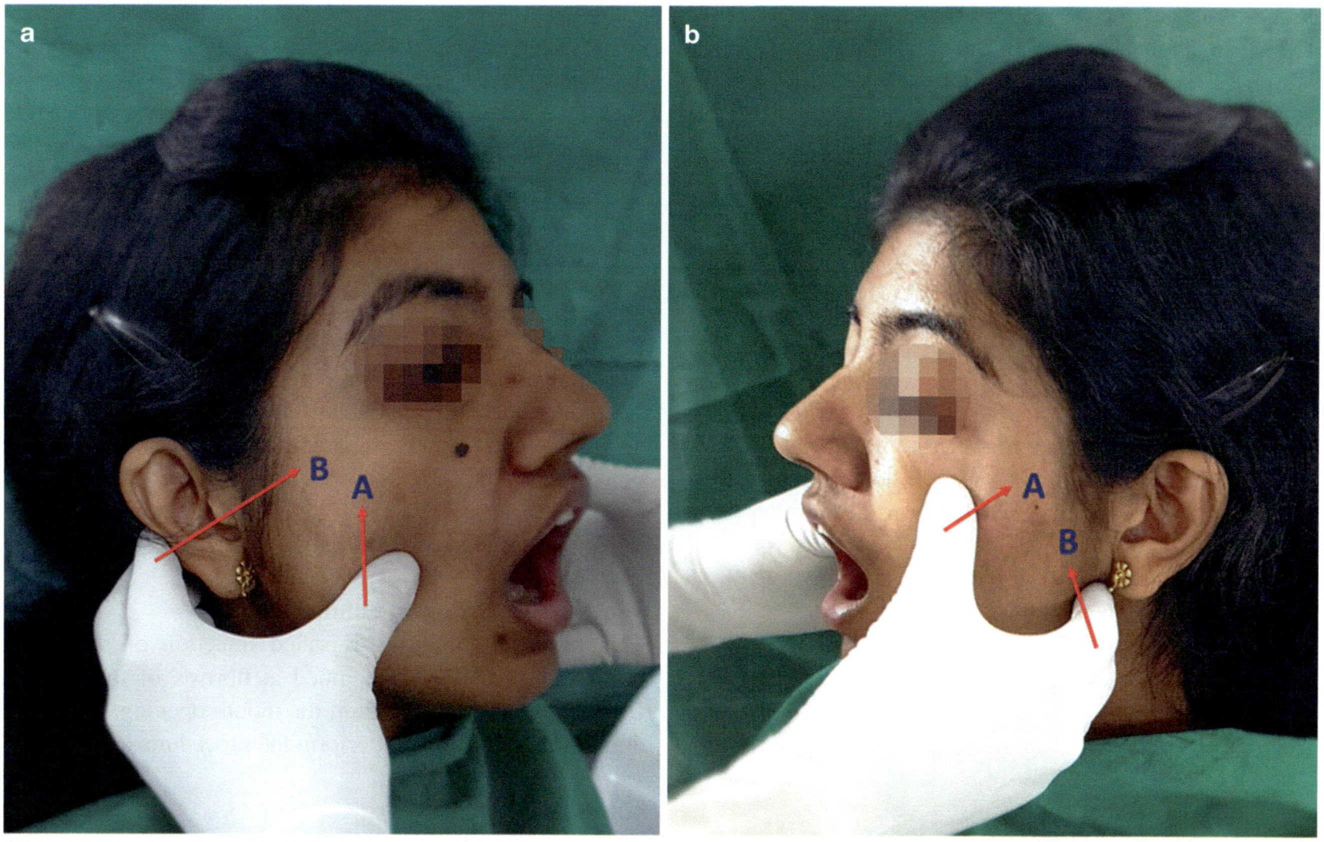

Fig. 64.9 (**a**, **b**) Extraoral method for reduction of dislocation. (**a**) A: Thumb on coronoid process. B: Other fingers on mastoid process. (**b**) A: Thumb on malar eminence. B: Other fingers on angle of the mandible

64.6.2 Management of Chronic Recurrent Dislocation/Subluxation (Box 64.5 and 64.6)

Box 64.5 Management of Chronic Recurrent Dislocation/Subluxation

Conservative
1. Physiotherapy
2. Intermaxillary fixation
3. Chin straps
4. Barton's bandage
5. Kinesio taping

Minimally invasive
1. Injection of sclerosing agents
2. Autologous blood injection
3. Prolotherapy
4. Botulinum toxin injection

Box 64.6 Management of Chronic Recurrent Dislocation/Subluxation

Surgical procedures
1. Capsular tightening procedure
   (a) Capsulorrhaphy
2. Creation of mechanical obstacle
   (a) Dautrey's procedure
   (b) Glenotemporal osteotomy
3. Removal of mechanical obstacle
   (a) Eminectomy
   (b) Condylectomy
4. Creation of new muscular balance
   (a) Temporalis scarification
   (b) Lateral pterygoid myotomy
   (c) Pterygoid dysjunction

Numerous treatment modalities have been described for TMJ dislocation, as it has multifactorial etiology. Miller and Murphy [9] proposed a comprehensive list of treatment options which targeted specific anatomical sites of the joint that exhibited abnormality: the capsule, eminence, and condylar head.

For practical purposes, the types of management may be broadly classified based on the degree of invasiveness as:

1. Conservative
2. Minimally invasive
3. Surgical

64.6.2.1 Conservative Methods

Conservative methods may be used following reduction of dislocation to prevent further dislocation, such as:

1. Physiotherapy
2. Intermaxillary fixation
3. Chin straps
4. Barton's bandage (Fig. 64.10)
5. Kinesio taping

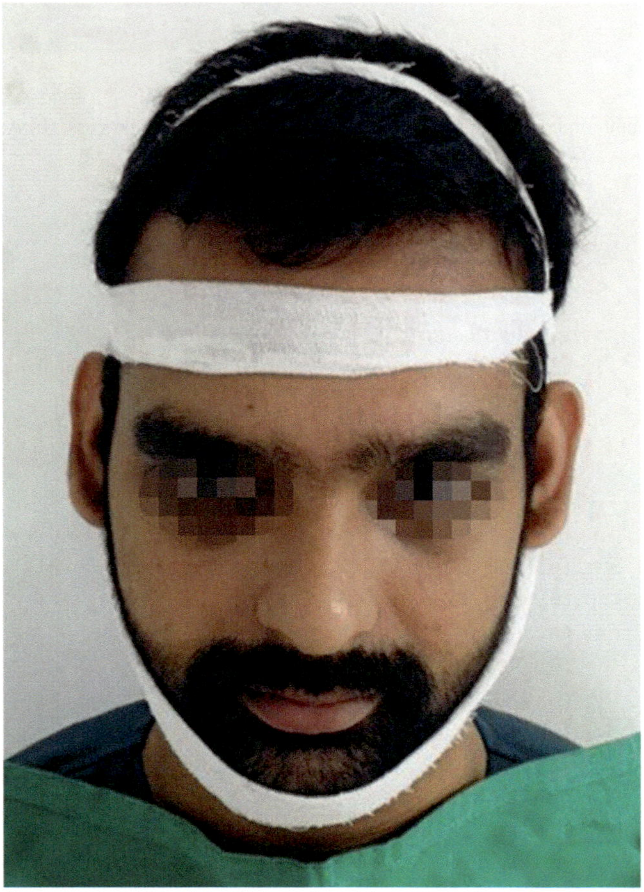

Fig. 64.10 Barton's bandage

Intermaxillary fixation, chin strap, and Barton's bandage are done for 4 weeks to induce fibrosis of soft tissues around the joint so that further dislocation is prevented. Physiotherapy including ultrasound and infrared therapy are advised to reduce pain. Isotonic and isometric exercise are advised to strength the muscle involved in TMJ function [9].

Kinesio Taping (Fig. 64.11)
In the year 1970, Dr. Kenzo Kase, a Japanese chiropractor, first described the techniques of Kinesio taping. The thin elastic tape acts by lifting the skin which increases the blood and lymphatic flow, thereby reducing inflammation and accumulation of pain mediators. It also helps in better muscle function and joint realignment which is utilized in reduction of TMJ dislocation.

64.6.2.2 Minimally Invasive Treatment

Injection of Sclerosing Solutions [9]
This procedure involves repeated injection of sclerosing solution into the capsule aimed at fibrosis of the capsule which would eventually limit the mouth opening. The solutions commonly used to perform the procedure are:

- Sodium psylliate
- Sodium tetradecylsulfate
- Sodium morrhuate
- Ethanolamine oleate 5%
- Tincture of iodine
- OK-432 (Picibanil)

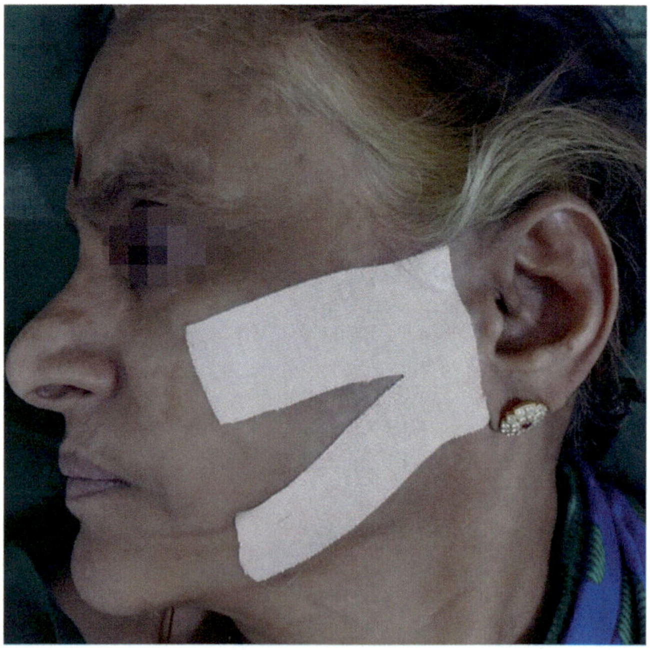

Fig. 64.11 Kinesio taping

These injections are usually given intra-articularly and in pericapsular region and can be repeated every 2–3 weeks till the fibrosis occurs. However, the outcome of this technique is not satisfactory and is also associated with complications such as TMJ ankylosis and facial nerve injury [9].

OK-432 which is a streptococcal derivative inactivated by penicillin G is used as sclerosing agent for the treatment of TMJ dislocation. A 21-gauge needle is used to inject 1.25 KE/ml concentration of OK-432 into the superior joint space and pericapsular region. 2 ml of the solution is injected in each region. This produces fibrosis in and around the joint by inducing local inflammation and formation of granulation tissue. Mouth opening is restricted for 4 days following injection by elastic bandage.

Autologous Blood Injection [1]

This procedure works by producing fibrosis which restricts the opening of the mouth wide. It involves injection of patient's own blood into the superior joint space and pericapsular region following two puncture arthrocentesis. Prior to the injection of blood into the joint, lavage should be done using two needles in the superior joint space, and then one needle is removed. Blood is injected through the other needle into the joint and around the joint. It may be injected either unilaterally or bilaterally. It can be given as a single or multiple injections with intervals.

Injection of Platelet Rich Plasma (PRP) (Refer suggested reading at the end of the chapter)

Platelet rich plasma is a yet another minimally invasive technique used to treat various Temporomandibular joint disorders. It is prepared from 10 ml of patient's own blood which was centrifuged at 3200 rpm for 12 minutes. The 2ml solution was then injected it to the superior joint space which was located 10 mm forward and 2 mm downward on the canthotragal line. Another 1ml of the solution was injected into the pericapsular tissues. Patients were advised for various mandibular movements for a minute following injection for the equal distribution of PRP in the joint. Elastic bandage is given for a week followed by mandibular exercise advised. PRP has 3-8 folds concentration of platelets and various growth factors such as platelet derived growth factor, transforming growth factor beta and vascular endothelial growth factor which helps in healing of the tissues. In a comparative study between autologous blood injection and PRP for TMJ dislocation demonstrated both groups were equally effective in decreasing mouth opening in TMJ dislocation.

Prolotherapy [1]

It is also called as regenerative injection therapy. This involves injection of solutions into the joint to stimulate regeneration potential. Various prolotherapy solutions are available such as psyllium oil, glycerin, phenol, etc. of which

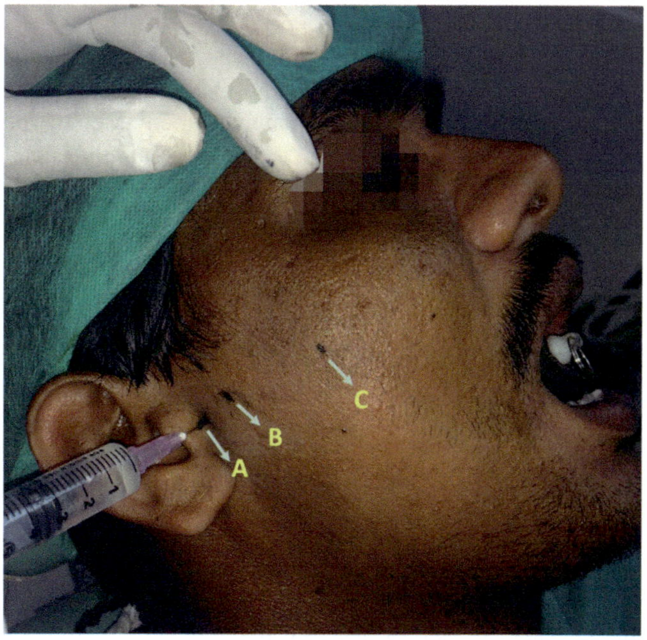

Fig. 64.12 Injection sites for prolotherapy. A: Posterior joint space. B: Anterior attachment of disc to lateral pterygoid muscle. C: Most tender point of masseter muscle

dextrose is the most commonly used solution. 2 ml of 10–50% dextrose can be injected in and around the joint space. Either single or multiple injections are needed based on severity of dislocation. This technique is indicated in laxity of the ligaments and capsule. It induces low-grade inflammation which releases growth factors. These growth factors stimulate fibroblasts which deposit new collagen fibers that strengthen ligaments and tendons.

Landmarks—prolotherapy solutions are given in the following three points (Fig. 64.12):

A. Posterior joint space—palpate the depression posterior to condyle when mouth is opened.
B. Attachment of disc to lateral pterygoid muscle—depression felt anterior to the condyle when mouth is closed.
C. Tender spot in the masseter tendon.

Injection of Botulinum Toxin [1]

The first reported use of botulinum toxin for TMJ dislocation was described by Daelen et al. in the year 1995. Botulinum toxin type A weakens the skeletal muscle when injected by preventing the release of acetylcholine at the neuromuscular junction. It can be injected into any of the masticatory muscle, but injection into lateral pterygoid muscle is effective because forward movement of condyle is prevented. The dosage used is 25–50 units of botulinum toxin. It can be injected either by extraoral or intraoral route with or without EMG guidance (Refer Chap. 33 on Botox injections).

Extraoral Technique

A 30-gauge needle is inserted into the skin 1 cm below the central zygomatic arch to the depth of 3–4 cm based on the measurements obtained from computed tomogram of the patient. The 25–50 units of toxin is deposited into the lateral pterygoid muscle following aspiration.

Intraoral Technique

Hypodermic needle electrode is inserted in the mucobuccal fold of distal root of upper second molar directed superiorly and posteriorly to the depth of 25–30 mm; the position of the needle in the lateral pterygoid muscle is confirmed by EMG reading. After aspiration, 25–50 units of toxin is deposited into the muscle.

The injection should be repeated every 3–6 months as the action of this toxin lasts within 6 months. Complications of this technique included dysphagia, dysarthria, and hemorrhage.

Arthroscopy [1] **(Refer** Chap. 63 **on Internal Derangements of TMJ)**

Arthroscopic capsulorrhaphy is done by using either laser or cautery which produces contractions. Sclerosing solutions may be injected into the joint and capsule under direct visualization using arthroscopy.

Arthroscopic Capsulorrhaphy

A 1.7 mm TMJ arthroscope is introduced into the fossa portal following the double puncture technique described by McCain. Once the arthroscope reached the anterior recess, the second puncture is done using triangulation technique. Deep lesional burns are created in the oblique protuberance, laterally and the posterior wall using either bipolar cautery or holmium laser which causes shortening of the capsule.

Arthroscopic Eminectomy

The arthroscope is introduced into the joint through inferolateral approach, and then the articular eminence is reduced by electronic shaver which is introduced by triangulation technique.

64.6.2.3 Surgical Treatment

The following is a brief description of surgical procedures which are commonly employed for treating TMJ dislocation.

Capsular Tightening Procedure

Temporomandibular joint is completely covered by capsule which is attached superiorly from all around the rim of the glenoid fossa and inferiorly till the neck of the condyle. This capsule holds the joint components in position, which is later-

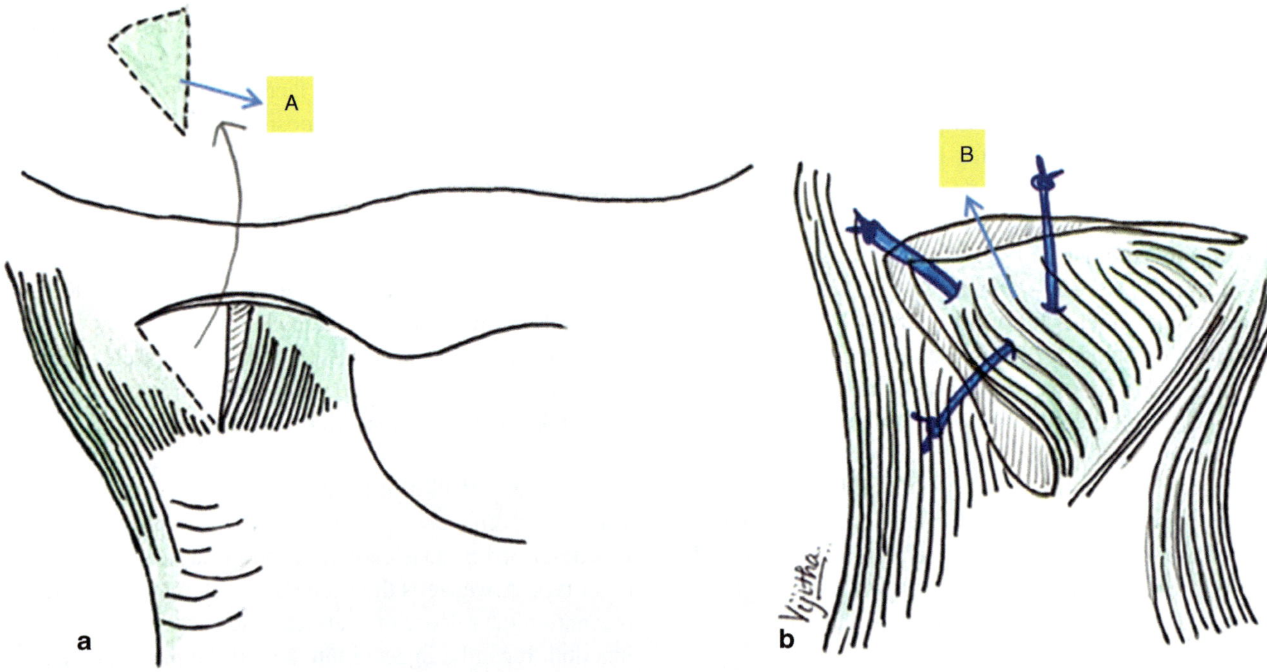

Fig. 64.13 (**a–b**) Capsulorrhaphy. Excised margin of the capsule. (**A**) Capsule is tightened by suturing it to the adjacent soft tissues (**B**)

ally strengthened by lateral ligament. Lax capsule is considered as one of the reasons for TMJ dislocation. So, capsular tightening procedures are done to address this problem.

Capsulorrhaphy (Fig. 64.13a, b)

This procedure was first implemented in the year 1907 by Perthes who excised a portion of the lateral capsule and sutured it together to increase the tautness of the capsule and thus restrain condyle. Later on, many modifications had been proposed including suturing of the capsule to zygomatic arch and overlapping of the capsule after making vertical incision on the capsule [9].

Creation of Mechanical Obstacle

Excessive translation of the condyle which is observed in dislocation is prohibited by creating impediment in the path of the condyle. Konjetzny (1921) had used articular disc as a mechanical impediment by bringing it forward and suturing it anteriorly. Lindemann and Mayer used articular tubercle to prevent condylar dislocation by either bending it down or placing a graft obtained from zygoma [9].

Dautrey's Procedure [10] (Fig. 64.14a, b)

Mayer (1933) created a mechanical obstacle by dislocating a part of the zygomatic arch down, in front of the articular eminence. Vertical osteotomy of the zygomatic arch and repositioning the osteotomized arch downward as a mechanical impediment has been described by LeClerc and Girard in the year 1943.

In 1967 Gosserez and Dautrey made an oblique osteotomy of the arch in front of the articular eminence extending from posterior-superior to the anterior-inferior direction. With gentle pressure towards inferior direction, a greenstick fracture was created at the zygomatico-temporal suture. The segment was then pushed downwards to create obstruction for the condylar movement. If this downfractured segment is unstable, plating can be done to prevent displacement (Fig. 64.15).

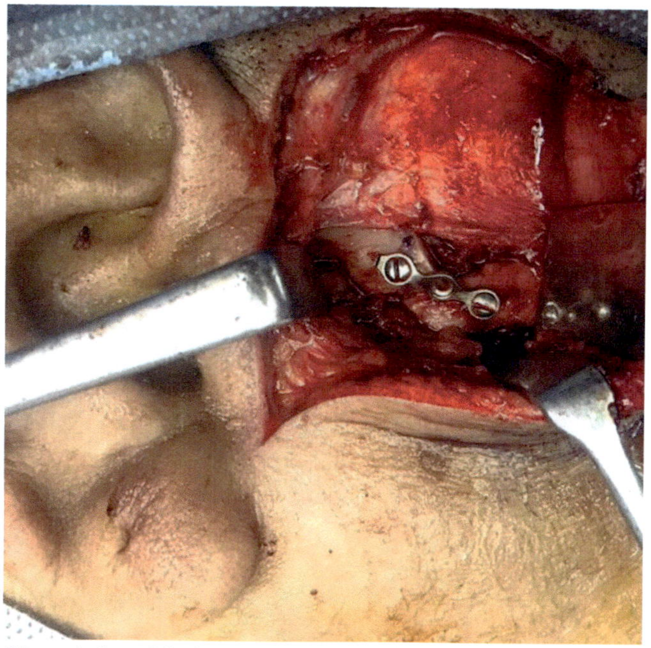

Fig. 64.15 Fixation of downfractured zygomatic arch segment using miniplates

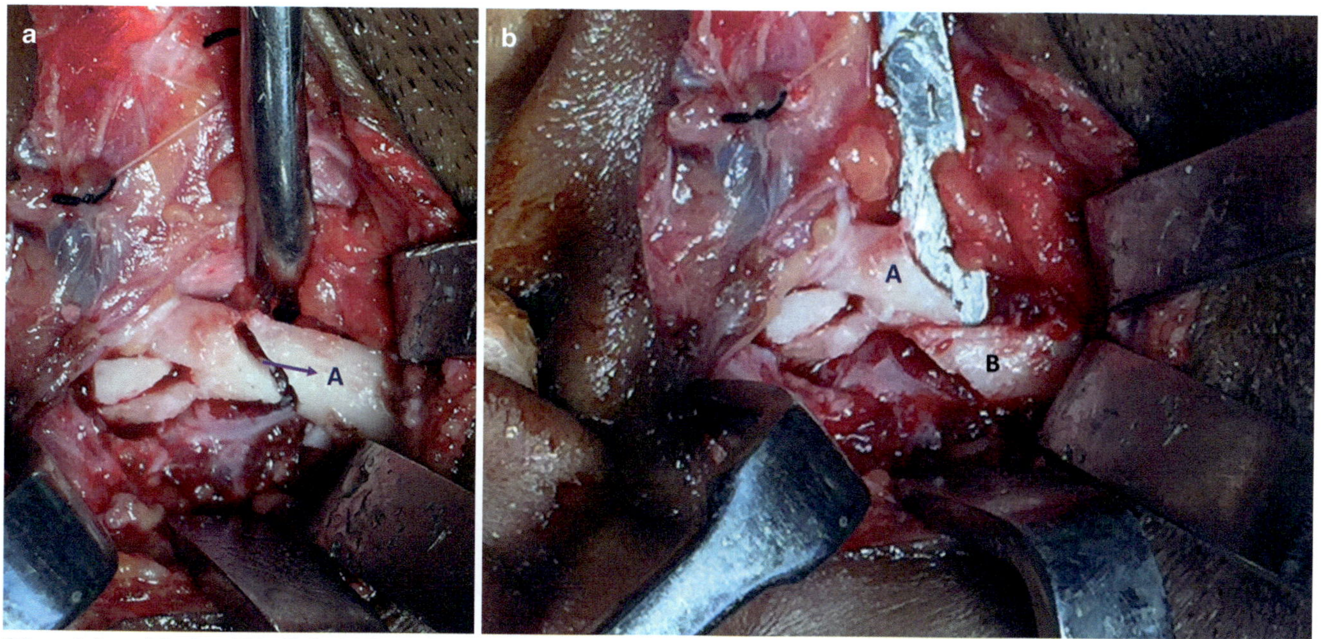

Fig. 64.14 (**a**, **b**) Dautrey's procedure. (**a**) A: Osteotomy of zygomatic arch (**b**) A: Proximal segment of zygomatic arch. B: Downfractured distal segment of zygomatic arch

The limitations of the technique include the following:

1. Not suitable for elderly individual as it may cause fracturing of the arch instead of greenstick fracture at the zygomatico-temporal suture.
2. Relocation of the fragments after repositioning [10].
3. Medial escape of the condyle as the width of the zygomatic arch is narrow.
4. Presence of a small condyle.

Glenotemporal Osteotomy (Fig. 64.16a, b and c)

Norman [10] described glenotemporal osteotomy as a definitive technique for dislocation. TMJ is exposed through any of the open surgical approaches described for TMJ, without violating the capsule. An oblique osteotomy on the articular eminence is made, following which the fragment is gently moved downwards to create a wedge-shaped defect which is grafted using bone taken from ilium, calvarium, symphysis, etc. Usually it is not necessary to fix these grafts as they stay in that wedge-shaped space created by osteotomy. Miniplates or screws can be placed on the eminence so that excessive condylar translation is prevented. Long-term results of this technique showed screw loosening and fracture of the plate.

Modifications of Norman's Procedure

Sharma et al. [11] added two modifications to the conventional glenotemporal osteotomy. Temporalis fascial flap was used to strengthen the capsule, and pterygoid dysjunction was performed to address the TMJ pain due to internal derangement which coexists with dislocation.

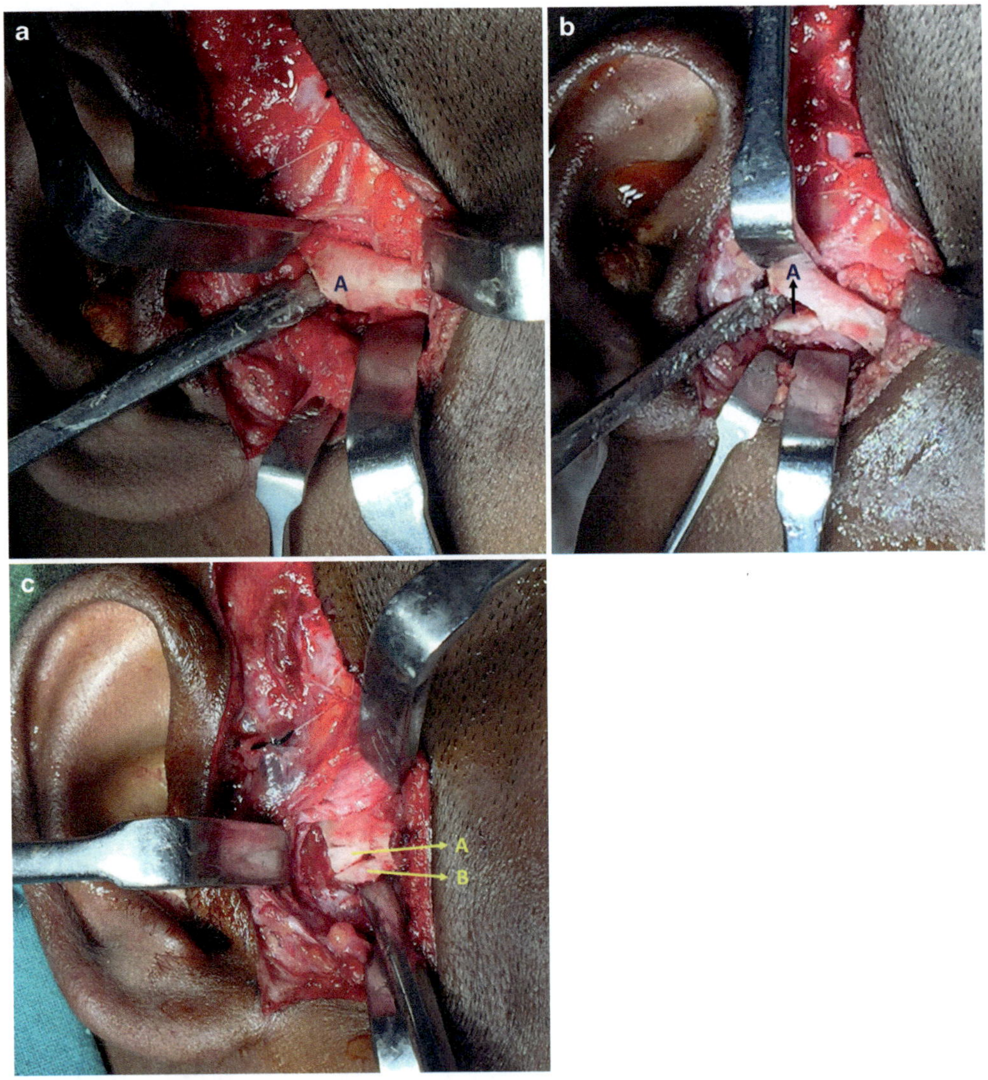

Fig. 64.16 (**a**, **b**, **c**) Glenotemporal osteotomy. (**a**) A: Articular eminence. (**b**) A: Osteotomy of articular eminence. (**c**) A: Chin graft in position. B: Downfractured articular eminence

Removal of Mechanical Obstacle

Eminectomy (Fig. 64.17a, b)
The first reported evidence of eminectomy for the treatment of TMJ dislocation was performed by Hilmar Myrhaug in the year 1951. This procedure is generally accomplished under general anesthesia or local anesthesia, or conscious sedation has also been used for patients with systemic conditions that prohibit general anesthesia. Though there are many techniques available to address this condition, this particular technique may be considered for those patients with neurological disorder, epilepsy, and advanced age [12].

Hall et al. [13] had studied the eminence configuration using 38 cadavers. The observations included the following:

1. Anteroposterior width of eminence—9–18 mm
2. Latero-medial width of eminence—16–25 mm
3. Articular tubercle to temporal bone measurement—5–14 mm
4. Deepest portion of the glenoid fossa thickness—0.1–8 mm

Articular eminence thicknesses in anterior and posterior regions were also mentioned [6]. These measurements provide guidelines while performing eminectomy procedure to avoid complications.

According to this technique, the joint may be approached through any of the incisions indicated for TMJ surgeries. Following exposure of the eminence, rotary instruments, osteotome, chisel, or piezo surgery device can be used to reduce the height of the eminence. Either total eminectomy or partial eminectomy may be done. Irregular bony surfaces and edges should be smoothened well. Segami et al. [14] described arthroscopic eminectomy where double puncture technique has been used. Motorized shaver was used to reduce the eminence.

Navigation system has also been used for accurate reduction of eminence especially on the medial side and superior surface to avoid intracranial exposure [6].

Eminectomy works by allowing free movement of the condyle over the eminence so that locking of the condyle is prevented. There are observations of reduced mouth opening following eminectomy that might be due to adhesions formed in and around the joint. This can be performed unilaterally or bilaterally [6].

The major problem associated with this technique is the excessive forward movement of the condyle than what is actually needed which leads to stretching of muscles and ligaments which is potentially injurious to the articular structures [11].

Condylotomy and Condylectomy (Fig. 64.18a, b)
Closed condylotomy is a blind procedure in which Gigli saw is used to cut the condyle as described by Kostecka [2].

Part of the condyle is removed to prevent the obstruction; at the same time, it allows the free translation of the condyle along the articular eminence.

Preauricular incision is used to approach the condyle, and then the condyle is sectioned at the inferior level of the articular eminence.

Creating New Muscular Balance

- *Temporalis Scarification* [1]
  A portion of the temporalis muscle is removed by this technique so that the scarring and fibrosis induced by surgery restrict the mouth opening.
- *Lateral Pterygoid Myotomy* [1] (Fig. 64.19a, b)

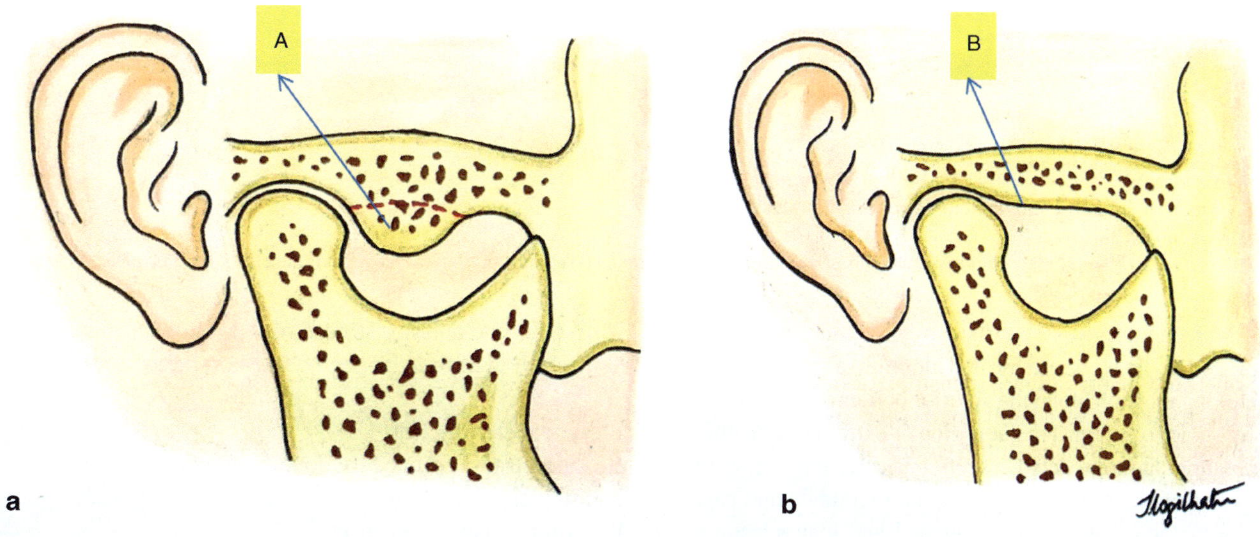

Fig. 64.17 (**a–b**) Eminectomy. (**A**) Articular eminence (**B**) Eminence removed

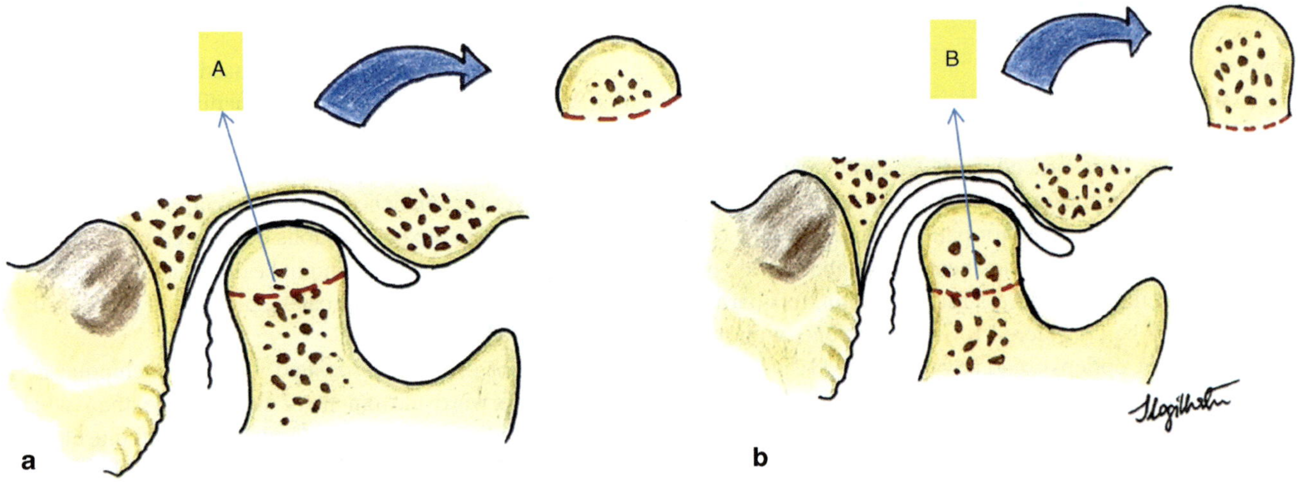

Fig. 64.18 (**a**–**b**) Condylectomy. (**A**) High condylectomy (**B**) Low condylectomy

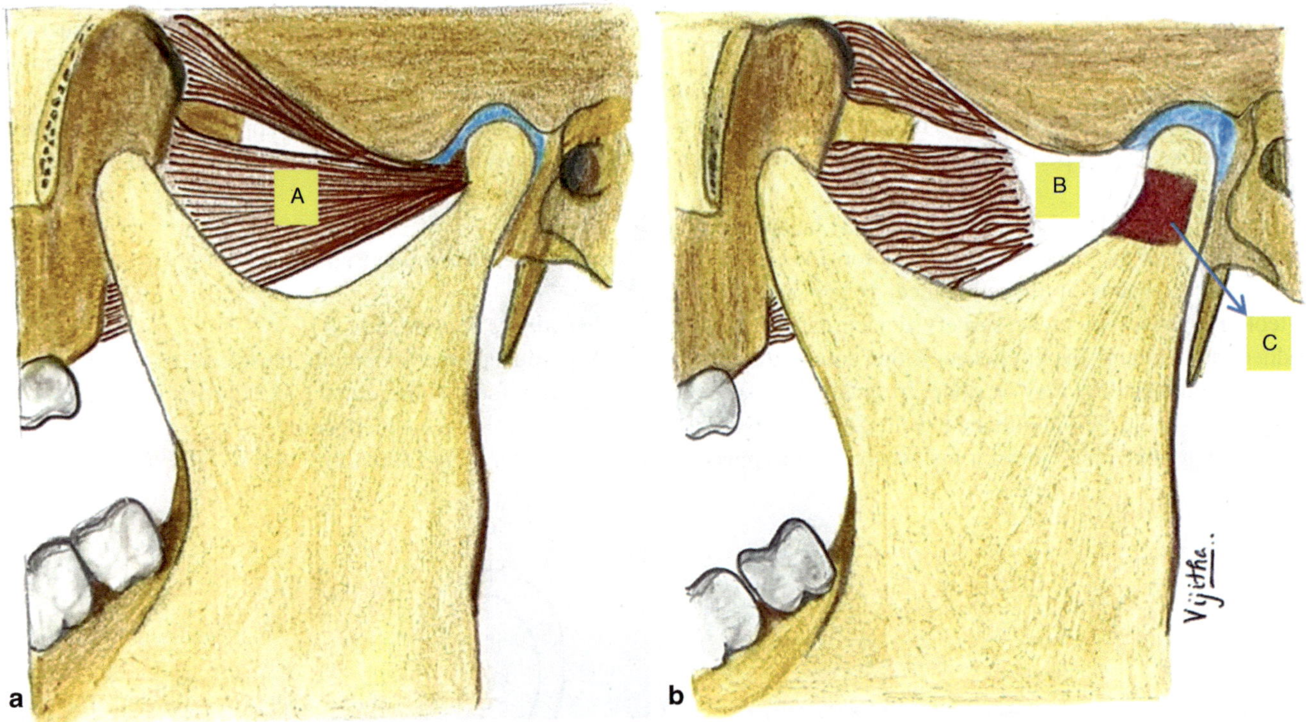

Fig. 64.19 (**a**–**b**) Lateral pterygoid myotomy. (**A**) Lateral pterygoid muscle (**B**) Part of the lateral pterygoid muscle excised (**C**) Barrier is placed

This technique was described by Bowman in 1949. This procedure may be performed through either intraoral by making incision along the anterior border of the ramus from coronoid to the third molar region or extraoral route through preauricular approach. Dissection is carried out to visualize the attachment of lateral pterygoid to condyle and capsule, and the attachment is then severed and then silastic sheet fixed to the anterior surface of the condyle. This results in restriction of mouth opening for short period of time.

Pterygoid Dysjunction

It is an intraoral procedure done to reduce the activity of the lateral pterygoid on the condyle so that forward movement of the condyle is reduced [11].

Intraoral vestibular incision is made in relation to the upper molars, and dissection is done to expose the posterolateral wall of the maxilla and pterygomaxillary suture. Pterygoid chisel is used to separate the pterygoid plates from maxilla, so that lateral pterygoid muscle along with pterygoid plate is detached.

64.6.3 Chronic Protracted Dislocation (Box 64.7)

Box 64.7 Management of Long Standing Dislocation

Conservative

1. Manual reduction
2. Continuous elastic traction using bite block
3. Indirect reduction
   (a) Using a wire passing in the mandibular angle region
   (b) Using a hook in the sigmoid notch

Surgical procedures

1. Joint procedures
   (a) Condylotomy, condylectomy
   (b) Myotomy
   (c) Joint prostheses
2. Procedures not involving the joint
   (a) Sagittal split osteotomy
   (b) Vertical ramus osteotomy
   (c) Inverted L osteotomy
   (d) Midline mandibulotomy

Initially conservative method is employed to reduce dislocation. Manual reduction is attempted either using local anesthesia, sedation, or general anesthesia. Continuous elastic traction may also be applied with the bite block in the posterior region which might reduce the dislocation [15].

Indirect reduction can be performed by inserting wire into the mandibular angle region, or bone hook is passed into the sigmoid notch through a small incision made on the angle region (Rowe and Killey 1968) [4]. Lewis in 1981 used Bristow's elevator for the reduction by giving downward and posterior force.

In long-standing persistent dislocation, patient might have functional movement due to pseudo joint formation in front of the articular eminence. In this scenario, the goal is to establish the occlusion by osteotomy procedures such as sagittal split osteotomy or vertical ramus osteotomy.

Adekeye (1976) [4] suggested inverted L osteotomy instead of vertical and horizontal osteotomies due to the coronoid hindrance. Lateral and medial surface of the ramus is exposed either through submandibular incision or intraoral incision extending from the coronoid process along the anterior border of the ramus to the vestibule of second molar region. Medial osteotomy (horizontal cut) is performed 4–5 mm above and posterior to the lingula and parallel to the occlusal plane. Vertical cut is performed from the distal aspect of the horizontal cut to the mandibular angle. Then the dentate segment is manipulated to get the desired occlusion. Proximal and distal segments are fixed with miniplates.

Other methods such as condylectomy, condylotomy, and myotomy (as described in previous sections) and TMJ prostheses are proposed to treat this condition [4].

Ratten et al. described midline mandibulotomy to reduce the dislocation [16].

Through the intraoral approach, the mandible is sectioned in the midline, and then each hemimandible is manipulated to reduce the dislocation on each side separately. Following reduction, mandibular midline is fixed with miniplates.

64.7 Recent Advances

64.7.1 Raja's Coronoid Repositioning Technique [17]

This is a new technique performed for the management of TMJ dislocation. Intraoral vertical incision extending from the coronoid process to the molar region is made, and the coronoid and anterior border of ramus is exposed, and then coronoid is osteotomized and inferiorly pulled along with temporalis muscle and fixed with miniplates on the lateral surface of the ramus. The advantage of this technique is that the temporalis is stretched to give new muscle balance and restricts the excessive opening of the mouth.

64.7.2 Wolford's Anchoring Technique [18] (Fig. 63.15)

This technique prevents the dislocation by using two Mitek screw with attached suture material. One screw is attached to the zygomatic arch and another to the posterolateral surface of the condyle, and the sutures are tied together to get the desired mouth opening. These suture materials act as artificial ligaments that control condylar movement.

Acknowledgment I would like to acknowledge Dr. Vijitha and Dr. Logitha for illustrations.

Disclosure Authors have no financial conflicts to disclose.

64.8 Case Scenarios

Case 1 (Fig. 64.20a–d)

Patient A 24-year-old male, with complaints of locking of the jaw after wide mouth opening

Preoperative open mouth OPG revealed bilateral TMJ dislocation (Fig. 64.20a)

OPG demonstrates:

- Displacement of condyle out of the glenoid fossa bilaterally
- Condylar head is antero-superior to articular eminence on both sides

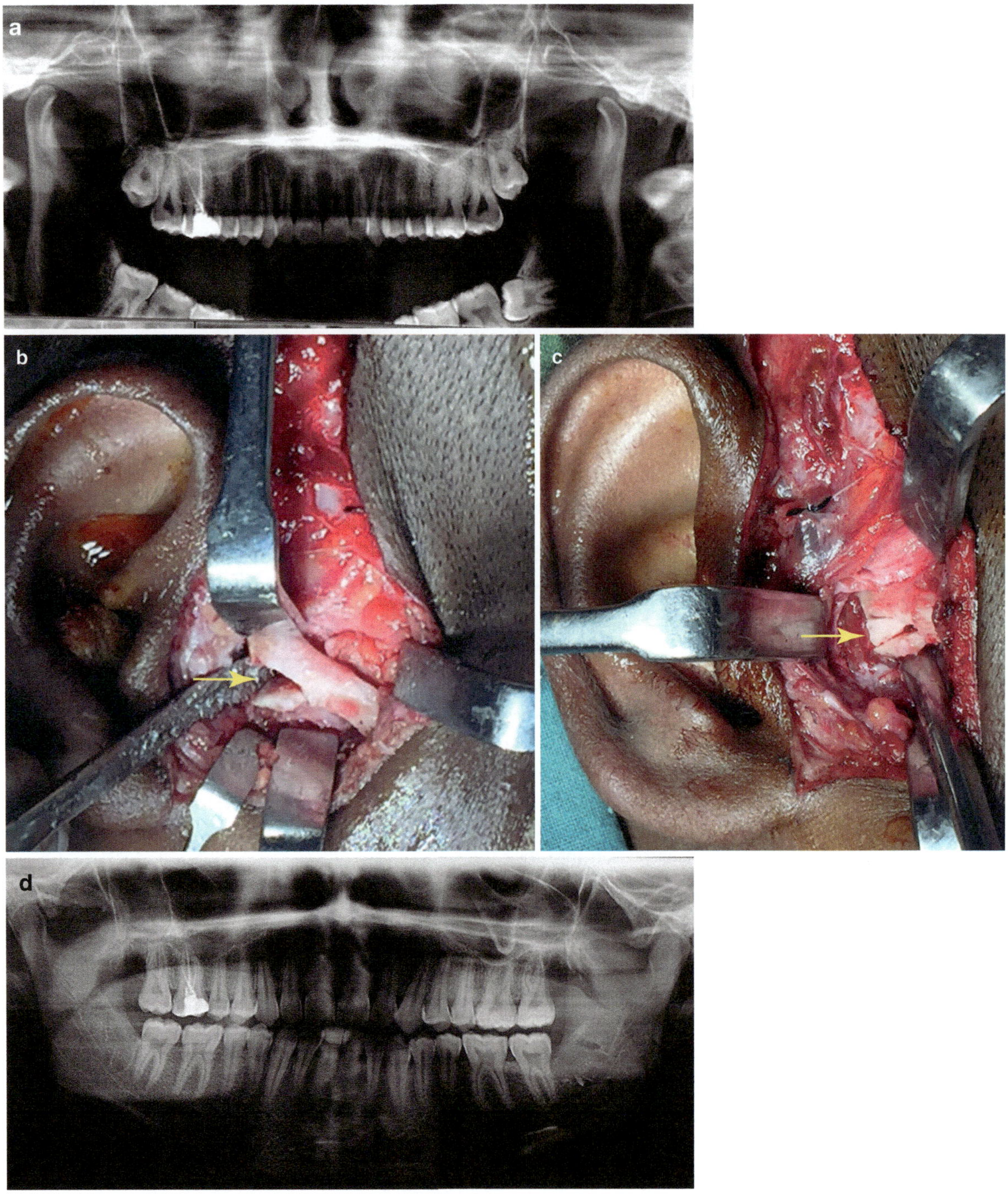

Fig. 64.20 Case scenario 1 (**a**) Pre op "open mouth "OPG showing bilateral dislocation of TMJ. (**b**) Osteotomy of articular eminence (yellow arrow). (**c**) Chin graft sandwiched between segments (yellow arrow). (**d**) Post op OPG showing increase in the height of articular eminence on right side

Surgical plan Augmentation of articular eminence by glenotemporal osteotomy on the right side. The right side was chosen for intervention as the symptoms were pronounced on that side

Surgical procedure

- Right TMJ was approached through preauricular incision with temporal extension
- Osteotomy of articular eminence (Fig. 64.20b)
- Wedging the chin graft between the osteotomy cut of articular eminence (Fig. 64.20c)

Postoperative OPG
OPG demonstrating increase in the height of articular eminence on the right side of TMJ (Fig. 64.20d)

Case 2 (Fig. 64.21a–d)

Patient A 54-year-old female, with pain in front of the ear and difficulty in closing the mouth following yawning

Preoperative open mouth OPG demonstrated bilateral TMJ dislocation (Fig. 64.21a)

OPG demonstrates:

- Displacement of condyle out of the glenoid fossa on both sides
- Condylar head is antero-superior to articular eminence

Surgical plan Inferior repositioning of the coronoid on the right side. The right side was chosen for surgery as the patient complained of more pain on that side

Surgical procedure

- Right coronoid was exposed through vestibular incision extending from lower second molar to anterior border of the ramus.
- Osteotomy cut was made from sigmoid notch to anterior border of the ramus (Fig. 64.21b).
- Trough was created on the lateral surface of the ramus just below the osteotomy cut.
- Coronoid was pulled down over the trough and fixed with miniplate (Fig. 64.21c).

Postoperative OPG (Fig. 64.21d)
Open mouth OPG demonstrating the condyle within the glenoid fossa on both the sides and coronoid fixed inferiorly on the right side

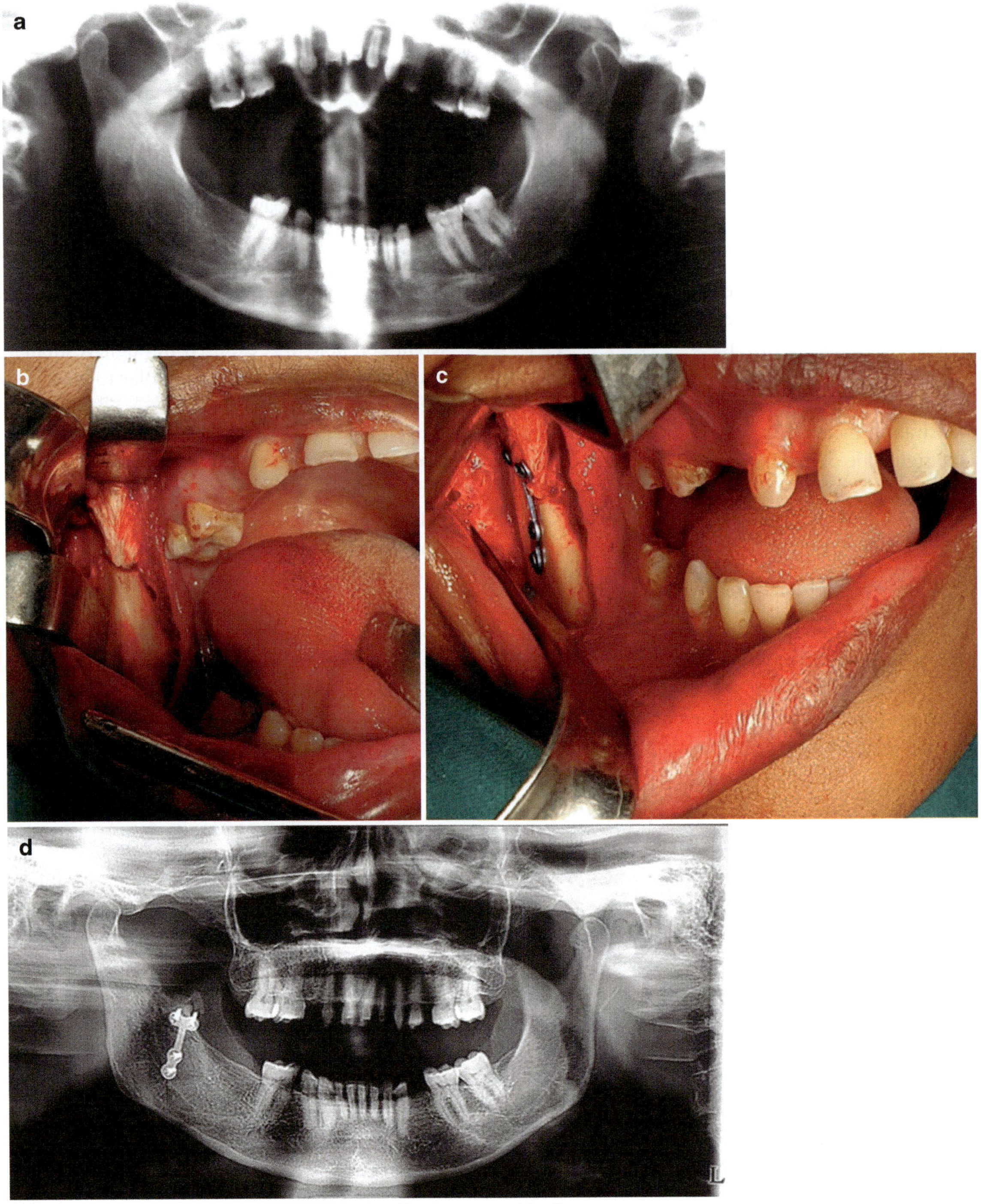

Fig. 64.21 Case scenario 2 (**a**) Pre- op "open mouth" OPG showing bilateral dislocation of TMJ. (**b**) Osteotomy of coronoid. (**c**) Inferiorly positioned coronoid fixed with 2 mm miniplate. (**d**) Post -op "open mouth" OPG showing normal positioning of condyle in relation to articular eminence

References

1. Liddell A, Perez DE. Temporomandibuar joint dislocation. Oral Maxillofac Surg Clin North Am. 2015;27(1):125–36.
2. Shakya S, Ongole R, Sumanth KN, Denny CE. Chronic bilateral dislocation of Temporomandibular joint. Kathmandu Univ Med J (KUMJ). 2010;8(30):251–6.
3. Awang MN. A new approach to the reduction of acute dislocation of the Temporomandibular Joint: a report of three cases. Br J Oral Maxillofac Surg. 1987;25:244–9.
4. Marqués-Mateo M, Puche-Torres M, Iglesias-Gimilio ME. Temporomandibular chronic dislocation: the long-standing condition. Med Oral Patol Oral Cir Bucal. 2016;21:e776–83.
5. Prechel U, Ottl P, Ahlers OM, Neff A. Clinical practice guideline: The treatment of temporomandibular joint dislocation—a systematic review. Dtsch Arztebl Int. 2018;115:59–64.
6. Undt G. Temporomandibular joint eminectomy for recurrent dislocation. Atlas Oral Maxillofac Surg Clin North Am. 2011;19(2):189–206.
7. Lowery LE, Beeson MS, Lum KK. The wrist pivot method, a novel technique for temporo-mandibular joint reduction. J Emerg Med. 2004;27:167–70.
8. Chen YC, Chen CT, Lin CH, Chen YR. A safe and effective way for reduction of temporo-mandibular joint dislocation. Ann Plast Surg. 2007;58:105–8.
9. Miller GA, Murphy EJ. External pterygoid myotomy for recurrent mandibular dislocation: review of the literature and report of a case. Oral Surg. 1976;42:705.
10. Norman J, Ede B, Bramley P. A textbook and colour atlas of the temporomandibular joint. London: Wolfe Medical; 1990. p. 136–50.
11. Sharma R. Modifications to Norman's procedure for hypermobility of the TMJ. Med J Armed Forces India. 2012;68(3):231–5.
12. Iwanaga J, Nakamura Y, Kusukawa J, Tubbs RS. Eminectomy for habitual luxation of the temporomandibular joint with sedation and local anesthesia: a case series. Case Rep Dent. 2016;2016:2505864.
13. Hall MB, Randall WB, Sclar AG. Anatomy of the TMJ articular eminence before and after surgical reduction. J Craniomandibular Pract. 1984;2:135–40.
14. Segami N, Kaneyama K, Tsurusako S, et al. Arthroscopic eminoplasty for habitual dislocation of the temporomandibular joint: preliminary study. J Craniomaxillofac Surg. 1999;27(6):390–7.
15. Pradhan L, Jaisani MR, Sagtani A, Win A. Conservative management of chronic TMJ dislocation: an old technique revived. J Maxillofac Oral Surg. 2015;14(Suppl 1):S267–70.
16. Lee SH, Son SI, Park JH, Park IS, Nam JH. Reduction of prolonged bilateral temporomandibular joint dislocation by midline mandibulotomy. Int J Oral Maxillofac Surg. 2006;35:1054–6.
17. Krishnakumar Raja VB, Balasubramanian S, Sridharan G, Tarun S, Panneerselvam E. Inferior Repositioning of Coronoid Process for the Treatment of Temporomandibular Joint Subluxation/Dislocation. Ann Maxillofac Surg. 2019;9(2):397–399. doi:10.4103/ams.ams_137_19
18. Wolford LM, Pitta MC, Mehra P. Mitek anchors for treatment of chronic mandibular dislocation. Oral Surg Oral Med Oral Pathol Oral Radiol Endod. 2001;92(5):495–8.

Suggested Reading

Yasso MM, Fahmy MH, Mohamad NS. Comparative study between Autologous Blood and Platelet Rich Plasma in Treatment of Recurrent Temporomandibular Joint Dislocation. Alex Dent J. 2018;43:101–107.

Temporomandibular Joint Ankylosis

65

Sonal Anchlia

65.1 Introduction and Etiopathogenesis

Temporomandibular joint (TMJ) ankylosis is defined as bony or fibrous adhesion of the anatomic joint components accompanied by limitation of mouth opening, causing difficulty in mastication, speech, and oral hygiene. This may also influence symmetry of the facial skeleton, especially in cases which occur when patient is still in the growth phase [1].

According to Kaban [2], trauma is the most common cause (31–98%), followed by local or systemic infection (10–49%), and lastly any systemic disease (10%). Infection occurring in the joint commonly occurs due to spread from otitis media or mastoiditis or from the hematogenous route—tuberculosis, gonorrhea, scarlet fever, etc. Systemic etiology may include ankylosing spondylitis, rheumatoid arthritis, or psoriasis.

Classically, hemarthrosis following trauma is the pathogenic factor for bone formation in TMJ ankylosis [3]. Condylar trauma may lead to hemarthrosis due to injury to the periosteum and capsular ligament. When this intracapsular hematoma organizes, hypertrophic bone is formed from the disrupted periosteum or metaplasia of non-osteogenic connective tissue. This may lead to hypomobility, and bony ankylosis may eventually develop.

Yan et al. in 2014 [4] put forth the hypotheses of hypertrophic nonunion. He described the sagittal fracture of condyle along with displacement of the disc. Herein, trauma also occurs in the glenoid fossa, thereby establishing the microenvironment in the articular surfaces for bone healing.

When the condylar trauma is recent, mouth opening will exert a dual effect on new bone formation. This is explained in Fig. 65.1. Restricted jaw movement is not a determinant but rather a promoting agent for ankylosis. Injuries to both the articular disc and the articular surfaces are prerequisites to TMJ ankylosis.

65.2 Clinical Features (Fig. 65.2)

In ankylosis, TMJ movements may be partially or completely restricted in opening, protrusion, and lateral excursions. Palpation of joint movements is better in fibrous than bony ankylosis. In children even in bony ankylosis, joint movements can be palpated because of stretching in the cranial sutures.

Ankylosis results in issues with mastication, digestion, speech, and oral hygiene. This may lead to caries, periodontitis, encumbered eruption of mandibular molars, crowding of teeth, and anterior open bite. Mandibular incisors often show supra-eruption and labial tipping as nature's compensation since the mandible is placed much posterior to the maxilla, thereby reducing lip competence. In severe cases, the lower lip may be trapped under the maxillary incisors.

As the vertical growth of the ramus is restricted, the lower face is significantly shortened. The digastric and mylohyoid muscles produce marked antegonial notching at the inferior part of the mandible just anterior to the insertion of the masseter and medial pterygoid. Failure of condylar growth impedes the forward and downward movement of mandible resulting in localized thickening of the bone at the angle due to subperiosteal apposition which accentuates the antegonion. The mandibular warping is caused due to this, as well as the obtuse angle between the inferior border of the mandible and the base of the skull [5]. The long-standing contractions of the masticatory muscles also give rise to elongation and thickening of the coronoid process, ramal shortening, and chin recession.

Electronic Supplementary Material The online version of this chapter (https://doi.org/10.1007/978-981-15-1346-6_65) contains supplementary material, which is available to authorized users.

S. Anchlia (✉)
Department of Oral and Maxillofacial Surgery, Government Dental College and Hospital, Ahmedabad, Gujarat, India

K. Bonanthaya et al. (eds.), *Oral and Maxillofacial Surgery for the Clinician*, https://doi.org/10.1007/978-981-15-1346-6_65

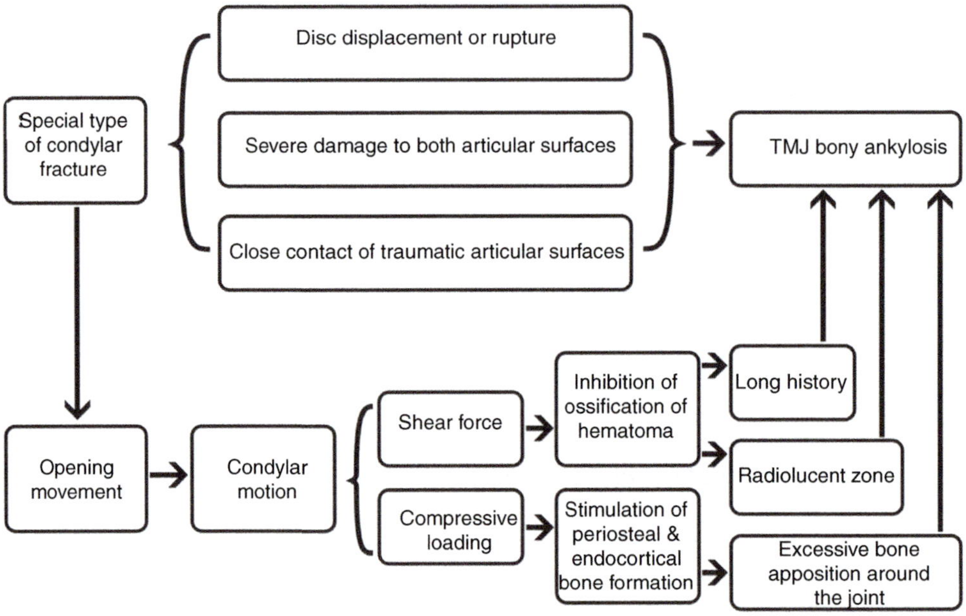

Fig. 65.1 Dual effect of mouth opening on new bone formation in recent condylar trauma

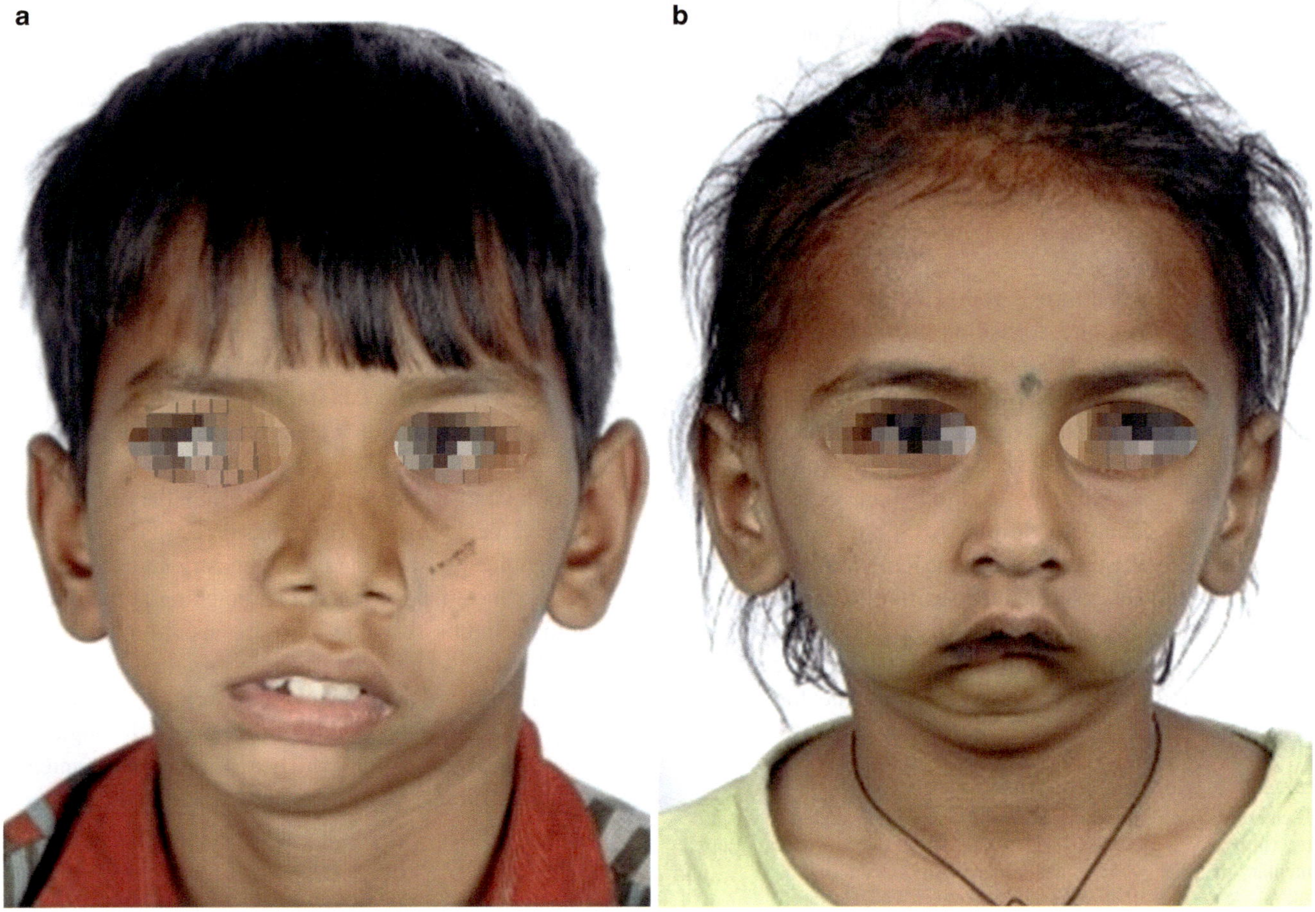

Fig. 65.2 (**a**) Unilateral ankylosis of the right side, (**b**) bilateral ankylosis

In unilateral cases, the chin deviates to the affected side due to restricted mandibular growth on the affected side and normal growth on the unaffected side. In growing patients, this may also restrict ipsilateral growth of the maxilla, although there is normal growth on the unaffected side. In some cases, the growth of the maxilla on the affected side may be normal but that on the unaffected side may be excess, due to uninhibited growth of the normal side. Both these phenomena result in a maxillary cant, though on opposite sides.

In bilateral cases, the mandible is visibly retruded, lacks a chin and the patient presents with an obtuse cervicomental angle. The posterior maxillary height is shortened, giving rise to steep occlusal planes. This convex facial profile or the bird face deformity is also described as the "Andy Gump deformity." Andy Gump was a cartoon character with a very insignificant chin, who first appeared in the Chicago Tribune in 1917, created by cartoonist Sidney Smith [6].

Worsened aesthetics of their appearance often becomes a reason for depressive disorders, psychological problems such as stubbornness, low self-esteem, and an inferiority complex.

The longer the duration of hypomobility, the more severe is the muscle atrophy and facial asymmetry. The prognosis for a favorable outcome with treatment is inversely related to the number of years of ankylosis.

65.2.1 Importance of Obstructive Sleep Apnea-Hypopnea Syndrome (OSAHS)

The presence of retruded mandible and micrognathia in patients with TMJ ankylosis creates narrowing of the pharyngeal airway space (PAS) with mechanical obstruction to respiration, more so in the supine position and during sleep. This process forms a complex syndrome of apneic episodes with significant reduction in the mean oxygen saturation levels and secondary cardiac and respiratory problems, known as OSAHS [7]. Therefore, for patients in whom the release of TMJ ankylosis is carried out without the advancement of the mandible for the correction of OSA, there is worsening of an already compromised airway. In such cases wide mouth opening during postoperative jaw exercises can lead to upper airway collapse—a sense of choking, bradycardia, and restlessness or apnea-like episodes, hence increasing chances of ankylosis [8].

65.2.2 Radiographic Features of Bony Ankylosis (Fig. 65.3)

According to Yan et al. [4], the deformed TMJ is characterized by an enlarged condyle, thickened temporal bone, excessive bone formation, and a radiolucent zone in the bony fusion area. No scattered calcified dots are found in the radiolucent zone, showing that ossification occurs only in the existing bones.

Bony fusion is located in the lateral part of the joint with decreased/absent bone marrow cavity and osteosclerosis. The medial non-bony fusion area shows the atrophic condylar head and rudimentary joint space. Here, the morphology of the bone marrow cavity and bone mineral density is similar to that of normal bone.

Wu et al. [9] demonstrated that in fibrous ankylosis, there is fibrous tissue intruding into the bone marrow of the condyle as well as degeneration of the condylar cartilage. In bony ankylosis, there occurs new bone formation on the rough ankylotic surface of the condyle and slight bone degeneration.

65.3 Classifications

Ankylosis has been classified by various authors according to its extent, site, development, heterotrophic bone formation, symptoms, and most recently, the extent of ankylosis guiding the treatment plan (Table 65.1).

65.4 Preoperative Assessment

65.4.1 Investigations

1. Detailed history, complete clinical examination, professional photographs, for documenting the:
   (a) Age of onset of ankylosis
   (b) Type, duration, and extent of ankylosis
   (c) Type of joint injury or infection
   (d) Maximal interincisal opening
   (e) Dental characteristics and occlusion
   (f) Type of facial deformity
   (g) Previous surgery
2. Routine hemogram and pre-op major investigations
3. Radiological examinations for evaluation of extent of ankylotic mass, discrepancy of jaws, and treatment planning (Fig. 65.4)
   (a) Orthopantomogram:
      (i) Decreased joint space
      (ii) Absence/presence of normal condylar and coronoid anatomy
      (iii) Prominent antegonial notch
      (iv) Markings for osteotomy cuts (for distraction)
   (b) PA cephalogram:
      (i) Chin deviation—Cg-ANS-Me (Crista Galli - Anterior Nasal Spine - Menton)
      (ii) Occlusal cant
      (iii) Grummon's analysis

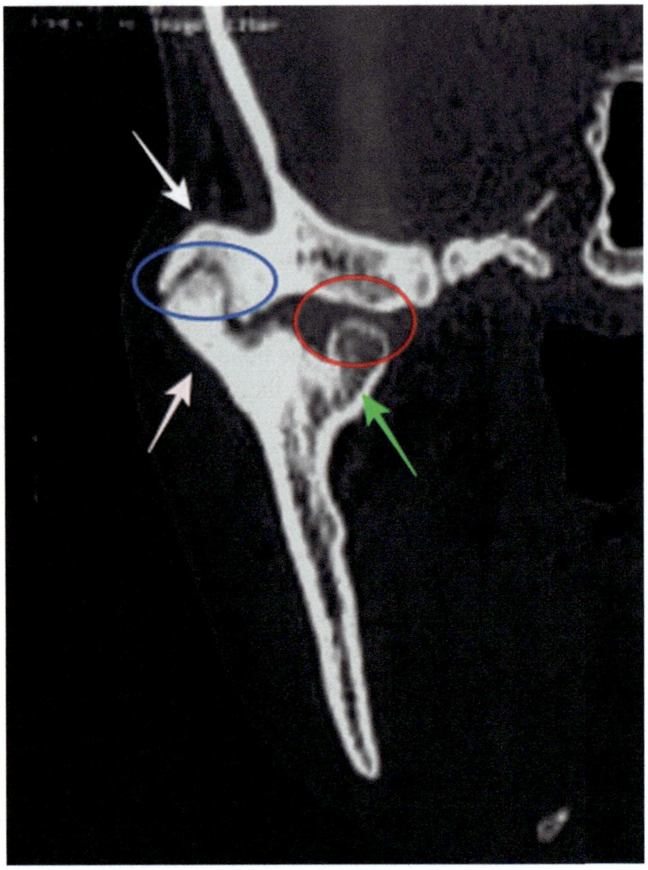

Fig. 65.3 The computerized tomographic features of TMJ bony ankylosis. The blue circle refers to the bony fusion area located in the lateral part of the joint; in this area, a radiolucent zone can be observed. The red circle refers to the atrophic condylar head and rudimentary joint space located in the medial part of the joint. The green arrow indicates that bone mineral density and morphology of the bone marrow cavity in the non-bony fusion area were normal. The white arrows indicate excessive bone formation around the joint

   (c) Lateral cephalogram:
      (i) Ramal length: Ar-Go (Articulare-Gonion)
      (ii) Corpus length: Go-Pog (Gonion-Pogonion)
      (iii) Pharyngeal airway space (PAS)
      (iv) N perpendicular to Pog (Nasion perpendicular to Pogonion)
   (d) Facial CT scan:
      (i) Three-dimensional anatomy of bony morphology
      (ii) Any anatomical measurements as and when required, e.g., size of ankylotic mass, location of ligula, airway space volume, etc.
   (e) CT Angiography may be required to assess the relationship of internal maxillary artery to the ankylotic mass. There are chances of the vessel being inside the bone, especially in re-ankylosis cases.
4. Assessment of OSA may be done using Epworth sleepiness scale, Pittsburgh sleep quality index, and polysomnography (PSG) for:
   (a) Apneic-hypopneic index (AHI)
   (b) Nocturnal desaturation episodes
   (c) Average respiratory disturbance index
   (d) Average lowest arterial oxygen saturation
5. 3D stereolithographic models printed, with the help of CT scan, may be used in treatment planning. Patient-specific surgical guides aid planning, precise control during operation, and thus more foreseeable treatment results.

65.4.2 Airway Implications of TMJ Ankylosis

65.4.2.1 Assessment

McNamara's airway analysis on lateral cephalogram helps to assess the PAS, CT provides volumetric assessment of the same, whereas PSG helps to assess the AHI. Moderate to severe AHI may require delayed extubation/tracheostomy.

65.4.2.2 Types of Intubation According to Clinical Situations

Blind nasal intubation was done historically, but it was traumatic, unpredictable, and unsafe. Tracheostomy is a traumatic experience, but nowadays, awake intubation is performed using midazolam and fentanyl [10]. Fiberoptic-assisted nasotracheal intubation has become the gold standard for such patients.

However, emergency tracheostomy during/after extubation may be required if:

(a) Bilateral ankylosis release is performed, but RCU reconstruction for ramal height rehabilitation has not been done.
(b) OSA is severe and release precedes mandibular advancement.

In these two situations, the mandible may fall back as there is no posterosuperior stop for the ramus and may impinge on the airway, causing further increase in OSA.

65.5 Surgical Anatomy [11]

65.5.1 Nerve Anatomy (Figs. 46.6 and 65.5)

65.5.1.1 Facial Nerve

The main trunk of the facial nerve exits from the skull at the stylomastoid foramen. Approximately 1.3 cm of the facial nerve is visible until it divides into temporofacial and cervicofacial branches.

According to Al-Kayat and Bramley (1979) [12], the distance from the lowest point of the bony external auditory canal (EAC) to this bifurcation measures 1.5–2.8 cm (mean 2.3 cm). The postglenoid tubercle to the bifurcation measures 2.4–3.5 cm (mean 3.0 cm). However, the point at which the upper trunk crosses the zygomatic arch is the most vari-

Table 65.1 Classifications

I. Topazian (1964)

- Stage 1: Ankylotic bone limited to the condylar process
- Stage 2: Ankylotic bone extending to the sigmoid notch
- Stage 3: Ankylotic bone extending to the coronoid process

II. Sawhney's classification (1986)

- Type 1: Minimal bony fusion but extensive fibrous adhesions around the joint
- Type 2: Bony fusion at the outer edge of the articular surface but no fusion on medial area of the joint
- Type 3: Bridge of bone between the mandible and temporal bone
- Type 4: Joint is replaced by a mass of bone

III. Turlington and Durr (1993)

According to heterotopic bone formation within the ankylotic mass

- Grade 0: No bone islands visible
- Grade 1: Islands of bone visible within the soft tissue around the joint
- Grade 2: Periarticular bone formation
- Grade 3: Apparent bony ankylosis

Grades 1, 2, and 3 are further classified as symptomatic (S) and asymptomatic (A)

IV. Recent advances: Dongmei He and Colleagues (2011)

Type of Ankylosis	Suggested Treatment Plan
• **Type A1**: Fibrous ankylosis without bony fusion of joint	• Ankylosis release temporalis muscle flap, costochondral graft
• **Type A2**: Bony fusion on lateral side of joint, residual condyle bigger than half of condylar head on medial side 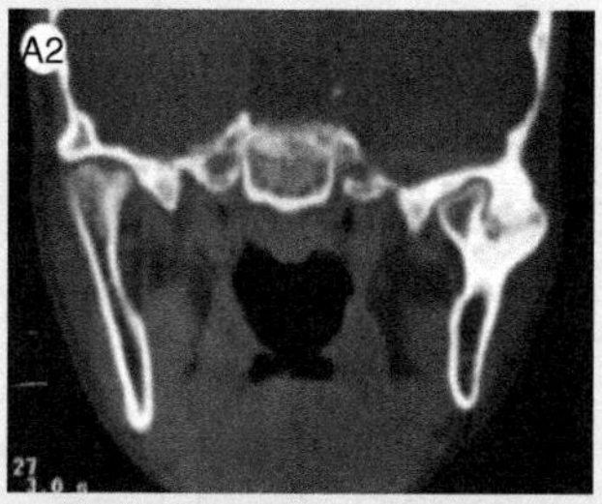	• Lateral arthroplasty
• **Type A3**: Similar to A2 but residual condylar fragment is smaller than half 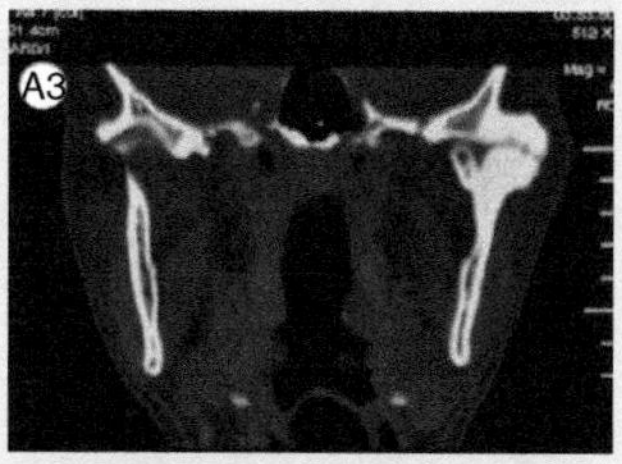	• Resection of ankylotic mass, costochondral graft
• **Type A4**: Ankylosis with complete bony fusion of joint 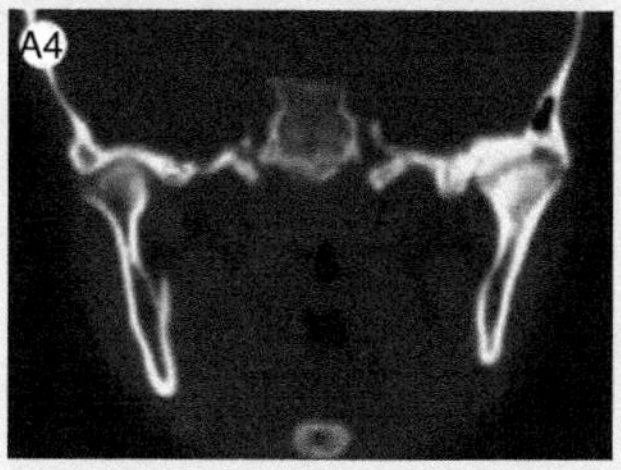	• Resection of ankylotic mass, costochondral graft

V. Recent advances: Yan and colleagues (2014)

Based on its development, ankylosis can be classified into three phases:

- Fibrous-chondral phase demonstrating fibrous tissue and chondrocytes occupied the joint gap
- Chondral-calcified cartilage phase manifesting abundant chondrocytes, cartilage matrix, and neo-formative endochondral ossification in the joint space
- Bone-cartilage phase showing compacted bone bridge in the lateral joint gap and cartilage in the medial joint gap

able in terms of distance. It may be anywhere from 8 to 35 mm anterior to the most anterior portion of the bony EAC (mean 2.0 cm). If the superficial layer of the temporalis fascia and the periosteum over the arch is incised within 8 mm, one can prevent injury to the upper trunk branches.

However, Miloro et al. [13] showed that the average distance anterior to bony EAC was 2.12 cm. (1.68–2.49 cm). His was an MRI-based study as compared to cadaveric dissection-based work of Al-Kayat and Bramley.

The temporal branch of the facial nerve emerges from the parotid gland and crosses the zygoma under the temporoparietal fascia to innervate the frontalis muscle in the forehead. Postsurgical palsy manifests as an inability to raise the eyebrow and ptosis of the brow. Damage to the zygomatic branch results in paralysis to the orbicularis oculi. Nerve damage may necessitate either tarsorrhaphy or gold weight implants into the upper eyelid for gravity-assisted closure. Transcutaneous nerve stimulation may be helpful in cases of neuropraxia.

65.5.1.2 Trigeminal Nerve

The auriculotemporal nerve courses from the medial side of the posterior neck of the condyle and turns superiorly, running over the zygomatic root of the temporal bone.

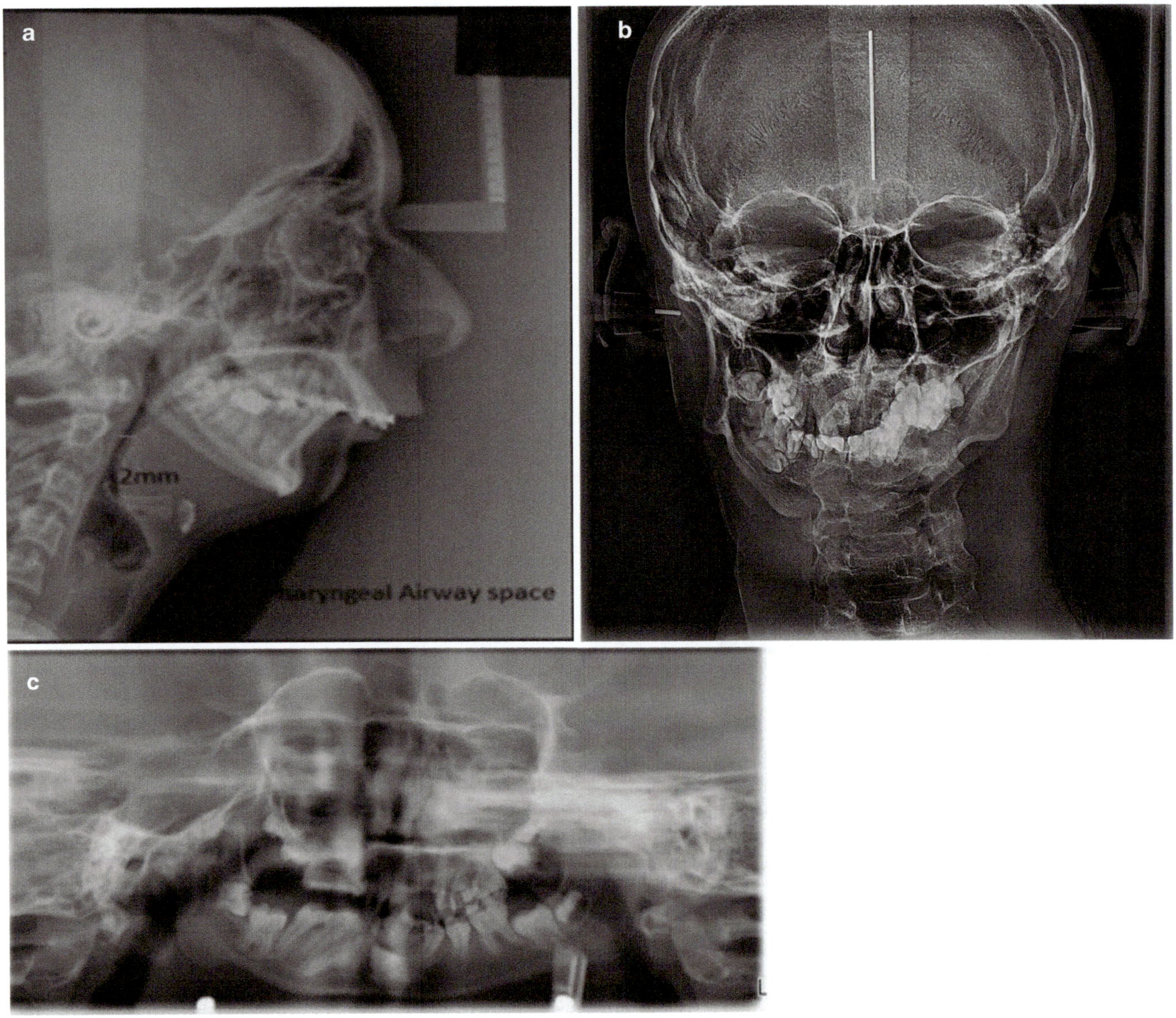

Fig. 65.4 (**a**) Lateral cephalogram, (**b**) PA cephalogram, (**c**) orthopantomogram, (**d**) facial CT scan, (**e**) facial cone beam CT, (**f**) volumetric assessment of pharyngeal airway space on CBCT

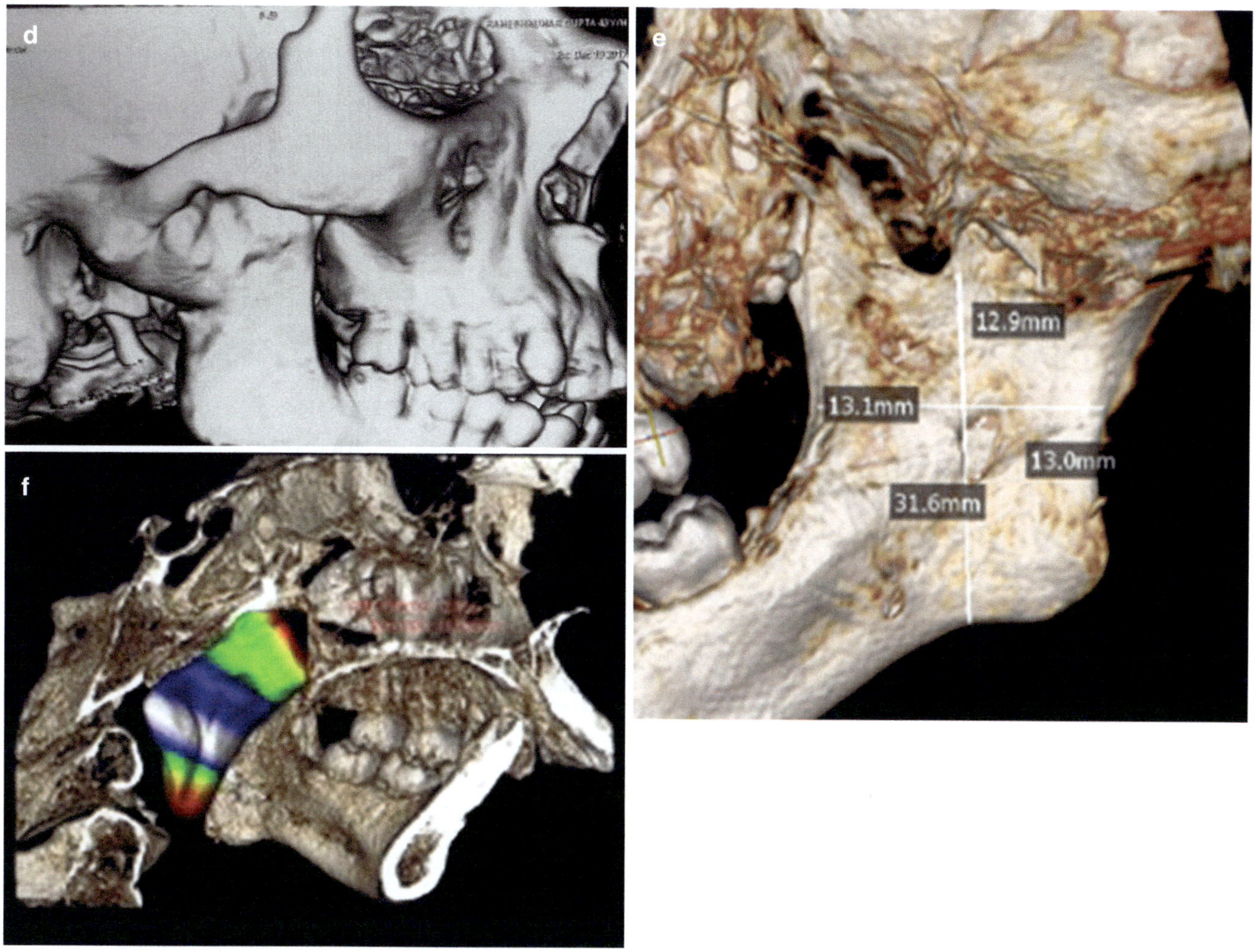

Fig. 65.4 (continued)

Preauricular exposure of the TMJ area invariably injures the nerve. Damage is minimized by incision and dissection in close apposition to the cartilaginous portion of the external auditory meatus.

65.5.2 Vascular Anatomy (Fig. 65.5)

The superficial temporal artery and internal maxillary artery are the terminal branches of the external carotid artery. In the preauricular approach, the internal maxillary artery runs about 3 mm medial to the mid-sigmoid notch.

The most commonly injured artery during temporomandibular procedures is the middle meningeal branch of the internal maxillary artery. Pogrel [14] in a cadaver study of structures medial to the temporomandibular joint found the middle meningeal artery to be a mean of 31 mm (21–43 mm) medial to the zygomatic arch and a mean of 2.4 mm (2–8 mm) anterior from the height of the glenoid fossa.

65.5.3 Incisions (Fig. 65.6) [5]

Dingman's Preauricular Approach
(Refer video on Pre auricular approach in Chap. 53 and Fig. 53.17**)**

It is the most commonly used incision with many variations. Classically, the incision begins along the course of the helix, just in front of the tragus till the attachment of the ear lobule. Going through the skin and superficial fascia, about 2 cm above the zygomatic arch, an oblique incision is made through the superficial layer of temporal fascia. Just above the arch, the periosteum of the zygomatic arch is incised and turned forward as one flap with the outer layer of the temporal fascia, superficial fascia containing nerves, and skin. The ankylotic mass now stands exposed.

65.5.3.1 Blair (1914)

It is like the Dingman's incision in preauricular fold, but unlike the former it bends in the region of the zygomatic arch

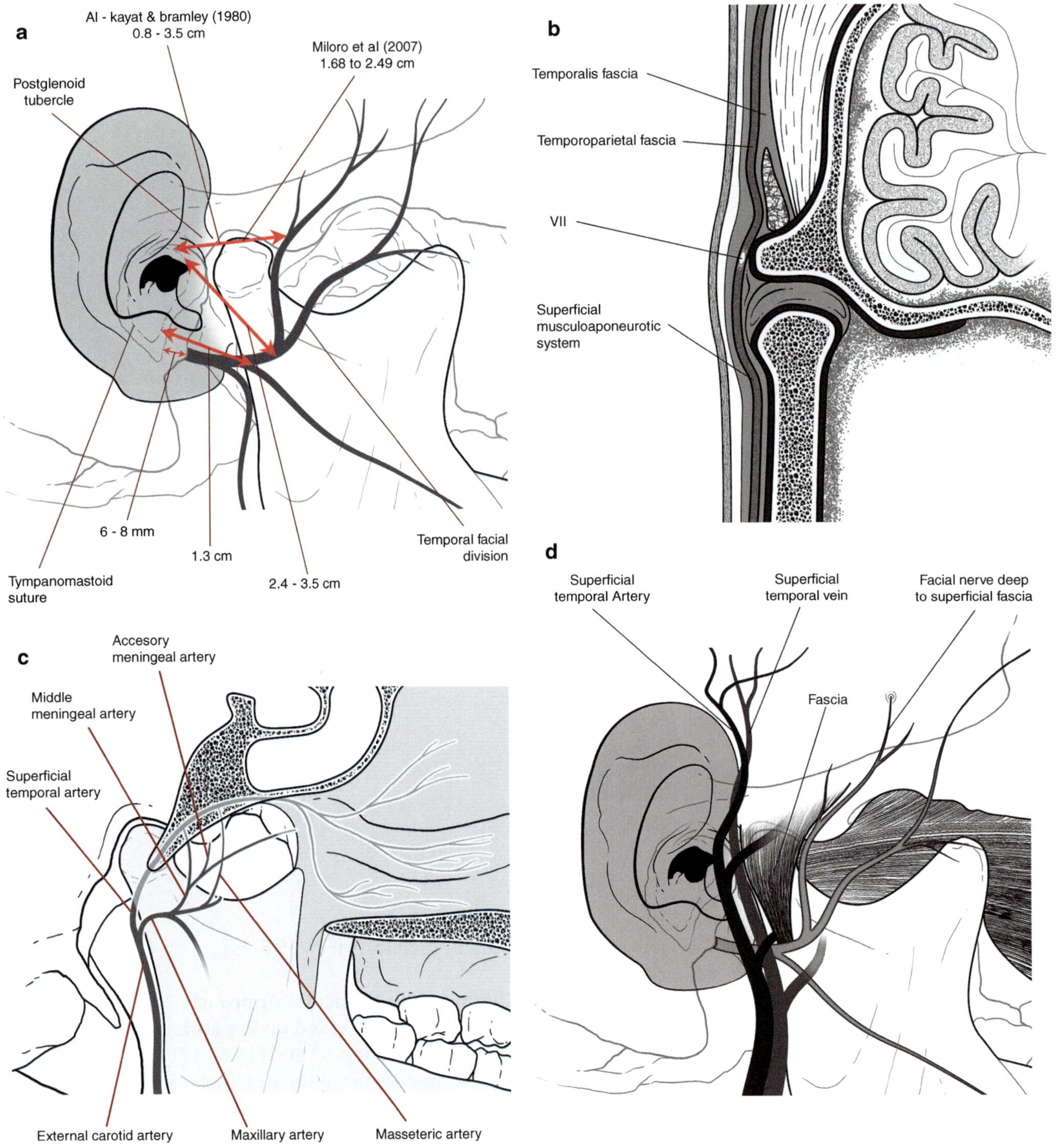

Fig. 65.5 (**a**) Surgical landmarks for identifying the location of main trunk of the facial nerve and the temporal-facial division during temporomandibular arthroplastic dissection. (**b**) Coronal diagram of the fascial layers and facial nerve at the level of the temporoparietal fascia. (**c**) View from medial aspect of the mandible. Note proximity of middle meningeal, external maxillary, and masseteric arteries. Care should be taken to protect these structures at the level of the condylar neck and sigmoid notch during osteotomies. (**d**) Relative position of the superficial temporal artery and vein and the temporal branch of the facial nerve

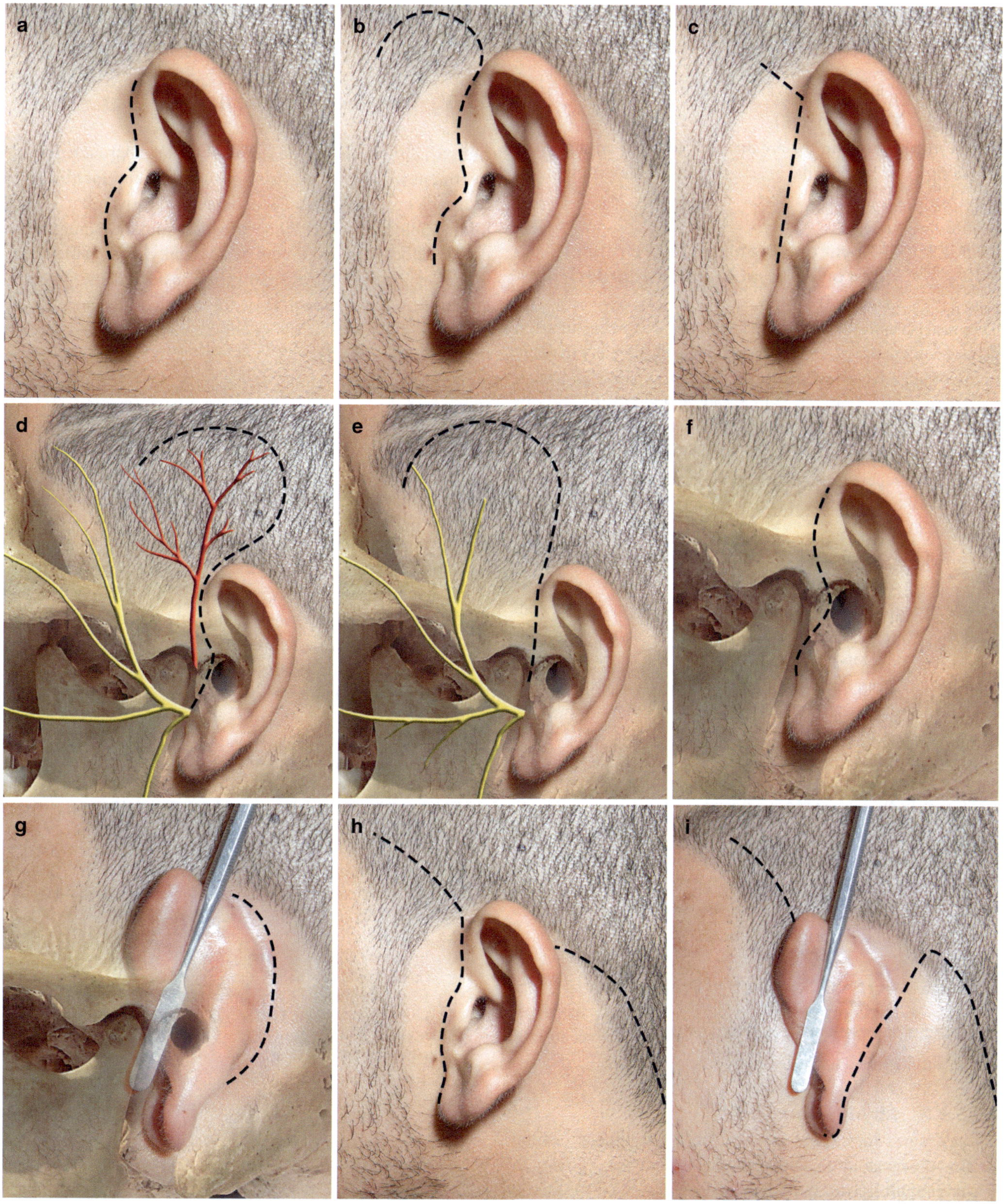

Fig. 65.6 (**a**) Dingman, (**b**) Blair's inverted hockey stick, (**c**) Thoma's, (**d**) Al-Kayat and Bramley. (**e**) Popowich's modification, (**f**) endaural, (**g**) postauricular, (**h**) rhytidectomy, (**i**) retro-auricular limb of rhytidectomy incision

like a hockey stick. The disadvantages include an unsightly scar and possible damage to the frontal branch of the facial nerve.

65.5.3.2 Thoma (1945)

The vertical limb is in the preauricular fold but angulated at 45° in the hairline near the bifurcation of the superficial temporal vessels.

65.5.3.3 Al-Kayat and Bramley (1979) (refer video on Al Kayat Bramley approach in Chap. 53)

This reverse question mark cosmetically acceptable incision gives excellent access to the TMJ without causing any damage to important anatomical structures. It starts superiorly through the scalp in the temporal region and extends to the inferior tragus. The superficial layer of the temporalis fascia is identified and incised at the root of the arch at 45° anterosuperiorly to avoid branches of the facial nerve. A vertical incision may be used if the temporalis fascia or muscle is to be used.

65.5.3.4 Popowich's Modification of Al-Kayat and Bramley [5]

This approach to the zygomatic arch and joint gives excellent visibility with safety. It is longer and wider than the conventional and question mark shaped and begins about a pinna's length away from the ear, anteroposterior just within the hair line, curves backward and downward well posterior to the main branches of the temporal vessels, till it meets the upper attachment of the ear.

65.5.3.5 Endaural [10]

This was first described by Rongetti in 1954, with the incision carried in the external ear. The advantages are good aesthetics and excellent access to the TMJ. However, the disadvantages include perichondritis, infection, paresthesia of the pinna, and deformity of the ear.

65.5.3.6 Coronal Extension of Preauricular Incision

The anterosuperior extension over the scalp of the preauricular incision gives a more aesthetic scar.

65.5.3.7 Rhytidectomy [10]

The endaural incision is extended in a curvilinear fashion around the mastoid tip, with an S-shaped extension ending in a submandibular incision. This allows access to the entire posterior border of the mandible and allows for identification of the main trunk of the facial nerve.

65.5.3.8 Postauricular

First described by Alexander [15] in 1975, its biggest advantage is that it avoids facial nerve injury and salivary fistula. However, possible complications include stenosis of external auditory canal, infection, and paresthesia of the pinna.

65.6 Treatment Protocol

Kaban [2] and colleagues described an approach for the treatment of TMJ ankylosis to minimize the incidence of re-ankylosis and produce satisfactory movement of the joint. Their study in 1990 became a landmark management protocol for the management of TMJ ankylosis (Table 65.2).

Yet again in 2009, Kaban [16] considered the potential effect of time and growth (i.e., the fourth dimension) on the outcome of TMJ ankylosis in children and presented another protocol (Table 65.2).

65.6.1 Surgical Options for Ankylosis Release (Fig. 65.7a–c)

History Ankylosis release surgeries, i.e., various ways of separation of the ramus from the skull have undergone great evolution during the nineteenth century. Esmarch [17] osteotomized the angle to release TMJ ankylosis in 1851. The first interpositional material was the pterygomasseteric sling, also developed by Esmarch. Condylectomy was first advocated by Humphrey in 1854. Abbe performed the first gap arthroplasty in 1880. But it was Topazian in the 1960s [18, 19] who signified the importance of interpositional grafts for reducing re-ankylosis.

65.6.1.1 Gap Arthroplasty

The conventional surgical treatment of TMJ ankylosis by gap arthroplasty includes complete resection of the ankylotic

Table 65.2 Kaban's protocols for TMJ ankylosis

1. Kaban's protocol for management of temporomandibular joint ankylosis (1990) [2]
(a) Aggressive resection of the ankylotic segment
(b) Ipsilateral coronoidectomy
(c) Contralateral coronoidectomy when necessary
(d) Lining the joint with temporalis fascia or cartilage
(e) Reconstruction of the ramus with a costochondral graft
(f) Rigid fixation of the graft
(g) Early mobilization and aggressive physiotherapy
2. Kaban's modified protocol for management of TMJ ankylosis in children (2009) [16]
(a) Aggressive excision of fibrous and/or bony mass
(b) Coronoidectomy on affected side
(c) Coronoidectomy on opposite side if steps 1 and 2 do not result in MIO of 35 mm or to point of dislocation of opposite side
(d) Lining of joint with temporalis fascia or the native disk, if it can be salvaged
(e) Reconstruction of RCU with either DO or CCG and rigid fixation
(f) Early mobilization of jaw; if DO used to reconstruct RCU, mobilize day of surgery; if CCG used, early mobilization with minimal intermaxillary fixation (not > 10 days)
(g) Aggressive physiotherapy

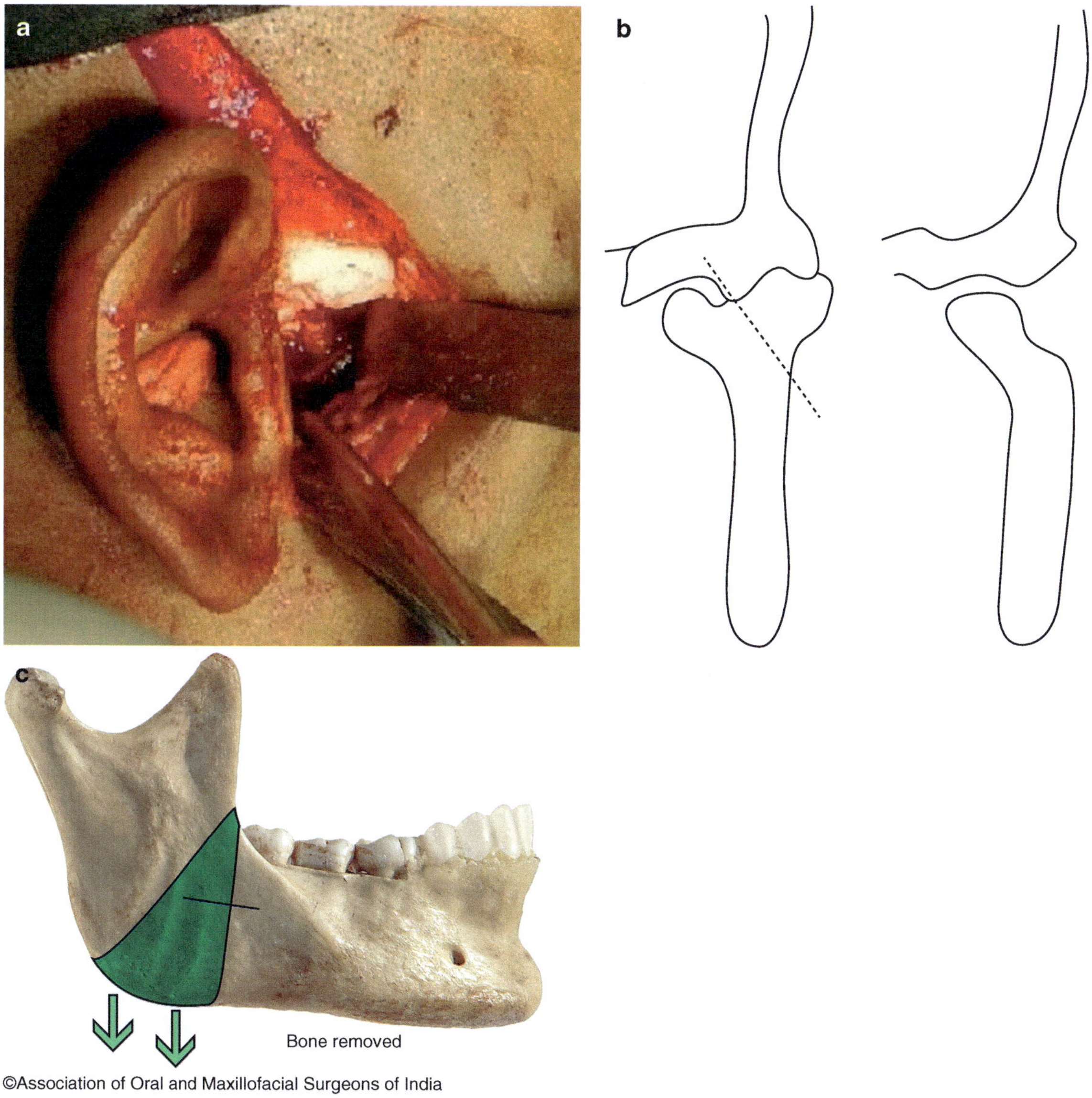

Fig. 65.7 (**a**) Gap arthroplasty, (**b**) Lateral arthroplasty (LAP), (**c**) Esmarch's procedure

mass with no soft tissue as an interposition between two cut ends. When a soft tissue is placed between the cut ends, it is known as interpositional arthroplasty. Gap arthroplasty is a relatively simple procedure requiring less operative time; however, it may cause ramal shortening, malocclusion, OSA, and, most distressingly, re-ankylosis. But it may still be used in certain adult patients, where the removal of a small ankylotic mass would not decrease the ramal height significantly.

Patients are operated under general anesthesia using a preauricular approach. After the ankylotic mass is exposed, the upper cut is marked, and the lower cut is placed 1.5 cm below it. In cases where normal architecture of the joint is maintained, the lower osteotomy cut is placed from the anterior to the posterior border of ramus just below the sigmoid notch. In cases where normal architecture is not clear, a cut is placed 1.5 cm below the lower border of zygomatic arch. Then the upper cut is completed, and the ankylotic mass is removed. The osteotomy is directed at 45° to prevent fracture of middle cranial fossa. The venous plexus if encountered medially needs only be packed to control bleeding.

A condylar retractor is kept below the ankylotic mass to prevent injury to the internal maxillary artery. Bone is cut initially using a bur/saw/piezoelectric unit through two thirds of its thickness. The remaining one thirds may be removed with an osteotome. A Piezoelectric unit if used, may cut bone till its very end. In case of a larger mass, it may also be removed in pieces. The ipsilateral coronoid process is always resected. Care is always taken to stop the application of Heister's mouth gag intraoperatively just before the opposite condyle dislocates.

In some patients with longstanding ankylosis, the coronoid process of the opposite site becomes hyperplastic. There may also occur fibrosis of the masseter, which would restrict jaw movements further. Thus, not only would the contralateral coronoidectomy be required, but the masseter attachment would also need to be completely dissected off the zygomatic arch. A coronoidotomy may not be adequate, as it may re form and attach again to the temporalis and subsequently cause decrease in mouth opening. An intact disc may not require another soft tissue interpositional graft but may itself be mobilized and repositioned into the new glenoid fossa.

R. F. Elgazzar [20] reviewed 101 patients (109 joints) and, on follow-up, reported that in comparison with other techniques of ankylosis release, gap arthroplasty had the least amount of mouth opening. Interpositional arthroplasty with temporalis gives better results in comparison.

Surgical navigation systems are useful in TMJ ankylosis surgery as they improve both the safety and accuracy of the surgery. The distance from the top of the glenoid fossa to the middle cranial fossa and that from the posterior margin of the fossa to the anterior border of the bony external auditory canal can be monitored via the navigation system. A safety distance of at least 3 mm from the middle cranial fossa and bony external auditory canal should be maintained to avoid injury. It reduces the risks of bleeding and CSF leak [21].

65.6.1.2 Esmarch's Procedure

This is of historical significance only. Esmarch [22] made a small incision posterior to the angle of the mandible and dissected the masseter and medial pterygoid muscles off the bone. A 2.5 cm wide wedge of bone, at the angle of the mandible with apex at upper border and base at the posteroinferior border, was removed. The muscles were then sutured back.

The disadvantage is that since the osteotomy is in the ramus, no ramal osteotomy or distraction can be done for correction of facial deformity. Hence, it is no longer used for ankylosis release.

65.6.1.3 Lateral Arthroplasty (LAP)

Nitzan hypothesized that in Sawhney's [3] Type II TMJ ankylosis or He's Type A2 [23], if the integrity and location of the displaced condyle and disc can be determined (despite morphological and positional alterations), both could be preserved to fulfill their roles in mandibular growth and function. Only the lateral part of the ankylosed mass was resected. Eight young patients were kept under observation for a period ranging from 6 to 60 months after surgery. She found significant improvement in facial symmetry and thereby concluded that the residual condyle retained its own growth potential and helped maintain normal mandibular movement function and occlusion [24].

Yang and Dongmei He evaluated long-term results after LAP in nine growing children and concluded that the residual condyle continues to grow after LAP. This then decreases the amount of further facial asymmetry [25].

65.6.2 Arthroplasty with Ramus-Condyle Unit (RCU) Reconstruction *(Details Covered Under "Hard Tissue Interposition")*

Interpositional arthroplasty with RCU reconstruction is the procedure of choice in recent times. The procedure consists of:

(i) Removal of the ankylotic mass.
(ii) Reconstruction of the RCU may be considered from amongst any of the following in costochondral graft, coronoid process graft, distraction osteogenesis (DO), total alloplastic joint replacement.

Early postoperative exercises and appropriate physiotherapy are essential to prevent re-ankylosis, adhesions, and soft tissue contracture and to regain normal function of the muscles. Dynamic mouth opening exercise initiated in the immediate postop period by achieving pain control using local infiltration of bupivacaine. Dynamic mouth exercises would have to be continued for at least 6 months after surgery.

65.7 Soft Tissue Interpositional Materials (Video 65.1)

65.7.1 Temporalis Myofascial Flap (Fig. 65.8d, e)

Historically, it has been the most commonly used material for interpositional arthroplasty as it is simple in technique and in the vicinity of the original area of surgery. An inferiorly based pedicled composite (fascia and muscle), temporalis myofascial flap is raised supraperiosteally which is finger shaped and about 5 × 2 cm. The flap is taken either over/under the zygomatic arch and sutured medially and posteriorly. However, its potential disadvantages include an extended incision, temporal hollowing, increased chances of facial nerve injury, inability to be used again in cases of re-ankylosis, and myofascial pain secondary to muscle flap compression.

Albert and Merril described the use of a posterior temporalis myofascial flap to prevent a visible anterior flap hollowing [26]. Pogrel and Kaban used an axial patterned temporalis myofascial flap, based on a branch of the middle temporal artery [27].

65.7.2 Dermal Fat Graft (Fig. 65.8a, b, c)

The abdominal dermal fat graft is harvested from the suprapubic area used an elliptical incision of around 7 × 3 cm. The fat is then de-epithelized to procure a volume of 6–20 ml. About 20–30% excess is taken than the actual requirement. The graft is folded onto itself with the dermis surfaces apposed.

It can be procured quickly and easily with a hidden scar. It is easy to sculpt into the gap after ankylosis release. Minimal heterotopic calcification is the advantage of dermal fat graft. However, since this is a non-vascularized graft, it may be prone to resorption.

Dimitroulis presented his study on dermal fat grafts. After a mean follow-up of 41.5 months, only 1 out of the 13 joints reported recurrence of ankylosis [28]. Thangavelu presented a review of eight ankylosed joints treated using full-thickness skin subcutaneous fat grafts and concluded that they were safe and effective [29].

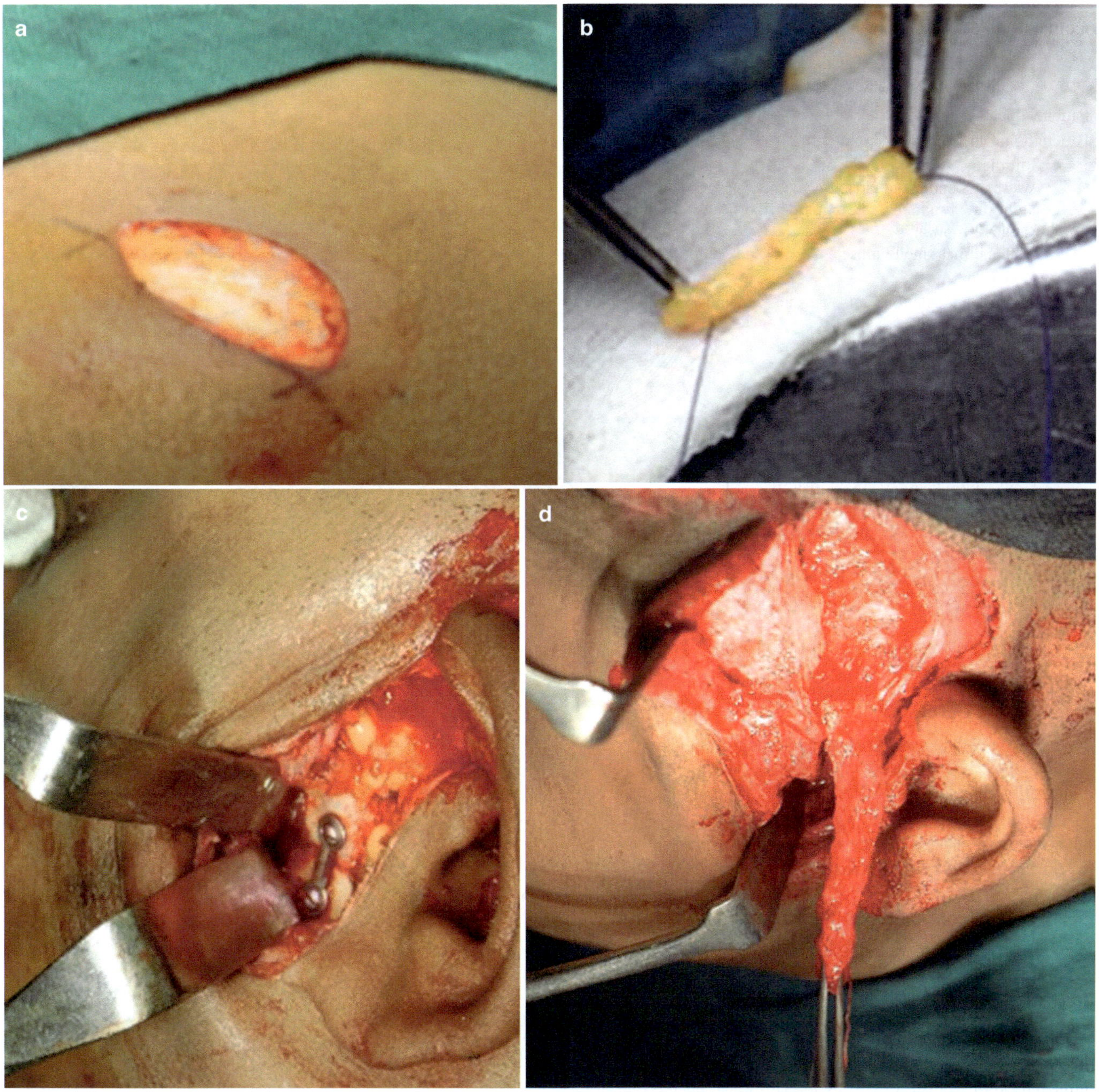

Fig. 65.8 (**a**) Abdominal fat graft donor site and (**b**) harvested graft, (**c**) abdominal fat graft in place, (**d**) harvested temporalis flap, (**e**) temporalis flap in place, (**f**) maneuver for harvesting buccal fat pad, (**g**) harvested buccal fat pad

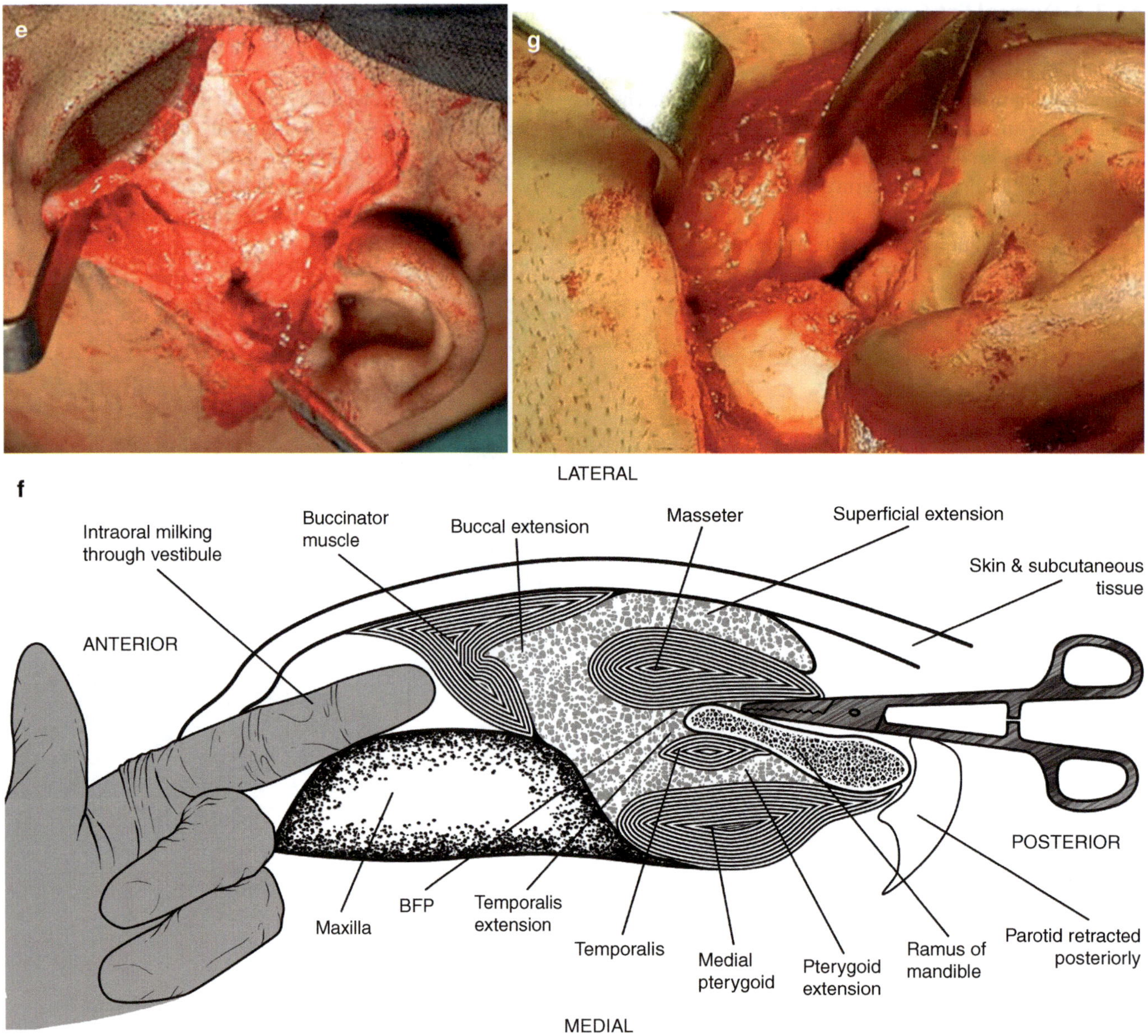

Fig. 65.8 (continued)

65.7.3 Buccal Fat Pad Graft (BFP) (Fig. 65.8f, g)

After the coronoid process is removed, dissection maybe performed along the anterior border of ramus. The main part and temporal extension of buccal fat pad are in close approximation to the coronoid process and tendon of the temporalis. Thus, incising through the periosteum and fascial envelope of BFP at the anterior most edge of the coronoid stump/superior most stump of anterior border of ramus exposes the yellowish buccal pad of fat.

Further blunt dissection is performed to herniate the BFP into the defect with a little teasing and simultaneous milking of maxillary buccal sulcus intraorally near second and third molar region. The main advantage is that its vascularity would maintain the volume of fat for a longer duration with minimal resorption.

Gaba et al. prospectively assessed the fate of BFP following interpositional arthroplasty in 23 joints. In 18 cases, BFP was viable even after 1 year [30]. Refer Chap. 24 for detailed anatomy of the Buccal fat pad.

65.7.4 Amniotic Membrane

The amniotic membrane, being a natural biologic entity, prevents inflammation, reduces scarring, and promotes healing and re-epithelialization. It also has pluripotent, non-antigenic properties. Akhter M. et al. used gamma radiation sterilized and freeze-dried amniotic membranes in 13 patients of TMJ ankylosis and showed that it prevented recurrence of ankylosis [31].

65.7.5 Auricular Cartilage

Parko in 1973 first published the use of aural cartilage to replace the meniscus. The biggest advantage of auricular cartilage graft is that it can be harvested from the same surgical field, remains viable and inert and takes the shape of the glenoid fossa.

However, there are studies that have reported adhesions between the auricular cartilage graft and the condyle, leading to re-ankylosis.

65.8 Hard Tissue Interpositional Materials (RCU Reconstruction)

65.8.1 Rationale for RCU Reconstruction

The goal of RCU reconstruction in TMJ ankylosis includes restoration of ramal height. This not only avoids occlusal discrepancies and deviation on mouth opening in unilateral cases but also anterior open bite in bilateral ankylosis. It also provides enough bone stock for future jaw corrective surgeries. The RCU may not contribute as much to facial aesthetics but impacts function greatly. In cases where RCU has not been reconstructed, the jaw deviates laterally when opening the mouth. When closing the mouth, tangential rather than vertical striking occurs on the occlusal surfaces, making mastication difficult.

Most importantly, in bilateral TMJ ankylosis after gap arthroplasty without RCU reconstruction, there are increased chances of OSA because the ramus falls back due to lack of posterosuperior stop. Also, it may be possible that restoring normal jaw movement and a symmetric mandible will allow future soft and hard tissue development. This would probably lead to decrease in facial asymmetry by giving as near normal anatomy as possible by restoration of growth spurts (Moss's functional matrix theory).

65.8.2 Options, Techniques, Advantages, and Disadvantages

65.8.2.1 Ankylotic Mass (Fig. 65.9a)

The ankylotic mass is recontoured and utilized to reconstruct the RCU and thereby restore the mandibular ramal height. All neocondyles after RCU reconstruction are fixed into position with miniplates/screws in the new glenoid fossa just 2 mm short of the soft tissue interpositional material after placing the patient into intermaxillary fixation (IMF).

R. Gunaseelan excised the ankylotic mass, recontoured and reimplanted it, and used it successfully for three cases of condylar reconstruction [32]. However, only if the ankylotic mass is resected as a whole (which poses greater risk to middle meningeal artery) can it be recontoured in an adequate size to reconstruct the RCU, hence the difficulty in routine use.

65.8.2.2 Coronoid Process Graft (Fig. 65.9b)

Khadka and Hu first reconstructed RCU using the coronoid process [33]. Reshaped, the coronoid process provides good bone of adequate quality and quantity to reconstruct the RCU. Its membranous origin leads to lesser resorption. Also, a secondary donor site is not utilized. However, as the coronoid is a nonvascular graft, there does exist a very real possibility of its resorption.

Gagan Mehta and Shadab Mohammad conducted a study on 20 cases and reported that there did occur resorption of the coronoid in most of the cases. However, that did not change mandibular function and occlusion [34].

Another method of using the coronoid process is to use it as RCU with its attachment to the temporalis kept intact. Most of the attachment may be stripped of, and only the anterior part of temporalis may be kept attached to the tip of the coronoid. It may cause less resorption as it would be a pedicled graft. Yiming Liu studied 48 patients and compared free vs. pedicled coronoid process grafts and proved that pedicled grafts showed less resorption on prolonged follow-up [35].

65.8.2.3 Costochondral Graft (CCG) (Fig. 65.9c)

Poswillo popularized the procedure for using CCG for TMJ ankylosis in 1987. In unilateral cases, CCG may be taken from the fifth rib using a submammary incision. If required on both the sides, alternate ribs, i.e., fifth and seventh, are used [36].

CCG has various benefits including its growth potential, its biological compatibility and the fact that it can remodel to form a new condyle. However, donor site morbidity, resorption or excessive growth on the treated side, and inability to catch up with the speed of growth on the normal side are its potential demerits. Perrott and Kaban [16] described two types of overgrowth—(a) linear overgrowth causing an

Box 65.1 Technical Tip

To maximize the chances of survival rate of CCG, the following techniques may be followed: meticulous dissection of periosteum and perichondrium, harvesting alternate ribs to prevent pain and pleural tear, retaining intact periosteum and perichondrium at costochondral junction, sectioning the chondral before the osseous part to reduce fracture at the costochondral junction, and only 2–3 mm chondral portion to prevent overgrowth.

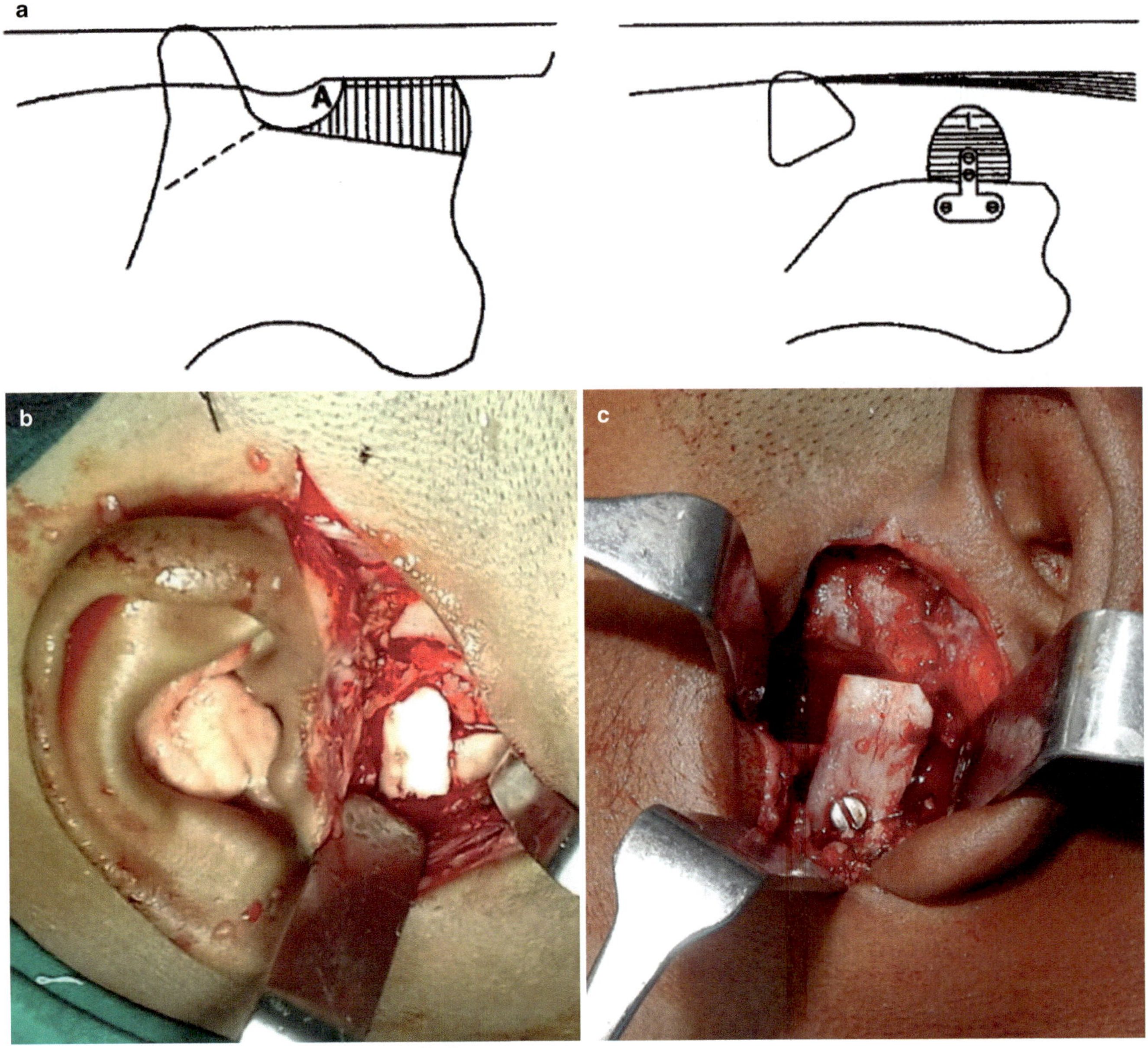

Fig. 65.9 (a) Ankylotic mass, (b) coronoid graft, (c) costocondral graft

asymmetric or bilateral prognathism and (b) tumor-like overgrowth causing re-ankylosis.

There are various controversies regarding which ribs and how much cartilaginous cap should be taken, how to fix, whether post-op IMF is required or not, and resorption vs. hypertrophy of the graft. Jean Salash reported that out of 72 cases, excessive growth occurred in 54% and equal growth occurred in 38% [37].

Hence, CCG may be used for RCU reconstruction in children less than 8 years of age with facial asymmetry. The justification is that it may help in growth. However, if it overgrows, the overgrowth may be treated like condylar hypertrophy, and the superior 2–3 mm may be cut off.

Children less than 8 years but without facial asymmetry would probably not need a growth impetus, in which cases, a coronoid graft would be sufficient. In children more than 8 years of age, vertical ramus osteotomies may be used to recreate the RCU.

65.8.2.4 Ramus Osteotomy Pedicled Grafts (Fig. 65.10a, b)

Y. Liu [38] used the method of total (Vertical ramus osteotomy—VRO) and partial (L- ramus osteotomy—LRO) sliding osteotomy on the posterior border of the ramus for reconstructing the mandibular condyle in TMJ ankylosis.

The chances of bony resorption and graft failure of the newly reconstructed RCU are greatly reduced as this segment is a pedicled graft with attachment to the medial pterygoid muscle and periosteum and is not a free graft. Hence the height of the ramus is maintained. This also leads to adequate bone stock for further corrective surgeries if and when so required.

For the VRO, the cut is made in a vertical direction starting from the sigmoid notch to the inferior border of the mandible just lateral to the lingula and parallel to the posterior border of the ramus. While retaining an adequate amount of medial pterygoid, the proximal segment is pushed upward to recreate the RCU and plated in the new position. A small triangular chunk of bone just anterior to the osteotomy cut is resected to reshape the lower border and mandibular angle.

For the LRO, an L-shaped cut is made from sigmoid notch parallel to the posterior border of the mandibular ramus, just lateral to the lingula, till 10 mm above the angle of the mandible. The osteotomized segment is shifted upward and fixed with a mini plate creating a gap between the osteotomized segment and remaining mandibular angle. The coronoid process on the affected side is resected, recontoured, and fixed in that gap with another mini plate. The upper part of the ramus is then reshaped like a condyle.

LRO and VRO differ in the residual height of the ramus left after ramal osteotomy. In LRO it is retained, and in VRO it decreases due to the removal of the step at the inferior bor-

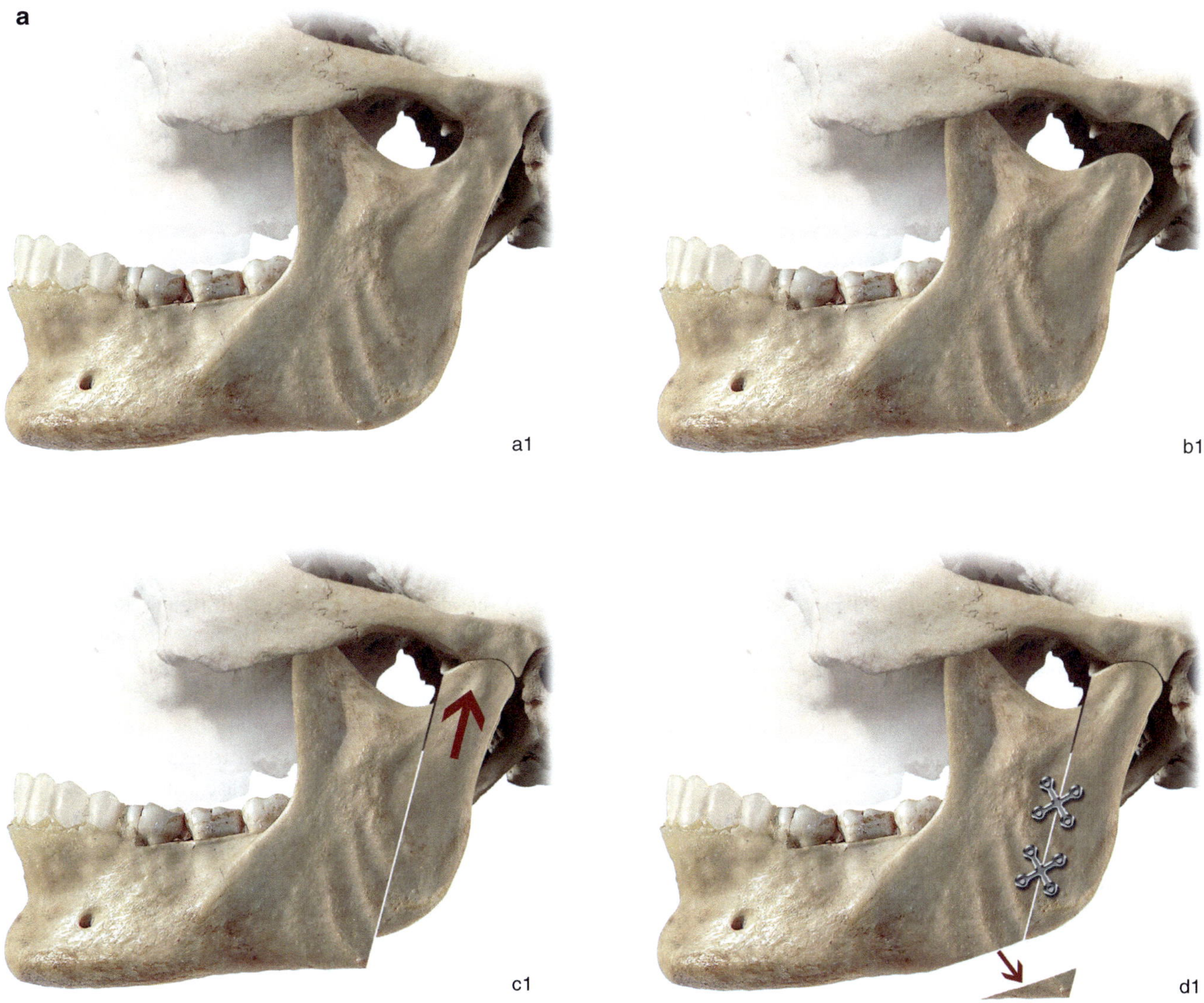

Fig. 65.10 (a) V Ramus osteotomy, (b) L Ramus osteotomy [38]

b

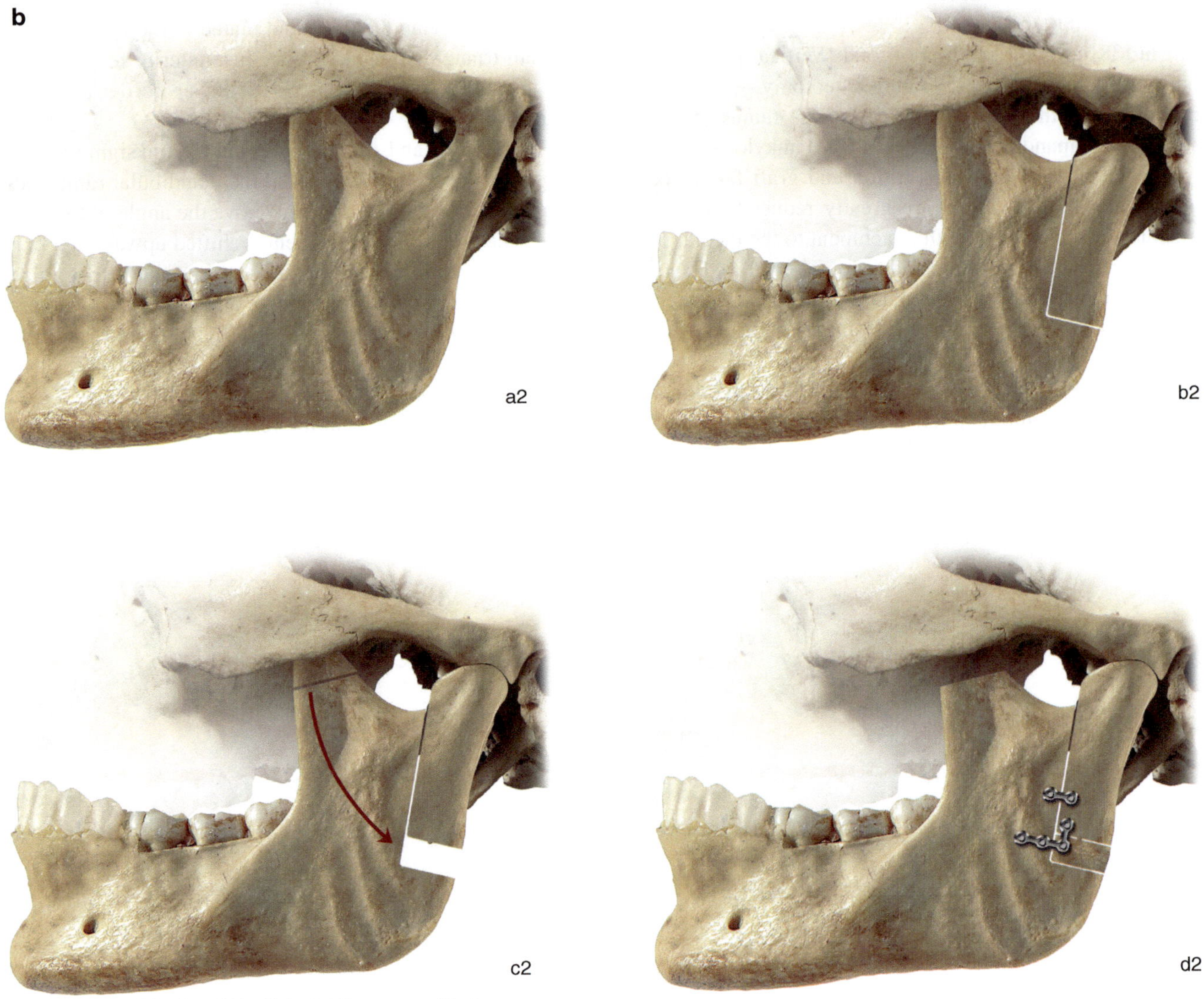

Fig. 65.10 (continued)

der. Thus, VRO may be performed in cases where a pronounced antegonial notch is present.

However, these osteotomies cannot be performed in patients less than 8 years because as observed on CBCT, the amount of bone behind the lingula is generally not enough to osteotomize the posterior border of the ramus.

65.8.2.5 Transport Distraction Osteogenesis (Fig. 65.11a, b) (Refer Chap. 87)

In multiple operated patients, scar tissue forms with each surgery, which may affect angiogenesis due to limited diffusion. Thus, free autogenous tissue grafts, such as costochondral and coronoid grafts often fail in such cases. Hence, transport distraction osteogenesis is considered as an option for RCU reconstruction, especially in re-ankylosis cases in children. The same L osteotomy cut may be used to fix the distractor.

When RCU reconstruction is performed by transport distraction, it forms a fibrous/pseudo-disc by compressing the connective tissue between the transport segment and the glenoid fossa. This disk decreases the chances of re-ankylosis [39]. Sharma et al. in 2019 carried out neocondyle distraction in five patients and reported adequate mouth opening and functional movements in all patients. None of them reported re-ankylosis [40]. But a long-term follow-up study found that the height of these condyles was unstable. Also, these mandibles exhibited some degree of asymmetry [41].

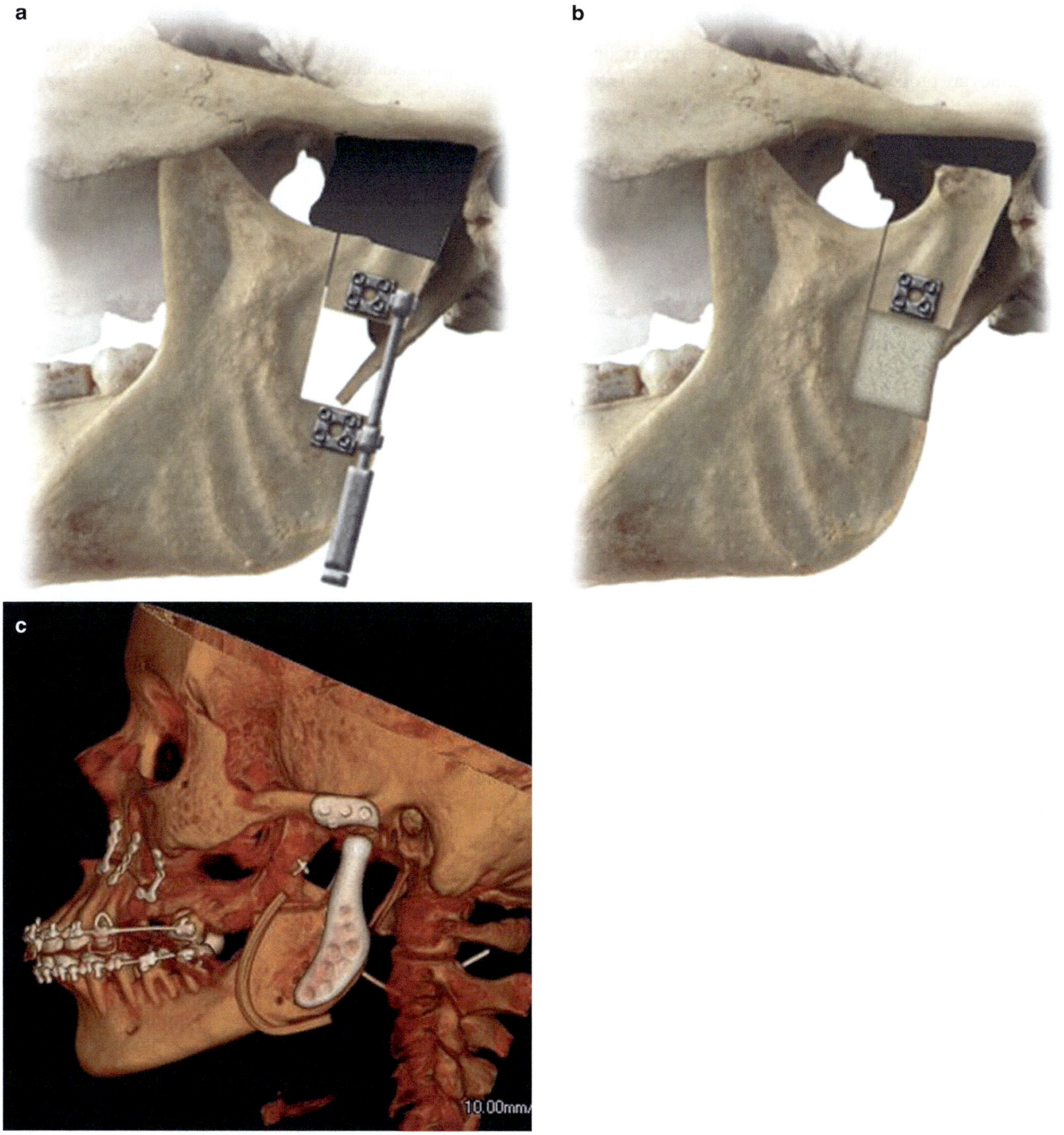

Fig. 65.11 (**a**) Transport distraction osteogenesis, (**b**) shows woven bone formation in place of callus in distracted gap, (**c**) alloplastic TMJ replacement with simultaneous release and OGS

65.8.2.6 Alloplastic Total TMJ Replacement (TJR) (Fig. 65.11c)

The alloplastic joint consists of a fossa component and a ramal component, as a stock or a custom-made prosthesis. Re-ankylotic scar tissue in an adult is best treated by total alloplastic TM joint replacement. Dongmei He and Yi Hui Hu reported that alloplastic TMJ prosthesis is a reliable method to treat recurrent TMJ ankylosis. It may be accompanied by bimaxillary osteotomies for simultaneous correction of secondary ankylotic deformity as well. Its distinct disadvantage is the fact that if used in children, it would need to be replaced [42].

Mercuri et al. [43] specified the indications of TJR (Box 65.2).

Based on all the above RCU reconstruction options, guidelines are proposed for technique of RCU reconstruction in various clinical situations (Table 65.3).

Box 65.2

1. Recurrent fibrous or bony ankylosis not responsive to the modalities of treatment which have been hitherto applied
2. Failed (bone and soft) tissue grafts
3. Loss of vertical mandibular height and occlusal relationship due to bone resorption, trauma, developmental abnormalities, or pathological lesions
4. Severe inflammation of TMJ involving damage to its structures and lack of response to other treatment methods.

Table 65.3 Guidelines for technique of RCU reconstruction in various clinical situations

	Situations		Technique	Justification
1.	<8 years	(a) With facial asymmetry	Costochondral Graft ± eventual high condylectomy	• Potential for growth • Treat overgrowth like condylar hypertrophy
		(b) Without facial asymmetry	Coronoid graft	• Potential for growth not required • Cannot do ramus osteotomy because of inadequate ramal width
2.	>8 years	(a) With prominent antegonial notch	Vertical ramus osteotomy	• Reduces antegonial notch
		(b) Without prominent antegonial notch	L-shaped ramus osteotomy	• Maintains height of ramus • Adequate ramal size
3.	Re-ankylosis	(a) Child	Ramal distraction	• Free graft will not take in scar tissue • Alloplastic joint will not grow
		(b) Adult	Total alloplastic TMJ replacement	• Best option for scarred tissue

Table 65.4 Treatment guidelines for different types of ankylotic deformities

Type I (presence of occlusal cant): treatment planning for both maxilla and mandible
1. Involved side is normal and other side is excess **(<6 mm deficiency)**
(a) Differential maxillary impaction
(b) Mandibular ramus osteotomy
(i) Sagittal split osteotomy
(ii) Inverted L ramus osteotomy
(c) ± Genioplasty
2. Involved side is deficient and other side is normal **(<6 mm deficiency)**
(a) Differential down fracture and bone grafting of maxilla
(b) Mandibular ramus osteotomy
(i) Sagittal split osteotomy
(ii) Inverted L ramus osteotomy
(c) ± Genioplasty
3. 6–8 mm discrepancy in maxilla **(6–8 mm in mandible)**
(a) Simultaneous maxillomandibular distraction
4. 6–8 mm discrepancy in maxilla **(>8 mm discrepancy in mandible)**
(a) Cant correction in maxilla
(b) Mandibular distraction as per type II-4, 5, 6
(c) Simultaneous OGS with TJR
Type II: (with minimal occlusal cant) treatment planning for mandible alone
1. Mandibular ramus osteotomy
2. Genioplasty
3. Orthomorphic osteotomy
4. Orthomorphic distraction
5. Unidirectional distraction
6. Bidirectional distraction
7. Simultaneous OGS with TJR

65.9 Facial Deformity Secondary to TMJ Ankylosis

TMJ ankylosis leads to mandibular deformity of varying magnitude and morphology in the form of decreased ramus and/or body length, deviation of chin, retrognathic/microgenia, bird face deformity, and narrow PAS leading to OSA (refer Fig. 68.18). Hence, establishing a single set treatment protocol for all clinical situations is not possible. Table 65.4 is an attempt to classify and thereby establish treatment guidelines for different types of ankylotic deformities.

Surgical Techniques and Indications:

65.9.1 Osteotomies (Fig. 65.12a–c)

They are indicated for movements of about 6–8 mm. For maxilla, Le Fort osteotomies and, for mandible, sagittal split osteotomy or inverted L ramus osteotomy may be performed.

65.9.1.1 Le Fort I Osteotomy (Refer Chap. 69)

It allows correction in three dimensions including roll, pitch, and yaw. For vertical maxillary excess, differential maxillary

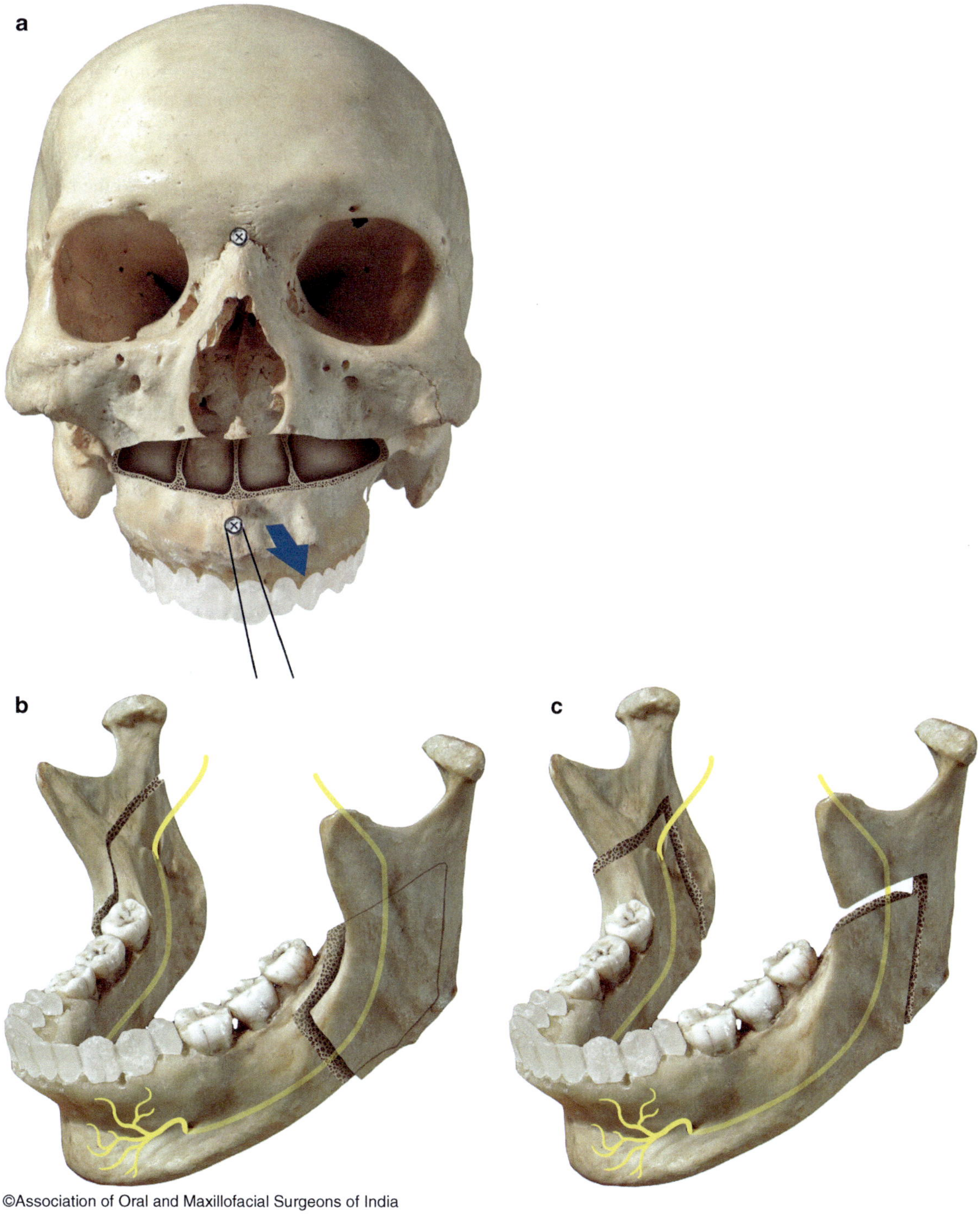

Fig. 65.12 (**a**) Le Fort I osteotomy, (**b**) sagittal split osteotomy (SSO), (**c**) inverted L ramus osteotomy (ILRO)

impaction may be performed, while for vertical maxillary deficiency, maxillary down fracture may be done along with bone grafting. Posterior maxillary height adjustments may also be required.

65.9.1.2 Sagittal Split Osteotomy (SSO) (Refer Chap. 68)

SSO is useful to differentially settle the occlusion according to the movement of the maxilla, as well as bring the retrognathic mandible forward. The procedure involves three corticotomies—the lingual horizontal, the buccal vertical, and the intermediate cuts. This osteotomy is generally done on the normal side in case of unilateral ankylosis. On the affected side, ramal contour and condylar anatomy distortions, reduced height of the ramus and steep mandibular plane angle make SSO difficult to perform.

65.9.1.3 Inverted L Ramus Osteotomy (ILRO) (Fig. 68.6)

ILRO can be better utilized for increasing the ramal height. This technique is advocated in cases which require significant counterclockwise movement to increase projection of the lower third of the face when the ramal anatomy is altered.

The cuts are placed using a submandibular and/or an intraoral approach, posterior and superior to the inferior alveolar canal. A horizontal cut is made above and behind the lingula and then joined to the vertical cut from the inferior border of the mandible.

65.9.1.4 Genioplasty (Figs. 68.29, 68.32 and 68.34)

Patients indicated for genioplasty have normal ramal height, functional occlusion, deficient or normal pharyngeal airway space, and chin deviation or retrusion up to a maximum of 10 mm, hence minimally deformed cases.

An extended genioplasty is performed with the osteotomy cuts extending up to the first molar on both sides. Advancement and translational movements in coronal and sagittal planes are carried out. Interpositional or onlay bone grafting may be done so as to achieve further symmetry wherever required.

Alloplastic chin implants made of PTFE, silicon, PEEK, or customized titanium are alternatives to the traditional genioplasty.

65.9.1.5 Orthomorphic Osteotomy

As opposed to conventional orthognathic surgery, an osteotomy used to restore morphology is termed "orthomorphic correction."

Patients who may undergo orthomorphic osteotomies are the ones having normal ramal height, functional occlusion, deficient or normal posterior airway space, and chin deviation or retrusion up to a maximum of 10 mm, but this can be done only in cases of unilateral ankylosis. Most importantly, the primary indication for this surgery is the presence of soft tissue depression over the mandibular ramus on the unaffected side resulting in a contour defect. The osteotomy cuts are placed on the unaffected side.

Paul Salins [44] designed the osteotomy as an eccentric genioplasty extending from the body to the buccal cortex of the mandible. The cut changes from full thickness from the body to the sagittal buccal cortical cut in the ramus. The segment is then repositioned in such a way that it corrects the midline, the anteroposterior deficit, as well as the lateral morphological contour defects Fig. 65.13a.

65.9.2 Distraction Osteogenesis (DO)

Traditional bone grafting and orthognathic surgery have disadvantages—bony resorption, necrosis, donor site morbidity, limited advancement, relapse, etc.

Advancement of the mandible using SSO generally is restricted to a maximum of 10–12 mm. In ankylotic patients, the mandible requires much greater movements. Kohn et al. have reported high relapse after SSO [45], especially when used for advancement of mandible. Patients with ankylosis may report higher relapse rate than others. All the above issues may be dealt with DO.

Mandible lengthening with distraction leads to increase in bone stock of the mandible as well as proportionate and harmonious growth of the surrounding soft tissues. This bony regeneration is principally dependent on intramembranous ossification. Also healing and mineralization need adequate vascularity. Therefore, the incision to perform the surgery may be kept as limited as possible.

Early distraction may have beneficial effects, on the facial harmony as well as on the TMJ. If the anatomy and thereby function of the soft and hard tissues of craniofacial skeleton is established early in life, it may be possible to regain as near normal growth of the face.

Distraction in TMJ ankylosis patients with obstructive sleep apnea has led to decrease in snoring, daytime somnolence, Apnoea Hypopnoea Index (AHI), and oxygen desaturation episodes. The disadvantage however is that the device may be costly and needs to remain in situ for several months.

65.9.2.1 Simultaneous Maxillomandibular DO

This technique was first described by Molina and Monasterio in 1997 [46]. The first stage of surgery comprises of a Le Fort I osteotomy and a unilateral mandibular osteotomy. The distraction device is fixed to the mandible on the affected site. Under IMF, as the mandible moves forward, the maxilla comes downward, thereby correcting the cant and, simultaneously, the anteroposterior deficiency of the mandible. As this whole procedure is done under IMF, occlusion is maintained. The second stage comprises of removal distraction device and an additional genioplasty if required.

This is indicated when the occlusal cant is such that there is vertical maxillary deficiency but with presence of functional occlusion. If the mandible alone is distracted, it may lead to occlusal disasters, hence the need to keep the patient under IMF while the distraction is being performed.

65.9.2.2 **Orthomorphic DO** (Figs. 65.13a–d, 78.23, 78.24 and 78.25)

As laid down by Manikandan et al. [47] , the concept of orthomorphic distraction of the mandible is a modification of Paul Salin's morphometric osteotomy. It involves the distraction of mandibular basal bone to correct the asymmetry in all dimensions, despite a deficient soft tissue capsule. It also provides more movement than that attainable via osteotomy.

The osteotomy design is similar to the one used in conventional orthomorphic surgery. Once the osteotomized segment is mobilized, an internal/external distractor may be placed. Maintenance of the periosteal attachment at the pterygomassetric sling region brings about a pivotal movement at the gonion facilitating the lateralization and advancement of the osteotomized segment. The mechanics of the mandibular asymmetry correction is based on the law of parallelogram of vectors.

65.9.2.3 **Genial Distraction**

Distraction of the chin may be performed either in isolation or simultaneously with ankylosis release. A case report on the latter has been published by Gunaseelan et al. [48] in 2007 wherein an extended genioplasty osteotomy was performed and external distractors placed and activated. They suggested that simultaneous genial distraction and arthroplasty may be performed in adults, as the mandible is no longer growing.

This is advocated in adults because they have functional stable occlusion. Therefore, distraction of the basal bone of the mandible without distracting the occlusion bearing segment will only correct the mandibular deformity and the OSAS, but not interfere with the occlusion. However, in children, dental relationships due to mandibular hypoplasia may be very severe and therefore this may not be the treatment of choice. Also, the eruption of the permanent teeth may interfere in osteotomy used in this technique.

Genial distraction is an option to gain larger advancements, although may be limited by an unsightly labiomental fold as advancement increases.

65.9.2.4 **Unidirectional DO** (Fig. 65.14a–i)

This procedure is indicated in patients with near normal ramal height but deficient corpus length, chin retrusion and deviation greater than 10 mm, and presence of mild to moderate OSA.

For deficient corpus length, osteotomy cut is placed in the body region, generally between second premolar and first molar or between first and second molars. If the patient has not undergone presurgical orthodontics or if distraction is being performed pre-ankylosis release, the cut depends on the distance between the roots of the teeth and presence of impacted teeth. Maria B. Papageorge [49] advised that the cut should be placed in such a manner that the integrity of mandibular angle is maintained as it forms a very important aesthetic component of the face.

According to Samchukov, the vector of distraction should always be parallel to the occlusal plane, regardless of the direction of the osteotomy, to prevent anterior open bite deformity. Kunz et al. [50] has stated it to be a well-known complication of mandibular distraction. Unidirectional distraction is contraindicated in patients exhibiting vertical growth pattern. This is because unidirectional distraction in patients with a steep mandibular plane angle and substantially deficient ramal height may again lead to anterior open bite.

Internal distraction has a definite edge over external distraction in terms of aesthetics and patient compliance. However, chances of postoperative infection are greater with internal distractors. Also, they have limitations in terms of the amount of distraction possible.

Unidirectional distractors may be placed through either intraoral or extraoral approach. Surgical splints may be prepared on 3D-printed models preoperatively. Upon exposure of the bone, these premarked splints are positioned. Using them as guides, corticotomy sites and sites for distractor pins/screws are marked. Buccal corticotomy and lower border full-thickness cuts are placed. Distractor is fixed and the osteotomy cuts are completed. In case impacted teeth are in the way of the osteotomy cuts, they may be removed intraoperatively itself.

The distractors are activated to check completeness of the cuts and then brought back. Latency period is of 5–7 days, depending on the patient's age. Larger movements require larger periods of consolidation to prevent relapse.

After distracting for around 8–10 days, shape of the regenerate may be changed (callus molding) during the distraction process. Complications may include infection, tooth fracture, change of vector, loosening of pin, anterior open bite, and parotid fistula, but all can be managed conservatively. Callous molding can take care of occlusal discrepancies to a large extent, except that if there is absolutely no overjet. However, with some amount of overjet present, differential distraction may be done on the superior and inferior borders of the mandible. Herein, with the help of callous molding using IMF screws/eyelets and elastics, the inferior border may be distracted more than the superior border.

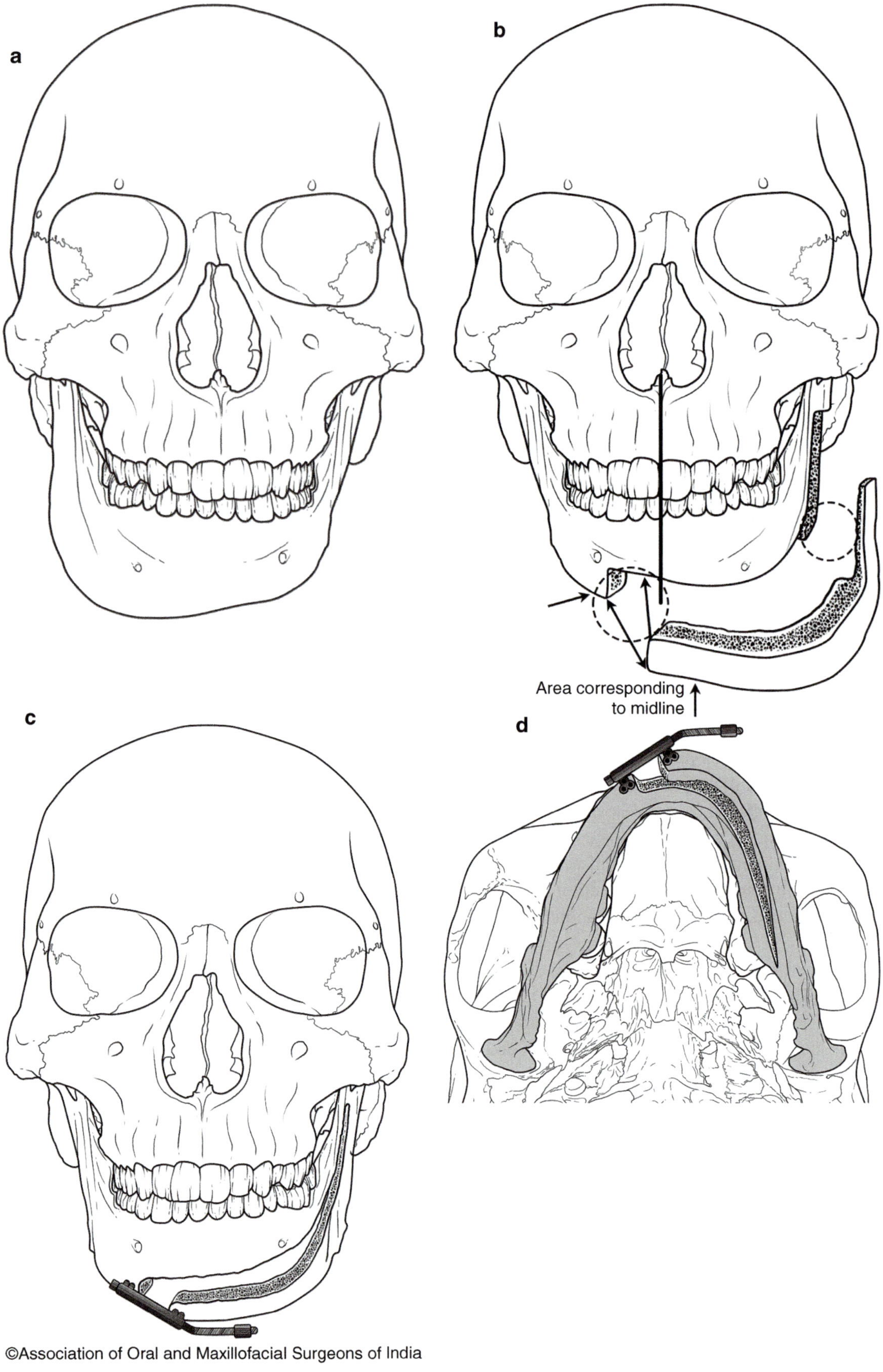

Fig. 65.13 (**a, b**) Orthomorphic osteotomy, (**c, d**) orthomorphic distraction

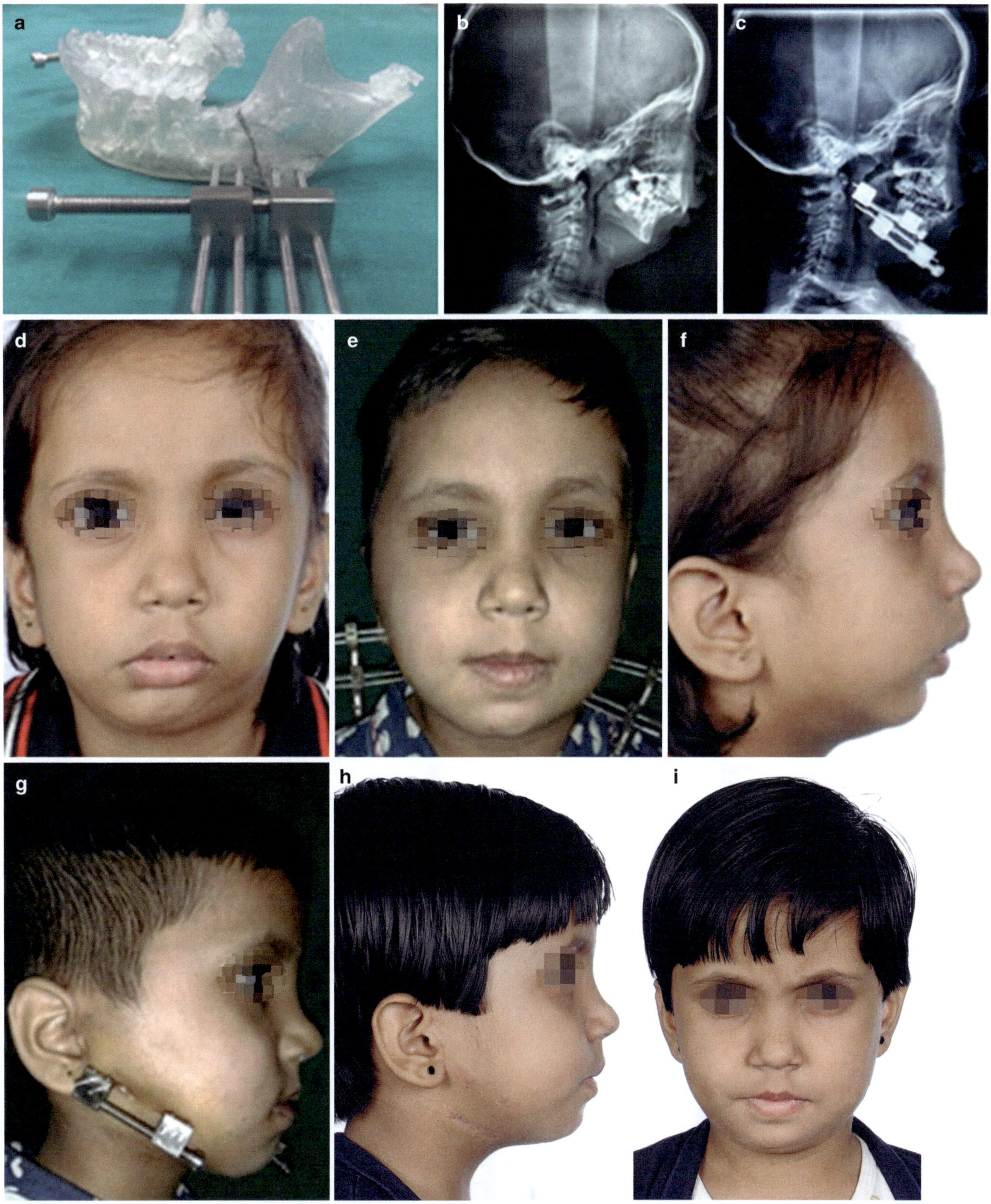

Fig. 65.14 (**a**) Uniplanar distractor fixed on the 3D stereolithographic model with osteotomy cut marked, (**b**) preoperative lateral cephalogram, (**c**) post-distraction lateral cephalogram, (**d**) preoperative frontal view, (**e**) post-distraction, frontal view (**f**) preoperative lateral view, (**g**) post-distraction lateral view, (**h**) six-month follow-up lateral, (**i**) six month follow-up frontal

Sometimes there may be occlusal locking thereby preventing the distracted regenerate from moving in the direction that is required. A composite block may be prepared on the tooth to first disocclude it and thereby get distraction in the favorable direction. Later occlusion may be regained by callous molding. The molding of the regenerate substantially reduces the time required for post operative orthodontics.

65.9.2.5 Bidirectional DO (Fig. 65.15a–g)

Bidirectional distractors are indicated for patients with severely shortened ramal height as well as corpal (body) length, requiring vertical as well as horizontal components of distraction. They are also indicated in cases with increased mandibular plane angle as well as for patients with moderate to severe OSA.

Surgical splints are prepared on 3D-printed models. Upon exposure of bone through a submandibular incision, two osteotomy cuts are placed on either side. One osteotomy cut is placed on the ramus and the other in the body region on either side of the angle, keeping the intermediate segment between 2.5 and 3 cm to avoid avascular necrosis. The device is secured to the mandible with six percutaneous pins (Schantz' pins)—one pair each at the ramus, angle, and corpus. The same procedure may be used for internal distractors as well.

The osteotomy site depends on position of teeth, lingula, mental foramen, and size of the intermediate segment. Vector of horizontal distraction should be parallel to occlusal plane, and vector of vertical distraction should be parallel to posterior border of ramus. In bilateral cases, horizontal and vertical components of either side should be parallel to each other. A 2–3 mm overcorrection is generally advisable. Callous molding may be used for occlusal adjustments. A single osteotomy cut may however be used for 3D or multivector distractors, thereby considerably reducing the surgical difficulty as well as the intraoperative time. Their main drawback is their prohibitive cost.

65.9.2.6 Impact of Mandibular DO on OSA

The ankylotic retruded mandible has an inefficient genial muscular apparatus as well, thereby causing retroglossal airway obstruction, therefore, OSAS. Mandibular advancement

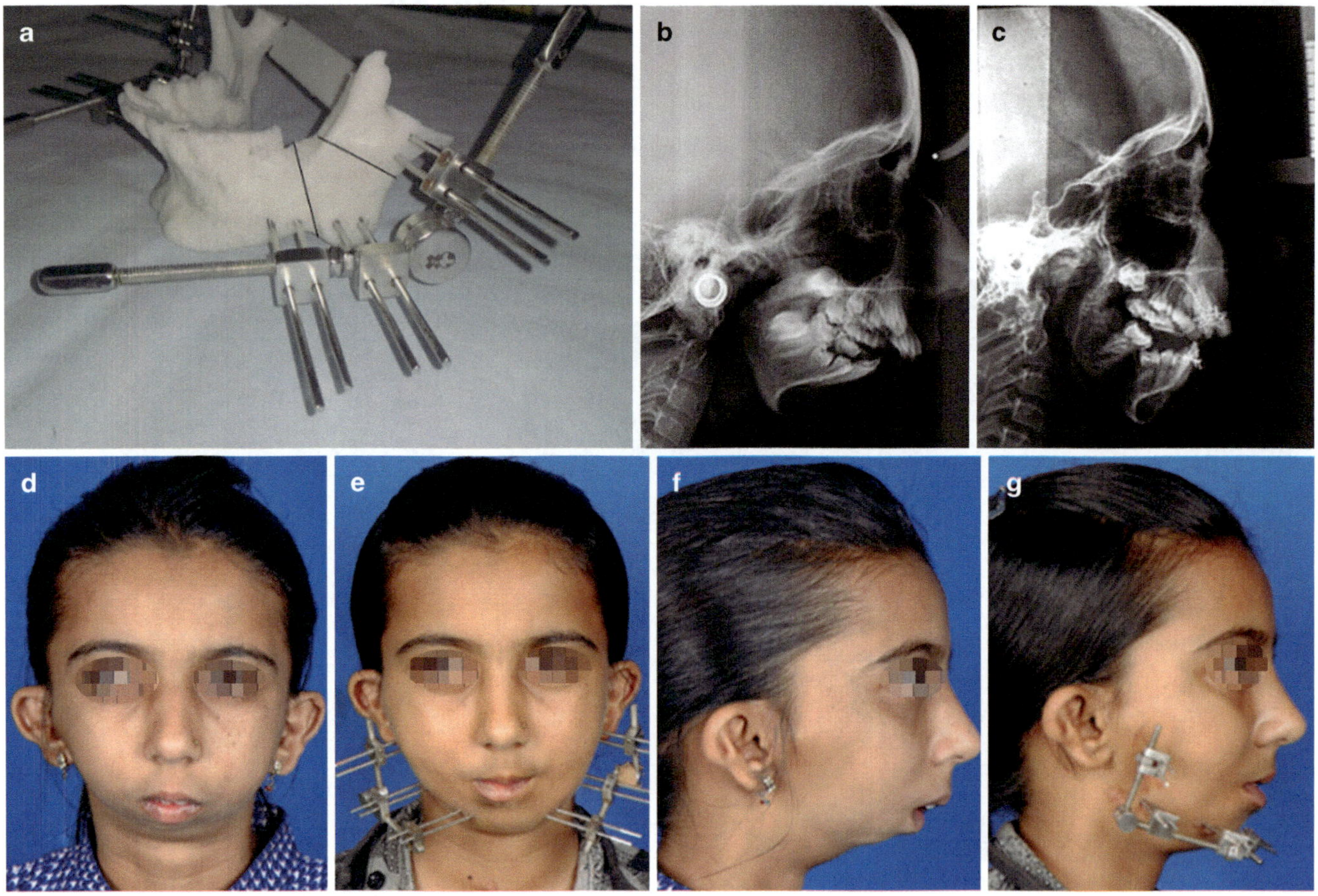

Fig. 65.15 (**a**) Biplanar distractor fixed on the 3D stereolithographic model with osteotomy cuts marked, (**b**) preoperative lateral cephalogram, (**c**) post-distraction lateral cephalogram (marked increase in PAS can be appreciated) (**d**) preoperative frontal view, (**e**) post-distraction frontal view, (**f**) preoperative lateral view, (**g**) post-distraction lateral view

in such cases has shown 97% success in pediatric and 100% success in adult patients. Decrease in OSAS may be evaluated by an AHI less than 50% decrease in the AHI with a near normal peripheral oxygen saturation.

65.10 Sequence of Release and Deformity Correction

OSA, in terms of AHI and PAS, is the principal factor that determines the sequence of release and deformity correction, i.e., whether to release first or distract first (refer Chap. 71 on OSAS and Figs. 71.8, 71.9, 71.10, 71.11, 71.12, 71.13 and 71.14).

Single-Stage vs. Multistage Procedure:

Treatment protocols can generally be categorized into single-stage or multistage treatments. Single-stage treatments institute ankylosis release and correction of secondary deformities (in the form of maxillary and mandibular osteotomies or distraction) all together. In the multistage protocol, ankylosis is released, and deformities are corrected in different stages.

65.10.1 Multistage Surgical Treatment

Severe secondary deformities are candidates for multistage procedures as a single-stage surgery may cause severe malocclusion. Correction of the same would require unrealistic amount of tooth movement.

Advantages: The multistage protocol is generally better for patients with significant medical comorbidity. This is so because a single-stage procedure obviously demands greater surgical time, thereby increasing the intraoperative risks. Multistage procedures facilitate early postoperative physiotherapy and, thus, a more stable postsurgical outcome. Also, the relapse monitoring is easier.

Disadvantages: Multiple surgeries, increased cost, and patient compliance issues

65.10.1.1 Multistage with Ankylosis Release First

According to López et al. [51], mandibular distraction should be performed after ankylosis release, as only then would be complete growth potential of the mandible be known. Releasing the ankylosis first would ensure adequate food intake, preparing the patients for subsequent, more complex surgeries. Also, surgeons could then formulate customized treatment plans based on individual clinical requirements and thereby provide more accurate correction of the deformity.

65.10.1.2 Multistage with Distraction First

Some surgeons recommend that distraction may be first used to restore the length and projection of the mandible. Later arthroplasty may be followed by orthognathic surgery to obtain mouth opening and settle the occlusion.

Advantages: The mandibular bone deficiency and the airway volume are both increased simultaneously. The subsequent intubation is much safer. Secondly, for patients with OSA, this treatment sequence reduces the incidence of postoperative airway issues—if ankylosis is released first, as the mandible falls back specially in bilateral cases, the already reduced airway space then gets further reduced, requiring reintubation or emergency tracheostomy. This incident can be avoided if distraction proceeds release.

65.10.2 Single-Stage Surgical Treatment

Patients with mild to moderate dental and skeletal deformities are ideal candidates for single-stage procedures. The minimal malocclusion may be treated by orthodontics alone. In these such cases, ankylosis release along with facial aesthetic surgeries which do not involve the occlusion may be performed, e.g., genioplasty, mandibular recontouring, and alloplastic implants.

Advantages: This corrects the restricted mouth opening as well as the secondary deformity simultaneously and avoids further surgeries. It provides low cost, immediate satisfaction, particularly in patients with psychological issues, and mild OSA.

Disadvantages: Maxillomandibular fixation often required after orthognathic surgery interferes with postoperative mouth opening exercises and therefore increases the chances of re-ankylosis. In case of internal distraction devices, there still arises the need for a second surgery to remove it. Also, the effect of distraction may be unsatisfactory because of the unstable condyle—if the osteotomy is placed in the ramus, the proximal segment may go up into the gap created after ankylotic mass removal, cause loss of vector and thereby re-ankylosis. Thus, to prevent this complication, while performing concomitant release and distraction, osteotomy cut may be placed only anterior to the angle, in the body region.

Another potential complication is the interference between physical exercises and distraction. A pseudo-joint may be formed in the callus area when the patient exercises, with the mouth opening force being directed toward the callus instead of the newly released joint. To prevent this complication, intensive active mouth opening exercise with wooden sticks/heisters may be started from postoperative day 1 itself. Mouth opening exercise from day 7 onward, i.e., once distraction is started, should exclude the use of the above.

65.10.2.1 Single-Stage Release with Orthognathic Surgery (OGS)

As mentioned earlier, in patients that exhibit mild dental and skeletal deformities, aesthetic surgeries not involving the tooth-bearing segments may be performed.

For the patients with moderate skeletal deformities, SSO along with ILRO and bone grafts may be used to lengthen the affected ramus. If necessary, Le Fort I osteotomy may be used to correct the occlusal cant in unilateral cases or bring the posterior maxilla down in bilateral cases.

Songsong Zhu [52] performed a study on 27 adult patients who underwent simultaneous ankylosis release and correction of secondary deformity as a single surgery. No relapse occurred.

Yi Hui Hu [42] studied 11 patients where CAD/CAM technique was utilized as a guide to determine level of removal of ankylotic mass and placement of TMJ prosthesis. Simultaneous Le Fort I osteotomy was performed in two patients guided by digital templates. Results showed that alloplastic TMJ prosthesis is a reliable treatment for recurrent ankylosis. The CAD/CAM technique produces accurate therefore stable results.

Many cases would require a custom-made prosthesis, typically fabricated with a stereolithographic model. Ryu et al. in 2016 reported a case where bilateral TM joints were replaced with a custom-made TMJ prosthesis. Virtual surgical planning (VSP) and STL model simulation helped in placing the mandible in a new improved occlusal and aesthetic profile [53]. This has become a routine procedure now in adult patients, i.e., custom-made joints based on VSP along with simultaneous OGS.

65.10.2.2 Single-Stage Release with DO

Simultaneous interpositional arthroplasty with DO for TMJ ankylosis, apart from increasing the length of the mandible, leads to the correction of gross facial asymmetry and midline shift and provides space for eruption of hitherto unerupted teeth. It helps reduce treatment time and need for an additional surgery and also alleviates the need for second tracheostomy, if the fiberoptic intubation is not possible.

Only unidirectional distraction in the mandibular body (in patients with AHI 15–30) may be performed along with release. If bidirectional distraction is performed, after placing the arthroplasty cuts, if two more cuts are placed in the body and the ramus, there are increased chances of avascular necrosis of the segments. Thus, bidirectional distraction may not be performed along with release; it may be performed either pre- or post-release, unless a 3D distractor is being used.

Krishna Rao et al. [54] performed a study on six patients and concluded that simultaneous release with DO should be used to correct ankylosis with facial asymmetry and reported satisfactory cosmetic correction of deformities. Girish B Giraddi et al. [55] performed a similar study with nine cases and concluded that it not only corrects the facial deformity but also saves the trauma of a second difficult intubation.

Lopez and Dogliotti [51] in 2004 asked a pertinent question—"Is it reasonable to perform ankylosis release and mandibular distraction simultaneously without knowing which patients will be able to experience growth with time? In that case it would be necessary to predict growth to apply the exact amount of mandibular distraction for obtaining stable results." This question can now be answered—in children, the only indications for simultaneous release with distraction would be moderate to severe OSA, with AHI 15–30 (however with normal ramal height) and extreme facial deformity causing issues with the child's psyche.

65.10.2.3 Single-Stage Release with Genioplasty

Most literature till date has either been looking at ankylosis in isolation from facial asymmetry and has been dealing with only ankylosis release or facial deformity as staged events or has been looking at correcting one of the biggest facial deformities, all at one go. There is no middle path mentioned in literature wherein ankylosis and a substantial part of its related deformities can be corrected without the following problems—a supra-major surgery under general anesthesia, extremely expensive 3D-printed splints and alloplastic joint replacements, expensive and protracted orthodontics requiring multiple hospital visits from the underprivileged, undernourished patients living in far-flung areas, and long-term patient noncompliance for distraction. Also, if osteotomies are performed before the TMJ attains stability, surgical outcome may be less than satisfactory as related to aesthetics and occlusion.

A suggested solution for the above problem in adults with mild to moderate OSA is a single-stage surgery—ankylosis release by interpositional arthroplasty simultaneously with genioplasty. It would provide a one-step solution to restoration of function and reasonable aesthetics within a reasonable amount of general anesthesia time, no occlusal discrepancies, no compliance for distraction, and no need for orthodontics. Most importantly, it would not interfere with any other secondary corrective procedure later, if the patient so desires.

The author has conducted a study on 43 ankylosed joints & set forth single-staged treatment guidelines—ankylosis release, RCU reconstruction, and extended advancement centering genioplasty for increase in mouth opening, restoration of ramal height, and improvement in facial asymmetry as well as OSA. Average mouth opening at maximum follow-up of 20 months was 34.36 mm with no reported recurrence. Average increase in N perpendicular to Pog was 7.16 mm, average decrease in neck-chin angle and labiomental angle was 31.6° and 35.4°; respectively, average increase in PAS was 2.92 mm. Average 50% improvement of AHI was seen in all 18 patients who had OSA [56].

65.11 Guidelines for sequencing of release and deformity correction

65.11.1 In Ankylosed Patients: To Decide Regarding Distraction Pre-/Post-/Simultaneously with Release (Table 65.5)

- AHI >30: Children and adults—distract first
- AHI <15
  - Children
    - Release first
    - Simultaneous release and unidirectional distraction
  - Adult
    - Release first
    - Simultaneous release with/without joint replacement and osteotomies
    - Simultaneous release and unidirectional distraction
- AHI 15–30
  - Short ramus (requiring bidirectional distraction)
    Children and adults: distract first
  - Normal ramus (requiring unidirectional distraction)
    - Children: simultaneous release and distraction
    - Adults
      - Joint replacement with osteotomies
      - Simultaneous release with distraction

Table 65.5 Relation of Apnea-hypoapnea index with PAS

PAS (mm)	AHI	Rating
>8	<5	Normal
8	5–10	Mild sleep apnea
5–7	15–30	Moderate sleep apnea
<4	>30	Severe sleep apnea

65.11.2 In Released Patients: To Decide Regarding Type of DO

- Only body deficiency with normal Mandibular Plane Angle (MPA)—unidirectional distraction
- Body and ramus deficiency with steep MPA—bidirectional distraction
- AHI >30—bidirectional distraction
- Asymmetry of mandibular angles—one side unidirectional, one side bidirectional distraction
- Dysmorphic asymmetry: orthomorphic distraction
- Functional occlusion in adults with normal ramus: genial distraction

65.12 Unfavorable Results in TMJ Ankylosis Surgery (Table 65.6)

Table 65.6

1. Issues in primary surgery
(a) ***Incomplete appreciation of the extent of the deformity***
(i) Unilateral or bilateral
(ii) Length of the coronoid process
(b) ***Anaesthesia-related issues***
(i) Excessive bleeding during fibreoptic intubation
(ii) Emergency tracheostomy
(c) ***Intra- and immediate postoperative issues***
(i) Surgical mishaps
1. Nerve traction
2. Inadequate exposure of the bony block
3. Bleeding from pterygoid venous plexus
4. Injury to the internal maxillary artery
(ii) Failure to achieve adequate mouth opening
1. Ipsilateral joint release → ipsilateral coronoidectomy → contralateral intraoral coronoidotomy
(iii) Severe bradycardia on mouth opening
(iv) Postoperatively open bite after bilateral arthroplasty/coronoidectomy
(d) ***Intermediate and long-term issues following primary surgery***
(i) Re-ankylosis—reasons
1. Incomplete or inadequate primary release
2. Inadequate mouth opening exercises
(ii) Growth alterations of costochondral graft
2. Issues related to secondary surgery of deformities
(a) No control of movement of proximal segment
(b) Careful calculation of the vector

65.13 Conclusion

- Traditionally, TMJ ankylosis and its associated micrognathia have been treated in multiple stages. Rehabilitation of mandibular function, prevention of re-ankylosis, and promotion of mandibular growth have been the main aims of treatment. The treatment has now advanced from only ankylosis release to total joint replacement as well as facial deformity correction, all simultaneously as far as possible.

- The patient at the time of presentation itself is looked at holistically. A more nuanced decision tree for treatment planning is formulated, be it for release, new joint reconstruction, distraction, osteotomies, or the sequencing of release vs. facial deformity correction. The most critical deciding factor in the treatment planning is obstructive sleep apnea, and the key for successful treatment is appropriate planning at each stage.
- Therefore, just because in the past, we were releasing all ankylosis first and doing corrective surgeries later, we cannot continue doing the same; albeit neither can we distract all patients first because that is the latest fad. An extensive review of literature as well as the vast experience of the author has helped lay down guidelines for most clinical scenarios of varying magnitude of deformities in TMJ ankylosis.
- In a few patients, some degree of facial imbalance may continue to persist even after surgical interventions. Additional aesthetic surgery, such as malarplasty reshaping of the chin, angle and lower border of the mandible, may be required to achieve the best results [57].
- Since TMJ ankylosis is generally a disease of the underprivileged and socioeconomically backward strata of society, it should be noted that the deformity cannot be the only criteria to select the surgical procedure. Patient's preference, the treatment cost, and compliance also need to be taken into consideration. Some patients are more concerned about their mouth opening and aesthetics rather than their occlusal disharmony.

Acknowledgment I wish to convey my deepest thanks and sincerest gratitude to my resident Dr. Hrushikesh Gosai, without whose observations, comments, and technical expertise this manuscript would have not been possible. A mere word of thanks is not sufficient to express the unflinching support and inestimable aid of my staff Dr. Jigar, Dr. Utsav, and Dr. Bipin and my residents Dr. Hiral, Dr. Philip and Dr. Nisha during the preparation of this chapter. I would be failing in my duty if I did not recognize the contribution of my biggest teacher in TMJ ankylosis, my Ex-Hod Dr. Babu Parmar.

Disclosure Authors have no financial conflicts to disclose

65.14 Case Scenarios

Case 1 (Fig. 65.16a–h)

A 23-year-old male patient presented with unilateral right-sided bony ankylosis with retruded and deviated chin with body and ramal length near normal. So, the patient was planned for advancement centering genioplasty and onlay bone graft along with TMJ ankylosis release.

Case 2 (Fig. 65.17a–f)

A 14-year-old male patient presented with facial asymmetry secondary to TMJ ankylosis with moderate OSA. Cephalometric analysis revealed deficiencies in the length of the mandibular ramus and corpus of the right side and the corpus alone on the left side. So, he was planned for biplanar distraction on right side and uniplanar distraction on left side.

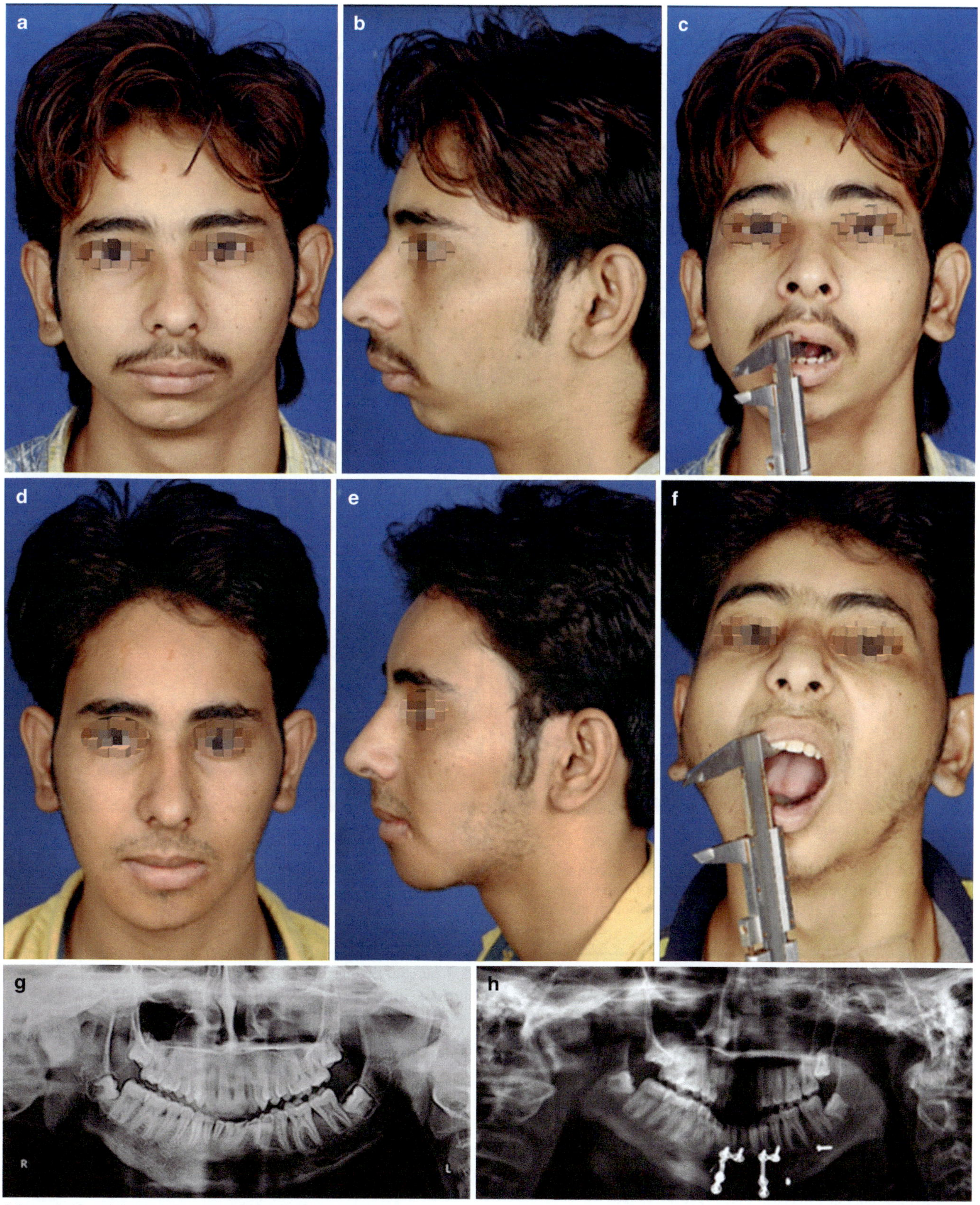

Fig. 65.16 (a–h) Case 1 Right side TMJ ankylosis (**a**) Preoperative frontal view, (**b**) preoperative lateral view, (**c**) preoperative mouth opening, (**d**) postoperative frontal view, (**e**) postoperative lateral view, (**f**) postoperative mouth opening, (**g**) preoperative orthopantomogram, (**h**) postoperative orthopantomogram (note the genioplasty and onlay bone graft fixations)

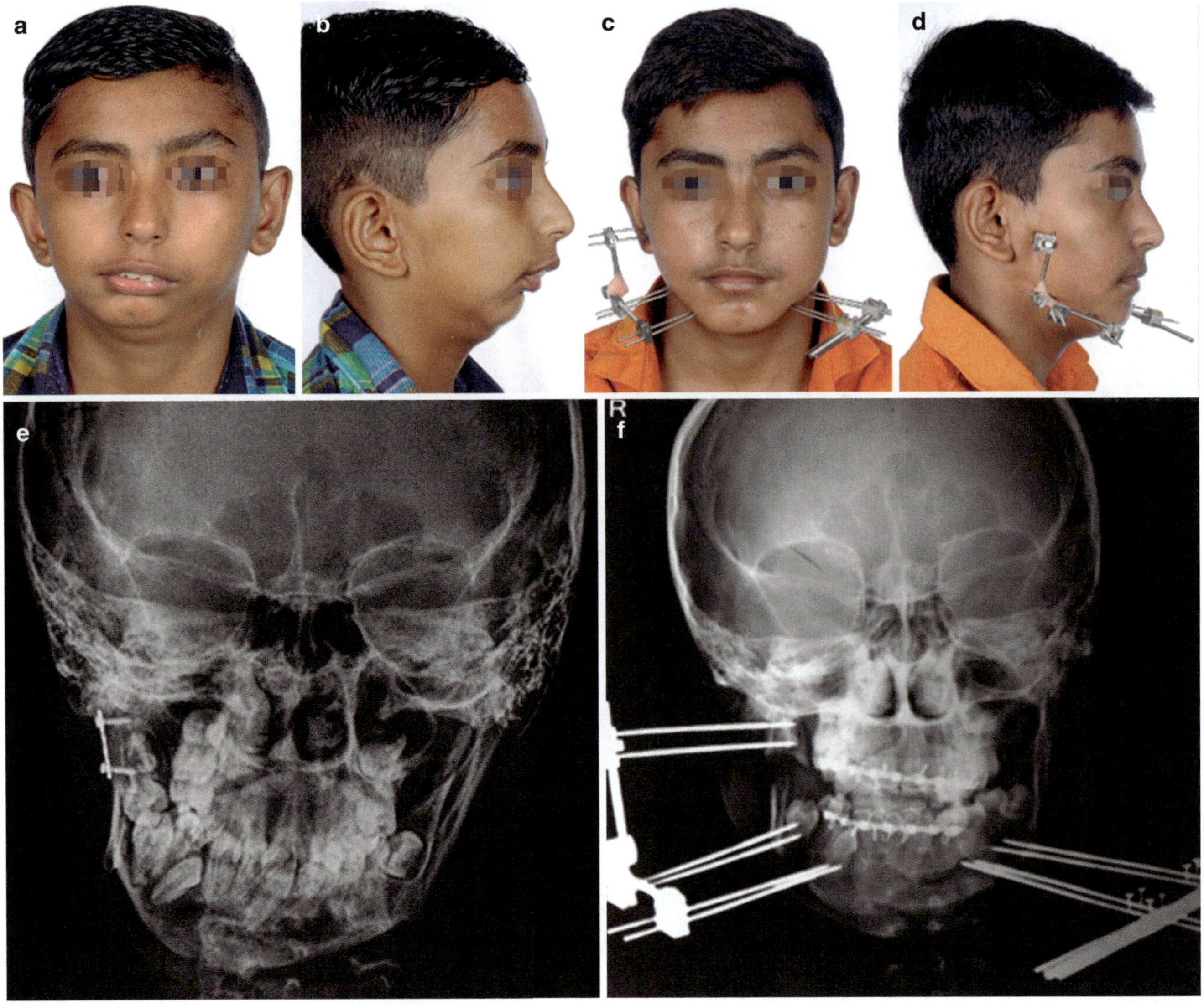

Fig. 65.17 Case 2 (**a**) Preoperative frontal view, (**b**) preoperative lateral view, (**c**) postoperative frontal view, (**d**) postoperative lateral view, (**e**) Pre-distraction PA cephalogram, showing implant on the right side from the earlier surgery for interposition arthroplasty, (**f**) postoperative PA cephalogram

References

1. Sporniak-Tutak K, Janiszewska-Olszowska J, Kowalczyk R. Management of temporomandibular ankylosis—compromise or individualization—a literature review. Med Sci Monit. 2011;17(5):RA111–6.
2. Kaban LB, Perrott DH, Fisher K. A protocol for management of temporomandibular joint ankylosis. J Oral Maxillofac Surg. 1990;48:1145–51.
3. Sawhney C. Bony ankylosis of the temporomandibular joint: follow—up of 70 patients treated with arthroplasty and acrylic space interposition. Plast Reconstr Surg. 1986;77:29–38.
4. Yan Y-B, Liang S-X, Shen J, Zhang J-C, Zhang Y. Current concepts in the pathogenesis of traumatic temporomandibular joint ankylosis. Head Face Med. 2014;10:35.
5. Mehrotra D, Sidebottom AJ. Management of ankylosis of the temporomandibular joint. In: Brennan P, Schliephake H, Ghali GE, Cascarini L, editors. Maxillofacial surgery. 3rd ed. Edinburgh: Churchill Livingstone; 2017.
6. Aziz SR. Andy Gump and his deformity. J Oral Maxillofac Surg. 2010;68(3):651–3.
7. Anantanarayanan P, Narayanan V, Manikandhan R, Kumar D, et al. Int J Pediatr Otorhinolaryngol. 2008;72:385–9.
8. Andrade NN, Raikwar KR. Management of patients with obstructive sleep apnoea induced by temporomandibular joint ankylosis: a novel 2-stage surgical protocol and report of 5 cases. Asian J Oral Maxillofac Surg. 2009;21:27–32.
9. Wu XG, Hong M, Sun KH. Severe osteoarthrosis after fracture of the mandibular condyle: a clinical and histologic study of seven patients. J Oral Maxillofac Surg. 1994;52(2):138–42.
10. Dhasmana S, Singh V, Pal US. Awake blind nasotracheal intubation in temporomandibular joint ankylosis patients under conscious sedation using fentanyl and midazolam. J Maxillofac Oral Surg. 2010;9(4):377–81.

11. Quinn PD, Granquist EJ ; Surgical approaches to temporomandibular joint; In: Quinn PD, Granquist EJ (eds) Atlas of temporomandibular joint surgery 2 Wiley Chichester 2015, 31–55.
12. Al-Kayat A, Bramley P. A modified pre-auricular approach to the temporomandibular joint and malar arch. Br J Oral Surg. 1979;17:91–103.
13. Miloro M, Redlinger S, Pennington DM, Kolodge T. In situ location of the temporal branch of the facial nerve. J Oral Maxillofac Surg. 2007;65:2466–9.
14. Talebzadeh N, Rosenstein TP, Pogrel MA. Anatomy of the structures medial to the temporomandibular joint. Oral Surg Oral Med Oral Pathol Oral Radiol Endod. 1999;88:674–8.
15. Alexander RW, James RB. Postauricular approach for surgery of the temporomandibular articulation. J Oral Surg. 1975;33:346–50.
16. Kaban LB, Bouchard C, Troulis MJ. A protocol for management of temporomandibular joint ankylosis in children. J Oral Maxillofac Surg. 2009;67(9):1966–78.
17. Clarkson P, Kenshole HH. Esmarch's operation for the relief of ankylosis and of pain in the temporomandibular joint; a modified operative technique. Br Dental J. 1949;87:257–64.
18. Topazian RG. Etiology of ankylosis of temporomandibular joint: analysis of 44 cases. J Oral Surg Anesth Hosp Dent Serv. 1964;22:227–33.
19. Topazian RG. Comparison of gap and interposition arthroplasty in the treatment of temporomandibular joint ankylosis. J Oral Surg Am Dent Assoc. 1966;24:405–9.
20. Elgazzar RF, Abdelhady AI, Saad KA, Elshaal MA, Hussain MM, Abdelal SE, Sadakah AA. Treatment modalities of TMJ ankylosis: experience in Delta Nile, Egypt. Int J Oral Maxillofac Surg. 2010;39:333–42.
21. He Y, Huang T, Zhang Y, An J, He L. Application of a computer-assisted surgical navigation system in temporomandibular joint ankylosis surgery: a retrospective study. Int J Oral Maxillofac Surg. 2017;46:189–97.
22. Ray PDA, Sundar Biswas DP, Chatterjee DA. Trismus—an old concept for successful treatment in the present era—case reports. IOSR J Dent Med Sci. 2016;15(9):12–6.
23. He D, Yang C, Chen M, Zhang X, Qiu Y, Yang X, Li L, Fang B. Traumatic temporomandibular joint ankylosis: our classification and treatment experience. J Oral Maxillofac Surg. 2011;69:1600–7.
24. Nitzan DW, Tair JA, Lehman H. Is entire removal of a post-traumatic temporomandibular joint ankylotic site necessary for an optimal outcome? J Oral Maxillofac Surg. 2012;70(12:e683–99.
25. Yang X, Lu C, Dong M, He D, Yang C, Hu Y. Evaluation of the condyle remodeling after lateral arthroplasty in growing children with temporomandibular joint ankylosis. Sci Rep. 2017;7:1–827.
26. Albert TW, Merrill RG. Temporalis myofascial for reconstruction of temporomandibular joint. Oral Maxillofac Surg Clin North Am. 1989;1:346.
27. Pogrel MA, Kaban LB. The role of a temporalis fascia and muscle flap in temporomandibular joint surgery. J Oral Maxillofac Surg. 1990;48:14–9.
28. Dimitroulis G. The interpositional dermis-fat graft in the management of temporomandibular joint ankylosis. Int J Oral Maxillofac Surg. 2004;33:755–60.
29. Thangavelu A, Thiruneelakandan S, Prasath CH, Chatterjee D. Fate of free fat dermis graft in TMJ interpositional gap arthroplasty: a long term MRI study. J Maxillofac Oral Surg. 2015;14(2):321–6.
30. Gaba S, Sharma RK, Rattan V, Khandelwal N. The long-term fate of pedicled buccal pad fat used for interpositional arthroplasty in TMJ ankylosis. J Plast Reconstr Aesthet Surg. 2012;65:1468–73.
31. Akhter M, Ahmed N, Arefin MRU, Sobhan MU, Molla MR, Kamal M. Outcome of amniotic membrane as an interpositional arthroplasty of TMJ ankylosis. Oral Maxillofac Surg. 2016;20(1):63–71.
32. Gunaseelan R. Condylar reconstruction in extensive ankylosis of temporomandibular joint in adults using resected segment as autograft. A new technique. Int J Oral Maxillofac Surg. 1997;26:405–7.
33. Khadka A, Hu J. Autogenous grafts for condylar reconstruction in treatment of TMJ ankylosis: current concepts and considerations for the future. Int J Oral Maxillofac Surg. 2012;41:94–102.
34. Mehta G, Mohammad S, Ram H, Singh V, Chak RK, Garg S, Vishwakarma K. Re-assessment of coronoid as a graft for condylar reconstruction in TMJ ankylosis patients: a prospective study and literature review. J Maxillofac Oral Surg. 2017;16(2):175–80.
35. Liu Y, Li J, Hu J, Zhu S, Luo E, Hsu Y. Autogenous coronoid process pedicled on temporal muscle grafts for reconstruction of the mandible condylar in patients with temporomandibular joint ankylosis. Oral Surg Oral Med Oral Pathol Oral Radiol Endod. 2010;109(2):203–10.
36. Poswillo DE. Biological reconstruction of the mandibular condyle. Br J Oral Maxillofac Surg. 1987;25(2):100–4.
37. Salash JR, Hossameldin RH, Almarza AJ, Chou JC, McCain JP, Mercuri LG, Wolford LM, Detamore MS. Potential indications for tissue engineering in temporomandibular joint surgery. J Oral Maxillofac Surg. 2016;74:705–11.
38. Liu Y, Khadka A, Li J, Hu J, Zhu S, Hsu Y, Wang Q, Wang D. Sliding reconstruction of the condyle using posterior border of mandibular ramus in patients with temporomandibular joint ankylosis. Int J Oral Maxillofac Surg. 2011;40:1238–45.
39. Cheung LK, Zheng LW, Ma L, Shi XJ. Transport distraction versus costochondral graft for reconstruction of temporomandibular joint ankylosis: which is better? Oral Surg Oral Med Oral Pathol Oral Radiol Endod. 2009;108(1):32–40.
40. Sharma R, Manikandhan R, Sneha P, Parameswaran A, Kumar JN, Sailer H. Neocondyle distraction osteogenesis in the management of temporomandibular joint ankylosis: report of five cases with review of literature. Indian J Dent Res. 2017;28(3):269–74.
41. Xiao E, Zhang Y, An J, Li J, Long-term YY. Long-term evaluation of the stability of reconstructed condyles by transport distraction osteogenesis. Int J Oral Maxillofac Surg. 2012;41:1490–4.
42. Hu YH, Zhang L, He DM, Yang C, Chen MJ, Zhang SY, Li H, Ellis E. Simultaneous treatment of temporomandibular joint ankylosis with severe mandibular deficiency by standard TMJ prosthesis. Sci Rep. 2017;7:45271.
43. Movahed R, Mercuri LG. Management of temporomandibular joint ankylosis. Oral Maxillofac Surg Clin NA. 2015;27(1):27–35.
44. Salins PC, Venkatraman B, Kavarody M. Morphometric basis for orthomorphic correction of mandibular asymmetry. J Oral Maxillofac Surg. 2008;66:1523–31.
45. Kohn MW. Analysis of relapse after mandibular advancement surgery. J Oral Surg. 1978;36:676–84.
46. Ortiz Monasterio F, Molina F, Andrade L, Rodriguez C, Sainz Arregui J. Simultaneous mandibular and maxillary distraction in hemifacial microsomia in adults: avoiding occlusal disasters. Plast Reconstr Surg. 1997;100:852–61.
47. Parameswaran A, Ramanathan M, Pendem S, Jeyakumar N. Orthomorphic distraction—a new concept and its mechanics. J Cleft Lip Palate and Craniofac Anomal. 2013;4:1.
48. Gunaseelan R, Anantanarayanan P, Veerabahu M, Vikraman B. Simultaneous genial distraction and interposition arthroplasty for management of sleep apnoea associated with temporomandibular joint ankylosis. Int J Oral Maxillofac Surg. 2007;36:845–8.
49. Kunz C, Hammer B, Prein J. Manipulation of callus after linear distraction: a "lifeboat" or an alternative to multivectorial distraction osteogenesis of the mandible? Plast Reconstr Surg. 2000;105:674–9.
50. Papageorge MB, Apostolidis C. Simultaneous mandibular distraction and arthroplasty in a patient with temporomandibular joint ankylosis and mandibular hypoplasia. Case Rep. 1999;57(3):328–33.

51. Lopez EN, Dogliotti PL. Treatment of temporomandibular joint ankylosis in children: is it necessary to perform mandibular distraction simultaneously? J Craniofac Surg. 2004;15:875–9.
52. Zhu S, Jiang Y, Pokhrel N, Hu J. Simultaneous correction of temporomandibular joint ankylosis and secondary dentofacial deformities in adult patients: surgical technique, treatment outcomes, and a consideration of the factors involved. J Craniofac Surg. 2015;26:2351–6.
53. Ryu J, Cho J, Kim HM. Bilateral temporomandibular joint replacement using computer-assisted surgical simulation and three-dimensional printing. J Craniofac Surg. 2016;27:e450–2.
54. Rao K, Kumar S, Kumar V, Singh AK, Bhatnagar SK. The role of simultaneous gap arthroplasty and distraction osteogenesis in the management of temporo-mandibular joint ankylosis with mandibular deformity in children. J Craniomaxillofac Surg. 2004;5182:38–42.
55. Giraddi G, Arora K, Sai Anusha A. Distraction osteogenesis in the treatment of temporomandibular joint ankylosis with mandibular micrognathia. Ann Maxillofac Surg. 2016;6:68.
56. Anchlia S, Vyas SM, Dayatar RG, Domadia HL, Nagavadiya V. Guidelines for single-stage correction of TMJ ankylosis, facial asymmetry and OSA in adults. J Maxillofac Oral Surg. 2018;18(3):419–27.
57. Zhu S, Wang D, Yin Q, Hu J. Treatment guidelines for temporomandibular joint ankylosis with secondary dentofacial deformities in adults. J Cranio-Maxillofac Surg. 2013;41:e117–27.

Part XVIII

Orthognathic Surgery

Diagnosis and Planning in Orthognathic Surgery

66

Johan P. Reyneke and Carlo Ferretti

66.1 Introduction

Over the last four decades, the scientific foundations for the art of changing facial appearance and improving orofacial function through orthognathic surgery were laid, and the value of treatment to improve lives is undisputed. The main treatment objective is currently not limited to achieving short-term improved occlusal function but also enhanced facial aesthetics and an open airway. Orthognathic surgery requires the combined skills of the specialities of orthodontics and oral and maxillofacial surgery; however, there remain major limitations relating to the uneven geographical distribution of experienced dedicated clinicians and financial barriers to the correction of dentofacial deformities. The treatment of some malocclusions combined with mild skeletal disharmony is possible by orthodontic compensation of the dentition with compromised facial aesthetics. Borderline cases therefore require meticulous assessment before finally deciding on orthodontic treatment alone or a combination of orthodontics and surgery as treatment approach.

Most compromised treatments lead to suboptimal results such as:

- Dental instability
- Skeletal instability
- Poor facial aesthetics
- Airway problems
- Periodontal problems

Which treatment plan to adopt should be discussed with the patient (and perhaps the parents or spouse) and all the advantages and disadvantages of each approach explained. The decision may also be influenced by factors such as the orthodontist's experience, financial insurance cover, available surgical expertise, and the patient's attitude and preferences [1].

Patients with dentofacial deformities are treated with four prime goals in mind:

1. *Function.* Apart from establishing normal masticatory function, the clinicians should also consider other problems caused by an abnormal jaw relationship such as speech defects, sleep apnea, attrition of the teeth, periodontal problems, and temporomandibular joint problems.
2. *Stability of results.* Definitive orthognathic treatment is a change for life, and it is important to achieve dental and skeletal stability following treatment.
3. *Aesthetics.* Facial appearance is often the patient's main concern, but patients are often reticent to voice these concerns. However, the surgeon should resist the temptation to determine unilaterally what a patient's aesthetic concerns are but should encourage the patient to express these.
4. *Airway.* The impact of jaw malalignment (and its correction) on the patency of the upper airways is a relatively recent addition to the treatment considerations in patients with dentoskeletal malocclusion. The support of the retropharyngeal soft tissues is determined to a large degree by the position of the anterior osseous attachments. Inadequate support for

J. P. Reyneke (✉)
Director of The Center for Orthognathic Surgery, Mediclinic, Cape Town, South Africa

Department of Oral and Maxillofacial Surgery, Faculty of Health Sciences, University of the Western Cape, Cape Town, South Africa

Department of Oral and Maxillofacial Surgery, University of Oklahoma, Oklahoma City, OK, USA
e-mail: johanrey@worldonline.co.za

C. Ferretti
Department of Maxillofacial and Oral Surgery, University of Pretoria, Pretoria, South Africa

Private practice, Johannesburg, South Africa

K. Bonanthaya et al. (eds.), *Oral and Maxillofacial Surgery for the Clinician*, https://doi.org/10.1007/978-981-15-1346-6_66

these soft tissues will contribute greatly to the development of sleep apnea especially as soft tissue laxity develops with aging. This consideration may influence treatment decisions particularly in Class III malocclusion. For example, we may be loath to unduly setback a mandible in a young adult due the future potential for sleep apnea development. Thus, in double jaw surgery, a treatment plan that favors greater maxillary advancement or in a single jaw surgery case a maxillary advancement may be preferable to a mandibular setback. These considerations add a further layer of complexity to the treatment algorithm as airway considerations may mean a compromise of aesthetics and vice versa [2, 3].

66.2 Systematic Aesthetic Facial Evaluation

The clinical assessment of the face is the most valuable of all diagnostic procedures and should be performed in a systematic fashion. The facial examination should start at the first instant a clinician meets the patient and continues during the initial informal discussion. During this period the patient is not self-aware, and facial function and features will be at their most natural. The focused facial examination follows and should be done while the patient is seated comfortably in natural head posture, the teeth in centric occlusion and the lips relaxed. The goal of the facial examination is to determine what components of the face are detracting from facial harmony and what functional problems may accompany the malocclusion and to make a tentative diagnosis.

It is helpful to structure the facial examination into frontal and profile views [4].

66.2.1 Frontal View

Facial appearance when viewed from the front is, not surprisingly, what a patient will value most.

A helpful first step is to assess the facial form.

- Facial form (Fig. 66.1a–h)—The relationship between the facial width and height has a strong influence on facial harmony. The ratio of facial width to facial height is more important than absolute values in establishing the overall facial type. Attractive faces tend to have proportions that fall within normative values. When evaluating facial form, the overall body build of the individual (corporo-facial relationship) should be considered (i.e., short and stocky versus long and thin). The height-to-width proportion (trichion to menton: bizygomatic width) is 1.3:1 for females and 1.35:1 for males. The bigonial width should be approximately 30% less than the bizygomatic dimension, and the width and shape of the chin should form a harmonious part of the overall facial contour. Leptoprosopic faces (long and narrow) are often associated with vertical maxillary excess, a narrow nose, mandibular anteroposterior deficiency, narrow gonial angles, microgenia, a high palatal vault, and an anterior open bite (Fig. 66.1a–c), while dolichoprosopic faces (short and square) are often associated with vertical maxillary deficiency, masseter hyperplasia, wide gonial angles, macrogenia, and Class III deep bite malocclusions (Fig. 66.1d, e). Individuals from Asia often have round oval faces (Fig. 66.1f). Patients with mandibular deficiency often have a tapered facial lower facial third and microgenia (Fig. 66.1g, h).
- Transverse facial dimensions (Fig. 66.2)—In general terms the *rule of fifths* is a convenient method used to evaluate the transverse proportions of the face. The face is sagittally divided into five equal parts, each the approximate width of the eye, from helix of the outer ears.
  - *Outer fifths:* Is measured from the lateral helix of the ear to the lateral canthus and is an indication of the width of the ears. Bat ears can be camouflaged by an appropriate hairstyle; however, otoplastic surgical procedures are relatively atraumatic and can improve the facial appearance dramatically. Otoplasty can be performed at the same time as orthognathic procedures.
  - *Medial fifths:* Are measured from the outer to the inner canthus of the eyes. The outer border should coincide with the gonial angles of the mandible. In patients with long and narrow faces, the gonial angles will fall medial to this line, while in patients with broad and square faces, the gonial angles will fall lateral to these lines. Within these fifths it should be noted that the distance between the inner margins of the irides of the eyes should be equal to the width of the mouth. Abnormal interpupillary and intercanthal distance are often observed in syndromic patients and can only be altered by means of craniofacial surgery.
  - *Middle fifth:* Is demarcated by the lines through the inner canthus of the eyes. In patients with hypertelorism, this fifth would be relatively larger than the others. The ala of the nose (alar base width) should coincide with these lines, while the nasal dorsum

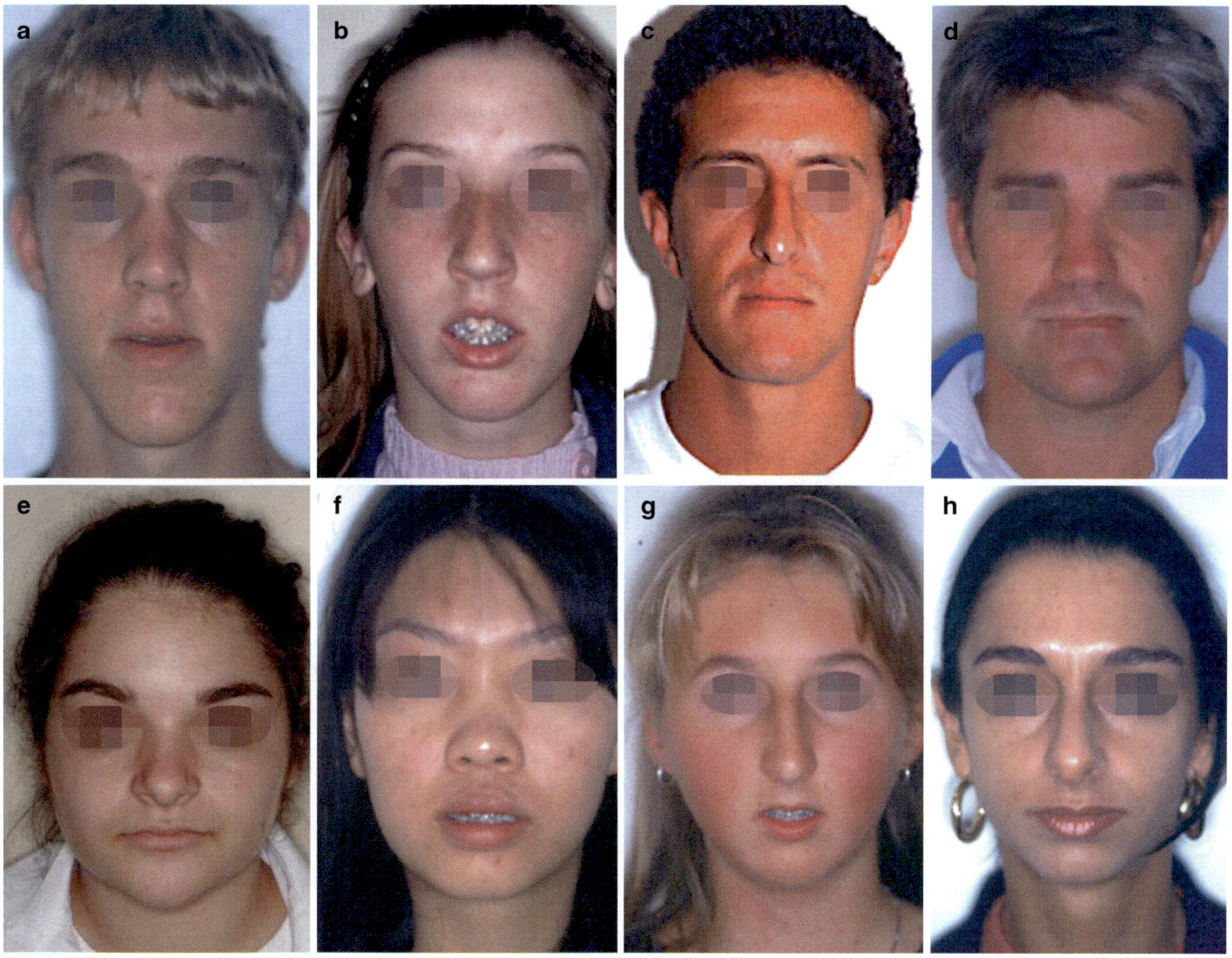

Fig. 66.1 The relationship between the facial height and width influences facial harmony. The variations of facial form: (**a**) narrow, (**b**) long, (**c**) tapered, (**d**) square, (**e**) round, (**f**) oval, (**g**) sharp, and (**h**) pointed, are demonstrated

should be approximately half of the intercanthal distance. For patients in whom maxillary advancement and/or superior repositioning is planned, this measurement should be considered and surgical control of the alar base may be indicated.

- Vertical evaluation (Fig. 66.3)—By convention the face is divided into three parts by horizontal lines adjacent to the hairline (trichion) to the soft tissue glabella, the nasal base (subnasale), and the lower border of the chin (menton). An aesthetically pleasing face should have approximate equivalence of the three parts.
  - *Upper third:* Deformities in this third can fortunately often be masked by an appropriate hairstyle; however, it is important to record deformities in this area as they may indicate craniofacial syndromes.
  - *Middle third:* Generally, no sclera is seen above and below the iris in a relaxed eyelid position. Individuals with midface deficiency tend to show sclera under the iris of the eye and will tend to have a long narrow nose. The cheekbone-nasal base-upper lip-lower lip contour line is a convenient indicator of the harmony of the structures of the midface (zygoma, maxilla, and nasal base) with the paranasal area and upper lip. This imaginary line starts just anterior to the ear, extends anteriorly across the cheekbone, and then curves antero-inferior over the maxilla adjacent to the alar

base of the nose, ending lateral and slightly below the commissure of the mouth. The line should form a smooth, continuous curve (Fig. 66.4a, c). A skeletal deformity will cause an interruption of the curve, and the area of interruption in the line is often an indication of a specific underlying deformity (Fig. 66.4b).

- *Lower third:* (Fig. 66.3) The middle to lower third vertical height of the face should have a 5:6 ratio. In the well-balanced lower third of the face, the upper lip makes up one third, while the lower lip and chin composes the lower two thirds. Normal upper lip length is 20 ± 2 mm for females and 22 ± 2 mm for males and measured from subnasale to upper lip sto-

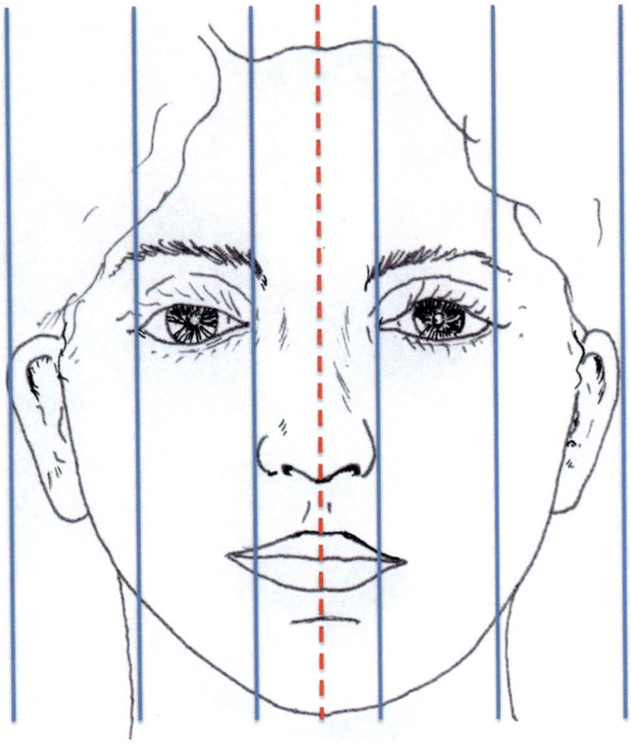

Fig. 66.2 Transverse facial proportions

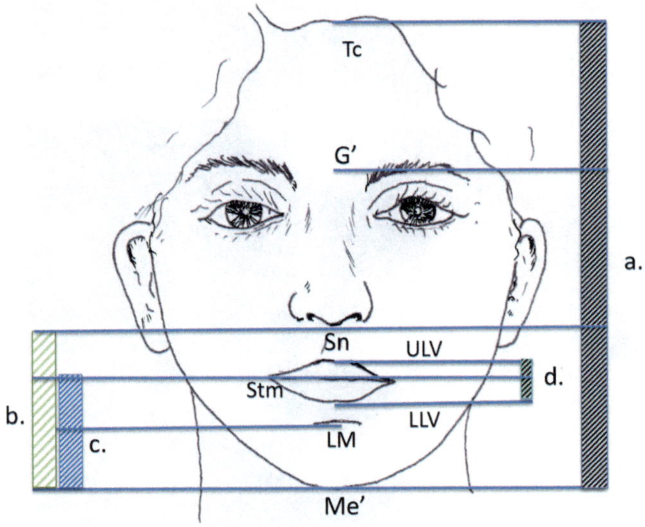

Fig. 66.3 Vertical facial proportions

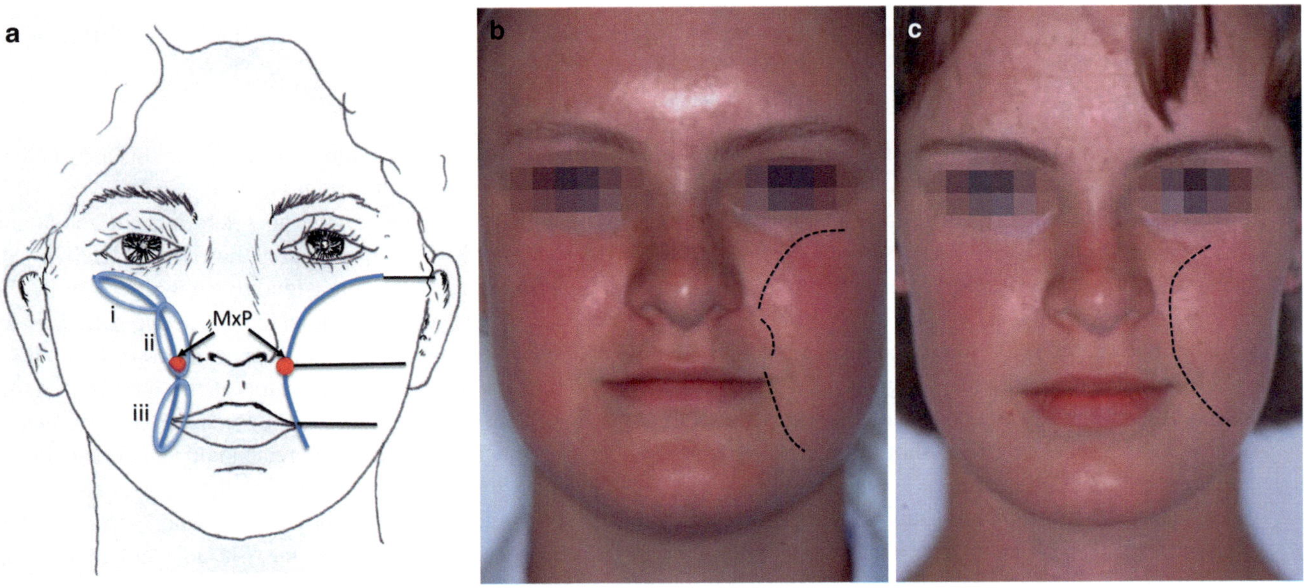

Fig. 66.4 (**a**) Cheekbone-nasal base-lip contour. (**b**) The interruption of the curve at MxP (maxillary plane) indicates maxillary anteroposterior deficiency. (**c**) Correction of the malocclusion establishes a smooth contour line

mion (stomion superius). When the upper lip is relatively short, there will be a tendency to an increased interlabial gap and excessive upper incisor exposure with normal facial height. This should not be confused with the same observations in patients with vertical maxillary excess (Fig. 66.8). Normal lower lip length is 40 ± 2 mm for females and 44 ± 2 mm for males. The lower lip may give the false impression of being short due to a deep bite. It is mandatory that the interlabial gap and tooth exposure be evaluated with the teeth in occlusion and the lips in repose (Fig. 66.8b). A gummy smile is not a definite indication of vertical maxillary excess as some patients may have a normal maxillary height but hyperactive upper lip when smiling. An increased interlabial gap (more than 3 mm), excessive upper incisor exposure (more than 4mm), and a gummy smile are typical characteristics of vertical maxillary excess (Fig. 66.9). For patients in whom the upper incisors are not visible under the upper lip, the tooth lip relationship should be evaluated with the mandible rotated open until the lips just separate (Fig. 66.8a). Lack of upper incisor exposure is indicative of vertical maxillary deficiency and usually occurs in combination with decreased lower facial height. The height of the lower face can also be influenced by the height of the mandible, and the height of the chin should be noted in any discrepancy in vertical facial height.

The arbitrary subdivision of the face into vertical thirds has a critical flaw. The effects of a deformity of one jaw and the correction thereof may stretch across two conventional facial thirds.

It is for this reason that the authors believe a more pragmatic approach to facial aesthetic assessment is to divide the face into zones of influence, i.e., zones which can be modified by orthodontics and orthognathic surgery.

The *Ferretti-Reyneke analysis* (Fig. 66.5) divides the face into five zones of influence, i.e., zones of soft tissue facial integument that are under the influence of the corresponding underlying skeleton:

- *The fore-head zone* (i). Extending from trichion (hairline) to a line connecting the eyebrows across glabella.
- *The oculonasal zone* (ii). Extending inferiorly from the eyebrow line to a line extending from the lower border of the zygomatic arch curving upward to the infraorbital foramen onto the nose above the supra tip break and continuing to the opposite side.

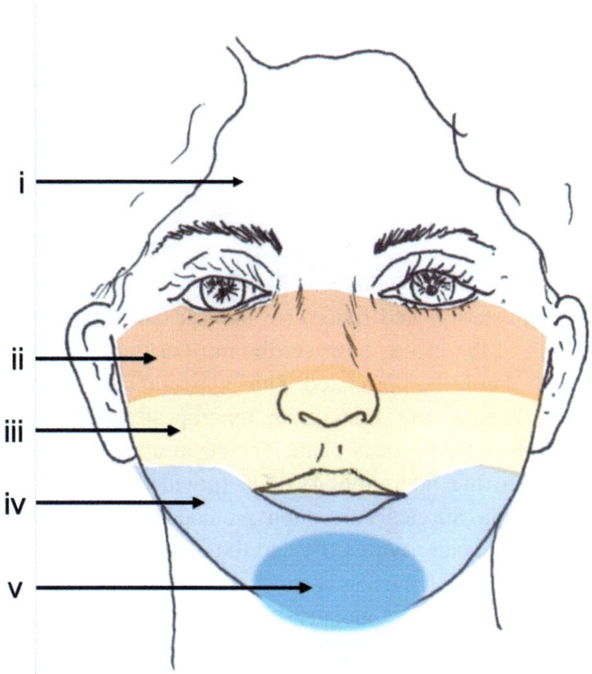

Fig. 66.5 The *Ferretti-Reyneke* analysis

- *The gnathic complex.* This subunit is subdivided into an upper *maxillary component* (iii) which extends from the lower aspect of the oculonasal complex to a curved line extending along the lower margin of the upper lip (or the incisal edge of exposed maxillary teeth) to the angle of the mouth and proceeding in a curvilinear fashion to the lower attachment of the auricle and a lower *mandibular component* (iv) which extends to the lower border of the mandible and contains in its anterior aspect the oval *mental subunit* (v) which delimits the soft tissue chin.

It is critical to remember that facial evaluation is not the search for deviation from the norm of a single subunit but the search for proportion. For example, a facial form diagnosed as vertically excessive means it is excessive in relation to its transverse dimension, *not* that it is longer than the norm. By increasing only the transverse or only the vertical dimension, facial harmony will be lost; however, harmony is re-established by increasing both the transverse and vertical dimensions.

Facial Symmetry

The facial midline is the reference line to evaluate the forehead (glabella), nasal dorsum, nasal tip, maxillary dental midline, columella of the nose, philtrum of the upper lip, mandibular dental midline, lower lip, and the chin (Figs. 66.2 and 66.6). In the initial overall assessment of facial asymmetry, we should establish whether the asymmetry involves the chin, the mandible or the maxilla, or a combination of the structures. Careful assessment of an occlusal cant of the maxilla is mandatory as it will play an important role in the correction of the asymmetry. Soft tissue asymmetry, either primary or secondary to skeletal asymmetry, should be noted. Finally, symmetry of the nose, orbits, and forehead should be evaluated (Figs. 66.2 and 66.6).

The face is a three-dimensional structure, and the symmetry of the face will be influenced by deformities in the vertical, anteroposterior, and transverse planes. Clinical frontal assessment of the face is however the most critical, and discrepancies should be correlated with posterior facial asymmetry by noting any transverse, anteroposterior, and/or sagittal cants in the occlusal plane. The occlusal plane should be parallel to the interpupillary line, provided there is no orbital dystopia. Surgical correction of an occlusal plane cant often corrects facial asymmetry, and the severity of the cant should correlate with the dental and facial asymmetry. During treatment planning the clinicians should assess if orthodontic or surgical correction of dental midlines is required. With skeletal asymmetry the dental midline should not be orthodontically coordinated but rather aligned in the center of each jaw to allow surgical correction of the skeletal asymmetry. Keep in mind that no face is perfectly symmetric.

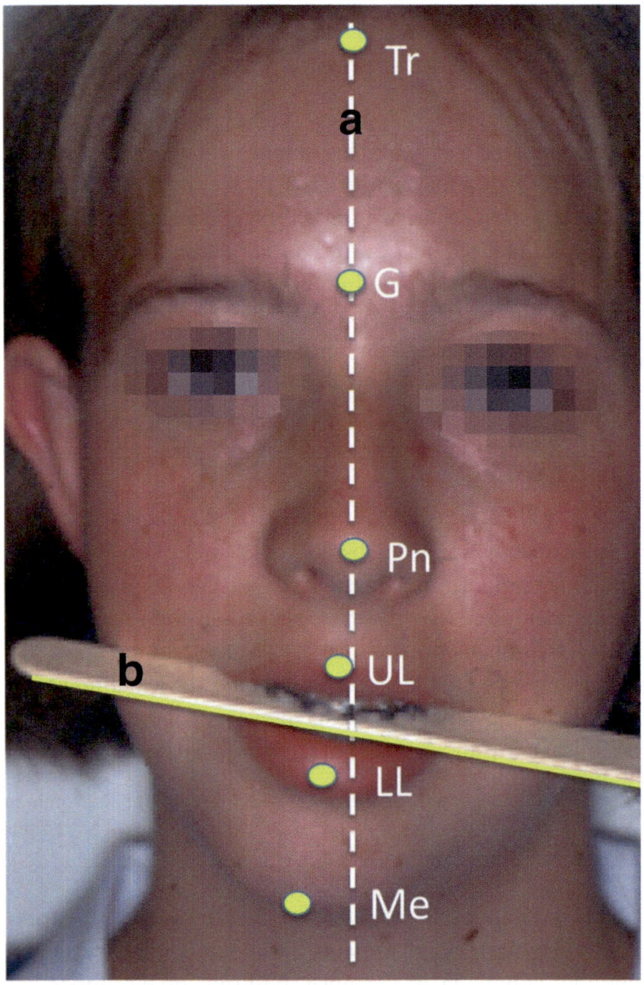

Fig. 66.6 The facial midline (**a**), and occlusal cant (**b**)

Lips

The lips play an extremely important role in the overall facial aesthetics, and careful assessment is required. Lip symmetry should be evaluated in the rest position as well as when the patient is smiling. Lip symmetry may be influenced by facial nerve dysfunction, underlying dentoskeletal deformities, scarring due to previous trauma, congenital clefting, microstomia, macrostomia, or hyperplasia. The lower lip generally exhibits 25% more vermillion than the upper lip. With the presence of an accentuated Cupid's bow, only the upper incisor may be visible under the upper lip and very little or even no lateral incisor (Fig. 66.7). An interlabial gap of 0 to 4mm and 1 to 4mm of upper incisor tooth exposure under the upper lip with the lips in repose are considered pleasing while the full crown of the incisor exposed when smiling.

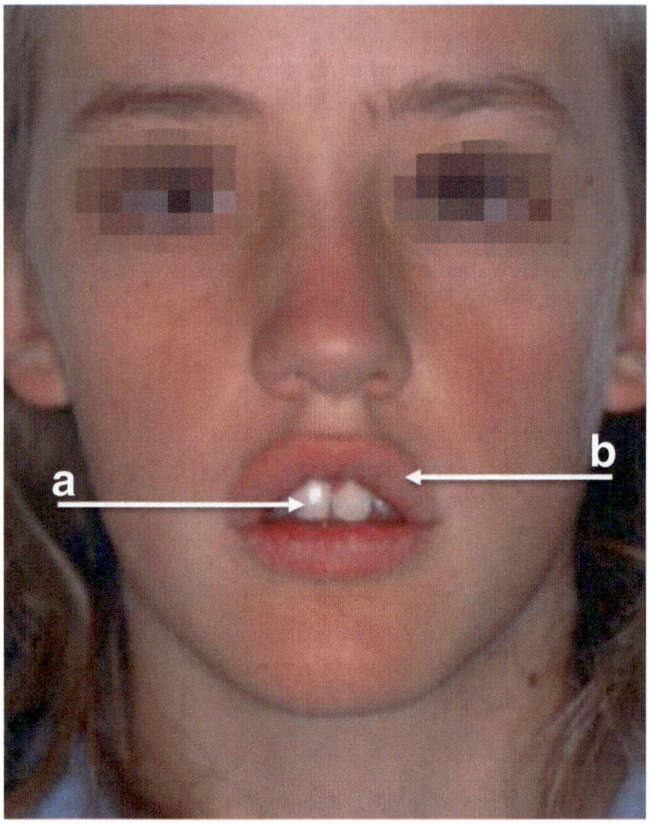

Fig. 66.7 An increased interlabial gap with excessive amount of upper incisor exposure under the upper lip (**a**). A poorly shaped upper lip (distorted Cupid's bow) and excessive amount of vermillion excessive exposure (**b**)

Note any asymmetry of the lips when smiling (Fig. 66.10). When vertical skeletal or dental corrections are contemplated, the vertical relationship of all four incisors to the upper lip should be clinically considered. Only the upper central incisors are visible on a lateral cephalometric radiograph and should not be used to plan vertical maxillary changes (c in Fig. 66.13).

66.2.2 Profile View

Although it is emphasized that the clinical assessment of the face is mandatory, the cephalometric analysis of the lateral cephalometric radiograph has been the predominant method of profile evaluation. Many orthodontists are accustomed to using the quantitative data obtained from the lateral cephalometric analysis as the main diagnostic tool. The contemporary orthodontist and facial surgeon rely on facial proportionality and more subjective aesthetic evaluation criteria than linear and angular measurements. Treatment decisions should rather be made by what is most aesthetically appealing rather than by what the cephalometric norms indicate. The plethora of cephalometric values available can lead to confusion and unnecessary complexity. The undermentioned cephalometric measurements are the most useful indicators to confirm a clinical diagnosis.

Nasolabial Angle (a in Fig. 66.11)

The angle is measured between the columella of the nose and the upper lip and should be between 85° and 105°. It is influenced by the position and angle of the upper incisor teeth and the anatomy of the nasal columella. Excessive orthodontic retraction of the upper incisor teeth (i.e., com-

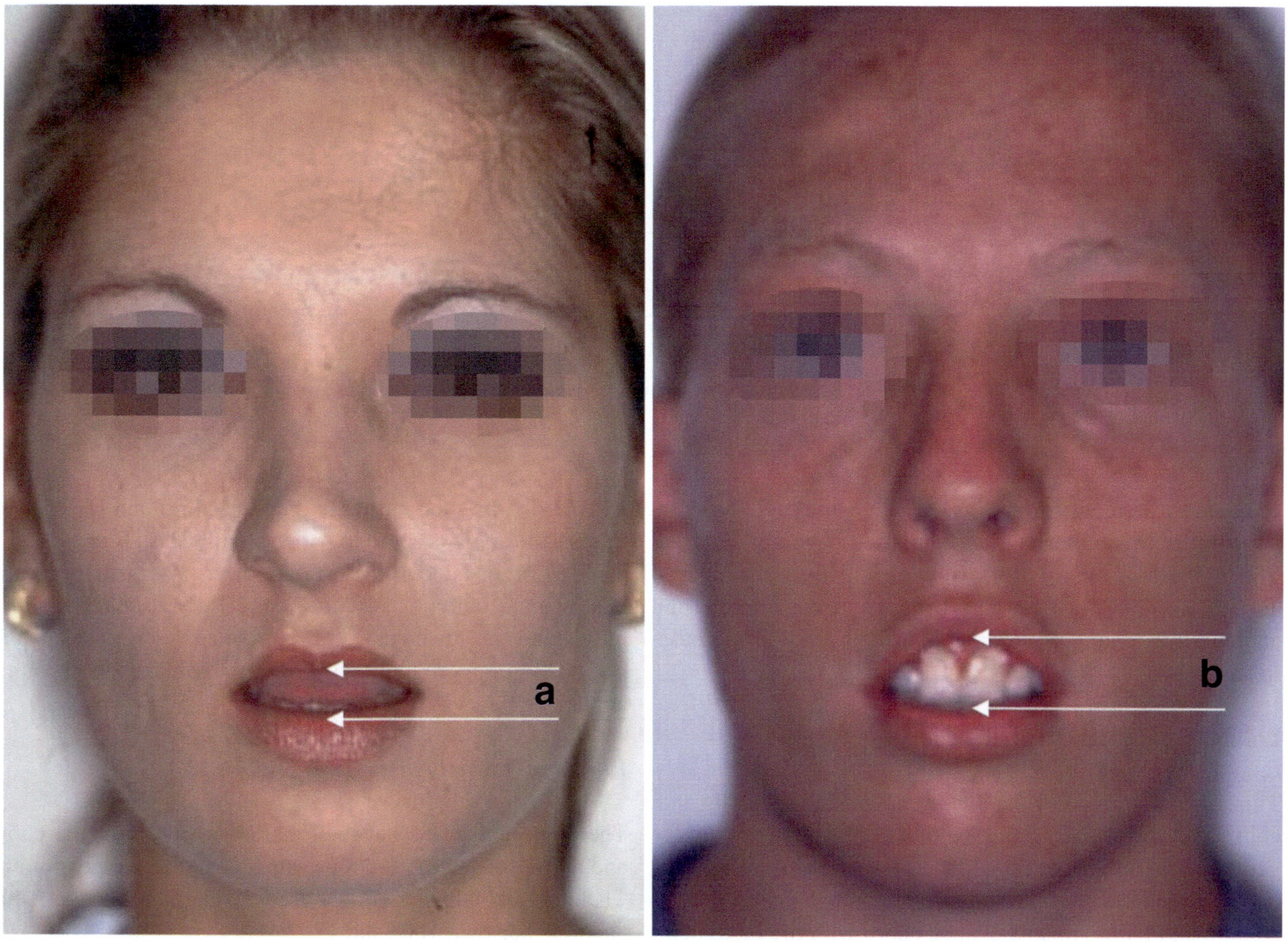

Fig. 66.8 No upper incisor exposure under the upper lip leads to a "toothless" look (**a**). An increased interlabial gap with excessive upper incisor exposure suggests vertical maxillary excess (**b**). The assessment should always be done with the lips in repose

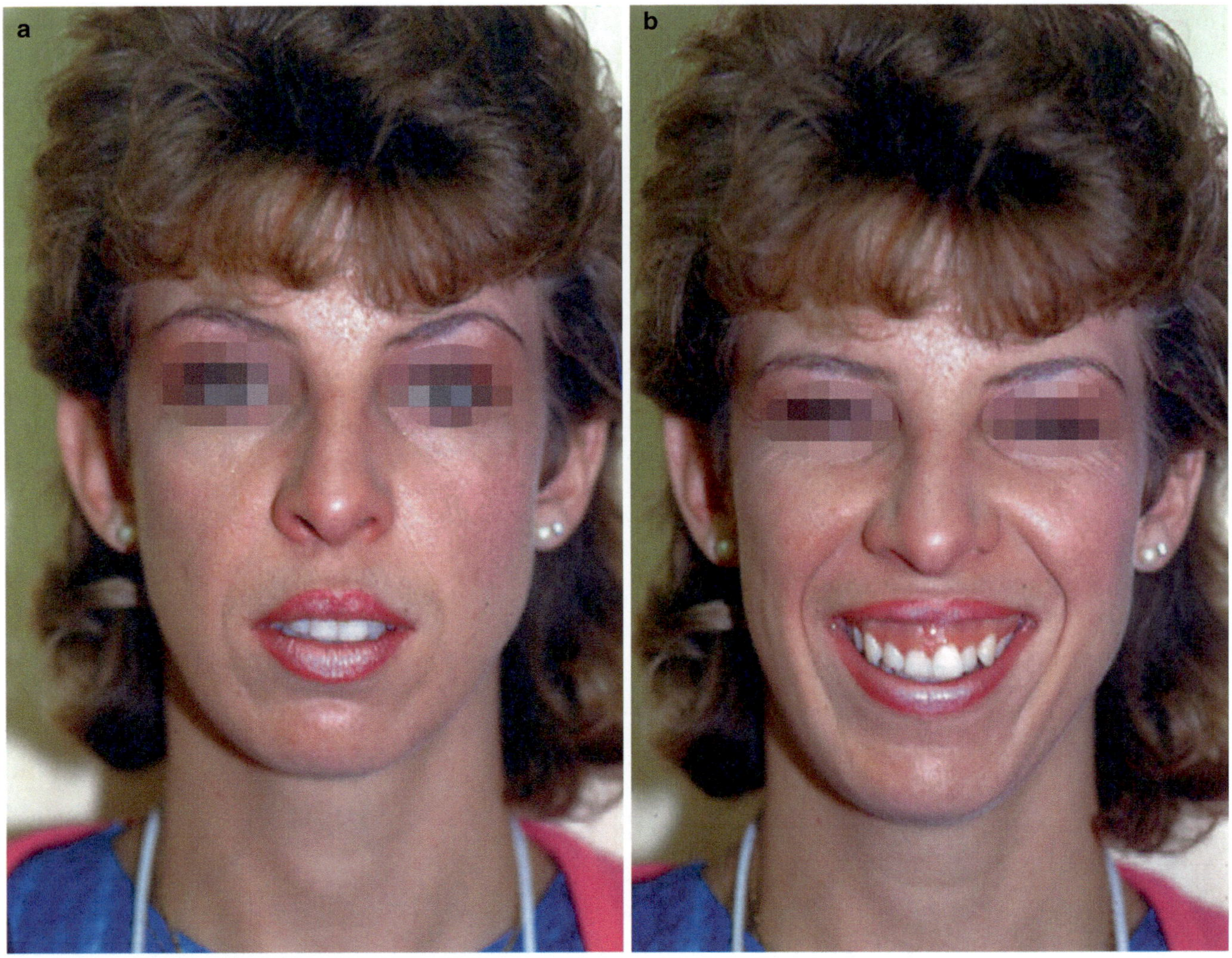

Fig. 66.9 A patient with vertical maxillary excess. Note the increased interlabial gap with the lips in repose (**a**) and gummy smile (**b**)

promised treatment for a Class II occlusion) will lead to poor upper lip support and an increased nasolabial angle. This will often lead to early wrinkling and an aging appearance of the lip. An over-closed bite will cause an acute angle, while a hanging columella of the nose will increase the angle.

Labiomental Angle (b in Fig. 66.11)

This angle is formed by the intersection of the lower lip and chin measured at the soft tissue of the chin. The angle is a gentle curve and should be 120° ± 10°. The lower lip, the depth of the labiomental fold, and chin button should form a smooth and harmonious S-shaped curve with the labiomental fold dividing the chin into an upper third and lower two thirds. The angle is acute in patients with Class II dentoskeletal deformities due to the everted lower lip or patients with macrogenia. Individuals with Class III dentoskeletal deformities and the lower incisors retroclined (compensated) or patients with microgenia will exhibit an obtuse labiomental angle.

Lip-Chin-Throat Angle ((i) in Fig. 66.12)

The angle is formed between the lower border of the chin and a line connecting the lower lip and soft tissue pogonion. The chin and submental area are considered attractive with an angle between 100° and 120°.

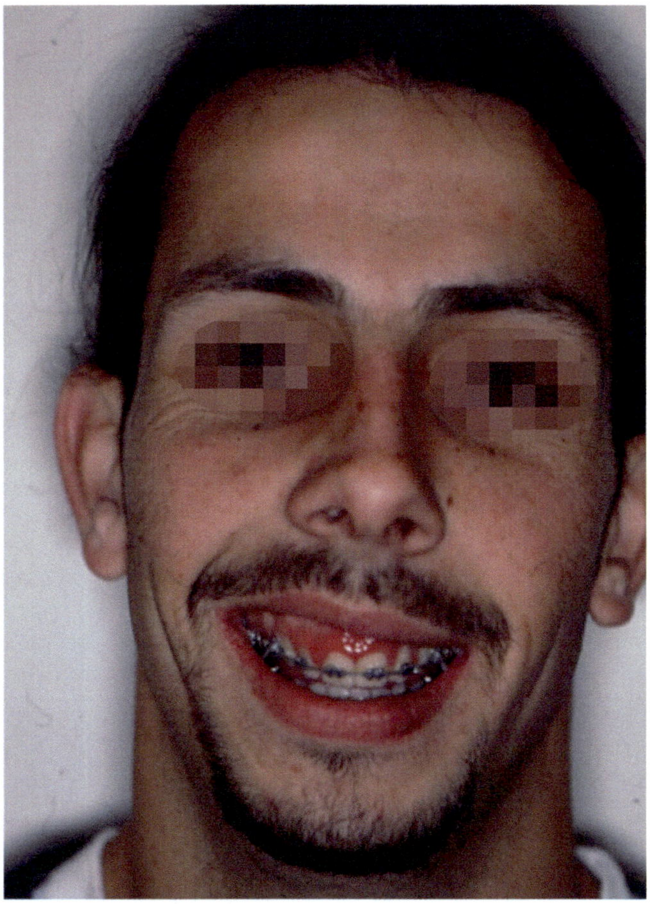

Fig. 66.10 An asymmetric smile

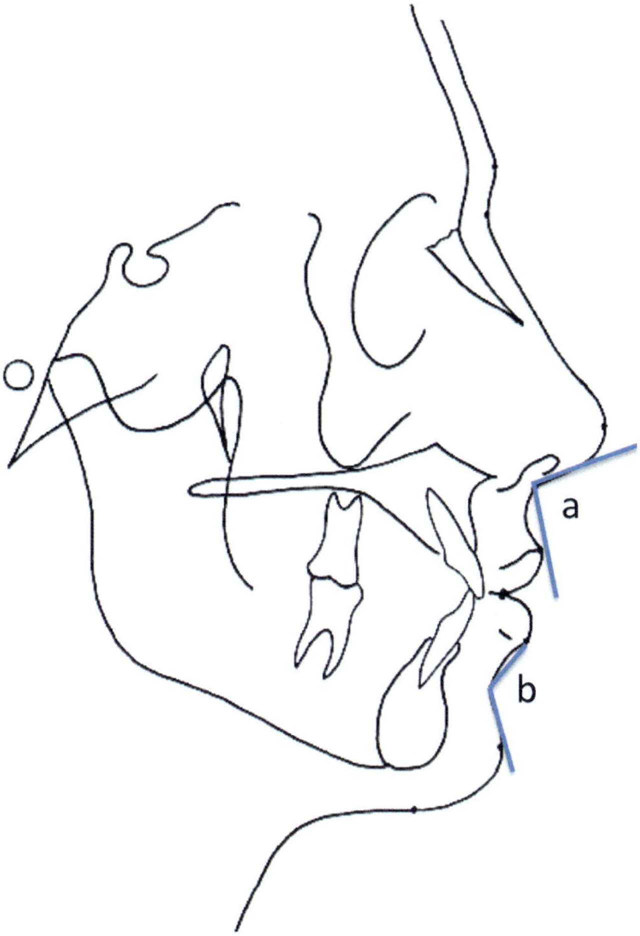

Fig. 66.11 (a) The nasolabial angle, measured between the inclination of the columella of the nose and the upper lip, should be 85°–105°. (b) Labiomental fold. The lower lip-chin angle should be 130°. However the general shape of the chin should be considered

Chin-Throat Length ((ii) in Fig. 66.12)

It is measured from the angle of the throat to the soft tissue menton. It is only meaningful when this angle is measured with the patient's head in natural posture. A length of between 38 and 48mm is considered to be normal and is significant when assessing mandibular length. This measurement is helpful for differentiating between mandibular anteroposterior excess and maxillary anteroposterior deficiency. For a patient with a Class III malocclusion and normal chin-throat length, maxillary deficiency should be suspected.

Upper Lip Length (b in Fig. 66.13)

The length of the upper lip is measured from subnasale to the lower border of the upper lip (stomion superius) and should be 18–22 mm in females and 20–24 mm in males. This measurement should be performed with the lips in repose. During the planning of tooth-lip relationship, it should be kept in mind that the upper lip will increase in length with age.

Interlabial gap (d in Fig. 66.13)

The interlabial gap should be assessed with the lips in repose and the teeth in occlusion. It is measured between stomion superius and stomion inferius (0–4 mm). If the lips touch when the teeth are in occlusion, the upper incisor-lip relationship should be evaluated with the lower jaw rotated open until the lips are slightly apart.

Facial Contour Angle (e in Fig. 66.13)

This measurement will give the clinician an indication of facial convexity or concavity and is influenced by the anteroposterior relationship between glabella, subnasale, and menton. The angle is formed between the upper facial plane (glabella-subnasale) and lower facial plane (subnasale-pogonion). The angle is recorded above subnasale and expressed as negative when the angle is ahead of the upper facial plane (in convex profiles) and as positive when the angle is behind the upper facial plane (usually in concave profiles). A pleasing facial profile for females will have a facial contour angle of $-13° \pm 4°$ and for males $-11° \pm 4°$. This measurement will also be influenced by the height of the maxilla. The mandible will rotate counterclockwise (upward and forward) with vertical maxillary deficiency leading to a more concave profile, while it will rotate clockwise (downward and backward) with vertical maxillary excess leading to a more convex profile.

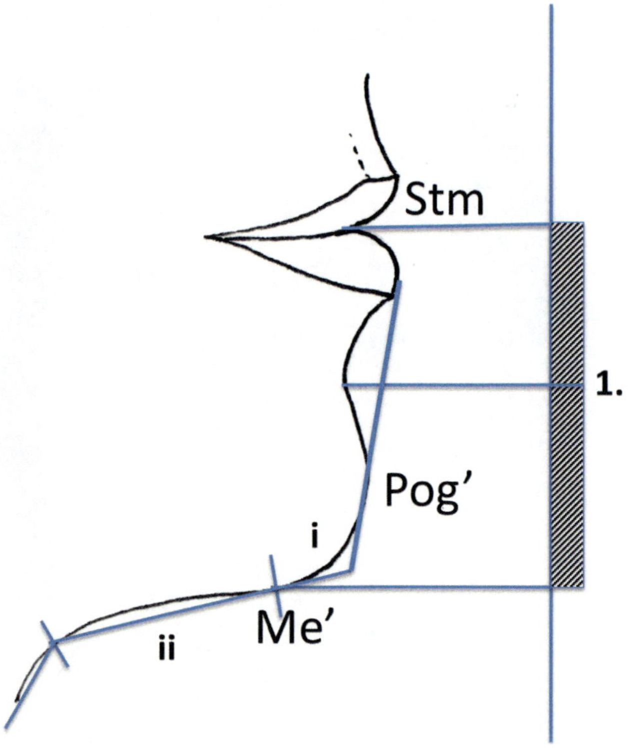

Fig. 66.12 The lip-chin-throat angle (i). Chin-throat length (ii)

Nose (Fig. 66.14)

This important anatomic structure is situated in the middle of the face, and its important influence on facial aesthetics has often been neglected by orthodontists and maxillofacial surgeons in the past. More focus is placed on the aesthetic evaluation of the nose by the fact that the relative nasal aesthetics can be influenced by orthodontic treatment and certainly by orthognathic surgery. The fact that rhinoplasty is now considered to be part of the field of treatment for many orthognathic surgeons has certainly made the careful aesthetic evaluation of the nose an important consideration. In many cases nasal reconstruction will form part of the orthognathic treatment plan, and in some cases, reconstruction can be performed concurrently with orthognathic surgery. The authors prefer to defer most nasal reconstructions to 6 months after orthognathic surgery due to the substantial relative effects orthognathic surgery has on nasal aesthetic.

The amount of nostril show in profile view may be affected by either a hanging columella or retracted alae (Fig. 66.14a). The shape of the dorsum should be noted as normal, convex, or concave. It is important to distinguish between a large dorsum and a turned-down nasal tip as the treatment would be entirely different. The relationship between the lengths of the nasal dorsum and the projection

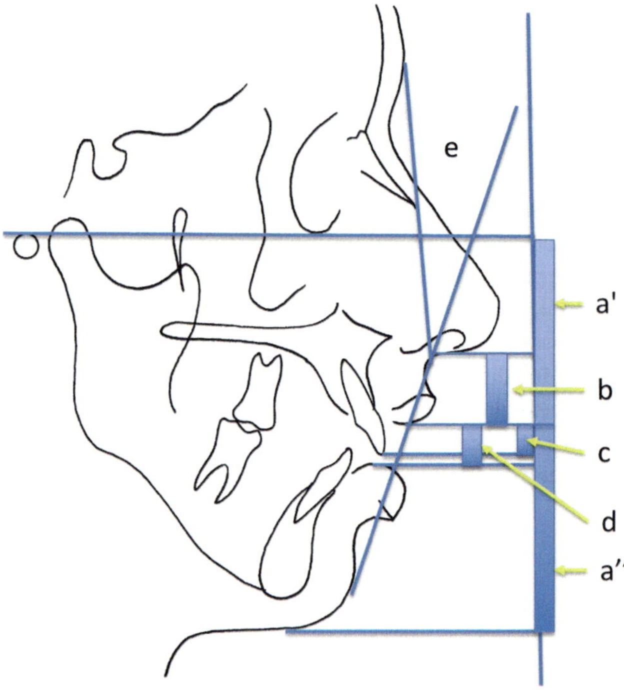

Fig. 66.13 Midface height (a'), lower facial height (a''), upper lip length (b), upper lip vermillion (c), interlabial gap (d), and facial contour angle (e)

of the nose can be evaluated by the method of Goode. According to Goode the length of the nose should be about 55–60% greater than the projection of the nose (Fig. 66.14b). From nasal base to the tip, the ratio of projection should be 1–2 (Fig. 66.14c). The nostrils and columella should be assessed from a "worm's eye" view (Fig. 66.14d). The nasal bridge should project about 5–8 mm in front of the globes of the eyes. The nasal tip should be noted as narrow, bulbous, asymmetric, or normal. The width of the nasal base, the acuteness of the supra tip break, the visibility of the nostrils,

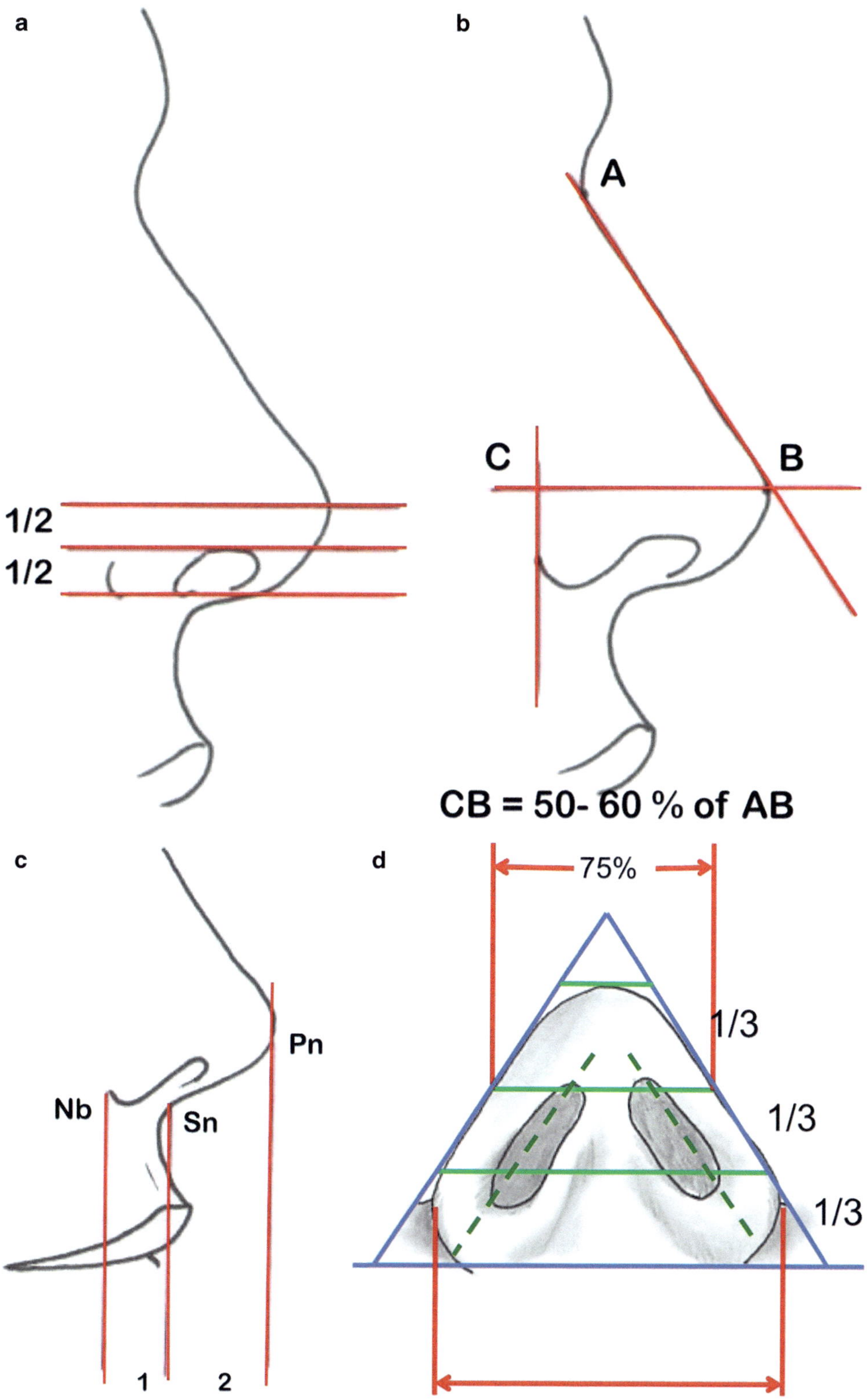

©Association of Oral and Maxillofacial Surgeons of India

Fig. 66.14 Assessment of nostril show (**a**). Nasal projection (CB) to nasal length (AB), according to Goode's ratio: CB:AB = 0.55:0.6 is normal (**b**). Horizontal assessment of nasal projection: from nasal base (Nb), the Pn-Sn to Sn-Nb should be 2:1 (**c**). Nasal base ("worm's eye") view assessment of the nose. The general shape of the alar base should resemble an isosceles triangle (**d**) and symmetry of the columella are important factors to consider when maxillary surgery (especially superior repositioning or advancement) is contemplated. Fortunately, adverse aesthetic effects as a result of maxillary surgery can be controlled during surgery [4].

Cheeks (Fig. 66.15)

As in the frontal evaluation, the *cheekbone-nasal base-upper lip-lower lip curve* contour line is also very helpful in the profile analysis. The line starts just in front of the ear, extending forward over the cheekbone, downward over the maxilla adjacent the ala of the nose, and ending lateral to the commissure of the mouth. The line should form a smooth continuous curve, and any interruption may indicate an underlying skeletal deformity (Fig. 66.15). The variations in interruptions in the curve and the possible underlying skeletal deformities responsible for the soft tissue deformities are demonstrated in Fig. 66.15b, c [5].

Orbit

The globes of the eye generally project 0–2 mm ahead of the infraorbital rims, while the lateral orbital rims lie 8–12 mm behind the most anterior projection of the globes. The bridge of the nose should be about 7 mm ahead of the globes although there is a significant ethnic difference in this measurement (Fig. 66.14) [6].

Paranasal Area

The flatness or fullness of the paranasal areas is an important indicator to distinguish between middle third deficiency and mandibular anteroposterior excess. Another useful indicator of midface deficiency is the ratio of the linear distance from the nasal tip to subnasale and from subnasale to the alar base crease. The ratio should be 2:1 (Fig. 66.14). A ratio closer to 1:1 will indicate maxillary anteroposterior deficiency, while an increased ratio will indicate decreased nasal projection.

Lips

The lips play an important part in the overall aesthetics of the face and should be carefully assessed before treatment. The effects of treatment as well as the aesthetic changes that may take place during the aging process should be considered. The upper lip usually projects slightly anterior to the lower lip, and the E-line and S-line are helpful guides to assess the projection of the lips (Fig. 66.16) [7].

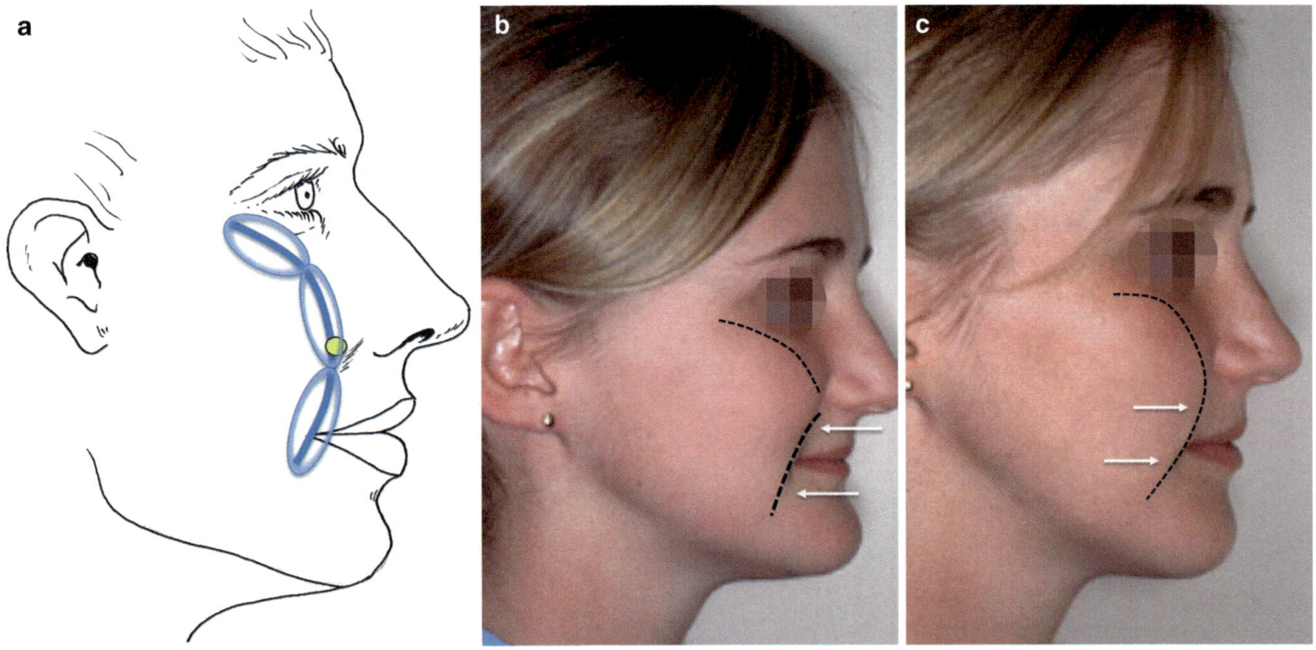

Fig. 66.15 (**a**) The cheekbone-nasal base-lip curve contour. The curve should be unerupted and smooth in an individual with good facial proportions. (**b**) The cheekbone-nasal base-lip curve contour. The interruption of the curve (arrows) indicates maxillary as well as mandibulae anteroposterior deficiency. (**c**) The cheekbone-nasal base-lip curve contour. Following maxillary and mandibular advancement, the curve is uninterrupted and smooth (arrows)

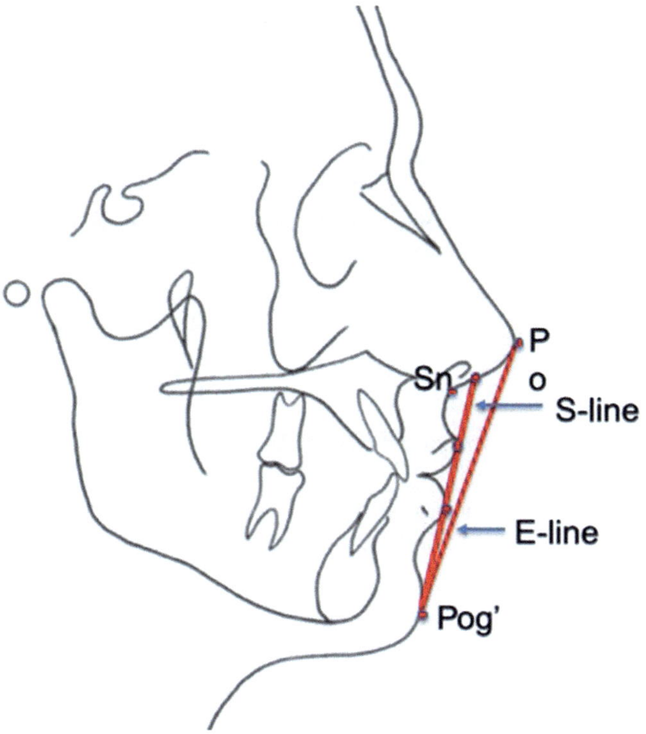

Fig 66.16 Lip prominence. Li should be 2 ± 2mm behind the E-line (Pn-Pog'). Li – Labrae inferioris and Ls – Labrae superioris should just touch the S-line (S-line follows Pog' to the point between Sn and Pn)

Chin

The chin is one of the most noticeable structures in the face and demands special evaluation. The shape of the chin is more important than the position of pogonion. Chin surgery should not be considered for patients requiring mandibular surgery. Performing an advancement genioplasty for a patient as compromise treatment for mandibular advancement may achieve correct chin projection; however, the balance and harmony of the chin will be poor. The authors use seven criteria for the aesthetic profile evaluation of the chin which also serve as a guide to surgical treatment planning (Figs. 66.11, 66.12, and 66.13) [8].

1. Height of the chin. The chin height is measured from lower lip stomion to soft tissue menton and should be equivalent to two thirds of the lower facial height. The linear height should be 40 ± 2 mm for females and 44 ± 2 mm for males. For individuals with deep bites, the measurement should be performed with the teeth apart and the lip separated (i in Fig. 66.12).
2. Vermillion exposure. The lower lip vermillion exposure should be 25% more than the upper lip. The lower lip will be everted with increased vermillion exposure when the lower incisors are proclined or in individuals with an increased overjet (Fig. 66.13).
3. The labiomental fold. The depth of the fold should divide the chin into an upper third and lower two thirds (Fig. 66.11).
4. Chin throat length. Patients with mandibular anteroposterior deficiency will have short chin-throat lengths and vice versa for individuals with mandibular anteroposterior excess. Normal length is considered to be 42 ± 6 mm. This measurement is important when considering setback or advancement of the chin (ii in Fig. 66.12).
5. Lower lip-chin-throat angle. The angle is considered pleasing at 110° ± 8° and tends to be acute in mandibular prognathism and obtuse in mandibular deficiency (Fig. 66.12).
6. S-shaped curvature. The profile of the chin should form a well-proportioned, harmonious and smooth curve (Fig. 66.12).
7. The lower lip position. A helpful guide to the lower lip position is the E-line (aesthetic line). The E-line is drawn from the nasal tip (pronasale) to pogonion. The lower lip should be 2 ± 2 mm behind the line. The measurement will be influenced by the projection of the nose and the anteroposterior position of the chin which should be kept in mind during this evaluation (Fig. 66.13).

Most of the aforementioned aesthetics parameters can also be assessed on a lateral cephalometric radiograph; however, there is no substitute for clinical evaluation of facial harmony. It is hoped that the short overview of the clinical assessment of facial aesthetics will increase the reader's acuity in the treatment of his/her patients. In most instances the orthodontist is the first professional to see patients with malocclusions. Some of these patients may require skeletal and/or soft tissue modification incorporated into the treatment plan, and the responsibility lies with the orthodontist to recognize the dental, skeletal, and soft tissue problems and then to appropriately inform the patient. The aesthetic outcome following orthodontic (and surgical) treatment should be a priority for the contemporary orthodontist.

66.3 Clinical Evaluation

The clinical assessment of the face is probably the most valuable of all diagnostic procedures. While an astute clinical diagnosis can be made at the chair side, photographs are essential for accurate assessment and record purposes. The face is systematically assessed from a frontal view, profile view, and three-quarter view. Figures 66.1, 66.2, 66.3, 66.4, 66.5, 66.6, 66.7, 66.8, 66.9, 66.10, 66.11, 66.12, and 66.13 illustrate some angular and linear parameters used during the clinical assessment of the face.

66.4 Special Investigations

Cephalometric and panoramic radiographs and dental casts are essential; however, temporomandibular joint investigations, Technetium bone scans, hand wrist radiographs, CT scans, etc. may be required. The lateral cephalometric radiograph taken in centric occlusion and the lips in repose allows the clinician to analyze and evaluate the soft tissue, skeletal, and dental relations of a dentofacial deformity.

66.5 Diagnosis and Problem List

A diagnosis is made following the clinical evaluation of the patient, a radiographic evaluation and cephalometric analysis, model analysis, and other indicated evaluations. The data base is used to compile a problem list.

66.6 Treatment Objectives

Clear orthodontic and surgical treatment objectives regarding soft tissue, skeletal, and dental structures should be identified and noted.

Development of a Visual Orthodontic and Surgical Cephalometric Treatment Objective The lateral cephalometric radiograph tracing is used to develop an orthodontic visual treatment objective to predict orthodontic tooth movements. This is followed by the development of a surgical visual treatment objective predicting the required jaw repositioning and expected soft tissue changes [10].

66.7 Treatment Plan

All the factors identified in the diagnosis and problem list as well as patient concerns and reasons for considering orthognathic surgery are considered to formulate a final treatment plan (Flowchart 1). The sequence of treatment and the treatment to be performed by all healthcare professionals concerned are outlined. When defining the treatment plan, a thorough knowledge of the many types of dentofacial deformities and the treatment modalities available to correct them is essential.

The flowchart (Fig. 66.17) summarizes the systematic gathering of data leading to diagnosis and, finally, the development of a treatment plan [9–11].

The basic treatment plan will consist of:

Presurgical Orthodontic Treatment

1. Alignment of both dental arches (with or without tooth extractions)
2. Levelling of both dental arches (in segments or one piece)
3. Deviation of tooth roots at planned interdental osteotomies areas
4. Decompensation of any dental compensations
5. Coordination of dental arches (or segments)

Surgery

The treatment of patients with dentofacial deformities can broadly be divided into four groups. The specific surgical procedure(s) will be indicated by the problem list as discussed:

1. Single jaw surgery—mandibular repositioning (advancement or setback)
2. Single jaw surgery—maxillary repositioning (advancement or setback or superior repositioning or downgraft and/or segmental surgery or a combination)
3. Double jaw surgery
4. Rotation of the maxillomandibular complex

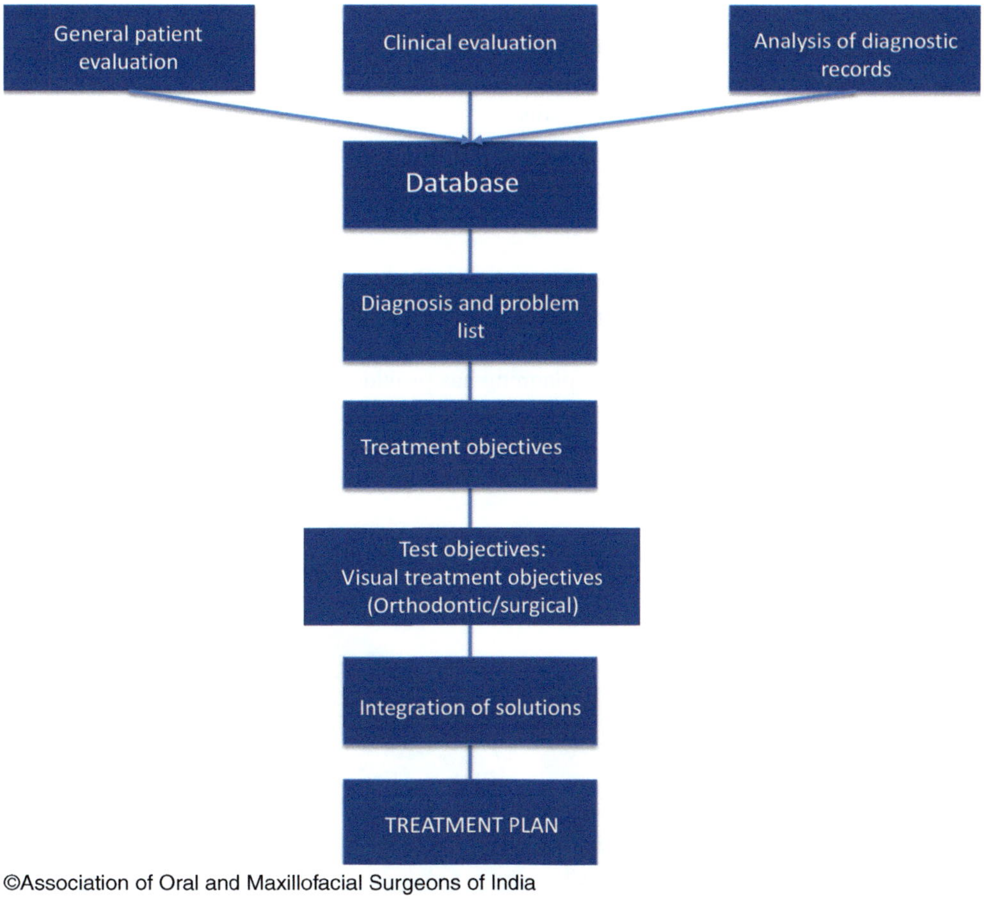

Fig. 66.17 Flowchart 1

For each of the above surgical treatment categories, the orthodontist and the surgeon will have specific responsibilities to make the treatment efforts occur smoothly and successfully. In most surgeries, conventional treatment planning using lateral cephalometric and PA cephalometric radiographs and cast model surgery with surgical splint fabrication is indicated. However the authors use 3D virtual treatment planning for more challenging surgeries such as facial asymmetries, rotation of the maxillomandibular complex, etc. [12, 13].

66.8 Treatment

Although the orthodontist and the oral and maxillofacial surgeon are the main role players, comprehensive correction of dentofacial deformities may involve several members of the healthcare team. The surgeon should understand the orthodontic decision-making process, while the orthodontist must understand the pre- and postsurgical orthodontic requirements. It is mandatory that the therapeutic management is carried out as planned and any problem or change in treatment plan should be communicated to the treatment team. Successful and knowledgeable practitioners always maintain good interprofessional communication and mutual respect to achieve the best treatment results.

66.9 Conclusion

Successful orthognathic surgery relies on understanding and interpreting a patient's desires, correlating these with the diagnosis, and finally developing a treatment plan and executing it accurately. While virtual 3D planning has provided another tool to aid in diagnosis and surgical planning, it behooves surgeons to continue to develop proficiency in traditional cephalometry-based treatment planning.

66.10 Case Scenarios

Case 1: A female patient suffering from hemifacial microsomia on the left (Figs. 66.18, 66.19, 66.20, 66.21, 66.22, 66.23 and 66.24).
Case 2: A male patient suffering from skeletal Class 3 malocclusion (Figs. 66.25, 66.26 and 66.27)

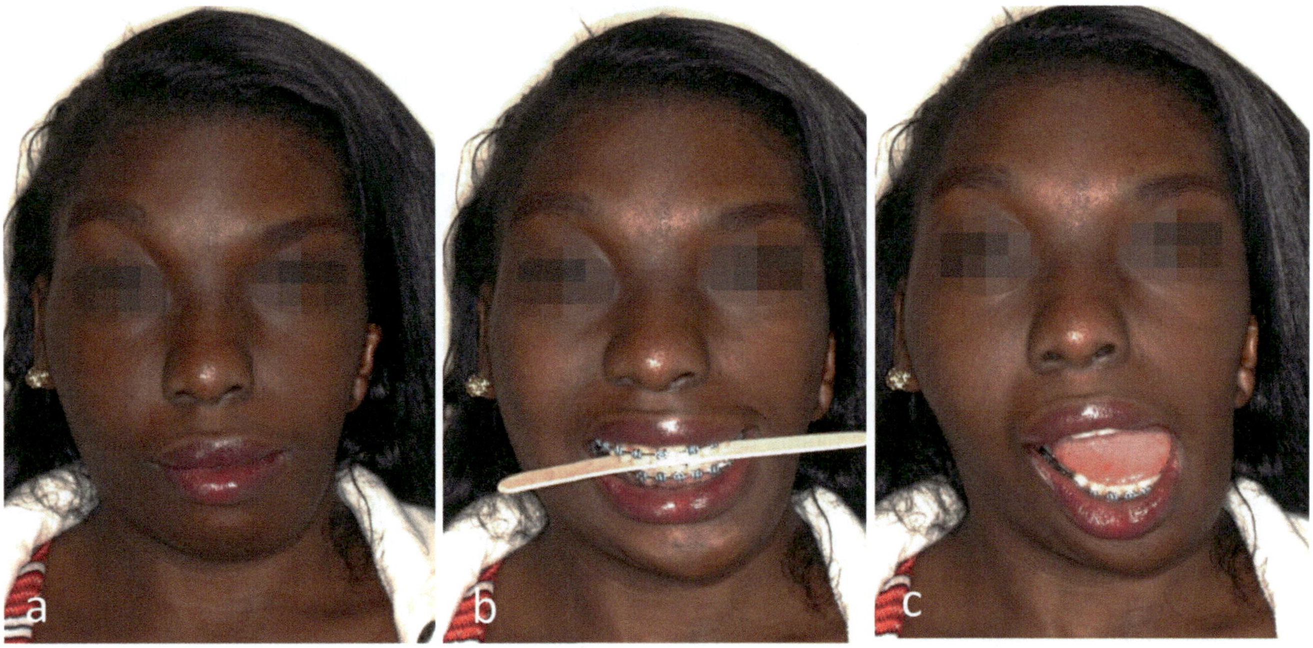

Fig. 66.18 (**a**) Frontal view; (**b**) note the occlusal cant; (**c**) the mandible swing to the affected side; (**d**) right side profile view; (**e**) left side three-quarter view, note the microtia; and (**f**) the left side profile view, note the microtia

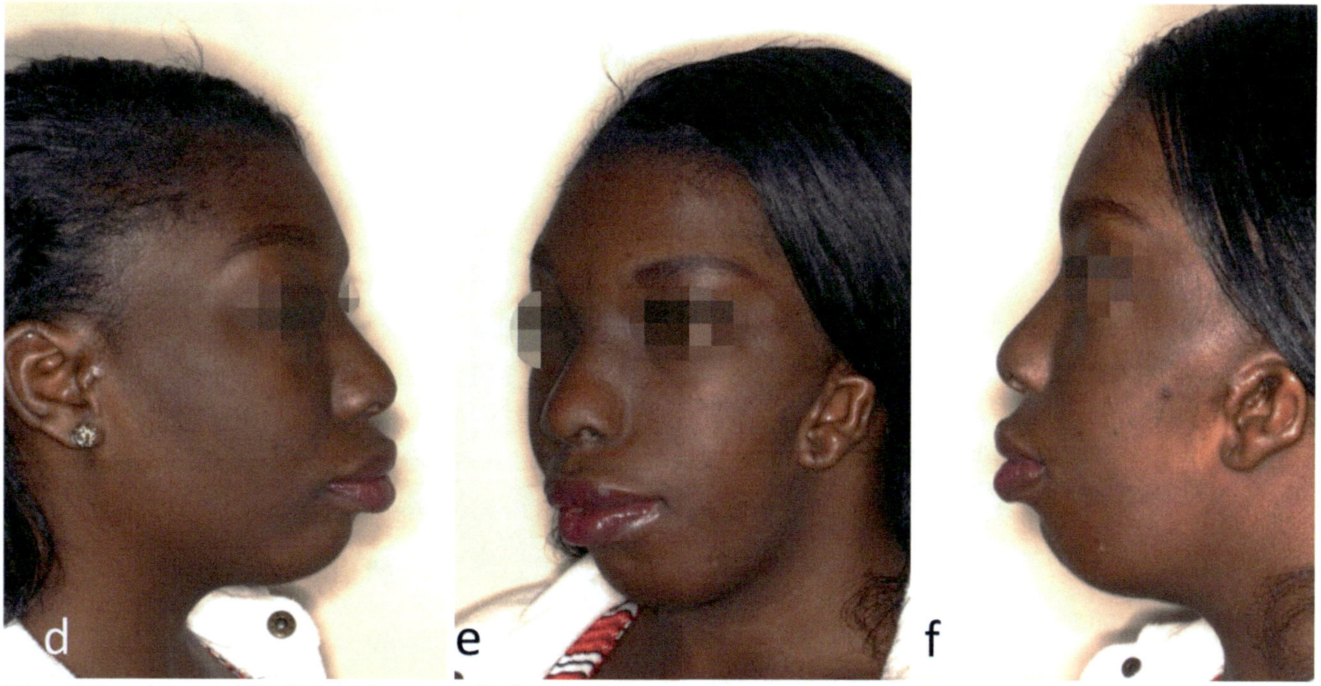

Fig. 66.18 (continued)

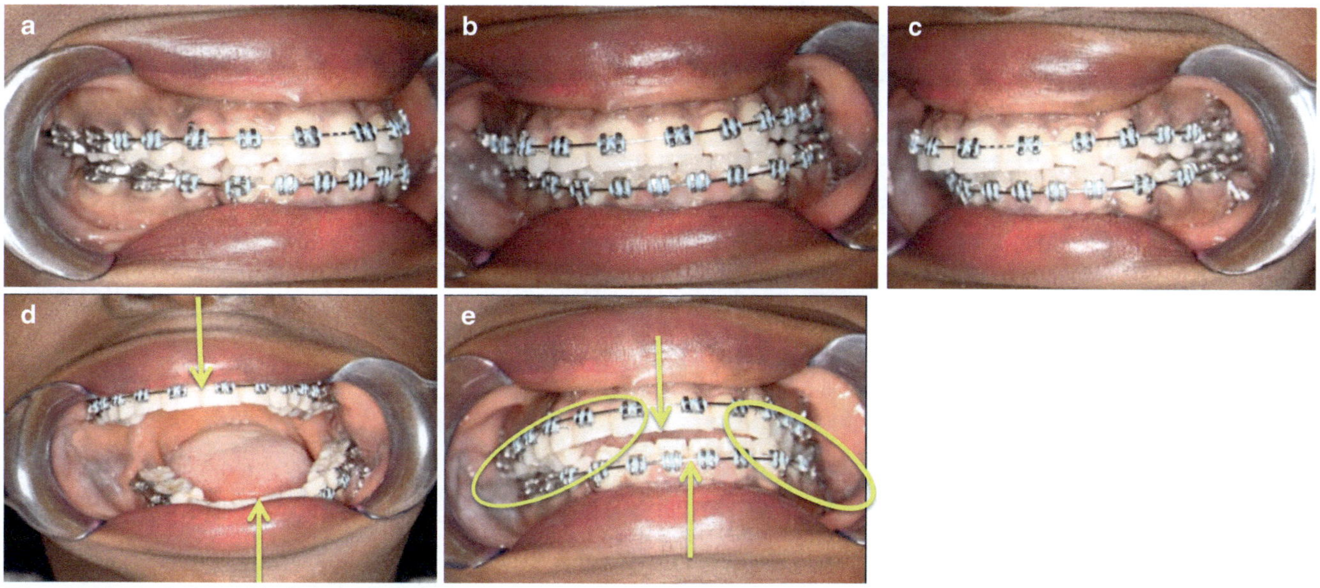

Fig. 66.19 (**a**–**c**) Presurgical occlusion, (**d**) the occlusion swings to the left on mouth opening, and (**e**) the lower dental midline is displaced to the left (arrows) and bilateral cross bites (circles)

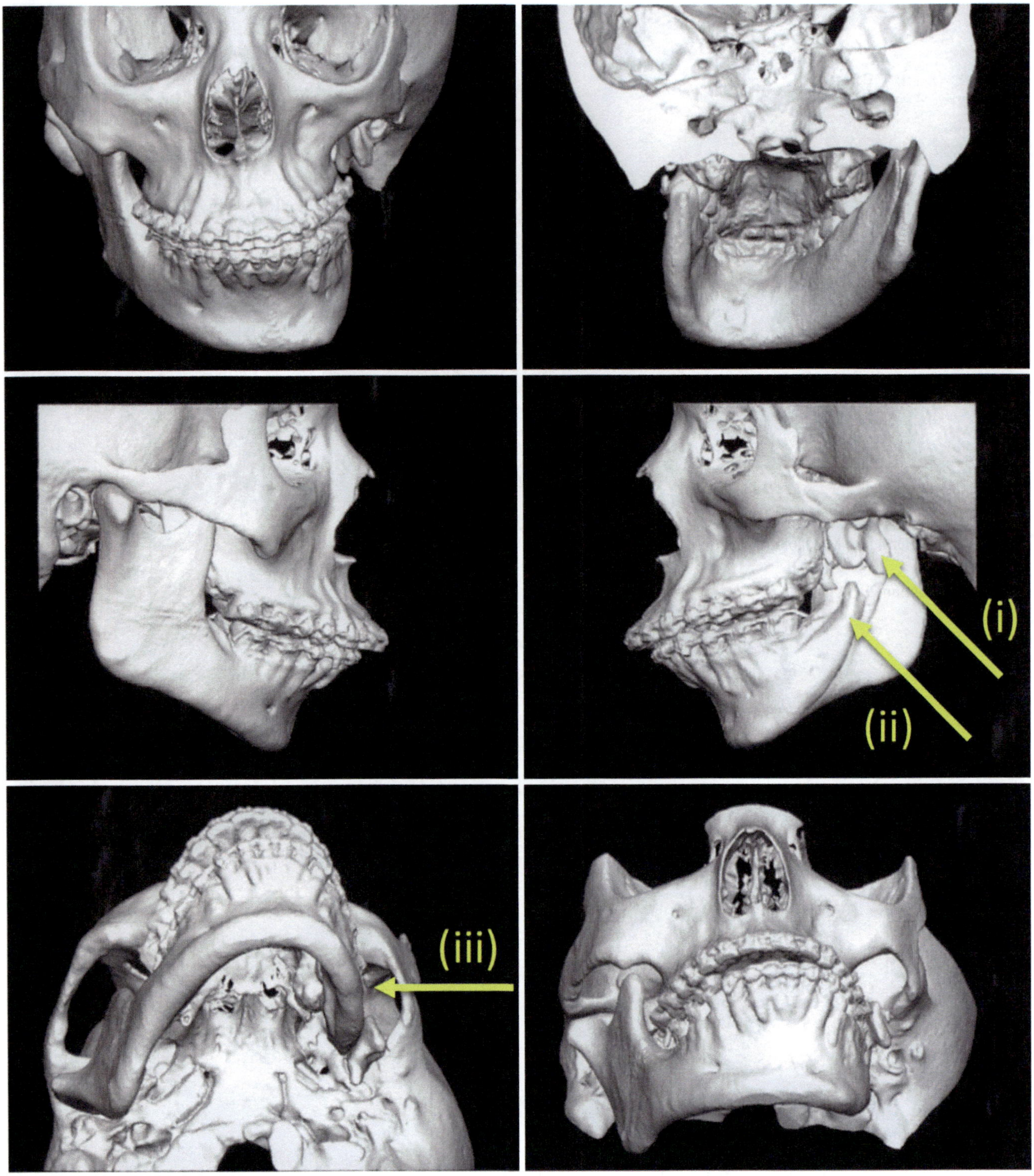

Fig. 66.20 3D images of the skeletal deformities. Note the absence of the left condyle and mandibular ramus (Kaban type III) (i) absence of glenoid fossa, (ii) absence of mandibular condyle, (iii) deficient mandibular ramus on the left side, basal view)

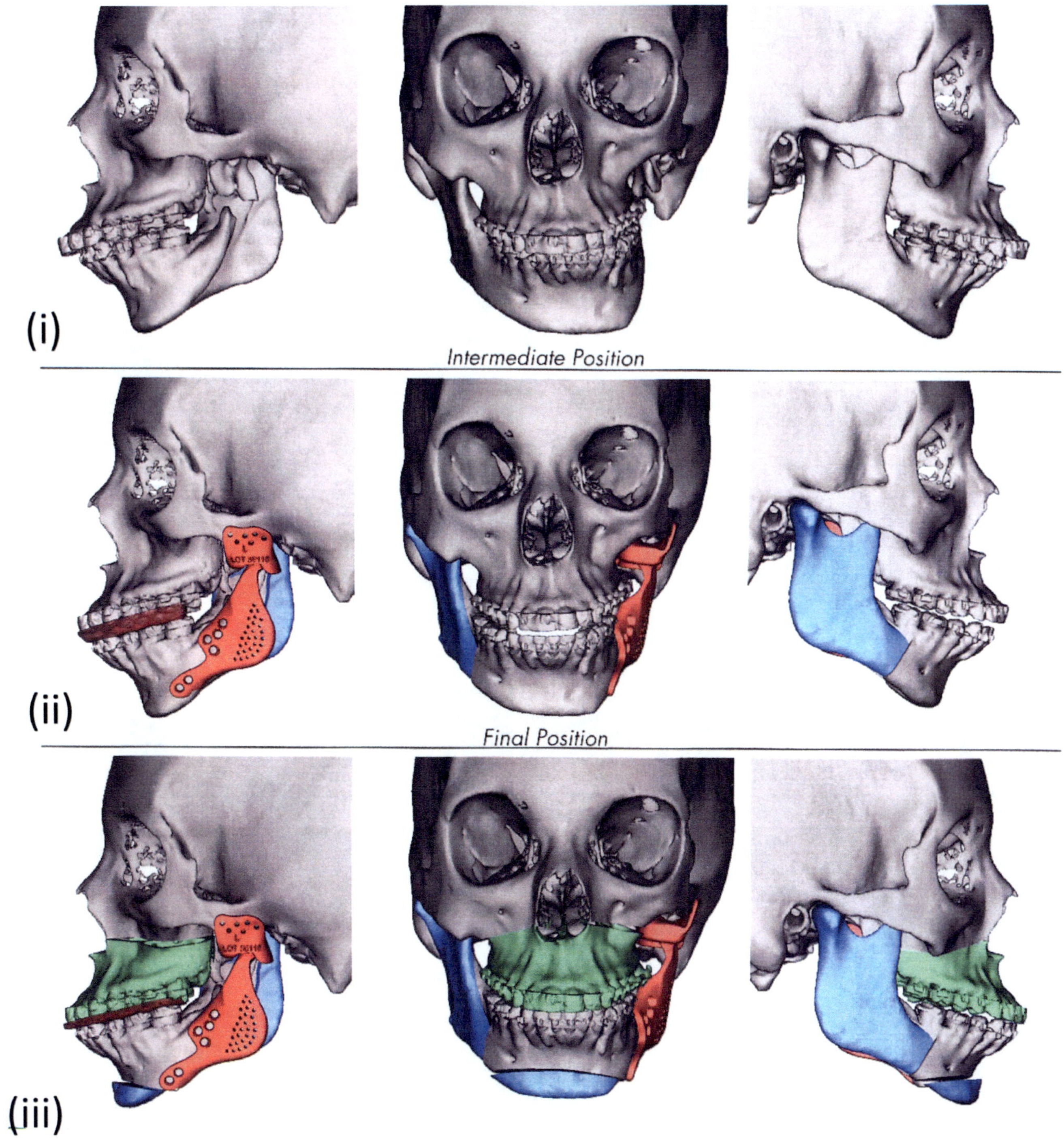

Fig. 66.21 The 3D orthognathic virtual surgical plan: Total joint reconstruction on the left, Le Fort I osteotomy correcting of the maxillary cant, unilateral sagittal split ramus osteotomy on the right, and an advancement genioplasty. (i) Pre-surgical, (ii) intermediate position after mandibular surgery, (iii) Final position after maxillary surgery and genioplasty

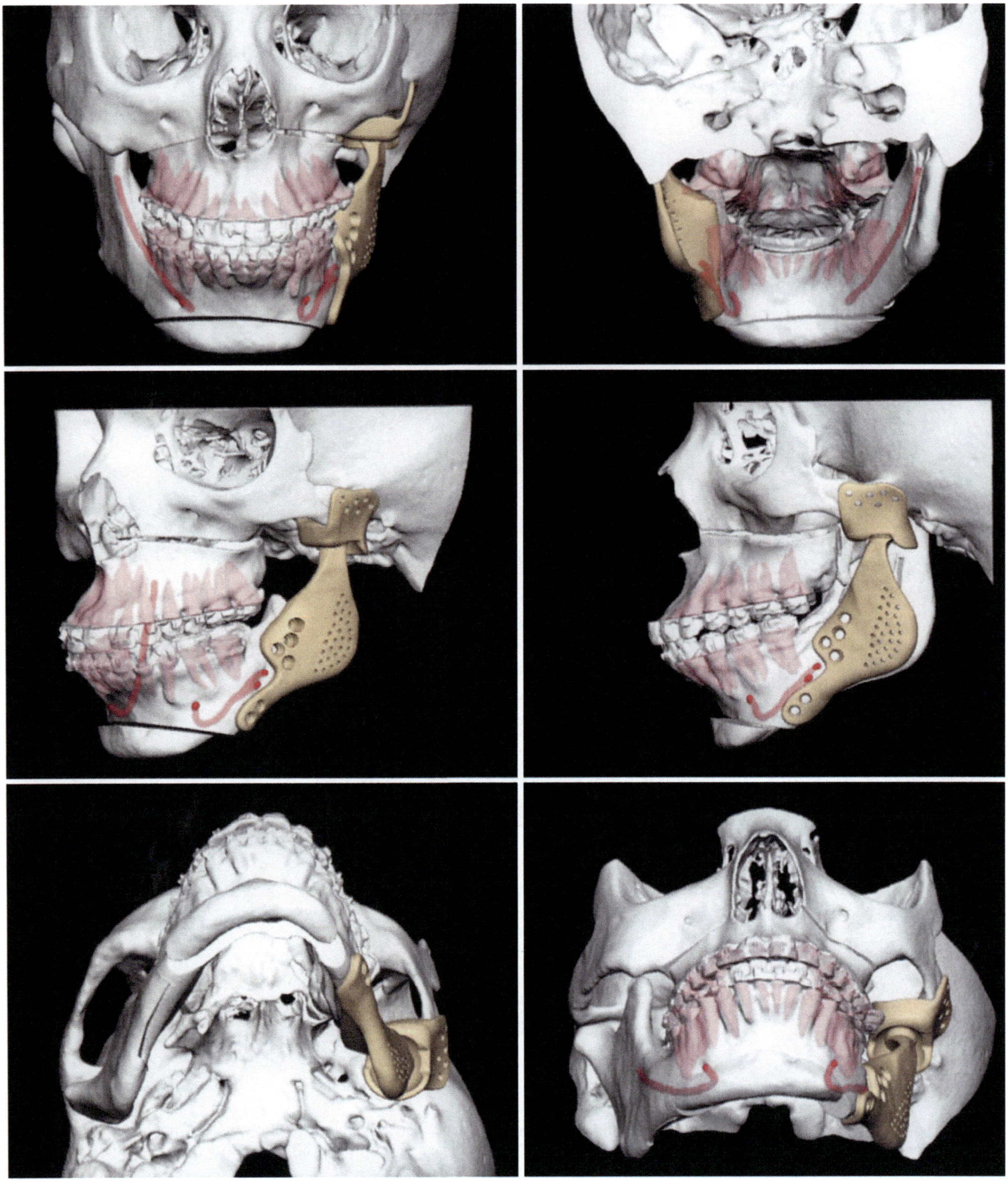

Fig. 66.22 The 3D surgical plan for patient-matched left alloplastic condyle, mandibular ramus and angle

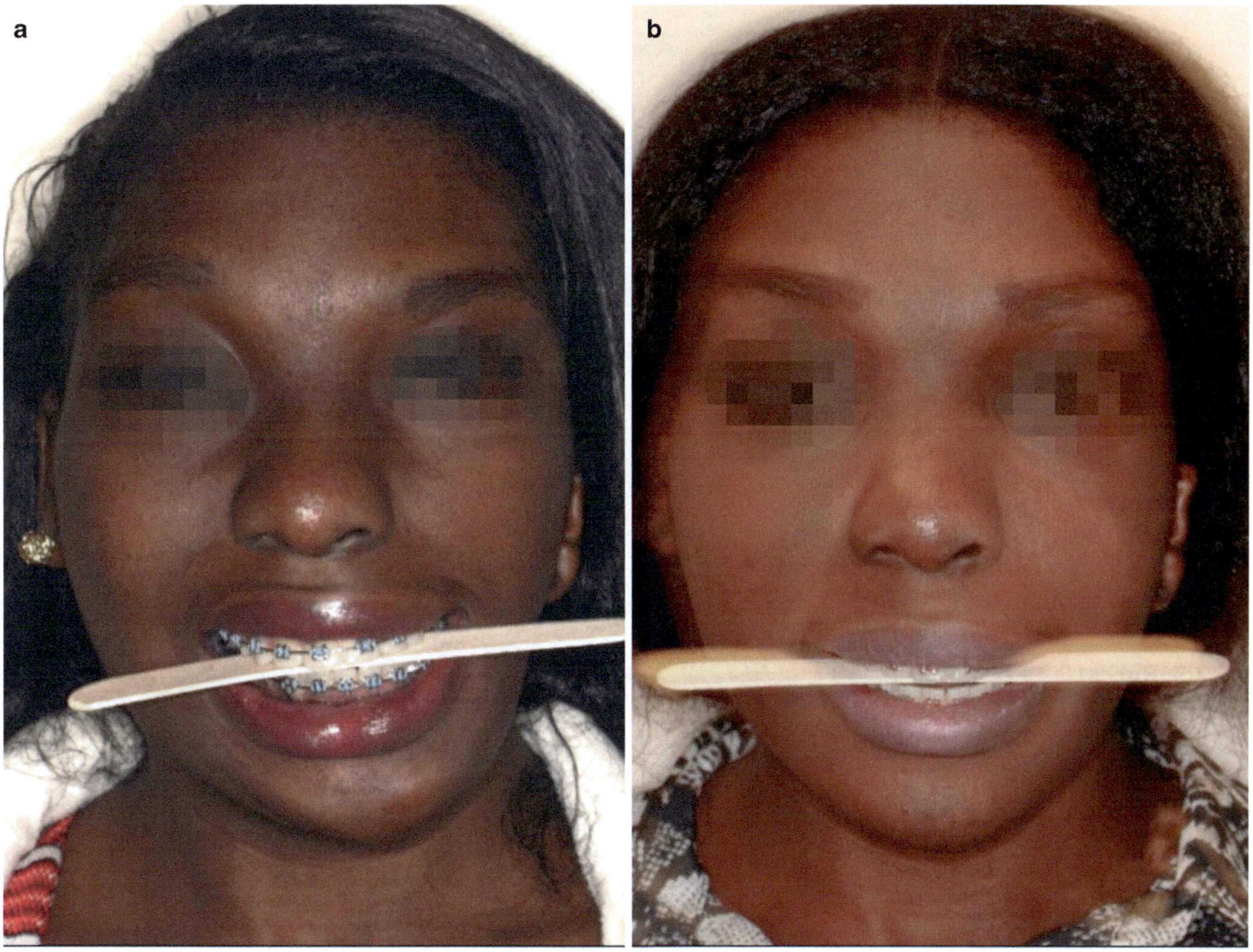

Fig. 66.23 (**a**) Presurgical frontal view, (**b**) postsurgical fontal view. Note the correction of the occlusal cant

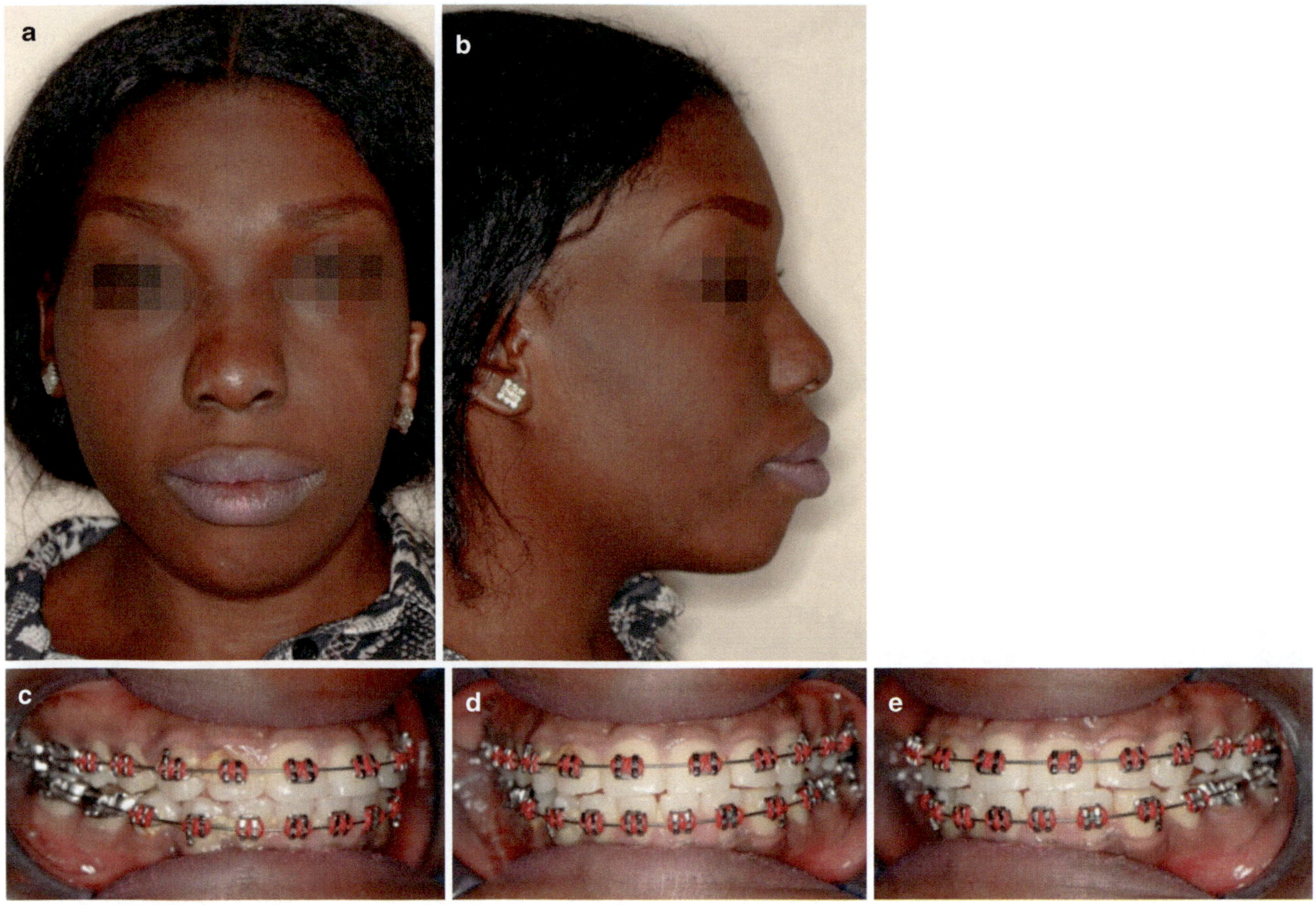

Fig. 66.24 (**a**–**e**) Postsurgical frontal and profile views and occlusion

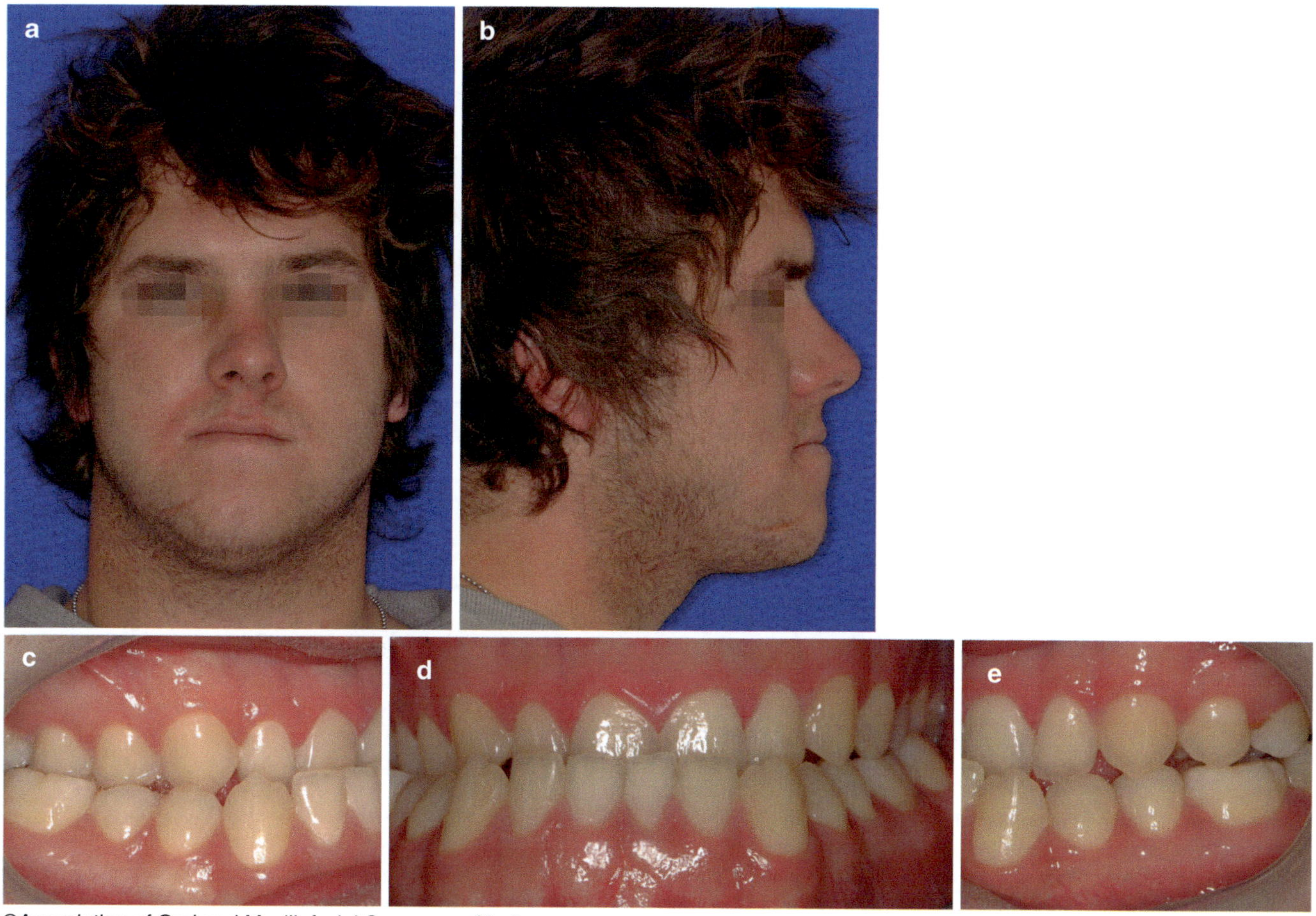

Fig. 66.25 (**a–e**) Frontal, profile, and intraoral views of patient with Class III malocclusion. Patient has paranasal flattening, mandible deviated to right, and flat facial profile. Negative overjet, Class III dental occlusion, and mandibular midline to the right

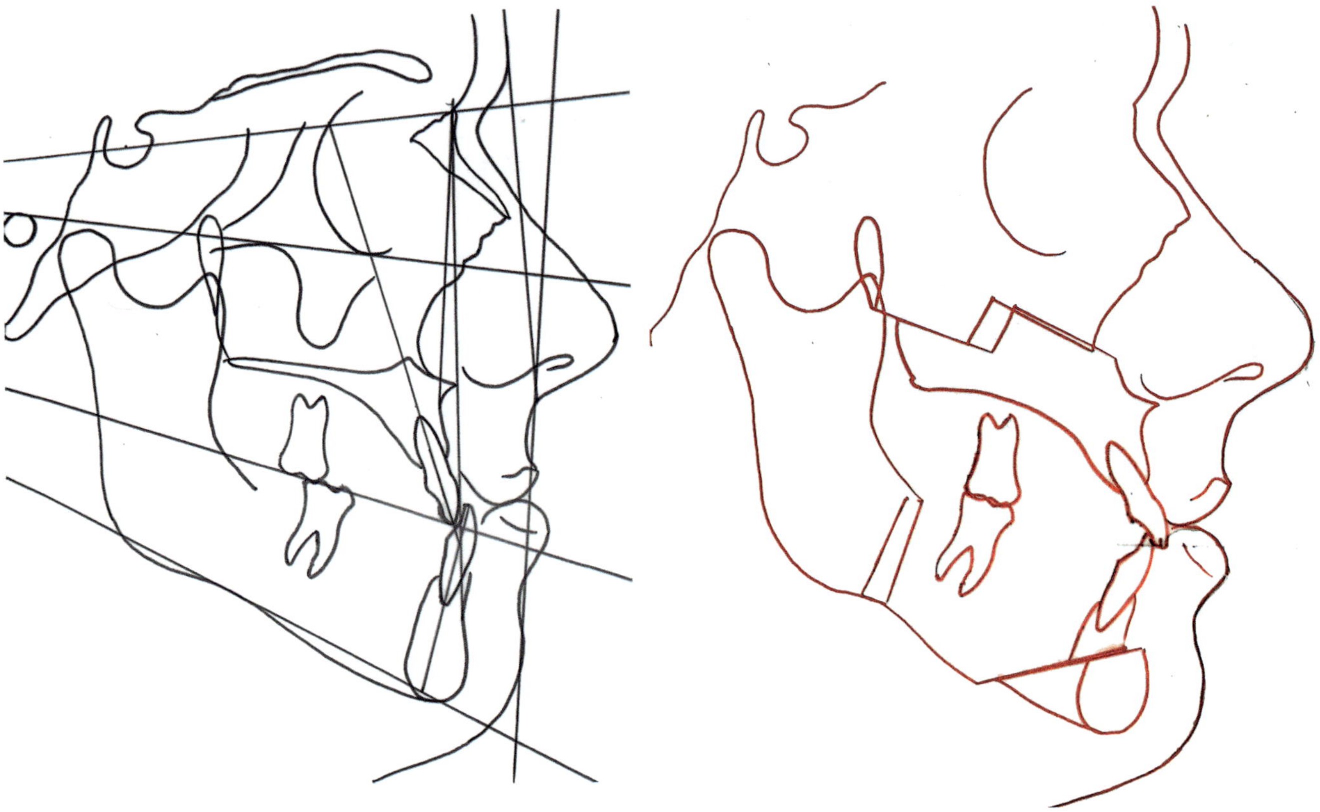

Fig. 66.26 2D cephalometric analysis and 2D surgical treatment planning. Surgical plan is Le Fort I downslide, mandibular setback, and advancement genioplasty

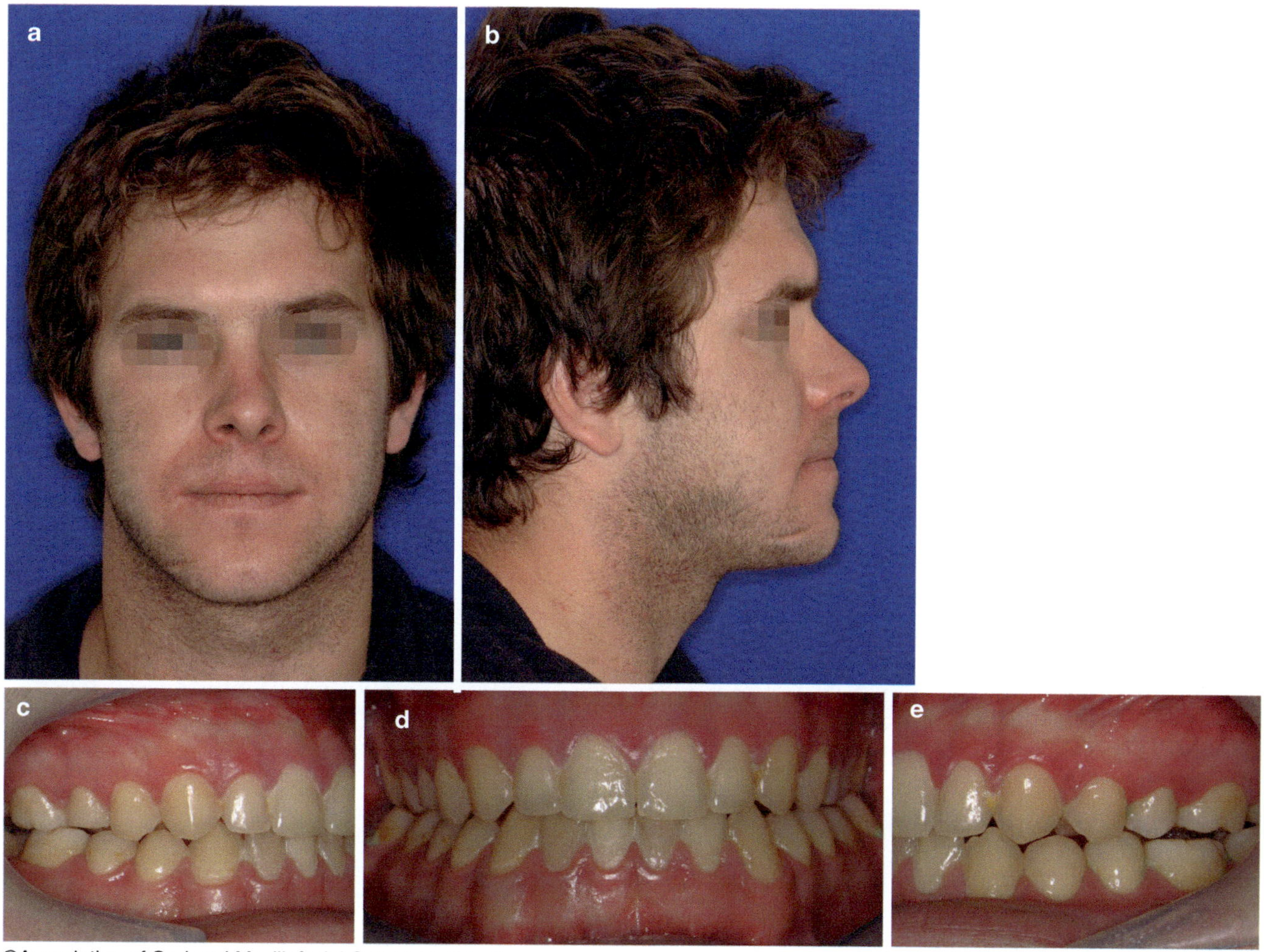

Fig. 66.27 (**a**–**e**) Postsurgical views show that the treatment planning goals have been achieved

References

1. Bell WH. Modern practice in orthognathic and reconstructive surgery, vol. 1. Philadelphia: Saunders; 1992.
2. Hart PS, McIntyre BP, Kadioglu O, Currier GF, Sullivan SM, Li J, et al. Postsurgical volumetric airway changes in 2-jaw orthognathic surgery patients. Am J Orthod Dentofacial Orthop. 2015;147:536–46.
3. Hernandez-Alfaro F, Guijarro-Martinez R, Marque-Bueno J. Effect of mono- and bimaxillary advancement on pharyngeal airway volume: cone-beam computed tomography evaluation. J Oral Maxillofac Surg. 2011;69:E395–400.
4. Naini FB. Facial aesthetics, concepts & clinical diagnosis, Ch. 14. In: The nose. London: Wiley-Blackwell. 2007. p. 214–36.
5. Naini FB, Gill DS. Patient evaluation and clinical diagnosis, Ch. 12. In: Naini FB, Gill DS, editors. Orthognathic surgery, principles, planning and practice. London: Wiley-Blackwell; 2017. p. 199–206.
6. Reyneke JP, Ferretti C. Diagnosis and treatment planning for orthognathic surgery. In: Anderson L, Khanberg K-E, Pogrrel MA, editors. Oral and maxillofacial surgery. London: Wiley-Blackwell; 2010. p. 973–1012.
7. Reyneke JP, Ferretti C. Correction of dentofacial deformities. In: Anderson L, Khanberg K-E, Pogrrel MA, editors. Essentials of oral and maxillofacial surgery. London: Wiley-Blackwell; 2014. p. 315–30.
8. Reyneke JP. Systematic evaluation of the chin. In: The art and science of the sliding genioplasty. Gainesville: REAeducation. 2018.
9. Sarver DM. Esthetic orthodontic and orthognathic surgery. St Louis: Mosby; 1998.
10. Posnick JC. Orthognathic surgery, principles & practice. St Louis: Elsevier; 2014.
11. Arnett GW, McLaughlin RP. Facial and dental planning for orthodontists and oral surgeons. St Louis: Mosby; 2004.
12. Reyneke JP. Esthetic facial evaluation in: essentials of orthognathic surgery. 2nd ed. Chicago: Quintessence; 2011.
13. Swennen GR, Mollemans W, Schutyser F. Three-dimensional treatment planning of orthognathic surgery in the era of virtual imaging. J Oral Maxillofac Surg. 2009;67:2080–92.

Surgery-First Orthognathic Approach

67

N. Viveka Vardhan Reddy and Abhinand Potturi

67.1 Introduction

Treatment philosophies for the management of dentofacial deformities are varied. Milder forms of dentofacial deformity not manifesting as a significant skeletal discrepancy can be corrected by orthodontic treatment alone called "orthodontic camouflage", but those presenting with significant skeletal discrepancy need the skills of both the orthodontist and the maxillofacial surgeon. Hence, correction of dentofacial deformities has come to be a confederate work between both specialties. The dentition and maxillomandibular skeletal complex (MMSC) are intertwined, and changes to one will invariably affect the other, especially more so when the MMSC positional and spatial relationships change. Over the years many new concepts have evolved in orthognathic surgery, and the odyssey between the surgical and orthodontic teams is only getting more inseparable and interesting.

67.2 Background

Looking back to 1960s when techniques of mandibular and maxillary orthognathic surgeries were still evolving from the works of Obwegeser and Trauner, surgeons often performed the procedures either before orthodontic treatment or well after the completion of orthodontic treatment, and rarely any surgeon depended on an orthodontist to move the teeth into certain relationship before undertaking surgery [1]. With time it was realized that the natural dental compensations became a hindrance to the optimal movement of MMSC, thus compromising the results and final outcome.

Poulton et al. [1] in 1963 reported few cases of excessive mandibular growth (mandibular prognathism) which were treated surgically without any pre-surgical orthodontics. In the process, the authors observed that the overjet relationship between the upper and lower anterior teeth limited the amount of mandibular setback, thereby compromising the overall treatment outcome. They concluded that proper alignment of teeth in upper and lower arches is a prerequisite to get adequate mandibular setback. This proposal had almost paved the way for the "orthodontics-first" concept for correcting dentofacial deformities. Worms et al. [2] in the 1970s popularized the concept of "orthodontics first" for all orthognathic surgeries which led to the split of orthodontic treatment into two phases: the pre-surgical orthodontics phase and post-surgical orthodontics phase with an intervening surgical phase.

The pre-surgical orthodontics phase, which essentially antecedes the orthognathic surgical phase, brings out the accurate skeletal discordance by decompensating the natural compensations which have occurred, thereby helping the surgeon to perform a more precise spatial relocation of the MMSC during surgery [3]. However, the pre-surgical phase of orthodontic treatment, also called reverse orthodontics, is a long-drawn process lasting anywhere between 1 and 2 years depending on the complexity of the discrepancy [4]. To add to the woes, during this phase there is gradual deterioration of facial form and dental function [5–7]. Worsening of the facial profile has become a great deterrent for the patients seeking orthognathic surgery because the very reason for seeking the orthognathic surgery for improving facial aesthetics stands defeated and therefore fails to address the patients' chief complaint. Also, the long preoperative preparatory phase can aggravate or initiate other dental problems like dental caries or periodontal problems. For all these reasons, the "orthodontics-first" concept can produce a negative influence on the patient's compliance [8] (Table 67.1).

N. V. V. Reddy (✉) · A. Potturi
SVS Institute of Dental Sciences, Mahabubnagar, Telangana, India

K. Bonanthaya et al. (eds.), *Oral and Maxillofacial Surgery for the Clinician*, https://doi.org/10.1007/978-981-15-1346-6_67

Table 67.1 Challenges associated with conventional "orthodontics-first" approach

1. Time-consuming
2. Deterioration of facial form
3. Difficulty to chew or masticate during pre-surgical phase
4. Psychosocial problems
5. Other complications like dental decay, gum recession and root resorption or root damage

67.3 Surgery-First Orthognathic Approach (SFOA)

In order to overcome the shortcoming of conventional orthognathic surgery, a new approach has been conceptualized called "surgery-first orthognathic approach (SFOA)".

Even though some surgeons expressed the necessity to reposition the MMSC before performing any orthodontics in the past, it did not gain much popularity. With the advent of skeletal anchorage system in orthodontics and rigid fixation system in orthognathic surgery, the problem of skeletal relapse due to unstable bony segments during post-surgical orthodontics has been significantly reduced, paving the way for popularization of SFOA [8, 9].

Correction of various skeletal deformities like Class III [10] and Class II [11] and facial asymmetry [12] using SFOA technique has been reported in the past, and all of them claimed shortening of the total treatment time as a significant and greatest advantage over the conventional technique. William Bell, the "godfather" of orthognathic surgery, during one of his clinical rounds with his residents, highlighted the changing trends in orthognathic surgery by contending that the present orthognathic surgical procedures remain too complicated, too invasive, too time-consuming, too expensive, and too unpredictable, and he literally set the tone for discussing "paradigm shifts in orthognathic surgery" [13]. After the clinical applications of advanced three-dimensional imaging and office-based surgery, the 2011 symposium on SFOA created a broader interest in complete elimination of time-consuming pre-surgical reverse orthodontics and paved the way for worldwide acceptance of this paradigm shift in orthognathic surgery [14, 15].

SFOA technique is fundamentally a "face-first" approach wherein the patient's chief complaint is taken care immediately by improving the facial soft tissue profile and thereby increasing the patient's compliance to overall treatment (Fig. 67.1). In SFOA, greater part of the dentition remains at the same position with respect to their respective arches as there is no pre-surgical orthodontic phase involved. Following the orthognathic surgery, MMSC will be in a Class I relationship, yet the upper and lower dentition may not fit perfectly into occlusion. A *treatable malocclusion*, called *transitional occlusion*, is set at the end of surgery which can be corrected by the orthodontists. Hence, the

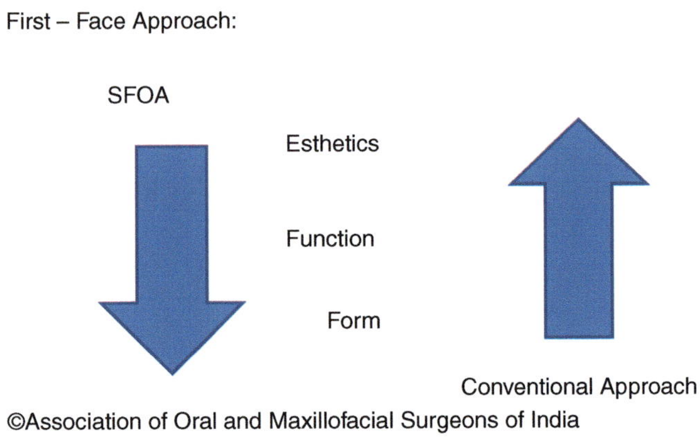

Fig. 67.1 The flow diagram demonstrating fundamental differences and the order of priority between the SFOA and conventional approach

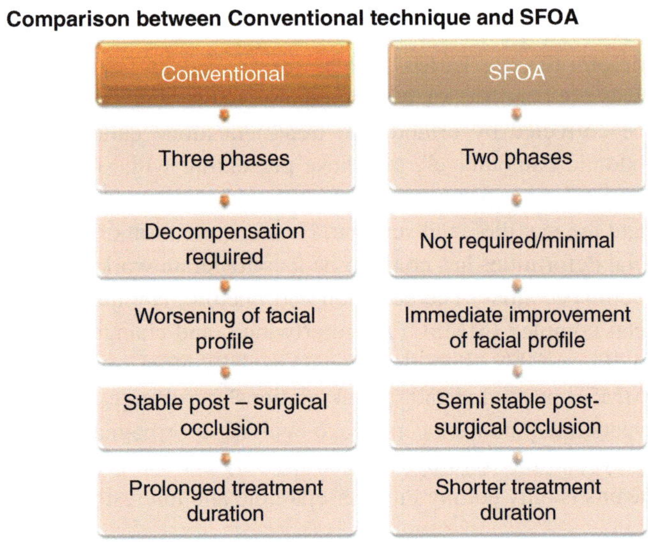

Fig. 67.2 The comparison chart demonstrating various steps for conventional technique and SFOA

orthodontist must actively participate in the treatment planning in SFOA so as to achieve a treatable transitional occlusion at the end of surgery. The orthodontist must be able to foresee the resulting occlusion even before the surgery, and this ability to plan and foresee the resultant transitional occlusion accurately is the linchpin of the entire SFOA technique. Therefore, in SFOA technique the orthodontic principles and guidelines must be established in advance so as to ensure that treatable malocclusions are attained.

Kim JH et al. [8] in their treatise called "Guidelines for "surgery first" orthodontic treatment" have emphasized caution when embarking on SFOA technique. The entire planning process (Fig. 67.2) is laborious since the skeletal changes should be preconceived and the casts should be mounted accordingly to determine the anticipated post-operative orthodontic teeth movements, and, even for the highly accomplished orthodontic and surgical team, it is challenging to pinpoint accurately the occlusal relationship that will balance ideal aesthetic and functional results. It should be remembered during planning that surgical movement should be adequate enough such that dental decompensation is possible after the surgery. Customarily, the dentition is bonded/banded and a passive arch wire is placed before surgery. Active orthodontic tooth movement begins within a relatively short period of time after the jaw(s) are repositioned to take advantage on the inherent phenomena called accelerated tooth movement [8].

67.4 Regional Accelerated Phenomena (RAP)

It is observed that the orthodontic tooth movement following orthognathic surgery is rapid and it is significantly rapid during initial 4–5 post-operative months. This rapid tooth movement post-surgery is attributed to RAP, and it is observed with all the three planes, sagittal, vertical and transverse.

It is an established fact that orthodontic tooth movement is a metabolic event of alveolar bone resorption in the areas of pressure and bone formation in the areas of tension [16, 17]. In order to analyse post-surgical changes in bone metabolism after orthognathic surgery and the corresponding response in the dento-alveolus, Liou et al. conducted a prospective clinical pilot study in 2011. All 22 adult patients who participated in their study underwent both maxillary LeFort I osteotomy and mandibular bilateral sagittal split osteotomy for repositioning of their jaws. Each of these patients was evaluated for serum alkaline phosphatase (ALP) and C-terminal telopeptide of type I collagen (ICTP) before and after surgery at sequential intervals for up to 4 months post-operatively [14].

ALP and ICTP are two bone markers which are indicative of bone turnover rate. ICTP is a bone resorption metabolite of type I collagen in bone and has been associated with the activities of osteoclasts [18]. ALP is an enzyme for bone formation and has been found to associate with osteoblasts function [19]. The results of Liou et al.'s study [14] showed transient increase in the levels of both ICTP and ALP in the immediate post-surgical period indicating burst in the activity of bone remodelling and turnover activity. It was observed from Liou et al.'s [14] study that the ICTP levels peaked from 1 week to 3 months and the ALP levels from 1 to 4 months post orthognathic surgery. This increase in bone turnover markers in the initial post-operative period is a clear indicator of high metabolic activity in the bone and therefore can be used to advantage in shortening the total treatment time in SFOA.

The RAP is not isolated to SFOA. Even in conventional, orthodontics-first approach, this phenomenon plays its role in post-surgical orthodontics. The only difference is that in conventional technique the surgery is done after the decompensation is achieved. The SFOA technique utilizes the golden opportunity of RAP by speeding up the decompensation process which occurs after the orthognathic surgery contrary to that in conventional technique. Therefore, in SFOA, the surgical procedure increases the bone metabolic rate of dento-alveolus in the first 4 post-operative months, which in turn accelerates the orthodontic tooth movement. Hence to make complete use of RAP in SFOA, the post-surgical orthodontic tooth movements have to be begun as early as 1st week and completed by the 4th month.

67.5 Indications

Though SFOA technique can be employed in any kind of maxillomandibular skeletal discrepancy, Liou et al. proposed the following indications in 2011 (Box 67.1) which could help in easy case selection and will act as a guide for the beginners.

67.6 Treatment Planning Considerations

67.6.1 General Guidelines

- The upper and lower dentition are bonded and banded before the surgery without placing any arch wire in order to keep the dentition undisturbed and solid during and after the surgery.
- When planning for SFOA, multiple treatment options must be taken into account. It is very important for the orthodontist to plan the resulting occlusion on the preoperative model set-up in order to achieve relatively stable occlusion on the table during surgery.
- The decompensation of the teeth to normal positions and angulations will be done after surgery, and hence transitional occlusion should allow any orthodontic teeth movement after the surgery. Since the incisors cannot be used as a guide to foresee the final form of occlusion in SFOA, the molar relationship can be utilized as a starting point to come up with a temporary occlusion.

Box 67.1 Proposed indications for SFOA technique

- Well-aligned to mildly crowded anterior teeth
- Flat to mild curve of Spee
- Normal to mildly proclined/retroclined incisors
- Minimal transverse discrepancies
- Cases in which decompensation is not required or minimal decompensation is required

- For the model surgery, the maxillary and mandibular casts are positioned in a proper molar relationship and with a positive overbite. The molar relation could be set up in Class I in cases of non-extraction or bimaxillary first premolar extraction, Class III in cases of lower first premolar extraction and Class II in cases of maxillary first premolar extraction. Once the molar relationship has been established, the overjet should also have been determined.
- The inclination and angulations of upper incisors determine the pattern of extractions. If upper incisors are excessively inclined, then premolar extraction needs to be planned in order to allow post-operative retraction of upper incisors. As a rule of thumb, if the upper incisor to occlusal plane angulation is less than 53–55°, extraction must be considered [20].
- The transverse dimension often creates a special challenge when performing model surgery in surgery-first cases. The upper and lower midlines must be coincident or close to it post-surgery, and proper buccal overjet must be established bilaterally.
- Once surgery is completed, the post-operative orthodontic treatment can begin anytime between 1 week and 1 month post-operatively in order to take the advantage of RAP.

Envisioning the final dental occlusion based on the present occlusion is the key factor in success of SFOA. The interim transitional occlusion achieved on preoperative model set-up must be stable enough to allow predictable splint preparation and skeletal movement. *It is highly recommended that at least three point contacts are achieved between upper and lower teeth when planning for interim transitional occlusion.* In situations where such transient occlusion cannot be established, it is advisable to commence some orthodontic movement in order to assuage some of the interferences and allow for a more stable transitional malocclusion to be established.

67.6.2 Specific Guidelines [15]

Anteroposterior and Vertical Decompensation in Class III Cases

- The sagittal decompensation for proclined upper incisors in a Class III case could be achieved by an anterior segmental osteotomy with removal of the maxillary first bicuspids or by clockwise rotation of the maxilla by LeFort I osteotomy to upright the maxillary incisor inclination.
- The anteroposterior decompensation for moderately retroclined and crowded lower incisors in a Class III case could be achieved by setting up the molars in a Class I relationship with an excessive incisor overjet, and then the mandibular incisors could be aligned after the surgery to obtain the desired overjet.
- The sagittal decompensation for severely retroclined and crowded lower incisors in a Class III situation could be achieved by extraction of the lower first bicuspid and anterior segmental osteotomy, setting up the molars in a Class III relationship with an excessive incisor overjet, and then the lower incisors could be aligned after the surgery to obtain a desired overjet.
- A moderate to deep mandibular curve of Spee in a Class III case is better levelled preoperatively or surgically by anterior segmental osteotomy to avoid the upward and forward rotation of the mandible post-operatively. Alternatively, the lower incisors could be intruded, and the upper incisors at the same time could be extruded post-operatively.

Anteroposterior and Vertical Decompensation in Class II Cases

- For a moderate to deep mandibular curve of Spee and proclined mandibular incisors in Class II mandibular retrognathism, the anterior segment of the lower jaw could be levelled and intruded surgically through anterior segmental osteotomy so that the mandible could be advanced accurately.
- Alternatively, the mandible could be surgically advanced to an edge-to-edge incisor relationship and without occlusal contact in the posterior teeth, and then post-surgically, the lower anterior teeth could be orthodontically intruded so that the mandible rotates upwards and forwards for posterior occlusal contact and a better chin projection.

67.7 Treatment Protocol (Table 67.2)

The protocol variations between the conventional orthognathic surgery and SFOA can be clearly appreciated in the Table 67.2 highlighted in Bold fonts. A simulation of pre-

Table 67.2 Treatment protocol comparing SFOA technique to conventional technique

Conventional technique	SFOA technique
1. Initial diagnosis	1. Initial diagnosis
2. Surgical planning—STO	2. Surgical planning—STO
3. Pre surgical orthodontic treatment	**3. Simulation of pre-surgical orthodontic treatment**
	Model mounting and model setup
	4. Simulation of orthognathic surgery
4. Surgical arch wire	5. Surgical arch wire
5. Fabrication of splints	6. Fabrication of splints
6. Orthognathic surgery and post-op care	7. Orthognathic surgery and post-op care
7. Orthodontic rediagnosis	8. Orthodontic rediagnosis
8. Orthodontic treatment	9. Orthodontic treatment
9. Finishing	10. Finishing

surgical orthodontic treatment using model mounting and set-up will compensate the pre-surgical orthodontic treatment.

67.8 Protocol Variations

Although the sequence of treatment is similar, different protocols are being used to prepare the patient for surgery, perform the operative procedure, and commence the orthodontic treatment.

67.8.1 Timing of Bonding

- Chung C Yu and Villegas [12]—1 week before orthognathic surgery
- Sugawara and Nagasaka [10, 11]; E Liou et al. [15]—Just before surgery
- Federico Hernandez [21]—brackets 10–14 days after surgery

67.8.2 Initial Arch Wires

- Liou et al. [15]—did not place any orthodontic arch wires before surgery
- Sugawara and Nagasaka [10, 11]—preferred 0.019″ × 0.025″ SS wires in 0.022″ slot

Placement of passive stainless steel arch wires bent and adapted to each tooth before surgery will preclude any untoward tooth movement during or immediately after the surgery. The authors wishing to capitalize on the RAP concept immediately after surgery prefer to place active nickel-titanium arch wires prior to surgery. Nonetheless, in doing so, the orthodontist loses an opportunity to observe the stability of the surgical correction prior to beginning of the tooth movement. The rapid acceleratory phenomenon not just influences the tooth movement but also can disturb the alveolar bone [8].

There are also protocol variations regarding the usage of surgical splints after the surgery among the various authors. While some authors suggested the use of the surgical splints only intraoperatively, others have advocated its use anywhere between 1 and 4 post-operative weeks. Nagasaka et al. have used removable Gelb-type splints post-surgery [10]. Kim's preference is to leave the splint in for about 1 month to 1 and a half months post-operatively and if an open bite is observed to use elastics between the splint and the mini-screws placed into the bone or to leave the splint for an even longer time period [8].

67.9 Procedural Guidelines for Model Mounting and Model Set-Up in SFOA (Fig. 67.3)

- Once the treatment planning and diagnosis is completed, impressions are made and customary model mounting is performed with bite registration to scrutinize the present state of the occlusion.
- In the model set-up, teeth that have adapted by natural compensation to the existing skeletal discrepancy are simulated and reorganized into anticipated occlusion similar to the preoperative orthodontic treatment plan. All the teeth on the set-up model are rearranged as if orthodontic treatment is done in the real patient in conventional orthognathic surgery technique into the desired preoperative occlusal relationship.
- Once the desired dental occlusion is set on the models, the amount of the skeletal movement required in the maxilla, mandible or both will become evident. Subsequently, a simulation of the actual orthognathic surgery is performed on the mounted models as in conventional technique. This will indicate the possible occlusal outcome of the standard approach.
- Intermediate and final splint can then be made on these mounted models as they are set up into the planned skeletal movements.
- With the advent of virtual planning and three-dimensional simulation softwares, the same set-up model surgery can be performed by scanning the physical models and bite registration details into the software, and the three-dimensional intermediate and final splints can be printed.

67.10 Surgical Procedures (Fig. 67.4)

The surgical procedures in the maxilla, mandible or chin are themselves performed using described standard techniques, whether it is the conventional technique or the SFOA technique.

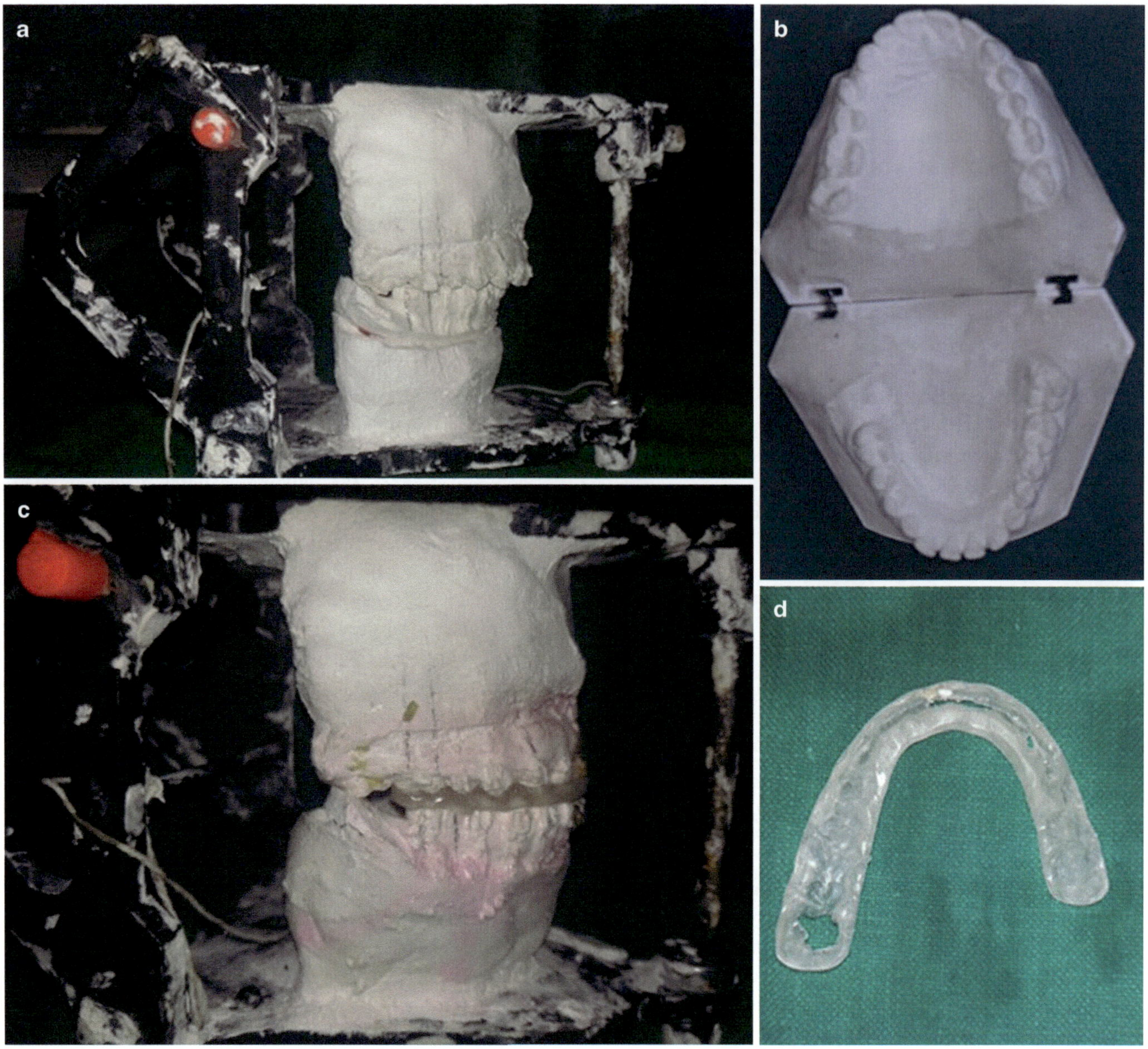

Fig. 67.3 (**a**) Standard model mounting. (**b**) Before the procedure, the teeth that have adapted to the skeletal discrepancy are simulated and reorganized into their predicted location, similar to real pre-surgical orthodontic treatment. (**c**) Simulation of actual orthognathic surgery is then performed. (**d**) Surgical splints fabricated to aid in real-time surgery

Fig. 67.4 Flow diagram showing various surgical procedures in each of the jaws

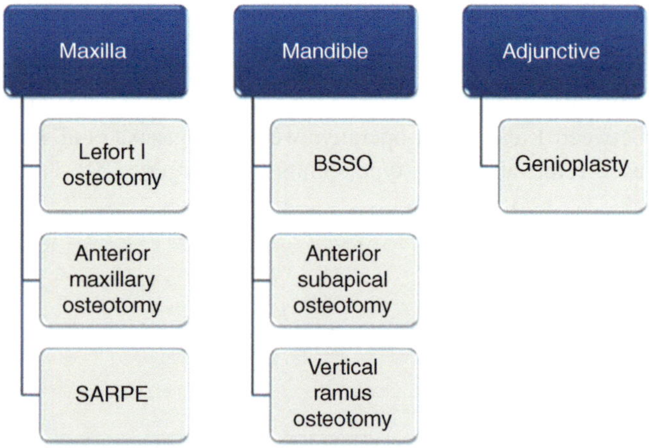

67.11 Advantages and Disadvantages of SFOA (Table 67.3)

Systematic review published by Peiró-Guijarro et al. [21] in 2006 reviewed 179 publications and finally selected 11 articles for final reporting. They found that the SFOA technique was most commonly reported in Class III skeletal malocclusion than in skeletal Class II malocclusion with prevalence of about 84.7%. The single largest advantage described was shortened treatment duration time owing to the RAP concept, and the disadvantage was potential error in predicting the post-operative occlusal outcome resulting in greater or lesser surgical movements of the jaws.

67.12 The Future of "Surgery-First" Approach

The future of SFOA technique lies in using augmented skull models, virtual orthodontic set-up to replace the mounted study model set-up and the computer-aided design and computer-aided manufacturing fabrication of intraoperative splints (Fig. 67.5). The 3D virtual orthodontic set-up will help the orthodontist to predict the eventual (at the end of orthodontic treatment) position and the axial inclination of each tooth scrupulously. This is a compelling step before the surgeon's skeletal base correction simulation, since the patient's prevailing occlusion

Table 67.3 Advantages and disadvantages of the surgery-first approach

Advantages
1. Total duration of treatment is shorter
2. The facial profile is improved from the commencement of treatment as a result of skeletal base correction
3. Patient and orthodontist satisfaction rates are high. High patient satisfaction is associated with improved cooperation during post-operative orthodontics
4. Orthodontic decompensation is efficient and effectual in response to the establishment of a proper maxillomandibular relationship and the regional acceleratory phenomenon
5. Surgical movements may not be curbed due to orthodontic constraints. There is more freedom to choose the surgical movement in accordance with the clinical requirement for individual patients
6. Patient recovery takes place expeditiously
7. When sleep-disordered breathing is the main indication for treatment, early maxillomandibular advancement increases the dimensions of the upper airway immediately
Disadvantages
1. Case selection is critical because the baseline occlusion cannot guide treatment objectives. Therefore, high clinical expertise, meticulous prediction of post-operative tooth movement and precise assessment of skeletal discrepancy are imperative
2. The bending procedure for a passive surgical wire is tedious and complex
3. Bonding and removal of the surgical wire are taxing; there is a relatively high bonding failure rate before and during surgery
4. The extent of surgical movements is necessarily greater, because surgical correction needs to make up for dental compensation
5. Impacted lower third molars could add difficulty to surgery
6. ost-surgical fluidity during bone healing could cause skeletal instability, and its impact on relapse has not yet been fully investigated
7. Orthodontic appointments should be scheduled more often than in a traditional approach. This could be stressful for the orthodontist
8. Constant correspondence between the surgeon and the orthodontist is indispensable

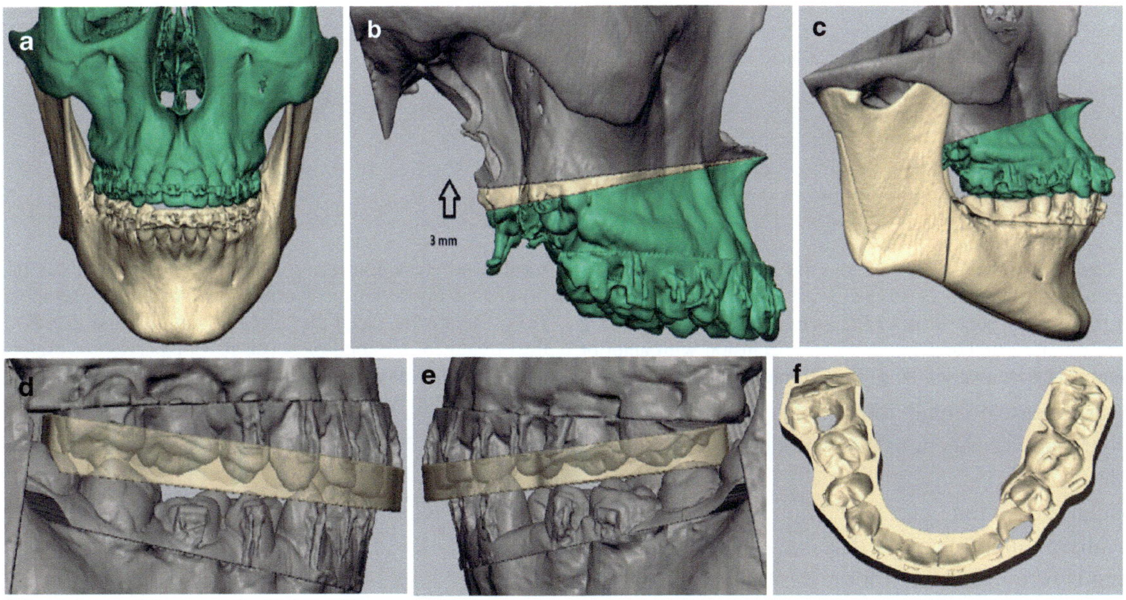

Fig. 67.5 The workflow demonstrating the pre-surgical orthodontic movement set-up (**a**), the surgical procedure on the maxilla (**b**), the procedure on the mandible (**c**), the post-operative ensuing dental occlusion with splint in situ (**d**, **e**) and the design of the final splint (**f**)

cannot serve as a guide for skeletal repositioning as it lies in a compensated state.

Usability of temporary anchorage devices (TAD) and interdental corticotomies is a factor which can add to the future of SFOA. The TAD permits a wider range of orthodontic vectors and avoids premature bracket loading with secondary troublesome dental extrusion. Interdental corticotomies can augment the RAP and further enhance the orthodontic treatment duration.

67.13 Conclusion

Performing orthognathic surgery even before any orthodontic tooth movement (SFOA) offers a unique advantage of addressing the patient's chief complaint at the very beginning, thereby improving the acceptance and compliance of the patient to overall treatment. It also offers the big advantage of significant decrease in total duration time by making use of the RAP. The final outcomes, in the way of facial aesthetics, dental occlusion and stability, are similar when using orthodontics-first and surgery-first approaches. However, it must be remembered that both the surgeon and the orthodontist must trend with care as there is a premium on patient selection and both should be involved as a team during every stage of the treatment, starting from diagnosis to debonding. Surgeon-orthodontist team should know the orthodontic principles and understand the limits of orthodontic teeth movement and must accommodate dental decompensation in their initial treatment planning. The surgeon should be capable of carrying out designated osteotomy and intermaxillary fixation with occlusion bite plate on misaligned dental arches and providing the stability after skeletal reposition. The future of orthognathic surgery is geared towards reducing the overall treatment duration without compromising the final outcome.DisclosureAuthors have no financial conflicts to disclose.

67.14 Case Scenarios

Case Scenario 1 (Fig. 67.6)

Case Scenario 2 (Fig. 67.7)

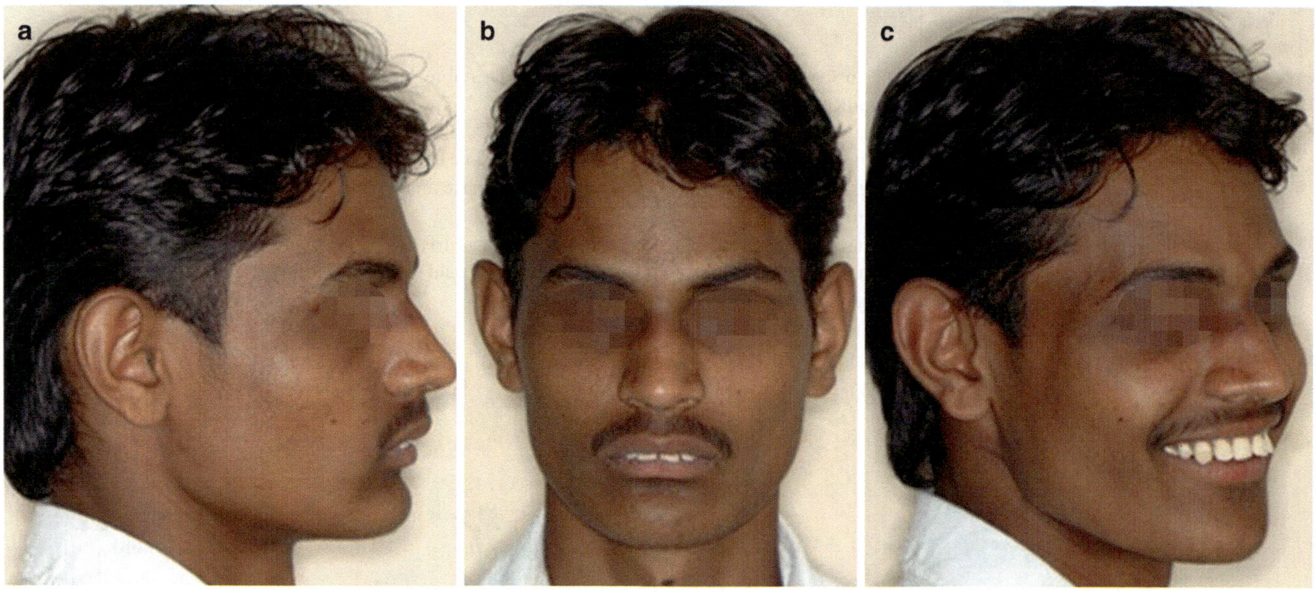

Fig. 67.6 Case Scenario 1. A 19-year-old male presenting with forwardly place upper front teeth. (**a**–**c**) Preoperative pics showing frontal, profile and right lateral views. (**d**, **e**) Preoperative occlusion showing end on molar relation and compensated dental occlusion with anterior deep bite and excessive overjet. (**f**, **g**) Post-surgical orthodontic treatment in progress. Excessive nature of curve of Spee can be noted, and the change in overjet and overbite post-surgery can be appreciated. (**h**–**j**) Post-treatment facial pics: frontal, smiling and lateral views. (**k**, **l**) Post-treatment intraoral pics. (**m**, **n**) Comparison of pre-operative and post-operative lateral cephalograms

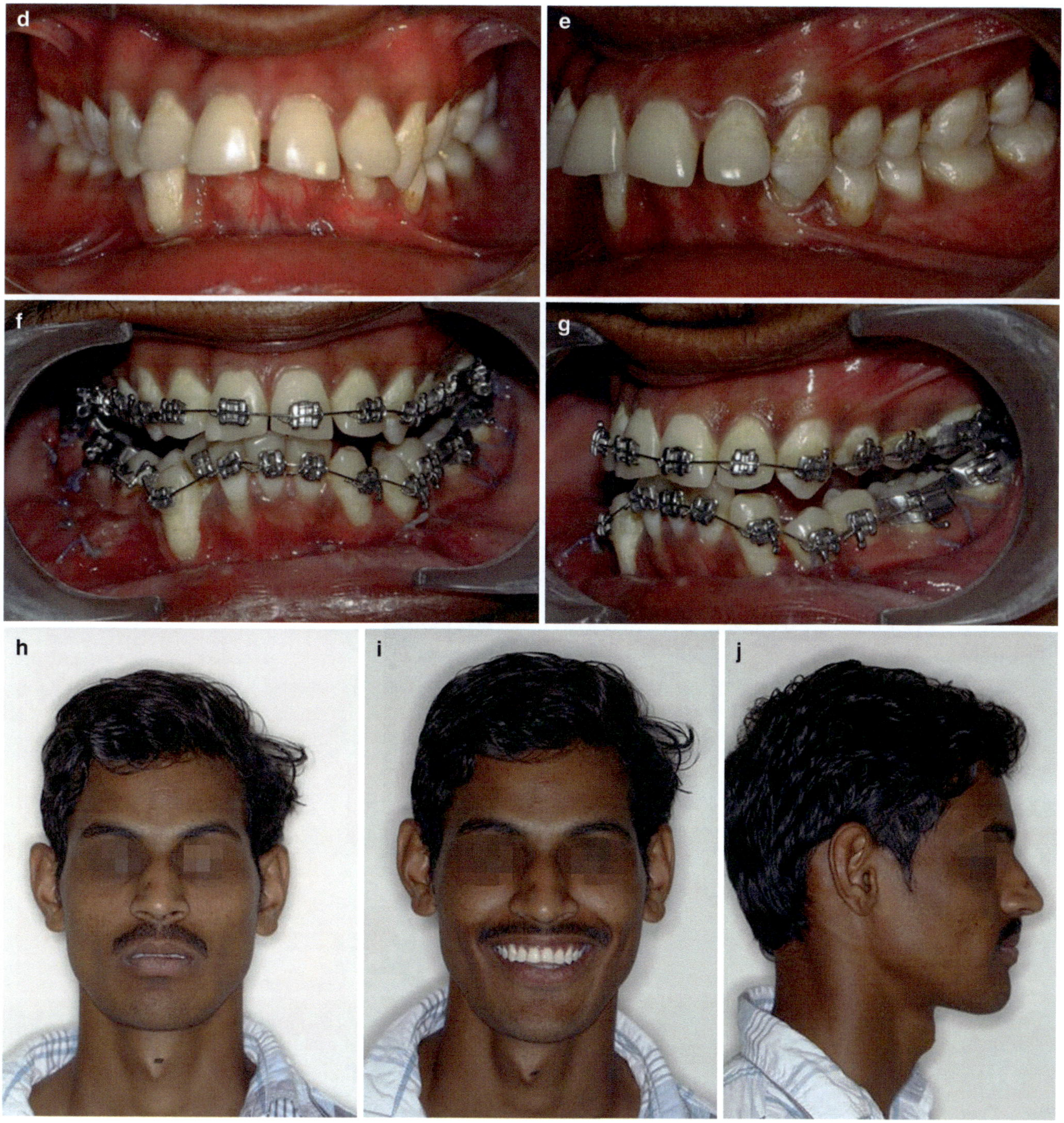

Fig. 67.6 (continued)

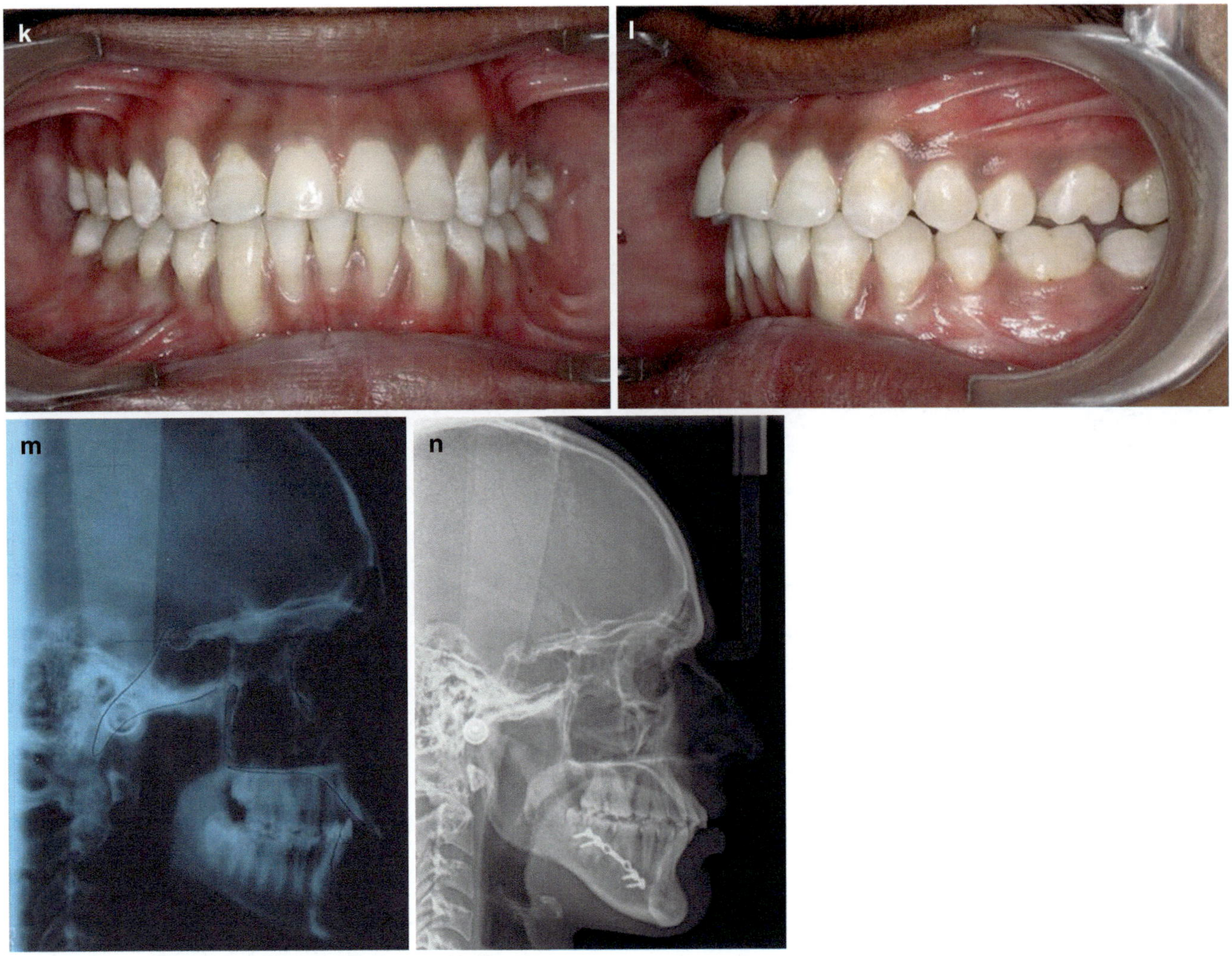

Fig. 67.6 (continued)

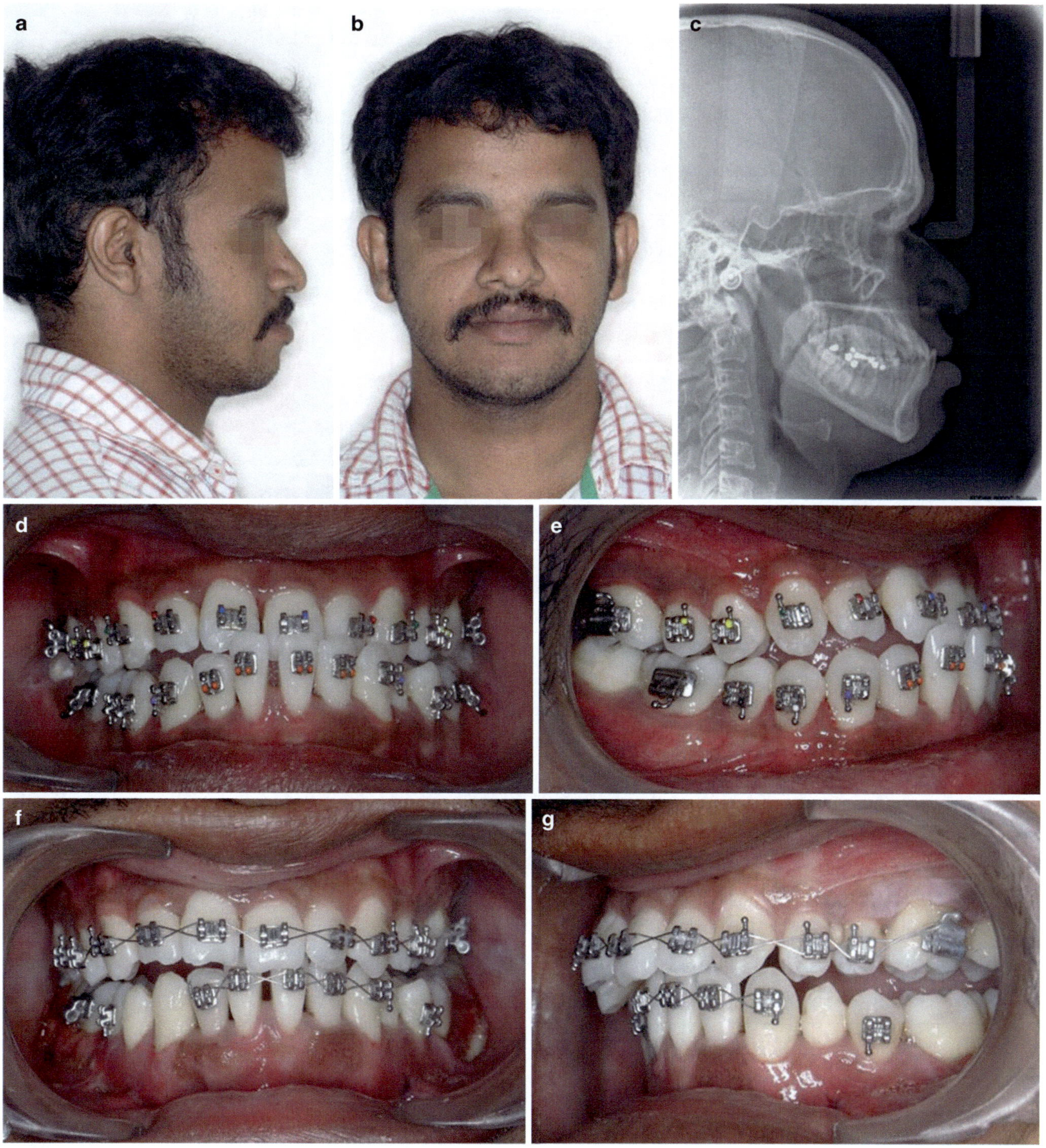

Fig. 67.7 Case Scenario 2. A 26-year-old male presenting with prominent lower facial appearance and mobile lower front teeth. (**a**, **b**) Clinical pics showing lateral and frontal views: Concave facial profile can be appreciated with acute nasolabial angle. (**c**) Lateral cephalogram showing skeletal Class III jaw bases with normodivergence. (**d**, **e**) Intraoral picture showing reverse overjet, Class III molar relationship and spacing in lower anteriors. (**f**, **g**) Post-surgical orthodontics in progress. Reversal of overjet can be noticed. (**h–J**) Post-treatment facial pics in profile and frontal. (**k**) Intraoral post-treatment pic showing occlusal relationship with normal overjet and Class I molar relationship. (**l**) Post-operative cephalogram

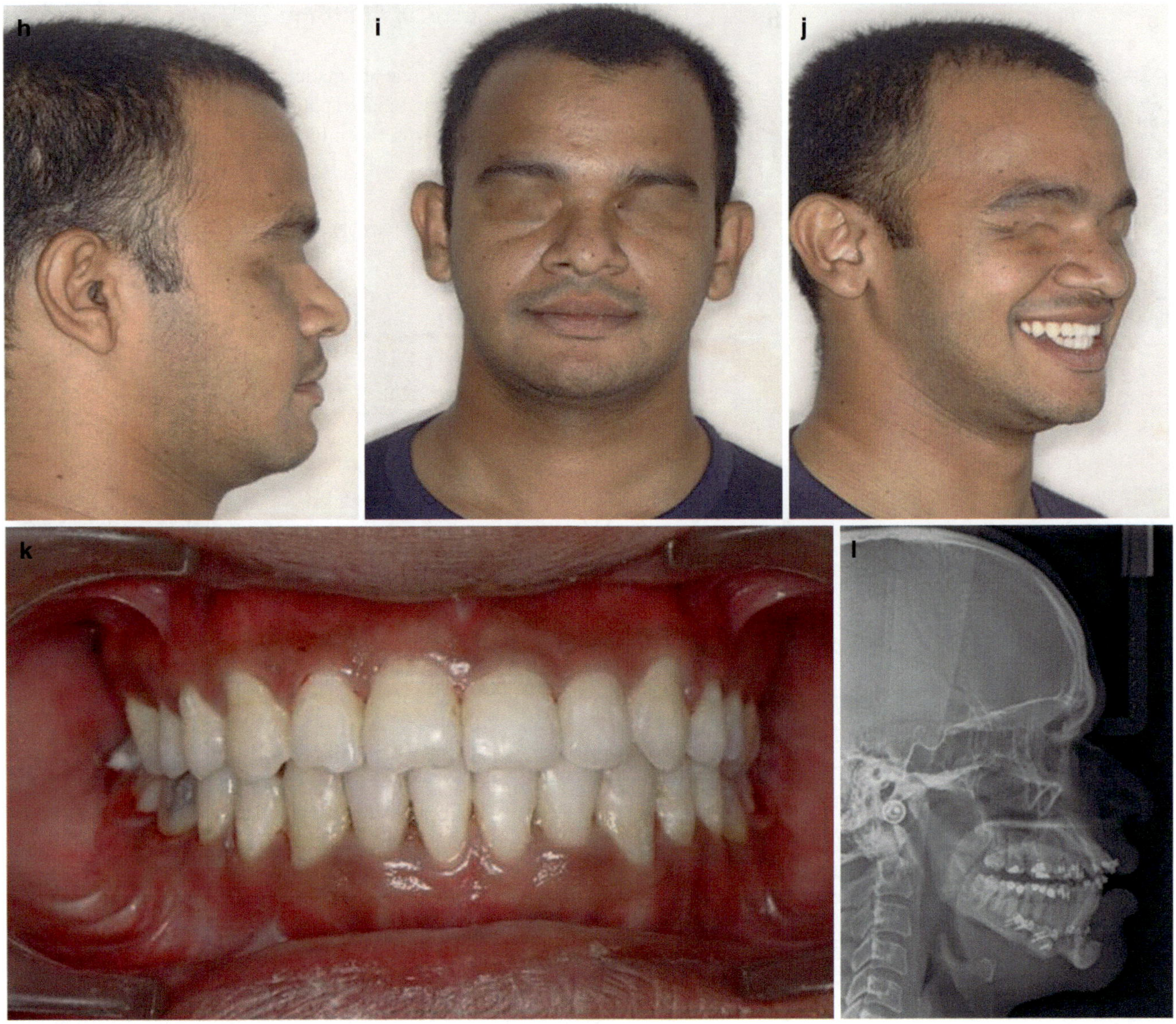

Fig. 67.7 (continued)

References

1. Poulton DR, Taylor RC, Ware WH. Cephalometric x-ray evaluation of the vertical osteotomy correction of mandibular prognathism. Oral Surg Oral Med Oral Pathol. 1963;16:807–20.
2. Worms FW, Isaacson RJ, Speidel TM. Surgical orthodontic treatment planning: profile analysis and mandibular surgery. Angle Orthod. 1976;46(1):1–25.
3. Sabri R. Orthodontic objectives in orthognathic surgery: state of the art today. World J Orthod. 2006;7(2):177–91.
4. Grubb J, Evans C. Orthodontic management of dentofacial skeletal deformities. Clin Plast Surg. 2007;34(3):403–15.
5. Bailey LTJ, Proffit WR. Combined surgical and orthodontic treatment. In: Sarver DM, Fields HW, Proffit WR, editors. Contemporary orthodontics. 3rd ed. Philadelphia, PA: Mosby; 1999. p. 674–709.
6. Jacobs JD, Sinclair PM. Principles of orthodontic mechanics in orthognathic surgery cases. Am J Orthod. 1983;84(5):399–407.
7. Proffit WR, White RP, Sarver DM. Combining surgery and orthognathics: who does what, when? In: Proffit WR, White RP, Sarver DM, editors. Contemporary treatment of dentofacial deformity. 1st ed. St Louis, MO: Mosby; 2003. p. 245–67.
8. Kim JH, Mahdavie NN, Evans CA. Guidelines for "surgery first" orthodontic treatment. In: Bourzgui F, editor. Orthodontics—basic aspects and clinical considerations. 1st ed. Casablanca: University Hassan II of Casablanca: IntechOpen; 2012. p. 265–300.
9. Huang CS, Chen YR. Orthodontic principles and guidelines for the surgery-first approach to orthognathic surgery. Int J Oral Maxillofac Surg. 2015;44(12):1457–62.
10. Nagasaka H, Sugawara J, Kawamura H, Nanda R. "Surgery first" skeletal class III correction using the skeletal anchorage system. J Clin Orthod. 2009;43(2):97–105.
11. Sugawara J, Aymach Z, Nagasaka DH, Kawamura H, Nanda R. "Surgery first" orthognathics to correct a skeletal class II malocclusion with an impinging bite. J Clin Orthod. 2010;44(7):429–38.

12. Villegas C, Uribe F, Sugawara J, Nanda R. Expedited correction of significant dentofacial asymmetry using a "surgery first" approach. J Clin Orthod. 2010;44(2):97–103.
13. Assael LA. The biggest movement: orthognathic surgery undergoes another paradigm shift. J Oral Maxillofac Surg. 2008;66(3):419–20.
14. Liou EJ, Chen PH, Wang YC, Yu CC, Huang CS, Chen YR. Surgery-first accelerated orthognathic surgery: postoperative rapid orthodontic tooth movement. J Oral Maxillofac Surg. 2011;69(3):781–5.
15. Liou EJ, Chen PH, Wang YC, Yu CC, Huang CS, Chen YR. Surgery-first accelerated orthognathic surgery: orthodontic guidelines and setup for model surgery. J Oral Maxillofac Surg. 2011;69(3):771–80.
16. Storey E. The nature of tooth movement. Am J Orthod. 1973;63(3):292–314.
17. Reitan K. Some factors determining the evaluation of forces in orthodontics. Am J Orthod. 1957;43(1):32–45.
18. Pellegrini GG, Gonzales CM, Somoza JC, Friedman SM, Zeni SN. Correlation between salivary and serum markers of bone turnover in osteopenic rats. J Periodontol. 2008;79(1):158–65.
19. Binder T, Goodson J, Socransky S. Gingival fluid levels of acid and alkaline phosphatase. J Periodontal Res. 1987;22(1):14–9.
20. Liao YF, Chiu YT, Huang CS, Ko EW, Chen YR. Presurgical orthodontics versus no presurgical orthodontics: treatment outcome of surgical-orthodontic correction for skeletal class III open bite. Plast Reconstr Surg. 2010;126(6):2074–83.
21. Peiró-Guijarro MA, Guijarro-Martínez R, Hernández-Alfaro F. Surgery first in orthognathic surgery: a systematic review of the literature. Am J Orthod Dentofac Orthop. 2016;149(4):448–62.

Orthognathic Surgery for Mandible

68

Varghese Mani

68.1 Introduction

Proper balance and harmony between the different parts of the face—forehead, eyebrows, eyes, nose, ears, cheeks, lips, mouth, jaws, chin, etc.—are the main factors deciding aesthetics. Aesthetic evaluation is mandatory to understand the problems systematically. During the primate evolution, jaws lost many functions, and the size suffered a gradual reduction, which resulted in an orthomorphic face. The facial muscles gained fine expression and smile, the exceptional features of *Homo sapiens*.

Mandible forms the movable lower part of the head. Mandible is attached to the upper part of the head by ligaments and musculature. It articulates with the glenoid fossa of temporal bone through temporomandibular joint, a synovial joint having translator and rotator movements (ginglymoarthrodial). These movements facilitate chewing and grinding functions. In our prehuman ancestors, the body of the mandible was parallel. In humans, since the brain case has expanded, the temporal bones were pushed apart, TMJ followed suit giving the lower jaw a parabolic contour. The Simian shelf reduced to genial tubercles to facilitate speech and to compensate and strengthen the jaw and the chin developed in humans. Metaphorically it is often stated that "the brain case has expanded at the expense of the jaws".

In some people, surgical repositioning of the mandible may be required to achieve an ideal facial form and restore functions such as mastication and breathing.

68.2 Surgical Anatomy of the Mandible (Fig. 68.1a, b)

Mandible is the sturdiest bone of the face with strong basal bone and the alveolar part housing the dentition. The near round protuberances seen bilaterally at the cephalic end of the mandible are called condyles, and they form its articulation with the TMJ. The mandibular condyles articulate with the temporal bone and help in the rotatory and translatory movements of the mandible as well as to transmit forces from the mandible to the skull base. A good understanding of the gross anatomy of the mandible is essential to understand its surgical implications. This needs to include the TMJ, the dentition, the supporting ligaments, and the muscles of mastication (Fig. 68.2a, b) and facial expression.

On the medial aspect of the vertical ramus is the mandibular foramen just posterior to halfway between the anterio-posterior width of the vertical ramus almost in line with the most concave part of the anterior border of the ramus. Just above is the lingula, a triangular prominence to which the sphenomandibular ligament is attached. Mandibular neurovascular bundle enters the mandibular foramen on the lingual side of the mandible and runs below the tooth roots in the body of the jaw, in the inferior alveolar canal. It curves upward and backward by about 2 mm and gives out the main branch, mental nerve, below the second premolar area, and gives sensory supply to the lower lip and chin [1].

Electronic Supplementary Material The online version of this chapter (https://doi.org/10.1007/978-981-15-1346-6_68) contains supplementary material, which is available to authorized users.

V. Mani (✉)
Department of Oral and Maxillofacial Surgery, Mar Baselios Dental College, Kothamangalam, Kerala, India

K. Bonanthaya et al. (eds.), *Oral and Maxillofacial Surgery for the Clinician*, https://doi.org/10.1007/978-981-15-1346-6_68

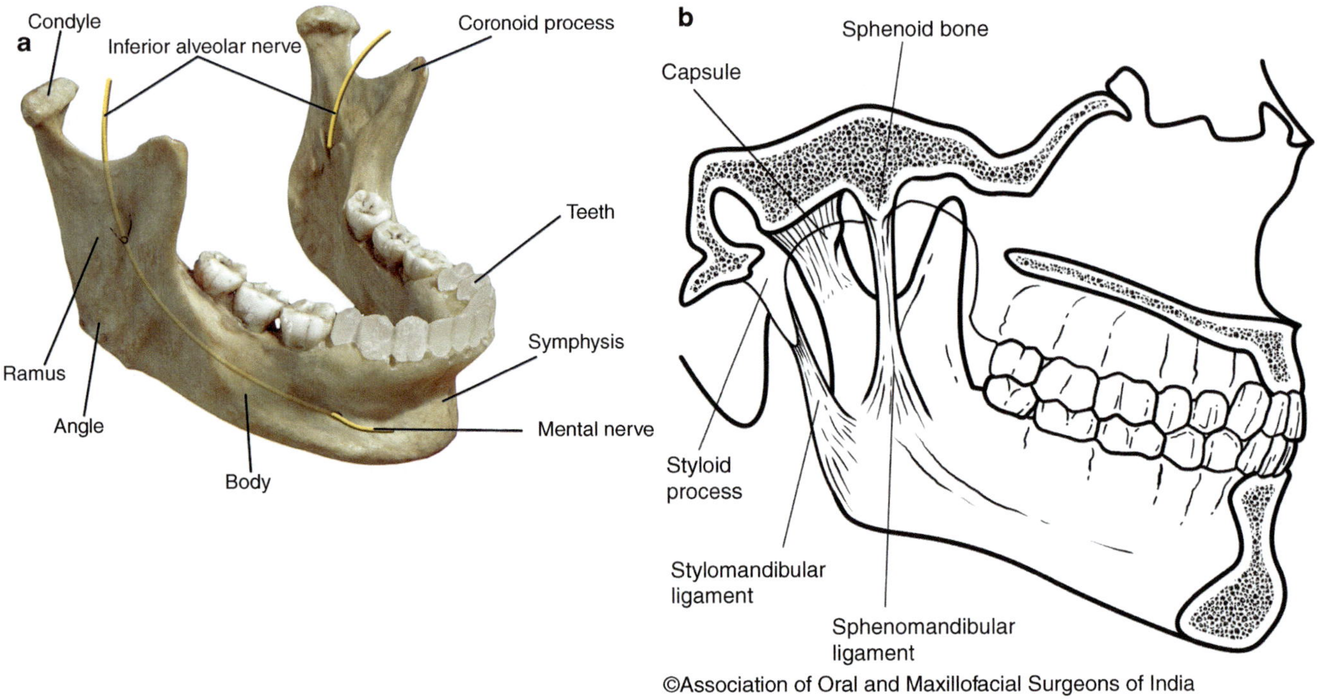

Fig. 68.1 (**a**) Gross anatomy of mandible, (**b**) ligaments attached to mandible

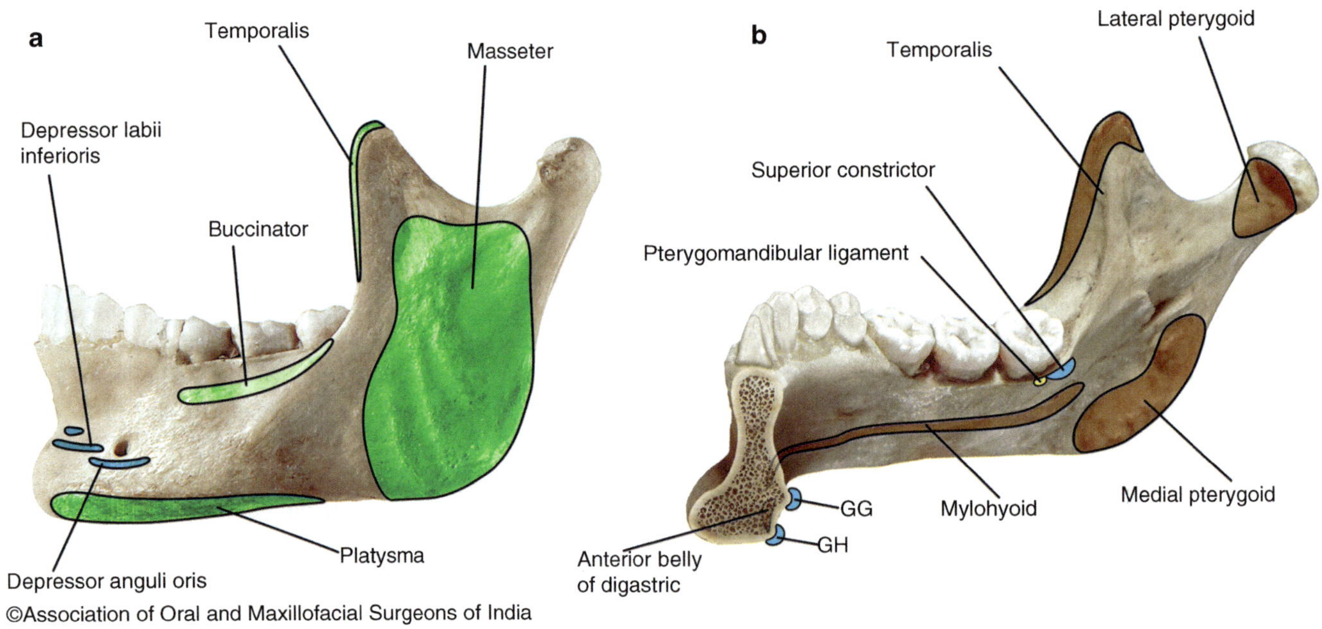

Fig. 68.2 Muscles attached to mandible. (**a**) Buccal aspect and (**b**) lingual aspect. (GG) Genioglossus and (GH) Geniohyoid

68.3 Classification of Deformities of the Mandible (Table 68.1)

Table 68.1 Classification of dentofacial deformities

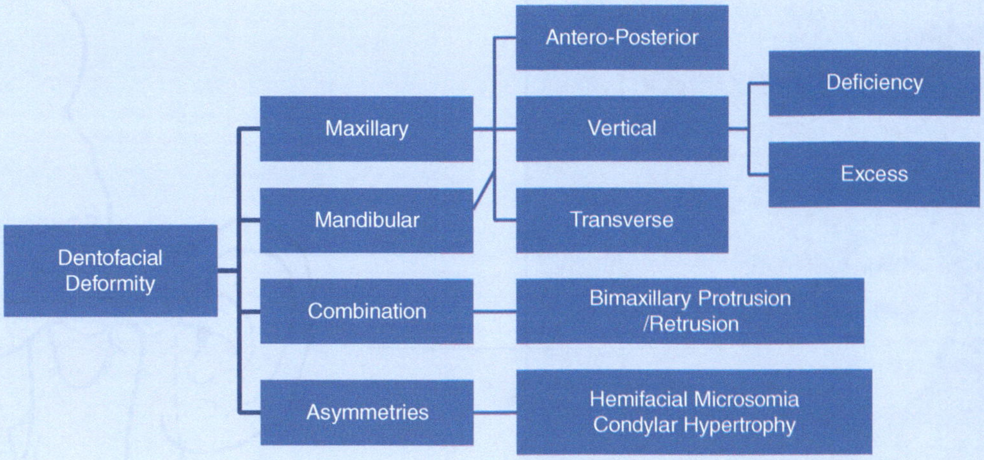

Deformities of the jaws can be associated with the dento-alveolar complex, the skeletal base or both.

They may be either an excess or a deficiency.

These problems can occur in three different vectors: Antero-posterior, Transverse and Vertical

Before venturing into the classification of the jaw deformities it will be appropriate to assess the relationship of the lower jaw to the rest of the face. Certain parameters are used to assess the deformity objectively. Clinical evaluation is the most important of them all. Face has to be assessed frontally and laterally.

Profile analysis of the face is the most important of them all—it could be convex, straight, or concave. Convexity can be due to protruded maxilla or retruded mandible/chin. Concave face can be due to retruded maxilla or prognathic mandible/chin (Fig. 68.3a, b, c).

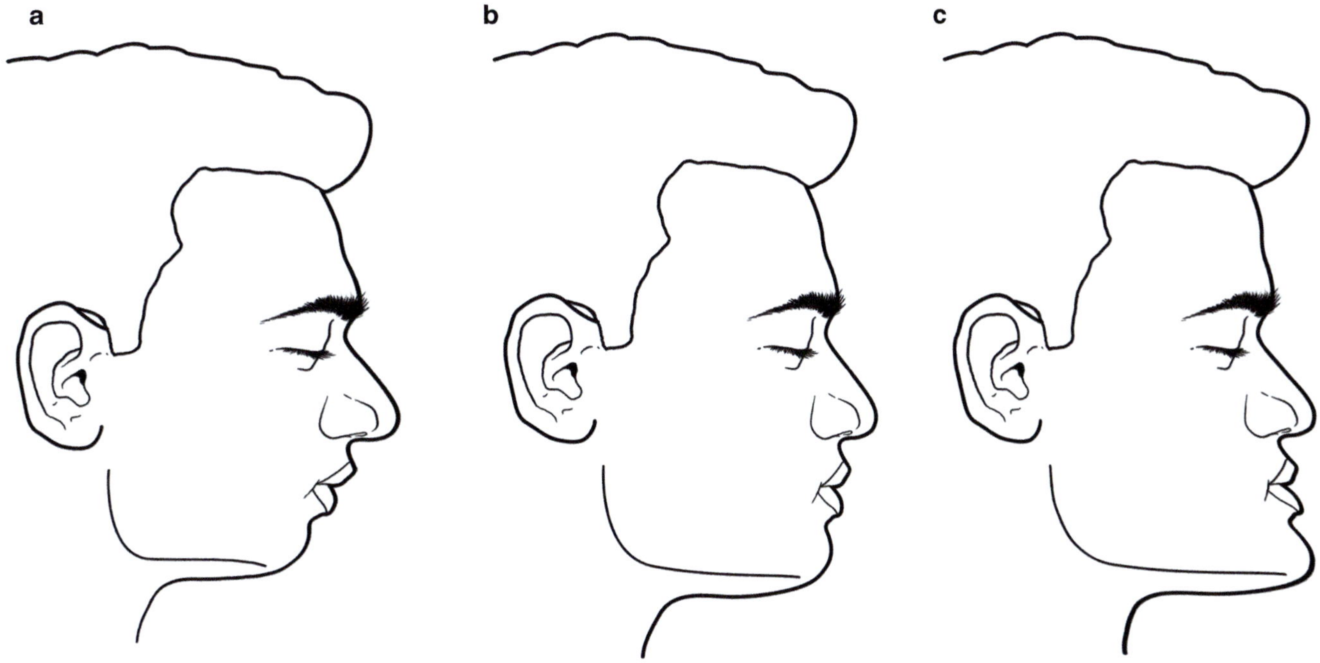

Fig. 68.3 On profile analysis face can be convex (**a**), straight (**b**), or concave (**c**)

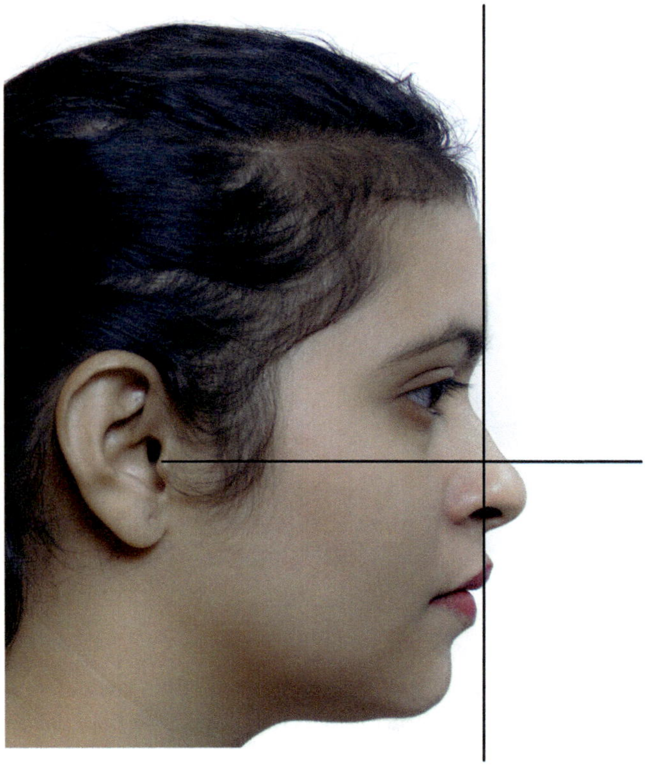

Fig. 68.4 Subnasale perpendicular to FH plane

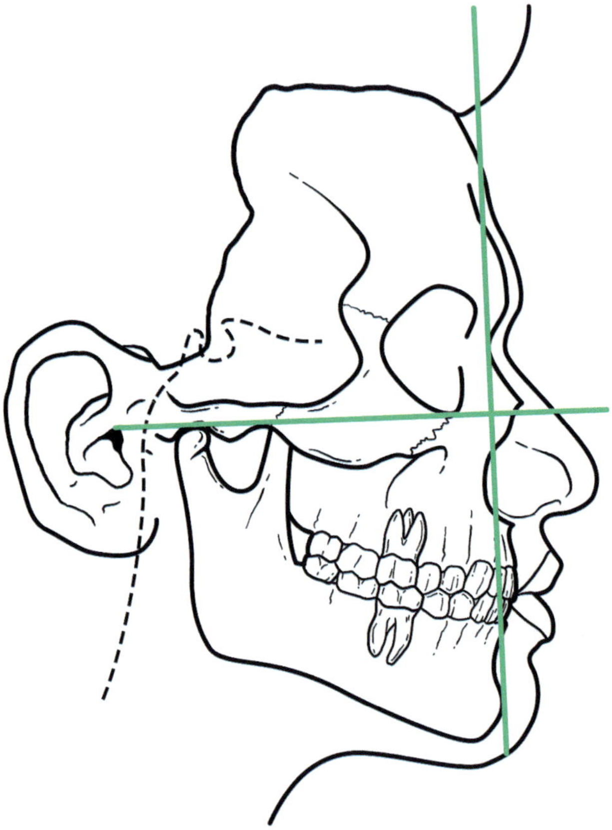

Fig. 68.5 Nasion perpendicular to FH plane

Subnasale perpendicular is another important tool for assessing the profile. A line is drawn perpendicular to the Frankfort horizontal plane through the point Subnasale. This line is expected to go through the upper vermilion border, 2 mm anterior to the lower vermilion border and 4 mm anterior to the soft tissue (Fig. 68.4) Pogonion. +/–2 mm is considered to be within normal limits. This is an important assessment tool for understanding the sagittal relationship of both the maxilla, mandible and dentition.

Likewise another perpendicular line is drawn from Nasion. (N. Perpendicular). This line is ahead by 5.3 ± 6.7 mm in males and 6.9 ± 4.3 mm in females. This indicates the position of mandible. Regarding the bony pogonion this line is ahead by 4.3 ± 8.5 mm in males and 6.5 ± 5.1 mm in females. This indicates the position of the chin. Angle SNB is 80 ± 2 normally. Less indicates retruded mandible and more indicates protrusion of mandible. All these measurements are in relation to the cranial base, the portion that is not changed in routine orthognathic surgery. (Fig. 68.5) (Refer Chap. 66 for further details).

- Mandibular prognathism
  - (a) Skeletal
  - (b) Dento- alveolar
- Mandibular retrusion
  - (a) Skeletal
  - (b) Dento- alveolar
- Mandibular Transverse Deformity
  - (a) Broad
  - (b) Narrow
- Chin Deformity-Excess
  - (a) Vertical
  - (b) Transverse
  - (c) Antero posterior
- Chin deformity deficient
  - (a) Vertical
  - (b) Transverse
  - (c) Antero posterior
- Deep bite deformity
- Open bite deformity(Apertognathia)
- Asymmetry

Specific conditions like presence of deep bites and open bites can occur with these clinical situations and may help us understand the dentoalveolar compensations that occur with them. Assessment of patients is done with facial analysis and cephalometrics.

68.3.1 Mandibular Excess

Common cause for mandibular excess is either developmental or genetic. Very large mandible may be associated with acromegaly.

The clinical features associated with mandibular excess are the following:

1. Prognathic mandible.
2. Anterior cross bite.
3. Elongated face.
4. Relatively long lower third of the face
5. Stomion-menton length—proportionately long.
6. Concave facial profile.
7. Lower lip and chin are more anteriorly placed than normal (SN perpendicular)
8. Class III relationship of occlusion.
9. Angle SNB—more than 82°.

68.3.2 Mandibular Deficiency

It is often due to genetical or developmental reasons. Ankylosis of temporomandibular joint, trauma to mandibular condyle and aplasia of condyle can also cause deficiency in mandibular growth.

Clinical features associated with mandibular deficiency are the following:

1. Bird face appearance.
2. Severe over jet.
3. Class II relationship of dentition.
4. Crowding of lower anterior teeth.
5. Flaring compensation of lower anterior teeth.
6. Face appears small.
7. Lower third of the face is short.
8. Stomion-menton is proportionately short.
9. Labiomental fold is usually absent.
10. Chin neck angle is obtuse.
11. Angle SNB—less than 78°.
12. Angle FHP N P—less than 82°.

68.3.3 Deformities of Chin

Deformities of chin could be three dimensional—vertical, anterio-posterior, or horizontal.

Vertical and anterio-posterior excess of chin are usually associated with mandibular prognathism. Though in prognathic mandible, chin appears prominent, it need not be so in objective analysis. Hence it is essential that the chin be assessed independently in relation to the other structures. To assess the vertical discrepancy, the best technique is to measure the length from stomion of the lower lip to the menton and compare this to the length obtained from measuring the subnasale to stomion of the upper lip, in rest position. The former should be double the latter normally.

68.3.4 Facial Asymmetry

The reasons for facial asymmetry are many.
A few of the etiological factors are the following:

1. Hemifacial microsomia/dysplasia
2. Unilateral cleft lip and palate, and other unilateral clefting syndromes
3. Childhood trauma especially to the condyle
4. Discrepancy in blood supply to the maxillofacial region
5. Habits
6. Early unilateral loss of teeth
7. Faulty use of functional appliances
8. Pathologies and childhood surgeries of the face

Asymmetry could be pan facial or limited to certain areas. Frontal analysis is the ideal method to assess asymmetries. Drawing vertical and horizontal parallel lines on the face will help to locate the area of asymmetry. This can also be done using a grid. PA cephalogram and frontal photographs are helpful in analyzing facial symmetry.

Orthognathic surgery to the mandible involves numerous procedures that facilitate the correction of deformities of the mandible and its dentoalveolar complex in all planes of space. This encompasses a wide array of techniques which may be classified based on the anatomical location they are applicable to.

Osteotomies of the Mandible

1. Dentoalveolar complex
   (a) Anterior subapical
   (b) Total subapical
2. Midline symphyseal osteotomy
3. Body osteotomy
4. Ramus Osteotomy
   (a) Vertical sub-sigmoid osteotomy—intra- and extraoral
   (b) Sagittal split ramus osteotomy (BSSO)
5. Subcondylar osteotomy

The discussion of all the techniques is beyond the scope of this chapter, and hence, detailed description of the vertical ramus osteotomy, the sagittal split ramus osteotomy, and theÚnterior subapical osteotomy are provided here.

68.4 Ramus Osteotomies

Movement of the mandible in the antero-posterior direction is usually achieved by ramus osteotomy. Limberg in 1925 reported subcondylar oblique osteotomy [2]. Thomas, Robinson, Shira, and others described buccal osteotomy which involved the ramus. Later, Caldwell and Letterman (1954) described vertical subcondylar osteotomy by extraoral approach, which became very popular [3]. This technique minimized trauma of the inferior alveolar neurovascular bundle.

In 1927 Wassmund described the inverted “L” osteotomy. Though the primary indication was mandibular prognathism, many surgeons advocated vertical osteotomy and certain modifications like inverted “L” osteotomy [4] and “C” osteotomy for advancement of the mandible [5]. Bone grafting has to be done to fill the gap created (Fig. 68.6).

In 1937 Lane described a sagittal osteotomy. Obwegeser modified the Lane’s technique in 1955, and the technique of sagittal split osteotomy is credited to him. Sagittal split is a versatile technique and has the following superiority over others [6]. It gives great flexibility in repositioning the distal tooth-bearing segment. There is better cancellous bone contact, which enhances healing. The alterations in the position of the condyles and muscles of mastication are minimal. There is no extraoral scar. Injury to the marginal mandibular nerve is avoided. However, chance of injury to the inferior alveolar neurovascular bundle is high [7].

Dal Pont made the modification to sagittal split by a vertical cut through the lateral cortex [8]. Hunsuck extended the medial cut only to a point above the lingula. This minimized trauma to overlying tissue [9].

68.4.1 Extraoral Vertical Ramus Osteotomy

This was one of the most popular procedures for correcting mandibular prognathism. Rigid internal fixation techniques and certain modifications like “C” osteotomy and inverted “L” osteotomy have been used for advancement of the mandible. After “C” or “L” osteotomy, the gap created while advancing or rotating the distal segment is filled with bone graft [10].

The major disadvantages are the external scar and the possible inadvertent damage to the marginal mandibular nerve. With judicious care, these problems can be minimized. Better visibility is the major advantage (Fig. 68.7).

Surgical Technique:
Submandibular skin incision is placed, about 1.5 cm below the angle of the mandible. The incision is taken down to the platysma, which is then divided. Marginal mandibular nerve lies below the platysma running parallel to and often below the lower border of the mandible, crossing the facial vessels superficially as it passes upward. Attempt should be made to identify this structure and preserve it.

After identification and protection of the marginal mandibular nerve, dissection is carried down to the bone. The periosteum is incised over the angle. The periosteum is reflected superiorly to the level of the sigmoid notch on the lateral aspect of the ramus. Coronoid process may be cut in cases when more than 1 cm of posterior movement is required (Fig. 68.8).

Lateral aspect of the ramus is inspected for a small bulge corresponding to the lingula. This helps to identify the mandibular foramen. Osteotomy is performed posterior to the anti-mandibular foramen bulge so that the mandibular nerve is not injured. (The position of the bulge is arbitrary and not definite.) A vertical bony cut is made starting at the sigmoid notch and progressing to the lower border near the angle of the mandible. Condylar segment is separated from the distal part of the mandible and is detached from the medial pterygoid muscle. The condylar part is

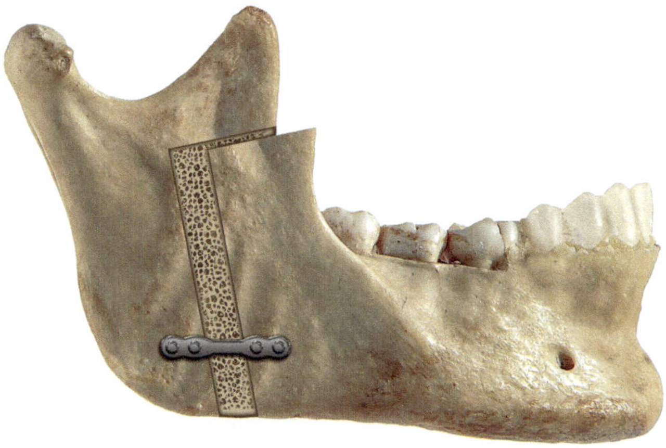

Fig. 68.6 Inverted “L” osteotomy of the ramus used for advancing the mandible

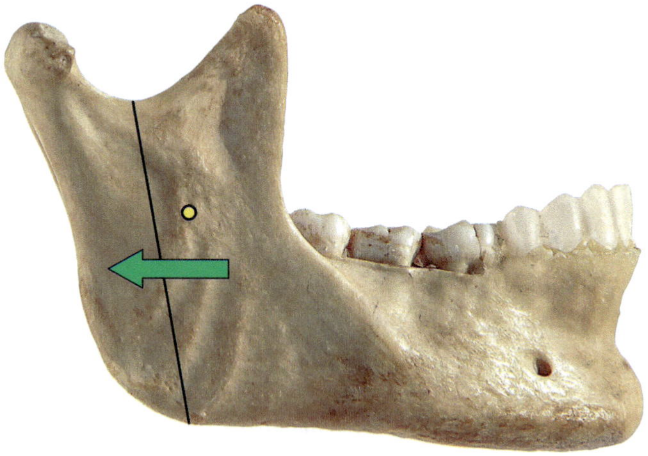

Fig. 68.7 Subsigmoid vertical osteotomy was the most popular technique before the introduction of sagittal split osteotomy. This technique is used for correcting mandibular prognathism

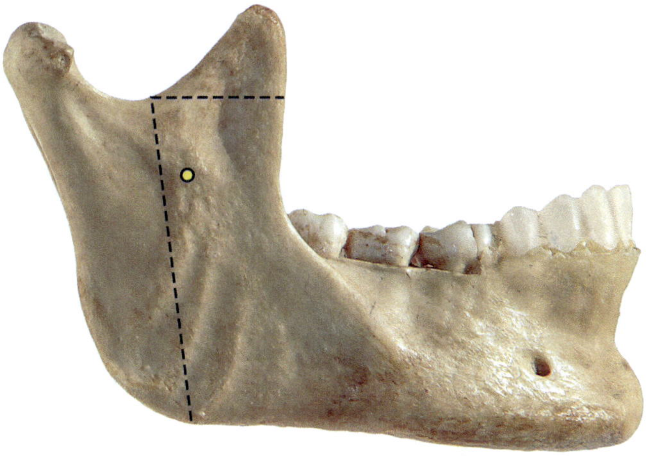

Fig. 68.8 When the push back required in subsigmoid vertical osteotomy is more than 1 cm, sectioning of the coronoid process helps in better stability

laterally placed on the distal segment. After packing the wound, the same steps are followed on the contralateral side.

The mandible is repositioned into the desired position with the help of the splint, and intermaxillary fixation is done. The site of surgery is again approached. Some surgeons prefer to leave the condyle as such on the lateral aspect without any transosseous wiring. There is no consensus regarding the decortication of the opposing surfaces.

Removal of bone or decortication may be done if it helps the condyle to achieve a proper position within the glenoid fossa with minimal displacement. Decortication helps better contact of the cancellous bone enhancing healing. Stabilization of the fragments by transosseous wires or screws and plates can be done. Rigid internal fixation eliminates intermaxillary fixation. Except in rigid internal fixation, intermaxillary fixation for a period of 4–6 weeks is mandatory. After the fixation is removed, elastics may be used to guide the movements.

Wound closure is done in layers. Skin may be closed by monofilament 6-0 or smaller sutures. A pressure dressing is applied for the first 24–48 h. Drain is usually not necessary and, if done, has to be done through a separate stab incision below the main incision. Sutures are removed after 5–7 days, and the wound is supported by dressing for a period of another 1 week, if required.

Complications are usually rare. Bleeding may occur due to injury to the retromandibular vein or masseteric artery where it crosses laterally through the sigmoid notch. Bleeding can be controlled by routine methods like pressure packs, ligation, etc. Injury to the marginal mandibular nerve is another possibility. A transitory deficiency in the function of the lower lip may be anticipated due to traction on the nerve. This often recovers completely. In case of sectioning of the nerve, micro-surgical repositioning is advised.

If care is taken in closure, and infection is avoided, scar formation is minimal. If scar is formed, revision may be done subsequently (Fig 68.9a–d).

68.4.2 Sagittal Split Osteotomy

Sagittal split osteotomy (SSO) can be employed for correcting both retrognathism and prognathism. Modifications by Dal Pont, Hunsuck, and Epker have made the procedure simpler and more acceptable biologically. Schuchardt and Lane described sagittal split osteotomy of the vertical ramus [11]. It was Obwegeser who popularized it. His medial cut was above the mandibular foramen, and his lateral cut was below that of Schuchardt's and extended to a part just above the angle, at least 25 mm below the lingual cortical cut. Obwegeser and Trauner in 1955 described the bilateral sagittal split osteotomy [6].

Dal Pont in 1961 made a major modification by extending the cut anteriorly and making the vertical cut just below the second molar [8]. Hunsuck in 1968 modified the cut in the medial cortex of the vertical ramus, limiting the cut to just behind the mandibular foramen. Postoperative complications got reduced [9] (Fig. 68.10a, b).

Bell and Schendel and Epker extended the vertical cut on the buccal side to the lower border of the mandible reducing the incidence of wrong splits [12, 13]. A reciprocating osteotomy saw, which is specifically meant for the inferior border (right and left) may be used to perform inferior border osteotomy [14].

Performing an inferior border osteotomy results in much lower incidence of persisting inferior border defects. Hence, during advancement of the mandible, it is advisable to exclude the lingual cortex in the split. Piezosurgery has been compared with conventional surgical drills/saws by several authors for BSSO. They have reported substantially longer surgery time for piezosurgery. Image-guided surgery has also become popular in the recent years, and this allows the surgeon to track the position of the instruments and segments during the operation in real time. Modern intraoperative navigation systems are being used in orthognathic surgery also [15].

A. Incision and Dissection:

Incision is placed over the region of the ramus to the mid ramus. It is carried over the external oblique ridge, extends up to the first molar region, and curves down to the buccal vestibule.

Initially only the mucosa is incised over the ramus region. Retracting the tissue buccally, before incision, prevents the exposure of the buccal pad of fat, a troublesome interference, during surgery. Sharp dissection at the ramus is continued to the periosteum, using scissors, knife, and periosteal elevators.

Periosteal elevation of the lateral aspect of the mandible at the molar region is performed down to the inferior border. On the ramus, lateral dissection may be kept minimal but enough to achieve proper visibility and access.

Medial dissection is done very carefully on the medial side of the ramus. The level of the lingula and the entry of the inferior alveolar nerve into mandibular foramen are visualized. This is usually in level with the deepest concavity along

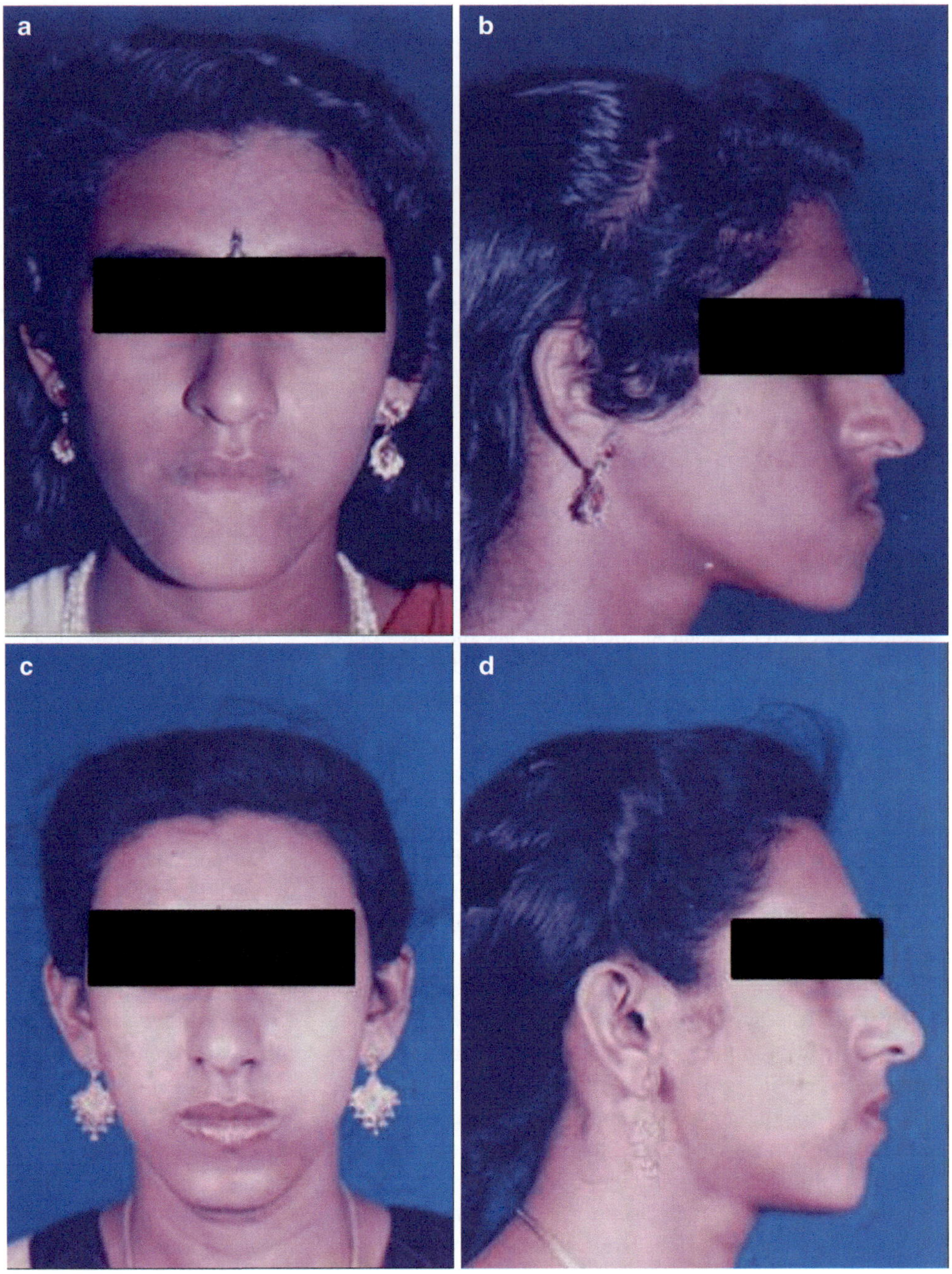

Fig. 68.9 Mandibular prognathism corrected by subsigmoid vertical osteotomy of the ramus on both sides to set back the mandible. (**a**, **b**) Preop pictures, (**c**, **d**) postop pictures

the anterior border of the coronoid and ramus. With a small flexible Freer Elevator, the tissue is dissected taking care not to perforate the periosteum on the medial aspect. Dissection should be above the level of the mandibular foramen. Using a bigger elevator, the medial aspect of the mandible above the lingula is exposed subperiosteally. (Perforation of the periosteum not only induces bleeding but may injure the mandibular nerve.) Sigmoid notch is identified for better orientation. Subperiosteal dissection should be minimal, but enough to retract the tissues medially without much traction on the mandibular neurovascular bundle [16].

B. Osteotomy (Videos 68.1 and 68.2):

Osteotomy is initiated by cutting the cortical bone above the lingula on the medial side. This cut should extend behind the mandibular foramen but need not be up to the posterior border of the ramus (about half to two-thirds of the antero-posterior dimension of the ramus). The cut is taken downward along the external oblique ridge to the second or first molar region. The depth of the cut should be minimal, just enough to reach the cancellous bone (Figs. 68.11 and 68.12).

Conventionally the vertical cut is made at the second molar region as the bone is thicker there. The CT analysis conducted by Y Tsuji et al. on prognathic mandible demonstrated that the mandibular thickness of the mandible increased along the mandibular foramen toward the mandibular body. The mandibular canal was located relatively lingually at all sites. They also observed that marrow space, located on the buccal side, was thicker at the region of mandibular body [17].

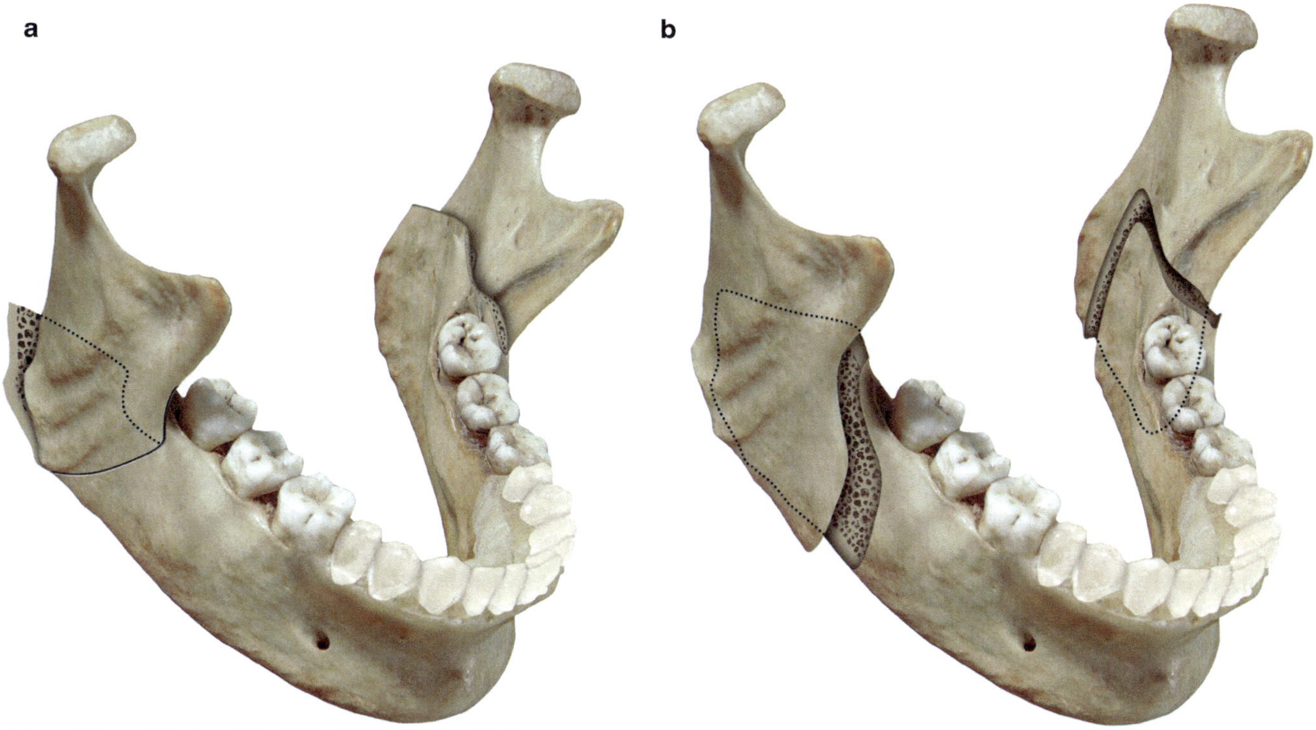

Fig. 68.10 Bilateral Sagittal Split Ramus Osteotomy (BSSO/BSSRO). (**a**) Obwegeser split: Initially the medial cut in sagittal split osteotomy extended up to the posterior border, and when the distal segment was pushed back, the margin used to jut out, which had disadvantages like relapse tendency and injury to the retromandibular tissues. (**b**) Hunsuck split: At present the medial cut is taken above the mandibular foramen much short of the posterior border but behind the foramen. The complications are much less (also see Fig. 65.12b)

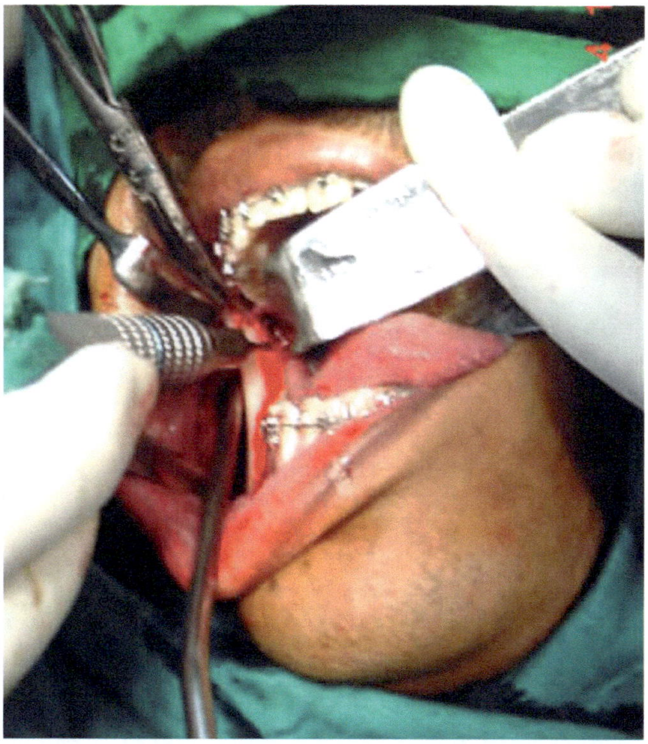

Fig. 68.11 The medial cut is taken above and behind the mandibular formen and deepened to the cancellous bone

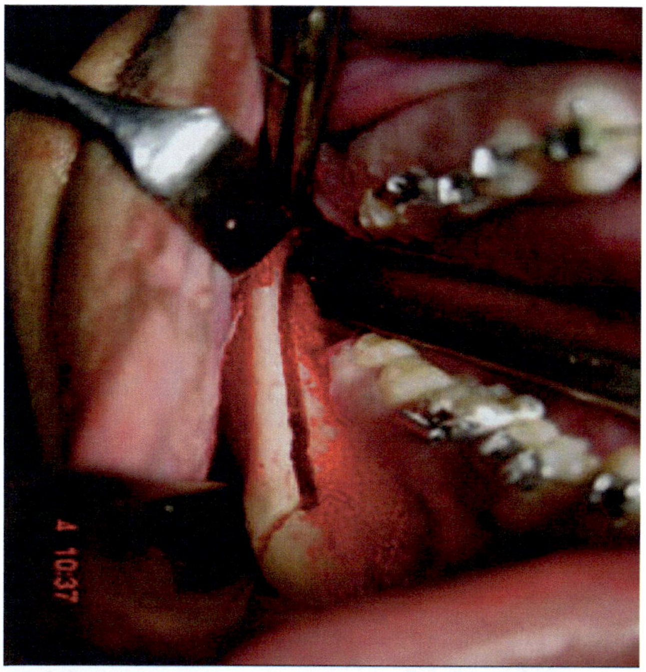

Fig. 68.12 The cut is extended obliquely through the anterior border of the mandible to the buccal plate and taken downward at the level of the first or second molar region, up to the inferior border. Only the cortex need be cut. Deeper cuts could injure the inferior alveolar nerve and may cause wrong splits (also see Figs. 69.31 a–c and 70.24 c, d)

A study on cadaveric mandible by Promma et al. reported that the thickness of buccal cortex to the mandibular canal is about 6.5 and 5 mm at the second molar and first molar regions, respectively [18].

Some surgeons prefer to take the cut more forward to the first molar region. This gives better accessibility for intraoral plating. When the vertical cut is made, it is mandatory to protect the soft tissue over the inferior border by using a channel retractor. If the vertical cut includes the inferior border, the direction of the split is controlled. A rotary instrument or a reciprocating saw is used for cutting. Once the cortical cut is completed, a small spatula osteotome is malleted to the site beginning from the medial cut to the vertical cut. Osteotome should be directed laterally just beneath the cortical plate so that the neurovascular bundle is not injured. Larger osteotomes are used, and slowly the fragments are pried apart using a smith spreader (Fig. 68.13).

As the splitting takes place, the neurovascular bundle is visualized, and care is taken to maintain it to the medial fragment. If it is attached to the proximal segment, the NV bundle is freed with a periosteal elevator. Next the fragments are pried apart using the spreader. The procedure is repeated on the opposite side.

Sagittal split osteotomy can be used for either mandibular advancement or setting back. If mandibular advancement is to be done, the medial pterygoid muscle is separated from the inferior border of the distal segment with a periosteal elevator. When the mandible is set back, medial pterygoid and masseter may have to be stripped, if needed, to prevent the displacement of the condylar segment posteriorly. Posterior stripping of the pterygomasseteric sling in SSO should be minimized to the antegonial notch. In excessive stripping, possibility for avascular necrosis increases [19].

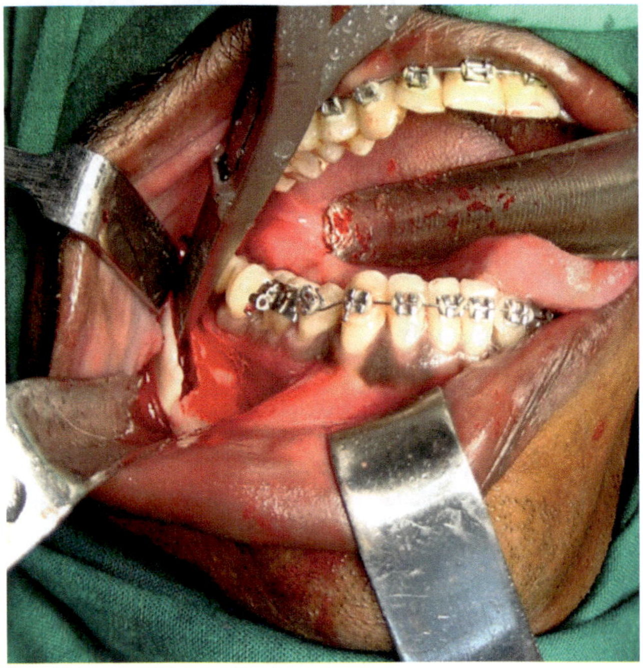

Fig. 68.13 A spreader is used to split the mandible at the ramus region

When the tooth bearing segment (distal segment) is pushed back, the buccal plate of the condylar segment (proximal segment) overlaps the distal. This overlapping part is excised, and the proximal segment is allowed to rest on the cancellous part without any tension (Fig. 68.14).

Pushing the mandible backward reduces the space in the oral cavity. The tongue may not have enough space, and sometimes this induces tongue thrusting, snoring, etc. Some authors advocate reduction glossectomy to improve function related to airway speech and mastication. They also opine that reduction glossectomy improves aesthetics and controls unfavorable mandibular growth [20].

Mommaerts reported that mandibular lengthening done through endoscopic surgery, with transoral osteosynthesis, reduced stripping of the periosteum and therefore consequent edema [21]. In certain clinical situations Unilateral sagittal osteotomy is performed. Refer case scenario in Fig. 69.31 (Maxillary orthognathic surgery Chap. 69) where an unilateral sagittal osteotomy was combined with maxillary osteotomy to correct canting of the maxilla.

C. Stabilization and Fixation:

Rigid internal fixation (RIF) using plates and screws or lag screws is the preferred way of fixation. Prior to RIF, the position of the jaw is adjusted, and intermaxillary fixation is done with splint in position. Both fragments are allowed to be in passive position before RIF is performed. Intermaxillary fixation (IMF) is removed after rigid fixation. However, some surgeons prefer to keep the IMF for 1 week. For rigid fixation 2.5 mm four-hole mini plate with gap is used for push back (Fig. 68.15). Longer plates are used for advancement. Multiple lag screws can also be used. Skeletal rigid fixation has been shown to reduce relapse following mandibular advancement [22–24] (Figs. 68.16a, b, c, and 68.17a, b, c).

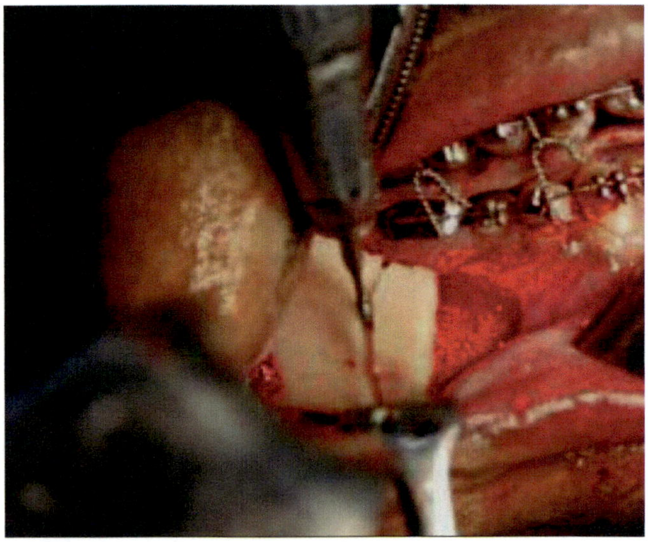

Fig. 68.14 Excess of the buccal plate is cut off when the intention is to push the mandible backward

Rachmiel et al. in their study found improved stability with four-hole plate and monocortical screws, with a relapse rate of about 18% only [25].

Based on a 10-year experience of using bioresorbable plates in orthognathic surgery, Laine P et al. opine that these devices are safe to be used. Relapse rate with bioresorbable screws is the same as with metal in SSO [26]. Another method of fixation is wiring. If resorting to wiring, intermaxillary fixation has to be kept for 5–6 weeks. Maturation of soft and bony tissues continues at the surgical site and approximates that of non-surgical sites at 12 weeks postoperatively [27–29].

The inferior alveolar nerve is less likely to get damaged when monocortical screws are used. These screws also allow for readjustment if there is any inadvertent malposition during surgery can be readjusted more easily [30]. An in vitro study on sheep mandibles found that both mini plates and bicortical screws resulted in a similar level of stability [31]. (Figs. 68.18a, b, c, d, 68.19a, b, c, and 68.20a, b, c).

D. Wound Closure:

Wounds are irrigated well and bleeding is controlled by routine methods. If there is continued bleeding drain is indicated. Wounds are closed by 3-0 Vicryl sutures.

E. Postoperative Sequelae:

Edema is expected after sagittal split osteotomy. It resolves within 2 weeks. Edema at the angle is the last to resolve. Suction drainage minimizes tissue edema following mandibular surgeries. Betamethasone administration significantly reduces postoperative edema. Widar H. et al. has also observed less bleeding intraoperatively, but no difference in neurosurgery disturbances [32].

Diminished sensation over the lip is experienced by most of the patients and is mainly due to traction on the neurovascular bundle. If there is no injury to the neurovascular bundle, sensation returns within a few weeks. More than two-thirds of the patients experience some sensory deficit even after 1 year. However, most of the patients get adjusted to this altered sensation and are satisfied with the overall result. Limitation of movements of jaw in all direction after osteotomy is often experienced. Sagittal split advancements often cause significant limitation of range of motion [33].

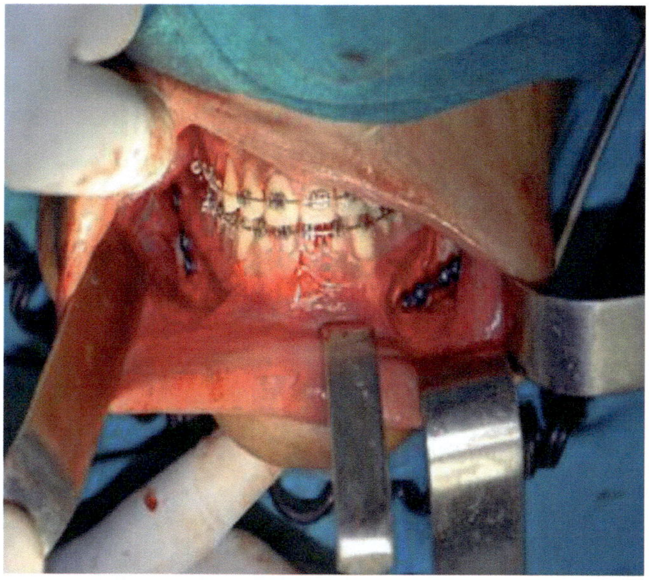

Fig. 68.15 Rigid fixation after sagittal split osteotomy of the mandible using mini plate

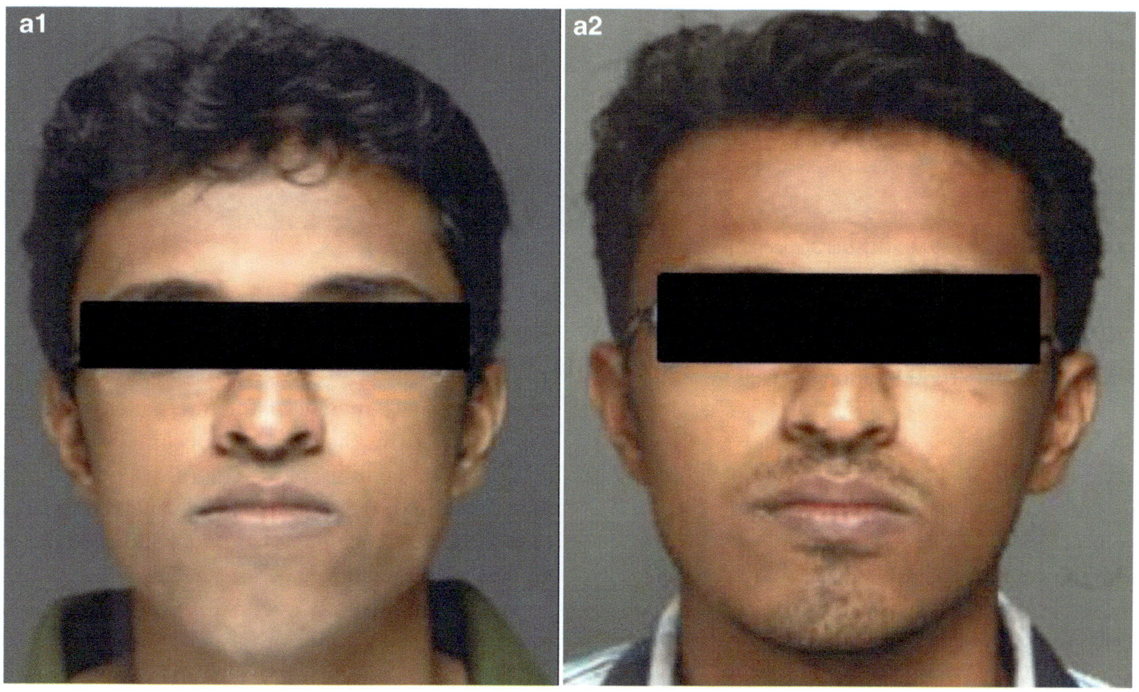

Fig. 68.16 Bilateral sagittal split osteotomy to set back the mandible, with rigid fixation. (**a1**, **b1**) Preoperative photographs. (**a2**, **b2**) Postoperative photographs. (**c1**, **c2**) Pre and post operative lateral cephalograms with superimposed tracings

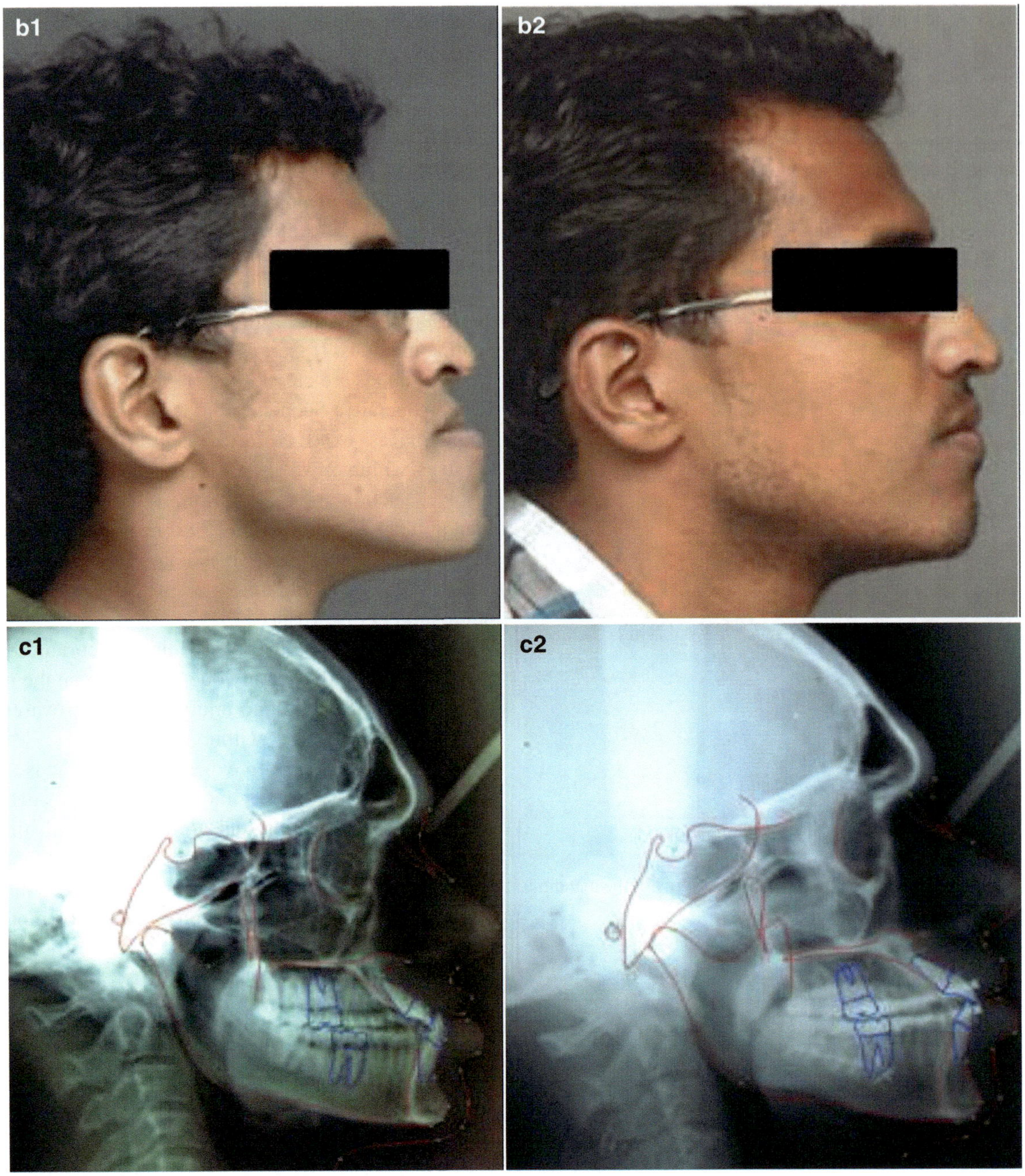

Fig. 68.16 (continued)

Physiotherapy following rigid fixation showed minimal limitation [34].

F. Complications:

Important complications associated with sagittal split osteotomy are:

1. Bad split
2. Injury to the neurovascular bundle
3. TMJ problems
4. Excessive bleeding
5. Relapse

1. Bad Split:

A systematic review of fracture patterns in sagittal split was analyzed by Steenen and Becking and reported 2.3% bad splits in sagittal splits. The most common was buccal plate fracture of the proximal segment and lingual plate fracture of the distal segment. Coronoid and condylar neck fractures were seldom [35].

Wrong split usually occurs in cases where the last molar is removed at the time of surgery. Hence it is advised to have the third molar removed (if needed) about 6 months

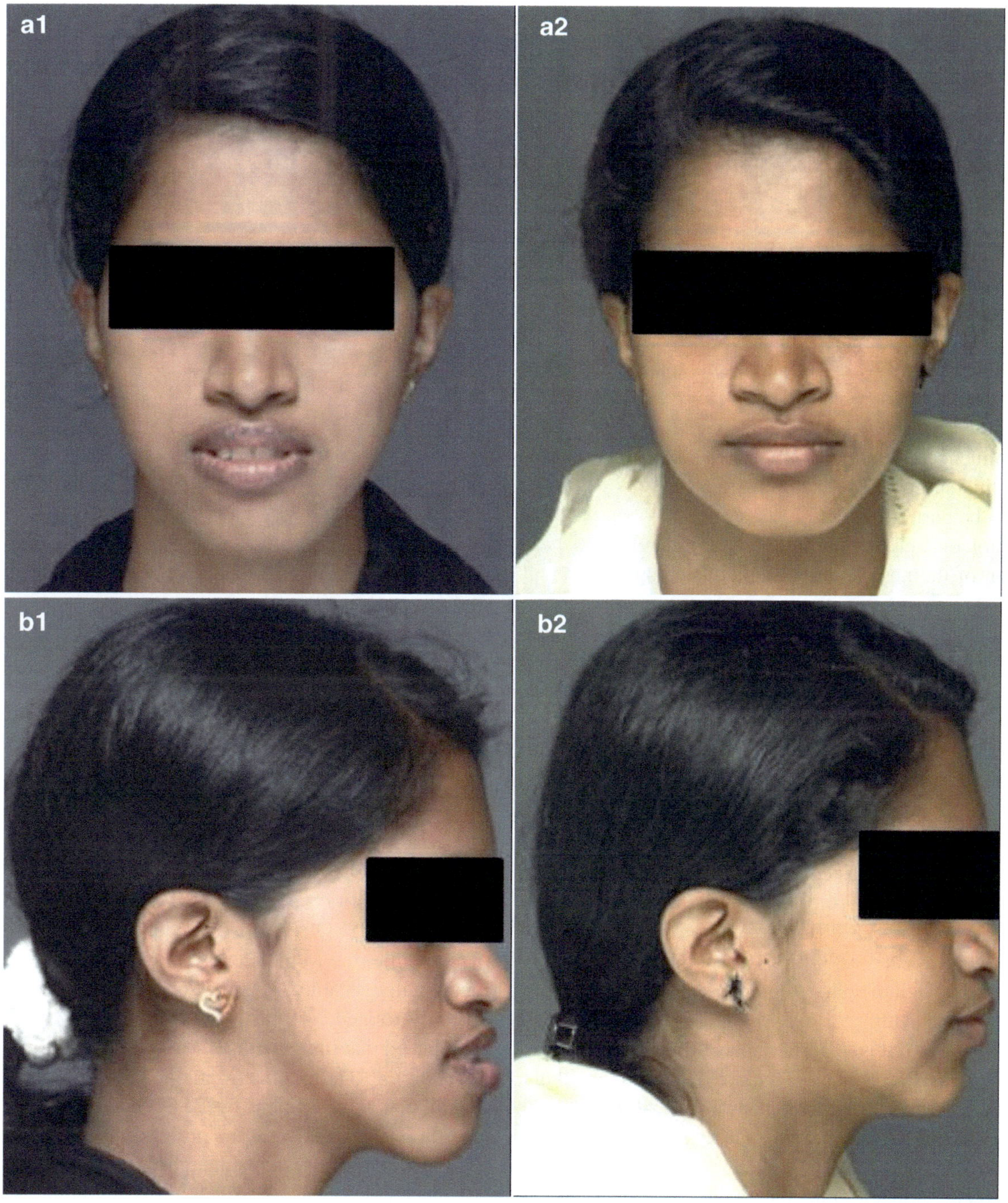

Fig. 68.17 Case of mandibular prognathism with maxillary deficiency, managed by maxillary advancement and mandibular set back by BSSO. (**a1**, **b1**) Preop pictures. (**a2**, **b2**) Postop pictures. (**c1**) Preop cephalogram. (**c2**) Postop cephalogram

prior to the osteotomy. If the lingual cortical plate is broken, soft tissue separation from the lingual plate should be kept to the minimum, so that the blood supply is not jeopardized. Patients with a shorter ramus and buccolingually thin mandible are more susceptible to wrong split during SSO [36]. Advanced age can increase the risk of a bad split. Use of a spreader helps to reduce the incidence of wrong splits.

2. Injury to the Neurovascular Bundle:

Care should be taken to maintain the continuity of the neurovascular bundle. If it is transected, ideally the cut ends are micro-anastomosed. However, in common practice, where a micro-surgeon may be unavailable, it is advisable to perform direct suturing to attain epineural approximation. With a repositioned and repaired neurovascular bundle, the sensation is recovered though the period it takes is longer.

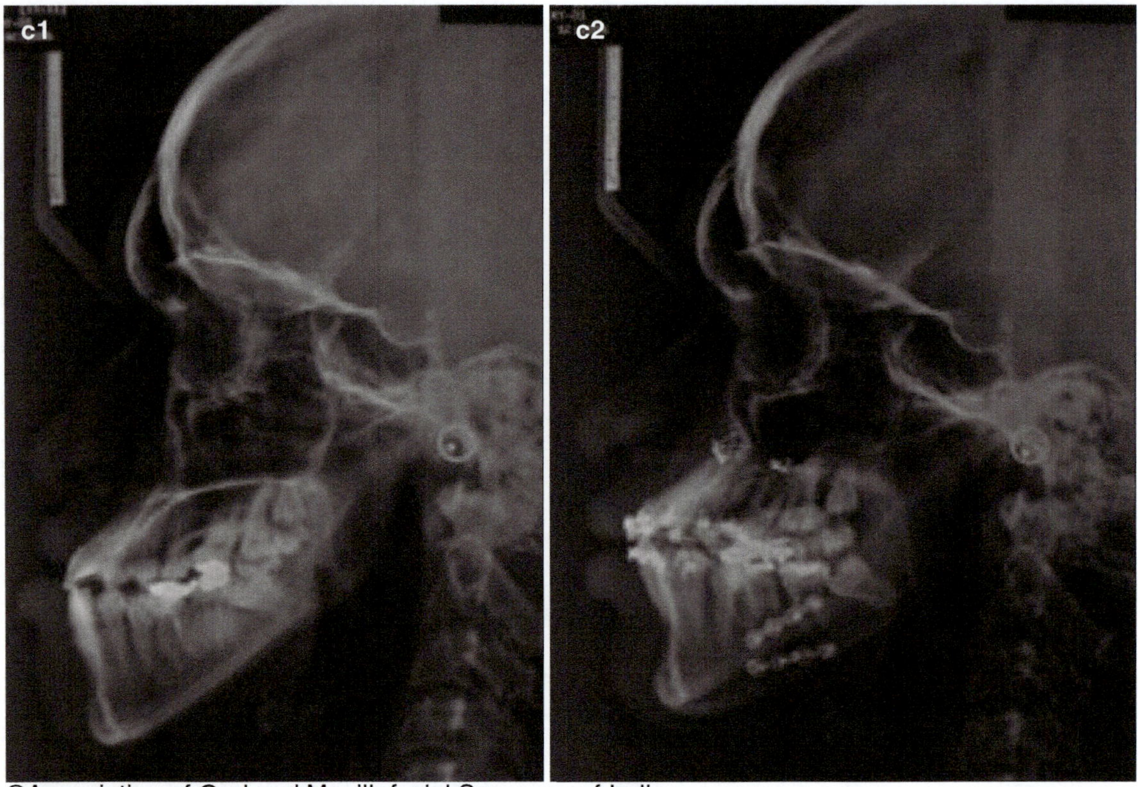

©Association of Oral and Maxillofacial Surgeons of India

Fig. 68.17 (continued)

Long-lasting neurosensory deficiency (NSD) was underestimated by the surgeons as compared to the patient's subjective symptoms. Long-lasting NSD was reported as 7.5% (Questionnaire) and 3.8% (Record), after intraoral vertical ramus osteotomy, and as 11.6% (Questionnaire) and 8.1% (Record) after sagittal split osteotomy [37]. Vertical subsigmoid osteotomy with rigid fixation may be considered as a viable alternative if it is important to avoid alterations in sensation, whereas BSSO maybe preferred if retromandibular scar is of concern. Neurosensory disturbance, after SSO with additional genioplasty, is more than after SSO alone [38].

3. TMJ Problems:

Care should be taken while plating the segments. Improper plating can pull or push the condyle to an untoward position. Postoperative X-rays are taken to assess the situation. If needed, the displacement has to be corrected by returning the patient to surgery. Displacement of the condyle from the fossa is one of the main reasons for relapse [24, 39] (Fig. 68.21).

Beukes J. et al. in 2016 studied condylar rotational tolerance in BSSO treatments and reported a range of 10°–15° after orthognathic surgery.

Unilateral SSO is a safe procedure in lateral prognathism of mandible due to unilateral condylar hyperplasia or traumatic malocclusions [40]. The condyle that was not operated on, only rotated 3–4° within the glenoid cavity, and it was established that this is within the range of functional articular adaptation [41]. Mendez-Manjon R. et al. observed that mandibular advancement by BSSO can positively displace the condyle especially on the posterior aspect [42].

In their study Borstlap et al. observed that in sagittal split advancement postoperatively, 8% of patients showed postoperative condylar resorption. Patients of relatively low age are at risk of condylar alterations or resorption. Occurrence of pain and TMJ sounds in the first few months postoperatively are highly indicative of condylar changes to occur in the preceding months [43]. Predisposition in females for condylar resorption after sagittal split osteotomy may be attributed to

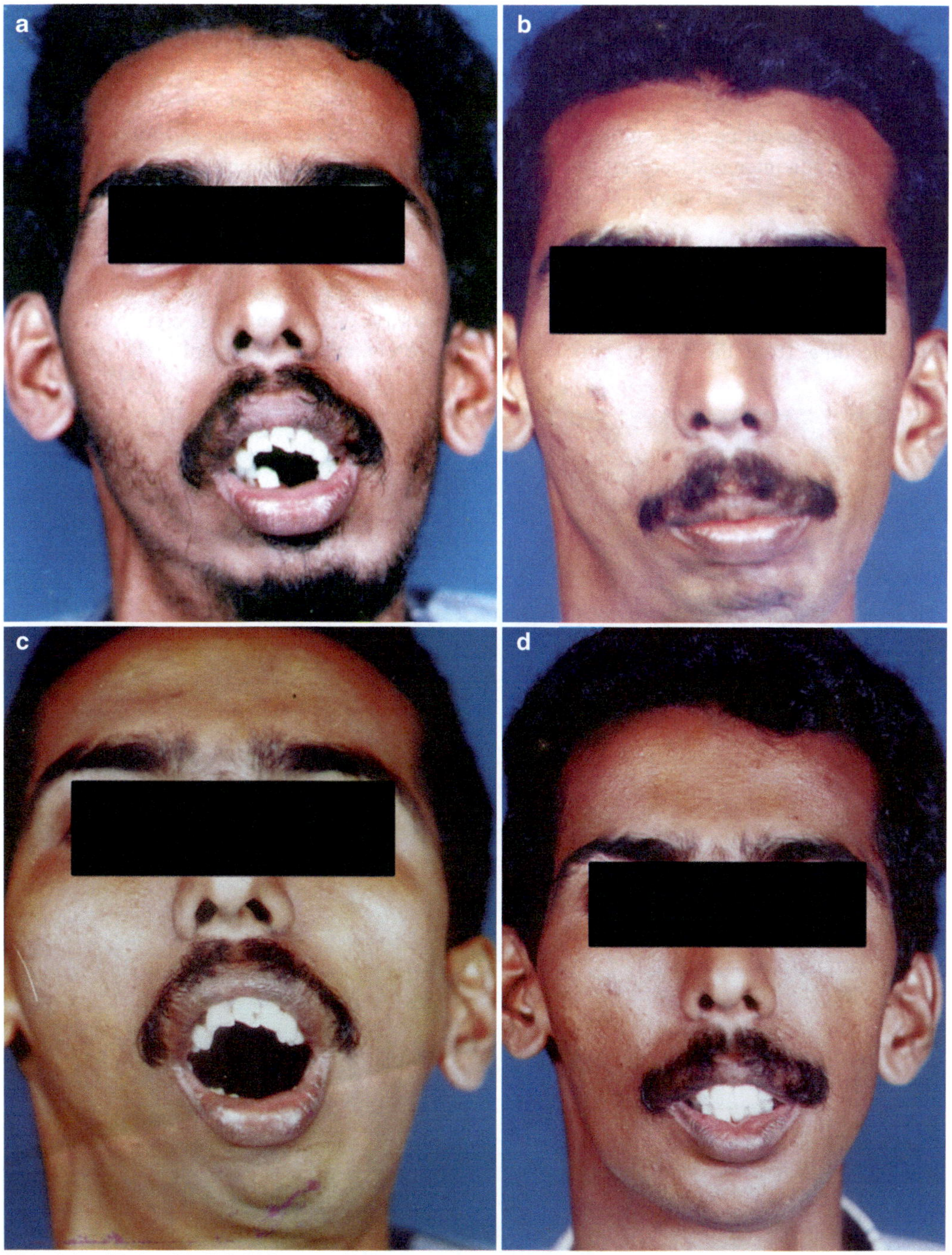

Fig. 68.18 A case of left unilateral ankylosis of the TMJ resulting in trismus and facial deformity. Treated by release of ankylosis by gap arthroplasty, temporal myofacial flap interposing, and extended lateral sliding genioplasty. (**a**) Pre operative picture before ankylosis correction (**b**) frontal view with facial asymmetry (**c**) after release of ankylosis, (**d**) after correcting facial asymmetry

the modulation of biologic response, by estrogen and prolactin [44]. Mobarak compared the skeletal stability of postoperative changes in low angle and high angle Cl II patients following mandibular advancement. High angle had more horizontal skeletal relapse due to condylar movement in a superior direction. Changes in intercondylar angle and width after BSSO advancement or set back may influence TMJ function [45–48].

4. Excessive Bleeding:

Bleeding can be from inferior alveolar neurovascular bundle, medullary bed, and facial vessels or rarely from retromandibular vein. Bleeding from the former two can be controlled by local measures; but the facial vessels will have to be clamped and tied, for which an extraoral incision may be required. Using the channel retractor with a cup to hold the inferior border and cutting with a Steiger-type carbide bur (this has side cutting and rounded cutting end and cuts bone with minimal injury to the soft tissue) prevents injury to the facial vessels.

Injury to the retromandibular vein is very rare and is due to inadvertent injury to the soft tissues behind the mandible. Bleeding can be controlled by absorbable gelatin sponge. Excessive oozing can cause significant edema, and if oozing is present, a drain may be placed.

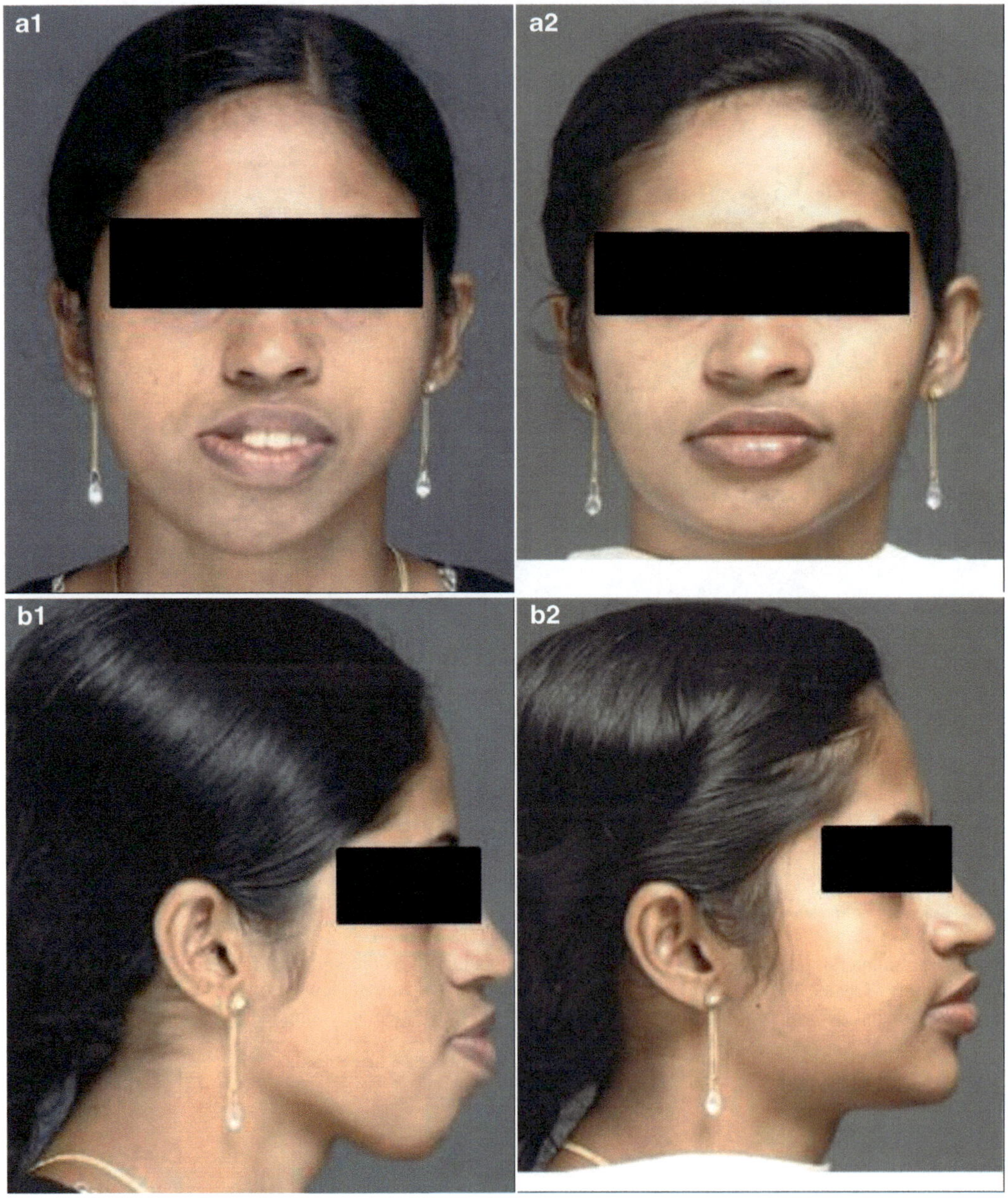

Fig. 68.19 Facial asymmetry and vertical and sagittal excess of maxilla corrected by LeFort1, anterior maxillary osteotomy, bilateral sagittal split osteotomy and advancement genioplasty. (**a1**, **b1**) Preoperative pictures. (**a2**, **b2**) Postoperative pictures. (**c1**) Preoperative lateral cephalogram. (**c2**) Postoperative lateral cephalogram

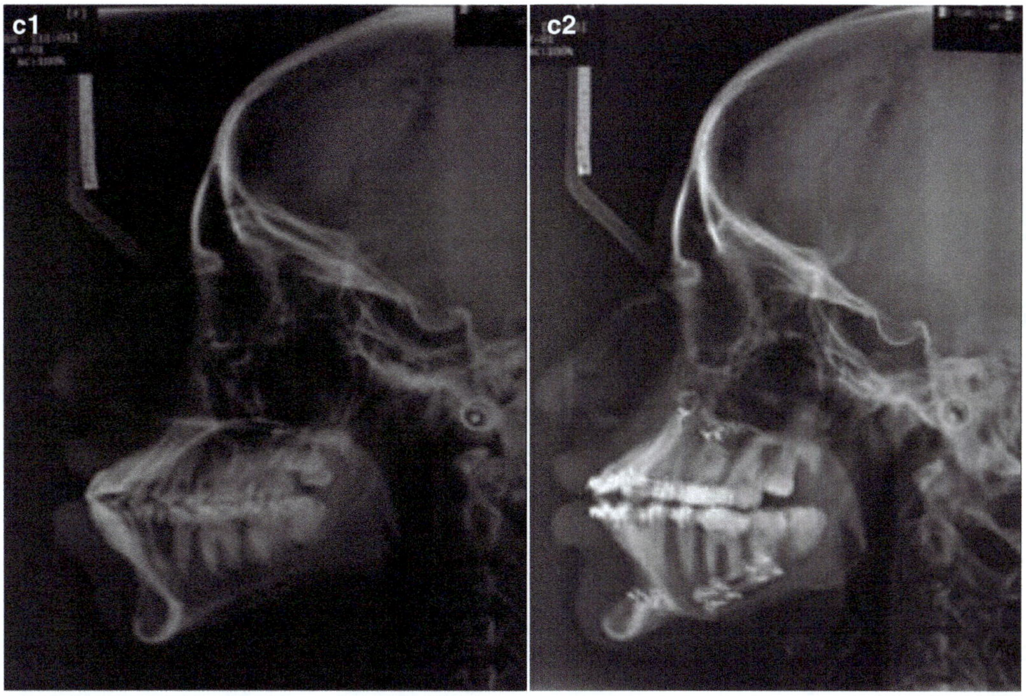

Fig. 68.19 (continued)

68.4.3 Vertical Ramus Osteotomy: Intraoral Approach

It was Caldwell and Letterman who developed the intraoral vertical ramus osteotomy in 1954 [3]. Later in 1964, this was described by Moose [49] and Winstanley in 1968 [50], and modifications have been suggested by many others. Intraoral approaches medially and laterally to ramus were described [49, 50]. Herbert and associates in 1970 described the use of special oscillating saw and popularized the intraoral technique to reach the ramus (Fig. 68.22).

The procedure overcomes the disadvantages of extraoral vertical ramus osteotomy. The advantages are the following: (1) external scar is avoided and (2) there is no injury to the marginal mandibular nerve. The advantages over sagittal split osteotomy are that injury to the mandibular neurovascular bundle is avoided. The main disadvantage is the difficulty in access and visualization of the area. However, there is a delay in healing and possibility of projection of antegonial notch [51]. Mandibular nerve hypoesthesia can be expected to improve faster in young patients than the older ones. So IVRO may be a better option for elder patients [52].

Surgical Technique

A mucosal incision is made along the anterior border of the mandibular ramus. This is extended to the coronoid process and extended laterally up to the first molar area and subperiosteally dissected to expose the sigmoid notch, inferior border, and the posterior border of the ramus. Two fibro-optic lit Bauer retractors (left and right) are used—one on the sigmoid notch and the other at the angle area to get excellent exposure of the ramus. An oscillating saw angled at 105° is used to do the osteotomy. The cut is made posterior to the ante lingula prominence and directed superiorly to the sigmoid notch and inferiorly to the mandibular angle.

If circummandibular wiring fixation is planned, the medial aspect of the ramus above the lingula is dissected subperiosteally to the posterior border. The width need only be enough to pass the wires.

Osteotomy, as in the extraoral approach, extends from the sigmoid notch to the inferior border behind the entry of the mandibular nerve. The intraoral vertical cut should be made no more than 5–7 mm anterior into the posterior border. This will be behind the mandibular foramen [53]. According to some, ante lingual prominence as a landmark is unpredictable [54].

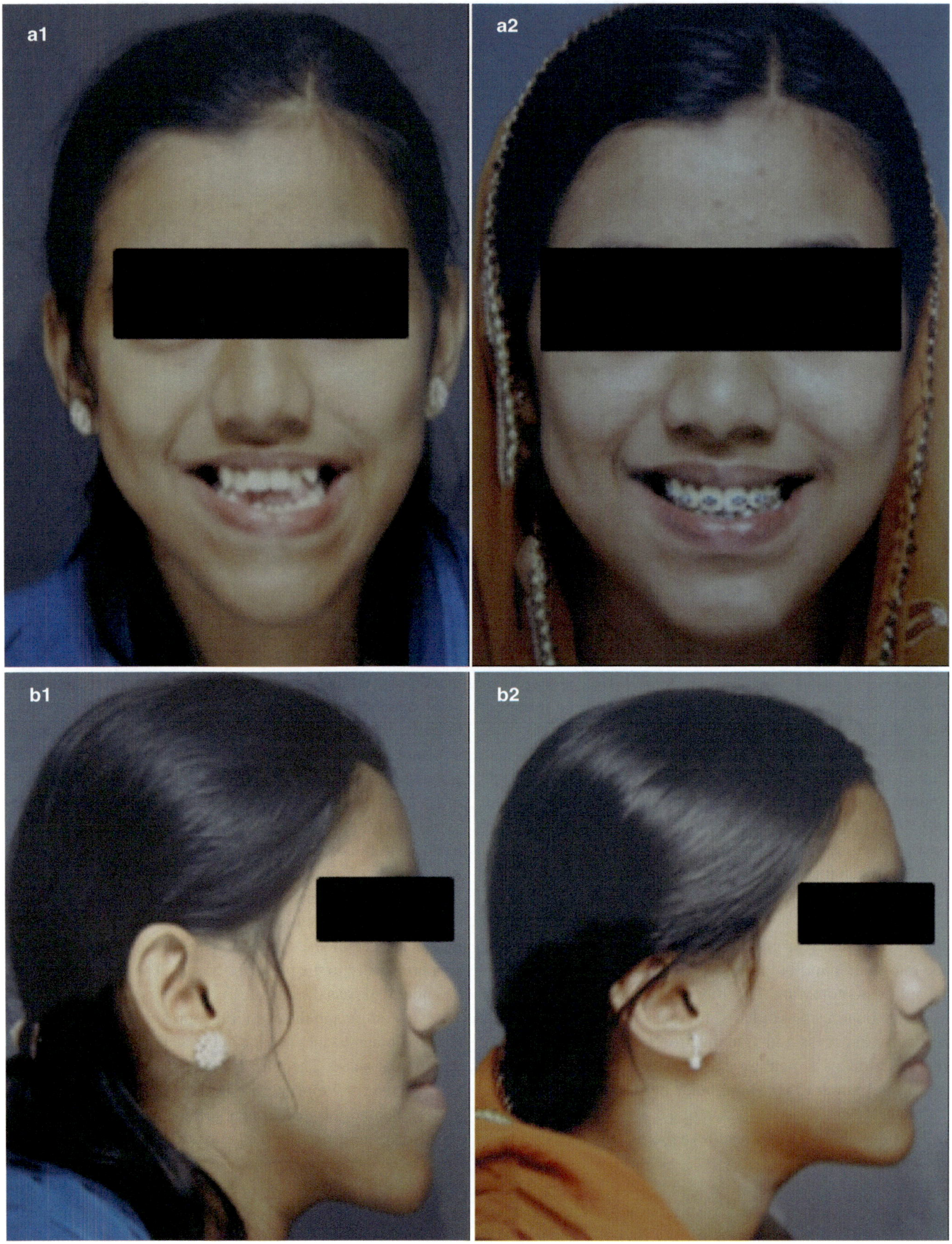

Fig. 68.20 Case of open bite managed by BSSO. (**a1**, **b1**) Preoperative pictures. (**a2**, **b2**) Postoperative pictures. (**c1**) Preoperative lateral cephalogram. (**c2**) Postoperative lateral cephalogram

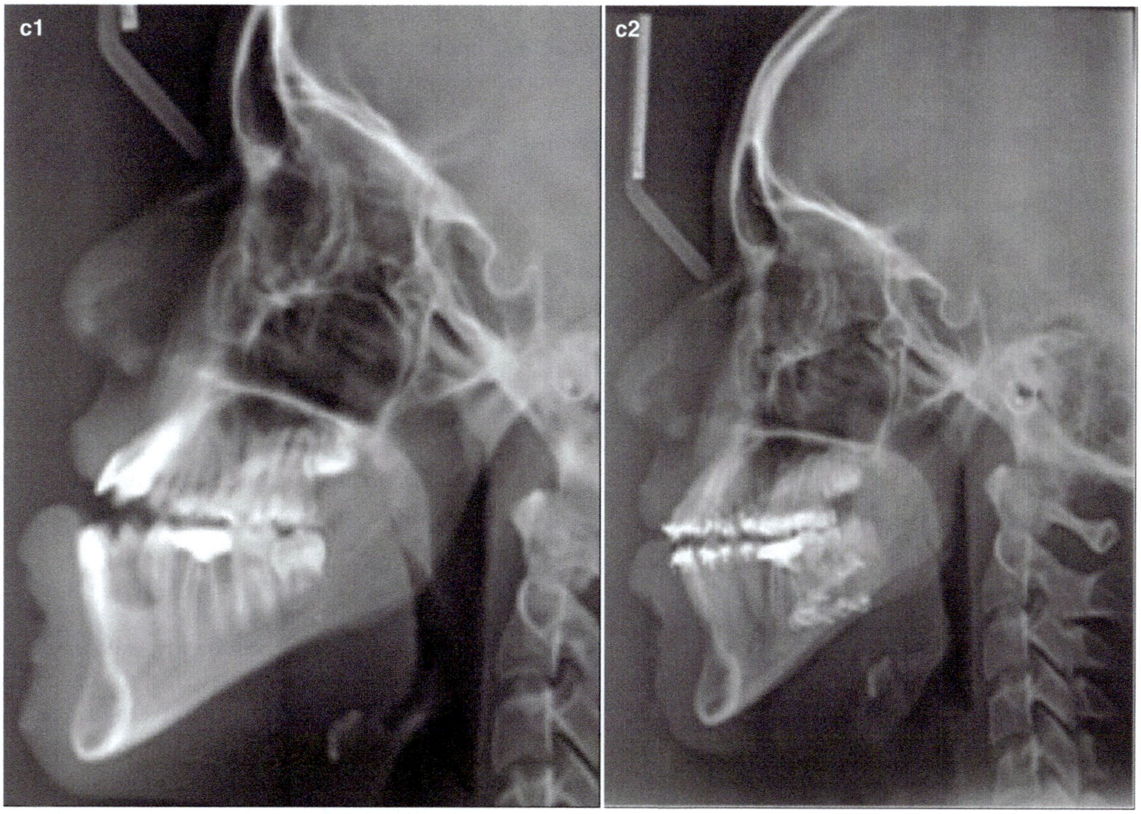

©Association of Oral and Maxillofacial Surgeons of India

Fig. 68.20 (continued)

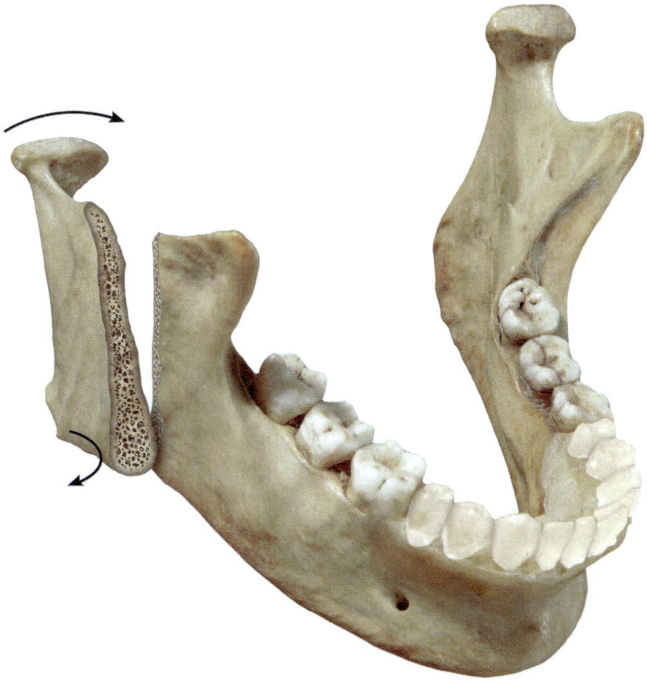

©Association of Oral and Maxillofacial Surgeons of India

Fig. 68.21 Displacement of the condyle due to torquing as demonstrated here in a vertical ramus osteotomy, is the most common reason for TMJ problems

For better access, as well as visibility and mobility of the fragments, the coronoid process can be separated using a reciprocating saw. The coronoid process is allowed to retract with the temporal muscle.

An appropriate retractor with a cup at the end can be held hooked to the posterior border, and the soft tissue is held retracted laterally. Care should be taken to orient the cut and also to prevent injury to the soft tissues.

After the osteotomy, the condylar segment is overlapped laterally over the mandible. Medial pterygoid attached to the medial aspect may be stripped in the anterior region of the segment to facilitate tension-free positioning of the condylar segment. The same osteotomy is performed on the opposite side, and intermaxillary fixation is maintained for 6 weeks. Extraoral approach for vertical subsigmoid osteotomy is advocated for large mandibular set back of greater than 10 mm [55, 56].

Over correcting the mandibular set back by 2 mm to provide compensation for relapse is also recommended [57]. The use of skeletal wire fixation seems to stabilize the initial movement, but does not influence long-term relapse [58].

Ghali and Sikes have reported that IVRO improves TMJ functions and relieves TMJ symptoms more effectively when compared with SSRO, due to the final position of the condyle more anteriorly and inferiorly which

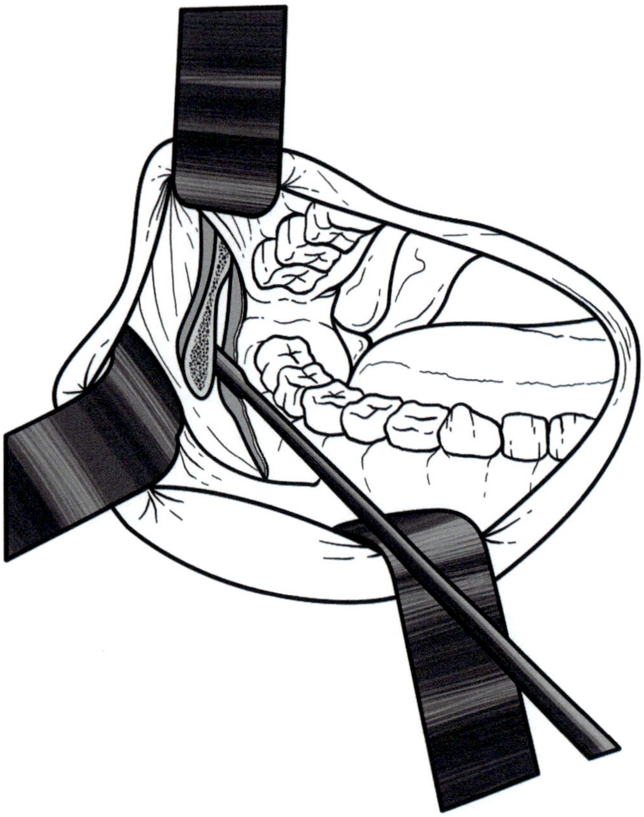

Fig. 68.22 Diagram for intraoral subsigmoid vertical osteotomy

results in an increased joint space and better disk-condyle relationship [59].

Raúl González-García described endoscopically assisted intraoral vertical ramus (IVRO) and subcondylar (ISCO) osteotomies for the treatment of symmetric mandibular prognathism. He claimed the use of saw and bone chisel under the continuous control of the endoscope provides a safer approach since the osteotomy is controlled during the whole process and provides complete visualization of the osteotomy site [60].

Stabilization, Fixation, and Wound Closure

Most surgeons use circummandibular or transosseous wires. Rigid internal fixation using plates is rather difficult to place and carries greater risk of injury to the mandibular nerve. Lag screws or mini plates are sometimes used.

Intermaxillary fixation for a period of 6 weeks is advised, if rigid fixation is not used. Wound closure is done as in sagittal split, adhering to the basic principles.

TMJ Considerations

Radiographically there is an anterior downward and forward movement of the condyle after ramus osteotomy. However, there is a tendency to return to its preoperative position [61–63]. Double contouring of the condyle after 6 months was reported which is attributed to condylar remodeling [64]. Remodeling of the glenoid fossa also has been documented [65]. Complications and their management are very much similar to those of sagittal split.

68.5 Body Osteotomy of Mandible

This was one of the earlier procedures used for mandibular prognathism. Blair reported a body osteotomy at the premolar level for mandibular prognathism in 1906 [19]. Since the advent of the ramus procedures, body osteotomy has lost its popularity. However, in certain conditions, body osteotomy may have to be resorted to.

Surgical Procedure

Depending on the site of osteotomy, soft tissue dissection varies. The basic principle is to reflect the buccal mucoperiosteum down to the inferior border taking care not to injure the mental nerve, but at the same time, exposing it.

The next step is to remove the buccal cortical plate from the mental foramen region backward to behind the osteotomy/ostectomy site for release of the neurovascular bundle. The tooth at the osteotomy site is extracted.

Using a fissure bur, the outer cortical plate is marked and a window is cut. Using curettes and chisels, the cancellous bone around the neurovascular bundle is removed. The nerve is released using a nerve hook. Anterior continuation of the inferior alveolar nerve (the incisal branch) is severed. This helps in better retraction of the nerve. Continuation of the mental nerve is preserved. Mucoperiosteum on the lingual aspect is elevated and protected by a periosteal elevator. Osteotomy is completed adhering to the basic principles. The same procedure is repeated on the contralateral side. Body osteotomy at the molar level is almost outdated since the advent of sagittal split osteotomy.

Body osteotomy anterior to the mental foramen can be resorted to in certain specific cases. The main indication of this procedure is lower dentoalveolar protrusion with anterior open bite. "V" osteotomy is done at the first premolar region. This will not reduce the total mandibular length but rotates the anterior segment upward and backward. Maintenance of the arch and occlusion is important. Rigid fixation is mandatory as tendency for relapse is very high due to the pull exerted by the genioglossus and geniohyoid muscles (Fig. 68.23).

Stabilization is achieved by arch bars or by orthodontic means. Fixation using two plates (each plate having a minimum of 4 holes) on each side is advised.

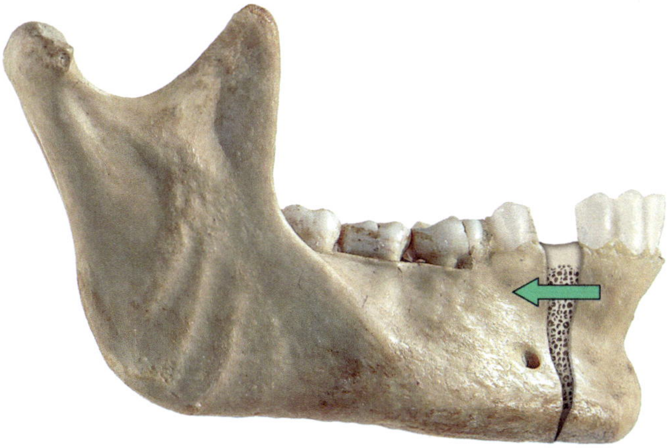

©Association of Oral and Maxillofacial Surgeons of India

Fig. 68.23 Body osteotomy at the level of the premolar region. Diagrammatic representation

68.6 Symphyseal Osteotomy

Midline osteotomy is used either to narrow or to expand the mandible. Expansion is more difficult than narrowing, due to tissue resistance. Before narrowing the mandible, a space must be created at the symphysis by extracting an anterior tooth (Fig. 68.24). Parasymphyseal step osteotomy approach with a hybrid mode of force application might be the most viable option for true mandibular arch expansion.

68.7 Lower Anterior Subapical Osteotomy

Hullihen performed the first ever anterior subapical osteotomy and published it in 1849 [66]. This procedure was done for a girl who had sustained burns and had the anterior segment of the mandible got distracted anteriorly by the traction of the scar resulting in everted lip, protrusion of teeth, and open bite.

Hofer used anterior subapical osteotomy to advance anterior teeth for correction of mandibular dentoalveolar retrusion [67]. Kole used this technique to correct an anterior open bite.

Lower anterior subapical osteotomy is widely used in the following conditions:

1. To retrude the lower anterior dentoalveolar segment; often used in conjunction with subapical osteotomy in bimaxillary protrusion
2. To close minimal anterior open bite
3. To intrude the anterior segment in deep bite deformity

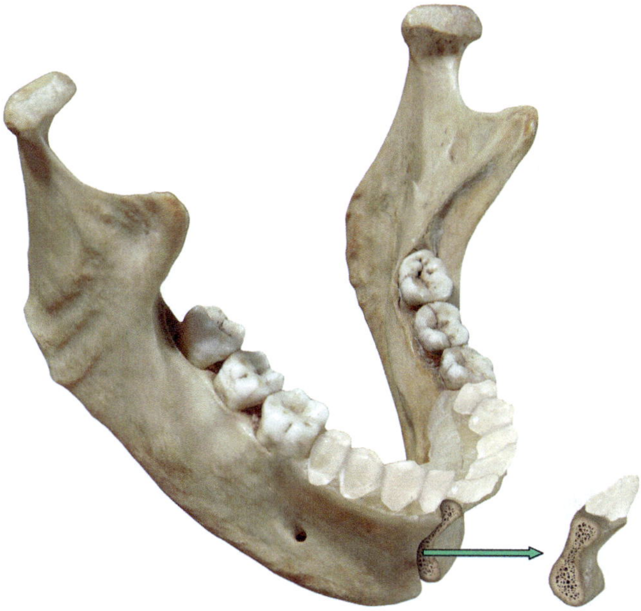

©Association of Oral and Maxillofacial Surgeons of India

Fig. 68.24 Midline osteotomy (Diagrammatic representation)

Surgery

Sulcus incision is made and the mucoperiosteal flap is reflected. Subperiosteal tunneling is done at the lingual aspect of the planned osteotomy site. Extraction of tooth (usually the first premolar) is done, if the intention is to retrude the dentoalveolar segment (Figs. 68.25a, b, c and 68.26a, b, c).

Osteotomy or ostectomy is done as planned. Stabilization and fixation are done in the preplanned position using prefabricated occlusal wafer splint or arch wires. Stabilization is done by using lag screws, position screws, or wires. Semi rigid bone plates are considered superior.

In cases where the anterior segment of the mandible is repositioned superiorly, a gap is created at the osteotomy site (subapically). Autogenous bone grafting is advised to fill this gap.

When the osteotomy is planned behind the mental foramen, the neurovascular bundle may be released from the mandibular canal and protected.

68.8 Total Subapical Osteotomy Mandible

Mcintosh in 1974 described total mandibular alveolar osteotomy. In 1942 Hofer [67] described horizontal osteotomy of mandible for horizontal deficiency or excess and asymmetry.

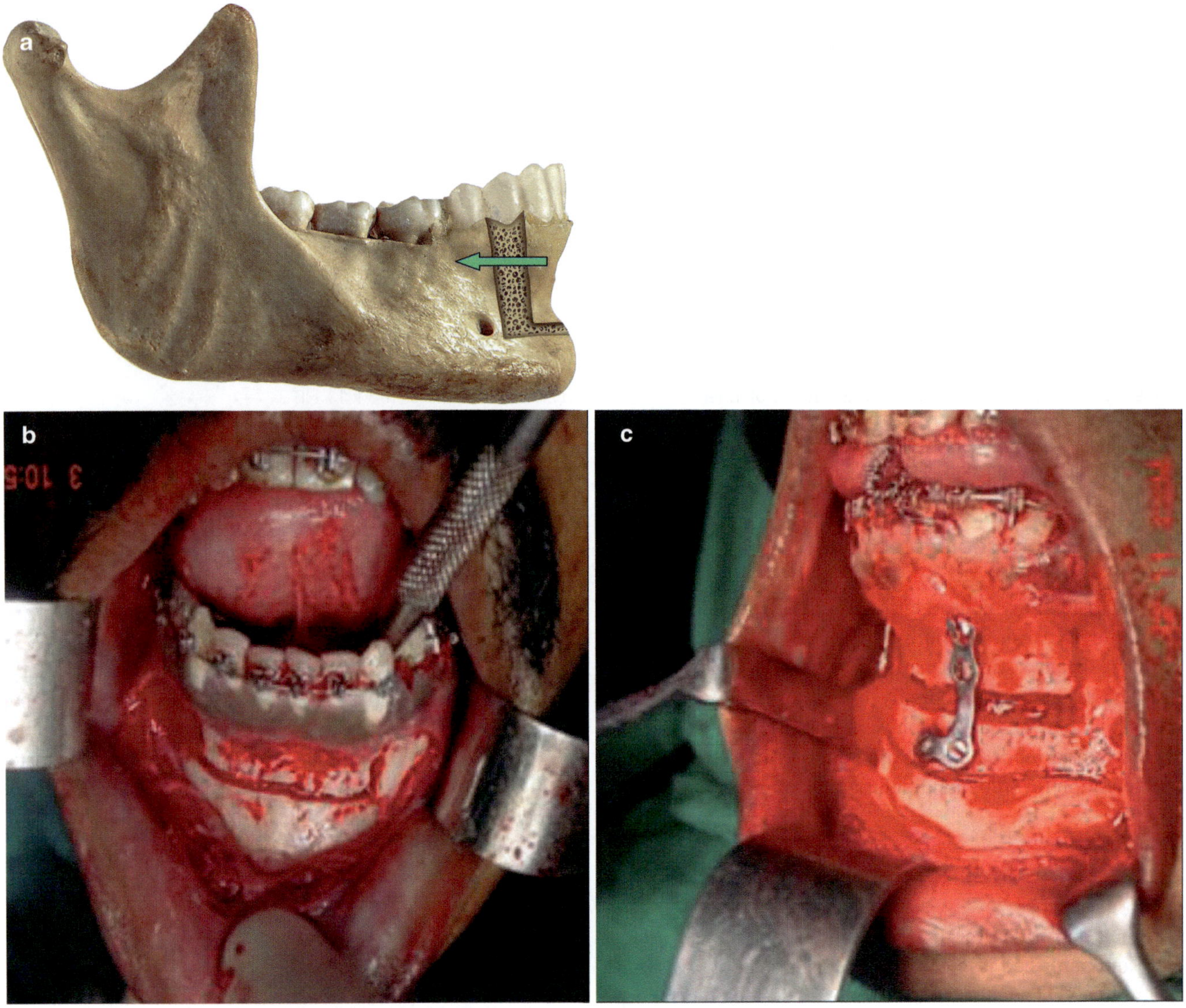

Fig. 68.25 Lower anterior subapical osteotomy. (**a**) Diagrammatic representation. (**b**) Photograph demonstrating the vertical interdental and the horizontal connecting osteotomies. (**c**) Lower subapical osteotomy can also be combined with genioplasty

Total subapical osteotomy of the mandible is used mailly for the following indications:

1. For repositioning the entire dentoalveolar segment.
2. When the mandibular length and chin position are compatible with the maxilla and its position, but the deformity is mainly in the dentoalveolar part.

Adequate bone should be present below the apices of the roots.

Surgery (Fig. 68.27a, b, c)

Mucoperiosteal flap is reflected. The neurovascular bundle is released as described earlier (under "Body Osteotomy of Mandible"). Osteotomy is started behind the most posterior teeth. The cut is made using reciprocating saw or bur. Care should be taken not to damage the lingual tissues. Osteotomy is continued anteriorly, without injuring the released neurovascular bundle. About 4 mm of bone should be left below the apices of the teeth to ensure proper blood supply. The dentoalveolar segment is freed and mobilized. Preplanned

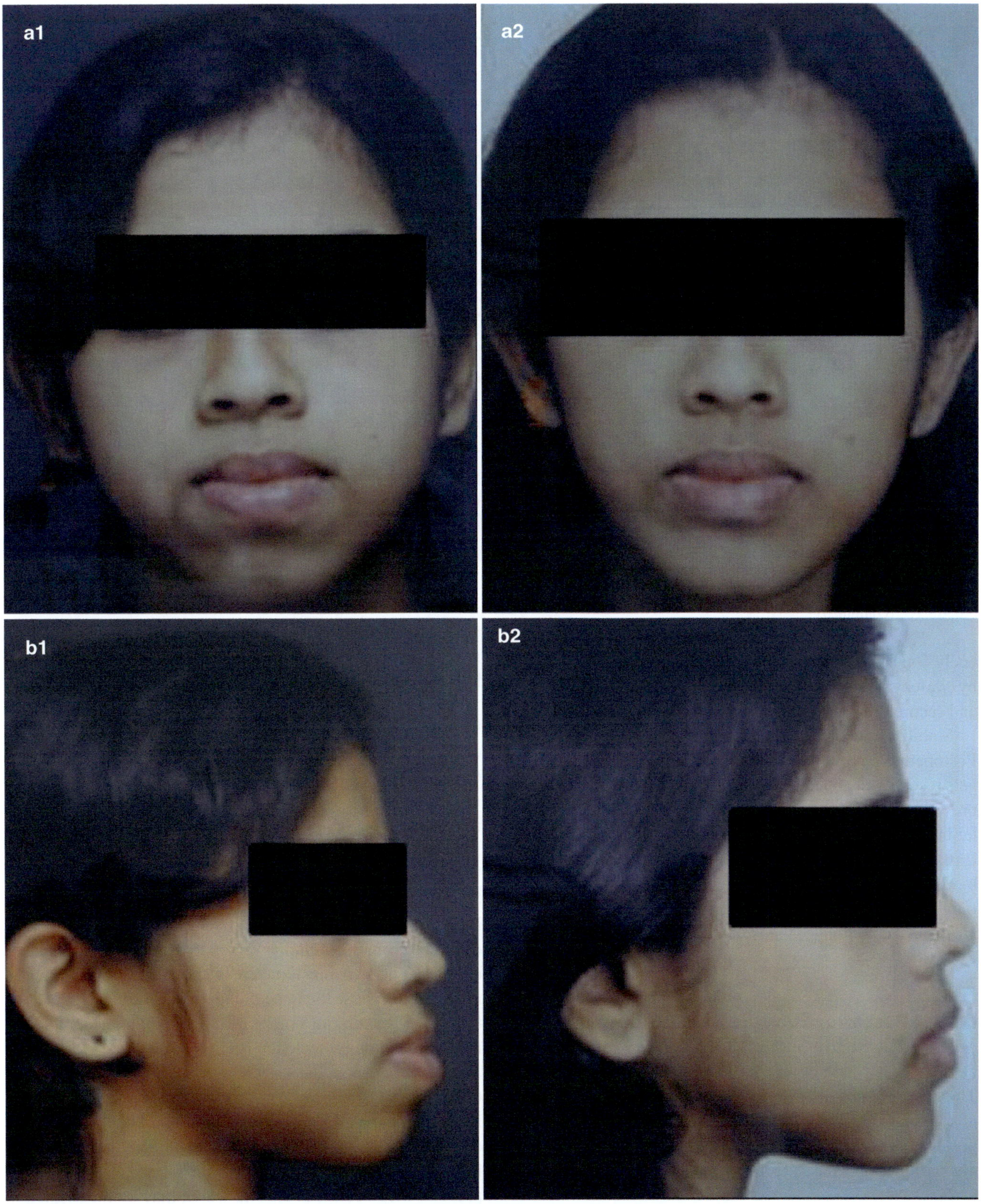

Fig. 68.26 Protrusion anterior dentoalveolar segment of mandible treated by lower anterior subapical osteotomy. (**a1**, **b1**) Preoperative pictures. (**a2**, **b2**) Postoperative pictures. (**c1**) Preoperative lateral cephalogram. (**c2**) Postoperative lateral cephalogram

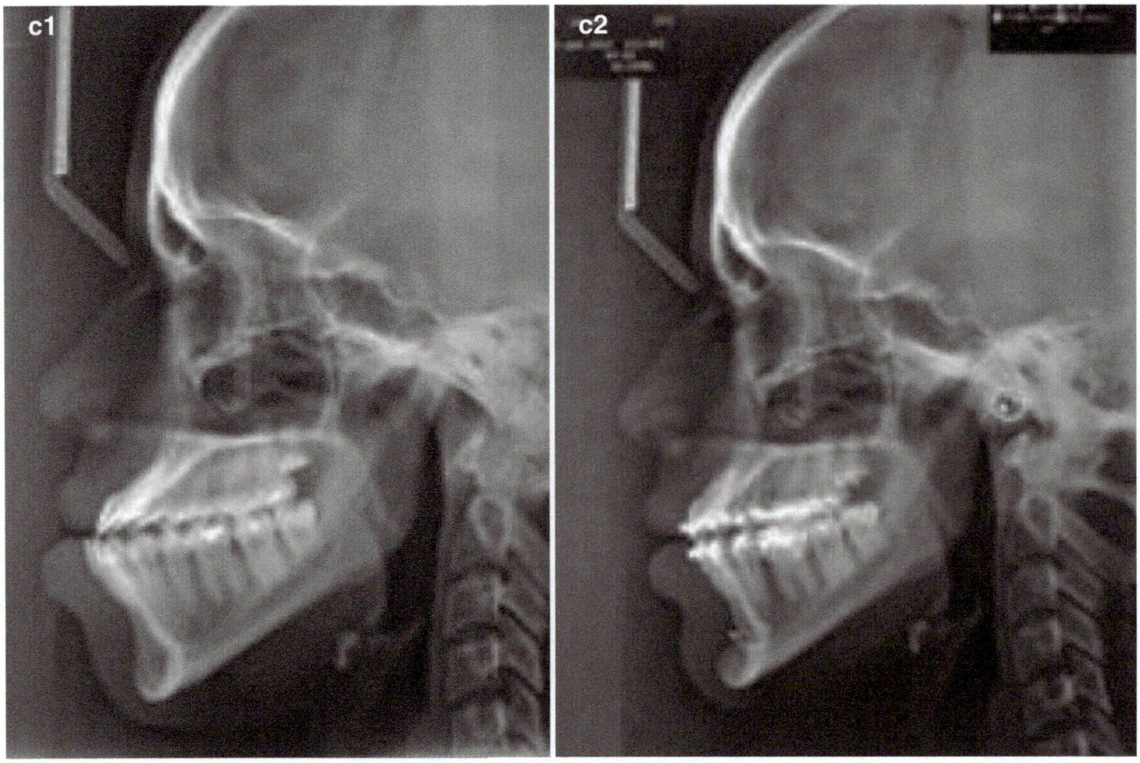

Fig. 68.26 (continued)

occlusion is established. Maxillomandibular fixation is aided by wafer splint. The neurovascular bundle is repositioned and secured in position using struts of bone [68].

Stabilization is done using rigid internal fixation. Postoperative sequelae are usually marked by edema which gets resolved in about 2 weeks. Sensory disturbances, though present, usually recover with time. Injury to the neurovascular bundle may cause permanent anesthesia.

Complications are usually rare. The importance of proper blood supply through the lingual pedicle is of utmost importance. This is mainly through the mylohyoid, genioglossus, and geniohyoid muscle attachments.

68.9 Posterior Subapical Osteotomy Mandible (Fig. 68.28)

The basic plan of the surgery is not very different from that of total subapical osteotomy. The incision is limited to the posterior area. The decompression of the neurovascular bundle is done, and the osteotomy is performed as described earlier.

The main indications are to shift the dentoalveolar segment in question to the required direction in all three dimensions of space, i.e., antero-posterior, vertical, or horizontal.

68.10 Genioplasty

Genioplasty is used for the correction of deformities of the chin. It is possible to reposition the chin in all the three dimensions of space. Hofer in 1942 introduced horizontal osteotomy of the symphysis [67]. By repositioning the inferior mandibular symphysis, a more stable and natural appearance can be attained [69].

Surgical Procedure (Fig. 68.29a, b) (Video 68.3)
Incision is made on the labial mucosa on the lower lip. It is extended from the premolar region to the opposite symmetrical site. The incision is taken to the periosteum, which is reflected to expose the bone. Subperiosteal dissection is done to expose the inferior border of the mandible. Mental nerve is identified and protected.

Osteotomy/Ostectomy
Bony cut is made on the chin about 4.5 mm below the apices of the teeth. The posterior end of the cut should taper to the inferior border, behind and below the mental foramen. (This prevents step defects at the site which may be manifested in the soft tissue also.) The segmented portion is freed from the rest of the mandible but remains pedicled to the digastric and geniohyoid. If the inferior segment is stripped off the periosteum, making it a free graft, intense inflammatory reaction

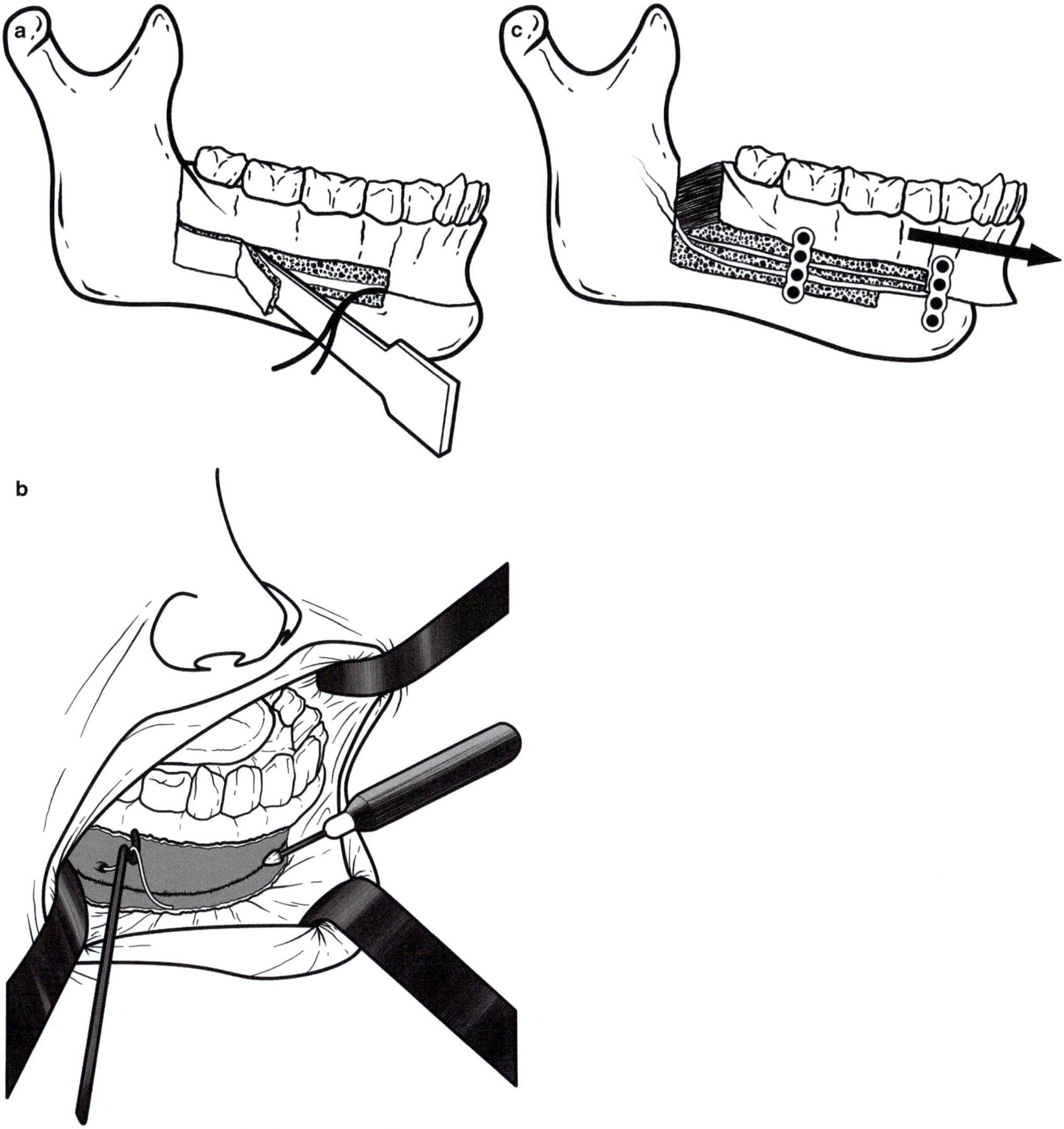

Fig. 68.27 Total subapical osteotomy. (**a**) Neurovascular bundle is released. (**b**) Osteotomy is done using bur or saw. (**c**) The dentoalveolar segment is positioned and fixed rigidly.

and necrosis may occur [70, 71]. The degree of bone resorption and necrosis is indirectly proportional to the amount of pedicle attached to the segment [72].

For vertical reduction, another horizontal cut is made below the original cut, and the measured segment of bone between the two cuts is removed. It is not advisable to cut off the bone from the inferior border as this can imperil the normal contour of the chin. Unilateral vertical reduction/augmentation can be done for correction of asymmetry, since the chin can be moved in all three dimensions (Fig. 68.31a, b).

Increase in the height of the chin can be achieved by bone grafting (preferably autogenous) and rigid internal fixation using plates. Unilateral height increase can be done in asymmetry. However, high morbidity is associated with bone graft and alloplastic materials, such as recurrence, infection, and resorption [73]. Chin can be augmented (augmentation genioplasty) (Fig. 68.30a–c) by bringing the cut inferior segment anteriorly and fixing it by rigid fixation. For major advancement, stepwise augmentation, slicing the inferior border into more than one horizontal segment is advocated (Figs. 68.32 and 68.33a, b, c) (Also refer Fig. 78.42).

Retropositioning of the chin can also be done, but the soft tissue adaptation following posterior positioning of the chin is not 100%. While positioning the inferior border posteriorly, the labiomental fold may get compromised (Fig. 68.34a, b).

Genioplasty can be used for widening and narrowing the chin in the horizontal direction. In mild mandibular asymmetry, the midpoint of the chin may be off the facial midline. By horizontal repositioning of the inferior border, the midpoint of the chin can be brought to the midline of the face, and the mandibular asymmetry can be camouflaged (Fig. 68.35).

Following surgery, the wound is closed adhering to the basic principles. Like in other osteotomies, 3–6 months are necessary for the lip to adapt to the new position and resume normal function. Complications are rare with this procedure. Wound dehiscence occurs in some cases. Meticulous irrigation and aseptic measures can reduce the chances of infection. Sensory loss for a period may be noticed due to traction on the mental nerve. Often sensation is regained within 3–6 months. Rigid fixation technique has reduced the chances shifting of position of the moved segment. Though the reported relapse rates vary in genioplasty, most authors agree that relapse occurs within the first year [38, 70].

68.11 Extended Genioplasty/Mandibular Basal Osteotomy

Mandibular basal osteotomy is an innovative predictable technique for correction of deficiency, excess, and/or asymmetry of the inferior mandibular border, decreasing morbidity, and many other complications of traditional bone grafts and alloplastic techniques [74].

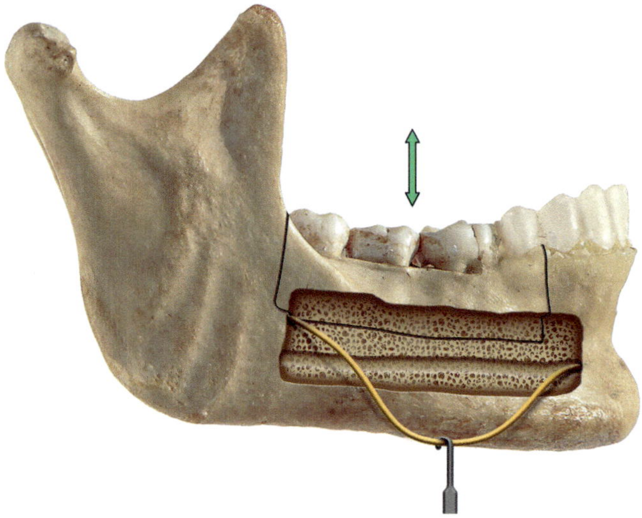

Fig. 68.28 Posterior subapical osteotomy

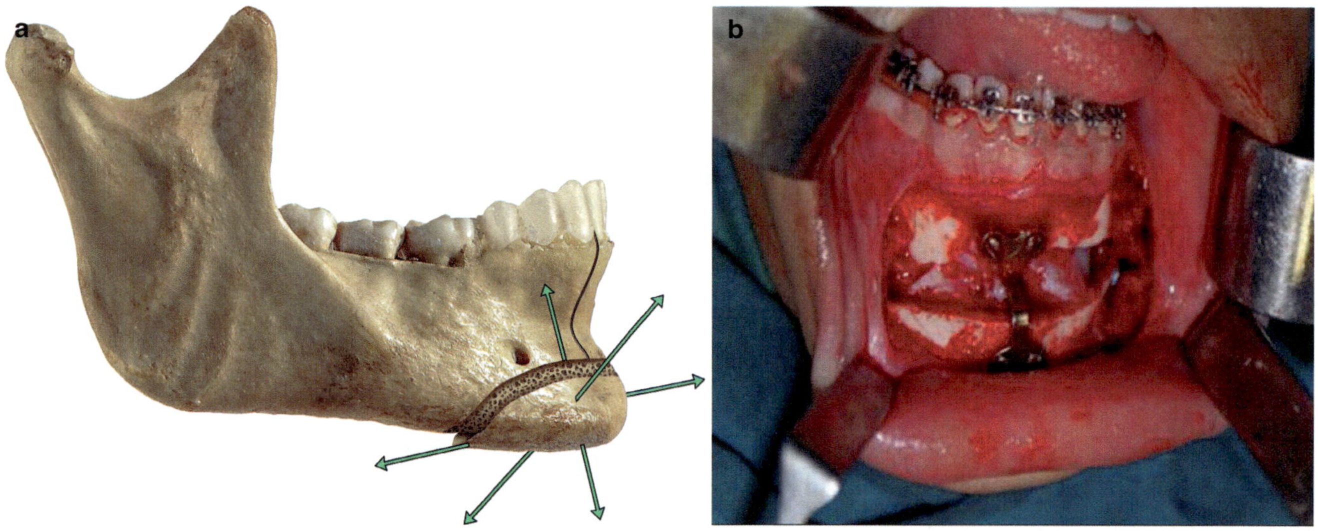

Fig. 68.29 (**a**) Osteotomized chin can be moved in all the three dimensions. (**b**) Advancement genioplasty

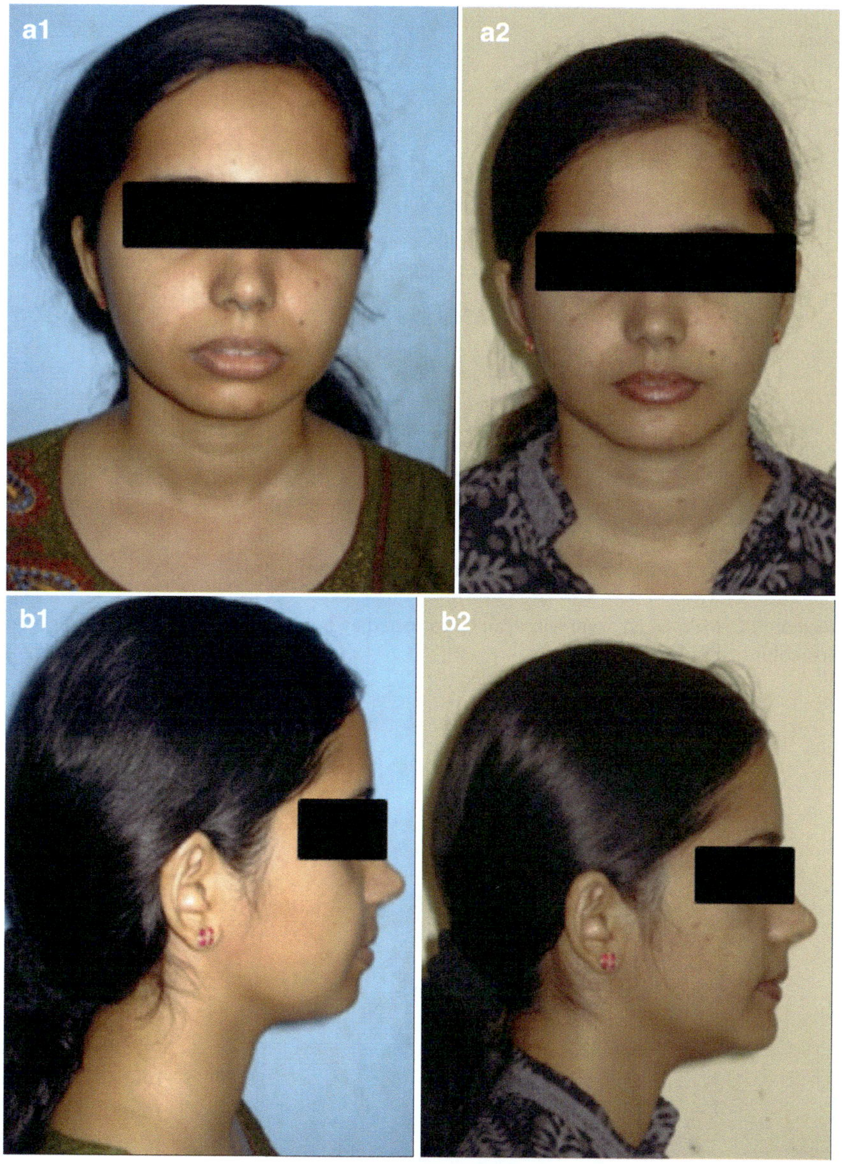

Fig. 68.30 Case of augmentation genioplasty. (**a1**, **b1**) Preoperative pictures. (**a2**, **b2**) Postoperative pictures. (**c1**) Preop lateral cephalogram. (**c2**) Post op lateral cephalogram

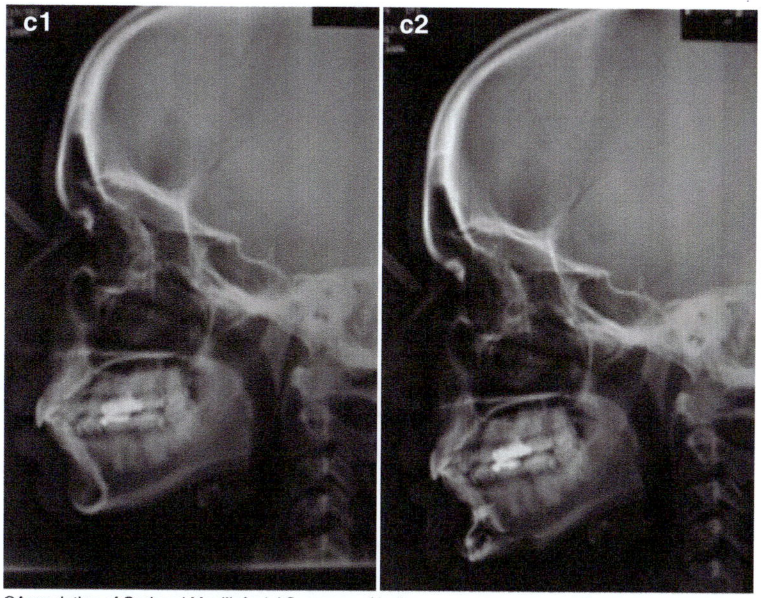

Fig. 68.30 (continued)

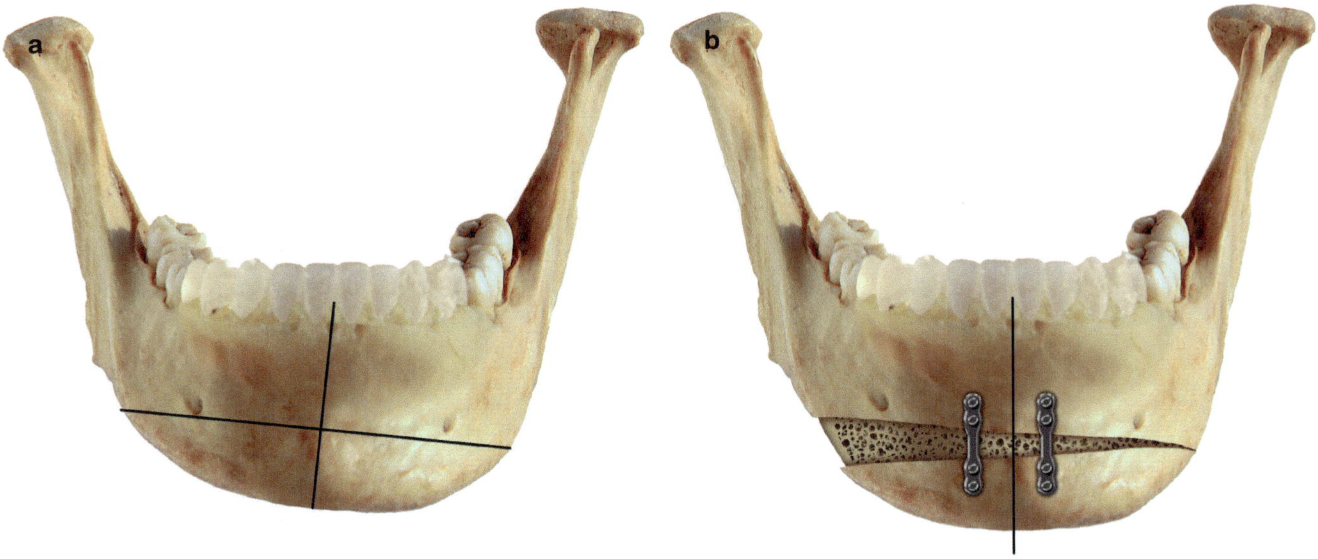

Fig. 68.31 Mild facial asymmetry can be corrected by bone grafting on one side, after osteotomy. (**a**) Pre-operative assessment and (**b**) treatment (osteotomy design)

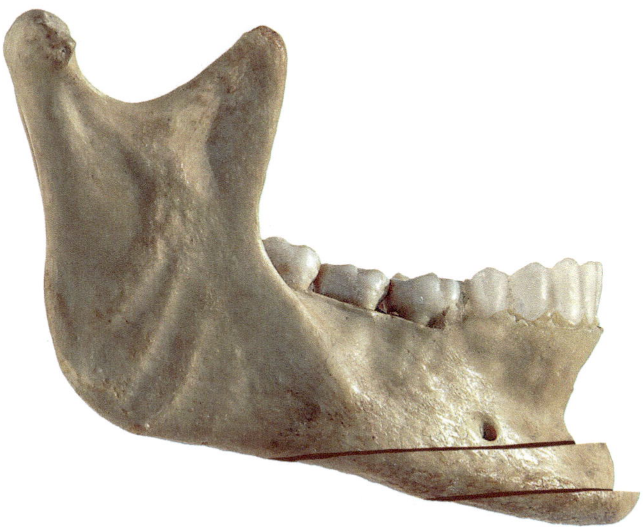

Fig. 68.32 Major advancement of the chin can be effected by a double sliding genioplasty, which is a step osteotomy of the lower border

In extended genioplasty dissection and exposure of the chin, mental nerve and body of the mandible is recommended by a degloving incision. With complete dissection and mobilization of nerves, an extended osteotomy to the antegonial angle may be carried out (Fig. 68.36a, b). The basal osteotomy below the inferior alveolar canal ensures proper proportionality between the advanced segment and the posterior mandible [75]. By laterally sliding the lower border (extended lateral sliding genioplasty), facial asymmetry can be corrected. This procedure can be used for minimal to moderate hemifacial microsomia and facial deformity resulting from unilateral ankylosis of the temporomandibular joint [76] (Fig. 68.37a, b).

68.12 Distraction Osteogenesis

Distraction osteogenesis is a recent introduction into the field of orthognathic surgery. This technique has revolutionized the possibilities of orthognathic surgery. It was Ilizarov, a Russian orthopedic surgeon, who popularized this technique. The first team to report gradual distraction of human mandible was McCarthy et al. in 1992 [77]. As bone has got regenerative capabilities, it is possible to create new bone and lengthen the bone in a cut segment by slowly distracting it. The technique is very useful in the management of deficiency of bone in the maxillofacial region as this is an excellent method to increase bone quantity. The spectrum of indications for distraction is widening and innovations are coming up in the field rapidly. During distraction certain important principles are to be followed.

It is advisable to complete the osteotomy and mobilize the segment as far as possible and then put back the segment to its original position and distract it gradually. During distraction directional stability should be ensured, in order to counteract the pull of the soft tissue and the muscles [78]. A new terminology “distraction histogenesis” has come into vogue as not only the bone but the surrounding tissues also get lengthened. Geniohyoid muscle can be lengthened to a maximum of 20% of its resting length [79]. It is possible to distract the inferior alveolar nerve as well [80]. It is important that the distracted tissue is attached to vital tissue to maintain

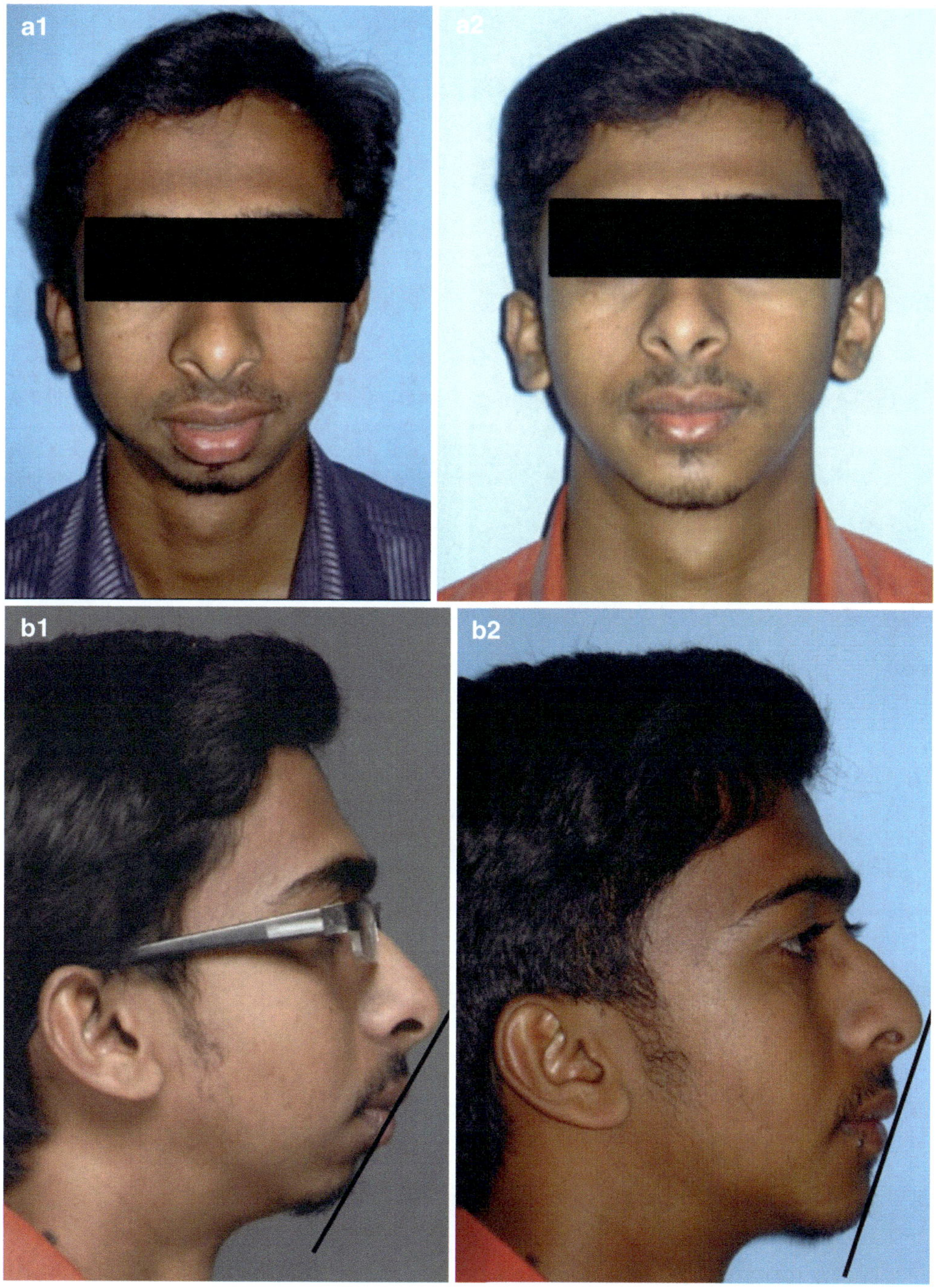

Fig. 68.33 Case of retruded chin corrected by double sliding advancement genioplasty. (**a1**, **b1**) Preoperative pictures. (**a2**, **b2**) Postoperative pictures. (**c1**) Preoperative lateral cephalogram. (**c2**) Postoperative lateral cephalogram

perfusion. Periosteum is rich in osteogenitor cells, and for callus distraction and bone lengthening, the periosteum should be intact, and hence it should be preserved [48].

After osteotomy a latency period of 4–7 days is advised to provide time for the soft tissue to heal. However other factors like age, stability of fixation, type of operative procedure that affects the formation process during the initial stages of distraction, etc. are to be considered before deciding on the latency period [81]. Certain other studies did not show any difference between no latency period and a latency period [82, 83].

Four stages are recognized in distraction osteogenesis—(a) fibrovascular hematoma formation, (b) formation of collagen fibers parallel to distraction vector, (c) bone formation and remodeling of new bone, and (d) formation of solid compact bone. In fast distraction collagen, fibers may lose contact, and bone formation may not take place. In slow

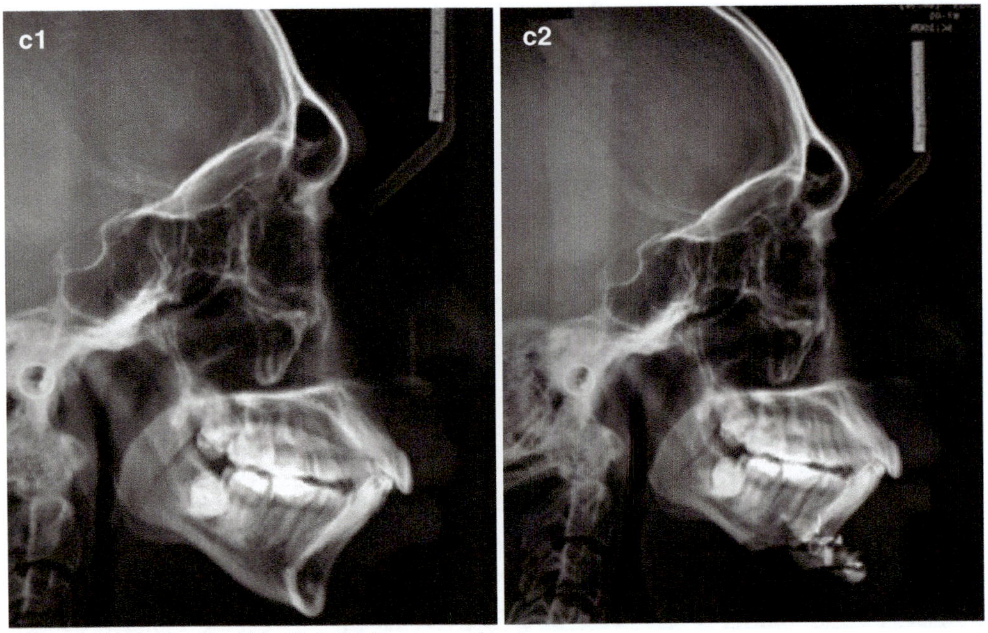

Fig. 68.33 (continued)

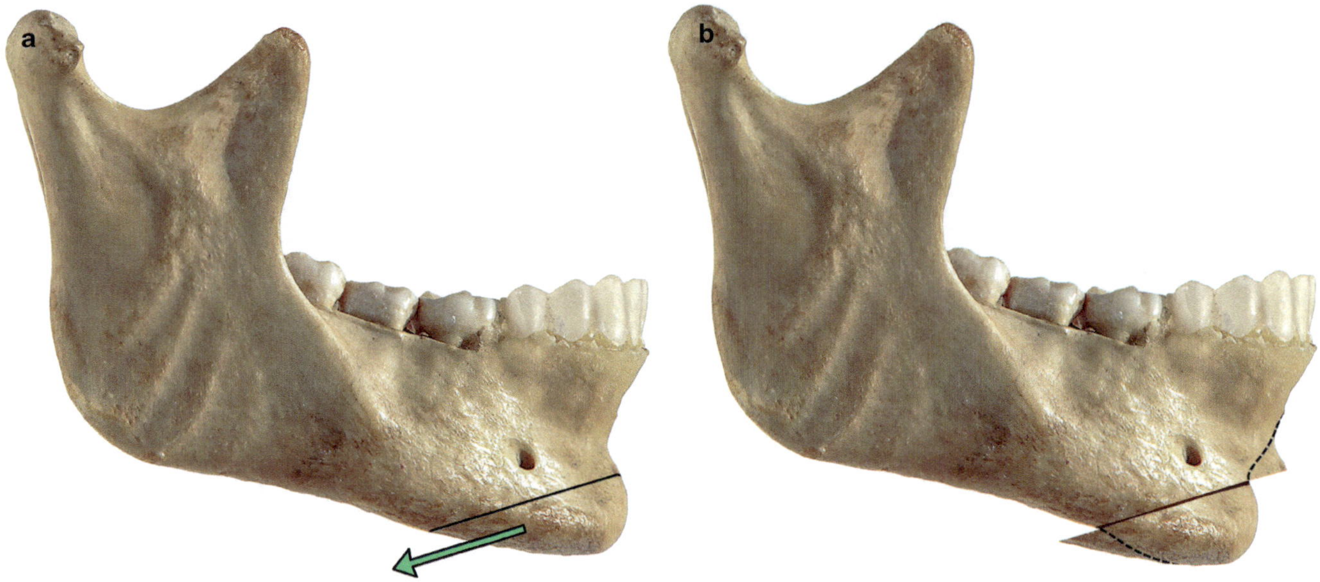

Fig. 68.34 Reduction of the chin can also be achieved. However, sharp margins are to be trimmed off. (**a**) Pre-operative planning and (**b**) treatment (osteotomy design)

distraction, consolidation of bone may occur earlier [84]. Karp et al. demonstrated that intramembranous ossification is what occurs predominantly [85]. Distraction of 1 mm per day is the widely accepted rate [86]. Direct current electrical stimulation may be useful in activation and consolidation period [87–89]. Insufficient distraction and defective vectors can compromise the final result. These complications can be, to some extent, managed by manipulating the regenerate bone by the application of orthodontic traction [79, 90–92]. OW and Cheung reported a lower incidence of persistent IAN disturbance (3%) after MDO compared with BSSO, of which the incidence was 28% [93]. In terms of skeletal stability in small to moderate advancements, there is no significant difference between BSSO and DO. DO requires a second surgery for removal of the distractor, which goes in favor of BSSO [94].

Distraction osteogenesis has got an important role in managing sleep apnea, in cases like micrognathia, Pierre Robin syndrome, hemifacial microsomia, Treacher Collins syndrome, etc. [4, 95]. Due to its complex nature, it is rather difficult to treat unilateral craniofacial microsomia, in growing children. Maxilla, zygoma, mandible, external and middle ear, facial and trigeminal nerves, muscles of mastication, and overlying soft tissues are the structures of the first and second arch which are involved [96] (Refer Chap. 78 on Hemifacial microsomia and Treacher Collins syndrome).

In severe cases, in neonatals, tracheostomy may become necessary. Mandibular distraction is an effective method in resolving upper airway obstruction and decannulation of tracheostomy [97–99]. Rachmiel A. et al. have reported an increase of mandibular volume by 28.4%, increase of upper airway volume

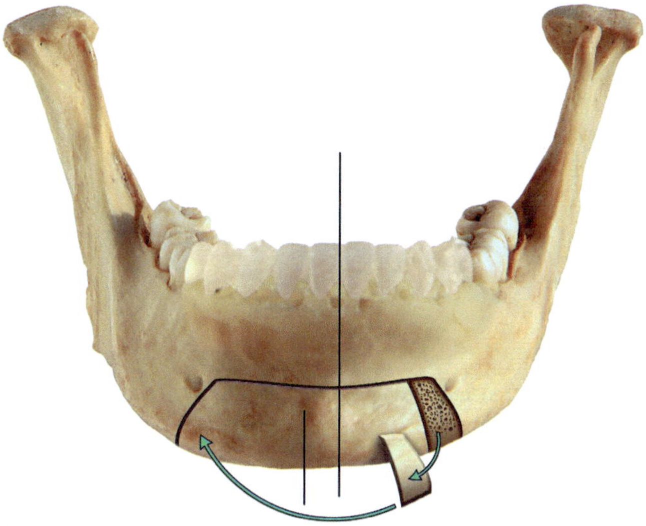

Fig. 68.35 Osteotomy plan for mild facial asymmetry pertaining to the chin

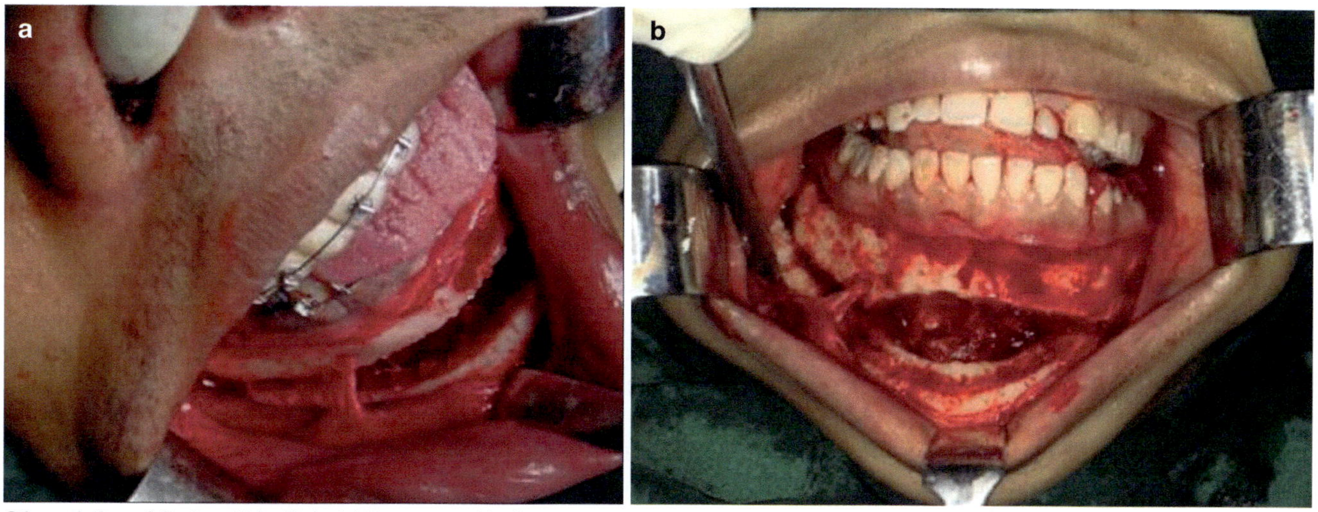

Fig. 68.36 After making a degloving incision an extended genioplasty may be done. it is possible to preserve the mental nerve. (**a**) Oblique view and (**b**) frontal view

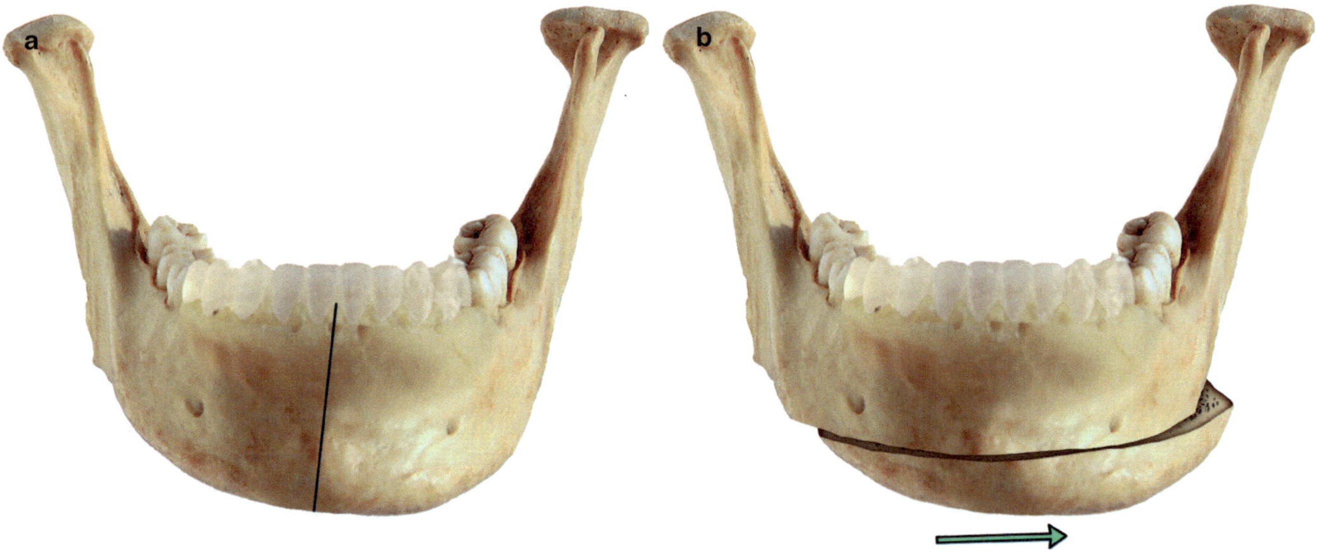

Fig. 68.37 Major asymmetry of the mandible can be corrected to a great extent by extended lateral sliding genioplasty. (**a**) Pre-operative plan and (**b**) treatment (osteotomy design)

by 71.92%, and increase in oxygen saturation. This study was conducted in children between 13 months and 7 years of age [25] (refer Chap. 87 on distraction osteogenesis).

In severely hypoplastic mandible multi-stage correction starting from young age may be considered for functional and psychological reasons. Less severe cases may be taken up for single stage correction after the permanent dentition is erupted [100].

68.13 Conclusion

Mandible is a horse shoe-shaped bone hinged to the skull and performs the major function, chewing, and forms the lower part of the mouth which houses the tongue and other musculature. All the muscles of mastication and many other muscles of facial expression are attached to the mandible. Hence mandible is an important structure in both function and aesthetics. Different osteotomies of mandible can move the jaw in almost all the three directions and change the size and shape of the jaw and face to achieve better function and aesthetics. This chapter is intended to elucidate various osteotomy techniques on the mandible.

Disclosure Authors have no financial conflicts to disclose.

68.14 Case Scenarios

Case 1 (Fig. 68.38a, b, c)

Patient aged 22 years, female, reported with complaint of facial deformity with a history of fall when she was about 8 years old. No deformity was noticed, and no treatment was taken at that time, and as she grew up, she started developing deviation of the face.

On examination she had facial asymmetry with deviation of the jaw to left side. She had class II occlusion and deficient chin. Radiographs revealed under developed and deformed condyle on the left side. The mandible was shifted to the left side due to underdevelopment of the mandible on left side (Fig. 68.38a1, b1, c1).

Treatment: Pre-surgical orthodontic treatment with sagittal split osteotomy and extended lateral sliding genioplasty with rib bone grafting on right side.

Postoperative pictures after 1 year (Fig. 68.38a2, b2, c2).

Case 2 (Fig. 68.19a, b, c)

Patient aged 19 years reported with complaint of protruded teeth and facial deviation with no relevant history.

On examination, she had vertical maxillary excess with mandibular prognathism. Other clinical findings included incompetent lips, convex facial profile, acute nasolabial angle, and facial asymmetry with deviation of chin toward right side. Radiographs revealed vertical and anterioposterior maxillary excess with mandibular prognathism and deficient chin.

Preoperative pictures (Fig. 68.19a1, b1, c1)

Treatment plan: Pre-surgical othodontic treatment followed by surgery.

Surgery: LeFort 1, anterior maxillary osteotomy, bilateral sagittal split osteotomy, and genioplasty were done for the patient under general anesthesia.

Postoperative pictures after 1 year (Fig. 68.19a2, b2, c2)

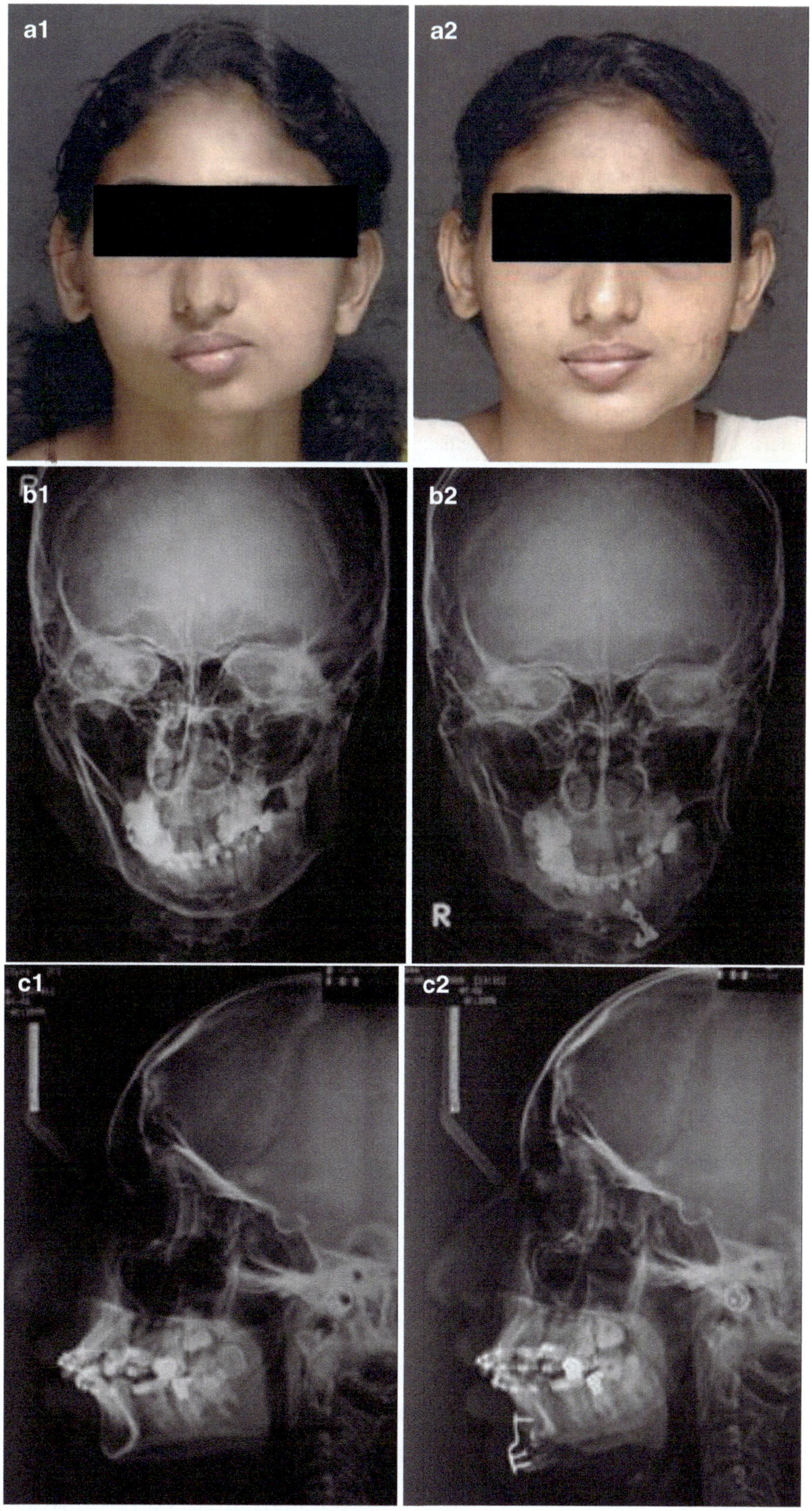

Fig. 68.38 Mandibular asymmetry corrected by extended lateral sliding genioplasty. (**a1**) pre operative frontal view. (**a2**) post operative frontal view. (**b1, b2**) pre and post operative Frontal cephalogram. (**c1, c2**) pre and post operative lateral cephalogram

References

1. Batra APS, Mahajan A, Gupta K. Marginal mandibular branch of the facial nerve: an anatomical study. Indian J Plast Surg. 2010;43(1):60–4.
2. Limberg A. Treatment of open bite by means of plastic oblique osteotomy of the ascending rami of the mandible. Dent Cosmos. 1925;67:1191–7.
3. Caldwell JB, Letterman GS. Vertical osteotomy in the mandibular rami for correction of prognathism. J Oral Surg. 1954;12:185–202.
4. Cosman B, Criilair G. Mandibular hyperplasia and the late development of glossopharyngeal airway obstruction. Plast Reconstr Surg. 1972;50:573–9.
5. Caldwell JB, Hayward JR, Lister RL. Correction of mandibular retrognathia by vertical L osteotomy: a new technique. J Oral Surg. 1968;26:259–64.
6. Obwegeser H, Trauner R. Zur Operationstechnik bei der progenie und anderen unterkieferanomalien. Dtsch Z Mund Kieferheilkd. 1955;23:H1–2.
7. Trauner R, Obwegeser H. Zur Operationstechnik bei der progenieund anderen unterkieferanomalien [The surgical correction of mandibular prognathism and retrognathia with consideration of genioplasty]. Dtsch Zahn Mund Kieferheilk. 1955;23(1):1–26.
8. DalPont G. Retromolar osteotomy for the correction of prognathism. J Oral Surg Anesth Hosp Dent Serv. 1961;19:42–7.
9. Hunsuck EE. Modified intraoral sagittal split technique for correction of mandibular prognathism. J Oral Surg. 1968;26:250–3.
10. Reitzik M, Barer PG, Wainwright WM, Lim B. The surgical treatment of skeletal anterior open-bite deformities with rigid internal fixation in the mandible. Am J Orthod Denthofac Orthop. 1990;97(1):52–7.
11. Hensel GC. The surgical correction of mandibular protection, retraction, and fractures of the ascending rami. Int J Orthodont Oral Surg. 1937;23:184.
12. Bell WH, Schendel SA. Biological basis for the modification of the sagittal ramus split operation. J Oral Surg. 1977;35:362–9.
13. Epker BN, Wolford LM, Fish LC. Mandibular deficiency syndrome: surgical considerations for mandibular advancement. Oral Surg. 1978;45:349–63.
14. Wolford LM. Influence of osteotomy design mandibular ramus sagittal split osteotomy. J Oral Maxillofac Surg. 2015;73(10):1994–2004.
15. Pietruski P, Majak M, Swiatek-Najwer E, Popek M, Szram D, Zuk M, Jaworowski J. Accuracy of experimental mandibular osteotomy using the image-guided sagittal saw. Int J Oral Maxillofac Surg. 2016;45:793–800.
16. Panula K, Finne K, Oikarinen K. Neurosensory deficits after bilateral sagittal split ramus osteotomy of the mandible—influences of soft tissue handling medial to the ascending ramus. Int J Oral Maxillofac Surg. 2004;33:543–8.
17. Tsuji Y, Muto T, Kawakami T, Takeda S. Computed tomographic analysis of the position and course of the mandibular canal: relevance to the sagittal split ramus osteotomy. Int J Oral Maxillofac Surg. 2005;34:243–6.
18. Promma L, Sakulsak N, Putiwat P, Amarttayakong P, Iamsaard S, Trakulsuk H, Hirunyakorn K, Suarbua S, Wattanaraeungchai Y. Cortical bone thickness of the mandibular canal and implications for bilateral sagittal split osteotomy: a cadaveric study Int. J Oral Maxillofac Surg. 2017;46:572–7.
19. Blair VP. Report of a case of double resection for the correction of protrusion of the mandible. Dent Cosmos. 1906;48:817–20.
20. Wolford LM, Cottrell DA. Diagnosis of macroglossia and indications for reduction glossectomy. Am J Orthod Dentofac Orthop. 1996;110:170–7.
21. Mommaerts MY. Endoscopically assisted sagittal split osteotomy for mandibular lengthening: technical note and initial experience. J Craniomaxillofac Surg. 2010;38:108–12.
22. Ellis E III, Gallo WJ. Relapse following mandibular advancement with dental plus skeletal maxillomandibular fixation. J Oral Maxillofac Surg. 1986;44:509–15.
23. Ellis E III, Reynolds S, Carlson DS. Stability of the mandible following advancement: a comparison of three post surgical fixation techniques. Am J Orthod Dentofac Orthop. 1988;94:38–49.
24. Schendel SA, Epkar BN. Result after mandibular advancement surgery: an analysis of 87 cases. J Oral Surg. 1980;38:265–81.
25. Rachmiel A, Aizenbud D, Pillar G, Srouji S, Peled M. Bilateral mandibular distraction for patients with compromised airway analyzed by three dimensional CT. Int J Oral Maxillofac Surg. 2005;34(1):9–18.
26. Laine P, Kontio R, Lindqvist C, Suuronen R. Are there any complications with bioabsorbable fixation devices? A 10 year review in orthognathic surgery. Int J Oral Maxillofac Surg. 2004;33:240–4.
27. Bell WH, Fonseca RJ, Kennedy JW III, Levy BM. Bone healing and revascularization after total maxillary osteotomy. J Oral Surg. 1975;33:253–60.
28. Bell WH, Levy BM. Revascularisation and bone healing after posterior maxillary osteotomy. J Oral Surg. 1971;29:313–20.
29. Bell WH. Revascularisation and bone healing after anterior maxillary osteotomy: a study using adult rhesus monkeys. J Oral Surg. 1969;27:249–55.
30. Stoelinga PJ, Borslap WA. The fixation of sagittal split osteotomies with mini plates the versatility of a technique. J Oral Maxillofac Surg. 2003;61:1471–6.
31. Foley WL, Beckman TW. In vitro comparison of screw versus plate fixation in the sagittal split ramus osteotomy. Int J Adult Orthodon Orthognath Surg. 1992;7:147–51.
32. Behrman SJ. Complications associated with orthognathic surgery. In: Irby WB, editor. Current advances in oral surgery. St Louis: CV Mosby; 1974. p. 109.
33. Storum KA, Bell WH. Hypo mobility after maxillary and mandibular osteotomies. J Oral Surg. 1984;57:7–12.
34. Aragon SB, VanSickels JE. Mandibular range of motion with rigid/no rigid fixation. Oral Surg. 1987;63:408–11.
35. Steenen SA, Becking AG. Bad splits in bilateral sagittal split osteotomy: systematic review of fracture patterns. Int J Oral Maxillofac Surg. 2016;45:887–97.
36. Aarabi M, Tabrizi R, Hekmat M, Shahidi S, Puzesh A. Relationship between mandibular anatomy and the occurrence of a bad split upon sagittal split osteotomy. J Oral Maxillofac Surg. 2014;72:2508–13.
37. Al Bishri A, Barghash Z, Rosenquist J, Sunzel B. Neurosensory disturbance after sagittal split and intra oral vertical ramus osteotomy: as reported in questionnaires and patients records. Int J Oral Maxillofac Surg. 2005;34:247–51.
38. Posnick JL, Qattan MM, Stepner NM. Alteration in focal sensibility in adolescents following sagittal split and chin osteotomies of the mandible. Plast Reconstr Surg. 1996;97:920–7.
39. Lake SL, McNeill RW, Little RM, West RA. Surgical mandibular advancement: a cephalometric analysis of treatment response. Am J Orthod. 1981;80:376–94.
40. Fariña R, Pintor F, Pérez J, Pantoja R, Berner D. Low condylectomy as the sole treatment for active condylar hyperplasia: facial, occlusal and skeletal changes. An observational study. Int J Oral Maxillofac Surg. 2015;44:217–25.
41. Lee SG, Kang YH, Byun JH, Kim UK, Kim JR, Park BW. Stability of unilateral sagittal split ramus osteotomy for correction of facial asymmetry: long-term case series and literature review. J Korean Assoc Oral Maxillofac Surg. 2015;41:156–64.
42. Mendez-Manjon I, Guijarro-Martınez R, Valls-Ontanon A, Hernandez-Alfaro F. Early changes in condylar position after

mandibular advancement: a three-dimensional analysis. Int J Oral Maxillofac Surg. 2016;45:787–92.
43. Borstlap WA, Steolinga PJW, Hoppenreijs TJM, Van't Hof MA. Stabilization of sagittal split advancement osteotomies with mini plates: a prospective multi centre study with two year follow up part III—condylar remodeling and resorption. Int J Oral Maxillofac Surg. 2004;33:649–55.
44. Arnett GW, Milam SB, Gottesman L. Progressive mandibular retrusion—idiopathic condylar resorption part I. Am J Orthod Dentofac Orthop. 1996;110:8–15.
45. Alder ME, Deahl ST, Matteson SR, Van Sickel JE, Tiner BD, Rugh JD. Short term change of condylar position after sagittal split osteotomy for mandibular advancement. Orrl Surg Oral Med Oral Pathol Oral Radiol Endod. 1999;87:159–65.
46. Ueki K, Nakagawa K, Marukawa K, Takazakara D, Shimada M, Takatsuka S, Yamanoto E. Changes in condylar long axis and skeletal stability after bilateral sagittal split ramus osteotomy with poly-L-lactic acid or titanium plate fixation. Int J Oral Maxillofac Surg. 2005;34:627–34.
47. Mobarak KA, Espeland L, Krogstad O, Lyberg T. Mandibular advancement surgery in high-angle and low-angle class II patients: different long-term skeletal responses. Am J Orthod Dentofac Orthop. 2001;119:368–81.
48. Kojimoto H, Yasin N, Goto T, Matsudo S, Shimomura Y. Bone lengthening in rabbits by callus distraction. The role of periosteum and endosteum. J Bone Joint Surg Br. 1988;70:543–9.
49. Moose SM. Surgical correction of mandibular prognathism by intra oral subcondylar osteotomy. J Oral Surg. 1964;22:197–201.
50. Winstanley RP. Subcondylar osteotomy of the mandible and the intra oral approach. Br J Oral Surg. 1968;6:134–6.
51. Rokutanda S, Yamada S, Yanamoto S, Omori K, Fujimura Y, Morita Y, Rokutanda H, Kohara H, Fujishita A, Nakamura T, Yoshimi T, Yoshida N, Umeda M. Comparison of osseous healing after sagittal split ramus osteotomy and intraoral vertical ramus osteotomy. Int J Oral Maxillofac Surg. 2018;47(10):1316–21.
52. Al-Moraissi EA, Ellis E 3rd. Is there a difference in stability or neurosensoy func-tion between bilateral sagittal split ramus osteotomy and intraoral vertical ramus osteotomy for mandibular setback? J Oral Maxillofac Surg. 2015;73:1360–71.
53. Hall HD, Chase DC, Payor LG. Evaluation and refinement of the intraoral vertical subcondylar osteotomy. J Oral Surg. 1975;33:333–41.
54. Tornes K, Wisth PJ. Stability after vertical subcondylar ramus osteotomy for correction of mandibular prognathism. Int Oral Maxillofac Surg. 1988;17:242–8.
55. Nystrom E, Rosenquist J, Astrand P, Nordin T. Intraoral or extra oral approaches in oblique sliding osteotomy of the mandibular ramus. J Maxillofac Surg. 1984;12:277–82.
56. Reitzk M, Griffiths RR, Mirels H. Surgical anatomy of the ascending ramus of the mandible. Br J Oral Surg. 1976;14(2):150–5.
57. Goldstein A. Appraisal of results of surgical correction of class III malocclusions. Angle Orthod. 1974;17(3-4):59.
58. Komiri E, Aigase K, Sugisaki M, Tanabe H. Skeletal fixation versus skeletal relapse. Am J Orthod Dentofac Orthop. 1987;92(5):412–21.
59. Ghali GE, Sikes JW Jr. Intraoral vertical ramus osteotomy as the preferred treatment for mandibular prognathism. J Oral Maxillofac Surg. 2000;58:313e315.
60. González-García R. Endoscopically-assisted subcondylar and vertical ramus osteotomies for the treatment of symmetrical mandibular prognathism. J Craniomaxillofac Surg. 2012;40:393–5.
61. Poulton DR, Taylor RC, Ware WH. Cephalometric x-rays evaluation of the vertical osteotomy correction of mandibular prognathism. Oral Surg Oral Med Oral Pathol. 1963;16:807–20.
62. Ritzau M, Wenzel A, Williams S. Changing in condyle position after bilateral vertical ramus osteotomy with and without osteosynthesis. Am J Orthod Dentofac Orthop. 1989;96:507–13.
63. Sund G, Eckerdal O, Astrand P. Changes in the temporomandibular joint after oblique sliding osteotomy of the mandibular rami: a longitudinal radiological study. J Maxillofac Surg. 1983;11(2):87–91.
64. Hollender L, Ridell A. Radiography of the temporomandibular joint after oblique sliding osteotomy of the mandibular ramis. Scand J Dent Res. 1974;82:466–9.
65. Sund G, Eckerdal O, Astrand P. Skeletal remodeling in the temporomandibular joint after oblique sliding osteotomy of the mandibular rami. Int J Oral Maxillofac Surg. 1986;15(3):233–9.
66. Hullihen SP. Case of elongation of the under jaw and distortion of the face and neck, caused by a burn, successfully treated. Am J Dent Sci. 1849;9:157.
67. Hofer O. Operation der prognathie und Mikrogenie. Dtsch Zahn Mund Kieferheilk. 1942;9:121–32.
68. Boye T, Doyle P, McKeown F, Sandler J. Total subapical mandibular osteotomy to correct class 2 division1, dento-facial deformity. J Craniomaxillofac Surg. 2011;40(3):238–42.
69. Bell WH, Gallagher DM. Versatility of genioplasty with broad pedicle. J Oral Maxillofac Surg. 1983;41:763–9.
70. Mercuri LG, Laskin DM. Avascular necrosis after anterior horizontal augmentation genioplasty. J Oral Surg. 1977;35:296–8.
71. Storum KA, Bell WH, Nagura H. Micro angiographic and histologic evaluation of revascularization and healing after genioplasty by osteotomy of the inferior border of the mandible. J Oral Maxillofac Surg. 1988;48:210–6.
72. Fitzpatrick BN. Reconstruction of the chin in cosmetic surgery (genioplasty). Oral Surg. 1975;39:522–35.
73. Cohen SR, Mardach OL, Kawawata HK. Chin disfigurement following removal of alloplastic chin implants. Plast Reconstr Surg. 1991;88:62.
74. Lopez PE, Guerrero CA, Mujica EV. Mandibular basal osteotomy: new designs and fixation techniques. J Oral Maxillofac Surg. 2011;69:786–97.
75. Troulis MJ, Kearns GJ, Perrott DH, Kaban LB. Extended genioplasty, long term cephalometric, nurpometric and sensory results. Int J Oral Maxillofac Surg. 2000;29:167–75.
76. Mani V, et al. Extended lateral sliding genioplasty for the correction of facial asymmetry. Asian J Oral Maxillofac Surg. 2004;16(2):84–90.
77. McCarthy JG, Schreiber JS, Karp NCH, Thorne CH, Grayson BH. Lengthening of the human mandible by gradual distraction. Plast Reconstr Surg. 1992;89:1–10.
78. Raghoebar GM, Heydenrijk K, Vissink A. Vertical distraction of the severely resorbed mandible. The Groningen distraction device. Int J Oral Maxillofac Surg. 2001;59:728–33.
79. Suhr MAA, Kreatsch T. Technical considerations in distraction osteogenesis. Int J Oral Maxillofac Surg. 2004;33:89–94.
80. Hu J, Tang Z, Wang D, Buckley MJ. Changes in the inferior alveolar nerve after mandibular lengthening with different rates of distraction. J Oral Maxillofac Surg. 2001;108(5):1103–14.
81. Aida T, Yoshioka I, Tominaga K, Fukuda J. Effects of latency period in a rabbit mandibular distraction osteogenesis. Int J Oral Maxillofac Surg. 2003;32:54–62.
82. Tavakoli K, Walsh WR, Bonar F, Smart R, Wulf S, Poole M. The role of latency in mandibular osteo-distraction. J Craniomaxillofac Surg. 1998;26(4):209–19.
83. Troulis MJ, Glowacki J, Perrott DH, Kaban LB. The effects of latency and rate on distraction osteogenesis of the procine mandible. J Oral Maxillofac Surg. 2000;58(5):507–14.
84. Koudstaal MJ, Poort Poort LT, Vandel Wal KGH, Wolvers EB, Prahl Anderson B, Schulten AJM. Surgically assisted rapid max-

illary expansion (SDRME) a review of the literature. Int J Oral Maxillofac Surg. 2005;34:709–14.
85. Karp NS, McCarthy JG, Schreiber JS, Sissions HA, Thorne CHM. Membranous bones lengthening: a serial histological study. Ann Plast Surg. 1992;29:2–7.
86. Al Ruhaimi KA. Comparison of different distraction rates in the mandible: an experimental investigation. Int J Oral Maxillofac Surg. 2001;30:220–7.
87. El-Hakin E, Azins AMA, El Hanson MFA, Maree SM. Preliminary investigation into the effects of electrical stimulation on mandibular distraction osteogenesis in goats. Int J Oral Maxillofac Surg. 2004;33:42–7.
88. Friedenberg ZB, Kohanin M. Effect of direct current on bone. Surg Gynecol Obstet. 1968;127:97–102.
89. Hagiwara T, Bell WH. Effect of electrical stimulation on mandibular distraction osteogenesis. J Craniomaxillofac Surg. 2000;28:12–9.
90. Hoffmeister B, Marks CH, Wolff KD. The floating bone concept in intraoral mandibular distraction. J Craniomaxillofac Surg. 1998;26:76–7.
91. McCarthy J, Hopper R, Hollier L, Peltomaki T, Katzen T, Grayson B. Molding of the degenerate in mandibular distraction—clinical experience. Plast Reconstr Surg. 2003;12:1239–46.
92. Peltonaki T, Greyson B, Venditelli B, Katzen T, McCarthy J. Moulding the generate to control open bite during mandibular distraction osteogenesis. Eur J Orthod. 2002;24:639–45.
93. Ow ATC, Cheung LK. Skeletal stability and complications of Bilateral Sagittal Split Osteotomies (BSSO) and Mandibular Distraction Osteogenesis (MDO): an evidence-based review. J Oral Maxillofac Surg. 2009;67:2344–53.
94. Baas EM, Bierenbroodspot F, de Lange J. Skeletal stability after bilateral sagittal split osteotomy or distraction osteogenesis of the mandible: a randomized clinical trial. Int J Oral Maxillofac Surg. 2015;44:615–20.
95. Sjolui S. Hypoplasia of the mandible as a cause of respiratory difficulties in the infant. Acta Paediatr Scand. 1950;39:255–6.
96. Keogh IJ, Troulis MJ, Monroy AA, Eavey RD, Kaban LB. Isolated microtia as a marker for unsuspected hemifacial microsomia. Arch Otolaryngol Head Neck Surg. 2007;13:997–1001.
97. Moore MH, Guzman-Stein G, Proudman TW, Abott AH, Netherway DJ, David DJ. Mandibular lengthening by distraction for airway obstruction in Treacher collins syndrome. J Craniofac Surg. 1994;5:22–5.
98. Morovic CG, Monasterio L. Distraction osteogenesis for obstructive apneas in patients with congenital craniofacial malformations. Plast Reconstr Surg. 2000;105:2324–30.
99. Perkins JA, Sie KCY, Miczuk K, Richardson MA. Airway management in children with cranio facial anomalies. Cleft Palate Craniofac J. 1997;34:135–40.
100. Pluijmers C, Caron JJM, Dunaway DJ, Wolvius EB, Koudstaal MJ, Posnick JC, Al-Quattan MM, Stepner NM. Alteration in facial sensibility in adolescents following sagittal split and chin osteotomies of the mandible. Plast Reconstr Surg. 1996;97:920–7.

Orthognathic Surgery for the Maxilla-LeFort I and Anterior Maxillary Osteotomy

69

Ashok Dabir and Jayesh Vahanwala

69.1 History of Maxillary Osteotomies

Maxillary Osteotomies
One does not know a science completely without knowing its history.

Auguste Comte (1798–1857) [1]

The Le Fort I-Type Maxillary Osteotomy
The development of modern maxillary orthognathic surgical procedures had diverse historical origins and contributions. The removal of nasal and nasopharyngeal polyps via hemi maxillary osteotomy was being undertaken in Europe in the mid-nineteenth century, notably by the German surgeon Bernhard Rudolf Konrad von Langenbeck (1810–1887) in Berlin [2]. The first maxillary procedure that would today be described as a total Le Fort I-type osteotomy appears to have been undertaken in 1868 by the American surgeon, David Williams Cheever (1831–1915) in Boston City Hospital to provide surgical access for removal of a large nasopharyngeal polyp [3]. One year prior to this, in 1867, Cheever had undertaken a down-fracture of the right hemimaxilla for similar surgical access in another patient, who had made a complete recovery [4]. The total down-fracture of the maxilla at the Le Fort I level performed in 1868, described as Cheever's "double operation," though technically successful, had an unfortunate postoperative outcome in that the patient subsequently died 5 days later, though probably not as a direct result of the maxillary procedure [5, 6].

In 1901, a French surgeon from Lille named René Le Fort (1869–1951) conducted experiments using blunt trauma to intact cadaveric faces, from different directions and varying magnitudes, and thereby described the natural planes of maxillary and facial fractures [7, 8] now known as the Le Fort classification of facial fractures. The names of the Le Fort I-, II-, and III-type osteotomies are due to their similarity to the Le Fort fractures.

In 1927, Wassmund carried out a maxillary osteotomy at the Le Fort I level, without pterygoid plate disjunction or mobilization at the time of surgery [9]. He used elastics to close an anterior open bite, without placing a bone graft, which subsequently relapsed. In 1934, Axhausen in Berlin described advancement of the maxilla at the Le Fort I level, which was incompletely mobilized, again with postoperative elastic traction [10].

Wassmund was the first to apply osteotomies at the Le Fort I level for correction of midfacial deformities [11]. The technique was subsequently modified by several surgeons including Axhausen [12], Schuchardt [13], and Willmar [14]. In 1965, Obwegeser improved the precision of the Le Fort I osteotomy by suggesting complete mobilization of the maxilla so that repositioning was achieved without tension [15, 16]. The operation was slow to gain popularity until 1973, till Bell's description of the remarkably resilient maxillary blood supply [17]. With advancement in technique and the introduction of safe hypotensive anesthesia, the Le Fort I osteotomy has been increasingly utilized over the last four decades. Over the years, various modifications of the osteotomies, ORIF methods and bone grafting to the mobilized maxilla, have continued to evolve and progress.

69.2 Surgical Anatomy

The paired maxillae are made up of a body and four projections: frontal, zygomatic, palatine, and the alveolar process. The maxilla forms the inferior and medial borders of the

Electronic Supplementary Material The online version of this chapter (https://doi.org/10.1007/978-981-15-1346-6_69) contains supplementary material, which is available to authorized users.

A. Dabir (✉)
D. Y. Patil University School of Dentistry, Nerul, Navi Mumbai, India

Breach Candy Hospital, Mumbai, India

J. Vahanwala (✉)
Department of Oral Surgery, Vaidik Dental College and Research Centre, Nani Daman, Daman, India

Breach Candy Hospital, Mumbai, India

K. Bonanthaya et al. (eds.), *Oral and Maxillofacial Surgery for the Clinician*, https://doi.org/10.1007/978-981-15-1346-6_69

orbits. The infraorbital foramen is located at an average distance of 7.8 mm, positioned inferiorly to the infraorbital rim in women and 8.5 mm in men [18]. The vascular and sensory supplies to the cheek, lateral aspect of the nose, and upper lip exit the bone from this foramen.

The anterior alveolar processes surround the piriform apertures and join to form the anterior nasal spine in the midline. The anterior nasal spine is the most anterior inferior attachment for the cartilaginous nasal septum, which extends posteriorly along the nasal crest and articulates with the vomer.

The maxillary sinuses are housed in body of maxilla. Anteriorly, palatine process of each maxilla and posteriorly, horizontal lamina of palatine bone form the hard palate. The greater palatine foramen is located on each side approximately 10 mm posteromedial to the second molar.

The nasolacrimal duct travels within the bony wall between the nasal cavity and the maxillary sinus before terminating below the inferior turbinate. It can be injured during the Le Fort I osteotomy or during an inferior turbinectomy performed to allow superior repositioning of the maxilla (Fig. 69.1) [19, 20].

Posterolaterally, the maxilla articulates with the pyramidal processes of the palatine bones and the pterygoid plates of the sphenoid bone. This pterygomaxillary junction extends superiorly as a fissure, which ends at the pterygopalatine fossa. The terminal portion of the internal maxillary artery traverses the pterygopalatine fossa and gives off several branches that can be encountered during a Le Fort I osteotomy (Fig. 69.2a, b). The average distance between the infe-

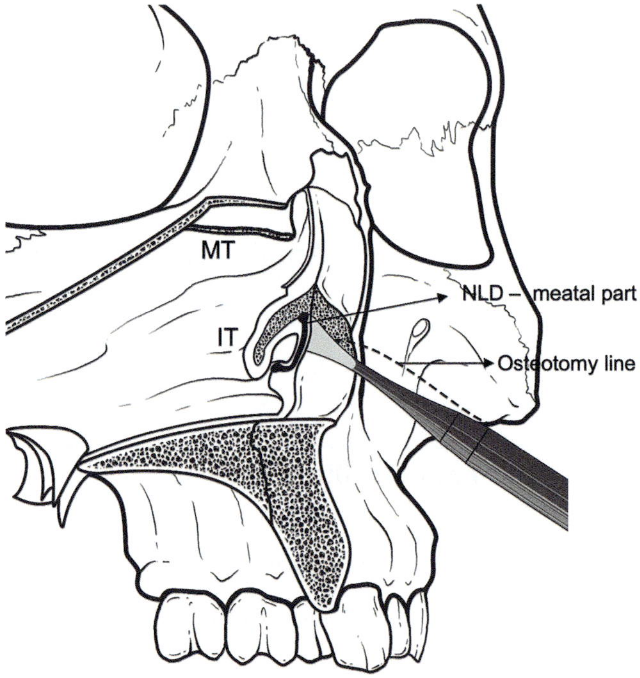

Fig. 69.1 Relationship of the nasolacrimal duct to the Le Fort I osteotomy cut. The meatus of the nasolacrimal duct is unlikely to be injured if the osteotomy is made just beneath the infraorbital foramen and into the piriform rim at the level of the inferior turbinate (IT). *MT* middle turbinate

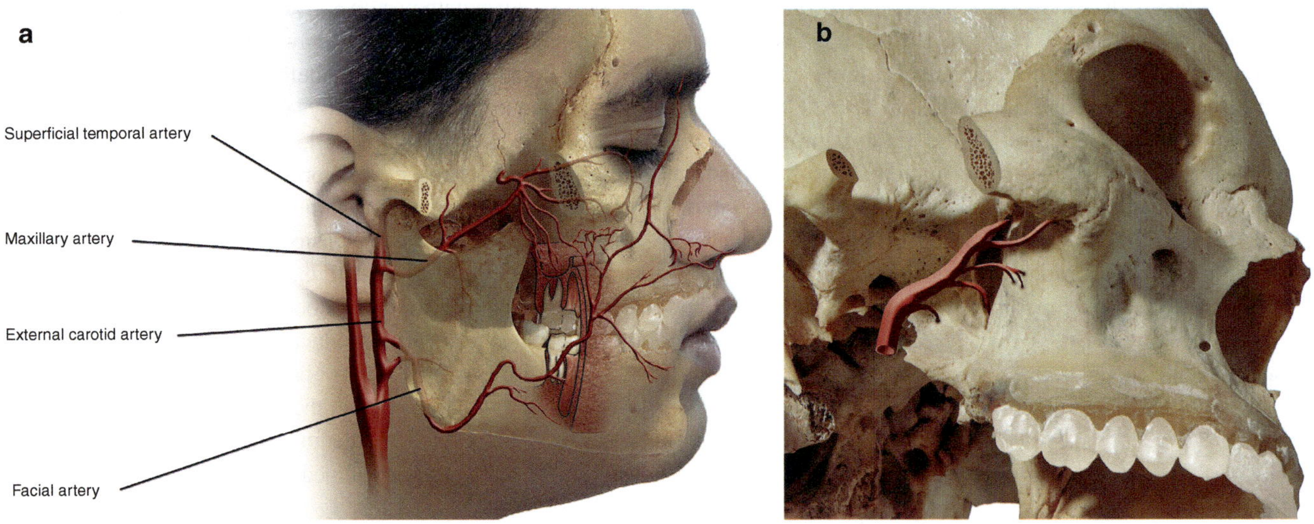

Fig. 69.2 (**a**) Branches of external carotid artery, (**b**) terminal branches of internal maxillary artery

rior extent of the pterygomaxillary junction and the posterior superior alveolar artery is 15 mm, the infraorbital artery is 32 mm, and the descending palatine artery is 25 mm. The descending palatine arteries travel through the perpendicular plate of the palatine bones and are located approximately 34 mm posterior to the piriform rims and within 10 mm medial to the pterygomaxillary fissures [21].

Osteotomies of the lateral nasal walls and at the pterygomaxillary fissures must be completed carefully to avoid injuring these vessels. The internal maxillary artery is 23–25 mm above the base of the junction of the maxilla with the pterygoid plates, with an average diameter of 2.5 mm. In addition to the direct vascular supply of the maxilla by the descending palatine arteries, there is a rich collateral vascular network from the soft palate supplied by the ascending pharyngeal arteries and the ascending palatine branches of the facial arteries (Fig. 69.3). The risk of damaging the artery can be minimized by ensuring the pterygoid osteotome is directed downward toward the palate and is less than 1.5 cm above the inferior part of the fissure [22, 23].

Bell's work revealed that ligation of the bilateral descending palatine arteries does not compromise the vascularity of the maxilla as long as the soft palate pedicle is preserved [24, 25].

The pterygoid plexus of veins is located between the temporalis and lateral pterygoid muscles and between the medial and lateral pterygoid muscles. It receives tributaries corresponding to the branches of the maxillary artery and drains into the maxillary vein. Venous bleeding from this plexus may be encountered during the posterolateral maxillary dissection and pterygomaxillary disjunction.

The risk of damaging the artery can be minimized by ensuring the pterygoid osteotome is directed downwards towards the palate and is less than 1.5 cm above the inferior part of the fissure [22, 23].

Bell's work revealed that ligation of the bilateral descending palatine arteries does not compromise the vascularity of the maxilla as long as the soft palate pedicle is preserved [24, 25].

S. Bruneder et al. studied a special type of arterial variation of the Le Fort I segment's blood supply. Individuals with this special arterial anatomy may clinically be at high risk for hypoperfusion and avascular segment necrosis after surgery. Individualized operation planning that takes the patient's arterial anatomy into consideration may help to prevent ischemic vascular complications of the Le Fort I segment and improve operative outcomes in at-risk patients [26].

S. Salmanet et al. studied Dynamic analysis of maxillary perfusion during Le Fort I osteotomy using indocyanine green and concluded that there was a statistically significant decrease in perfusion, as assessed by intraoperative dynamic angiography, to the anterior maxilla following maxillary down-fracture. Patient age, conventional versus segmental Le Fort I osteotomy, changes in mean arterial pressure and/or heart rate, and preservation of the descending palatine vessels had no statistically significant effect on perfusion [27].

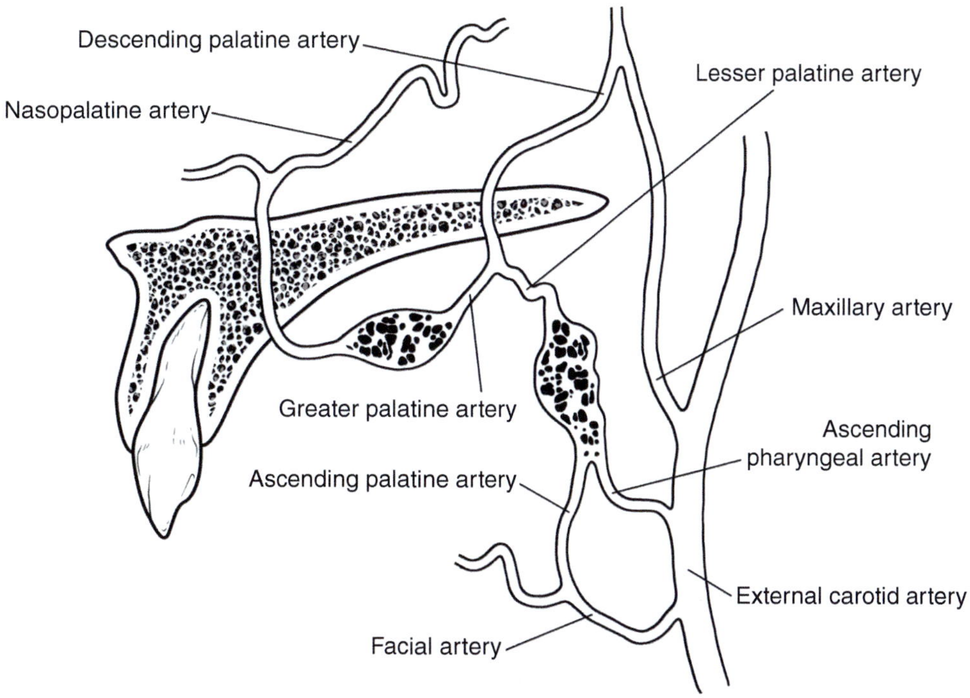

Fig. 69.3 The vascular supply of the osteotomised LeFort I segment. The ascending pharyngeal arteries and the ascending palatine branches of the facial artery

The patient's sex and aspects of the skeletal and craniofacial pattern have an influence on the pterygomaxillary area and descending palatine canal anatomy. A preoperative computed tomography analysis involving this evaluation could reduce the risk of surgical complications. A preoperative CT analysis should be performed on an individual basis and should identify the differences between the two sides in the same patient to allow a safer surgical procedure during Le Fort I osteotomy [28].

69.3 The Anterior Segmental Maxillary Osteotomy

The first anterior segmental maxillary osteotomy (ASMO) was reported at the beginning of the twentieth century by Günther Cohn-Stock [29], wherein he tried to surgically "correct a marked overjet and overbite of the central maxillary teeth." In his pioneering article in 1921, he described the evolution of his idea to perform an osteotomy of the anterior segment of the maxilla while preserving the vestibular pedicle and, in a later design, also the palatal artery [29].

After Cohn-Stock's original report, three variations of the procedure were developed by Wassmund [9], Wunderer [30], and Cupar [31]. These variations were designed to maintain sufficient blood supply to the maxilla while giving adequate access for instrumentation [32, 33].

In 1927 Wassmund [9] improved Cohn-Stock's design by creating a direct approach to the labial premaxillary cortex using three vertical incisions and subperiosteal tunnelling for completion of the labial osteotomy without reflection of labial or palatal flaps. Both the labial and palatal blood supply are maintained; however, the osteotomy is made in a relatively blind fashion. This method may be indicated for closure of multiple interdental spaces [33] and for anteroposterior repositioning of the premaxilla [34]. It was found to maintain the best vascularity of the repositioned segment in comparison to all other ASMO methods [35].

In 1954 Cupar [31] described a different approach for down-fracture of the anterior maxilla: exposure of the labial aspect of the maxillary bone by a vestibular circumferential cut and labial flap to facilitate the labial osteotomy under direct vision. A palatal osteotomy was performed through a tunnel, maintaining the palatal blood supply. This technique is indicated for superior repositioning of the anterior maxilla in cases of vertical maxillary excess.

In 1963 Wunderer [30] advocated reflection of a palatal flap without fracturing of the anterior maxilla and maintenance of the labial blood supply. Direct access for the palatal osteotomy is the main advantage of this technique, especially if posterior segments of the premaxilla must be removed.

Therefore, this technique may be indicated for setback of the anterior part of the maxilla. Blood flow studies have demonstrated that the transpalatal approach causes the greatest decrease in blood supply to the anterior maxilla [36]. However, transpalatal soft tissue incision and labial osteotomies impair vascular supply to the anterior maxilla from the greater palatine vessels and the superior alveolar vessels, respectively, leaving the labial collaterals as the sole blood supply to the anterior maxilla [37].

In 1977 Epker modified the Cupar technique for down-fracture of the anterior maxilla. He used only labial flaps and vertical tunnels labial to the teeth to be extracted, which were usually premolars on both sides [38]. Epker's modification enables repositioning of the anterior maxilla superiorly, posteriorly, and inferiorly. The main advantages of the Epker modification include preservation of the palatal pedicle, ease of placement of internal fixation, provide access to the nasal septal structures to prevent buckling of the nasal septum with superior repositioning of the maxilla, and a direct approach for removal of palatal bone. When required, bone grafting for stabilization of an inferiorly positioned anterior maxilla may also be done using this method.

The segmental Le Fort I osteotomy should not be excluded from the technical armamentarium in orthognathic surgery. On the contrary, the literature consulted suggests it to be a useful tool for the three-dimensional surgical correction of maxillary malposition [39].

69.3.1 Technique (Video 69.1)

Anaesthetic and Positioning Considerations: Controlled hypotensive anesthesia has been shown to reduce bleeding from mucosal and bone edges that contain a rich network of small vessels, which cannot easily be identified and controlled with surgical techniques. In healthy patients, a reduction in mean arterial pressure (MAP) of 30% below the patient's baseline with a minimum MAP of 50 mmHg is safe [40]. In bimaxillary surgery, postoperative blood transfusions are necessary in 13–48% of patients who do not have controlled hypotension during the operation [41, 42]. The need for transfusion has been nearly eliminated by using this technique. Placement of an indwelling bladder catheter for intraoperative monitoring of urine output as a marker of renal perfusion should be considered when using controlled hypotension. After induction of general anesthesia, the patient is nasally intubated. Because intraoperative maxillomandibular fixation is essential to establish the postoperative position of the anterior maxilla, oral intubation is less desirable and should be avoided. The endotracheal tube must be sufficiently below the level of the vocal cords to prevent unintended dislodgement during premaxillary manipulation. A shoulder roll is inserted to extend the neck without creating hyperextension. A sterile preparation and draping is performed, leaving the orbits and nasion exposed. After the planned mucosal incision is marked, local anaesthetic with vasoconstrictor (lidocaine with 1:100,000 epinephrine) is infiltrated in the labial sulcus. Palatal injection should be avoided so as not to induce vasoconstriction in the palatal pedicle.

69.3.2 Exposure

A horizontal buccal sulcus incision is made by diathermy or a #15 scalpel blade in one strike to the bone in the deepest section of the buccal vestibule, circumferentially from right to left second premolar. Next, the periosteum is reflected superiorly to expose the entire canine fossa and piriform aperture bilaterally. Inferiorly, minimum mucoperiosteal stripping should be done, to maximize blood supply to the osteotomized maxilla. The alveolar mucoperiosteum should be undermined to the crestal bone only at preplanned osteotomy or ostectomy sites. The nasal mucoperiosteum should be carefully separated from the nasal cavity floor to prevent intraoperative bleeding, postoperative oronasal communication, and fistula formation. The cartilaginous nasal septum is separated from the nasal groove of the maxilla to facilitate its manipulation later.

69.3.3 Extractions and Horizontal Osteotomies

As per surgical plan, maxillary premolars are extracted on each side. Then, a reciprocating saw or piezo-surgical saw is used to perform horizontal osteotomies. These bone cuts should run posteriorly from each side of the piriform rim, including the lateral maxillary walls and the lateral nasal cavity walls. The nasal mucosa is protected with a curved periosteal elevator. Due care should be taken to avoid injury to the infraorbital nerve during retraction of the upper mucoperiosteal flap. The posterior limit for these osteotomies is the planned vertical osteotomy/ostectomy, usually the first or second premolar (Fig. 69.4a–d).

Figure 69.4b and Fig. 69.5 indicates the horizontal and vertical osteotomies/ostectomies that are performed using a #701 bur, mini-saw, or piezo. Precise bone removal should be done to ensure an accurate postoperative position and sufficient intersegmental bony contacts.

Meticulous tissue handling is of paramount importance at this stage. Failure to preserve buccal mucosa may lead to an impaired blood supply to the down-fractured maxilla or establishment of an oroantral fistula, in addition to periodontal compromise of the adjacent teeth.

69.3.4 Final Osteotomy and Down-Fracture of the Premaxilla

After completion of the planned osteotomies and ostectomies under direct visualization, the final osteotomy is done using an osteotome. Neither a palatal incision nor a mucosal undermining is done at this stage. A palpating finger is positioned on the palatal mucosa, and the transpalatal osteotomy is completed with an osteotome. Down-fracture of the premaxilla is accomplished with a bone hook. Additional transpalatal and nasal ostectomies may be necessary at this stage and should be finalized under direct access gained to the nasal aspect of the down-fractured premaxilla. Careful separation of the mucoperiosteum from the posterior segment of the palate facilitates setback of the anterior segment and prevents it from becoming detached from the anterior segment, compromising the blood supply (Fig. 69.6a, b).

69.3.5 Midpalatal Osteotomy

If indicated for transverse widening or narrowing of the premaxilla or closure of a diastema, a midpalatal osteotomy is performed with an osteotome or piezo-surgical saw (Fig. 69.7a, b).

69.3.6 Fixation

After completion of the ostectomies, maxillary teeth are placed into a preformed acrylic occlusal wafer, which is wired to the maxillary dentition. Temporary maxillomandibular fixation then is done, and a standard 1.5 or 2.0 maxillary plating system is used at the maxillary buttresses to fixate the bone segments in their planned postoperative position (Fig. 69.8a–c).

69.3.7 Closure

After thorough irrigation of the surgical site with saline, the mucosal incisions are closed with 3-0/4-0 vicryl suture. If indicated, alar cinch and V-Y closure of the buccal incision are performed at this stage. Maxillomandibular fixation is removed at the end of the procedure. The maxillary surgical wafer may be kept in place for 6 weeks for additional stability of the maxillary segments and occlusal guidance (Fig. 69.9a, b).

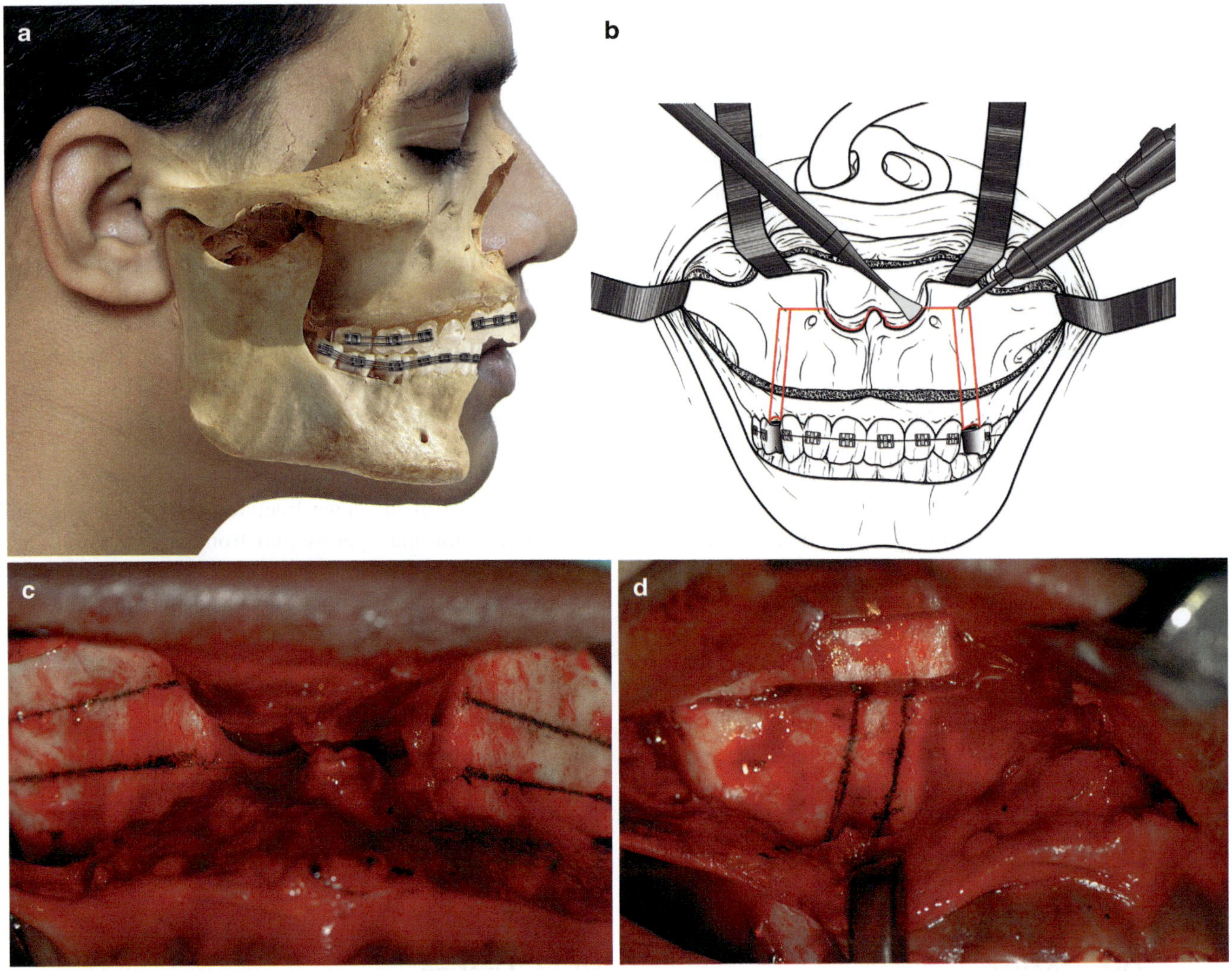

Fig. 69.4 (**a–d**) Epker's modificaiton of Cupar's down-fracture anterior maxillary osteotomy. (**a**) Anterior maxillary excess with first premolar to be extracted, not bonded othodontically, (**b**) vestibular incision (5 mm superior to mucogingival junction). Osteotomy marked, which includes a horizontal cut beginning at the pyriform rim, going lateral above the apices of the anterior teeth and vertical cuts to complete the bone removal at the site of the extraacted premolar, (**c**, **d**) Osteotomy marking with autoclaved pencil and cuts for anterior maxillary segmental osteotomy. (see Fig. 69.10a2 for clinical profile view)

69.4 Le Fort I Osteotomy

69.4.1 Operative Technique (Video 69.2)

There are many acceptable modifications to the Le Fort I osteotomy, and the sequence of steps may vary from surgeon to surgeon. Figures 69.10a, b and 69.11a, b demonstrate a patient who has undergone a Lefort 1 with anterior maxillary osteotomy and mandibular subapical osteotomy for addressing her Vertical Maxillary Excess and dento-alveolar protrusion. The following is a description of the authors' preferred approach.

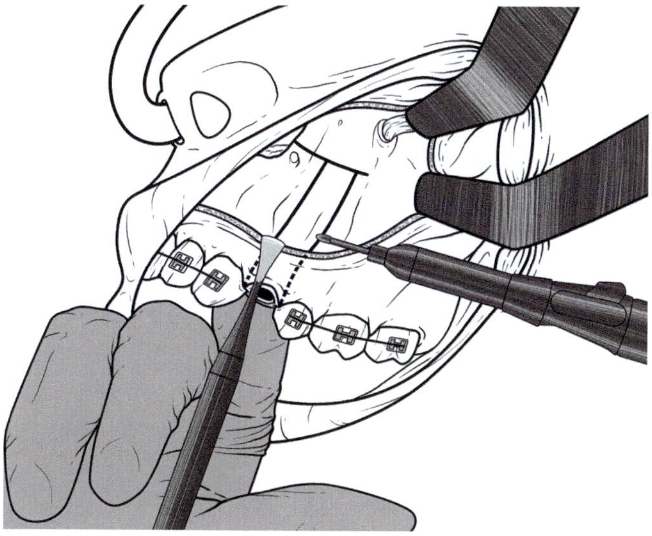

Fig. 69.5 Horizontal and Vertical Osteotomy Cuts (5 mm superior to mucogingival junction) Osteotomy marked, Horizontal cut 5 mm above the canine root tip, Vertical osteotomy marked approximate mesiodistal width of premolar

Anaesthetic and Positioning Considerations:
Anaesthetic and positioning considerations must be followed as previously discussed in the anterior segmental maxillary osteotomy technique.

69.4.2 External Reference Marker

An external reference marker is placed at the nasion to facilitate proper positioning of the maxilla in the vertical plane (Fig. 69.12a). Common techniques include insertion of a Kirschner wire or a bone fixation screw. Less invasive methods include marking with a skin scribe, a suture or tape, but these may be less reproducible due to skin mobility at the site. Occasionally a soft tissue landmark such as the medial canthus can also be used as a guide to measure from the incisal edge of the anterior teeth (Fig. 69.12b)

External reference points have been shown to be superior to internal references (lines or burr holes placed on the maxilla above and below the osteotomy), which are prone to inaccuracy due to the complex three-dimensional movement of the maxilla [43, 44]. Preoperative measurements are then obtained from the reference site to reproducible midline and lateral maxillary landmarks, typically the maxillary dental midline and the bilateral canine cusp tips or orthodontic brackets.

69.4.3 Surgical Exposure

Local anesthesia with vasoconstrictor is infiltrated labially and buccally from the pterygoid plate region, forward to the midline bilaterally. A full-thickness mucosal and periosteal

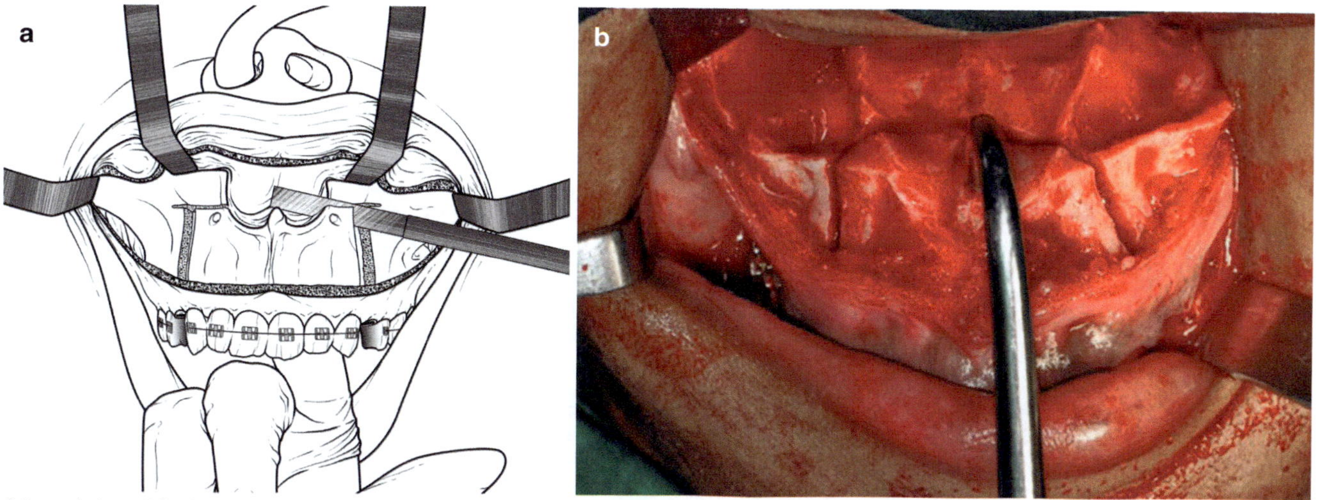

Fig. 69.6 (**a**, **b**) Final palatal bone cut with osteotome, palatal mucosa protected with non-dominant hand for tactile sensation

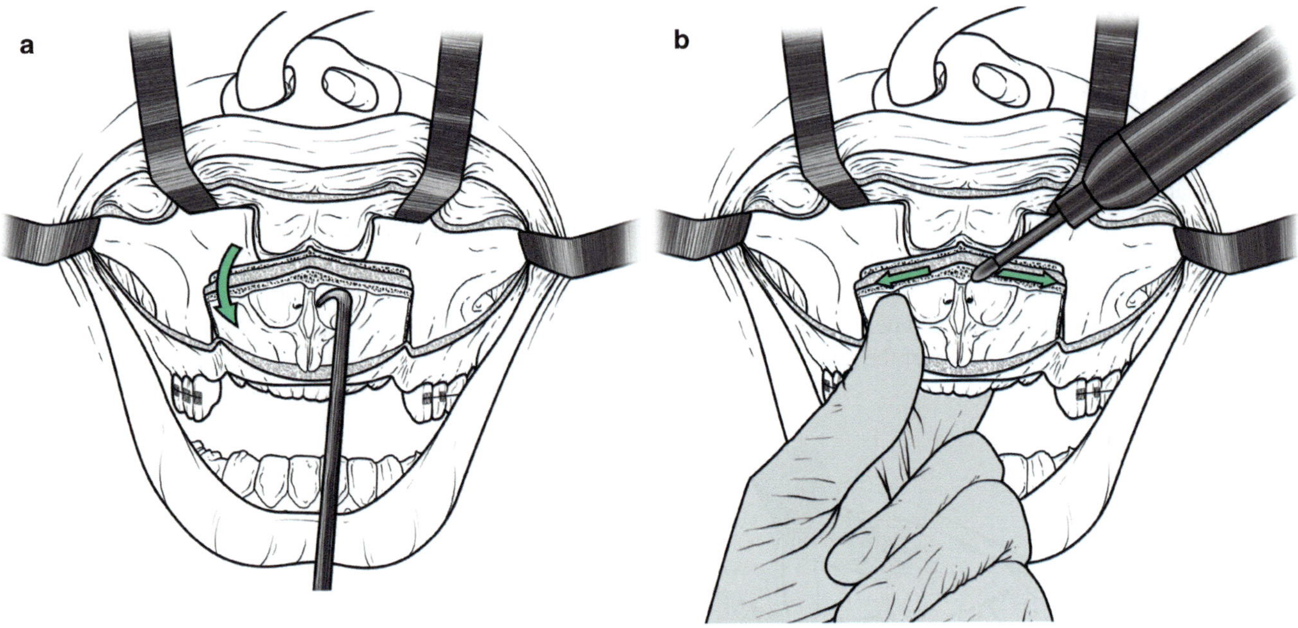

Fig. 69.7 (**a**) Down-fracture anterior segment of maxilla and maintaining palatal mucosa. (**b**) Midline or paramidline osteotomy for horizontal movement

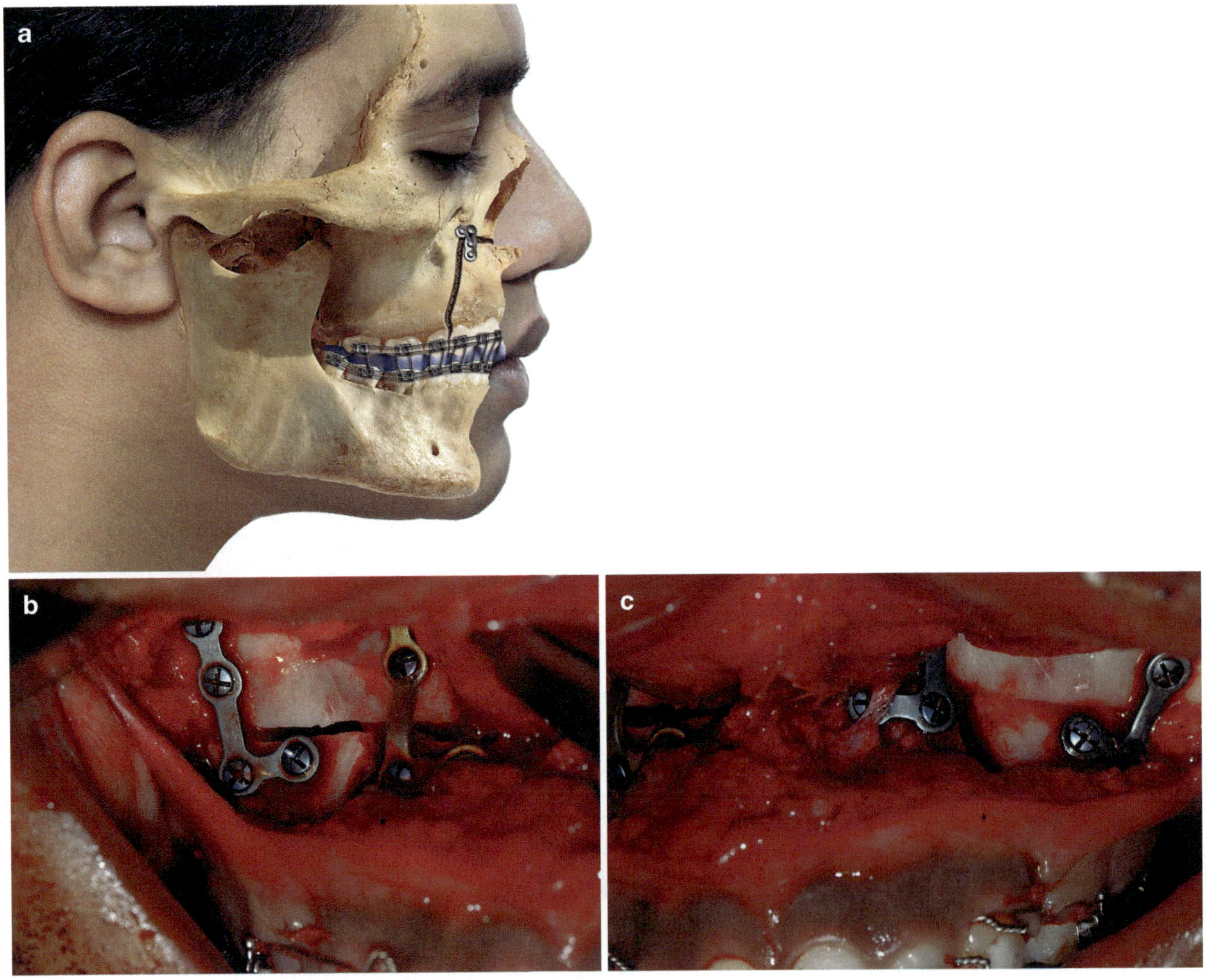

Fig. 69.8 (**a–c**) Maxillary plating system used at the maxillary buttresses and pyriform region to fixate the bone segments in their planned post-operative position in case of Le Fort I with AMO, (**b**) right side (**c**) left side

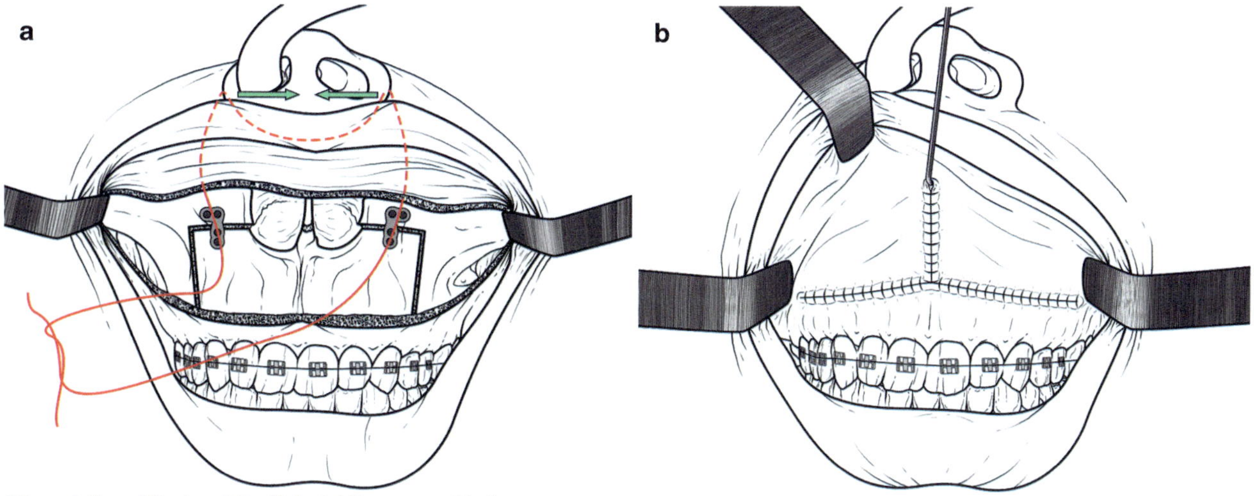

Fig. 69.9 (**a**, **b**) (**a**) Alar cinch placement to control alar base, (**b**) V-Y closure of mucosa to maintain upper lip length

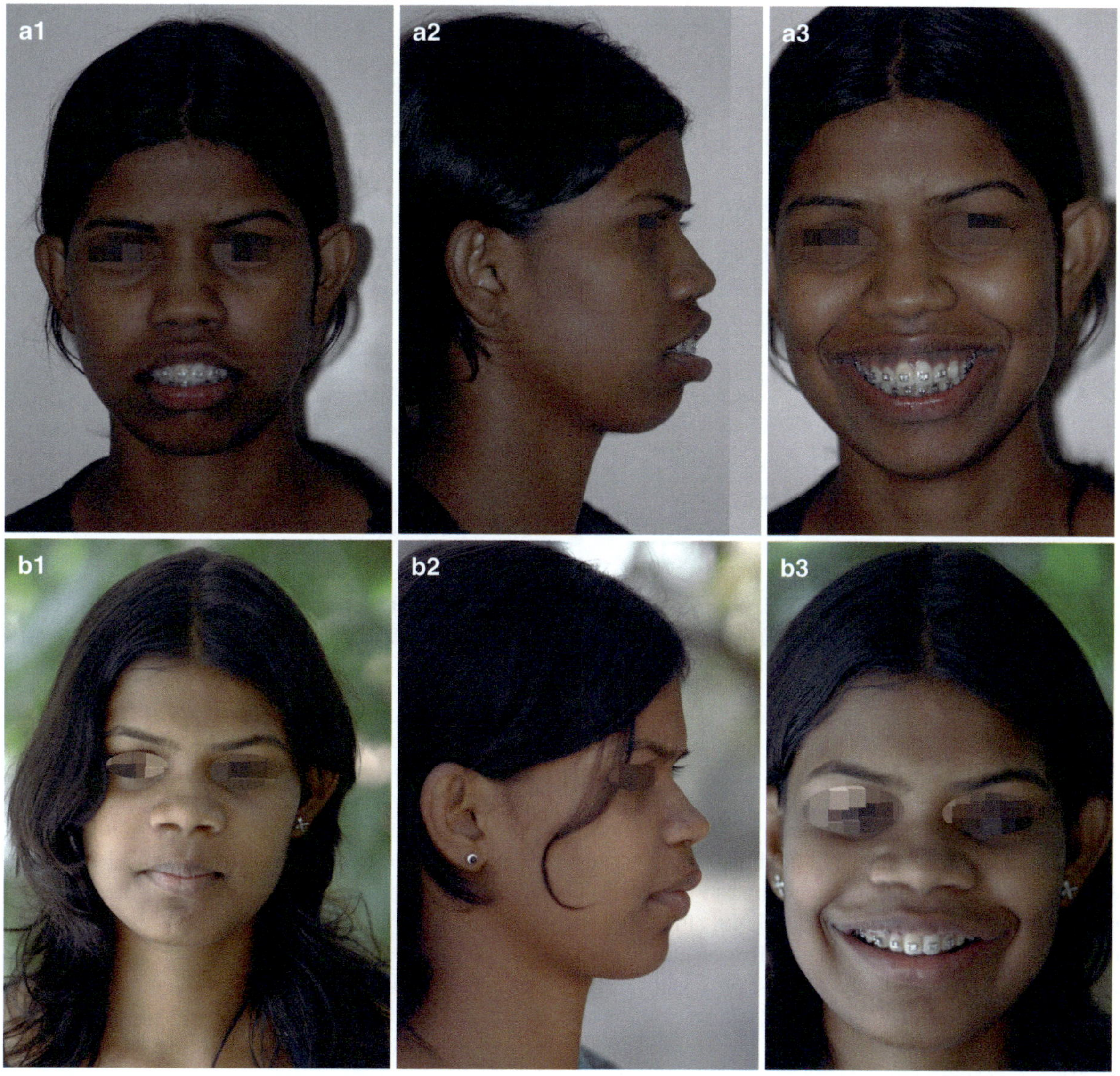

Fig. 69.10 (**a**, **b**) (**a1, a2, a3**) Pre-surgical images of the patient. (**b1, b2, b3**) Post Le Fort I and anterior maxillary osteotomy images of the patient

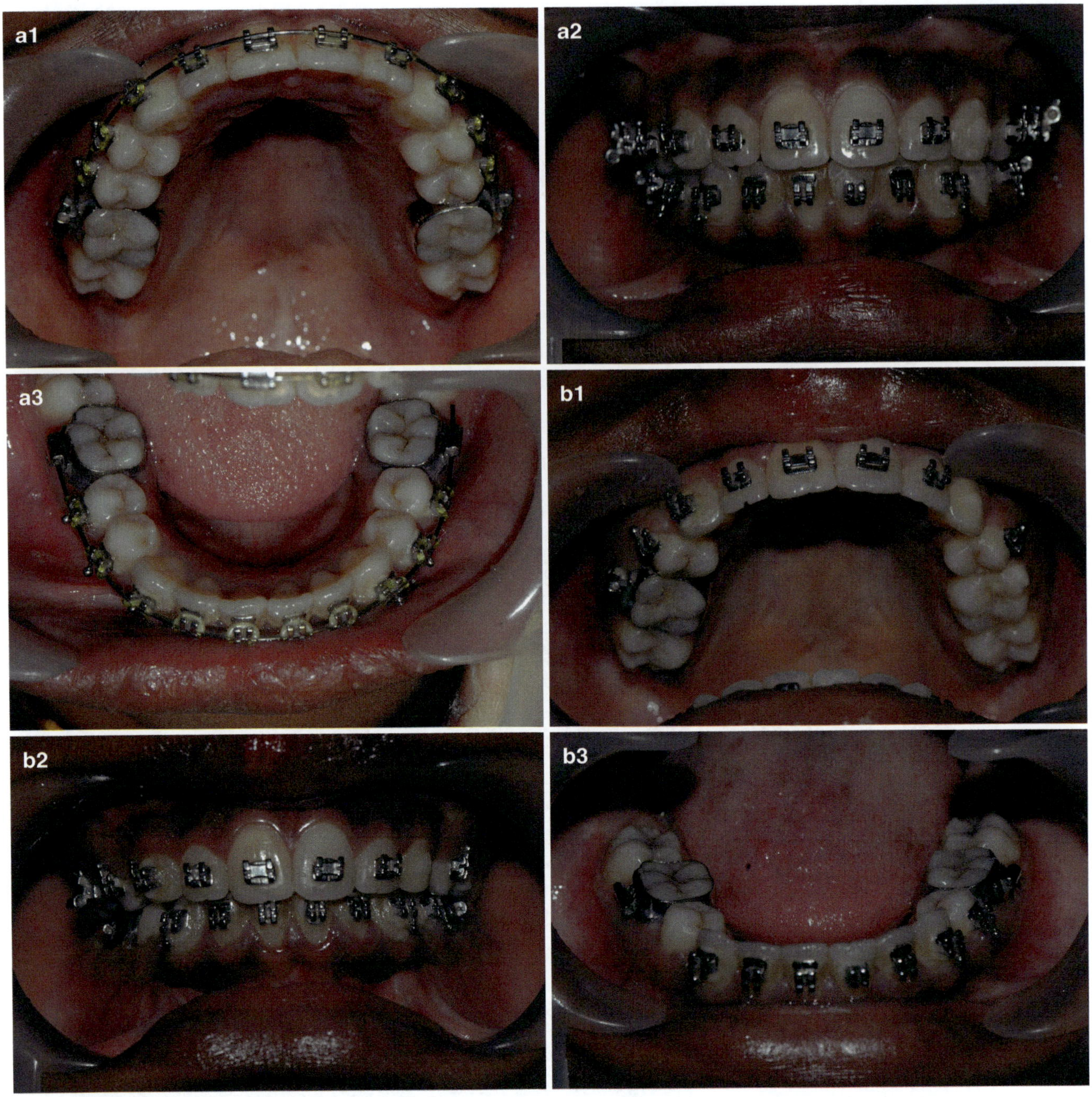

Fig. 69.11 (**a**, **b**) Intra oral photos of the same patient as in Fig. 69.10. (**a1, a2, a3**) Pre-surgical images of the occlusion. (**b1, b2, b3**) Post anterior maxillary osteotomy images of the occlusion. A mandibular sub-apical osteotomy was also done for this patient (**b2, b3**)

incision is made in the soft tissue extending from the buttress of the zygoma on the either side, 3–4 m above the mucogingival junction with attention in the midline to a V-shaped incision to allow for aesthetic closure [45, 46] (Fig. 69.13). The incision can be made with a scalpel or electrocautery Colorado needle. While layered incisions serve no advantage for the dissection, electrocautery seems to control some hemorrhage at the time of the incision.

Retraction is maintained with down-turned Obwegeser retractors, and the superior mucoperiosteal flap is elevated with a #9 Molt periosteal elevator. The anterior nasal spine, piriform rim, infraorbital foramen, lateral maxillary wall, and zygomaticomaxillary junction are exposed. Exposure of the posterior maxillary wall and pterygomaxillary junction is next performed with a Molt periosteal elevator, placed parallel to the maxillary teeth and advanced posteriorly below

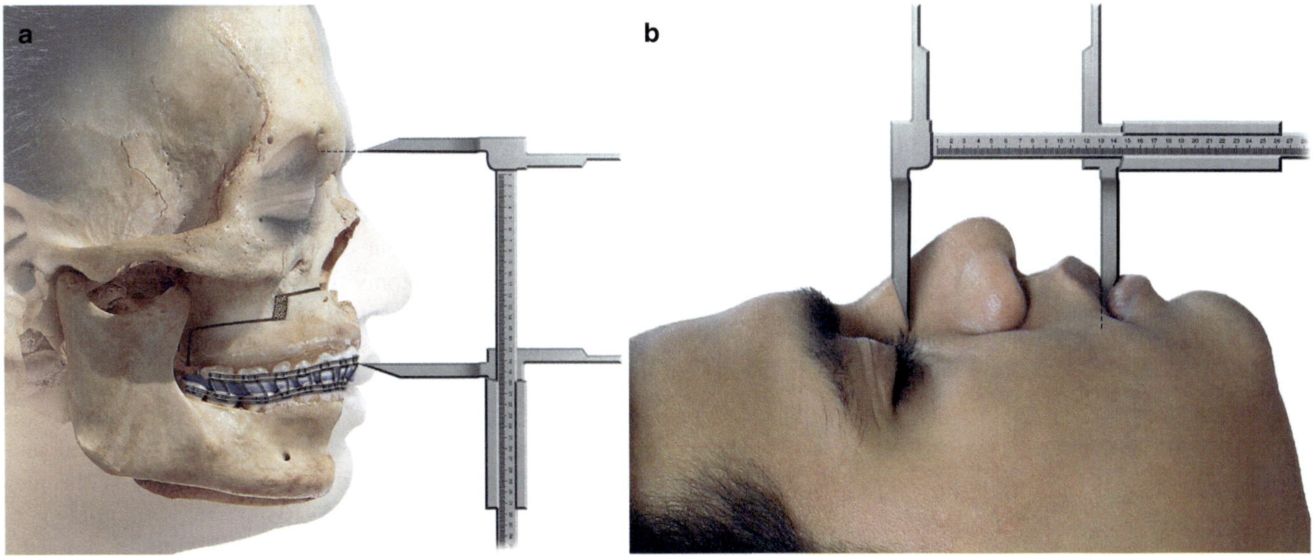

Fig. 69.12 (**a**, **b**) (**a**) External reference marker (skeletal landmark). A stable extraoral reference point is established with a 0.035-inch K-wire placed in the nasion. A caliper is used to measure the vertical distance from the K-wire to the brackets of the central incisor teeth, and these measurements are recorded. (**b**) A extraoral reference point at medial canthal (soft tissue landmark). A caliper is used to measure the vertical distance from medial canthal to the brackets of the central incisor teeth

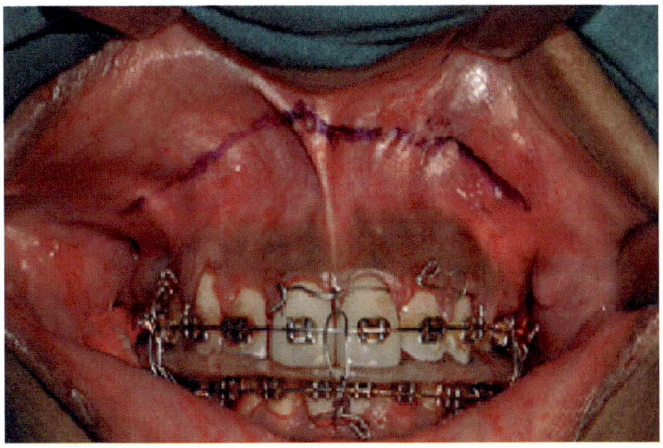

Fig. 69.13 Maintain a small inverted "V" shape over the midline frenum, with the lateral extension of the incision being 5mm above the muco-gingival junction, from first molar one side to the other

periosteum until the pterygomaxillary junction is encountered. The periosteal elevator on the bone and in a subperiosteal plane is maintained with angulation as it proceeds posteriorly to incline inferiorly or toward the hamular process of the sphenoid bone. This alleviates the potential problem of entering the pterygomaxillary fissure and concomitant increased hemorrhage [23, 47].

The nasal/septal mucosal dissection is performed after the bilateral maxillary osteotomies have been completed and involves elevation of the nasal mucosa with a curved freer elevator to the posterior palatine bone (Fig. 69.14).

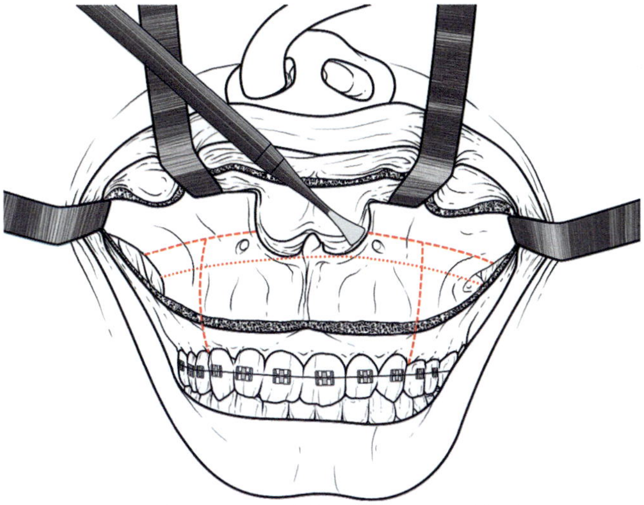

Fig. 69.14 Exposure of the maxilla is achieved with a full horizontal vestibular incision superior to the mucogingival junction. With appropriate retraction, the infraorbital nerves, piriform rims, posterior maxilla, and anterior nasal spine will be identified

As may be preferred by some surgeons, reference marks are placed vertically in the lateral wall of the maxilla, or bone reference holes are placed a standardized distance apart (15 mm seems to be a reasonable distance) vertically in the buttress and in the pyriform rim region (Fig. 69.15) [48–50].

Alternatively, a non-threaded Kirschner wire or Steinmann pin is placed in the nasal dorsum, and a reference measurement is taken from that Kirschner wire to the anterior dentition to allow for determination of the amount of superior repositioning of the anterior maxilla [51, 52].

With the use of a Tessier caliper, the vertical distance (height) between the medial canthus and the mid-maxillary incisor crown is measured on the left and right sides and recorded; this generally measures between 55 and 70 mm (Fig. 69.12). This is a reproducible relative measure of the anterior vertical maxillary height [53].

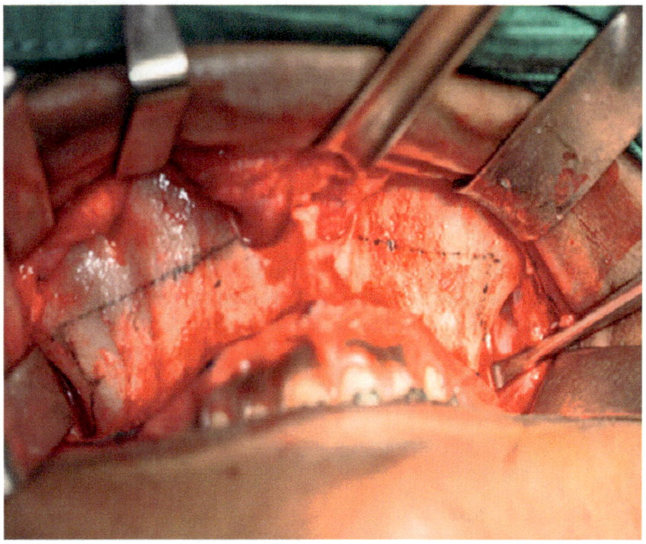

Fig. 69.15 Marking of osteotomy cuts, horizontal cut minimum of 5 mm above the apices of the teeth, step or sloping downward and backward toward to maxillary pterygoid plates or Le Fort I level with step-ladder cut

69.4.4 Bony Osteotomies

69.4.4.1 Lateral Osteotomies

A 701 straight fissure bur or reciprocating saw creates the lateral maxillary osteotomy from the lateral nasal rim to the zygomaticomaxillary junction. The osteotomy starts 3–4 m above the nasal floor and is carried to the depth of the maxillary sinus, back to the pterygomaxillary junction, approximately 30–35 mm above the bracket on the first molar tooth. Cuts are made at least 5 mm above the roots of the teeth and can be made higher as needed. A vertical step at the first molar is carried inferiorly for 5–10 mm (step osteotomy permits grafting in the zygomaticomaxillary buttress area subsequently, if required) [54], and then it is continued in a horizontal plane to the posterior maxilla ending in front of the pterygomaxillary junction (Fig. 69.16a, b).

69.4.4.2 Pterygoid Plate Separation

A 6- to 8-mm-wide, curved osteotome is placed in the pterygomaxillary junction, with the leading edge angled inferior, medial, and anterior. It is positioned in the junction with the horizontal osteotomy centered over the middle of the osteotome.

A finger can be placed palatally at the junction of the hamulus with the tuberosity, and the mallet is used to drive the chisel through the junction. The end of the osteotome should be palpated on the palatal side as it comes through the junction, but it should not penetrate through

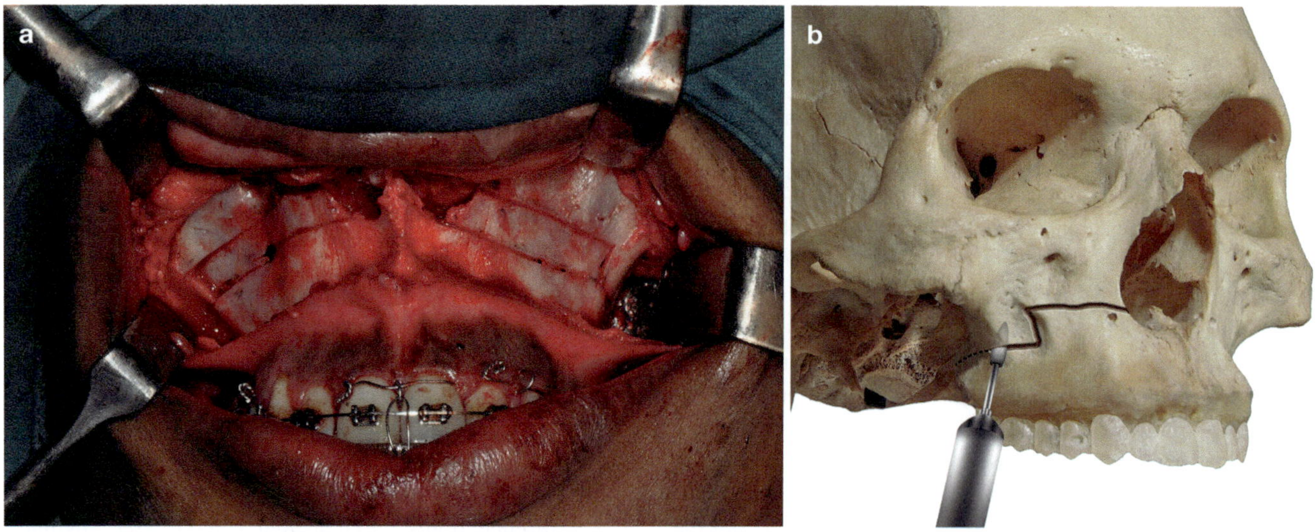

Fig. 69.16 (**a**, **b**) (**a**) The lateral maxillary wall osteotomy is carried posteriorly from the piriform rim to the pterygomaxillary junction, (**b**) with a vertical step ladder cut in the first molar region. The osteotomy is placed at least 5 mm superior to the root apices

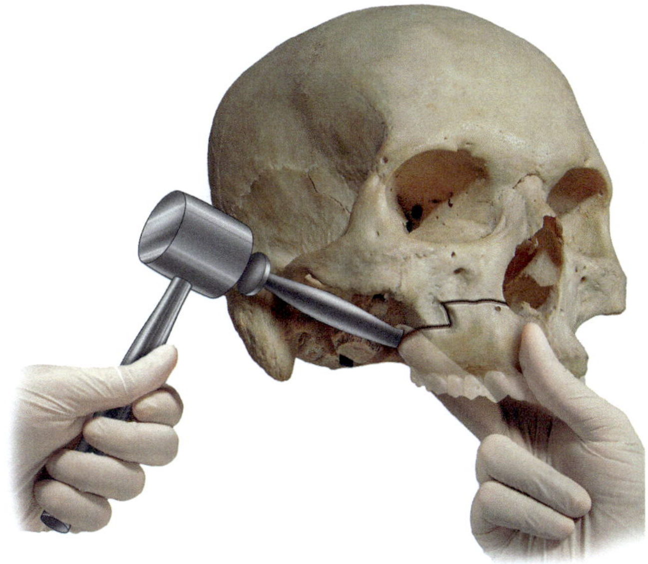

Fig. 69.17 A curved osteotome is placed in the pterygomaxillary junction, with the superior edge of the osteotome just above the horizontal osteotomy. A finger is placed on the palatal side of the junction, and the osteotome is gently tapped through the junction until palpated on the palatal side, without perforating the soft tissue

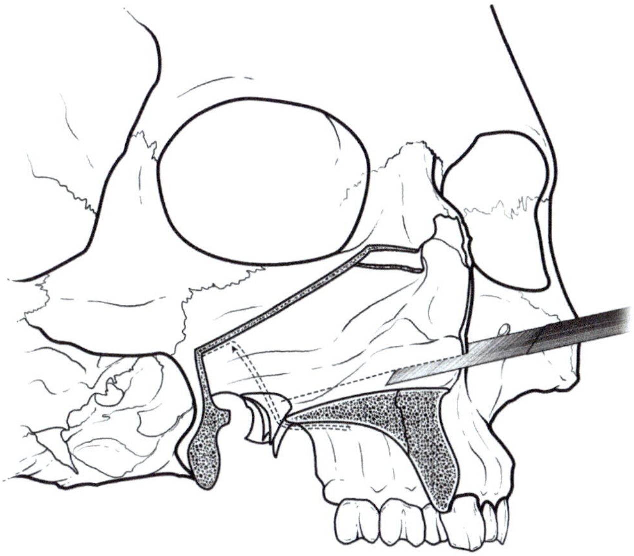

Fig. 69.18 The lateral nasal wall osteotomy is completed from the inferior piriform rim to the anterior portion of the pyramidal process of the palatine bone. Care is taken to avoid a complete osteotomy through the pyramidal process in order to prevent injury to the greater palatine artery and nerve. The right maxilla has been removed to show the desired cross-section clearly

the palatal tissue. There should be minimal resistance to separation, and if significant resistance is encountered, the osteotome position should be evaluated and repositioned (Fig. 69.17).

The scientific literature cites examples of damage to the cranial nerves during the Le Fort I osteotomy [55–58].

69.4.4.3 Lateral Nasal Wall and Septal Osteotomies

A small safe-sided osteotome initiates the lateral nasal osteotomy at the piriform rim in the anterior extension of the lateral maxillary osteotomy. A mallet drives the osteotome posterior, parallel to the nasal floor, below the inferior turbinate. One must take care not to go beyond 25 and 30 mm in depth during osteotomy. The lateral nasal wall diverges (widens) posteriorly, and the osteotome must follow that divergence. Minimal resistance will be encountered until the pyramidal process of the palatine bone is encountered. At this resistance point, the osteotome can be driven another few millimeters to influence the fracture plane through this structure during down-fracture (Fig. 69.18). The nasal septum osteotomy is next performed with a guarded U-shaped osteotome. The osteotome is introduced at the top of the nasal spine and is driven inferiorly and posteriorly along the nasal floor to separate the maxilla and palatine bone from the septum (Fig. 69.19).

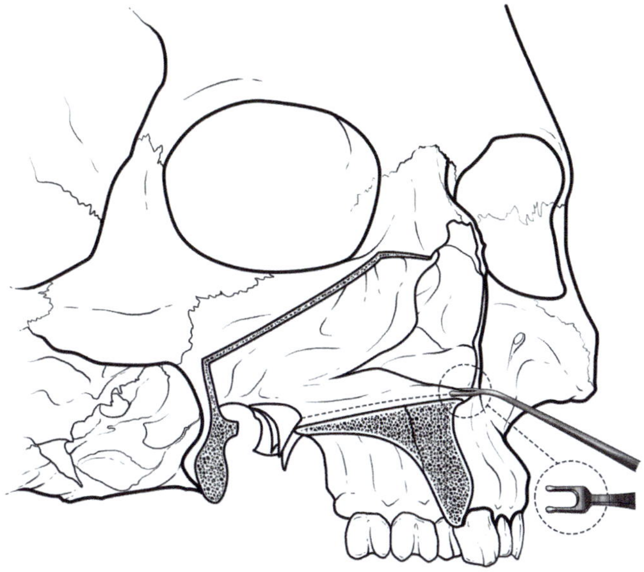

Fig. 69.19 The septal osteotomy is completed from the anterior nasal spine through the vomer bone posteriorly, with the guarded prongs on the septal osteotome angled inferiorly. Care is taken to retract the nasal mucosa to minimize injury and bleeding to the soft tissue. The right maxilla has been removed to show the desired cross-section clearly

69.4.5 Down-Fracture and Mobilization

Once the osteotomy cuts have been completed, some mobility should be readily evident, and down-fracturing be easily

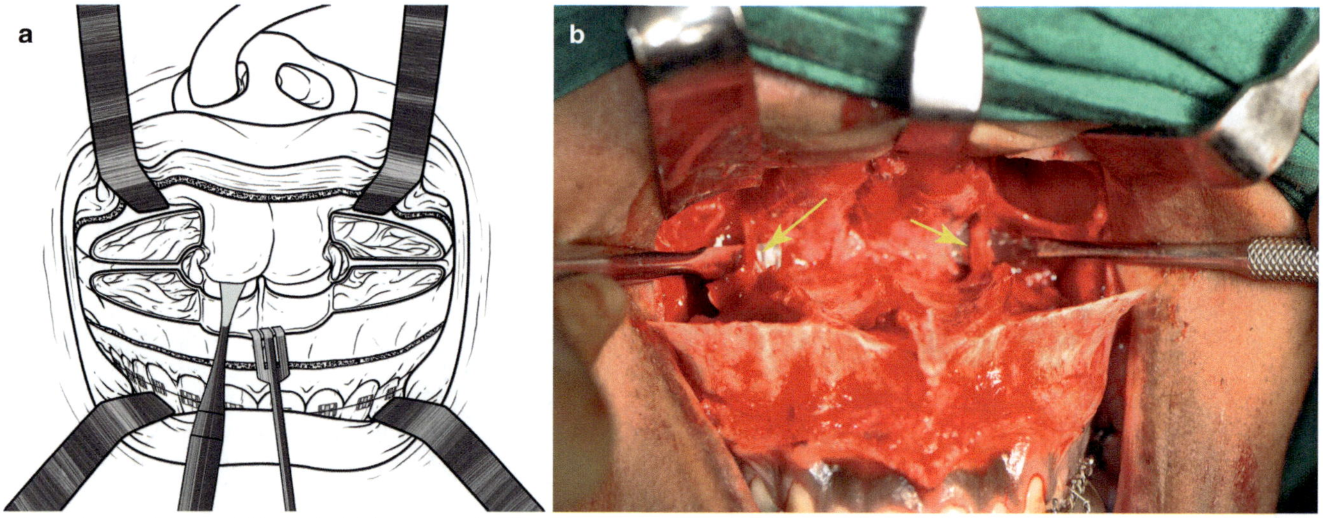

Fig. 69.20 (**a**, **b**) (**a**) Once the maxilla is mobilized, the nasal mucosa can be completely freed from the maxilla in the piriform rim region, (**b**) The greater palatine nerve and artery can be visualized and protected during posterior bone removal from the lateral nasal wall area (yellow arrows) (also see Fig. 65.12a)

done with either bilateral manual digital pressure in the canine fossa or with instrumentation support at the piriform rim. Slowly separate the maxilla by pulling the anterior portion inferiorly while observing the nasal mucosa to avoid tears. If significant resistance is encountered, revise the osteotomy cuts thoroughly to ensure complete separation. To avoid complications related to pterygomaxillary disjunction, we prefer to extract maxillary third molar and make a vertical osteotomy cut through the socket connecting the horizontal cut on the posterolateral surface of maxilla.

Precious et al. (1991) did a study of 138 consecutive Le Fort I osteotomies with successful down-fracture of the maxilla by digital pressure alone (with no serious complications except transient epistaxis that responded to local packing) [59, 60].

Once the down-fracture is completed, place a Seldin elevator or tongue depressor behind the tuberosity, and pull the posterior maxilla forward. This will fully mobilize the maxilla from its attachments. For large advancements, freeing the tissue from the nasal side of the posterior maxilla in the soft palate area will provide significantly more forward mobility. In addition, in repeat maxillary surgery, mobilizing the maxilla will most likely be more difficult, and time must be spent freeing hard and soft tissue attachments to ensure passive movements and surgical stability.

69.4.6 Removal of Posterior Interferences

Removal of posterior interferences should be done immediately after down-fracture which will make it easier to set the maxillary position later. The maxillary bony septum is reduced most easily with a bur. The lateral nasal wall can be reduced with a rongeur, bur, or reciprocating saw. While protecting the descending palatine nerve and artery with a curved freer (Fig. 69.20a, b), the pyramidal process of palatine bone is most safely reduced with the reciprocating saw or bone file. Sometimes a thin spatula osteotome can be used. Finally, the posterior tuberosity, anterior pterygoid plate, and posterior lateral maxillary wall can be reduced with a bur or reciprocating saw (Fig. 69.21). If the superior movement of the maxillary is more that 6 or 7 mm, a partial inferior turbinectomy may be indicated to allow a passive impaction. The nasal mucosa is incised with a scalpel blade along its inferior surface in an anterior-posterior direction. The inferior half of the turbinate is grasped with a large curved hemostat, and a dean scissor is used to excise this portion. Complete removal of the inferior turbinate is rarely necessary and can result in unpleasant clinical side effects. Electrocautery is used to coagulate the incised edge of the turbinate to minimize bleeding. The nasal mucosa is then sutured with a running 4-0 vicryl suture.

69.4.7 Placement of Surgical Guide

A prepared surgical guide is necessary to ensure accurate positioning of the maxilla. The guide is generally ligated to the upper teeth with 26–28 gauge wire. The upper and lower teeth are then wired together with 26–28 gauge wire, elastics, or power chain (Fig. 69.22).

69.4.8 Removal of Anterior Interferences

With the maxilla now fixed to the mandible, it is rotated into position by applying posterior and superior pressure on the

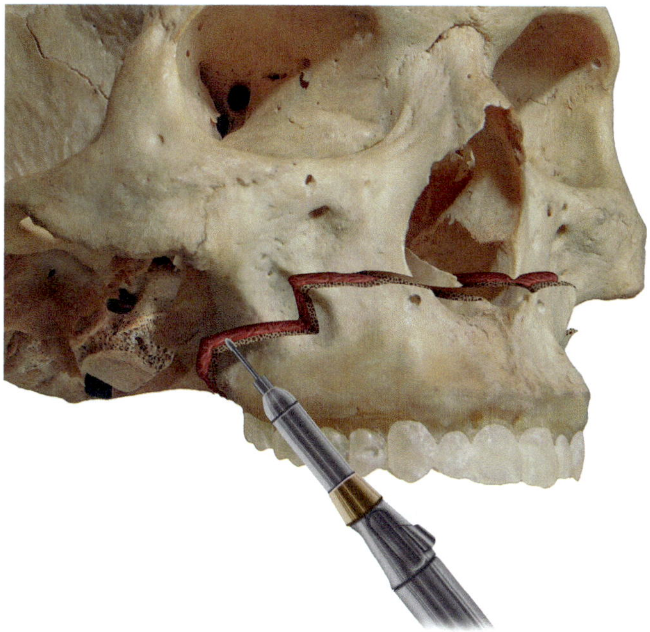

Fig. 69.21 Posterior interferences are initially removed from the posterior septum, lateral nasal walls, pyramidal processes of the palatine bones, and lateral maxillary walls. This allows for passive seating of the maxilla without posterior pivoting

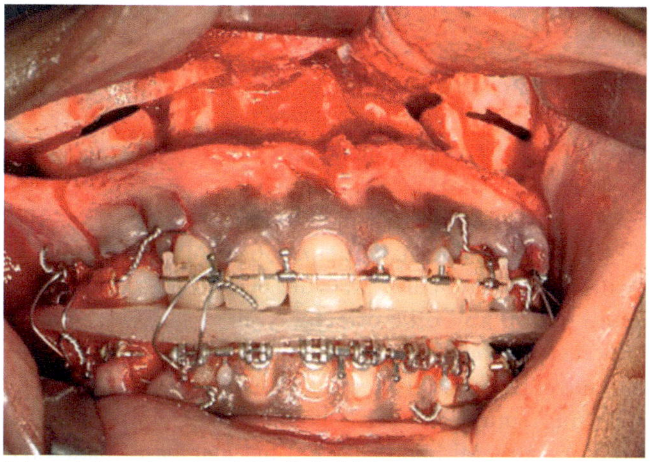

Fig. 69.22 Placement of surgical guide and achieve desire stable occlusion. The lefort I osteotomy and AMO cuts are visible

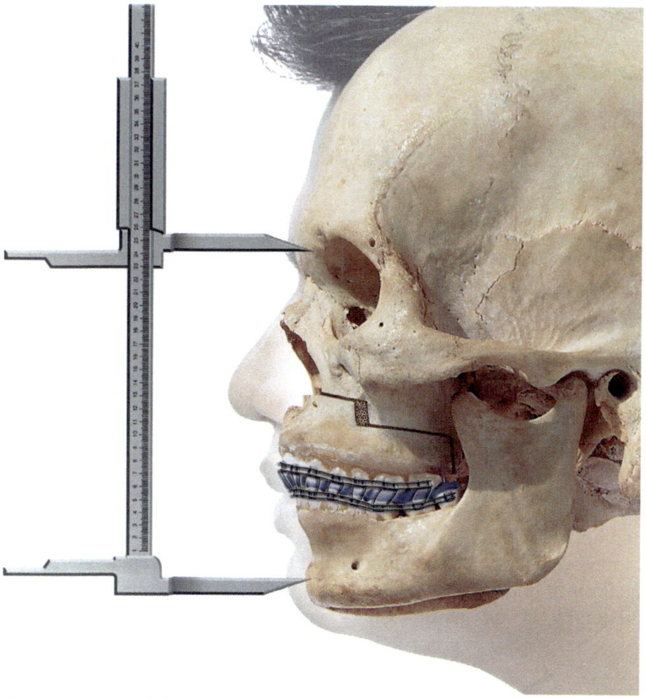

Fig. 69.23 The maxilla is rotated into place and anterior interferences are removed to ensure full seating of the condyles at the desired vertical position. Seating of the condyles of the mandible is achieved with superior pressure at the gonial notches and posterior pressure at the chin. Once the correct vertical maxillary positioning is achieved, the mandibular-maxillary complex can be reproducibly rotated with the condyles in the fossa without any bone or soft tissue pre maturities (Also see Fig. 69.12a, b)

mandible. To properly rotate the mandible, the surgeon places two fingers at the gonial notch regions of the mandible and the thumb of the same hand at the chin. Upward pressure is exerted with the two fingers at the gonial notches, and the thumb exerts a posterior and downward pressure. This "triangular" finger formation ensures full seating of the condyles during mandible rotation and maxillary positioning. The surgeon then rotates the mandible and maxilla upward, keeping pressure on the two fingers and thumb (Fig. 69.38a–c). Upward rotation is stopped as soon as the first contact is detected, and this interference is reduced accordingly. Anterior interferences can be easily reduced with a bur. The caliper is used to check the vertical distance from the anterior brackets to the K-wire and interferences are reduced accordingly. Closely observe the nasal septum for early inferences and deviation. When all the bony interferences have been completely removed, utilizing the "triangular" finger formation, the mandible and maxilla can be easily rotated up into a stable reproducible position, with the condyles fully seated (Fig. 69.23).

69.4.9 Fixation, Grafts, and Final Measurements

With the maxilla positioned, four miniplates are accurately bent to passively fit across the osteotomy in the piriform and anterior buttress areas of the maxilla. Typically, there are two fixation holes above and below the osteotomy in each bone plate, for placement of four screws. Thin bone or large bone gaps may require more fixation screws in each plate or even require additional plates. Bone grafts can be adapted into the

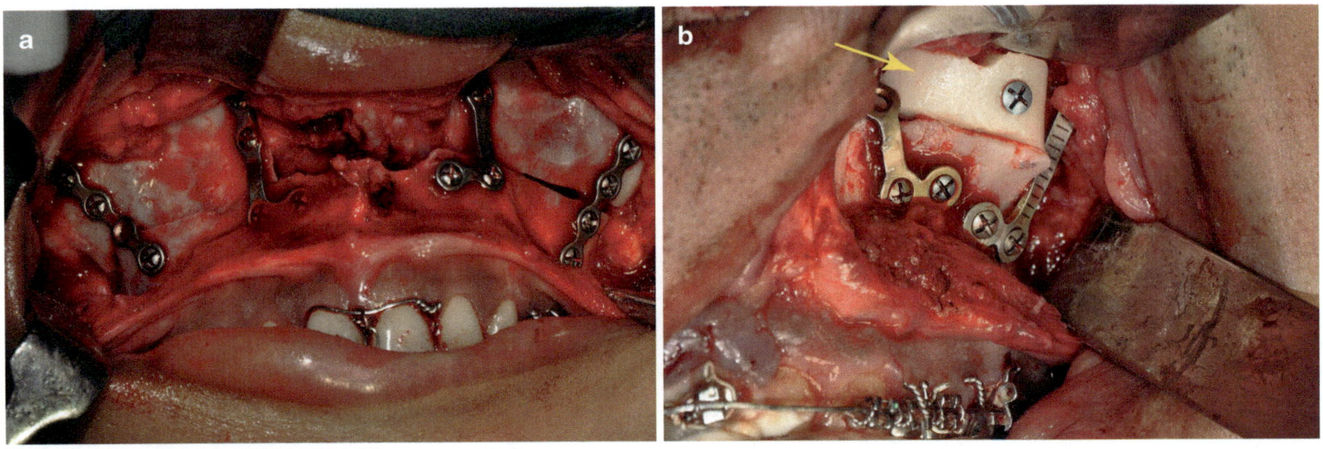

Fig. 69.24 (**a**, **b**) (**a**) Rigid fixation with four plates provides vertical and horizontal stability to the maxilla. The nasal septum should be free of deviation, and the occlusion should be reproducible once interdental fixation is released. Bone plates are used to stabilize the osteotomy bilaterally at the nasomaxillary and zygomaticomaxillary buttress areas. (**b**) Autogenous bone grafts have been adapted and fixated in the osseous gaps to optimize bone healing and minimize postsurgical relapse. Grafting may be indicated in complex movements, especially large advancements and down grafting cases (yellow arrow)

osteotomy gaps, and press-fit into position, or rigidly fixed if necessary [61]. Once the fixation has been competed, final measurements with calipers are made to confirm proper vertical placement (Fig. 69.24a, b).

69.4.10 Checks to Be Made Before Plate Fixation of the Maxilla

1. Ensure there are no bony interferences.
2. Check that the teeth are occluding into the splint correctly (particularly posteriorly, ensure the tongue is out of the way) and the condyles are seated correctly.
3. Check there are no soft tissue/septal interferences.
4. Check the nasal septum is in center (suture or cut groove into anterior nasal spine). Ensure that tears in the nasal mucosa if any are sutured.
5. Check any septal adjustment and piriform aperture bony adjustments have been made.
6. Make sure the maxillary dental midline and transverse maxillary occlusal plane cant are correct.
7. Ensure facial appearance, incisor exposure and aesthetics are optimal.
8. Check occlusion.

Once the maxillary fixation is completed, the intermaxillary fixation is released. The mandible is hinged with the condyles fully seated using the "triangular" finger formation. Retractors should be used to hold the cheeks away from the posterior teeth, and the mandible is rotated upward such that the teeth fit into the maxillary splint. The tongue is also manipulated out of the way if it is interfering with closure. There should be a smooth closure into the splint without any shifting or deviation of the occlusion. Contact should occur simultaneously in the anterior and posterior areas.

69.4.11 Closure

Proper closure occurs in three steps.

69.4.11.1 Nasal Cinch Suture (Alar-Base Suture) [62]

With the dissection and exposure of the paranasal musculature during Le Fort I osteotomy, the nasal cinch suture provides appropriate repositioning of the soft tissue to minimize postoperative nasal base widening. A slowly resorbing suture (e.g., 2-0 polyglycolic acid) is placed from an intraoral approach into the alar base bilaterally, pulling the alar bases toward each other when tightened (Fig. 69.25a, b). If properly done, tightening should result in an equal or shorter alar base width when compared to the preoperative width. This will frequently result in an immediate upturned appearance of the nose, a protruded positioning of the upper lip, and edema. These immediate changes are transient and will disappear within a few weeks. Following healing, the procedure results in minimal widening of alar base from the preoperative measurement (Fig. 69.26a, b).

69.4.11.2 V-Y Closure [63]

Typical movements of the maxilla and normal healing of the circumvestibular incision can result in lip shortening,

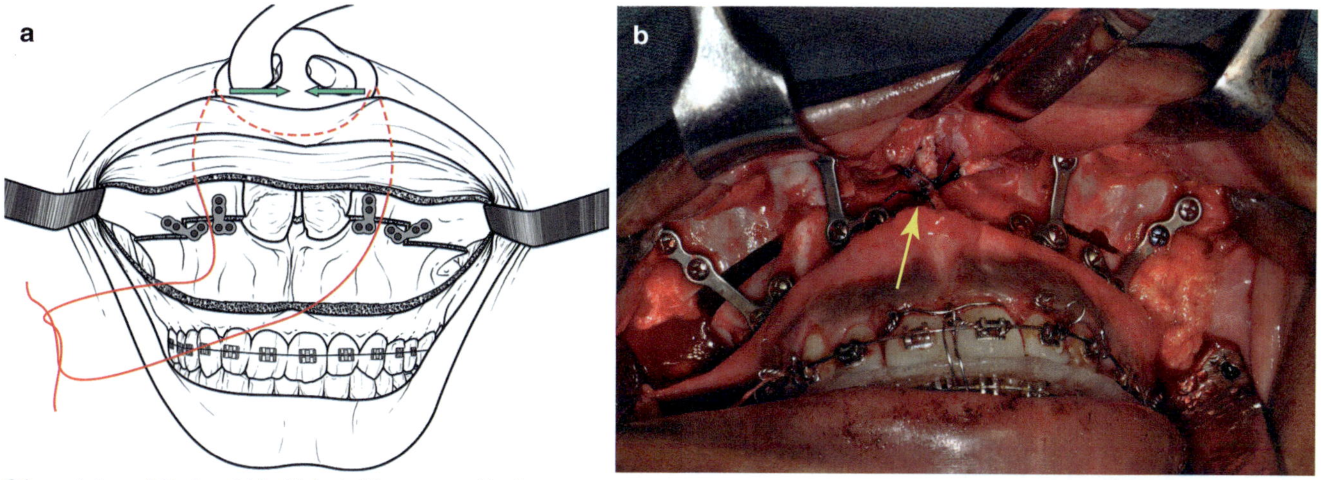

Fig. 69.25 (**a**, **b**) An alar base cinch suture controls the alar base width and counteracts postsurgical widening of the alar base. Care is taken to correctly place the suture in the fibro adipose tissue and transverse nasalis muscle at the lateral nasal base, allowing medial positioning of the alar base during suture tying (yellow arrow)

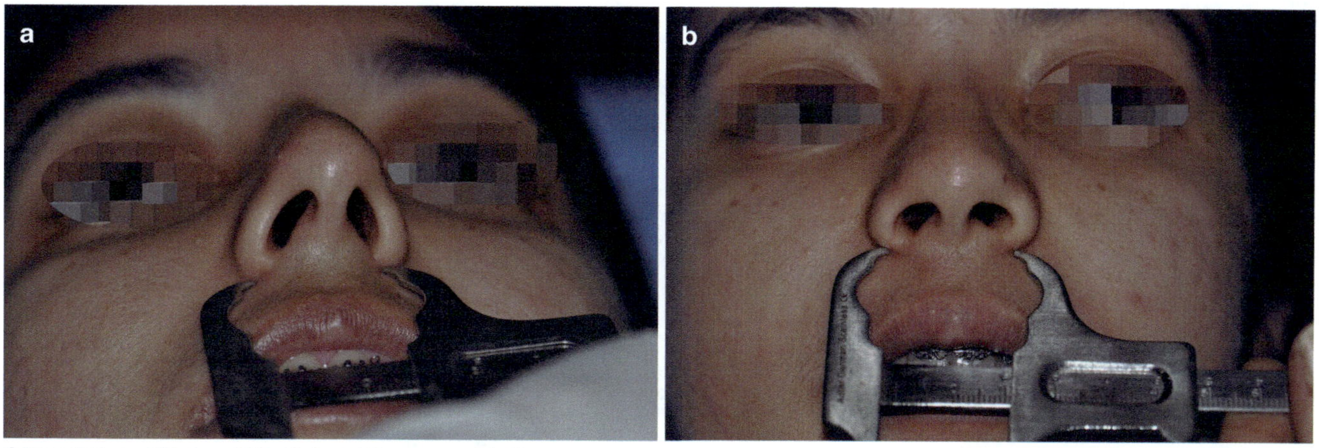

Fig. 69.26 (**a**, **b**) Measuring the alar base pre-surgically (**a**) and post-surgically (after edema subsides and soft-tissue settles) (**b**) and confirming that the size remains same

lip thinning, and decreased vermillion show. The Le fort I incision transects various components of the midface musculature, including the transverse part of the nasalis muscle, the myrtiformis muscle), and the levator anguli oris muscle.

It is important to correctly suture the deep muscular layers in proper anatomic orientation, so that the facial contour may be maintained [64].

The V-Y closure is performed to combat these undesirable changes. With the use of a skin hook, the tissue of the midline vestibular incision is grasped and pulled superiorly. Using a resorbable suture (e.g., 4-0 vicryl), the incision is closed vertically by grasping the tissue 1 cm away from the midline on either side of the skin hook and advancing these edges together by tightening the suture. This provides for a 1 cm V-Y closure. The remaining closure is completed with either a continuous suture or interrupted sutures. The closure generally requires four or five throws of the suture (Fig. 69.27, Fig. 69.9b).

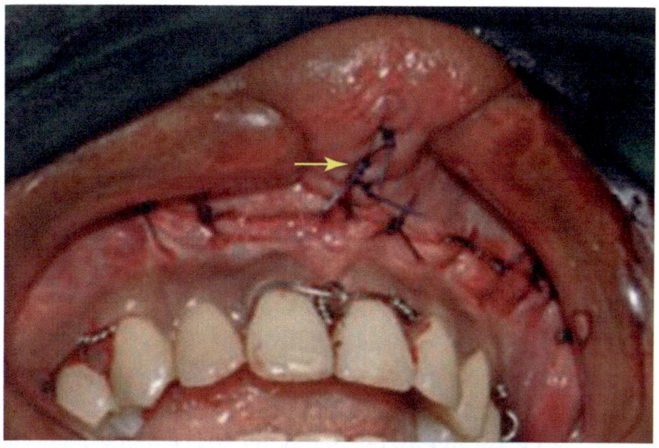

Fig. 69.27 Vestibular soft tissue closure is performed with a running resorbable suture. A midline V-Y closure provides support to the upper lip and rolls the vermillion upward and outward, gives fullness to the lip, and makes a prominent white-roll. Closure is started posteriorly and moved anterior to bring the labial side mucosa forward, which is then, closed in the midline in the form of an inverted "Y" (yellow arrow)

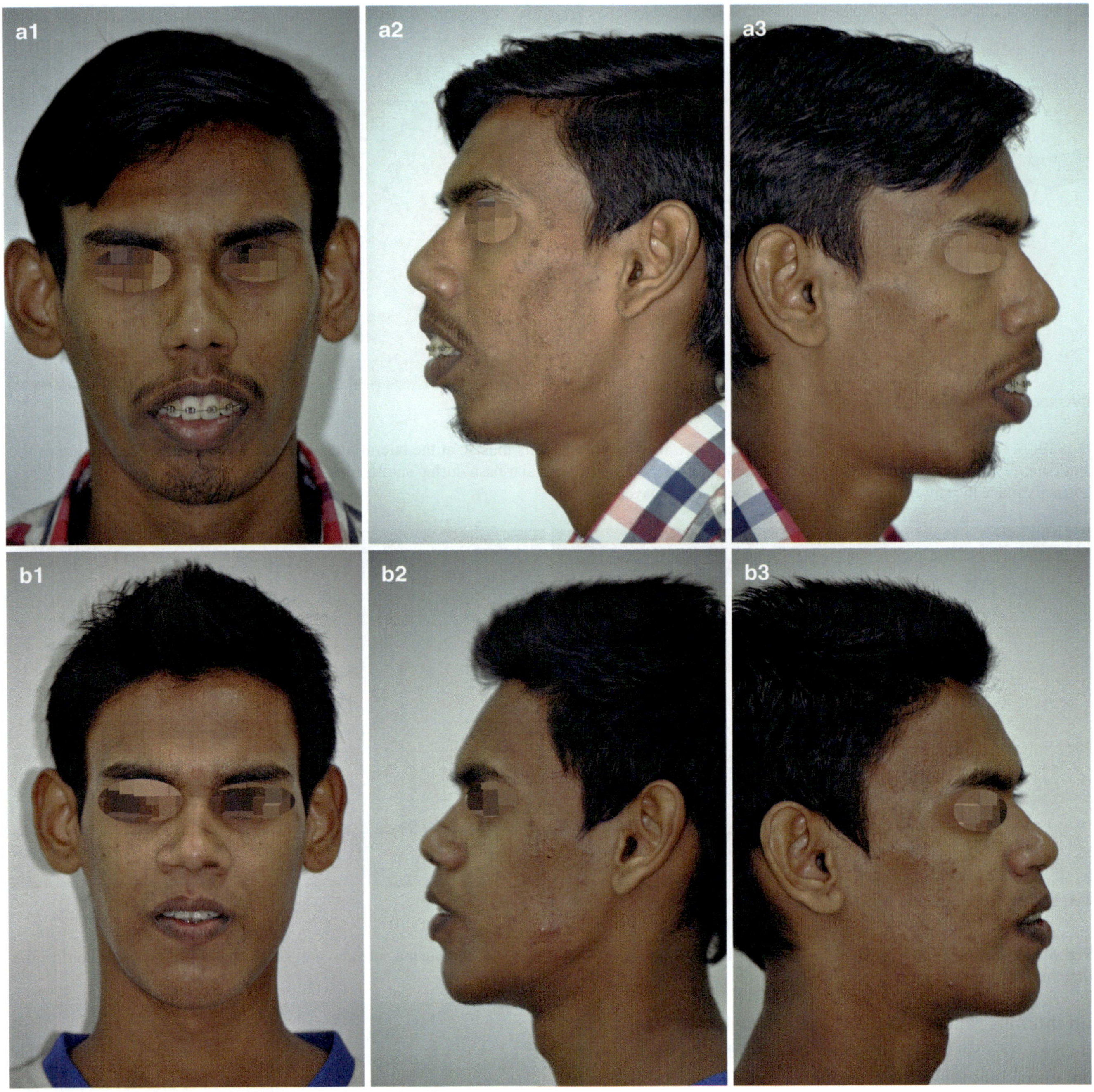

Fig. 69.28 (**a, b**) A case of vertical maxillary excess treated with superior positioning of the maxilla showing frontal, right lateral and left lateral views. (**a1, a2, a3**) Pre-surgical photos of the patient; (**b1, b2, b3**) post-surgical photos of patient (Also see Figs. 69.29 and 69.39 for the full case series images)

69.4.11.3 Vestibular Closure

The remaining vestibular closure continues from the posterior portion of the incision. A running resorbable suture (e.g., 4-0 vicryl) is passed in a simple running fashion. Figures 69.10, 69.11, 69.28a, b, 69.29a, b, 69.30a, b and 69.32a, b depict the results achieved by the technique described above for different clinical indications. Figure 69.31 demonstrates steps involved in peforming a Lefort I osteotomy in a bimaxillary setting.

69.5 Quadrilateral (Quadrangular) Osteotomy

This high-level osteotomy is a variant of the Le fort I osteotomy and extends up to the lower part of the zygoma, to a point just below the infraorbital nerve bilaterally.

The indications for this osteotomy are midface retrusion, including excessive scleral exposure.

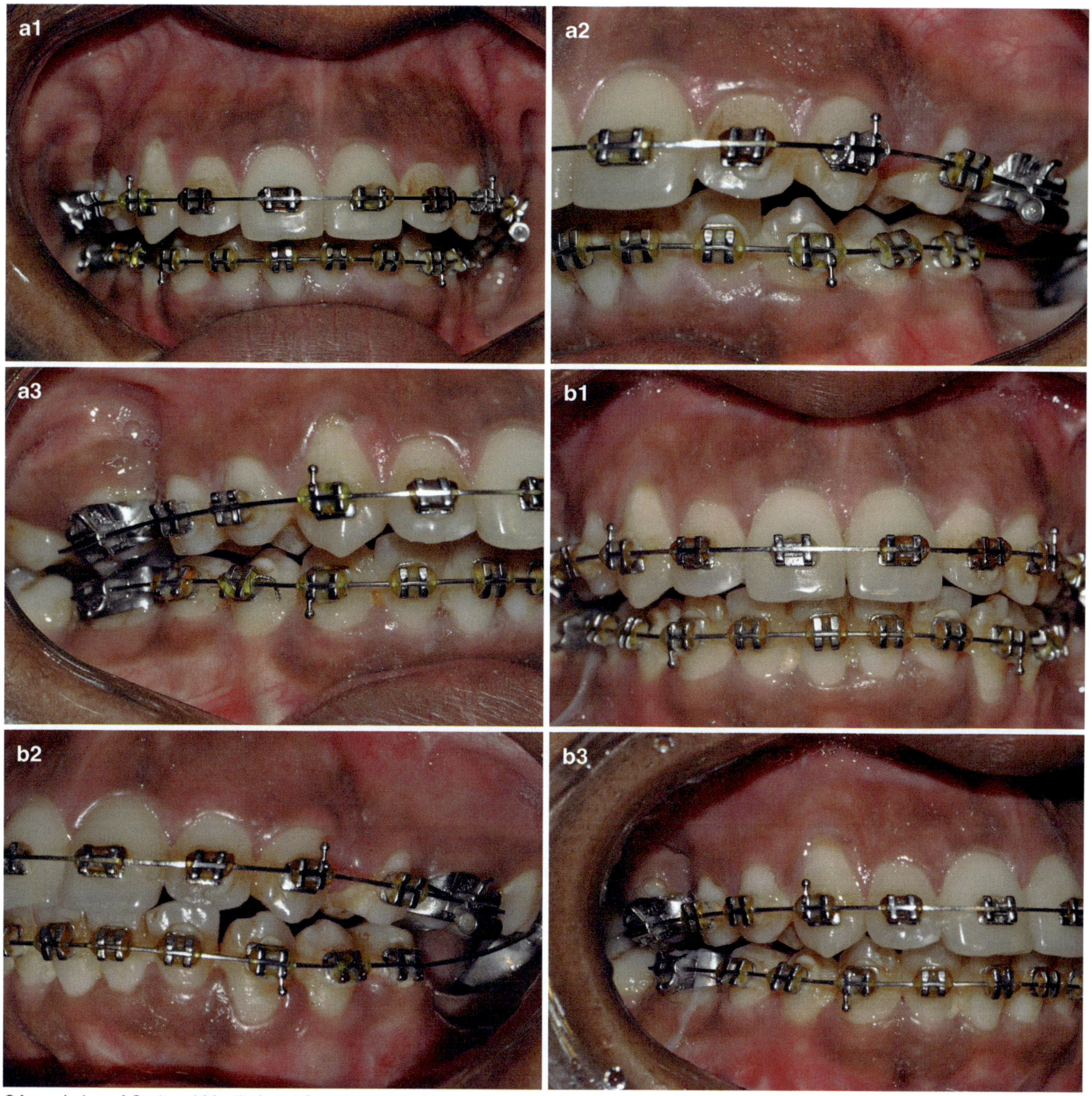

Fig. 69.29 (**a, b**) (**a1, a2, a3**) Pre-surgical occlusion of the same patient as in Fig. 69.28, treated with LeFort I superior repostioning. (**b1, b2, b3**) Post-surgical occlusion of the same patient

The benefits of the quadrangular osteotomy are that it improves the appearance of midfacial retrusion and flattening and improves zygomatic prominence and support for the lower eyelid. This osteotomy has minimal surgical morbidity and has acceptable outcomes. This may therefore be considered, especially in Asian patients, as a viable treatment alternative for midfacial advancement without augmentation of the malar region [65].

If the cuts are made from high to low a significant inferior movement of the maxilla can be achieved thus reducing the necessity for an interpositional bone graft (which would be required following a maxillary set down) and alloplastic onlay grafts for the zygomatic regions. It is more stable than conventional inferior positioning of the maxilla as there is good bone contact with native bone and no bone graft. This osteotomy also produces less rotation of the nasal tip than the conventional Le Fort I osteotomy. However, it is important to recognize that if there is a mild facial asymmetry in the maxillary region, this asymmetry can be emphasized with this high-level cut as the maxilla is advanced. The surgical technique is the same as for the conventional Le Fort I osteotomy, but significant sharp dissection of the masseter muscle from

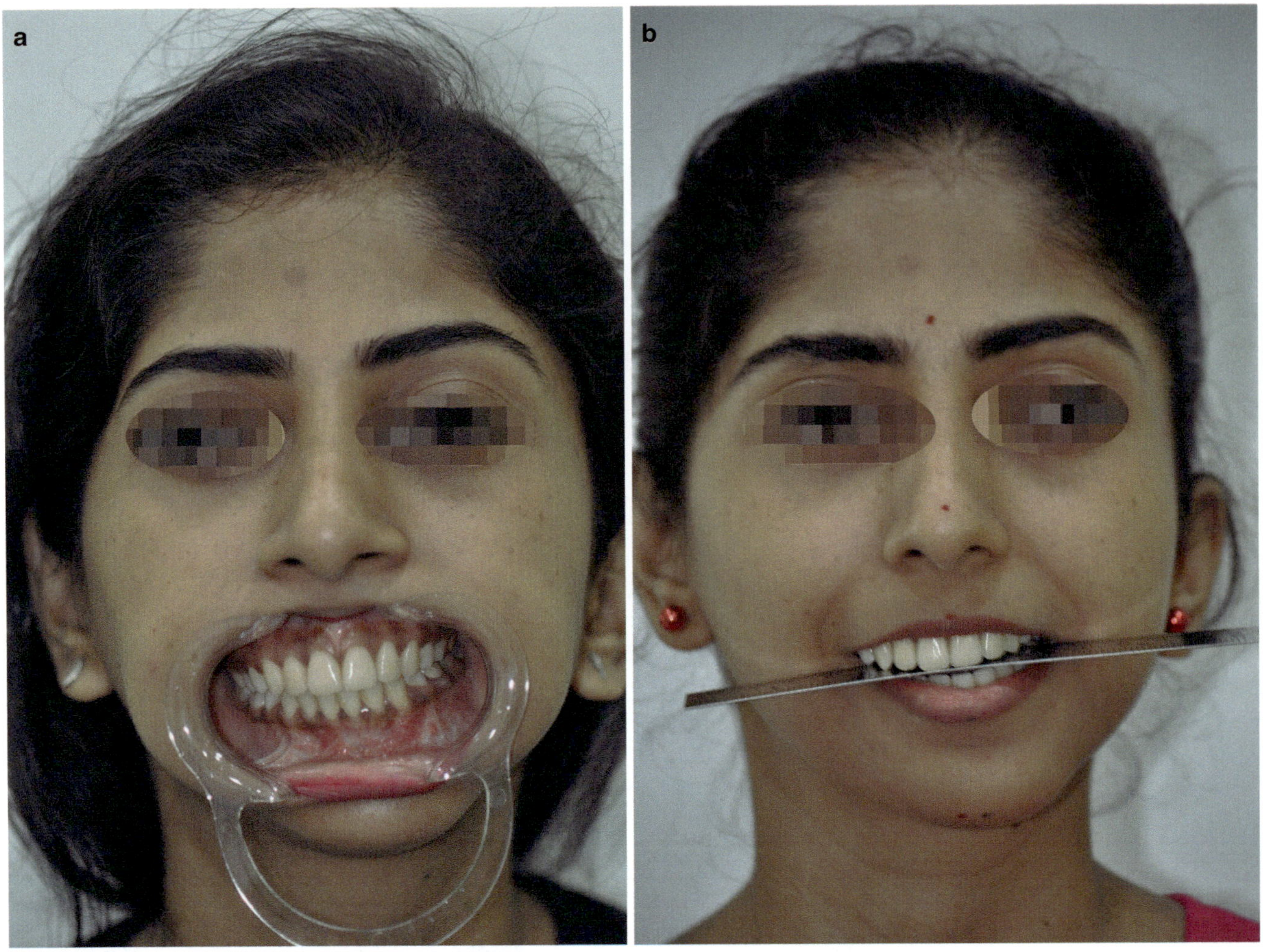

Fig. 69.30 (**a**, **b**) Patient with maxillary occlusion cant and asymmetry (also see Figs. 69.31, 69.32 and 69.40)

the zygoma is required to expose the prominence of the zygomatic bone. The bony cuts are demonstrated in Fig. 69.33. The cuts are made just below the infraorbhital nerves.

The bone over the zygomatic prominence is thick, and control over the shape of the cuts is easier using a burr and a saw. This ensures that the bony cut does not propagate upward to the cranial base but instead is directed downward to the normal pterygomaxillary disjunction level. The other steps to complete the bony cuts and down-fracture the Le Fort I cut are made as above. Fixation is with miniplates. However, care must be taken to ensure the plates are not palpable in the infraorbital regions.

69.6 Surgically Assisted Rapid Palatal Expansion (SARPE)

SARPE is a combination of orthodontic and surgical techniques to expand the maxillary arch. This is ideal in patients with of transverse maxillary deficiency, where the palatal suture has completely fused. This concept initially was met with skepticism but later was repopularized through the works of several clinicians, including Issacson and Ingram [66] and Haas [67], as a viable method of treating maxillary transverse deficiency. SARPE is indicated in cases where skeletal maturity has been achieved, transverse maxillary deficiency is present, excessive display of buccal corridors when smiling, and presence of anterior dental crowding. It has been shown that the midpalatal suture undergoes ossification at a wide range of ages [68]. In general, SARPE is recommended for patients who are over 16 years of age [69]. Nonsurgical expansions can be a reasonable consideration for patients younger than 12 years of age.

Before starting the surgery, it is important to confirm the secure placement of the appliance and also the presence of the device key to activate the appliance.

This procedure follows Le Fort I single piece osteotomy.

The maxilla is *not* down-fractured. Relieving of the osteotomies present at the zygomaticomaxillary buttresses is done, as this allows clearance during separation. The midline

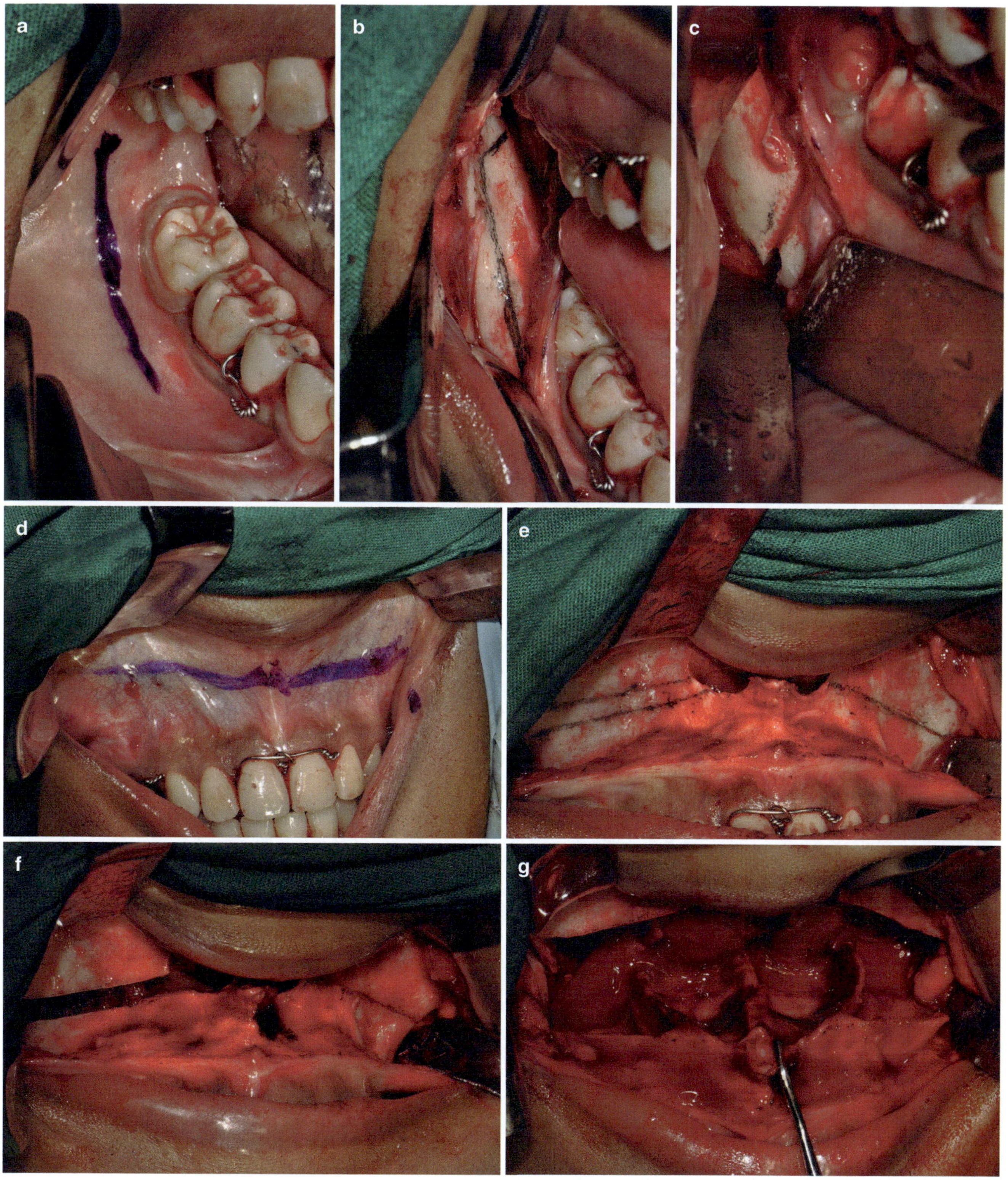

Fig. 69.31 (**a–m**) Surgical procedure for correcting the maxillary occlusion cant (also see Figs. 69.30, 69.32 and 69.40). (**a–c**) Sagittal split osteotomy cuts. (**d**) Incision marking for le fort Osteotomy. (**e, f**) Osteotomy cuts marked and made for asymmetric superior repositioning of maxilla. (**g**) Down-fracture of maxilla. (**h**) Superior repositioning of maxilla. (**i**) Fixation of maxilla with mini plates and screws. (**j**) Open bite on right side of occlusion because of asymmetric superior repositioning. (**k**) Unilateral sagittal split osteotomy of mandible split and fixed with mini plates and screws. (**l**) New Occlusion achieved. (**m**) Closure of wound done

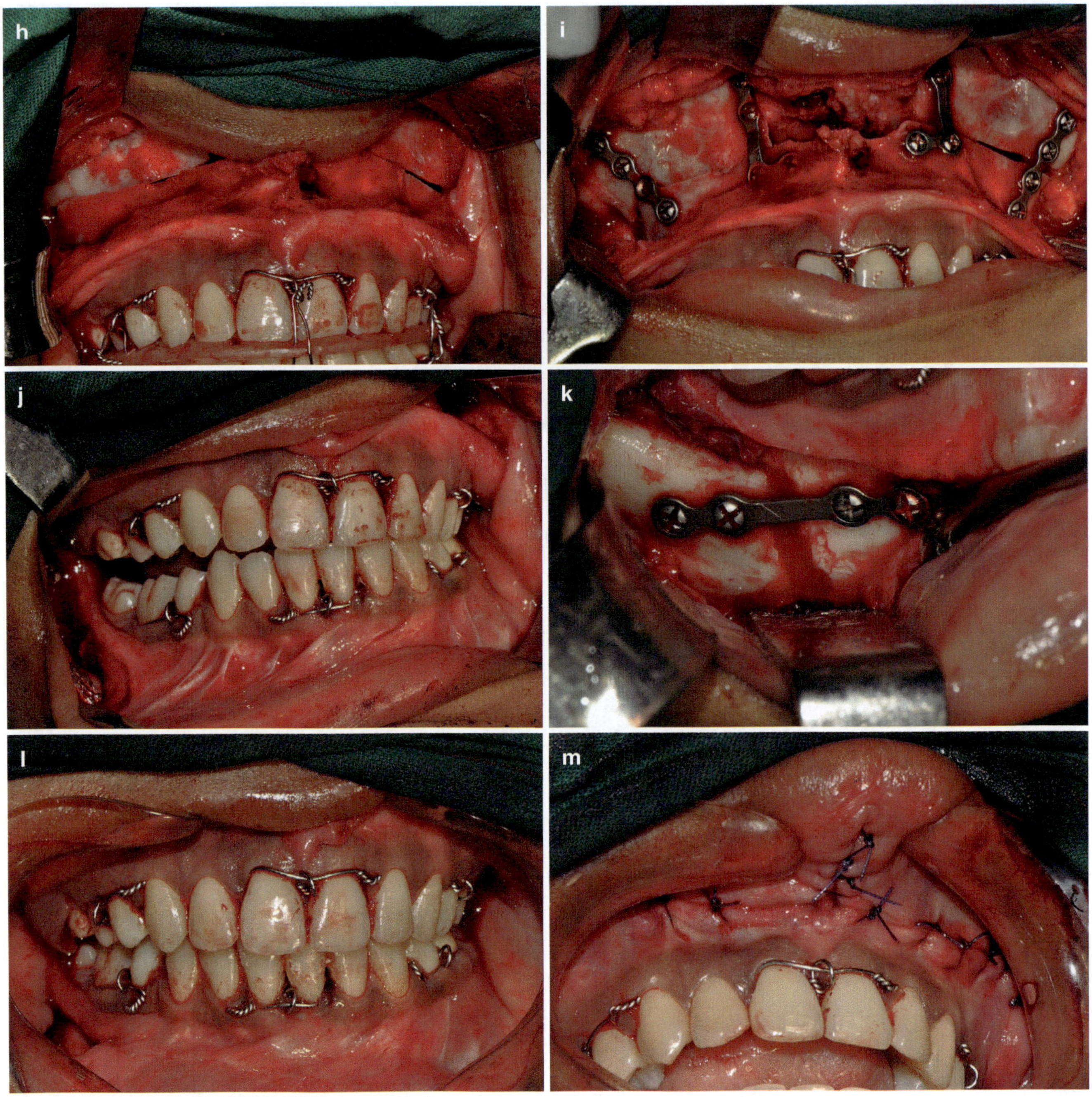

Fig. 69.31 (continued)

gingiva is elevated to expose the alveolus. The midline osteotomy is carried out using a sagittal or piezo saw from the piriform rim of the nose, to the alveolus. The mid-palatal suture osteotomy is completed with chisels. The zygomaticomaxillary buttresses clearance is confirmed intraoperatively by activating the palatal appliance (Fig. 69.34a–c). The remainder of the procedure is according to Le Fort 1 single piece osteotomy [70].

Salient Features of SARPE

1. SARPE is usually performed on arches that are V shaped.
2. The scope of orthodontics is limited in masking a skeletal transverse discrepancy that is greater than 5 mm. A segmental Le Fort expansion cannot be carried out for movements greater than 7 mm. If a significant amount of maxillary expansion is required, presumably greater than

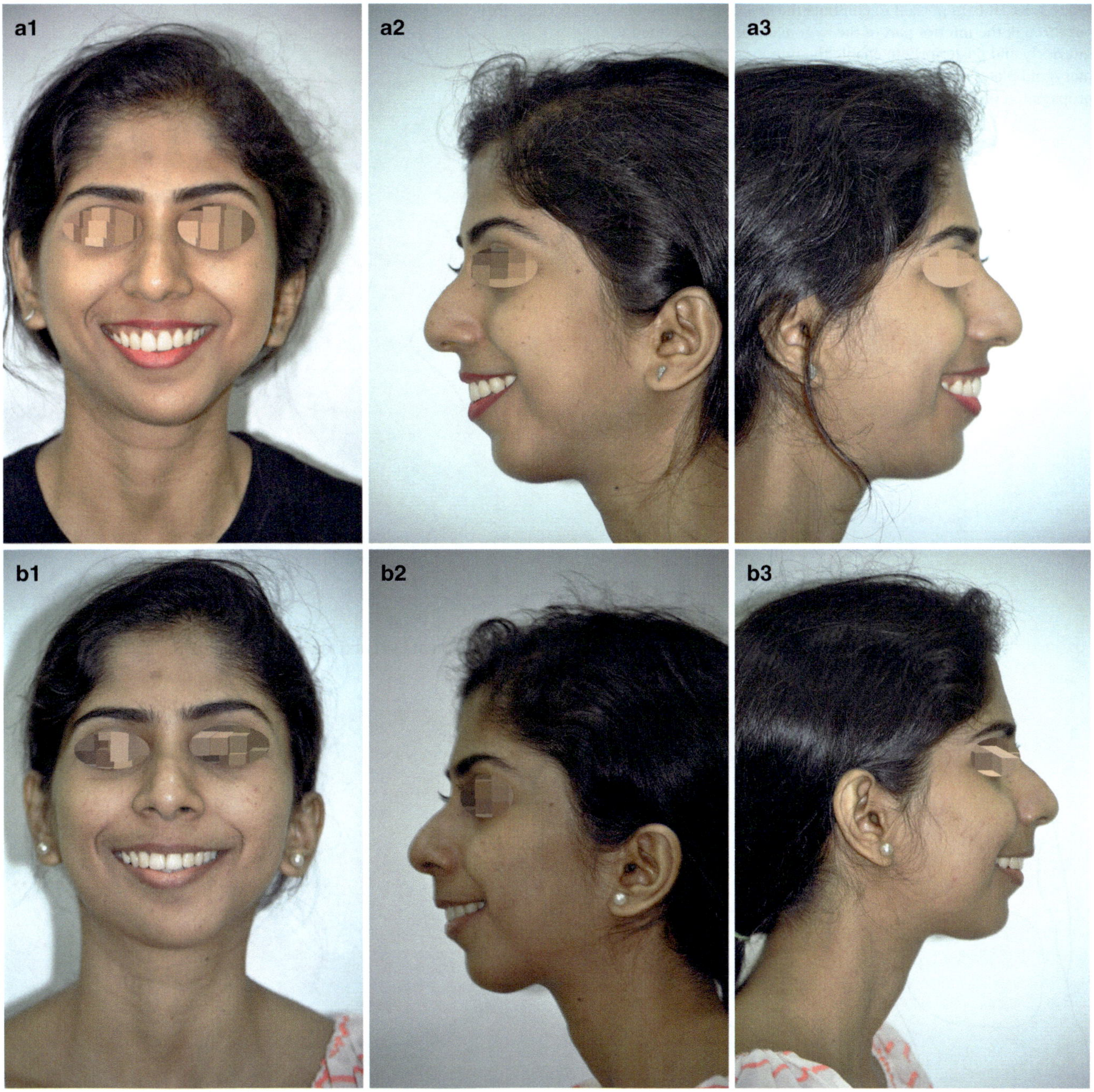

Fig. 69.32 (**a**, **b**) (**a1, a2, a3**) Pre-surgical pictures of patient with cant; (**b1, b2, b3**) postoperative asymmetric superior repositioning of maxilla and unilateral sagittal split osteotomy of the mandible to close the open bite created (Also see Figs. 69.30, 69.31 and 69.40)

7 mm, a SARPE procedure is preferred as it would offer more stability.

3. An IOPA X-ray is taken to ensure that sufficient space exists for an interdental osteotomy.
4. Osteotomies performed during a Le Fort I are replicated for the SARPE procedure, without down-fracturing the maxilla.
5. Pterygoid plates are separated for the posterior expansion of maxilla.
6. The zygomaticomaxillary buttresses offer greatest resistance to maxillary expansion. Activation of the palatal appliance must be done within the operating room. This will ensure that the maxilla is able to expand bilaterally, in a symmetric fashion, with no interferences.

Fig. 69.33 It is important to continue the saw or cut with a fissure bur through the inferior part of the zygomatic arch and extend it inferiorly and posteriorly to enable the important back cut to the pterygoid plates. This reduces the possibility of unwanted propagation of fractures to the cranial base

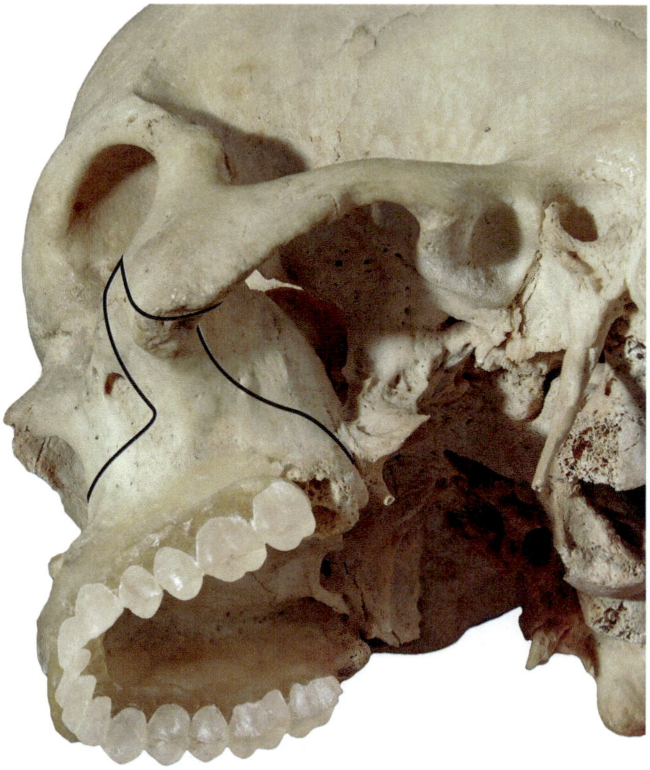

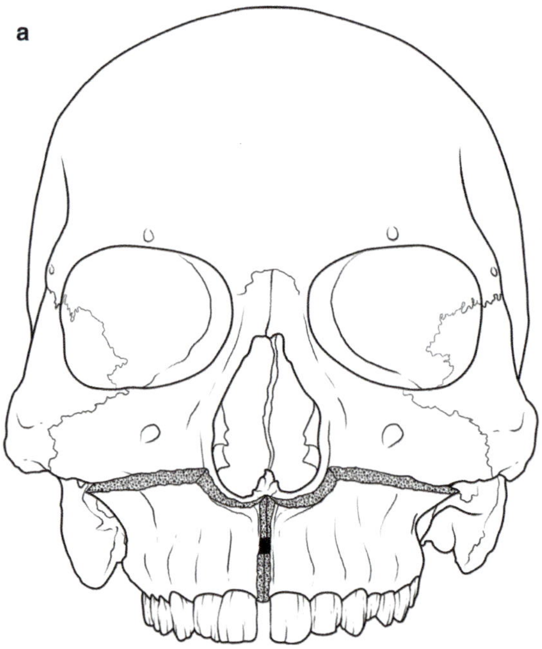

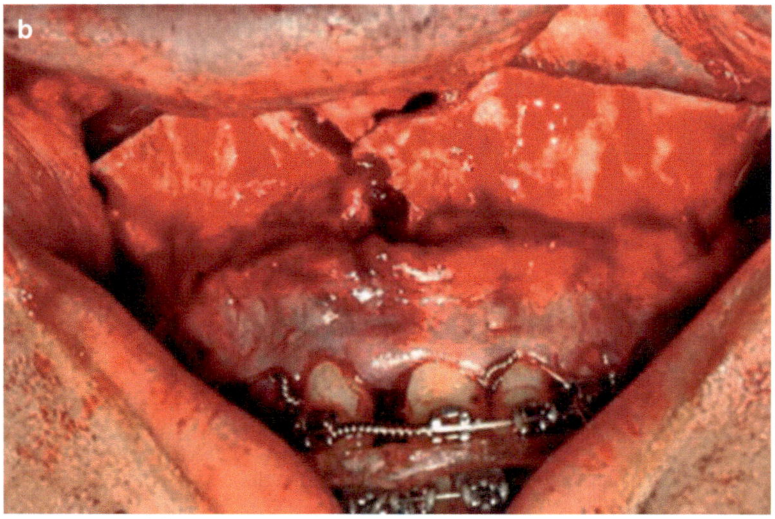

Fig. 69.34 (**a**) Maxilla down-fracture, paramedial osteotomy, palatal expansion device in situ, and checking for the horizontal segmental movement. (**b**) Midline palatal osteotomy, device for palatal expansion, (**c**) Tooth- borne Haas & Hyrax Appliance

c

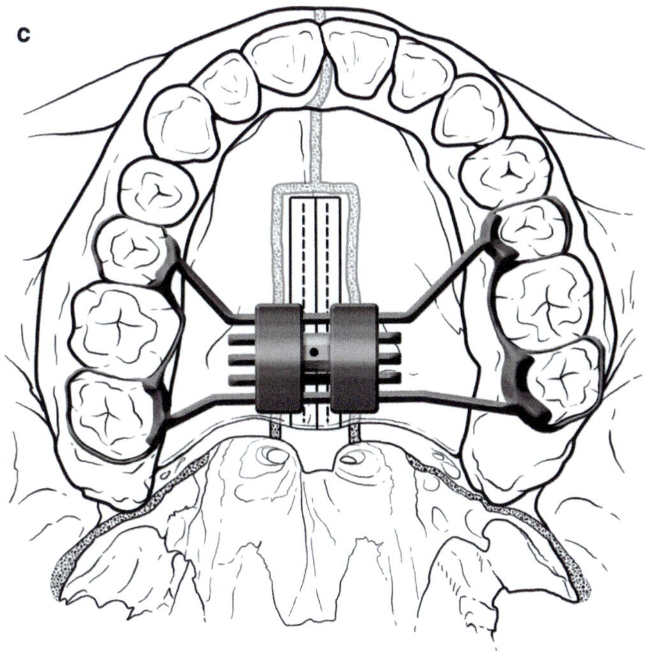

Fig. 69.34 (continued)

7. Overcorrection is recommended to allow for relapse. This is because maximum instability is associated with transverse maxillary expansion.
8. Either a tooth-borne appliance (Haas and Hyrax appliance) or a bone-borne palatal appliance may be used. The tooth-borne appliances may be more acceptable for patients, as they are less invasive and more hygienic. The disadvantage of these appliances is that they can create an occlusal tipping effect at the level of the alveolar bone and teeth. This may be minimized by engaging at least three posterior teeth. On the other hand, a bone-borne appliance offers better control over orthopedic movements at the level of the palate, but it requires a steep palatal vault for anchorage and is more invasive [71, 72].

69.7 Sequence of Bimaxillary Surgery (Fig. 69.31a–m)

A single surgical procedure can be employed to correct skeletal deformities of the mandible and the maxilla as well. The surgeon generally determines the preferred sequence. The authors personal preference is provided below.

1. The mandibular bony cuts are usually performed first, without splitting the mandible. This is followed by completion of the maxillary osteotomy, repositioning and fixation. In the past, fixation was only by trans-osseous wiring. Hence, when the mandible was performed first, its position was arbitrary as it incorporated the mobile proximal fragment (due to the TMJ) based on which the final maxillary position was determined. To avoid this the maxilla was completed first.
2. The mandible is exposed, and the bony osteotomy cuts are completed. However the formal split is not completed.
3. The maxilla is exposed, osteotomy completed and fixed in its final position.
4. The split for the mandible is completed, followed by the reposition of the mandible to the desired position. The mandible is then stabilised and fixed in its final position. This eliminates the possibility of any undesired maxillary movement as the movement of the maxilla is completed based on a stable intact mandible.
5. Finally, the genioplasty cuts are stabilized.
6. The same order must be considered during model surgery and when fabricating the intermediate and final splints for guidance.

The authors personal preference has been detailed above. Alternatively, mandibular splitting may be performed first, and an intermediate splint may be used to to fix the mandible to the unoperated maxilla. The maxilla may then be stabilized to the operated and repositioned mandible. However, it must be noted that stabilization and fixation of the mandible are more challenging than for the maxilla. Rigid fixation may be more challenging if an improper or misdirected split occurs. The procedure may even need to be aborted altogether. However, by stabilizing the maxilla first, the mandible can use appropriately positioned maxilla for stabilization. Therefore, we have always preferred to complete the maxillary surgery before mandibular surgery.

Having listed a general guide above, we reiterate that no dogma should be given regarding the sequence of maxillary or mandibular surgery. Proper planning and preparation will in turn logically dictate the sequence, which must be kept flexible [73].

69.8 Soft Tissue Changes with Le Fort I Osteotomy

Changes in the jaw position in turn lead to changes in the position of soft tissues such as the lips, cheeks, and nose [74]. The lips may show thinning, reduced vermillion show, and may lack adequate lip support [46]. The nasal tip may be upturned, the alar base width may increase, and the nasolabial angle may widen [75] (Fig. 69.35a–c). Soft tissue swelling

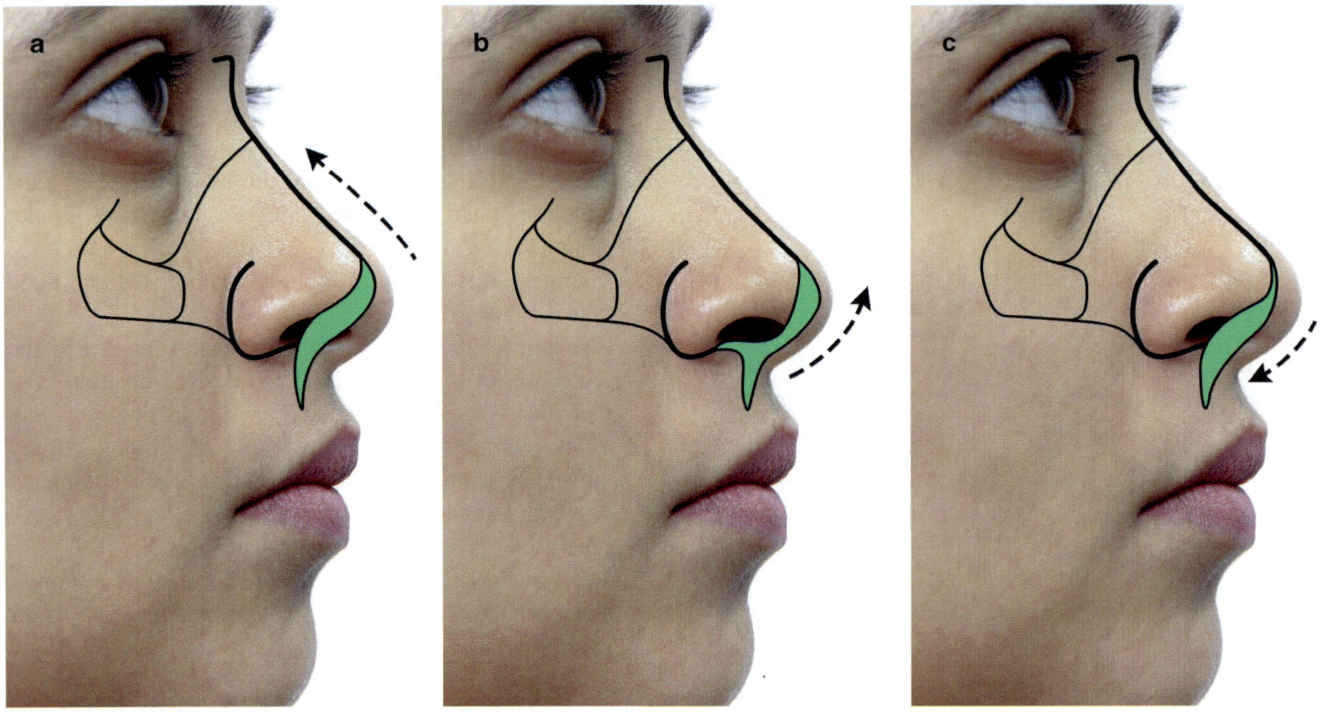

Fig. 69.35 (**a–c**) (**a**) reduction of a strip along the caudal septum will shorten the nose; (**b**) reduction involving the nasal tip as shown will increase the nasolabial angle; (**c**) wedge reduction predominantly at the septal base will reduce the nasolabial angle

may take up to a year to resolve, so these changes may not be apparent immediately [76]. In some regions, such as the subnasale, and the lips, greater than 10% change has been documented over 5 years [4]. Nasal changes are quite complex and are therefore unpredictable. Both the structure of the nose (including nasal cartilage connective tissue, anterior nasal spine, and the other nasal cartilages) and the degree of movement of the maxilla play a role in nasal changes. Other patient-related factors, including thickness and morphology of the soft tissue, postoperative healing, age, and ethnicity, can also affect nasal changes, which may either be favorable or unfavorable or beneficial. The nasal width alone increases predictably in Le Fort I osteotomies, and the increase in width depends on the extent of maxillary movement. Adjunctive procedures to limit widening of the nasal width may be performed intraoperatively. These include alar cinch suture and piriform aperture sculpting. Alternatively, the changes may be accepted and later procedures can be performed if necessary. The disadvantage of this is the need for an additional surgical procedure, e.g., alar wedge resection rhinoplasty. The alar cinch suture and V-Y closure (ACVY) is efficient and less invasive in controlling nasolabial changes. Its long-term results need to be evaluated. One study showed that the alar base cinch suture reduced the inter-alar width to its preoperative width following a Le Fort I osteotomy. The suture was stable when evaluated at 12 months and 3 years postoperatively [77]. There have been studies comparing nasal and maxillary vermilion morphology after Lefort osteotomies by simple primary closure, Single VY closure and Double VY closure. The results indicated that better aesthetics are seen in double VY closure cases (See Hackney et al. 1989, Ledezma et al. 2014, in Additional reading provided). However a systematic review in 2014 couldn't reach a conclusion regarding the efficacy of various methods of closure in Lefort Osteotomies.

69.9 Specific Considerations

1. Attempts to study the nasal changes resulting from maxillary movements have demonstrated very variable results. The general consensus is that nasal changes are unpredictable after Le Fort I osteotomy [78].
2. The ascending pharyngeal artery and ascending palatine artery maintain blood perfusion to the down-fractured maxilla.
3. Impacted, unerupted, or erupted wisdom teeth may be removed during the Le Fort I surgery. The curved pterygoid osteotome must be placed posterior to the impacted teeth or through the socket. The technique of pterygoid separation through the socket of the third molar was described by Trimble et al in 1983 (Refer additonal reading).
4. If posterior bony interferences are present, they may cause condylar displacement, condylar distraction, asym-

metrical jaw movements (deviations), malocclusion, and aberrant maxillary position.
5. If the maxilla is not mobilized sufficiently prior to fixation, this may hinder optimal advancements.
6. The zygomaticomaxillary and nasomaxillary buttresses consist of thick struts of bone and are ideal for securing fixation [79].
7. Blood loss is variable but rarely warrants transfusion. A review of over 500 osteotomies concluded an average loss of just under 300 mL, greater for bimaxillary osteotomies and less for single jaw surgery [80].

69.9.1 Adjustment to the Anterior Nasal Spine and Piriform Aperture

Mommaerts et al. reported that the anterior nasal spine is a significant component of nasal tip projection and may be reduced to limit the degree of nasal tip rotation [81]. Betts et al. also stated that changes in the lateral part of the piriform aperture significantly affected the soft tissue of the nasal base and nasal tip projection [82].

It is important not to remove too much of the septum as this can produce a retracted columella, which is a potentially unattractive feature.

Osseous recontouring of the nasal crest of the maxilla and/or resection of a portion of the caudal extent of the cartilaginous septum is recommended to keep interference at bay. Placement of a suture through the anterior nasal spine and cartilaginous septum to prevent its displacement upon removal of the nasoendotracheal tube is beneficial.

69.9.2 Effect of Changing the Inclination (Slope) of the Osteotomy Cut

If the osteotomy cut is made in a parallel direction to the occlusal plane and the maxilla is advanced, the maxillary incisor exposure will increase but the face height will not change. However, if the osteotomy cut starts high posteriorly and slopes downwards toward the piriform aperture, the maxilla will move down the slope as it is advanced, thus increasing the maxillary incisor exposure. The mandible will subsequently rotate in a clockwise direction and the lower anterior face height will increase (Fig. 69.36a, b). The opposite is true for the osteotomy cuts that start low posteriorly and slopes upward toward the piriform aperture (Fig. 69.37a, b).

69.9.3 Impacted Wisdom Teeth

If an impacted maxillary wisdom tooth is indicated for removal, this is done through the sinus floor. Using a rotary drill with a rosette bur, the bone from the sinus floor, which lies above the impacted tooth, is removed. Next, a tapered fissure bur is used, and the bone just adjacent to the impacted tooth is removed. The impacted wisdom teeth may also be sectioned if necessary

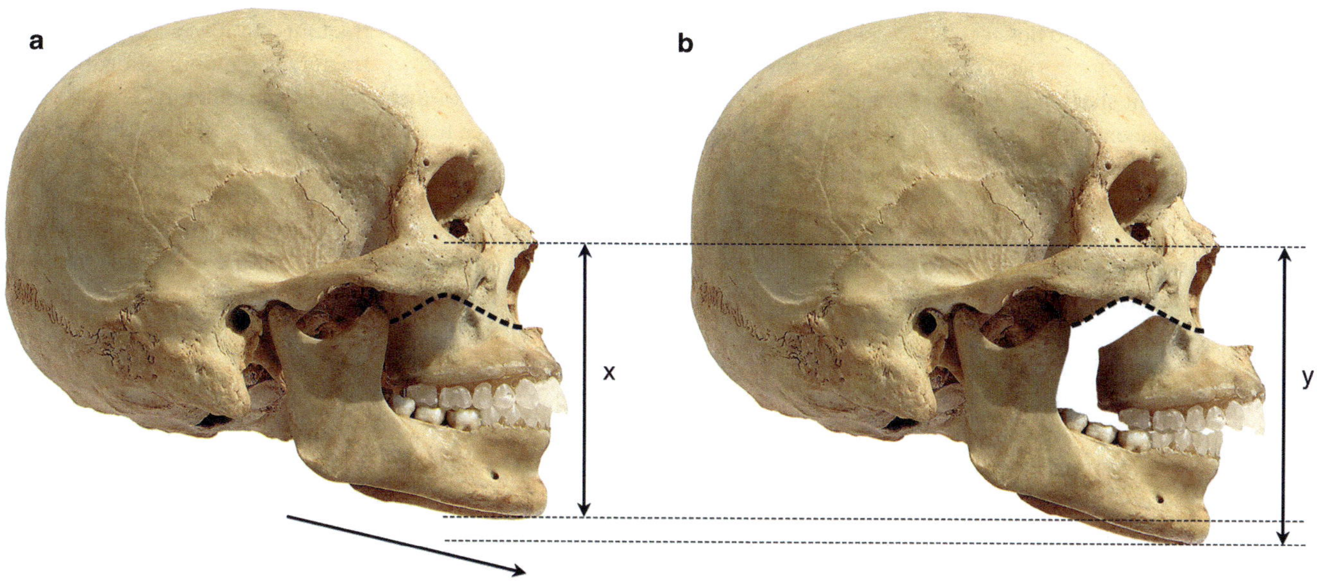

Fig. 69.36 (**a**, **b**) Diagram showing effects of the inclination (high to low postero-anteriorly) of the osteotomy cut when advancing the maxilla—(**a**) osteotomy inclination to increase incisor exposure and potentially increase lower face height, (**b**) advancement of maxilla producing increase of lower facial height due to downward ramp effect

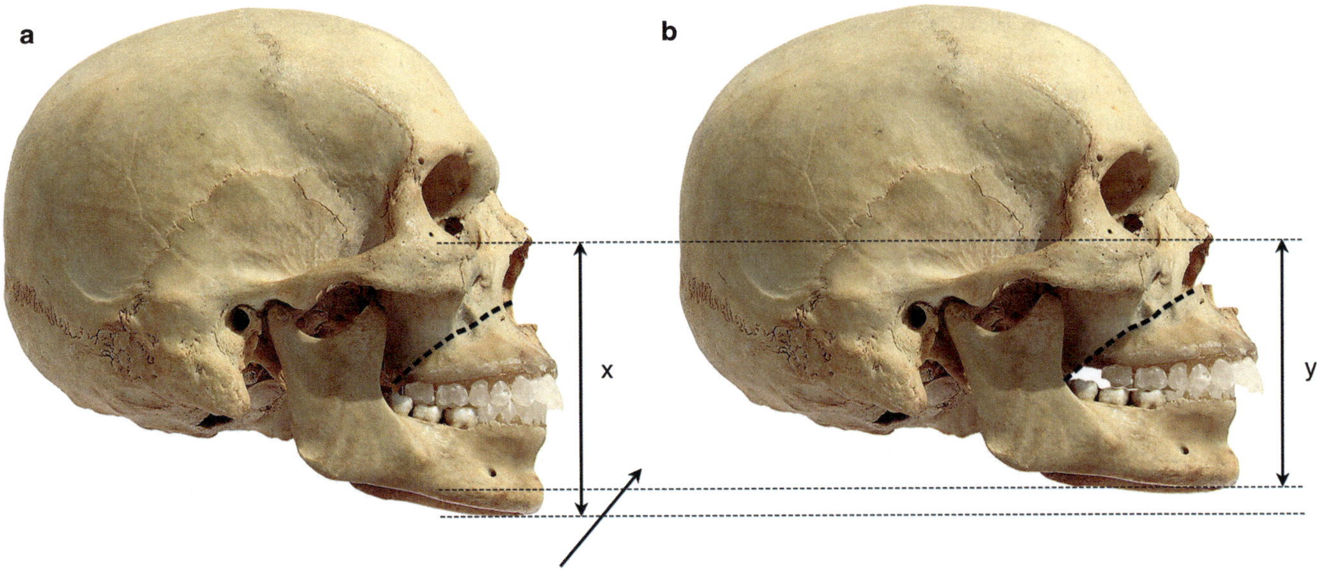

Fig. 69.37 (**a**, **b**) Diagram showing effects of the inclination (low to high postero-anteriorly) of the osteotomy cut when advancing the maxilla—(**a**) osteotomy inclination to reduce incisor exposure and potentially reduce lower face height, (**b**) advancement of maxilla producing reduction of lower facial height due to upward ramp effect

to aid in removal; this usually depends on the developmental stage. The tooth is delivered using a dental elevator. Rarely, perforation through the palatal mucosa may occur.

69.9.4 Erupted Wisdom Teeth

If the maxillary wisdom tooth is completely erupted, this may be extracted prior to down-fracture. This will allow the operator to have a stable "workbench" during extraction. In order to maintain the blood supply to the down-fractured maxilla, the adjacent palatal and labial mucosa must be preserved carefully at the time of extraction.

69.9.5 Considerations of Pre-operative Difficulties

The pre-surgical workup and planning of patients who require corrective jaw surgery required detailed analysis of clinical features, study models, and plane radiographs. Radiographic analysis includes comprehensive assessment of lateral cephalograms, postero-anterior cephalograms, and orthopantomograms. The need for multiple individual planar views has been replaced by the advent of cone beam technology.

69.9.6 Considerations of Operative Difficulties

Horizontal osteotomy of the maxilla should result in a clean pterygomaxillary separation to subsequently allow for down-fracture and mobilization. At this step, the pterygoid plates should ideally remain intact and attached to the skull base. However, in some exceptional cases, such as patients with cleft maxilla, the pterygoid plates are unusually thick and well buttressed. On the other hand, some patients have thin and almost translucent pterygoid plates [83]. Pterygomaxillary synostosis (fusion) may be seen in up to 12% of all patients [21].

If the pterygoid plates fracture at a lower level, this may cause difficulties in down-fracture and mobilization, because of the attachment of the pterygoid musculature. On the other hand, if the plates fracture at a higher level, the fracture may propagate into and along the skull base, which can potentially cause neuro-ophthalmic complications.

On postoperative CT scans, the incidence of pterygoid plate fracture after a Le Fort I osteotomy was found to range from 58 to 75% [84, 85]. However, despite this high incidence, the incidence of fractures propagating to the skull base/orbit is low [83].

Lanigan et al. carried out a study on unfixed fresh cadavers and found that 26% of cases were "difficult down-fracture." They stated that this was probably due to the presence of "thick bony maxillary walls" [83].

These authors stated that if a difficult down-fracture was encountered after a routine Le Fort I osteotomy, then the posterior walls of the maxilla must be sectioned completely using an osteotome. Alternatively, sectioning through the tuberosity could be performed, using a micro-oscillating saw or straight osteotome, as this would avoid the thick posterior walls and aid in pterygomaxillary separation. However, these authors have stated that it would not be possible to totally prevent untoward fractures that could occur during pterygomaxillary disjunction and down-fracture. We emphasize that thorough CBCT imaging should be undertaken preoperatively, as this would familiarize the surgeon with the maxillary morphology.

The following maneuvers may help if the surgeon finds difficulty in down-fracture following osteotomy and disjunction:

1. Revise the osteotomy cuts at all accessible sites, including anteromedial antral, lateral antral, and superior-nasal crest.
2. The maxilla may be "hinged down" to directly visualize the posterior maxilla, after which the cuts in this region may be completed, using a straight 4 mm osteotome.
3. Down-fracture can then be undertaken under direct vision.

O'Regan and Bharadwaj stated that an osteotome or saw must never be used blindly in these situations [86].

69.9.7 Proper Positioning

- Proper positioning can be difficult in isolated maxillary surgery, usually due to unrecognized posterior bony interferences.
- With an unrecognized posterior interference and inadequate effort or improper seating of the condyles, the maxilla can rotate around this interference, resulting in an anterior open bite after release of intermaxillary fixation. The maxillomandibular complex should be rotated with pressure seating the condyles in the glenoid fossa (Fig. 69.38a, b, c).
- Looking for the posterior interferences and eliminating them will result in the intended postoperative occlusion. Prior to any attempt to position the maxilla, effort is devoted to removing bone in the most likely areas of potential posterior interference, that being the area posterior to the second molar and along the perpendicular process of the palatine bone.
- Whether or not there is a potential for interference in the region of the pterygoid plates, per se, depends upon the

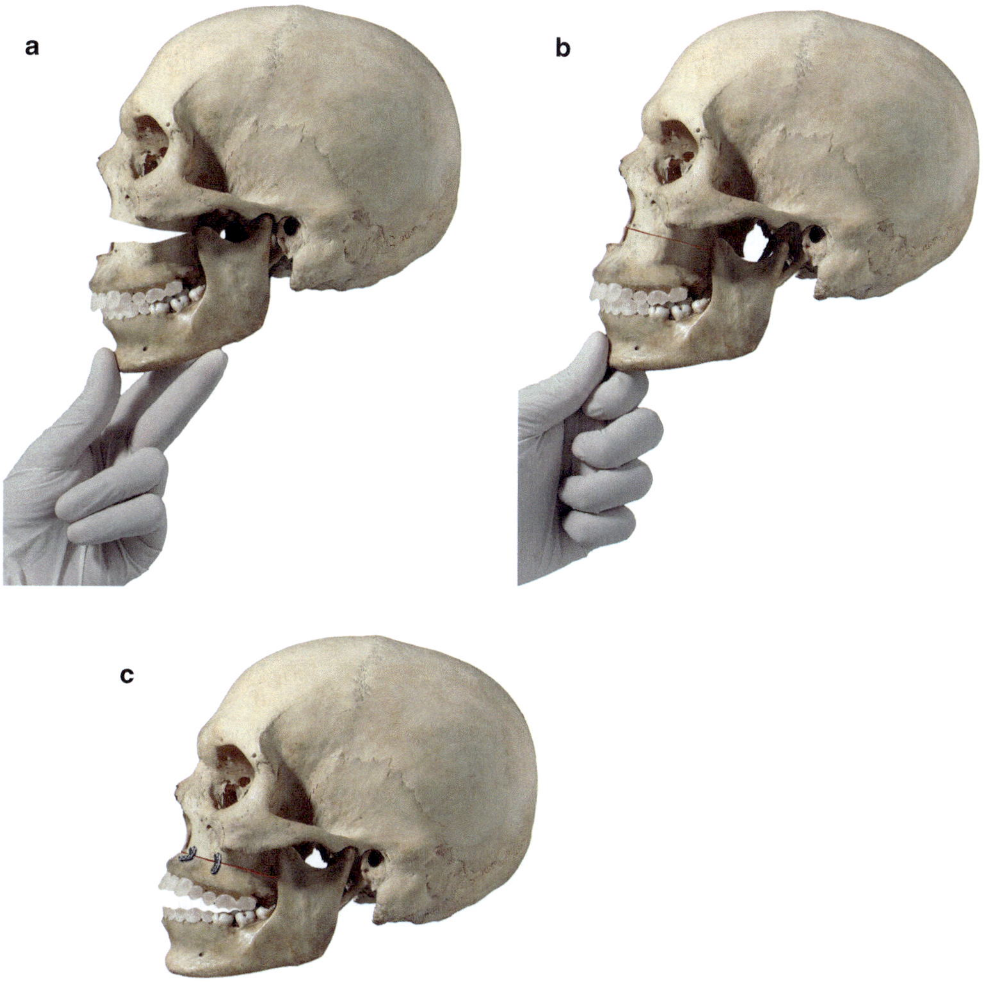

Fig. 69.38 (a–c) (a) The proper method for condylar seating at the time of maxillary positioning prior to fixation. Posterior prematurities are best appreciated with this method. (b) Pressure on the chin to push the anterior aspect of the maxillary osteotomy together may rotate the condyles inferiorly and posteriorly while maxillary fixation is applied. (c) Upon release of intermaxillary fixation, the condyles may return to the fosse, and an open bite may appear. Unfortunately, this open bite may not appear immediately, especially if postoperative elastics are used to "guide" the occlusion

surgical move. This is much less likely with advancement than it is with other moves such as impaction.

- It is often easiest to adapt the plates for fixation with Le Fort osteotomy and initially secure them only to the inferior fragment. Once all the plates are properly bent and secured to the inferior fragment, the maxillomandibular complex and condyles can be positioned with great care, and the shape and bending of the plates critically evaluated and secured to the superior fragment in succession, while the maxillomandibular complex is held in position.

69.9.8 Nutritional Support

Orthognathic surgery throws up many physiological challenges. These include postoperative facial swelling and catabolism which increase the nitrogen requirements. If these are not met, wound healing may be compromised. A diet fortified with macro- and micronutrients and adequate hydration is therefore essential [87].

Mandibular movements may be restricted in the postoperative period, owing to facial swelling and pain. Meeting the daily nutritional needs and hydration requirements (Table 69.1) may therefore be difficult. Studies have shown that in 6 weeks following surgery, patients can lose between 3.1 and 6.8 kg of weight [88].

It is important to adapt the diet to suit these needs, to promote wound healing, and to minimize postoperative complications. Another important factor in patient recovery is the patient's mood. Adequate nutrition and hydration will serve to improve the patient's mood, thereby diminishing postoperative irritability or depression [89]. Dietician assessment of nutritional status is essential to ensure that the above goals are achieved.

The modification of the diet is a sequential process. This aims at reducing the masticatory forces on the underlying healing bone, which in turn optimizes the conditions for healing.

1. The first 7 days following surgery should consist of a diet rich in energy and protein. This must be in a liquid form, and foods may be completely blended in a food processor to a smooth liquid consistency.
2. After the first week, patients can start consuming food with a small spoon or fork. It is still advised to minimize chewing, and foods may be mashed. The high-energy-high-protein diet must be continued.
3. After the second week, light chewing may be done, and a soft diet is recommended. The jaw muscles may fatigue easily at first, but gradually the muscles adapt to the new position. The soft diet is continued for two months, after which regular diet may be resumed [87, 90–98].

Table 69.1 Recommended postoperative nutrition requirements for patients above 16 years, undergoing orthognathic surgery [87]

	Energy (kcls)	Protein (g)	Fluid (ml)
Male	2500	1 g/kg/day	35 mL/kg/day
Female	2000	1 g/kg/day	35 mL/kg/day

69.9.9 Complications

1. *Hardware failure*: Unstable orthoappliance, splints/wafer, must be tried separately on each arch pre-operatively. Hardware exposure or fracture, palpable hardware, and loosening of screws are certain complications in hardware failure. Management involves removal of hardware with or without replacement, depending on the amount of bone union and time duration after surgery.
2. *Unanticipated fracture of maxilla*: A occlusal splint with a palatal vault extension is essential to counter this complication.
3. *Hemorrhage*: Bleeding commonly occurs from the descending palatine artery and pterygoid plexus. Injury to pterygoid plexus may happen while performing pterygomaxillary disjunction. This may lead to arteriovenous malformations which may cause life-threatening bleeding 2–4 weeks post-surgery. It needs to be managed with selective embolization. Hemorrhage may occur in patients with undiagnosed bleeding disorders.
4. *Deviated nasal septum*: This can occur when inferior septoplasty is inadequate during superior repositioning of the maxilla. It is managed postoperatively with adjunctive septoplasty.
5. *Damage to apices of teeth*: The horizontal osteotomy should be placed at least 5 mm above the apices of the maxillary teeth to avoid damage to the apices.
6. *Malunion and nonunion*: This can occur if fixation is inadequate fixation or has failed.

Rigid fixation with plates provides the initial stability until bone has united. Bone first unites in the pterygoid region [99]. The most stable maxillary movement is superior repositioning, followed by advancement, and the least stable is inferior repositioning. However, the studies looking at the inferior positioning of the maxilla have been based on the need for bone grafting. Studies have reported relapse rates for maxillary superior repositioning of the maxilla ranges from a mean of 0–18% for the anterior maxilla and 6–7% for the posterior maxilla. Relapse rates for maxillary advancement range from 5 to 15%. As with most orthognathic surgery, relapse is greater with increase in the maxillary advancement. With inferior maxillary repositioning (using bone grafts), there may be 28% anterior relapse and up to 70% posterior relapse [100]. Nonunion is rare and probably associated with failure of the initial plate fixation and poor bony contact. If this persists for greater than 6 months, further surgery with rigid fixation and autogenous bone grafting is recommended [101]. Maxillary advancement and posterior and superior movements are shown to be stable, whereas inferior and transverse movements are unstable [99–110]. The use of autogenous bone grafts and/or hydroxyapatite has been proposed to improve the stability of inferior repositioning of the maxilla [101, 111–117].

7. *Unfavorable aesthetic result*: This results from poor treatment planning or unrealistic patient expectations.
8. *Infection*: Infection may occur in rare cases and is managed with systemic antibiotics with or without placement of a drain and the causative hardware removal. Septic complications have been recorded in 1.1% of osteotomy operations [55].
9. *Dental problems:* As a result of the osteotomy cut, the maxillary teeth lose their nerve supply. Generally, the nerve supply is re-established after 18 months to 2 years [118]. The teeth maintain their viability from the collateral blood supply. Patients should be warned that their teeth and gingivae may be numb for up to 2 years [119]. Osteotomy cuts should be a minimum of 5 mm above the root apices to avoid complications.
10. *Trigeminocardiac reflex (TCR):* The stimulation of trigeminal nerve branches during Le Fort I osteotomy can be a possible cause of the TCR, and transient cessation of the procedure is adequate to allow the heart rate and blood pressure to normalize and dysrhythmia to stop [120].

69.10 Recent Advances (Refer Figs. 66.21 and 78.51)

(a) *Virtual planning in Orthognathic Surgery:* the last decade has seen a tremendous evolution in the field of surgical planning. Computer Assited Virtual Surgical Planning and the use of CAD-CAM designed splints have significantly improved intra-operative accuracy of maxillary repositioning in orthognathic surgery [121].

(b) *Waferless Orthognathic Surgery:* Another technique which has created a paradigm change is the design of custom-fabricated cuttiing stents and patient specific implant for fixation, which help not only perform the osteotomy but also fix the segment in the desired position without the use of occlusal wafers [122].

69.11 Conclusion

The development of modern maxillary orthognathic surgical procedures had diverse historical origins and contributions. With advancement in technique and the introduction of safe hypotensive anesthesia, the Le Fort I osteotomy has been increasingly utilized over the last four decades. Over the years, various modifications of the osteotomies, ORIF methods and bone grafting to the mobilized maxilla, have continued to evolve and progress. The Le Fort I osteotomy of the maxilla is one of the core procedures in orthognathic surgery for the management of facial skeletal deformities. The surgery, often used in conjunction with the bilateral sagittal split osteotomy, is used to correct functional and cosmetic irregularities in all three planes of space and can be utilized in the treatment of a wide range of malocclusions. Traditionally, the surgery has been known for its low technical difficulty and dependable results. Changes in the soft tissue of the nose, lips, and cheeks due to this surgical procedure need due consideration.

The risk of complications is higher in patients with segmental Le Fort 1 osteotomies or anterior movements greater than 9 mm. Efforts to minimize maxillary movement (e.g., with two-jaw surgery) are recommended to reduce complications. An emphasis should be placed on proper pre-surgical orthodontics and solid pre-surgical planning to ensure predictable and stable results. It is also imperative to plan and provide for optimal nutrition as Orthognathic surgery throws up many physiological challenges that may compromise the nutritional status including catabolism, postoperative facial swelling, and increased nitrogen requirements to promote wound healing. The premise of maxillary orthognathic surgery is therefore a multidimensional approach through planning, execution, and postoperative management.

Disclosure Authors have no financial conflicts to disclose. Authors have written consent and reconfirmation from the patients for the use of clinical pictures.

69.12 Case Scenarios

Case Scenario 1 (Figs. 69.28, 69.29 and 69.39a–h)

(A) Chief Complaints

Gummy smile
Long face
Deficient chin
Protruding upper front teeth

(B) Postoperative Result

Competent lips
Normal chin projection
Balanced face

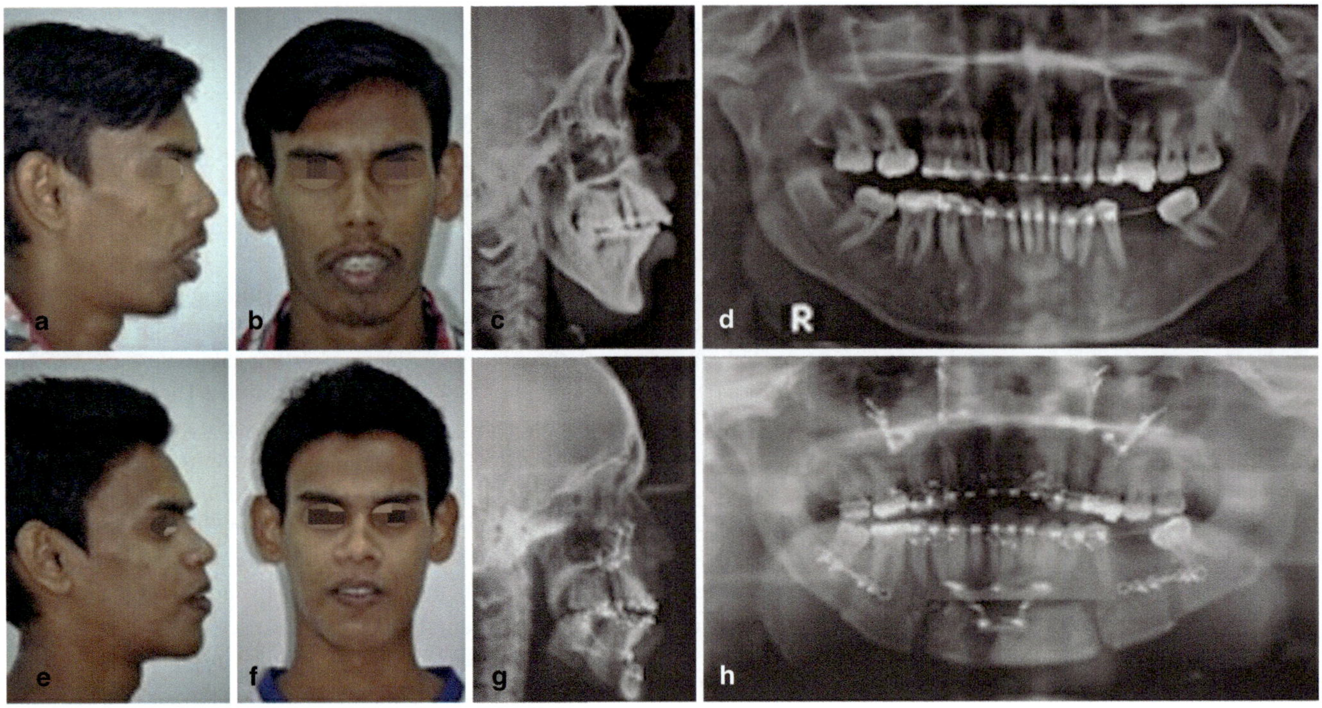

Fig. 69.39 (**a–h**) Vertical maxillary excess with mandibular deficiency. Treatment: Le fort I with superior repositioning of maxilla; bilateral sagittal split ramus osteotomy advancement; advancement genioplasty. (**a**) Pre-operative profile picture; (**b**) pre-operative frontal view; (**c**) pre-operative lateral cephalogram. (**d**) Pre-operative OPG; (**e**) postoperative lateral profile; (**f**) postoperative frontal view; (**g**) postoperative lateral cephalogram; (**h**) postoperative OPG showing the implants and the osteotomy cuts in mandible. (Also see Fig. 69.28)

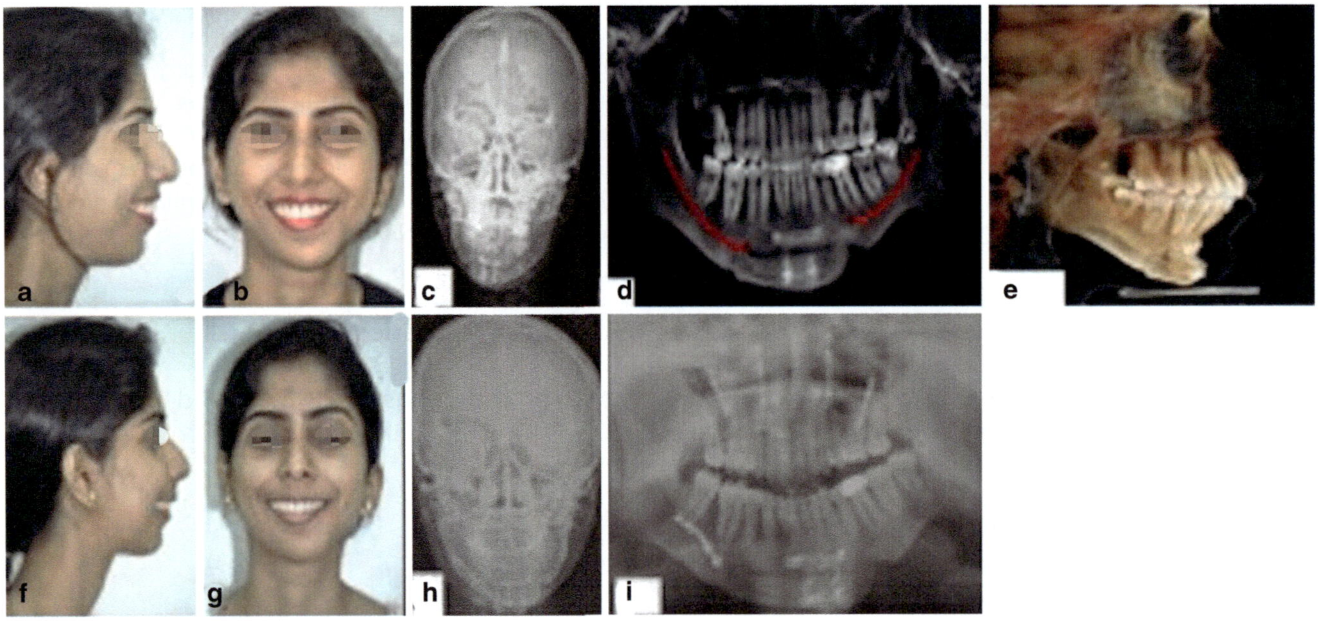

Fig. 69.40 (**a–i**) Facial asymmetry with maxillary occlusal cant, deviation of chin (surgery for left TMJ ankylosis and genioplasty done previously elsewhere). Treatment: Le fort I osteotomy for correction of maxillary occlusal cant; right unilateral sagittal split ramus osteotomy to close the open bite. (**a**) Pre-operative profile picture; (**b**) pre-operative frontal view; (**c**) pre-operative PA skull; (**d**) pre-operative OPG; (**e**) pre-operative lateral cephalogram; (**f**) postoperative profile picture; (**g**) postoperative frontal view; (**h**) postoperative PA skull; (**i**) Post-operative OPG (Also see Figs. 69.30, 69.31 and 69.32)

Surgical Procedure

Le fort I osteotomy for superior repositioning of maxilla

Bilateral Sagittal Split Ramus osteotomy for advancement of mandible

Advancement genioplasty

Later rhinoplasty was done.

Case Scenario 2 (Figs. 69.30, 69.31, 69.32, and 69.40a–i)

Chief Complaints

Facial asymmetry

Deviation of chin to left

Incisal/occlusion cant (Fig. 69.30)

Facial asymmetry was secondary to ankylosis of left TMJ. Left side treated with costochondral graft when patient was younger.

Pre-operative Findings

Occlusal cant

Asymmetry of face

The patient presented with occlusal canting visible at the anterior region. This needed to be addressed as it is clinically evident and may affect visual cosmesis.

Judge the incisal cant by drawing an imaginary interpupillary line and its inclination with incisal cant represented by the metal scale held in incisors

Surgical Plan (Figs. 69.31 and 69.32)

Le Fort I osteotomy for superior repositioning of maxilla on right side by 5 mm

Sagittal split osteotomy on right side of mandible to match mandible to maxilla

References

1. Comte A. The positive philosophy of Auguste Comte. Freely translated and condensed by Harriet Martineau (1855). London: George Bell & Sons; 1896.
2. Von Langenbeck B. Beitrange zur osteoplastik. In: Goschen A, editor. Die osteoplastiche resektion des oberkierers. Deutsche Klinik. Berlin: Reimer; 1859.
3. Cheever D. Displacement of the upper jaw. Med Surg Rep Boston City Hosp. 1870;1:156.
4. Cheever D. Nasopharyngeal polypus, attached to the basilar process of occipital and body of the sphenoid bone successfully removed by a section, displacement, and subsequent replacement and reunion of the superior maxillary bone. Boston Med Surg. 1867;8:162.
5. Moloney F, Worthington P. The origin of the Le Fort I maxillary osteotomy: Cheever's operation. J Oral Surg. 1981;39:731–4.
6. Halvorson EG, Mulliken JB. Cheever's double operation: the first Le Fort I osteotomy. Plast Reconstr Surg. 2008;121:1375–81.
7. Le Fort R. Etude experimentale sur les fractures de la machoire superieure. Rev Chir. 1901;1:208, 260, 479.
8. Le Fort R. Experimental study of fractures of the upper jaw (paper of 1901 translated by Paul Tessier). Plast Reconstr Surg. 1972;50:497–506.
9. Wassmund M. Frakturen und luxationen des gesichtsschädels. Leipzig: Meusser; 1927.
10. Axhausen G. Zur behandlung veralteter disloziert geheilter oberkieferbruche. Dtsch Zahn Mund Kieferheilk. 1934;1:334–9.
11. Wassmund M. *Frakturen und Lurationen des Gesichtsschadels*. Berlin: Meusser; 1927.
12. Axhausen G. Zur Behandlung veralteter desloziert verheilter Oberkieferbrunche. Dtsch Zahn Mund Kieferheilk. 1934;1:334.
13. Schuchardt D. Ein Beitrag zur chirurgeschen Kieferorthopadie unter Berucksichtigung ihrer Bedertung fur die Behandlung angeborener und erworbener Kieferdeformitaten bei Soldaten. Dtsch Zahn Mund Kieferheilk. 1942;9:73.
14. Willmar K. On Le Fort I osteotomy: a follow-up study of 106 operated patients with maxillo-facial deformity. Scand J Plast Reconstr Surg. 1974;12(Suppl 12):11–68.
15. Obwegeser H. Surgery of the maxilla for the correction of prognathism. SSO Schweiz Monatsschr Zahnheilkd. 1965;75:365–74.
16. Obwegeser HL. Surgical correction of small or retrodisplaced maxillae. The "dish-face" deformity. Plast Reconstr Surg. 1969;43:351–65.
17. Bell WH. Biologic basis for maxillary osteotomies. Am J Phys Anthropol. 1973;38:279–89.
18. Aziz SR, Marchena JM, Puran A. Anatomic characteristics of the infraorbital foramen: a cadaver study. J Oral Maxillofac Surg. 2000;58:992–6.
19. Demas PN, Sotereanos GC. Incidence of nasolacrimal injury and turbinectomy—associated atrophic rhinitis with Le Fort I osteotomies. J Craniomaxillofac Surg. 1989;17:116–8.
20. You ZH, Bell WH, Finn RA. Location of the nasolacrimal canal in relation to the high Le Fort I osteotomy. J Oral Maxillofac Surg. 1992;50:1075–80.
21. Cheung LK, Fung SC, Li T, et al. Posterior maxillary anatomy: implications for Le Fort I osteotomy. Int J Oral Maxillofac Surg. 1998;27:346–51.
22. Choi J, Park H. The anatomy of the maxillary artery in the pterygopalatine fossa. Int J Oral Maxillofac Surg. 1999;28(Suppl 1):133.
23. Turvey TA, Fonseca RJ. The anatomy of the internal maxillary artery in the pterygopalatine fossa: its relationship to maxillary surgery. J Oral Surg. 1980;38:92–5.
24. Bell WH. Revascularization and bone healing after anterior maxillary osteotomy: a study using adult rhesus monkeys. J Oral Surg. 1969;27:249–55.
25. Bell WH, Fonseca RJ, Kenneky JW, et al. Bone healing and revascularization after total maxillary osteotomy. J Oral Surg. 1975;33:253–60.
26. Bruneder S, et al. Anatomy of the Le Fort I segment: are arterial variations a potential risk factor for avascular bone necrosis in Le Fort I osteotomies? J Craniomaxillofac Surg. 2018;46:1285–95.
27. Salman S, Fattahi T, Fernandes R, Steinberg B. Dynamic analysis of maxillary perfusion during Le Fort I osteotomy using indocyanine green. Int J Oral Maxillofac Surg. 2018;47:1311–5.
28. Oliveira GQV, Rossi MA, Vasconcelos TV, Neves FS, Crusoé-Rebello I. Cone beam computed tomography assessment of the pterygomaxillary region and palatine canal for Le Fort I osteotomy. Int J Oral Maxillofac Surg. 2017;46:1017–23.
29. Cohn-Stock G. Die Chirurgische Immediatregulierung der Kiefer, Speziell die Chirurgische Behandlung der Prognathie. Vjschr Zahnheilk. 1921;37:320.

30. Wunderer S. Erfahrungen mit der Operativen Behandlung Hochgradiger Prognathien. Dtsch Zahn Mund Kieferheilk. 1963;39:451.
31. Cupar I. Die chirurgisehe Behandlung der Form- und Stellungsveranderungen des Oberkiefers. Ost Z Stomatol. 1954;51:565.
32. Bell WH. Revascularization and bone healing after anterior maxillary ostectomy. J Oral Surg. 1969;27:249.
33. Bell WH. Correction of maxillary excess by anterior maxillary osteotomy. Oral Surg Oral Med Oral Pathol. 1977;43:323.
34. Gunaseelan R, Anantanarayanan P, Veerabahu M, et al. Intraoperative and perioperative complications in anterior maxillary osteotomy: a retrospective evaluation of 103 patients. J Oral Maxillofac Surg. 2009;67:1269.
35. Rosenquist B. Anterior segmental maxillary osteotomy: a 24-month follow-up. Int J Oral Maxillofac Surg. 1993;22:210.
36. Meyer MW, Cavanaugh CD. Blood flow changes after orthognathic surgery: maxillary and mandibular subapical ostectomy. J Oral Surg. 1976;34:495.
37. Epker NB. Vascular considerations in orthognathic surgery: maxillary osteotomies. J Oral Surg. 1984;57:473.
38. Epker NB. A modified anterior maxillary ostectomy. J Maxillofac Surg. 1977;5:35.
39. Haas Junior OL, Guijarro-Martıínez R, de Sousa Gil AP, da Silva Meirelles L, de Oliveira RB, Hernaíndez-Alfaro F. Stability and surgical complications in segmental Le Fort I osteotomy: a systematic review. Int J Oral Maxillofac Surg. 2017;46:1071–87.
40. Rodrigo C. Induced hypotension during anesthesia with special reference to orthognathic surgery. Anesth Prog. 1995;42:41–58.
41. Zellin G, Rasmusson L, Palsson J, et al. Evaluation of haemorrhage depressors on blood loss during orthognathic surgery: a retrospective study. J Oral Maxillofac Surg. 2004;62:662–6.
42. Carlos E, Monnazzi MS, Castiglia YM, et al. Orthognathic surgery with or without induced hypotension. Int J Oral Maxillofac Surg. 2014;43:577–80.
43. Van Sickels JE, Larsen AJ, Triplett RG. Predictability of maxillary surgery: a comparison of internal and external reference marks. Oral Surg Oral Med Oral Pathol. 1986;61:542–5.
44. Ferguson JW, Luyk NH. Control of vertical dimension during maxillary orthognathic surgery. A clinical trial comparing internal and external fixed reference points. J Craniomaxillofac Surg. 1992;20:333–6.
45. Hackney FL, Nishioka GJ, VanSickels JE. Frontal soft-tissue morphology with double V-Y closure following LeFort I osteotomy. J Oral Maxillofac Surg. 1988;46:850–5.
46. Schendel SA, Williamson LW. Muscle reorientation following superior repositioning of the maxilla. J Oral Maxillofac Surg. 1983;41(4):235–40.
47. Newhouse RF, Schow SR, Kraut RA, et al. Life-threatening haemorrhage from a Le Fort I osteotomy. J Oral Maxillofac Surg. 1982;40(2):117–9.
48. Epker BN, Fish LC. *Dentofacial deformities, integrated orthodontic and surgical correction*, vol. 1. St Louis: Mosby; 1986.
49. Epker BN. Superior surgical repositioning of the maxilla: long-term results. J Maxillofac Surg. 1981;9(4):237–46.
50. Maloney F, West RA, McNeill W. Surgical correction of vertical maxillary excess: a re-evaluation. J Maxillofac Surg. 1982;10(2):84–91.
51. Johnson DG. Intraoperative measurement of maxillary repositioning: an ancillary technique. Oral Surg Oral Med Oral Pathol. 1985;60(3):266–8.
52. Nishioka GJ, Van Sickels JE. Modified external reference measurement technique for vertical repositioning of the maxilla. Oral Surg Oral Med Oral Pathol. 1987;64(1):22–3.
53. Posnick JC. 15: Sequencing of orthognathic procedures: step-by-step approach. In: Posnick JC, editor. Orthognathic surgery: principles & practice. St Louis: Saunders; 2014.
54. Bennett MA, Wolford LM. The maxillary step osteotomy and Steinmann pin stabilization. J Oral Maxillofac Surg. 1985;43:307.
55. Kramer FJ, Baethge C, Swennen G, Teltzrow T, Schulze A, Berten J, Brachvogel P. Intra- and perioperative complications of the Le Fort I osteotomy: a prospective evaluation of 1000 patients. J Craniofac Surg. 2004;15:971–9.
56. Aldridge T, Gulati A, Baker N. Theories of acquired blindness following Le Fort 1 osteotomy. Br J Oral Maxillofac Surg. 2013;51:e86.
57. Bays RA, Bouloux GF. Complications of orthognathic surgery. Oral Maxillofac Surg Clin North Am. 2003;15:229–42.
58. Richardson D. Avoiding surgical complications in orthognathic surgery. In: Ward-Booth P, Schendel S, Hausamen J, editors. Maxillofacial surgery. 2nd ed. London: Churchill Livingstone; 2006. p. 1259–74.
59. Breeze J, et al. comReview Is an osteotome necessary for pterygomaxillary dysjunction or dysjunction through the tuberosity during Le Fort I osteotomy? A systematic review. Br J Oral Maxillofac Surg. 2016;54:248–52.
60. Precious DS, Morrison A, Ricard D. Pterygomaxillary separation without the use of an osteotome. J Oral Maxillofac Surg. 1991;49:98–9.
61. Mehra P, Hopkin JK, Castro V, Freitas RZ. Stability of maxillary advancement using rigid fixation and bone grafting: cleft lip versus non-cleft patients. Int J Adult Orthodon Orthognath Surg. 2001;16:193.
62. Muradin MS, Seubring K, Stoelinga PJ, et al. A prospective study on the effect of modified alar base cinch sutures and V-Y closure versus simple closing sutures on nasolabial changes after Le Fort 1 intrusion and advancement osteotomies. J Oral Maxillofac Surg. 2011;69:870.
63. Peled M, Ardekian L, Krausz AA, Aizenbud D. Comparing the effects of V-Y advancement versus simple closure on upper lip esthetics after Le Fort 1 advancement. J Oral Maxiillofac Surg. 2004;62:315.
64. Vercruysse H Jr, et al. The effect of a Le Fort I incision on nose and upper lip dynamics: unraveling the mystery of the "Le Fort I lip". J Craniomaxillofac Surg. 2016;44:1917–21.
65. Lee H-J, Park H-S, Kyung H-M, Kwon T-G. Soft tissue changes and skeletal stability after modified quadrangular Le Fort I osteotomy. Int J Oral Maxillofac Surg. 2015;44:356–61.
66. Issacson R, Ingram A. Forces produced by rapid maxillary expansion: forces present during treatment. Angle Orthod. 1964;34:256.
67. Haas AJ. The treatment of maxillary deficiency by opening the midpalatal suture. Angle Orthod. 1965;35:200.
68. Persson M, Thilander B. Palatal suture closure in man from age 15 to 35 years of age. Am J Orthod. 1977;72:42.
69. Epker BN, Wolford LM. Transverse maxillary deficiency dentofacial deformities: integrated orthodontic and surgical correction. St Louis: Mosby; 1980.
70. Spalding PM. Craniofacial growth and development: current understanding and clinical considerations. In: Miloro M, editor. *Peterson's principles of oral and maxillofacial surgery*. 2nd ed. London: BC Decker; 2004. p. 1051–86.
71. Suri L, Taneja P. Surgically assisted rapid palatal expansion: a literature review. Am J Orthod Dentofac Orthop. 2008;133:290–302.
72. Verquin M, Daems L, Politis C. Short-term complications after surgically assisted rapid palatal expansion: a retrospective cohort study. Int J Oral Maxillofac Surg. 2017;46:303–8.

73. Turvey T. Sequencing of two-jaw surgery: the case for operating on the maxilla first. J Oral Maxillofac Surg. 2011;69:2225.
74. Guymon M, Crosby DR, Wolford LM. The alar base cinch suture to control nasal width in maxillary osteotomies. Int J Adult Orthodon Orthognath Surg. 1988;3:89–95.
75. Betts NJ, Vig KW, Vig P, Spalding P, Fonseca RJ. Changes in the nasal and labial soft tissues after surgical repositioning of the maxilla. Int J Adult Orthodon Orthognath Surg. 1993;8:7–23.
76. Hack GA, de Mol van Otterloo JJ, Nanda R. Long-term stability and prediction of soft tissue changes after LeFort I surgery. Am J Orthod Dentofac Orthop. 1993;104:544–55.
77. Raithatha R, Naini FB, Patel S, Sherriff M, Witherow H. Long-term stability of limiting nasal alar base width changes with a cinch suture following Le Fort I osteotomy with submental intubation. Int J Oral Maxillofac Surg. 2017;46:1372–9.
78. Schendel SA, Carlotti AE. Nasal considerations in orthognathic surgery. Am J Orthod Dentofac Orthop. 1991;100:197–208.
79. Perciaccante VJ, Bays RA. Maxillary orthognathic surgery. In: Miloro M, editor. *Peterson's principles of oral and maxillofacial surgery*. 2nd ed. London: BC Decker; 2004. p. 1179–204.
80. Moenning JE, Bussard DA, Lapp TH, Garrison BT. Average blood loss and the risk of requiring perioperative blood transfusion in 506 orthognathic surgical procedures. J Oral Maxillofac Surg. 1995;53:880–3.
81. Mommaerts MY, Abeloos JV, De Clercq CA, Neyt LF. The effect of the subspinal Le Fort I-type osteotomy on interalar rim width. Int J Adult Orthodon Orthognath Surg. 1997;12:95–100.
82. Betts NJ, Vig KW, Vig P, Spalding P, Fonseca RJ. Changes in the nasal and labial soft tissues after surgical repositioning of the maxilla. Int J Adult Orthod Orthognath Surg. 1993;8:7–23.
83. Lanigan DT, Guest P. Alternative approaches to pterygomaxillary separation. Int J Oral Maxillofac Surg. 1993;22:131–8.
84. Renick BM, Symington JM. Postoperative computed tomography study of pterygomaxillary separation during the Le Fort I osteotomy. J Oral Maxillofac Surg. 1991;49:1061–5.
85. Robinson PP, Hendy CW. Pterygoid plate fractures caused by the Le Fort I osteotomy. Br J Oral Maxillofac Surg. 1986;24:198–202.
86. O'Regan B, Bharadwaj G. Prospective study of the incidence of serious posterior maxillary haemorrhage during a tuberosity osteotomy in low level Le Fort I operations. Br J Oral Maxillofac Surg. 2007;45:538–42.
87. Gustafsson UO, Scott MJ, Schwenk W, Demartines N, Roulin D, Francis N, McNaught CE, MacFie J, Liberman S, Soop M, Hill A, Kennedy RH, Lobo DN, Fearon K, Ljungqvist O. Guidelines for perioperative care in elective colonic surgery: enhanced recovery after surgery (ERAS) society recommendations. Clin Nutr. 2012;31:783–800.
88. Robinson RC, Holm RL. Orthognathic surgery for patients with maxillofacial deformities. Assoc Periop Regist Nurs. 2010;92:28–52.
89. Hoffman GR, Islam S. The difficult Le Fort I osteotomy and downfracture: a review with consideration given to an atypical maxillary morphology. J Plast Reconstr Aesthet Surg. 2008;61:1029–33.
90. Kendell BD, Fonseca RJ, Lee M. Postoperative nutritional supplementation for the orthognathic surgery patient. J Oral Maxillofac Surg. 1982;40:205–13.
91. Olejko TD, Fonseca RJ. Preoperative nutritional supplementation for the orthognathic surgery patient. J Oral Maxillofac Surg. 1984;42:573–7.
92. Chidyllo SA, Chidyllo R. Nutritional evaluation prior to oral and maxillofacial surgery. N Y State Dent J. 1989;55:38–40.
93. Kehlet H. Multimodal approach to control postoperative pathophysiology and rehabilitation. Br J Anaesth. 1997;78:606–17.
94. Fearon KC, Luff R. The nutritional management of surgical patients: enhanced recovery after surgery. Proc Nutr Soc. 2003;62:807–11.
95. Younis J, Salerno G, Fanto D, Hadjipavlou M, Chellar D, Trickett JP. Focused preoperative patient stoma education, prior to ileostomy formation after anterior resection, contributes to a reduction in delayed discharge within the enhanced recovery programme. Int J Colorect Dis. 2011;27:43–7.
96. Aarts MA, Okrainec A, Glicksman A, Pearsall E, Victor JC, McLeod RS. Adoption of enhanced recovery after surgery (ERAS) strategies for colorectal surgery at academic teaching hospitals and impact on total length of hospital stay. Surg Endosc. 2012;26:442–50.
97. Larsson J, Akerlind I, Permerth J, Hornvist JO. The relation between nutritional state and quality of life in surgical patients. Eur J Surg. 1994;160:329–34.
98. Nygren J, Thacker J, Carli F, Fearon KCH, Norderval S, Lobo DN, Ljungqvist O, Soop M, Ramirez J. Guidelines for perioperative care in elective rectal/pelvic surgery: enhanced recovery after surgery (ERAS) society recommendations. Clin Nutr. 2012;31:801–16.
99. Piecuch J, Tideman H, DeKoomen H. Short face syndrome: treatment of myofascial pain dysfunction by maxillary disimpaction. Oral Surg. 1980;49:112.
100. Baker DL, Stoelinga PJ, Blijdorp PA, Brouns JJ. Long-term stability after inferior maxillary repositioning by miniplate fixation. Int J Oral Maxillofac Surg. 1992;21:320.
101. Wardrop RW, Wolford LM. Maxillary stability following downgraft and/or advancement procedures with stabilization using rigid fixation and porous block hydroxyapatite implants. J Oral Maxillofac Surg. 1989;47:336.
102. Proffit WR, Phillips C, Turvey TA. Stability following superior repositioning of the maxilla by LeFort I osteotomy. Am J Orthod Dentofac Orthop. 1987;92(2):151–61.
103. Proffit WR, Turvey TA, Phillips C. Orthognathic surgery: a hierarchy of stability. Int J Adult Orthodon Orthognath Surg. 1996;11:191.
104. Dowling PA, Espeland L, Sandvik L, Mobarak KA, Hogevold HE. Le Fort I maxillary advancement: 3-year stability and risk factors for relapse. Am J Orthod Dentofac Orthop. 2005;128:560.
105. Louis PJ, Waite PD, Austin RB. Long-term skeletal stability after rigid fixation of LeFort I osteotomies with advancements. Int J Oral Maxillofac Surg. 1993;22:82.
106. Nimkarn Y, Miles PG, Waite PD. Maxillomandibular advancement surgery in obstructive sleep apnea syndrome patients: long-term surgical stability. J Oral Maxillofac Surg. 1995;53:1414.
107. Bishara SE, Chu GW. Comparisons of postsurgical stability of the LeFort I maxillary impaction and maxillary advancement. Am J Orthod Dentofac Orthop. 1992;102:335.
108. Bailey LJ, Phillips C, Proffit WR, Turvey TA. Stability following superior repositioning of the maxilla by LeFort I osteotomy: five-year follow-up. Int J Adult Orthodon Orthognath Surg. 1994;9:163.
109. Emshoff R, Scheiderbauer A, Gerhard S, Norer B. Stability after rigid fixation of simultaneous maxillary impaction and mandibular advancement osteotomies. Int J Oral Maxillofac Surg. 2003;32:137.
110. Mogavero FJ, Buschang PH, Wolford LM. Orthognathic surgery effects on maxillary growth in patients with vertical maxillary excess. Am J Orthod Dentofac Orthop. 1997;111:288.

111. Hedemark A, Freihofer HP. The behavior of the maxilla in vertical movements after LeFort I osteotomy. J Maxillofac Surg. 1978;6:244.
112. Ellis E III, Carlson DS, Frydenlund S. Stability of midface augmentation: an experimental study of musculoskeletal interaction and fixation methods. J Oral Maxillofac Surg. 1989;47:1062.
113. Rosen HM. Definitive surgical correction of vertical maxillary deficiency. Plast Reconstr Surg. 1990;85:215.
114. Major PW, Philippson GE, Glover KE, Grace MG. Stability of maxilla downgrafting after rigid or wire fixation. J Oral Maxillofac Surg. 1996;54:1287.
115. de Mol van Otterloo JJ, Tuinzing DB, Kostense P. Inferior positioning of the maxilla by a LeFort I osteotomy: a review of 25 patients with vertical maxillary deficiency. J Craniomaxillofac Surg. 1996;24:69.
116. Chow J, Hagg U, Tideman H. The stability of segmentalized LeFort I osteotomies with miniplate fixation in patients with maxillary hypoplasia. J Oral Maxillofac Surg. 1995;53:1407.
117. Junger TH, Krenkel C, Howaldt HP. LeFort I sliding osteotomy: a procedure for stable inferior repositioning of the maxilla. J Craniomaxillofac Surg. 2003;31:92.
118. Gulabivala K, Naini FB. The orthodontic-endodontic interface. In: Gulabivala K, Ng YL, editors. Endodontics. 4th ed. St Louis: Mosby; 2014.
119. El Deeb M, Wolford L, Bevis R. Complications of orthognathic surgery. J Clin Plast Surg. 1989;16(4):825–40.
120. Kiani MT, Tajik G, Ajami M, Fazli H, Kharazifard MJ, Mesgarzadeh A. Trigeminocardiac reflex and haemodynamic changes during Le Fort I osteotomy. Int J Oral Maxillofac Surg. 2016;45:567–70.
121. Chen Z, Mo S, Fan X, et al. A Meta-analysis and Systematic Review Comparing the Effectiveness of Traditional and Virtual Surgical Planning for Orthognathic Surgery: Based on Randomized Clinical Trials. Journal of Oral and Maxillofacial Surgery: Official Journal of the American Association of Oral and Maxillofacial Surgeons. 2020 Sep. https://doi.org/10.1016/j.joms.2020.09.005.
122. Heufelder M, Wilde F, Pietzka S, et al. Clinical accuracy of waferless maxillary positioning using customized surgical guides and patient specific osteosynthesis in bimaxillary orthognathic surgery. Journal of Cranio-maxillo-facial Surgery: Official Publication of the European Association for Cranio-maxillo-facial Surgery. 2017;45(9):1578–85.

Additional Readings

Laster Z, Ardekian L, Rachmiel A, Peled M. Use of the 'shark-fin' osteotome in separation of the pterygomaxillary junction in Le Fort I osteotomy: a clinical and computerized tomography study. Int J Oral Maxillofac Surg. 2002;31(1):100–3.

Cheng LH, Robinson PP. Evaluation of a swan's neck osteotome for pterygomaxillary dysjunction in the Le Fort I osteotomy. Br J Oral Maxillofac Surg. 1993;31(1):52–3.

Stajcić Z. Altering the angulation of a curved osteotome—does it have effects on the type of pterygomaxillary disjunction in Le Fort I osteotomy? An experimental study. Int J Oral Maxillofac Surg. 1991;20(5):301–3.

Trimble LD, Tideman H, Stoelinga PJ. A modification of the pterygoid plate separation in low-level maxillary osteotomies. J Oral Maxillofac Surg. 1983;41(8):544–6.

Perez D, Ellis E 3rd. Sequencing bimaxillary surgery: mandible first. J Oral Maxillofac Surg. 2011;69(8):2217–24.

Hackney FL, Timmis DP, Van Sickels JE. Esthetic evaluation of frontal labial morphology after double V-Y closure following Le Fort I osteotomy. J Oral Maxillofac Surg. 1989;47(12):1277–80; discussion 1281.

Khamashta-Ledezma L, Naini FB. Systematic review of changes in maxillary incisor exposure and upper lip position with Le Fort I type osteotomies with or without cinch sutures and/or VY closures. Int J Oral Maxillofac Surg. 2014;43(1):46–61.

Facial Asymmetry

70

Neelam N. Andrade, Paul Mathai, and Neha Aggarwal

70.1 Introduction

Physical appearance is of much significance to the humans, as the human mind perceives the slightest form of deviation from normal form, function, and symmetry of the body and especially of the face as it is easily discernible [1]. Facial asymmetry could be defined as a clinically perceptible and significant difference between the two halves of the face. Every individual has some degree of asymmetry which may provide a uniqueness to the face. However, the magnitude and acceptability of the same depend on the location of the asymmetry and the patient's perception of disproportion. Facial asymmetry may also adversely affect the patient's nutritional and psychosocial development [2].

Any abnormality of the soft or hard tissues can lead to asymmetry. This could be a consequence of a congenital anomaly, a developmental, or an acquired defect. Asymmetry can be progressive in nature, while those acquired due to trauma or ablative surgeries are non-progressive [2, 3]. It is prudent for the clinician to consider the aetiology of the asymmetry, the extent, and its severity in all three dimensions in order to provide an optimal treatment plan. Besides, it is important to take into consideration factors such as growth, timing of treatment, and psychological aspirations of the patients when deciding the treatment plan [3, 4].

The present chapter will discuss the etiopathogenesis and classifications, clinical considerations, and diagnosis, evaluation, and treatment planning of facial asymmetries. Few interesting case scenarios will also be discussed for a better understanding of clinical presentations and their management.

N. N. Andrade (✉) · P. Mathai · N. Aggarwal
Department of OMFS, Nair Hospital Dental College, Mumbai Central, Mumbai, India

70.2 Classification

Understanding the etiopathogenesis and classification of facial asymmetry allows for accurate diagnosis, optimal treatment planning, and improved surgical outcomes. Facial asymmetries are most commonly classified according to aetiology or morphology. Other classifications are based on time of onset, structures involved, and surgical planning outcomes and may even be restricted to the mandible alone. Table 70.1 is a summary of the various classification systems available to us today [5–19].

We have identified three classifications that are essential for the evaluation and treatment planning of facial asymmetries [Table 70.2 by Cheong et al. (2011) [13], Table 70.3 by Wolford et al. in (2009) [11], Table 70.4 by Wolford et al. (2014) [2, 19–21]].

70.3 Diagnostic Evaluation

Facial asymmetry is usually the least at the cranial base level and increases toward the lower levels of the face, with the mandible and chin commonly exhibiting the greatest asymmetry. Hence, the cranial base is used as a reference plane for assessing the type and severity of the asymmetry in the middle and lower thirds of the face. Conditions where the cranial base is also involved like syndromic or non-syndromic craniosynostosis, tumors of the cranium, and midface and Tessier's craniofacial clefts cannot be assessed in a routine manner. The presence of orbital dystopia, unequal pupillary heights, and/or unequal ear heights will make the assessment more challenging [2, 20, 22, 23].

Every clinical examination begins with identifying the chief complaint of the patient followed by a detailed physical and medical evaluation of the patient. In order to better understand the facial asymmetry, it is studied in the sagittal, coronal, and vertical dimensions with the cranial base as the reference plane. Common facial planes that represent the

K. Bonanthaya et al. (eds.), *Oral and Maxillofacial Surgery for the Clinician*, https://doi.org/10.1007/978-981-15-1346-6_70

Table 70.1 Summary of the various classification systems

Author	Based on	Classification subsets
Pirttiniemi, 1994 [5]	Time of onset	Pre-natal [further divided into embryonal and fetal] and post-natal
Bishara, 1994 [6]	Structures	Dental, skeletal, muscular, functional, and combination
Lundstrom, 1961 [7]	Etiology	Genetic, non-genetic, and combination
Plint, 1974 [8]	Etiology	Laterocclusion [apparent asymmetry due to occlusal disharmony] and laterognathism [true facial asymmetry]
Chia, 2008 [9]	Etiology	Pathological, functional, traumatic, and developmental
Haraguchi, 2008 [10]	Etiology	Hereditary factors of pre-natal origin and acquired factors of post-natal origin
Wolford, 2009 [11]	Etiology	Pseudo-asymmetry, normal facial asymmetry [non-pathologic], unilateral overdevelopment, and unilateral underdevelopment
Reyeneke, 2010 [12]	Etiology	Congenital, developmental, post-traumatic, and pathology-related
Cheong, 2011 [13]	Etiology	Congenital [pre-natal origin], acquired [injury or disease], and developmental [unknown origin]
Waite, 2012 [4]	Etiology	Congenital [malformation, deformities, and disruptions], developmental [primary and secondary growth deformities], acquired [trauma and pathology], and idiopathic
Obwegeser, 1986 [mandible only] [15]	Morphology	Hemi-mandibular elongation, Hemi-mandibular hyperplasia, combined/hybrid forms
Cohen, 1995 [16]	Morphology	Hemi-hyperplasia [hemifacial hypertrophy], Hemi-hypoplasia [hemifacial microsomia], Hemi-atrophy [Parry Romberg syndrome], and miscellaneous entities [hemi-maxillofacial dysplasia]
Kim, 2014 [mandible only] [17]	Morphology centric surgical outcome	TML system for optimal surgical planning in mandibular prognathism cases only: menton deviation with transverse asymmetry [T], maxillary cant [M], and lip cant [L]
Hwang, 2007 [mandible only] [8]	Morphology	Based on deviation of the chin and bilateral difference between mandibular rami length
Wolford, 2014 [mandible only] [19]	Morphology, imaging, etiology, histology	Restricted to condylar hyperplasia [CH] only: Type 1 CH [prolonged accelerated growth], Type 2 CH [osteochondroma], Type 3 CH [benign tumors other than osteochondroma], and Type 4 CH [malignant tumors]

Table 70.2 Major etiological factors of facial asymmetry, according to Cheong et al. (2011) [13]

Congenital factors	Acquired factors	Developmental factors
Cleft land cleft palate	TMJ ankylosis	Unknown cause
Tessier's clefts	Facial trauma	
Hemifacial Microsomia	Children's radiotherapy	
Neurofibromatosis	Fibrous dysplasia	
Congenital muscular torticollis	Facial tumors	
Craniosynostoses	Unilateral condylar hyperplasia	
Vascular disorders	Parry Romberg syndrome	
Others	Others	

cranial base are the pupillary plane, the ear plane, and the clinical Frankfort horizontal plane. It is also important to note that patients may hold the head in an abnormal position or use hairstyles and mannerisms to mask the extent of the asymmetry [e.g., a patient with a deficient mandible may tip his head upward in order to improve chin projection]. It is important to identify these compensatory mechanisms during the treatment planning process. Similarly, it can be beneficial to study the lower or middle third individually in comparison with the unaffected upper third [cranial base] by blocking out the part not being studied with an opaque sheet [e.g., card board] [20, 23].

70.3.1 Clinical Evaluation: Frontal, Axial, and Profile

Frontal View

The patient's head is positioned such that the interpupillary plane or ear plane [passing through the bottom of the ear lobes or tragi of the ears] is parallel to the floor. The pupillary plane can also be used for assessing bilateral vertical discrepancies by measuring height differences from the plane to the mandibular angles, chin, nose, and commissures (Fig. 70.1). The facial midline is represented by a vertical plane passing through the nasion or glabella, perpendicular to the pupillary plane and ear plane (Fig. 70.2). It allows to compare the degree of left-to-right asymmetry and transverse facial width discrepancies of various facial structures [e.g., orbits, pupils, malar eminences, nose, commissures, and mandibular angles]. In case of some imbalance in the frontonasal region [e.g., past naso-orbito-ethmoidal trauma], other landmarks can also be used as a reference to identify the facial midline, e.g., half the interpupillary or inter-canthal distance, the subnasal point, or the philtrum [20, 22].

Table 70.3 Wolford's classification of facial asymmetry 2009 [11]

	Normal facial	Unilateral	
Pseudo-asymmetry	**asymmetry**	Overdevelopment	Underdevelopment
Occlusal interferences	Genetics	Condylar hyperplasia / Mandibular hyperplasia/Deviant prognathism	Acquired: trauma, infection, TMJ ankylosis, and iatrogenicities [due to tumor resection, radiation, unstable orthognathic procedures and adverse surgical events], failed TMJ alloplastic implants, and failed autogenous tissue grafts
Neuromuscular dysfunction	Intrauterine moulding	Osteochondroma/osteoma	
Habitual posturing	Natural growth variance	Unilateral muscle hyperplasia [masseteric muscle hypertrophy]	
Condylar dislocation		Other benign/malignant tumors	
Temporary unilateral facial swelling due to trauma/infection		Neuromuscular disorders [facial nerve trauma, Bell's palsy, Ramsey-Hunt syndrome, Mobius syndrome, mastoid infections, and cerebral vascular accidents affecting the facial nerve]	Congenital deformities [unilateral cleft lip and palate, hemifacial microsomia, and Treacher Collins syndrome]
			Adolescent idiopathic condylar resorption
			TMJ reactive [inflammatory] arthritis
			Connective tissue and autoimmune diseases

Table 70.4 Wolford's classification of condylar hyperplasia [CH] 2014 [2, 19–21]

CH type	Age at onset	Clinical findings	Imaging	Histology
CH Type 1 [similar to hemi-mandibular elongation]: Type 1A and Type 1B	Puberty	Type 1A Bilateral [BL] or Type 1B Unilateral [UL] accelerated growth; self-limiting; Class 3 occlusion; prognathic mandible	UL/BL elongated condylar head, neck and body; normal condylar head shape	Normally growing condyle; may show chondrocyte proliferation during initial and active phases, with normal bone after growth ceases
CH Type 2 [similar to hemi-mandibular hyperplasia]: Type 2A and Type 2B	Two-thirds of cases begin in 2nd decade	UL vertical elongation of face and jaws; non-self-limiting; ipsilateral posterior open bite; occlusal cant occasionally	Unilateral vertical enlarged condylar head, neck, ramus and body; Type 2A: Enlargement without horizontal exophytic growth of the condyle; Type 2B: enlargement with exophytic growth of the condyle	Osteochondroma; cartilaginous cap similar to that seen in a normal growth cartilage; endochondral ossification; cartilaginous islands in the sub- cortical bone; thickened irregular bony trabeculae
CH Type 3	No specific age	UL facial enlargement	Varies from normal anatomy of condyle; usually presenting as condylar enlargement	Benign tumors, e.g., osteoma, neurofibroma, giant cell tumor, fibrous dysplasia, chondroma, chondroblastoma, and arterio-venous malformation
CH Type 4	No specific age	UL facial enlargement	Varies from normal anatomy of condyle; usually presenting as condylar enlargement with lytic lesions	Malignant tumors, e.g., chondrosarcoma, multiple myeloma, osteosarcoma, metastatic lesion, and Ewing's sarcoma

The patient should be reminded to relax the peri-oral musculature for assessing the tooth to upper lip relation at rest [e.g., patients with vertical maxillary excess will constantly purse their lips to reduce excessive gum and teeth show]. The smile needs to be assessed for the amount of gingival show on either side, tooth to upper lip relation, comparison of dental midline with facial midline and symmetry by comparing parallelism of commissural and pupillary lines. Finally, a tongue blade or thin ruler can be placed between the maxillary and mandibular canines and premolars to assess the presence of a cant in relation to the pupillary plane (Fig. 70.2). Comparing the vertical heights from the pupillary plane to the canine tips on either side can help quantify the cant. An occlusal plane inclination of greater than 4° is said to cause significant perceptible asymmetry.

Assessment of midline structures such as nasal bridge, nasal tip, philtrum, and the chin point should also be carried out. Submental [worm's-eye] (Fig. 70.3) and superior [bird's-eye] views (Fig. 70.4) are very useful in assessing deviation of the abovementioned structures. We can also assess symmetry

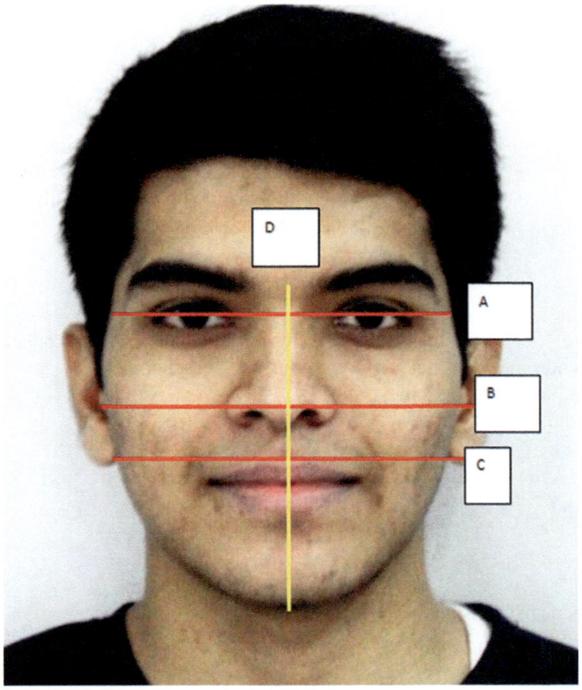

Fig. 70.1 Various facial planes **A** horizontal plane (interpupillary plane) **B** horizontal plane (inter tragal plane) **C** horizontal plane (plane marked through ear lobes) **D** vertical plane (mid-sagittal plane)

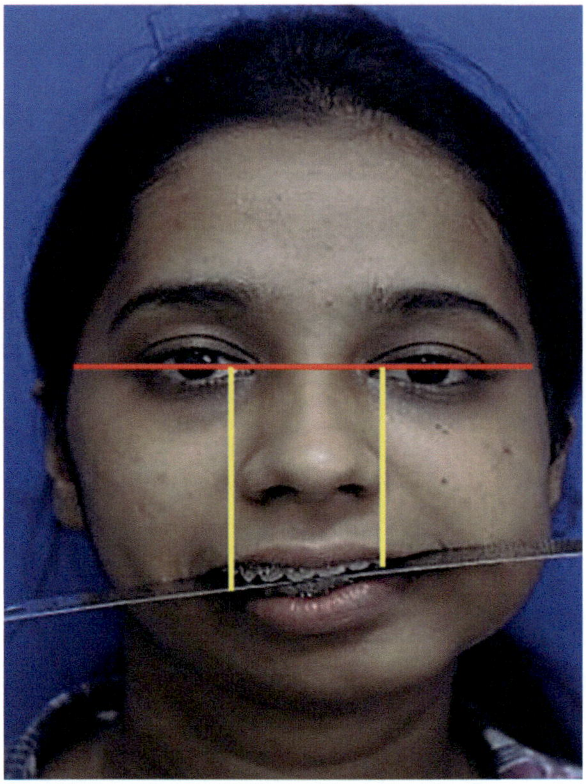

Fig. 70.2 Occlusal cant in relation to the pupillary plane and asymmetry marked from medial canthi to the oral commissure

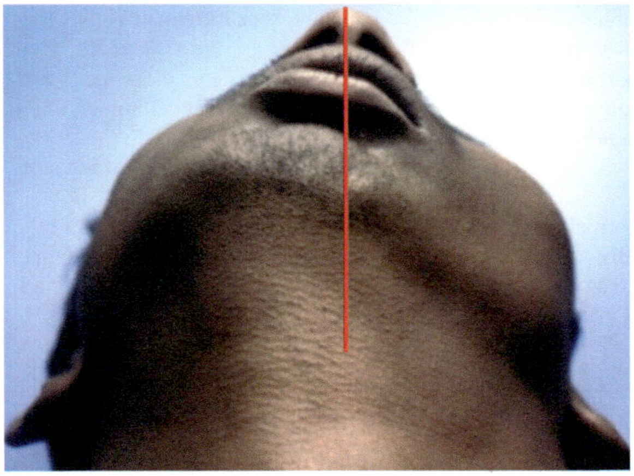

Fig. 70.3 Submental (worm's-eye) view exhibiting asymmetry in the lower facial third and skeletal midline

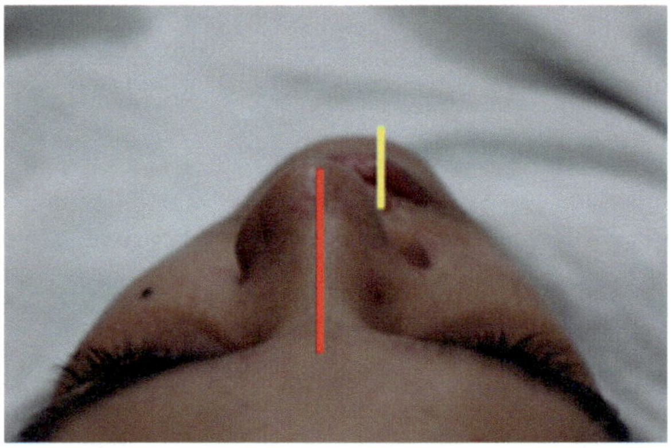

Fig. 70.4 Superior (bird's-eye) view exhibiting midline discrepancy and rotation of the face

and projection of the anterior cranial vault, orbital areas, nose, cheeks, malar eminences, and mandibular body contours.

Profile View

In order to avoid underestimating the severity of the facial asymmetry due to compensatory head postures, it is essential to position the head so that the clinical Frankfort horizontal plane (a line from the tragus of the ear through the palpable bony infraorbital rim) is parallel to the floor (Fig. 70.5). The patient should also be reminded to relax the peri-oral musculature to better assess the tooth to upper lip relation at rest. Evaluating the left and right sides from the profile view will allow assessment of discrepancies in the antero-posterior and vertical dimensions [e.g., maxilla, mandible, and chin] rather than asymmetry evaluation.

70.3.2 Oral Examination

Orthodontic study models mounted in centric relation by face-bow transfer onto a semi-adjustable anatomic articulator help in dento-alveolar and occlusal assessment with a further advantage of studying the occlusion from the lingual aspect. The dental arches are evaluated for overdevelopment, underdevelopment, presence of yaw, and asymmetry in the antero-posterior, transverse, and vertical planes. The dental examination should include the presence or absence of missing, deformed, carious, impacted, or ankylosed teeth; dental midline shift; dental crowding or spacing; congenital deformity [e.g., cleft alveolus in a case of cleft lip and palate]; habitual pattern [e.g., tongue thrusting or thumb sucking]; pathology; and size of tongue and trauma (Figs. 70.6, 70.7, and 70.8). These findings can be incorporated into the treatment planning.

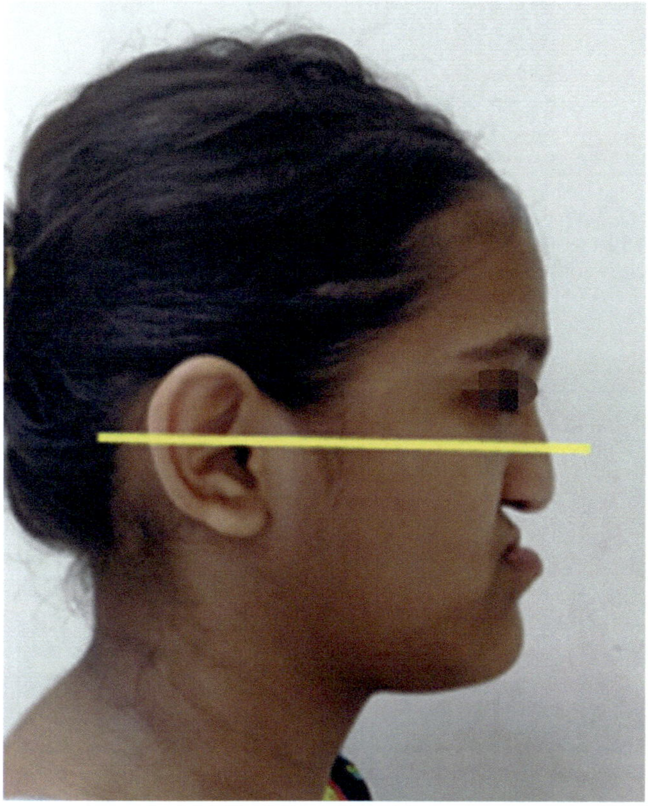

Fig. 70.5 Orientation of FH plane parallel to the floor

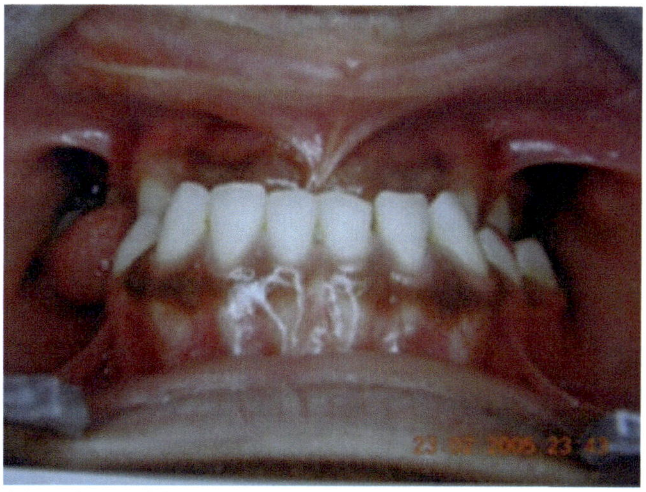

Fig. 70.6 Complete telescoping of the maxilla

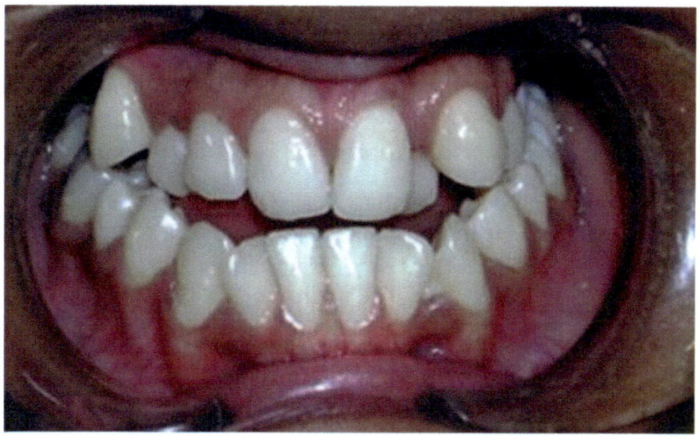

Fig. 70.7 Crowding in both arches along with a reverse overjet

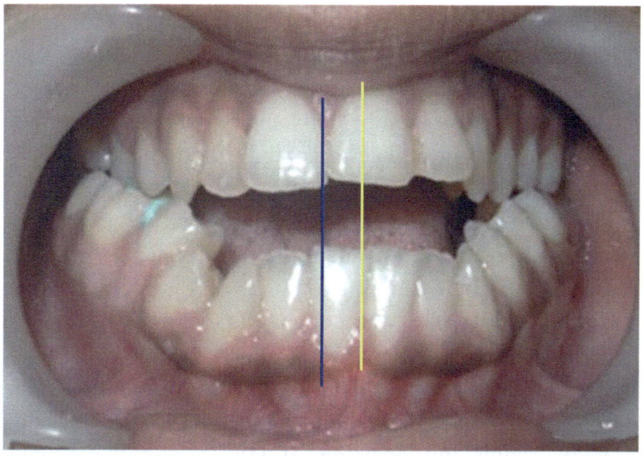

Fig. 70.8 Non co-incident dental midlines (blue-upper dental mid line, yellow-lower dental midline)

70.3.3 Photographic Examination

A dedicated photography room where extra-oral and intra-oral photographs are taken under standardized settings [e.g., lighting, background, focal length, and distance-to-subject] is ideal. Extra-oral photographs of the frontal [with and without smile, occlusal and mandibular inferior border cant], three-quarter, submental, and superior views are essential for the assessment of facial asymmetry. Intra-oral frontal, lateral, superior [45° to the occlusal plane from above], and inferior [45° to the occlusal plane from below] views with the teeth in occlusion are essential for dento-alveolar assessment [11, 23–26].

70.3.4 Radiographic Examination

The three primary radiographic examinations performed in the assessment of facial asymmetry are lateral cephalometry, postero-anterior cephalometry, and orthopantomography. They have been described briefly below. As a rule, serial cephalometric assessment every 6 months for a minimum duration of 1 year may be helpful in determining if the asymmetry is static and stable or if it is progressive [24, 25].

1. Lateral Cephalometry:
   It is used to assess hard tissue and soft tissue relationships in 2D, i.e., antero-posterior and vertical dimensions. This tool is less commonly used to assess facial asymmetry. The head is placed into a reproducible position within the cephalostat with the help of the nasal bridge indicator and ear roads which closely approximates the clinical Frankfort horizontal plane. The patient keep should also be instructed to keep the jaws in centric relation with the teeth lightly touching and the lips slightly parted or relaxed. The ability of the cephalostat to reproduce the near about the same position every time allows for comparative cephalometric analysis and super-imposition of tracings. Bilateral vertical discrepancies [e.g., increased vertical dimension of the body and ramus-condyle unit of the mandible in unilateral condylar hyperplasia type 2] can usually be assessed in a lateral cephalogram. The right and left sides are presented as two separate non-super-imposing lines, and this can be measured as a discrepancy between the two images of the occlusal plane and inferior borders of the mandible (Fig. 70.9).
2. Orthopantomograph [OPG]:
   The OPG is an excellent tool to evaluate mandibular asymmetry and dental status. The anatomy of the condyle—ramus unit, body, and inferior border of the mandible is readily discernible. Increase or decrease in dimensions or changes in mandibular morphology can be studied. In cases of unilateral asymmetry, the affected side can be compared to the normal side. The course of the inferior alveolar nerve can also be assessed and is of vital importance if an inferior border osteotomy is being performed [e.g., inferior border osteotomy in cases of unilateral condylar hyperplasia type 2 where the inferior alveolar nerve might be coursing near the lower border of the mandible] (Fig. 70.10). The OPG is also an excellent tool for the screening of maxillofacial pathology that may cause facial asymmetry, e.g., tumors and fibro-osseous lesions.

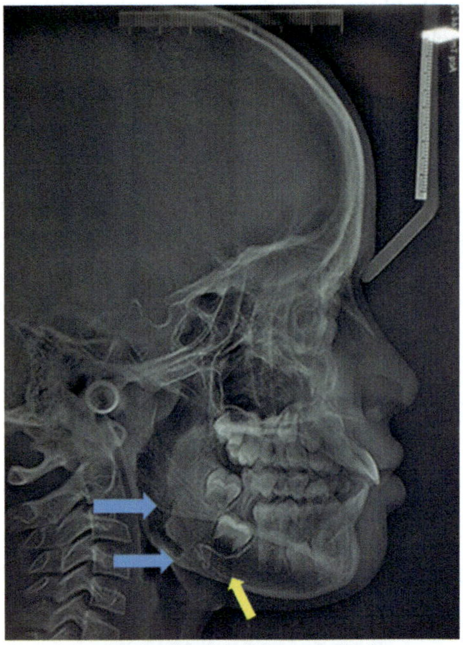

Fig. 70.9 Lateral cephalogram showing double images of the inferior border of the mandible (blue arrows) along with displaced IAN canal (yellow arrow) in a case of type 2 condylar hyperplasia

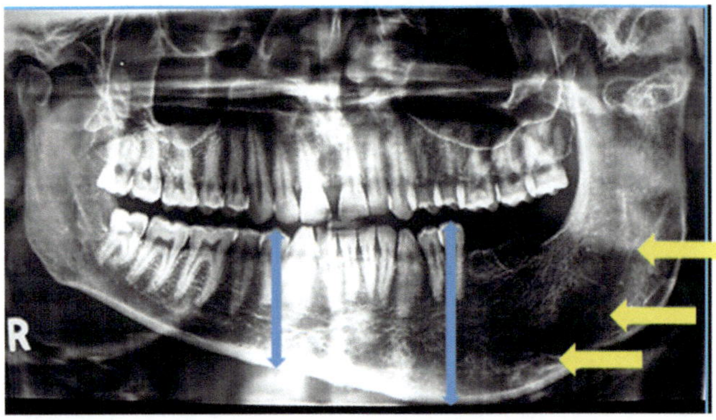

Fig. 70.10 OPG demonstrating the difference in height of the mandibular body (blue arrows), displacement of the IAN canal toward the inferior border (yellow arrows)

3. Postero-antero Cephalometry:
   The PA cephalogram allows a comparative study of the symmetry between the structures of the right and left sides. Projections can be obtained in both open mouth position and centric occlusion with head oriented in natural head position to identify the full extent of static and dynamic [functional] asymmetry. The horizontal reference plane is represented by a line passing through the bilateral zygomatico-frontal sutures. The vertical reference plane is a line perpendicular to the horizontal plane passing through crista galli. Transverse and vertical distances of various facial structures are measured by drawing perpendicular lines drawn from the structures in question to the vertical and horizontal reference planes. By comparing the distances measured bilaterally, the type and extent of the underlying asymmetry can be assessed. Additionally, a shift in the dental midlines can be assessed by comparing them to the skeletal midline. The Grummons and Ricketts analyses are commonly used PA cephalometric analyses for the evaluation of facial asymmetry (Fig. 70.11).
4. Computed Tomography/Cone Beam CT with 3D Reconstruction:
   The main advantage of the 3D CT scan is that it helps in visualization and treatment planning of complex facial asymmetry in cases like craniosynostosis, Treacher Collins syndrome, hemifacial microsomia (Figs. 78.4, 78.5 and 78.6), TMJ ankylosis, and unilateral condylar hyperplasia (Fig. 70.12a, b). Unlike cephalometric and panoramic radiographs, there is no superimposition of structures, the absolute position of anatomical landmarks can be defined, and viewing is possible from any angle. It is also an excellent tool for patient education. The CT scan data can be used for fabrication of stereolithographic

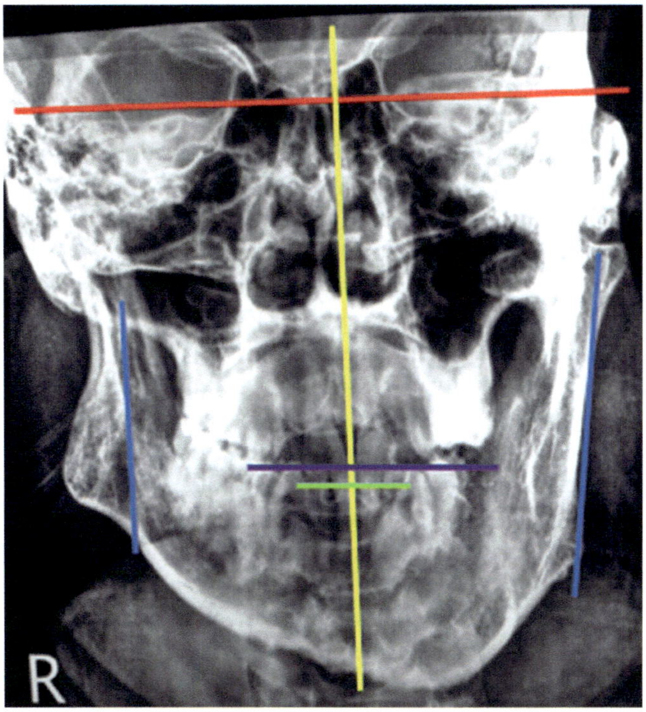

Fig. 70.11 Grummons and Ricketts analysis using PA Cephalogram for evaluating the facial asymmetry. Horizontal reference plane (red); vertical reference plane (yellow); ramal height (blue); intercuspid width (green); intermolar width (purple). Refer to additional reading

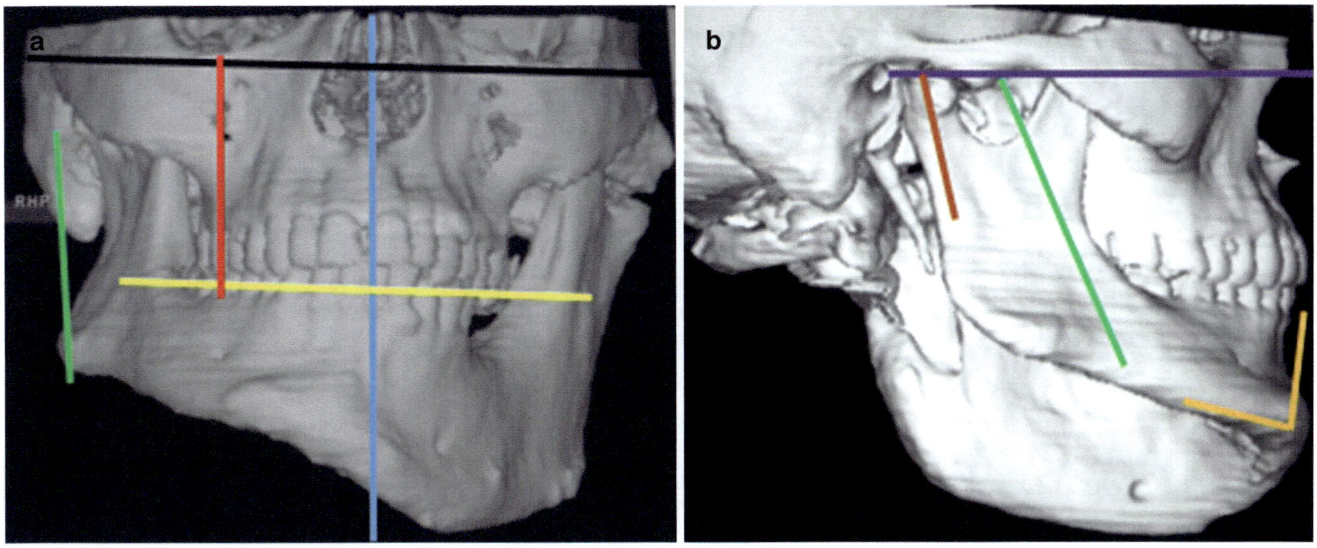

Fig. 70.12 (**a**, **b**) 3DCT face analysis for assessing the facial asymmetry. Various parameters include, Arbitrary horizontal reference plane assuming orbits are normal (black); FH plane (purple); mandibular height [canine to mandibular plane (orange)]; maxillary height (first molar to FH) (red); ramal length (Co superior to Go inferior) (green); occlusal plane (yellow); lateral ramal inclination (Co superior to Go posterior to FH) (brown); midsagittal plane (light blue)

medical models which help make surgical planning even easier. The disadvantage of the CT scan is the exposure to a high radiation dose; with the introduction of the CBCT, the amount of radiation exposure has been greatly reduced. 3D reconstruction, stereolithographic model printing and integration with 3D stereo photogrammetry data allows for treatment planning, treatment simulation, and assessment customized according to the patient [e.g., Dolphin 3D, IPS by KLS Martin]. Lastly, both CT and CBCT provide valuable information regarding the hard tissue status of the TMJ and aid in the diagnosis of reactive [inflammatory] arthritis of the TMJ, osteoarthritis of the TMJ, idiopathic condylar resorption, avascular necrosis, and degenerative remodeling of hard tissues of the TMJ in dentofacial asymmetries [24, 25].

5. Magnetic Resonance Imaging:
   MRI is primarily used to study the soft tissues of the TMJ [e.g., disc, capsule, ligaments] and combined with the CT/CBCT scan data is able to accurately diagnose reactive [inflammatory arthritis] of the TMJ, internal derangements, condylar resorption, and degenerative remodeling of soft tissue of the TMJ in dentofacial asymmetries (Fig. 70.13a, b) [e.g., thinning and displacement of the disc of the contralateral unaffected TMJ in cases of unilateral condylar hyperplasia] [24, 25].

70.3.5 Stereophotogrammetry

It is the construction of a three-dimensional model based on the positions of recognizable points or landmarks in several different photographs. It utilizes two or more cameras configured to capture a pair of stereo images of the surface of patient's face which are then used to generate a 3D image of the face by triangulation performed through sophisticated stereo algorithms. The technique is minimally invasive and has an expanded coverage of close to 360° of the structure being studied with quick capture speeds (often under 1 second). These advantages make it is particularly useful when working with young children [with craniofacial deformities] for whom quantification of facial features can be challenging [25, 26]. The ability to store images for subsequent use, accurate reproduction of the surface geometry of the face, and ability to map realistic color and texture data onto the recorded geometric shape make this technique the preferred facial surface imaging modality over older conventional imaging modalities like laser scanning [26].

70.3.6 Stereolithographic [SLA] Models

Medical modelling involves first acquiring a CT, CBCT, or MRI. This data consists of a series of cross-sectional images of the region being studied. The selected part is now created in a layer-by-layer fashion using photopolymerization ultimately forming a three-dimensional solid. The use of such models in maxillofacial surgery has significantly improved predictability of clinical outcomes in facial asymmetry cases when compared to similar treatments without its use. The models facilitate direct visualization of complex 3D facial asymmetry, decrease operating time due to better treatment planning, and can also be used as an educational tool for patients (Fig. 70.14) [27].

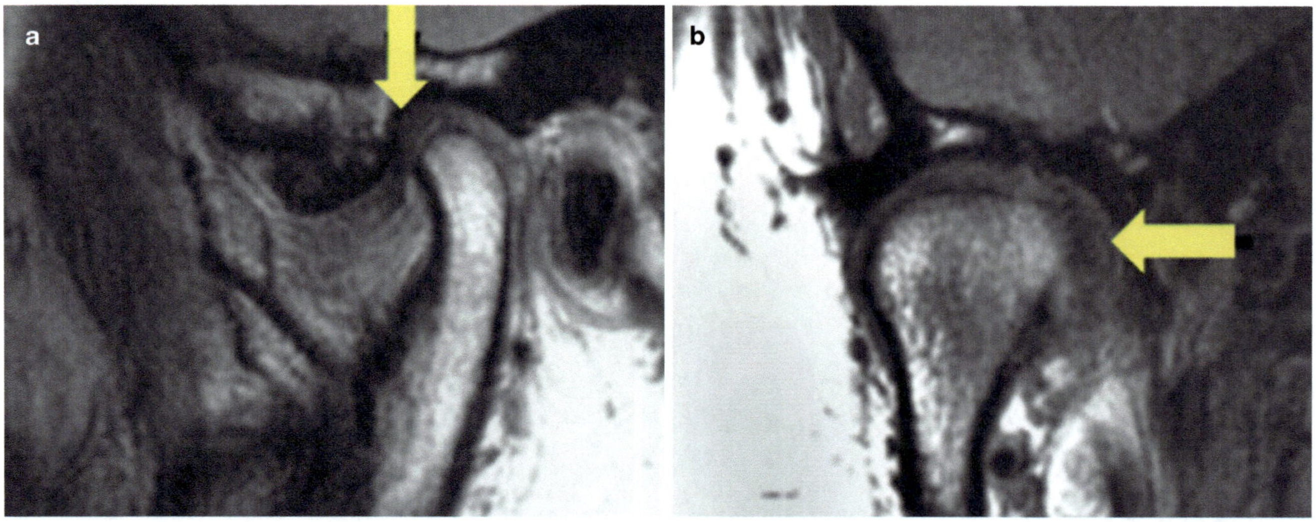

Fig. 70.13 (**a**, **b**) MRI of TMJ showing anteromedial disc displacement (yellow arrows)

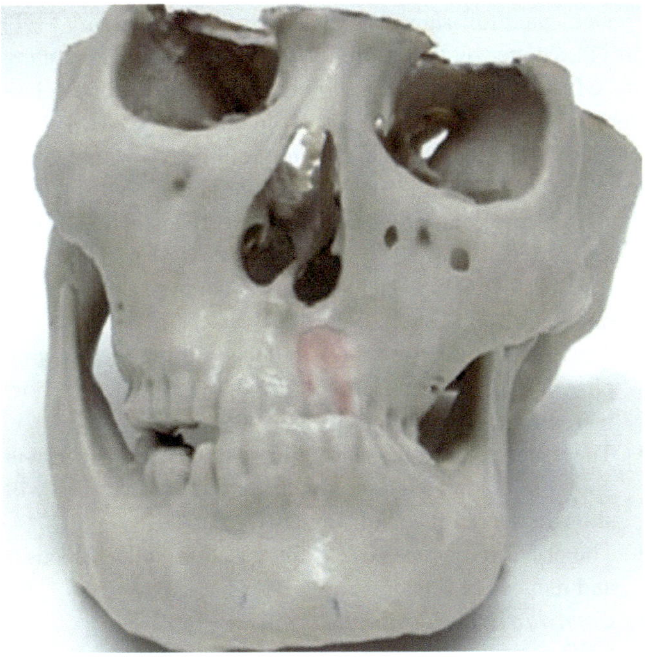

Fig. 70.14 Facial asymmetry demonstrated on STL model involving both the midface and mandible with hyperplasia involving the right side

70.3.7 Virtual Surgical Planning [VSP]/ Computer-Aided Surgical Simulation [CASS]

VSP/CASS involves four key stages demonstrated in Box 70.1.

Figure 70.15 shows the sequence involved in VSP/CASS. The advantages are an increased dental relationship accuracy, reduced OR time, increased patient satisfaction, and decreased costs. Simulating surgery preoperatively allows measurements to the 1/100th of a millimeter, and when combined with 3D-printed splints and customized pre-bent plates, the reconstructive and aesthetic outcome is supe-

Box 70.1 Four key stages in virtual surgical planning

- Data collection and pre-surgical workup
- Virtual treatment planning
- Splint fabrication
- Surgery and accuracy

Data collection and presurgical work-up

Clinical examination
Occlusal record (casts)
Centric relation record
CBCT or CT scan
Final occlusion established by surgeon
Data transfer to planning center
Planning specifics – order from (osteotomy design, order of osteotomy, and anticipated movements)

Virtual treatment planning – web meeting/video conferencing (for sequence of treatment planning)

Natural head position based on clinical examination

Frontal planning – midline/yaw or cant/roll correction

Profile planning – repositioning of central incisor/pitch changes (anteroposterior and vertical)

Occlusal plane changes (clockwise or counterclockwise)

Based on 2-D imaging programs

Yaw/ orientation of proximal and distal segments

Segment orientation/ interferences

Splint design

Surgery

Transfer of virtual planning to operating room

Occlusal splints

Cutting guides to aid in orientation of bony osteotomy

Occlusal borne guides to aid in repositioning of bony segment

Templates to aid in contouring of bone grafts

Predictive hole placement for custom plating of osteotomies

Accuracy

Merger of postoperative scans to virtual plan

CASS more accurate than traditional model surgery

Improved clinical outcomes with CASS

Fig. 70.15 Flow chart outlining the steps involved in virtual surgical planning has been reproduced after permission from the article "Farrell BB, Franco PB, Tucker MR. Virtual surgical planning in orthognathic surgery. Oral Maxillofac Surg Clin North Am. 2014; 26(4):459–73" [28]

rior to traditional 2-dimensional (2D) modelling and cephalometric tracing [28].

70.3.8 TMJ Examination

TMJs must be healthy for predictable orthognathic surgery outcomes. The TMJ must be assessed before and after orthognathic surgery for joint noises (clicking and popping), localized tenderness, radiating facial [e.g., headaches] and neck pain, and limitation of mouth opening and jaw locking. The literature reports a higher incidence of TMD in patients with retrognathic mandibles and in those with steep occlusal planes [29, 30].

There is no conclusive evidence regarding the effect of orthognathic surgery on TMD with opinions split between improvement, no change, or worsening of signs and symptoms. However, high-angle, class II patients with pre-existing TMD undergoing counterclockwise rotation or large mandibular advancement procedures are known to experience worsening of symptoms. Figure 70.16 is the Boston University Protocol for the management of facial asymmetry requiring orthognathic surgery with pre-existing TMD [29].

70.3.9 Nuclear Medicine Imaging Modalities (Scintigraphy)

A bone scan is a nuclear imaging test that involves injecting a small amount radiotracer that into the bloodstream. The radiotracer travels through the area being examined and gives off radiation in the form of gamma rays which are detected by a special gamma camera and a computer to create images of your bones. Thus, skeletal scintigraphy offers the potential to identify disease in its earliest stages as it is able to identify any abnormal increases in metabolic activity [31].

Cisneros first used bone scintigraphy to study mandibular asymmetry in patients [31]. There are two types of bone scan techniques commonly used: skeletal scintigraphy [subtypes: planar bone scanning and single-photon emission-computed tomography] using technetium-99m methylene diphosphate and positron emission tomography [subtypes: with and without CT, full ring and half ring] using radiolabeled 18F-2-fluoro-2-deoxyglucose [glucose analog].

Planar [regular] scintigraphy is not very accurate as it is only a two-dimensional assessment of three-dimensional anatomy. On the other hand, SPECT [single-photon emission computed tomography] allows three-dimensional assessment as the isotope is dispersed in the subject's body thus allowing spatial localization of the pathology in the mapped body organ.

Dedicated/full-ring PET [as compared to half-ring PET] provides better spatial resolution than a planar bone scanning and SPECT (Refer Fig. 78.13) because of its narrower electronic collimation [full width half maximum (FWHM) central resolution for PET being 6 mm compared with 11 mm for SPECT] [21, 32, 33]. As the condylar growth plate is thin, PET gives an advantage to identify pathologies like condylar hyperplasia.

Important factors to be taken into account when assessing a bone scan:

- The efficacy of bone scan is reduced during the growing phase as condyles are growth centers and both will show increased metabolic activity.
- The efficacy of bone scan is increased after the growth phase is completed as only the affected condyles will show increased metabolic activity.
- The efficacy of bone scan is increased in unilateral cases and reduced in bilateral cases.
- *Condylar Hyperplasia Type 1*
  - The growth in type 1 condylar hyperplasia is only slightly faster than the normal condylar growth rate. Therefore, the difference in intensity of radiotracer uptake between a normal and affected condyle is negligible.
  - The cellular growth activity is confined to a narrow band at the normal growth center resulting in low uptake of the radiotracer.
  - Condylar hyperplasia type 1A cases: It is difficult to differentiate CH type 1A from normal growth as it a bilateral condition with both joints involved.
  - Condylar hyperplasia type 1B cases: As this is a unilateral condition, it is easy to identify clinically. There has to be a difference in activity of at least 10% between the affected side and the normal side for a diagnosis of asymmetric growth activity/unilateral condylar involvement to be made.
- *Condylar Hyperplasia Type 2*
  - It is easy to diagnose on the bone scan as it is usually a unilateral condition with a tumorous rate.
  - There is diffuse cellular activity throughout the tumor in the condylar head which makes it easier to diagnose on the bone scan.

70.4 Clinical Considerations

70.4.1 Occlusal and Orthodontic Considerations

Asymmetries with congenital and developmental etiology are commonly associated with dental compensations in all three dimensions as growth ensues. Rotations and crowding are

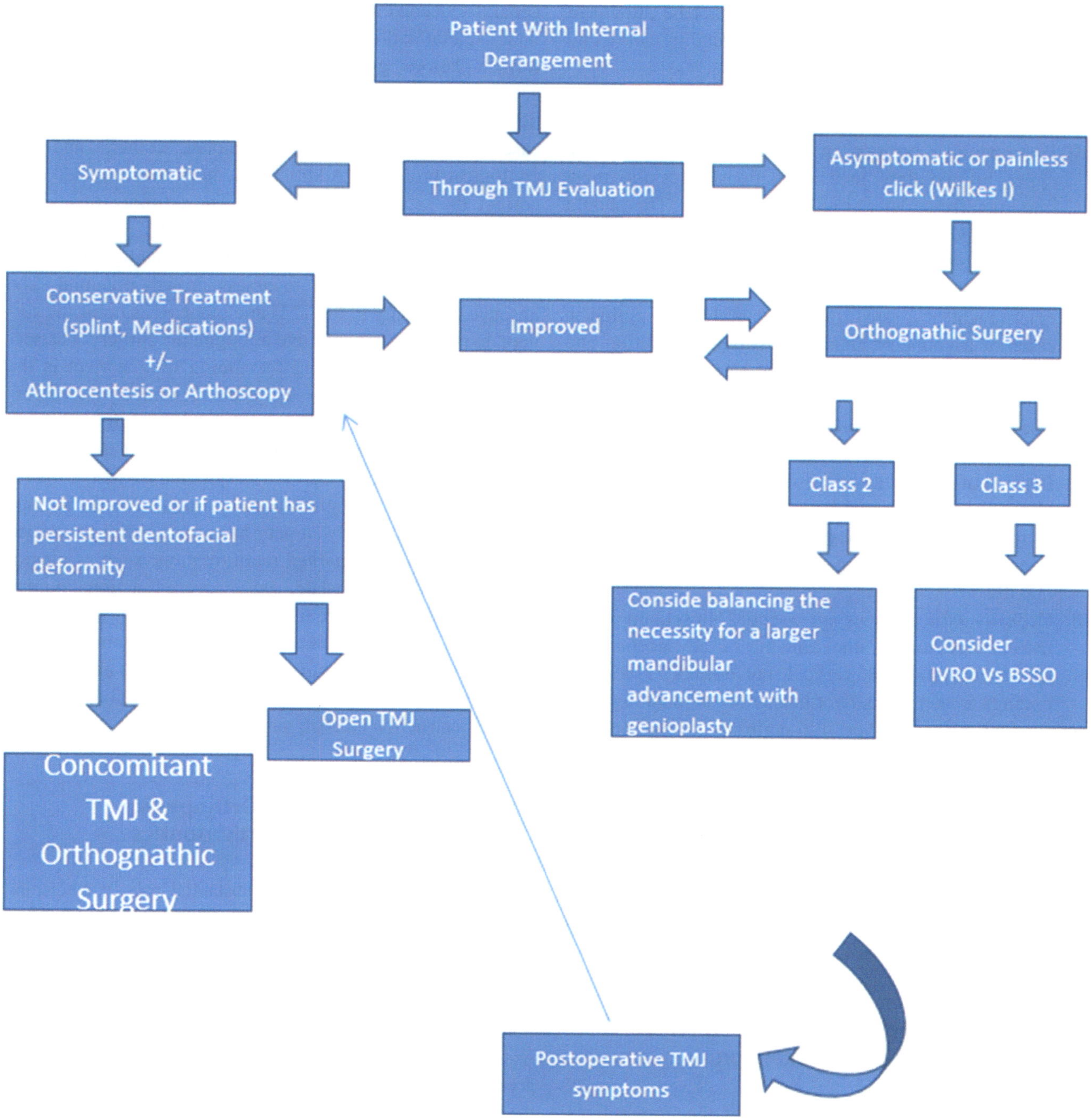

Fig. 70.16 The flow chart outlines the Boston University Protocol for the management of temporomandibular disorders in patients who present for orthognathic surgery and has been reproduced from the article "Nadershah M, Mehra P. Orthognathic Surgery in the Presence of Temporomandibular Dysfunction. What Happens Next? Oral Maxillofac Surg Clin North Am. 2015; 27(1):11–26" [29]

seen in hypoplasia cases such as hemifacial microsomia, and spacing and cross bites can be encountered in case of overdevelopment such as condylar hyperplasia. Transverse growth discrepancies also result in different arch shapes and Bolton discrepancy. Also, the extent of maxillary asymmetry should be accounted for, as maxilla tends to be ignored in obvious mandibular asymmetry. Thus, pitch, yaw, and roll need to be adjusted or decompensated keeping the surgical movement in mind [34]. Pre-surgical orthodontic treatment in patients with facial asymmetry must include the following:

(a) The presence of a dental and facial midline mismatch indicates a discrepancy in the yaw of the affected jaw[s]. Midline correction at the time of orthognathic surgery provides the best results.

(b) Any occlusal cant correction should not be attempted orthodontically. Cant is evidently skeletal in nature and should be corrected surgically.
(c) Levelling and alignment of the dental arches should be done.
(d) Post-operative position of the upper incisor and the upper lip-maxillary incisor relationship is the most important factor determining surgical result. This should be checked intra-operatively before fixation of the maxilla.
(e) Position of the symphysis similarly is another important determinant of a satisfactory postsurgical correction in cases of asymmetry; thus the anatomical position and surgical limits of symphysis correction should be determined pre-surgically.
(f) The facial midline reference should be taken from the unaffected jaw.
(g) In cases of hemifacial microsomia and temporomandibular joint ankylosis, a unilateral open bite is created after increasing the ramus height. This is done to correct the skeletal cant by allowing the vertical alveolar growth of maxilla.
(h) Cephalometric analyses are essential but seldom definitive in determining the amount of advancement in antero-posterior and vertical movements. Prediction tracings are helpful but not mandatory in planning post-surgical outcome. Specific norms available are not always applicable especially in asymmetry cases as the etiology is variable. The etiology and duration of asymmetry influence the extent and severity of the case.
(i) Based on the severity of crowding, the amount of retraction and uprighting needed; upper second bicuspid extraction [minimal decompensation] or upper first bicuspid extraction [greater decompensation] is indicated.

70.4.2 Growth and Development of the Craniofacial Skeleton

Importance of understanding growth of the maxillofacial skeleton in an individual presenting with asymmetry cannot be emphasized enough. Almost half of the asymmetries are either due to an underdevelopment or an overdevelopment of the TMJ resulting in a deviated mandible in the vertical or antero-posterior direction or both of the involved side or the contralateral side. If this development takes place in the growing period, the maxilla follows the deviation of the mandible. Interceptive orthodontics can be applied in growing areas to arrest or limit the extent of asymmetry of the maxilla and mandible [35]. However, surgical intervention is generally needed after completion of growth period for the final skeletal and dental correction. Surgical treatment performed before growth completion is unpredictable on account of the continual growth that the patient experiences till skeletal maturity and as such is reserved only for those cases suffering from extreme functional, aesthetic, and psychological problems. Additional surgery may be needed to correct the recurrent asymmetry. Thus, timing of surgery relies very much on the growth completion.

Serial cephalometric radiographs, scintigraphy, and SPECT scans are useful to assess growth potential. The absence of activity in the TMJ and other areas helps the surgeon to proceed for corrective orthognathic surgery. The second factor for determining the timing of treatment is the progression of the asymmetry. If the asymmetry is progressive like condylar hyperplasia, it is better to wait or perform high condylectomy to check any further asymmetric growth. On the contrary, non-progressive asymmetries such as hemifacial microsomia, treatment can be initiated in early years [36]. Comparably, early surgery has usually been performed for individuals with marked malformations such as plagiocephaly, cleft lip and palate, and/or severe functional burden (e.g., increased intracranial pressure, severe obstructive sleep apnea, etc.). Lastly, in few cases of acquired asymmetry such as tumor resection, "wait-and-watch" policy needs to be adopted to eliminate chances of recurrence before a definitive reconstruction can be planned.

70.4.3 Role of Functional Orthopedics and Interceptive Orthodontics

Functional orthopedics play a substantial role in congenital asymmetries, the greatest example being nasoalveolar molding in cleft lip and palate cases to bring the maxillary segments into a more desirable position prior to surgery. Growth modification with the use of functional appliances is directed toward eruption of the dentition in a more favorable position and prevents worsening of the skeletal asymmetry exacerbated during growth period. Functional therapy is also aimed at maintaining the condyle in a more anatomical position to allow further growth in a symmetrical pattern. Studies have shown that an asymmetric lateral force during the growth period results in growth modification by influencing the morphology of the mandibular bone and the overlying masseter muscle. Occlusal splints can be fabricated to allow for mandibular shifts toward midline, and open bite can be created to eliminate canting. This is especially helpful in hemifacial microsomia and TMJ ankylosis cases. Patient compliance is a prerequisite in functional therapy cases. Also, keeping in view the growth potential, long-term follow-up is always warranted.

70.4.4 Role of TMJ and Considerations for Treatment

TMJ is the driving force in the development of an asymmetry. Although the role of condylar cartilage has been proved to be secondary in mandibular growth and development, any pathological change leading to under- or overdevelopment can cause severe progressive asymmetry. As mentioned, TMJ-related asymmetries can be categorized as underdevelopment or overdevelopment of the condyle and in some cases both. Pseudo-asymmetry occurs due to lateral shifts on account of dental pre-maturities. Kaban and Pruzanksy have also graded hemifacial microsomia (Refer Chap. 78) based on the anatomy of the ramus condyle unit [RCU] and the glenoid fossa which make up the TMJ [36, 37]. Management of the TMJ pathology should be performed initially following which any skeletal correction should be attempted. Failure to do so has led to relapse due to the unpredictability of TMJ behavior and growth. Clinical and diagnostic imaging should be performed prior to any asymmetry correction to assess the status of TMJ. CT scans are a must for assessment in all three axes, as TMJ tumors like osteochondroma may not be discernible on 2D imaging. High or low condylectomy, ankylosis release, and RCU reconstruction should be done prior or simultaneously with orthognathic surgery. Distraction osteogenesis has also been used for neo-condyle formation. Alloplastic reconstruction of the TMJ is the most recent advancement with stable long-term results. The rationale for TMJ reconstruction is to provide a functional stable and reproducible movement which is harmonious with the stomatognathic system. Asymmetrical patients have also been found to have a higher incidence of condylar morphological changes and temporomandibular disorders on the affected side. Over time, due to the imbalance of masticatory loads and poor jaw function, the TMJ of the unaffected side also displays similar pathological changes [38].

70.5 Treatment Planning

Following issues need to be considered before planning orthognathic surgery (Box 70.2):

Box 70.2 Issues that need to be considered before planning orthognathic surgery

1. Single jaw versus bi-jaw surgery
2. Mandible first versus maxilla first approach
3. Surgery first approach
4. Traditional planning versus virtual planning
5. Modifications in surgical technique for asymmetry cases

70.5.1 Single Jaw Versus Bi-Jaw Surgery

Facial asymmetries are rarely corrected by single jaw surgery. When the amount of discrepancy is excessive, it is best treated by dividing the overjet as well as the cant between the two jaws to achieve optimal results. During growth in congenital and developmental cases, maxilla follows and is equally involved as the mandible. Thus, it is prudent to do a bi-jaw surgery. Also, in cleft maxillary hypoplasia cases, differential maxillary advancement with simultaneous setback is the treatment of choice. We have presented a case where simultaneous maxillary distraction was done with mandibular setback. Owing to the presence of a cleft, maxilla has severely deviated midline with an extreme reverse overjet. In such cases, maxillary distraction allows slowly advancing the maxilla and simultaneously correcting the midline by distracting more on the deficient side [39] (Fig. 70.17a–c). Segmental osteotomies or differential surgically assisted rapid palatal expansion (SARPE) might also be needed in some cases to correct transverse asymmetry (Fig. 70.18a–c). Additionally, bone contouring of the mandible and zygoma may be needed to reduce the hyperostotic bone to achieve a harmonious facial contour. This is true in case of hemifacial hypertrophy and hemi mandibular hyperplasia. Similarly, additional augmentation of paranasal areas, malar prominence, and angle of mandible augmentation are frequently indicated in hypoplasia cases.

70.5.2 Mandible First Versus Maxilla First Approach

Either of the surgical sequences can produce similar outcomes when properly planned and executed in the vast majority of bimaxillary cases. Mandible first approach is specially mentioned here as it is important in Class 3 asymmetries. Firstly, in cases where maxilla may be hypoplastic, especially in the syndromic cases of mandibular hyperplasia, rigid fixation of maxilla and down-grafting may not give stable results. Thus mandible should be fixed first, then maxilla. Secondly, because of differential load on the TMJ, CO-CR discrepancy exists, and it is difficult to achieve a stable centric. In such cases fixing the mandible first is beneficial [40]. Lastly, Class 3 asymmetries are associated with concomitant TMJ pathologies, hence TMJ surgeries such as high condylectomy may be needed to be performed simultaneously, in such cases, and mandible first approach is generally the preferred choice.

70.5.3 Surgery First Approach (Refer Chap. 67)

The surgery first approach [SFA] came about as there was a need for immediate aesthetic improvement with shortening of the overall duration of treatment. However, it should be known that not all cases fulfil the criteria for SFA [e.g., flat curve of Spee and minimal crowding and rotations]. The total treatment duration can be shorter than the conventional three-staged surgical orthodontic treatment owing to the lack of need of pre-operative orthodontics and the subsequent post-surgical "regional acceleratory phenomenon." However, reliability of SFA is still questionable, especially in more complex dentofacial deformities, like facial asymmetry.

Park et al. reported no significant differences in postoperative stability between SFA and OFA after bimaxillary surgery in skeletal class III malocclusion patients [41]. In SFA, vertical dimension in surgical occlusion can increase due to occlusal interference and lead to postoperative counter clockwise rotation of the mandible as occlusal settling progresses during the postoperative orthodontic period. This may contribute toward greater postoperative mandibular forward movement.

70.5.4 Modifications in Surgical Technique for Asymmetry Cases

The bilateral sagittal split osteotomy is the commonly used technique in asymmetry cases. It is highly flexible and adaptable in all movements. The three-dimensional anatomy of the mandible must be retained when planning a BSSO. According to Schwartz, three types of surgical move-

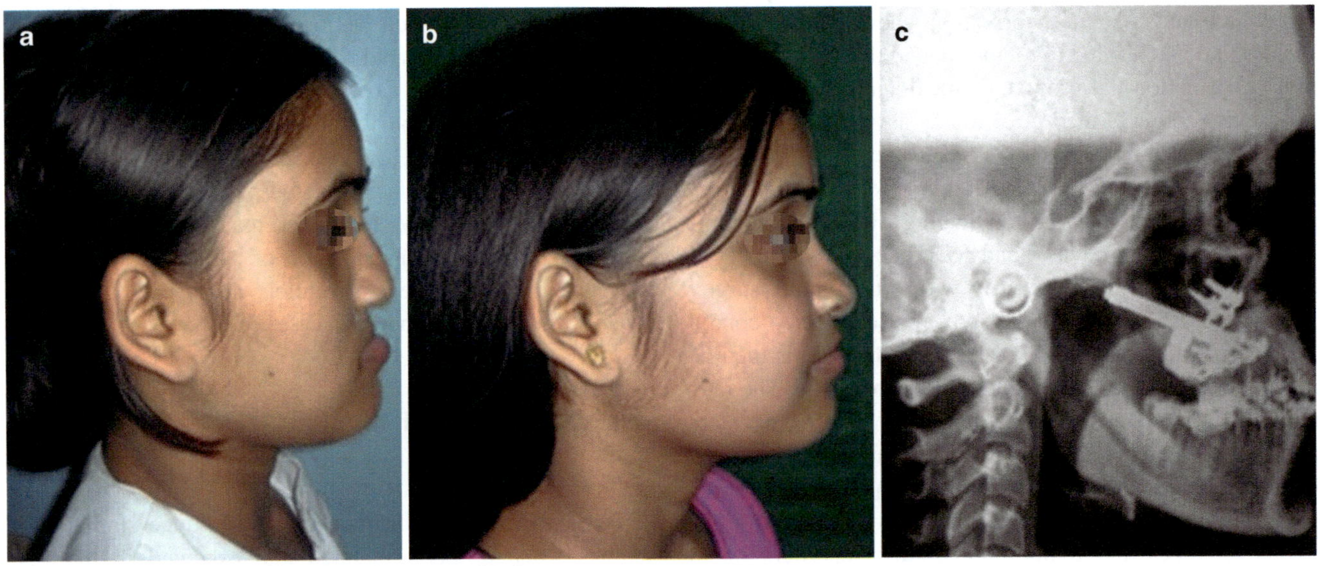

Fig. 70.17 Case of cleft maxillary hypoplasia who underwent maxillary distraction using internal device. (**a**) Pre-operative profile photo showing retruded midface, (**b**) post-operative profile photo showing good midface fullness, (**c**) post-distraction lateral cephalogram showing distractor in-situ

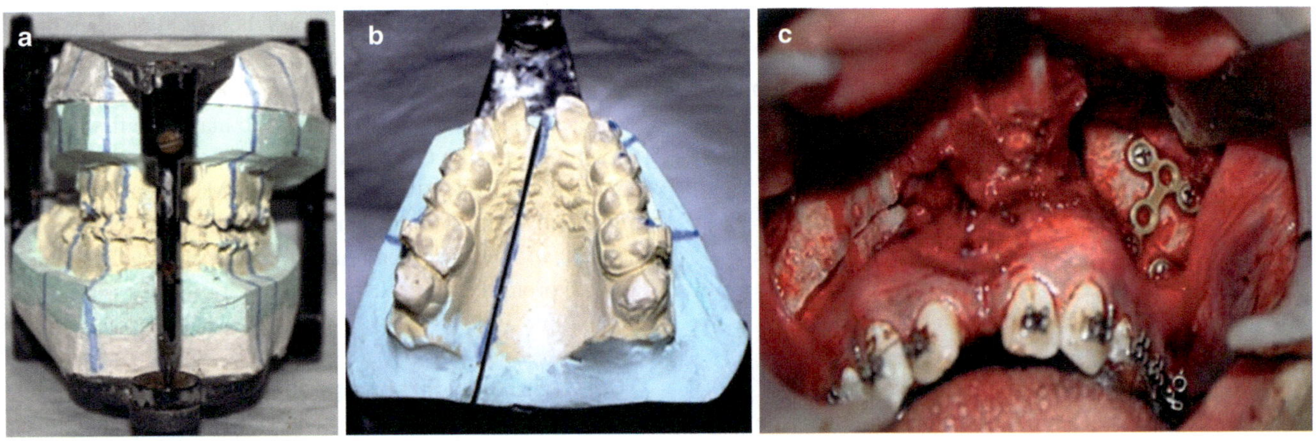

Fig. 70.18 (**a**) View of the maxillary study model. (**b**) Osteotomy cut marked for SARPE. (**c**) Fixation done using miniplate only on left side. This is done to ensure expansion of the only the right side on activation of appliance

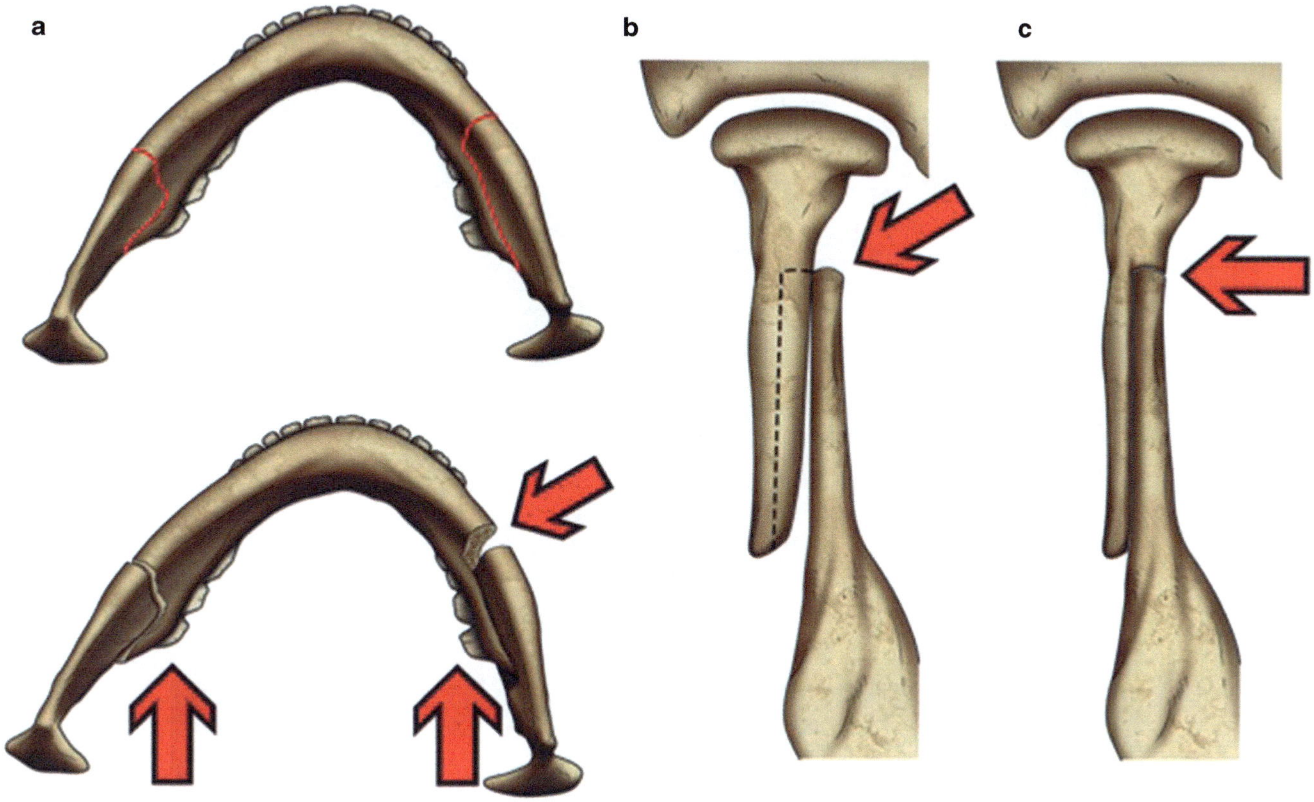

Fig. 70.19 (**a**) When an asymmetric case is viewed along the vertical axis, areas that require immediate bone removal become obvious. Heavy interferences will take place anteriorly on the long side and posteriorly on the short side; (**b**) After the condyle is seated, premature bone contact is noted posteriorly. The area proposed for additional bone removal is indicated by the dotted line; (**c**) Good bone contact has been achieved. Image Source: Schwartz HC. Efficient surgical management of mandibular asymmetry. J Oral Maxillofac Surg. 2011 Mar;69(3):645–54. doi: 10.1016/j.joms.2009.03.009. Epub 2010 Oct 8. PubMed PMID: 20934795 [42]

ments can be planned with BSSO in asymmetry cases: in case of a normal overjet and overbite, differential movements will be made that is setback on the long side and advancement on the short side. In Class II asymmetry, in order to achieve symmetrical advancement, there will be a longer advancement on the short side than on the long side and lastly in Class III cases, there will be a larger setback on the long side than on the short side. During surgery, the distal segment rotates from the short side to the long side as the midline is corrected (Fig. 70.19a). Selective bone removal from the area of interferences should be done before the distal segment has been passively repositioned. Bone is removed from the anterior and medial aspects of the proximal segment until there is broad contact along segments. On the short side, first contact will occur posteriorly [42]. Bone is removed from the medial aspect of the proximal segment posteriorly (Fig. 70.19b, c). This is done to reduce condylar torque during rigid internal fixation to ensure stability of the movement. Figures 70.20a–d and 70.21a, b show a case of unilateral condylar elongation treated with differential BSSO.

70.5.5 Soft Tissue Interventions

The asymmetrical growth of soft tissues may lead to residual soft tissue asymmetry even after correction of the underlying bony deformity. Furthermore, some asymmetrical craniofacial regions cannot be corrected by means of conventional surgical techniques. Adjunctive soft tissue procedures [e.g., dermis fat transplant, autologous fat transfer, microvascular adipose free flaps] might be indicated to achieve bulk in deficient soft tissue deformities such as Parry Romberg syndrome, TMJ ankylosis, etc. Alloplasts such as Medpore, silicone, nanogels, tissue expander, etc. have also been used with varying degrees of success (Sect. 70.7 "Case Scenarios").

70.5.6 Distraction Osteogenesis (Also refer Chap. 87)

Distraction osteogenesis is the process of native bone formation via traction of osteotomized segments. On account of distraction histogenesis, simultaneous soft tissue and

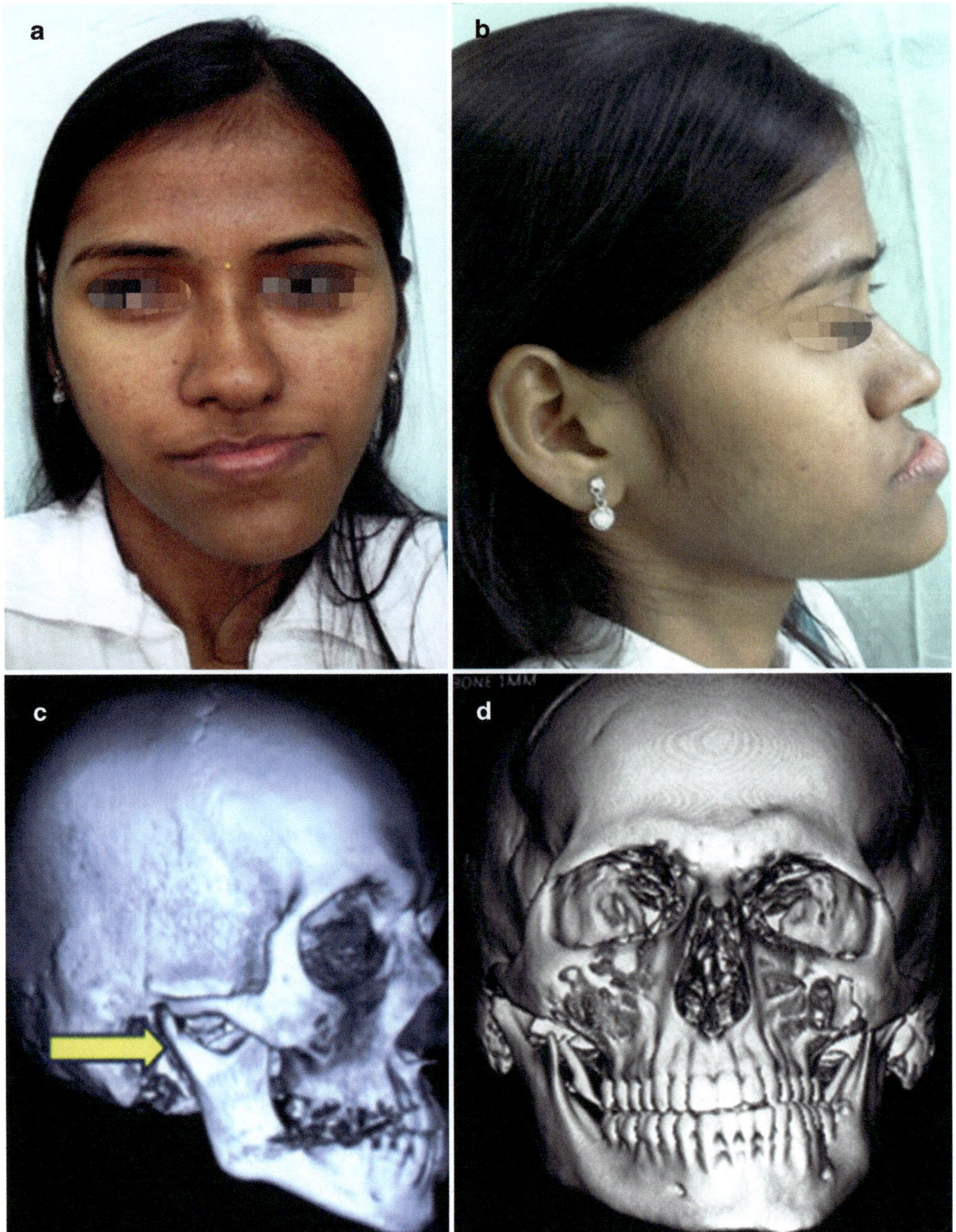

Fig. 70.20 (**a–d**) Clinical and radiographic images showing a case of image showing severe facial asymmetry with unilateral condylar elongation on the right side. (**a**) frontal photo, (**b**) profile photo, (**c, d**) lateral and frontal views on volume rendered 3D CT scan

hard tissue augmentation can be achieved. Adequate amounts of advancements can be achieved without any soft tissue limitations. Various cases have been treated successfully with DO that are presented in this chapter. DO has various advantages over conventional osteotomies in complex facial asymmetries. Pre-arthroplastic distraction in ankylosis-related asymmetries has been reported to have excellent results [43]. This is because simultaneous distraction of skin, muscle, and tissue takes place with bone regeneration. Thus, better esthetics are achieved without any need for additional soft tissue procedures. Distraction is often the only procedure of choice in large advancements, rate of relapse is significantly lower, and results are much stable. Figures 70.22a–e, 70.23a, b, 70.24a–d and 70.25a–g show a case of facial asymmetry secondary costochondral graft resorption in a case of TMJ ankylosis, treated with stage one distraction osteogenesis followed by definitive correction with BSSO.

(Also refer Figs. 78.43, 78.44, 78.45, 78.46, 78.47, 78.48, 78.49, 78.50, 78.51, 78.52, and 78.53 for management of facial asymmetry cases due to Hemifacial microsomia and Traecher Collins syndrome).

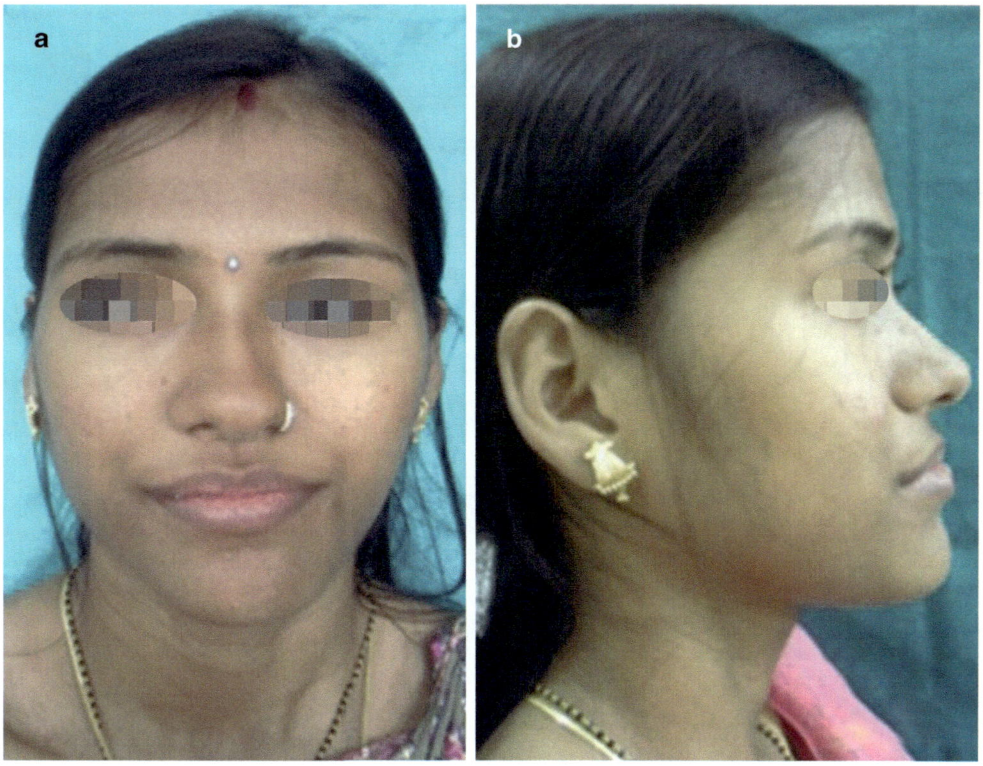

Fig. 70.21 Same patient as in Fig. 70.20 demonstrating corrected facial midline and mandibular prognathism postoperatively (**a**) frontal view, (**b**) profile view

70.6 Conclusion

Facial asymmetry is a three-dimensional facial deformity having multiple etiologies. Complete and thorough knowledge of the etiological factors, the progressive nature of the asymmetry plays a crucial role in formulating a treatment plan. Growth and development of the individual and timing of intervention is the single most important factor affecting the stability of results in any form of asymmetry. Severe relapses could occur if the exact cause of asymmetry is overlooked and treatment is attempted before completion of growth [44, 45].

Acknowledgment Gratitude and acknowledgments to Dr. Harsh Desai and Dr. Shibani Nerurkar for their sincere efforts in collection of data and editing of the contents.

DisclosureAuthors have no financial conflicts to disclose.

70.7 Case Scenarios

Case 1: Condylar Hyperplasia with Concomitant Masseteric Hypertrophy (Figs. 70.26a, b, c, 70.27a, b, 70. 28a, b and 70. 29a, b)

A 27-year-old female patient reported with a complaint of a progressive facial asymmetry and an appearance of fullness over the left angle of the mandible.

On examination, the patient had a tapered, triangular shape of the face with an obvious facial asymmetry which was evident along with elongation of the right side of the face and fullness over the left angle region (Fig. 70.26a). The mandible revealed bowing on the right side with a mild symphysis kink. TMJ on palpation revealed mild clicking on the right side and otherwise equal movements along with unrestricted mouth opening was noted. On assessing the left angle region, an outward projection was noted due to the underlying hyper functioning of the masseter muscle. On clenching, significant enlargement of the involved muscle was seen as compared to the contralateral side (Fig. 70.26b).

Intraoral examination did not reveal any occlusal cant (Fig. 70.26c). There was an absence of cross bite/open bite, on either side, along with a stable occlusal relationship. The dental midlines were coincident with the skeletal midline and with each other too. No other dental abnormalities were evident on examination.

Imaging studies revealed mild degree of deflection of the chin and mandible toward the left side (Fig. 70.27a, b). Transverse mandibular asymmetry was reported. The condylar head appeared to be irregularly deformed, while the neck on the right side appeared broader as compared to the left side. The ascending ramus appeared elongated with a rounded gonial angle. The mandibular lower border was bowed downward and positioned lower on the right side as compared to the left side. The distance between the tooth

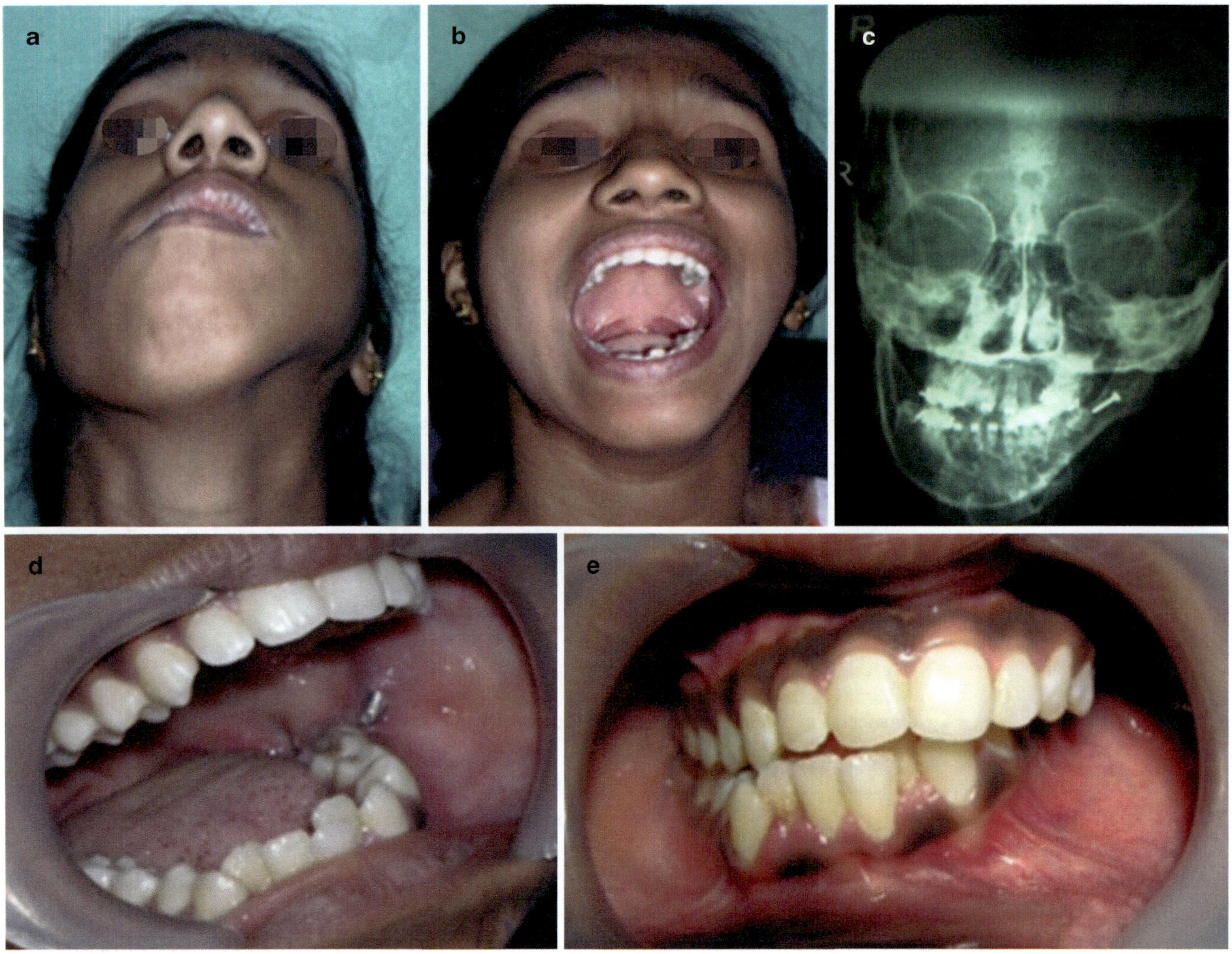

Fig. 70.22 (**a–e**) Case of facial asymmetry post-TMJ ankylosis treatment, due to resorption of costochondral graft. Note the exposed screw intraorally. Left side of mandibular arch fully telescoped inside the maxilla. (**a**) basal view showing gross asymmetry, (**b**) patient retaining good mouth opening after surgery for anlykosis, (**c**) Antero-posterior skull view showing asymmetry on the left side with screw from earlier costo-chondral graft fixation, (**d**) photograph showing trans-oral exposure of screw and (**e**) malocclusion with midline shift to the right, dental crowding and left sided lingual cross-bite

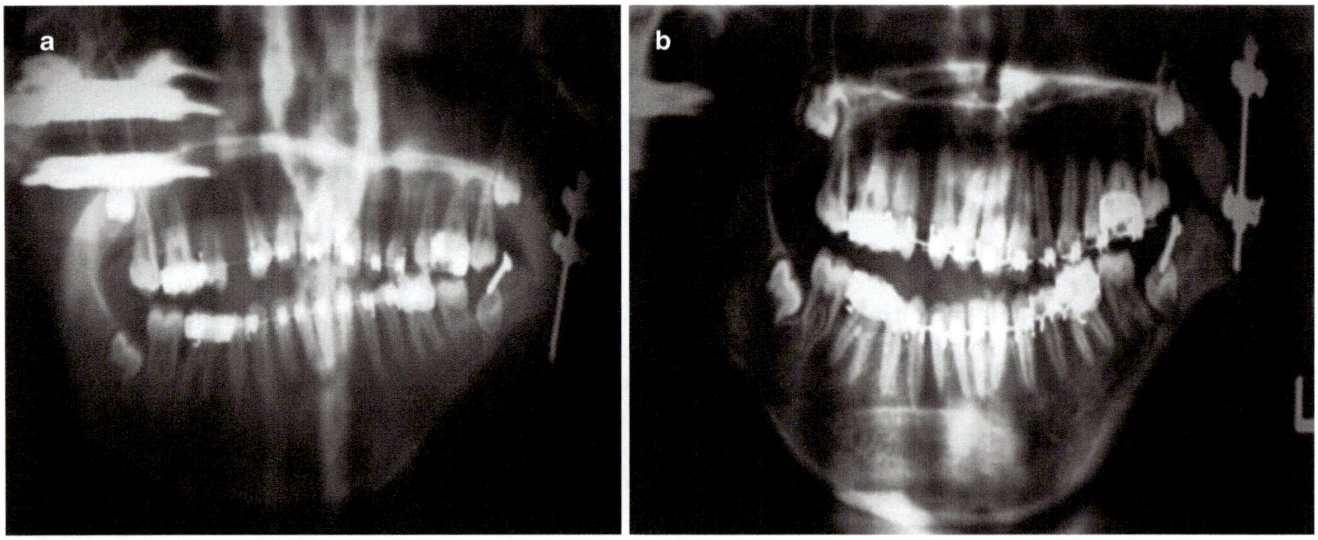

Fig. 70.23 (**a**, **b**) Stage 1 treatment in the same patient as in Fig. 70.22, left side vertical ramus distraction to establish equal ramal height. (**a**) Initial height of ramus prior to beginning distraction, (**b**) vertical lenghtening of ramus after completion of distraction

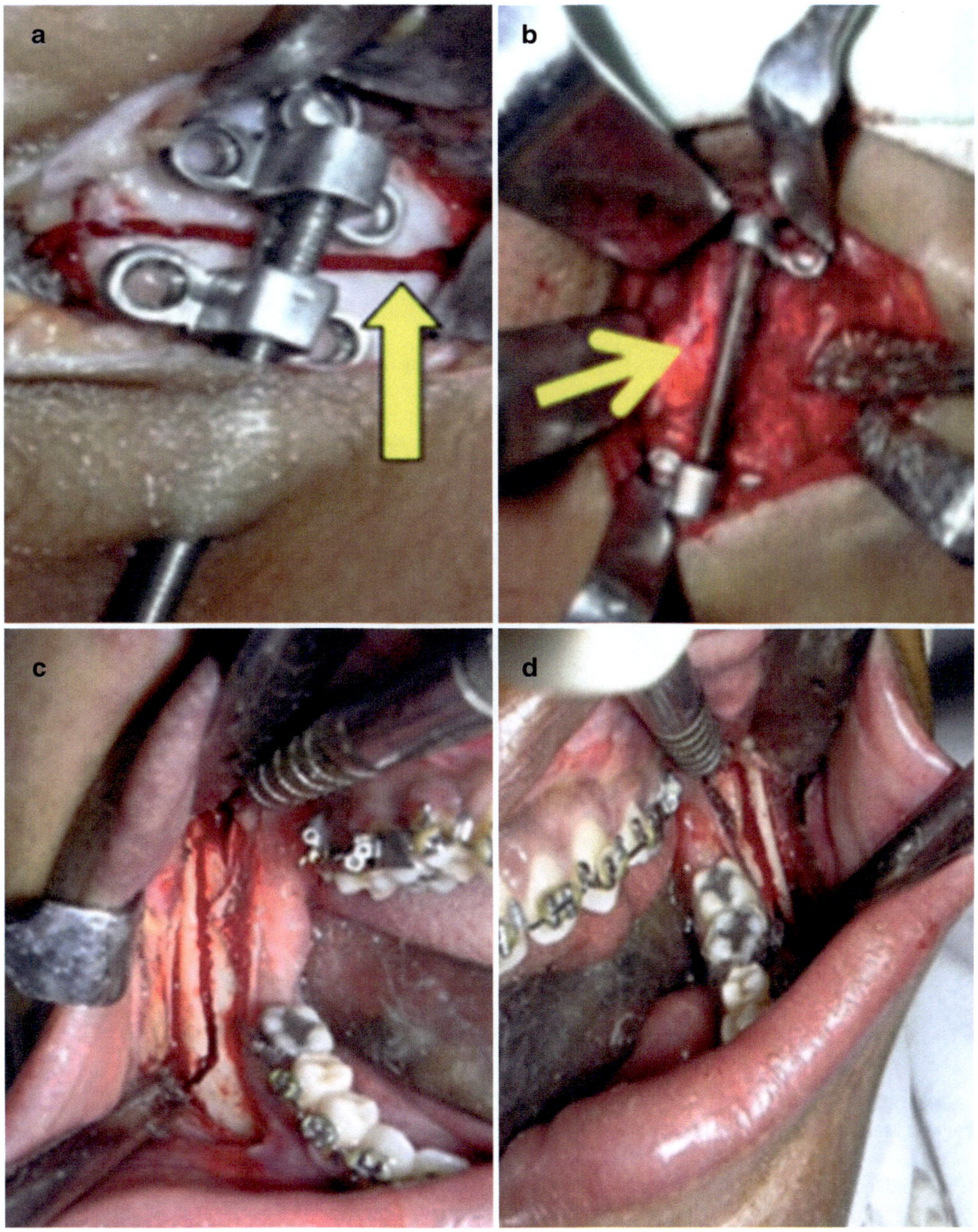

Fig. 70.24 (**a**–**d**) Second stage treatment in same patient as in Fig. 70.22: distractor removal with differential BSSO. (**a**) intra-operative photo from stage 1 surgery, showing osteotomy line for distraction (yellow arrow), (**b**) intra-operative photo during distractor removal demonstrating new bone formation(yellow arrow), (**c, d**) intra-operative photos showing osteotomy cuts for BSSO

roots and mandibular canal was increased with displacement of the latter towards the lower border of the mandible on the right side. The right side vertical ramus appeared relatively increased height as compared to the left. Thickened trabecular pattern was also evident on the right side.

Management

Following preparation for the administration of GA and a scintigraphy report which did not reveal an active mandibular hyperplastic condyle on the right side, the patient was prepared to be taken up for the procedure of an intraoral inferior border osteotomy. An intraoral vestibular incision was taken from 33 regions up to the external oblique ridge on the right side. Complete degloving was done to expose the inferior border in the anterior, body, and angle region of the mandible on the right side. Care was taken to identify the mental foramen and salvage the nerve. Methylene blue ink was used to mark the osteotomy line extending from the right central incisor posteriorly up to the angle region (Fig. 70.28a). It was correlated with the position of the neu-

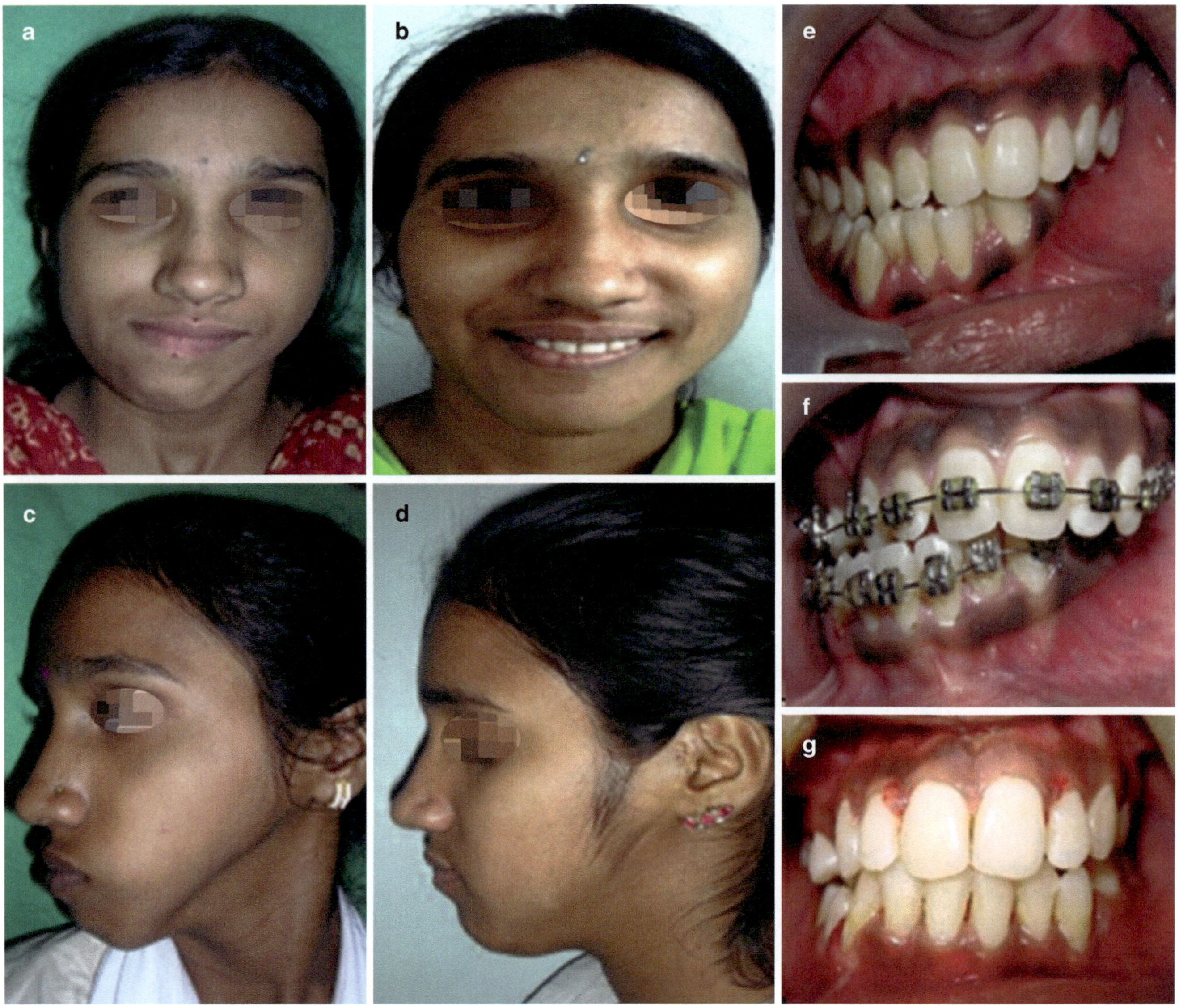

Fig. 70.25 (**a–g**) Pre- and postoperative photographs of the same patient as in Fig. 70.22, showing restoration of symmetry and midline (**a, b**) pre and post-operative frontal photographs showing correction of asymmetery, (**c, d**) pre and post-operative profile photographs demonstrating increased vertical height of ramus, (**e**) pre-treatment intra oral occlusion demosntrating severe shift in the dental midline with lingual crossbite on the left side, (**f**) orthodontic strap-up for dental and arch alignment, (**g**) post-treatment occlusion showing good dental rehabilitation

rovascular bundle, so as to prevent any damage to the same. The cut was initiated with a fine fissure bur under copious saline irrigation extending from buccal cortical plate to lingual cortical plate. With the help of an osteotome, the anterior cut was completed, and the lower inferior hyperplastic border was removed in one piece (Fig. 70.28b). The raw surface was smoothened with a vulcanite bur, and contouring was done to match the normal left side. The wound was closed in two layers with interrupted sutures using 3-0 vicryl. The surgical site was flushed with 2% povidone iodine solution.

For the masseteric hypertrophy on the left side, Botox [botulinum toxin Type A, Allergan™] powder was reconstituted with normal saline solution, pushed within the vial, and 30 units of it were administered using an insulin syringe and 30 gauge needle within the substance of the muscle, divided equally at three sites in a triangular fashion (Refer Chap. 33 and Fig. 33.10 for details on Botox injection to treat masseteric hypertrophy).

Complete correction of facial asymmetry with left side masseteric hypertrophy and right side condylar hyperplasia features was achieved with this surgical method (Fig. 70.29a, b).

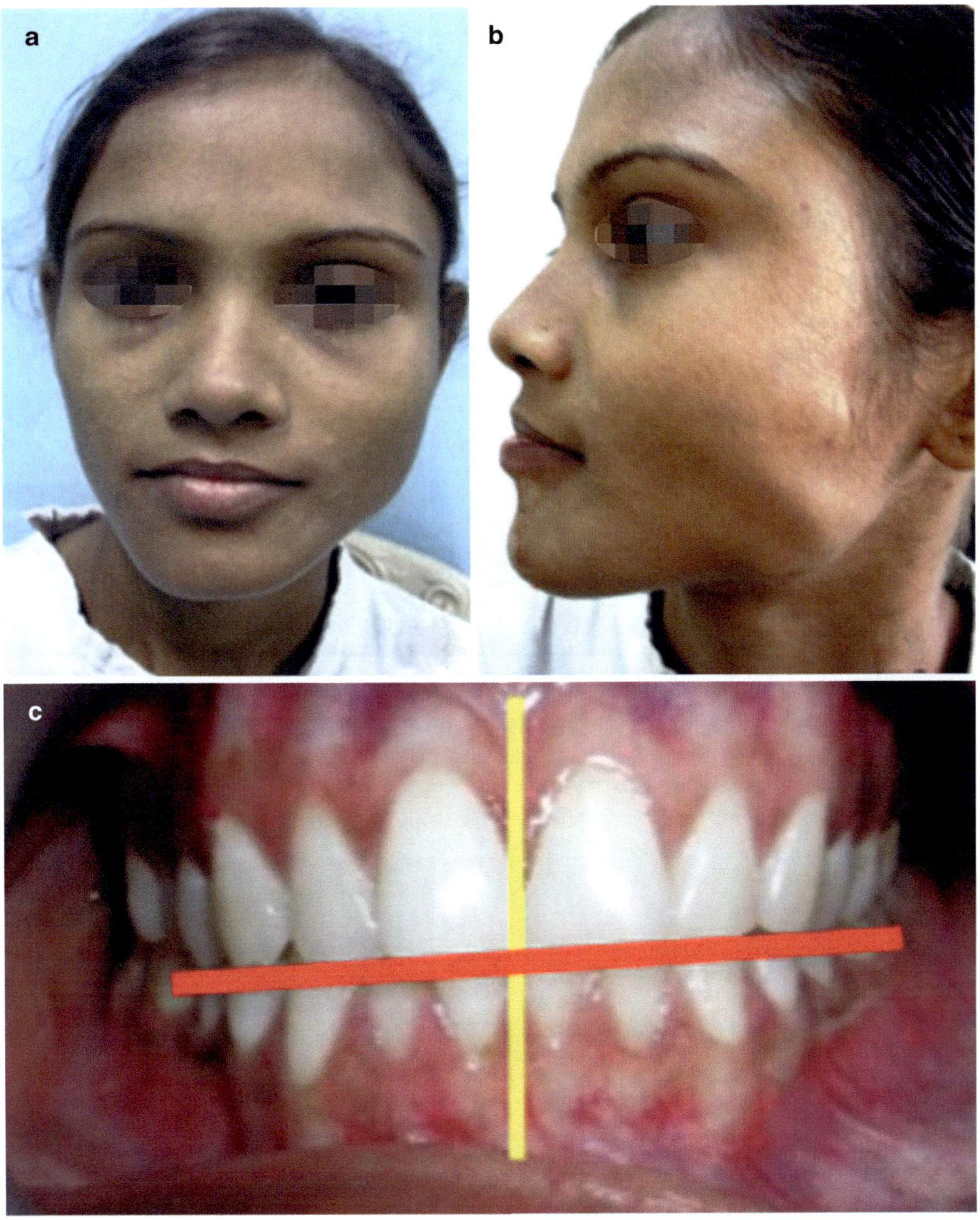

Fig. 70.26 (**a**, **b**) Frontal and profile views showing facial asymmetry due to condylar hyperplasia of the right side. (**c**) Occlusal view showing dental cant on account of condylar hyperplasia

Case 2: Parry Romberg Syndrome (Figs. 70.30a, b, 70.31a, b, 70.32a, b, c, 70.33a–h and 70.34a–f)

An 18-year-old female patient reported with gradual disfigurement and shrinkage of the right side her face since last 8–9 years.

Clinical examination revealed an asymmetry of the face on the right side with a marked atrophy of facial soft tissue (Fig. 70.30a). Significant orbital dystopia along with a hypoplastic soft tissues in the right, evident on worm's view (Fig. 70.30b). Clinically, a deformed and hypoplastic upper lip was seen with an increased vermillion show of the lower lip, resulting in a slanting rima oris. The right commissure, right ala of the nose, and the right supraorbital ridge region revealed obvious depression.

Intraoral examination revealed a missing upper right permanent canine along with crowding in the premolar region. Alveolar height in the maxillary right premolar region was reduced which was a pathognomonic sign of Parry Romberg (Fig. 70.31a, b). The occlusion was deranged, with a shift of the dental midline to the right.

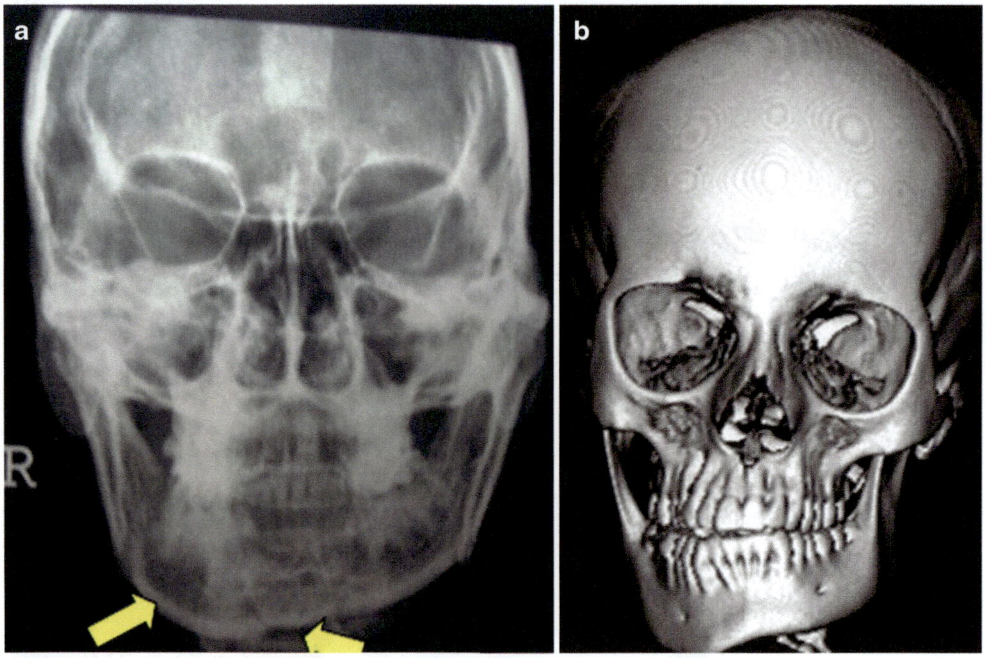

Fig. 70.27 (**a**) PA mandible showing inferior border bowing on the right side and kink in chin region (yellow arrows) which stops at the midline. (**b**) 3D CT shows mild degree of tilting of chin and mandible toward the left side

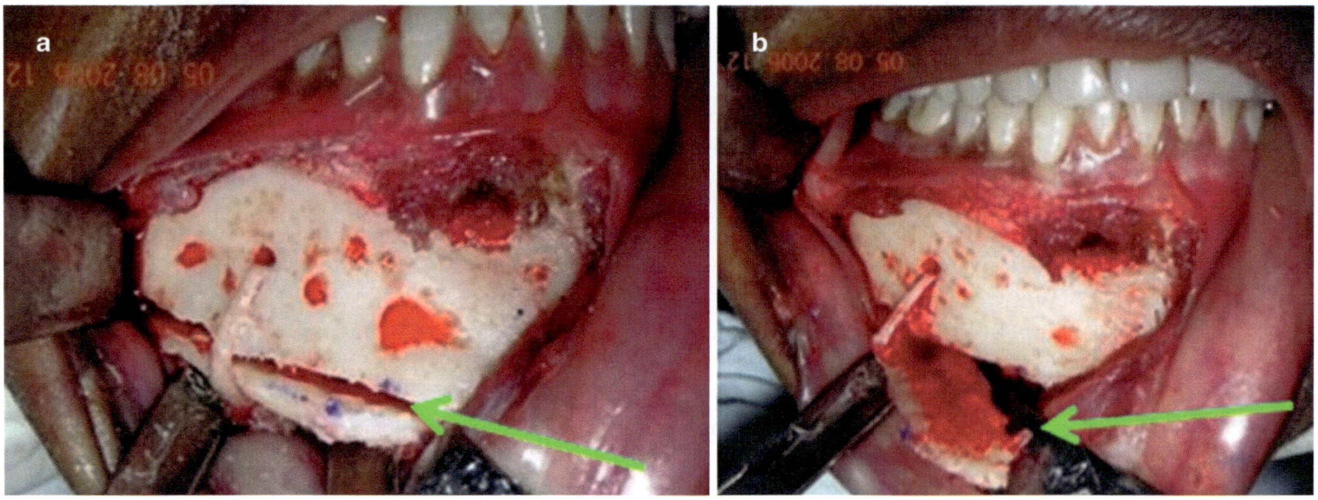

Fig. 70.28 (**a**, **b**) Inferior border osteotomy to remove the excessive contour below the mental nerve

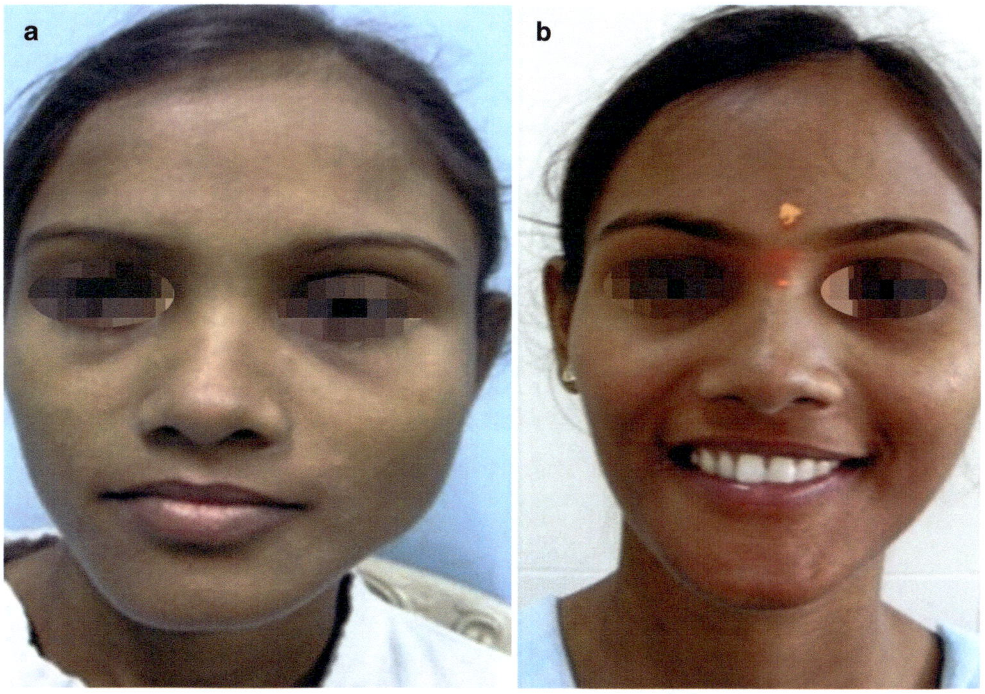

Fig. 70.29 (**a**) Pre- and (**b**) post-op correction in facial asymmetry. Reduction of fullness on left side and centralization of chin

Imaging studies revealed some degree of hypoplasia of mandible, zygoma, and maxilla on the right side. Presence of impacted permanent right maxillary canine was evident. The body-angle ramus, coronoid, and condylar process however appeared normal. Alveolar height was reduced in the right maxillary premolar region (Fig. 70.32a, b, c).

Management

The patient was prepared for GA administration for correction of facial asymmetry. A camouflage technique was planned wherein multiple Medpore© implants were used to fill up the deficient areas on the right side of her face in the right supraorbital, right maxillary alveolar region in the canine, and premolar areas right parasymphysis region of the body of mandible and right side chin along with autologous lipo transfer to increase the volume of the upper lip. Two separate small incisions were taken in the submandibular region anteriorly and posteriorly keeping the intervening skin and tissues intact. Layerwise dissection was done to reach the angle, body, and the anterior regions of the mandible. Tunnelling was done between the two incisions so as to receive the pre-shaped Medpore© implant, which was inserted from the anterior site and was pushed posteriorly to sit on the body, angle, and a portion of the ramus. The implant was notched in the superior aspect, in the region of the mental nerve to prevent impingement of the same. Four long titanium screws were used to fix the Medpore© implant on the body of the mandible on the right side (Fig. 70.33a). An additional half chin implant was placed to augment the deficient chin on the right side for achieving symmetry and was fixed with 2 long titanium screws (Fig. 70.33b). The incision sites were closed in two layers.

Another lateral eyebrow incision was taken on the right side (Fig. 70.33e). Dissection was done to expose the supraorbital rim. Supraorbital foramen and nerve were identified. An infra-orbital rim Medpore© implant for the right side was inverted and placed on the right supraorbital region to augment this deficient area. Two long titanium screws were used to stabilize the Medpore© implants.

Intra-orally a vestibular incision was taken in the right premolar and canine region. A full-thickness mucoperiosteal flap was raised. The infra-orbital nerve was identified and protected. A paranasal Medpore© implant was fixed with 1 long titanium screw to give fullness in this region. The wound was sutured in two layers with 3-0 vicryl.

Periumbilical and medial thigh regions were prepared to harvest fat cells. Manual aspiration of the fat cells was done. Following the simple method of sedimentation, the fat cells were separated from the blood components (Fig. 70.33f). 2 mm incisions were taken on either side of the oral commissure. A large 16 gauge epidural needle attached to 10cc syringe was used to push the fat within the substance of the upper lip from either side (more on right side than on the left) increasing the

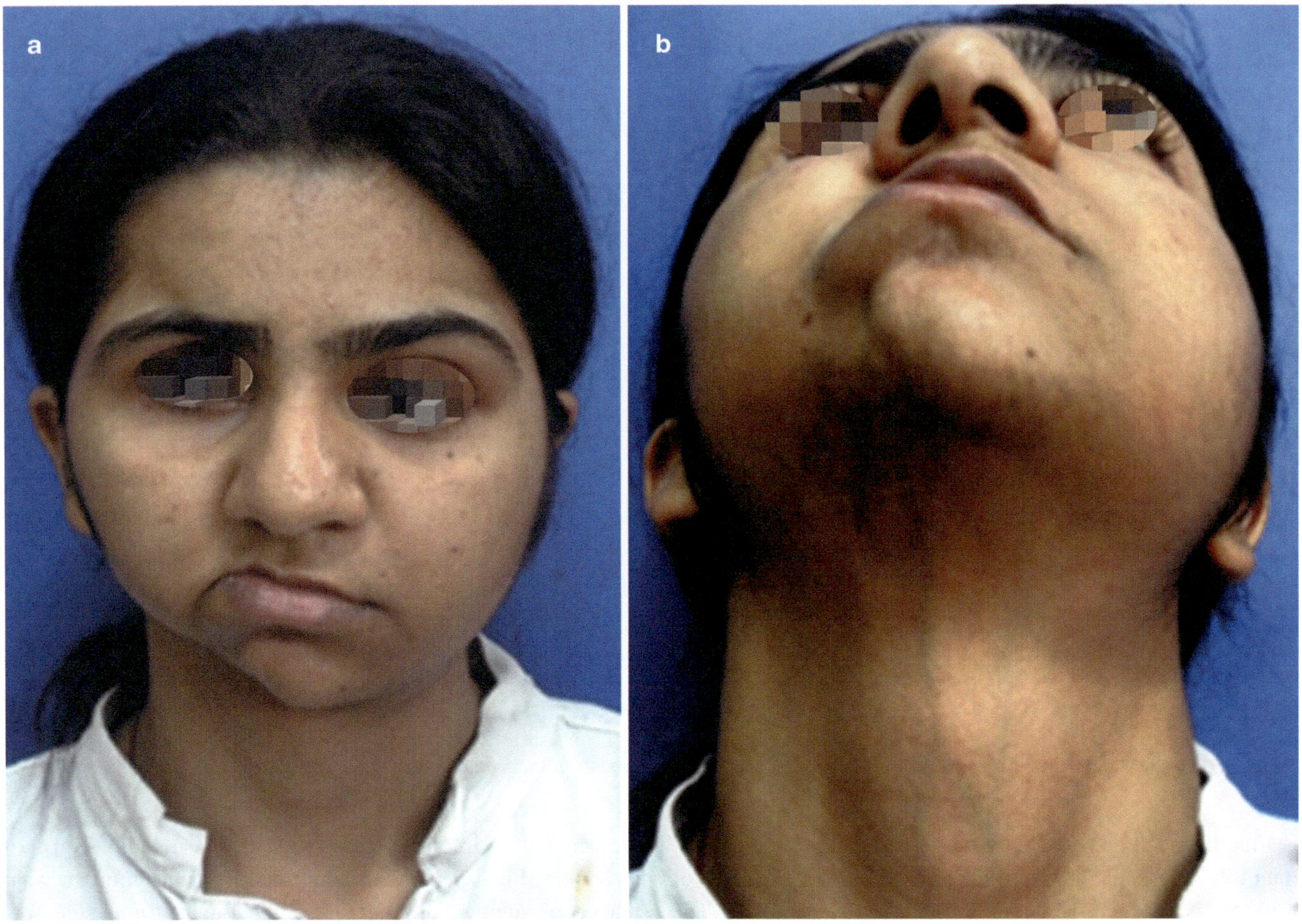

Fig. 70.30 (**a**) Frontal view—right side reveals marked atrophy in the distribution of all three branches of trigeminal nerve. (**b**) Asymmetry of the inferior border evident on worm's-view involving soft and hard tissue

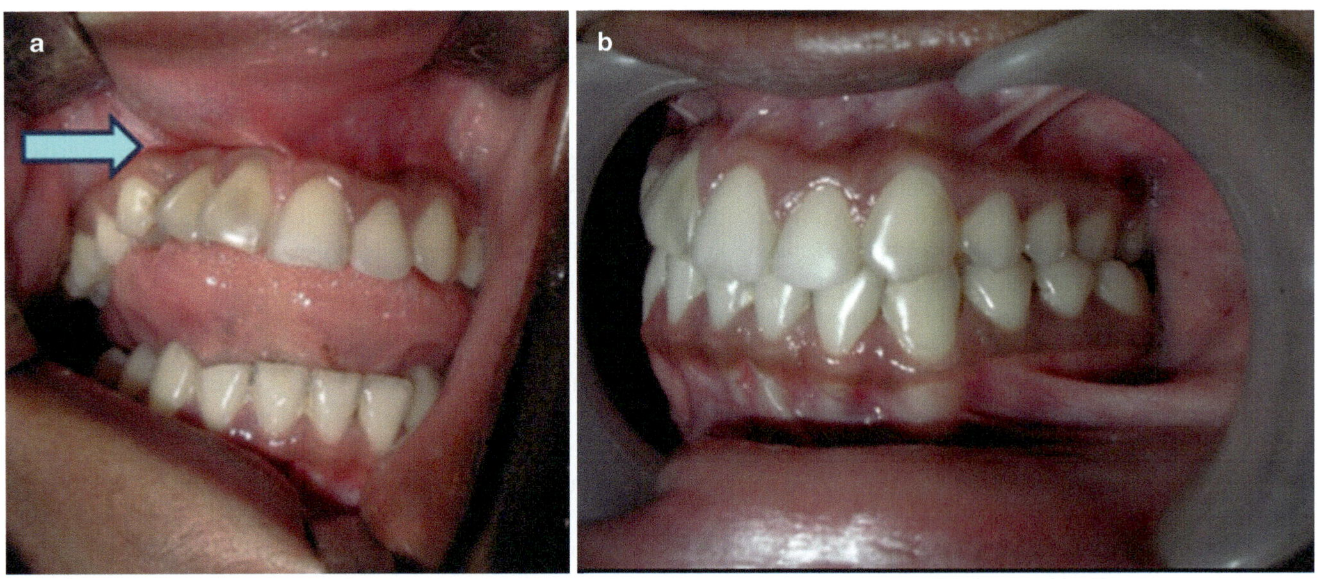

Fig. 70.31 (**a, b**) Intraoral examination of the same patient as in Fig. 70.30, reveals reduced alveolar height (blue arrow) in the right premolar region (**a**), as compared to the left side (**b**). Alveolar height reduction is an important clinical finding in Romberg's disease

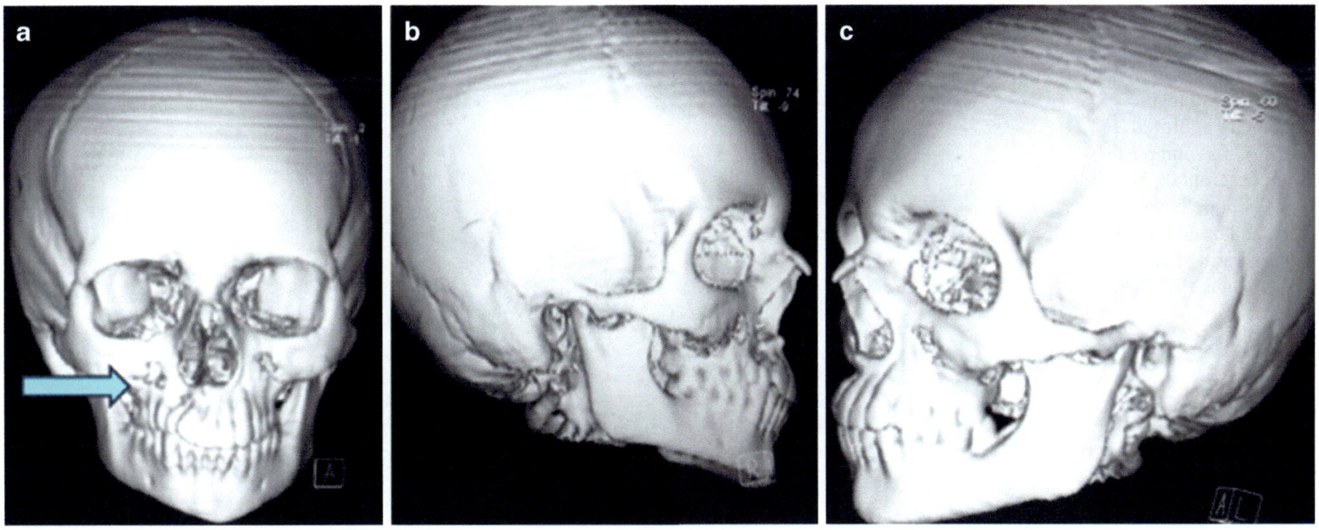

Fig. 70.32 (**a**, **b**) 3D CT of the patient in Fig. 70.30 reveals skeletal deficiency of alveolar height on right side (blue arrow), and reduction in vertical height of the ramus and body of the mandible on right side, (**c**) left side shows normal anatomy

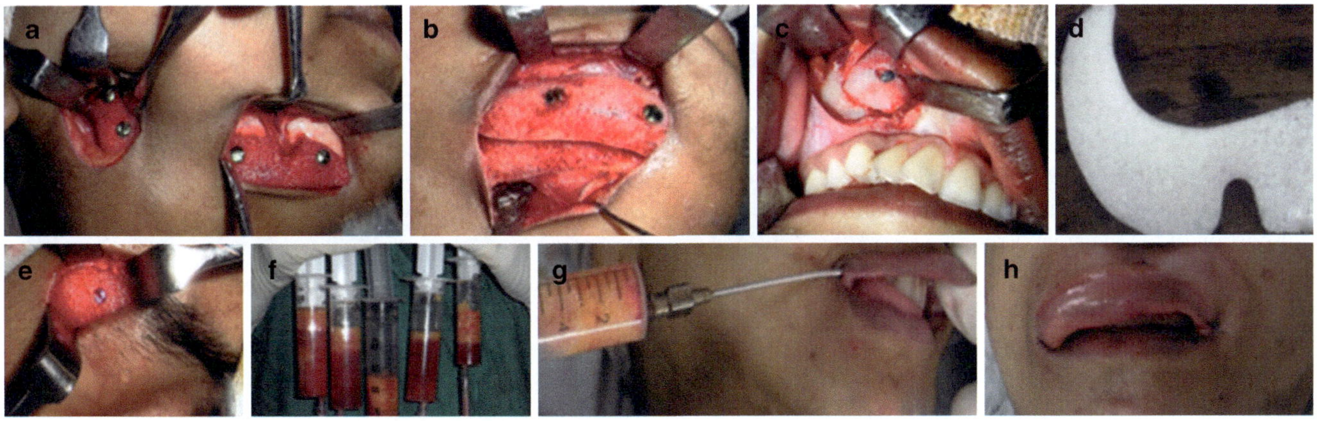

Fig. 70.33 (**a**) Extra-oral incisions—submandibular incisions made anteriorly and posteriorly. Medpore implant in ramus and body fixed with four titanium screws. (**b**) Additional half chin implant fixed with two titanium screws on right side of chin region. (**c**) Paranasal and alveolar Medpore implant fixed through intra-oral approach with titanium screws. Infraorbital nerve protected. (**d, e**) Use of Medpore implant for right side supra orbital rim. Notch placed superiorly to protect the supraorbital nerve. (**f**) Sedimentation to separate fat cells from blood components. Harvesting autologous fat grafts. (**g**) Introduction of fat cells into the upper lip through needle prick in right commissure. (**h**) Overcorrection achieved on table

volume of upper lip (Fig. 70.33g). A stitch on either side of the commissure was taken to prevent escape of fat cells (Fig. 70.33h). Overcorrection was done on table. Postoperatively, good facial symmetry was achieved with fullness at the deficient site using fat and implant (Fig. 70.34a–f).

For further case scenarios on management of facial asymmetry refer Figs. 68.19 and 68.38, in Chap. 68 on mandibular orthognathic procedures and Figs. 69.30, 69.31, 69.32 and 69.40 in Chap. 69 on maxillary orthognathic procedures.

Fig. 70.34 (**a–f**) Comparison of pre and post op results after 4 years. Satisfactory correction in facial asymmetry achieved. Pre (Fig. 70.30a) and post treatment frontal photographs (**a, b**) oblique facial views (**c, d**) and basal views (**e, f**) demonstrating better soft tissue balance and symmetry

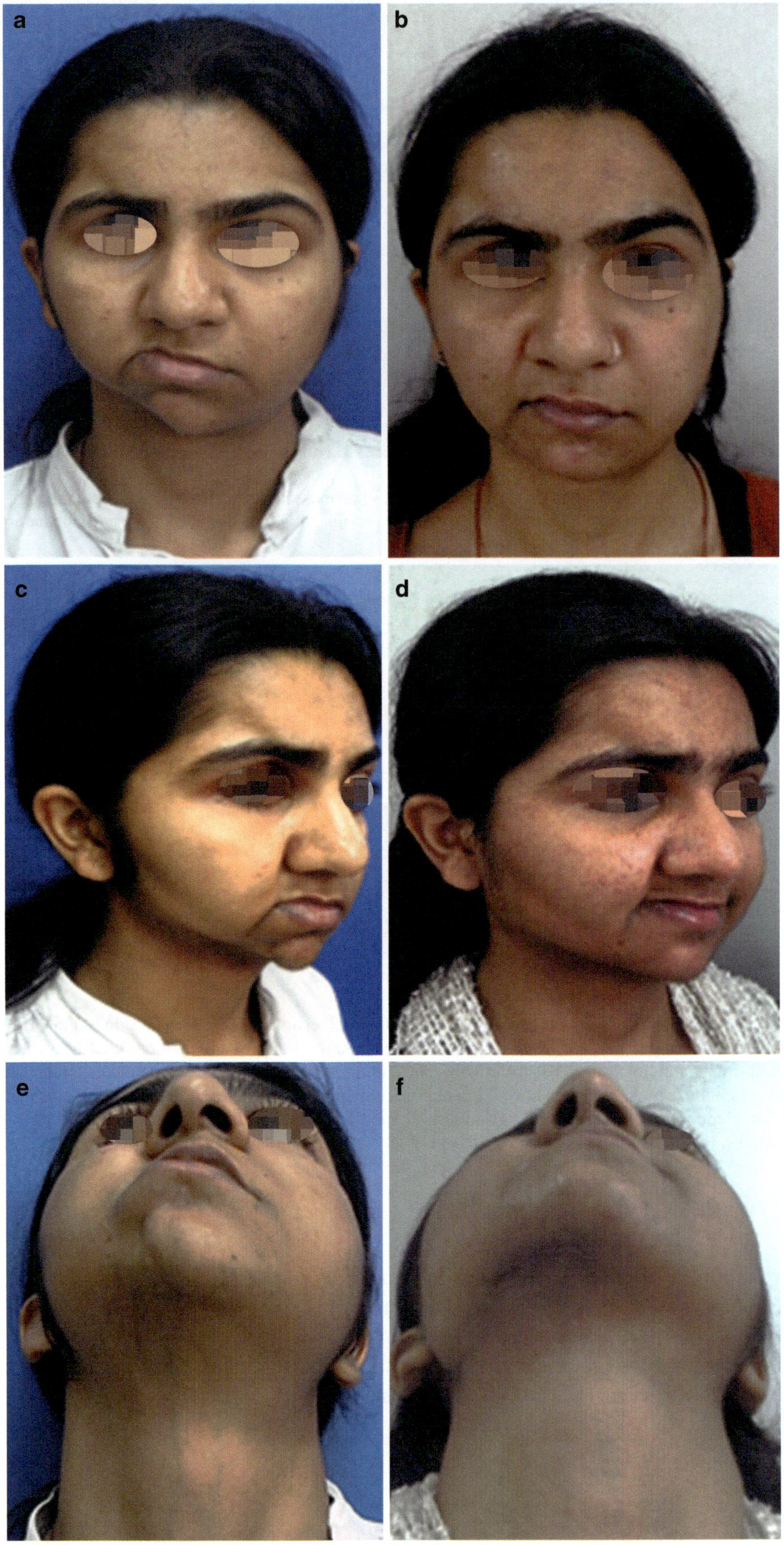

References

1. Little AC, Jones BC, De Bruine LM. Facial attractiveness: evolutionary based research. Philos Trans R Soc Lond Ser B Biol Sci. 2011;366(1571):1638–59.
2. Thiesen G, Gribel BF, Freitas MPM. Facial asymmetry: a current review. Dental Press J Orthod. 2015;20(6):110–25.
3. Chouinard AF, Kaban LB, Peacock ZS. Acquired abnormalities of the temporomandibular joint. Oral Maxillofac Surg Clin North Am. 2018;30(1):83–96.
4. Wolford LM, Gonçalves JR. Condylar resorption of the temporomandibular joint: how do we treat it? Oral Maxillofac Surg Clin North Am. 2015;27(1):47–67.
5. Pirttiniemi PM. Associations of mandibular and facial asymmetrieseview. Am J Orthod Dentofac Orthop. 1994;106:191–200.
6. Bishara SE, Burkey PS, Kharouf JG. Dental and facial asymmetries: a review. Angle Orthod. 1994;64:89–98.
7. Lundström A. Some asymmetries of the dental arches, jaws, and skull, and their etiological significance. Am J Orthod. 1961;47(2):81–106.
8. Plint DA, Ellisdon PS. Facial asymmetries and mandibular displacements. Br J Orthod. 1974;5:227–35.
9. Chia MS, Naini FB, Gill DS. The aetiology, diagnosis and management of mandibular asymmetry. Ortho Update. 2008;1(1):44–52.
10. Haraguchi S, Iguchi Y, Takada K. Asymmetry of the face in orthodontic patients. Angle Orthod. 2008;78(3):421–6.
11. Wolford LM. Facial asymmetry: diagnosis and treatment considerations. In: Fonseca's oral and maxillofacial surgery, vol. III. 3rd ed. St. Louis, MO: Saunders; 2017.
12. Reyeneke JP. Basic guidelines for the diagnosis and treatment of specific dentofacial deformities. 2nd ed. New Malden: Quintessence Publishing; 2010.
13. Cheong YW, Lo LJ. Facial asymmetry: etiology, evaluation, and management. Chang Gung Med J. 2011;34(4):341–51.
14. Waite P, Urban S. Facial asymmetry. In: Peterson's principles of oral and maxillofacial surgery. 3rd ed. New York: McGraw-Hill Medical; 2012.
15. Obwegeser HL, Makek MS. Hemimandibular hyperplasia: hemimandibular elongation. J Maxillofac Surg. 1986;14(4):183–208.
16. Cohen MM Jr. Perspectives of craniofacial asymmetry. Part IV. Hemi-asymmetries. Int J Oral Maxillofac Surg. 1995;24:134–41.
17. Kim JY, Jung HD, Jung YS, Hwang CJ, Park HS. A simple classification of facial asymmetry by TML system. J Craniomaxillofac Surg. 2014;42(4):313–20.
18. Hwang HS. A new classification of facial asymmetry. In: McNamara JA, editor. Early orthodontic treatment: is the benefit worth the burden? Craniofacial growth series, vol. 44. Ann Arbor: University of Michigan; 2007. p. 269–94.
19. Wolford LM, Movahed R, Perez DE. A classification system for conditions causing condylar hyperplasia. J Oral Maxillofac Surg. 2014;72(3):567–95.
20. Srivastava D, Singh H, Mishra S, Sharma P, Kapoor P, Chandra L. Facial asymmetry revisited: part I-diagnosis and treatment planning. J Oral Biol Craniofac Res. 2018;8(1):40–3.
21. Rodrigues DB, Castro V. Condylar hyperplasia of the temporomandibular joint. Types, treatment, and surgical implications. Oral Maxillofac Surg Clin North Am. 2015;27(1):155–67.
22. Srivastava D, Singh H, Mishra S, Sharma P, Kapoor P, Chandra L. Facial asymmetry revisited: part I-diagnosis and treatment planning. J Oral Biol Craniofac Res. 2018;8(1):7–14.
23. Cheong Y-W, Lo L-J. Facial asymmetry: etiology, evaluation, and management. Chang Gung Med J. 2011;34(1):341–51.
24. Choi KY. Analysis of facial asymmetry. Arch Craniofac Surg. 2015;16(1):1.
25. Photogrammetry [Internet]. Available from: https://en.wikipedia.org/wiki/Photogrammetry
26. Heike CL, Upson K, Stuhaug E, Weinberg SM. 3D digital stereophotogrammetry: a practical guide to facial image acquisition. Head Face Med. 2010;6(1):1–11.
27. Stereolithography [Internet]. Available from: https://en.wikipedia.org/wiki/Stereolithography
28. Farrell BB, Franco PB, Tucker MR. Virtual surgical planning in orthognathic surgery. Oral Maxillofac Surg Clin North Am. 2014;26(4):459–73.
29. Nadershah M, Mehra P. Orthognathic surgery in the presence of temporomandibular dysfunction. What happens next? Oral Maxillofac Surg Clin North Am. 2015;27(1):11–26.
30. Saridin CP, Raijmakers PGHM, Tuinzing DB, Becking AG. Bone scintigraphy as a diagnostic method in unilateral hyperactivity of the mandibular condyles: a review and meta-analysis of the literature. Int J Oral Maxillofac Surg. 2011;40(1):11–7.
31. Cisneros GJ, Kaban LB. Computerized skeletal scintigraphy for assessment of mandibular asymmetry. J Oral Maxillofac Surg. 1984;42(8):513–20.
32. Oron A, Arieli I, Pritsch T, Even-Sapir E, Halperin N, Agar G. SPECT versus planar scintigraphy as a clinical aid in evaluation of the elderly with knee pain. ISRN Orthop. 2013;2013:1–11.
33. Laverick S, Bounds G, Wong WL. [18F]-fluoride positron emission tomography for imaging condylar hyperplasia. Br J Oral Maxillofac Surg. 2009;47(3):196–9.
34. Srivastava D, Singh H, Mishra S, Sharma P, Kapoor P, Chandra L. Facial asymmetry revisited: part II-conceptualizing the management. J Oral Biol Craniofac Res. 2018;8(1):15–9.
35. Costello BJ, Rivera RD, Shand J, Mooney M. Growth and development considerations for craniomaxillofacial surgery. Oral Maxillofac Surg Clin North Am. 2012;24(3):377–96.
36. Pruzansky S. Not all dwarfed mandibles are alike. Birth Defects. 1969;5:120.
37. Kaban LB, Padwa BL, Mulliken JB. Surgical correction of mandibular hypoplasia in hemifacial microsomia: the case for treatment in early childhood. J Oral Maxillofac Surg. 1998;56:628–38.
38. Al-Moraissi EA, Wolford LM, Perez D, Laskin DM, Ellis E III. Does orthognathic surgery cause or cure temporomandibular disorders? A systematic review and meta-analysis Q2 Q24. J Oral Maxillofac Surg. 2017;75(9):1835–47.
39. Bawane SS, Andrade NN. Hard and soft tissue changes following maxillary distraction osteogenesis and mandibular setback with bilateral sagittal split osteotomy. J Maxillofac Oral Surg. 2016;15(4):491–500.
40. Posnick JC, Ricalde P, Ng P. A modified approach to "model planning" in orthognathic surgery for patients without a reliable centric relation. J Oral Maxillofac Surg. 2006;64(2):347–56.
41. Guo J, Wang T, Han JJ, Jung S, Kook MS, Park HJ, Oh HK. Corrective outcome and transverse stability after orthognathic surgery using a surgery-first approach in mandibular prognathism with and without facial asymmetry. Oral Surg Oral Med Oral Pathol Oral Radiol. 2018;126(1):22–30.
42. Schwartz HC. Efficient surgical management of mandibular asymmetry. J Oral Maxillofac Surg. 2011;69(3):645–54.
43. Andrade NN, Aggarwal N, Mathai P, Nerurkar S. Versatility of uniplanar prearthroplastic distraction osteogenesis in the correction of post-ankylosis facial deformities—a report of five different cases. Oral Maxillofac Surg. 2018;22(4):463–74.

44. Wolford LM, Karras SC, Mehra P. Considerations for orthognathic surgery during growth, part 1: mandibular deformities. Am J Orthod Dentofac Orthop. 2001;119(2):95–101.
45. Wolford LM, Karras SC, Mehra P. Considerations for orthognathic surgery during growth, part 2: maxillary deformities. Am J Orthod Dentofac Orthop. 2001;119(2):102–5.

Additional Reading

Grummons DC, Kappeyne van de Coppello MA. A frontal asymmetry analysis. Journal of Clinical Orthodontics: JCO. 1987;21(7):448–465.

Obstructive Sleep Apnea Syndrome

71

Suresh Menon

71.1 Introduction

Obstructive sleep apnea (OSA) is a condition that affects 2–4% of the adult population. This disease has reached a proportion of increasing importance due to its neurological and cardiological consequences. Abnormal pharyngeal anatomy and altered activity of the upper airway musculature dilator physiology are primarily responsible for the collapse of the pharyngeal walls during sleep.

71.2 Definition

OSA is defined by the occurrence of daytime sleepiness, loud snoring, witnessed breathing interruptions, or awakenings due to gasping or choking in the presence of at least five obstructive respiratory events (apneas, hypopneas, or respiratory effort-related arousals) per hour of sleep [1].

When OSA is accompanied by excessive daytime sleepiness, it is termed Obstructive Sleep Apnea Syndorme.

The common terms that are used in OSA are apnea, hypopnea, apnea hypopnea index (AHI), and respiratory distress index (RDI) [2].

1. *Apnea* is the cessation of airflow, exceeding 10 seconds.
2. A *hypopnea* is reduced airflow exceeding 10 seconds accompanied by a desaturation of 3% or more of oxygen and/or electroencephalographic evidence of arousal.
3. *The apnea hypopnea index* (AHI) is the number of apneas and hypopneas per hour of sleep. A value of 5–15 represents mild sleep apnea, 15–30 moderate, and greater than 30, severe.
4. *Respiratory distress index* (RDI) includes other parameters in addition to apnea and hypopnea like respiratory effort-related arousals (RERAs). This is characterized by increasing respiratory effort for 10 or more seconds leading to an arousal from sleep but not meeting the criteria of an apnea or hypopnea [3].

71.3 Etiopathogenesis

The upper airway is a flexible structure consisting of muscle and fat tissue and is usually only passively supported by bones. Therefore, it can be easily influenced by soft tissue factors like fat deposition in the parapharyngeal structures, edema/inflammation of the parapharyngeal region, hypertrophy of adenotonsillar tissues, or enlarged tongue.

The primary actor in the pathophysiology of OSA is the narrow, floppy upper airway. There is increased resistance of the upper airway due to anatomic factors that creates a negative airway pressure. This results in impaired function of airway-dilating muscles, thus increasing collapsibility. During sleep, the loss of skeletal muscle tone narrows the upper airway, making it floppier, especially during rapid eye movement (REM) sleep when muscle relaxation is intense. This results in two significant actions:

- The turbulent flow patterns that occur lead to vibration of structures causing snoring.
- The pharynx collapses due to the Bernoulli effect. This causes an obstruction which could be partial or complete. This tends to persist until sleep is interrupted and muscle tone is restored. These interruptions usually last less than 15 seconds, and the individual is unaware of them. Sometimes, the obstruction results in an awakening, and the individual complains of suddenly waking with a snort or a snore. Breathing is reestablished on arousal, and after a few breaths deeper sleep resumes with repetition of the cycle during muscle relaxation.

S. Menon (✉)
Department of Oral and Maxillofacial Surgery, Vydehi Institute of Dental Sciences and Research Centre, Bangalore, India

K. Bonanthaya et al. (eds.), *Oral and Maxillofacial Surgery for the Clinician*, https://doi.org/10.1007/978-981-15-1346-6_71

Additional factors that can increase the severity of upper airway resistance during sleep are mouth opening or a supine posture which allows the gravitational forces to push the tongue and soft palate back. Upper airway resistance can occur anywhere from the nasopharynx to the hypopharynx but primarily involves the oropharynx (Fig. 71.1).

71.4 Risk Factors for OSA

71.4.1 Age

The disease prevalence increases steadily with age and reaches a stable level after the age of 60 years. The probable explanations for the age-related increase in prevalence include increased fat deposition in the parapharyngeal area, soft palate lengthening, etc.

71.4.2 Excess Body Weight

Body weight is an important risk factor for OSA, and studies have endorsed the positive effects of dieting and surgical weight loss on reducing OSA. Body weight increase can affect normal upper airway mechanics during sleep through:

1. Reduction of upper airway by increased parapharyngeal fat deposition.
2. Changing neural compensatory mechanisms that maintain patency of airway.
3. Instability of respiratory control system.
4. Reduction in functional residual capacity.

71.4.3 Gender

It is an established fact that men are more vulnerable than women toward developing OSA. The differences exist not only in prevalence but also in polysomnographic characteristics of sleep and breathing patterns. Women were seen to have a lower AHI in non-rapid eye movement (non-REM) sleep. Disordered breathing events in women have a shorter duration and are associated with less oxyhemoglobin desaturation than in men.

71.4.4 Craniofacial Anatomy

The mechanical properties of the upper airway and the tendency to collapse during sleep can be influenced by both hard and soft tissues in the region. Findings in the craniofacial region like large tongue or soft palate, reduced mandibular size, or tonsillar hypertrophy in addition to inferiorly placed hyoid, maxillary, and mandibular retropositioning can narrow upper airway dimensions and leading to episodes of apneas and hypopneas during sleep.

71.4.5 Familial and Genetic Predisposition

Inheritance and familial factors also play a major role in OSA. First-degree relatives of OSA patients seem to be at risk more likely than others. The familial susceptibility tends to increase directly with the number of affected relatives.

Heredity and genetic factors also have been found to have a role in determining the volume of the lateral parapharyngeal

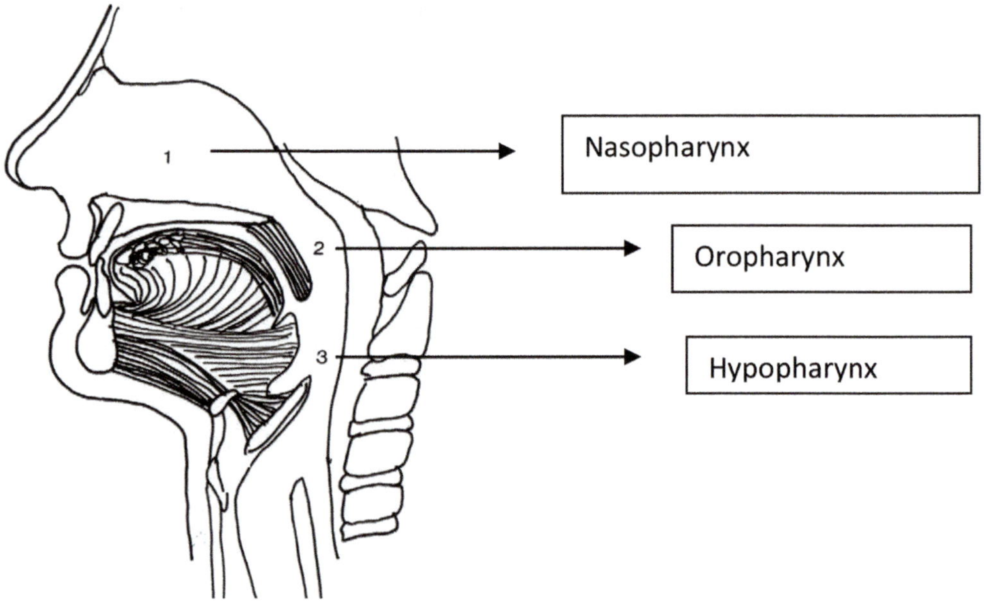

Fig. 71.1 Areas causing OSA

walls, tongue, and total soft tissue structures. A detailed family history can help in identifying those that have the disorder but remain undiagnosed.

71.4.6 Smoking and Alcohol Consumption

Cigarette smoking and alcohol are also possible risk factors for obstructive sleep apnea. Airway inflammation can occur due to cigarette smoke that could modify the properties of upper airway and increase its collapsibility during sleep. Alcohol consumption before sleep increases upper airway collapsibility and the precipitate apneic and hypopneic episodes during sleep. Another effect of alcohol is to inhibit respiratory motor output to the upper airway, causing hypotonia of the oropharyngeal muscles.

71.4.7 Medical Comorbidity

There is enough evidence to suggest that OSA can be a factor in the development of hypertension, coronary artery disease, congestive heart failure, and stroke [4].

OSA is also associated with diabetes mellitus, Therefore, diagnosing the condition and intervening early could directly or indirectly enhance glycemic control [5]. The role of positive airway pressure (PAP) therapy could result in reduced day time fatigue, better physical activity, resulting in improved metabolic control.

71.5 Clinical Sequelae [6]

71.5.1 Endocrine and Metabolic Effects

The central effects of sleep fragmentation and hypoxemia have been seen to induce a reversible neuroendocrine defect in growth hormone and testosterone secretion. This may explain impaired growth seen in children with upper airway obstruction which seems to get better after adenotonsillectomy.

71.5.2 Neuropsychological and Social Consequences

The classic feature of OSA prevalent as excessive daytime sleepiness may lead to both impaired work performance and driving. OSA patients seem to perform poorly on psychometric tests, and improvement has been seen after nasal CPAP therapy.

71.5.3 Cardiovascular Sequelae

There are two serious consequences of OSA involving the cardiovascular system. Initially acute cardiovascular changes occur during an apnea. This is followed by more chronic cardiovascular conditions like hypertension, myocardial infarction, stroke, and death.

71.6 Epidemiology [7, 8]

OSA has no specific age predilections, but a study by Young et al. estimated the prevalence in middle age to be 4% for men and 2% for women. Their study estimated that 1 of every 5 adults has at least mild OSA and 1 of every 15 has at least moderate OSA.

71.7 Diagnosis [1]

A detailed study of clinical signs and symptoms established during a comprehensive sleep evaluation and findings identified by sleep testing lead to the diagnosis of OSA.

71.7.1 History and Physical Examination

The diagnosis of OSA begins with a sleep history in one of three settings:

1. Part of routine health maintenance evaluation.
2. Part of an evaluation of symptoms of OSA.
3. Part of the comprehensive evaluation of patients at high risk for OSA.

Of the available, the Epworth sleepiness scale (ESS) (Table 71.1) is a popular subjective-based self-assessment of sleepiness that determines the degrees of sleepiness [9]. When scores are greater than 10, further investigations are recommended. However as about 10% of the population have a score of 11 or more, this score should be complemented by a narrative confirmation of intrusive somnolence.

71.7.2 Polysomnography (PSG)

This is an overnight sleep study monitored by a sleep technologist and is considered the "gold standard" in sleep medicine (Fig. 71.2). The physiologic parameters measured during PSG include simultaneous monitoring of

Table 71.1 Epworth sleepiness scale

Name:	Date:
Age:	Sex:
How likely are you to doze off or fall asleep in the following situations, in contrast to feeling just tired?	
Use the following scale to choose the most appropriate number for each situation:	
0—Would never doze	
1—Slight chance of dozing	
2—Moderate chance of dozing	
3—High chance of dozing	
Situation	*Chance of dozing (0–3)*
1. Sitting and reading.	----------
2. Watching TV.	----------
3. Sitting inactive in a public place like theatre/ meeting.	----------
4. As a passenger in a car for an hour without break.	----------
5. Lying down to rest in the afternoon when circumstances permit.	----------
6. Sitting and talking to someone.	----------
7. Sitting quietly after lunch without alcohol.	----------
8. In a car, while stopped for a few minutes in traffic.	----------

brain wave activity continuously, eye movements, muscle activity of the legs and mandible, body position, heart rate and rhythm, blood pressure, snoring, and respiratory activity including breathing patterns and oxygen saturation. A detailed analysis of these can reveal apneic, hypopneic activities, etc.

Presence of obesity or signs of upper airway narrowing should also be documented.

Patients at High Risk for OSA and Who all should be evaluated for OSA Symptoms [1]

1. Obesity (BMI > 35).
2. Congestive heart failure.
3. Atrial fibrillation.
4. Treatment refractory hypertension.
5. Type 2 diabetes.
6. Nocturnal dysrhythmias.
7. Stroke.
8. Pulmonary hypertension.
9. High-risk driving populations.
10. Alcohol consumption.
11. Preoperative for bariatric surgery.

OSA Symptoms That Should Be Evaluated During a Comprehensive Sleep Evaluation

1. Witnessed apneas.
2. Snoring.
3. Gasping/choking at night.
4. Excessive sleepiness not explained by other factors.
5. Non refreshing sleep.
6. Total sleep amount.
7. Sleep fragmentation/maintenance insomnia.
8. Nocturia.
9. Morning headaches.
10. Decreased concentration.
11. Memory loss.
12. Decreased libido.
13. Irritability.

71.7.3 Imaging Aids

71.7.3.1 Cephalometrics

There is a plethora of imaging aids to help diagnose and plan the management of OSA. Cephalometrics has been the oldest imaging modality in the diagnosis of OSA. However, its role in quantification of the pharyngeal volume is controversial as the image that is two-dimensional is used to evaluate a three-dimensional structure [3].

It is a known fact that the lateral pharyngeal wall collapse has a bigger influence on severe sleep apnea than retropalatal and retrolingual collapse as studied with dynamic MRI, and this would not appear evident on a lateral cephalogram [10]. Another shortcoming of lateral cephalograms is that they are taken with the patient upright and awake and therefore do not characterize the asleep or supine airway.

Cephalometric images however have other advantages that can be used to predict OSA. It can be used to measure the upper airway length (UAL) (Fig. 71.3). UAL is significantly longer in OSA patients due to the relation between UAL and airflow resistance. Since the part of the airway is primarily composed of the soft tissues compared to the more rigid, cartilaginous, subglottic airway, this region may predispose to collapse. Studies have proved that male patients with UAL $\geq$ 72 mm have an eightfold increase in the probability of OSA while females with UAL $\geq$ 62 mm have a fivefold increase in OSA probability [11].

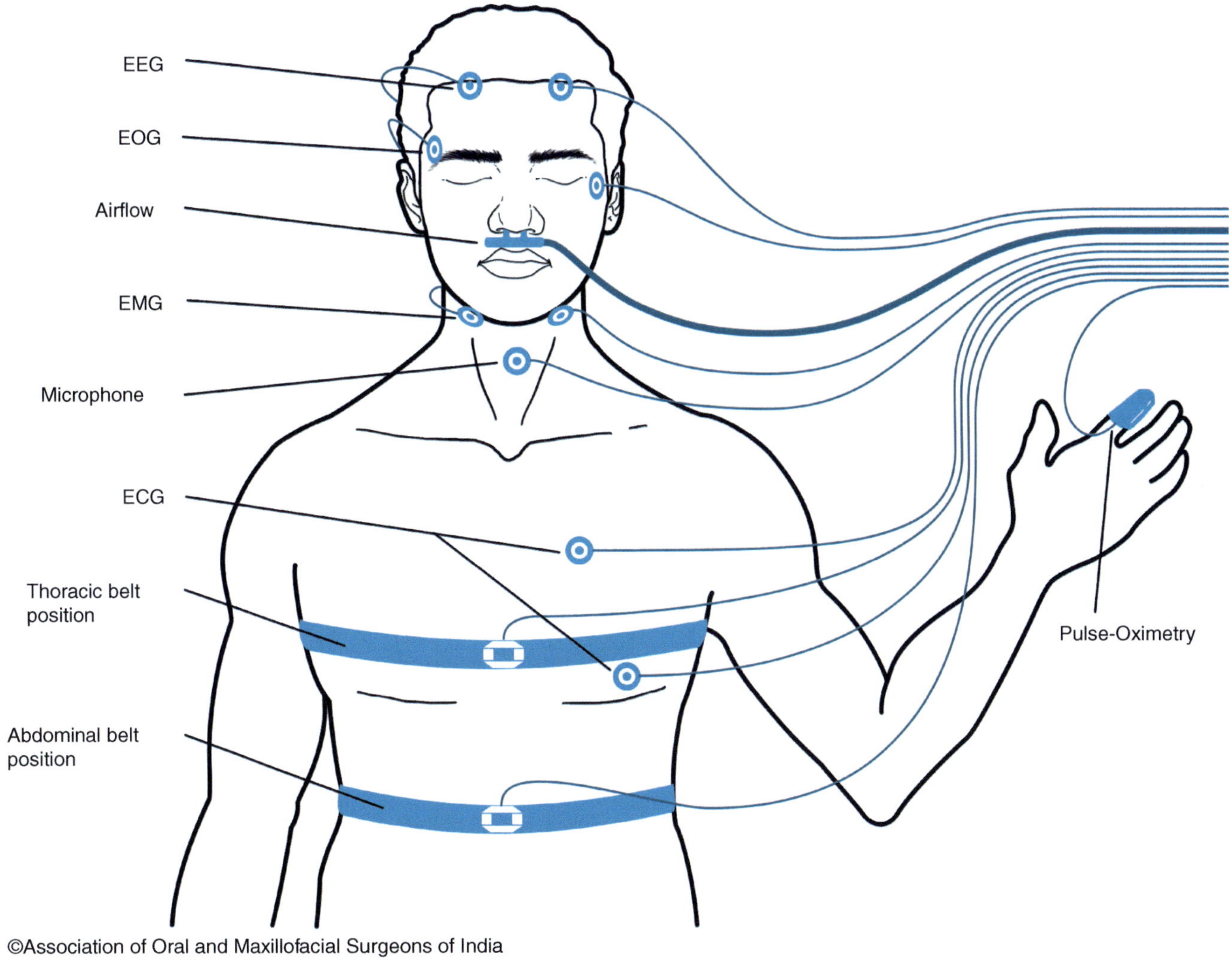

Fig. 71.2 Polysomnography leads and parameters. *EEG* Electroencephalogram, *EOG* Electrooculography, *EMG* Electromyography, *ECG* Electrocardiography

Cephalometrics can also be used to predict the success in multilevel phase I therapy for patients. Skeletal class II patients with a more retrognathic mandible are poor responders. Other patients who could be poor responders include those with hyperdivergent vertical pattern with a larger mandibular plane angle, longer lower facial height, and steeper occlusal plane [9].

71.7.3.2 Dynamic Upper Airway Imaging [12]

Dynamically assessment of the level of upper airway obstruction in OSA patients will allow targeted intervention and allow planning a specific surgical procedure by allowing a delineation of the site and specifying degree and pattern of obstruction. It can also be used to exclude pathology like tumors. Dynamic sleep MRI and drug-induced sleep CT scan characterize the airway in OSA with the advantage of ability to evaluate the airway in a multiplane fashion in the sleeping state or a simulated sleep state.

Drug-induced sleep endoscopy (DISE) is an alternative to conventional endoscopy with the goal of more accurately representing patterns of collapse during the sleeping state.

71.7.3.3 Acoustic Reflex Ion Test

In this test, sound waves are projected into the airway and are reflected into the tube to a computer which creates an image that determines the location of obstruction. This can also predict the effect of mandibular advancement and protrusion on upper airway.

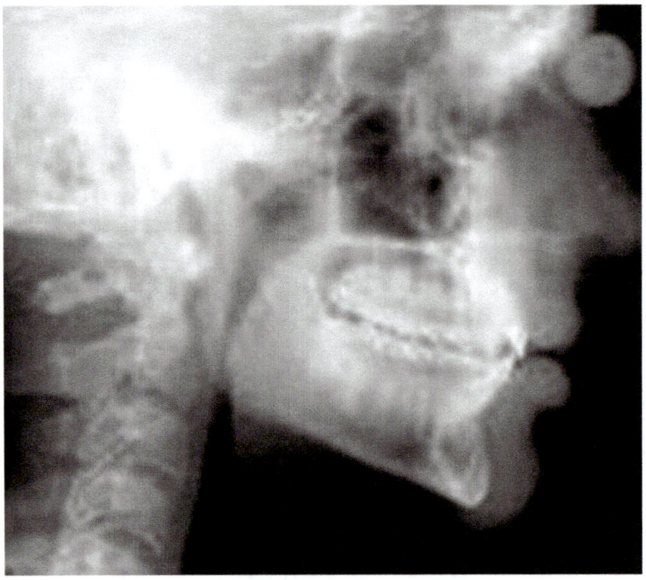

Fig. 71.3 Narrowing of oropharynx and long upper airway length in OSA

Table 71.2 Symptoms of OSAS

Adult	Children
Heavy snoring	Snoring
Excessive daytime sleepiness	Restless sleeping
Apneas	Somnolence
Sudden awakenings with 'choking'	Aggression/behavioral problems
Accidents related to sleepiness	Hyperactivity
Poor memory/concentration	Odd sleeping postures
Delirium	Frequent coughs/colds
Gastroesophageal reflux	
Mood/personality changes	
Nocturnal sweating	
Restlessness during sleep	
Nocturia	
Enuresis	
Dry mouth on awakening	
Nocturnal or morning headache	
Impotence	
Nocturnal epilepsy	

Table 71.3 Signs of OSAS

Edematous soft palate or uvula
Long soft palate and uvula
Decreased oropharyngeal dimensions
Nasal obstruction
Maxillary hypoplasia
Retrognathia
Central adiposity/increased neck circumference
Hypertension and other cardiovascular consequences

71.8 Clinical Features (Tables 71.2 and 71.3)

71.9 Treatment Modalities

OSA is a chronic condition that would require multidisciplinary management over a long period of time. There is a myriad of options to treat the condition ranging from behavioral to medical to surgical options. The success of treatment would have to ensure the voluntary active participation of the patient.

71.9.1 Positive Airway Pressure [13]

Continuous positive airway pressure (CPAP) is usually the first line of treatment for OSA. It works on the principle of binding the upper airway in an open position to improve patency during sleep (Fig. 71.4).

This was first described by Sullivan [14] in 1981. The pneumatic splinting action is effective in reducing the AHI. PAP may be delivered in either continuous (CPAP), bilevel (BPAP), or auto titrating (APAP) modes. CPAP is the first line of treatment for moderate to severe OSA and may be used occasionally in mild OSA. CPAP has also found to be effective as an adjunctive therapy to alter blood pressure in OSA patients having hypertension.

Some of these patients may elicit intolerance for CPAP therapy. In these cases, BPAP, pressure relief, or APAP can be considered as an alternative. In addition to its splinting action, CPAP increases vagal tone, cardiac output, and stroke volume and decreases systemic vascular resistance, and there is reduced risk of cardiovascular mortality.

Compliance with nasal CPAP (nCPAP) ranges from 50 to 89% [15]. Reasons for noncompliance are usually due to tolerance problems like dry mouth, conjunctivitis, rhinorrhea, skin irritation, pressure sores, nasal congestion, and epistaxis. Other less common causes of noncompliance include aerophagia, chest discomfort, and bed partner intolerance or psychological problems arising from lack of motivation, claustrophobia, and anxiety.

Though there is no established known lower limit of nightly use below which nCPAP therapy is ineffective, it is suggested that 3.4 h per night of nCPAP use may be adequate to improve cognitive function and quality of life.

71.9.2 Behavioral Strategies [16]

Behavioral strategies have also been used as treatment methods in OSA. These include weight loss, regular exercise, positional therapy, and sleep hygiene which involves alcohol abstinence and consumption of sedatives before sleep.

Sleep position while supine can decrease the lateral upper airway dimensions, particularly while in the supine position.

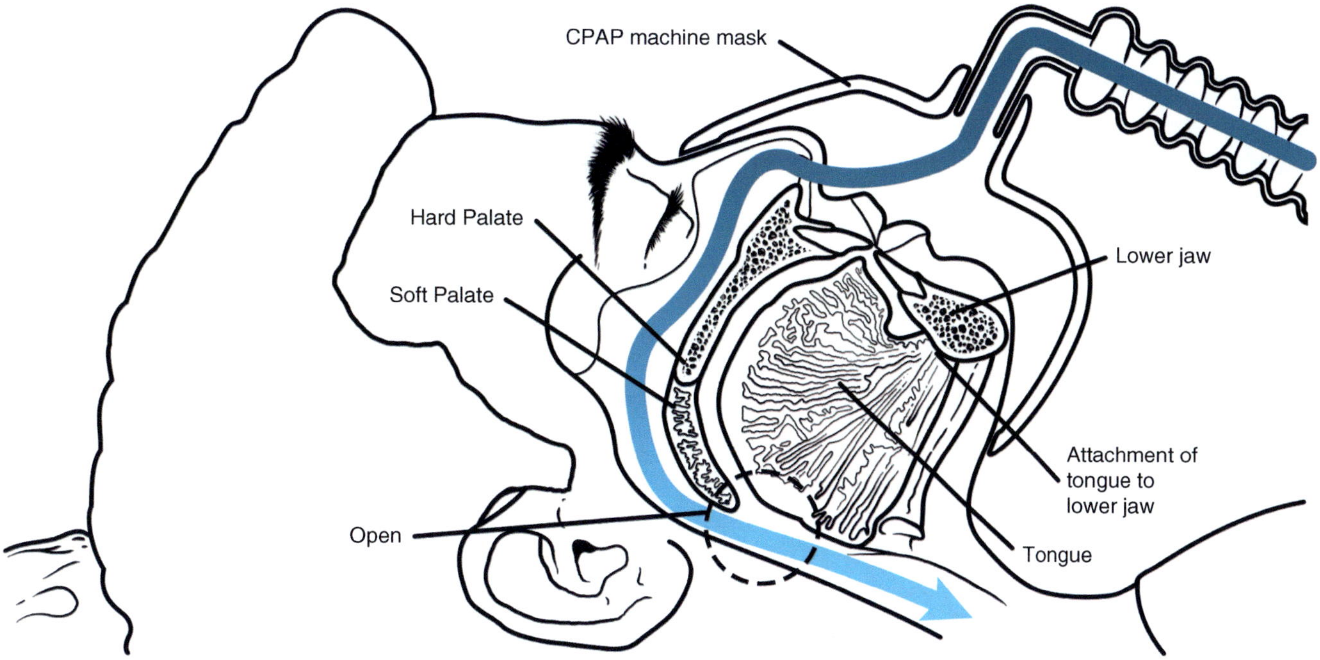

Fig. 71.4 CPAP usage

Therefore, in positional therapy, the patient is kept in a non-supine position.

71.9.3 Oral Appliances [17]

The primary role of oral appliances (OAs) is to enlarge the posterior oropharyngeal airway space, leading to reduction of chances of the upper airway collapsing during sleep. They are ideally indicated in mild and moderate cases of OSA who are noncompliant/poorly compliant to nasal CPAP. Oral appliances are of two types: tongue retaining or mandibular repositioning.

- *Tongue retaining devices* [18]: These appliances position the tongue anteriorly by means of negative pressure and are indicated for patients who have few teeth or are edentulous, have macroglossia, or who are unable to adequately advance their mandible. The result is increase of the volume of the upper airway.
- *Mandibular repositioning devices (MRD)* [19]: As the name suggests, they reposition the mandible and structures attached to it like the tongue and hyoid bone anteriorly, thus increasing the upper airway dimensions in both sagittal and transverse planes, especially at the level of the velopharynx (Fig. 71.5). The appliances completely cover the maxillary and mandibular dentition and hold the mandible forward with respect to the resting position. The amount of advancement is titrated depending on the symptoms not exceeding 80% of the patient's maximum protrusive capacity. This is followed by polysomnography to check the efficacy.

It is mandatory for patients using MRD to have adequate number of teeth to seat the appliance. There should not be any deleterious TMJ disorder, and the patients should have an adequate range of jaw motion and adequate manual dexterity and should be motivated to use the appliance.

The MRD device is customized and the material used is flexible polyamide.

In general, OAs are either titratable or non-titratable. Titratable OAs permit varying amounts of mandibular protrusion. Non-titratable OAs hold the mandible in a single protrusive position without any possibility to change the position during treatment. Some of the non-titratable devices are a simple splint, bionator, Karwatsky activator, or Herbst appliance [20].

71.9.4 Surgical Treatment of Obstructive Sleep Apnea [21] (Table 71.4)

Surgical procedures to correct or treat OSA essentially provide site-specific treatment to increase airway size and decrease airway resistance, thus reducing the effort required in breathing. The site of obstruction is specific to each patient and is as unique as fingerprints. Therefore, one needs to know which the most appropriate procedure is to guarantee success. Since no single factor is predictive of OSA, the significance of a thorough physical examination and imaging to

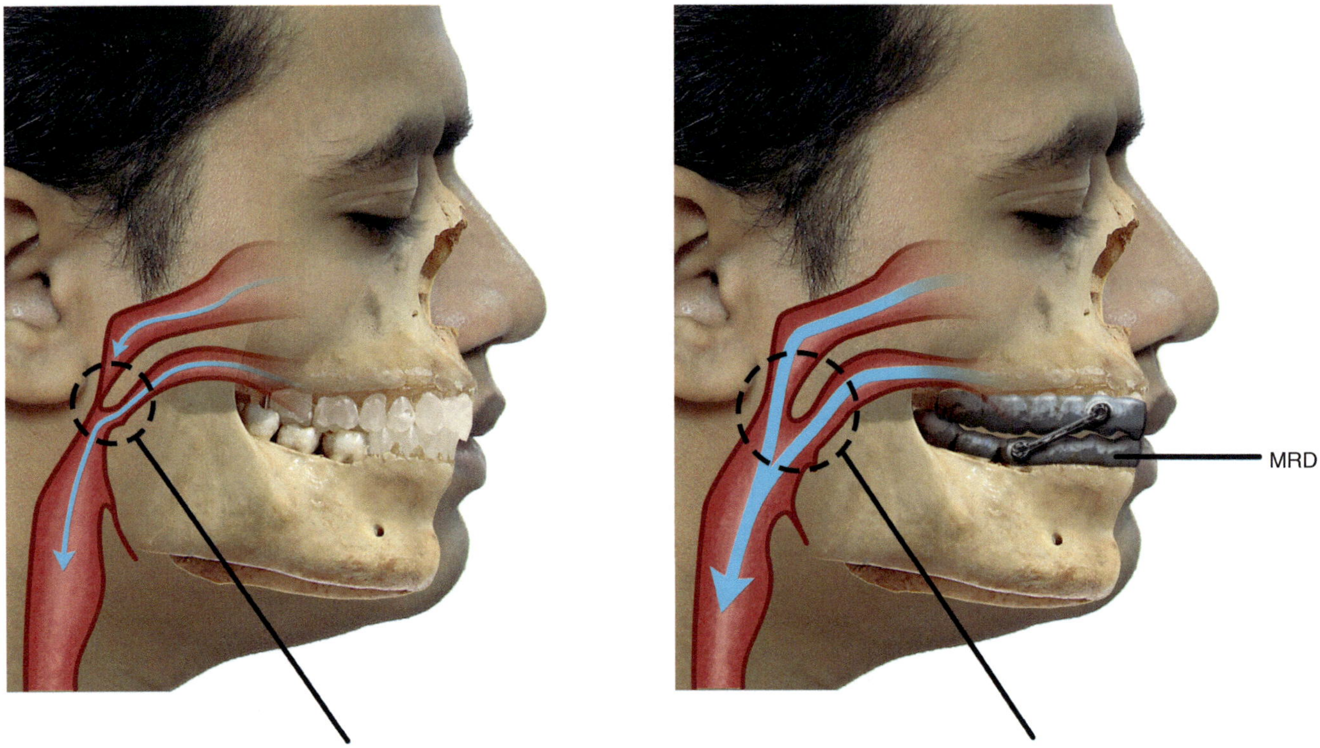

Fig. 71.5 Mandibular repositioning device

Table 71.4 Common surgical procedures for OSA by site

Procedures that bypass the upper airway	Tracheostomy
Nasal procedures	Septoplasty
	Functional rhinoplasty
	Nasal valve surgery
	Turbinate reduction
	Nasal polypectomy
	Endoscopic procedures
Oral, oropharyngeal, and nasopharyngeal procedures	uvulopalatopharyngoplasty
	Palatal advancement pharyngoplasty
	Tonsillectomy/adenoidectomy
	Tori mandibularis excision
Hypopharyngeal procedures	Tongue reduction
	Lingual tonsillectomy
	Genioglossus advancement
	Hyoid suspension
	Mandibular advancement
Laryngeal procedures	Epiglottoplasty
	Hyoid suspension
Global airway procedures	Maxillomandibular advancement
	Bariatric surgery

identify the target site of airway resistance cannot be over emphasized.

Tracheostomy has been used to bypasses the upper airway and is thus a successful modality in treatment, but the morbidity associated with it limits its application.

Factors in the nasal cavity may also play a role in influencing the pharyngeal stability through abnormalities like septal deviation and inferior turbinate. *Nasal surgery* to remove these abnormalities can improve nasal airflow, thus having a positive effect on OSA.

Multiple surgical procedures of the palate like uvulopalatopharyngoplasty (UPPP), which involves removal of the tonsils, uvula, and posterior velum in patients with large tonsils and relatively normal palatal position, are also good adjunctive procedures.

UPPP can also be done assisted by lasers allowing more precise incision and excision than conventional surgery. It also has the advantages of avoiding the need for general anesthesia and with minimal bleeding.

Tonsillectomy with adenoidectomy is the usually first line of surgery for children with OSA without significant craniofacial anomalies.

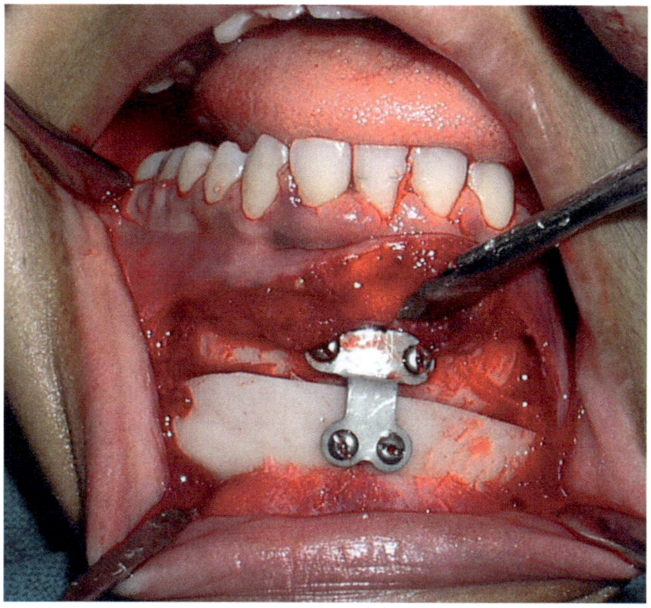

Fig. 71.6 Genioglossal advancement

Tongue reduction is also a part of the surgical option in enlarges tongue cases where partial glossectomy can reduce the tongue volume.

Surgical procedures of the genial segment of the mandible like *Genioglossal advancement* moves the genial tubercles forward along with the genioglossus muscle, resulting in a more forwardly positioned base of tongue. In addition, it also causes the forward movement of the hyoid bone. This shift increases the posterior airway space and avoids the collapse of its walls during the REM phase of sleep. There are a lot of modifications of the genial advancement procedures.

The standard procedure moves the whole genial segment including the chin. A modified technique allows the surgeon to advance the genial tubercle without altering the normal anatomic position or shape of a patient's chin by only moving the rectangular bony component involving the tubercle (Fig. 71.6).

Hyoid myotomy involves the detachment of infrahyoid muscles and moving the hyoid forward and upward and fixing it with sutures. Another procedure moves the hyoid forward and downward with excision of the lesser cornu and fixing the hyoid anterior to the thyroid cartilage by sutures.

Surgical procedures can also be performed at different levels either concomitantly or in a staged manner. This is done when patients have more than one site of obstruction.

Hypoglossal nerve stimulators (HGNS) are a new addition to the armamentarium for treatment of OSA. It was approved by the FDA for treatment of moderate to severe OSA in 2014 [22].

The device which acts like a pacemaker monitors the breathing patterns and gets activated during sleep to stimulate the hypoglossal nerve, thus controlling upper airway muscles.

Maxillomandibular advancement (MMA) is undoubtedly the most successful surgical technique in OSA. This advantage of this procedure is the effect in correcting airway obstruction at multiple levels. The surgical advancement of the maxillomandibular skeletal framework corrects the airway collapsibility at the nasopharyngeal and oropharyngeal levels and is ideal in patients with moderate and severe OSA who exhibit multilevel obstruction.

The Le Fort I osteotomy of the maxilla along with mandibular sagittal split osteotomy is performed for advancing maxilla and mandible, thus increasing the airway space as it draws the base of the tongue and soft palate forwards (Fig. 71.7).

Achieving *MMA by distraction* is another alternative technique, especially in cases of TMJ ankylosis (Figs. 71.8 and 71.9) where a deficient mandible in the sagittal plane is primarily responsible for the obstructed airway.

The dimensions of maxilla and mandible can also be increased in the transverse plane by distraction resulting in increase in the dimensions of nasopharynx, oropharynx, and the nasal cavity along with movement of tonsillar pillars and the musculature of the velum. Maxillomandibular transverse distraction osteogenesis can be concomitantly be performed with their sagittal advancement for a more effective form of treatment MMA alone.

71.10 Adjunctive Therapies

71.10.1 Bariatric Surgery [23]

Weight loss procedures through bariatric surgery is indicated in patients with a body mass index (BMI) $\geq$ 40 kg/m^2 or those with a BMI $\geq$ 35 kg/m^2 with important comorbidities especially when dietary attempts are ineffective.

71.10.2 Medications [23]

Pharmacologic agents can on occasion be used with some degree of success in treating OSA by increasing glossopharyngeal neurologic activity or decreasing REM sleep.

Protriptyline, a tricyclic antidepressant reduces the frequency of apnea and desaturation in non-REM sleep and suppressing REM activity. It also increases the tone of the upper airway muscles. The anticholinergic activity of the drug however limits its use.

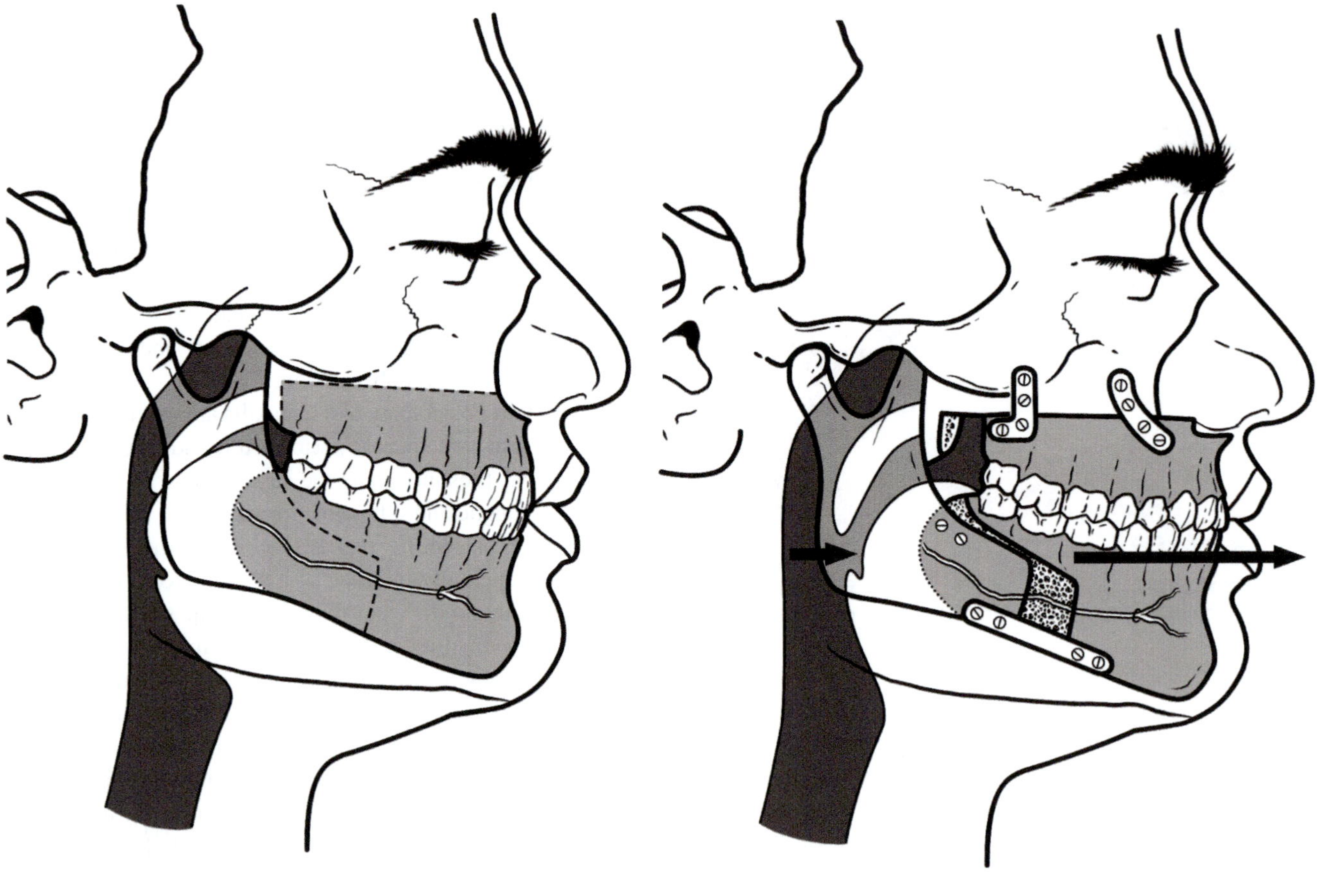

Fig. 71.7 Maxillomandibular advancement and its effect on the airway

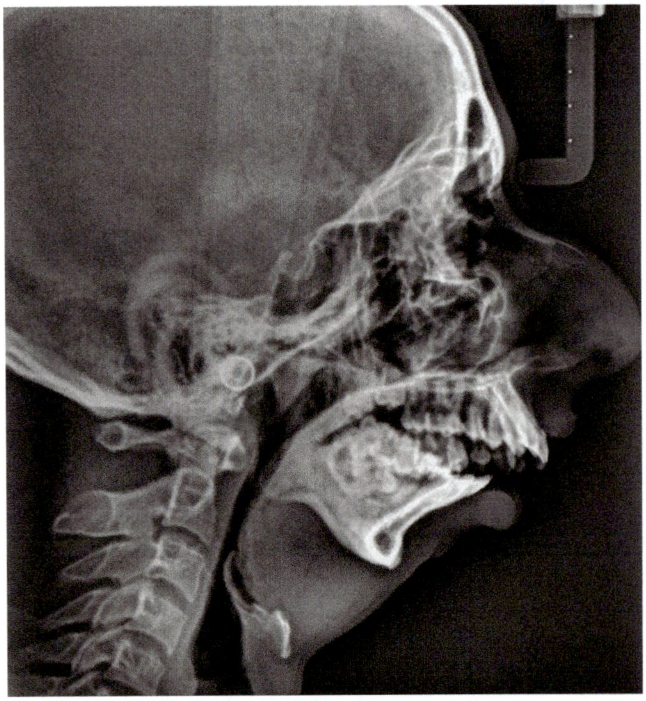

Fig. 71.8 Compromised airway in ankylosis

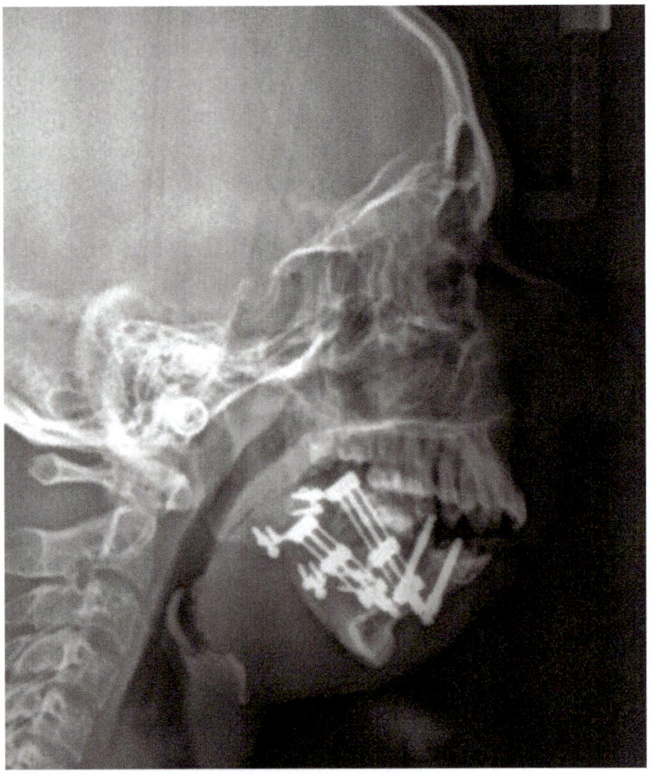

Fig. 71.9 Improved airway after mandibular distraction in a TMJ ankylosis case

Theophylline reduces the episodes of apneas and hypopneas, but the quality of sleep deteriorates.

Modafinil is a wake-promoting medication that can improve residual daytime sleepiness in OSA patients despite regular use of CPAP. It is however avoided in patients who are noncompliant with CPAP. The adverse effects of these drugs are headache and nervousness.

Topical nasal corticosteroids have also been recommended in patients suffering from concurrent rhinitis.

71.11 Conclusion

Obstructive sleep apnea is a multi-factorial and multi-level condition whose management needs to be customized for every patient after a correct diagnosis. Treatment is regulated starting with the non-surgical options and moving to specific site surgical procedures depending on the area of involvement.

71.12 Case Scenario

A 12-year-old female patient with history of sleeping difficulty due to airway obstruction.

Clinical features: Retruded chin, incompetent lips, dry mouth, short chin throat distance (Fig. 71.10).

Preoperative radiographic findings: Deficient mandible, posteriorly placed menton, narrowed oropharynx (Fig. 71.11).

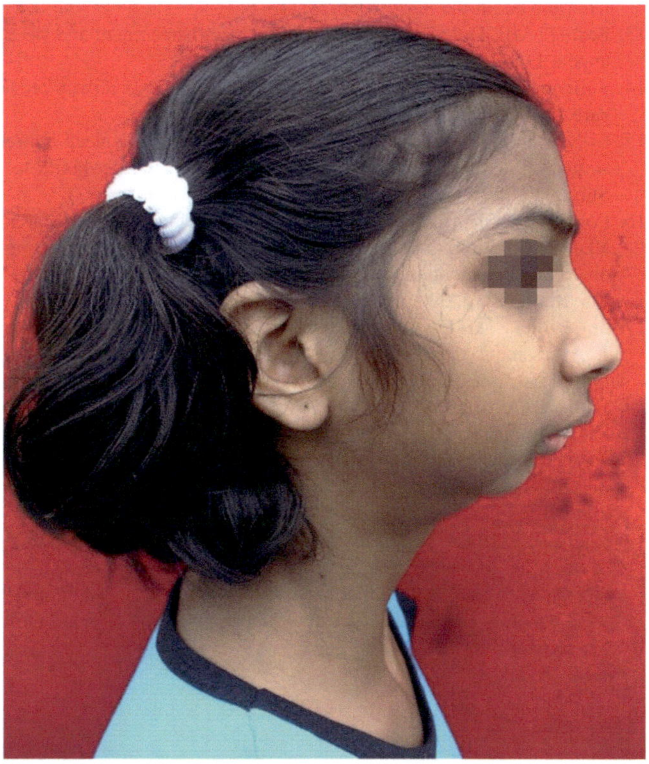

Fig. 71.10 Patients profile

PSG report: Episodes of 33 apneas and 76 hypopneas confirming OSA (Box 71.1).

Treatment plan: Mandibular advancement of 10 mm by distraction (Fig. 71.12).

Post op findings: Improved profile, no episodes of apneas hypopneas (Figs. 71.13, 71.14 and Box 71.2).

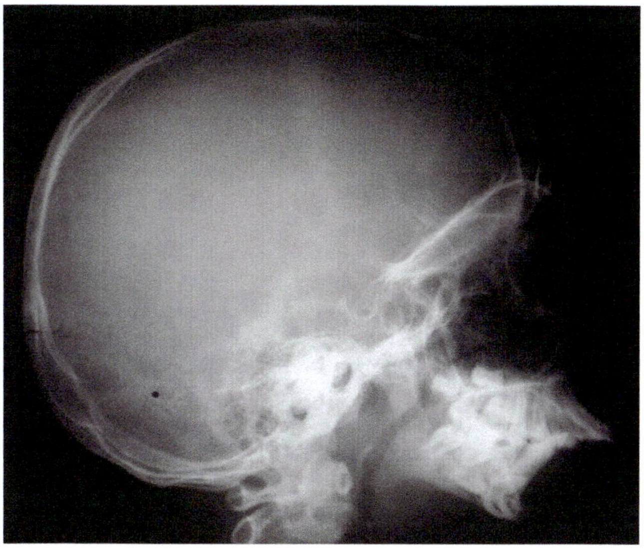

Fig. 71.11 Preoperative cephalogram

Box 71.1 Preoperative PSG report

Events	Number
Apnoeas	33
Hypopnoeas	76

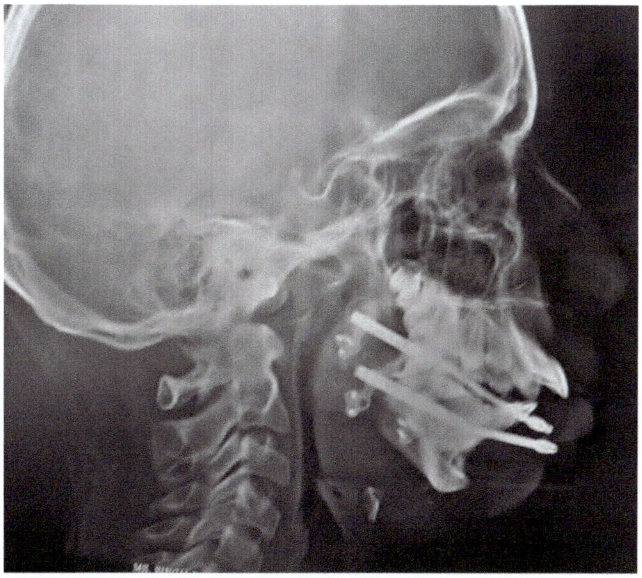

Fig. 71.12 Mandibular distraction

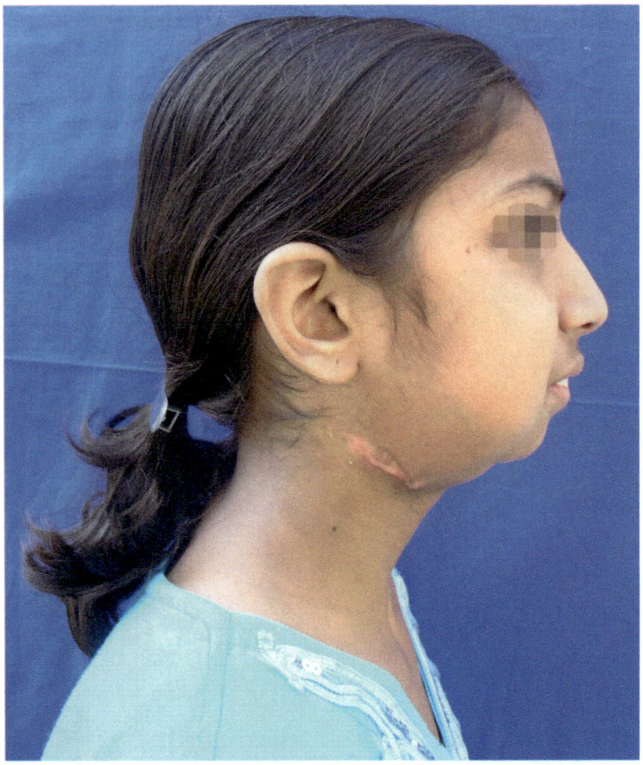

Fig. 71.13 Postoperative profile of the patient

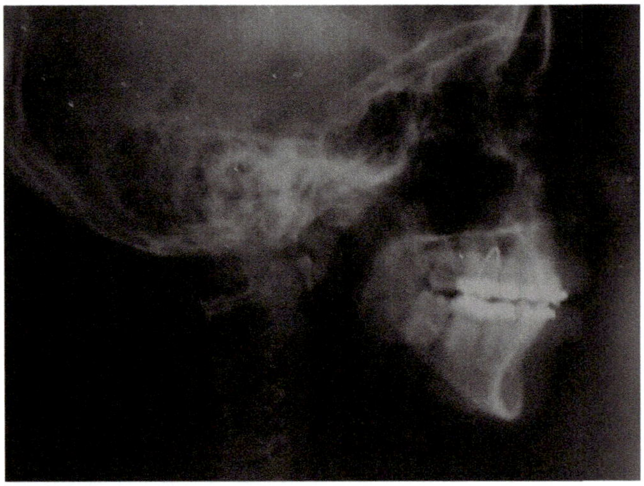

Fig. 71.14 Postoperative cephalogram showing improved airway

Box 71.2 Post distraction PSG report

Events	Number
Apnoeas	0
Hypopnoeas	0

References

1. Epstein LJ, Kristo D, Strollo PJ, Friedman N, Malhotra A, Patil SP, et al. Clinical guideline for the evaluation, management and long-term care of obstructive sleep apnea in adults. J Clin Sleep Med. 2009 Jun 15;5(3):263–76.
2. Susarla SM, Thomas RJ, Abramson ZR, Kaban LB. Biomechanics of the upper airway: changing concepts in the pathogenesis of obstructive sleep apnea. Int J Oral Maxillofac Surg. 2010;39:1149–59.
3. Carolyn C, Brookes D, Boyd SB. Controversies in obstructive sleep apnea. Surg Oral Maxillofac Surg Clin N Am. 2017;29:503–13.
4. Javaheri S, Barbe F, Campos-Rodriguez F, Dempsey JA, Khayat R, Javaheri S, et al. Sleep apnea types, mechanisms, and clinical cardiovascular consequences. J Am Coll Cardiol. 2017;69(7):841–58.
5. Kaur A, Mokhlesi B. The effect of OSA therapy on glucose metabolism: it's all about CPAP adherence! J Clin Sleep Med. 2017 Mar 15;13(3):365–7.
6. Yee B, Liu P, Phillips C, Grunstein R. Neuroendocrine changes in sleep apnea. Curr Opin Pulm Med. 2004 November;10(6):475–81.
7. Young T, Palta M, Dempsey J, Skatrud J, Weber S, Badr S. The occurrence of sleep disordered breathing among middle aged adults. N Engl J Med. 1993;328:1230.
8. Young T, Peppard PE, Gottlieb DJ. Epidemiology of obstructive sleep apnea. Am J Respir Crit Care Med. 2002;165:1217.
9. Kim S-J, Kim Y-S, Park J-H, Kim S-W. Cephalometric predictors of therapeutic response to multilevel surgery in patients with obstructive sleep apnea. J Oral Maxillofac Surg. 2012;70:1404–12.
10. Tangugsorn V, Krogstad O, Espeland L, Lyberg T. Obstructive sleep apnoea: multiple comparisons of cephalometric variables of obese and non-obese patients. J Cranio Maxillofac Surg. 2000;28:204–12.
11. Gotsopoulos H, Kelly JJ, Cistulli PA. Treatment of OSA oral appliance therapy reduces blood pressure in obstructive sleep apnea: a randomized, controlled trial. Sleep. 2004;27(5):934–41.
12. Herford AS, Finn R. Single-stage CO2 laser assisted uvuloplasty for treatment of snoring and mild obstructive sleep apnoea. J Cranio-Maxillofac Surg. 2000;28:213–6.
13. Barbick MB, Dolwick MF. Genial tubercle advancement and sleep apnea. J Oral MaxillofacSurg. 2009;67:1767–70.
14. Sullivan C, Berthon-Jones M, Issa F. Nocturnal nasal-airway pressure for sleep apnea. N Engl J Med. 1983;309:112.
15. Li KK, Riley RW, Powell NB, Troell RJ. Obstructive sleep apnea surgery: Genioglossus advancement revisited. J Oral Maxillofac Surg. 2004;59:1181–4.
16. Foltan R, Hoffmannova J, Pretl M, Donev F, Marek VLK. Genioglossus advancement and hyoid myotomy in treating obstructive sleep apnoea syndrome – a follow-up study. J Cranio-Maxillofac Surg. 2007;35:246–51.
17. de Ruiter MHT, Apperloo RC, Milstein DMJ, de Lange J. Assessment of obstructive sleep apnoea treatment success or failure after maxillomandibular advancement. Int J Oral Maxillofac Surg. 2017;46:1357–62.
18. Scott Conleya R, Leganb HL. Correction of severe obstructive sleep apnea with bimaxillary transverse distraction osteogenesis and maxillomandibular advancement. Am J Orthod Dentofac Orthop. 2006;129:283–92.
19. Louro RS, Calasans-Maia JA, Mattos CT, Masterson D, Calasans-Maia MD, Maia LC. Three-dimensional changes to the upper airway after maxillomandibular advancement with counterclockwise rotation: a systematic review and meta-analysis. Int J Oral Maxillofac Surg. 2018;47:622–9.

20. Jayan B, Prasad BNBM, Bhattacharya D, Rajput AK, Dhiman RK. Management of a case of severe obstructive sleep apnoea with acrylic Herbst splint appliance: a case report Indian. J Sleep Med. 2006;1(3):157–60.
21. Fleisher KE, Krieger AC. Current trends in the treatment of obstructive sleep apnea. J Oral Maxillofac Surg. 2007;65:2056–68.
22. Hochban W, Podszus T, Eisele DW, Schwarz AR, Smith PL, Erickson D, Testerman R. Hypoglossal nerve stimulation for obstructive sleep apnoea. Int J Oral Maxillo fac Surg. 1997;26:156.
23. W Keith Thornton and D Heath Roberts. Non-surgical management of the Obstructive sleep apnea patient. J Oral Maxillofac Surg. 1996;54:1103–8.

Suggested Reading

Carolyn C. Dicus Brookes, Scott B. Boyd: Controversies in Obstructive Sleep Apnea Surgery. Oral Maxillofacial Surg Clin N Am 29 (2017) 503–513.

Kasey K Li: Maxillomandibular advancement for Obstructive Sleep Apnea. J Oral Maxillofac Surg 69:687–694, 2011.

Lawrence J. Epstein, David Kristo, Patrick J. Strollo, Norman Friedman, Atul Malhotra, Susheel P. Patil et al. Clinical Guideline for the Evaluation, Management and Long-term Care of Obstructive Sleep Apnea in Adults. J Clin Sleep Med. 2009 Jun 15; 5(3): 263–276.

Part XIX

Developmental Deformities of the Oral and Maxillofacial Region

72 Cleft Lip

Pritham N. Shetty, Jaideep Singh Chauhan, Mamatha Patil, Neha Aggarwal, and Dipesh Rao

72.1 Introduction

A cleft lip [CL] is defined as a congenital defect in lip continuity due to an embryological malformation. Cleft lip and palate [CLP] have an overall incidence of 1 in 1000 live births [1]. For different ethnicities, the incidence varies. Like other facial deformities, cleft lip and palate produce a considerable degree of disfigurement and functional impairment. A comprehensive treatment involving a cleft surgeon, otolaryngologist, geneticist, speech pathologist, orthodontist and others are required at multiple stages right from infancy to adulthood. A successful lip repair requires careful consideration of presentation of the cleft, the availability of tissues or the lack thereof and effect of intervention on growth and function. We have tried to simplify this concept, keeping certain key points in mind necessary for comprehension of the subject. In this chapter, we have discussed embryology, anatomy and clinical presentation of cleft as an integrated phenomenon for better understanding of cleft lip. The author's technique of cleft lip is discussed in a stepwise manner.

Electronic Supplementary Material The online version of this chapter (https://doi.org/10.1007/978-981-15-1346-6_72) contains supplementary material, which is available to authorized users.

P. N. Shetty (✉)
OMFS, Bangalore Institute of Dental Science, Bangalore, India

J. S. Chauhan
Department of Maxillofacial Surgery and the Smile Train, CHL Hospital, Indore, India

M. Patil
Sparsh Hospital Bommasandra Industrial Area, Bangalore, India

N. Aggarwal
Cleft and Craniofacial Surgery, Meenakshi Cleft and Craniofacial Centre, Chennai, India

D. Rao
Bhagwan Mahaveer Jain Hospital, Bangalore, Karnataka, India

72.1.1 History of Cleft Lip Repair

The enigma of cleft lip and the historic journey to repair the defect has been well described in the narrative book by Millard [2].The excerpts from it illustrates the documentation of the first cleft lip repair in the year 390 AD where an unidentified Chinese physician cut the edges of the cleft and stitched it together with a postoperative order of limited lip movements for the next 100 days. The need to identify an ideal technique was derived on the basis of the anatomical outcome of the repair and also the postoperative scarring. The concepts of cleft lip repair have evolved from straight line repairs to a variety of techniques using various cutbacks, triangles, z-plasties and other flaps.

The techniques for cleft lip can be broadly classified into:

- Straight line repairs.
- Geometric designed techniques.
- Rotational advancement techniques.

We will discuss certain techniques to explain the evolution from a historical point of view. The rotation-advancement technique with its modifications will be discussed later in this chapter.

72.2 Embryology

72.2.1 Development of the External Face

The face is derived from two sources: the frontonasal process that covers the forebrain (neural crest origin) and the tissues of first pharyngeal arch (mixed mesoderm and neural crest origin). These tissues surround the oropharyngeal membrane. From the frontonasal process, two medial nasal processes and lateral nasal processes arise [3]. The first pharyngeal arch gives

K. Bonanthaya et al. (eds.), *Oral and Maxillofacial Surgery for the Clinician*, https://doi.org/10.1007/978-981-15-1346-6_72

rise to a pair of mandibular processes and a pair of maxillary processes from which palatal processes arise [3]. The maxillary prominences continue to grow medially, compressing the medial nasal prominences towards the midline, subsequently meeting the lateral nasal processes and then the lower part of the medial nasal processes (Figs. 72.1, 77.1). This lower part is known as the globular or premaxillary process. The components derived from various parts are given in Table 72.1.

Abnormalities throughout this complicated developmental process occur in the most severe congenital forms if they develop early in facial embryogenesis (4–8 weeks) to the relatively minor problems developing later (8–12 weeks). Cleft lip varies from a notch in lips red border to extending into the floor of nostril and the alveolar ridge. It may be unilateral or bilateral (Fig. 72.2). Some other forms of facial clefts have also been described in a pictorial form as a result of failure of fusion of the same processes but in a different trajectory and various permutations and combinations (Fig. 72.3).

1. Unilateral cleft lip—due to the failure of the maxillary prominence to join with the merged median nasal prominences which results in a cleft.
2. Bilateral cleft lip—due to failure of fusion of the maxillary prominences with merged nasal prominences bilaterally. The extent of clefting may or may not be similar on both sides.

Table 72.1 Components of face derived from various prominences

Prominence	External face derivatives
Frontonasal	The forehead, the bridge of nose, median and lateral nasal processes
Medial nasal	The philtrum of the upper lip, crest and tip of the nose
Lateral nasal	Alae of the nose
Maxillary process (first pharyngeal arch)	Lateral portion of the upper lip
Mandibular process (first pharyngeal arch)	The lower lip

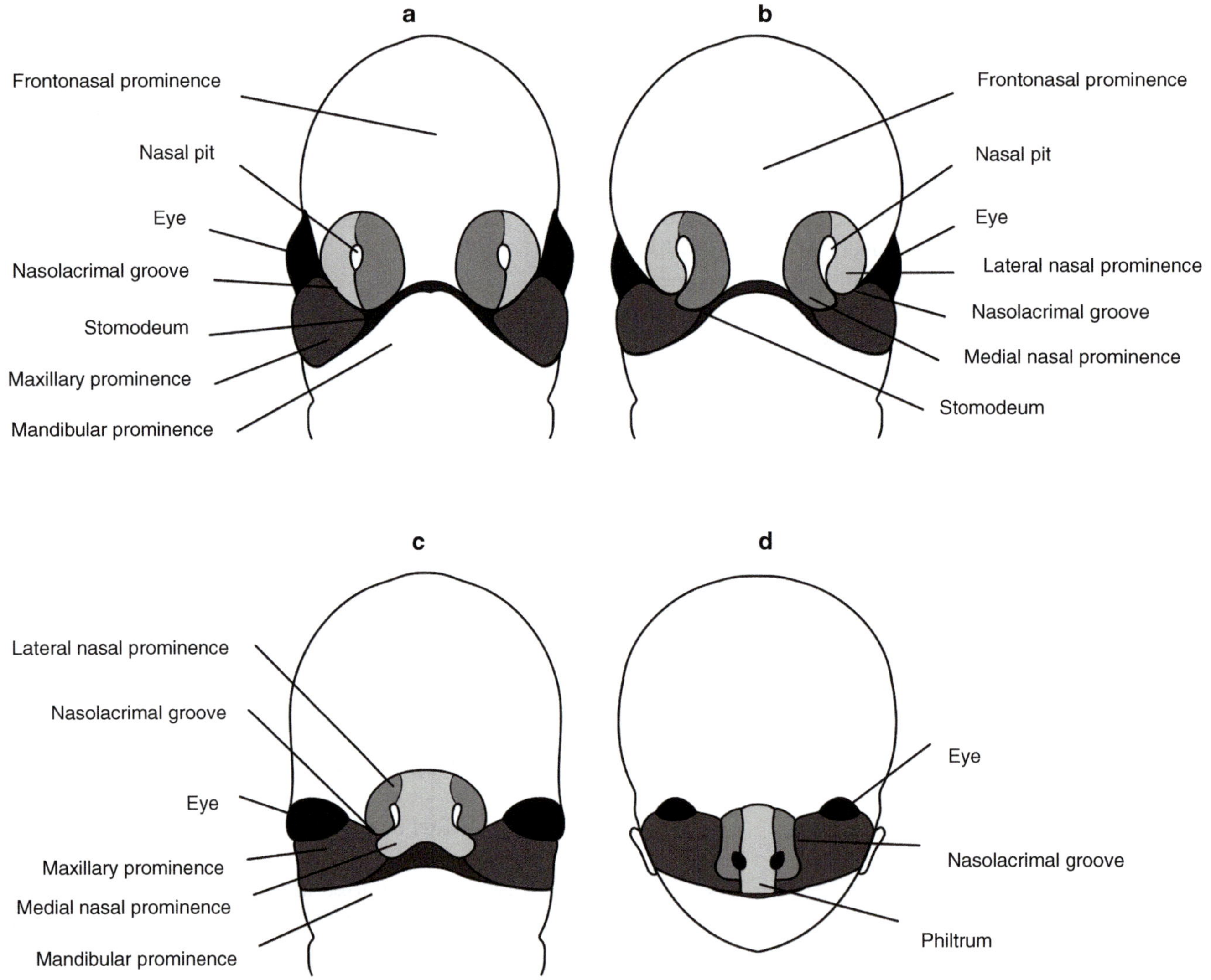

Fig. 72.1 (**a–d**) Development of the face. (**a**) Lateral nasal and medial nasal swellings that surround the nasal placodes appear on the frontonasal process (**b**) Paired maxillary processes grow medially, compressing the medial nasal prominences towards the midline. (**c**) Medial nasal processes fuse with each other, lateral nasal processes and the maxillary processes. (**d**) Complete development of the nose and upper lip

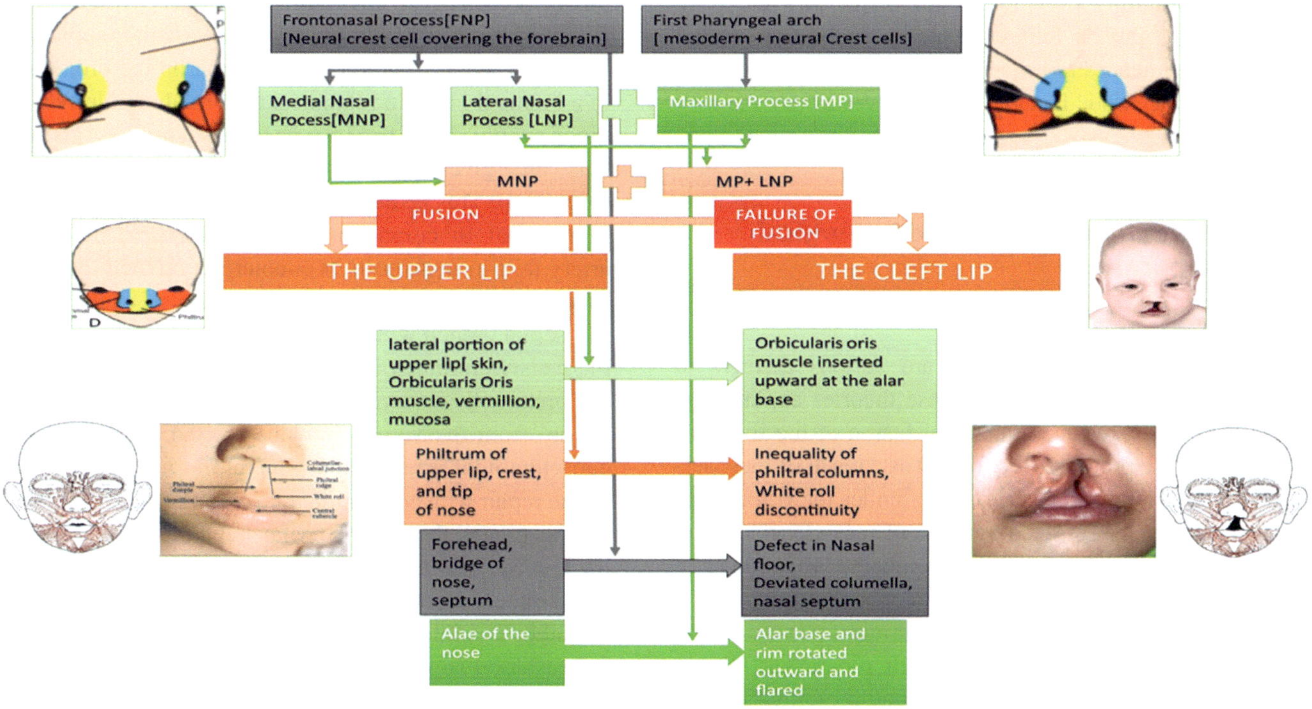

Fig. 72.2 Relation of embryological derivative to the anatomical and clinical description of cleft lip

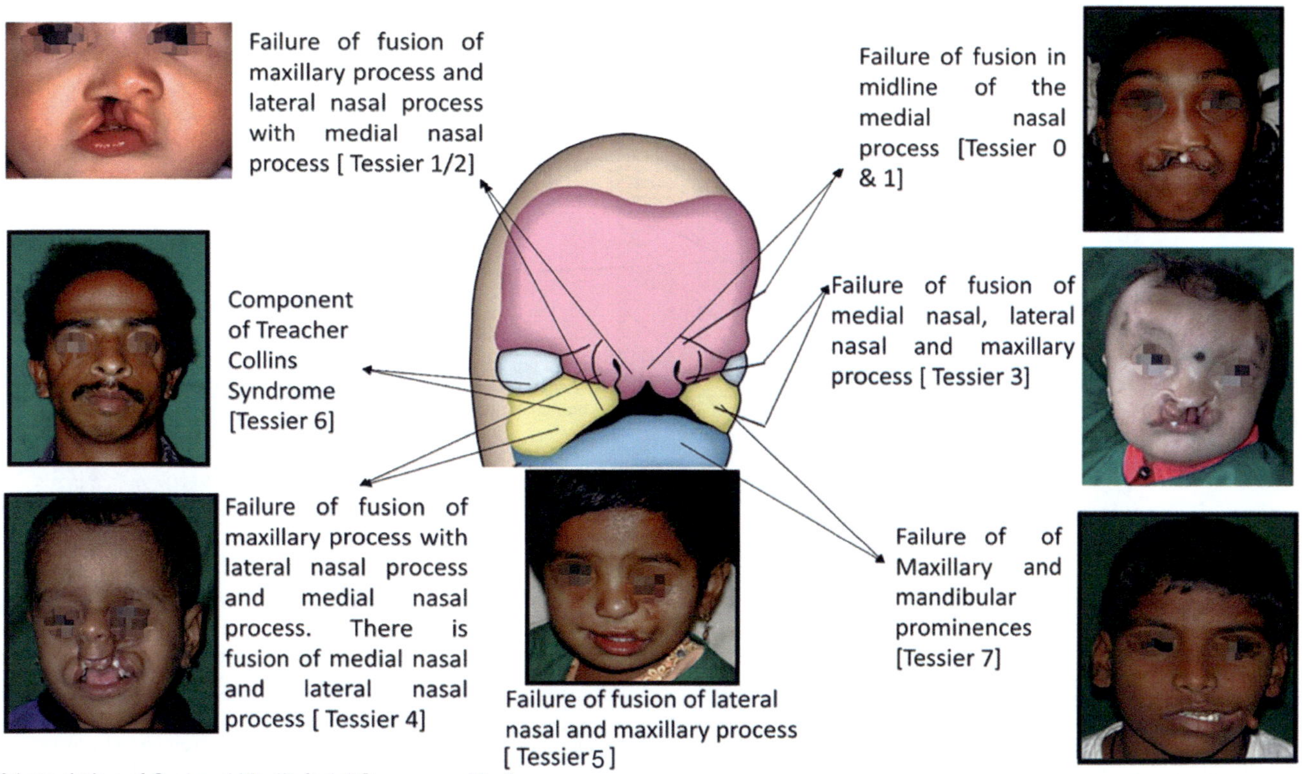

Fig. 72.3 Embryology of various facial clefts

3. Median cleft lip—a very rare condition. Occurs due to the partial or complete failure of fusion of the two medial nasal prominences to form the intermaxillary segment. It is the characteristic feature of Mohr's syndrome.

72.2.2 Embryology of Cleft and its Surgical Implications

1. Mesodermal Migration: There are various theories to describe how a cleft occurs. These theories explain that cleft rises as a result of failure of fusion of the five processes. These processes are formed as a result of mesodermal migration resulting in heaping under the ectodermal layer. Insufficient or late migration of mesoderm leads to partial or total cleft as a result of epithelial breakdown.

   Mesoderm gives rise to the fibromuscular layer of the lip. The importance of mesodermal migration carries in itself an important principle of cleft repair, i.e. muscle approximation. The author's technique presented later in this chapter describes this step as an important step in functional cleft repair. Also the mesoderm has chondrogenic potential which explains the accompanying deficit in the development of nasal capsule [4].
2. Vascular Supply: The philtrum and premaxilla derive their blood supply from the posterior septal artery and terminal branches of the ethmoidal artery (Fig. 72.4). Knowledge of this embryological vascular supply is important while designing the incision on the prolabium in a bilateral cleft lip repair. As the prolabium derives its blood supply solely from the frontonasal process, no back cuts are given during dissection of prolabial flap (Fig. 72.4). This is discussed again in surgical technique.
3. Premaxilla: In complete bilateral cleft lips, the labial artery fails to unite with its counterpart on the other side. In addition the arcade made by anastomosis of the posterior septal branch with the greater palatine artery through the incisive foramen is absent. Thus the blood supply of the premaxilla is derived from three sources: periosteal supply from the vomer, branches of the sphenopalatine and ethmoidal artery. This principle is used in anterior palate repair with concomitant lip repair in bilateral clefts. It is postulated that anterior palate repair using the vomerine flap can lead to premaxillary necrosis due to cutoff of blood supply from the posterior septal arteries. However, in author's opinion and experience, the premaxilla has a robust blood supply even after using vomerine flaps for anterior palate repair [5].
4. The maxillary process carries within itself the superior labial artery which supplies the orbicularis oris muscle. During muscle dissection, the artery is encountered within the muscle going upward. This vessel should be identified throughout the length of incision and muscle dissection and should be carefully cauterised.

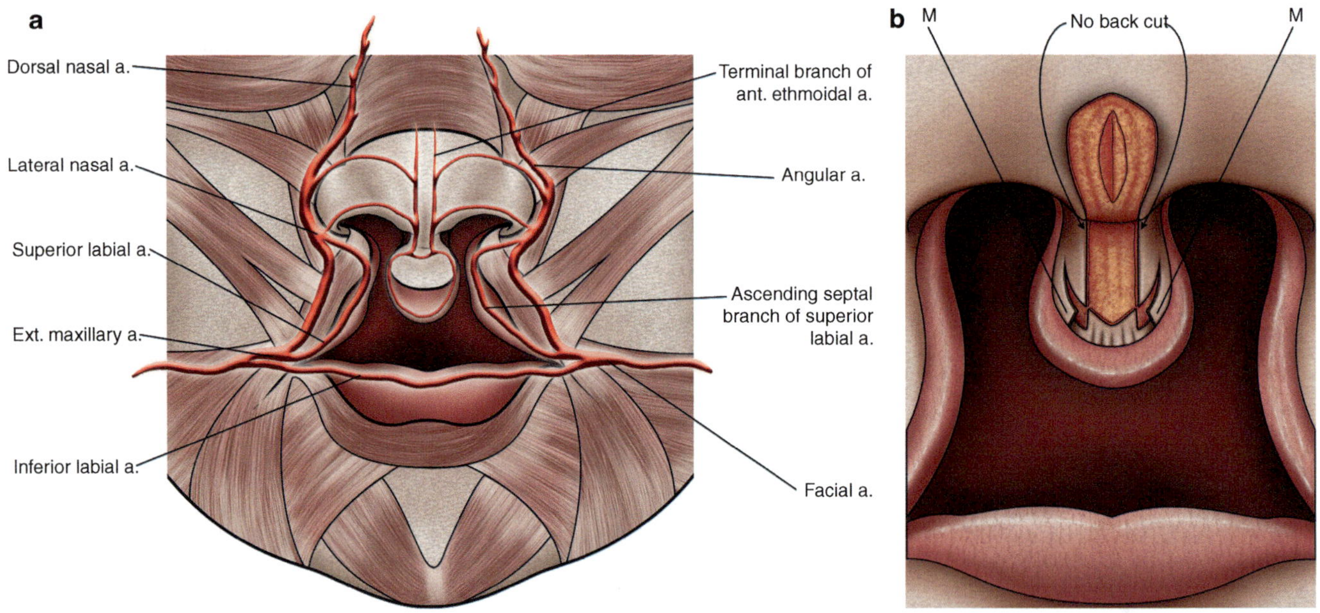

Fig. 72.4 (**a**, **b**) As the philtrum and premaxilla are derived from the frontonasal process, their blood supply is from the posterior septal artery and terminal branches of the ethmoidal artery (**a**). As the prolabium derives its blood supply solely from the frontonasal process, no back cuts are given during dissection of prolabial flap (**b**)

72.2.3 Prenatal Diagnosis in Cleft Lip

Cleft lip can be diagnosed in the intrauterine stage with the help of routine ultrasound scanning at different intervals of gestation. The prenatal diagnosis is usually established during the second and third trimester [6]. Recent data suggests that during the 11–13 gestational weeks, a midsagittal view of the fetal head, face and brain, in addition to certain measurable abnormalities, such as a smaller palatino-maxillary diameter, can make grounds for an underlying CLP. 3D sonography can construct a computerized volumetric rendering of the foetus, similar to 3D CT volumetric reconstructions. Detection rates of up to 75% have been described by specialist maternal-fetal medicine [MFM] physicians and radiologists. Thus, prenatal counselling continues to be important with evolving diagnostic procedures. Although there is currently no intrauterine treatment of cleft lip and palate, research has indicated that both mother and child benefit from early diagnosis and counselling. Prenatal counselling has positive psychological implications on the parents of a child with cleft as they are better prepared and motivated for treatment.

72.3 Surgical Anatomy

Anatomy of the cleft lip patient includes two major components: the lip and the nose. Both the structures vary greatly in a unilateral and bilateral cleft lip deformity and are discussed individually here.

The upper lip is attached above to the nose and blends laterally into the cheek, curving into the lower lip at the commissures. It is formed of muscles and glands covered superficially with skin and lined internally with mucous membrane. These layers are tightly adherent to the muscles and are sealed along the free margin (Box 72.1).

Box 72.1 Components of an Upper Lip
Normal upper lip anatomy

1. Skin, mucous membranes and vermillion with lbial mucosal glands.
2. Muscles: orbicularis oris insertion is displaced in unilateral and bilateral cleft patients.
3. Vascular supply: superior labial artery, inferior labial artery and septal arteries are the major blood supplies of the lips and the nose.

72.3.1 Surface Anatomy

The following anatomical surface components of the upper lip are to be kept in mind when assessing a patient with cleft lip (Fig. 72.5). Anatomical equal repositioning of these features is essential for an aesthetic and functional outcome (Box 72.2).

Box 72.2 Anatomic Landmarks
Philtral columns: They are paired bilateral vertical lip bulges created by the dermal insertion of orbicularis oris fibres into the skin of the upper lip.

Philtral dimple: It's a concavity between the philtral columns created by relative deficiency of muscle fibres.

White roll: The white roll is a prominent ridge just above cutaneous-vermillion border. It appears very distinct and white/light in colour due to reflection of light off the skin. This is due to insertion of pars maginalis of orbicularis muscle and absence of hair in this region.

Vermillion: It's the red mucosal portion of lip divided into dry (keratinized) and wet (nonkeratinized) mucosa.

Red line: It's the junction between wet and dry vermillion mucosa.

Cupid's bow: A curvature of central white roll, formed by the two lateral peaks as the philtral columns extend inferiorly.

Tubercle: Vermillion fullness at central inferior apex of Cupid's bow.

In the normal lip, the columella is a central straight column reaching up to the nasal tip. At its base the columella blends into the nostril sill in front of the nasal floors laterally towards the alar bases. The arches of the alae are symmetrical with equal bulges of the alar cartilages. The eversion of the upper lip places it slightly out in front of the lower lip at the mucocutaneous junction of the upper lip. There is a continuous 1–2 mm rounded roll from commissure to commissure which tops the vermilion and picks up white light it coincides in its curves with the peaks of the Cupid's bow of the vermilion which has central tubercle flanked by, each arch of the bow. The abundance of eleidin in the epithelial cell layers increases the translucency, and the numerous rich capillaries of the papillae create the red colour of this area [5].

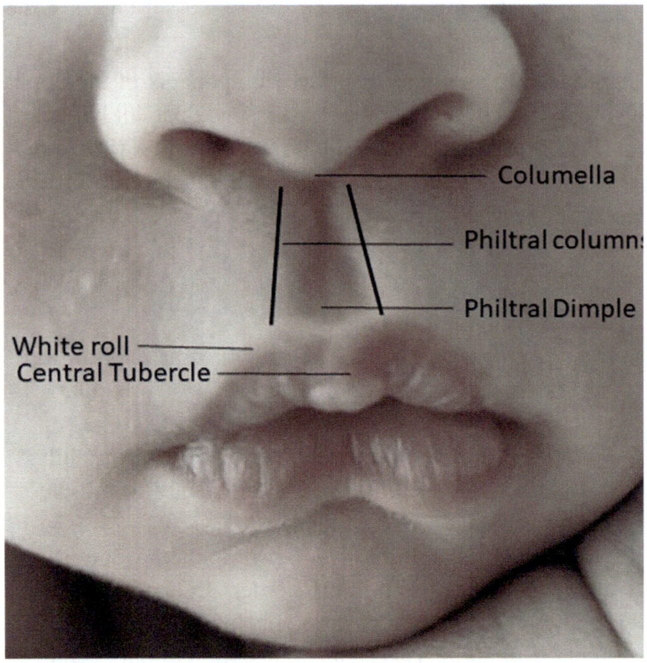

Fig. 72.5 Surface landmarks of a normal lip and nose

72.3.2 Muscles

The *orbicularis oris* consists of numerous layers of muscle fibres surrounding the rima oris traversing in different directions. It is partly derived from muscle fibres of the other facial muscles which are inserted into the lips and partly fibres of its own inserted into the skin near the midline. The main fibres of the lips are oblique and pass from the skin to the mucous membrane, throughout the lip thickness. In the upper lip, these fibres group into two bands bilaterally, lateral and medial [total of four bands]: the *lateral band* originating from the alveolus of the lateral incisor tooth and the *medial band* connecting the upper lip to the septum of the nose. The area between the two medial bands forms the *philtrum*, below the septum of the nose. The additional fibres for the lower lip arise on either side of the midline lateral to the mentalis and merge with the other muscles at the commissure [7].

Orbicularis oris derives from eight muscle components with their origins in the modiolus at each angle of the mouth. Orbicularis fibres of one side end by decussating in the median line with fibres from the opposite side. The orbicularis is composed of four pars peripheralis extending from the rima oris on the right and left side. Intimately associated with the pars peripheralis is the pars marginalis with its two right and left components lying in a plane superficial to the pars peripheralis and confined to the area beneath the vermillion. Pars marginalis is responsible for fine movement (speech) and pars peripheralis for gross movement of the lips (Fig. 72.6a–c). In the presence of cleft, the orbicularis oris muscle fibres do not decussate transversely across the midline but tend to go parallel to the cleft edges towards the base of the nose with their integrity divided. In addition, the transverse nasalis muscle, levator labii superioris and depressor septi do not insert and are prolapsed laterally. They often contract abnormally which has a ripple effect of the lip and the nose. Muscles make the most of their advantage exerting unnatural lateral lifting and distortion of the lip elements in both incomplete and complete clefts. They play a role in displacement of alar base to the side of cleft and the nasal septum on non-cleft healthy side.

72.3.3 Vascular Supply

The major vascular supply to the lip and nose area is derived from the facial artery, branch of the external carotid artery. Other additional sources are from the ophthalmic and the infraorbital arteries. The facial artery gives off inferior and superior labial branches which arise near the corner of the mouth and course as the coronary vessels beneath the free border of the lips deep to the muscle and close to the mucous membrane. The right and left labial arteries freely anastomose to form a circle surrounding the oral aperture. The facial artery then proceeds upwards along the nasolabial fold and gives off the lateral nasal branch and then becomes the angular artery proceeding up to anastomose with the dorsal nasal branch of the ophthalmic artery. The posterior septal artery arising from the sphenopalatine artery in the roof of the nasal cavity courses down the vomerine groove to the incisive foramen anastomosing with the major palatine and ascending septal branches of the superior labial arteries (Fig. 72.7a, b).

Near the inferior lateral attachment of the ala, the lateral nasal artery divides to run one branch along the lower border and another along the superior margin of the lower lateral cartilage. These branches anastomose in the midline with the terminal branches of the anterior ethmoidal artery. It enters the nose and passes along the undersurface of the nasal bone continuing distally over the upper lateral cartilages to the tip of the nose. It joins the lateral nasal branches to continue into the columella anastomosing with the ascending septal branches of the superior labial artery [5].

Vascular anatomy in a cleft lip has been described pictographically in Fig. 72.8. There is an interruption in the usual arcade in the upper lip in unilateral clefts. However, there is sufficient blood supply to both lip elements and the nose to ensure adequate healing.

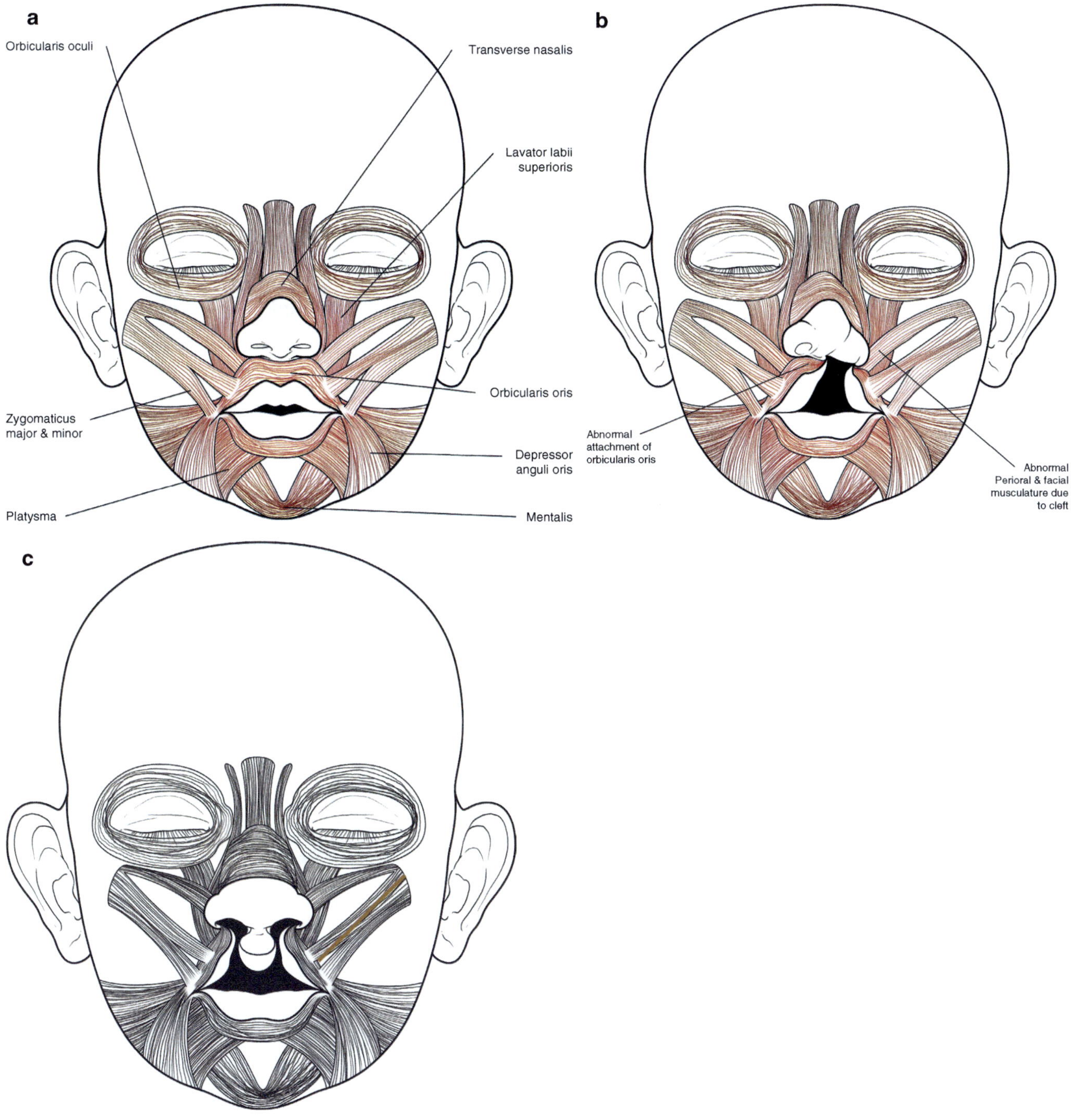

Fig. 72.6 (**a–c**) Concentric band of orbicularis oris forming oral sphincter. Upper and lower fibres arise from each modiolus and decussate in the midline. Superficial fibres upper lip criss-cross at midline to attach to the dermis of the overlying skin at the philtrum. Deeper fibres attach to the anterior nasal spine [left]. Note the abnormal attachments in unilateral and bilateral clefts [middle and right]

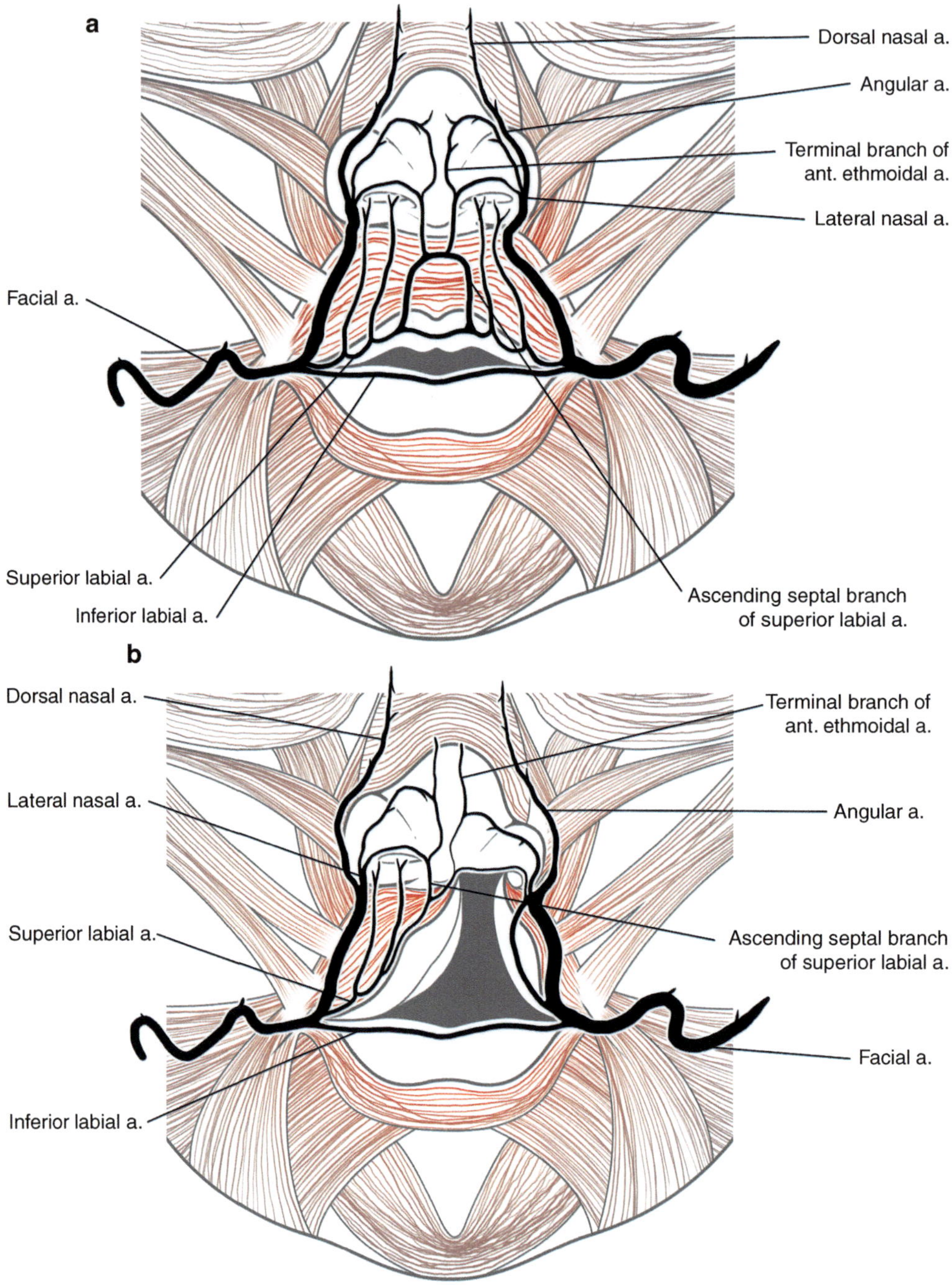

Fig. 72.7 (**a**, **b**) Vascular anatomy of a complete lip (**a**) and a unilateral cleft lip (**b**)

72.3.4 Nerve Supply

The sensory nerve supply to the involved areas of the lips and nose comes from branches of the fifth cranial nerve, trigeminal nerve surfacing through the infraorbital foramen as the infraorbital nerve and through the mental foramen as the mental nerve The motor nerve supply to the muscles of the lips and nose comes from the seventh or facial nerve through its zygomatic, buccal and mandibular branches.

72.3.5 Anatomy of the Unilateral Cleft Lip

A thorough knowledge of the normal lip anatomy can help us understand the abnormal anatomy in cleft. Displacement of muscle insertions and deformation and functional hypotrophy leading to paucity of tissues result in a distorted anatomy of labial clefts (Fig. 72.9). The following are the characteristics of the cleft lip and nose deformity (Table 72.2):

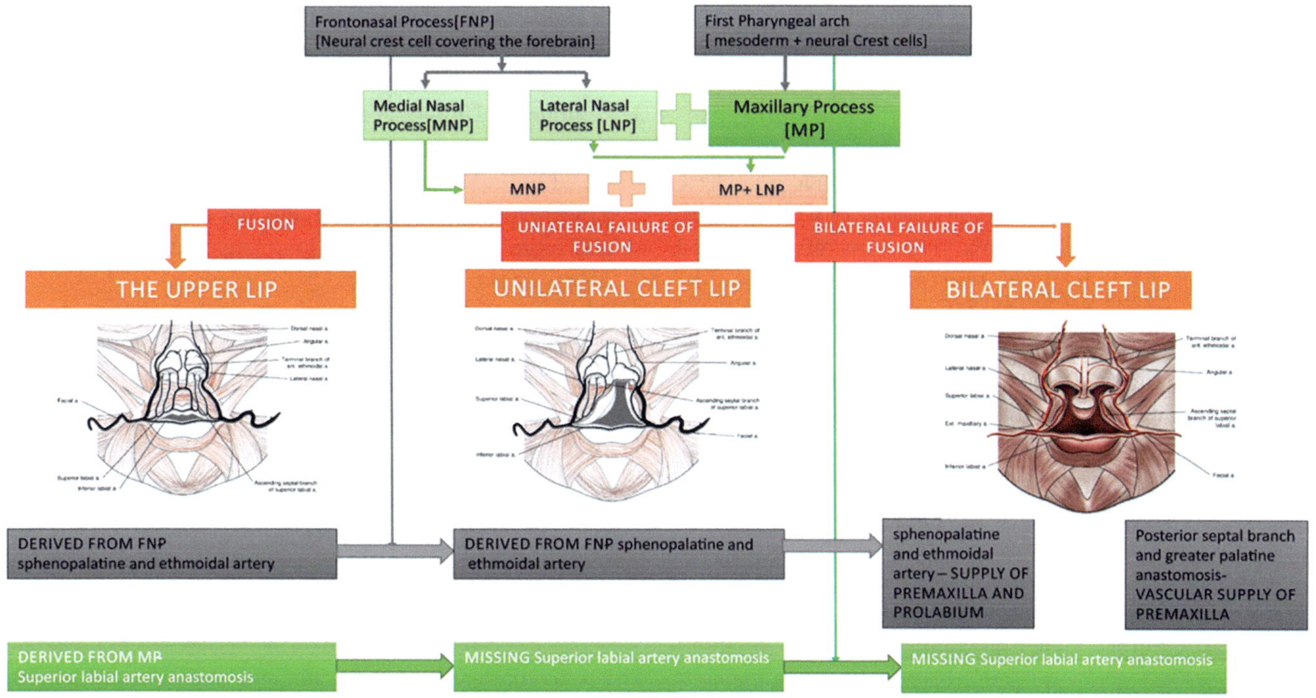

Fig. 72.8 Embryological basis of vascular anatomy in unilateral and bilateral cleft lip

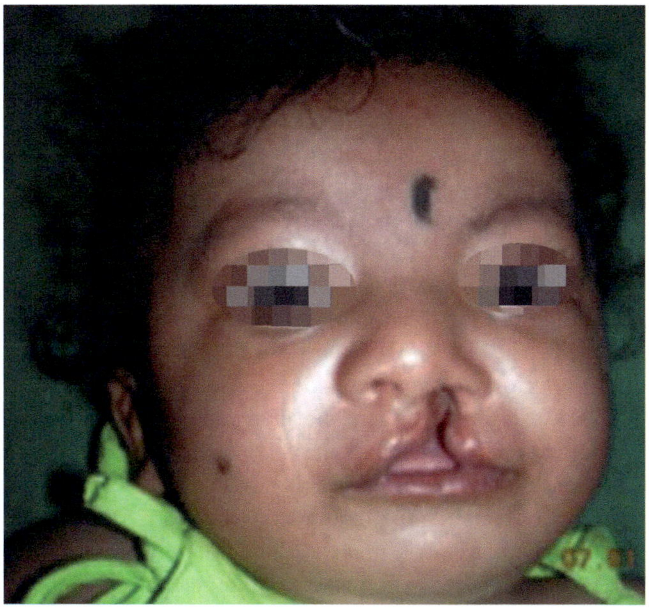

Fig. 72.9 Presentation of a unilateral cleft lip. Note the abnormal anatomy of the lip and nose compared to the non-cleft side

Table 72.2 Comparison of normal and cleft anatomy

Normal anatomy	Unilateral cleft anatomy	Bilateral cleft anatomy
Labial skin	Non-fusion of the lip, the skin on both sides of the lip is less projected or drawn out	One prolabium and bilateral lip elements. The prolabium is the central lip element that has severe paucity of tissues
Philtral columns	Philtral columns are on the non-cleft side, obliquity and discrepancy in their length	No philtral columns present on any element
White roll	Lateral side, the white roll gradually diminishes to about 2–3 mm before it disappears. On the medial side, the demarcation of the white roll is less clear	The white roll on the prolabium is rounded and indistinct
Mucosa	Absence of a labial glandular bed, paucity of compressor muscles, thinner and finer mucosa	Absence of a labial glandular bed, paucity of compressor muscles, thinner and finer mucosa
Orbicularis oris	No muscle decussating in the midline. Abnormal attachment at alar base	Muscle runs bilaterally up into the alar bases, no muscle on the median lip element

1. Labial skin: Apart from the non-fusion of the lip, the skin on both sides of the lip is less projected or drawn out. This leads to a hypoplastic or decreased cutaneous length of the skin. However, the skin is thicker than in normal individuals. The lip consists of the skin, orbicularis oris muscle, minor salivary glands and the labial mucosa. These anatomical planes are important to identify while dissecting the muscle layer. Only 1–2 mm of subdermal dissection should be done, whereas on the mucosal side, the plane of dissection is between the muscle on one side and minor salivary glands and mucosa as a single layer.
2. Unequal philtral columns: The philtral columns are on the non-cleft side, with an obliquity due to discrepancy in their length leaning towards the contralateral sides.

   Matching of the philtral columns of both sides is central to a successful lip repair. The philtral columns are the paired elevated soft tissue structures of the face which make an important aesthetic subunit. Various surgical manoeuvres have been used to achieve symmetry of the philtral columns. The surgical design of rotation-advancement technique is also based on making the philtral columns of the same height.
3. White roll abnormality: From the lateral side, the white roll gradually diminishes to about 2–3 mm before it disappears. On the medial side, the demarcation of the white roll is less clear. Identifying the white roll is pivotal in making incision markings during surgery. A practical tip is to identify maximum width of the dark/dry mucosa; it is generally the most pertinent area to mark the point where the white roll starts diminishing. This is discussed again in the surgical technique.
4. Mucosa: In cleft lip, due to absence of a labial glandular bed and the paucity of compressor muscles, the mucosa of the cleft side is thinner and finer. Also, the mucosa merges with the skin closer to the nose and rolls inward. This mucosa of the cleft region is considered redundant and excised frequently. However, in author's clinical judgement, this tissue can be converted into a flap to close the nasal floor, thus precluding the need for any vestibular releasing incision.
5. Nostril skin on the lip: The skin of the lateral alar part, the columella and part of nasal vestibule intrudes onto the lip in the upper part. Distinction can be made between nostril skin and labial skin as the former is finely stippled while the latter is finely striated and has hair.

72.3.5.1 Nose

1. Platform: The base, i.e. the premaxilla, is projected and rotated outwards, whereas the lateral maxillary segment is retropositioned. Consequently, there is nasal asymmetry at the base.
2. Septum: Lower border of the septum is dislocated out from the vomerine grove, thus twisting the nasal tip and columella.
3. Columella: Unilateral shortness in vertical dimension is seen with deflection towards the non-cleft side.
4. Nasal floor: Has a defect in the skin, muscle and bone.
5. Lower lateral cartilage: The cleft alar cartilage is flattened and more horizontal in its long axis and stretched at an obtuse angle.
6. Alar crease: Due to the absence of alar cartilage bulge, alar crease continues across the tip to produce a disjointed effect.
7. Alar base: Rotated outwardly in a flare.
8. Alar rim: There is a skin curtain of ala that is without cartilage further reducing the apparent length of the columella on the cleft side (Fig. 72.9).

72.3.6 Anatomy of the Bilateral Cleft

The following are the salient anatomical features of a bilateral cleft:

- Prolabium and premaxilla: The prolabium and premaxilla isolated from lateral segments (lip and maxilla). The premaxilla is not found in the alveolar arch and either protruded or deviated or rotated. This is probably because of the excessive forward growth of the premaxillary-vomerine suture and uninhibited forward growth of the cartilaginous nasal septum (Fig. 72.10).
- The prolabium is the central lip element that has paucity of tissues. The prolabium has no muscle, is non-mobile and has a limited blood supply. The white roll on the prolabium is rounded and indistinct.
- Nasal deformity depends on the premaxilla and size and position of the prolabium. The columella is very short or absent. The base of the ala is positioned laterally and posteroinferiorly. There is a wide nasal base. The deformity in LLC is presented by the elongated lateral crus and shorter medial crus. The nasal tip is flat with increased distance between alar domes. Only in cases of asymmetric bilateral clefts, the septum is deviated.
- The orbicularis oris muscle runs bilaterally up into the alar bases. There is no muscle on the median lip element (Fig. 72.4).
- In complete bilateral cleft lips, the labial artery fails to unite with its counterpart on the other side. In addition the arcade made by anastomosis of the posterior septal branch with the greater palatine artery through the incisive foramen is absent. The philtrum and premaxilla therefore derive their blood supply from the posterior septal artery and terminal branches of the ethmoidal artery.

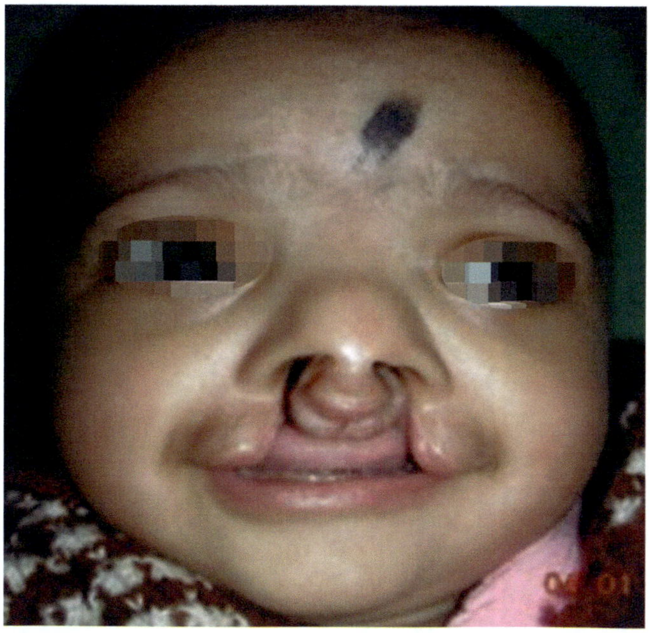

Fig. 72.10 Presentation of a bilateral cleft lip

72.4 Classification and Presentations of Cleft

As we discussed in embryology, insufficient or late migration of mesoderm leads to epithelial breakdown resulting in a cleft. Thus, a cleft lip presents in various forms, and the management differs slightly for all forms of cleft. The basic classification is based on the side of presentation, i.e. left and right and complete and incomplete (Figs. 72.11 and 72.12). The incomplete cleft lip can be further classified into various types (Box 72.3).

Box 72.3 Presentation of Incomplete Clefts

Incomplete clefts can be further divided on the basis of extent of involvement of the mucosa, skin and nasal floor.

1. Incomplete cleft lip with mucosal notch not extending into the skin.
2. Incomplete cleft lip with mucosal and skin notching.
3. Incomplete cleft lip involving the mucosa and skin extending upwards but not up to the nasal floor.
4. Incomplete cleft lip with Simonart's band. Simonart's band is a bridge of tissue between the premaxilla and the lateral lip element. Its prevalence is approximately 20%.

Similarly, bilateral cleft lip can be divided into complete and incomplete clefts. Complete clefts can be further divided on the basis of status of the premaxilla. The premaxilla can be severely, moderately or mildly protruded. However, this is a clinical classification and helps in deciding treatment of a bilateral cleft lip.

72.4.1 Classification

Throughout history, many surgeons have attempted to classify cleft lip and palate in their own ways. Classifications made have been on three bases: laterality, severity and morphology of the cleft. At the least any classification system should be able to specify the laterality, extent and severity of

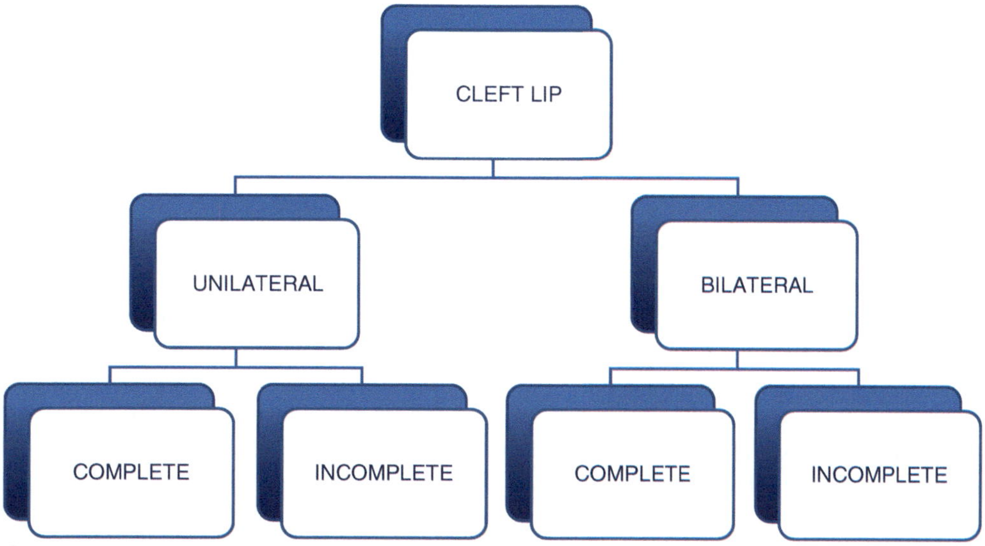

Fig. 72.11 Basic classification of cleft lip

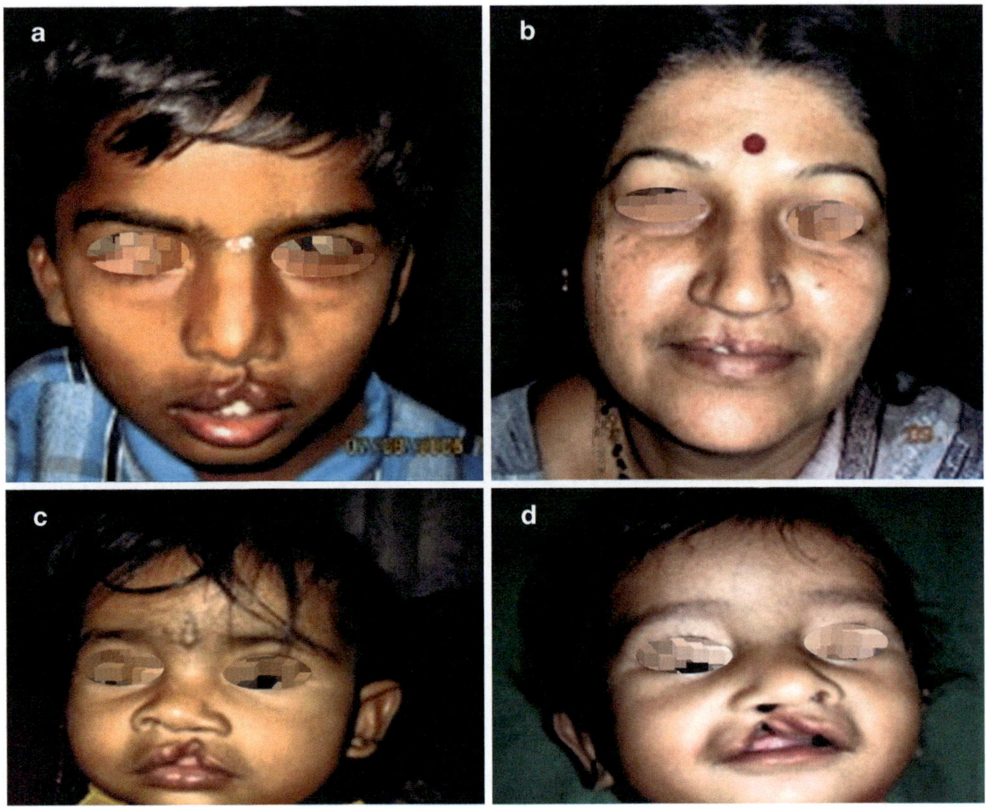

Fig. 72.12 Incomplete cleft lip with mucosal notch not extending into the skin. (**a**) Incomplete cleft lip with mucosal and skin notching. (**b**) Incomplete cleft lip involving the mucosa and skin extending upwards but not up to the nasal floor. (**c**) Incomplete cleft lip with Simonart's band

the labial cleft and the palatal cleft necessary for treatment planning or outcome assessment (Tables 72.3 and 72.4).

Apart from the above-mentioned classifications, there are various reports of individual classifications by many international and Indian surgeons based on their experience and perspective. An ideal classification should be simple, clear and universally acceptable for purpose of communication and documentation.

72.5 Treatment of Cleft Lip

72.5.1 Timing of Intervention

Cleft lip repair constitutes the first surgical step in cleft lip and palate. Each cleft protocol team advocates different timings for lip reconstruction, with slight variations from the neonatal period to 6 months and later. Timing of intervention can be broadly categorised based on chronological age of the cleft patient or based on certain dental age milestones and status of dentition (Tables 72.5 and 72.6). There are a number of protocols adopted by various centres around the world. Proponents of traditional repair at the chronological age of 10–12 weeks argue that it poses a decreased risk of anaesthesia-related complications and provides improved aesthetic outcomes and positive psychological assurance to the parents. Surgery was traditionally delayed for several weeks based on the "rule of tens", i.e. infant weighing a minimum of 10 pounds, having a haemoglobin level of 10 g/mL and reaching an age of 10 weeks. This rule was based on the fact that the musculature of the lip is more evolved by this age and thus allows for proper reconstruction [23]. Another important milestone is the neck holding capacity of the baby. It is generally present at 3–4 months of age. It is prudent to wait till this milestone is achieved. This is crucial in cautious transfer of the infant as he/she is transferred to the operating room, recovery or intensive care unit and is handled by various healthcare personnel.

72.5.2 Basic Treatment Algorithm

We have devised a basic treatment algorithm for unilateral and bilateral cleft lip repair that we follow at our centre. Due to lack of awareness, prenatal and postnatal counselling and the social taboo, many patients in India do not report at the correct age for surgery. As a result, the treatment methods have been modified based on the age of presentation of the cleft patient to provide the optimal outcome (Figs. 72.13 and 72.14).

72.5.3 Presurgical Nasoalveolar Moulding

Wider, extensive clefts and bilateral clefts are associated with significant deformities of nasolabial complex, presenting a greater surgical challenge in approximating anatomic struc-

Table 72.3 Summary of all classifications given so far

Year	Author		Foundation point
1922	Davis and Ritchie [8]	Group I: Prealveolar process cleft (clefts affecting the Lip) 1. Unilateral (right/left: Complete/incomplete) 2. Bilateral (right, complete/incomplete; left, complete/incomplete) 3. Median (complete/incomplete) Group II: Postalveolar process cleft (clefts affecting the palate) 1. Soft palate 2. Hard palate Group III: Alveolar process cleft (any cleft involving the alveolar process) 1. Unilateral (right/left: Complete/incomplete) 2. Bilateral (right, complete/incomplete; left, complete/incomplete) 3. Median (complete/incomplete)	Alveolus
1921–1923	Brophy [9]	16 categories of distinct morphological forms of cleft palate with/without cleft lip	Based on morphology
1931	Veau [10]	I. Clefts of the soft palate II. Clefts of the soft and hard palate, up to the incisive foramen III. Clefts of the soft and hard palate extending unilaterally through the alveolus IV. Clefts of the soft and hard palate extending bilaterally through the alveolus	Extent, laterality and morphology
1958	Kernahan and Stark [11]	1. Clefts of structures anterior to the incisive foramen 2. Clefts of structures posterior to the incisive foramen 3. Clefts affecting structures anterior and posterior to the incisive foramen	Incisive foramen
1962	American Cleft Palate-Craniofacial Association Classification [12]	1. Clefts of the prepalate (cleft of lip and embryologic primary palate) (a) Cleft lip (cheiloschisis) (b) Cleft alveolus (alveoloschisis) (c) Cleft lip, alveolus and primary palate (cheiloalveoloschisis) 2. Clefts of the palate (cleft of the embryologic secondary palate) (a) Cleft of the hard palate (uranoschisis) (b) Cleft of the soft palate (staphyloschisis or veloschisis) (c) Cleft of the hard and soft palate (uranostaphyloschisis) 3. Clefts of the prepalate and palate (alveolocheilopalatoschisis) 4. Facial clefts other than prepalatal and palatal (a) Cleft of the mandibular process (b) Naso-ocular clefts (c) Oro-ocular clefts	Two principal anatomical landmarks: The “prepalate”, anterior to the incisive foramen and the “palate”, posterior to the incisive foramen
1969	International Classification (Broadbent et al., 1969)	1. Clefts of the anterior (primary) palate 2. Clefts of the anterior (primary) and posterior (secondary) palates 3. Clefts of the posterior (secondary) palate	Categorization of clefts of the lip, alveolus and palate based on embryologic origin and rare facial clefts based on topographic findings

(continued)

Table 72.3 (continued)

Year	Author		Foundation point
1971	Kernahan pictographic form [13]	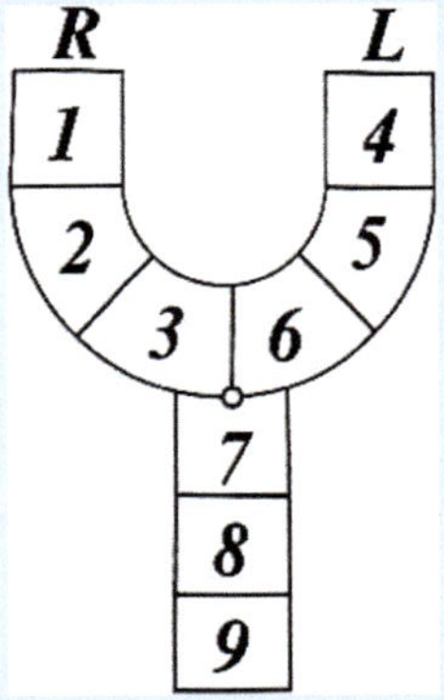	Striped Y Most accepted
1973	Spina [14]	Modified international classification: Renamed group 1 as preforaminal clefts, group 2 as transforaminal clefts	
1973 and 1976	Kernahan's striped Y modified by Elsahy (1973), Millard (1976), Friedman and Smith [15–19]	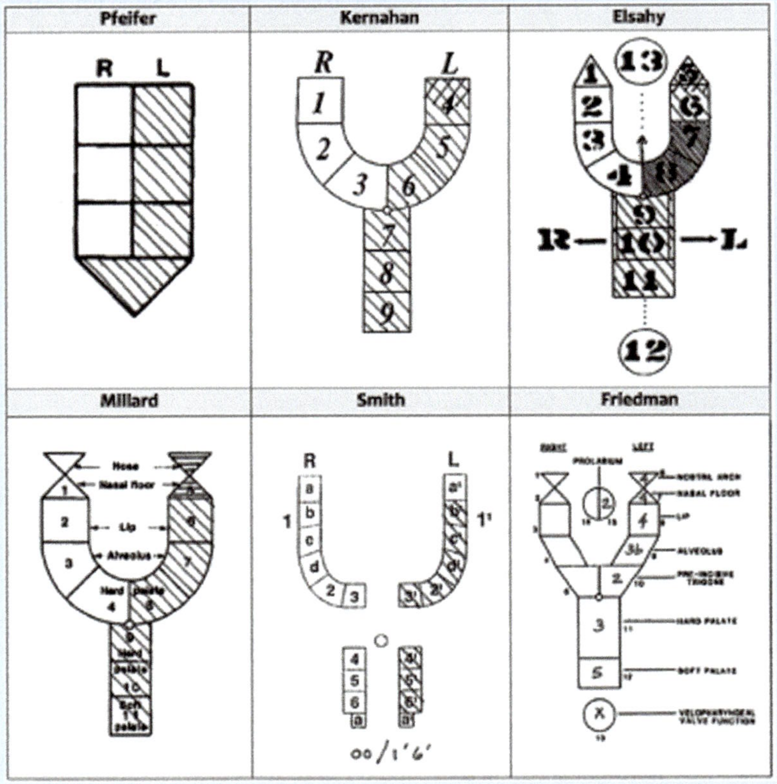	Most accepted classification

<table>
<tr><td>1975</td><td>Balakrishnan [20]</td><td>
<table>
<tr><th>Cleft type</th><th>Original abbreviation</th></tr>
<tr><td>Cleft lip</td><td>Gp1</td></tr>
<tr><td>Cleft palate</td><td>Gp2</td></tr>
<tr><td>Cleft lip, alveolus and palate</td><td>Gp3</td></tr>
<tr><td>Right</td><td>R</td></tr>
<tr><td>Left</td><td>L</td></tr>
<tr><td>Midline</td><td>M</td></tr>
<tr><td>Alveolus</td><td>A</td></tr>
<tr><td>Additional abbreviations</td><td></td></tr>
<tr><td>Partial</td><td>P</td></tr>
<tr><td>Submucosal</td><td>S</td></tr>
<tr><td>Simonart's band</td><td>sb</td></tr>
<tr><td>Microform</td><td>micro</td></tr>
</table>
</td></tr>
<tr><td>1987</td><td>Kreins O (cited by Hodgkinson et al) [21]</td><td>LAHSAL system is a diagrammatic classification of cleft lip and palate
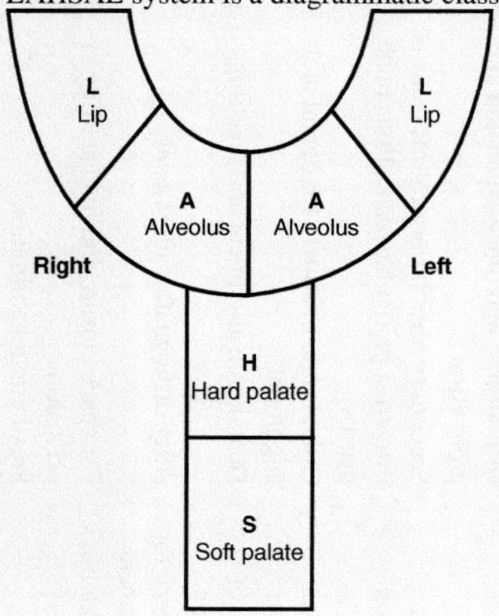
</td></tr>
</table>

Table 72.4 Incomplete cleft lip can be further divided into minor-form, microform and mini-microform [22]

Minor-form	Microform	Mini-microform
1. Notched vermilion-cutaneous junction extending 3 mm or more above the normal Cupid's bow peak 2. Deficient vermilion on the medial cleft side 3. Cutaneous groove and muscular depression that is evident on puckering 4. Hypoplastic median tubercle 5. Nasal deformity	1. Medial vermilion-cutaneous point less than 3 mm above the normal Cupid's bow peak 2. Deficient vermilion on the medial cleft side 3. Lower cutaneous lip shows a variable glabrous strip 4. Philtral line shows muscular depression, with a prominent medial component of the philtral ridge 5. Nearly normal length of the hemicolumella, the sill shows a small depression, slight slump of the alar genu and 1 to 2 mm lateral displacement and outward flare of the alar base	1. Discontinuous vermilion-cutaneous junction 2. Level Cupid's bow peaks 3. Notched free mucosal margin 4. Variable muscular depression 5. Variable nasal deformity; mostly a depressed sill

Table 72.5 Timing of intervention based on chronological age

Timing	Procedure
After 16 weeks of pregnancy	Cleft lip diagnosis by USG images
Prenatal	Discussion with surgeon Consultation with a geneticist
Neonatal	Presurgical orthopaedics Feeding instructions
12 weeks of age	Cleft lip surgery
6–12 months of age	Cleft palate repair with intravelar veloplasty
14 years or later	Orthognathic surgery
Adulthood	Secondary rhinoplasty

Table 72.6 Timing of intervention based on status of dentition

Timing	Procedure
Prior to cleft lip repair	Presurgical orthopaedics [NAM]
Primary dentition	Orthodontic maxillary expansion
Mixed dentition	Orthodontic maxillary expansion and protraction
Before eruption of permanent dentition	Secondary alveolar bone graft using iliac crest particulate cancellous bone marrow
Permanent dentition	Orthodontic treatment for dental arch alignment
After full eruption of permanent dentition	Dental arch alignment and levelling
Orthognathic surgery for maxillary advancement	After orthognathic alignment
Postsurgical orthodontics	For space closure and final settling of occlusion Prosthetic rehabilitation

tures, thus obtaining an optimum functional and aesthetic result. The basic goal of any surgical technique is to restore normal anatomy and function. Thus in such cases, where it is difficult to achieve goals of primary repair due to wide discrepancies, presurgical maxillofacial orthopaedic appliances mould the nasolabial structures through specifically directed forces, thus reducing the deformity before surgery for an easy repair.

Currently, presurgical nasal alveolar moulding (PNAM) is a widely used orthopaedic technique for presurgical cleft deformity correction [23, 24]. PNAM theory is based on the theory that increased hyaluronic acid content is present in the infant cartilage, which makes the cartilaginous structure more pliable and plastic. By the age of 3 months, the cartilage becomes more rigid with less plasticity. PNAM can significantly improve the nasal symmetry, by elongating the columella, bolstering the alae, narrowing the cleft and restoring the alveolar arch form, thus demonstrating favourable immediate and long-term outcomes.

PNAM is based on the principles of negative sculpting and passive moulding of the alveolus, lip and nasal tissues. An initial impression is obtained, and custom-made plates are fabricated. A series of modifications are made to the surface of the appliances with the addition and deletion of materials in certain areas. This process is called negative sculpting [25]. The purpose of this is achieving approximation and symmetry of the two maxillary alveolar segments and addressing the nasal deformity by moulding the cartilage in anatomical position [26, 27] (Fig. 72.15). The process should be explained to the parents; insertion of the appliance should be carefully taught and made to practice. Parents should be explained the importance of this exercise through videos and photos of previous patients.

Impression Making A heavy-bodied polyvinyl siloxane impression material should be used for the first impression. The infant is held in prone position to keep the tongue forward and to allow any material or saliva to drain out of the oral cavity and prevent aspiration. This should be done in a hospital setting to manage any airway emergency in the presence of an anaesthetist available if needed. Once impression is made, the mouth should be examined for any residual material.

Device Fabrication The moulding plate is made with clear methyl methacrylate lined with a soft denture material on the dental stone model. The borders should be trimmed and smoothened to prevent any ulceration. The oral surface should be smooth and polished with good retention and no extensions into the cleft area.

Insertion and Moulding The moulding plate is to be worn full-time by the patient. It should be removed for cleaning and routine hygiene practices to prevent infection and check for any ulceration. Suckling should be checked with the plate in position and to check gagging. The plate is secured to the

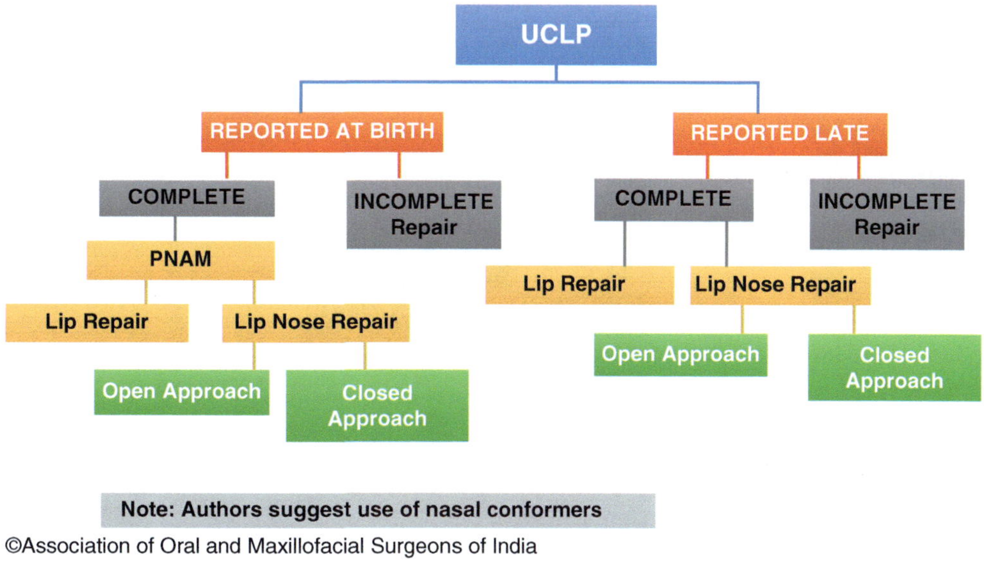

Fig. 72.13 Basic treatment algorithm for unilateral cleft lip

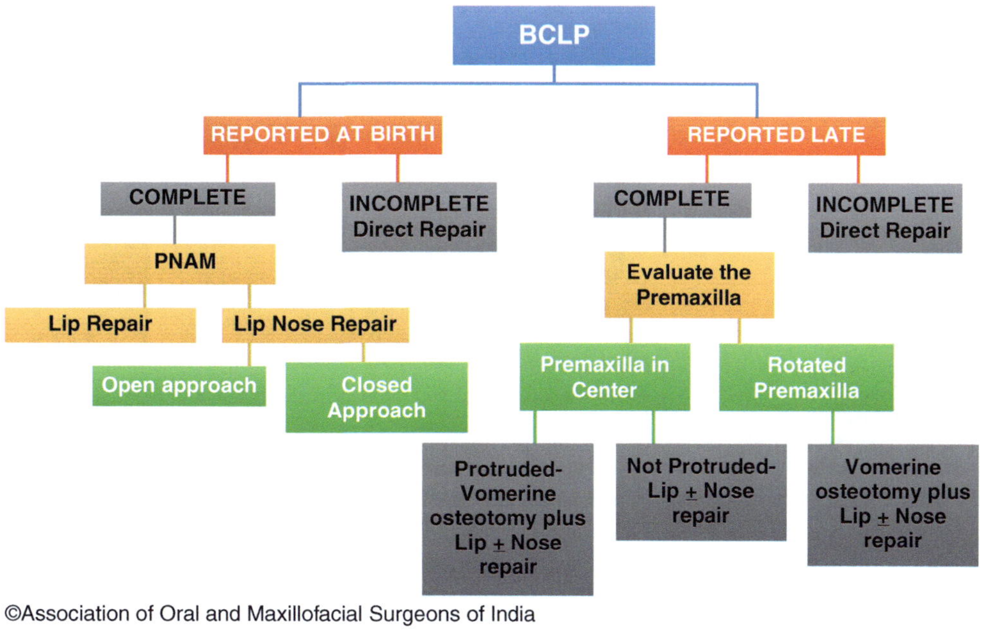

Fig. 72.14 Basic treatment algorithm for bilateral cleft lip

cheek bilaterally using orthodontic elastics going to the opposite side and secured with surgical tapes. The elastic loop extends from the retention arm approximately in a 40–45 degree angle, thus pulling the anterior flange of the plate posterosuperior vector for activation. 2 ounces of traction force is given by stretching the elastic to twice its original. The surgical tape is applied to a layer of wound dressing material like micropore tape and not the skin directly. The tape is to be changed once a day. The tape should be applied to the non-cleft side first and then pulled over to the cleft side. Weekly follow-ups should be made to evaluate the moulding plate for retention and changes in the alveolar segments.

Moulding Plate Modification Selective grinding of acrylic material is done from the region into which the alveolar segments are to move. At the same time, soft denture lining material is selectively added to the plate to direct the alveolar segments to the midline, as desired. In a patient with bilateral cleft, the premaxilla is retracted and derotated, to bring to a normal maxillary arch alignment. An ideal surgical result may be obtained when 1–2 mm gap remains between alveolar segments.

Nasal Stent When the maxillary alveolar segment approximation has been achieved, the nasal moulding should begin. The nasal stent is added to the existing moulding plate in the form of a stainless steel wire projecting out of the plate outwards going into the nose like a "swan neck". A small wire loop can be made on which a bilobed intranasal acrylic component is made with a layer of soft denture liner. Nasal stent is placed 3–4 mm inside the ala and gently lifted towards dome until slight blanching is noted.

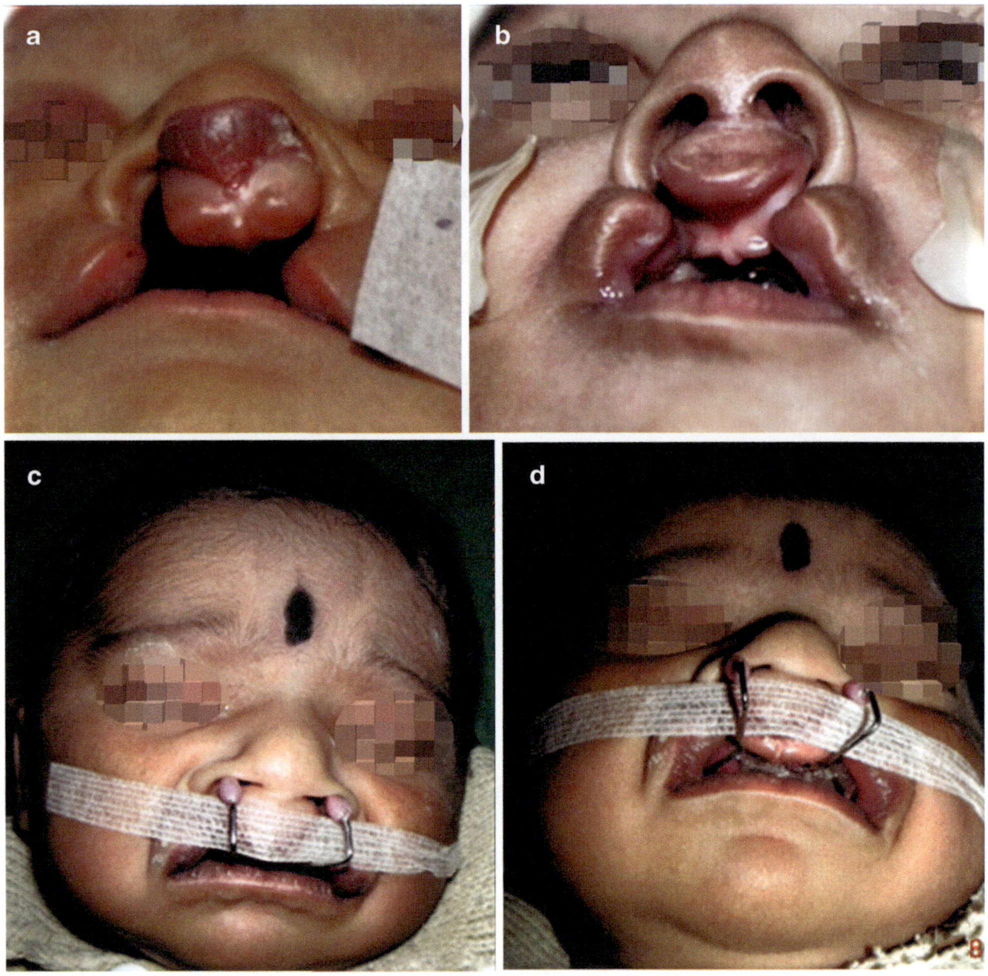

Fig. 72.15 PNAM treatment in a case of bilateral lip. (**a** and **b**) Pre- and postoperative PNAM. Note the changes in the nasal tip, alar cartilages and position of the premaxilla. (**c** and **d**) PNAM device with the nasal stent and lip taping

Blanching of the nasal tip as the baby suckles activates the appliance. Lip taping is continued after the nasal stent appliance is added.

In a follow-up study over 6–9 years, Bennum et al. observed that patients treated with PNAM within 15 days after birth maintained satisfactory nasal symmetry [28]. Ezzat et al. compared 12 unilateral cleft lip and palate patients with PNAM treatment and found narrowing of the alveolar cleft, increased posterior width of the dental arch, uprighting of the columella and improved nasal symmetry [29]. Yang et al. reported similar results from 45 unilateral complete cleft lip and palate patients [30]. In a large multicentre study sample, Ross argued that orthopaedic correction of the premaxilla failed to stimulate maxillary growth and thus was not necessary [31].

The authors conducted a study to evaluate the nasolabial aesthetics on two-dimensional photographs at 6 months post cheiloplasty. Cupid's bow, vermilion symmetry, vermilion notching, premaxillary show at rest, scar aesthetics, columella height and bialar width were all significantly better in the PNAM group [32].

72.5.4 Protocols

There is no universal protocol for management of cleft lip, and there is a striking diversity of clinical practice. There is a paucity of higher-level evidence (i.e. systematic reviews and randomized controlled trials) on cleft lip and palate. There have been few RCTs comparing individual treatment steps. The Eurocleft study showed that among the 201 European centres, 194 different treatment protocols existed for unilateral clefts [33]. Listed below are some standard protocols followed worldwide.

- Rule of tens.
- IOWA Protocol [34].
- Dallas Protocol [35].
- Warsaw Protocol [36].
- Oslo Protocol [37].
- Malek Protocol [38].
- American Cleft Protocol [39].
- Australian Cleft Craniofacial Society Protocol [40].
- European Studies and results [41, 42].

Discussion of each protocol is beyond the scope of this chapter. However, we have tried to compare and discuss in detail few protocols for a comprehensive understanding of cleft lip and palate repair

The basic protocols of cleft lip repair can also be classified as follows:

1. Primary cleft lip repair.
2. Primary cleft lip and anterior palate repair.
3. Primary cleft lip and soft palate repair.
4. Primary cleft lip and palate repair.

Primary Cleft Lip Repair Only: This protocol of early lip repair at 3–4 months of age following the rule of tens is followed popularly at various centres. The author's centre also follows the same protocol. The timing of intervention has been discussed previously in the chapter.

Primary lip and anterior palate repair: was proposed by Abyholm in Oslo protocol [37]. In the first operation, cleft lip repair using Millard technique with simultaneous anterior hard palate closure using a single layer vomer flap. The mean age for first surgery was 3.3 months. The soft palate was closed at a mean age of 17.2 months (Fig. 72.16).

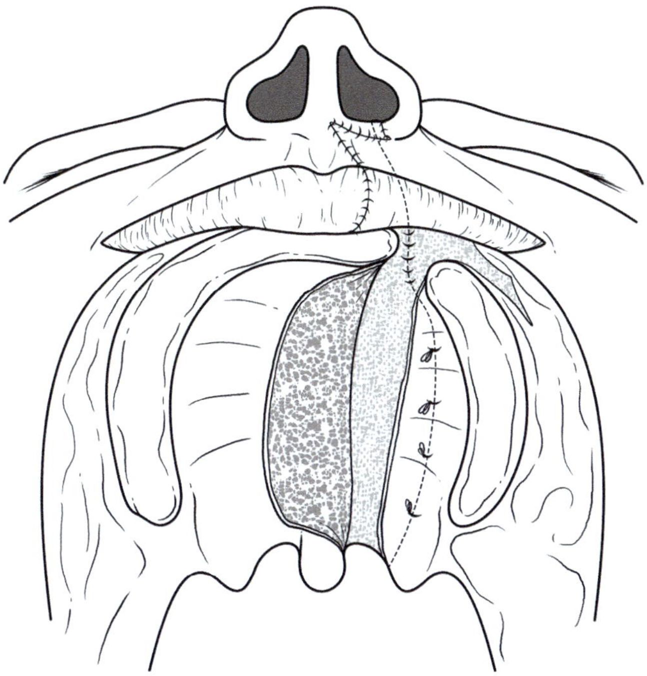

Fig. 72.16 Cleft lip and anterior palate repair: Veau's vomer flap (Veau. 1931). An incision was made on the medial side of the cleft along the border line between oral and nasal mucosae or in bilateral clefts, along the free edge of the vomer. A mucoperiosteal flap is raised from the vomer and turned across the cleft. The lateral edge of the cleft is incised, and the palatal mucoperiosteum is elevated, allowing the vomer flap to be put under the mucoperiosteum and fixed with mattress sutures. In the alveolar area, and in continuity with the vomer flap plasty, the nasal mucoperiosteum is mobilised on both sides and joined across the cleft to complete the nasal floor anterior to the vomer flap. Towards the oral cavity, the raw surfaces of the vomer and of the flap are left uncovered

Primary lip and soft palate repair: It is a well-established early palatal closure which causes maxillary hypoplasia. Because of this reason, many surgeons used to perform palate repair in two stages, i.e. soft palate first followed by hard palate. At the time of introduction of this protocol, the soft palate was repaired along with the lip at around 4–6 months of age, and the hard palate was repaired at the age of 10–12 years. This was later reduced to 4–5 years.

Complete Lip and Palate Repair: one-stage simultaneous repair of the entire cleft is a simple and economic treatment of complete unilateral cleft lip and palate [43]. The concept of one-stage repair was first introduced in 1958, when Farina (1958) described the surgical technique. A decreased risk associated with general anaesthesia, better healing, lower incidence of fistulae and reduced hospitalization costs has been the rationale for performing such repair. This repair performed in children above 10 months of age has been claimed by surgeons with extremely good results without any complications. Overall, the cleft teams from Brussels, Belgium; Konya and Zonguldak, Turkey; and Warsaw, Poland, found that their protocols employing one-stage closure of UCLP produced favourable morphological results [36, 37, 44, 45].

72.6 Unilateral Cleft Lip Repair

72.6.1 Techniques of Cleft Lip Repair

The evolution of cleft repair was bound to happen mainly due to the nature of the aesthetics that had to consider the anatomical parameters, namely:

(a) Cupid's bow.
(b) White roll continuity.
(c) Vermillion continuity.
(d) Muscle continuity.
(e) Philtral columns and equality of length on both cleft and non-cleft sides.
(f) Minimizing scarring on the anatomical unit of the lip, i.e. philtral column, philtral dimple and nasal base.

Broadly over the period of cleft history, lip repair can be divided into three basic types depending on the design of flap used (Fig. 72.17). These are straight line repairs (Box 72.4), geometric flap repairs (Box 72.5) and rotation-advancement flap.

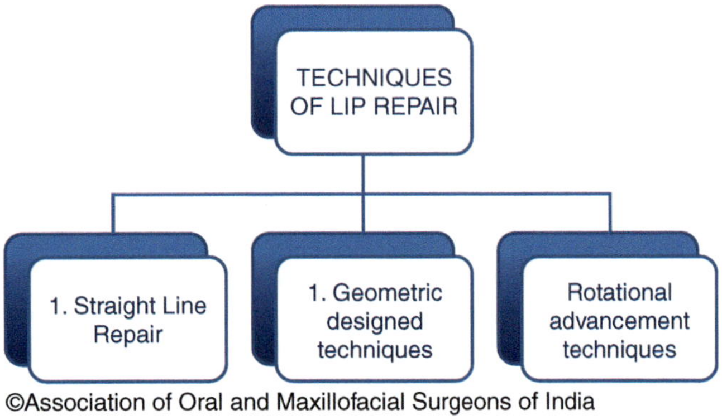

Fig. 72.17 Basic techniques of lip repair

Box 72.4 Straight Line Repairs
- Rose [1981] [46].
- Thompson [1912] [47].
- Veau [1925] [48].
- Pfeifer [1970].
- Delaire [1975] [49].
- Chaid [2007] [50].
- Nakajima [2008] [51].

Box 72.5 Geometric Flap Repairs
- Joseph Malgaigne [1843] [52].
- G Mirault [1844] [52–54].
- Triangular flap.
- Le Mesurier [1849] [55, 56].
- Tennison [1952] and Randall [1959] [57, 58].
- Skoog [1969] [59].

Millard's Rotation-Advancement Flap.

Ralph Millard (1957) [2] revolutionized the cleft repair technique with most of its principles applicable and widely used in current day practice. His innovation was in designing the incisions without disrupting the aesthetic subunits. The cut as you go technique was simplified further by understanding the anatomy of the lip. He realized that two thirds of the Cupid's bow, complete with tubercle, white roll of the mucocutaneous junction, one column and the dimple of the philtrum, were all present in the non-cleft side but askew and thus had to be rotated down to normal position [60].

72.6.1.1 Basic Components of Millard's Repair (Video 72.1)

Labelling of the Flaps

A—Non-cleft side (with Cupid's bow and dimple—rotation). In Millard's original description, the incision for the rotation flap begins at the peak of the Cupid's bow [cleft side], marked along the cleft edge up to the junction with the columella, and curves under the base, crossing the midline, but doesn't cross the contralateral philtral column. Millard later added a back cut at the end of the incision, to allow for adequate rotation of the medial lip element and less tension on the repair [61, 62].

B—Cleft side (advancement).

The incision on the lateral lip element of cleft forms the advancement flap. It is made along the cleft edge, extending up to the nasal floor. This incision should match the length of the incision on the medial side of the cleft.

C—A small triangular flap attached to the columella from the non-cleft side left after the incision.

72.6.1.2 Points Marked: The Following Points are Marked in a Classic Millard's Technique (Fig. 72.18a, b)

1. Deepest point on the Cupid's bow.
2. Bow peak on the non-cleft side (distance usually 4 mm).
3. Bow peak on the cleft side (equal to distance between point 1 and 2 from point 1).
4. The alar base on normal side.
5. Final extent of the incision following a rotational curve, skirting the columella-lip junction and extending past the midline of columella base almost as far as the philtrum column on the normal side but no farther.
6. Commissure of the lip on the non-cleft side.
7. Commissure of the lip on the cleft side.
8. Equidistant point from 6 to 2 marked on the mucocutaneous junction (usually 20 mm), and distance between 10 and 8 is equal to 4 and 2.

   The vertical distance from the alar base on the normal side 4 to the height of the non-cleft peak of the bow 2 gives the distance that must be matched ultimately on the cleft side from its alar base 10 to its peak 8 (usually around 10 mm).
9. Most medial point or leading point of the advancement flap.
10. The alar base on the cleft side.

Despite being seemingly complicated, a simple exercise of carrying out the points over an illustration of complete cleft lip shall allow the reader to completely understand the simplicity of the description (Fig. 72.19). Complete surgical technique of Millard's cleft lip repair with the author's modification is discussed later in this chapter.

Once the markings are made, the rotation and advancement flaps are designed. The basic aim is to achieve symmetry of the philtral columns. This can be achieved by the following methods in a Millard's repair:

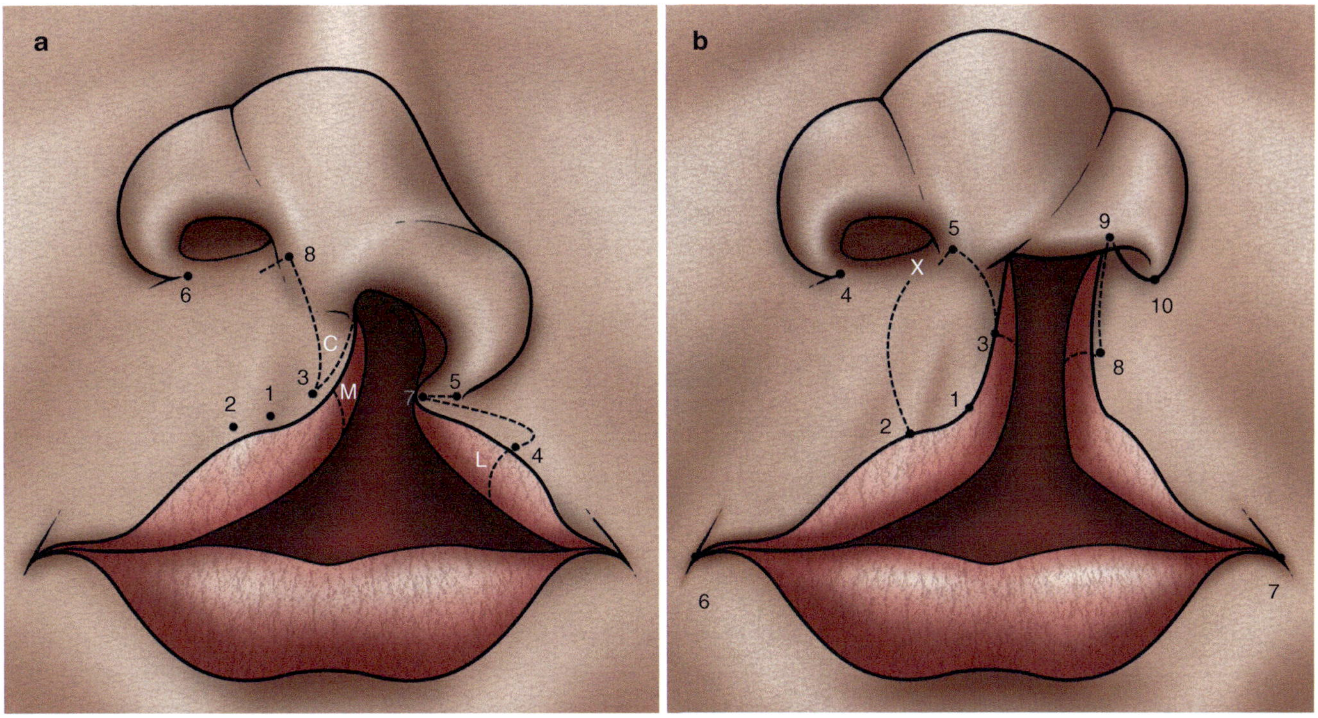

Fig. 72.18 (**a**, **b**) Basic design of Millard's technique

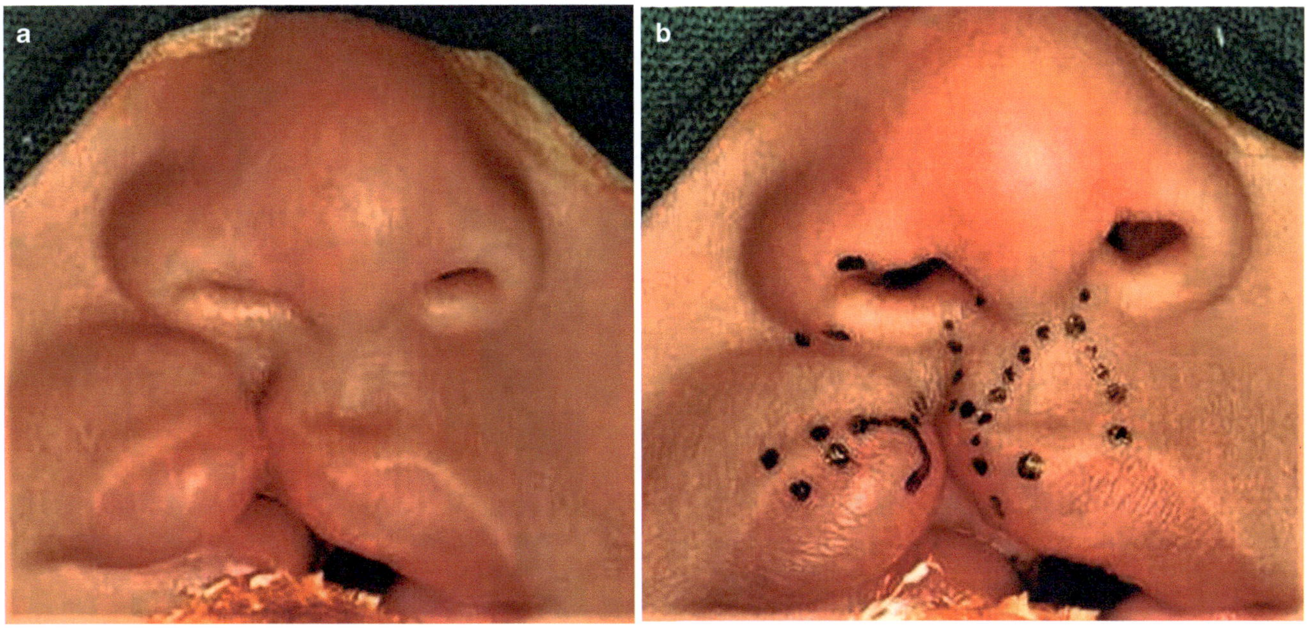

Fig. 72.19 (**a**, **b**) Marking of incisions

1. Curve the incision on the rotation side; this helps in gaining length on the cleft side philtral column.
2. Back cut: The role of the back cut comes into force when the rotation is not adequate to provide enough length to match the normal philtral column. It can be made to cross the midline or made parallel to the normal side philtral column as in Mohler's modification.
3. Role of "C" flap: The "C" flap can be designed to accomplish either of the following goals: closure of nasal sill, columellar lengthening or back into the defect created by rotation of the flap [63].

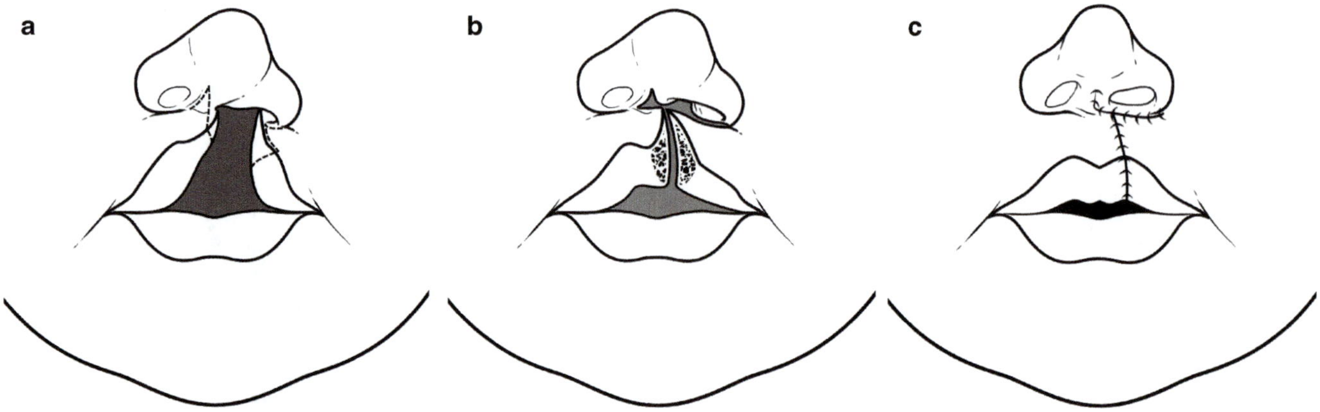

Fig. 72.20 (**a–c**) Mohler's modification of Millard's technique

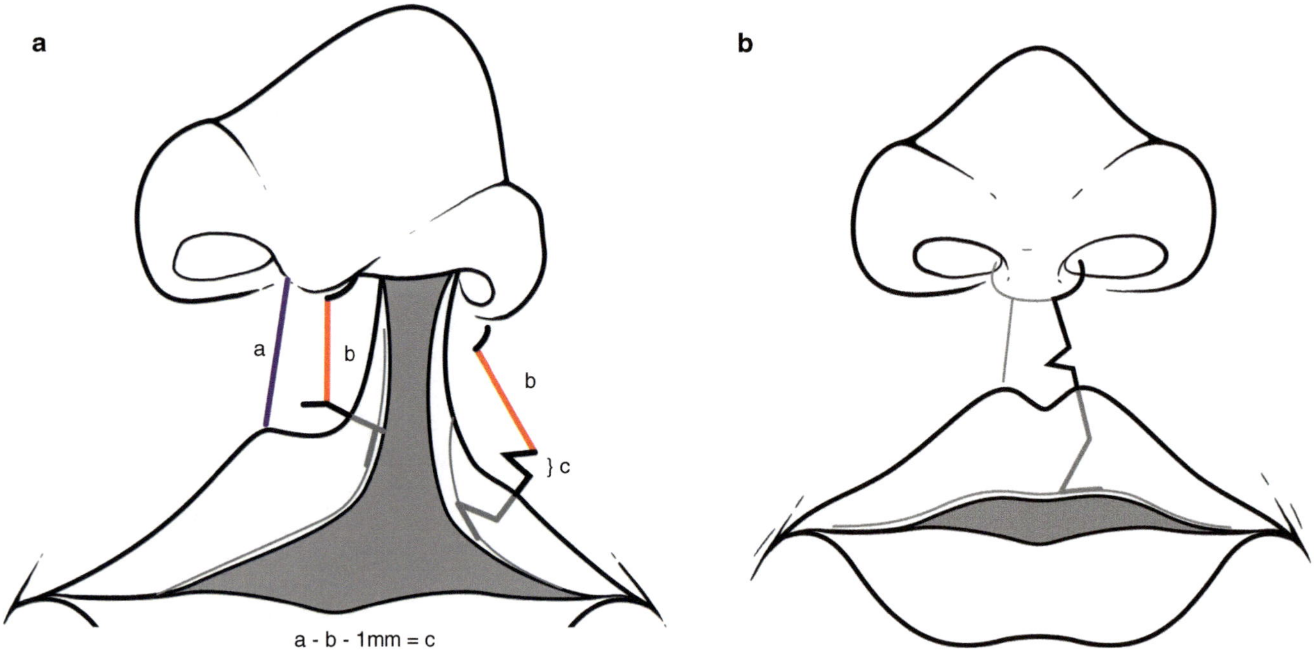

Fig. 72.21 (**a**, **b**) Fischer's modification

72.6.1.3 Modifications to Millard's Technique

In the original Millard's technique, the advancement flap often disrupts the upper third of the cleft side philtral column. Also, in wider clefts the advancement flap results in an unaesthetic scar around the alar base. This led to a series of modifications to the conventional Millard's rotational advancement technique:

External Scar Placement

1. *Mohler (1987)* [64]: The medial lip rotation incision was modified to extend onto the columella. The back cut was added which was confined to the columella. The C flap is used to fill the defect created by rotating the medial lip element at the base of the columella. Thus it is used for lengthening the shortened columella (Fig. 72.20).
2. *Fisher (2005)* [65] merged techniques of the Tennison triangle repair and rotation-advancement from Millard. It uses a small triangle above the white roll at the outset and avoids the use of rotation incision allowing most scar to be placed along the ideal philtral column (Fig. 72.21a, b).
3. *Vermilion Repair/Noordhoff's* [66] technique:

   In Noordhoff's words the essential features of this technique are as follows:

   (a) No dissection over the maxillary base.
   (b) No "back cuts" in rotation flap.

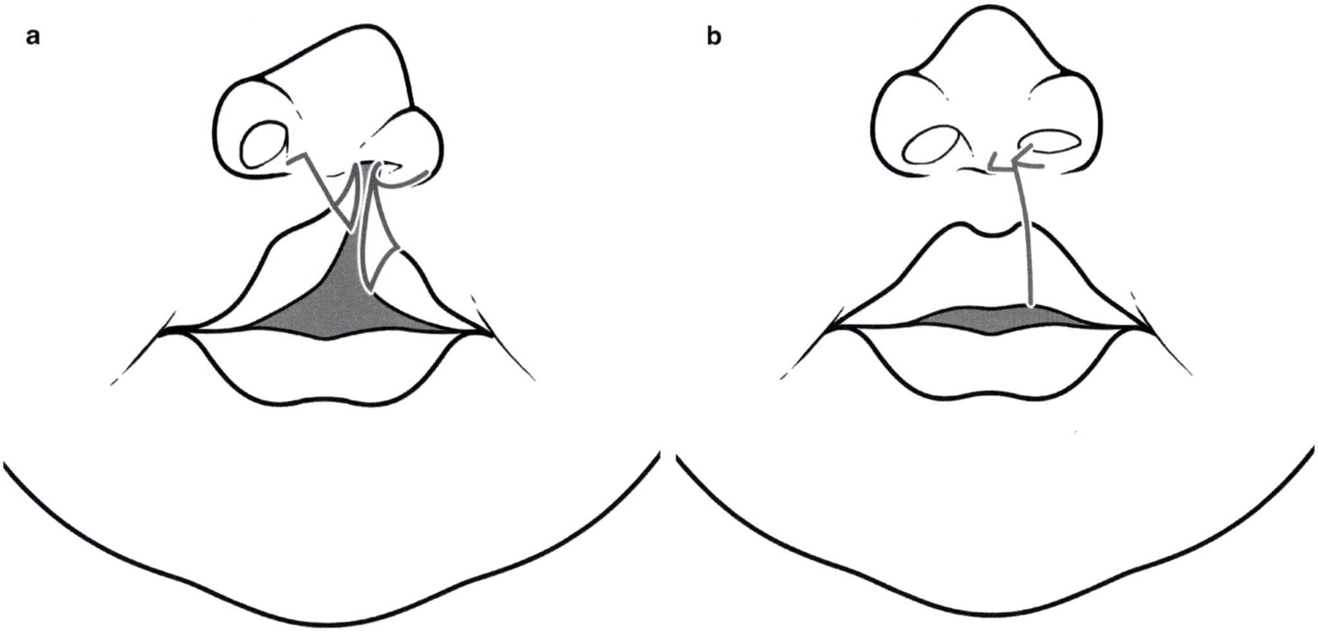

Fig. 72.22 (**a**, **b**) Cutting's modification

(c) In cases where the rotation is inadequate, the use of a small triangular flap of the skin above the "white roll" will be used to achieve adequate rotation without distorting the philtral column. These flaps heal well and are aesthetic.
(d) A lateral vermilion flap used for reconstruction of deficient vermilion on the cleft side Cupid's bow.
(e) Muscle reconstruction.
(f) Complete closure of mucosa of all areas using inferior turbinate mucosal flap that allows for repositioning of the lower lateral cartilage and adds mucosa wherever there is a deficiency.
(g) Fixation of the lower lateral cartilage to the upper lateral cartilage at its base and to the skin with alar transfixion sutures.
(h) Delayed upper limb rotation-advancement incisions limiting scars around the ala and nostril floor.
(i) The alar groove should be defined well.
(j) Postoperative splinting with a nasal silicone conformer to limit wound contracture.

4. *Columella Flap/Cutting* Repair: Cutting uses a technique that does not curve the incision towards the cleft and extends up onto the columella 1.5 to 2.0 mm slightly to the non-cleft side [67]. This yields a wider C flap thus filling the entire medial defect, allowing for a straight line closure (Fig. 72.22a, b).
5. *Muscle Repair*:

   The following modifications have been made in muscle repair:

   (a) *Cutting* [67]: Interposition orbicularis muscle repair.
   (b) *Mulliken* [68]: Vertical mattress sutures for end-to-end muscle repair to evert the orbicularis.
   (c) *Fischer* [65]: On both medial and lateral cleft elements, dissection of the overlying skin from the orbicularis. Dissection on the medial lip is limited to 1 mm from cut edge whereas of the lateral lip extends to the alar base to eliminate orbicularis bulge.

72.6.2 Step-by-Step Technique of Unilateral Cleft Lip Repair: Author's Technique (Figs. 72.23, 72.24, 72.25, 72.26, 72.27, 72.28, 72.29, 72.30, 72.31, 72.32, 72.33 and 72.34)

Lip Repair:

The authors have presented their technique of lip repair in a stepwise manner.

The following steps have been described:

- Markings: The most important principle of cleft lip repair is to identify the normal and abnormal structures. This includes the length of the philtral columns and the width of wet and dry mucosa. All the soft tissues should be kept in mind while designing the flap. No soft tissue should be discarded or considered redundant.

  Non-Cleft Side.

  Deepest point on cupid's bow, peak on non-cleft side and normal philtral column. (To make the philtral column prominent, one may use a two-pronged nasal hook to pull and retract the columella.)

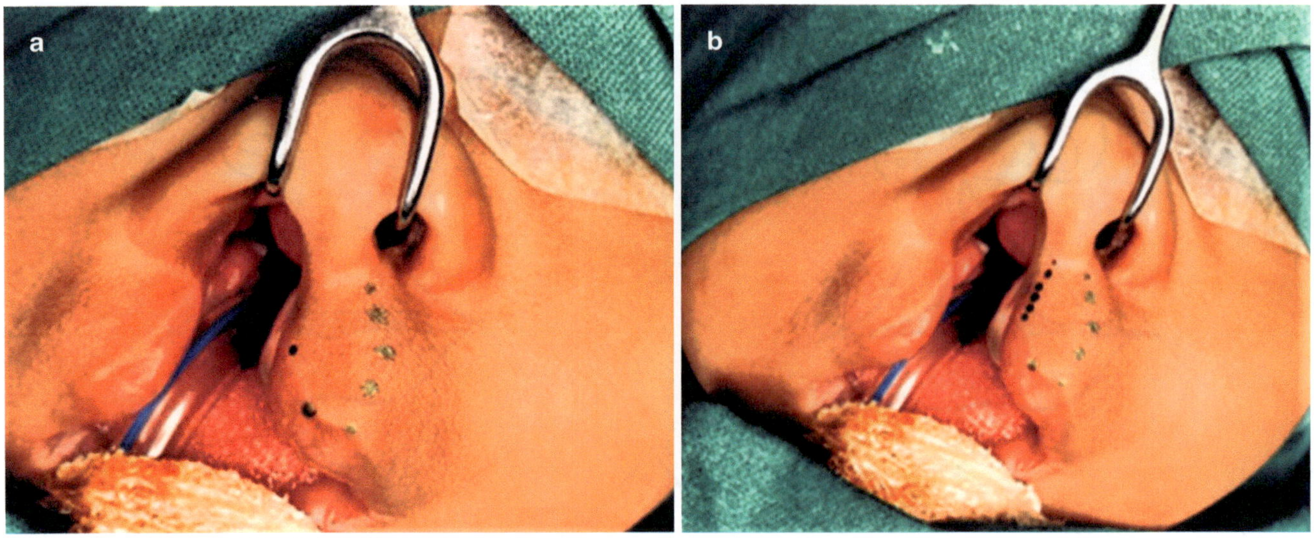

Fig. 72.23 (**a**) Mark the highest point on the Cupid's bow (cleft side), and also notice the philtral dimple. (**b**) Mark the future philtral column, and continue it up to the columella without cutting across the columella

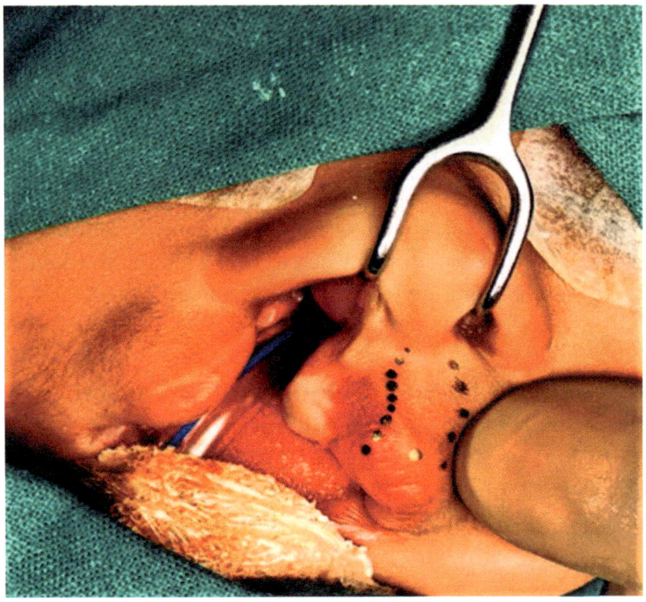

Fig. 72.24 From the peak of Cupid's bow on the cleft side, mark the incision on the dry mucosa till the junction of wet and dry mucosa

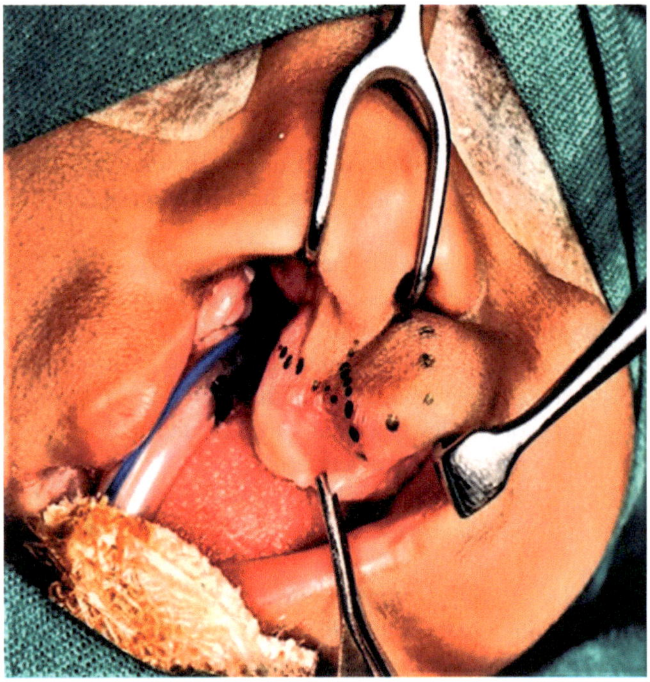

Fig. 72.25 *Marking of C flap*: A triangular flap between the mucosa and the future philtral column

- Mark the highest point on the Cupid's bow (cleft side), and also notice the philtral dimple (Fig. 72.23a).
- Mark the future philtral column, and continue it up to the columella without cutting across the columella (Fig. 72.23b).
- At this point the surgeon should compare the mark with the philtral column on the normal side. It might appear shorter; however, it will increase in length once the muscle is dissected from the abnormal attachment. The back cut discussed previously is used for adequate rotation of the cleft side philtral column. The back cut should be made after the muscle closure.
- From the peak of Cupid's bow on the cleft side, mark the incision on the dry mucosa till the junction of wet and dry mucosa (Fig. 72.24).
- Marking of C Flap: A triangular flap between the mucosa and the future philtral column. Continue between the skin

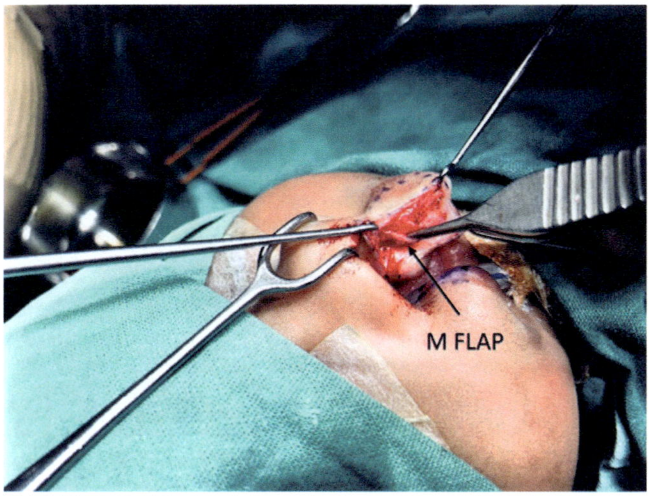

Fig. 72.26 M flap: The mucosal element on the non-cleft segment after raising the C flap becomes the M flap and is raised to expose the underlying muscle

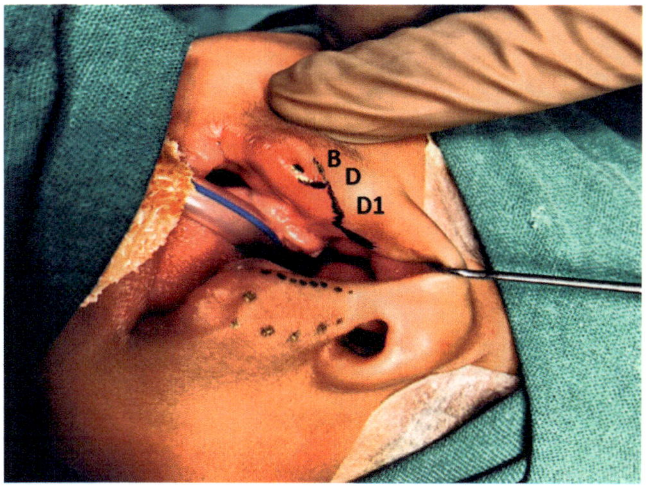

Fig. 72.27 On the side of the cleft, mark the point B. From the B point, extend the incision along the mucocutaneous junction till point D. From point D, marking goes into the nose to separate the nasal mucosa and the skin [D1]

and mucosa junction down to the mucosa to keep enough mucosa for nasal layer closure (Fig. 72.25).

- C flap originally described by Millard was used to augment the lateral lip at the insertion of alar base. We use the C flap either to create the nasal sill or if a back cut is given; it can be used to reconstruct the columella-lip junction.
- M Flap: The mucosal element on the non-cleft segment after raising the C flap becomes the M flap and is raised to expose the underlying muscle (Fig. 72.26).
- Rotational Flap: The muscle is now exposed, and the preparation of the lateral element can be divided into three easy steps:
- Oral mucosal layer: Separation of this layer from the muscle bulk can be identified with the plane where the minor salivary glands exist. Bleeding is generally encountered in this plane and should be managed early to reduce blood loss and keep a good plane of dissection.
- Skin-muscle dissection: The incision between this plane is to ensure just adequate separation to provide room for suturing the muscle bulk. Overexposing the muscle not only leads to excessive swelling postoperatively but also distorts the natural anatomical curves of the non-cleft element. On the cleft side, only 1–2 mm of subdermal dissection should be done. Closure of the skin later reinforced by the underlying muscle gives better elevation of the future philtral column as compared to overzealous separation of the muscle from the overlying skin.
- Release of abnormal muscle attachment: The abnormal attachments are usually near the alveolus and the base of the columella. At this point blunt dissection can be done to straighten out the septum.

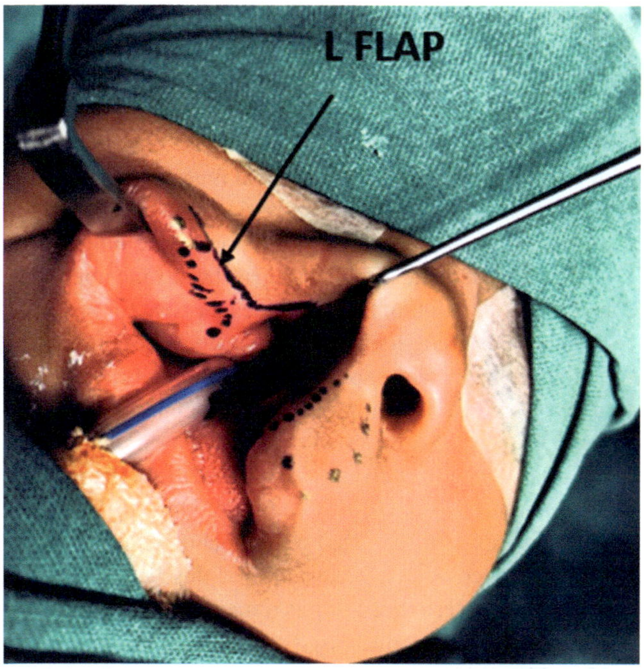

Fig. 72.28 Marking of L flap

Cleft Side:

- On the side of the cleft, mark the point B. First identify the white roll, and look for the point where the white roll starts to diminish; that is the exact point to join the Cupid's bow. Drop an imaginary line from this point to the junction of dry and wet mucosa. The maximum mucosal width is present at this point.

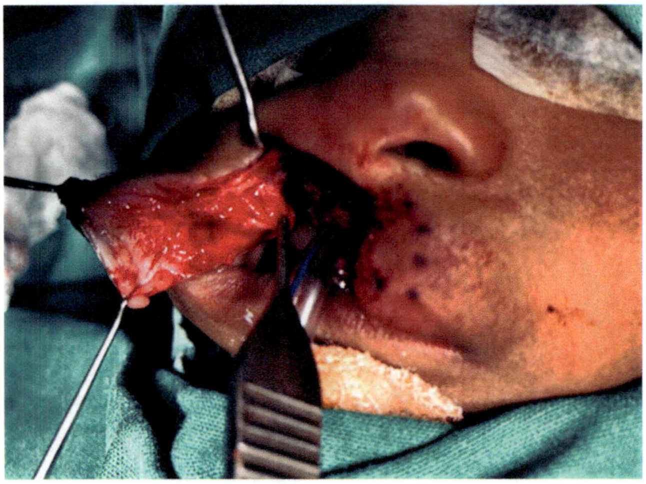

Fig. 72.29 Incision starts from the deepest point of the Cupid's bow till the columella base. The plane of dissection is just above the muscle

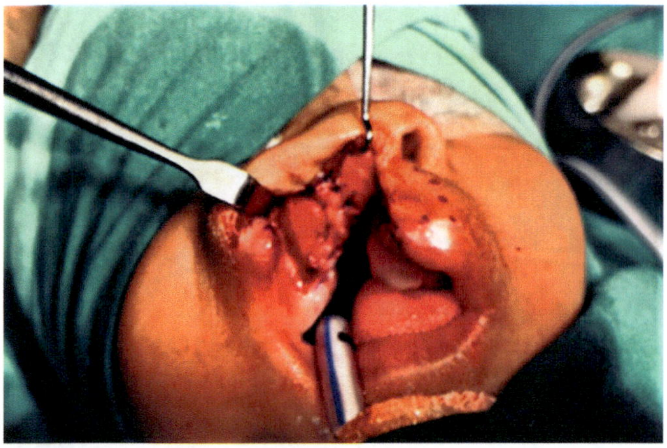

Fig. 72.30 Nasal layers are now sutured from both the cleft and non-cleft sides and sutured using a 4.0 Vicryl

- From the B point, extend the incision along the mucocutaneous junction till point D. Point D is a point at the edge of the lip at the junction of the skin and mucosa. From point D, marking goes into the nose to separate the nasal mucosa and the skin (Fig. 72.27).
- After marking the L flap, the incision is continued down to the alveolus, to free the abnormal muscle attachment at the base of the alveolus. In a classic Millard's technique, additional incision is given into the vestibule on the cleft side to get adequate mobilization of the advancement flap and medicalization of the cleft side alar base for nasal sill closure. Few surgeons also advocate subperiosteal or supraperiosteal dissection, through the intraoral incision at the pyriform region. However, in the author's experience, the need for this vestibular incision is not always necessary. An "L" flap can be designed from the mucosa of the cleft side as shown in the figure. This flap is continued upwards into the nasal mucosa and not towards the alveolar mucosa. The importance of this lies in the fact that, once harvested, the flap is retracted upwards into the nasal base and is thus used for closure of nasal sill. Moreover, due to this upward pull, the abnormal alar base attachment that leads to flattening of the alar rim is corrected. Thus, it helps in reducing the nasal symmetry (Fig. 72.28).
- Incision starts from the deepest point of the Cupid's bow till the columella base. The plane of dissection is just above the muscle. On the mucosa the incision continues till the junction of the dry and wet mucosa to expose the muscle. Insert a skin hook which will stretch the lip and aid in further dissection. *Note*: The superior labial artery can be encountered at this point and may need cauterization (Fig. 72.29).
- Begin the incision from the point where the white roll diminishes, and carry it along the marking between the skin and mucosa to reach the junction between the nasal skin and mucosa.
- A small mucosal triangle containing the dark mucosa is maintained, and incision is then carried out to raise the L flap.
- Once the L flap is raised, the muscle of the cleft side element is exposed.
- Incision is made between the mucosa and muscle similar to the non-cleft side in the plane of existing minor salivary glands.
- The incision between the skin and muscle is similar to the lateral element.
- The abnormal muscle attachments on this side are at the base of the alar and the pyriform region that would require subperiosteal dissection to release the attachment.
- *Insertion of Flaps and Suturing*.
- The final step of closing the flaps into desired position begins with insetting the L and M flaps.
- *Step 1*
- Using the M flap is optional. The author generally discards the M flap but occasional uses it to reduce tension while doing the nasal floor repair in very wide clefts.
- The L flap is used to create the nasal layer on the cleft side by lining it between the nasal skin and the nasal floor.
- *Step 2*
- *Creating the Nasal Floor*: Nasal layers are now sutured from both the cleft and non-cleft sides and sutured using a 4.0 Vicryl (Fig. 72.30).
- At this point of time, the septum is exposed. When the nasal layer is being raised, if required the septum can be straightened.
- *Step 3*

- *Suturing the Oral Mucosa*: Begin at the point where the wet and dry mucosae meet. The alignment of these two points from both elements is crucial for good mucosal repair. The rest is completed till the alveolar base. The suture material used here is 4.0 Vicryl. The dry mucosa will be closed last (Fig. 72.31).
- *Muscle Suturing*: The preference is to suture the muscle at the junction of white roll and Cupid's bow. The suture allows reassessment of adequate rotation of the flap to create equal length of the philtral columns. A back cut can now be placed to accommodate for discrepancies. The back cut is made parallel to the existing philtral column at the base of the columella.
- Muscle layer suturing is then completed carefully reorienting the fibres at equal height and bites from both elements. At this stage the lip anatomy should correspond to final anatomy, and the skin should be passively seated over the muscle layer. The suturing is completed using 4.0 Vicryl, and the knots are cut flush to prevent any extrusion of sutures on the skin surface (Fig. 72.32).
- *Skin Suturing*: The first step in suturing the skin is to evaluate the area where the C flap is going to be utilized and also the dimension of the flap needed. The excess flap can be trimmed or in some instances completely discarded (Fig. 72.33a).
- The preference of the C flap is to use it as a hemi-columella or nasal sil. Using the C flap into the back cut defect creates an unnatural scar across the cutaneous lip and columella junction.
- Once the C flap is tucked beneath the skin, excess skin tissue if any is trimmed, and suturing begins from the base of the columella down to the vermilion. The suture

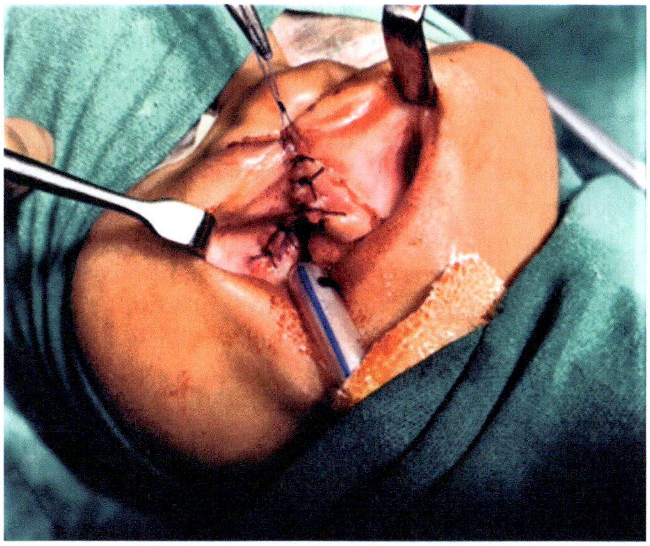

Fig. 72.31 Suturing of the oral mucosa

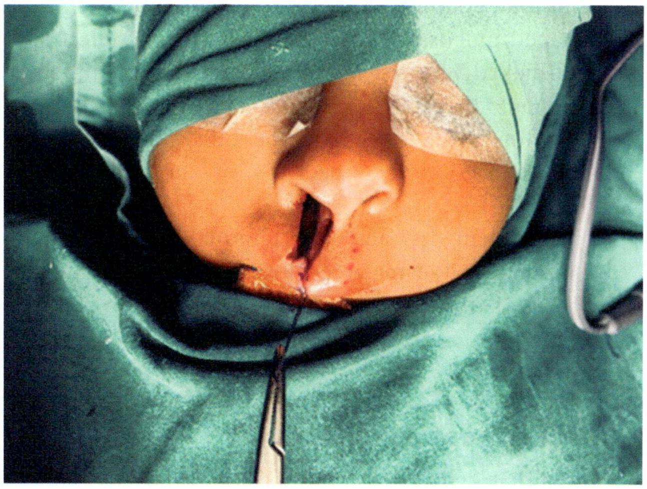

Fig. 72.32 Muscle suturing

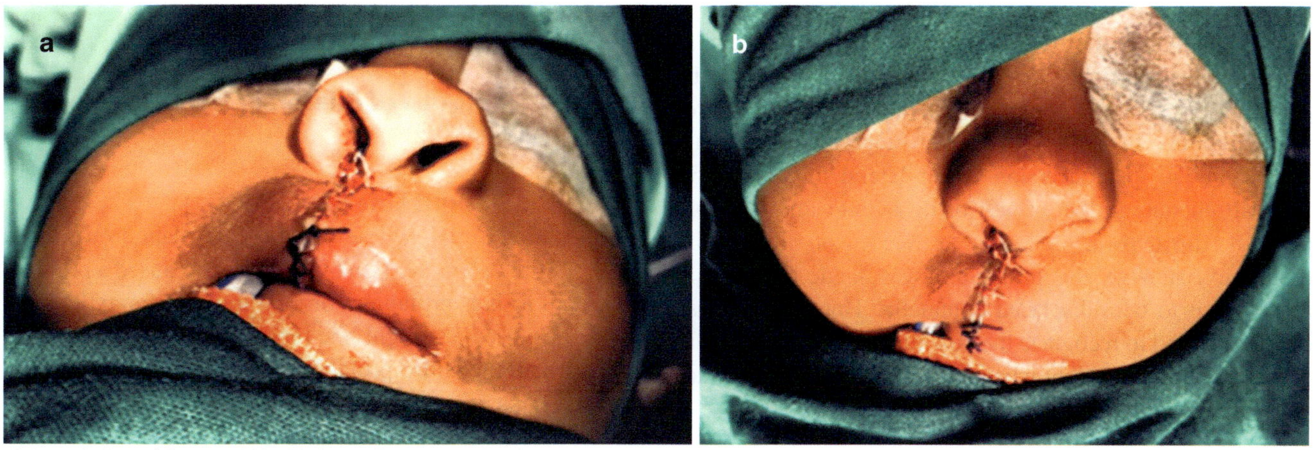

Fig. 72.33 (**a**) Skin suturing. (**b**) Note the matching of the white roll

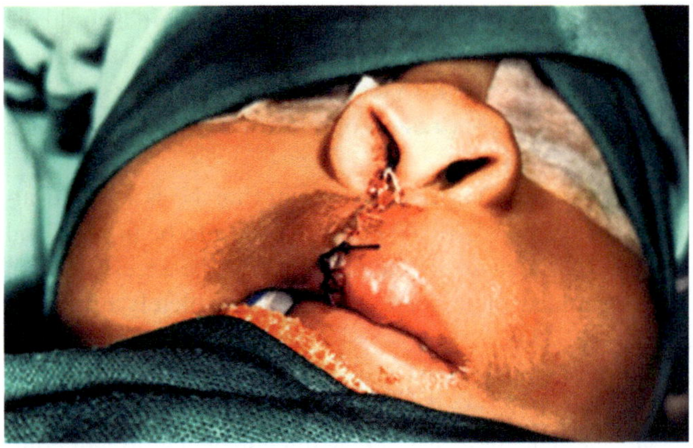

Fig. 72.34 Dry mucosa suturing

used here is 5.0 Vicryl Rapide or 6.0 Vicryl Rapide (Fig. 72.33b).

- *Dry Mucosa Suturing*: At the end of skin suturing, the vermilion continuity is established by using the V-shaped mucosal flap established from the cleft segment tucked into the non-cleft mucosa. At this stage care should be taken to secure a suture beneath the vermilion for muscle repair, and the mucosal stitch should be passive to reduce necrosis of the mucosal tip (Fig. 72.34).
- A good repair depends upon minimal handling of the tissues and a tension-free closure of all layers especially the skin as the muscle bears the stress of tension forces.

72.7 Bilateral Lip Repair

James Barrett Brown said "Bilateral clefts are twice as hard as unilateral clefts, and the results are less than half as good" [69]. Bilateral cleft lip repair can be one-stage or two-stage. Proponents of one-stage repair stress on creating a symmetric, balanced lip. This is indicated in cases of complete or incomplete symmetric bilateral clefts or where the premaxilla is within the arch. Two-stage repair is indicated in the presence of a small prolabium, an asymmetric cleft or a protruded premaxilla. Proponents of two-stage repair advocate this technique for conversion of a bilateral into unilateral cleft, to encourage the growth of prolabium and to avoid excessive lip tension. In earlier techniques of bilateral lip repair, excision of the prolabium was made mistakenly assuming it to be a displaced columella. This was because surgeons failed to recognize the potential of the prolabium to grow in width and height when attached to the dynamic lateral lip elements.

Principles of Bilateral Cleft Lip Repair: Certain key points and landmarks need to be kept in mind while considering a bilateral cleft lip repair. The following principles of bilateral cleft lip repair should be adhered to:

1. Symmetry must be established. In case of staged repairs, this is hindered which lead to asymmetrical results.
2. The surgeon should anticipate a fourth dimensional changes that occur with growth. Failure to account for this may result in a widened philtrum. This is attributable to slower-growing areas such as the lengthening columella and projection of the nasal tip, compared with faster-growing areas such as the philtral width [70] Thus, there is a need to undercorrect fast-growing areas and overcorrect the slow-growing structures.
3. Prolabium: No matter how small it is, the prolabium is always sufficient for reconstruction. It should always be used for reconstruction of the midportion and not used for partial reconstruction of the philtrum and columella. When white line is present in the prolabium, it must be used, however, a short prolabium pulls down nasal tip creating a secondary nasal deformity.
4. Premaxilla: Presurgical orthopaedic treatment should be done only to expand the maxillary segments. Closure and joining the muscle at the midline create enough pressure to retroposition the protruding premaxilla. Sometimes, resection of the vomer behind the vomerine-premaxillary suture can be done, and the premaxilla can be repositioned using plating or K-wire with or without bone graft.
5. Vermillion: There is a very narrow strip of vermillion present in a bilateral cleft lip. A vermillion flap from lateral lip elements should be taken for fullness and protrusion of the lip.
6. Muscle repair: As the prolabium is without muscle fibres, muscle continuity under the prolabium is necessary for a functional lip. There is a need to release the abnormal attachment at the base of the ala from the vertical to horizontal and functional attachment.
7. The nasal deformity can be addressed either primarily or secondarily.

72.7.1 Techniques of Bilateral Cleft Lip Repair (Video 72.2)

72.7.1.1 Straight Line Repair

Bardach used a straight line repair. The prolabium was used for the entire central portion of the lip. This caused a problem in case of a short prolabium or a protruded premaxilla [71]. Salyer also used a straight line repair. In his repair, no tissue is discarded, the entire prolabium is lengthened and philtral and skin flaps are used for vestibular lining [72].

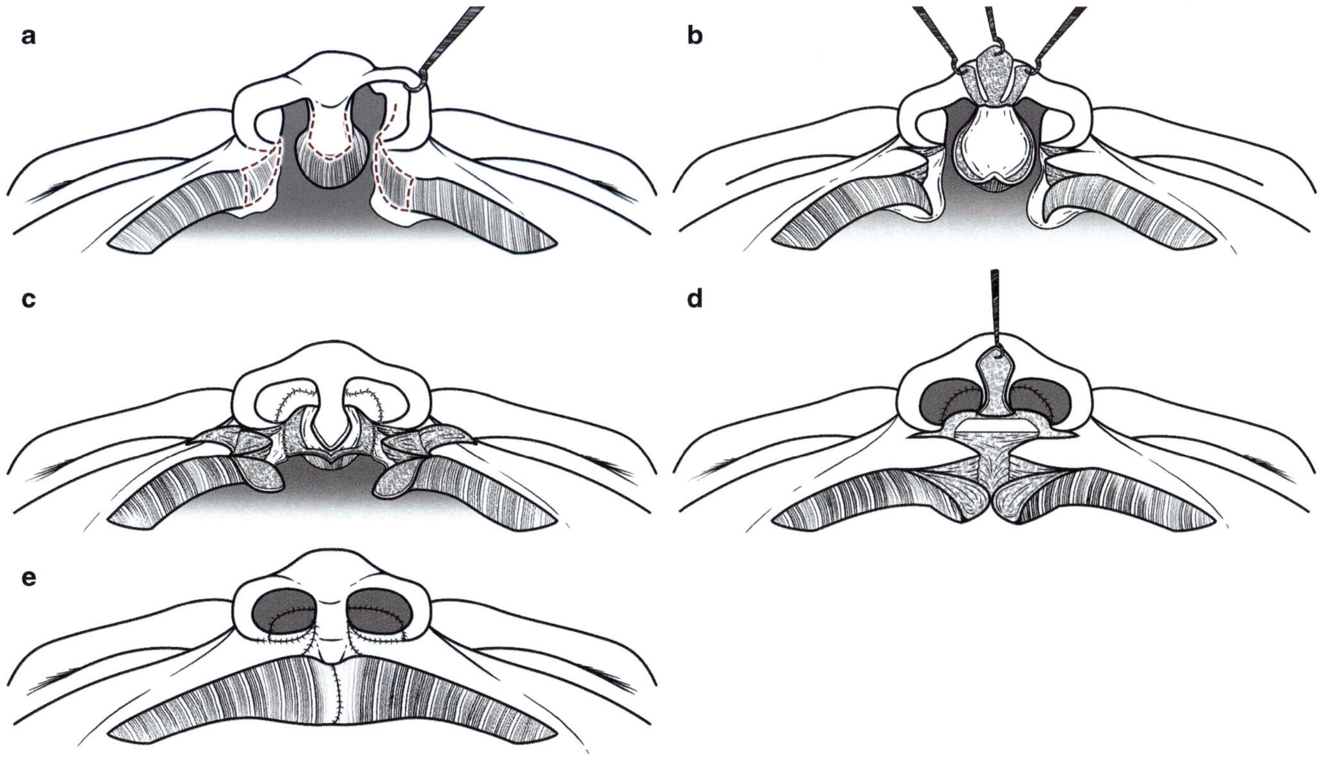

©Association of Oral and Maxillofacial Surgeons of India

Fig. 72.35 (**a**–**e**) Millard's technique of bilateral lip repair

72.7.1.2 Millard's Repair

Millard's repair allowed rotation of the Cupid's bow with the gap filled from skin advanced from the lateral element [73]. It allowed complete elevation of the prolabium and suturing of the orbicularis across the premaxilla. In addition, Millard created lateral segments of the prolabium as "forked flaps". These flaps were banked to add columellar height at a later stage, thus addressing the vertical height deficiency, and it also corrected the wide alar bases (Fig. 72.35a–e). The key elements of bilateral lip repair are given in Box 72.6.

72.7.1.3 Mulliken's Repair

Mulliken designed a narrow prolabial flap with slightly concave sides; 2; 2.5 mm at base and 3.5–4 mm between Cupid s bow peak. The surgical stratagem is symmetrical labial repair and synchronous anatomic positioning of the alar cartilages with sculpturing/draping of the nasal soft tissues. It consists of following elements:

- Suture of the orbicularis oris in the midline.
- Fixation to anterior nasal spine.
- Positioning dislocated lower lateral cartilages: interdomal suture.
- Suspension over ipsilateral upper lateral cartilage with intercartilaginous suture.
- Suture of the orbicularis oris in the midline.
- Fixation to the anterior nasal spine.
- Positioning dislocated lower lateral cartilages: interdomal suture.
- Suspension over the ipsilateral upper lateral cartilage with intercartilaginous suture.

Box 72.6 Key Elements of Bilateral Lip Repair

- Bringing in a new white roll from the lateral lip elements.
- The prolabium parings are banked for future columella lengthening.
- Bringing lateral vermilion flaps beneath the prolabium.
- Reconstructing the orbicularis muscle beneath the elevated prolabium.

72.7.2 Bilateral Lip Repair: Author's Technique

Markings: Fig. 72.36 shows the marking of the prolabial flap and the lateral flaps.

- Once all incisions are designed, the lip is infiltrated with 1:100.000 epinephrine. We can start with either the prolabium or lateral flaps. Grab the lip between fingers for better control during incision and bloodless field.

- Incision starts on the prolabium following the previous markings, the medial flap is for philtral reconstruction, and two laterals segments of the skin are discarded (Fig. 72.37a).
- The philtral flap is dissected, leaving a generous amount of deeper soft tissues attached. The flap is raised in a pre-periosteal plane off the premaxilla and up to the base of the columella (Fig. 72.37b).
- Next step is creation of mucosal flap from the prolabium for sulcus reconstruction and exposure of anterior nasal spine.
- Incision in lateral lip following the marks in the skin and mucosa of the vermillion is made (Fig. 72.38).
- Incision is carried on the vermilion-cutaneous junction, dissecting the vermilion to the point where the peak of the Cupid's bow is marked.
- Full thickness cuts are made through the orbicularis oris and the oral mucosa of the upper lip.
- Incision in the sulcus to aid in the detachment of the abnormal lateral lip element, especially the muscle.
- Those incisions facilitate mobilization of the lateral lip elements so they can be brought up and over the premaxilla which aids in decreasing tension.

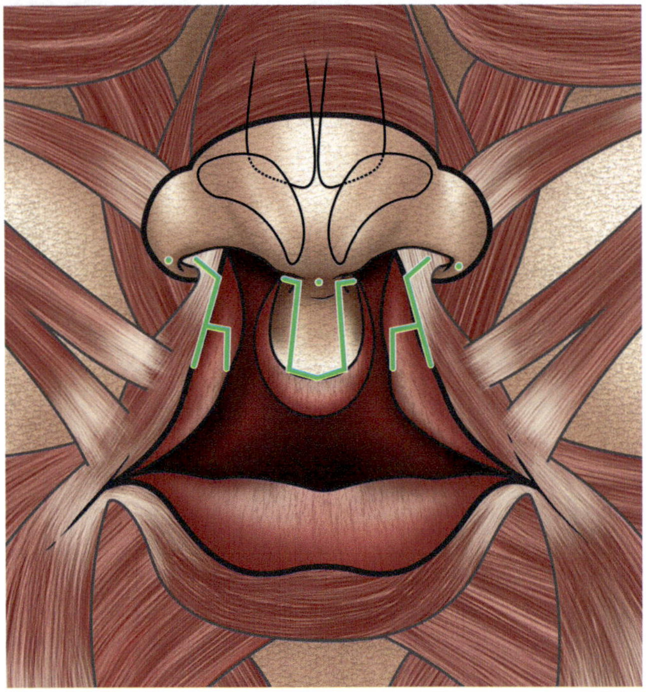

Fig. 72.36 Markings for bilateral lip repair

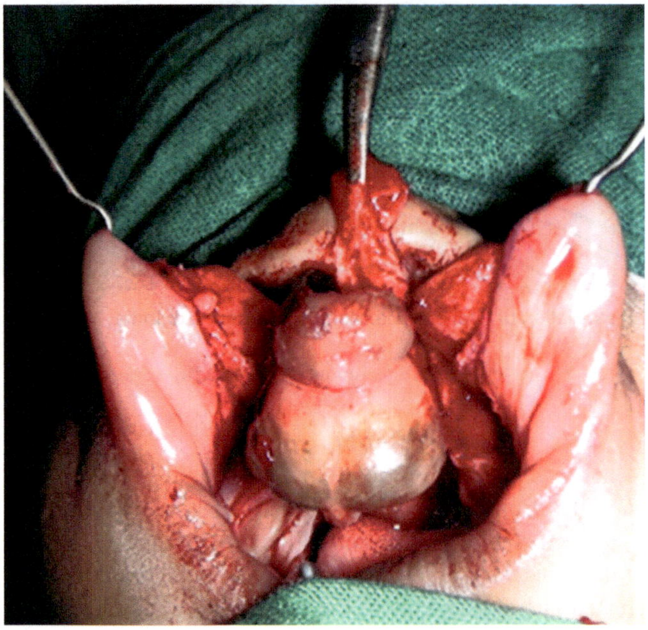

Fig. 72.38 Dissection of the lateral flaps

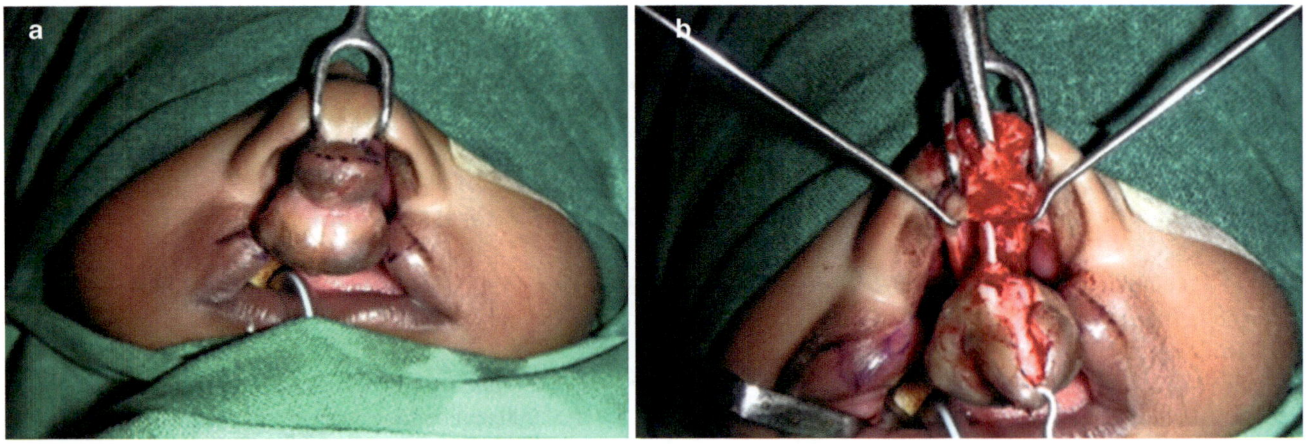

Fig. 72.37 (**a**) Marking of the prolabium flap and lateral flap. (**b**) The prolabium flap dissected

- The muscle is dissected as a separate layer from the mucosa not from the skin. Undermining of the soft tissue, dissection and release are carried up to the inferior orbital nerve.
- Subperiosteal dissection of the pyriform aperture towards the frontomaxillary pillar, to release the ala from its abnormal insertions.

Release and repositioning of the following structures from their abnormal attachment:

- Alar base.
- Muscular, ligamentous and lining attachments.
- Fibrous attachments with the accessory chain of the lateral crus.
- Full-thickness cut is made along the nasal lining at the pyriform aperture. This release creates a lining defect that will be filled with the septal flap.
- Dissection of mucoperiosteal flap from lateral nasal wall.
- Liberation of the orbicularis oris, freeing it from its abnormal attachment around the base of the nose.
- Reposition of the orbicularis from vertical to horizontal position with retrograde dissection without dissection of the muscle and the skin in the free border.

  Suturing

  (a) Nasal Floor
  - Mucoperiosteal flap from lateral nasal wall and mucoperichondrial flap from the nasal septum are sutured to form the nasal floor. This helps to bring the base of the ala medially, thus narrowing the width of the nostril.

  (b) Recreating the Sulcus
  - Advance prolabial mucosal flap superiorly to establish the lining of the labial sulcus, trimmed as needed, and fixing it to the periosteum inferiorly to the nasal spine.
  - Medial advancing of mucosal flaps and fixation to the mucosal flap of the prolabium, previously fixed. Then they are sutured together in the middle line from inferior to superior, starting in the red line (key stitch).

  (c) Muscle Repair
  - Medial advanced musculocutaneous flaps from the lateral lips.
  - Muscle is brought across the midline below the prolabium.
  - Apposition of the muscle is done from distal (key stitch) to proximal area (Fig. 72.39).
  - Proximal segment fixed to the periosteum of the anterior nasal spine in the middle line.

  (d) Vermillion Repair
  - The midportion of the vermilion is reconstructed by bringing lateral vermilion flaps below the philtrum flap (Fig. 72.40).

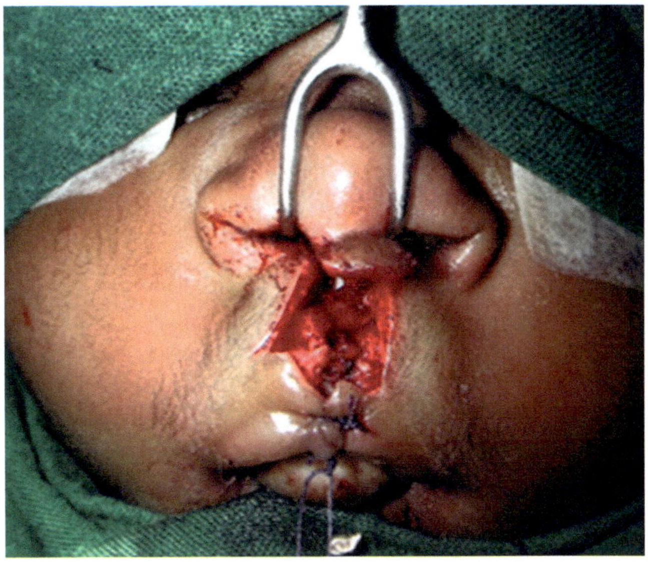

Fig. 72.39 Lateral flaps sutured beneath the prolabium. Muscle sutured to create the continuity

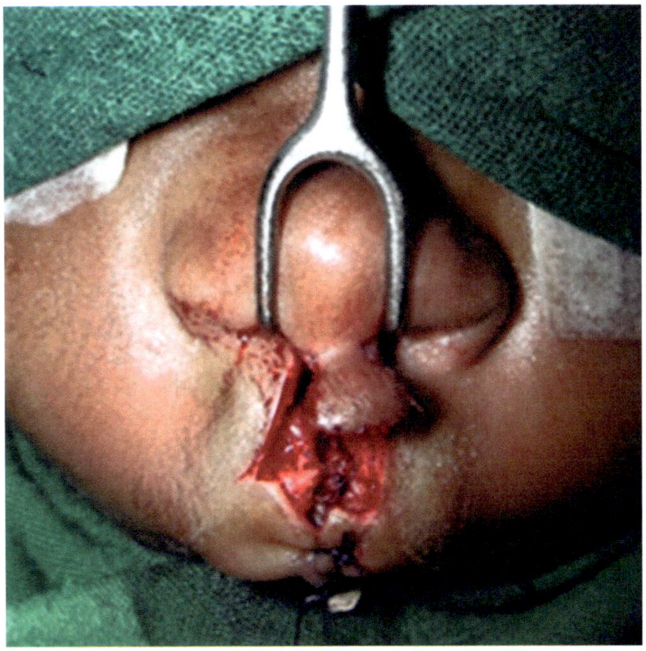

Fig. 72.40 Position of the prolabium to create the future philtral column

  (e) Skin
  - Preventing or minimizing lip tension is the key to successful bilateral cleft repair (Fig. 72.41).
  - Excessive tension: tethering of the columella, increased scarring and facial growth problems.
  - Attention is given to construction of the Cupid's bow.

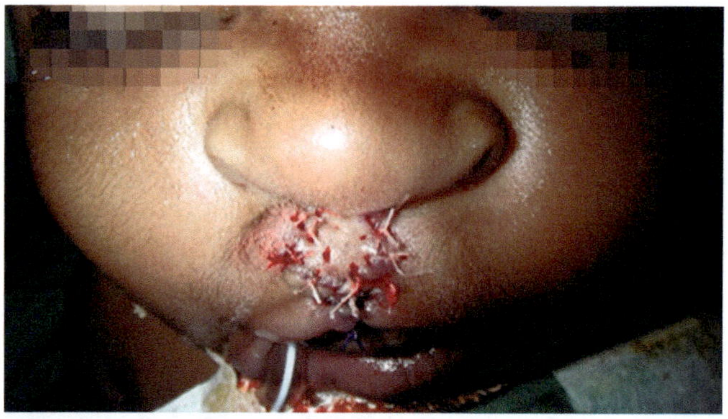

Fig. 72.41 Skin suturing done

72.8 Primary Chielorhinoplasty

A variety of options exists to address the nasal deformity with cleft lip. These include preoperative nasoalveolar moulding, overcorrection of the nostril width and alar cartilage at the time of lip repair and postoperative use of nasal conformers. Primary treatment of the nose at the time of lip repair has become popular, in order to gain early restoration of the symmetry by repositioning the alar cartilage and lengthening the columella. However, relapse is frequent due to the elastic deformed alar cartilage. Various theories and opinions have been popularized regarding correction of the septum, to either straighten the septum or leave for later correction. A study done by Mancini et al. involves three-dimensional analysis of unilateral cleft lip and palate patients treated with PNAM and primary rhinoplasty, which demonstrated significant improvements in nasal projection, columellar length, nasal symmetry and nasal width [74].

72.9 Postoperative Wound Care and Outcome Assessment

Postoperative wound care is extremely important in determining the results of lip repair and is often a factor resulting in the need of a lip revision.

1. Suture area should be cleaned daily with saline and baby soap twice; topical application of antibiotics is recommended for 10 days.
2. 3 weeks post-op, we recommend to massage the scar towards the mucosa to prevent scar contracture.
3. Massage can be done with vitamin E cream/silicone gel/oil. It is recommended to massage for at least 6 months.

72.9.1 Outcomes

Improper surgical technique and tissue dissection can lead to certain undesirable outcomes. Other factors such as wide deformities, severely displaced premaxilla, inadequate postoperative care, poor healing and infection can also lead to aesthetic results. Understanding the process and severity of the outcome helps in addressing the problem in secondary lip repair or lip scar revisions. The outcomes can be divided into the following types:

- Mucosal notching—As pointed above, the mucosal dissection should always be in the plane between the muscles and the mucosa plus minor salivary glands. Failure to maintain that results in a thin mucosa that inverts after suturing. This leads to mucosal notching. As a trainee, one can also give mattress sutures to achieve mucosal eversion. In case of very mild mucosal notching presenting at 3 weeks, it is advised to continue the massage. If notching persists after 6 months of lip repair, it can be treated by surgically improving placement of muscle; thus we recommend a lip revision.
- Scarring—A scar can present in various forms. A scar can be linear but hypertrophic in appearance. Such scars can be avoided if proper massaging is done in the postoperative phase. If the scar has keloid tendency, triamcinolone injections are to be given at an interval of 15 days followed by vigorous massage.
- Contracture—A scar can also present as a gross or mild vertical contracture. This usually results due to inadequate rotation, thus pulling the lip towards the nose resulting in vertical shortening of cleft side philtral column. Improper muscle closure or overzealous separation of the skin from the muscle can lead to scarring of the skin.
- Inadequate philtral column matching—This again results due to lack of a proper design and improper mobilization of the rotation flap.
- Complete breakdown of the surgical wound may be the most severe adverse outcome in the immediate post-operative phase.

72.10 Indications for Lip Revision

Scarred fibrous tissues with poor vascularity always make secondary surgery more challenging. Dissection and re-approximation of surgical landmarks are difficult in such cases. The basic surgical principles that should be followed are identification and preservation of all the vital anatomic structures.

The basic indications for a lip revision surgery are:

1. Unilateral.
   - The scar is not in line with the natural philtral column.
   - The lip length is short.
   - There is a mucosal notching.
   - There is a white roll to Cupid's bow mismatch.
   - There is a nasolabial fistula.
2. Bilateral.
   - There is a wide philtral column.
   - Mucosal notching.
   - Whistling defect.
   - No sulcus depth.

72.11 Conclusion

In our course of learning of cleft, we often understand embryology, anatomy and the surgical technique as separate concepts. In this chapter, we have tried to integrate them and tried to explain the rationale behind the surgical steps. Embryological basis of normal anatomy and then of cleft is pivotal to understand the arrangements of muscles, the vascular supply and thus the basis of incisions. We have described our surgical technique of cleft lip repair with long-term follow-ups. In the congenital deformity of cleft where there is paucity and deformation of tissues, preserving the tissues during surgery is one of the important principles of lip repair.

72.12 Case Scenarios

Figures 72.42, 72.43, 72.44, 72.45 and 72.46 represent cases of operated unilateral and bilateral cleft lip with long-term follow-ups.

Figures 72.47, 72.48, 72.49 and 72.50 represents cases of lip revisions with follow-ups.

Disclosure: Authors have no financial conflicts to disclose.

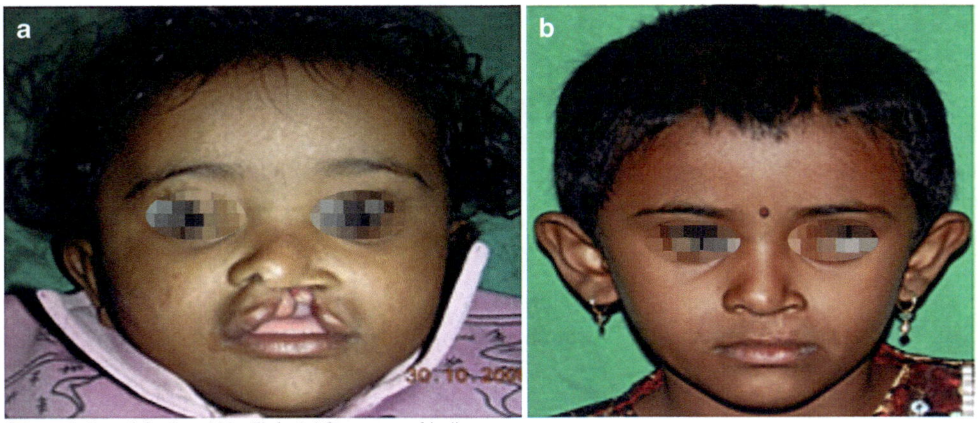

Fig. 72.42 (**a**, **b**) Pre operative (**a**) and postoperative (**b**) Photograph of repair of unilateral cleft lip using author's technique of lip repair [7-year follow-up]

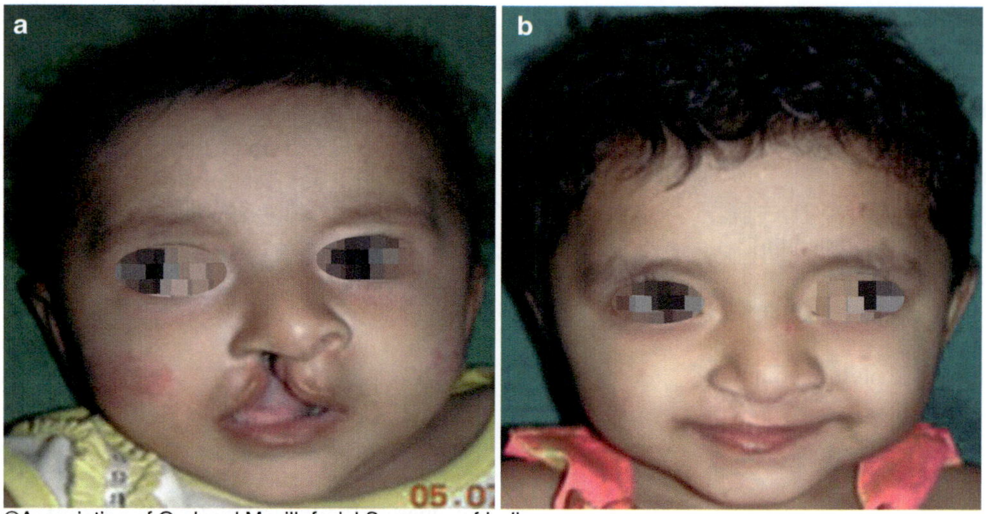

Fig. 72.43 (**a**, **b**) Another case of a 3-month-old female of complete unilateral cleft lip repaired. Left, preoperative; right, postoperative after a 4-years follow-up

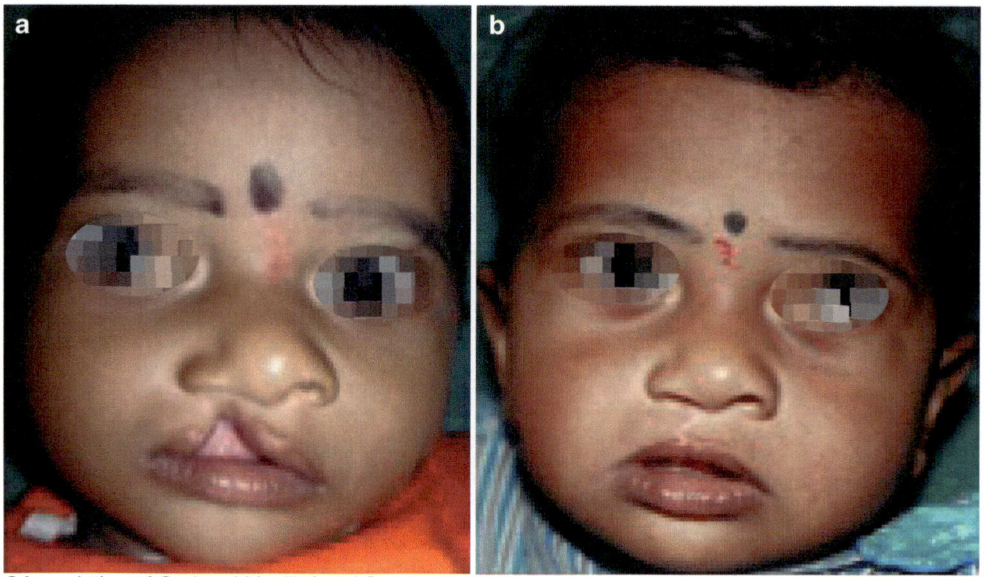

Fig. 72.44 (**a**, **b**) Operated case of an incomplete cleft lip, 2-year follow-up

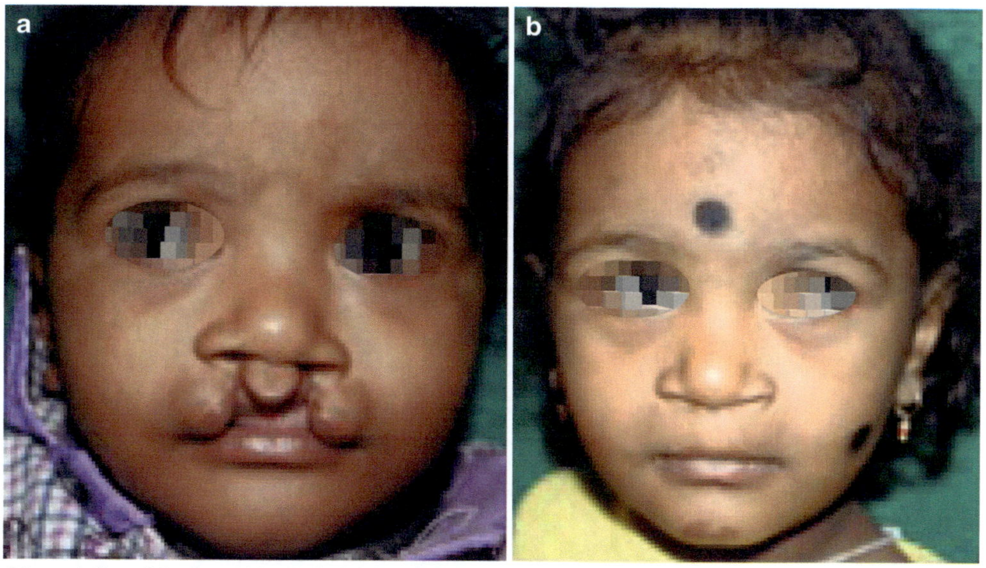

Fig. 72.45 (**a**, **b**) Pre-op and post-op photograph of a case of bilateral cleft lip repair, 5-year follow-up

Fig. 72.46 (**a**, **b**) Another case of operated bilateral cleft lip

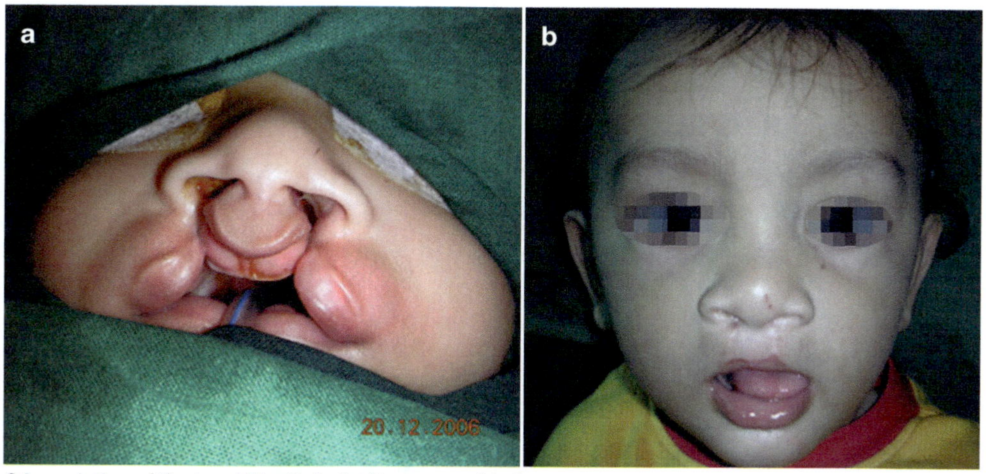

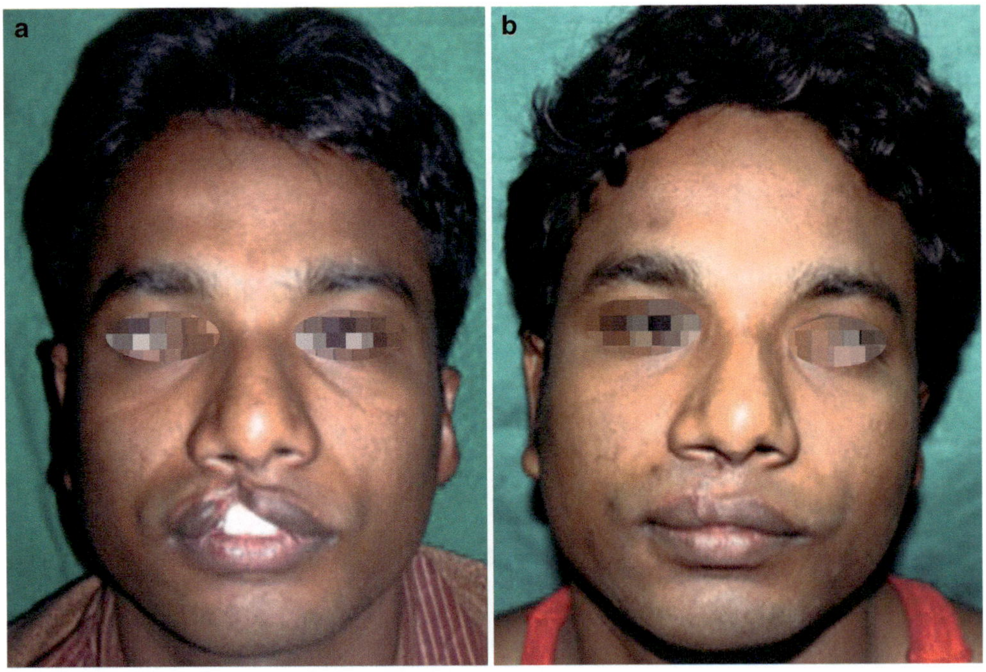

Fig. 72.47 (**a**, **b**) A case of mucosal notching in an adult lip (**a**) Postoperative image after a 2-year follow-up (**b**)

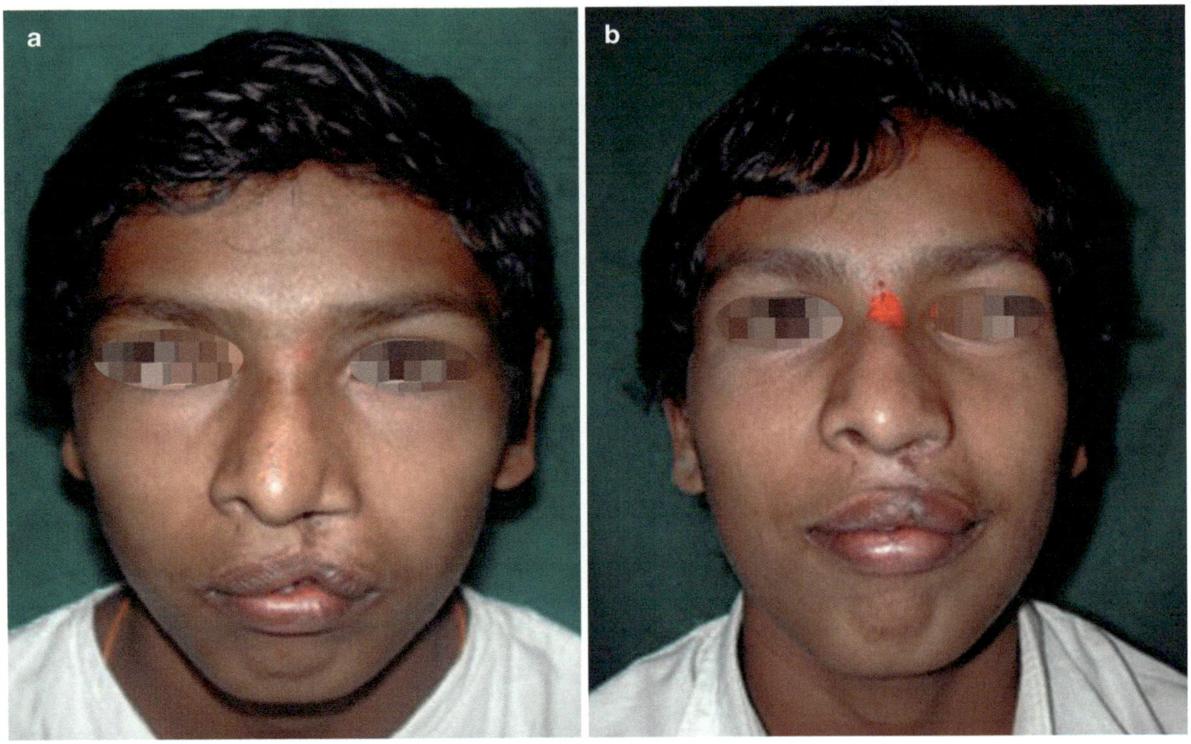

Fig. 72.48 (**a**, **b**) A case of operated unilateral cleft lip with mucosal notching and vertical scar contracture (**a**) Postoperative image after lip revision (**b**)

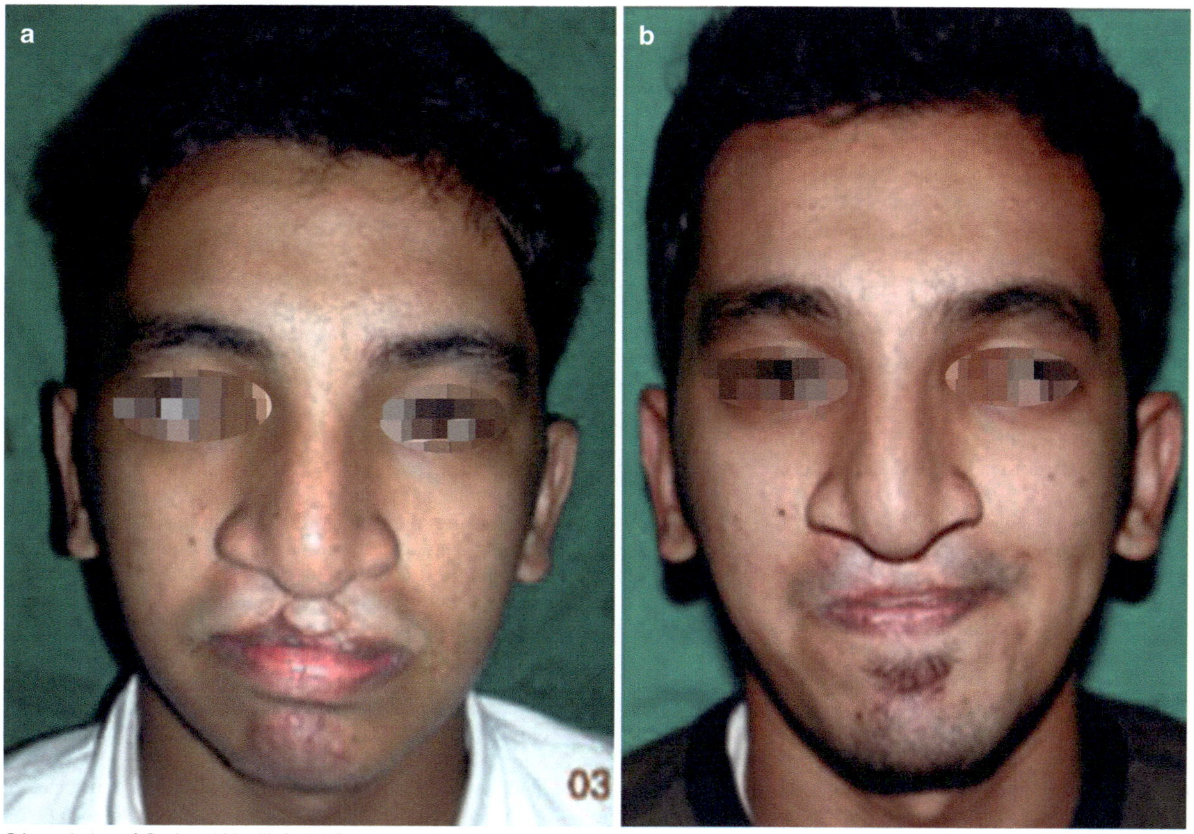

Fig. 72.49 (**a**, **b**) An operated case of bilateral cleft lip before (**a**) and after (**b**) lip revision

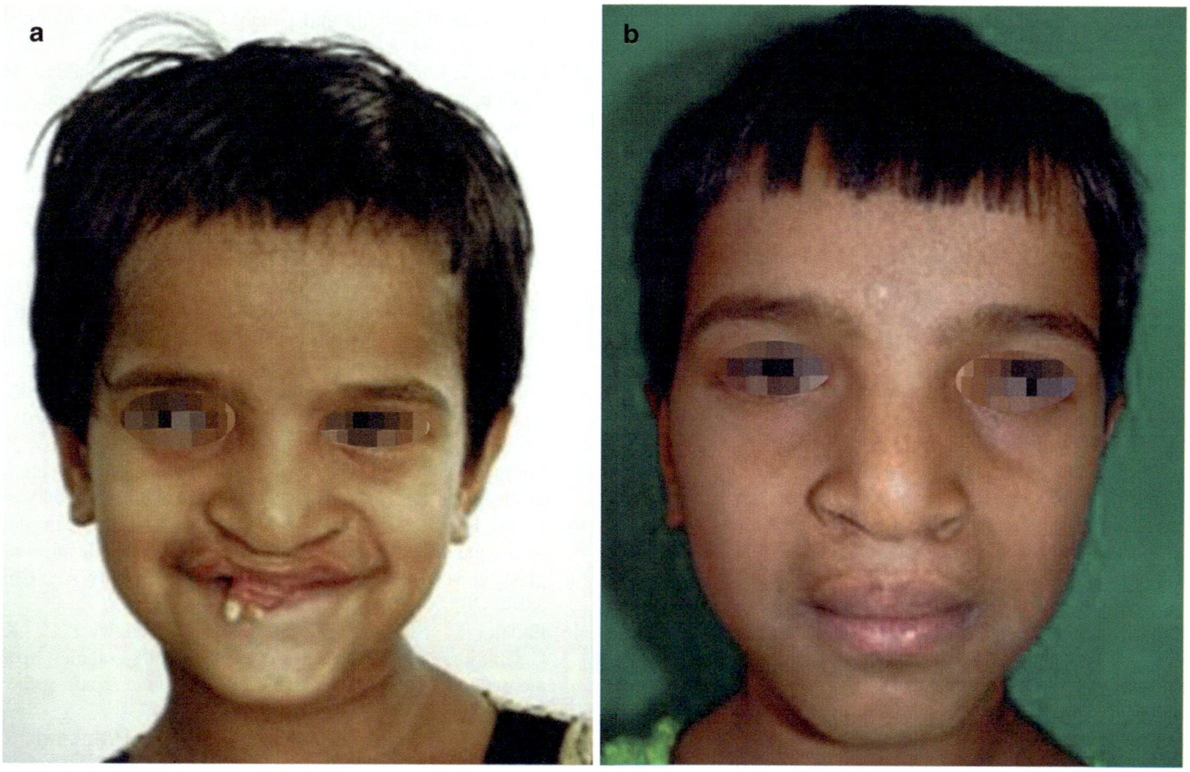

Fig. 72.50 (**a**, **b**) A case of an operated bilateral cleft lip with protruding premaxilla and a wide lip (**a**) Postoperative image (**b**) after lip revision and premaxillary repositioning

References

1. Kadir A, Mossey PA, Blencowe H, Moorthie S, Lawn JE, Mastroiacovo P, et al. Systematic review and meta-analysis of the birth prevalence of orofacial clefts in low- and middle-income countries. Cleft Palate Craniofac J. 2017;54:571–81.
2. Millard DR Jr. Cleft craft: evolution of its surgery. In: The unilateral deformity, vol. 1. Boston: Little, Brown; 1976.
3. Sadler TW, Langman J. Langman's medical embryology. 12th ed. Philadelphia: Wolters Kluwer Health/Lippincott Williams & Wilkins; 2012.
4. Millard DR Jr. Cleft craft: evolution of its surgery. In: Embroyological theories, vol. 1. Boston: Little, Brown; 1976.
5. Millard DR Jr. Cleft craft: evolution of its surgery. In: Anatomy in multiple dimensions, vol. 1. Boston: Little, Brown; 1976.
6. Ghi T, Perolo A, Banzi C, et al. Two-dimensional ultrasound is accurate in the diagnosis of fetal craniofacial malformation. Ultrasound Obstet Gynecol. 2002;19:543–51.
7. Drake RL, Vogl W, Mitchell AWM, Gray H. Gray's anatomy for students. Philadelphia: Elsevier/Churchill Livingstone; 2005.
8. Davis JS, Ritchie HP. Classification of congenital clefts of the lip and palate. JAMA. 1922;79:1323–7.
9. Brophy TW. Cleft palate and harelip procedures. Int J Orthod Oral Surg. 1921;7:319–30.
10. Veau V. Division Palantine. Paris: Masson et Cie; 1931.
11. Kernahan DA, Stark RB. A new classification for cleft lip and cleft palate. Plast Reconstr Surg Transplant Bull. 1958;22:435–41.
12. Harkins CS, Berlin A, Harding RL, Longacre JJ, Snodgrasse RM. A classification of cleft lip and cleft palate. Plast Reconstr Surg Transplant Bull. 1962;29:31–9.
13. Kernahan DA. The striped Y – a symbolic classification for cleft lip and palate. Plast Reconstr Surg. 1971;47:469–70.
14. Spina V. A proposed modification for the classification of cleft lip and cleft palate. Cleft Palate J. 1973;10:251–2.
15. Elsahy NI. The modified striped Y – a systematic classification for cleft lip and palate. Cleft Palate J. 1973;10:247–50.
16. Millard DR Jr. Cleft craft, vol. I. Boston: Little, Brown and Company; 1977. p. 41–55.
17. Friedman HI, Sayetta RB, Coston GN, Hussey JR. Symbolic representation of cleft lip and palate. Cleft Palate Craniofac J. 1991;28:252–9.
18. Kernahan DA. On cleft lip and palate classification. Plast Reconstr Surg. 1973;51:578.
19. Smith AW, Khoo AK, Jackson IT. A modification of the Kernahan "Y" classification in cleft lip and palate deformities. Plast Reconstr Surg. 1998;102:1842–7.
20. Balakrishnan C. Indian classification of cleft lip and palate. Indian J Plast Surg. 1975;8:23.
21. Kriens O. Lahshal: a concise documentation system for cleft lip, alvolus and palate diagnoses. In: Kriens O, editor. What is cleft lip and palate? A multidisciplinary update workshop, Bremen 1987. Stuttgart: Thieme; 1989.
22. Yuzuriha S, Mulliken JB. Minor-form, microform, and mini-microform cleft lip: anatomical features, operative techniques, and revisions. Plast Reconstr Surg. 2008;122(5):1485–93.
23. Bhuskute AA, Tollefson TT. Cleft lip repair, Nasoalveolar molding, and primary cleft rhinoplasty. Facial Plast Surg Clin North Am. 2016;24(4):453–466.
24. Cutting C, Grayson B, Brecht L, Santiago P, Wood R, Kwon S. Presurgical columellar elongation and primary retrograde nasal reconstruction in one-stage bilateral cleft lip and nose repair. Plast Reconstr Surg. 1998;101:630–9.
25. Smith KS, Henry BT, Scott MA. Presurgical Dentofacial orthopedic management of the cleft patient. Oral Maxillofac Surg Clin North Am. 2016;28(2):169–176.
26. Santiago PE, Grayson BH, Cutting CB, et al. Reduced need for alveolar bone grafting by presurgical orthopedics and primary gingivoperiosteoplasty. Cleft Palate Craniofac J. 1998;35(1):77–80.
27. Wood RJ, Grayson BH, Cutting CB. Gingivoperiosteoplasty and midfacial growth. Cleft Palate Craniofac J. 1997;34(1):17–20.
28. Bennun RD, Perandones C, Sepliarsky VA, et al. Nonsurgical correction of nasal deformity in unilateral complete cleft lip: a 6-year follow-up. Plast Reconstr Surg. 1999;104(3):616–30.
29. Ezzat CF, Chavarria C, Teichgraeber JF, et al. Presurgical nasoalveolar molding therapy for the treatment of unilateral cleft lip and palate: a preliminary study. Cleft Palate Craniofac J. 2007;44(1):8–12.
30. Yang C, Huang N, Shi B. [Clinical research of presurgical orthodontic treatment of complete cleft lip and palate infant.] Hua Xi Kou Qiang Yi Xue Za Zhi. 2011;29(4):396–399. Chinese.
31. Ross RB. Growth of the facial skeleton following the Malek repair for unilateral cleft lip and palate. Cleft Palate Craniofac J. 1995;32(3):194–8.
32. Bonanthaya K, Nayak T, Bitra S, Rachwalski M, Shetty PN. An assessment and comparison of nasolabial aesthetics in bilateral clefts using the anatomical subunit-based scale: a nasoalveolar moulding versus non-nasoalveolar moulding study. Int J Oral Maxillofac Surg. 2019;48(3):298–301.
33. de Ladeira PR, Alonso N. Protocols in cleft lip and palate treatment: systematic review. Plast Surg Int. 2012;2012:562892.
34. https://medicine.uiowa.edu/iowaprotocols/cleft-lip-and-palate-protocols
35. Salyer KE, Xu H, Genecov ER. Unilateral cleft lip and nose repair; closed approach Dallas protocol completed patients. J Craniofac Surg. 2009;20 Suppl 2:1939–1955.
36. Dudkiewicz Z. Ocena jednoetapowego chirurgicznego leczenia jednostronnych rozszczep_ow podniebienia pierwotnego i wt_ornego. Probl Chir Dziec. 1991;18:8e19. [in Polish]
37. Åbyholm F. Primary closure of cleft lip and palate. In: Turvey TA, KWL V, Fonseca RJ, editors. Facial clefts and craniosynostosis. Philadelphia: WB Saunders; 1996. p. 370–83.
38. Ross RB. Growth of the facial skeleton following the Malek repair for unilateral cleft lip and palate. Cleft Palate Craniofac J. 1995 May;32(3):194–8.
39. Russell K, Long RE Jr, Hathaway R, Daskalogiannakis J, Mercado A, Cohen M, et al. The Americleft study: an inter-center study of treatment outcomes for patients with unilateral cleft lip and palate part 5. General discussion and conclusions. Cleft Palate Craniofac J. 2011;48:265–70.
40. http://www.wch.sa.gov.au/services/az/divisions/psurg/craniofacial/documents/management_cleft_lip_palate.pdf.
41. Shaw WC, Brattström V, Mølsted K, Prahl-Andersen B, Roberts CT, Semb G. The Eurocleft study: intercenter study of treatment outcome in patients with complete cleft lip and palate. Part 5: discussion and conclusions. Cleft Palate Craniofac J. 2005;42:93–8.
42. Shaw WC, Semb G, Nelson P, Brattström V, Mølsted K, Prahl-Andersen B. The Eurocleft project 1996–2000. Standards of care for cleft lip and palate in Europe. Amsterdam: IOS Press; 2000.
43. Lehman JA Jr, Douglas BK, Ho WC, Husami TW. One-stage closure of the entire primary palate. Plast Reconstr Surg. 1990;86:675–81.
44. Farina R: Total unilateral harelip: correction of severe deformity of the palate and lips in a single operation; Le Mesurier's cheiloplasty & Veau-Ernst's gnathourano- staphyloplasty. Ann Chir Plast. 3:199–205. 1958 In French.
45. Fudalej P, Surowiec Z, Offert B, Dudkiewicz Z, Katsaros C. Craniofacial morphology in complete unilateral cleft lip and palate patients consecutively treated with 1-stage repair of the cleft. J Craniofac Surg. 2010;21:1468–73.
46. Rose W. On harelip and cleft palate. London: H.K. Lewis; 1891.
47. Thompson JE. An artistic and mathematically accurate method of repairing the defect in cases of hairlip. Surg Gynecol Obstet. 1912;14:498–504.

48. Veau V. Le role tubercle median dans la constitution de la face. Ann Anat Pathol (Paris). 1926;3:305–48.
49. Pfeifer G. Lip corrections following earlier cleft surgery by way of wave-line incisions. Dtsch Zahnarztl Z. 1970;25:569–76.
50. Delaire J. Primary cheilorhinoplasty for congenital unilateral labio-maxillary fissure. Trial schematization of a technic. Rev Stomatol Chir Maxillofac. 1975;76:193–215.
51. Chait L, Kadwa A, Potgieter A, et al. The ultimate straight line repair for unilateral cleft lips. J Plast Reconstr Aesthet Surg. 2009 Jan; 62:50–55. [Epub 2007 Nov 26].
52. Mirault G. Deux lettres sur l'operation du bec-de-lievre. J Chir Paris. 1844:1–12.
53. Blair VP, Brown JB. Mirault operation for single harelip. Surg Gynecol Obstet. 1930;51:81.
54. Brown JB, McDowell F. Simplified design for repair of single cleft lip. Surg Gynecol Obstet. 1945;80:12.
55. LeMesurier AB. The quadrilateral mirault flap operation for hare-lip. Plast Reconstr Surg (1946). 1955;16:422–33.
56. Hagedorn W. Uber eine Modifikation der Hasenschartenoperation. Zentralbl Chir. 1884;11:756.
57. Tennison CW. The repair of unilateral cleft lip by the stencil method. Plast Reconstr Surg. 1952;9:115.
58. Randall P. A triangular flap operation for the primary repair of unilateral clefts of the lip. Plast Reconstr Surg Transplant Bull. 1959;23:331–47.
59. Millard DR Jr. A primary camouflage of the unilateral Harelook. In: Skoog T, editor. Transactions of the first international congress of plastic surgery, stockholm, 1955. Baltimore: Williams & Wilkins; 1957. p. 160–6.
60. Millard DR. Complete unilateral clefts of the lip. Plast Reconstr Surg. 1960;25:595–605.
61. Millard DR. A radical rotation in single harelip. Am J Surg. 1958;95:318–22.
62. Millard DR. Refinements in rotation-advancement cleft lip technique. Plast Reconstr Surg. 1964;33:26–38.
63. Stal S, Brown RH, Higuera S, Hollier LH Jr, Byrd HS, Cutting CB, Mulliken JB. Fifty years of the Millard rotation-advancement: looking back and moving forward. Plast Reconstr Surg. 2009;123(4):1364–77.
64. Mohler LR. Unilateral cleft lip repair. Plast Reconstr Surg. 1987;80:511–7.
65. Fisher DM. Unilateral cleft lip repair: an anatomical subunit approximation technique. Plast Reconstr Surg. 2005;116:61–71.
66. Noordhoff MS. Reconstruction of vermilion in unilateral and bilateral cleft lips. Plast Reconstr Surg. 1984;73:52.
67. Cutting CB, Dayan JH. Lip height and lip width after extended Mohler unilateral cleft lip repair. Plast Reconstr Surg. 2003;111:17–23.
68. Mulliken JB, Martinez-Perez D. The principle of rotation advancement for repair of unilateral complete cleft lip and nasal deformity: technical variations and analysis of results. Plast Reconstr Surg. 1999;104:1247–60.
69. Wolfe SA. Repair of bilateral incomplete cleft lip: techniques and outcomes. Plast Reconstr Surg. 2014;134(1):166e–168e.
70. Zhang JX, Arneja JS. Evidence-based medicine: the bilateral cleft lip repair. Plast Reconstr Surg. 2017;140(1):152e–165e. Review.
71. Bardach J, Cutting C. Anatomy of the unilateral and bilateral cleft lip and nose. In: Bardach J, Morris HL, editors. Multidisciplinary Management of Cleft lip and Palate. Philadelphia: Saunders; 1990. p. 150–9.
72. Salyer KE, Bardach J. Salyer & Bardach's atlas of craniofacial & cleft surgery: craniofacial surgery. Philadelphia: Lippincott-Raven Publishers; 1999.
73. Trier WC. Repair of bilateral cleft lip: Millard's technique. Clin Plast Surg. 1985 Oct;12(4):605–25.
74. Mancini L, Gibson TL, Grayson BH, Flores RL, Staffenberg D, Shetye PR.Three-dimensional soft tissue nasal changes after Nasoalveolar molding and primary Cheilorhinoplasty in infants with unilateral cleft lip and palate. Cleft Palate Craniofac J. 2019;56(1):31–38.

Cleft Palate

73

P. V. Narayanan and H. S. Adenwalla

73.1 Introduction

It was Kilner who said, "Ask not for a spatula and torch to check your cleft palate repair, but listen to your patient speak." By this obvious but profound statement, he drew the cleft surgeons' attention to the fact that gone are the days of breakdowns and fistulae and that if your child does not speak well, your operation is a failure, for such a child would be out of the mainstream of life forever. In spite of the advances in technique and execution, experienced cleft surgeons all over the world still struggle to obtain perfect speech in a large percentage of cases.

In view of the obvious difficulties of intraoral surgery, it is not surprising that cleft lips were repaired way before anyone tried to repair a cleft palate. Credit for the first successful repair of a cleft palate goes to Le Monnier, a French dentist from Roven. Le Monnier in 1766 cauterized to freshen the cleft edges and sutured them successfully [1].

Cleft surgery then passed through a stormy period of uncertainty in the hands of giants like Ferdinand von Graefe [2], Roux, Dupuytren [3], Dieffenbach [4], and Warren [5]. Mucosal flaps were used, and even lateral osteotomies were tried to move the hard palate medially. In 1859, almost a hundred years after the first hard palate was repaired, von Langenbeck [6] emphasized the need to raise mucoperiosteal bipedicled flaps to repair a palate. Langenbeck procedure was a fundamental breakthrough, and with this major advance, breakdowns of the palate were reduced. In its wake refinements followed. In 1931, Victor Veau [7] parted from the bipedicled flap to single pedicled flaps based on the greater palatine vessels. Veau stressed the importance of repairing the nasal lining of the palate and the need to lengthen it.

In 1937, Kilner [8] working in Oxford and Wardill [9] working in Newcastle on Tyne independently used a four flap procedure for the complete cleft palate.

The weakness of this procedure was a high fistula rate at the junction of the four flaps. In the 1940s, Dorrance [10], Cronin [11], and others used various flaps to lengthen the palate. In 1966 Millard [12] introduced his island flaps based on the greater palatine arteries to lengthen the nasal lining. Ravin Thatte [13] went a step further and took two island flaps one for lining and one for cover and used a tongue flap on the denuded hard palate. All these procedures had their day but were short lived in popularity. However, special mention must be made of the buccal myomucosal flap originally called the cheek flap by Padgett [14]. This flap was revived 30 years later by Murari Mukherjee [15] of Calcutta. He changed the direction of the flap. Recently Ian Jackson has introduced muscle into this mucosal flap to make it more robust, and he calls it a myomucosal flap. He uses it in all his palates to lengthen the nasal lining by 1.5 cm and believes that as a result he achieves better speech. Robert Mann [16] does a Furlow's and coves the residual raw areas with two buccal flaps. His rationale is that there is deficiency of tissue in the palate and therefore, on first plastic surgical principles, bring in tissue from outside. This may become the philosophy of the future.

73.2 Embryology and Anatomy (Figs. 72.1 and 77.1)

73.2.1 Embryology

The primary palate is derived from the intermaxillary segment derived from the frontonasal and medial nasal

Electronic Supplementary Material The online version of this chapter (https://doi.org/10.1007/978-981-15-1346-6_73) contains supplementary material, which is available to authorized users.

P. V. Narayanan (✉)
Consultant Plastic Surgeon, Jubilee Mission Medical College and Research Institute, Thrissur, Kerala, India

H. S. Adenwalla
Department of Plastic Surgery, Burns and the Charles Pinto Centre for Cleft Lip, Palate and Craniofacial Anomalies, Jubilee Mission Medical College and Research Institute, Thrissur, Kerala, India

K. Bonanthaya et al. (eds.), *Oral and Maxillofacial Surgery for the Clinician*, https://doi.org/10.1007/978-981-15-1346-6_73

prominences. The main part of the definitive palate is formed by two shelf-like outgrowths from the maxillary prominences. These outgrowths, the *palatine shelves,* appear in the sixth week of development and are directed obliquely downward on each side of the tongue (Fig. 73.1a and b).

In the seventh week, however, the palatine shelves ascend to attain a horizontal position above the tongue and fuse, forming the *secondary palate* (Fig. 73.2a and b). Anteriorly, the shelves fuse with the triangular primary palate, and the *incisive foramen* is the midline landmark between the primary and secondary palates. At the same time as the palatine shelves fuse, the nasal septum grows down and joins with the cephalic aspect of the newly formed palate (Fig. 73.3a and b).

The secondary palate lies posterior to the incisive foramen and consists of the bony hard palate anteriorly and the soft palate posteriorly, terminating at the uvula. The hard palate consists of the palatine bony shelves on either side, attached to the vomer in the midline. The soft palate consists of a sandwich of muscles enveloped by oral and nasal mucosa.

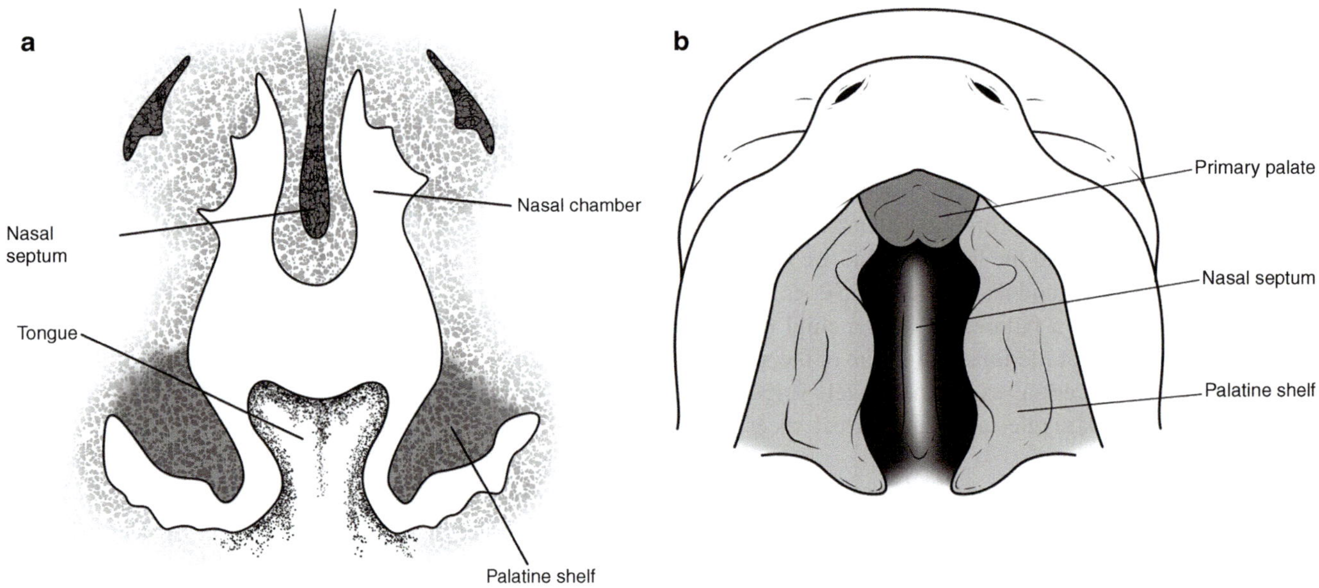

Fig. 73.1 (**a**, **b**) Embryology of palate—primary palate

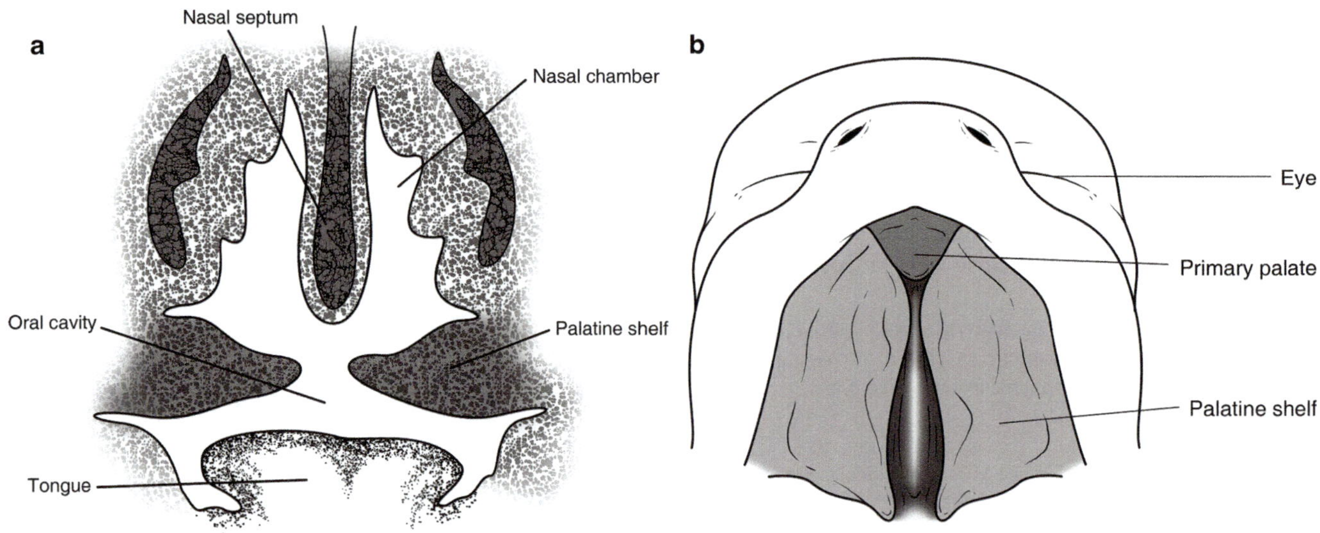

Fig. 73.2 (**a**, **b**) Embryology of palate—secondary palate

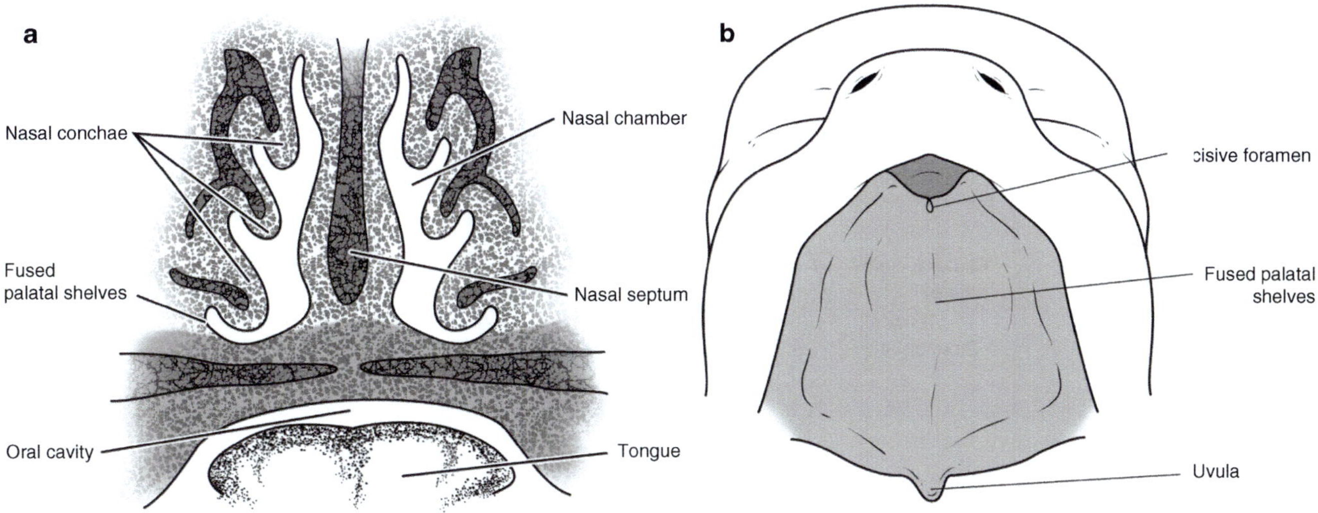

Fig. 73.3 (**a**, **b**) Embryology of palate—completion of palate

73.2.2 Muscles

The muscles of the soft palate include intrinsic muscle, i.e., musculus uvulae, and the insertions of several extrinsic muscles. Apart from this, large amount of.glandular material is present in the anterior inferior portion of the velum and an anterior aponeurosis. Extrinsic muscles of the velum include the tensor veli palatine, levator veli palatini, palatopharyngeus, palatoglossus, and fibers of the superior constrictor. Pharyngeal muscles usually described as having functional role in velopharyngeal movement include the superior constrictor and the salpingopharyngeus (Fig. 73.4).

Following is a tabular summary for the muscles of palate and their abnormal anatomy in a cleft palate (Table 73.1).

From functional standpoint, it is apparent that the levator veli palatini muscle is the principal and quite possibly the only muscle to function for elevation of the velum in speech. The differences between the normal and the cleft arrangement of the muscles of velopharyngeal closure occur because the muscles extending toward the central line of the soft palate cannot attach themselves in the midline of the velum so they insert at some substitute points. These points prevent the muscles from becoming fully functional, and therefore their development is retarded. With the preservation of normal origins, the atypical insertions and hypoplasia of the muscles are the main pathological features in the cleft palate. The abnormal insertions of levators in clefts illustrate that the function of these muscles in cleft palate is almost opposite to that in normal one. While the muscles of both sides normally join in the raphe to form a sling lifting the palate upward, in cleft palate each muscle pulls its own half of the soft palate in an entirely different direction, i.e., superolaterally, causing further widening of the cleft.

73.2.3 Vascular Supply (Fig. 73.5a and b)

The internal maxillary artery gives off the descending palatine artery, which in turn gives off several branches to the tonsils and soft palate. It then passes through the posterior palatine foramen, just above the periosteum, and proceeds forward close to the alveolar margin on each side as the greater major palatine artery to the incisive fossa. At that point it sends terminal branch through the incisive foramen to anastomose with the terminal branch of the sphenopalatine artery. The vascular supply of importance is discussed under two headings, anterior and posterior palate.

73.2.3.1 Vascular Supply of the Anterior Palate/Premaxilla

The blood supply to the anterior alveolar process of the maxilla comes from the arterial complex composed of the major palatine, anterior and superior alveolar, and branches of the sphenopalatine artery. The posterior septal artery arises from the sphenopalatine artery in the roof of the nasal cavity and courses down the groove of the vomer to the incisive foramen. In the complete bilateral cleft lip and palate, the union of the superior labial arteries is lacking; thus they do not contribute to the blood supply of the philtrum. Also the anastomosis of the posterior septal artery with the major palatine artery is absent. Therefore premaxilla and philtrum must derive their blood supply from the posterior septal artery and to some degree from the lateral and terminal branches of the anterior ethmoid vessels which pass through the columella. There is usually one well-developed vessel on either side of the premaxilla in the region where the incisive foramen should have been. Each of these vessels moves anteriorly and inferiorly into

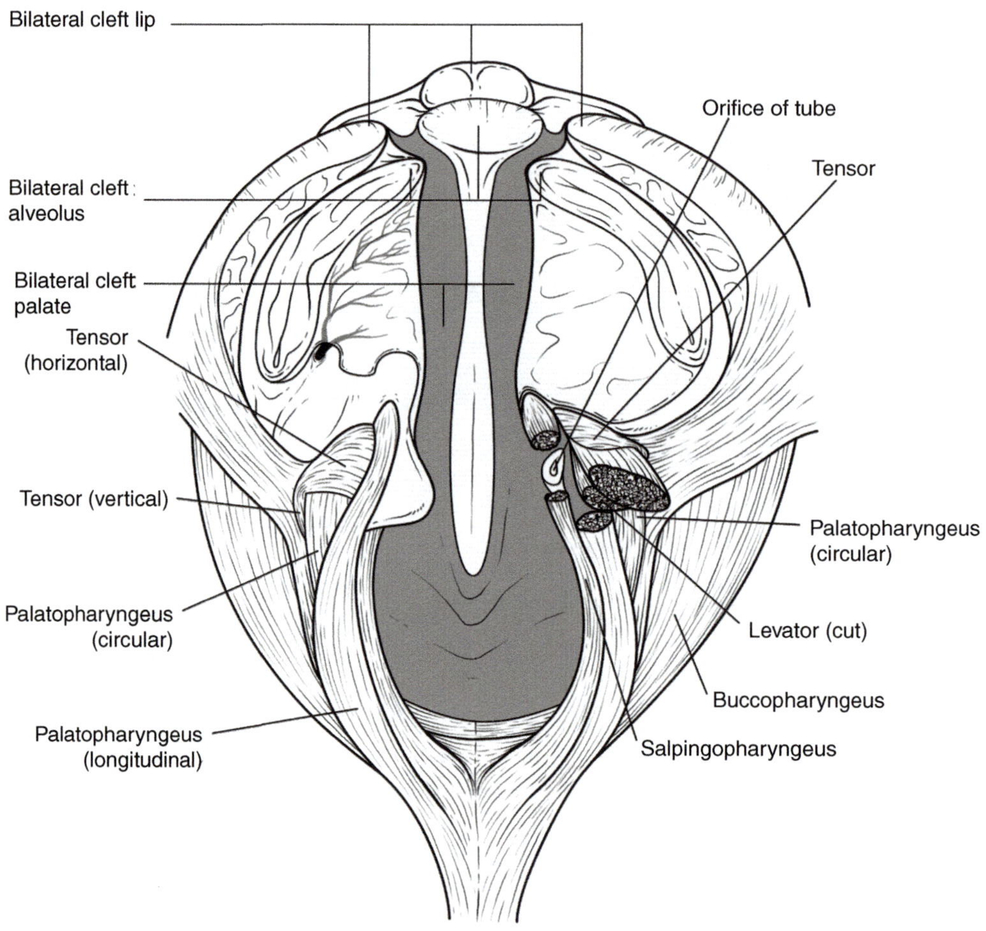

Fig. 73.4 Muscles of the palate demonstrated in a complete cleft of the lip, palate and alveolus (bilateral)

Table 73.1 Muscles of soft palate

Muscle	Origin	Insertion	Function	Pathological anatomy in cleft palate
Tensor veli palatini	Originates from the scaphoid fossa at the base of the medial pterygoid plate, spina angularis of the sphenoid and from the cartilaginous part of the auditory tube	The muscle descends anteroinferiorly and winds around the pterygoid hamulus, to which some fibers are attached, and passes into a tendon that fans out to form the palatine aponeurosis few fibers are attached to the maxillary tuberosity	The main role of the tensor is to dilate the Eustachian tube and its role in speech is insignificant	In a cleft palate child, the palatine aponeurosis is deficient, especially medially
Levator veli palatini	Arises from the petrous part of the temporal bone and from the cartilaginous part of the Eustachian tubes	The muscle descends on either side, enters the intermediate 40% of the soft palate, and forms a muscular sling with its counterpart on the other side	When the paired muscle contracts, it elevates the soft palate superiorly and posteriorly to enable closure of the velopharyngeal sphincter. The latter is formed by the soft palate anteriorly, the posterior pillars of the fauces on either side, and the posterior pharyngeal wall posteriorly	In a cleft child, as there is obviously no continuity across the midline due to the cleft, there are abnormal attachments of the levator muscle to the palatopharyngeus muscle posteriorly, to the edge of the cleft medially, to the tensor veli palatini, and to the posterior edge of the hard palate anteriorly

Table 73.1 (continued)

Muscle	Origin	Insertion	Function	Pathological anatomy in cleft palate
Palatopharyngeus	Has a palatine portion, a pterygopalatine portion and the salpingopharyngeal part. It arises from the lateral and posterior part of pharynx and attaches into the velum. Its superior fibers arise from complex intermingling with the superior constrictor muscle. Lower fibers of the palatopharyneus arise from the inferior part of the lateral wall of the pharynx, medial to the middle and inferior constrictor muscles. Some fibers may arise from the thyroid cartilage. These lower fibers pass through the palatopharyngeal arch to insert into the velum	It is found in the posterior pillar of the fauces. The fibers pass horizontally into the posterior three fourths of the soft palate inferior to the fibers of the levator palatini muscle	The muscle helps to narrow the velopharyngeal opening by bringing the palatopharyngeal arches together	The muscle is relatively well developed in the cleft palate child and ends partly along the cleft edge and partly along the posterior edge of the hard palate. Some fibers pass along the edge of the cleft along with the levator to form the muscle of veau
Palatoglossus	Arises from the tongue	Inserts into the soft palate	The paired muscle forms the anterior part of the sphincter and narrows the isthmus. It is antagonistic to the levator in its action, drawing the palate inferiorly	This muscle doesn't play a major role in cleft palate anatomy
Musculus uvulae	Arises from the posterior nasal spine and the palatine aponeurosis	Passes posteriorly along either side of the midline and inserts into the junction of the proximal and middle thirds of the uvula. The rest of the uvula contains only mucous glands	Contraction of the muscle aids the levator in forming the levator eminence, which is a hump like projection formed proximal to the uvula and aids in closure of the velopharynx during speech	The presence and extent of the muscle in a cleft palate child is disputed. It is also supposed to be absent in occult submucous cleft patients
Superior pharyngeal constrictor	Quadrangular muscle in the upper third of the posterior pharyngeal wall. Origin at the hamulus and the adjacent pterygomandibular raphe	Merges with the palatopharyngeus.. Fibers pass around and through the lateral pharyngeal wall, and merge with the corresponding fibers of the opposite side forming a tendinous strip- the pharyngeal raphe, which runs in the midline from the pharyngeal tubercle of the occipital bone through the entire length of the pharynx	The upper most fibers are responsible for the formation of the passavant's ridge, which is a projection on the posterior pharyngeal wall during speech. However, the edge is usually below the level of closure of the velopharyngeal sphincter, and in only about one third of the patients, it is believed to contribute to closure of the sphincter (the mistake of passavant)	

the philtrum and forms an arcuate anastomosis across the midline in the inferior part of the philtrum.

73.2.3.2 Vascular Supply of Posterior Palate

The greater palatine artery supplies the oral surface of the hard palate and gives off a few fine branches which perforate the horizontal plate of the maxilla to supply the nasal mucosa. It also sends twigs to the gingiva and the palatoglossal arch. The lesser palatine artery supplies the anterior half of the oral surface of the soft palate. A branch of the facial artery, the ascending palatine artery, is the largest vessel entering the soft palate. It ascends on the lateral side of the superior constrictor muscle to turn downward and forward into the soft palate, between the tensor and levator palati giving small branches to these muscles. Twigs from the tonsillar and ascending pharyngeal arteries also reach the soft palate. In the secondary palate, the existence or absence of cleft makes little difference to the vascular pattern. The palatal mucoperios-

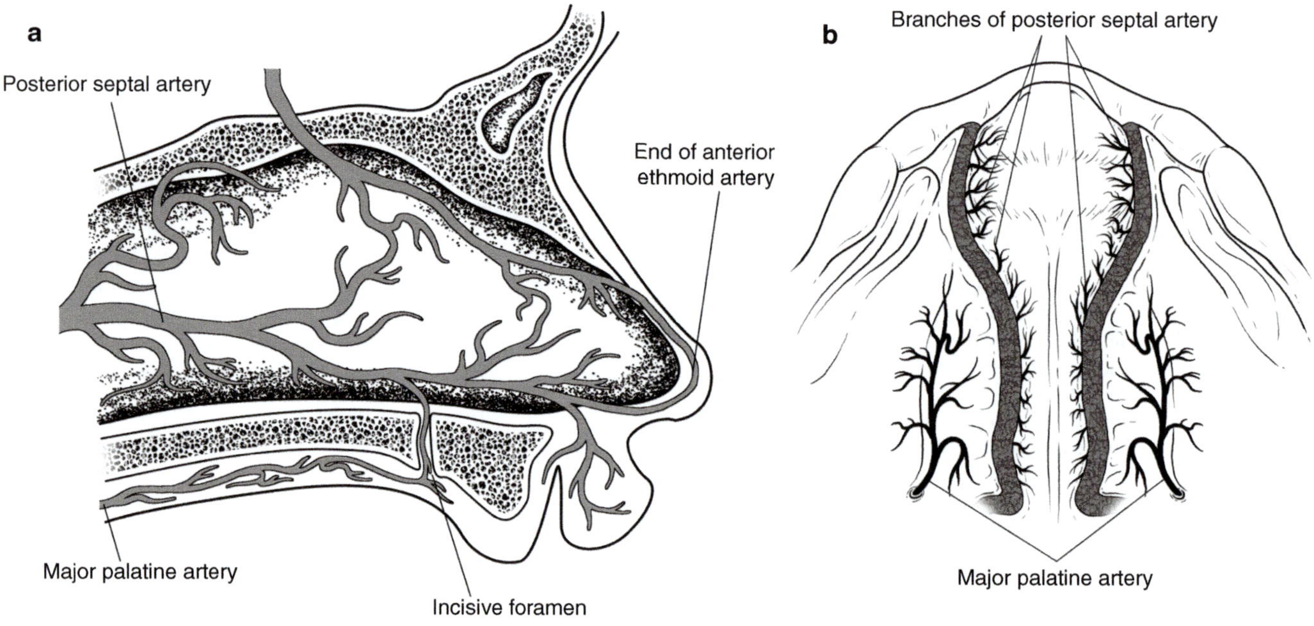

Fig. 73.5 (**a**, **b**) Vascular supply of the palate

teum is detached from its bony base in the palatal pedicle flap, and as a result the recurrent bony branches are severed. These branches result in bleeding from their cut stumps at the bony surface. This may be judged insignificant at the time of surgery; however, after the flap is repositioned, should bleeding continue, blood may pool beneath the repositioned flap [17].

73.3 Classification and Presentations of Cleft Palate

Many of the historical and contemporary classifications have been discussed in brief in the Chap. 72 on cleft lip. However, Veau's classification for palate is the most practical and therefore is mentioned again here.

Submucous cleft palate exhibits at least one of Calnan's three criteria [17]:

(a) A palpable notch on the posterior border of the hard palate.
(b) Zona pellucida or a bluish tinge in the midline of the soft palate due the paucity of muscle bulk at this level.
(c) Bifid uvula- this may extend from a mere groove on the uvula to complete bifidity.

Table 73.2 Veau's classification of cleft palate

I.	Cleft of the soft palate alone
II.	Complete cleft of the palate up to the incisive foramen
III.	Unilateral complete cleft of the palate and pre-palate. In these the vomer is attached to the maxilla on the non-cleft side
IV.	Complete bilateral cleft of the palate and pre-palate. These patients have a protruding premaxilla, and the vomer is in the midline

Victor Veau (1931) has classified cleft palates into four groups [7] (Table 73.2)

Clefts of the palate that are less extensive in magnitude include the submucous cleft palate and the occult submucous in cleft palate.

Sommerlad has devised a grading system for the submucous cleft palate with three points for each of the above criteria [18]. A lesser score in this system naturally denotes more trivial clefting. However, paradoxically a lower score reflects a poorer prognosis for speech according to this study. An occult submucous cleft does not exhibit any of Calnan's criteria but shows a trough-like depression on the superior surface of the soft palate as seen in nasoendoscopy. Croft believed that in these patients, the musculus uvulae is absent. It is suspected when a child with a normal palate speaks with nasal emission.

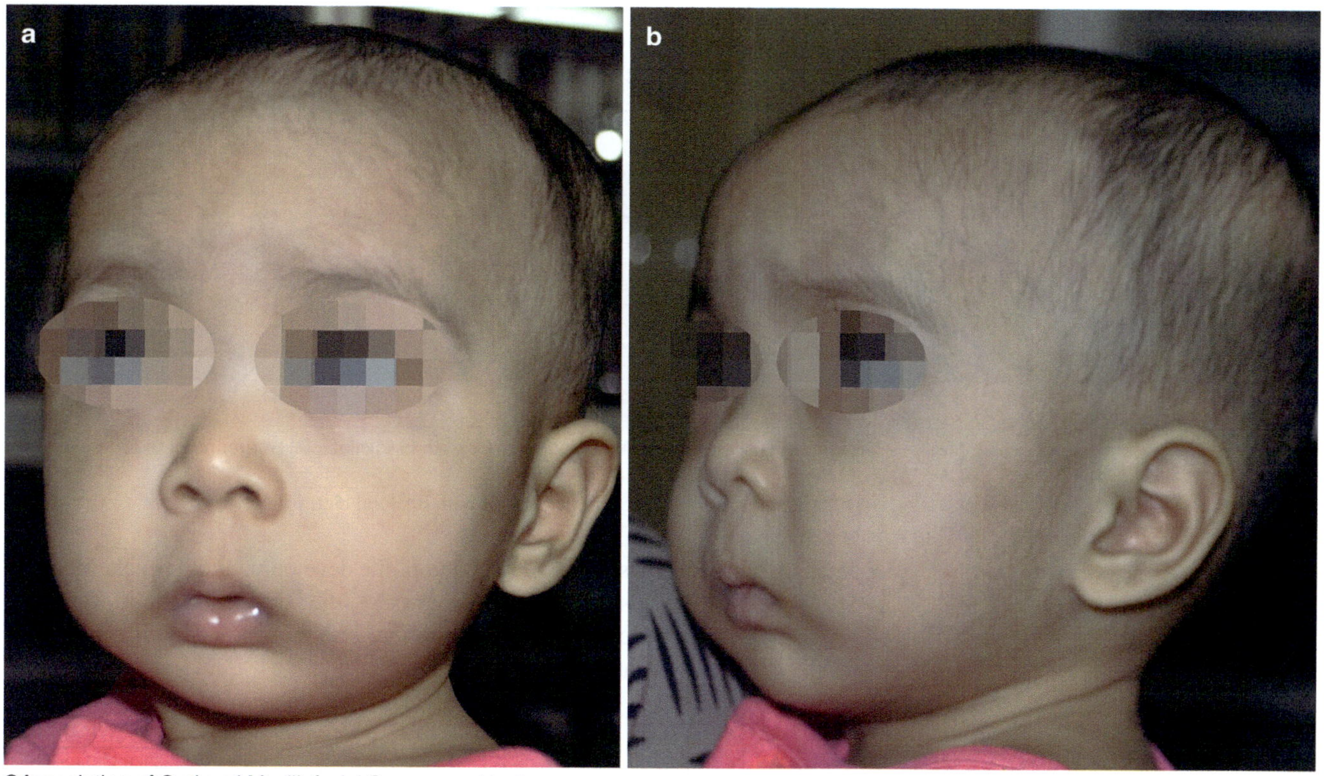

Fig. 73.6 (**a**, **b**) Picture of child with Pierre Robin Sequence

73.4 Clinical Evaluation of the Cleft Palate Patient

73.4.1 General Examination

A routine per-oral examination of the neonate reveals the cleft of the palate with or without cleft lip. The extent of clefting is noted. General examination is mandatory as it is important to identify syndromic patients. These are more common in isolated cleft palate patients [19]. Pierre Robin sequence is a fairly common presentation with micrognathia or retrognathia (Fig. 73.6 and b). As the bony abnormalities are believed to be the cause of the non-descent of the tongue in utero leading to the clefting of the palate, this is now believed to be a sequence and not a syndrome. Syndromic patients include Treacher Collins syndrome, Goldenhar syndrome, etc.

73.4.2 Clinical Assessment of the Cleft

The first clinical visit usually happens soon after birth. The extent cleft is assessed, i.e., the length of the palate and the width of the cleft. Randall has classified cleft palate on the basis of length into four types [20]. Clefts may be partial or complete. A partial cleft of the secondary palate is confined to the soft palate (Fig. 73.7).

A complete cleft includes both the soft and the hard palate up to the incisive foramen (Fig. 73.8). In patients with bilateral cleft lips, the associated cleft palate usually presents with a central vomer and clefting on either side of the vomer (Fig. 73.9).

A pediatric assessment is made for other anomalies, weight of the baby is noted, and feeding instructions are given during this visit. A squeezable feeding bottle is usually advisable to overcome child's difficulties in sucking. The child is fed with the head held slightly higher. Parents are counselled about the need for immunization. They are also explained about the need for surgery and are shown results of the procedure on similar patients. It is very important to allay their anxiety as they are very often crestfallen on seeing the deformity in their baby. Subsequent visits, possibly at monthly intervals, aim to assess the growth and development of the baby. Associated cardiac or other anomalies if present need investigation.

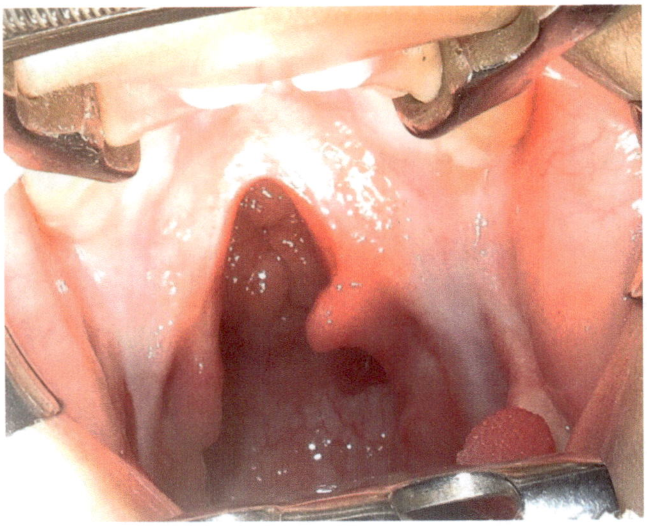

Fig. 73.7 A child with partial cleft palate

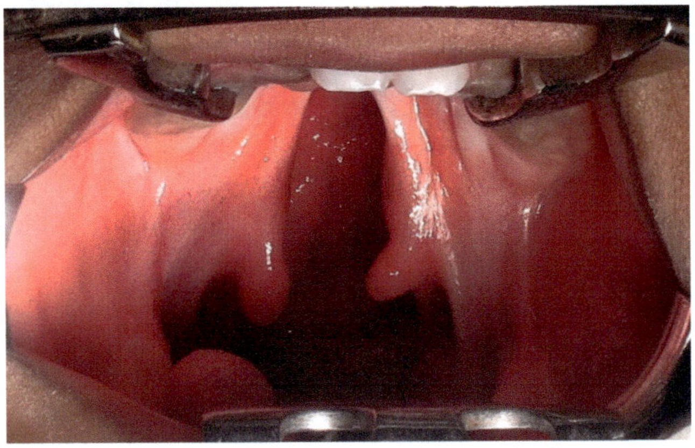

Fig. 73.8 A child with complete cleft palate

73.4.3 Imaging and Other Investigations

Routine imaging is not generally practiced in the evaluation of cleft palate patients. Syndromic patients require other investigations as part of the various manifestations of their syndromes. For instance, children with velocardiofacial syndrome may require echocardiogram in view of the associated cardiac anomalies. Children with delayed development, microcephaly, etc. will require neurological assessment and will usually need an MRI of the brain. Rarely a child may have a meningoencephalocele presenting behind the palate. MRI has been used to evaluate submucous clefts with a view to help in the planning of the management. If it can be shown that there is not adequate muscle continuity across the midline, an early decision can be taken to operate on the child at the usual time of cleft palate repair. On the other hand, if there is good muscle across the midline, these repairs can be justifiably delayed until the development of speech. MRI has also been used to assess the Eustachian tube function. Hearing assessment should be mandatory in all cleft palate patients.

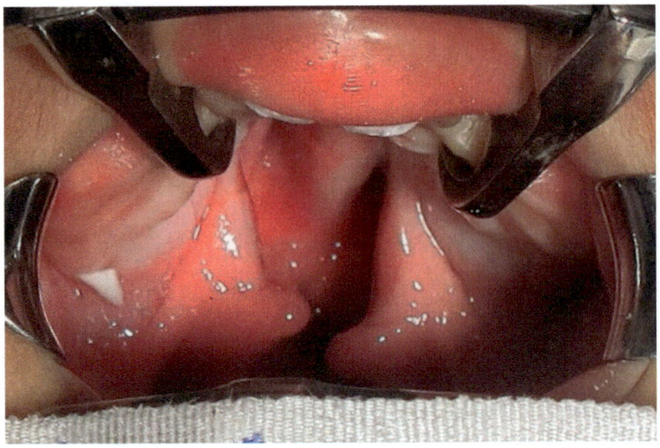

Fig. 73.9 A child with bilateral cleft palate

73.5 Preoperative Factors (Box 73.1)

Box 73.1 Preoperative Considerations

- Timing of repair.
- One stage or two stage repair.
- Anatomy of the cleft.
- Airway.
- Feeding.
- Pediatric consultation.
- Cardiac consultation.
- Neuro consultation.
- Ent consultation.
- Anesthesia.

1. Timing and Age of the Patient.

   The dilemma regarding the timing of repair is between earlier repair with better prognosis for speech, but worse prognosis for maxillary growth, and late repair which is exactly the opposite. Most surgeons today agree that the cleft palate is to be operated close to 1 year. Some prefer 9 months, where others wait for up to a year and 4 months. At our center we have been operating on these children at about 11 months of age. The Oslo school of surgeons [21, 22] devised a protocol of operating on the lip with the soft palate in the first stage and operating on the hard palate much later. In some centers, the palate has been repaired first at initial presentation, and the cleft lip is repaired, subsequently, in view of the fact the children may not be brought back for treatment of the palate once the lip is repaired [23].

2. Airway.

   Airway management is important at the time of birth in cleft palate patients, as most of isolated cleft palates may be associated with a smaller airway at birth. This may be due to associated sequence or syndromes, such Pierre Robin sequence or Treacher Collins syndrome. Such patients might require emergency tracheostomy or tongue lip adhesion to secure airway. Definitive management for mandibular advancement and cleft palate repair can be undertaken at a later stage.

3. Feeding.

   As mentioned already, the parents are counselled about feeding practices during the first visit itself. Expressed breast milk is to be preferred. Special feeding bottles like the Haberman feeding bottle are used when the common methods like the use of simple squeezable bottles are not effective. As a cleft child swallows air along with the milk, frequent burping is essential to avoid regurgitation of feeds.

4. Anesthesia.

   The operation is performed under general anesthesia with an endotracheal tube. RAE tubes are preferred for cleft palate patients. Previously, Oxford red rubber tubes were used. These were well adapted to the needs of the cleft children but often caused laryngeal edema presumably due to the latex in the tubes. At our center we have given up the use of these otherwise very useful tubes.

   Preoperatively, the child must be assessed by a good pediatrician and also by a senior anesthetist. Respiratory infections are common in these children and must be treated if significant. X-ray of the chest is usually done to rule out heart or lung anomalies. Cardiology clearance is required when there are suspected cardiac anomalies. We have come across one case with a congenital absence of the lung.

   The anesthetist should be experienced in pediatric anesthesia. In patients with Pierre Robin sequence or other anomalies like shoulder or spinal anomalies, difficult intubation is to be anticipated, and appropriate equipment such as intubating endoscopes, etc. should be at hand, and the anesthetist must be familiar with its use.

73.6 Principles and Methods of Repair

There are various surgical techniques described in literature. The techniques have been mentioned (Box 73.2), with the author's surgical technique described in detail (Figs. 73.23, 73.24, 73.25, 73.26, 73.27, 73.28, 73.29, 73.30, and 73.31).

The major objectives of a cleft palate operation are:

- To produce anatomical closure of the defect.
- To create an apparatus for development and production of normal speech.
- To minimize the maxillary growth disturbances.

The basic principles of cleft palate repair are:

- Closure of the defect.
- Repositioning of the abnormal position of the muscles of the soft palate.
- Reconstruction of the muscle sling.
- Favorable retro positioning of the soft palate and uvula so as to achieve velopharyngeal closure during speech.
- Last and most important is tension-free suturing [24, 25].

Box 73.2 Methods of Cleft Palate Repair

Methods of repair

- *Von Langenbeck's bipedicle flap technique* (Fig. 73.10).
- *Veau-Wardill-Kilner Pushback technique* (Fig. 73.11).
- *Bardach's-Pinto-Wardill two-flap technique.*
- *Furlow double opposing Z-Plasty.*
- *Two-stage palatal repair.*
- *Whole in one repair.*
- *Palatoplasty.*
- *Alveolar extension palatoplasty (AEP).*
- *Primary pharyngeal flap.*
- *Intravelar veloplasty.*
- *Vomer flap.*
- *Buccal myomucosal flap.*

73.7 Surgical Technique (Figs. 73.12, 73.13, 73.14, 73.15, 73.16, 73.17, 73.18, 73.19, 73.20, 73.21, 73.22, 73.23, 73.24, 73.25, 73.26, 73.27, and 73.28)

Once intubated, the child is placed with the neck extended for adequate visualization of the palate. A pillow under the shoulder helps in this positioning. A suitable mouth gag is used. We use the Dott's gag (Fig. 73.12) with the Kilner suture carrier. A popular gag used widely is the Dingman's gag.

Infiltration: A solution of lignocaine with 1 in 200,000 adrenaline is infiltrated under the mucoperiostem of the hard

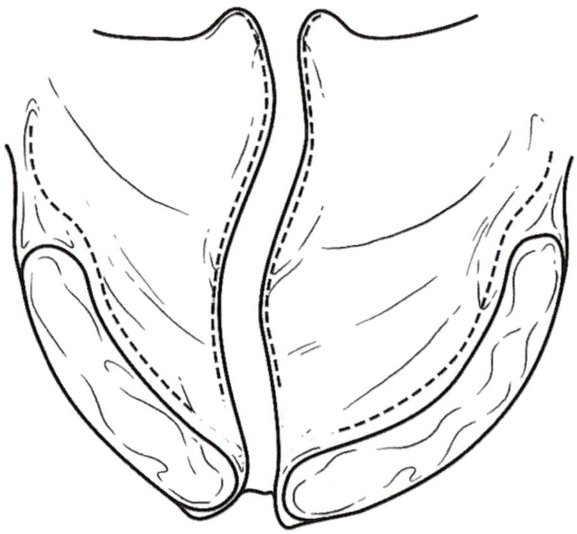

Fig. 73.10 Langenbeck procedure. Incisions are placed to raise flaps which remain attached in the anterior palatal region

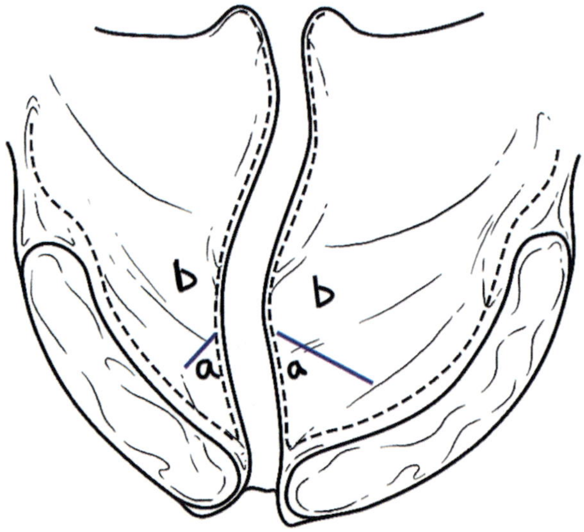

Fig. 73.11 Wardill's four flap palate repair. (**a**) are the anterior flaps while (**b**) form the posterior flaps that are closed in a "V to Y" fashion to gain length for the "push-back"

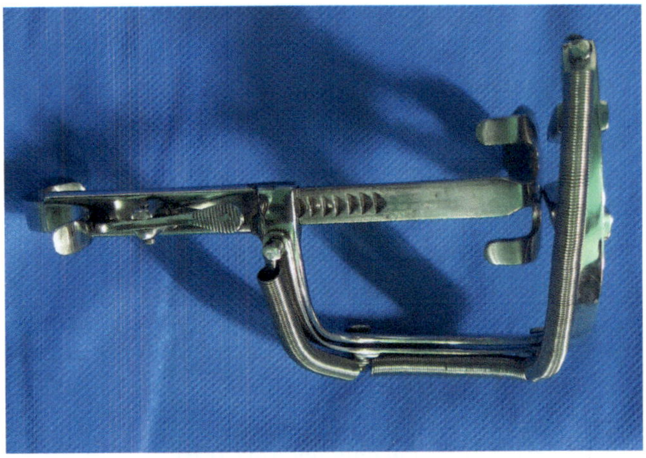

Fig. 73.12 Dott's gag

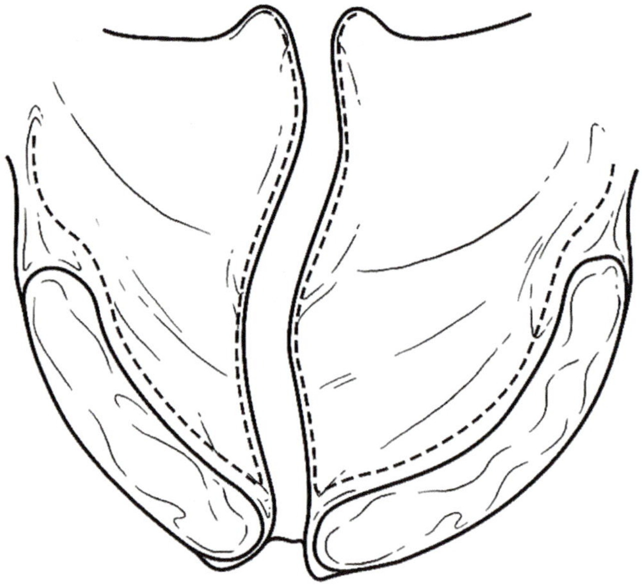

Fig. 73.13 Pinto Wardill (Bardach) two long-flap procedure. Classical method of raising two flaps detached at the anterior pedicled on the greater palatine artery

palate and above the nasal mucosa in the soft palate. A dental syringe with a short-beveled needle is very useful for this purpose.

Surgical procedure: At our center, we use the two long-flap technique popularized in India by Charles Pinto and the world over by Bardach (Fig. 73.13). The technique was originally used by Veau. The cleft edges are pared (Fig. 73.14).

The lateral incision is made from the maxillary tuberosity area toward the retromolar area posteriorly. The pterygoid hamulus is dissected, fractured, and detached (Fig. 73.15a and b).

This aids in mobilization of the nasal layer subsequently. However, there are many surgeons nowadays who do not believe in fracturing the hamulus. It has, however, been shown in different studies that fracture of the hamulus does not cause any deleterious effects on hearing [26].

The lateral incision is then carried anteriorly and the oral mucoperiosteal flap is lifted off till the medial edge of the hard palate using Kilner's palate elevators (Fig. 73.16a and b).

An incision is then made on the medial border of the hard palate, and the flap is also divided anteriorly taking care to secure the end of the greater palatine vessels. The oral flap is then raised till the posterior border of the hard palate. Laterally, the greater palatine vessel is identified and skeletonized, after incising the cone of periosteum which binds the vessel behind it (Fig. 73.17a, b, c and d).

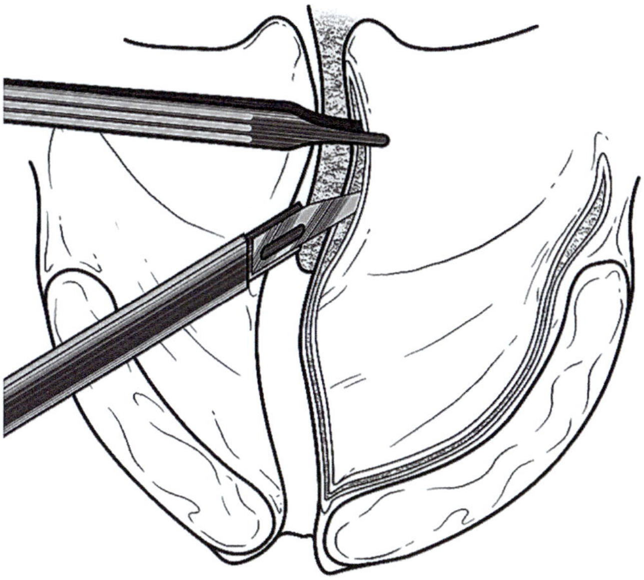

Fig. 73.14 Pared cleft edges

After the hamulus is fractured, the medial pterygoid plate is denuded of any soft tissue attachments (Fig. 73.18).

Similarly, the posterior border of the hard palate is also cleared of muscular attachments (Fig. 73.19a and b).

A Cumine Scaler is introduced over the bare medial pterygoid plate and then turned anteriorly to separate the nasal layer from the hard palate in one clean sweep. This dissection is then completed on a deeper plane with a Wallace's finisher (Fig. 73.20a and b).

This practice of separating the nasal layer from behind forward was originally introduced by Kilner [8] but has somehow not been followed widely. It is much easier than the alternative method of separating the nasal layer from the hard palate starting anteriorly. Very often this results in tearing of the nasal layer.

Similar dissection is performed on the other side also, raising a long oral mucoperiosteal flap. The vomer flap is raised (Fig. 73.21) and used when accessible and necessary.

Rarely, the vomer is receding and cannot be used. In a bilateral cleft lip patient, the vomer is in the midline, and a central incision on the vomer is made to raise two mucoperiosteal flaps, one on each side, to be sutured to the corresponding side in nasal layer of the hard palate.

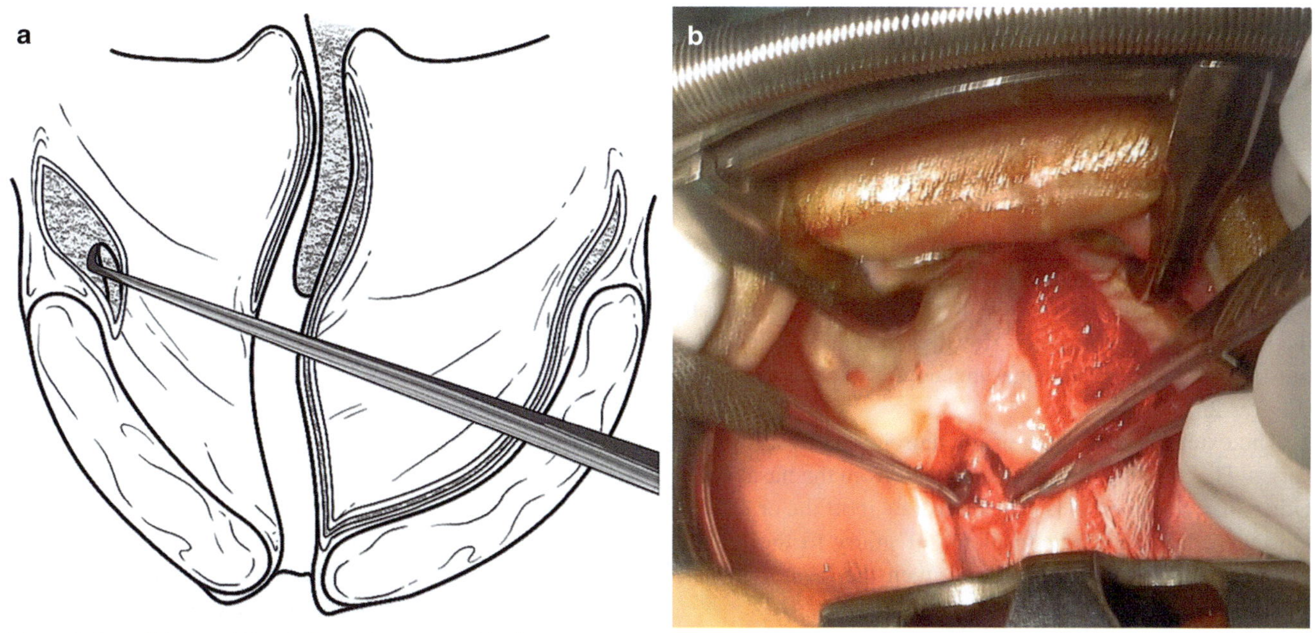

Fig.73.15 (**a**, **b**) Fracture of the pterygoid hamulus

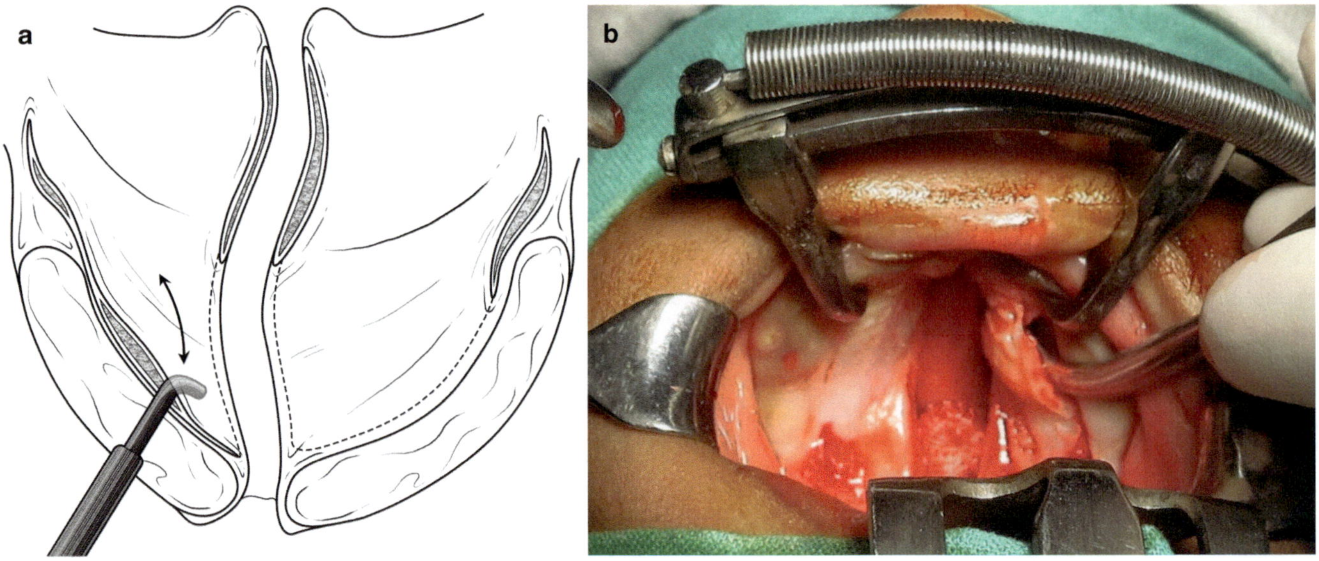

Fig. 73.16 (**a**, **b**) Elevation of the oral flap with Kilner's elevator

73.7.1 Dissection of the Soft Palate

The early techniques of cleft palate repair only detached all false attachments of muscles from the posterior border of the hard palate (Fig. 73.22).

Surgeons like Braithwaite [27] and Kriens [28] emphasized the importance of the dissection and retroposition of the levator veli palati muscle. This was popularized by Sommerlad [29] and Tambewekar in India.

Infiltration of lignocaine with 1:200,000 adrenaline is made between the nasal mucosa and the muscle (Fig. 73.23).

A transverse incision is made on the aponeurotic layer just beyond the hard palate (Fig. 73.24).

Then the muscle is dissected off the underlying mucosa leaving behind enough tissue on the nasal layer, to avoid its tearing during suturing. Also, a narrow layer of muscle is retained along the cleft edges to hold the sutures. The muscle is dissected till just short of the uvula. The muscle contains the levator veli palati mostly. However, it also contains other muscles like the palatopharyngeus ("muscle of Veau") (Fig. 73.25).

The extent of dissection of the muscle on the soft palate varies. The authors [30] only separate it from the nasal layer. Others like Sommerlad [29] also separate it off the oral layer. However, if there is any suspicion of injury to the greater palatine vessels during dissection, then the levator muscle should not be dissected free of the oral mucosa.

73.7.2 Suturing

Suturing commences on the nasal layer from anteriorly, proceeding backward. The sutures are not tied but held on the Kilner suture carrier.

73.7.2.1 Uvula

The last suture on the nasal layer is a mattress suture (Fig. 73.26) [30].

Next, an apical mattress suture is placed on the tip of the uvula, and this suture is left long and held on an artery forceps, thus turning the uvula over, providing access to the nasopharyngeal aspect of the uvula. Two or three simple sutures are placed between the mattress suture and the apical stitch (Fig. 73.27a).

Then two or three mattress sutures are placed on the oral aspect of the uvula (Fig. 73.27b).

The nasal layer sutures are then tied from behind forward.

"A" suture: this is the suture placed at the junction of the hard and soft palate. It goes through the nasal mucosa and later crisscrosses into the oral mucosa, resembling the letter A, but is like the figure of "8" when tied.

Anterior sutures are also tied but retained long.

Suturing of the oral layers then proceeds from behind forward, with every suture picking up a bite on the nasal layer to obliterate dead space. The dissected levator mus-

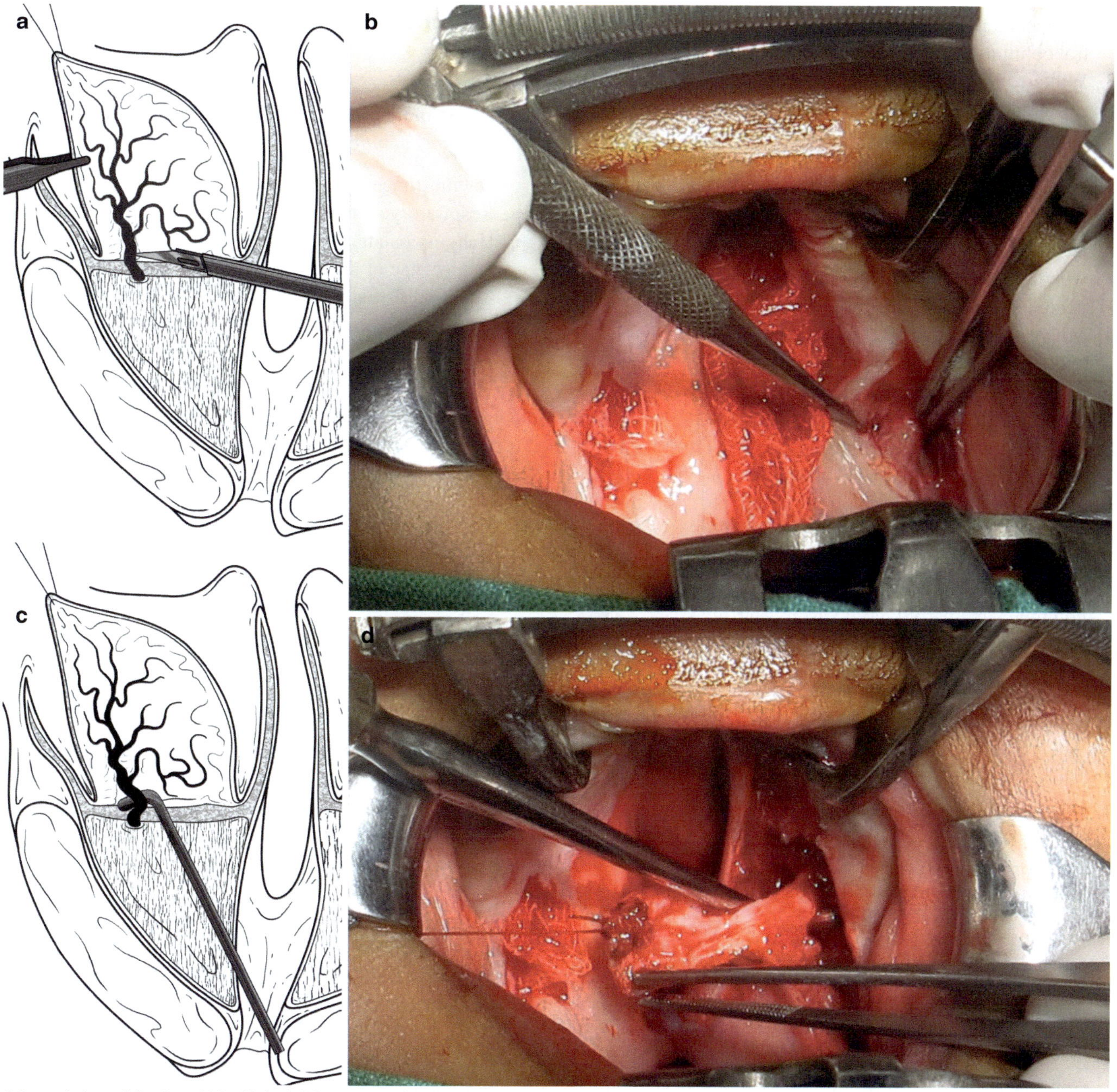

Fig. 73.17 (**a, b**) Incising the Periosteal cone to free the greater palatine artery. (**c, d**) Hooking out the greater palatine vessels (the vessel is pulled out like a bird pulls a worm out of the ground). This reduces the tension on the flaps on suturing

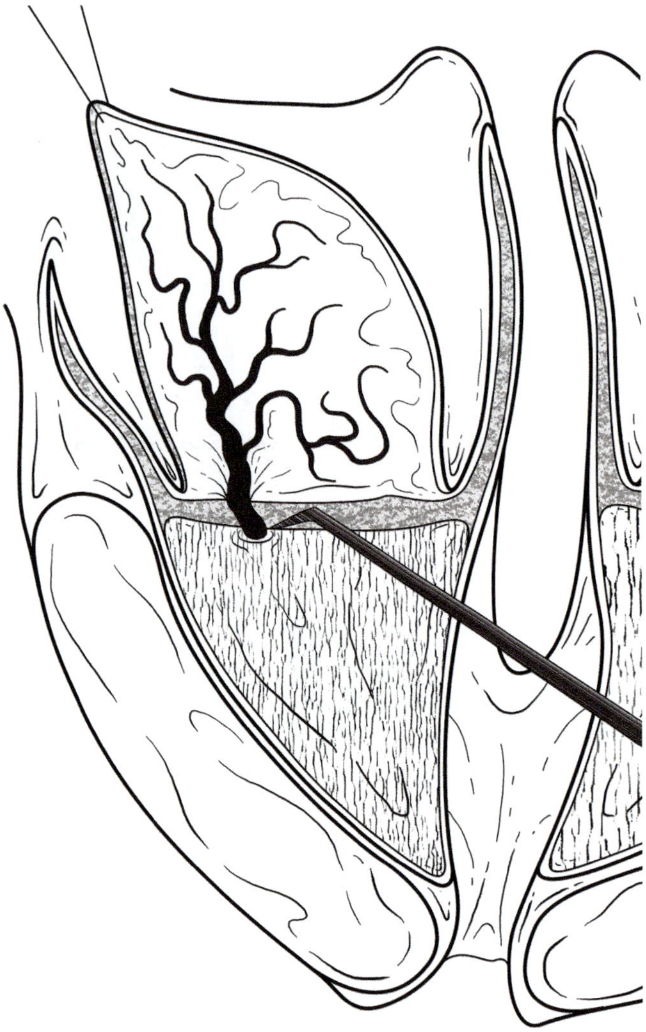

Fig. 73.18 Medial pterygoid plate dissection

cle is also included in these oral sutures. Some surgeons close the levator muscle as a separate layer. The anterior sutures are then brought through the oral layer also, helping in anchoring the oral layer. In the absence of the anchoring, the oral layer may sag postoperatively causing a "fallen palate."

Laterally the raw areas are sutured with interrupted sutures without tension. This helps in hemostasis (Fig. 73.28).

Previously, this area used to be packed with different materials, but there was often bleeding from the areas on removal of the pack postoperatively.

Buccal pad of fat harvested through a stab incision on the buccal aspect bilaterally has also been used to fill large lateral raw areas.

73.8 Complications: (Box 73.3)

Box 73.3 Complications

Immediate complications.

- Haemorrhage.
- Respiratory obstruction.
- Hanging palate.
- Dehiscence of the repair.
- Oronasal fistula formation.

Late complications.

- Bifid uvula.
- Velopharyngeal incompetence.
- Abnormal speech.
- Maxillary hypoplasia.
- Dental malpositioning and malalignment.
- Otitis media.

73.8.1 Early Complications

Hemorrhage

This is often from the apices of the long flaps, from the cut ends of the greater palatine vessels. Arterial bleeding points need to be ligated or cauterized using diathermy. Small venous bleeding areas can be controlled by the use of pressure with fingers or by the use of crushed ice or topical hemostatic agents like tranexamic acid.

Respiratory Obstruction

This may be from tongue fall and can be avoided by use of a tongue stitch at the time of palate repair. The tongue stitch has to be placed well posteriorly and must include a good bulk of the tongue tissue to avoid the sutures from tearing through.

When a wide cleft palate is closed, the child may have difficulty in learning to breathe adequately through the nose. Laryngeal edema due to endotracheal tube-related trauma may present with a hoarse cry and, in severe cases, chest retraction. Early detection is important, and this can be reversed by intravenous steroids and nebulization.

Breakdown of the Repair

It may result in fistulas or complete breakdown of the repair. The most common cause of these, especially at the junctional area, is suturing of the cleft edges under tension due to inadequate mobilization.

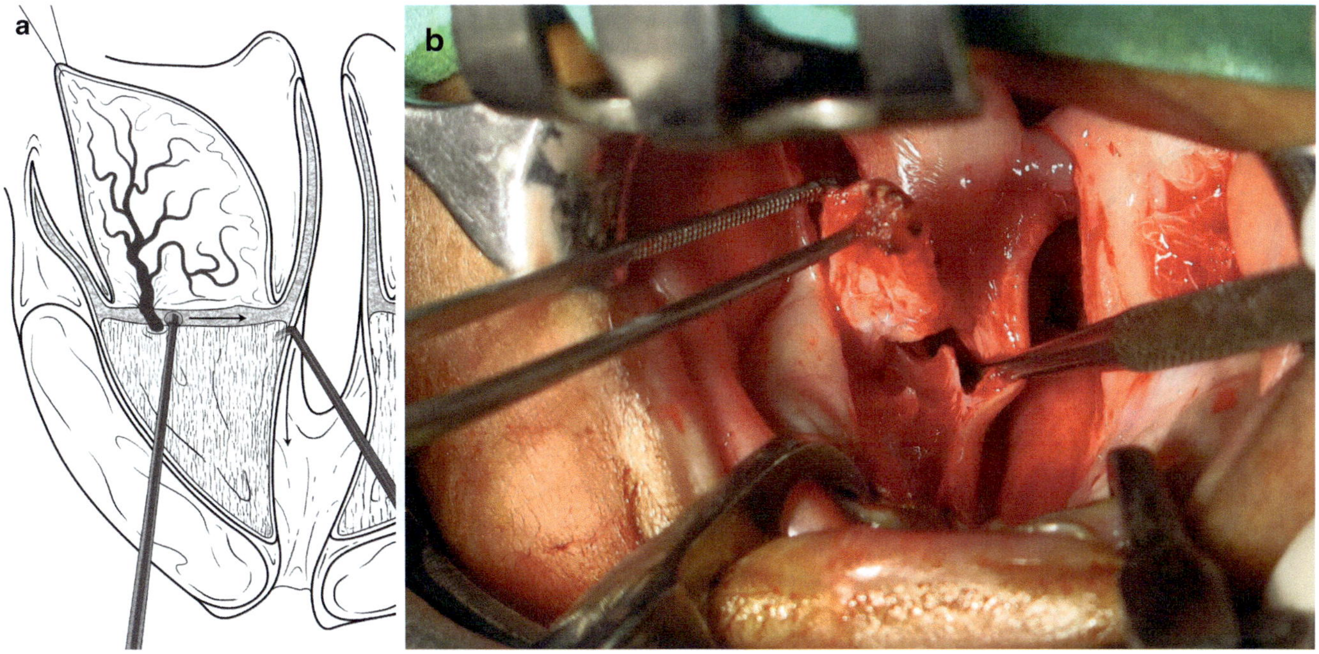

Fig. 73.19 (**a**, **b**) Dissection of the posterior end of the hard palate

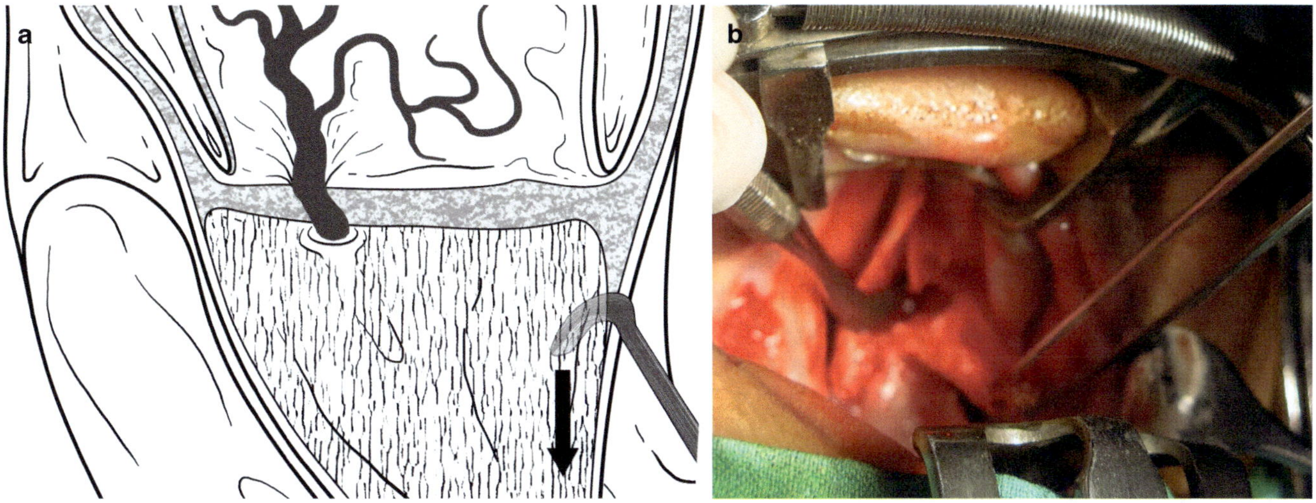

Fig. 73.20 (**a**, **b**) Completion of nasal layer dissection with Wallace's Finisher

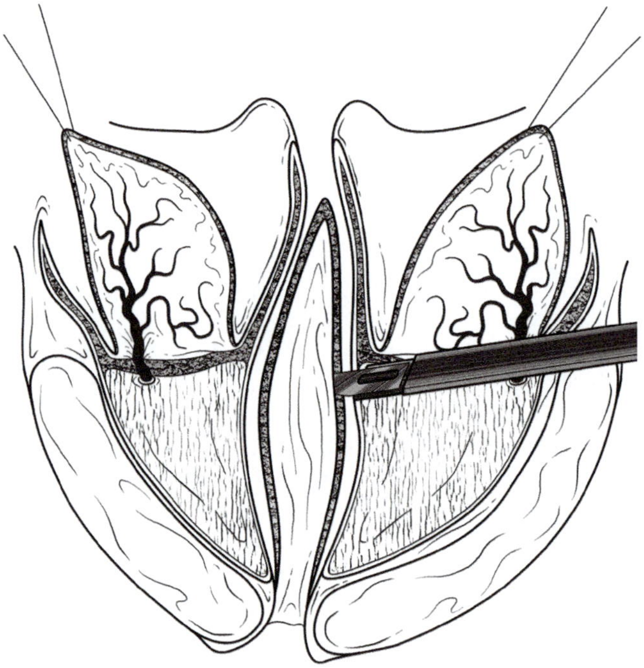

Fig. 73.21 Posterior incision on the vomer

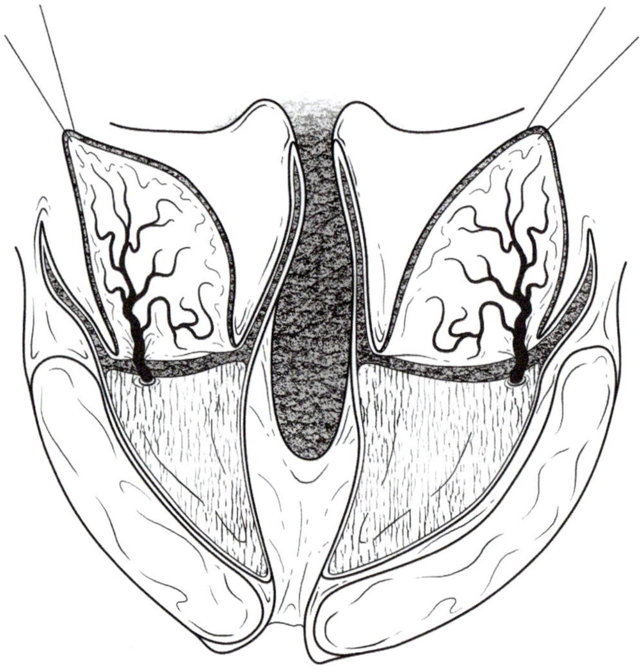

Fig. 73.22 Complete dissection of the oral and nasal layers

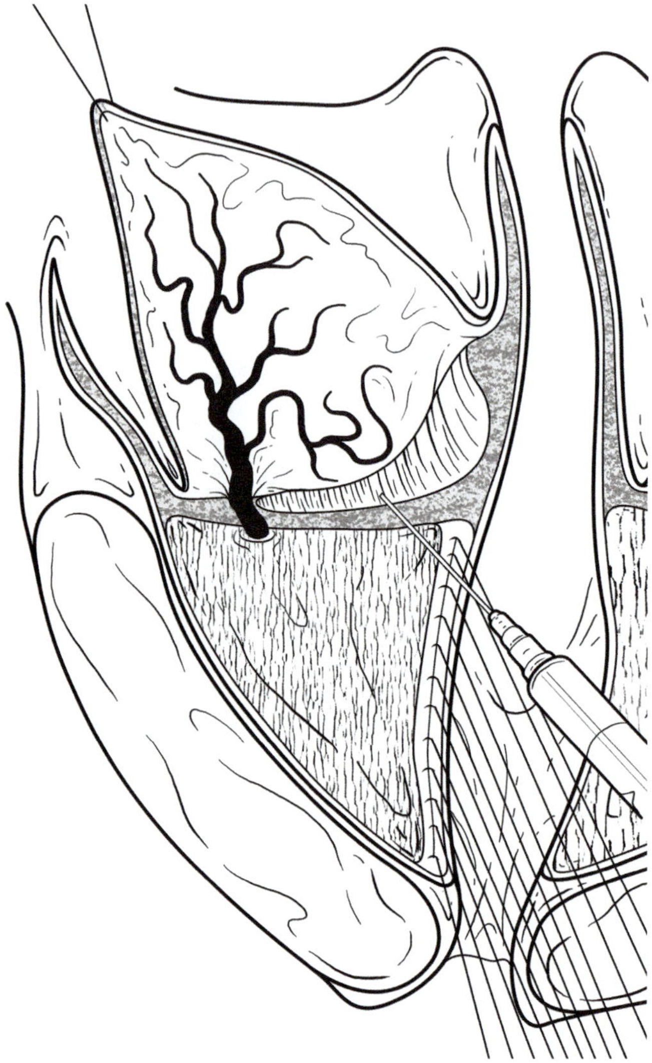

Fig. 73.23 Infiltration of adrenaline beneath the palatine aponeurosis

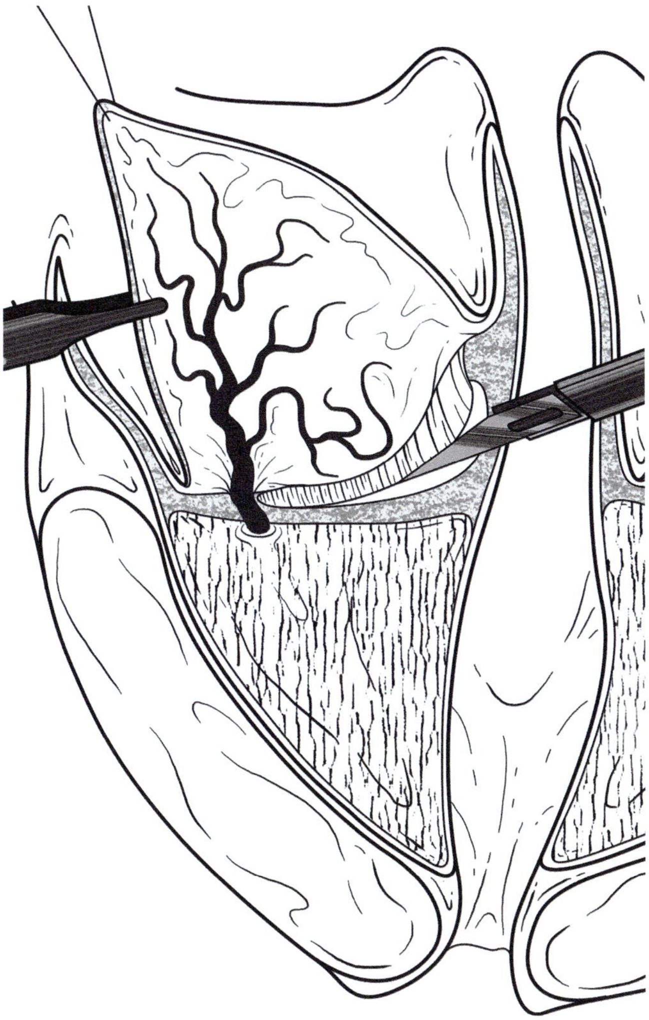

Fig. 73.24 Incision of the palatine aponeurosis

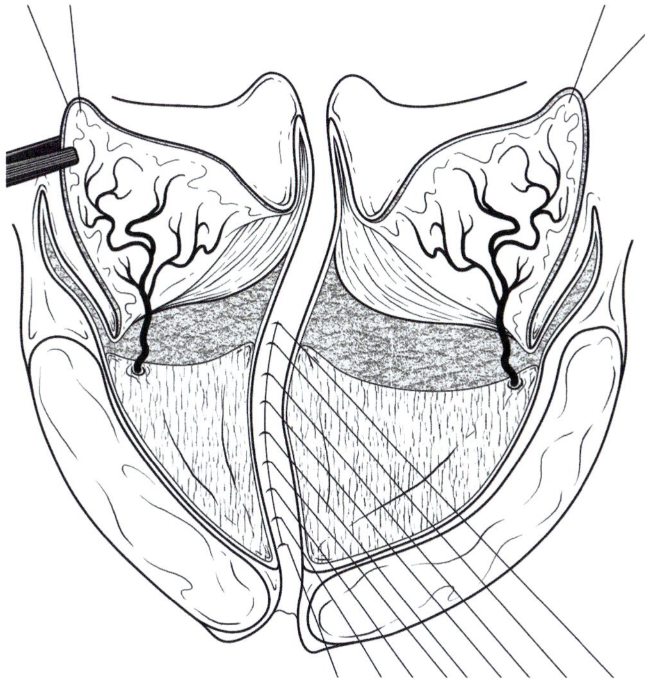

Fig. 73.25 Complete dissection and retroposition of the levator palati muscle

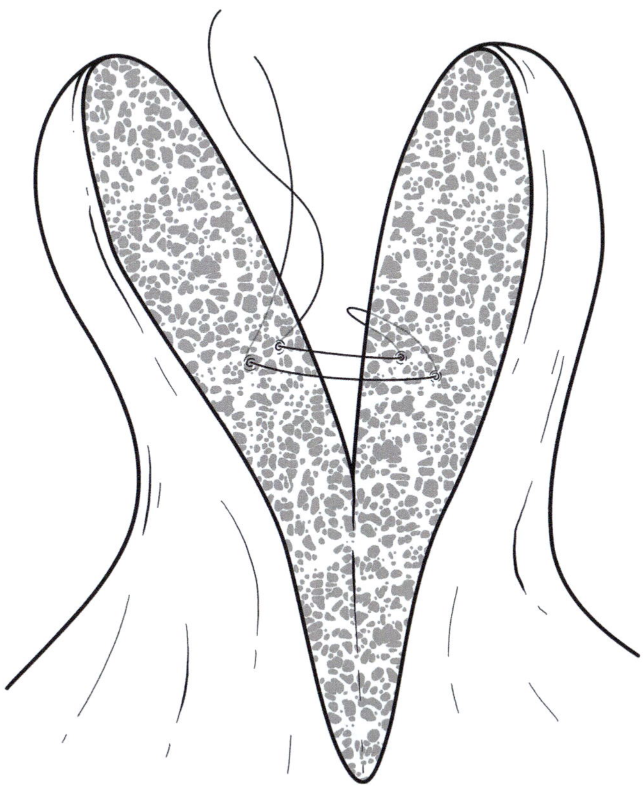

Fig. 73.26 Mattress suture at the base of uvula

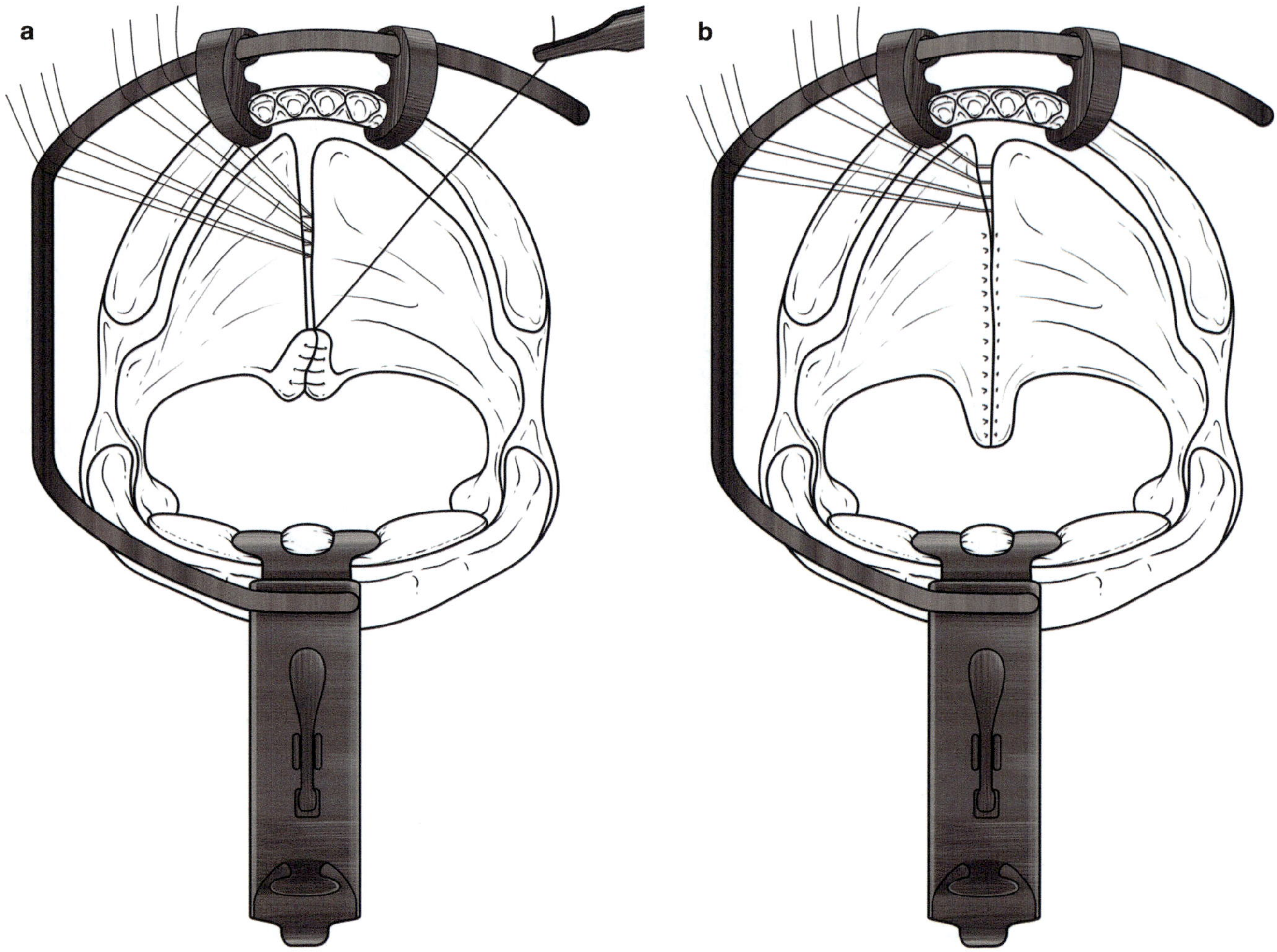

Fig. 73.27 (**a**) Apical suture on uvula turned over and posterior sutures placed. (**b**) Completion of uvular reconstruction

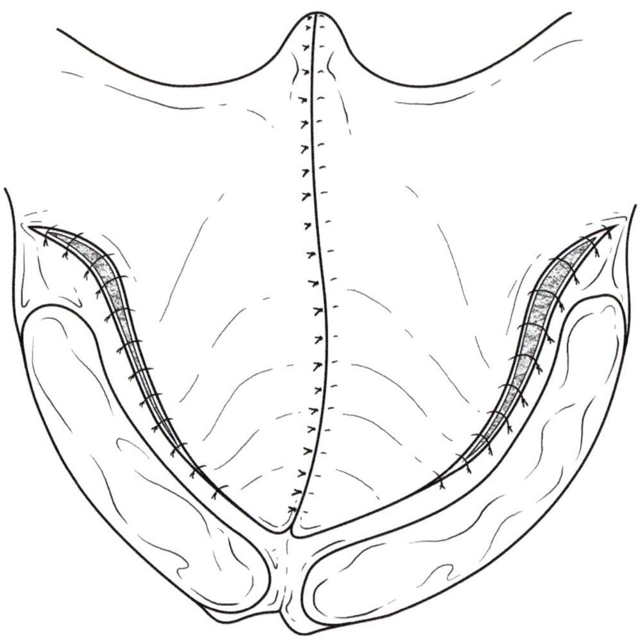

Fig. 73.28 Completed suturing of the palate and the lateral raw areas

73.8.2 Long-Term Complications

Long-term complications include poor speech. Adequate muscle repair has helped in better speech results. Nonetheless, speech is an enigma that has not been adequately understood and mastered. The variables like width of the cleft, the gap between the uvula and the pharynx, and the adequacy of the muscle repair all have a bearing on the speech results. Despite all the advancements in the repair of the cleft palate, no surgeon can truly claim to achieve perfect speech results in all patients consistently.

73.9 Long-Term Results

The long-term evaluation of cleft palate patients should include the presence or absence of a fistula, the quality of speech, and the growth parameters of the maxilla, i.e., whether there is maxillary hypoplasia.

At present, many centers are able to produce fistula-free palates in a majority of patients. Tension-free closure of the palate and meticulous suturing are the key factors in the prevention of fistulas. A review of literature reveals a huge range in the incidence of fistula after cleft palate repair. The range is from 2.6 to 58%. In between these extremes, many have reported around 10%, some 15 and 23% [31, 32].

The emphasis on good levator veli palatini dissection and repair has led to improved speech results overall. However, one can never perfectly predict the speech outcome, as speech itself is an enigma. Probably as a result of the variation in the presentation, mode of repairs and age at the time of repair, etc., the published literature notes a VPI rate of 5.9–70% [32].

Maxillary growth continues to be a problem. Operations like these of Robert Mann show promise in this direction. Again, owing to variability involved in the type and extent of cleft, the time of repair and the nature of the surgery, the need for maxillary advancement may range from 10 to 40% in non-syndromic cleft patients [32].

73.9.1 Secondary Repair and Revision

The age old saying that primary surgery is the best chance for the surgeon to obtain optimal results is very apt in the repair of the cleft palate. A badly repaired cleft palate sometimes leaves behind a grossly scared palate with paucity of tissue. Small soft palate fistula can be repaired by freshening of the edge and two-layered closure. Small hard palate fistulas can be repaired by local turn over flaps for lining and oral mucoperiosteal flaps for the oral layer. Larger ones and those with poor speech will require revision palate repair. When there is gross deficiency of tissue, flaps like the tongue flaps, or temporalis musculocutaneous flap, facial artery muscle mucosal (Famm) flap may be necessary [33, 34].

Secondary palate repair is also required for velopharyngeal incompetence (VPI). A detailed discussion about the management of such incompetence is beyond the scope of this chapter. Diagnosis of VPI is by speech assessment, nasoendoscopy, or videofluoroscopy. Once a diagnosis is made, treatment modalities will include redo palate repair, sphincter pharyngoplasty, or flap pharyngoplasties, depending on whether it is the palate, lateral wall (palatopharyngeus) or the posterior wall, or a capacious pharynx as seen on investigations.

Subsequent interventions will be required for maxillary hypoplasia when significant. This is again out of the scope of this chapter. In brief, anterior maxillary distraction is done if the maxillary advancement required is significant and the facial bones are still growing. Some of these do require a LeFort 1 osteotomy later on if there is relapse. When the growth is completed, then a LeFort 1 osteotomy is required when there is significant maxillary hypoplasia. When the advancement required is more than in 1 cm, bi-jaw surgery is needed, with a LeFort 1 advancement in the maxilla and a bilateral sagittal split osteotomy of the mandible.

73.10 Recent Techniques

The use of the buccal mucosal flap in primary repair was pioneered by Padgett [14] and then used extensively by Murari Mukherjee [15]. Later Ian Jackson incorporated buccinator muscle into the flap and used it on the nasal layer transverse to provide for lengthening of the soft palate.

Furlow's Double Opposing Z plasty described by Furlow [35] is increasingly used both for primary and secondary repair of cleft palates. This illustrated in the figure (Fig. 73.29a, b, c and d). Robert Mann has described the extensive use of the double opposing "Z" plasty with the buccal flaps over the nasal and/or oral layers to avoid lateral incisions and to promote for better bony growth. This is probably the method of the future as it shows promise of good speech and good maxillary growth. However, extensive suturing of the buccal flaps is involved and this is not the optimal surgery for the novice to try. The Mann procedure is for the experienced cleft surgeons [36].

73.11 Case Scenario

Case 1

This is a patient with a partial cleft of the secondary palate (Fig. 73.30). The hard palate is intact. The cleft palate was repaired at the age of 11 months using the Veau-Wardill V-to-Y repair and radical muscle dissection in the soft palate. Subsequently the child is undergoing regular follow-up and speech assessment.

Case 2

This is a child with a complete cleft of the primary and secondary palate on the (Fig. 73.31). The cleft lip was repaired at 6 months of age using the Millard's rotation advancement technique. At 11 months, the cleft palate was repaired using the two long-flap procedure popularized in India by Charles Pinto, the mentor of the senior author, and, worldwide, by Bardach. The child is now being subjected to constant follow-up and speech therapy.

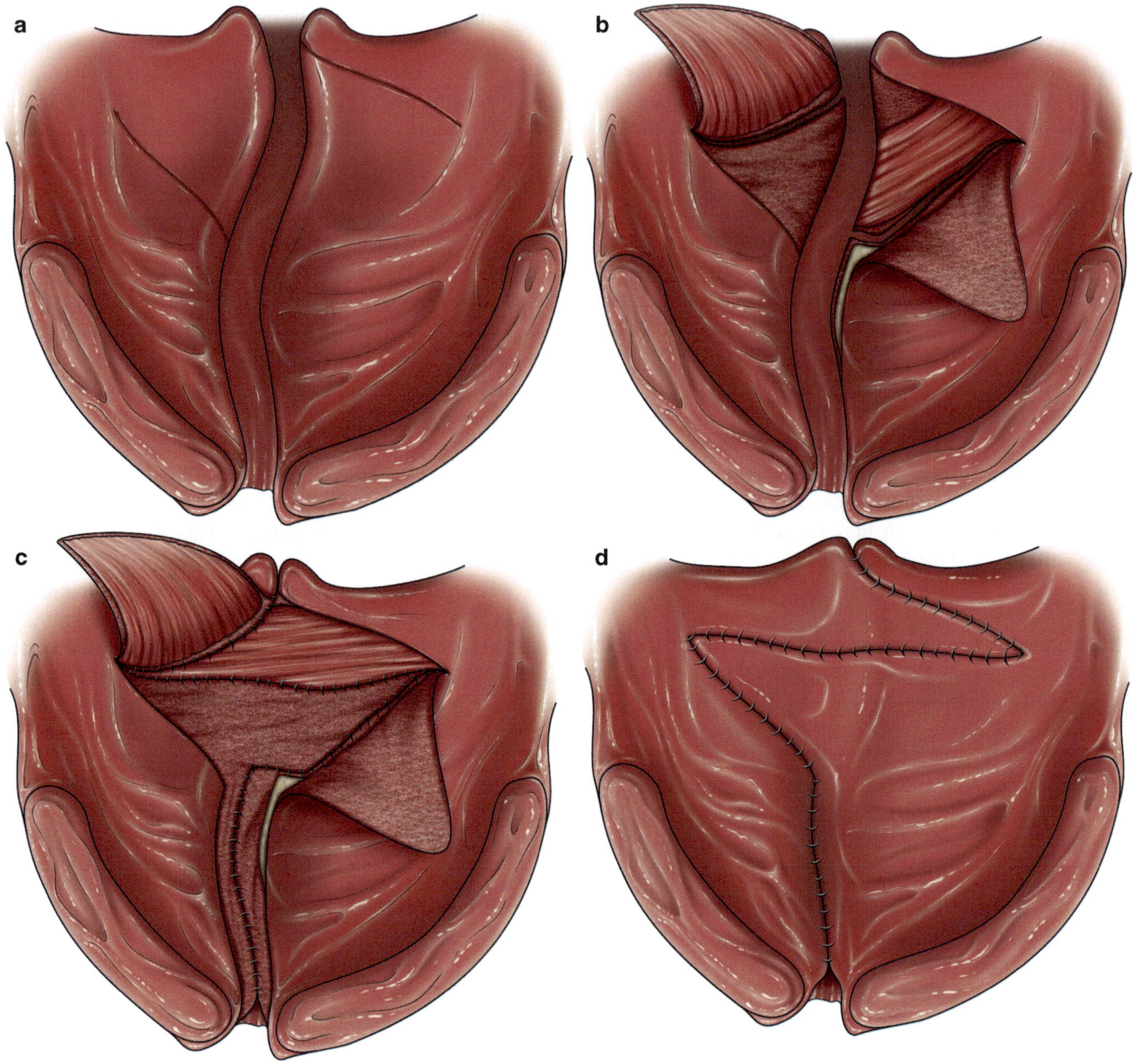

Fig. 73.29 (**a**, **b**) Furlow's double opposing "Z" plasty (**a**) incision, (**b**) flaps raised and mucosal incisions placed, (**c**) double opposing Z plasty completed and (**d**) oral flaps inset

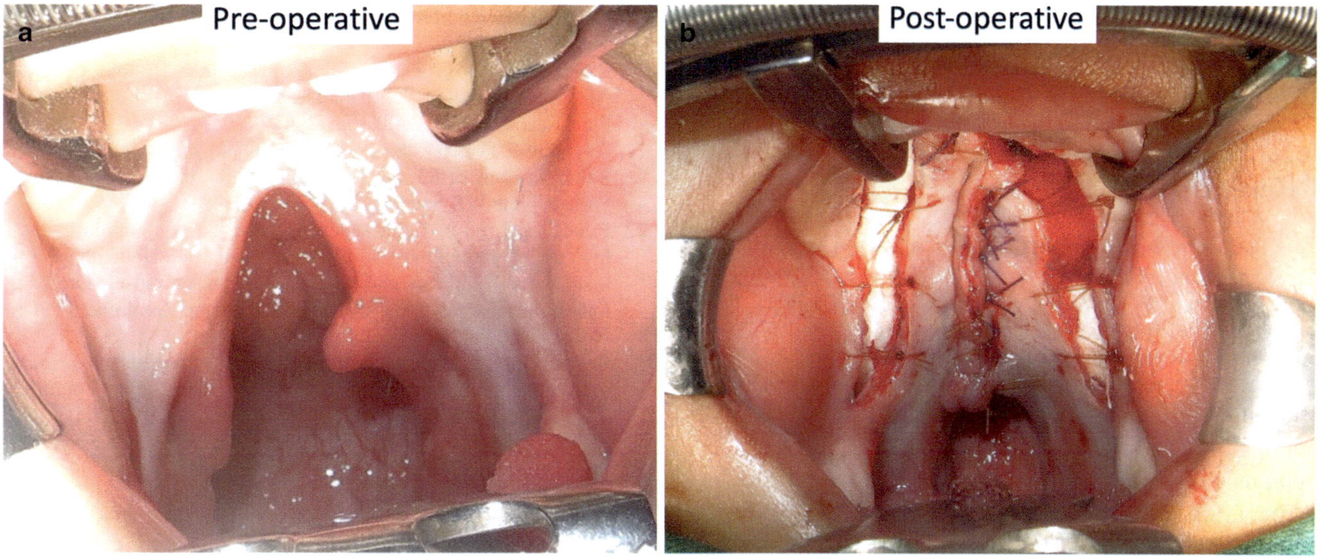

Fig. 73.30 Repair of incomplete cleft palate

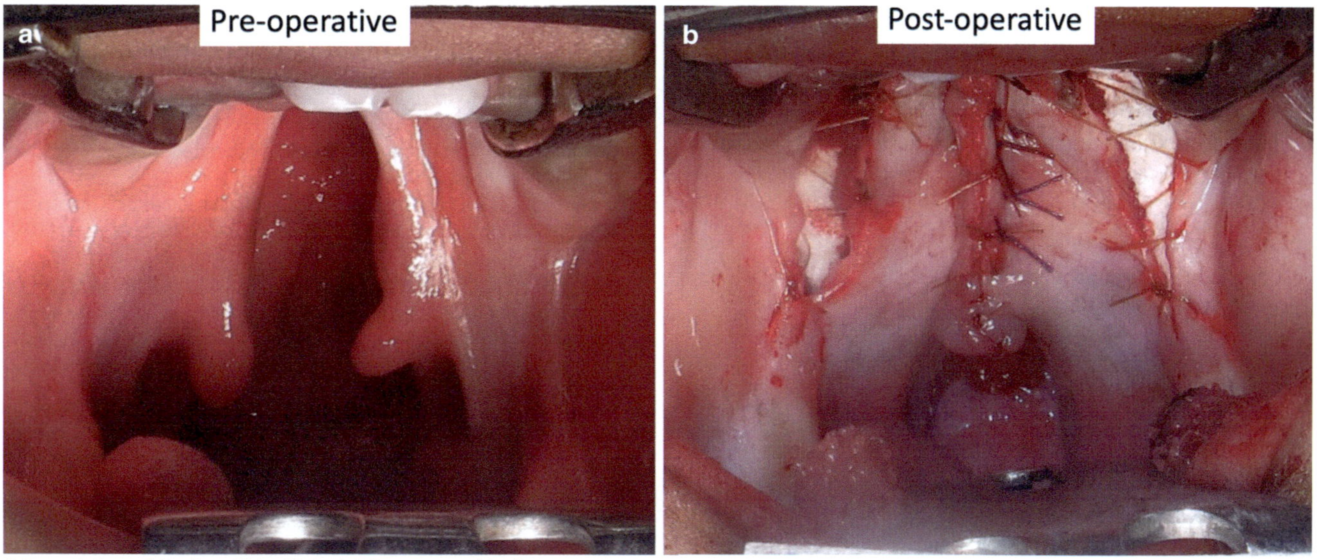

Fig. 73.31 Repair of complete Cleft palate

73.12 Disclosure

Authors have no financial conflicts to disclose.

References

1. Holdsworth WG. Cleft lip and plate, vol. 82. London: William Heinemann; 1957.
2. Von Graefe CF. Kurze nachrichten and auszuge. J Pract Azneck Wundarzk. 1817;44:116.
3. Randall P, Rossa D. Cleft palate in plastic surgery. In: JC MC, editor. Cleft lip, palate and craniofacial anomalies, vol. 4. Philadelphia: Saunders; 1990. p. 2723–4.
4. Dieffenbach JF. Die operative chirurgie, vol. 1. Leipzig: F.S. Brockhaus; 1845.
5. Warren JM. Operations for fissures of the soft and hard palate. Am J Med Sci. 1843;6:257.
6. Von Langenbeck B. Beitrage zur osteoiplastik. Deutsche Klin. 1859;2:471.
7. Veau V. Division palatine, anatomie, chirurgie, phonetique. Paris: Masson et cie; 1931.
8. Kilner TP. Cleft lip and palate repair technique. St Thomas Hosp Rep. 1937;2:127.
9. Wardill WEM. Techniques of operation for cleft palate. Br J Surg. 1937;15:117.
10. Dorrance GM, Bransfield JW. The pushback operation for repair of cleft palate. Plast Reconstr Surg. 1946;1:145.
11. Cronin TD. Pushback palatorrhaphy with nasal mucosal flaps. In: Grabb WC, Rosenstein SW, Bzoch KR, editors. Cleft lip and palate: surgical, dental, and speech aspects. Boston: Little, Brown And Company; 1971.
12. Millard DR Cleft craft, vols. i, ii, iii. Boston: Little, Brown and Company; 1976, 1977, 1980.
13. Thatte R, Govilkar P, Patel J. The tongue flap in the primary treatment of cleft palate: a report of 19 cases. Br J Plast Surg. 1992;45(2):150–4.
14. Padgett EC. The repair of cleft palates after unsuccessful operations. Arch Surg. 1930;20:453–72.
15. Mukherji MM. Cheek flap for short palates. Cleft Palate J. 1969;6:415–20.
16. Mann RJ, Fisher DM. Bilateral buccal flaps with double opposing z-plasty for wider palatal clefts, Plast Reconstr Surg. 1997 Oct;100(5):1139–1143; discussion 1144-5.
17. Calnan J. Submucous cleft palate. Br J Plast Surg. 1954;6(4):264–82.
18. Sommerlad BC, Fenn C, Harland K, Sell D, Birch MJ, Dave R, Lees M, Barnett A. Submucous cleft palate: a grading system and review of 40 consecutive submucous cleft palate repairs. Cleft Palate Craniofac J. 2004 Mar;41(2):114–23.
19. Cohen MM. Syndromes with cleft lip and cleft palate. Cleft Palate J. 1978;15:306–28.
20. Randall P, La Rossa D, McWilliams BJ, Cohen M, Solot C, Jawad AF. Palatal length in cleft palate as a predictor of speech outcome. Plast Reconstr Surg. 2000;106:1254–9.
21. Åbyholm F. Primary closure of cleft lip and palate. In: Turvey TA, KWL V, Fonseca RJ, editors. Facial clefts and craniosynostosis. Philadelphia: WB Saunders; 1996. p. 370e383.
22. Friede H, Lilja J, Lohmander A. Long term, longitudinal follow up of individuals with UCLP after the Gothenburg primary early veloplasty and delayed hard palate closure protocol: maxillofacial growth outcome. Cleft Palate Craniofac J. 2012 Nov;49(6):649–56.
23. Agrawal K, Panda K ,A modified surgical schedule for primary management of cleft lip and palate in developing countries. Agrawal K, Panda K. Cleft Palate Craniofac. J. 2011;48(1):1–8.
24. Peet E. The Oxford technique of cleft palate repair. Plast Reconstr Surg Bull. 1961;28:282–94.
25. Lehman JA Jr, Douglas BK, Ho WC, Husami TW. One-stage closure of the entire primary palate. Plast Reconstr Surg. 1990;86:675–81.
26. Kane AA, Lo LJ, Yen BD, Chen YR, Noordhoff MS. The effect of hamulus fracture on the outcome of palatoplasty: a preliminary report of a prospective, alternating study. Cleft Palate Craniofac J. 2000 Sep;5:506–11.
27. Braithwaite F, Maurice DG. The importance of the levator palatini muscle in cleft palate closure. Br J Plast Surg. 1968;21:60–2.
28. Kriens OB. Anatomy of velopharyngeal area in cleft palate. Clin Plast Surg. 1975;2:261.
29. Sommerlad BC. A technique for cleft palate repair. Plast Reconstr Surg. 2003 Nov;112(6):1542–8.
30. Adenwalla HS, Narayanan PV. Primary cleft palate repair, surgical correction, facial deformity varghese mani. Kochi: Jaypee; 2010.
31. Lindsay WK, Witzel MA. Cleft palate repair: Von Langenbeck technique. In: Bardach J, Morris HL, editors. Multidisciplinary management of cleft lip and palate. Philadelphia: W.B. Saunders Company; 1990. p. 303.
32. Pomerantz JH, Hoffmann WM. In: Nelegan P, editor. Chapter 23 cleft palates in plastic surgery. 4th ed. Philadelphia: Elsevier; 2010. p. 579.
33. Gue-Santos J, Altamirano JT. The use of lingual flaps in repair of fistulas of the hard palate. Plast Reconstr Surg. 1966;38(2):123–8.
34. Pribaz J, Stephens W. Crespol, Gifford G. a new intraoral facial artery musculomucosal (Famm) flap. Plast Reconstr Surg. 1992;90(3):421–9.
35. Furlow LT Jr. Cleft palate repair by double opposing Z-plasty. Plast Recostr Surg. 1986;78:724–38.
36. Mann RJ, Martin MD, Eichhorn MG, Neaman KC, Sierzant CG, Polley JW, Girotto JA. The double opposing z-plasty plus or minus buccal flap approach for repair of cleft palate: a review of 505 consecutive cases. Plast Reconstr Surg. 2017 Mar;139(3):735e–44e.

Alveolar Bone Grafting

74

Veerabahu Muthusubramanian
and Kalarikkal Mukundan Harish

74.1 Introduction

Attempts to graft the alveolus started in the early 1900. The rationale for the procedure however has changed over the period. From its use as a procedure for establishing continuity over a defect, it has evolved and made itself indispensable in both cleft-related orthodontics and orthognathic surgery. Over the years, the technique has evolved, and the materials used have also been constantly studied and improved upon. This chapter aims to elaborate on the morphology of the alveolar cleft, its implications on dentition as well as facial skeleton, and the various management strategies and evolving trends.

74.2 Normal Anatomy of Alveolus

The alveolar process is that part of the jaw that contains the tooth sockets and forms a bridge between the teeth and the basal bones. The alveolar process is present in both the maxilla and the mandible. The status of the alveolar process and its development depends on the status of the teeth; if the teeth are absent or lost in later life, it reduces in size, eventually disappearing completely.

74.2.1 Development of Alveolar Process (Figs. 72.1, 73.1, and 77.1)

The alveolar process begins to form in the end of the second month of fetal life. The maxilla and mandible develop a groove-like structure that opens toward the surface of the oral cavity. This groove contains the tooth germs, the dental nerves, and vessels. Gradually, bony septa begin to develop between adjacent tooth germs. Later the primitive mandibular canal is separated from the dental crypts through a horizontal plate of bone. The alveolar process remains fused to the body of the maxilla and mandible, and its formation is completed during tooth eruption.

74.2.2 Structure of Alveolar Process

There is no distinct boundary between the body of the maxilla or mandible and their corresponding alveolar processes. In conditions where the alveolus is not functionally related to teeth, it may be fused with and partly masked by bone.

Based on function, the alveolar process consists of two parts:

1. *Alveolar bone proper*: It consists of a thin lamella of bone which surrounds the root of the tooth and gives attachment to the periodontal membrane.
2. *Supporting bone*: It is the structure which surrounds the alveolar bone and gives support to the socket. The latter, in turn, consists of two parts.
   (i) The compact bone/cortical plate forming the vestibular and oral plates of the alveolar processes.
   (ii) The spongy bone between these plates and the alveolar bone proper.

The cortical plates are usually much thinner in the maxilla than in the mandible. They are thickest in the bicuspid and molar region of the mandible especially on the buccal side. In the maxilla, the outer cortical plate is perforated by many small openings through which blood and lymph vessels pass. In the mandible, the cortical bone of the alveolar process is dense and, occasionally, shows small foramina. In the region of the anterior teeth of both jaws, the supporting bone is, usually, very thin. No spongy bone is found here and the cortical plate is fused with the alveolar bone proper.

The interdental and interradicular septa contain the perforating canals of *Zuckerkandl and Hirschfeld*, which house

V. Muthusubramanian (✉) · K. M. Harish
Department of Oral and Maxillofacial Surgery, Ragas Dental College, Uthandi, Chennai, India

K. Bonanthaya et al. (eds.), *Oral and Maxillofacial Surgery for the Clinician*, https://doi.org/10.1007/978-981-15-1346-6_74

the interdental and interradicular arteries, veins, lymph vessels, and nerves. The alveolar bone proper which forms the inner wall of the socket contains many openings which transmit branches of the interalveolar nerves and blood vessels into the periodontal membrane. It is named cribriform plate or lamina dura.

74.2.3 Functions of Alveolar Bone

The primary functions of the alveolar bone are highlighted in (Box 74.1).

74.3 Alveolar Anatomy in Cleft Patients

The alveolar cleft is usually represented either by a notch in the alveolus on the labial aspect or as a complete gap between the alveolar segments. In unilateral alveolar clefts, the cleft side of the maxilla (referred to as the lesser segment) is underdeveloped, causing abnormalities of the alveolus, as well as the lip, nose, and palate.

74.3.1 Abnormalities of the Alveolus and Dentition

The abnormalities of the alveolus and the dentition are projected in (Box 74.2).

74.3.2 Abnormalities of the Lip-nasal Complex

- The pyriform rim on the cleft side, when viewed sagittally, appears retrusive.
- The nasal floor is displaced inferiorly, and there is transverse constriction of the anterior bony nasal aperture.
- The nasal tip is asymmetrical.

Box 74.1 Primary Functions of the Alveolar Bone

1. Protection: Alveolar bone forms and protects the dental roots.
2. Attachment: It gives the attachment for periodontal ligament fibers, which are the principle fibers. These fibers which enter into the bone are called as Sharpey's fibers.
3. Support: It supports tooth roots on the facial and the palatal/lingual sides.
4. Shock absorber: It helps to absorb forces placed upon the tooth by disseminating the force to underlying basal bones.

Box 74.2 Abnormalities of the Alveolus and the Dentition

- There is medial collapse of the arch, producing dental crossbites (Fig. 74.1a).
- The position of the premaxilla may be altered with the arch being normal or rotated toward the non-cleft side. There is change in the position of the premaxilla.
- The central incisor is usually rotated toward the cleft side (Fig. 74.1b).
- The lateral incisor may be congenitally absent or hypoplastic or at times resemble a supernumerary tooth. It may also protrude through the nasal floor and lie within the cleft (Fig. 74.1c).
- The periodontal attachments of the central incisor and canine on the cleft side are poor and have high risk of future bone loss.

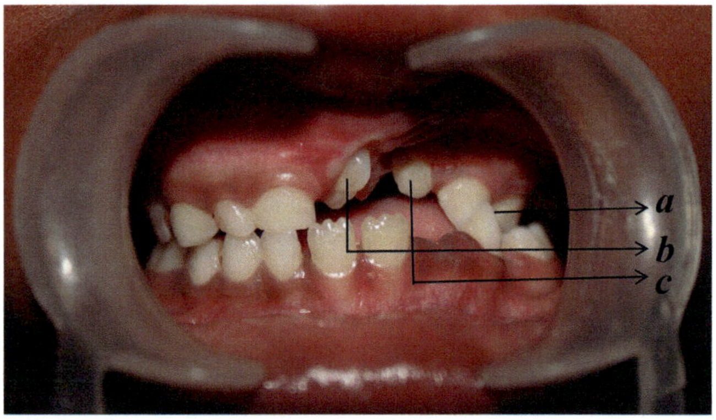

Fig. 74.1 Intraoral frontal picture demonstrating clinical features of cleft alveolus (left side). (Refer to Box 74.2 for description of a, b and c)

- The medial crus of the nasal cartilage is short, and the upper and lower lateral cartilages do not overlap. There is a mismatch in the level of lower lateral cartilages (Fig. 74.2a).
- The columella, caudal septum, and anterior nasal spine tend to deviate to the non-cleft side.
- The above factors result in lack of support for the external nose, especially around the alar base, which is displaced laterally, inferiorly, and posteriorly, widening the nasal aperture (Fig. 74.2b).
- The fibers of the orbicularis oris muscle do not run transversely and instead turn upward along the margins of the cleft, to terminate beneath the base of the columella medially and below the alar base and periosteum of the pyriform rim laterally. Due to the abnormal muscle attachment, there will be a bulge on the unrepaired cleft lip, distortion of the ala of the nose, and deflection of the nasal septum and anterior nasal spine.

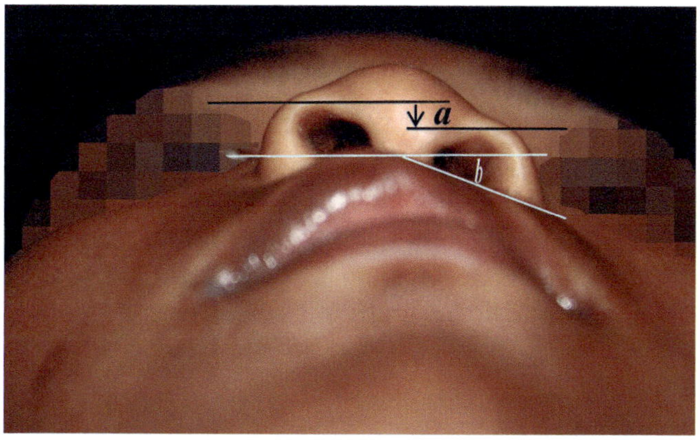

Fig. 74.2 Basal view picture demonstrating abnormalities of the lip-nasal complex (**a**) mismatch of the lower lateral cartilages and (**b**) widening of the nostril due to lack of support for the cleft side alar base

Box 74.3 Goals of Orthodontics in Alveolar Bone Grafting (ABG)

1. Alignment of arches in preparation for ABG.
2. Stabilize the arches.
3. Arch expansion to correct the transverse discrepancy.
4. Align the teeth.
5. Increase the cleft width in preparation to receive the graft.

74.4 Role of the Orthodontist in Patients with Alveolar Cleft (Box 74.3)

The objective of alveolar bone grafting (ABG) primarily involves restoring the structural and functional integrity of maxillary alveolar arch. This would further facilitate the eruption of the canine or lateral incisor into their respective position in the maxillary alveolar arch. The further employment of orthodontic treatment would help in stabilizing the arches and achieving proper alignment of misaligned teeth, The aim of orthodontics in ABG are highlighted in Box 74.3.

The orthodontist must be involved at all stages of dental development, namely, infancy, primary, mixed dentitions, and the permanent dentition stages.

74.4.1 Infancy

1. Pre-surgical orthopedics can be done with the use of appliances such as Latham's appliance, etc. It consists of a pin-retained device that is inserted into the palate with acrylic extensions onto the alveolar ridges. Further a screw mechanism is then used to manipulate the segments as desired.
2. Primary bone grafting is also an option, which is done in some cases, as it was believed that defect, which when corrected earlier, would allow normal development and function. However, it remains controversial, as there are no important benefits compared to secondary bone grafting done. In addition, scarring can cause deleterious effects and retard growth.
3. Gingivoperioplasty can also be done to improve the closure. It involves creation of a mucoperiosteal bridge across alveolar cleft region, thus creating a subperiosteal tunnel. This in turn facilitates bone generation.

   In case of untreated clefts, the maxillary development was found to be normal. Which indicates that early lip repair may affect maxillary growth.
4. In case of a bilateral cleft repair, posterior alveolar segments behind the premaxilla are collapsed leading to a protruded and superiorly positioned premaxilla.
5. Orthodontist's role would be to reposition the maxilla and expand the collapsed alveolar segments.

   Jackscrew and spring-loaded appliance are some of the orthopedic appliances used. However, the effect of these appliances are still controversial.

74.4.2 Primary Dentition

1. In a primary dentition, the orthodontist has no role to play unless the children have crossbites.
2. Routine dental screening is advised to detect any caries.

74.4.3 Mixed Dentition

1. Standard records for orthodontic diagnosis are procured for the patient. Some of them being OPG, IOPA, and occlusal radiographs.
2. Missing teeth, supernumerary teeth, and bone requirement are assessed with these radiographs.
3. Presence of posterior crossbite, malaligned upper incisors, and bone defects at the cleft area are documented.
4. Bone grafting should be done prior to any orthodontic treatment, which is to prevent root exposure or periodontal defects.
5. Arch expansion done should be limited if the patient is supposed to undergo orthognathic surgery later.
6. The expansion is usually limited by the zygomatic buttress and scar tissue present.
7. The direction of the expansion, its extent, the presence or absence of teeth, the resistance of tissue (which can

be high in scarring), surgical access to cleft area, and compliance of the patient are factors that determine the selection of appliance.

8. Spring appliances offer lighter forces with quad helix providing better control in the expansion.
9. Any fistulae that are present in the patient should be corrected during bone grafting.
10. In case of bilateral cleft, the mobile premaxilla is stabilized by grafting, and orthodontic treatment is started only after the bony union is complete, which may be a range between 2 and 6 months.
11. Orthopedic appliances like headgears can be given to patients with mild maxillary deficiencies.
12. Distraction osteogenesis or orthognathic surgery should be chosen depending on the patient's growth status (refer Chap. 69 on maxillary orthognathic surgeries, Chap. 75 on cleft maxillary hypoplasia and Chap. 87 on distraction osteogenesis).

74.4.4 Permanent Dentition

1. Fresh set of diagnostic records are obtained.
2. Most common problems which are seen are missing or malformed teeth.
3. Sometimes teeth may be present but compromised. Most often it is the lateral incisor. One must decide whether this has to be treated with canine substitution or prosthetic replacement.
4. In cases where there is (i) deviation of the dental midline toward the non-cleft side, with the canine erupted mesially with favorable root position, or (ii) the canine is small and wide with both premolars present on the cleft side, and the molar and canine relationships on same side are *class* II, the right choice of treatment would be canine substitution. It involves extraction of the malformed lateral incisor with poor periodontal support, followed by facilitating the eruption of canine in the place of lateral incisor.
5. In cases in which both the maxillary canine and the first molar have a class I relationship, or the canine is positioned with the crown mesially and root distally, with a shift of the maxillary midline to the cleft side, prosthetic replacement is ideal. Adequate space should be planned to accommodate the prosthesis.
6. Comprehensive orthodontic treatment starts almost a year or 2 prior to surgery.
7. Dental decompensation for cleft maxillary osteotomy surgery must be planned and executed. Surgical preparation should include wire placements, retentive hooks for IMF, and plans for post-surgical retention.
8. If relapse is noticed post-surgically, it is immediately addressed with class III elastics or a reverse pull headgear.

74.5 Alveolar Bone Grafting Procedure

74.5.1 History [1]

Attempts to graft the alveolus started in the early 1900s. In the beginning, the goal was to prevent collapse of the alveolar ridge. Therefore, it was done during infancy. In 1970, reconstructive surgeons like Boyne [2, 3] stated that the ideal age for grafting the cleft was between 9 and 11 years. This was done to allow eruption of the canine.

74.5.2 Classification

Alveolar bone grafting procedures are classified into four types based on the age and timing of the procedure:

- *Primary*—This is performed in infancy, with the patient being below 2 years of age. This is done following lip repair but before the palate is repaired.
- *Early secondary*—This is done between 2 and 5 years of age, prior to the eruption of incisors.
- *Secondary*—Performed between 8 and 11 years of age, prior to eruption of the maxillary permanent canine.
- *Late secondary*—Performed above 12 years of age, after the canine has erupted.

The advantages and disadvantages of the various methods are highlighted in Table 74.1.

74.5.3 Materials Used in Alveolar Bone Grafting

A variety of materials have been used in grafting in secondary cleft deformities.

These include autogenous, allogenic, or alloplastic materials.

The success rate differs for each type, but fresh autologous cancellous bone is considered to be superior because it allows cells that are immune-compatible and integrate fully into the maxilla and trigger osteogenesis. In addition, it is the only bone source which possesses all the properties that promote bone formation—osteogenesis, osteo-conduction, and osteo-induction.

74.5.3.1 Bone Grafts

- Cortical:
  Cortical bone refers to the compact outer part of the bone. This is generally less vascular, and so establishment of nutritional supply to cortical cells is a slow pro-

Table 74.1 Comparison of advantages and disadvantages of different ABG techniques

Procedure	Advantage	Disadvantage
Primary grafting	Limited dissection. Reduced maxillary growth discrepancy	Alveolar segments have to be aligned orthopedically. Requires additional surgeries. Reduced success rates [4]
Early secondary grafting	Possibly could facilitate eruption of lateral incisor as well	Not accepted widely in literature [4]
Secondary grafting	Minimal influence in maxillary growth as most of the maxillary growth is completed by 6–7 years [4]. Sufficient quantity of bone at donor site is available. Better patient cooperation. Orthodontic treatment acceptance is good. Allows eruption of permanent teeth through the graft, thus maintaining good periodontal health	Earlier intervention could result in eruption of lateral incisors as well
Late secondary grafting	No significant advantage. Mandibular symphysis could be considered as good donor site as the chances of damaging unerupted teeth are less	Less success rate. Loss of osseous support to teeth adjacent to cleft. Less chances of salvaging lateral incisor. Delay in orthodontic correction of underlying deformity

cess. Therefore, this graft generally resorbs and is replaced by invasion of bone cells originating from the recipient site. The rate of metabolic turnover and cortical bone remodeling is much slower than in cancellous bone. Therefore, keeping the tooth-bearing function in mind, cortical grafts may not be feasible for the alveolar process.

- Cancellous:
  Cancellous bone refers to the softer trabecular bone that is more vascular. This allows better ingrowth from the recipient site. The formation of new bone starts at the surface of the existing cancellous bone. Cancellous bone theoretically heals by osteogenesis, followed by bone resorption and deposition. This graft is harvested as a particulate form, so it may be difficult to stabilize it in the recipient site.
- Cortico-cancellous:
  A combination of the two produces good results and enables good vascularization to help incorporate bone with surrounding structures. It also adds good mechanical strength.

74.5.3.2 Autogenous Materials

The following sites are commonly used as sources for autogenous material used in alveolar bone grafting:

1. Cranium [5]
   - The cranium, or calvarial bone, is a source of both cortical and cancellous bone.
   - This site is associated with low morbidity and minimum postoperative pain.
   - Scar will be unseen within the hair with early discharge and good prognosis.
   - It has poor outcomes as compared to iliac crest bone.
2. Iliac Crest [6]
   - It has huge quantity of cancellous bone which aid osteogenesis. The process of condensing bone chips into the defect increases the reliability of this bone.
   - Bone from this region may be harvested using a trephine or through an open approach.
   - Approach needs to be planned well as it may leave an unacceptable scar.
   - The main disadvantage of using iliac crest is postoperative pain, which may require extended hospitalization, which can be surmounted by regional anesthetic techniques for post-surgical pain control.
   - This is the most preferred donor site and is used by 87% of European surgeons and 83% of North American surgeons performing ABGs [6].
3. Mandibular Symphysis [7]
   - Bone provided is more cortical and is limited compared to the ilium.
   - Damage to the adjacent teeth and mental nerve has been reported.
   - It is used by 4% of surgeons in Europe [7].
4. Tibia [8]
   - It has sufficient bone which is quick to harvest.
   - There is minimal scarring, and patient may be mobilized early but is restricted from sports for 3 weeks.
   - In children where the tibia is usually small, there is a possibility of damage to the epiphyseal cartilage.
   - Used by 3% of European and 2% of North American surgeons [8].
5. Rib [9]
   - This is rarely used, as it provides limited amount of bone.
   - Postoperative risk of chest infections and prolonged discomfort may be present.
   - Esthetically identical scar to other sources.
   - 0.5% of European and 3% of North American surgeons use this method [9].
6. Femur
   - Bone may also be harvested from the intermedullary canal of the femur, but it carries the risk of high morbidity.

74.5.3.3 Alloplastic Materials

Alloplastic materials that have been used for ABG include rhBMP-2 (recombinant human bone morphogenetic protein), undecalicified freeze-dried bone, TEOM (tissue-engineered osteogenic material), and bioglass.

1. rhBMP-2
   - This is recombinant bone morphogenic protein, with superior bone quality reported in BMP-2 group [10].
   - Studies have shown that this material, when used for ABG, had high chances of successful grafting as is considered very effective in situations involving a larger bony defect, and does not demonstrate any detrimental effect on neighboring anatomical structures and no evidences of ectopic bone formation [11].
2. TEOM
   - This material contains MSC (mesenchymal stem cells), PRP (platelet-rich plasma), human thrombin, and mixed air.
   - Available in a gel form.
   - Claimed rate of success is about 70%.
3. Bioactive Glasses
   - This commercially available material is made up of silicone dioxide, sodium dioxide, calcium oxide, and phosphorus pentoxide.
   - It binds both to the soft tissue and bone.
   - Designed to engender surface reaction, which leads to osseointegration.

74.5.3.4 Allogenic Materials

These materials are comparable to autogenous materials and allow for eruption of teeth while avoiding donor site morbidity. However, they do not have osteogenic potential, which causes delayed graft incorporation.

These materials include:

- Undecalcified freeze-dried bone.
- Allograft CTBA [Cells and Tissuebank Austria].
- Osteograft.
- Maxgraft.

Most of the abovementioned products involve bone obtained from genetically dissimilar individuals. These allogenic bone particles are subjected to various processes to ensure the allogenic graft material is devoid of any microbial contamination however retaining the organic matrix and the inorganic components. They are available in various particle sizes or as block grafts or can even be milled for specific patients using CAD CAM technology.

Box 74.4 Goals of ABG

- To allow closure of the oronasal fistula.
- To provide tension-free, watertight closure to retain the graft and establish soft tissue continuity.
- To pack adequate volume of graft in the defect and restore bony continuity.
- Aid in the eruption and alignment of teeth.
- Add stability to the maxilla as a single unit while planning for orthognathic surgery.

74.5.4 Technique for Alveolar Bone Grafting

The technique of alveolar bone grafting must be performed with the following goals in mind (Box 74.4).

Alveolar bone grafting procedure is performed under general anesthesia. It can be performed comfortably using both naso-tracheal and oro-tracheal intubation. When iliac crest is the chosen donor site, a two-team approach can be followed simultaneously. The surgical sequence for unilateral ABG (Figs. 74.3a–f and 74.4a–f) and bilateral ABG (Fig. 74.5) are detailed below.

Surgery in the oral cavity is begun with infiltration of local anesthesia containing adrenaline to assist hemostasis. It has to be borne in mind that the reconstruction of cleft alveolus involves neat and precise development of labial/palatal/nasal layers and creating of a pocket for placement of graft, as this will ensure creation of structural and functional integrity of the alveolar arch. A fine needle gauge is used to probe the bony edges of the cleft in order to identify the site of the first incisions (Fig. 74.5b). The initial incision must be made through the mucosa lying over the cleft and must pass down to the bony margins (Fig. 74.3a, b). Try to preserve the soft tissue on the labial and palatal sides. Adequate (and sometimes excess) tissue is usually present within the oronasal fistula, which may be sacrificed after planning for the oral layer closure. In the region of the pyriform aperture, there is no bony margin. Hence, at this site the soft tissue is divided to provide a layer for the superior most extent of the nasal closure. A similar kind of division of the mucosa is necessary on the palatal side too (Fig. 74.3c).

Next, incisions are made around the cervical region of the teeth on the labial aspect of the alveolus. The incisions should extend several teeth posteriorly from the cleft with the exact distance determined by the width of the cleft. A full-thickness mucoperiosteal dissection should be begun to raise a large advancement flap. A similar procedure is carried out on the palate, where incisions are made around the neck of the teeth followed by full-thickness mucoperiosteal dissection. As an alternative oblique sliding flaps can also be raised (Fig. 74.3a, b). As these dissections are proceeding,

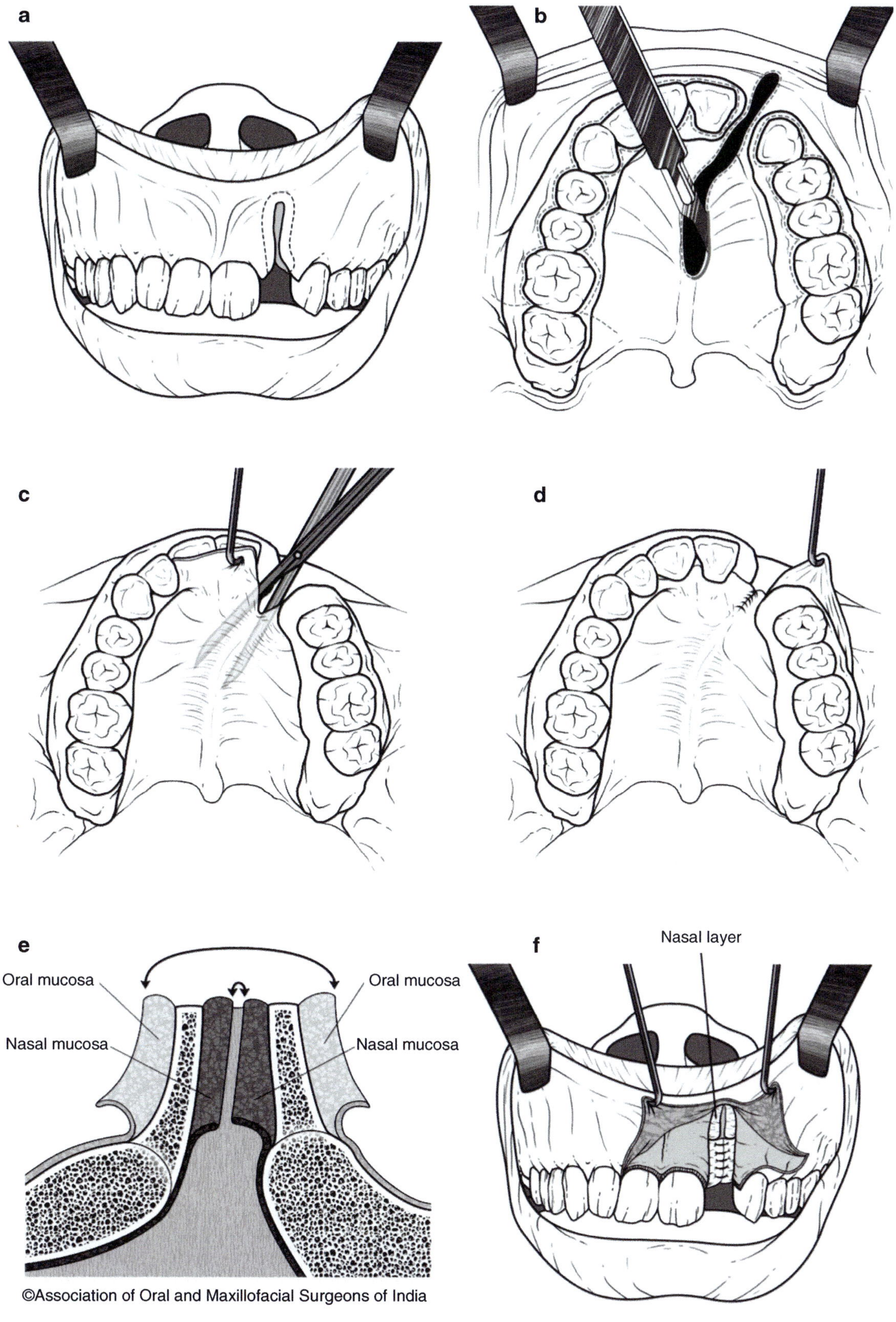

Fig. 74.3 (**a–f**) (**a** and **b**) Incisions around the cleft margin and for developing oblique sliding flaps (dashed lines), (**c**) Palatal flaps are developed sharply with scissors. This also separates the nasal mucosa from the palatal tissue. (**d**) Palatal closure. This can be done before or after the nasal mucosa is closed. (**e**) Depiction of the nasal mucosal flap along with the closure of the oral mucosa. (**f**) Nasal mucosal flaps are reflected from the bony walls of the cleft. The palatal flap facilitates packing and protects the palatal closure [4]

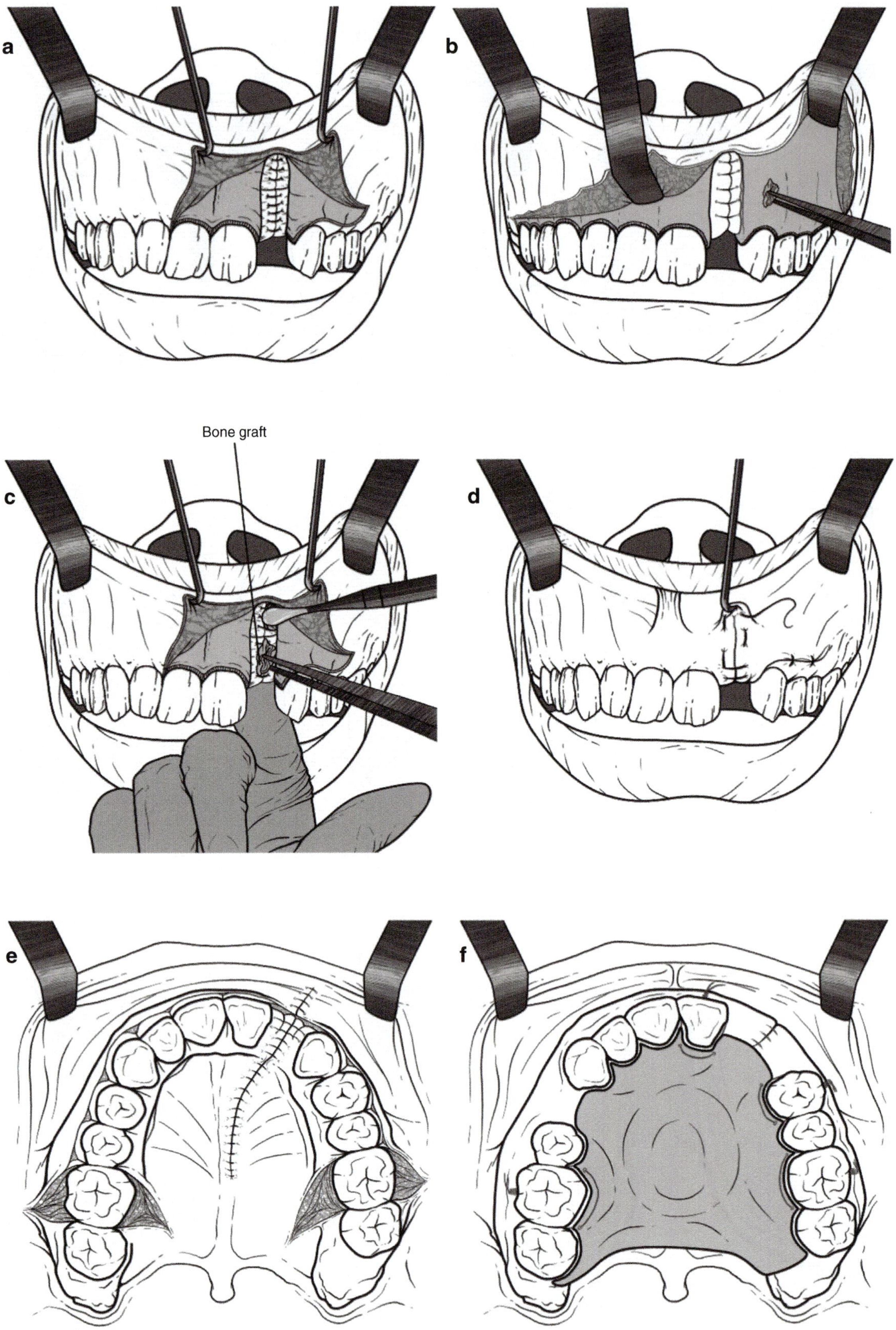

Fig. 74.4 (a–f). (a) Nasal flaps are approximated with sutures burying the knots when possible. (b) The closure of the nasal mucosa and the introduction of the bone graft to the alveolar defect. (c) Bone is packed into the defect with a periosteal elevator or orthodontic band pusher. Digital pressure against the palatal flap facilitates packing and protects the palatal closure [4]. (d) Closure of the labial oblique sliding flap. (e) Final mucosal closure of the labial and palatal oblique sliding flaps. (f) A palatal splint placed over the closure area to prevent formation of a hematoma and stabilize the bone graft

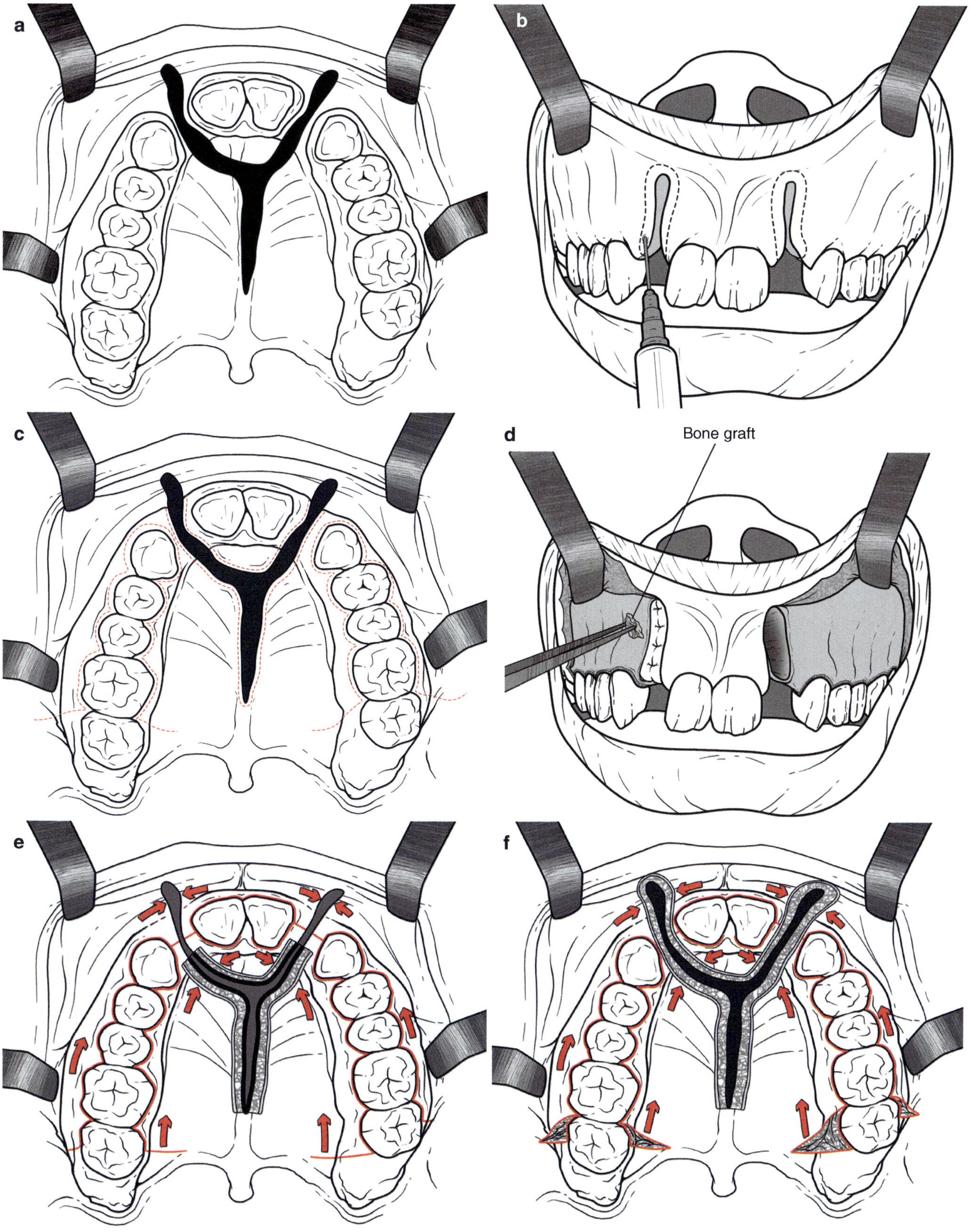

Fig. 74.5 (**a–i**) (**a**) A bilateral alveolar cleft palate. (**b**) Needle palpation of the bony edges of the alveolar cleft while injecting local anesthesia. (**c**) The incision line (dashed line). (**d**) Elevation of the nasal mucosa on the left and closure of the nasal mucosa on the right. Placement of the bone graft. (**e**, **f**) Palatal depiction of the movement of the adjacent mucosa in the oblique sliding flap technique. (**g**) Mucosal closure in a bilateral alveolar cleft. (**h** and **i**) Final closure of the bilateral alveolar cleft repair using an oblique sliding flap technique

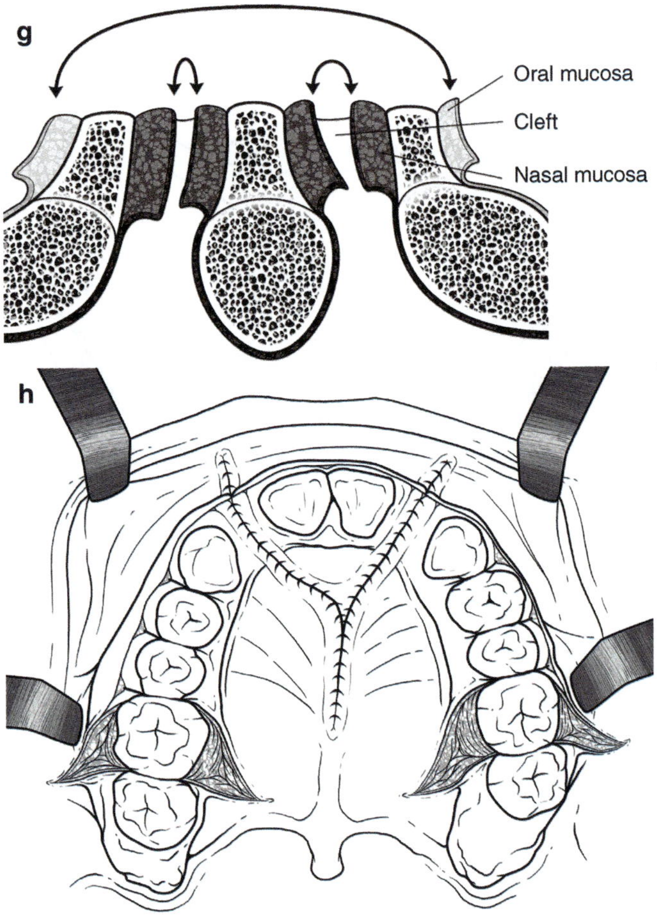

Fig. 74.5 (continued)

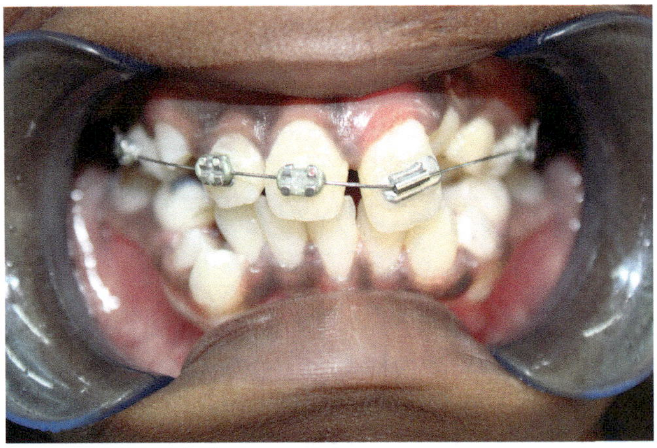

Fig. 74.6 Pre-operative intra oral picture demonstrating collapsed maxillary arches with hidden oro-nasal fistula

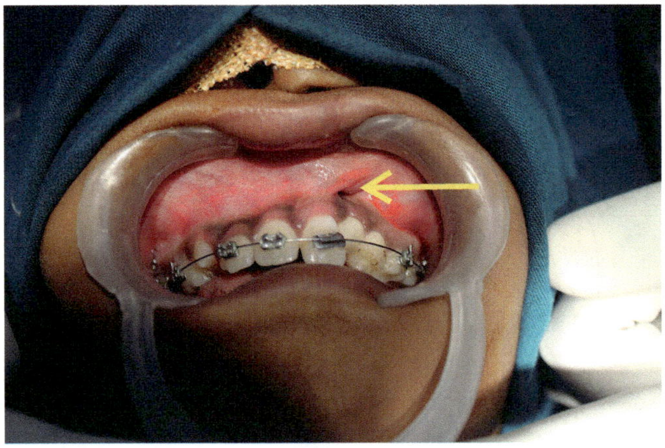

Fig. 74.7 Pre-operative intra-oral maxillary arch view of the same patient in Fig. 74.6, providing good visualisation of the oro-nasal fistula

the periosteal elevator may be carried around the cleft to allow the mucoperiosteum within the fistula to be rotated superiorly. This allows the full extent of the bony cleft to be visualized. Excess tissue within the nasal portion of the cleft can be trimmed, and then the nasal flaps are sutured to provide closure of the nasal floor. This helps in the closure of a persistent oro-nasal fistula (Figs. 74.6, 74.7, and 74.8). It is ideal to evert these flaps into the nose and to use inverted

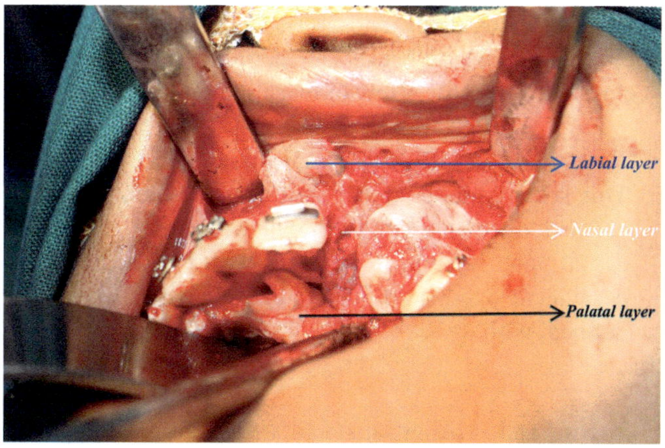

Fig. 74.8 Clinical picture demonstrating labial and palatal flap reflection and closure of nasal layer

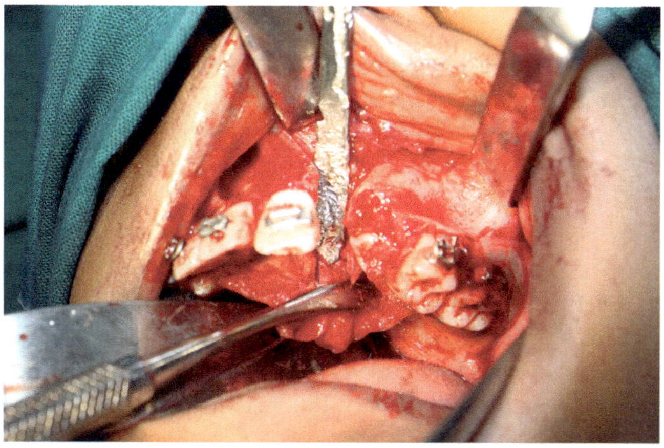

Fig. 74.9 Clinical step in which a periosteal elevator is used to define the alveolar cleft after closure of the nasal layer

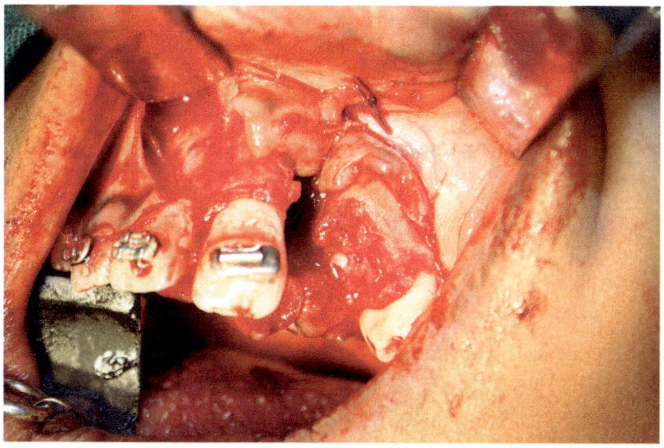

Fig. 74.10 Creation of a pouch with closure of the labial flaps in the alveolar cleft region to facilitate bone grafting

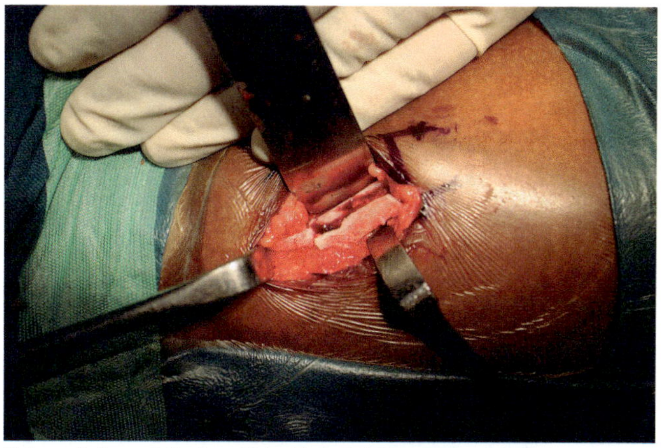

Fig. 74.11 Exposure of the iliac crest to harvest bone graft

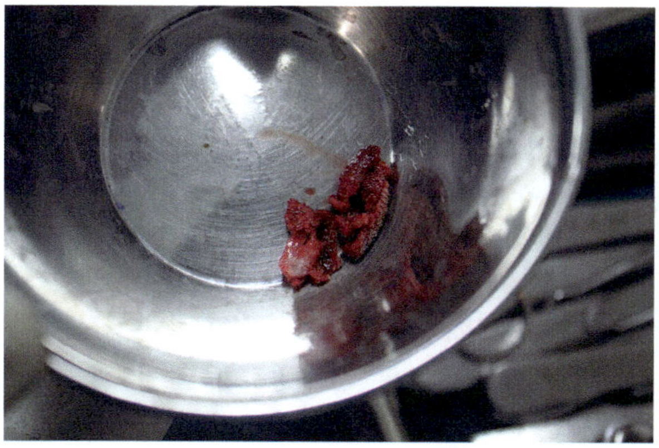

Fig. 74.12 Cancellous bone graft harvested from iliac crest

sutures so that the knots are on the nasal side. One should mobilize the palatal flaps toward the cleft (Fig. 74.8), utilizing releasing incisions if necessary. The palatal flaps may be sutured using interrupted sutures (Figs. 74.9 and 74.10).

The harvested bone is then (Figs. 74.11 and 74.12) condensed into a syringe prior to placement and packed tightly into the exposed bony cleft. While placing the bone graft, it is important to establish a normal contour to the pyriform aperture region. The labial flaps can be then advanced over the graft. This usually requires the utilization of the periosteal-releasing incisions made perpendicular to the direction of the advancement. A tension-free closure is mandatory for this technique (Fig. 74.13).

The two palatal and two labial flaps are then closed, utilizing a suture that simultaneously approximates all four corners. The final closure is completed with interrupted sutures closing the labial flaps and the interdental releases (Fig. 74.14). Closure is performed in a way that retains the attached gingiva overlying the reconstructed alveolus. Rarely, it may not be possible to obtain adequate advancement of flaps which necessitate the use of a cheek flap or a free gingival graft.

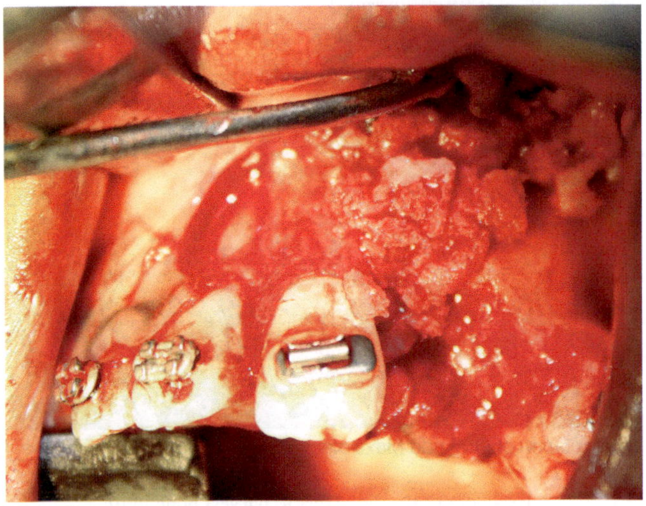

Fig. 74.13 Grafting of the alveolar cleft using harvested cancellous bone from the iliac crest

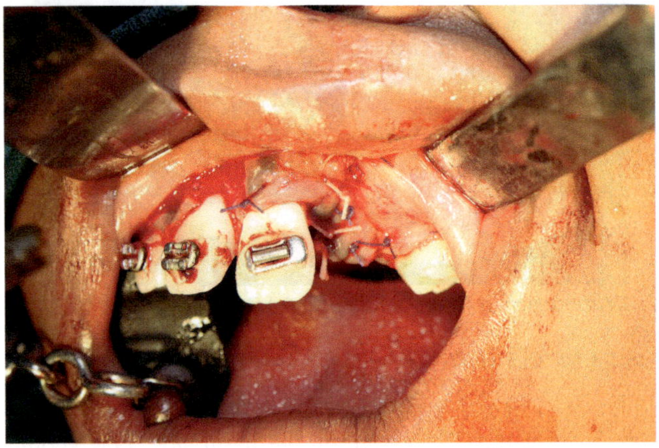

Fig. 74.14 Watertight closure of the alveolar cleft after grafting

74.5.5 Postoperative Assessment of Alveolar Bone Grafting

The success of alveolar bone grafting depends on certain outcomes, which include Box 74.5.

Box 74.5 Factors Determining Success of ABG
1. Closure of the oronasal fistula.
2. Adequate bone support that allows eruption of the canine and support for adjacent teeth.
3. Architecture of the grafted bone.

Several scales are used to assess the success based on the above criteria. These scales use periapical, panoramic, or occlusal radiographs. A few of these scales are given below:

- *Bergland scale* [12] (Fig 74.15a–d).
  This scale is the gold standard of assessment, and success is judged based on the height of the post-graft interdental bone septum. It is assessed after the eruption of permanent canine. Four categories of success are defined, with

Types I and II being satisfactory outcomes and Types III and IV being unsatisfactory:
Type I: Interdental septum height is almost normal (<25% of bone resorption).
Type II: Interdental septum height is equal to or greater than ¾ of the normal height (bone resorption 25%–50%).
Type III: Interdental septum height is less than ¾ of the normal height (bone resorption 50%–75%).
Type IV: Bone graft failure; no continuous bony bridge is visible across the cleft (bone resorption ≥75%) (Fig. 74.15).

- *Chelsea scale* [14] (Fig 74.16a–f).
  This scale evaluates the presence of bone in relation to the teeth adjacent to the cleft. Based on this, six categories have been identified. Only Types A and C represent satisfactory outcomes.

Type A: Bone tissue is present at the cementoenamel junction of the teeth adjacent to the cleft. At least 75% of roots on either side are covered by bone.
Type B: Bone tissue is present at the cementoenamel junction of the teeth adjacent to the cleft. At least 25% of roots on either side are covered by bone.
Type C: Bone tissue is present and surrounds at least 75% of the roots on either side of the cleft, in an apical direction.
Type D: Bone tissue surrounds at least 50% of roots on either side of the cleft, with an apical to coronal direction.
Type E: Bone tissue bridge is present in the cleft, except in the apical and coronal directions.
Type F: Less than 25% of bone tissue is present around both roots in the apical direction (Fig. 74.16).

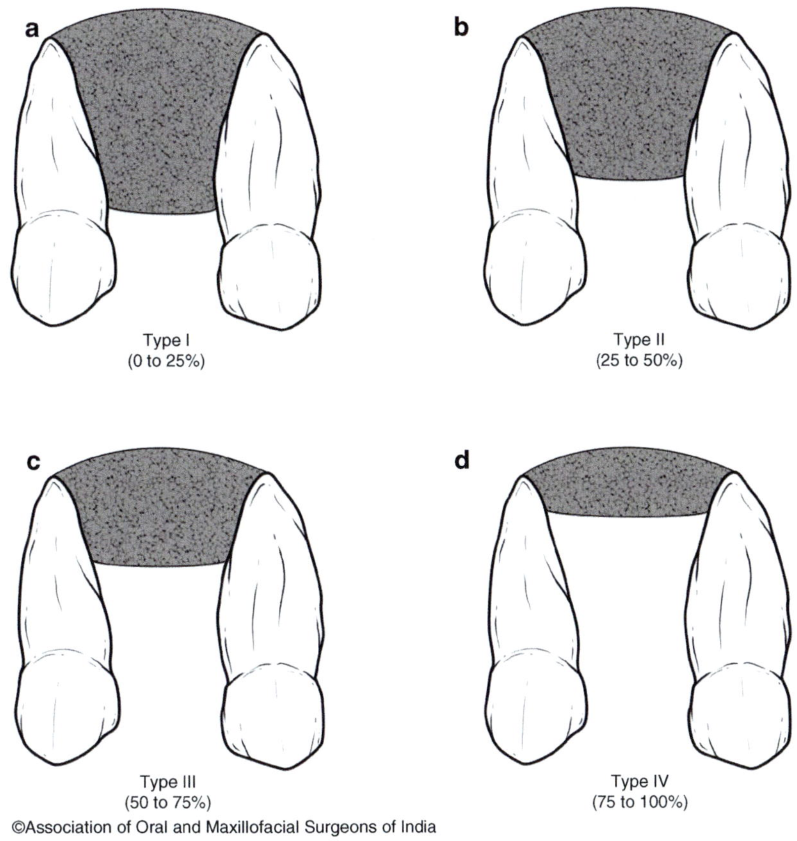

Fig. 74.15 (**a**–**d**) Bergland scale [13]

- *Trindade-Suedam scale* [15].
  These authors modified the Bergland scale described above and used alphabets to describe success or failure:

> *E (Excellent)*: Interdental septum height is normal.
> *G (Good)*: The bony septum is visible, with minimal disability.
> *R (Regular)*: Bone graft is enough to allow for canine eruption. However, tooth movement is deficient, or a defect that is more than 25% of root length is seen.
> *B (Bad)*: Deficient bone in the nasal region, which does not permit tooth movement.
> *F (Failure):* Bone graft is completely resorbed.

- *Kindelan scale* [16].
  This scale compares pre-operative and postoperative occlusal radiographs, to assess the percentage of bone fill. This also considers the eruption of the canine.

> Grade 1—Bone fill >75% (Fig. 74.17).
> Grade 2—Bone Fill 50–75%.
> Grade 3—Bone fill <50%.
> Grade 4—Complete absence of bone.

74.6 Complications of Alveolar Bone Grafting

The complications of alveolar bone grafting may be witnessed at the donor as well as the recipient site.

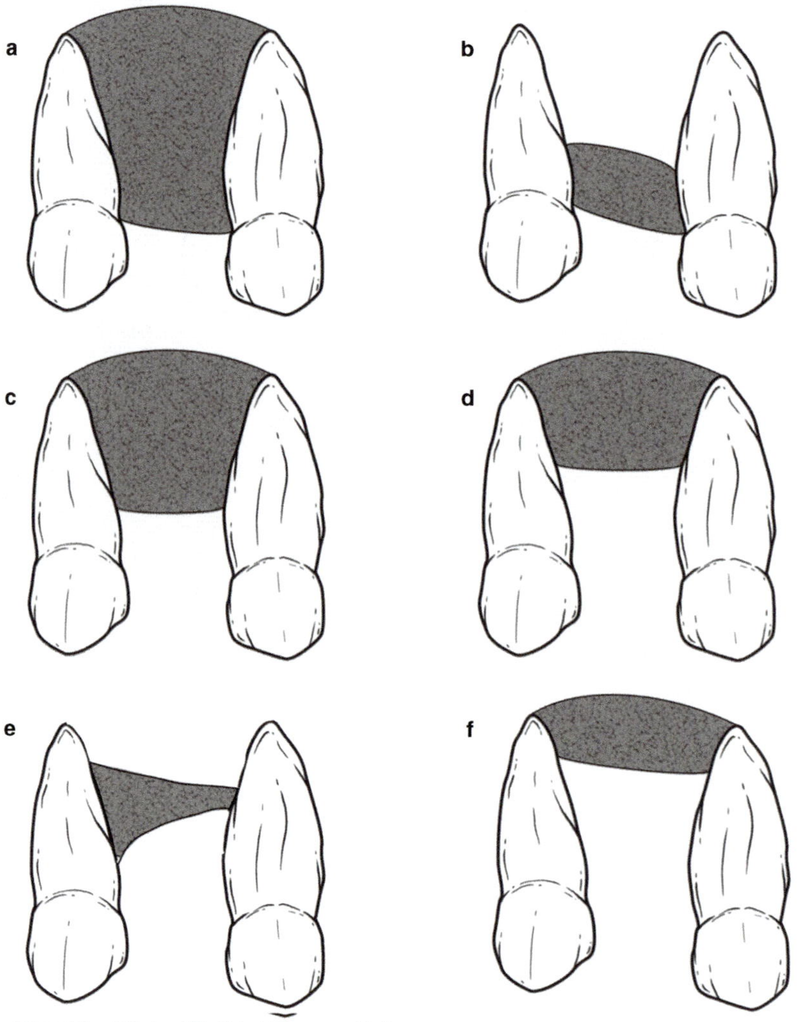

Fig. 74.16 (**a–f**) Chelsea scale [13]. (**a**) bone present at the Amelo-cemental Junction (ACJ) and covering 75% of both the roots, (**b**) bone present at the ACJ covering atleast 25% of both the roots, (**c**) bone covering atleast 75% of both the roots from the apical direction, (**d**) bone covering atleast 50% of the roots from the apical direction, (**e**) bony bridge present across cleft but no bone apically or coronally and (**f**) less than 25% bone cover from the apical direction

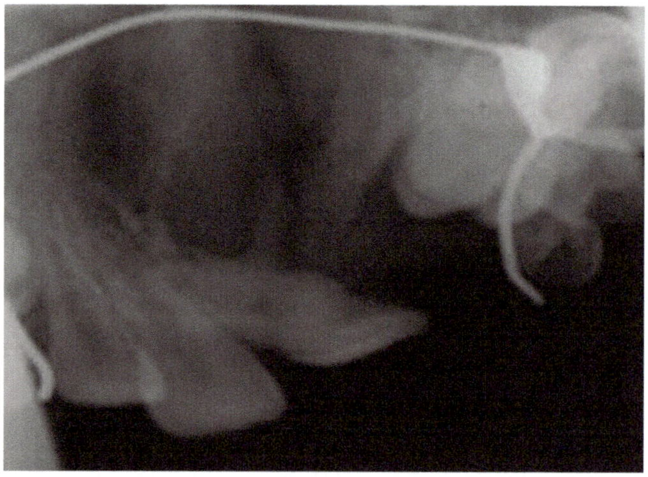

Fig. 74.17 Occlusal radiograph after bone graft with a Kindlean score of 1

74.6.1 Donor Site Complications

The site-specific donor site complications are highlighted in Box 74.6.

74.6.2 Recipient Site Complications

1. Damage to canine or central incisor roots.
2. Graft resorption: Graft resorption signifies complete failure of ABG, which can occur due to the following reasons:
   (a) Osteoresorptive cells and an environment suitable for bone resorption—this occurs with deciduous tooth extraction.
   (b) Excessive tension or trauma after surgery, resulting in exposure and loss of the graft.
   (c) Overpacking of the graft, causing alveolar notching and graft resorption. (d) Poor oral hygiene.

74.7 Conclusion

Alveolar bone grafting aims at restoring the functional integrity of the alveolar arch. In addition, they facilitate the eruption of teeth through the grafted bone into their respective positions. The timing of alveolar bone grafting is very crucial and can be effectively assessed by evaluating the thickness of bone covering the crown (of the lateral incisor or of the canine), rather than the degree of root formation of these teeth. The usage of autologous cancellous bone from the iliac crest is the most widely accepted graft in the mixed dentition period. In recent years, bone substitutes have also been used because of a tendency toward limited bone harvesting. These allograft or alloplastic sources of bone graft are especially useful in case of deficient donor autogenous bone material or to minimize donor site morbidity or in complicated cases. However, autologous bone is still the ideal choice for alveolar bone grafting, and none of the currently available methods can replace autologous bone completely. The future trend in alveolar bone grafting could be related to the usage of stem cells for bone regeneration; however many long-term clinical trials have to be conducted using stem cells to ensure its wide usage and cost-effectiveness.

Box 74.6 Donor Site Complications

(a) Iliac crest:
- Excessive blood loss.
- Hematoma.
- Delayed wound healing.
- Long and adherent and scars under belts or clothing which may be painful.
- Hypoesthesia or anesthesia over the lateral femoral cutaneous nerve and in its distribution areas.

(b) Cranium:
- Risk of inner table penetration.

(c) Rib grafts:
- Postoperative chest infection.
- Pneumothorax.

(d) Mandible grafts:
- Injury to mental nerve.

Disclosure Authors have no financial conflicts to disclose.

74.8 Case Scenarios

Case 1 (Fig. 74.18a–f)

An 11-year-old female patient who was treated for unilateral cleft lip and palate on the left side presented with the complaint of leakage of fluid from the nose and escape of air from the oral cavity. She had undergone primary unilateral lip repair when she was 6 months old, and a palatal repair was done when she was 2 years old.

Procedures, which were performed at this stage—fistula closure and alveolar bone grafting.

A sulcular incision along with incision around the fistula was performed both on the labial and palatal side so to enable direct access to the fistula and bony defect. Oral and nasal layers were separated. The nasal layer was initially closed in a watertight manner. Cancellous bone graft was obtained from the iliac crest, and the bone graft was placed into the defect, and watertight closure was obtained.

Future treatment required—pre-surgical orthodontics, orthognathic surgery, post-surgical orthodontics, and rhinoplasty (if required).

Case 2 (Fig. 74.19a–j)

Case Presentation

A 10-year-old female patient who was diagnosed with unilateral cleft lip and alveolus on the left side (Fig. 74.19a, b) reported to us with a chief complaint of leakage of fluid from the nose. She had previously undergone primary lip repair at 8 months of age. An OPG and IOPA revealed the extent of alveolar cleft (Fig. 74.19c, d). Pre-surgical orthodontic treatment was started to align the teeth and facilitate the eruption of 23 (Fig. 74.19e).

Procedures, which were performed at this stage—fistula closure and alveolar bone grafting.

A sulcular incision was placed around the involved teeth both on labial and palatal sides which exposed the fistula and the alveolar defect. A careful dissection was performed so as to separate the nasal layer and oral layer. The nasal layer was initially closed in a watertight manner. An adequate quantity of cancellous bone graft was harvested from the iliac crest. Thus obtained bone graft was placed into the alveolar defect, and a watertight closure was performed (Fig. 74.19f). The alveolar bone graft was assessed 6 months post-surgery using IOPA (Fig. 74.19g). The orthodontic treatment was completed after facilitating the eruption of canine and achieving leveling and alignment of teeth (Fig. 74.19h, i, j).

Future treatment required—Patient has to be assessed after growth completion, and if required the following treatment will have to be carried out:

- Pre-surgical orthodontics.
- Orthognathic surgery.
- Post-surgical orthodontics.
- Rhinoplasty.

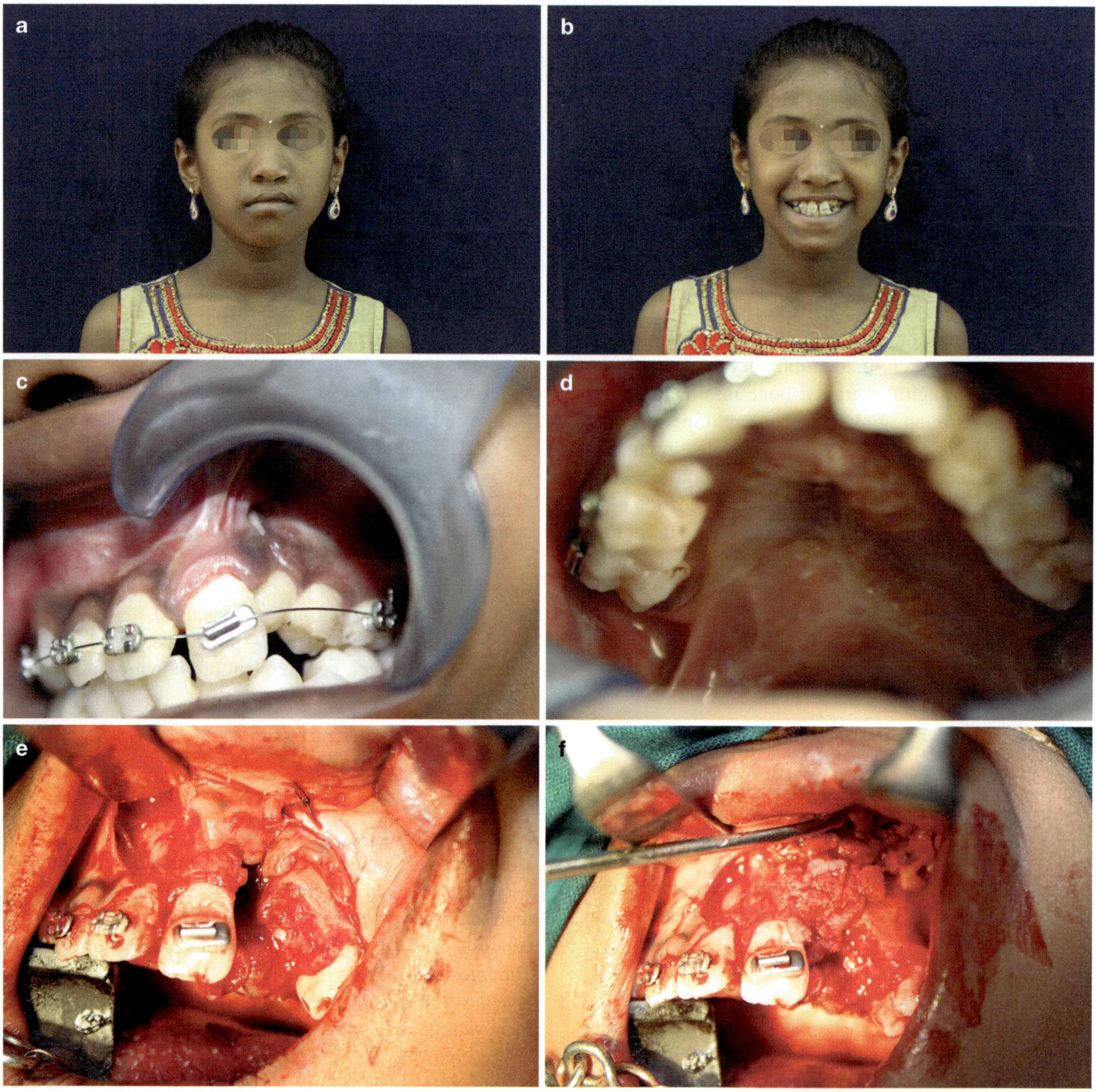

Fig. 74.18 (**a–f**) (**a**) Extraoral frontal picture at rest. (**b**) Extraoral frontal picture at smile. (**c**) Intraoral picture demonstrating fistula. (**d**) Palate post-repair. (**e**) Creation of a pouch in the alveolar cleft region to facilitate bone grafting. (**f**) Grafting of the alveolar cleft using harvested cancellous bone from the iliac crest. (Fig. 74.14 shows Watertight closure of the alveolar cleft case shown in Fig. 74.18, after grafting)

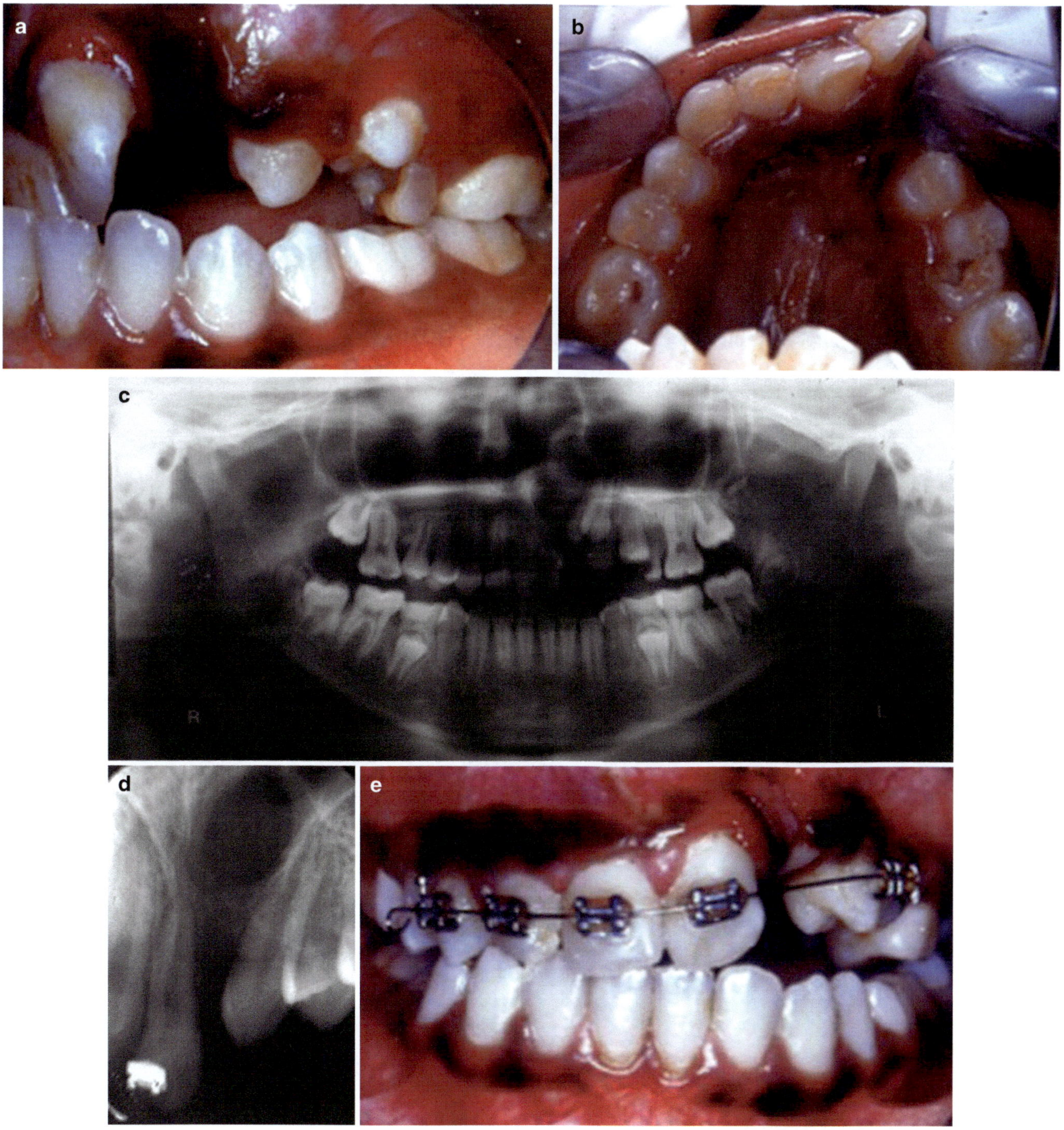

Fig. 74.19 (**a–j**) (**a**) Intraoral frontal picture demonstrating alveolar cleft on the left side of maxilla and associated fistula. (**b**) Intraoral maxillary occlusal picture demonstrating alveolar cleft and fistula. (**c**) OPG demonstrating the alveolar cleft on the left side and the eruptive status of the upper left permanent canine. (**d**) IOPA demonstrating the presence of alveolar cleft between upper left central incisor and upper left canine. (**e**) Intraoral frontal picture. Orthodontic treatment to facilitate tooth alignment and eruption of permanent upper left canine. (**f**) Intraoral picture demonstrating the completion of alveolar bone grafting. (**g**) IOPA demonstrating the uptake of alveolar bone graft in the region of alveolar cleft between upper left central incisor and upper left canine. (**h**) Intraoral frontal picture demonstrating orthodontic treatment. The permanent canine on the left side has been clinically moved to the occlusal plane. (**i**) Intraoral maxillary occlusal photograph post-orthodontic treatment demonstrating the eruption and alignment of upper left canine in the alveolar arch. (**j**) Intraoral photograph post-orthodontic treatment demonstrating the eruption and alignment of upper left canine in the alveolar arch

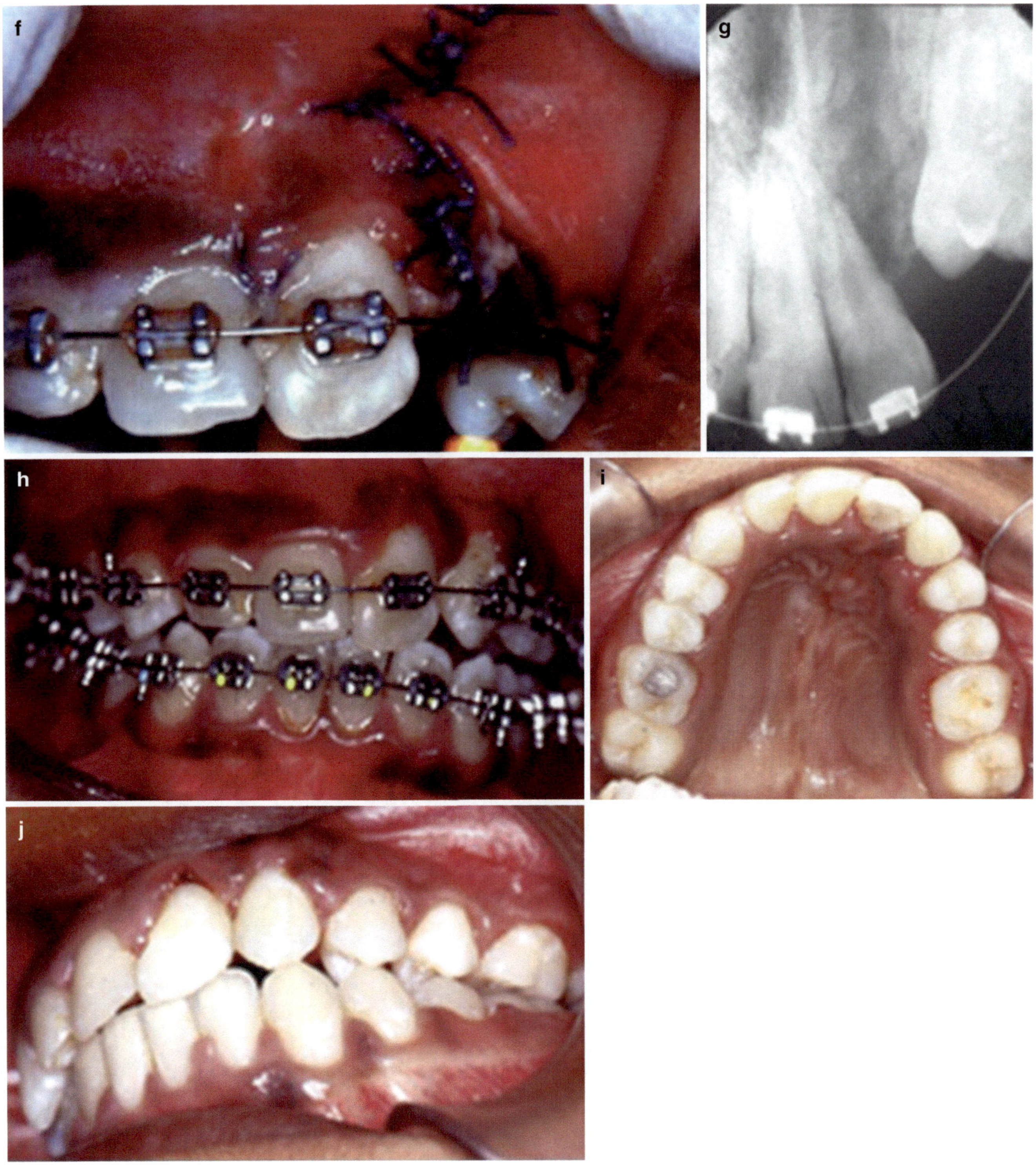

Fig. 74.19 (continued)

References

1. Mccarthy JG, editor. Plastic surgery. vol 1, General principles. Philadelphia: Saunders. p. 77.
2. Boyne PJ, Sands NR. Combined orthodontic-surgical management of residualpalato-alveolar cleft defects. Am J Orthod 1976 Jul;70(1):20–37. PubMed PMID:782258.
3. Boyne PJ, Sands NR. Secondary bone grafting of residual alveolar and palatal clefts. J Oral Surg 1972 Feb;30(2):87–92. PubMed PMID: 4550446.
4. Peterson's principles of Oral and Maxillofacial surgery, chapter 43, 2:867.
5. Deatherage J. Bone materials available for alveolar grafting. Oral Maxillofac Surg Clin North Am. 2010 Aug;22(3):347–52.
6. Swan MC, Goodacre TEE. Morbidity at the iliac crest donor site following bone grafting of the cleft alve. Br J Oral Maxillofac Surg. 2006;44:129–33.
7. Enemark H, Jensen J, Bosch C. Mandibular bone graft material for reconstruction of alveolar cleft defects: long-term results. Cleft Palate Craniofac J. 2001, March;38(2):155–63.
8. Hughes CW, Revington PJ. The proximity tibia donor site in cleft alveolar bone grafting: experience of 75 consecutive cases. J Cranio Maxillofac Surg. 2002;30:12–6.
9. Borstlap WA, Heidbuchel KLWM, Freihofe HPM, Kuijpers-Jagtman AM. Early secondary bone grafting of alveolar cleft defects – a comparison between Chin and Rib grafts. J Cranio Max Fac Surg. 1990;18:205.
10. Hibi H, Yamada Y, Ueda M, Endo Y. Alveolar cleft osteoplasty using tissue-engineered osteogenic material. Int J Oral Maxillofac Surg. 2006;35:551–5.
11. Chin M, Ng T, Tom WK, Carstens M. Repair of alveolar clefts with recombinant human bone morphogenetic protein (rhBMP-2) in patients with clefts. J Craniofac Surg. 2005;16(5):778–89.
12. Bergland O, Semb G, Abyholm F. Elimination of residual alveolar clefts by secondary bone grafting and subsequent orthodontic treatment. Cleft Palate J. 1986;23:175–205.
13. Khalil W, De Musis C, Volpato L, Veiga KA, EMM V, Aranha A. Clinical and radiographic assessment of secondary bone graft outcomes in cleft lip and palate patients. Int Sch Res Notices. 2014;2014:1–8.
14. Witherow H, Cox S, Jones E, Carr R, Waterhouse N. A new scale to assess radiographic success of secondary alveolar bone grafts. Cleft Palate Craniofac J. 2002;39(3):255–60.
15. Trindade-Suedam IK, da Silva Filho OG, Carvalho RM, et al. Timing of alveolar bone grafting determines different outcomes in patients with unilateral cleft palate. J Craniofac Surg. 2012;23(5):1283–6.
16. Kindelan JD, Nashed RR, Bromige MR. Radiographic assessment of secondary alveolar bone grafting in cleft lip and palate patients. Cleft Palate Craniofacial J. 1997;34:195–8.

Cleft Maxillary Hypoplasia

75

Philip Mathew, Mustafa. K, and Paul Mathai

75.1 Introduction

Studies of adult patients with unoperated cleft lip and palate (CLP) indicate that the maxilla in the unoperated patient is normally positioned or protruded. There are two major factors contributing to the protruded maxilla. The first is the absence of normal functional forces that are provided by the perioral muscle and tissue continuity. The tongue pressure pushes the teeth and the alveolus forward while the pressure from the cleft lip and affected perioral tissues is insufficient to balance this force out. The second factor contributing to the prognathic maxilla is the missing surgical scar [1–3].

Studies comparing unoperated cleft lip cases versus those with cleft lip repair show minimal difference in the growth of the maxilla. Thus, it has been proven that cheiloplasty has little effect on the growth of the maxilla and its dentition. On the other hand, palatal surgery has been identified as the main cause of inhibition of midface growth. Scar tissue forms across sutural areas as a result of palatoplasty surgery. This scar tissue interferes in the downward and forward translation of the maxilla that plays a major role in normal development. Furthermore, the scar tissue across the palate causes the constriction of the maxilla leading to a collapsed bite or crossbite [1–3].

Maxillary hypoplasia is a secondary deformity that occurs as a result of cleft lip and palate surgery with a reported incidence of about 9–45% with isolated cleft lip cases having the lowest incidence. The need for surgical correction of the same can be identified as early as age 10. Factors frequently associated with maxillary hypoplasia are congenitally missing maxillary teeth, revision palatoplasty procedures, pharyngeal flaps, and delayed orthodontic care [4–7]. However, recent evidence has suggested that presence of a pharyngeal flap does not affect maxillary growth [8].

75.2 Features of Cleft Maxillary Hypoplasia

Cleft maxillary hypoplasia presents as a three-dimensional deficiency. The degree of deficiency increases with the severity of orofacial clefting and affects different anatomical subunits, e.g., dentoalveolar, para-nasal, infra-orbital, and zygomatic regions. The clinical features associated with cleft maxillary hypoplasia are described in Boxes 75.1–75.3 [1–3, 7].

The presence of the cleft alveolus causes the dentoalveolar segment to collapse palatally on the affected side(s) leading to the creation of anterior and posterior crossbites. The failure to perform an alveolar bone grafting and orthodontics during the growing phase increases the severity of the malocclusion [9, 10]. The extent of this abnormal growth of the midface varies from mild to severe and is also affected by genetic endowment, the severity of clefting (extent of orofacial and labio-palatal involvement), timing of surgery, surgeon skills, and the number of primary and revision surgeries performed in the process of re-habilitating the patient. It has not been conclusively proven if any particular palate closure technique or if a staged technique has reduced effects on maxillary growth. It is the author's opinion that techniques that leave a raw area on the palate like push-back palatoplasty are generally associated with greater maxillary regression [1–3, 11–15].

Disclosures: The authors have no financial conflicts to disclose

Electronic Supplementary Material The online version of this chapter (https://doi.org/10.1007/978-981-15-1346-6_75) contains supplementary material, which is available to authorized users.

P. Mathew (✉)
Head of Department of Oral and Maxillofacial Surgery, Jubilee Mission Medical College and Hospital, Thrissur, Kerala, India

Mustafa. K
Department of Craniofacial Surgery, Kanachur Institute of Medical Sciences, Mangalore, Karnataka, India

P. Mathai
Senior Resident cum Fellow of Orthognathic Surgery, Department of Oral and Maxillofacial Surgery, Jubilee Mission Medical College and Hospital, Thrissur, Kerala, India

K. Bonanthaya et al. (eds.), *Oral and Maxillofacial Surgery for the Clinician*, https://doi.org/10.1007/978-981-15-1346-6_75

Box 75.1: Primary Features of Cleft Maxillary Hypoplasia

- Concave facial profile
- Class 3 skeletal relationship,
- Increased scleral show,
- Lack of normal cheek contour,
- Inadequate support of nasal tip and upper lip,
- Short upper lip and Acute nasolabial angle [subject to variability],
- Steep mandibular plane angle,
- Retruded chin,
- Decreased posterior facial height,
- Increased anterior facial height,
- Anterior and posterior cross bites,
- Increased mandibular plane – cranial base angle,
- Anterior open bite [less common],
- Chin and mandibular skeletal asymmetry [less common].

Box 75.2: Secondary Residual Deformities in Cleft Lip and Palate Patients

- Speech and hearing impairments (chronic otitis and velopharyngeal insufficiency)
- Residual oronasal fistula
- Residual bony defects
- Obstructive nasal breathing (septum deformity/ enlarged inferior turbinates/intranasal strictures/ enlarged tonsils and adenoids/pharyngeal flaps)

Box 75.3: Dental Anomalies in Cleft Lip and Palate Patients

- Delayed eruption of teeth, severe crowding of arches (with impacted, malformed and supernumerary teeth)
- Palatally collapsed dentoalveolar segments (cleft side)
- Anterior and posterior crossbites
- Anomalous or missing lateral incisor, infra-erupted, rotated, and tipped cleft-adjacent teeth

In most cases, photographic and cephalometric analysis reveals that the mandibular plane-cranial base angle is increased leading to a more backwardly placed mandible. Thus, the mandible tends to have a mild retrognathic appearance in spite of having normal dimensions. An anterior open bite is observed if the patient has an underlying tongue thrust habit as well. In certain rare cases, the chin and mandible may also exhibit a degree of skeletal asymmetry [1–3] (Box 75.2).

The need for orthognathic surgery should be based not only on occlusion and jaw relationship but also on facial proportions, midface projection, and complaints of the patient [1–3].

75.3 Objectives of Treatment (Box 75.4)

Box 75.4: Objectives of Treatment in Cleft Maxillary Hypoplasia

1. To improve facial aesthetics
2. To improve psychological health
3. Achieve adequate occlusion for efficient mastication
4. Improve phonation and airway dimensions
5. Avoid deterioration of velopharyngeal insufficiency

75.4 Sequencing Treatment in CMH (Box 75.5)

Box 75.5: Sequencing Treatment in CMH

1. Growth modulation—7–16 years.
2. Phase 1 orthodontics—7–11 years
3. Alveolar bone grafting—8–11 years
4. Phase 2 orthodontics—12–17 years
5. Anterior maxillary distraction—after 12 years
6. Orthognathic surgery at 17 years and up
7. Phase 3 orthodontics after orthognathic surgery

75.5 Orthodontics in Cleft Lip and Palate Patients

Owing to the severity of the condition, period of orthodontics can be prolonged and is carried out in three phases. Sometimes patients with CLP have a limited ability to open their mouth further increasing the difficulty of orthodontic treatment.

Phase 1 Treatment It is carried out between 7 and 12 years of age. Maxillary transverse expansion is carried out in cases that present with maxillary constriction. Maxillary protraction may be carried out in cases with significant midface regression. This phase also involves monitoring facial growth, space management, monitoring eruption of permanent teeth, and preventing ectopic eruption of permanent teeth [1–3].

In preparation for secondary alveolar bone grafting, extractions of supernumerary teeth and deciduous teeth on either side of the cleft and closure of oronasal fistulae are performed [16]. Box 75.6 outlines the controversy regarding whether maxillary expansion should be performed before or after alveolar bone grafting [17–19].

Box 75.6: Arch expansion, before or after Alveolar Bone Grafting (ABG)

Expansion before ABG	Expansion after ABG
Greater expansion can be achieved with the lower bony resistance between the maxillary segments	Though expansion is possible, the degree of expansion obtained is less predictable
Nasal floor mucosa layer can be easily visualized and reconstructed as the cleft has been widened	Difficult to visualize and reconstruct the nasal floor mucosa layer as the cleft is narrow
Widening of the cleft alveolus leads to increased tension on the overlying suture site after grafting, which increases the risk of wound dehiscence and graft failure	As the cleft is narrow at the time of grafting, there is lesser tension on the overlying suture site after grafting, which reduces the risk of wound dehiscence and graft failure
Increased risk for cleft-adjacent teeth moving into the cleft alveolus while widening, thus compromising their periodontal support	Decreased risk of loss of periodontal support as the teeth will move into an already grafted cleft alveolus
Clinical studies have shown that there is minimal risk for graft loss when expansion was performed before grafting	Clinical studies have shown that bone graft was not lost when expansion was performed after grafting; instead, some degree of stimulation of graft took place

Phase 2 (Presurgical phase) Treatment It is carried out between 12 and 17 years of age. It involves maintaining the previously attained expansion and further expanding the arch in cases of relapse or if no prior expansion was done. In case the skeletal discrepancy is minimal, we can also consider camouflage orthodontics to correct the occlusal discrepancy. Camouflage orthodontics involves correction of crowding and rotations, extraction of teeth that have erupted ectopically and cannot be accommodated, proclination of maxillary incisors, and retraction of mandibular incisors.

In case the skeletal discrepancy is moderate to severe, then we will have to consider surgical correction (distraction osteogenesis or orthognathic surgery) of the deformity. Presurgical fixed orthodontics is started to facilitate the planned skeletal movements and is described in Box 75.7.

Box 75.7: Objectives of Pre-surgical Orthodontics

- Removal of dental compensations
- Alignment of teeth, de-crowding and de-rotation of teeth
- Flattening of the curve of Spee
- Incorporating divergence in roots for segmental osteotomies
- Co-ordination of dental arches

In case the lateral incisor is missing, the decision to maintain space for prosthetic rehabilitation or substitute it with the adjacent canine needs to be made during this phase [1–3]. There is also a need to extract the mandibular third molars in case a bilateral sagittal split osteotomy is planned. There is an increased risk for bad splits associated with un-erupted and impacted mandibular third molars in the age group of less than 20 years on account of thinner and immature cortical bone [20].

Phase 3 (Postsurgical Phase) Treatment It is performed after surgical correction of the facial deformity (orthognathic surgery or distraction osteogenesis). It involves fine-tuning of the occlusion and maintaining achieved results in the long term through retentive appliances. One may have to consider re-creating dental compensations to accommodate for increased rates of relapse after cleft-orthognathic surgery.

75.6 Considerations Before Surgery

75.6.1 Timing of Surgery

Facial growth is normally completed by 16 years of age in females and by 17 years of age in males. It is advisable to perform orthognathic surgery only after skeletal maturity is achieved, in order to increase stability of the surgical results in the long term. In selective cases, orthognathic surgery is performed during growth for psychosocial or functional reasons. However, this has shown unpredictable results because of continued growth of the mandible with relapse rates in the range of 50–70% when operated before 18 years of age [2, 21, 22].

As an alternative, one may consider distraction osteogenesis prior to 17 years of age. A study by Meazzini et al. [23] reported a relapse rate of 26% in the long term when distraction osteogenesis of the maxilla was carried out during the growing phase. A systematic review by Liu et al. [24] reported a relapse rate 12–46% at "point A" and 26–77% for the SNA angle in the long term. Thus, the patient will require additional surgery after skeletal maturity for correction of the residual facial deformity, irrespective of whether distraction osteogenesis or orthognathic surgery was performed.

75.6.2 Status of Alveolar Bone Grafting and Oronasal Fistulae

Patients with cleft lip and palate usually present with a cleft alveolus. This cleft communicates with the nasal cavity, thus, creating an oronasal fistula. The cleft is also a source of weakness in the maxillary arch and increases the risk of arch collapse, thus, creating dentoalveolar deformities (e.g., crossbites) which make later surgical procedures like orthognathic surgery unstable. Lastly, the permanent teeth that erupt into the cleft will have a poor prognosis due to lack of bony support and inadequate periodontium. Thus, it is of utmost importance to graft the cleft alveolar region, and the benefits associated with it are described in Box 75.8 [9, 25].

Box 75.8: Benefits of Alveolar Bone Grafting

Reduction of oronasal fistula, creation of continuity of the maxillary alveolar arch, eruption of permanent teeth into the cleft site, elevation of the alar nasal base, and stability for future surgical procedures like orthognathic surgery and rhinoplasty

A prerequisite to a successful alveolar bone grafting is the closure of oronasal fistulae. Small fistulae can be closed at the time of grafting. However, the presence of a large fistula requires a staged reconstruction with the fistula closure initially and alveolar bone grafting later.

It is not rare to see a patient with a complaint of maxillary regression who presents at a later age (17 years and above) with a history of no alveolar bone grafting or failed alveolar bone grafting. If we proceed with a LeFort I osteotomy in this clinical scenario, the difficulty of the surgical procedure increases significantly as the maxilla is not a single unit. There are three possible treatment protocols that we can follow:

1. The patient is willing to undergo a staged approach with alveolar bone grafting followed by orthognathic surgery at later stage. Though this is the ideal approach, it adds to the cost and time of overall treatment. It is important to note that tertiary alveolar bone grafting has an overall lower success rate [26, 27].
2. The patient is willing to undergo alveolar bone grafting as long as it is done simultaneously with orthognathic surgery. This approach saves time and cost of overall treatment. Keeping in mind that tertiary alveolar bone grafting already has a lower success rate; it is the author's opinion that risk for graft failure might increase when this step is combined with orthognathic surgery. This is on account of the compromise in vascularity that occurs as extensive mucoperisoteal flap refelction is performed to accomodate orthognathic surgery.
3. In case the patient wants to avoid bone grafting, one can use the modified LeFort I osteotomy approach by Posnick et al. [3, 28, 29]. It allows for simultaneous correction of maxillary hypoplasia, cleft dental gaps, alveolar defects, and small residual oronasal fistulas through the use of modified skeletal osteotomies. The cleft alveolar defect is closed by differential repositioning of the cleft maxilla segments. This technique requires a transverse plate to be placed across the cleft site just below the pyriform aperture so as to convert the cleft-maxilla into a single unit. In a study by Posnick et al. [30], the modified LeFort I osteotomy technique had stable results in more than 90% of the subjects at 1 year with a low complication rate. It is the author's opinion that along with the midline transverse plate, one can also use a dental prosthesis (fixed partial denture) spanning the cleft alveolus site to add stability to the cleft maxilla. However, there is a risk for failure of the prosthesis and loss of abutment teeth in the long term due to increased movement across the cleft alveolus site.

75.6.3 Velopharyngeal Insufficiency (VPI)

If air or sound is allowed to leak through or resonate in the nasal cavity during the production of the non-nasal sounds (all phonemes except /m/, /n/, and /ng/), speech will be marked by hyper-nasality (nasal twang) and nasal air emission. VPI describes a structural or anatomic defect that prevents closure of the velopharyngeal mechanism during function. It is most commonly observed in patients with an overt cleft palate (unoperated > operated cases) and submucous cleft palate. In operated cleft palate patients, the incidence of VPI can range between 20 and 50% [31]. Chua et al. [32] and Pereira et al. [33] proposed the usage of perceptual speech assessment, acoustic measurement with nasometer, video nasoendoscopy (or video fluoroscopy), and cephalometric analysis for the assessment of preoperative speech and VPI.

When the maxilla is advanced in operated cases of the cleft palate, speech articulation is improved on account of improved lip competency and correction of previous dental malocclusion [34, 35]. There is also an associated increase in the velopharyngeal cavity depth [36]. As compared to the normal palate, the scarred cleft palate has decreased ability to adapt to such changes as it is unable to stretch adequately [37] This leads to an increase in the risk for worsening of preoperative VPI. The effect of maxillary advancement on VPI, especially in cleft palate patients, is still a controversial topic [34, 38].

There are two methods that are commonly used to advance the maxilla as given in Box 75.9.

Box 75.9: Methods Used for Maxillary Advancement

1. Distraction osteogenesis: total maxillary distraction and anterior maxillary distraction
   (a) Total maxillary distraction: internal maxillary distraction and rigid external distraction
2. Conventional orthognathic surgery

The theoretical advantage of distraction is that the maxilla is advanced slowly which allows the patient to adapt to the changes in the velopharyngeal dimensions through increased velar muscle activity. Furthermore, distraction can be halted at any point of time that speech begins to deteriorate. Orthognathic surgery, unlike distraction, creates an immediate surgical advancement of the maxilla and does not allow speech to be assessed incrementally or allow for gradual adaption of the palate to the increase in the velopharyngeal cavity depth.

A randomized controlled trial by Chua et al. [32] for moderate maxillary advancement (4–10 mm) in cleft patients demonstrated that distraction osteogenesis had no advantage over orthognathic surgery for the purpose of preventing velopharyngeal incompetence and speech disturbance. Furthermore, no correlation was found between the amount of advancement and speech parameters. However, it should be noted that extreme advancements of the maxilla (greater than 10 mm) were excluded from the study.

A study by McComb et al. [37] helped identify predictors for worsening of VPI in cases of cleft maxillary advancement using conventional orthognathic surgery. Short preoperative soft palate, large postoperative velopharyngeal cavity depth, preoperative perceptual speech assessment, nasometry, and video nasoendoscopy were identified as clinically significant predictors. Preoperative velopharyngeal cavity depth was not considered a satisfactory predictor as changes in the velopharyngeal space did not correspond proportionally to maxillary advancement [39]. Lastly, the span of maxillary advancement (2–16 mm) did not show a significant association with the worsening of VPI [37].

Janulewicz et al. [35], Philips et al. [40], Alaluusua [41], Smedberg [42], Seok-Kwun Kim et al. [43], Kelly Schultz et al. [44], and Pereira et al. [33] studied the relation between postoperative worsening of VPI and maxillary advancement using conventional LeFort I osteotomy in cleft patients. They established that preoperative borderline and higher grades of VPI were highly prone to worsening in the postoperative phase. Absent to negligible VPI pre-operatively, carries minimal risk of worsening during the post-operative period. Furthermore, the amount of maxillary advancement and the cleft type did not influence the degree of worsening of VPI. In the author's opinion, the only confounding factor in the above studies was that some of the patients already had a preoperative pharyngeal flap.

A study by Trindade et al. [45] suggested that deterioration in the VPI after orthognathic surgery was transient and improved over time. Compensatory changes are known to occur in the velopharyngeal region during that time as documented by the study of Yu Wu et al. [36]. The velar length and angle and the velopharyngeal depth all increased. However, velar thickness, posterior pharyngeal wall thickness, and velar motility remained unchanged. During certain phonations, the motion of the posterior pharyngeal wall and the thickness of the Passavant's ridge increased significantly. Thus, it is advisable to wait for at least 1 year prior to considering surgical correction for VPI [35].

Poole et al. [46] and James et al. [47] suggested alternative surgical approaches to the routine LeFort I maxillary advancement which involved transecting the palatal mucosa followed by mobilizing the soft palate lying distal to the incision. This was combined with strategically placed vertical incisions in the maxillary buccal mucosa to avoid circulation injury. The advantage of the procedure was that the maxilla could be advanced by large amounts without worsening of speech and VPI as the soft palate did not move anteriorly with the maxilla. The disadvantage of the procedure was that a significant portion of the palate was left denuded and was expected to heal secondarily. Though the results were promising, the techniques did not become mainstream.

Anterior maxillary distraction (AMD) is a versatile, stable, and simple technique that can be used to correct the maxillary dentoalveolar regression in the cleft maxilla after the mixed dentition phase (Video 75.1). As the osteotomy is anterior to the junction of the hard and soft palate, the velopharyngeal dimensions and soft palate activity are not affected. Thus, it is considered optimal for the correction of cleft maxillary regression in cases with preoperative moderate to severe VPI. When used in the age group of 10–16 years, there is also an associated posterior movement of the distal maxilla owing to the elasticity of the bone which may also reduce preoperative VPI to a certain extent. An added advantage is that the increased arch length can be used to accommodate un-erupted teeth and correct crowding [48–53].

In case postoperative VPI develops, it is advisable to wait and watch for at least 1 year prior to resorting to surgical correction. During this period, one can try conservative methods like speech therapy and bulb palatal lift prosthesis and minimally invasive methods like autologous fat injections into the soft palate and the posterior pharyngeal wall [31, 54, 55]. If the VPI does not improve to a clinically acceptable level even after a year, then surgical options need to be considered.

In terms of risk of development of postoperative obstructive sleep apnea, Furlow palatoplasty and buccal myomucosal flaps have the least adverse effect followed by sphincter pharyngoplasty and finally pharyngeal flap which has the most adverse effect [56, 57]. Nonetheless, the pharyngeal flap is the most commonly used method, and a recent paper by Dentino et al. [58] demonstrated that the superiorly based pharyngeal flap was highly successful in correcting VPI after cleft maxillary advancement.

75.6.4 Degree of Maxillary Hypoplasia

The classification of cleft maxillary hypoplasia is given in Box 75.10.

Box 75.10: Classification of Maxillary Hypoplasia

- Mild cases—reverse overjet below 6 mm
- Moderate cases—reverse overjet between 6 and 10 mm
- Severe cases—reverse jet between 11 and 16 mm
- Extreme cases—reverse overjet equal to or greater than 17 mm

The above classification of maxillary hypoplasia needs to be combined with the age at which the patient presents for optimal treatment planning. It should be noted that the regression is calculated only on the basis of reverse dental overjet. The presence or severity of para-nasal hollowing is not accounted for in the above classification.

75.7 Treatment Plans

75.7.1 Pearls for Treatment Planning

- If surgical treatment (distraction osteogenesis or orthognathic surgery) is performed prior to the skeletal maturity, there is a high chance of relapse due to continued skeletal growth. Thus, additional surgery will be required to correct the residual skeletal deformity. Nonetheless, distraction osteogenesis is preferred over orthognathic surgery in the growing patient.
- Time constraints and patient's needs might require you to modify the ideal treatment plan. Though the overall facial profile is important, it is equally essential to establish a functional occlusion with positive overjet and good intercuspation as they go a long way in preventing relapse.
- Procedures like camouflage orthodontics, face mask protraction, and anterior maxillary distraction produce a greater change at the dentoalveolar level and fail to significantly improve para-nasal hollowing. In case of AMD, the anterior maxillary osteotomy does not extend sufficiently enough in to the posterior and superior aspect of the zygomaticomaxillary buttress region.
- Orthognathic surgery and total maxillary distraction (TMD; subtypes, internal maxillary distraction and rigid external distraction) can both correct para-nasal hollowing when combined with a modified high-level LeFort I osteotomy.
- While operating, the facial profile and occlusion can be immediately appreciated during orthognathic surgery. Results can similarly be approximated in total maxillary distraction (TMD) by activating the distractor to the desired extent on the operating table. This is possible as the posterior extent of a conventional LeFort I osteotomy lies in the region of the more mobile soft palate.
- While performing anterior maxillary distraction, the final facial profile and occlusion cannot be immediately appreciated on the OT table as the posterior extent of the maxillary osteotomy lies anterior to the permanent first molar. The palatal mucosa in this region is firmly attached to the underlying bone, and excessive activation of the distractor can lead to stripping of the mucosa from the underlying bone.
- Masticatory efficiency is not significantly compromised during AMD, as the device is fairly rigid and the posterior limit of the osteotomy is anterior to the permanent first molars. A complete LeFort I osteotomy, like that used in total maxillary distraction (TMD), reduces masticatory efficiency on account of increased mobility of the whole maxilla on the application of masticatory loads.
- One needs to take into account that a reverse overjet of "x mm" requires a net advancement of "$x + 2$ mm" to obtain adequate overjet and overbite. Hence, a reverse overjet of 8 mm requires a net advancement of 10 mm for adequate correction. If one wants to accommodate for expected relapse, then one needs to overcorrect by at least 20%. Hence, the actual amount of advancement required would be 10 + 2, i.e., 12 mm.
- Limits of movements with orthognathic surgery: Conventional orthognathic surgical advancement of the maxilla beyond 10 mm increases the risk of relapse on account of the scar tissue in the soft palate and upper lip

regions. As the mandible is usually unaffected in cleft maxillary hypoplasia, a setback beyond 8 mm leads to a poor aesthetic result and is also associated with higher relapse rates.

- A reverse overjet of 16 mm in cleft maxillary hypoplasia requires a net advancement of 18 mm. The maxilla can be advanced by 10 mm, and the mandible can be setback by 8 mm to achieve the desired correction. Thus, a reverse overjet of 16 mm can be treated by orthognathic surgery with acceptable stability in the long term. Although it is possible to treat a reverse overjet greater than 16 mm with orthognathic surgery, it is associated with a higher relapse rate.
- When the cleft maxilla is advanced > 10 mm, there is an increased risk of damage to the palatal vascular pedicle on account of the inability of the scarred soft palate to stretch and accommodate the change [59]. Furthermore, there is also risk of suture site dehiscence in the maxillary labial vestibule as this region would be closed under tension on account of the presence of scarred tissue with minimal elasticity [37, 60].
- Distraction osteogenesis (AMD/TMD) can be used for all spans of maxillary advancement and is preferred for advancements > 10 mm on account of the stability of results in the long term [61, 62]. There is also minimal risk of damage to the palatal vascular pedicle as the advancement is gradual and a certain degree of histogenesis accompanies the distraction osteogenesis.
- The span of movement (small or large) or mode of advancement (total maxillary distraction or orthognathic surgery) is not to be associated with an increased risk for deterioration of preoperative VPI.
  - Determining preoperative speech and VPI status is a must: perceptual speech assessment, acoustic measurement with nasometer, video nasoendoscopy (or video fluoroscopy), and lateral cephalometric analysis.
  - If there is no preoperative VPI, then there is minimal risk for worsening of speech and occurrence of VPI postoperatively.
  - If there is borderline (or greater) VPI preoperatively, then there is a high risk for worsening of VPI postoperatively.
  - Wait for at least 1 year before considering surgical correction of postoperative VPI.

75.7.2 Age Group of 6–11 Years (Fig. 75.1)

The patient has a mixed dentition during this phase. There are multiple un-erupted dental follicles present that can pose a problem to certain surgical procedures. Alveolar bone grafting is preferably performed during this phase as it is associated with higher success rates [26]. Large oronasal fistulae, if present, need to be closed prior to secondary alveolar bone grafting.

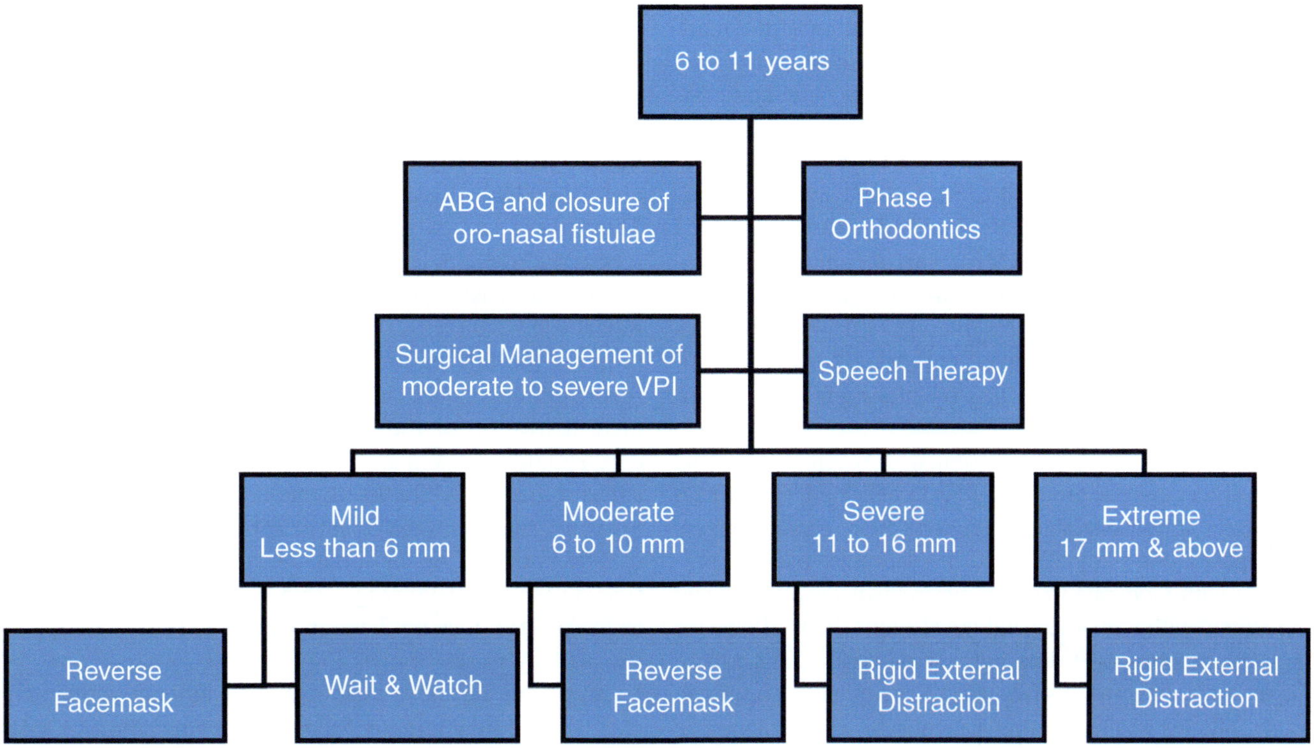

Fig. 75.1 Treatment plan for age group 6–11 years

If the child presents with a mild regression, one can choose to wait and watch or proceed with dentofacial orthopedics using a reverse pull headgear to achieve protraction of the maxilla. If the child presents with moderate regression, then one must proceed with reverse pull headgear therapy to achieve some degree of correction.

The usage of reverse facemask therapy requires considerable patient co-operation and works by stimulating growth at the various maxillary suture sites (Fig. 75.2a–c). It is usually combined with a maxillary expansion appliance that helps disrupt the circum-maxillary sutural system and increase the effects of the orthopedic face mask. The general effect produced is that of a downward and forward movement of the maxilla, backward rotation of the mandible, and a net increase in the lower facial height. However, the response varies widely from individual to individual, and long-term stability is also questionable [7, 63–66].

The stability and extent of correction with reverse facemask therapy reduces with increasing severity of labiopalatal clefting and absence (or failure) of prior alveolar bone grafting [63–66]. The degree of ossification of the zygomaticomaxillary buttress also plays an important role in the results of facial protraction therapy. Earlier stages (younger age group) of ossification are associated with a greater span of movement and skeletal and dental changes. Later stages of ossification (older age group) are associated with a smaller span of movement and mainly dentoalveolar changes [67, 68]. Today, skeletal anchorage is slowly replacing traditional tooth borne anchorage on account of better control of degree of rotation of the mandible and greater potential for skeletal movements [69, 70]. In patients who are less co-operative, one can consider using a modified technique with inter-maxillary elastics between a miniplate secured to the zygomaticomaxillary buttress region posteriorly and another miniplate secured to the mandible anteriorly (Bone-anchored maxillary protraction - BAMP). This technique has provided promising results which are comparable to traditional reverse facemask therapy. However, this modification can be performed only after the eruption of the mandibular canine to allow for plating in the anterior mandible [69, 71, 72].

Very rarely will a child present with severe or extreme regression in this age group. Rigid external distraction (RED) is the only option available for the correction of such a severe discrepancy and is mainly used in syndromic patients presenting with moderate to severe obstructive sleep apnea and in patients with a poor psychological status. RED allows for high osteotomies as it does not rely on rigid fixation techniques to secure the distractor. This helps avoid injury to tooth follicles in the growing patient while simultaneously correcting para-nasal hollowing. On the contrary, internal total maxillary distraction (ITMD) and anterior maxillary distraction (AMD) cannot be used as the lower-level osteotomies used in these procedures will damage the un-erupted dental follicles. The plates of the internal distractor also need to be secured to the bone with screws, which will also cause damage to the tooth follicles.

In spite of the above treatments, it is difficult to maintain results in the long term on account of continued mandibular growth. Thus, surgery will mostly be required once the patient reaches skeletal maturity to correct any residual skeletal deformity. However, the final amount of maxillary advancement will be much lesser resulting in increased post-operative stability of the cleft maxilla.

75.7.3 Age 12–16 Years (Fig. 75.3)

All permanent teeth (except the third molars) have erupted. The absence of un-erupted dental follicles makes procedures like AMD and ITMD (internal total maxillary distraction) feasible in this age group. Due to deficient arch length, there may be moderate to severe crowding. Some permanent teeth may have remained un-erupted, impacted, or erupted ectopically adding to the complexity of the treatment. If alveolar bone grafting has not been done prior or has failed, it needs to be performed during this phase. Large oronasal fistulae, if present, also need to be closed in preparation for orthognathic surgery.

If the regression is mild to moderate, one can consider camouflage orthodontics, maxillary protraction therapy, or AMD in order to create an acceptable occlusion. Alternatively, we can choose to wait and watch and directly correct the maxillary hypoplasia once growth is complete (Fig. 75.4a, b).

Severe to extreme maxillary regression is preferably treated with AMD. The available span of most commercially available hyrax screws does not exceed 13 mm. Thus, there are two options available to the clinician: repeat the AMD twice in a single stage or in a two-staged manner (at least 1 year apart) [50]. The author prefers to repeat the AMD activation twice, in a single stage. This requires the fabrication and immediate application of a fresh appliance, once the first appliance has attained complete activation of the incorporated Hyrax screw. Great care should be taken to avoid excessive pressure on the anterior maxilla while fitting the new appliance as the callus is not fully mature and large forces may easily destroy it. Alternatively, we can consider total maxillary distraction (ITMD or RED) (Figs. 75.5a–d and 75.6a–f) as long as the patient does not have moderate to severe preoperative VPI (Also see Fig. 70.17).

In spite of the above treatments, it is difficult to maintain results in the long term on account of continued mandibular growth. Thus, surgery will mostly be required once the patient reaches skeletal maturity to correct any residual skel-

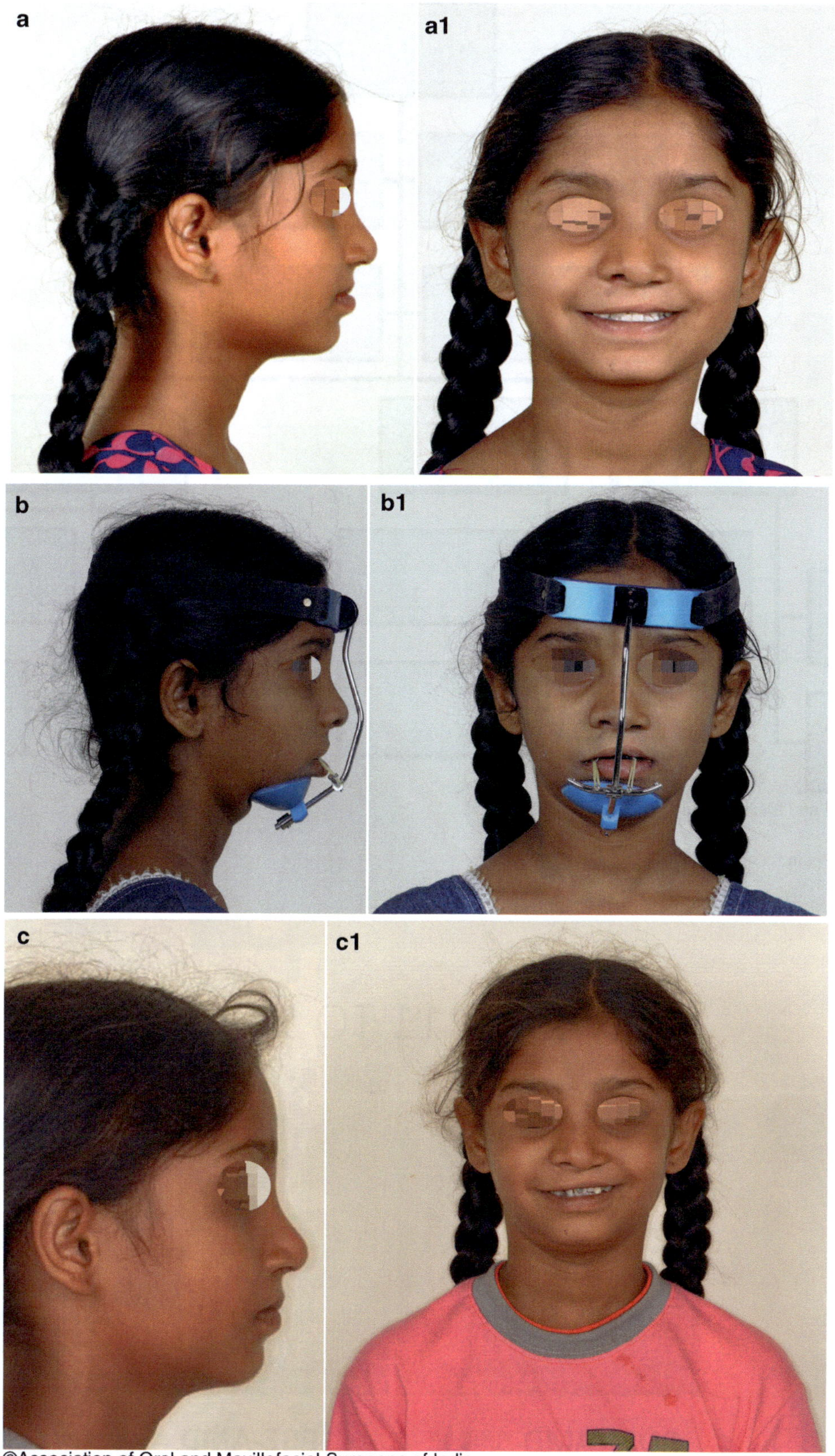

Fig. 75.2 (**a–c**) Reverse pull headgear therapy in a growing child with cleft maxillary hypoplasia. (**a**, **a1**) Pre-treatment profile and frontal photographs, (**b**, **b1**) Profile and frontal photographs of patient after application of "reverse-pull headgear", (**c**, **c1**) Post-treatment profile and frontal photographs demosntrating an improvement in the patient's profile

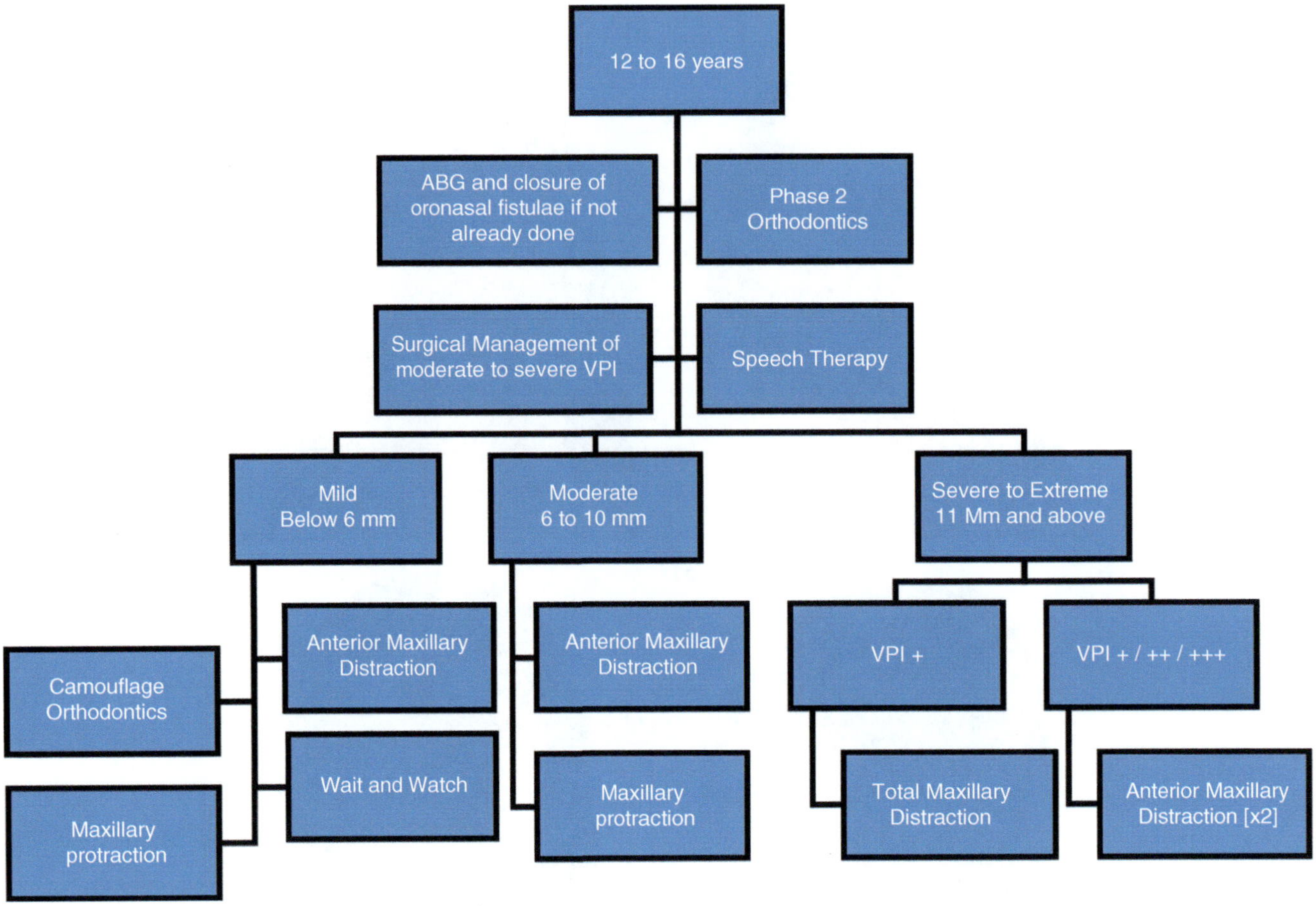

Fig. 75.3 Treatment plan for age group 12–16 years

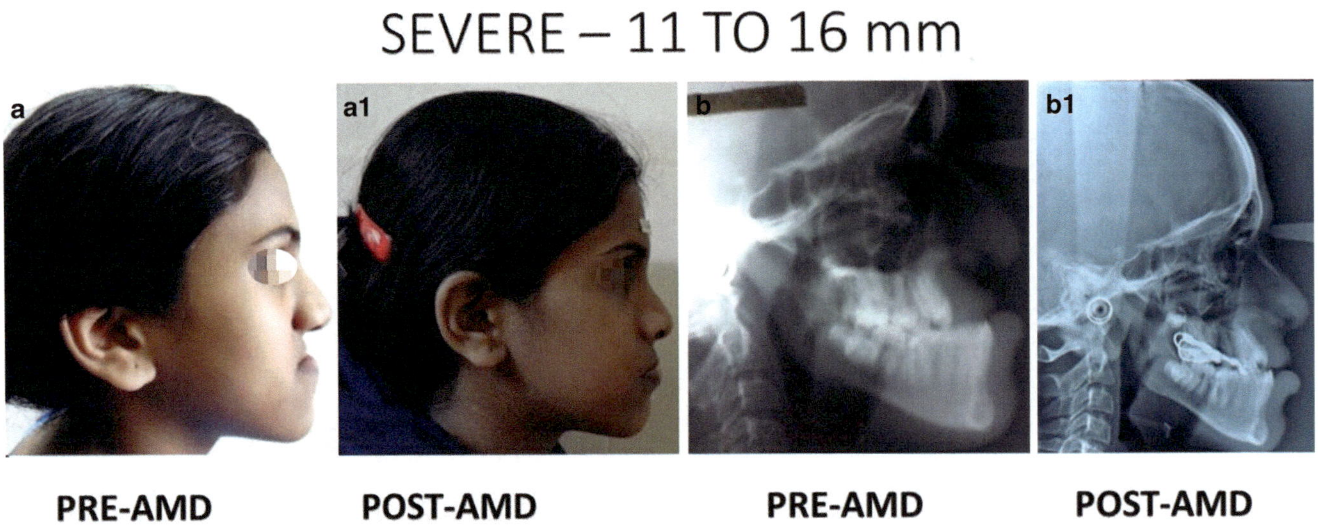

Fig. 75.4 (**a**, **b**) Severe reverse overjet at 14 years of age and mild VPI. Anterior maxillary distraction was performed (AMD). Final correction with orthognathic surgery to be done after 16 years of age

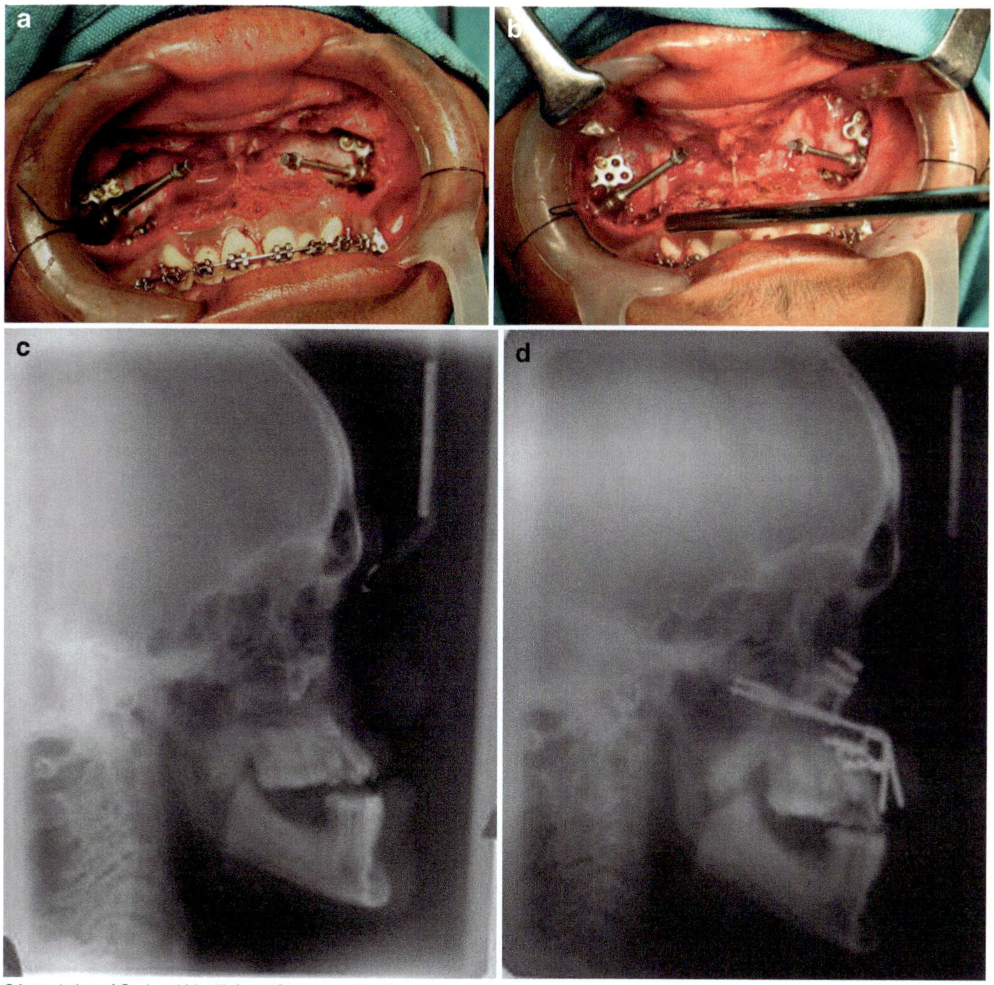

Fig. 75.5 (**a**–**d**) Use of internal maxillary distraction in the management of CMH. (**a**) Intra-operative positioning of internal maxillary ditractors, (**b**) post-distraction picture prior to the removal of distractor devices, (**c**) Pre-operative lateral cephalogram and (**d**) Post-operative lateral cephalogram demonstrating ditractor in-situ

etal deformity. However, the final amount of maxillary advancement will be much lesser resulting in increased post-operative stability of the cleft maxilla.

75.7.4 Age 17 Years and Above (Fig. 75.7)

If prior alveolar bone grafting has failed or has not been performed, a decision should be made as to whether it needs to be performed or not. Large oronasal fistulae, if present, need to be closed in preparation for orthognathic surgery.

If the regression is mild to moderate and VPI is absent or negligible, then either total maxillary distraction, AMD, or orthognathic surgery can be performed. Orthognathic surgery is preferred in this scenario as we can achieve immediate improvement in facial profile and occlusion (Figs. 75.8a–h, 75.9a–h). If there is moderate to severe VPI preoperatively, then it is advisable to perform AMD to avoid further deterioration of the same.

If the regression is severe to extreme and the VPI is absent or negligible, then either orthognathic surgery (Fig. 75.10a–f), AMD, or TMD can be performed. AMD may have to be repeated twice in the same sitting or in a stage manner as described previously. If optimal esthetics is the goal, then AMD followed by conventional LeFort I maxillary advancement is the ideal treatment plan (Fig. 75.11a–g). The only drawback of this procedure is the prolonged treatment duration as a minimum waiting period

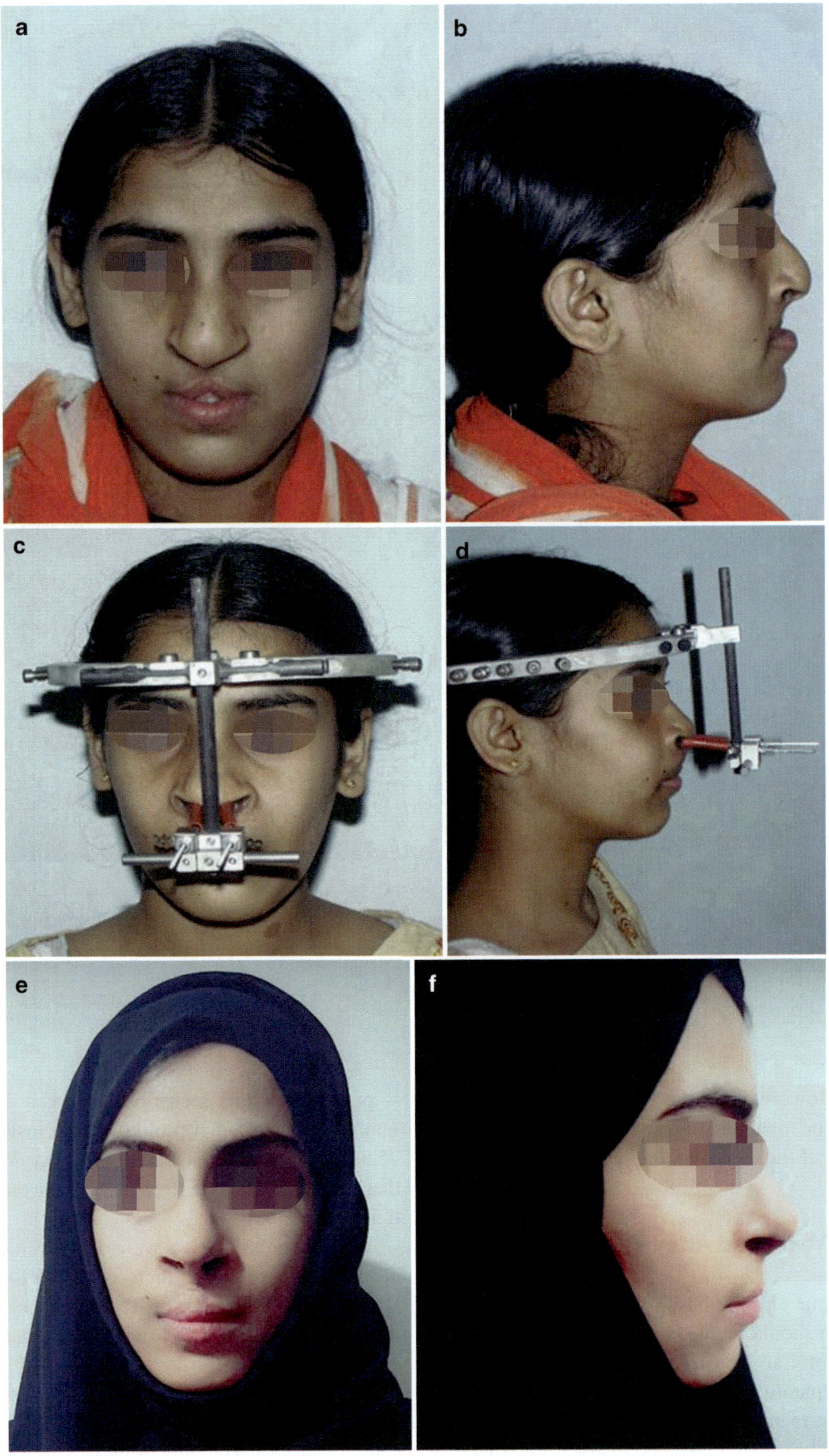

Fig. 75.6 (**a–f**) Patient treated with rigid external distractor (RED). (**a**, **b**) Pre-operative frontal and profile photographs, demonstating hypoplastic midface and concave profile. (**c**, **d**) Frontal and profile photographs showing RED in situ. (**e**, **f**) Post-operative frontal and profile photographs demonstrating good midface fullness and a convex facial profile

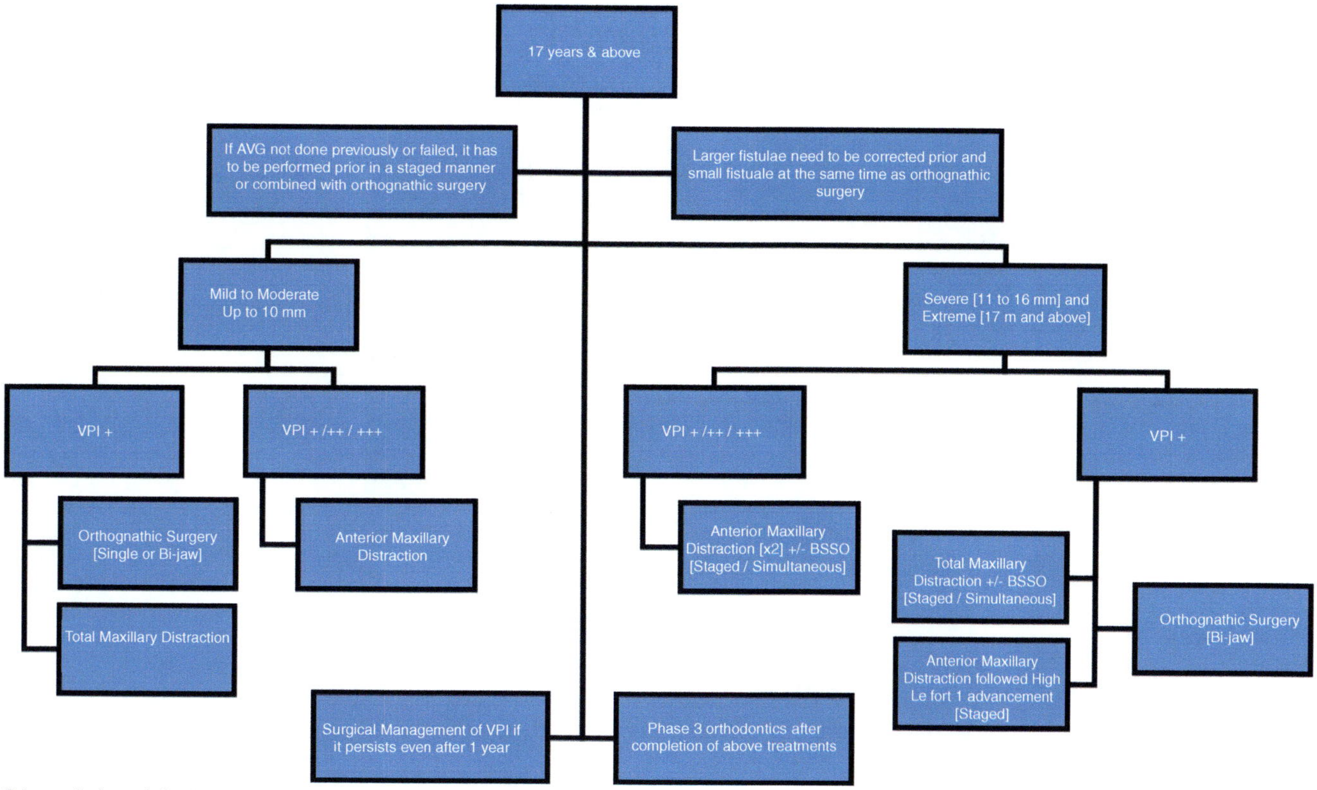

Fig. 75.7 Treatment plan for age group 17 years and above

of 1 year is needed between both surgeries. If there is moderate to severe VPI preoperatively, then it is advisable to perform AMD to avoid further deterioration of the same. As a means of saving time or if the mandible is truly prognathic, AMD and TMD can be combined with a mandibular setback (using bilateral sagittal split osteotomy) in a simultaneous or staged manner to reduce the span needed to be distracted [73].

75.8 LeFort I Procedure for Cleft Maxillary Hypoplasia

The protocol preferred by the authors is described below.

75.8.1 Preoperative Investigations

The preoperative investigations are described in Box 75.11.

Chronic Maxillary Sinusitis Most CLP patients suffer from chronic maxillary sinusitis on account of the presence of nasal obstructions and residual oronasal fistulae. It is the author's opinion that such patients need to be referred to an ENT specialist at least 3 months prior as active sinusitis affects the quality of the bone in the maxilla.

Box 75.11: Preoperative Investigations

Primary Investigations

Clinical diagnosis, pre-anesthetic assessment (blood investigations, chest x-ray, ECG, additional investigations for any significant medical history), facial photographs, cephalometric analysis (lateral cephalogram and postero-anterior cephalogram), articulated study models with bite registration and facebow transfer, dental model analysis, orthopantomogram, perceptual speech assessment, video nasoendoscopy (or video fluoroscopy) for velopharyngeal insufficiency, psychological screening, and patient education regarding realistic expectations

Adjunctive Investigations

3D computed tomography scans, stereolithographic model, sleep studies, and 3D virtual surgical planning

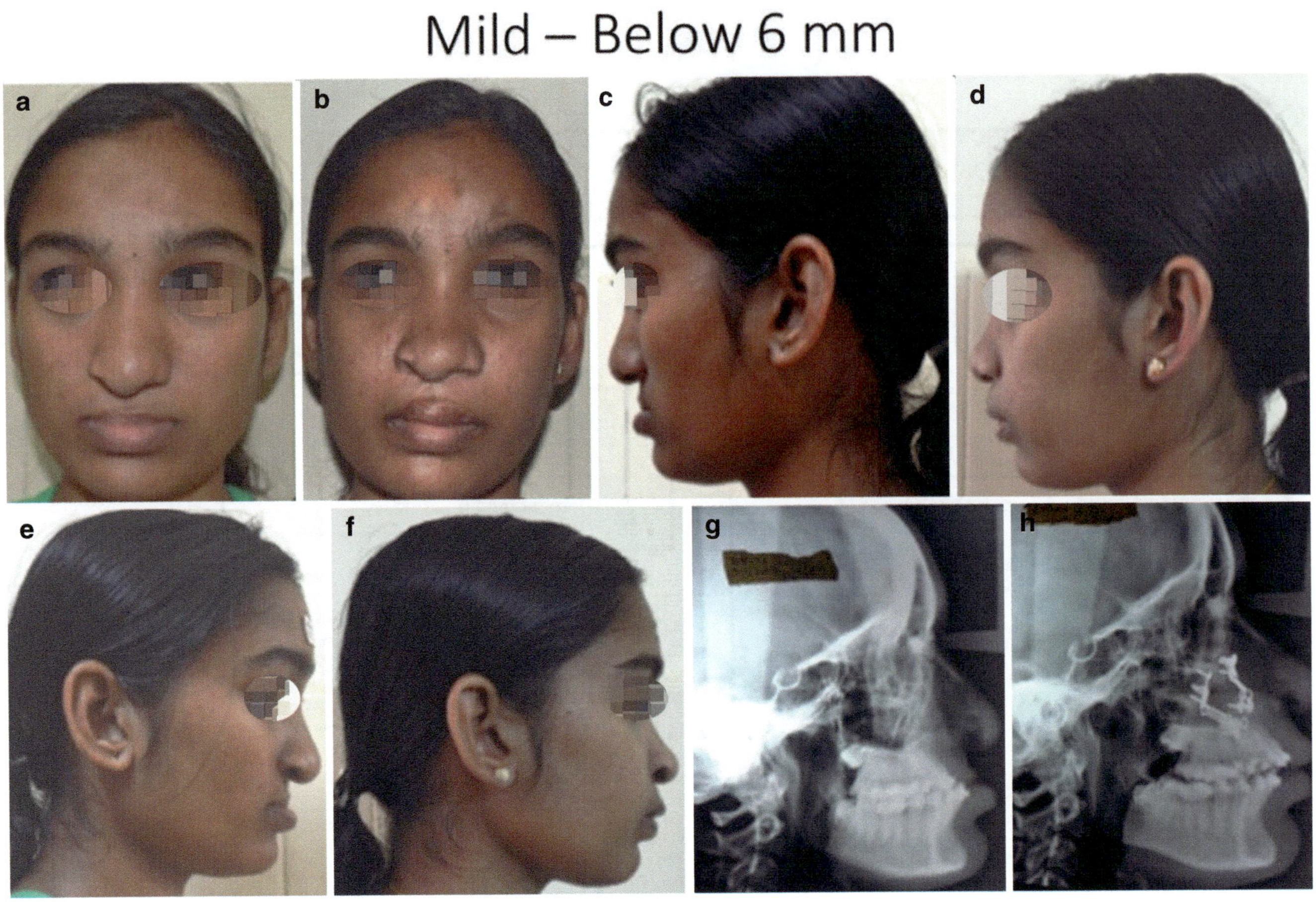

Fig. 75.8 (**a–h**) Mild reverse overjet and no preoperative VPI. The patient was treated with single jaw orthognathic surgery (maxillary advancement). (**a**, **b**) Pre and post-operative frontal photographs. (**c**, **d**) Pre and post operative profile photographs (left side). (**e**, **f**) Pre and post-operative profile photographs (right side). (**g**, **h**) Pre and post-operative lateral cephalograms

75.8.2 Preoperative Preparation

A single dose of 8 mg dexamethasone (half-life of 36–54 h) is given preoperatively to help reduce postsurgical airway and maxillofacial edema. It also has a synergistic analgesic effect when combined with postoperative analgesics. As a only a single dose is given, it is associated with minimum side effects [74, 75]. A single dose of 1 gm tranexamic acid is given 1 h preoperatively as it helps reduce intraoperative blood loss [76].

75.8.3 Intubation

Nasal intubation is preferred followed by submental intubation. In case a pharyngeal flap or nasal obstruction (enlarged inferior turbinates or deviated nasal septum) is present, it is advisable to perform fiber-optic assisted awake intubation. Alternatively, it may be necessary to pass a more rigid tube or catheter initially after which the endotracheal tube is passed over it.

The author always prefers to use a flexometallic naso-endotracheal tube as the tube is able to maintain its integrity even if damaged during the LeFort I osteotomy on account of the additional strength imparted by the metal coils.

75.8.4 General Anesthesia

The author commonly uses hypotensive anesthesia during orthognathic surgery as it provides a clean hemostatic field, reduces blood loss, and shortens hospital stay. There is an association between hypotensive anesthesia, forces generated during pterygomaxillary dysjunction, and optic nerve damage. Risk for optic nerve damage increases when hypotensive anesthesia is used in head and neck surgery which is

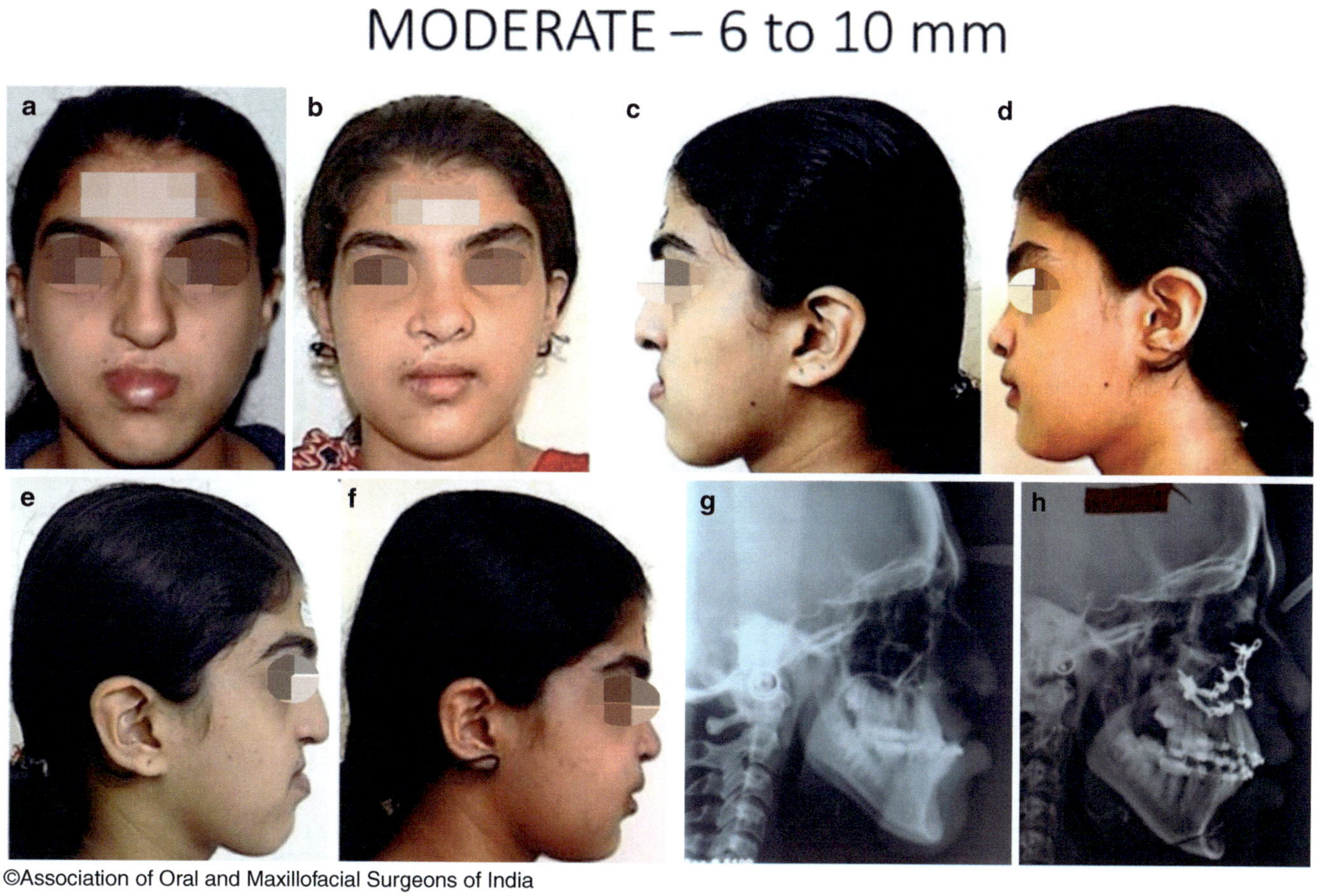

Fig. 75.9 (**a**–**h**) - Moderate reverse overjet and mild preoperative VPI. The patient was treated with orthognathic surgery alone (maxillary advancement and advancement genioplasty). (**a**, **b**) Pre and post-operative frontal photographs. (**c**, **d**) Pre and post operative profile photographs (left side) (**e**, **f**) Pre and post-operative profile photographs (right side). (**g**, **h**) Pre and post-operative lateral cephalograms

prolonged (>6 h) and large amount of blood loss (> 1 l) has taken place [77–82].

A larger amount of force is needed for pterygomaxillary dysjunction in CLP patients on account of the thicker pterygomaxillary junction. The stray forces, generated as a result of the dysjunction, can dissipate toward the orbital cavity and optic foramen with a magnitude potent enough to cause damage to the optic nerve. This is possible due to the orbital extensions of the palatine and sphenoid bones [7, 83, 84]. Thus, the author prefers to maintain hypotensive anesthesia during the entire orthognathic surgery except during pterygomaxillary dysjunction.

75.8.5 Cleft LeFort I Osteotomy (Video 75.2)

In cases of unilateral CLP, a routine incision in the height of the maxillary vestibule is used, and care should be taken that it extends only to the mesial surface of the first maxillary molars on both sides [7, 30, 85] (Refer Chap. 69 on Maxillary orthognathic procedures).

In cases of bilateral CLP, the incision is modified such that it extends from the lateral incisor to mesial surface of the first molar on both sides. A vertical stab incision is made in the midline to allow for placement of the nasal septal osteotome. This is to preserve blood supply to the pre-maxillary segment as most of its blood supply comes from the upper lip [2, 7, 28, 30].

Frequent surgery in the cleft maxilla leads to creation of scar tissue in the buccal, palatal, and upper lip regions. This scar tissue has compromised vascularity and healing ability. Therefore, it is essential to maintain an adequate soft tissue pedicle. There have also been suggestions to use modified vertical incisions instead of circumvestibular incisions, but it increases the difficulty of the procedure manyfold due to poor access and visualization [2, 3, 86]. Careful and gentle retraction of tissues (especially the pedicles) is essential throughout the procedure and especially during the down-fracture process.

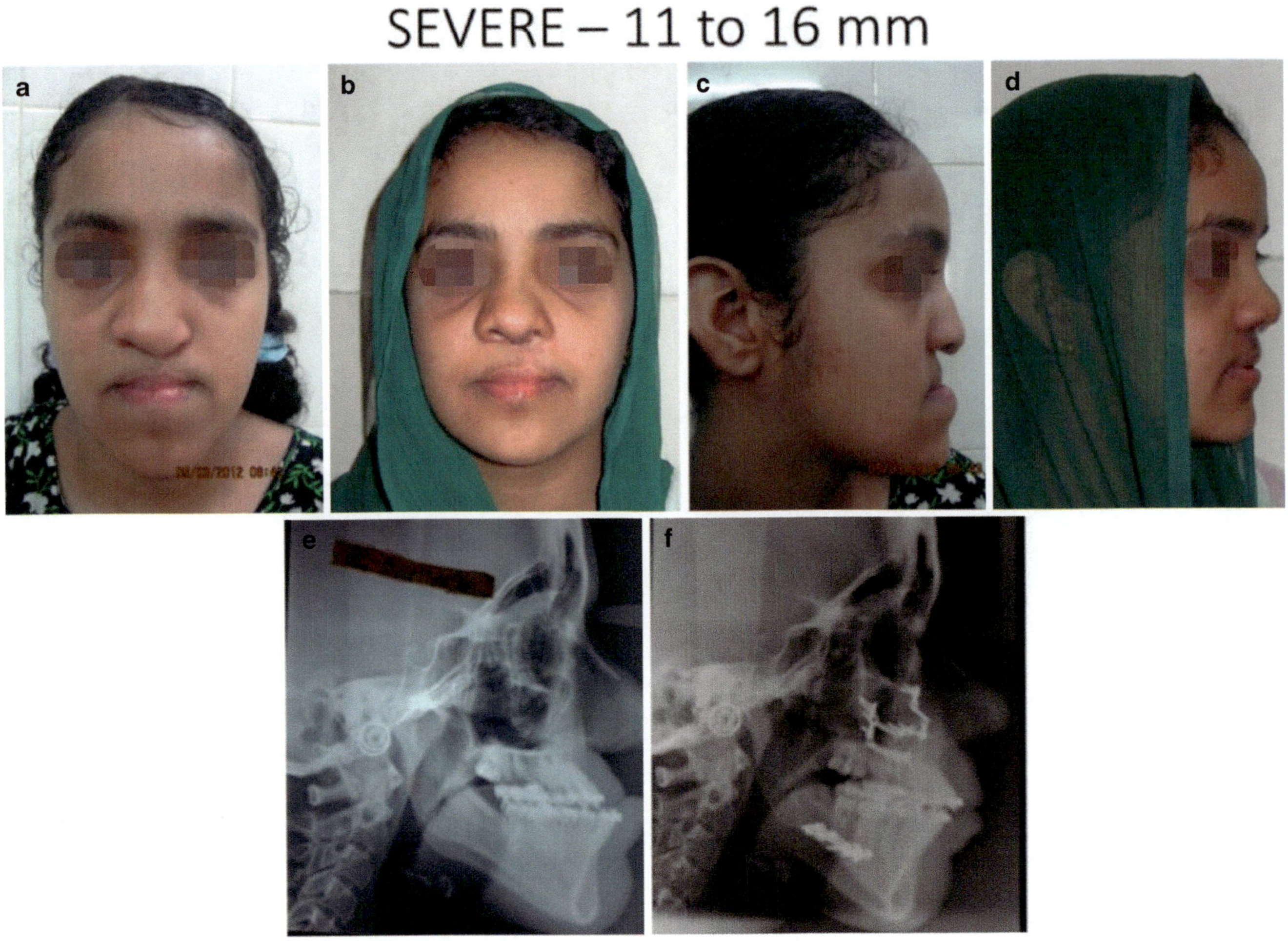

Fig. 75.10 (**a–f**) Severe reverse overjet and mild preoperative VPI. The patient was treated with bi-jaw orthognathic surgery. (**a**, **b**) Pre and post operative frontal photographs. (**c**, **d**) Pre and post operative profile photographs. (**e**, **f**) Pre and post operative lateral cephalograms

The nasal mucosa is routinely elevated from the walls and floor of the nasal cavity prior to starting the LeFort I osteotomy. In the cleft maxilla, there is no intervening bone between the oral and nasal cavity in the region of the cleft; instead, the nasal mucosa is fused to the palatal mucosa due to the previously performed palatoplasty. This tissue should be sharply dissected close to the nasal floor, and care should be taken to avoid perforating the palatal mucosa. This step also aids in the down-fracture and mobilization of the maxilla.

The cleft maxilla usually exhibits para-nasal hollowing. Hence, the routine LeFort I osteotomy may not suffice for complete correction of cleft maxillary hypoplasia. Instead a high LeFort I osteotomy is used which has the added advantage of correcting the para-nasal hollowing as well [7, 30, 86]. Care should be taken to avoid damage to the tooth roots and the infra-orbital nerve as it exits from the infra-orbital foramen (Fig. 75.12). One should keep in mind that the descending palatine artery is closer to the lateral pyriform rim while performing the lateral nasal wall osteotomy.

To completely mobilize the maxilla during a LeFort I osteotomy, it is necessary to perform a pterygomaxillary dysjunction which separates the maxilla from the pterygoid plates. The maneuver is essentially blind and involves orienting a pterygoid chisel (curved osteotome) in a downward, medial, and anterior direction such that it engages the lower part of the pterygomaxillary fissure while maintaining a safe distance from the internal maxillary artery [87–89].

Studies have revealed that the medial pterygoid plate is shorter and the pterygomaxillary junction is thicker in cleft patients as the region around the hamular notch is fre-

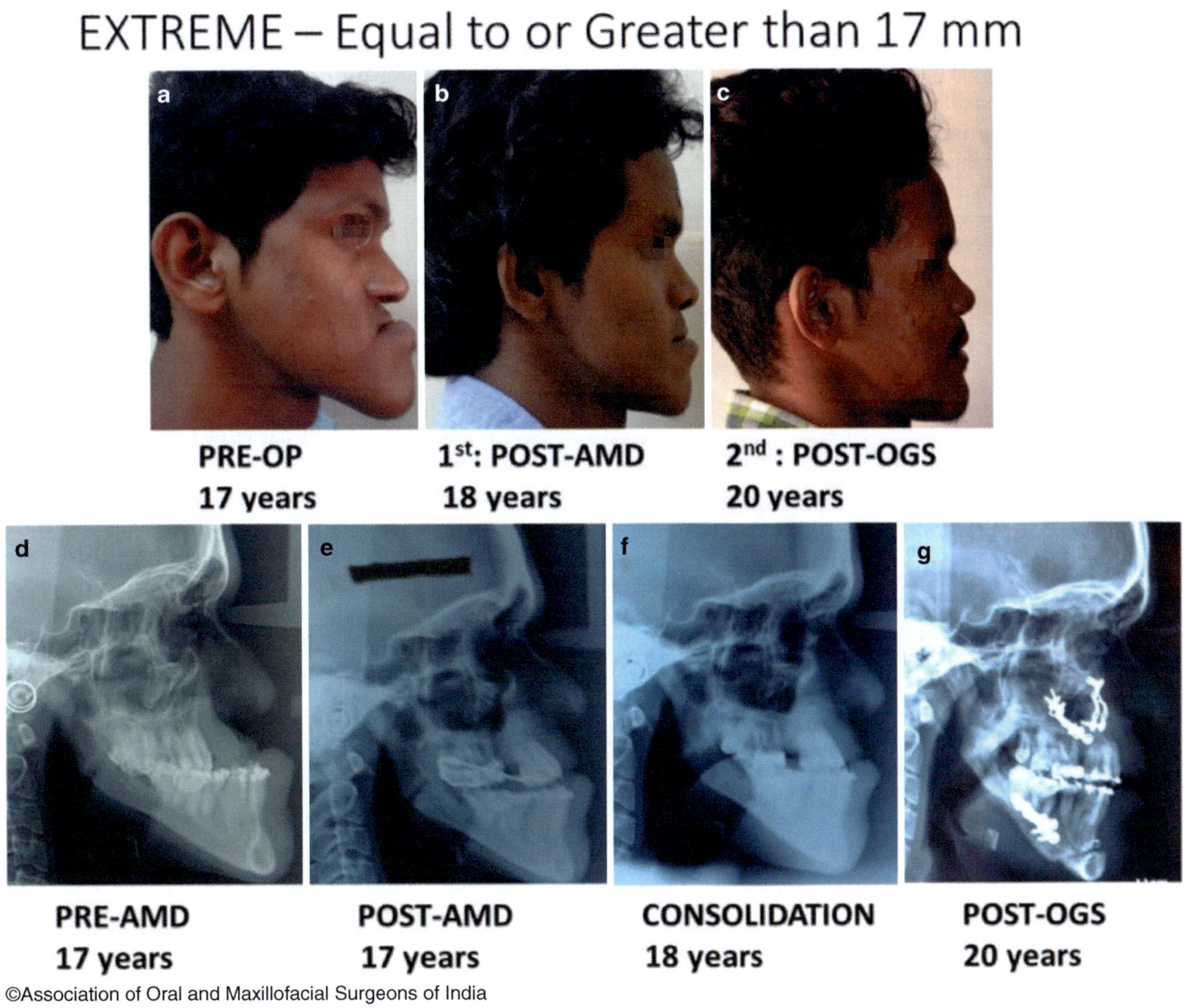

Fig. 75.11 (**a**–**g**) Extreme reverse overjet and mild preoperative VPI. 1st stage corrected by anterior maxillary distraction (AMD). Note the persistent para-nasal hollowing that is only partially corrected by AMD. 2nd stage completed by bi-jaw orthognathic surgery (OGS) with improvement in para-nasal hollowing. (**a**) Pre-operative profile photograph. (**b**) Profile after stage 1 correction wthe AMD. (**c**) Profile after stage 2 correction with orthognathic surgery. (**d**) Pre-operative lateral cephalogram. (**e**) Lateral cephalogram after stage 1 - AMD. (**f**) Post-consolidation lateral cephalogram. (**g**) Lateral cephalogram after stage 2 -orthognathic surgery

quently manipulated during palatoplasty. The shorter medial pterygoid plate, by virtue of its smaller dimensions, may be more prone to fracture which increases the risk for vascular complications [87, 88]. Furthermore, the thicker pterygomaxillary junction requires a larger magnitude of force to achieve adequate separation. The usage of greater force leads to less control over this blind manoeuvre, thus increasing the risk for vascular complications (internal maxillary artery damage, carotid cavernous sinus) and neurologic (optic nerve damage) and skull base fractures (sphenoid fractures) [84].

There have been many modifications suggested to the original technique with an intention to reduce complications [87, 88, 90–95]. However, their use has never been documented widely in CLP cases. One may also attempt to use a piezo-surgical instrument or sequentially increase the size of the osteotomes to help reduce the force required for final pterygomaxillary separation [96, 97]. Another important consideration would be the preference of a third molar vertical osteotomy cut instead of a pterygomaxillary disjunction. This manoeuvre is anatomically less hazardous, allows greater mobility of the segments, allows a larger vascular pedicle to be maintained and permits the use of interpositional bone graft in the osteotomised area, after the advancement in order to prevent relapse.

Once pterygomaxillary dysjunction has been performed, the maxilla is down-fractured using leverage or specialized instruments like the Smith's spreader. If the nasal mucosa has not been dissected from the palatal mucosa previously, then it has to be done at this point [2, 7, 30]. After the down-fracture, it is important to suture the divided edges of the nasal mucosa to regain continuity of nasal lining. In the author's opinion, the edges of the divided nasal mucosa are a common source of bleeding postoperatively if left un-sutured (Fig. 75.13a, b). The presence of nasal obstructions like enlarged inferior turbinates can be corrected at this time.

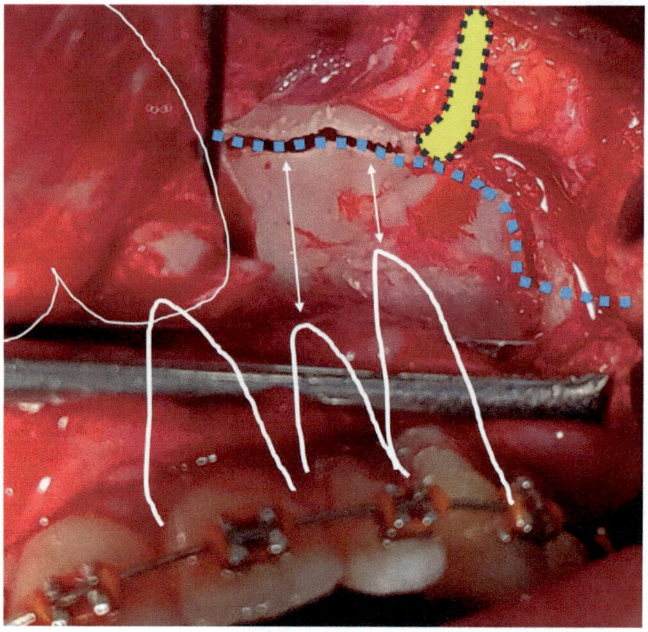

Fig. 75.12 Modified high LeFort I osteotomy (blue) cut to help correct para-nasal hollowing. Avoid damage to the infra-orbital nerve (yellow) and roots of teeth (white) while making the osteotomy. The pyrifiorm rim is marked in orange

After the down-fracture, the process of mobilizing the maxilla is done in a gradual progressive manner as the scarred tissues are less compliant. Specialized instruments like the Tessier's mobilizer can be used. If a pharyngeal flap is present and is impeding maxillary advancement, it may need to be incised. The maxilla is finally advanced to its desired position and should be seated in a passive manner. Signs of resistance at this point may indicate that the maxilla has not been adequately mobilized, and the previous steps need to be revisited. If resistance to the desired maxillary position persists, then one must consider to switch to maxillary distraction or set-back the mandible to avoid postoperative relapse. In situations where an alveolar bone grafting procedure has not been performed, or where the take of the grafting is sub-optimal, the cleft maxilla may present as a two-piece (unilateral cleft) or a three-piece (bilateral) maxilla. This may necessitate the use of transverse maxillary plating (Fig. 75.14a, b), for stabilization of the segmented bone.

There may also be need for segmental osteotomies as it is difficult to completely co-ordinate both arches with presurgical orthodontics on account of the variable anatomy of the cleft maxilla. The cleft alveolar gap can be opened or closed

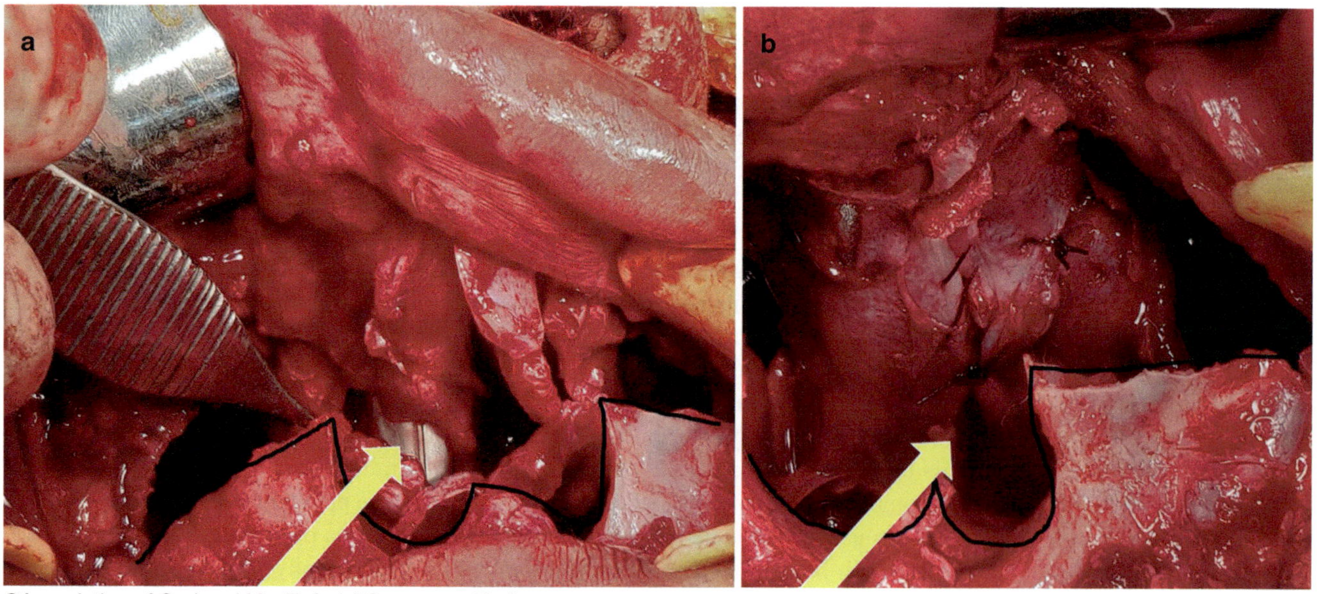

Fig. 75.13 (**a**) Torn nasal floor mucosa after down-fracture of maxilla. The endotracheal tube is visible. (**b**) The torn edges should be sutured back to prevent postoperative bleeding

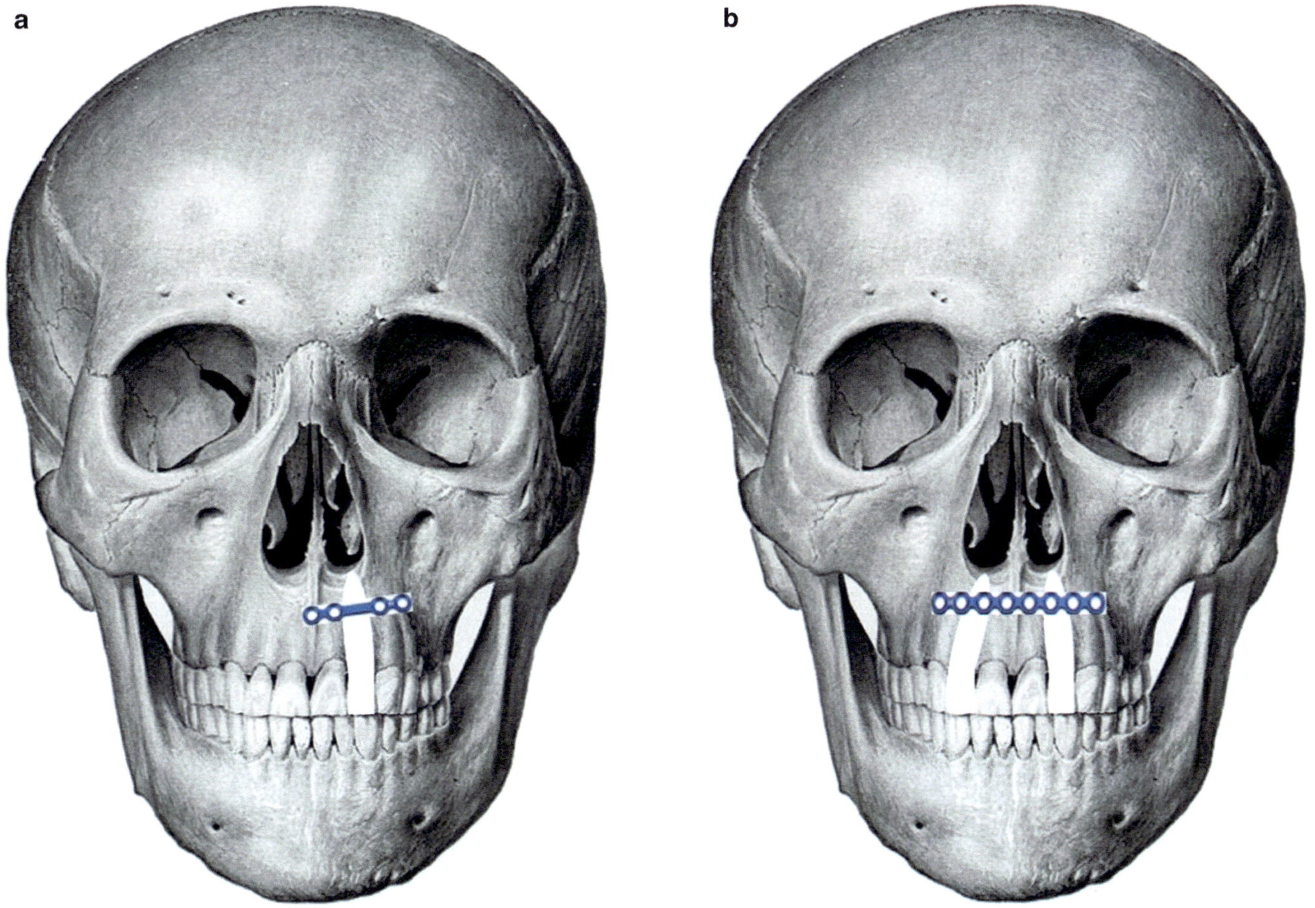

Fig. 75.14 Transverse plate across maxilla for stability during LeFort I osteotomy in a cleft. (**a**) Unilateral cleft of maxilla (**b**) Bilateral cleft of maxilla

to facilitate alveolar bone grafting or close alveolar fistulas. It can widen the maxillary arch within acceptable limits, allow differential movement of greater and lesser segments, align the occlusal plane, and maximize intercuspation to improve postoperative stability [98].

The presence of a persistent oronasal fistula and alveolar cleft defect requires careful soft tissue closure and bone grafting. One can also augment the deficient area along the lateral piriform rim on the cleft side to improve the contour of the alar base. The maxilla can fracture at the cleft alveolus site into two segments during the down-fracture and mobilization, even when the alveolar cleft site has been previously grafted. A preoperatively fabricated surgical palatal stent helps stabilize the maxilla in this situation.

Rigid fixation with mini plates and screws is preferred to stabilize the maxilla in its final position with a preference for the lateral pyriform rim and zygomaticomaxillary buttress regions as the bone here is thicker [83, 99]. One should pay attention while suturing and prevent entrapment of soft tissues into the osteotomy sites. The soft tissue of the upper lip may be tight with a shallow vestibular depth and deficient vermilion show that may become worse following maxillary advancement. "V-Y" closure can be used to reduce lip shortening.

75.8.6 Additional Steps Performed on a Case-to-Case Basis

75.8.6.1 Deciding the Level of Midface Advancement (Fig. 75.15a–f)

In most of the cases, a traditional LeFort I (Fig. 75.15a) osteotomy is advocated. However, in some rare instances, it may need a LeFort II (Fig. 75.15b) or LeFort III (Fig. 75.15c) osteotomy depending on the severity and the extent of the involvement. As the CMH involves the pyriform, the paranasal, and the zygomatic areas, though not symmetrical, the LeFort I osteotomy design in such situations may need modification to involve the para-nasal (Fig. 75.15d) and/or zygomatic (Fig. 75.15e) areas unilaterally (Fig. 75.15f) or bilaterally as the case may be.

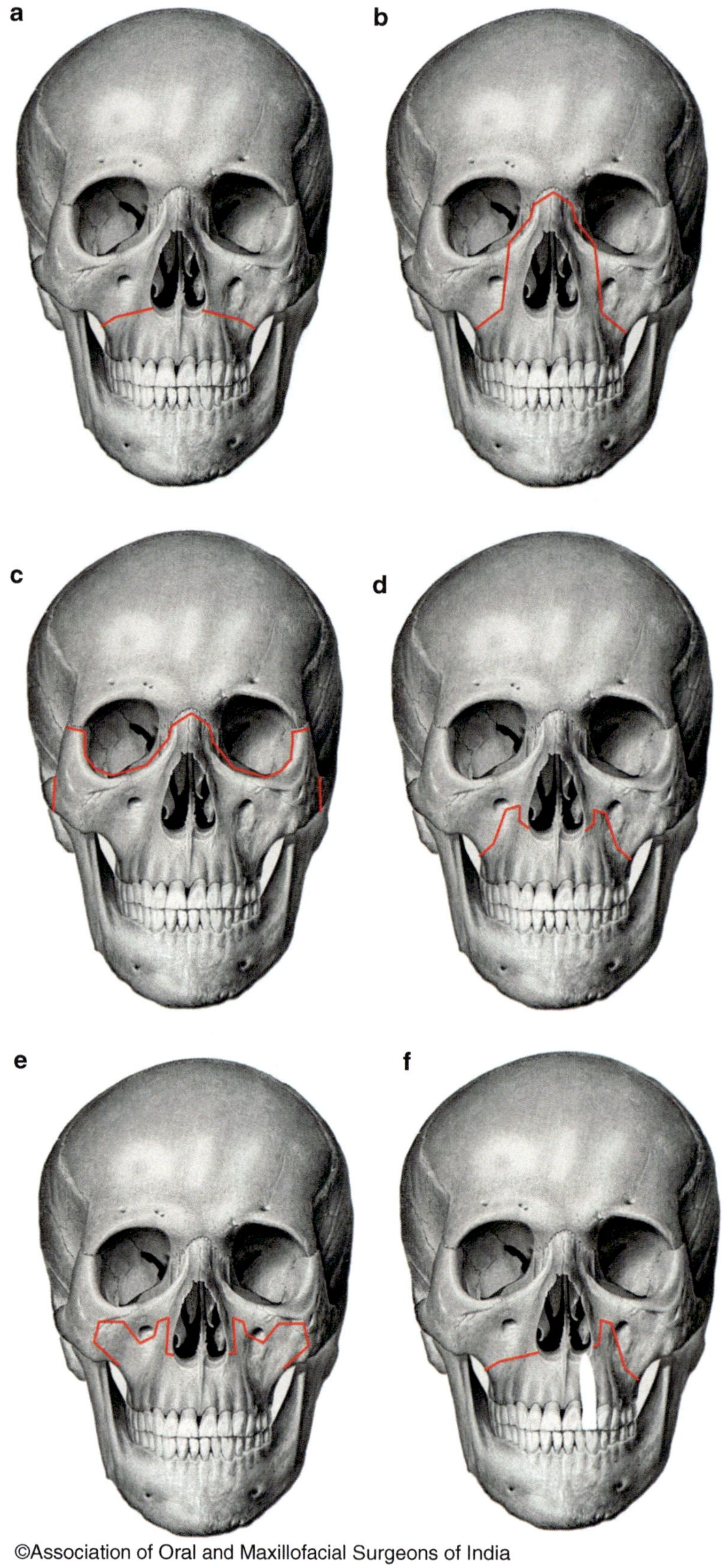

Fig. 75.15 Levels of midface advancement (**a**) LeFort I, (**b**) LeFort II, (**c**) LeFort III osteotomies. Modifications of LeFort I osteotomy (**d**), para-nasal extension, (**e**) para-nasal and zygomatic extensions, and (**f**) conventional LeFort I on the unaffected side and para-nasal extension on the affected side

75.8.6.2 Preserving the Descending Palatine Artery

Studies by Bell et al. established that the descending palatine artery did not contribute significantly to the re-vascularization of the maxilla after a total maxillary osteotomy in routine cases [100, 101]. However, the greater palatine arterial network in CLP patients may become narrow and develop vascular anomalies because of the presence of scar tissue created by the palatoplasty procedure [7, 60, 83]. Considering the unique scenario of the cleft maxilla, it is advisable that efforts should be made to preserve the descending palatine artery and secure it as an additional source blood supply for the osteotomized maxilla [7, 102]. Techniques to identify and preserve the descending palatine artery have been documented in the literature [103–108]. However, the above technique needs to be tailored to the cleft maxillary anatomy as it is highly variable. Studies have established that the distance between the lateral pyriform aperture and the descending palatine artery is on an average 3–4 mm lesser in CLP patients. Similarly, the posterior and lateral distances to the descending palatine artery were greater on in CLP patients on account of the thickened pterygomaxillary junction [7, 83, 84]. The perpendicular process of the palatine bone surrounding the descending palatine artery is also of the dense cortical type adding to the difficulty of isolating the vessel [99]. The author reserves this step only when the patient has undergone a large number of revision surgeries in the palate.

75.8.6.3 Grafting of the Osteotomy Site

The cleft maxilla is deficient in all three dimensions, and hence its correction requires complex large movements. Cortico-cancellous bone grafts can be placed across the gap created in the region of the lateral osteotomy [2, 3, 7, 86, 109]. The ideal source of autogenous bone grafting is the anterior iliac crest [110]. As an alternative, one can also use autogenous genial grafts, allogenic grafts, or synthetic hydroxyapatite bone blocks [111–114]. The author prefers to graft the osteotomy site only when down-grafting the maxilla or advancing the maxilla more than 10 mm.

75.9 Clinical Morbidity and Psychological Response

According to Stork et al. and Chua et al., there was no major difference between clinical morbidity between distraction osteogenesis and orthognathic surgery and between grafted and non-grafted patients, the source of graft being the anterior iliac crest [115–117].

Patients undergoing distraction osteogenesis experienced greater levels of stress in the short term. Over time, the distraction group had a higher satisfaction with life [118–120]. This may be because of the better stability of the distraction osteogenesis in the long term as well as the self-perceived contribution of the patients to the success of their treatment. There is also an aspect of superior soft tissue response to distraction as compared to orthognathic surgery which may improve the final aesthetic result (refer Chap. 87 to read more about Distraction Osteogenesis) [121].

Nonetheless, psychological support from family and friends is recommended for patients undergoing either distraction or orthognathic surgery so as to achieve a better life satisfaction in the long term.

75.10 Stability of Results

The postoperative stability after orthognathic surgery in cleft patients is lower than non-cleft patients [2, 3, 7, 86]. Maximum relapse in cleft orthognathic surgery occurs in the first 6 months, and the situation stabilizes 2 years postoperatively [122].

75.10.1 Soft Tissue Envelope

The presence of scarred tissue in the palate and the lip prevents the maxilla from being adequately mobilized. Though the maxilla might be secured into its desired position with the help of rigid fixation and bone grafting, the excess stress placed on the maxilla due to the scarred soft tissue envelope leads to relapse in both the sagittal and vertical dimensions [2, 3, 7, 86, 123]. The severity of labio-palatal clefting and history of multiple revision surgeries increase the risk for relapse.

75.10.2 Magnitude of Planned Surgical Movement

The amount of surgical movement is the most important factor that determines the degree of relapse in cleft and non-cleft cases. Thus, most surgeons tend to overcorrect by an additional 20% to account for the possible relapse [2, 3, 7, 86, 124].

However, a recent study by Watts et al. [125] suggested that amount of linear advancement was not a major cause for skeletal and dental relapse rate in cleft orthognathic. Studies by Bhatia et al. [59] and Hoffman et al. [126] suggested the same. Nonetheless, the general trend is to perform bi-jaw orthognathic surgery or distract the maxilla if more than 10 mm advancement is needed.

75.10.3 Status of Alveolar Bone Grafting

Lack of alveolar bone grafting increases the difficulty of performing cleft orthognathic surgery. However, though alveolar bone grafting contributes to transverse stability of the maxillary arch and improve outcomes in orthodontia, it does not improve stability of sagittal, vertical, or rotational movements [122, 124].

75.10.4 Intraoperative Factors

Inadequate separation at the pterygomaxillary junction due to its thicker form in CLP patients, the presence of a pharyngeal flap, a shallow overbite, and the absence of multiple teeth leading to poor intercuspation may contribute to relapse as well [2, 3, 7, 86, 124]. Segmentation of the maxilla as compared to one-piece maxilla was not associated with greater relapse rates in CLP patients and instead could correct orthodontic and occlusal problems that were distinctive to the cleft maxilla. Nonetheless, no attempt should be made to significantly widen the cleft maxilla as using a segmental osteotomy is a highly unstable procedure [98, 127, 128].

In the author's opinion, poor-quality bone in the cleft maxilla makes rigid fixation difficult and increases the risk for relapse [2, 3, 7]. Thus, it is advisable to always secure plates in the region of thick cortical bone, i.e., the zygomaticomaxillary buttress region posteriorly and the lateral pyriform aperture anteriorly (Fig. 75.16a–c). Bony fenestrations can be encountered in cases with prior AMD during maxillary orthognathic surgery; extra care must be taken during plating the same (Fig. 75.17).

Owing to the large advancements commonly performed in cleft orthognathic surgery, the gap between the osteotomized segments is large. When the contact area between the bony shelves is small, there may be instability or fibrous union between segments which increases the risk for relapse. By grating these gaps, there is increased bony contact which helps in optimal healing. Rarely, the space posterior to the maxillary tuberosity after advancement of the maxilla is also grafted to help prevent relapse [46]. Owing to the hostile environment of the cleft maxilla, it is general consensus that autogenous bone grafts provide the best results in terms of take up of the graft and significantly lower complication rates. It is interesting to note that a recent study by Stork et al. [115] suggested that grafting was not a major factor in preventing postoperative skeletal relapse in cleft and non-cleft patients contrary to the currently accepted methodology. A study by Hoffman et al. [129] in non-cleft patients suggested the same. The author's opinion is in line with both the above authors and grafts the osteotomy site only when advancing the maxilla more than 10 mm or down-grafting the maxilla.

75.10.5 Timing of Surgery

As previously mentioned, surgery performed before skeletal maturity is associated with a higher relapse rate in both horizontal and vertical dimensions due to continued growth. This is applicable irrespective of the type of surgery being performed: orthognathic surgery or distraction osteogenesis [21, 23, 24]. Secondary surgery for the correction of residual growth deformities is required after growth is complete. It is

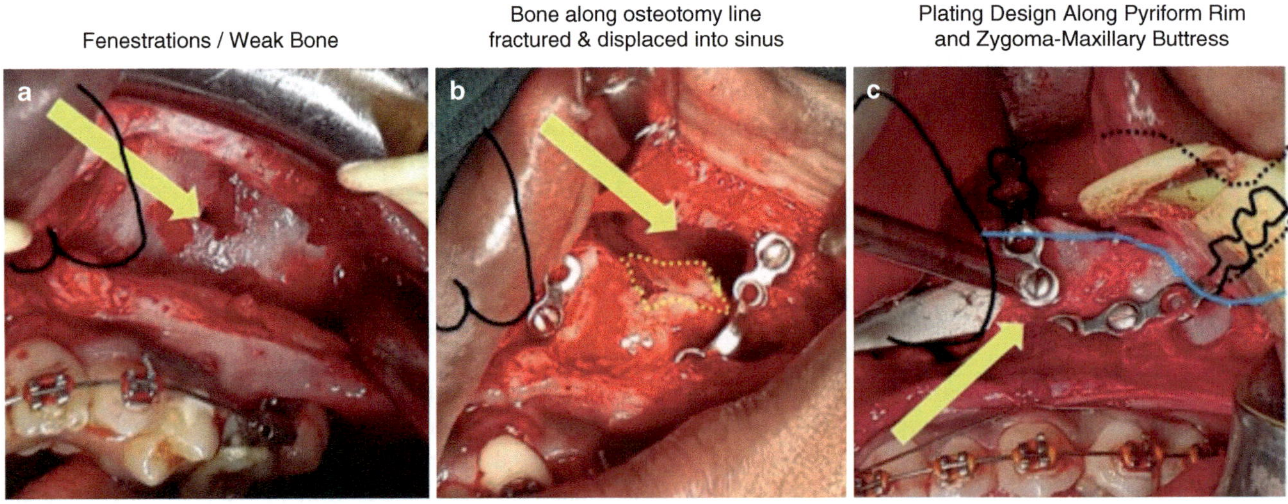

Fig. 75.16 (**a–c**) Poor-quality bone seen in the anterolateral and posterolateral walls of the maxilla. Always plate along the lateral pyriform rim and zygomamaxillary buttress (dotted) region which are known to have good-quality bone. Part of the miniplate obscured by the retractor and tissues has been traced for better understanding of the plate position. Blue line denotes line of osteotomy on the dental side

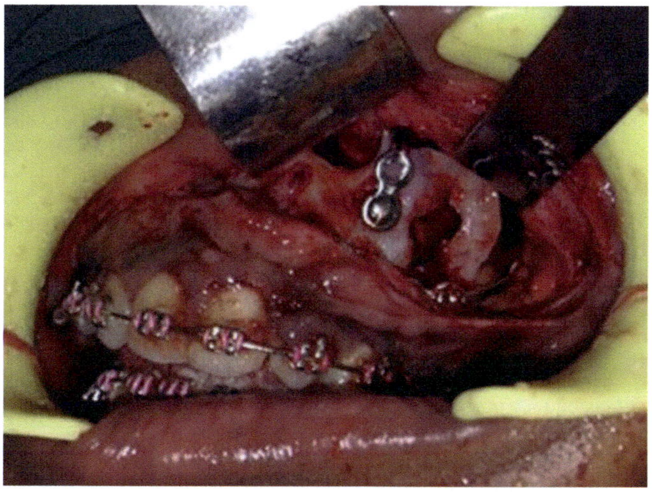

Fig. 75.17 Large bony fenestration in anterolateral wall of the maxilla at the time of orthognathic surgery. It is commonly found where prior anterior maxillary distraction was done. The presence of such a large fenestration can make plating difficult

important to note that distraction osteogenesis was more commonly preferred in the growing patient [2, 3, 7, 22, 130, 131].

75.10.6 Degree of Relapse

A review by Kloukos et al. [120] established that results obtained with distraction osteogenesis were more stable as compared to conventional orthognathic surgery 5 years postoperatively. A review by Saltaji et al. [132, 133] reported average horizontal relapse rates of 10 % in distraction cases and 25–30 % in orthognathic cases for cleft patients. Vertical relapse rates in cleft orthognathic patients were high with an average rate of 40–50 %. Similar results have been documented in other studies and reviews with up to 5-year follow-ups [134–140]. The rate for re-operation in cleft orthognathic surgery was approximately 12.2% [140]. Internal distractors were also found to be more stable than external distractors. This can be attributed to the rigidity provided by the internal distractor during the consolidation phase. The use of rigid fixation with miniplates was attributed with the least amount of relapse in cleft orthognathic surgery [2, 3, 7, 132].

Based on the above evidence, distraction osteogenesis has become the mainstay for the management of severe to extreme cleft maxillary hypoplasia (reverse overjet greater than 11 mm) as the slow distraction of bone and the accompanying histogenic abilities help reduce skeletal relapse. Orthognathic surgery is preferred for mild to moderate cleft maxillary hypoplasia (reverse overjet lesser than 11 mm).

75.10.7 Clinical Suggestions to Avoid Relapse

Commonly used methods to prevent or control relapse are as follows: overcorrection of the final surgical result by 20%, prolonged intermaxillary fixation during the postoperative phase, using face masks with reverse traction of the maxilla, interpositioning bone grafts between the gaps created by maxillary advancement, and performing bi-jaw surgery or distraction when advancements greater than 10 mm are required [114]. A study by Tabrizi et al. [141] established that the use of rigid fixation after the consolidation phase of cleft maxillary distraction did not increase stability of results. In anterior maxillary distraction, it is essential to lock the appliance with wire or acrylic plug during the consolidation phase to prevent backward rotation of the hyrax screw.

75.11 Complications

A study by Metalwala et al. [142] established that there is increased risk for infection and prolonged hospital stay in patients with craniofacial anomalies undergoing orthognathic surgery. The incidence of complications in non-cleft patients has been reported at 6.4% as compared to 25.2% in cleft patients [83].

Studies by Yamaguchi et al. [140] and Moran et al. [143] revealed that an average of 15–30 % of patients present with perioperative complications. The most common complications were closure failure of pre-existing palatal fistula, velopharyngeal impairment, temporary paresthesia of the infra-orbital nerve, and surgical site infection. A review by Santos et al. [144] established that cleft maxilla patients present with the highest incidence of cranial nerve damage on account of the anatomically higher modified LeFort I osteotomy cut and excessive forces needed at the time of pterygomaxillary dysjunction. Rare and severe complications like arteriovenous fistula, maxillary aneurysm, cavernous sinus thrombosis, skull base fractures, and maxillary necrosis blindness are more common among patients with craniofacial anomalies but have an incidence of lesser than 0.5% [140, 143, 145]. It has been suggested by Eduardo et al. [146] that the use of piezo-electric surgical instruments in orthognathic surgery is associated with a lower complication rate.

With the author's experience (PM) of approximately 900 cleft orthognathic cases while using the traditional dysjunction technique, there has been no major vascular complication or skull base fractures. However, two patients experienced transient blindness with partial recovery of vision in the long term [79].

75.12 Conclusion

Skeletal surgery is a critical component of surgical management of CLP. On account of the unique anatomy of the cleft maxilla that has been subjected to previous lip & palate interventions, the conventional LeFort I osteotomy technique and orthognathic surgical principles need to be adapted accordingly. The ultimate goal of treatment should be to achieve intelligible speech and an acceptable appearance with good balance of facial skeleton, soft tissues, and occlusion. Distraction osteogenesis is a useful technique in the management of severe maxillary deficiency, but does not replace conventional orthognathic surgery. Maxillofacial surgeons who treat these deformities should be part of a craniofacial team to provide interdisciplinary care for the patient. The aim of the team should be to help the child to develop into a confident young adult.

Acknowledgment Dr. Rahul Tiwari (M.D.S Oral and Maxillofacial Surgery) for manuscript preparation

Designation: Fellow of Orthognathic Surgery

Institutional Address with pin code: Jubilee Mission Medical College and Hospital, Thrissur 680005

References

1. Shetye PR. Facial growth of adults with unoperated clefts. Clin Plast Surg. 2004;31(2):361–71.
2. Chigurupati R. Orthognathic surgery for secondary cleft and craniofacial deformities. Oral Maxillofac Surg Clin North Am. 2005;17(4):503–17.
3. Posnick JC, Ricalde P. Cleft-orthognathic surgery. Clin Plast Surg. 2004;31(2):315–30.
4. Oberoi S, Chigurupati R, Vargervik K. Morphologic and management characteristics of individuals with unilateral cleft lip and palate who required maxillary advancement. Cleft Palate Craniofac J. 2008;45(1):42–9.
5. Oberoi S, Hoffman WY, Chigurupati R, Vargervik K. Frequency of surgical correction for maxillary hypoplasia in cleft lip and palate. J Craniofac Surg. 2012;23(6):1665–7.
6. Good PM, Mulliken JB, Padwa BL. Frequency of Le Fort I osteotomy after repaired cleft lip and palate or cleft palate. Cleft Palate Craniofac J. 2007;44(4):396–401.
7. Chigurupati R. Cleft lip and palate: Timing and approaches to reconstruction. In: Saunder, editor. Current therapy in oral and maxillofacial surgery. 1st ed. Elsevier; 2012. p. 726–50.
8. Jones CM, Mackay AFJ, Mackay DR, Long RE. Do pharyngeal flaps restrict early midface growth in patients with clefts? Cleft Palate Craniofacial J. 2016;53(6):629–33.
9. Abyholm FE, Otaki S. Cleft lip and palate. 3rd ed. Berkowitz S, editor. Berlin: Springer; 2013. p. 601–12.
10. Gopinath VK, Samsudin AR, Noor SNFM, Sharab HYM. Facial profile and maxillary arch dimensions in unilateral cleft lip and palate children in the mixed dentition stage. Eur J Dent. 2018;11(1):76–82.
11. Lee Y, Liao Y. Hard palate-repair technique and facial growth in patients with cleft lip and palate: a systematic review. Br J Oral Maxillofac Surg. 2013;51(8):851–7.
12. Campbell A, Costello BJ, Ruiz RL. Cleft lip and palate surgery: an update of clinical outcomes for primary repair. Oral Maxillofac Surg Clin North Am. 2010;22(1):43–58.
13. Yang I, Liao Y. Cleft lip and palate the effect of 1-stage versus 2-stage palate repair on facial growth in patients with cleft lip and palate: a review. Int J Oral Maxillofac Surg. 2010;39(10):945–50.
14. Stein S, Dunsche A, Gellrich NC, Härle F, Jonas I. One- or two-stage palate closure in patients with unilateral cleft lip and palate: Comparing cephalometric and occlusal outcomes. Cleft Palate Craniofac J. 2007;44(1):13–22.
15. Xu X, Kwon HJ, Shi B, Zheng Q, Yin H, Li C. Influence of different palate repair protocols on facial growth in unilateral complete cleft lip and palate. J Cranio Maxillofac Surg. 2015;43(1):43–7.
16. Santiago PE, Schuster LA, Levy-Bercowski D. Management of the alveolar cleft. Clin Plast Surg. 2014;41(2):219–32.
17. Da Silva Filho OG, Boiani E, Cavassan ADO, Santamaria M. Rapid maxillary expansion after secondary alveolar bone grafting in patients with alveolar cleft. Cleft Palate Craniofac J. 2009;46(3):331–8.
18. Emodi O, Noy D, Hazan-Molina H, Aizenbud D, Rachmiel A. Secondary bone grafting of the cleft maxilla following reverse quad-helix expansion in 103 patients. Ann Maxillofac Surg. 2015;5(1):32.
19. Uzel A, Benlidayı ME, Kürkçü M, Kesiktaş E. The effects of maxillary expansion on late alveolar bone grafting in patients with unilateral cleft lip and palate. J Oral Maxillofac Surg. 2019;77(3):607–14.
20. Reyneke JP, Tsakiris P, Becker P. Age as a factor in the complication rate after removal of unerupted/impacted third molars at the time of mandibular sagittal split osteotomy. J Oral Maxillofac Surg. 2002;60(6):654–9.
21. Wolford LM, Cassano DS, Cottrell DA, El Deeb M, Karras SC, Goncalves JR. Orthognathic surgery in the young cleft patient: preliminary study on subsequent facial growth. J Oral Maxillofac Surg. 2008;66(12):2524–36.
22. Wolford LM, Karras SC, Mehra P. Considerations for orthognathic surgery during growth, Part 2: Maxillary deformities. Am J Orthod Dentofac Orthop. 2001;119(2):95–101.
23. Meazzini MC, Basile V, Mazzoleni F, Bozzetti A, Brusati R. Long-term follow-up of large maxillary advancements with distraction osteogenesis in growing and non-growing cleft lip and palate patients. J Plast Reconstr Aesthetic Surg. 2015;68(1):79–86.
24. Liu K, Zhou N. Long-term skeletal changes after maxillary distraction osteogenesis in growing children with cleft lip/palate. J Craniofac Surg. 2018;29(4):e349–52.
25. Turvey TA, Golden BA, Brookes CD. Techniques in bone grafting of cleft maxilla. In: Saunders, editor. Atlas of oral and maxillofacial surgery. 1st ed. 2015. p. 569–78.
26. Dempf R, Teltzrow T, Kramer F-J, Hausamen J-E. Alveolar bone grafting in patients with complete clefts: a comparative study between secondary and tertiary bone grafting. Cleft Palate Craniofac J. 2002;39(1):18–25.
27. Kaura AS, Srinivasa DR, Kasten SJ. Optimal timing of alveolar cleft bone grafting for maxillary clefts in the cleft palate population. J Craniofac Surg. 2018;29(6):1551–7.
28. Posnick JC, Tompson B. Modification of the maxillary Le Fort I osteotomy in cleft-orthognathic surgery: The bilateral cleft lip and palate deformity. J Oral Maxillofac Surg. 1993;51(1):2–11.
29. Posnick JC, Tompson B. Modification of the maxillary Le Fort I osteotomy in cleft-orthognathic surgery: the unilateral cleft lip and palate deformity. J Oral Maxillofac Surg. 1992;50(7):666–75. Discussion 675–6
30. Posnick JC, Tompson B. Cleft-orthognathic surgery: complications and long-term results. Plast Reconstr Surg. 1995;96(2):255–66.
31. Glade RS, Deal R. Diagnosis and management of velopharyngeal dysfunction. Oral Maxillofac Surg Clin North Am. 2016;28(2):181–8.

32. Chua HDP, Whitehill TL, Samman N, Cheung LK. Maxillary distraction versus orthognathic surgery in cleft lip and palate patients: effects on speech and velopharyngeal function. Int J Oral Maxillofac Surg. 2010;39(7):633–40.
33. Pereira VJ, Sell D, Tuomainen J. Effect of maxillary osteotomy on speech in cleft lip and palate: Perceptual outcomes of velopharyngeal function. Int J Lang Commun Disord. 2013;48(6):640–50.
34. O'Gara M, Wilson K. The effects of maxillofacial surgery on speech and velopharyngeal function. Clin Plast Surg. 2007;34(3):395–402.
35. Janulewicz J, Costello BJ, Buckley MJ, Ford MD, Close J, Gassner R. The effects of Le Fort I osteotomies on velopharyngeal and speech functions in cleft patients. J Oral Maxillofac Surg. 2004;62(3):308–14.
36. Wu Y, Wang X, Ma L, Li Z. Velopharyngeal configuration changes following Le Fort I osteotomy with maxillary advancement in patients with cleft lip and palate: A cephalometric study. Cleft Palate Craniofac J. 2015;52(6):711–6.
37. McComb RW, Marrinan EM, Nuss RC, Labrie RA, Mulliken JB, Padwa BL. Predictors of velopharyngeal insufficiency after Le Fort i maxillary advancement in patients with cleft palate. J Oral Maxillofac Surg. 2011;69(8):2226–32.
38. Chanchareonsook N, Samman N, Whitehill TL. The effect of cranio-maxillofacial osteotomies and distraction osteogenesis on speech and velopharyngeal status: A critical review. Cleft Palate Craniofac J. 2006;43(4):477–87.
39. Satoh K, Nagata J, Shomura K, Wada T, Tachimura T, Fukuda J, et al. Morphological evaluation of changes in velopharyngeal function following maxillary distraction in patients with repaired cleft palate during mixed dentition. Cleft Palate Craniofac J. 2004;41(4):355–63.
40. Phillips JH, Klaiman P, Delorey R, MacDonald DB. Predictors of velopharyngeal insufficiency in cleft palate orthognathic surgery. Plast Reconstr Surg. 2005;115(3):681–6.
41. Alaluusua S, Turunen L, Saarikko A, Geneid A, Leikola J, Heliövaara A. The effects of Le Fort I osteotomy on velopharyngeal function in cleft patients. J Cranio Maxillofac Surg. 2019;47(2):239–44.
42. Smedberg E, Neovius E, Lohmander A. Impact of maxillary advancement on speech and velopharyngeal function in patients with cleft lip and palate. Cleft Palate Craniofac J. 2014;51(3):334–43.
43. Kim SK, Kim JC, Moon JB, Lee KC. Perceptual speech assessment after maxillary advancement osteotomy in patients with a repaired cleft lip and palate. Arch Plast Surg. 2012;39(3):198–202.
44. Schultz KP, Braun TL, Hernandez C, Wilson KD, Moore EE, Wirthlin JO, et al. Speech outcomes after LeFort I advancement among cleft lip and palate patients. Ann Plast Surg. 2019;82(2):174–9.
45. Trindade IEK, Yamashita RP, Suguimoto RM, Mazzottini R, Trindade AS. Effects of orthognathic surgery on speech and breathing of subjects with cleft lip and palate: Acoustic and aerodynamic assessment. Cleft Palate Craniofac J. 2003;40(1):54–64.
46. Poole MD, Robinson PP, Nunn ME. Maxillary advancement in cleft palate patients. Plast Reconstr Surg. 1987;80(1):154.
47. James DR, Brook K. Maxillary hypoplasia in patients with cleft lip and palate deformity-the alternative surgical approach. Eur J Orthod. 1985;7(4):231–47.
48. Richardson S, Seelan NS, Selvaraj D, Khandeparker R V., Gnanamony S. Perceptual speech assessment after anterior maxillary distraction in patients with cleft maxillary hypoplasia. J Oral Maxillofac Surg. 2016;74(6):1239.e1–9.
49. Richardson S, Agni NA, Selvaraj D. Anterior maxillary distraction using a tooth-borne device for hypoplastic cleft maxillas—a pilot study. J Oral Maxillofac Surg. 2011;69(12):e542–8.
50. Richardson S, Krishna S, Bansal A. Use of repeat anterior maxillary distraction to correct residual midface hypoplasia in cleft patients. J Korean Assoc Oral Maxillofac Surg. 2018;43(6):407.
51. Richardson S, Selvaraj D, Khandeparker R V, Seelan NS, Richardson S. Tooth-borne anterior maxillary distraction for cleft maxillary hypoplasia: our experience with 147 patients. J Oral Maxillofac Surg. 2016;74(12):2504.e1–14.
52. Richardson S, Krishna S, Khandeparker RV. A comprehensive management protocol to treat cleft maxillary hypoplasia. J Cranio Maxillofacial Surg. 2018;46(2):356–61.
53. Tahmasbi S, Jamilian A, Showkatbakhsh R, Pourdanesh F, Behnaz M. Cephalometric changes in nasopharyngeal area after anterior maxillary segmental distraction versus Le Fort I osteotomy in patients with cleft lip and palate. Eur J Dent. 2018;12(3):393–7.
54. Takahashi K, Dahy KG, Saito K, Masuoka H, Suzuki S, Bessho K. Patient with cleft maxillary hypoplasia who underwent distraction osteogenesis and conservative therapies to postoperative velopharyngeal insufficiency. J Craniofac Surg. 2017;28(5):1302–4.
55. Gart MS, Gosain AK. Surgical management of velopharyngeal insufficiency. Clin Plast Surg. 2014;41(2):253–70.
56. Denadai R, Sabbag A, Raposo-Amaral CE, Filho JCP, Nagae MH, Raposo-Amaral CA. Bilateral buccinator myomucosal flap outcomes in nonsyndromic patients with repaired cleft palate and velopharyngeal insufficiency. J Plast Reconstr Aesthetic Surg. 2017;70(11):1598–607.
57. Abdel-Aziz M, Hussien A, Kamel A, Azooz K, Fawaz M. The impact of velopharyngeal surgery on the polysomnographic parameters after cleft palate repair. J Craniofac Surg. 2018;29(3):717–9.
58. Dentino KM, Marrinan EM, Brustowicz K, Mulliken JB, Padwa BL. Pharyngeal flap is effective treatment for post maxillary advancement velopharyngeal insufficiency in patients with repaired cleft lip and palate. J Oral Maxillofac Surg. 2016;74(6):1207–14.
59. Bhatia S, Bocca A, Jones J, Sugar AW. Le Fort I advancement osteotomies of 1 cm or more. How safe or stable? Br J Oral Maxillofac Surg. 2016;54(3):346–50.
60. Drommer R. Selective angiographic studies prior to Le Fort I osteotomy in patients with cleft lip and palate. J Maxillofac Surg. 1979;7(C):264–70.
61. Rachmiel A. Treatment of maxillary cleft palate: distraction osteogenesis versus orthognathic surgery-part one: maxillary distraction. J Oral Maxillofac Surg. 2007;65(4):753–7.
62. Rachmiel A, Even-Almos M, Aizenbud D. Treatment of maxillary cleft palate: Distraction osteogenesis vs. orthognathic surgery. Ann Maxillofac Surg. 2012;2(2):127–30.
63. Zhang Y, Jia H, Fu Z, Huang Y, Wang Z, Guo R, et al. Dentoskeletal effects of facemask therapy in skeletal Class III cleft patients with or without bone graft. Am J Orthod Dentofac Orthop. 2018;153(4):542–9.
64. Ahn HW, Kim KW, Yang IH, Choi JY, Baek SH. Comparison of the effects of maxillary protraction using facemask and miniplate anchorage between unilateral and bilateral cleft lip and palate patients. Angle Orthod. 2012;82(5):935–41.
65. Zhang Y, Fu Z, Jia H, Huang Y, Li X, Liu H, et al. Long-term stability of maxillary protraction therapy in Class III patients with complete unilateral cleft lip and palate. Angle Orthod. 2019;89(2):214–20.
66. Tindlund RS. Skeletal response to maxillary protraction in patients with cleft lip and palate before age 10 years. Cleft Palate Craniofac J. 1994;31(4):295–308.
67. Angelieri F, Franchi L, Cevidanes LHS, Hino CT, Nguyen T, McNamara JA. Zygomaticomaxillary suture maturation: A predictor of maxillary protraction? Part I—A classification method. Orthod Craniofac Res. 2017;20(2):85–94.
68. Angelieri F, Ruellas AC, Yatabe MS, Cevidanes LHS, Franchi L, Toyama-Hino C, et al. Zygomaticomaxillary suture maturation: Part II—The influence of sutural maturation on the response to maxillary protraction. Orthod Craniofac Res. 2017;20(3):152–63.
69. Hino CT, Cevidanes LHS, Nguyen TT, De Clerck HJ, Franchi L, McNamara JA. Three-dimensional analysis of maxillary changes

associated with facemask and rapid maxillary expansion compared with bone anchored maxillary protraction. Am J Orthod Dentofac Orthop. 2013;144(5):705–14.

70. On SW, Baek SH, Choi JY. Effect of long-term use of facemask with miniplate on maxillary protraction in patients with cleft lip and palate. J Craniofac Surg. 2018;29(2):309–14.
71. Jahanbin A, Kazemian M, Eslami N, Pouya IS. Maxillary protraction with intermaxillary elastics to miniplates versus bone-anchored face-mask therapy in cleft lip and palate patients. J Craniofac Surg. 2016;27(5):1247–52.
72. Faco R, Yatabe M, Cevidanes LHS, Timmerman H, De Clerck HJ, Garib D. Bone-anchored maxillary protraction in unilateral cleft lip and palate: a cephalometric appraisal. Eur J Orthod. 2019:1–7.
73. Susami T, Mori Y, Ohkubo K, Takahashi M, Hirano Y, Saijo H, et al. Changes in maxillofacial morphology and velopharyngeal function with two-stage maxillary distraction–mandibular setback surgery in patients with cleft lip and palate. Int J Oral Maxillofac Surg. 2018;47(3):357–65.
74. Dan AEB, Thygesen TH, Pinholt EM. Corticosteroid administration in oral and orthognathic surgery: A systematic review of the literature and meta-analysis. J Oral Maxillofac Surg. 2010;68(9):2207–20.
75. Jean S, Dionne PL, Bouchard C, Giasson L, Turgeon AF. Perioperative systemic corticosteroids in orthognathic surgery: a systematic review and meta-analysis. J Oral Maxillofac Surg. 2017;75(12):2638–49.
76. Olsen JJ, Skov J, Ingerslev J, Thorn JJ, Pinholt EM. Prevention of bleeding in orthognathic surgery—A systematic review and meta-analysis of randomized controlled trials. J Oral Maxillofac Surg. 2016; 74:139–150.
77. Choi WS, Samman N. Risks and benefits of deliberate hypotension in anaesthesia: a systematic review. Int J Oral Maxillofac Surg. 2008;37(8):687–703.
78. Rodríguez-Navarro A, Gonzalez-Valverde FM. Unilateral blindness after orthognathic surgery: hypotensive anaesthesia is not the primary cause. Int J Oral Maxillofac Surg. 2018;47(1):79–82.
79. Mathew P, Adenwalla HS, Narayanan PV, Nyamu E. A report of 2 patients with transient blindness following Le Fort I osteotomy and a review of past reported cases. Indian J Plast Surg. 2015;48(3):297–300.
80. Lo L-J, Hung K-F, Chen Y-R. Blindness as a complication of Le Fort I osteotomy for maxillary distraction. Plast Reconstr Surg. 2002;109(2):688–98. Discussion 699–700
81. Ettinger KS, Yildirim Y, Weingarten TN, Van Ess JM, Viozzi CF, Arce K. Hypotensive anesthesia is associated with shortened length of hospital stay following orthognathic surgery. J Oral Maxillofac Surg. 2016;74(1):130–8.
82. Lin S, McKenna SJ, Yao CF, Chen YR, Chen C. Effects of hypotensive anesthesia on reducing intraoperative blood loss, duration of operation, and quality of surgical field during orthognathic surgery: a systematic review and meta-analysis of randomized controlled trials. J Oral Maxillofac Surg. 2017;75:73–86.
83. Watanabe M, Watanabe A, Takano N, Saito C, Shibahara T. Morphologic evaluation for safe le fort I osteotomy in cleft lip and palate. Cleft Palate Craniofac J. 2018;55(5):728–35.
84. Lee SH, Lee SH, Mori Y, Minami K, Park HS, Kwon TG. Evaluation of pterygomaxillary anatomy using computed tomography: Are there any structural variations in cleft patients? J Oral Maxillofac Surg. 2011;69(10):2644–9.
85. Hoffman GR, Islam S. The difficult Le Fort I osteotomy and downfracture: a review with consideration given to an atypical maxillary morphology. J Plast Reconstr Aesthetic Surg. 2008;61(9):1029–33.
86. Phillips JH, Nish I, Daskalogiannakis J. Orthognathic surgery in cleft patients. Plast Reconstr Surg. 2012;129(3):535e–48e.
87. Precious DS, Goodday RH, Bourget L, Skulsky FG. Pterygoid plate fracture in Le Fort I osteotomy with and without pterygoid chisel: a computed tomography scan evaluation of 58 patients. J Oral Maxillofac Surg. 1993;51(2):151–3.
88. Precious DS, Morrison A, Ricard D. Pterygomaxillary separation without the use of an osteotome. J Oral Maxillofac Surg. 1991;49(1):98–9.
89. Turvey TA, Fonseca RJ. The anatomy of the internal maxillary artery in the pterygopalatine fossa: its relationship to maxillary surgery. J Oral Surg. 1980;38(2):92–5.
90. Laster Z, Ardekian L, Rachmiel A, Peled M. Use of the "shark-fin" osteotome in separation of the pterygomaxillary junction in Le Fort I osteotomy: A clinical and computerized tomography study. Int J Oral Maxillofac Surg. 2002;31(1):100–3.
91. Trimble LD, Tideman H, Stoelinga PJW. A modification of the pterygoid plate separation in low-level maxillary osteotomies. J Oral Maxillofac Surg. 1983;41(8):544–6.
92. Kanazawa T, Kuroyanagi N, Miyachi H, Ochiai S, Kamiya N, Nagao T, et al. Factors predictive of pterygoid process fractures after pterygomaxillary separation without using an osteotome in le Fort i osteotomy. Oral Surg Oral Med Oral Pathol Oral Radiol. 2013;115(3):310–8.
93. Breeze J, Linares CV, Stockton P. Is an osteotome necessary for pterygomaxillary dysjunction or dysjunction through the tuberosity during le Fort i osteotomy? A systematic review. Br J Oral Maxillofac Surg. 2016;54:248–52.
94. Dadwal H, Shanmugasundaram S, Krishnakumar Raja VB. Preoperative and postoperative CT scan assessment of pterygomaxillary junction in patients undergoing Le Fort I osteotomy: comparison of pterygomaxillary dysjunction technique and Trimble technique—a pilot study. J Maxillofac Oral Surg. 2015;14(3):713–9.
95. Hernández-Alfaro F, Guijarro-Martínez R. "Twist technique" for pterygomaxillary dysjunction in minimally invasive Le Fort I osteotomy. J Oral Maxillofac Surg. 2013;71(2):389–92.
96. Ueki K, Nakagawa K, Marukawa K, Yamamoto E. Le Fort I osteotomy using an ultrasonic bone curette to fracture the pterygoid plates. J Cranio Maxillofac Surg. 2004;32(6):381–6.
97. Ueki K, Hashiba Y, Marukawa K, Okabe K, Alam S, Nakagawa K, et al. Assessment of pterygomaxillary separation in Le Fort I osteotomy in class III patients. J Oral Maxillofac Surg. 2009;67(4):833–9.
98. Watts GD, Antonarakis GS, Forrest CR, Tompson BD, Phillips JH. Single versus segmental maxillary osteotomies and long-term stability in unilateral cleft lip and palate related malocclusion. J Oral Maxillofac Surg. 2014;72(12):2514–21.
99. James JN, Costello BJ, Ruiz RL. Management of cleft lip and palate and cleft orthognathic considerations. Oral Maxillofac Surg Clin North Am. 2014;26(4):565–72.
100. Bell WH, Fonseca RJ, Kenneky JW, Levy BM. Bone healing and revascularization after total maxillary osteotomy. J Oral Surg. 1975;33(4):253–60.
101. Bell WH, Levy BM. Revascularization and bone healing after maxillary corticotomies. J Oral Surg. 1972;30(9):640–8.
102. Lanigan DT. Ligation of the descending palatine artery: pro and con. J Oral Maxillofac Surg. 1997;55(12):1502–4.
103. Regan BO, Bharadwaj G. The identification and protection of the descending palatine artery in Le Fort I osteotomy: a forgotten technique? Br J Oral Maxillofac Surg. 2007;45(5):412–4.
104. Omura S, Iwai T, Honda K, Shibutani N, Fujita K, Yamashita Y, et al. U-shaped osteotomy around the descending palatine artery to prevent posterior osseous interference for superior/posterior repositioning of the maxilla in le Fort i osteotomy. J Craniofac Surg. 2015;26(5):1613–5.
105. Omura S, Iwai T, Murata S, Tohnai I. Use of a simple handmade retractor to protect the descending palatine artery during removal

of posterior osseous interferences for maxillary impaction in le fort i osteotomy. J Craniofac Surg. 2013;24(3):978–9.
106. Johnson LM, Arnett GW. Pyramidal osseous release around the descending palatine artery: a surgical technique. J Oral Maxillofac Surg. 1991;49(12):1356–7.
107. Betts NJ, Fonseca RJ. Location of the descending palatine artery in relation to the Le Fort I osteotomy. J Oral Maxillofac Surg. 1996;54(7):826–7.
108. Li KK, Meara JG, Alexander A. Location of the descending palatine artery in relation to the Le Fort I osteotomy. J Oral Maxillofac Surg. 1996;54(7):822–5.
109. Waite PD, Tejera TJ, Anucul B. The stability of maxillary advancement using Le Fort I osteotomy with and without genial bone grafting. Int J Oral Maxillofac Surg. 1996;25(4):264–7.
110. Posnick JC, Gray JA. Is it safe to re-harvest the anterior iliac crest to manage Le Fort I interpositional defects in young adults with a repaired cleft? J Oral Maxillofac Surg. 2015;73(12):S32–9.
111. Wardrop RW, Wolford LM. Maxillary stability following downgraft and/or advancement procedures with stabilization using rigid fixation and porous block hydroxyapatite implants. J Oral Maxillofac Surg. 1989;47(4):336–42.
112. Mehra P, Castro V, Freitas RZ, Wolford LM. Stability of the Le Fort I osteotomy for maxillary advancement using rigid fixation and porous block hydroxyapatite grafting. Oral Surg Oral Med Oral Pathol Oral Radiol Endod. 2002;94(1):18–23.
113. Mehra P, Wolford LM, Hopkin JK, Castro V, Frietas R. Stability of maxillary advancement using rigid fixation and porous-block hydroxyapatite grafting: cleft palate versus non-cleft patients. Int J Adult Orthodon Orthognath Surg. 2001;16(3):193–9.
114. Gomes KU, Martins WDB, Ribas M de O. Horizontal and vertical maxillary osteotomy stability, in cleft lip and palate patients, using allogeneic bone graft. Dental Press J Orthod. 2013;18(5):84–90.
115. Stork JT, Kim RH, Regennitter FJ, Keller EE. Maxillary quadrangular le Fort i osteotomy: Long-term skeletal stability and clinical outcome. Int J Oral Maxillofac Surg. 2013;42(12):1533–46.
116. Cheung LK, Chua HDP, Hägg MB. Cleft maxillary distraction versus orthognathic surgery: clinical morbidities and surgical relapse. Plast Reconstr Surg. 2006;118(4):996–1008. Discussion 1009
117. Cheung LK, Chua HDP. A meta-analysis of cleft maxillary osteotomy and distraction osteogenesis. Int J Oral Maxillofac Surg. 2006;35(1):14–24.
118. Kwong Cheung L, Ser Pheng Loh J, Ho SMY. The early psychological adjustment of cleft patients after maxillary distraction osteogenesis and conventional orthognathic surgery: a preliminary study. J Oral Maxillofac Surg. 2006;64(12):1743–1750.
119. Chua HDP, Ho SMY, Cheung LK. The comparison of psychological adjustment of patients with cleft lip and palate after maxillary distraction osteogenesis and conventional orthognathic surgery. Oral Surg Oral Med Oral Pathol Oral Radiol. 2012;114(5 Suppl):S5–10.
120. Kloukos D, Fudalej P, Sequeira-Byron P, Katsaros C. Maxillary distraction osteogenesis versus orthognathic surgery for cleft lip and palate patients. Cochrane Database Syst Rev. 2018;8(8):CD010403.
121. Chua HDP, Cheung LK. Soft tissue changes from maxillary distraction osteogenesis versus orthognathic surgery in patients with cleft lip and palate—A randomized controlled clinical trial. J Oral Maxillofac Surg. 2012;70(7):1648–58.
122. Thongdee P, Samman N. Stability of maxillary surgical movement in unilateral cleft lip and palate with preceding alveolar bone grafting. Cleft Palate Craniofac J. 2005;42(6):664–674.
123. Precious DS. Treatment of retruded maxilla in cleft lip and palate—orthognathic surgery versus distraction osteogenesis: the case for orthognathic surgery. J Oral Maxillofac Surg. 2007;65(4):758–61.
124. Hirano A, Suzuki H. Factors related to relapse after Le Fort I maxillary advancement osteotomy in patients with cleft lip and palate. Cleft Palate Craniofac J. 2001;38(1):1–10.
125. Watts GD, Antonarakis GS, Forrest CR, Tompson BD, Phillips JH. Is linear advancement related to relapse in unilateral cleft lip and palate orthognathic surgery? Cleft Palate Craniofac J. 2015;52(6):717–23.
126. Hoffman GR, Brennan PA. The skeletal stability of one-piece Le Fort 1 osteotomy to advance the maxilla Part 2. The influence of uncontrollable clinical variables. Br J Oral Maxillofac Surg. 2004;42(3):226–30.
127. Haas Junior OL, Guijarro-Martínez R, de Sousa Gil AP, da Silva Meirelles L, Scolari N, Muñoz-Pereira ME, et al. Hierarchy of surgical stability in orthognathic surgery: overview of systematic reviews. Int J Oral Maxillofac Surg. 2019;48:1415.
128. Proffit WR, Turvey TA, Phillips C. The hierarchy of stability and predictability in orthognathic surgery with rigid fixation: An update and extension. Head Face Med. 2007;3(1):1–11.
129. Hoffman GR, Brennan PA. The skeletal stability of one-piece Le Fort 1 osteotomy to advance the maxilla Part 1. Stability resulting from non-bone grafted rigid fixation. Br J Oral Maxillofac Surg. 2004;42(3):221–5.
130. Kanno T, Mitsugi M, Hosoe M, Sukegawa S, Yamauchi K, Furuki Y. Long-term skeletal stability after maxillary advancement with distraction osteogenesis in nongrowing patients. J Oral Maxillofac Surg. 2008;66(9):1833–46.
131. Wolford LM, Karras SC, Mehra P. Considerations for orthognathic surgery during growth, Part 1: Mandibular deformities. Am J Orthod Dentofac Orthop. 2001;119(2):95–101.
132. Saltaji H, Major MP, Altalibi M, Youssef M, Flores-Mir C. Long-term skeletal stability after maxillary advancement with distraction osteogenesis in cleft lip and palate patients: A systematic review. Angle Orthod. 2012;82(6):1115–22.
133. Saltaji H, Major MP, Alfakir H, Al-Saleh MAQ, Flores-Mir C. Maxillary advancement with conventional orthognathic surgery in patients with cleft lip and palate: Is it a stable technique? J Oral Maxillofac Surg. 2012;70(12):2859–66.
134. Andersen K, Svenstrup M, Pedersen TK, Küseler A, Jensen J, Nørholt SE. Stability after cleft maxillary distraction osteogenesis or conventional orthognathic surgery. J Oral Maxillofac Res. 2015;6(2):e2.
135. Serafin B, Perciaccante VJ, Cunningham LL. Stability of orthognathic surgery and distraction osteogenesis: options and alternatives. Oral Maxillofac Surg Clin North Am. 2007;19(3):311–20, v.
136. Hirjak D, Reyneke JP, Janec J, Beno M, Kupcova I. Long-term results of maxillary distraction osteogenesis in nongrowing cleft: 5-years experience using internal device. Bratisl Lek Listy. 2016;117(12):685–90.
137. Gürsoy S, Hukki J, Hurmerinta K. Five-year follow-up of maxillary distraction osteogenesis on the dentofacial structures of children with cleft lip and palate. J Oral Maxillofac Surg. 2010;68(4):744–50.
138. Chua HDP, Hgg MB, Cheung LK. Cleft maxillary distraction versus orthognathic surgery-which one is more stable in 5 years? Oral Surgery. Oral Med Oral Pathol Oral Radiol Endodontol. 2010;109(6):803–14.
139. Figueroa AA, Polley JW, Friede H, Ko EW. Long-term skeletal stability after maxillary advancement with distraction osteogenesis using a rigid external distraction device in cleft maxillary deformities. Plast Reconstr Surg. 2004;114(6):1382–92.
140. Yamaguchi K, Lonic D, Lo LJ. Complications following orthognathic surgery for patients with cleft lip/palate: A systematic review. J Formos Med Assoc. 2016;115(4):269–77.
141. Tabrizi R, Tumer K, Shafiei S, Rashad A. Can use of rigid fixation after consolidation increase stability in cleft patients fol-

lowing distraction osteogenesis? J Oral Maxillofac Surg. 2018;76(6):1309–15.
142. Metalwala Z, Okunseri C, Fletcher S, Allareddy V. Orthognathic surgical outcomes in patients with and without craniofacial anomalies. J Oral Maxillofac Surg. 2018;76(2):436.e1–8.
143. Moran I, Virdee S, Sharp I, Sulh J. Postoperative complications following LeFort 1 maxillary advancement surgery in cleft palate patients: A 5-year retrospective study. Cleft Palate Craniofac J. 2018;55(2):231–7.
144. dos Santos Alves JM, de Freitas Alves BW, de Figueiredo Costa AC, Carneiro BGDS, de Sousa LM, Gondim DV. Cranial nerve injuries in Le Fort I osteotomy: a systematic review. Int J Oral Maxillofac Surg. 2018;10–2.
145. Ohrmann D, Hoyte-Williams PE, Chen PK-T. Update on complications in cleft orthognathic surgery. Curr Opin Otolaryngol Head Neck Surg. 2018;1
146. Eduardo Charles Pagotto L, de Santana Santos T, Juliana de Abreu de Vasconcellos S, Silva Santos J, Saquete Martins-Filho PR. Piezoelectric versus conventional techniques for orthognathic surgery: Systematic review and meta-analysis. J Cranio Maxillofacial Surg. 2017;45(10):1607–13.

Cleft Rhinoplasty

76

Sunil Richardson and Rakshit Vijay Sinai Khandeparker

76.1 Introduction

Rhinoplasties in cleft lip and palate (CLP) patients are considered one of the most difficult and challenging surgeries to carry out. The reasons understood for this are twofold: the principal reason being the simultaneous involvement of all the layers of the nose, including the skin, cartilage, skeleton and vestibular lining, and the other the significant scarring that accompanies multiple previous surgical interventions. The deformity has a major impact on nasal aesthetics as well as function and can range from being absolutely inconspicuous to catastrophic.

The literature is flooded with numerous techniques for ultimate correction of unilateral and bilateral cleft lip-nasal deformities. More recently, most cleft surgeons have started opting for primary rhinoplasties at the time of lip repair with or without presurgical orthopaedics. These early interventions have definitely improved the nasal deformity and the overall nasal symmetry; however, definitive rhinoplasty may still be required at a later date as the child grows. Despite all the recent developments in cleft surgery, an optimal surgical modality that addresses the issues of desired nasal form coupled with long-term stability for correction of cleft lip-nasal deformity still fails to exist.

Disclosure: Authors have no financial conflicts to disclose

Electronic Supplementary Material The online version of this chapter (https://doi.org/10.1007/978-981-15-1346-6_76) contains supplementary material, which is available to authorized users.

S. Richardson (✉)
Richardson's Dental and Craniofacial Hospital,
Chunkan Kadai, Nagercoil, Tamil Nadu, India

R. V. S. Khandeparker
Department of Oral and Maxillofacial Surgery, Goa Dental College and Hospital, Bambolim, Goa, India

76.2 Pathologic Anatomy

A clear understanding of the associated complex anatomical and pathological abnormalities is paramount to obtaining desired nasal form and function [1].

76.2.1 Unilateral Cleft Nasal Deformity

The hallmark of unilateral cleft nasal deformity is a three-dimensional asymmetry of the nasal tip and the alar base (Fig. 76.1a–c). The characteristic features include:

1. **Asymmetric nasal tip**: This is principally due to a shorter medial crus and longer lateral crus of the lower lateral cartilage (LLC) on the cleft side as compared to the non-cleft side. This contributes to a poorly defined nasal tip with less projection [2]. Furthermore, the angle between the medial and lateral crura on the cleft side is increased.
2. **Alar dome is flat and wider on the cleft side** due to posterolateral displacement of the alar dome [2].
3. **Deviation of the columellar base to the non-cleft side**: The unilateral cleft results in a discontinuous insertion of the orbicularis oris muscle into the columellar base on the non-cleft side rather than a horizontal insertion and continuous decussation as seen in the normal lip. The contraction of the orbicularis oris muscle results in an unopposed pull of the columella, caudal septum and premaxilla to the non-cleft side [3].
4. **Alar base on the cleft side is directed laterally, posteriorly and inferiorly**: Two factors contribute to this: one being the insertion of the orbicularis oris into the alar base and the other the deficient maxillary skeletal framework at the alar base [3].
5. **Hypoplastic maxilla on the cleft side.**
6. **Wide and horizontally directed nostril on the cleft side**: This is brought about by a combination of vector of

K. Bonanthaya et al. (eds.), *Oral and Maxillofacial Surgery for the Clinician*, https://doi.org/10.1007/978-981-15-1346-6_76

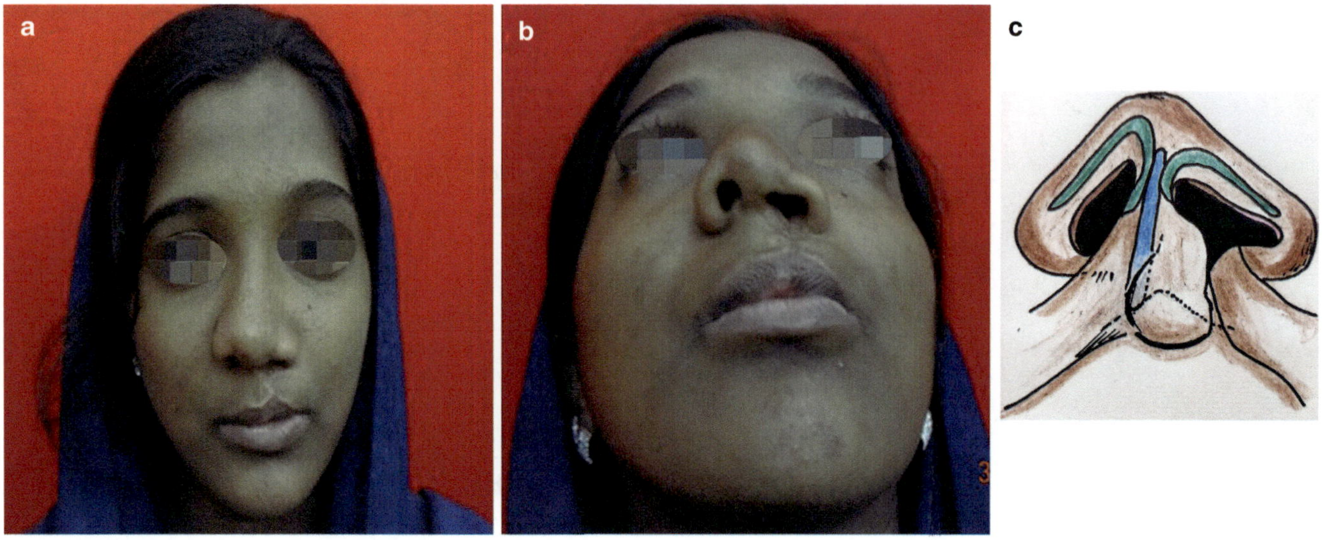

Fig. 76.1 (**a–c**) Photographs depicting the pathologic anatomy as observed in unilateral cleft nasal deformity. (**a**) Frontal view showing the deviation of the nasal root towards the non-cleft side with asymmetrical appearing nasal tip. (**b**) Basal view depicting the deviation of the base of the columella to the non-cleft side. Also, observe the wide and horizontally directed nostril on the cleft side. Furthermore, the alar base on the cleft side is directed laterally, posteriorly and inferiorly. (**c**) Pictorial depiction of deviation of the caudal nasal septum (blue) towards the non-cleft side

orbicularis oris muscle pull and asymmetric LLC on the cleft side [4, 5].

7. **Deviation of the caudal septum to the non-cleft side:** The unopposed pull of the orbicularis oris muscle due to its improper insertion into the columellar base results in deviation of the caudal septum to the non-cleft side [3]. This force affects only the caudal septum and results in deflection of the cartilaginous and bony septum into the cleft side posteriorly. This alone or in association with hypertrophied nasal turbinates significantly narrows the opening of the nasal airway and contributes to nasal airway obstruction [6].
8. **Compromised external nasal valve:** This is the consequence of two related factors: introversion of the nasal ala and webbing of the nasal vestibule. Due to the position of the columella and alar base on the cleft side, the LLC is subjected to distortional forces that causes it to rotate posteroinferiorly and brings about introversion of the cleft side nasal ala [7]. This leads to hooding and thickening of the ala and together with surgical scarring forms an oblique fold and contributes to webbing of the nasal vestibule. This tissue bulk has an influence on the nasal airflow and significantly alters the relationship of upper lateral cartilages (ULCs) and LLCs.
9. **Weakened upper lateral cartilages (ULC) and abnormal relationship to LLCs:** On the cleft side, the ULC displays side-to-side relationship rather than the typical overlap type of relationship seen on the non-cleft side. The ULC on the cleft side is also weakened by inadequate skeletal support [8]. The consequence of both these factors is reduced support and collapse of the ULC with deep inspiration.
10. **Compromised internal nasal valve on the cleft side:** This is primarily because of septal bowing into the cleft side at the internal nasal valve together with weakened support of the ULC at the cleft side which causes the cartilage to collapse with respiration.

76.2.2 Bilateral Cleft Nasal Deformity

The bilateral cleft lip nasal deformity is grossly symmetrical and shares similar clinical characteristics as observed in unilateral cleft deformity [9, 10] (Fig. 76.2a–c). The clinical characteristics include:

1. **Under-projected and bifid nasal tip**: The lateral crus of the LLC is long, and the medial crus is short which leads to under-projection of the nasal tip. The medial crura are typically splayed, producing a poorly defined, bifid tip [11]. The nose is wide and depressed.
2. **Blunting of the alar dome with a more obtuse angle** due to posterolateral displacement of the alar domes [11].

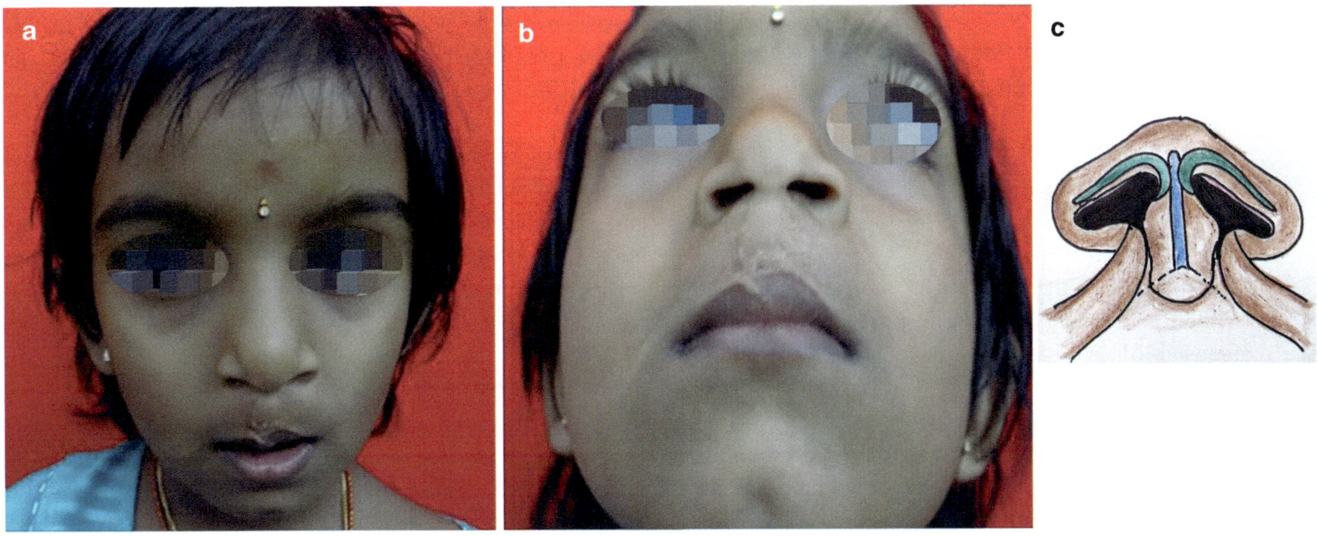

Fig. 76.2 (**a–c**) Photographs depicting the pathologic anatomy as observed in bilateral cleft nasal deformity. (**a**) Frontal view demonstrating a more or less symmetrical deformity with bifid nasal tip and blunting of the alar dome. (**b**) Basal view depicting symmetrical position of the caudal nasal septum, short columella and bilateral displacement of the alar bases laterally, posteriorly and inferiorly with wide and horizontally directed nostrils bilaterally. (**c**) Pictorial depiction of the classical midline position of the caudal nasal septum

3. **Short columella with a wider base:** The columella is short or nearly absent as a consequence of decreased soft tissue and skin between the nasal tip and the upper lip [12].
4. **Alar bases are displaced laterally, posteriorly and inferiorly.** This brings about flaring of the alar bases and widening of the nostrils.
5. **Hypoplastic maxillae bilaterally.**
6. **Nostrils are wide and horizontally directed with margins buckling inwards.**
7. **Classical midline positioning of the septum.** The nasal septum is classically midline; however, in case of a slight discrepancy, the septum deviates to the less affected side [13, 14].
8. **The external nasal valve is compromised by** introversion of the LLCs and webbing of the nasal vestibules bilaterally.
9. **The ULCs are weakened and display abnormal relationship to LLCs** similar to that seen in the unilateral cleft nasal deformity.
10. **The internal nasal valve is compromised by weakened support of the ULC:** It is important to note that midline positioning of the nasal septum in bilateral cleft nasal deformity results in compromise of the internal nasal valve to a lesser significant degree as compared to the unilateral cleft nasal deformity.

76.3 Surgical Timing

The timing of cleft lip nasal repairs can be divided into primary, intermediate and secondary or definitive repairs.

76.3.1 Primary Rhinoplasty

Initially, most surgeons were sceptical with early nasal interventions at the time of cleft lip repair following demonstrations of impairment of nasal and midfacial growth in experimental studies that resulted after large submucosal resections of the nasal septum. However, studies by McComb and Coghlan [7] have dispelled this philosophy and demonstrated that early interventions seldom interfere with growth provided the lower lateral cartilage is only repositioned and not resected. Primary rhinoplasties are now increasingly accepted, and their positive effects on secondary rhinoplasties are well documented.

Primary cleft rhinoplasty is typically carried out at 3 months of age at the time of primary cheiloplasty [15]. An early intervention improves the existing cleft nasal deformity by achieving better symmetry, allowing the nose to grow in a symmetric fashion and potentially improving long-term appearance and the final outcome.

The definite goals of the procedure are highlighted in Box 76.1.

Box 76.1: Definite Goals of Primary Cleft Rhinoplasty

- To bring about approximation of the nasal floor to establish a muscle and soft tissue sill across the nasal base
- Symmetrical positioning of the abnormally positioned LLC
- Providing nasal tip support
- Repositioning of the alar base and correction of the webbed lateral alar mucosa by plicating skin and mucosa [16]

The addition of presurgical naso-alveolar moulding device is advocated by some authors in conjunction with primary surgery. The technique delivers continuous low-level pressure on the alveolar segments and is highly successful in shaping the nasal cartilage within the initial 6 weeks due to high levels of circulating maternal oestrogen that makes the cartilage increasingly elastic [17].

The technique helps in bringing the alveolar segments closer thereby narrowing the cleft gap, improving the alar base symmetry, expanding the soft tissue envelope and elongating the columella [18, 19].

76.3.2 Intermediate Rhinoplasty

Intermediate rhinoplasty is reserved for procedures that are carried out prior to completion of nasal growth, in the time interval spanning between definitive lip repair and secondary rhinoplasty. The procedures are planned on the lines of conservation with the singular aim to achieve symmetry during continued nasal growth, ultimately creating a definitive platform for a more successful definitive repair.

The primary goal of surgery is to correct the abnormal position of the LLC on the cleft side so that there is no exacerbation of the deformity following nasal growth in future. It is imperative to perform a septorhinoplasty or cartilage grafting procedures in the post-adolescence age so that the nasal growth proceeds unimpeded [11].

Intermediate rhinoplasty can be carried out at two distinct time intervals [20]. One corresponds to 4–6 years of age, and this age group coincides with the timing of lip revision if required and also helps in achieving a better nasal symmetry. Also, this is the time when the peer pressure starts to mount necessitating the need for intermediate rhinoplasty in this age group. Furthermore, any lateral vestibular webbing can be dealt with preventing the obstruction of the external nasal valve.

The other instance when an intermediate rhinoplasty can be carried out is after completion of orthodontic alignment and secondary alveolar bone grafting (8–12 years). This helps in creating a solid skeletal platform to affect a long-lasting correction of severe nasal deformities.

76.3.3 Secondary or Definitive Rhinoplasty

Secondary or definitive rhinoplasty is performed once the maxillary and nasal growth ceases, which corresponds to 14–16 years of age in females and 16–18 years of age in males [21]. The procedure has to be definitive and provides an opportunity to introduce aggressive surgical interventions like septorhinoplasty, nasal osteotomies and cartilage grafting manoeuvres without fear of jeopardising the maxillary or nasal growth.

The goals of definitive rhinoplasty are mentioned in Box 76.2.

Box 76.2: Goals of Definitive Rhinoplasty

- Create a lasting symmetry and definition of the nasal base and tip.
- Relieve nasal obstruction.
- Manage nasal scarring and webbing.
- Correct short columellar skin if present, and augment the nasal dorsum in cases of bilateral cleft nasal deformities [1].

Most CLP patients present with maxillary hypoplasia and therefore require maxillary advancement surgery in the form of either LeFort I osteotomy, total maxillary distraction or anterior maxillary distraction. The maxillary projection can be improved with these procedures without affecting the nasal dorsum adversely [22]. These procedures also allow for forward movement of LLC and improvement of the tip projection. In scenarios such as this, definitive rhinoplasty is often carried out after addressing the skeletal discrepancies.

76.4 Preoperative Evaluation

Prior to carrying out a rhinoplasty surgery, it is prudent to carry out a thorough evaluation of the nose in a meticulous manner. This when backed up with sound knowledge of nasal anatomy can bring about aesthetically pleasing results in cleft rhinoplasty.

76.4.1 History

It is imperative to address any patient concerns as related to symmetry of the lip and nose, nasal airway, etc. prior to carrying out a rhinoplasty surgery. Any previous nasal surgeries have to be documented accurately. The effects of such surgeries on the postoperative outcomes have to be explained to the patient beforehand.

76.4.2 Physical Examination

A thorough physical examination involves examining both the external appearance and the internal nasal structures.

External examination of the nose must be carried out in accordance with its position on the facial skeleton. Measurements as traced on preoperative photographs can provide a guide in the surgical planning (Fig. 76.3a–d).

Internal nasal examination proceeds in a systematic and repeatable manner and is performed using a nasal speculum to evaluate for the nasal function.

When performing the physical examination of the nose, the clinical characteristics of unilateral and bilateral cleft nasal deformities as previously described are looked up for in a systematic manner. Gunter diagrams can be a valuable aid for the purpose of preoperative planning [21].

76.4.3 Photographic Documentation

76.4.3.1 Two-Dimensional Photographs

Appropriate documentation of the deformity is made possible by taking preoperative photographs in all views, viz. frontal, basal, lateral and oblique views (Fig. 76.4a–f). These photographs serve diagnostic purpose as well as help in protecting the surgeon in cases of medico-legal implications. The photographs also help in explaining the goals of surgery adequately to the patient. Furthermore, the photographs can serve as a visual guide to the surgeon intraoperatively, helping in implementing the planned surgical goals precisely.

76.4.3.2 Three-Dimensional Imaging

This method requires a set of devices, viz. an optical system, digital communication network and a computer with a calculation program which helps in determining the shape of the three-dimensional object by transforming the image from analogue to digital form (Fig. 76.5a). The technique is reliable, can be safely employed in child patients due to its non-ionising nature and offers both qualitative and quantitative assessments, and the digital model can be employed in the clinical setting immediately. The disadvantages include the cost, long time that is required for patient preparation and data acquisition and inability to measure bony or interactive landmarks.

76.4.4 Radiographic Assessment

76.4.4.1 Cephalometric Analysis

Cephalometric analysis aids in evaluating the maxillary position and its possible implications on the patient's nose [21] (Fig. 76.5b). The need for any maxillary advancement surgery and the importance of performing it before any rhinoplasty surgery should be conveyed to the patient. Cephalometric analysis also allows for evaluation of chin position [21].

76.4.4.2 Computed Tomography (CT)/Cone Beam Computed Tomography (CBCT)

CT scans of the paranasal sinuses in axial and coronal views help in defining the deformation of the septum as well as other intra-nasal structures. CBCT is an attraction alternative to CT with regard to decreased ionising radiation to the patient and image quality for hard tissues on par with CT. No modalities other than CT/CBCT allow for evaluation of nasal septum objectively [23] (Fig. 76.5c).

76.4.5 Facial Casts

Facial casts have been employed by authors to study the nasal morphology by direct anthropometry [24] (Fig. 76.5d). The technique is found to be objective and cost-effective and

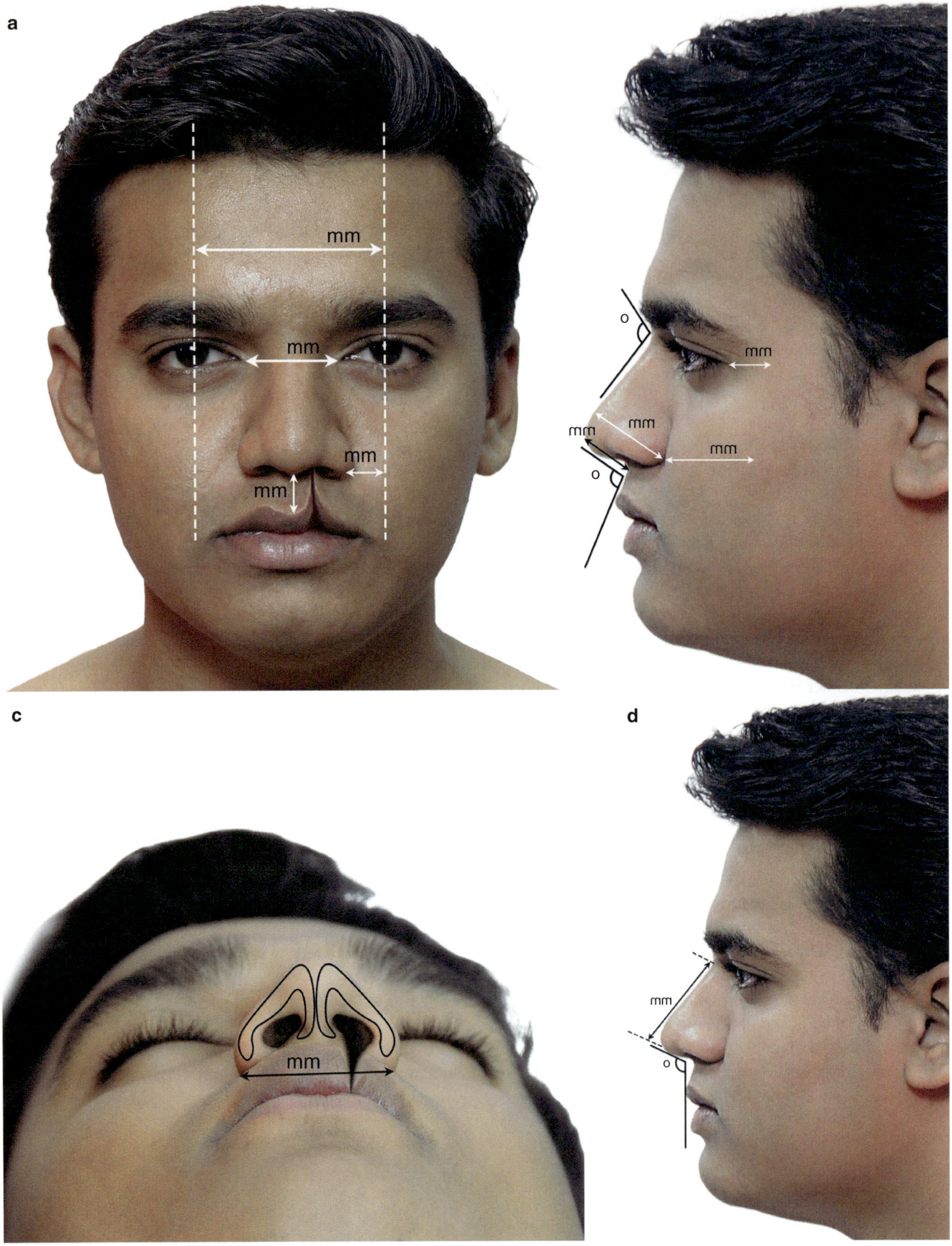

Fig. 76.3 (**a–d**) Important angular and linear measurements as traced from preoperative photographs can serve as a guide for preoperative surgical planning

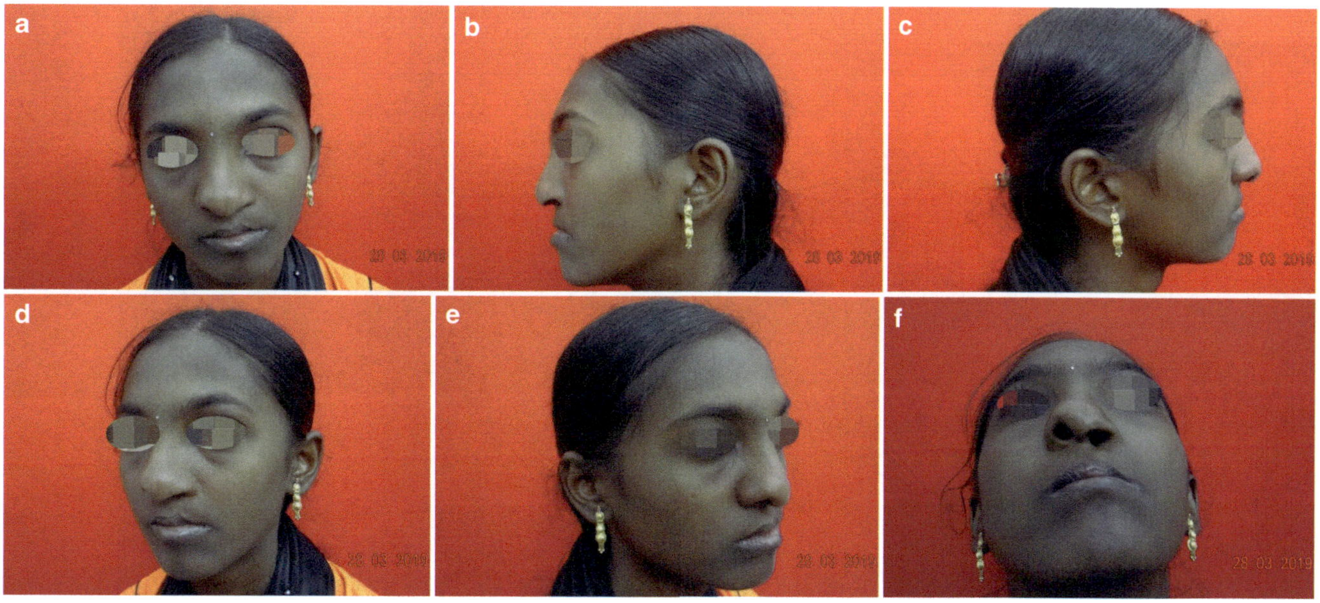

Fig. 76.4 (**a–f**) Standard photographic views for cleft rhinoplasty. (**a**) Frontal view. (**b**) Left lateral view. (**c**) Right lateral view. (**d**) Left lateral oblique view. (**e**) Right lateral oblique view. (**f**) Basal view

allows precise recording of selected parameters as the soft tissues are not deformed.

76.4.6 Video Recording

Some authors [25, 26] have also resorted to video recordings that make assessment of movements possible and eliminates the need for clinical photographs as these can be generated from the video records. The disadvantages include increased time and need for trained personnel with considerable cooperation from the patients.

76.4.7 Functional Assessment

Function is as important as nasal aesthetics. Functional assessment can be established using rhinomanometry; however the usefulness of such an evaluation is limited.

76.5 Surgical Correction

76.5.1 Surgical Approaches

Cleft rhinoplasty can be accomplished using either an open or closed approach.

While primary rhinoplasty can be carried out using either of the two approaches, definitive rhinoplasty is almost always accomplished using an open approach.

The open approach allows for both superior visual control and enhanced surgical exposure of all the abnormal components facilitating their anatomical reconstruction under direct vision. Furthermore, the approach facilitates nasal sculpting either by suturing or by introduction and fixation of different types of grafts. The approach also helps in saving time when compared to the closed approach. When employing the open approach, a combination of bilateral marginal incisions with an inverted V mid-columellar incision is preferred among most surgeons [27] (Fig. 76.6a, b).

Sometimes, additional skin needs to be recruited in the columella. In such cases, the typical external columellar incision can be modified. When addressing the unilateral cleft nasal deformity, columellar lengthening can be achieved with the help of an asymmetric V to Y incision on the side of the cleft. The V to Y incision is made in the midline, recruiting the skin from the upper lip into the columella in cases of bilateral cleft nasal deformity. A viable alternative incision in cases of bilateral cleft noses is an upper lip forked flaps which achieve columellar lengthening together with narrowing of the central segment [28].

Other viable options include the use of prolabium advancement flap together with an Abbe flap, composite graft of skin and auricular cartilage and skin rim rotation flap [29].

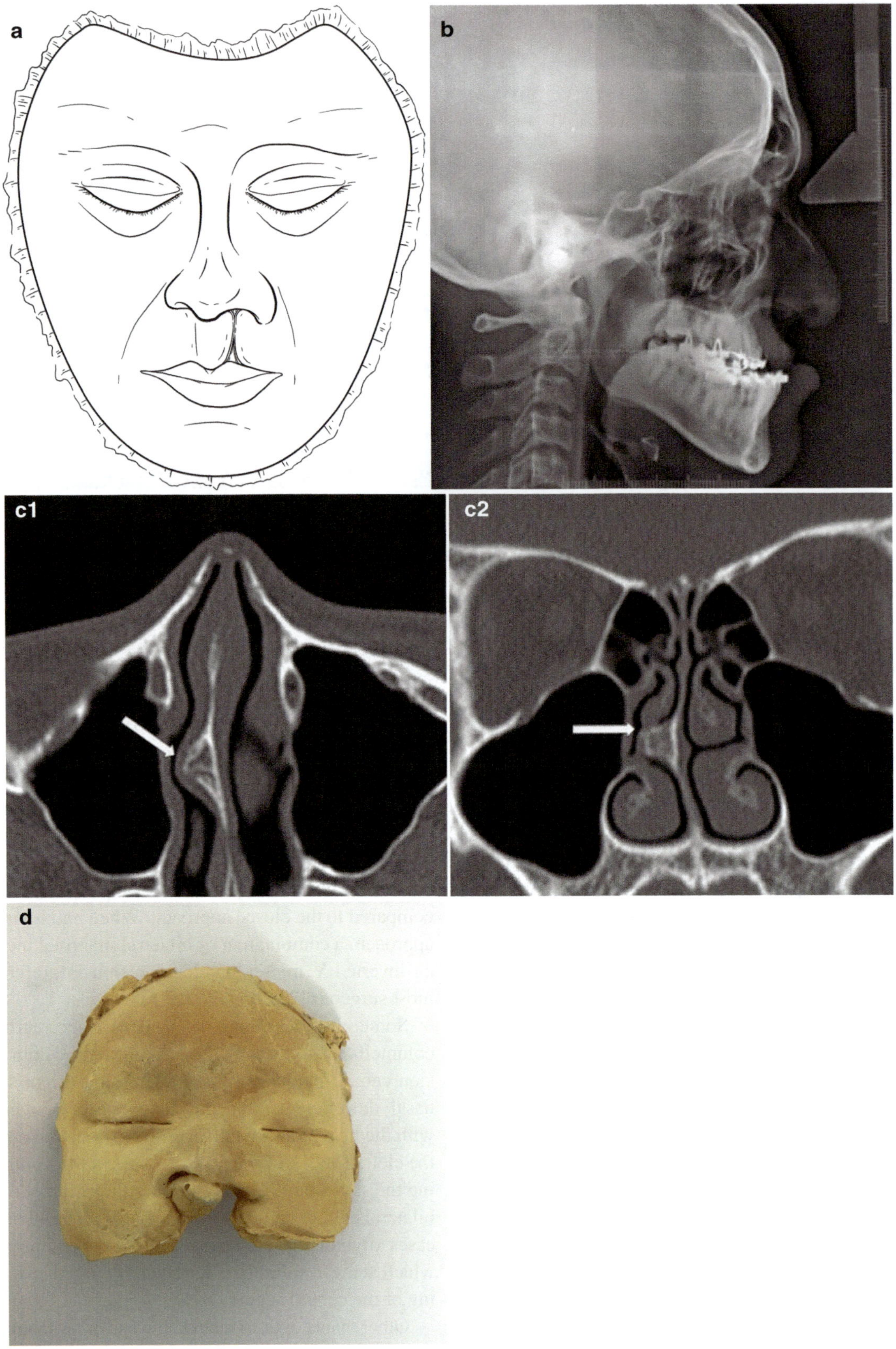

Fig. 76.5 (**a–d**) Tools for preoperative patient evaluation for cleft rhinoplasty. (**a**) Three-dimensional model of the face. (**b**) Lateral cephalogram for cephalometric analysis for evaluating the maxillary and chin position prior to cleft rhinoplasty. (**c**) (1 and 2): Axial and coronal CT scan views allow for evaluation of the nasal septal deviation objectively (white arrows). (**d**) Facial cast for evaluating the nasal morphology

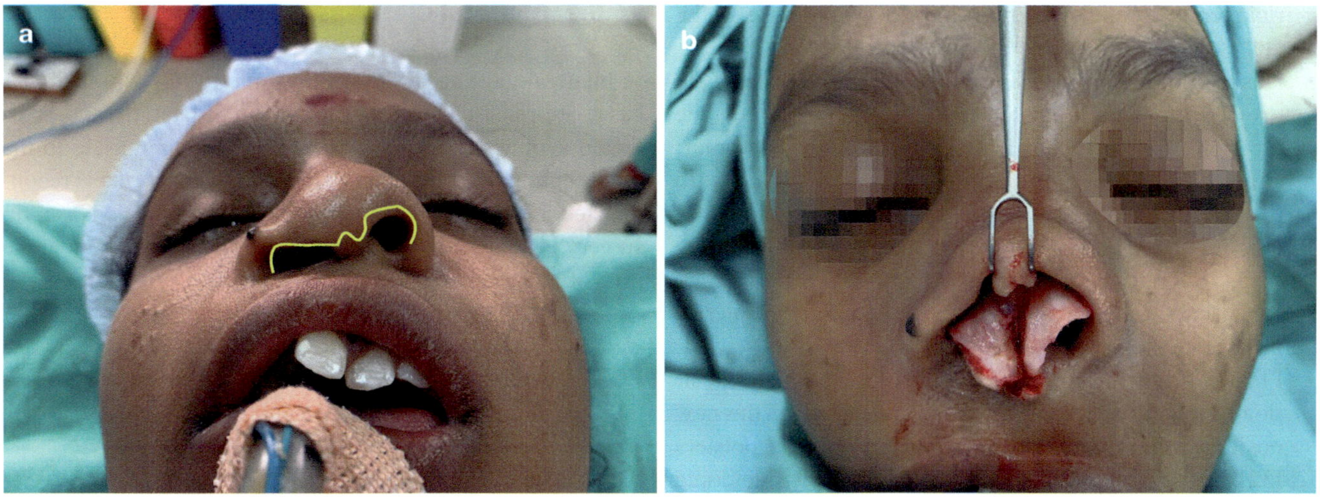

Fig. 76.6 Open approach for cleft rhinoplasty. A combination of inverted V (**a**, **b**) transcolumellar and bilateral marginal incisions is typically employed. (**a**) Marking of the incision. (**b**) Skeletonisation of the nose using the above incision

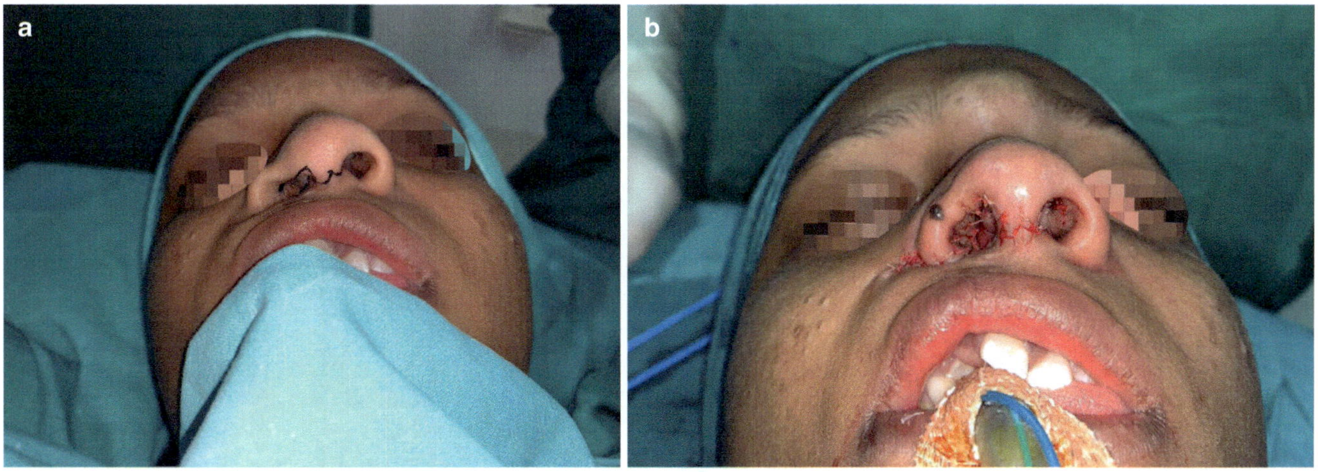

Fig. 76.7 (**a**, **b**) Tajima and Maruyama reverse U incision for correction of nostril asymmetry. (**a**) Marking of the reverse U incision on to the external nasal skin on the right side of the nostril. (**b**) Correction of nostril asymmetry following closure (also see Fig. 76.17)

Most patients with unilateral cleft nasal deformity are often disturbed with the nostril asymmetry that accompanies such a deformity. This has been addressed using a reverse U incision as described by Tajima and Maruyama in 1977 [30]. The technique involves extending the marginal incision into a rim incision at the point of the alar web. The skin of the web is incorporated with the LLC flap and vestibular skin, and the flap is suspended both medially and cephalically from the LLC to the ipsilateral ULC and the septum using sutures (Fig. 76.7a, b). This helps in recruiting the external skin of the alar web to the vestibular lining which also helps in addressing the issue of deficient vestibular skin associated with unilateral cleft noses. This incision is well accepted among surgeons for correction of nostril asymmetry.

76.6 Primary Rhinoplasty

The aim of the surgery is to attain symmetry of the nasal tip and alar base.

76.6.1 Unilateral Cleft Nasal Deformity

The literature has reported a number of techniques for achieving symmetry in unilateral cleft nasal deformities primarily [15, 31]. The salient points that are common to most of these techniques include:

- Completely freeing the soft tissue attachments of the alar base from the pyriform aperture and maxilla for symmetrical repositioning of the retro-positioned alar base on the cleft side.

- Nasal tip plasty is carried out to increase the nasal tip projection. This is made possible by utilising the incisions for lip repair. Dissecting through these incisions, the skin overlying the LLC's is dissected with the help of medial and lateral tunnels, and the cutaneous attachments of the lateral crura are separated [1] (Fig. 76.8a).
- Repairing the caudal septum by attaching it to the anterior nasal spine.
- Finally, following complete closure of the lip and repositioning of the alar base, the LLC is secured in the new position using either transnasal sutures or nasal bolsters [32]. These sutures help in recreating the cleft side dome thereby increasing the nasal tip projection and improving the tip symmetry (Fig. 76.8b).

76.6.2 Bilateral Cleft Nasal Deformity

In bilateral cleft nasal deformities, the retro-positioned alar bases are released from the nasal lining laterally and positioned symmetrically by securing the nasalis muscle to the nasal septum on both sides. The nasal muscular ring is reconstructed as performed in the unilateral cleft noses. Nasal tip surgery is not performed at this stage but is carried out at the time of intermediate rhinoplasty [21].

76.7 Intermediate Rhinoplasty

76.7.1 Unilateral Cleft Nasal Deformity

The intermediate rhinoplasty addresses two issues in unilateral cleft nose: the asymmetric position of LLC on the side of the cleft and vestibular webbing laterally (Fig. 76.9a–d).

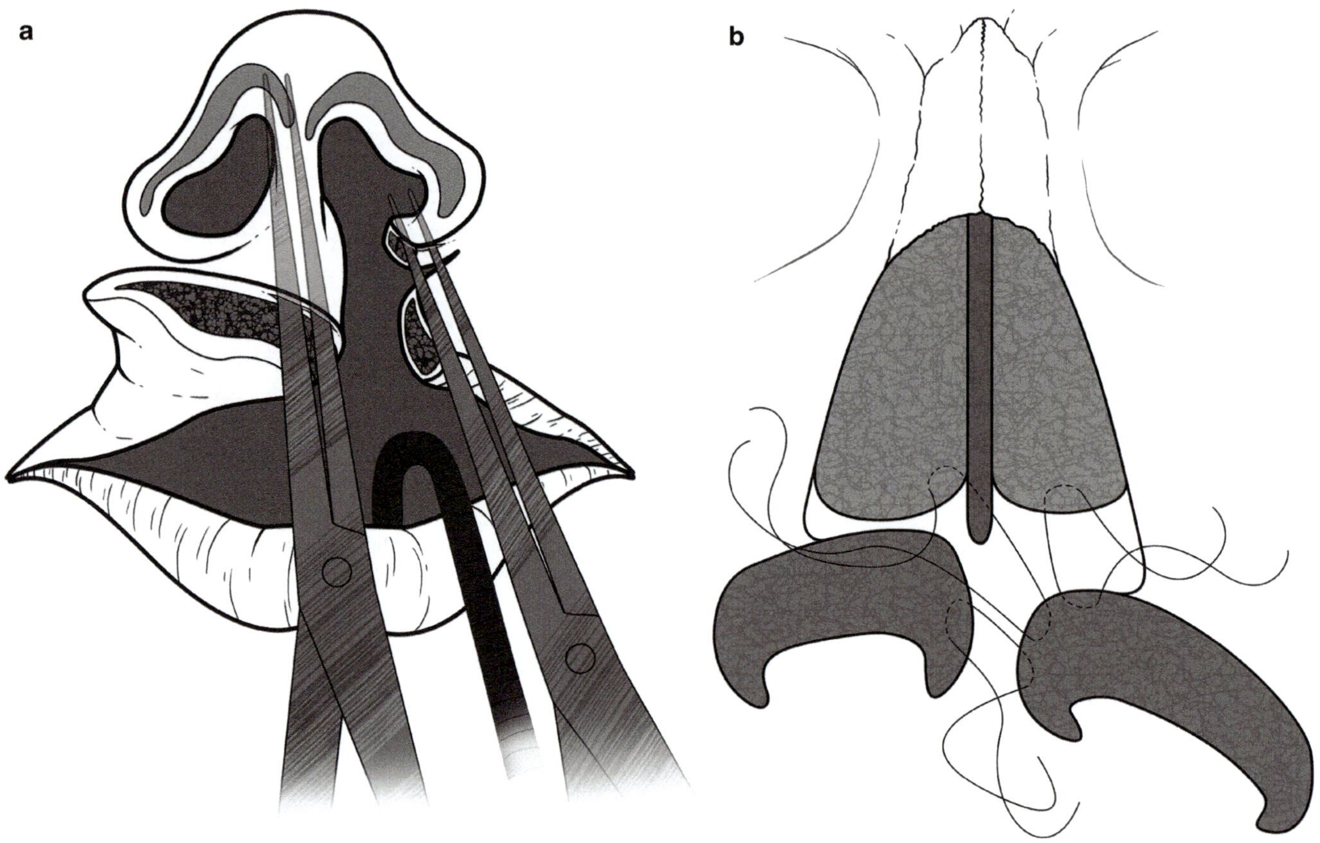

Fig. 76.8 (a, b) Schematic representation of primary rhinoplasty in a unilateral cleft lip nasal deformity case. (a) Dissection for access to crura utilising the incisions for lip repair. (b) Recreating the cleft side nasal dome using transnasal sutures for better symmetry and projection. The sutures are made to pass through the nose, vestibular lining and LLCs and through the nasal skin before being reintroduced through the nasal skin and ULC and sutured down within the nasal vestibule. It is important to reintroduce them through the same hole they exited to prevent necrosis of the nasal skin

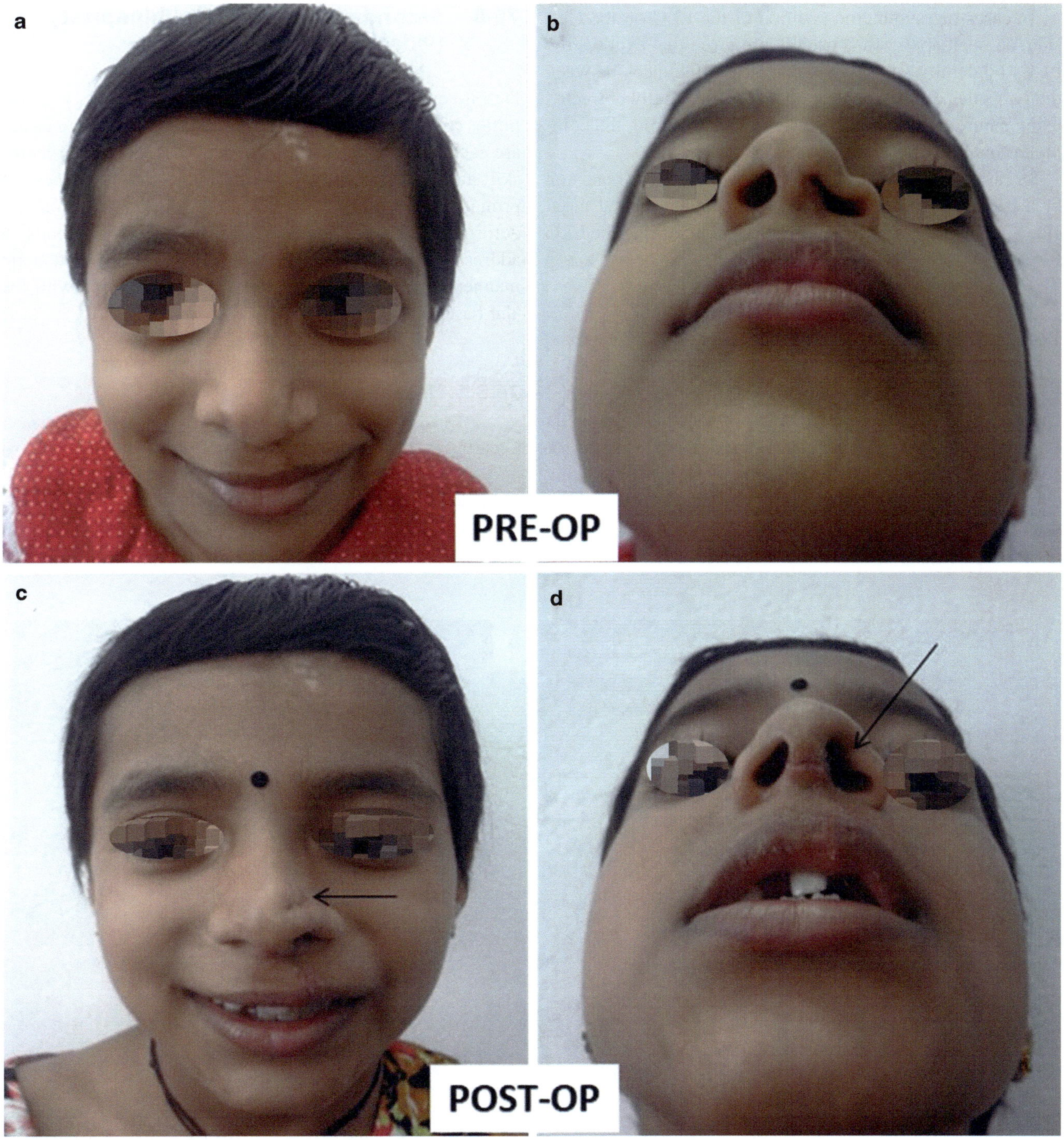

Fig. 76.9 (**a–d**) A case of unilateral cleft nasal deformity in a 6-year-old child managed using intermediate rhinoplasty. (**a**) Preoperative frontal view. (**b**) Preoperative basal view showing the abnormal position of LLC on the cleft side (Left). (**c**) Postoperative frontal view. The abnormal position of the LLC on the cleft side is corrected using an open approach (inverted V transcolumellar incision) and transnasal sutures (black arrow). (**d**) Postoperative basal view showing symmetrical positioning of the LLC on the cleft side (black arrow)

In cases of asymmetric position of the LLC on the cleft side, an open approach is usually preferred that exposes the LLCs bilaterally so that the geometric differences between the two sides can be appreciated and subsequently corrected using suture techniques followed by closure along the columellar incision [33].

In cases of lateral vestibular webbing, a V/Y-type incision or a back cut can be carried out to affect the lateral nasal sidewall lengthening which will subsequently bring the LLC forward [1].

76.7.2 Bilateral Cleft Nasal Deformity

In such cases, intermediate rhinoplasty corrects the depressed LLCs as well as affects lengthening of the short columella [1, 34] (Fig. 76.10a, b). An open approach is employed for correction of the above-mentioned scenarios. Following exposure of the LLCs, the angle of divergence between the domes is decreased using transdomal suture, helping in increasing the projection of the nasal tip [34].

76.8 Secondary or Definitive Rhinoplasty (Video 76.1)

Despite an excellent primary rhinoplasty, secondary deformities coupled with scarring are bound to occur. These issues are tackled upon by definitive rhinoplasty. The surgeon's skill and his expertise will ultimately decide the success of primary cleft lip nose repair and the severity of secondary deformities. The success of definitive rhinoplasty depends on addressing every component of the deformity in a systematic manner beginning with the nasal base and ending with the alar base reduction.

76.8.1 Nasal Base

Creating a strong base for the nose represents the preliminary step in correction of either unilateral or bilateral cleft nasal deformity, the foundation for which is laid down at the time of primary cheilorhinoplasty with the approximation of the nasal floor with the lip. This is followed by addressing

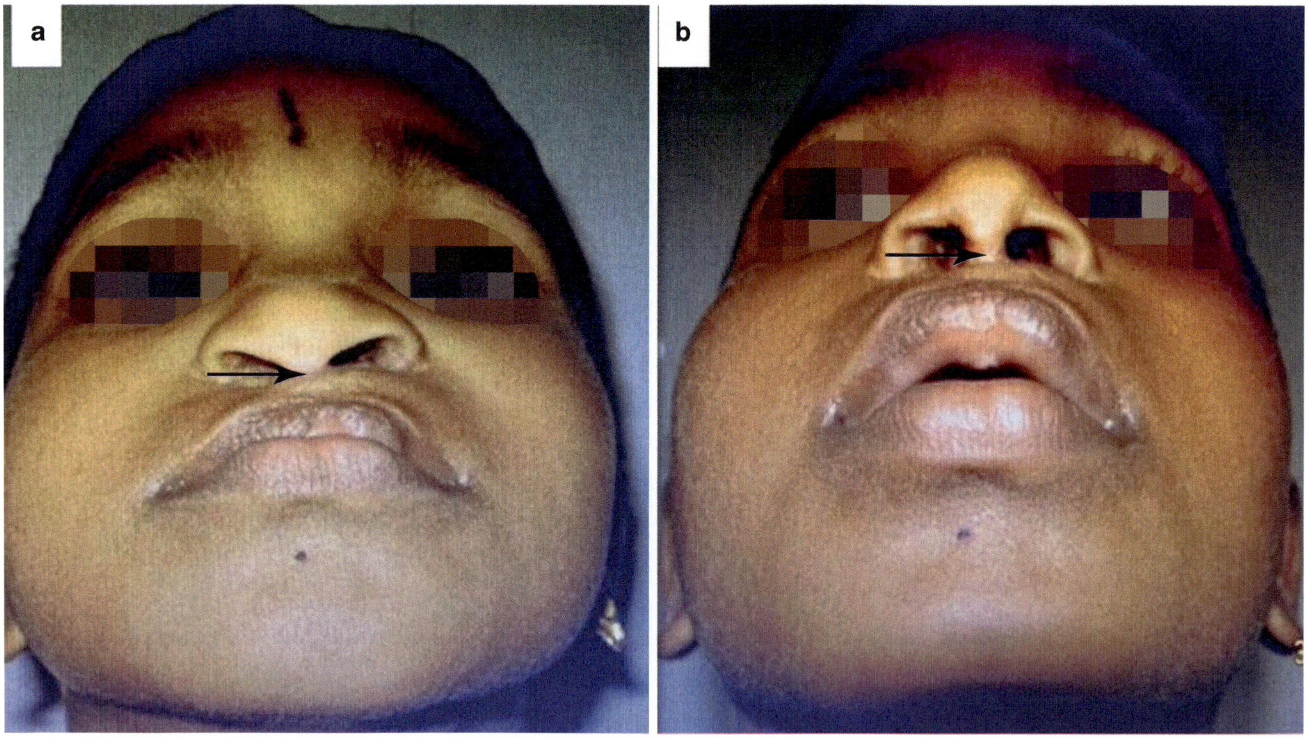

Fig. 76.10 (**a**, **b**) A case of bilateral cleft nasal deformity in a 5-year-old managed using intermediate rhinoplasty. (**a**) Preoperative basal view showing the abnormal position of the LLCs as well as short columella (black arrow). (**b**) Postoperative basal view. One can appreciate lengthening of the columella that is achieved (black arrow). The correction of LLCs is also affected bilaterally. An open approach was utilised with bilateral reverse U incision to correct the horizontal orientation of the nostrils

the skeletal deficiency in the maxilla and premaxilla and correction of the retro-positioned alar base. In some cases, the nasal sill and the nasal base might still have to be augmented at the time of secondary rhinoplasty using local tissue flaps [35].

76.8.2 Septum

The caudal septum is seen to deviate to the non-cleft side, bowing away from the anterior nasal spine with resultant nasal airway obstruction. This requires resection of this portion of the septum, maintaining at least 1 cm dorsal, and caudal septal segments in the form of a L strut to help in preserving the nasal tip and the dorsal support [21] (Fig. 76.11a–i). When doing so, more than 40% contact point must be allowed between the crest of the maxilla and L strut which helps by subjecting the septum to decreased load forces thereby preventing nasal deformities like saddle nose deformity or ptosis of the nasal tip from developing in the future. It is observed in most cases that despite resecting the deviated portion of the septum, the L strut continues to remain deviated due to residual memory that is present in the L strut. In such cases, sutures can be placed through the ULC and the septum applying force in the direction opposite of the deviation to aid in correcting the asymmetry [36]. In cases of severe septal deviation, one needs to resort to using caudal septal extension graft as struts along the dorsal margins followed by surgical repositioning of the caudal septum [37, 38] (Fig. 76.11). The resected portion of the septal cartilage can itself be used as a spreader graft. In cases where the resected septal cartilage is inadequate, one can use rib cartilage as a spreader graft. The caudal portion of the L strut is secured to the anterior nasal spine with the help of sutures. Some surgeons also prefer to make a notch in the anterior nasal spine to which the L strut can be secured. If there exists any residual memory in the septal cartilage after securing it to the nasal spine, it can be relieved by cartilage scoring with the help of a no. 15 blade.

Access to the caudal nasal septum is achieved using an open approach and by dissecting between the medial crura of the LLCs [21]. From this point onwards, a sub-perichondrial flap can be developed. Make sure that the dissection is in the proper plane. The blue appearance of the septal cartilage serves as a guide to correct plane of dissection. The mucoperichondrial flap should be cautiously raised without perforating the surrounding mucosa to provide superior coverage for a large septal extension graft especially from the rib.

76.8.3 Middle Third of the Nose

The middle third of the nose has poor support on the side of the cleft and therefore the ULCs tend to collapse resulting in internal valve dysfunction which affects the patient's ability to breathe normally. In such instances, spreader grafts placed between the septum and ULCs on either side and stabilised using sutures can help open the internal nasal valve and improve breathing [39, 40] (Fig. 76.11i).

76.8.4 Nasal Tip or LLCs

Once the caudal septum is stabilised, attention is shifted to the correction of asymmetric LLC and the nasal tip complex. Various techniques are advocated for the same.

- **Cephalic trimming:** Wide LLCs can make the nose appear asymmetric. In such cases, following surgical exposure of the LLCs via an open approach, small cephalic strips of LLCs can be excised advocating more excision on the larger side and leaving at least 5 mm for support. This manoeuvre narrows a bulbous nasal tip and improves symmetry. Cephalic trimming is followed by correction of the septal deviation by resection and replacement (Fig. 76.12a).
- **Septal extension graft:** A strong septal extension graft helps in providing support to the nasal tip and improves the tip projection by rotating an acute nasolabial angle which is the consequence of tip ptosis back to normal [22, 41]. The graft is ideally sutured in between the medial crura of LLCs and the caudal septum (Fig. 76.12b). Prior to suture stabilisation of the septal extension graft, the medial crus of LLC on the cleft side is advanced superiorly to match the vestibular dome height of the non-cleft side. This is then secured to the extension graft using mattress sutures (Fig. 76.12c). In cases where spreader grafts are used to relieve the internal nasal valve collapse, the extension graft can be secured to the spreader grafts. In such cases, the base of the nose is fortified with bolster sutures from medial crus to the septal extension graft. The strut (extension graft) is ideally placed slightly behind the medial crura to prevent the columella from either looking too wide or feeling too firm for the patient [39]. A good tip support entails extension of the septal extension graft for at least 4–5 mm beyond the septum maintaining a thickness of at least 1 mm. This also helps to resist deprojection from the resulting scar tissue that will form in this region.

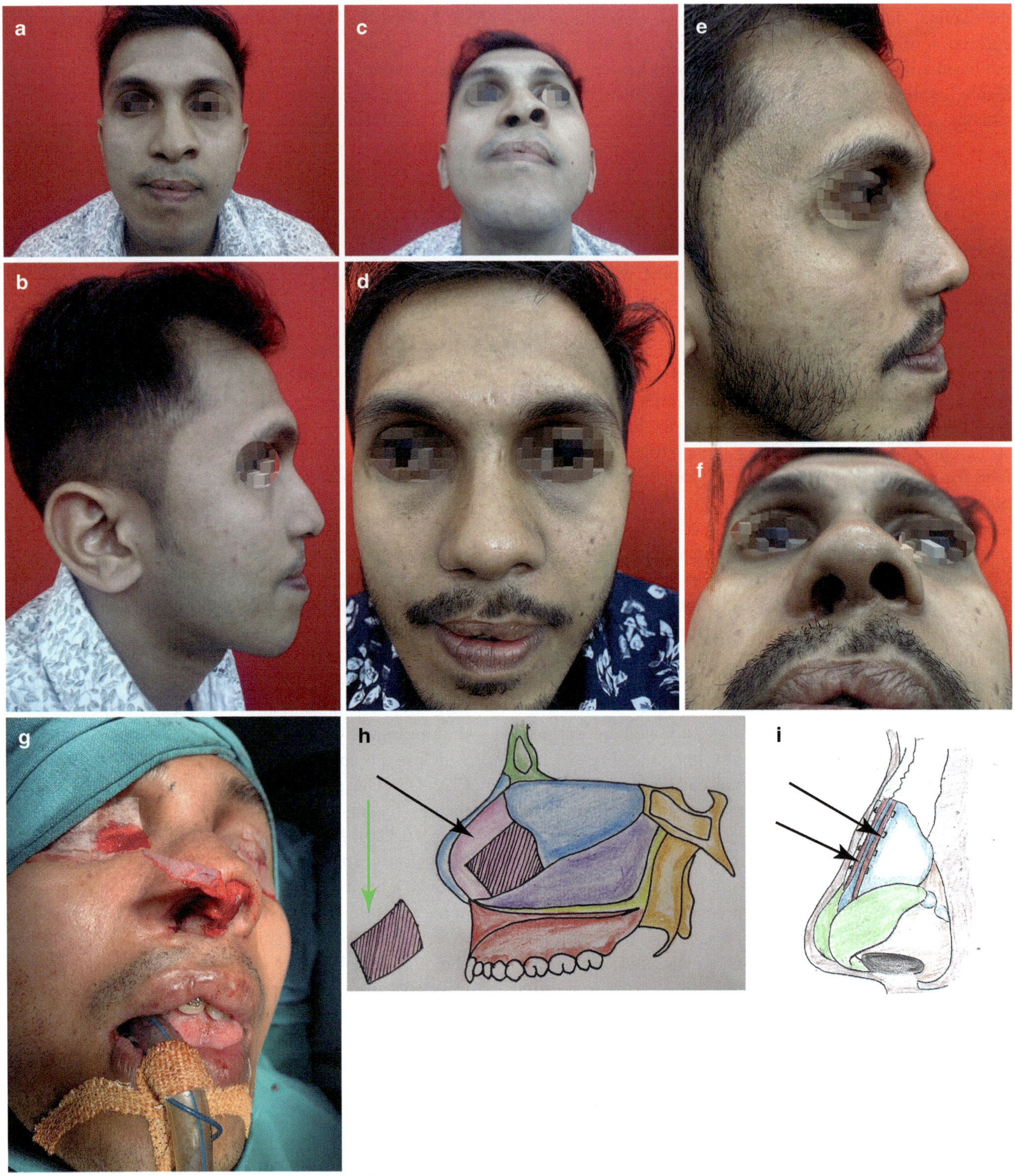

Fig. 76.11 (**a-i**) 22-year-old patient with unilateral cleft lip and palate before (**a–c**) and 2 months after (**d–f**) open rhinoplasty performed to correct the severely deviated caudal septum. (**g**) Intraop picture showing batten grafting. (**h**) Resection of septal cartilage in cases of severely deviated nasal septum, maintaining an L shaped contact (black arrow) for preserving tip and dorsal support. The resected portion can be utilised as a septal extension graft (green arrow). (**i**) Spreader grafts placed between ULCs and nasal septum (black arrows)

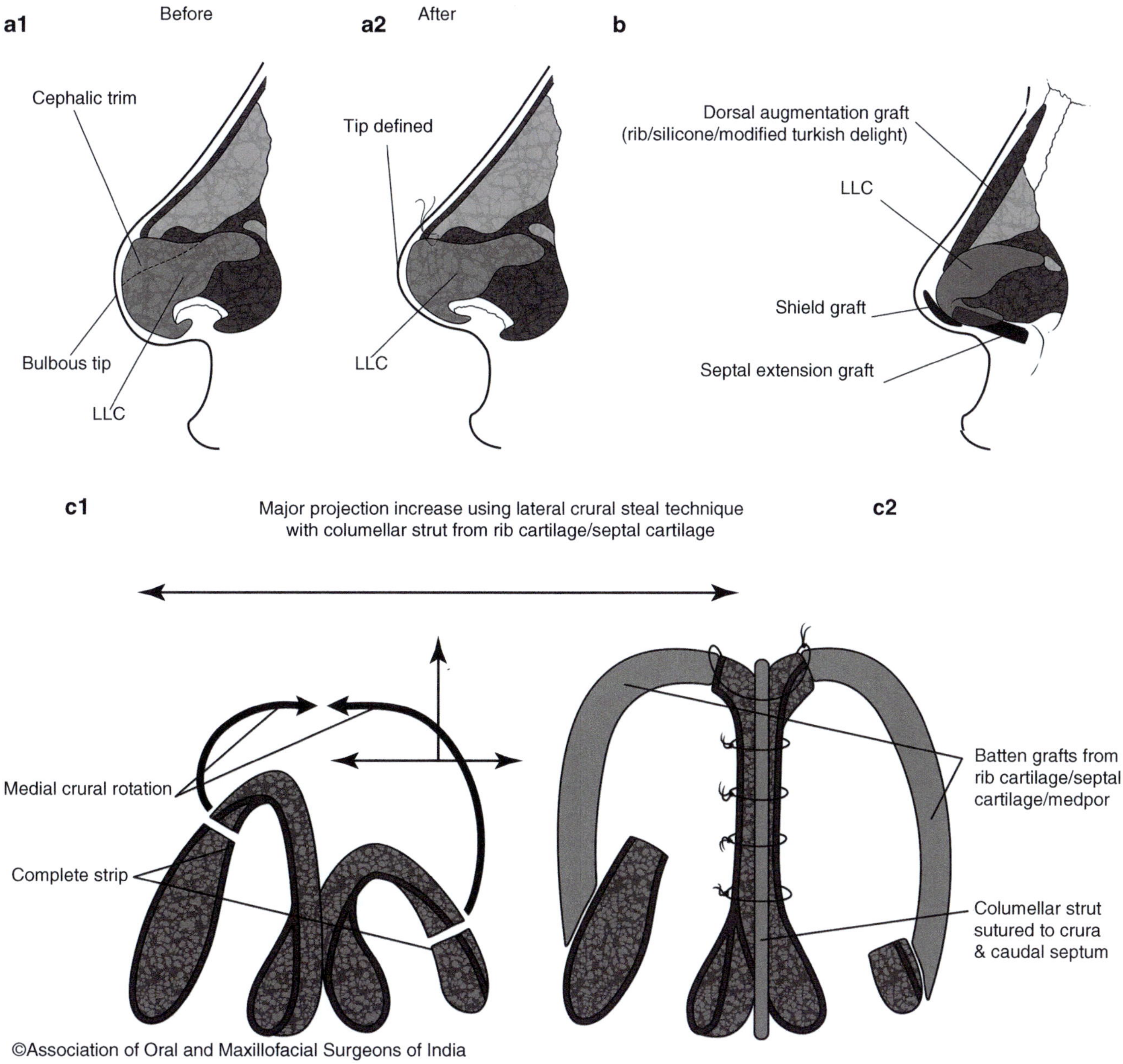

Fig. 76.12 (**a–c**) Schematic representation of techniques for correction of asymmetric LLCs and nasal tip complex. (**a1**, **a2**) Cephalic trimming (before and after). (**b**) Shield grafts, caudal septal extension grafts for improving the symmetry and projection of the nasal tip. Dorsal nasal augmentation is also been shown. (**c1**, **c2**) Lateral crural steal technique

- **Lateral crural steal or advancement flaps:** The medial crus of the LLC on the cleft side is shorter in vertical length, whereas the lateral crus is longer with a horizontal orientation as compared to the non-cleft side. In such cases, lengthening of LLC on the cleft side is achieved using the lateral crural steal technique which requires cutting of the longer part of the lateral crus of the LLC on the cleft side and shorter part of the lateral crus of LLC on the non-cleft side [39] (Fig. 76.12b). This facilitates utilisation of the longer crural flap on the side of the cleft for increasing the nasal tip projection on the cleft side thereby contributing to improved nasal tip symmetry. The lateral crura are then reconstructed using either robust cartilage struts or batten grafts in onlay or inlay fashion.
- **Shield graft:** These grafts are utilised to accentuate the tip projection further as well as improve the symmetry and tip shape (Fig. 76.12b).

In bilateral cleft nasal deformities, LLCs of either side need repositioning with tip suture techniques. In cases of weak cartilages, septal extension grafts as columellar struts as well as in onlay position need be used for ideal projection [42]. Large nasal tip can benefit from cephalic trimming of both LLCs. The goal is to decrease the angle of divergence between the domal points of the lower lateral cartilages, create a more defined nasal tip and provide a strong nasal framework for better tip projection.

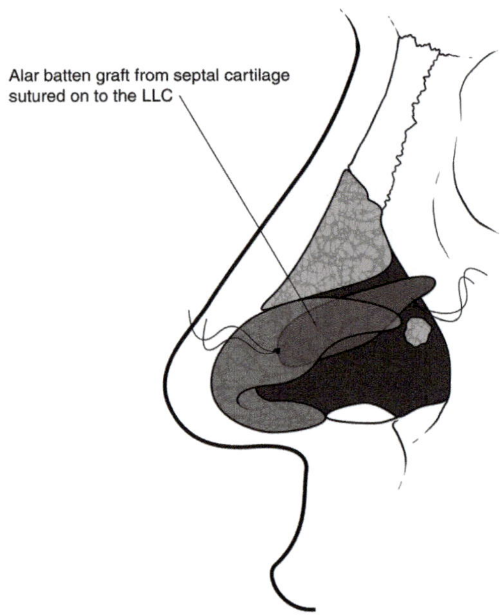

Fig. 76.13 Alar batten grafting demonstrated in a case of unilateral cleft nasal deformity. The graft fortifies the LLC and removes the concavity of the same (Refer Fig. 76.17i)

76.8.5 Alar Rim (Lateral Crus of LLC)

The LLC on the cleft side has poor skeletal support on the medial and lateral sides which makes the LLC concave with an introverted contour to the ala [43]. This concavity can be managed with different techniques, viz. suture techniques using horizontal mattress sutures, underlay alar batten grafts, onlay grafts and autocartilage flaps [44]. The lateral crus of LLC can also be dissected from the underlying vestibular skin, removed, flipped and resutured in a convex fashion.

Alar batten grafts either are placed below the residual lateral crus as underlay graft or can be placed above it as an onlay graft. This graft strengthens the lateral crus of the LLC and removes the concavity of LLC [39] (Fig. 76.13). Suture techniques such as horizontal mattress sutures also strengthen and flatten the lateral crus of the LLC. Lastly, the cephalic margin of the LLC can be made into an advancement flap which can be advanced to provide support to the remaining LLC. Each of these techniques provides support to the lateral crus of the LLC and fortifies the external nasal valve.

76.8.6 Nasal Dorsum and Nasal Osteotomies

The following issues are observed when addressing this area in definitive rhinoplasty.

- **Flat and under-projected dorsum deviating away from the cleft:** The authors' preferred technique for addressing this issue is by using a dorsal onlay graft from rib or modified Turkish delight. In modified Turkish delight technique, the authors use morselised Medpor mixed with autogenous blood and wrapped in Surgicel to affect dorsal nasal augmentation [45] (Figs. 76.12b and 76.14a–d). This cancels out the need to carry out harvesting of the rib cartilage and there eliminates the donor site complications associated with the same. Although silicone implant can also be used for this purpose, there is increased possibility of infection, graft migration or displacement or possible extrusion. It should be noted that the dorsal nasal pocket dissected should just accommodate the implant so that the implant fits snugly without much displacement or migration.
- **Dorsal humps:** The dorsal hump usually peaks at the region of the rhinion where the nasal bones and ULC join.

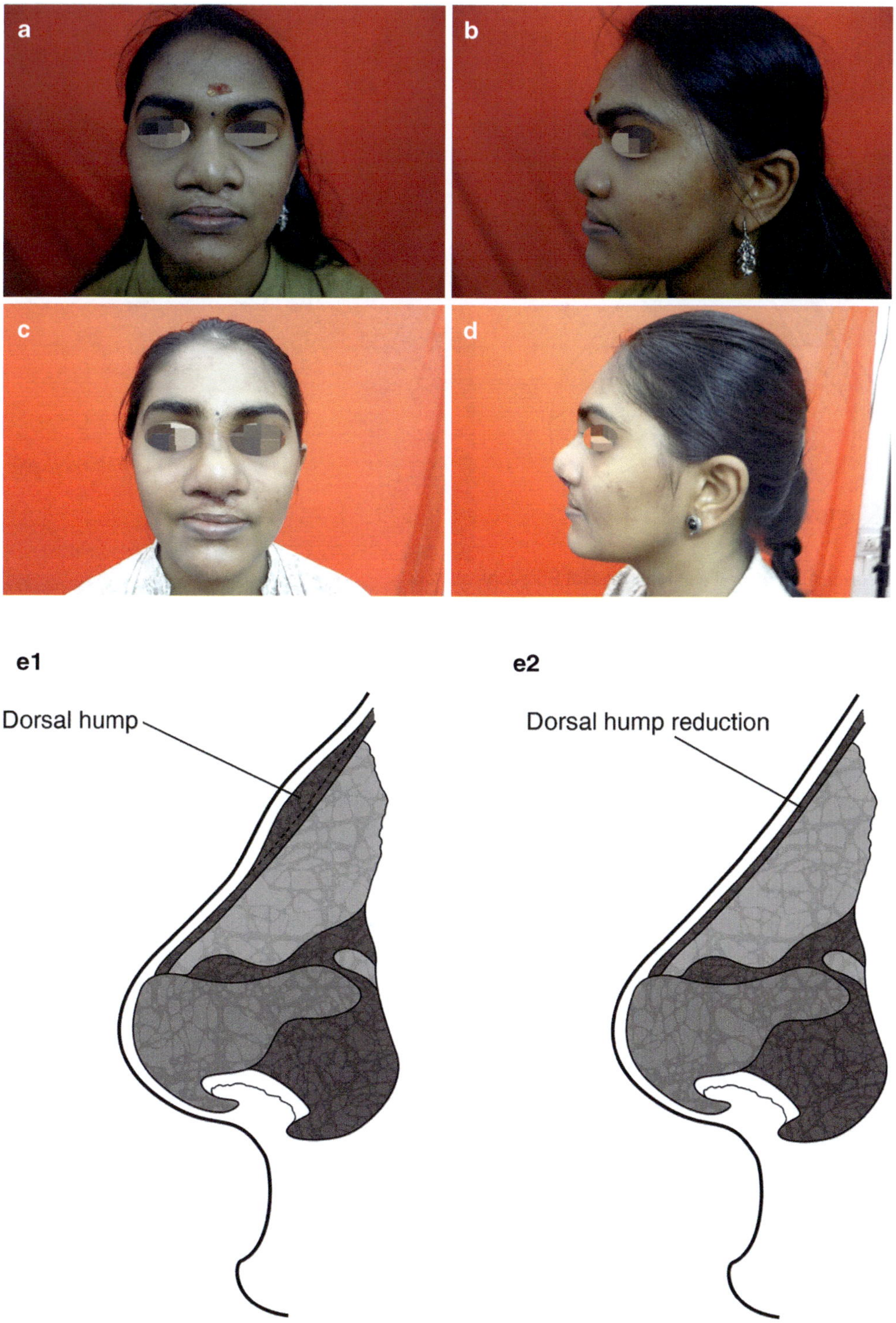

Fig. 76.14 Addressing the nasal dorsum and nasal osteotomies. A case of flat and under-projected dorsum managed using modified Turkish delight technique. (**a**, **b**) Pre op frontal and lateral. (**c**, **d**) Post op frontal and lateral. (**e1**, **e2**) Schematic representation of dorsal hump reduction. (**f**, **g**) Schematic and clinical lateral nasal osteotomies

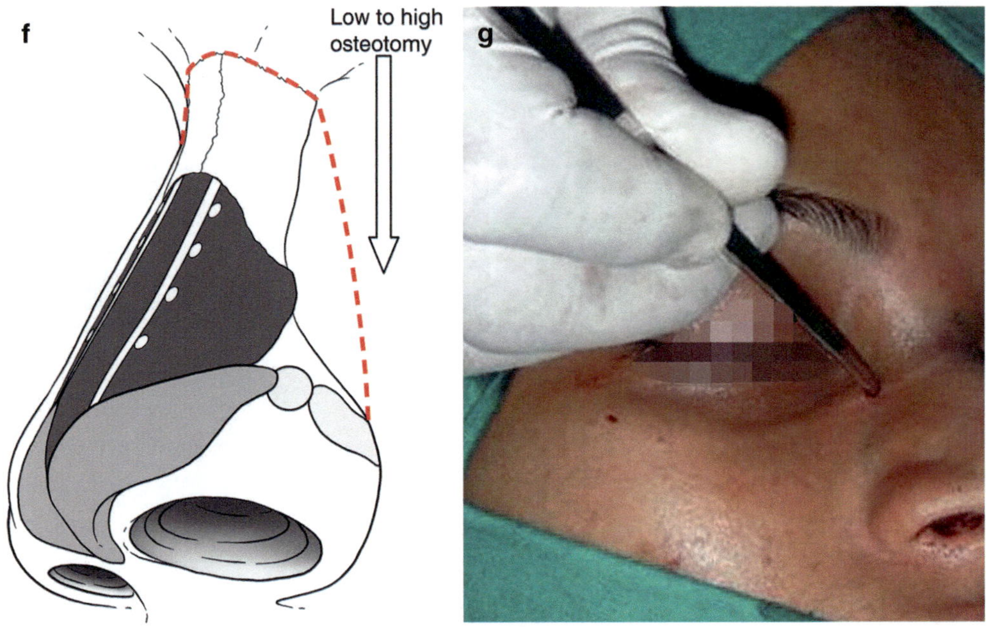

Fig. 76.14 (continued)

Dorsal hump should be addressed in conjunction with other aspects of the nose, or else an open roof deformity will be the consequence. The correction is carried out by reduction of the bone by rasping and the ULC using either scissors or number 15 blades (Fig. 76.14e).

- **Thick and wide nasal bones with deviation towards the non-cleft side with wide dorsum:** Such cases require either lateral or paramedian osteotomies to narrow the dorsal width and bring about symmetry. The authors' preferred technique for lateral osteotomies is by introducing a 2–3 mm osteotome transcutaneously to create micro punctures along the planned osteotomy going from low to high [42] (Fig. 76.14f, g). The same can also be carried out by introducing the osteotome transnasally. If this does not affect narrowing of the dorsum adequately, then the authors resort to paramedian osteotomies to create an open roof deformity followed by in-fracturing the nasal bones. This manoeuvre almost always requires placement of spreader grafts to prevent collapse of the internal nasal valve.

76.8.7 Piriform Rim and Pre-maxilla Augmentation

Cleft noses whether unilateral or bilateral present with skeletal deficiency in the region of the premaxilla and piriform rim which brings about posteroinferior displacement of the nose. If this area is left unattended, the final result is bound to be asymmetric despite addressing all the other aspects of rhinoplasty well [39]. This area can be augmented using a portion of the rib graft and securing it with a screw (Fig. 76.15). This allows for improving the anterior projection. Other options include the use of silicone implant, cortical one or fat grafting [21].

76.8.8 Nasal Alae

The nasal alae in cleft noses as discussed previously are usually displaced in a lateral and inferior direction. Correcting the abnormal orientation of the nasal alae represents the concluding steps in definitive rhinoplasty. This is usually achieved using two techniques, viz. V to Y advancement and Weir procedure (alar resection) along the alar facial groove [46–48]. These two procedures need to be supplemented with augmentation of the piriform rim as well as vertical enlargement of the nostril on the cleft side in order to achieve true symmetry. Vertical enlargement of the nostril can be achieved using skin grafts or composite grafts just inside the ala. Superior results are possible despite not addressing the nostril except from the basal view which will make the vertical height discrepancy of the nostril evident. Weir procedure is used in cases of excess skin laterally and allows for symmetrical correction of the alar base on the cleft side nostril which is usually longer and elongated (Fig. 76.15a–g). It also provides access for carrying out augmentation of the piriform rim using grafts. Nostril retainers are often sutured in place for the purpose of helping in moulding and maintaining the nasal sill.

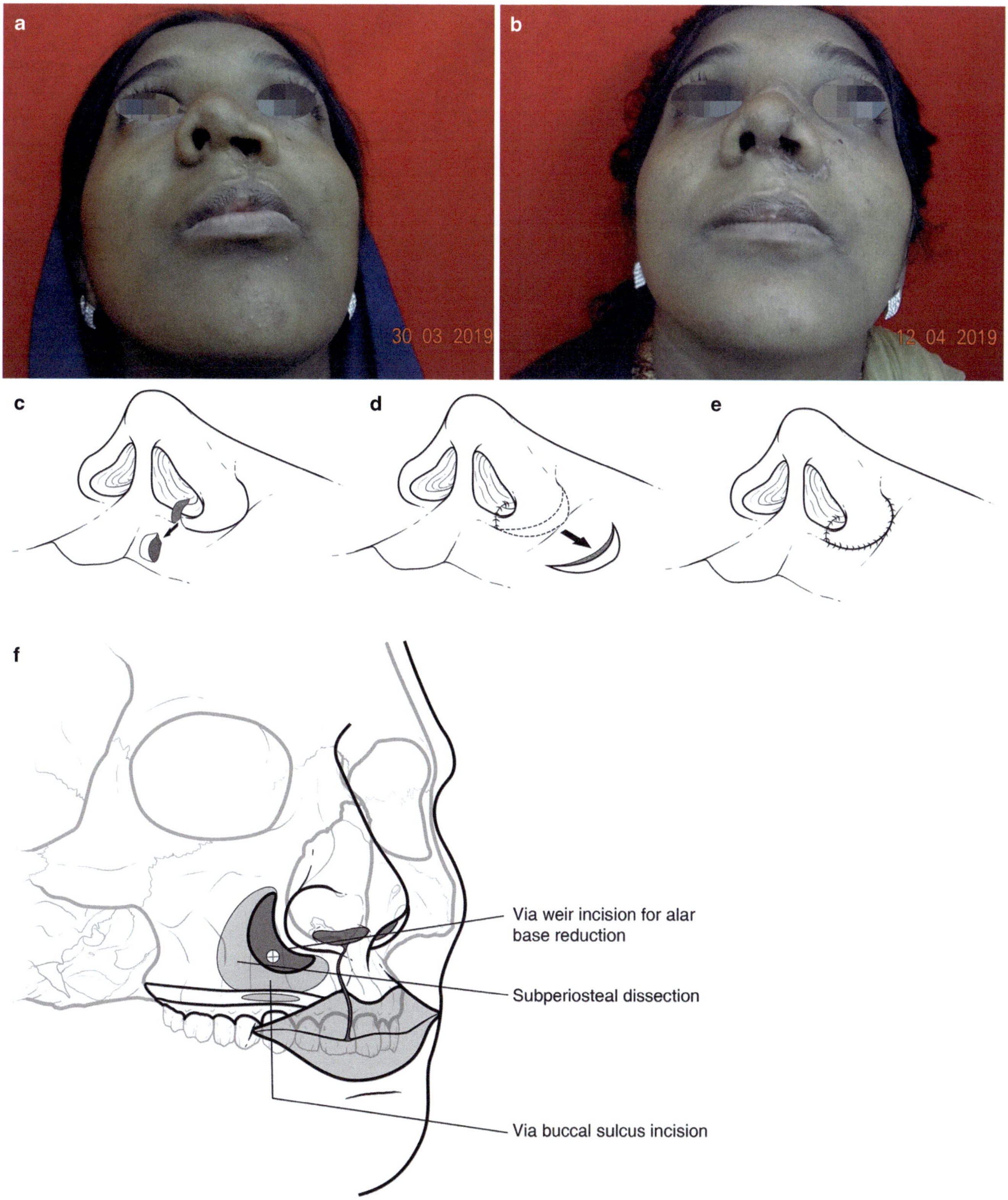

Fig. 76.15 (**a–f**) Piriform rim augmentation and alar base reduction using Weir procedure. (**a**, **b**) Pre op and post op basal views. (**c**) Alar base resection. (**d**) Peri alar resection. (**e**) Closure. (**f**) Piriform rim augmentation

76.9 Use of Grafts in Definitive Rhinoplasty

Grafts are pivotal to the long-standing success of definitive rhinoplasty in terms of nasal aesthetics and function. Autologous tissue is the norm and always preferred over synthetic substitutes like Medpor and silicone which presents with higher incidences of infection, displacement as well as possible extrusion. Among the autologous options available, cartilage (harvested from septum, auricle or rib) and bone (harvested from cranium, rib or iliac crest) are widely used.

Cartilage grafts harvested from the septum have the advantage of being located in the same surgical field, requiring no additional incisions and therefore preventing any additional donor site morbidity. Furthermore, simultaneous correction of septal deviations is possible with the use of this graft. The disadvantages include minimal amounts of cartilage available for grafting and presence of residual memory subjecting it to deformation. When the amount of available septal cartilage is inadequate, auricular cartilage can be the source of grafting. It may offer a large area for graft harvesting, and usually does not induce local sequelae. When larger amount of cartilage is needed especially for the purpose of dorsal augmentation, rib cartilage is an excellent source especially from the right seventh, eighth or ninth rib. This cartilage is present in abundance, is quite sturdy and robust, resists deformation by scar contracture, is easy to shape and also provides superior support for optimising the nasal projection [39]. The disadvantages include graft warpage, increased operating time, visible external scar, post-operative pain and risk of pneumothorax. Another disadvantage is ossification of cartilage in older patients [39].

Cartilage grafts are classically divided into contouring grafts and structural grafts.

76.9.1 Contouring Grafts

These grafts are added to the native osteocartilaginous nose in the coronal plane to improve upon the existing nasal aesthetics. Two most common sites for placement of these grafts are the dorsum and the infratip regions of the nose which help in optimising the tip projection. These grafts are stabilised using either resorbable or non-resorbable sutures or glue. Examples of contouring cartilage graft include dorsal onlay graft or shield-type tip graft.

- **Dorsal onlay graft**: It is used for dorsal nasal augmentation. The rib cartilage is the obvious choice. We have also utilised the modified Turkish delight (diced Medpor mixed with autologous blood and wrapped in Surgicel) for the same purpose with reasonable success.
- **Shield-type tip graft:** Onlay shield grafts help in defining the nasal tip better, optimise the tip projection as well as provide support and hide any minor tip asymmetries.

76.9.2 Reconstructive Grafts

These grafts strengthen the cartilaginous framework of the nose which improves upon the existing nasal function. These grafts are placed in the sagittal plane and display long-term stability especially when an open approach is used to secure the same. They allow structural and functional reconstruction of the nasal tip in cases of definitive rhinoplasty. Examples include spreader grafts, alar batten grafts, columellar strut grafts, etc.

- **Spreader graft:** Spreader grafts serve to open the internal nasal valve and improve nasal breathing. Options for harvest include the septal or rib cartilages. The graft can also be made to extend more caudally making it to function like a strut for improved nasal tip support as well as to straighten and stabilise the septum. Severe septal deviation can be also corrected by placing the grafts along the dorsal septum while reattaching the caudal strut to the nasal spine between the medial crura by suture fixation.
- **Alar batten graft:** Batten grafts serve to strengthen the lateral crura of the LLC. The curved portion of the rib cartilage can be used to the advantage for harvesting these grafts. They are stabilised to the LLC and the strut to mimic the natural convex form of the external nasal valve and provide structural support. These grafts are critical for the correcting alar retraction whenever present.
- **Columellar strut graft or septal extension graft:** Such a graft provides support to the nasal base and can be a platform upon which the nasal tip can be suture stabilised. It can be harvested from the septal cartilage or from the interior of the rib cartilage.

76.10 Treatment Strategy for Unilateral and Bilateral Cleft Nasal Deformities

Nakamura N has devised a treatment strategy for both unilateral and bilateral cleft noses that addresses each anatomical and pathological abnormality that is seen in either scenarios [49].

76.10.1 Unilateral Cleft Nasal Deformity

The pathologic abnormalities that have been previously mentioned are best explained by Nakamura N by comparing the unilateral cleft nose to a house that is been built on a slope. The mid-pole of the house can be thought to be nasal septum, whereas the roof is the LLC and skin, the lateral pole is the vestibule and the base of the house is the maxillary bone. As the house is present on the slope, the mid-pole and the roof incline towards the downward side. In such cases, a straight house can be built on the slope by up righting the centre pole in the centre of the pillar with expansion of the lateral pole and by lifting the roof upward [49] (Fig 76.16a).

Nakamura N's treatment strategy addresses each anatomical and pathological abnormality that causes the main deformities in unilateral cleft nasal deformity listed in Table 76.1. The author's steps in definitive rhinoplasty consist of an open approach; septoplasty; repositioning of the lower lateral cartilage; medial and upward advancement of the lip and nose components, the nasal vestibular tissues, the nasal ala, nasalis muscle and the upper part of the lip including orbicular oris muscle; and nasal vestibular expansion with or without bone graft [50].

76.10.2 Bilateral Cleft Nasal Deformity

The pathologic abnormalities that have been previously mentioned are best explained by Nakamura N by likening the bilateral cleft nose to a house that is compressed by stress. In such cases, normal form of the nose can be created by extending the centre pole at the centre, advancing the roof upwards and extension of the lateral poles on each side (Fig. 76.16b). It is very critical to relieve the stress which in other words means relieving the pull on the nasal tip due to columellar skin shortage [49].

The treatment strategy devised by Nakamura N is based on the principle that the ideal technique of definitive rhinoplasty should minimise damage to either or both the upper and lower lip tissue. This strategy also addresses each anatomical and pathological abnormality that causes the main deformities of the bilateral cleft lip-nose as shown in Table 76.2. Therefore, the author's secondary correction involves open rhinoplasty, repositioning of the lower lateral cartilages, a caudal septal extension graft, medial and upward advancement of the lip and nose components, nasal vestibular expansion and columella lengthening using a nostril rim rotation flap, if necessary [51].

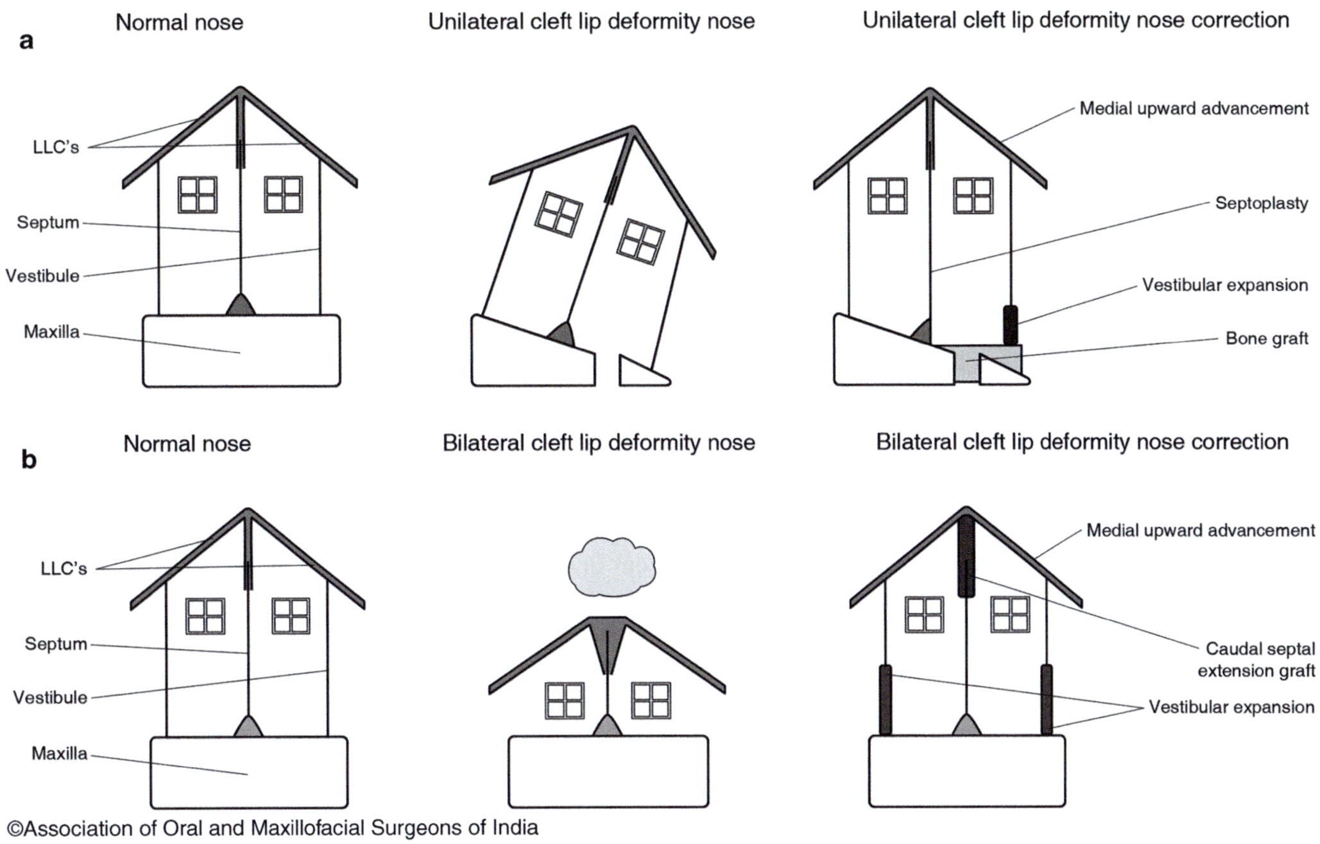

Fig. 76.16 (**a**, **b**) Simplifying cleft nasal anatomy by Nakamura N. (**a**) Unilateral cleft nasal anatomy. (**b**) Bilateral cleft nasal anatomy

Table 76.1 Treatment strategy for unilateral cleft nasal deformity

Nasal deformities	Anatomical pathological abnormalities	Secondary correction
Deviated columella	• Deviation of maxillary midline • Deviated septal cartilage	• Dissection around anterior nasal spine • Reposition of the inferior base of septal cartilage if necessary
Depressed and deviated nasal tip	• Distally and downwardly dislocated LLC on the cleft side • Growth disturbances of septal cartilage	• Freeing and repositioning of LLC by overlapping on ULC • Caudal septal extension graft
Wide and snub nasal ala on the cleft side	• Retro-positioned anterior maxillary wall • Dislocation of the attachment of nasalis muscle	• Secondary bone graft if necessary • Supra-periosteal dissection around piriform margin • Reposition of the nasalis muscle by medial upward advancement of nasolabial components
Flat and V shaped nostril	• Webbing of the rim skin • Shortage of nasalis vestibular lining • Disconnection of orbicularis oris muscle	• Bilaterally symmetric reverse U incision • Expansion of the nasal vestibule • Overlapped suturing of orbicularis oris muscle

Nakamura N et al., J Oral Maxillofac Surg 2010; 68: 2248 [50]

Table 76.2 Treatment strategy for bilateral cleft nasal deformity

Nasal deformities	Anatomical pathological abnormalities	Secondary correction
Short columella	• Shortage of columellar skin • Tightness of subcutaneous tissue in the columella	• Bilateral reverse U incision • Nostril rim rotation flap if necessary • V-Y elongation of fibrous tissue
Flat and flared nasal tip	• Growth disturbance of septal cartilage • Lateral and downward dislocation of LLC • Thin skin envelope of nasal tip	• Caudal septal extension graft. • Freeing and reposition of LLC by overlapping on ULC • Molding of fibrous tissue on nasal tip
Wide and snub nasal ala	• Dislocation of the attachment of nasalis muscle	• Supra-periosteal dissection around piriform margin • Reposition of the nasalis muscle by medial upward advancement of nasal alar component
Flat and V shaped nostril	• Webbing of the rim skin • Shortage of nasalis vestibular lining • Disconnection of orbicularis oris muscle	• Bilateral reverse U incision • Free mucosal graft in the nasal vestibule • Reposition of orbicularis oris muscle

Nakamura N et al, J Cranio Maxillofac Surg 2011; 39: 305 [51]

76.11 Outcomes in Cleft Rhinoplasty

Over the past few years, there has been an increased emphasis on the functional rather than aesthetic outcomes in cleft rhinoplasty [52]. Techniques like primary cleft rhinoplasty and naso-alveolar moulding have also been laden with complications. Although several studies have compared the different techniques of rhinoplasty to determine which technique offers the best surgical outcome, these studies lack standardised objective measurements to draw any meaningful conclusions.

The data regarding functional outcomes in cleft rhinoplasty is also sparse. In one of the prospective studies with 68 cleft patients, the authors evaluated aesthetic and respiratory outcomes at two intervals, viz. pre- and 6 months postoperatively using an active anterior rhinomanometry, rhinoresistometry and acoustic rhinometry [53]. The study showed significant improvement in many parameters. The authors concluded that while aesthetic improvement of the cleft nose is a goal, which can be achieved with regularity, nasal respiration still seems to be a challenge in cleft patients. This study highlights the need of recording functional data to study about the effects of surgery.

The outcome that is clearly documented in literature is the high satisfaction rates in patients undergoing surgery for cleft nose deformity. A study incorporating 35 patients with cleft nasal deformity was carried out by Sandor and Ylikontiola [54]. An open approach of rhinoplasty followed by alar base relocation and asymmetric nasal tip augmentation with auricular cartilage grafts was carried out in all patients. The patients' level of satisfaction was recorded in the form of a survey and interview 2 years post-surgery. A visual analogue scale (VAS) numbered 0–10 was also used by the patients to grade outcome compared to preoperative appearance at four anatomic sites. The study demonstrated highest improvements in VAS score for the tip, followed by alar position and dorsum and symmetry of nostrils. They noted that all patients were willing to undergo such procedure for a second time, if necessary. Two more studies have also reported high patient satisfaction rates for patients undergoing surgery for cleft nasal deformities [55, 56].

76.12 Further Revisions in Cleft Rhinoplasty

Although secondary cleft rhinoplasty is considered the ultimate revision rhinoplasty, in certain cases like those involving asymmetries or scarring, the patient's overall functional and aesthetic outcome may be compromised necessitating further revisions. It is important to remember that the principles that are followed in revision rhinoplasties are similar to those followed in primary and secondary rhinoplasties. The emphasis should be on early recognition after the definitive rhinoplasty so that revision is possible before scarring sets in.

76.13 Complications

The complications noted in cleft rhinoplasty are similar to those noted in the traditional open rhinoplasty in non-cleft patients. As cartilage grafts are employed, there exists a possibility of infection. Over the long term, the grafts, whether autologous, allogenous or alloplastic, can demonstrate failure. There is no difference in the risk of bleeding between cleft rhinoplasty and traditional rhinoplasty. All patients should be made aware of possible need for secondary rhinoplasty, need for revision either major or minor, existence of nostril asymmetry, visible scars, necrosis of the skin, nasal system dysfunction and morbidity associated with the donor site. One can fail to create the nasal contour as desired as well as fail in creating a normal looking appearance, and these are very common findings in cleft rhinoplasty.

76.14 Conclusion

Cleft rhinoplasty as a surgical procedure is often complex and complicated due to multiple surgical procedures that the patient needs over the years. Despite all the challenges that the procedure offers, the final surgical outcome could serve as a life changer for the patient in terms of aesthetics, function as well as symmetry. One should stick to the concepts of restoring symmetry and definition to the nasal tip and alar base, realigning and re-establishing the patency of nasal airway and preventing scarring and webbing from jeopardising the outcome. All cases have to be thoroughly planned preoperatively using the right assessment tools, and the surgery should be executed to near perfection. An increased emphasis should be placed on carrying out a primary rhinoplasty procedure keeping in mind that a definitive rhinoplasty will almost always be required to fine-tune the results.

76.15 Case Scenarios

Case 1 Figure 76.17 represents a case of right unilateral cleft nasal rhinoplasty in a 20-year-old female managed with definitive rhinoplasty. The patient presented with the chief complaint of crooked nose and difficulty in breathing from the right nostril. The patient was subjected to thorough clinical examination of both the external and internal nasal anatomy. The following features of the cleft nose were noted: deviated nasal dorsum away from the cleft in frontal view and horizontally oriented right nostril in basal view with deviated base of columella to the left. Deviated caudal septum was also noted with difficulty in breathing in the right nostril. Concavity of the right LLC was also observed in the basal view. In the lateral view, tip ptosis was observed. The patient was subjected to open rhinoplasty approach using inverted V transcolumellar incision with incorporation of the reverse U incision on the right side to correct the right nostril asymmetry. Following skeletonisation of the nose, dissection was carried between the medial crura of LLCs to expose the caudal septum which was resected to correct the septal deviation. *The authors would like to stress on the importance of addressing the nasal septum almost always in all cases when performing a definitive rhinoplasty in a unilateral cleft nasal deformity*. Substantial amount of septal cartilage was harvested to be used as a caudal extension graft to correct septal deviation as well as to improve tip projection. The cartilage was also utilised as an alar batten graft sutured to the lateral crura of LLC of the right side to correct the concavity of the right LLC. Bilateral spreader grafts were sutured between the ULC and the septum to improve the nasal breathing by improving the internal nasal valve function. Lateral crural steal was performed on the right side to maximise the projection of the nose, and further tip projection was achieved using

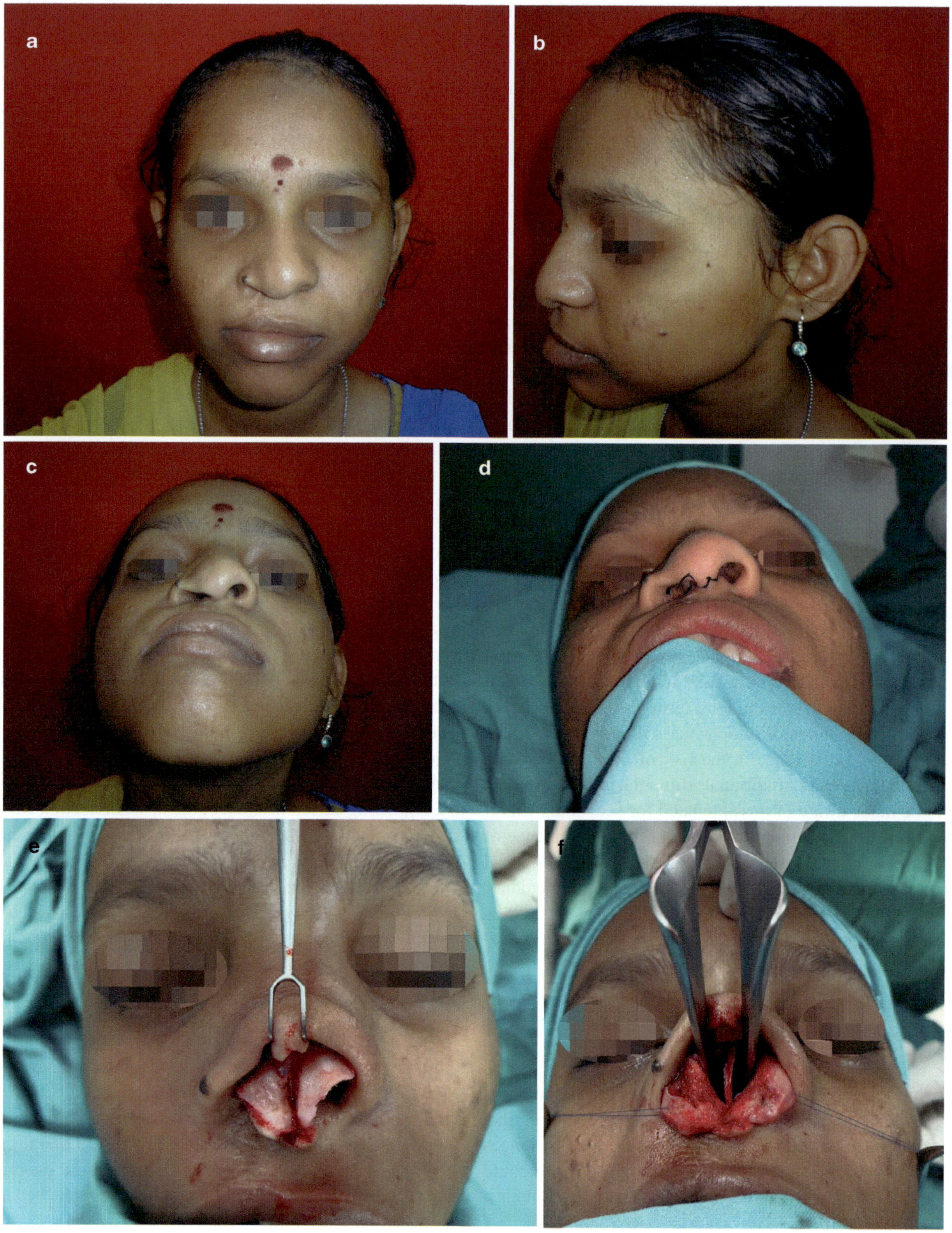

Fig. 76.17 (**a**–**n**) Clinical Scenario 1: A case of unilateral cleft nasal deformity in a 20-year-old female managed with definitive rhinoplasty. (**a**) Pre op frontal. (**b**) Pre op lateral. (**c**) Pre op basal. (**d**) Incision marking (inverted V with Tajima modification). (**e**) Exposure of lower lateral cartilages. (**f**) Exposure of nasal septum. (**g**) Spreader grafts placement bilaterally. (**h**) Columellar strut. (**i**) Columellar reconstruction and alar batten graft. (**j**) Intra op frontal. (**k**) Intra op basal. (**l**) Post op frontal. (**m**) Post op lateral. (**n**) post op basal

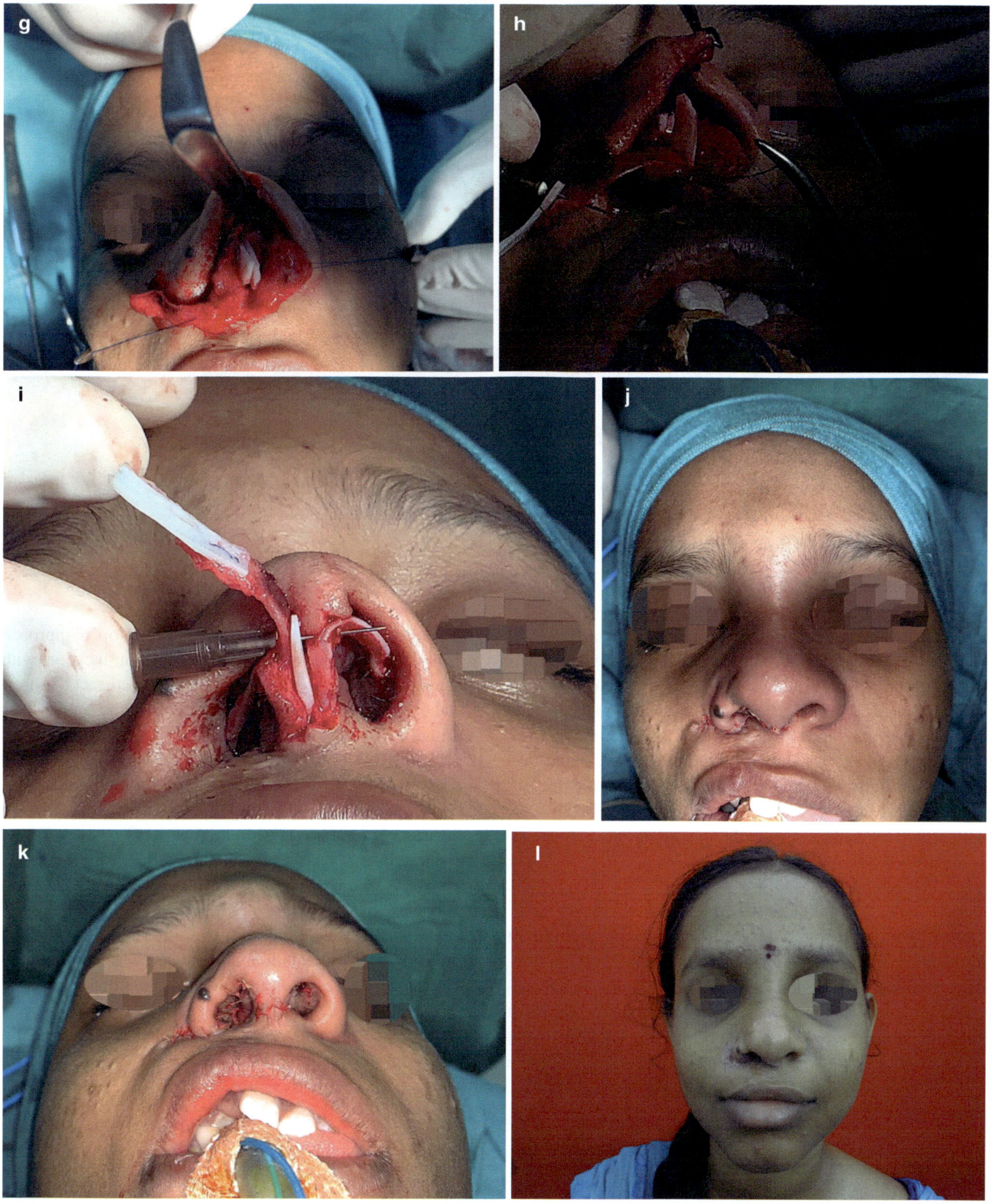

Fig. 76.17 (continued)

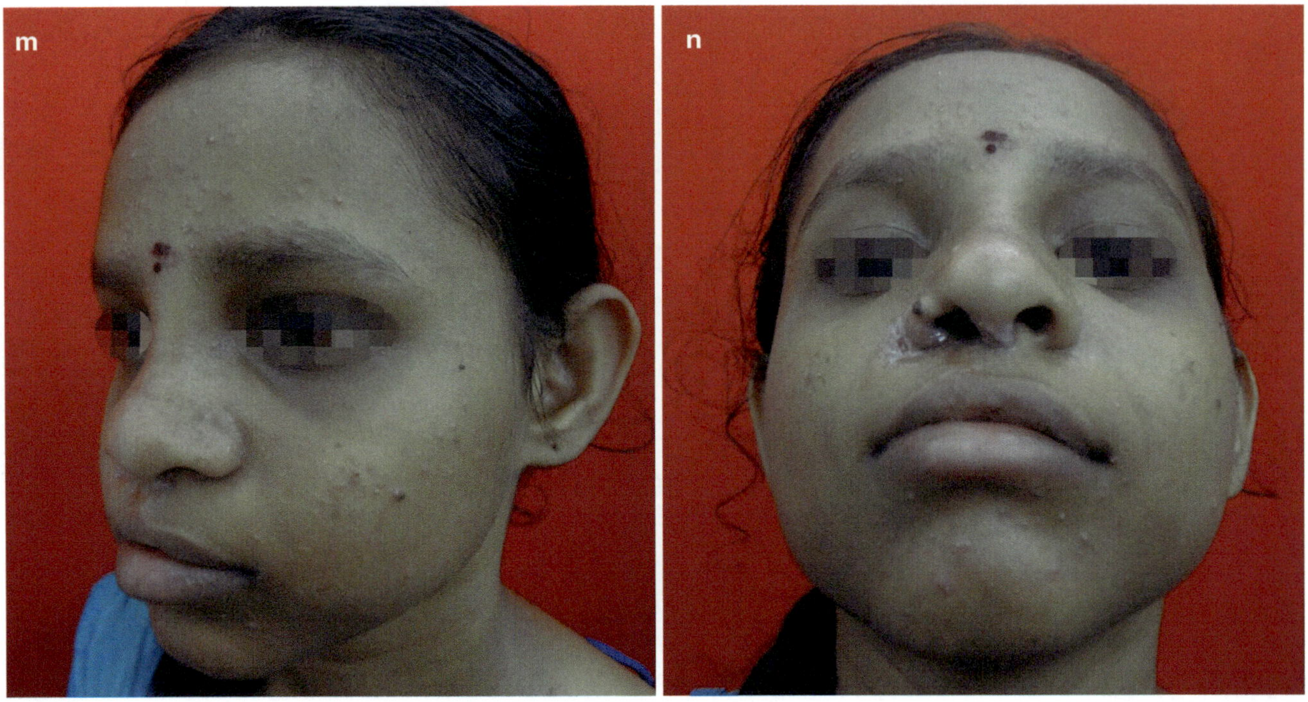

Fig. 76.17 (continued)

interdomal sutures. The deviated nasal dorsum away from the cleft was corrected using transcutaneous lateral osteotomies bilaterally in a low to high fashion. Lastly, right alar base reduction using a Weir procedure was carried out to achieve symmetry between the two alar bases. Closure of the incision was carried out using 4-0 Vicryl Rapide sutures. Comparison of the pre- and 4 weeks postoperative photographs demonstrate significant improvement in the nasal aesthetics. The patient is very satisfied with the overall result and has no complains of difficulty in breathing.

Case 2 Figure 76.18a–k represents a case of bilateral cleft nasal deformity in a 6-year-old male managed with intermediate rhinoplasty. On clinical examination, all the features characteristic of bilateral cleft nasal deformity was evident some of which included wide dorsum with bifid nasal tip, horizontally oriented nostrils, tip ptosis and short columella with a wide base. The septum was classically midline. Intermediate rhinoplasty was planned via an open approach in this case. An inverted V transcolumellar incision with bilateral reverse U incisions was planned to correct the horizontal orientation of the nostrils. The goal of the surgery was to primarily affect symmetric positioning of LLCs as well as to increase the length of the columella. Following exposure, dissection of the LLCs was carried out. A columellar strut from medpor was utilised which served to increase the tip projection. Symmetric positioning of LLC's was affected and sutured in place using horizontal mattress sutures. Transdomal sutures were also added to correct the bifid tip and decrease the angle of divergence between the alar domes. A modified Turkish delight graft was utilised for the purpose of dorsal nasal augmentation, and closure was affected with vicryl rapide sutures. It is important to note that any septal procedures were avoided to prevent growth disturbances. The pre- and 2 months postoperative photographs reveal a dramatic improvement and achievement of the preoperative goals.

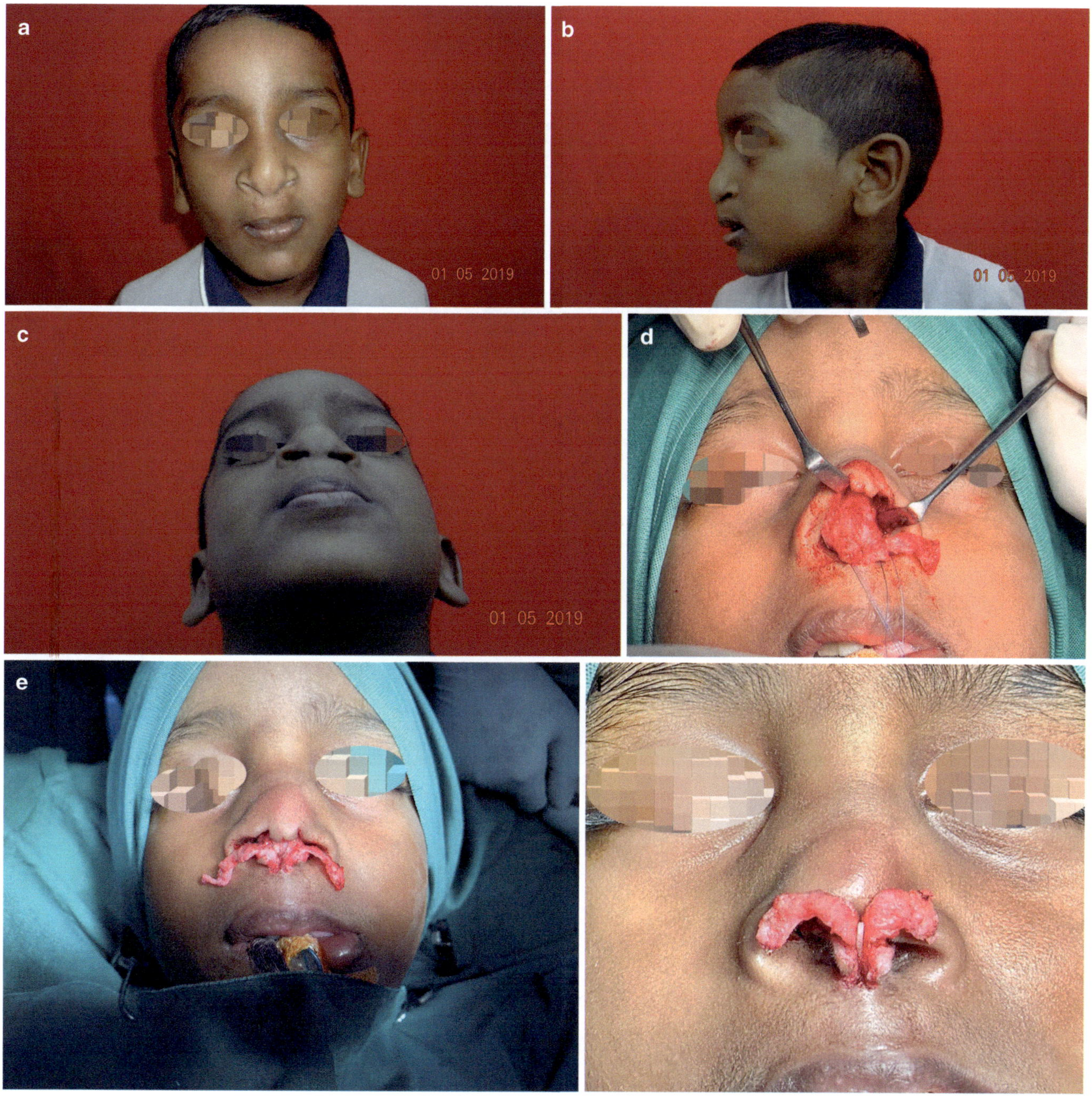

Fig. 76.18 (**a**–**k**) Clinical Scenario 2: A case of bilateral cleft nasal deformity in a 6-year-old male managed with intermediate rhinoplasty. (**a**) Pre op frontal. (**b**) Pre op lateral. (**c**) Pre op basal. (**d**) Exposure of lower lateral cartilages. (**e**) Cartilage delivery after lower lateral steal. (**f**) Columellar strut for columellar reconstruction. (**g**) Modified Turkish delight for dorsal augmentation. (**h**) Closure. (**i**) Post op frontal. (**j**) Post op lateral. (**k**) Post op basal

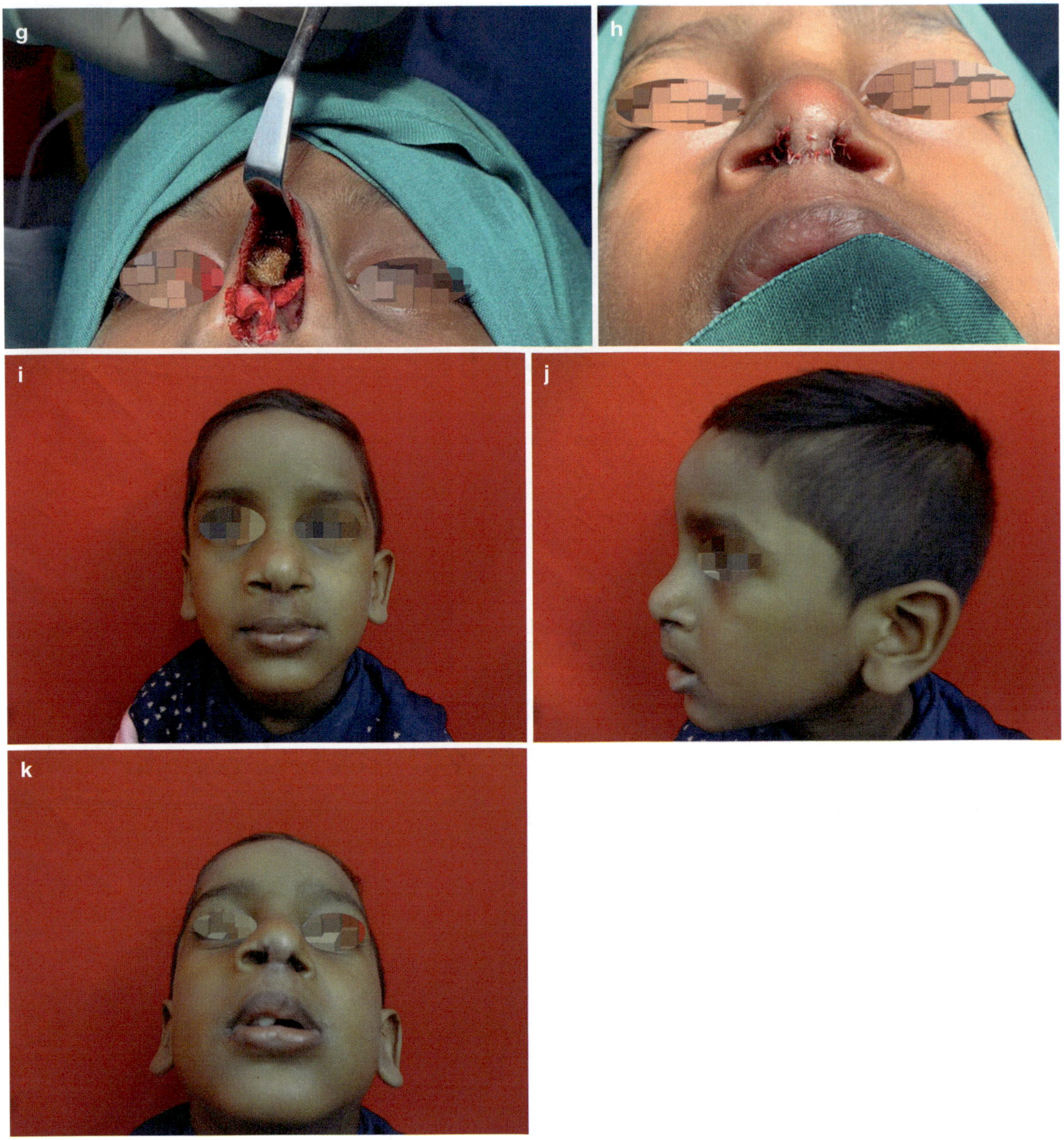

Fig. 76.18 (continued)

References

1. Shih CW, Sykes JM. Correction of cleft lip nasal deformity. Facial Plast Surg. 2002;18:253.
2. Bryd HS, El-Musa KA, Yazdani A. Definitive repair of the unilateral cleft lip nasal deformity. Plast Reconstr Surg. 2007;120:1348–56.
3. Fisher DM, Sommerlad BC. Cleft lip, cleft palate and velopharyngeal insufficiency. Plast Reconstr Surg. 2011;128:342e–60e.
4. Huffman WC, Lierle DM. Studies on the pathologic anatomy of the unilateral hare-lip nose. Plast Reconstr Surg. 1949;4:225–34.
5. Avery JK. The nasal capsule in cleft palate. Anat Anz. 1962;109(Suppl):722.
6. Latham RA. The pathogenesis of skeletal deformity associated with unilateral cleft lip and palate. Cleft Palate J. 1969;6:404–14.
7. McComb HK, Coghlan BA. Primary repair of the unilateral cleft lip nose. Completion of a longitudinal study. Cleft palate Craniofac J. 1996;33:23–31.
8. Bernstein L. Early submucous resection of nasal septal cartilage. A pilot study in canine pups. Arch Otolaryngol. 1973;97:272–85.
9. Sykes JM, Senders CW. Surgery of the cleft lip and nasal deformity. Oper Tech Otolaryngol Head Neck Surg. 1990;1:219–24.
10. Sykes JM, Senders CW. Surgical treatment of the unilateral cleft nasal deformity at the time of lip repair. Facial Plast Surg Clin North Am. 1995;3:69–77.
11. Fisher DM, Mann RJ. A model for the cleft lip nasal deformity. Plast Reconstr Surg. 1998;101:1448–56.
12. Penfold C, Dominguez-Gonzalez S. Bilateral cleft lip and nose repair. Br J Oral Maxillofac Surg. 2011;49:165–71.
13. Mulliken JB. Correction of the bilateral cleft lip nasal deformity. Evolution of a surgical concept. Cleft Palate Craniofac J. 1992;29:540–5.
14. Noordhoff MS. Bilateral cleft lip reconstruction. Plast Reconstr Surg. 1986;78:45–54.
15. Morovic CG, Cutting C. Combining the Cutting and Mulliken methods for primary repair of the bilateral cleft lip nose. Plast Reconstr Surg. 2005;116:1613–9. Discussion 1620–2
16. Cronin TD. The bilateral cleft lip with bilateral cleft of the primary palate. In: Converse JM, editor. Reconstructive plastic surgery. Philadelphia: WB Saunders; 1964.
17. Subramanian CS, et al. A modified presurgical orthopaedic (nasoalveolar molding) device in the treatment of unilateral cleft lip and palate. Eur J Dent. 2016;10:435–8.
18. Mulliken JB, Martinez-Perez D. The principle of rotation advancement for the repair of unilateral complete cleft lip and nasal deformity: Technical variations and analysis of results. Plast Reconstr Surg. 1999;104:1247–9.
19. Cronin TD. Lengthening columella by use of skin from nasal floor and alae. Plast Reconstr Surg Transplant Bull. 1958;21:417–26.
20. Wang TD. Secondary rhinoplasty in unilateral cleft nasal deformity. Facial Plast Surg. 2007;23:123–7.
21. Kaufman Y, Buchanan EP, Wolfswinkel EM, Wethers WM, Stal S. Cleft nasal deformity and rhinoplasty. Semin Plast Surg. 2012;26:184–90.
22. Garri JI, O'Leary K, Gabbay JS, et al. Improved nasal tip projection in the treatment of bilateral cleft nasal deformity. J Craniofac Surg. 2005;16:834–9.
23. Li J, Shi B, Liu K, Zheung Q. A preliminary study of hard-soft tissue relationships among unoperated secondary unilateral cleft nose deformities. Oral Surg Oral Med Oral Pathol Oral Radiol. 2012;113:300–7.
24. Duskova M, Kristen M, Smahel Z. The anthropometric verification of corrective surgery outcome in cleft secondary deformities. J Craniofac Surg. 2006;17:447–53.
25. Trottman CA, Faraway JJ, Losken HW, van Aalst JA. Functional outcomes of cleft lip surgery: Part II: Quantification of nasolabial movement. Cleft Palate Craniofac Surg. 2007;44:607–16.
26. Morrant DG, Shaw WC. Use of standardised video recording to assess cleft surgery outcome. Cleft Palate Craniofac J. 1996;33:134–42.
27. Sykes JM, Senders JW, Wang TD, Cook TA. Use of the open approach for repair of secondary cleft lip-nasal deformities. Facial Plast Surg. 1993;1:111–26.
28. Millard DR Jr. Columella lengthening by a forked flap. Plast Reconstr Surg. 1958;22:545.
29. Nakamura N, Sasaguri M, Okawachi T, Nishihara K, Nozoe E. Secondary correction of bilateral cleft lip nose deformity. Clinical and three-dimensional observations on pre- and postoperative outcome. J Craniomaxillofac Surg. 2011;39:305–12.
30. Tajima S, Maruyama M. Reverse U incision for secondary repair of cleft lip nose. Plast Reconstr Surg. 1977;60:256–61.
31. Haddock NT, McRae MH, Cutting CB. Long term effect of primary cleft rhinoplasty on secondary cleft rhinoplasty in patients with unilateral cleft lip cleft palate. Plast Reconstr Surg. 2012;129:740–8.
32. Tajima S. Follow up results of unilateral primary cleft lip operation with special reference to primary nasal correction by the author's method. Facial Plast Surg. 1990;7:97–104.
33. Bryd HS, Salomon J. Primary correction of the unilateral cleft nasal deformity. Plast Reconstr Surg. 2000;106:1276–86.
34. Mulliken JB. Primary repair of bilateral cleft lip and nasal deformity. Plast Reconstr Surg. 2001;108:181–6.
35. Park SS. Treatment of the internal nasal valve. Facial Plast Surg. 1999;7:333–45.
36. Teymoortash A, Fasunla JA, Sazgar AA. The value of spreader grafts in rhinoplasty: A critical review. Eur Arch Otorhinolaryngol. 2012;269:1411–6.
37. Jablon H, Sykes JM. Nasal airway problems in the cleft lip population. Facial Plast Surg Clin North Am. 1999;7:391–403.
38. Crockett D, Burnstead R. Nasal airway, otologic and audiologic problems associated with cleft lip and palate. In: Bradach J, Morris HL, editors. Multidisciplinary management of cleft lip and palate. Philadelphia: WB Saunders; 1990.
39. Cuzalina A, Jung C. Rhinoplasty for the cleft lip and palate patient. Oral Maxillofac Surg Clin North Am. 2016;28:189–202.
40. Ingels KJ, Orhan KS, Van Heerbeek N. The effect of spreader grafts on nasal dorsal width in patients with nasal valve insufficiency. Arch Facial Plast Surg. 2008;10:354–6.
41. Cho BC, Choi KY, Lee JH et al. The correction of a secondary bilateral cleft lip nasal deformity using refined open rhinoplasty with reverse U incision, V plasty and selective combination with composite grafting: Long term results. Arch Plast Surg 2012; 39:190–7.
42. Guyuron B. MOC-PS(SM) CME article. Late cleft lip nasal deformity. Plast Reconstr Surg. 2008;121(4, Suppl):1–11.
43. Park BY, Lew DH, Lee YH. A comparative study of the lateral crus of alar cartilage in unilateral cleft lip nasal deformity. Plast Reconstr Surg. 1998;101:905–19.
44. Chand MS, Toriumi DM. Treatment of the external nasal valve. Fac Plast Surg. 1999;7:347–55.
45. Richardson S, Agni NA, Pasha Z. Modified Turkish delight: morselized polyethylene dorsal graft for rhinoplasty. Int J Oral Maxillofac Surg. 2011;40:979–82.
46. Yan W, Zhao ZM, Yin NB, et al. A new modified forked flap and a reverse V shaped flap for secondary correction of bilateral cleft lip nasal deformities. Chin Med J (Engl). 2011;124:3993–6.
47. Rikimaru H, Kiyokawa K, Koga N, et al. A new modified forked flap with subcutaneous pedicles for adult cases of bilateral cleft lip nasal deformity: from normalisation to aesthetic improvement. J Craniofac Surg. 2008;19:1374–80.

48. Cheon YW, Park BY. Long term evaluation of elongating columella using conchal composite graft in bilateral secondary cleft lip and nose deformity. Plast Reconstr Surg. 2010;126:543–53.
49. Nakamura N. Surgical strategy for surgical correction of unilateral and bilateral cleft lip nose deformities. In: Brenner MJ, editor. Rhinoplasty. Croatia: In Tech; 2011.
50. Nakamura N, Okawachi T, Nishihara K, Hirahara N, Nozoe E. Surgical technique for secondary correction of unilateral cleft lip nose deformity—Clinical and three-dimensional observations of pre- and post-operative nasal forms. J Oral Maxillofac Surg. 2010;68:2248.
51. Nakamura N, Okawachi T, Nishihara K, Hirahara N, Nozoe E. Surgical technique for secondary correction of unilateral cleft lip nose deformity—Clinical and three-dimensional observations on pre- and post-operative nasal forms. J Cranio Maxillofac Surg. 2011;39:305.
52. Lee TS, Schwartz GM, Tatum SA. Rhinoplasty for cleft and hemangioma related nasal deformities. Curr Opin Otolaryngol Head Neck Surg. 2010;18:526–35.
53. Huempfner-Hierl H, Hemprich A, Hierl T. Results of prospective anthropometric and functional study about aesthetics and nasal respiration after secondary rhinoplasty in cleft lip and palate patients. J Craniofac Surg. 2009;20(Suppl 2):1863–75.
54. Sandor GK, Ylikontiola LP. Patient evaluation of outcomes of external rhinoplasty for unilateral cleft lip and palate. Int J Oral Maxillofac Surg. 2006;35:407–11.
55. Chaithanyaa N, Rai KK, Shivakumar HR, Upasi A. Evaluation of the outcome of secondary rhinoplasty in cleft lip and palate patients. J Plast Reconstr Aesthet Surg. 2011;64:27–33.
56. Pitak-Arnnop P, Hemprich A, Dhanuthai K, Pausch NC. Outcome research on secondary cleft rhinoplasty: The Leipzig experience. J Plast Reconstr Aesthet Surg. 2011;64:277–8.

Part XX

Craniofacial Anomalies

Rare Facial Clefts

77

Srinivas Gosla Reddy and Avni Pandey Acharya

77.1 Introduction

Since ages, congenital deformities were considered evil and wizard, and infants were abandoned to die in isolation. Jean Yperman (1295–1351) valued the congenital origin of the clefts. He additionally characterized the different types of the condition and set out the standards for their treatment. Fabricius ab Aquapendente (1537–1619) and William His of college of Leipzig independently researched and published embryological premise of clefts [1].

Laroche was the first to separate between common cleft lip or harelip and clefts of the cheek. Further qualification was made in 1864 by Pelvet, who isolated oblique clefts including the nose from the other cheek clefts, and drawing on Ahlfeld's work, in 1887 Morian gathered 29 cases from the writing, contributing 7 instances of his own. Morian perceived three unique groups of oblique facial clefts. From that point forward, astounding audits have been composed by Griinberg in 1913, Boo-Chai in 1970, Paul Tessier in 1976 [2] and Millard in 1977 [3].

Craniofacial cleft by definition is "a fissure of the soft tissues that corresponds as a general rule with a cleft of the bony structures." [1] The greatest research on craniofacial clefts was finished by Tessier and is credited for the formation of the craniofacial surgery for establishing the framework of the advanced craniofacial surgery by fundamentally breaking down facial clefts and portraying facial osteotomies [4].

Craniofacial clefts are significant clefts affecting the face, cranium, or both. These clefts cause distortion of the face and cranium with lacks or abundances of tissue that cleave anatomic planes in a straight fashion [2]. Craniofacial clefts exist in changing degrees of seriousness, and practically every one of them happens along the anticipated embryologic lines. These clefts can be either complete or incomplete and can seem alone or in relationship with other facial clefts. Seriousness of craniofacial clefts fluctuates extensively, running from a scarcely distinguishable indent on the lip or on the nose or a scar-like structure on the cheek to an extensive partition of all layers of facial structures. Notwithstanding one parted sort can show on one side of the face, while an alternate kind is available on the other side [2, 3].

Craniofacial clefts need comprehensive rehabilitation. Past the physical consequences for the patient, they have monstrous mental and financial impacts on both patient and family, prompting disturbance of psychosocial working and diminished nature of life [4, 5].

Cleft repair is a necessary part of the modern craniomaxillo-facial surgical spectrum and remains a challenge on account of inadequate and contorted tissue (minor to major) at the site of the deformity [6]. The outcomes are additionally impacted by the short and long haul aesthetic (soft tissue and facial skeletal appearance) [7] and useful (occlusal and discourse) outcomes [8]. What's more, the kind of careful fix, the specialist's abilities and the compliance of the patient likewise, affects the stylish [9] and utilitarian [10]outcomes. The real test isn't just understanding the hereditary qualities [11], in addition to plan the standard conventions for the surgery in these phenomenal kinds of clefts [12].

77.2 Incidence

Craniofacial clefts are a lot rarer than the simple cleft lip/palate deformity [13]. The precise occurrence of craniofacial clefts has not been exactly documented in view of their rarity. However, the reported frequency of craniofacial clefts is 1.5–6.0 per 100,000 live births [14]. The occurrence of uncommon craniofacial clefts contrasted with ordinary cleft lip and palate may vary from 9.5 to 34 for every 1000 [15].

Disclosure: Authors have no financial conflicts to disclose.

S. Gosla Reddy (✉) · A. P. Acharya
GSR Institute of Cranio-maxillofacial & Facial Plastic Surgery, Hyderabad, Telangana, India

K. Bonanthaya et al. (eds.), *Oral and Maxillofacial Surgery for the Clinician*, https://doi.org/10.1007/978-981-15-1346-6_77

Lateral or transverse clefts of the lip are very uncommon and have commonly archived to have a rate of 0.3% of 1.0% of all of the facial cleft deformity spectrum (Boo-Chai 1969; Hawkins et al. 1973; Bauer et al. 1982; Verheyden 1988; Gleizal et al. 2007), or of 0.02% of live births (Kuriyama et al. 2008) [16]. Median clefts of the lower lip are very rare and only 68 cases have been accounted for till date [17].

77.3 Embryology

Successful treatment of innate craniofacial defects depends on an intensive comprehension of the embryologic procedures prompting their development [18]. There are various interesting highlights that plainly recognize craniofacial improvement from the advancement of different tissues in the body.

One of these novel highlights is the double starting point of craniofacial tissues: the skeletal framework and the vast majority of the connective tissues, including veins, begin from a gathering of cells called the cranial neural crest, while the musculature and some parts of the skull begin from mesoderm.

A second one of a kind component is the unit of intricate, complementary tissue interactions between the neuroectoderm, the mesenchyme, and facial ectoderm that drive ordinary advancement.

A third novel element is the extravagantly arranged morphogenetic developments—brought about by both uninvolved cell removal and dynamic cell movement—that characterize head advancement. Any procedure that upsets the rate, the planning, or the degree of these complex cell conduct can result in a craniofacial birth imperfection.

77.3.1 The Initiation of Craniofacial Development

77.3.1.1 Establishment and Fusion of the Facial Prominences (Figs. 77.1 and 72.3)

The basic morphology of the face is established between the 4th and 10th week of human development. The face is formed as a result of fusion of the midline frontonasal prominence and three paired prominences, the maxillary, lateral nasal, and mandibular prominences. Each of these prominences is filled with cranial neural crest cells that originated at different positions along the neural tube.

77.3.1.2 The Frontonasal Prominence

The frontonasal prominence gives rise to the forehead, midline of the nose, the philtrum, the middle portion of the upper lip, and the primary palate. Interruptions in frontonasal growth often result in a bilateral cleft lip, where the primary palate frequently "everts." In the mildest cases, clefts involving frontonasal prominence-derived structures may be limited to a notch in the vermillion border of the lip. In more severe cases, frontonasal clefts involve all of the tissues of the lip, and these cases may most likely occur because of a failure of fusion between the frontonasal and maxillary prominences.

77.3.1.3 The Lateral Nasal Prominences

The lateral nasal prominences give rise to the alae of the nose. Clefts that involve the side of the nose often result from a failure in the fusion between the lateral nasal prominences and either the frontonasal or the maxillary processes.

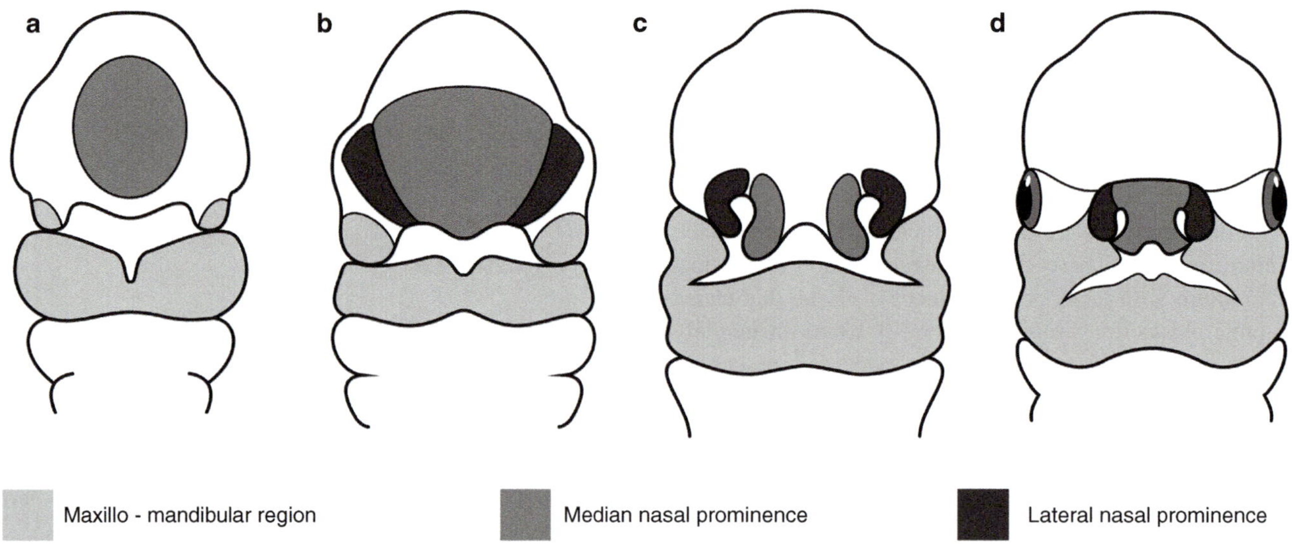

Fig. 77.1 (a–d) Embryological representation of fusion of nasal prominences

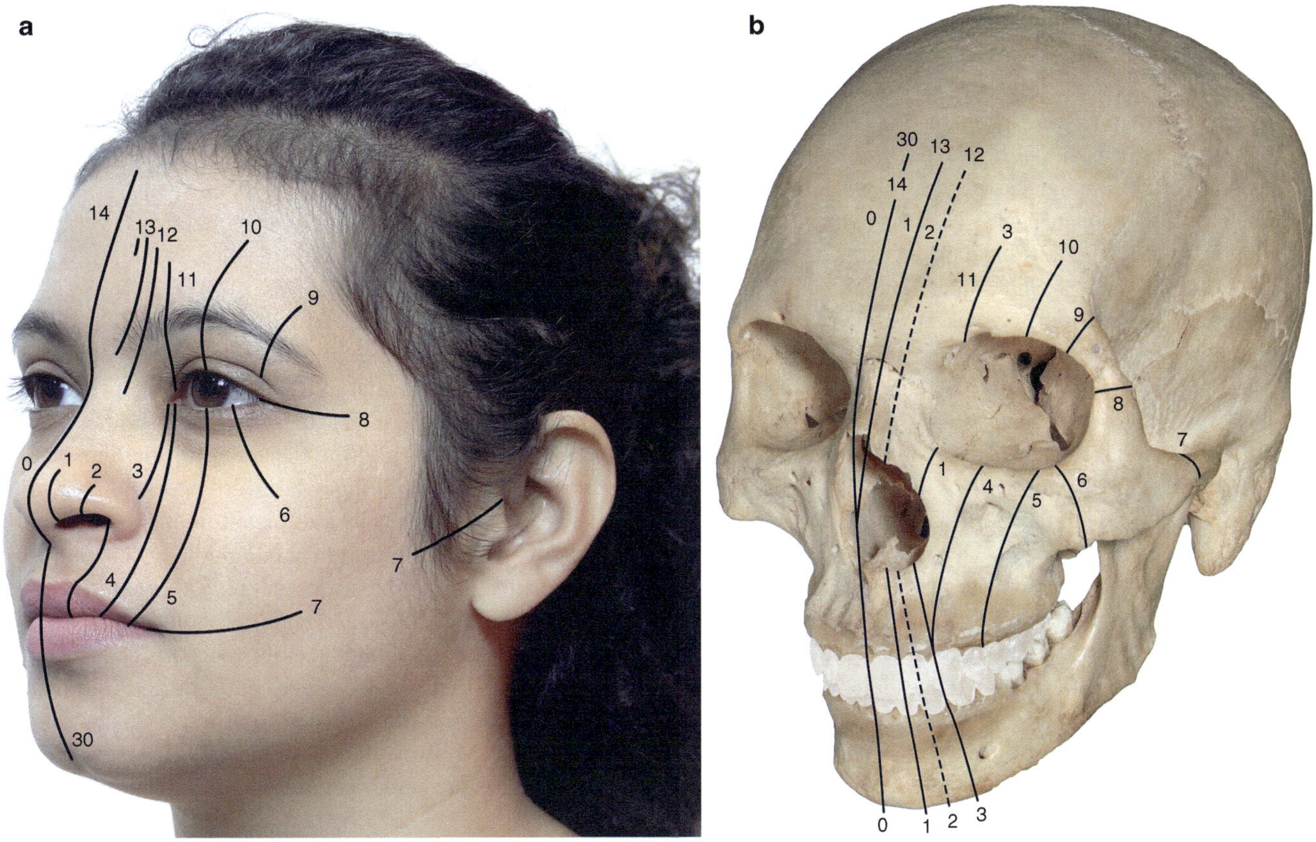

Fig. 77.2 (**a**)Tessier classification for soft tissue clefting. (**b**) Tessier classification for bony clefting

77.3.1.4 The Maxillary Prominences

The maxillary prominences develop into the upper jaw, the facial halves, the upper lips, and the secondary palate. The nasal passage is divided from the pharynx by the secondary palate, which is formed from the neural crest cells. The palatal shelves first drop vertically and then rotate into a horizontal plane on the dorsal side of the tongue before fusing. The epithelium of the palatal shelves sloughs off, with only the basal layer of epithelium remaining to cover the later palate.

77.3.1.5 The Mandibular Prominences

This develops into the lower jaw and lower lip. Clefts of the lower jaw are very rare, presenting with a wide variety of phenotypes, ranging from a vermillion notch on the lip to a complete cleft involving the anterior mandible, chin, tongue, and lower lip and occasionally involving midline structures of the neck up to the manubrium sterni [19].

77.4 Etiology and Pathogenesis

Development of the head and face contains a standout among the most mind-boggling events among embryonic advancement. Disturbance of this firmly controlled course can result in a facial cleft where the facial primordia fail to meet and form the suitable structures [20]. The definite instrument of the cause of facial clefts is obscure, yet they are accepted to have a multifactorial etiology including a mix of natural and hereditary causes during embryonic development [21, 22]. In India affiliation and healthful inadequacies in pregnant mothers are the main cause of clefts [23].

The discussion is as yet in contention between the supporters of Meckel who trusted that clefts were brought about by a developmental arrest and Geoffroy St. Hilaire (1832) who felt that amniotic groups were responsible [15].

Fogh-Andersen previously characterized hereditary factors in clefting, which have been affirmed by segregation analysis [23]. Research in molecular genetics have identified genes responsible for rare facial clefts which may be syndromic and also for complex non-syndromic variants [24].

The non-syndromic types of orofacial clefts are likely due to secondary gene-environment interactions [25]. Non-syndromic cleft is a heterogeneous disease entity with candidate clefting loci on chromosomes [1, 2, 4, 6, 11, 14, 17, 19].

Four general classes of natural "cleftogens" have been distinguished to date, as follows [26]:

Radiation. Huge dosages of radiation have been associated with microcephaly.

Infections. The offspring of mothers with toxoplasmosis, rubella, or cytomegalovirus diseases display expanded frequencies of facial clefts.

Maternal idiosyncrasies. Mothers of children with CLP display an increased rate of phenylketonuria. The oculo-auriculovertebral range has been seen with strange recurrence among neonates with mothers who are diabetic. Numerous examinations have proposed maternal factors, for example, age, weight, and general well-being, as potential reasons for distortions.

Chemicals. Nutrient deficiencies are related with expanded rates of CLP, which might be decreased with vitamin supplementation for expectant mothers. Vitamin A, its subsidiaries, and related compounds, for example, isotretinoin, have been involved in the developments of facial clefts and hemifacial microsomia [26].

Any maternal liquor consumption during pregnancy increases the frequency of orofacial clefting [27]. The impact of maternal smoking also may be responsible [28]. Multiple studies have demonstrated that folate deficiency is related with clefts. Pre-birth folic acid supplementation has shown to diminish this hazard. At present, folic acid supplementation is the main empirical safeguard to diminish the frequency of facial clefting [2].

77.5 Classification

An all-round grouping plan that completely envelops, precisely depicts, and coordinates all the different types of orofacial and craniofacial clefts does not exist [2]. Soemmering (1791), Morian in 1886, Degenhardt (1961), the American Association of Cleft Palate Rehabilitation (AACPR) (1962), and Boo-Chai have made huge contributions in building up a classification [29–32].

77.5.1 Tessier Classification

In 1976, Paul Tessier depicted an anatomical order framework in which a number is doled out to every abnormality based on its position with respect to the sagittal midline [33].

This framework has moved towards global acknowledgment and allows reliable correspondence among clinicians [34].

This classification involves the orbit as the principle reference point. Fifteen areas of clefting have been demonstrated with discussion of their soft tissue and hard tissue involvement [33] (Fig. 77.2a, b).

The numbered clefts relate the soft tissue features to underlying bony involvement.

These have been verified by operative findings and more recently preoperative 3D CT assessments [35]. The clefts are radially distributed around the orbit with the midline 0 cleft named as median facial dysrhaphia [33].

77.5.1.1 Number Zero

The no. 0 cleft is the most widely recognized of the craniofacial clefts [36]. No. 0 and 14 is also called as midline craniofacial dysrhaphia. Clinically, this cleft shows up as an absence of conclusion of the front neuropore [33].

It shows two variants: a true and false middle congenital cleft, with or without related hypo- or hypertelorism [36]. Developmental cause of Tessier no. 0 isn't evident; however, it is realized that midline facial deformities can be followed to a period relating to the third week of gestation [36]. The cleft expresses as a duplication of the crista galli in frontal bone ("skull bifidum" and middle encephalocele), and as nasal septal duplication, and cleft through the columella, maxilla, and lip [33]. This form of cleft may have either a deficiency or abundance of tissue: with tissue agenesis and holoprosencephaly toward one side and frontonasal hyperplasia and inordinate tissue (the hyperplasias) at the opposing end. Midway inconsistencies with normal tissue volume possess the center segment of the spectrum [37].

Features of true midline congenital fissure:

1. Split upper lip with renal duplication
2. Bifid nose with wide columella and a wide furrow in the nasal dorsum
3. Duplication of the nasal septum
4. Overprojected nose due to fibromuscular connection of the alar ligaments and the frontal bone
5. Hypertelorism
6. Low placed cribriform plate of the ethmoid bone
7. Occasional midline encephalocele [38]

Features of the pseudo midline congenital fissure include:

1. Hypotelorism
2. Absence of the philtrum of the lip, premaxilla, nasal septum, columella, and the crista galli [33]
3. Clefting along the entire length of the upper lip
4. Hypoplastic nasal septum
5. Holoprosencephaly
6. Hypoplastic ethmoid bones [37]
7. Widened body of the sphenoid bone with separation of the pterygoid plate [35]

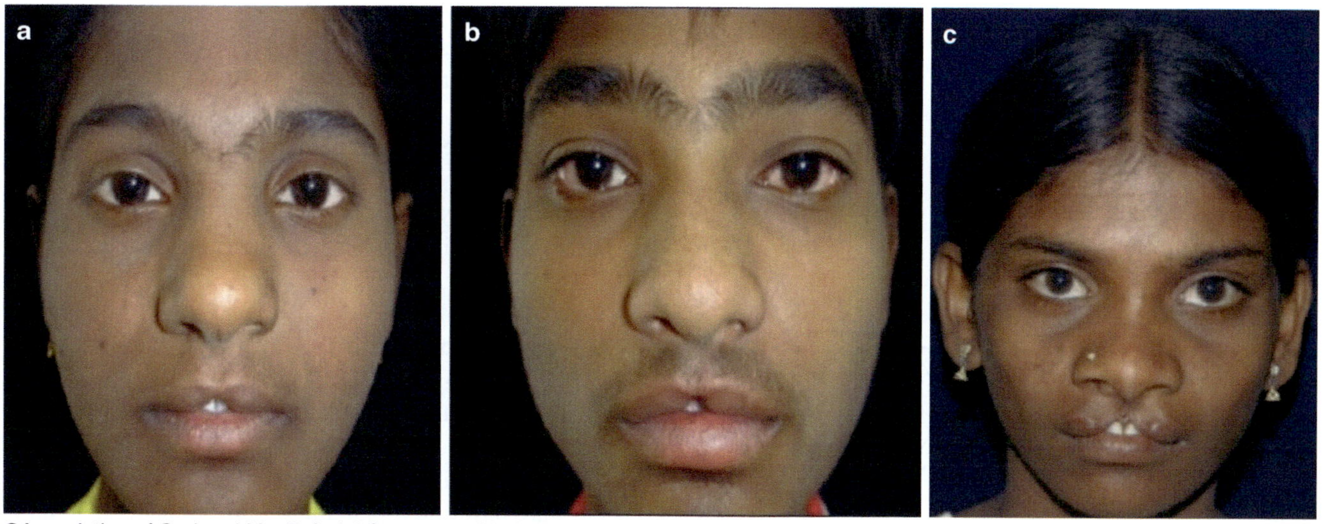

Fig. 77.3 (**a–c**) Clinical subclassification of Tessier number 0. (**a**) Type I—Involving only vermillion not involving the white roll. (**b**) Type II—Involving vermillion and white roll. (**c**) Type III—Involving vermillion, white roll, and philtrum

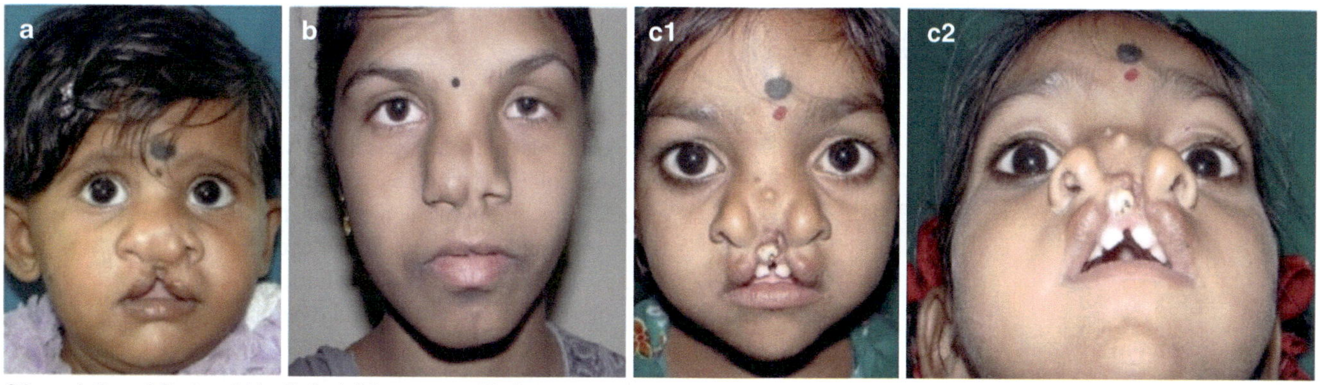

Fig. 77.4 (**a–c**) Clinical subclassification of Tessier no. 0. (**a**) Type IV—Involving vermillion, white roll, philtrum, columella. (**b**) Type V—Involving columella and tip, supratip, and dorsum of the nose. (**c1, c2**) Type VI—Involving columella, tips, supratip, dorsum of the nose and frontonasal area

Millard [39] classified a middle split of the lip as any vertical cleft through the focal point of the upper lip, paying little heed to the degree (Fig. 77.3a–c). Middle clefts have been isolated into two gatherings by Millard and Williams [39]. The principal bunching includes agenesis of the frontonasal procedure, and the second gathering is portrayed as separated to the middle component. The last is related with different degrees of nasal bifurcation and cranial malformations including hypertelorism [40–42] (Fig. 77.4a–c).

77.5.1.2 Number 1 Cleft

The number 1 cleft is also called as a paramedian cleft. Skeletally it passes through the frontal bone affecting the olfactory groove along the ethmoid producing hypertelorism (Fig. 77.5). It also widens the area between the nasal bone and the frontal process of maxilla. The soft tissue component involves the dome of the nose and may involve the alveolus and the lip. It may have a cranial counterpart in No 13 cleft. [33]

Soft Tissue Characteristics:

Soft tissue characteristics of No 1 cleft include:

1. Alar clefting that produces deviation of the nose to the opposite
2. Vertical ridges and furrows on the nasal dorsum
3. Vertical orbital dystopia and telecanthus
4. Tongue-shaped frontal hairline which is indicative of no. 13 cleft [35]

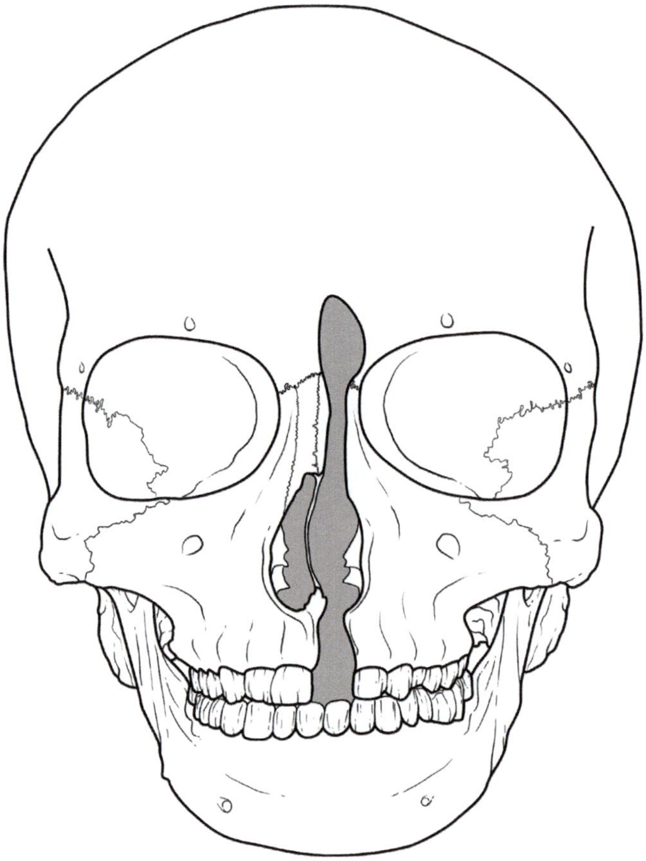

Fig. 77.5 Tessier 1

Skeletal Involvement:

Skeletal features are as follows:

1. Clefting of the maxilla extending posteriorly as a total cleft of the hard palate.
2. Hypoplastic maxilla.
3. Nasal dorsum is deviated.
4. Asymmetry of the pterygoid plates and increased prominence of the lesser wing of the sphenoid bone.
5. Mild plagiocephaly may also be an associated feature [35].

77.5.1.3 Number 2 Cleft

Tessier no. 2 clefts are found parallel to the midline Tessier No. 0 clefts [33]. The deformation of the middle third of the nostril rim is a characteristic feature of the Tessier 2 cleft. This produces widening of the nasal bridge and flattening of the lateral side of the nose (Fig. 77.6a–e).

Skeletal features of Tessier 2 clefts are as follows:

1. Alveolar dysplasia from the lateral incisor to the pyriform aperture.
2. Palatal cleft may or may not be seen.
3. Deviated nasal septum.
4. A bony indentation is seen near the naso-maxillary suture [35].
5. Dysplasia of the lateral ethmoid region with orbital hypertelorism [43].
6. Cranial base asymmetry.
7. Dislodged medial canthus with intact lacrimal duct [44].

77.5.1.4 Number 3 Cleft

No. 3 is the oculo-nasal cleft (Morian I). This is also called "medial" orbito-maxillary cleft which passes through the lacrimal segment of the lower eyelid. This paranasal cleft occurs obliquely involving the lacrimal groove [33]. The patient may have microphthalmia [35] but anophthalmia is rare [45] (Figs. 77.7a–c and 77.8a–c).

Soft Tissue Characteristics [35, 46]

The important soft tissue features of the Tessier 3 cleft are:

1. Soft tissue hypoplasia of the face in the vertical direction [35]
2. Clefting of the alar base involving the nasolabial groove
3. Alveolar cleft with cleft of the lip
4. Displacement of the medial canthal apparatus and the lacrimal punctum of the lower eyelid
5. No patency of the lacrimal duct into the nose
6. Normal globe with orbital dystopia

Skeletal involvement include the following features:

1. Absence of the frontal process of the maxilla and medial wall of the maxillary sinus [33]
2. Deviated nasal septum
3. Cleft lip and palate
4. Continuity of the nasal cavity into the maxilla with no bony lateral nasal wall [35]
5. Hypoplastic maxilla
6. Narrowing of the ethmoid body and sinus on the affected side [35]
7. May be associated with a cranial cleft No 10 or 11 [33]

77.5.1.5 Number 4 Cleft

The No 4 Tessier cleft is a rare, complex, and gruesome craniofacial malformation [47]. No. 4 is the oculofacial separated I (Morian II). This is a "focal" orbito-maxillary cleft [33].

It may range from a unilateral notch paramedially to large bilateral tissue defects extending from the mouth to the eyes with huge bony fissures [47] (Fig. 77.9a–f).

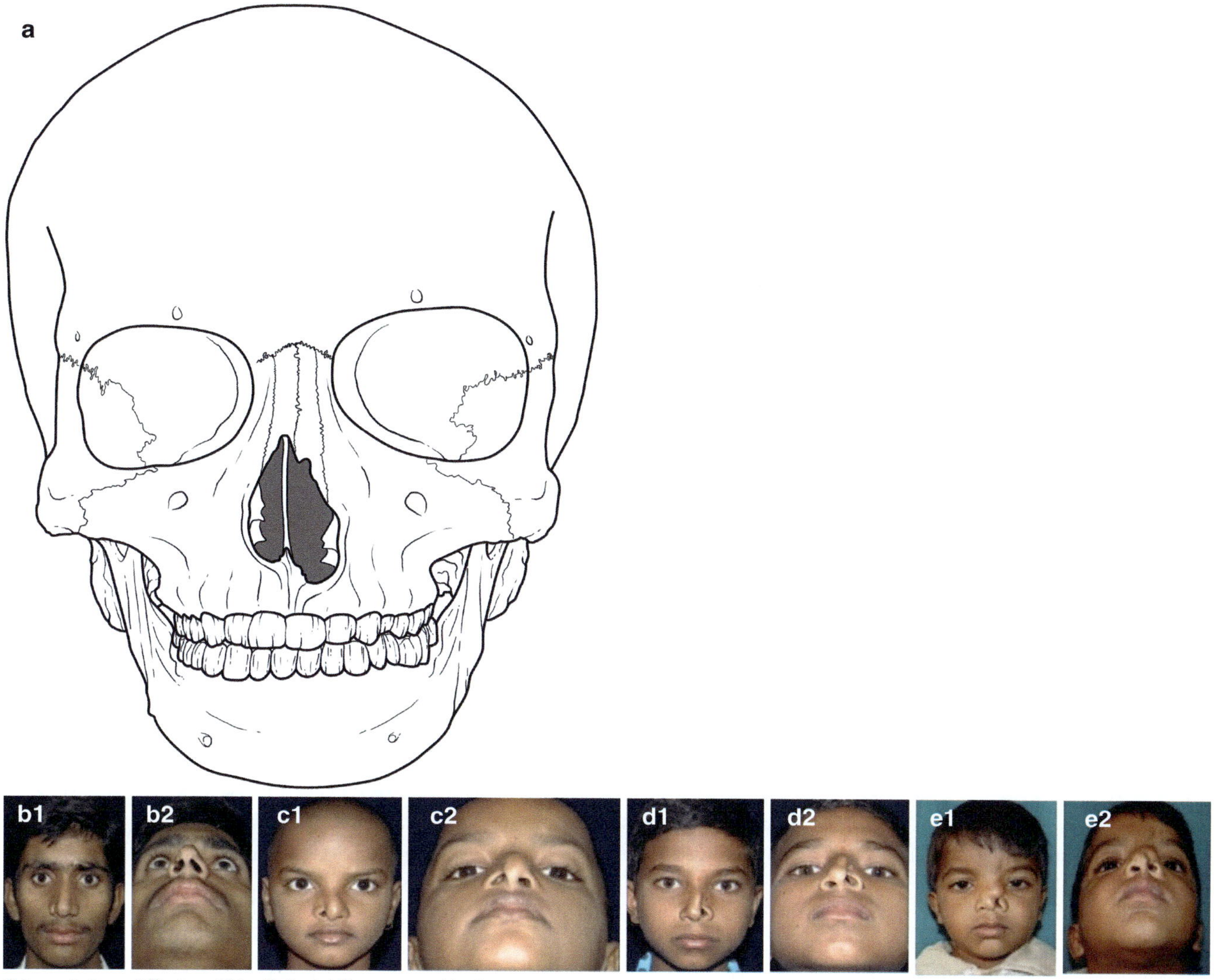

Fig. 77.6 (**a**–**e**) Tessier 2 clefts ranging from microform defect to more severe

Soft tissue characteristics include:

1. Clefting extending halfway between the philtral crest and the labial commissure
2. Extreme degree of vertical tissue deficiency extending from the labial cleft to the ocular separation in the lower eyelid [35]
3. Decreased oro-ocular distance
4. Microphthalmia with exposure keratitis secondary to eyelid deficiency [47]
5. Dystopia and inferior placement of the involved globe

Skeletal characteristics are enumerated below:

1. Bony cleft starting caudally between the lateral incisor and the canine proceeding cephalically medial to the infra-orbital foramen onto the orbital floor.
2. Prolapse of the orbital contents into the maxillary sinus due to the orbital defect.
3. Naso-lacrimal duct is intact, but the inferior lacrimal canaliculi may be hypoplastic or absent [47].
4. This may be associated with a cranial cleft no 12.

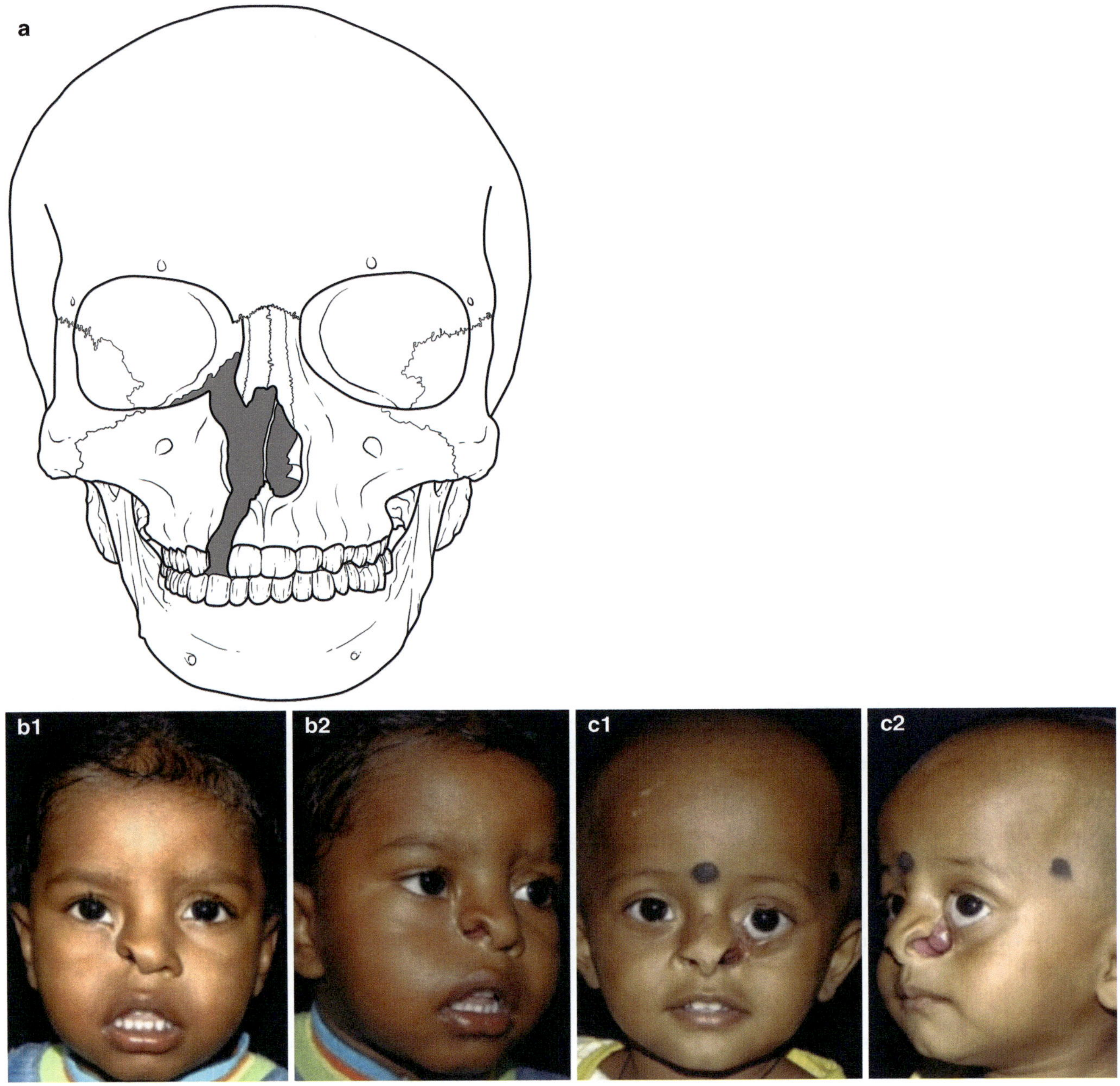

Fig. 77.7 (a–c) Tessier 3 cleft with ocular involvement

77.5.1.6 Number 5 Cleft

The Tessier No 5 cleft is a very uncommon malformation and is also referred as the oculofacial cleft II (Morian III). This lateral orbito-maxillary cleft gets through the medial third of the lower eyelid [33] (Fig. 77.10a, b).

Soft tissue involvement demonstrates:

1. Clefting immediately medial to the commissure which courses along the cheek lateral to the ala of the nose, ending in the lateral half of the lower eyelid.
2. The globes are usually normal but may occasionally show microphthalmia [35].

Skeletal involvement:

1. The alveolar cleft starts lateral to and travels lateral to the infra-orbital foramen and ends in the lateral part of the orbital floor. There may be associated hypoplasia of the maxillary sinus [48].

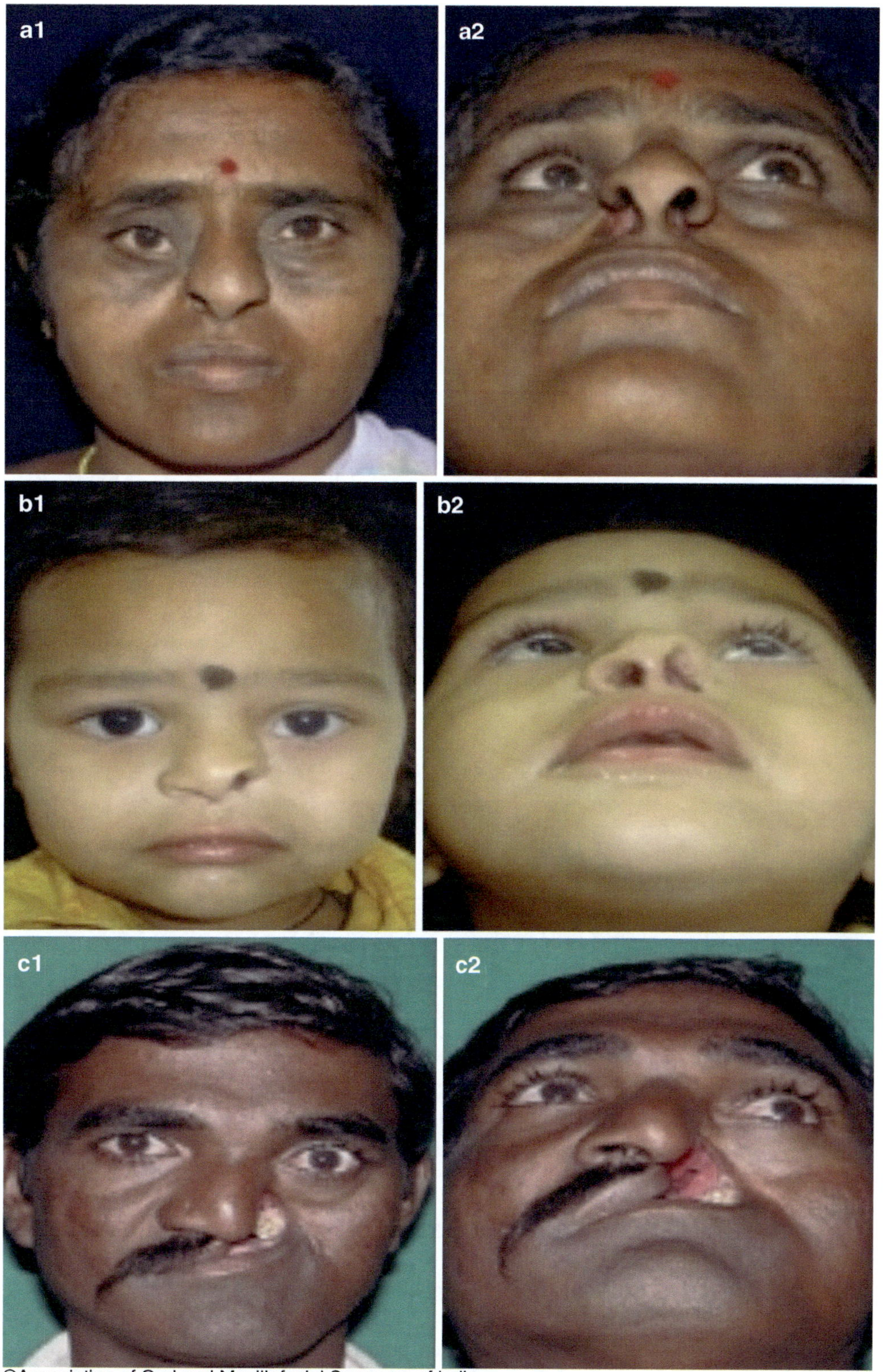

Fig. 77.8 (**a**–**c**) Tessier 3. (**a**) With bilateral involvement (**b**) without ocular involvement (**c**) with oral involvement

2. Vertical orbital dystopia due to prolapse of the orbital contents.
3. Thickened lateral orbital wall and abnormal greater wing of the sphenoid bone.
4. Cranial base may be generally normal [35].

77.5.1.7 Number 6 Cleft

This is otherwise called as zygomaticomaxillary cleft which may form an incomplete variant of the Treacher Collins syndrome (Fig. 77.11a, b). It was named as maxillozygomatic dysplasia by Van der Meulen [33, 49].

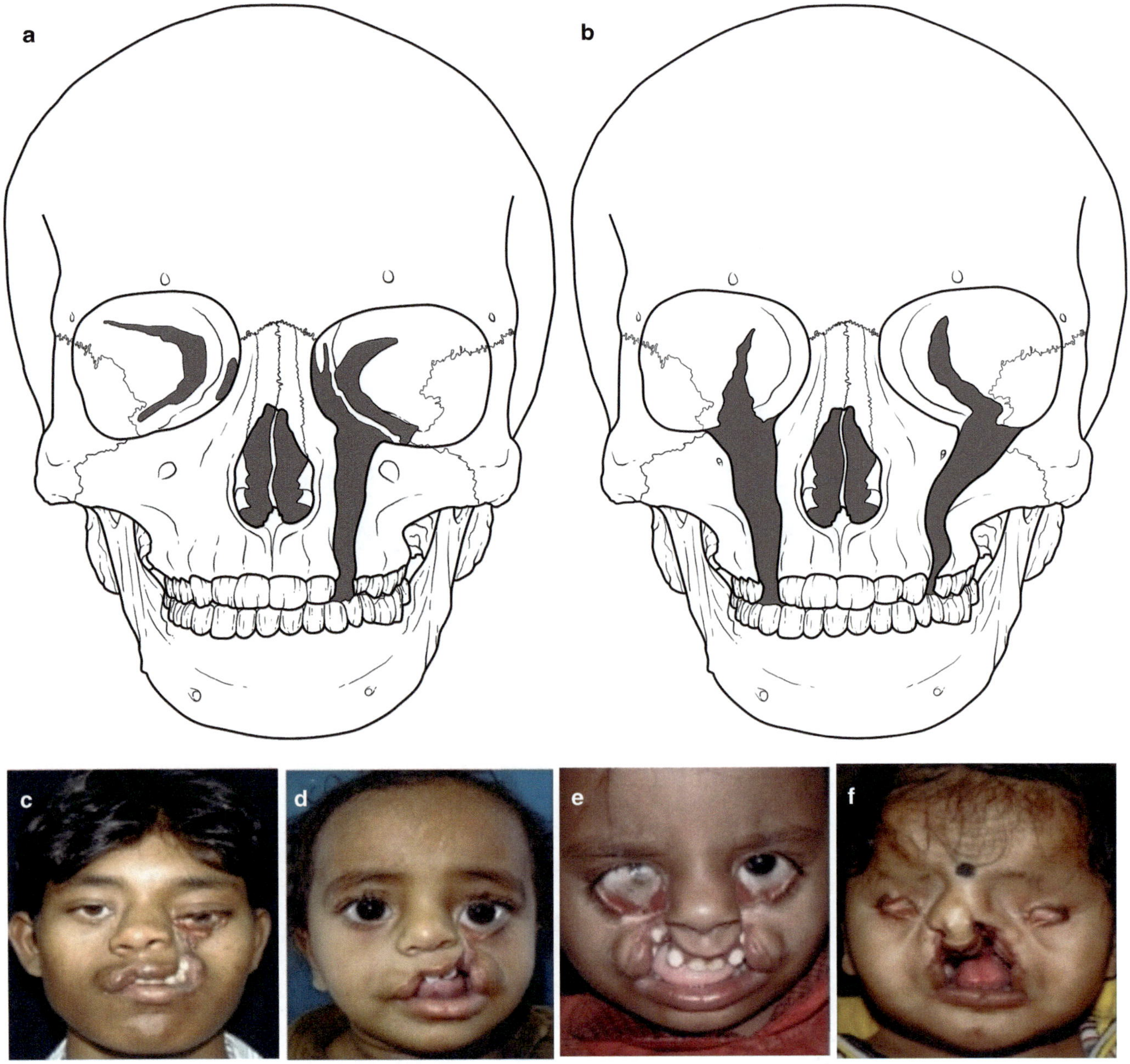

Fig. 77.9 (**a–f**) Tessier 4. (**a**, **b**) Skeletal Tessier 4. (**c**, **d**) Unilateral Tessier 4. (**e**, **f**) Bilateral Tessier 4

Soft tissue involvement of the No 6 cleft is detailed below:

1. Vertical cleft furrow extending from the oral commissure to the lateral aspect of the lower eyelid.
2. This also involves the zygomatic eminence pulling the lateral aspect of the palpebral fissure down with inferior displacement of the lateral canthus [33].
3. This gives the appearance of an anti-mongoloid slant and lower lid ectropion.
4. Colobomas may be seen in the lateral lower eyelid region [33].

Skeletal involvement is as follows:

1. A bony split is seen along the zygomaticomaxillary suture separating the maxilla and the zygoma [33].
2. Usually there is no alveolar cleft.
3. The maxilla may be shorter antero-posteriorly.
4. The cleft enters the orbit at the lateral orbital floor.
5. The zygoma is hypoplastic with change in the cheek contour.
6. The anterior cranial fossa is narrow but sphenoid is normal [35].

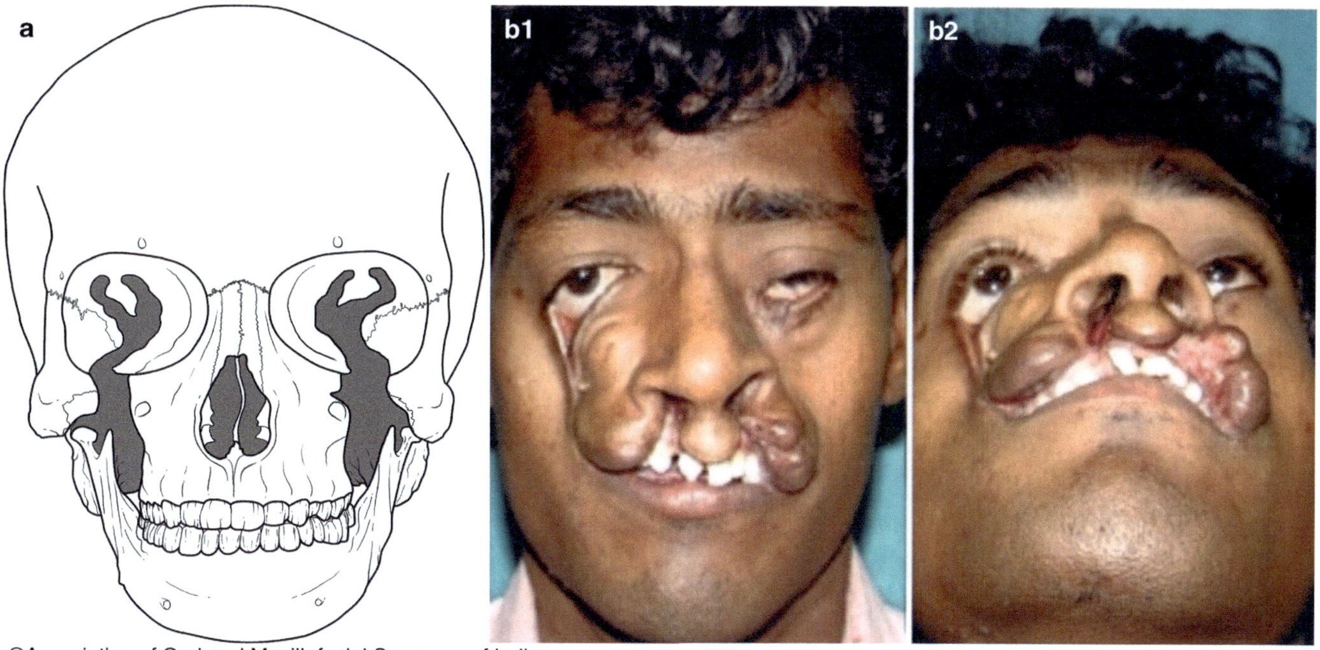

Fig. 77.10 (**a**, **b**) Tessier 5

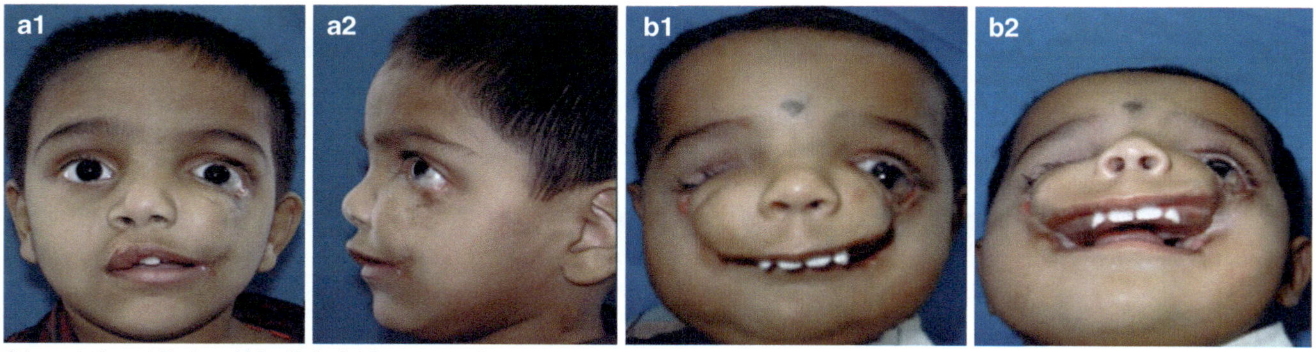

Fig. 77.11 (**a**, **b**) Tessier 6. Skeletal Tessier 6. (**a**) Unilateral Tessier 6. (**b**) Bilateral Tessier 6

77.5.1.8 Number 7 Cleft

This is a temporo-zygomatic cleft and is the most well-known of all the craniofacial clefts [35] (Figs. 77.12 and 77.13a–d). It may occur along with hemifacial microsomia.

Soft tissue features include:

1. Soft tissue clefting from the oral commissure to the pre-auricular hairline.
2. It may range from a mild broadening of the oral commissure with pre-auricular skin tags to a complete fissure ending in a microtic ear [35].
3. There may be deficiency of the ipsilateral tongue, soft palate, and muscles of mastication.
4. There may be absence of the parotid gland and duct.
5. There may be external and middle ear abnormalities [50–52].
6. Abnormal pre-auricular hair form in hemifacial microsomia and Treacher Collins disorder [35].

Skeletal qualities include [35, 53, 54]:

1. Skeletal cleft involves the pterygo-maxillary junction.
2. Hypoplasia of the posterior maxilla, mandibular ramus, coronoid, and condylar process with occlusal canting [33].

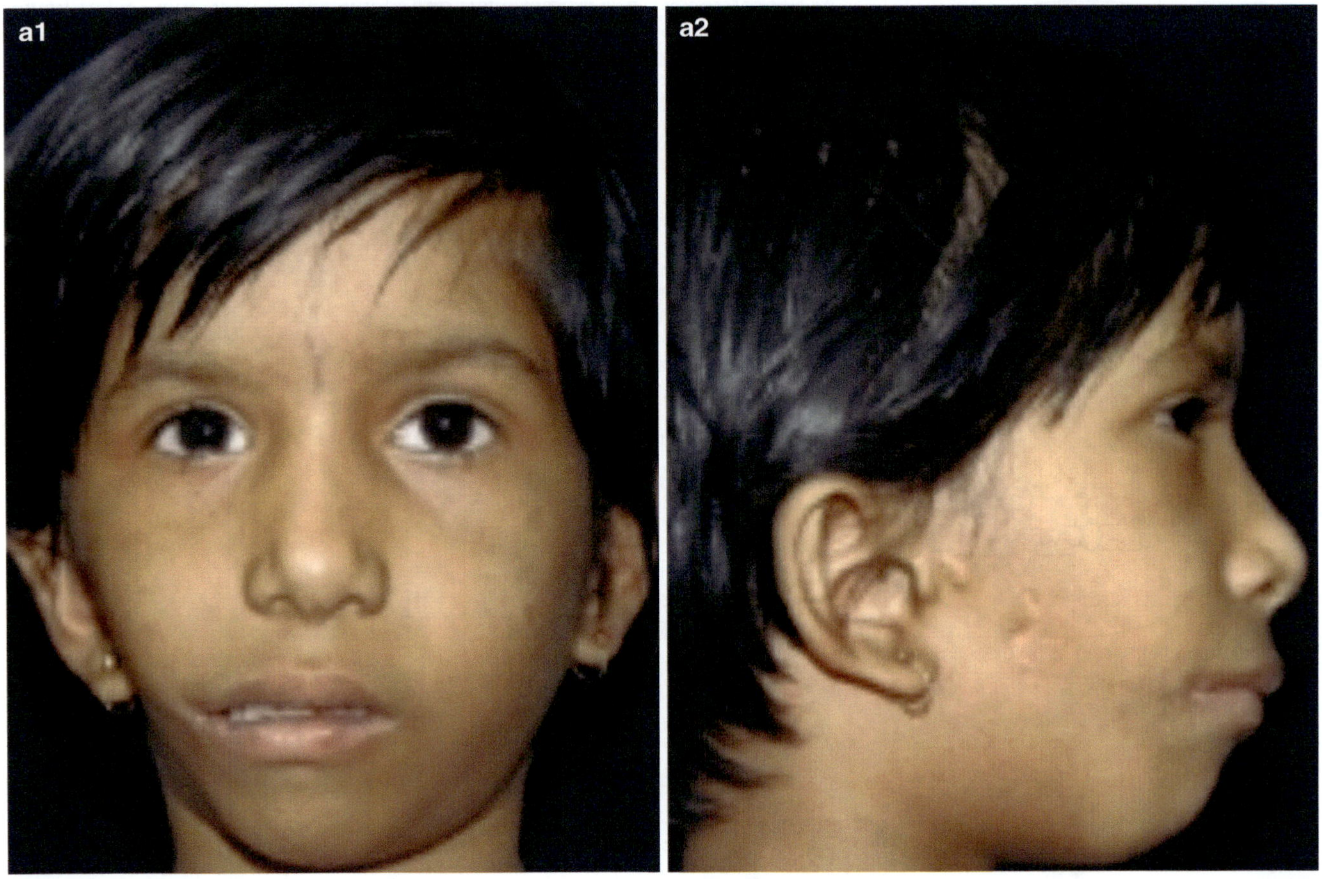

Fig. 77.12 Tessier 7

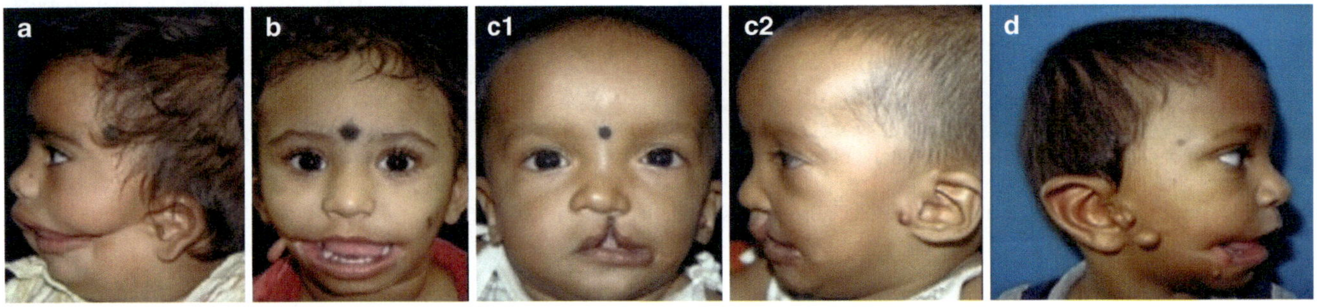

Fig. 77.13 (**a**–**d**) Subclassification of Tessier 7. (**a**) Oro-aural Tessier 7. (**b**) Bilateral Tessier 7. (**c**) Tessier 7 with cleft lip. (**d**) Tessier with ear tag

3. Hypoplasia of the zygoma with displacement and deformation. In extreme cases the arch may manifest as a little stump alone.
4. There may be true orbital dystopia in severe cases.
5. There may be a tilt of the cranial base [35].

77.5.1.9 Number 8 Cleft (Fig. 77.2)

This fronto-zygomatic cleft situated at the lateral canthus forms the equator of the Tessier craniofacial cleft sphere. It is a part of the zygomatico-frontal dysplasias [49]. The number 8 cleft seldom occurs in isolation and usually occurs as a part of other craniofacial clefts. It corresponds to the cranial occurrence of the No 6 cleft. In bilateral occurrences it is associated with numbers 6 and 7. This shows features similar to the Treacher-Collins and the Goldenhar's disorder with the former showing more skeletal deformities and the latter soft tissue ones [55].

Soft tissue features include [56, 57]:

1. Cleft extends from the lateral canthus to the temporal region.
2. They may present with dermatoceles and colobomas with absence of the lateral canthal apparatus.
3. Abnormal hair patterns may be present between the temporal area and the lateral canthus.
4. Globe may show eye bulbar dermoids.

Skeletal involvement includes [58, 59]:

1. Bony clefting at the fronto-zygomatic suture [58].
2. Features of the Goldenhar's or Treacher-Collins syndromes may be seen with the zygoma being hypoplastic or missing along with the lateral orbital wall [59].
3. The palpebral fissure shows a lateral descent due to the absence of the zygoma.

77.5.1.10 Number 9 Cleft

No. 9 is a form of the upper "lateral" orbital cleft. The clefting is seen in the lateral third of the upper eyelid and the lateral supra-orbital angle (Fig. 77.14). It is the cranial extension of the number 5 facial cleft [52]. There may be a deficient greater sphenoid wing in this type [60].

Soft tissue involvement shows:

1. Anomalies of the lateral third of the upper eyelid and the eyebrow.
2. Distortion of the lateral canthus.
3. Severe cases show microphthalmia.
4. The superolateral bony deficiency in the orbit may be the cause of lateral displacement of the globes.
5. Anterior displacement of the temporal hairline with temporal projection.
6. Palsy of the 7th cranial nerve with temporal and eyelid signs may be common.

Skeletal involvement:

1. Cleft extending through the superolateral aspect of the orbit.
2. The greater wing of the sphenoid may be distorted affecting morphology of the orbital wall.

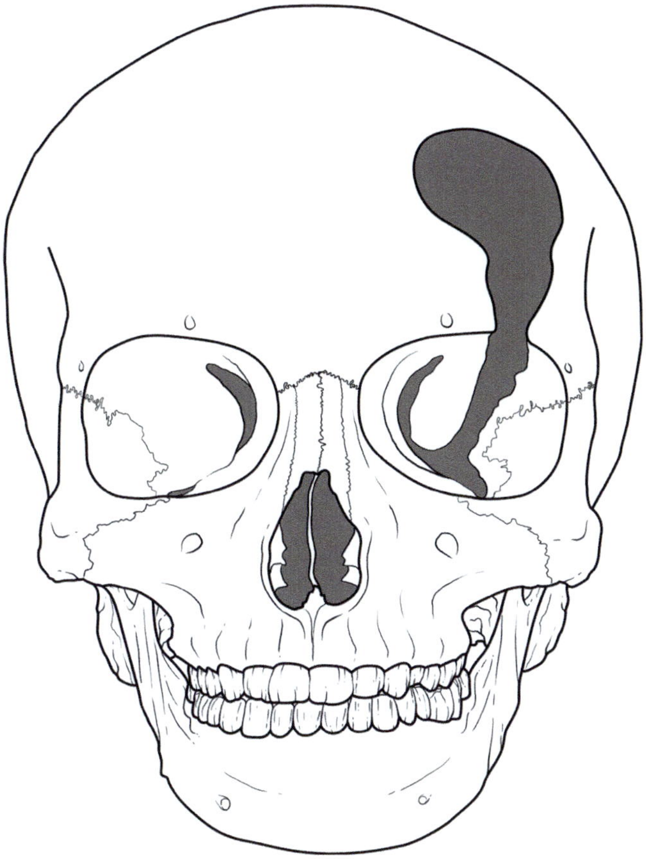

Fig. 77.14 Tessier number 9

3. Hypoplasia of the pterygoid plates.
4. Decrease in the antero-posterior dimensions of the anterior cranial fossa [35].

77.5.1.11 Number 10 Cleft

No. 10 is an upper "central" orbital cleft with the cleft happening in the middle third of

the supra-orbital edge, lateral to the supra-orbital nerve (Fig. 77.15a, b) [33]. This is the cranial counterpart of the No 4 cleft. Both present with similar ocular deformities and may show colobomata of the iris [33].

This cleft causes a large defect in the frontal bone [46].

Soft tissue features include:

1. Elongated palpebral fissure
2. Amblyopia with inferior and laterally displaced eye [35]
3. Eyebrow which is deficient medially and is more dispersed laterally [46]
4. Occurrence of frontal encephalocele involving the middle third of the frontal bone and the orbital roof [35]

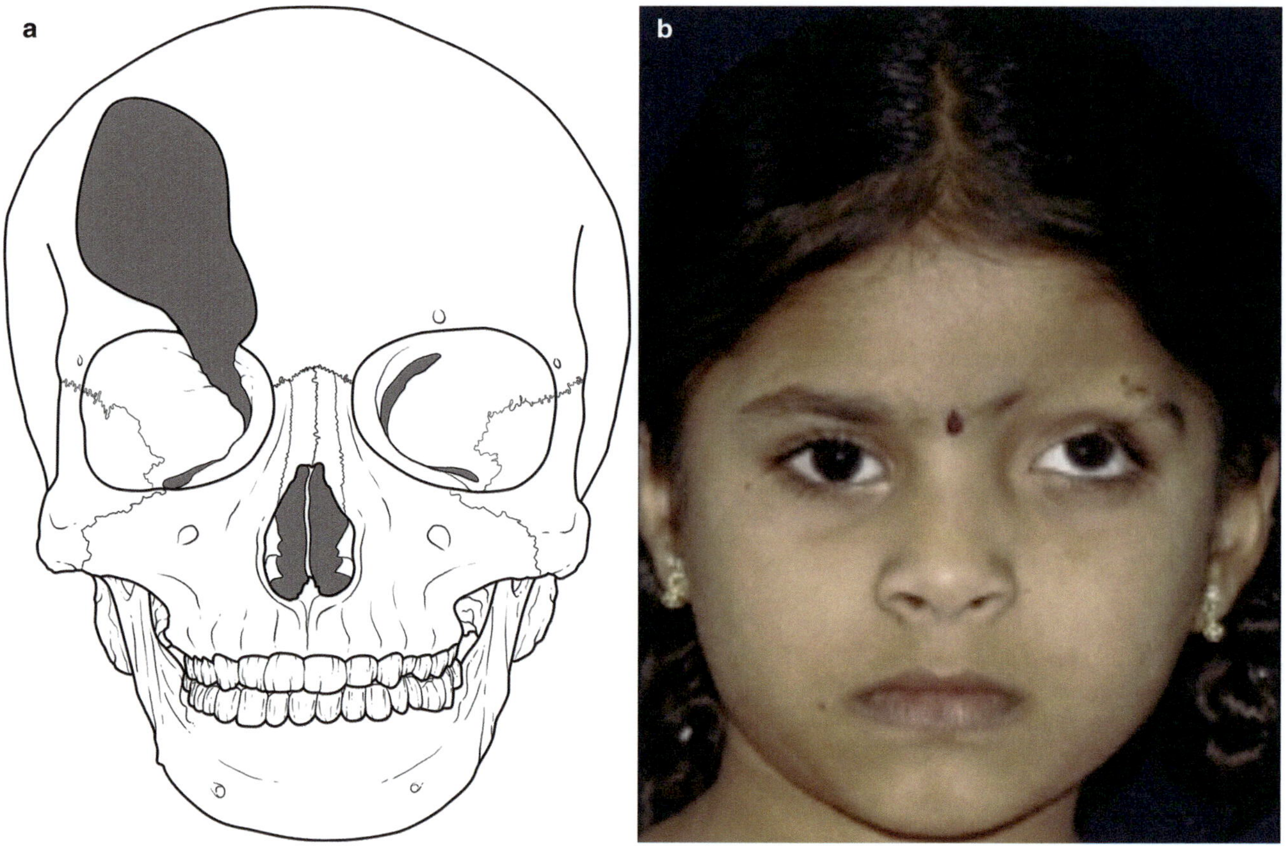

©Association of Oral and Maxillofacial Surgeons of India

Fig. 77.15 (**a**, **b**) Tessier number 10

Skeletal involvement:

1. Cleft defect on the lateral aspect of the supra-orbital rim which may involve an encephalocele.
2. Orbital deformity with a latero-inferior rotation.
3. Orbital hypertelorism may be a feature in severe cases with distortion of the anterior cranial base [35].

77.5.1.12 Number 11 Cleft (Fig. 77.2)

No. 11 is the upper "medial" orbital cleft. This shows coloboma of the medial third of the upper eyelid, with stretching of the eyebrow [33]. This cleft is often associated with the facial cleft No 3 [35]. Van der Meulen incorporated this deformity in his frontal dysplasia group [49].

Soft tissue involvement includes:

1. Coloboma of the upper eyelid in the medial third
2. Disturbance in the upper eyebrow with a tilt toward the frontal hairline
3. Tongue-like projection of the frontal hairline [35]

Skeletal involvement:

1. Frontal bone defect medial to the supra-orbital nerve and lateral to the ethmoid and lacrimal bones
2. Bony defect of the medial orbit
3. Fronto-ethmoid encephalocele with resultant orbital dystopia
4. Deficiency of the lacrimal bone with associated lacrimal stenosis [46]

77.5.1.13 Number 12 Cleft

The No 12 cleft shows deficiencies in the ethmoid labyrinth and the glabella [46]. This cleft is usually found medial to the medial canthus [35] (Fig. 77.16).

Soft tissue characteristics include:

1. Soft tissue dehiscence medial to the medial canthal apparatus [33]
2. Lateral displacement of the medial canthus with aplasia of the medial eyebrow

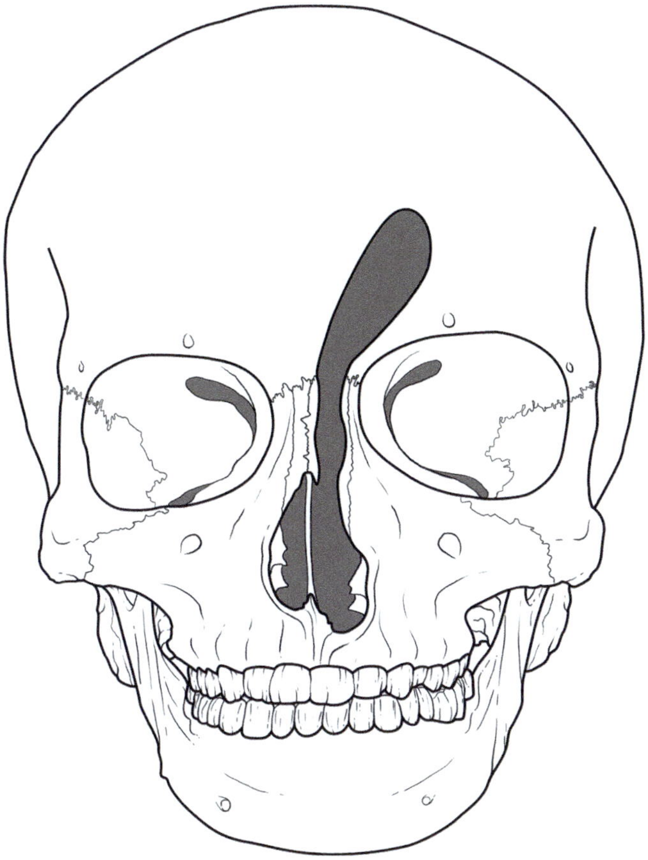

Fig. 77.16 Tessier number 12

3. Presence of a V-shaped frontal hairline in the paramedial region of the forehead [35]

Skeletal involvement:

1. There is a flattened widening of the affected bone.
2. May present with grades of hypertelorism or telecanthus.
3. Normal sphenoids with mild hyper-pneumatization of the frontal sinus.
4. Obtuse fronto-nasal angle.
5. Low incidence of associated encephaloceles.

77.5.1.14 Number 13 Cleft

The number 13 cleft is the cranial counterpart of the paramedian facial cleft 1.

It is situated between the nasal bone and the frontal process of the maxilla passing through the frontal bones and along the olfactory groove [36] (Fig. 77.17).

Soft tissue characteristics include the following:

1. This occurs medial to the eyebrow which remains undivided [36].
2. The cleft produces a paramedian widows peak [35].
3. The cleft may descend and pass through the intersection of the nasal skin and alar skin and results in an alar cartilage cleft [46].

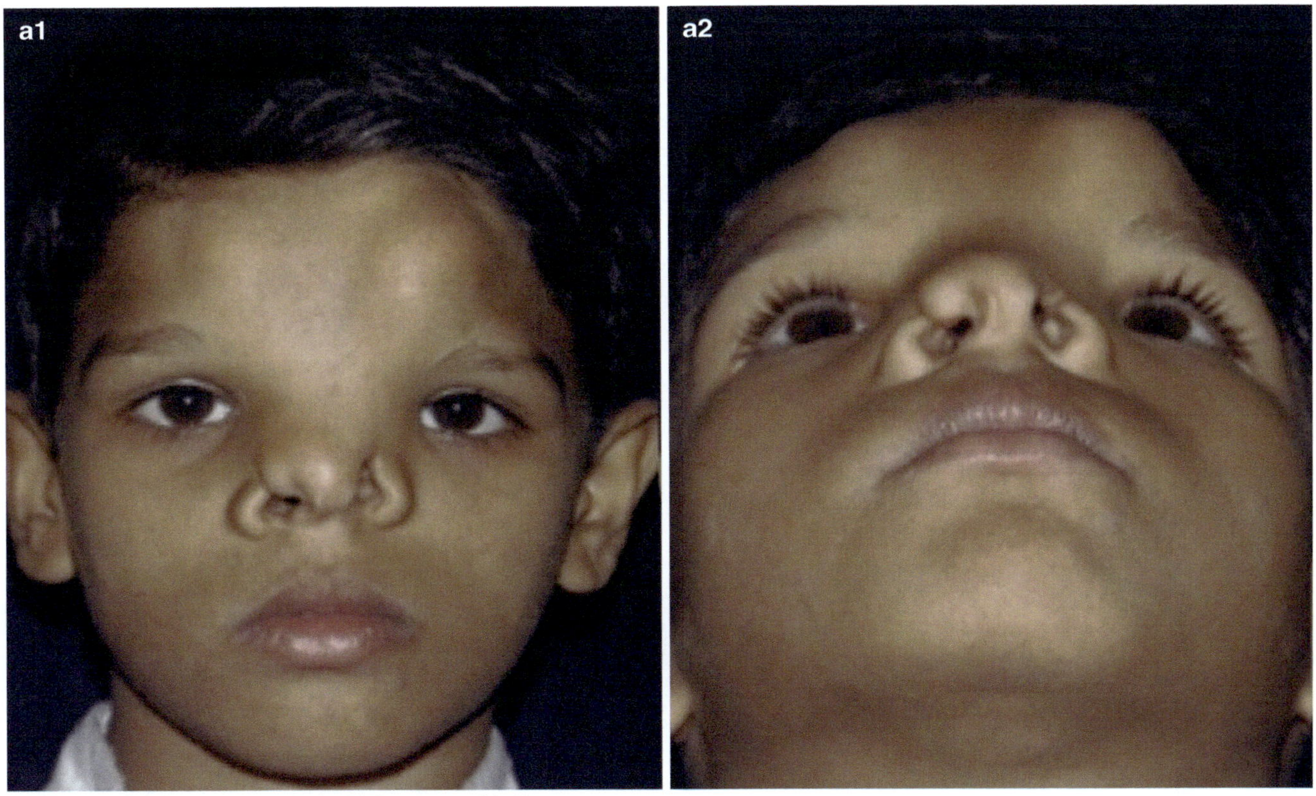

Fig. 77.17 Tessier number 13

Skeletal involvement:

1. Deformities of the medial aspect of the cribriform plate [46].
2. There may be olfactory groove widening with associated widening of the cribriform plate and the ethmoid sinus with resultant hypertelorism.
3. Paramedian frontal encephalocele may cause inferior displacement of the cribriform plate with orbital dystopia.
4. Unilateral and bilateral types of the number 13 cleft exist with bilateral demonstrating the most extreme forms of hypertelorism [4].

77.5.1.15 Number 14 Cleft

No. 14 is the cranial congener of the cleft no. 0, which is the median craniofacial dysrhaphia. The terms frontonasal and frontonasoethmoid dysplasia were utilized by Van der Meulen for this group of deformities [49] (Fig. 77.18a–g).

Soft tissue characteristics:

1. Severe lateral displacement of the medial canthal apparatus bilaterally.
2. Glabellar flattening.
3. The periorbita including the eyelids and eyebrows is generally normal.

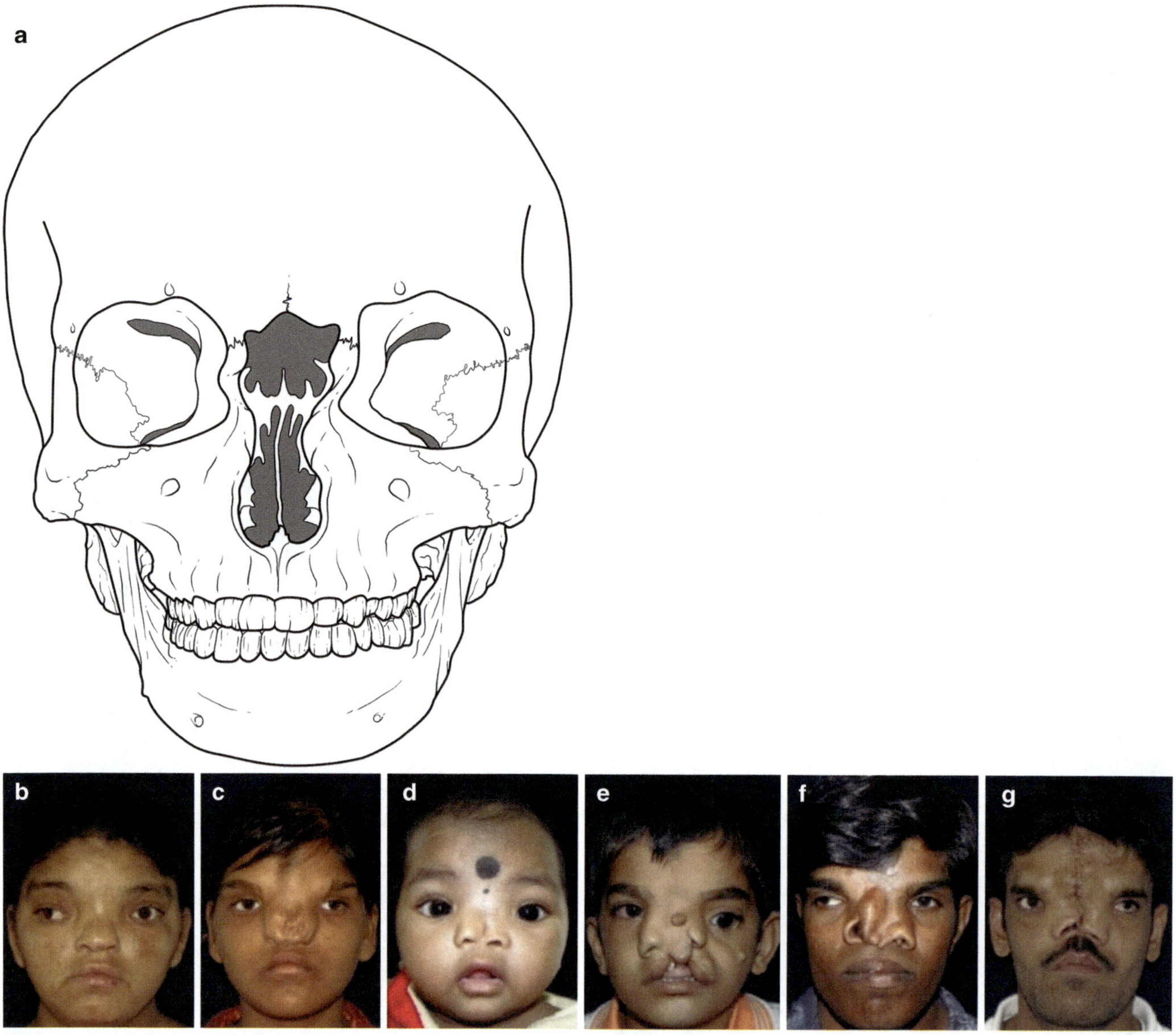

Fig. 77.18 (**a–g**) Tessier number 14 with variable degree of nasal duplication and hypertelorism

4. Midline projection of the frontal hairline [35].
5. There is distortion of the nasal capsule and the developing forebrain stays in a lower position.

Skeletal characteristics:

1. Severe hypertelorism.
2. Frontal encephalocele may be seen herniating through the midline frontal bone defect.
3. Caudal flattening of the frontal bone is flattened with flattened glabellar region
4. Absence of frontal sinus pneumatization.
5. The crista galli and the perpendicular plate of the ethmoid are bifid, and there is an expanded separation between the olfactory grooves [35].
6. The crista galli and ethmoids are widened with caudal dislodgement.
7. There may be a shortening of the middle cranial fossa.
8. The anterior cranial fossa is tilted upward, producing a harlequin eye disfigurement on plain radiographs [35].

77.5.1.16 Number 30 Cleft

Tessier 30 cleft otherwise known as lower midline facial cleft or median mandibular cleft is a rarity (Fig. 77.19). Median cleft of the lower jaw was first described in 1819 by Couronne [30].

It is generally constrained to a deformity in the soft tissue of the lower lip.

In its severe form, it may groove or split the mandibular symphysis and at times involve the midline structures of the neck including the hyoid bone, the thyroid, and even the strap muscles. The anterior part of the tongue may be bifid, showing ankyloglossia [54], with one case of absence of tongue being reported [55].

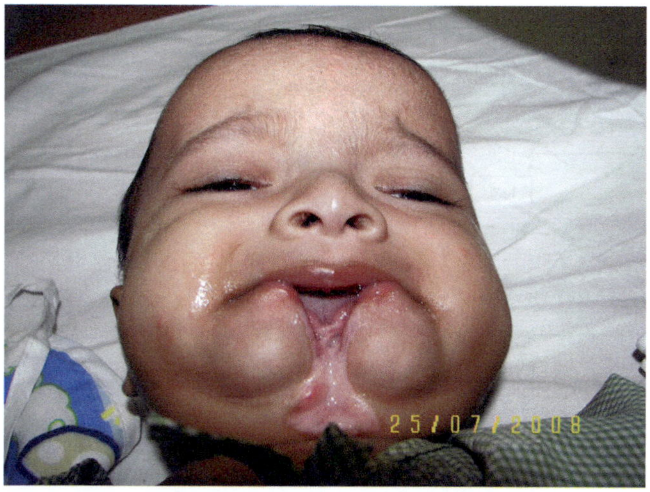

Fig. 77.19 Tessier no 30

77.6 Treatment of Craniofacial Clefts

Surgery for facial deformities involves the best balance of art and science. The restoration of the malformed anatomy requires artistic creativity, while the science lies in the reestablishment of impaired function [57].

From a careful perspective, even microform clefts might deform. Contingent upon the level of distortion, an arranged strategy has been viewed as the treatment of choice [58]. Due to their multifaceted nature; the individual level of cleft involves successful reconstruction and the rehabilitation in practically every one of the cases request multistep and multi-proficient procedure [59]. Besides cautious examination, imaging methods are important to evaluate the individual level of skeletal inclusion. For correct determination current imaging frameworks seen in systems, for example, CT, MRI, and 3D CT, permit better preoperative comprehension of the issue and planning of the surgeries. Analysis ought to be founded on a classification relying upon the site and types of defects (morphology) which helps in foundation of a legitimate treatment plan [60] (Figs. 77.20, 77.21, and 77.22a–e).

Institutionalized treatment plans are not constantly conceivable in light of the assortment of craniofacial clefts and dimensions of seriousness. Be that as it may, core values are useful in deciding the best possible planning and stages for restorative surgery [30]. The Australian Craniofacial Unit Treatment Protocol, which is a pioneering center with international acclaim, has recommended the following:

- Early repair of the soft tissue defects and preventing exposure keratitis
- Orthodontic intervention interceptive orthodontics and speech therapy for the school-going years (4–10 years)
- Reconstruction of the orbital floor, orthognathic surgery, and rhinoplasty to be done after growth completion [30]

77.6.1 Tessier No. 0–14 Cleft

Literature reveals that the midline Tessier 0 and 14 clefts are among the most common encountered [5], while the combination of 0 and 14 is the most common combination of non-isolated clefts [61].

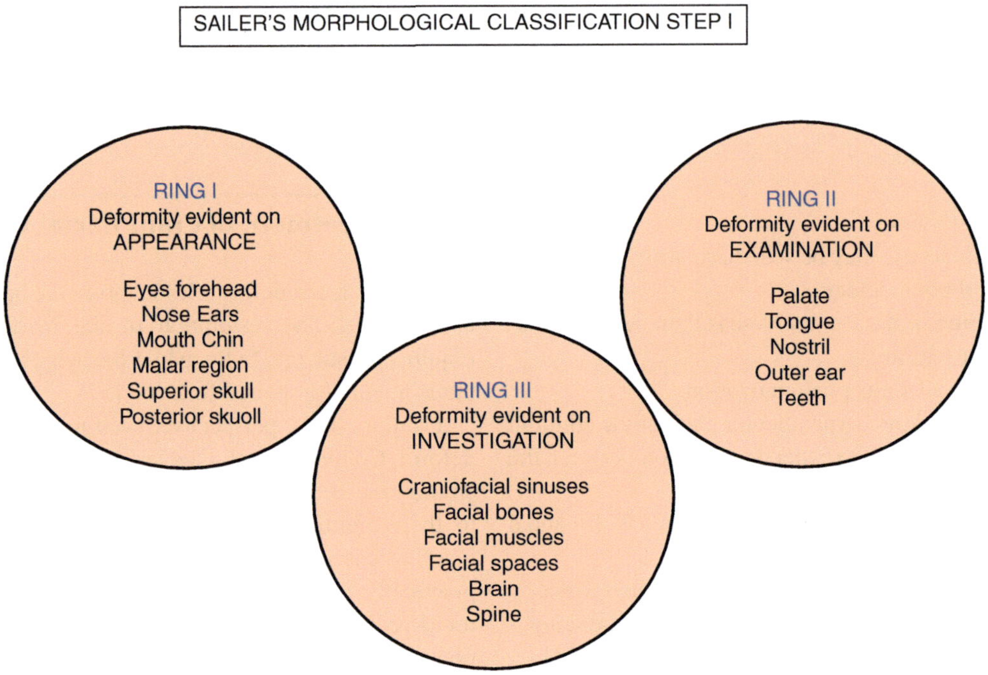

Fig. 77.20 Sailer's morphological classification step I

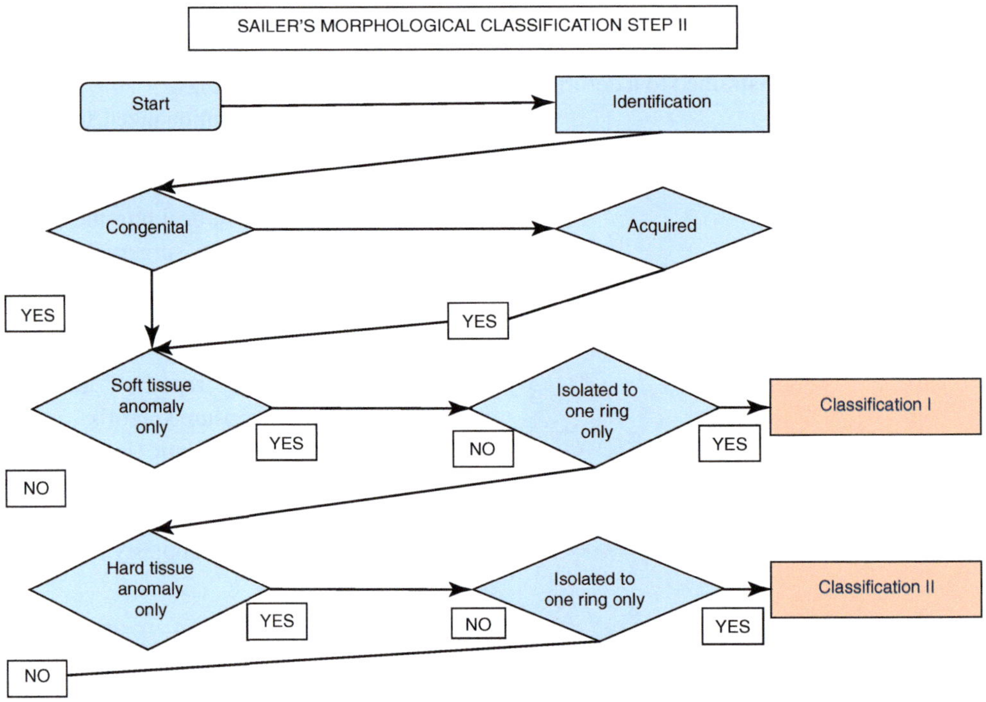

Fig. 77.21 Sailer's morphological classification step II

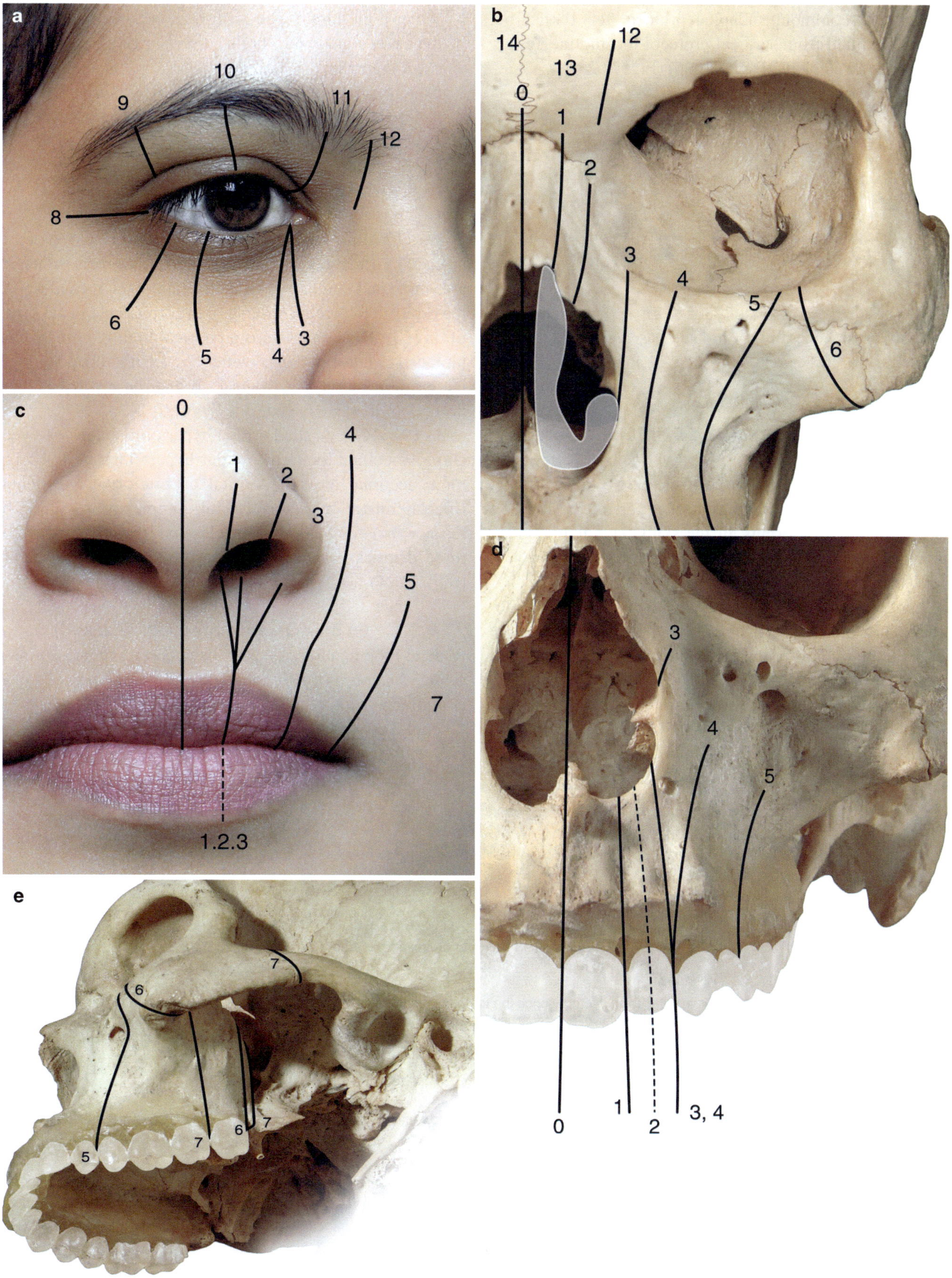

Fig. 77.22 (**a–e**) Anatomical classification of facial, craniocalvarial clefting

The most commonly adapted protocol for Tessier no. 0–14 is modified from surgical protocol for midline Tessier 0–14 craniofacial clefts (David 2006) (Fig. 77.23).

As per Sailer's morphological classification, Tessier 0–14 clefts involve:

(i) The medial orbital zone
(ii) The zone of the maxilla, oral cavity, and lips
(iii) The zone of the nose

Treatment is generally formulated based on the degree of involvement of these zones (Figs. 77.20 and 77.21).

77.6.2 The Orbital Zone and Skull Bone Defect

77.6.2.1 Resection of Encephalocele

An encephalocele is a herniation of a part of the cerebral matter through a deformity in the skull. This may contain meninges (meningocele), or meninges, cerebrum, and ventricle (meningoencephalocystocele) [61].

Tessier no. 0–14 is most generally connected with fronto-ethmoidal gathering of encephaloceles group which can be subdivided into nasofrontal, nasoethmoidal, and nasoorbital types.

The objectives of repair involve:

1. Meticulous repair of skin deformities. This helps prevent contamination and desiccation of brain tissue.
2. Water-tight dural repair with removal or invagination of the non-functional brain tissue which is present extra-cranially.
3. Complete craniofacial reconstruction of skeletal components. Care taken to prevent appearance of a long nose [62].

77.6.3 Orbital Hypertelorism

Hypertelorism is the most common indication for major craniofacial correction in a Tessier 0–14. Treatment strategies are varied and range from medialization of the medial wall of the orbits to total repositioning of the orbital and facial bipartition [63]. Hypertelorism is a physical finding in many craniofacial malformations, which is characterized by an increase in interorbital distance. It may be a part of a syndrome but it is not a syndrome by itself.

In 1924, Greig called orbital hypertelorism as "ox-eyed" and also coined the term "ocular hypertelorism" [64]. The more accurate term of "orbital hypertelorism" to denote true lateralization of the orbital complex was coined by Tessier in 1972 [65]. Tessier classified hypertelorism into three degrees based on the interorbital distance [65, 66] (Fig. 77.24).

77.6.3.1 En Bloc Osteotomies (Fig. 77.25a–d)

Radical mobilization of the orbits to correct increased interorbital distance is one of the most challenging procedures in craniofacial surgery [67].

Paul Tessier was the first to perform orbital mobilization using a trans-cranial approach [53]. This surgical intervention was planned to eliminate undue risk to the

Fig. 77.23 Surgical protocol for midline Tessier 0–14 craniofacial clefts

Adapted Surgical Protocol for Midline 0–14 Tessjer Craniofacial Clefts (David, 2006) [16, 17]

Birth to 1 year
- Preserve the essential functions of the airway, feeding, sight, and; hearing
- Repair any encephaloceles
- Craniosynostosis correction by fronto-orbital advancement at 3–6 months

5 years
- Orbital box osteotomy once the tooth buds can be reliably preserved
- As an alternative, a medial faciotomy (facial bipartition) can be performed slightly later
- Possible use of tissue expanders beneath the zygomatic periosteum in extreme hypertelorism
- Temporary nasad reconstruction, as this will not be repeated later

5 to 10 years
- Orthodontic management is commenced when enough permanent teeth are present
- Alveolar bone grafting is carried out to correcti the more extensive defects in the maxilla that may to present

10 years until the completion of growth
- Maintenance of the orthodonitic therapy with retainers
- Further preservation of the eyes and hearing if required

Completion of growth
- Orthodontic preparation for midface surgery
- Midface surgery performed at any level, with or without bone grafting/mandibuloar surgery depending on need
- After establishment of the facial platform, platform, definitive nasal reconstruction is performed
- Further secondary surgery is performed if necessary

HYPERTELORISM		
Degree		Interorbital distance (mm)
I.	Slight	30 to 34
II.	Moderate	35 to 39
III.	Severe	40 +

Fig. 77.24 Hypertelorism

optic nerve [65]. Converse described in 1968 preservation of the olfactory nerves by performing subcranial U-shaped osteotomy [68]. Schmid described the extra-cranial circumferential orbital osteotomies for medializing the orbits [68], while Jacques van der Meulen described the facial bipartition in 1983 [69]. Medialization of the medial orbital walls and hemifacial rotation do not interrupt midfacial growth and thus were performed before age 5 in the majority of patients. Orbital translocation causes growth disturbances and thus is to be performed after attaining skeletal maturity [63].

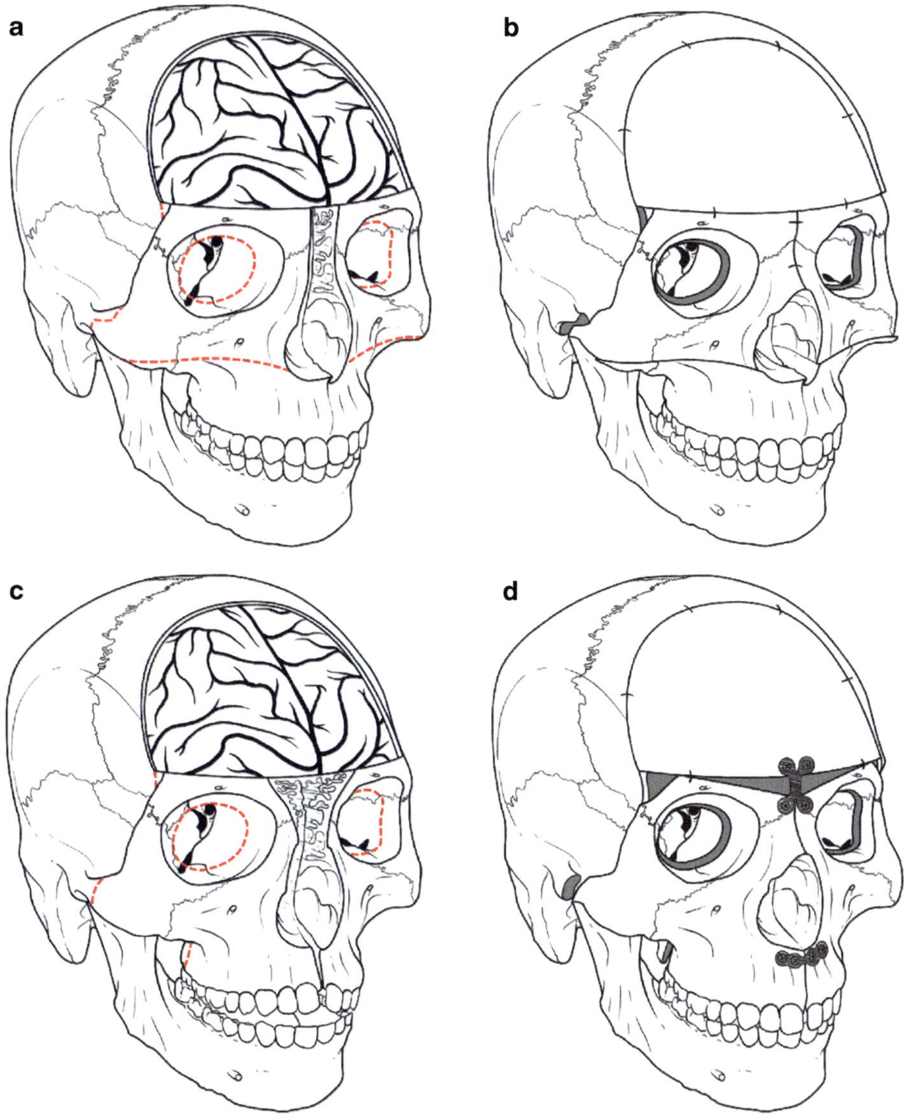

Fig. 77.25 En bloc osteotomies (**a**–**d**)

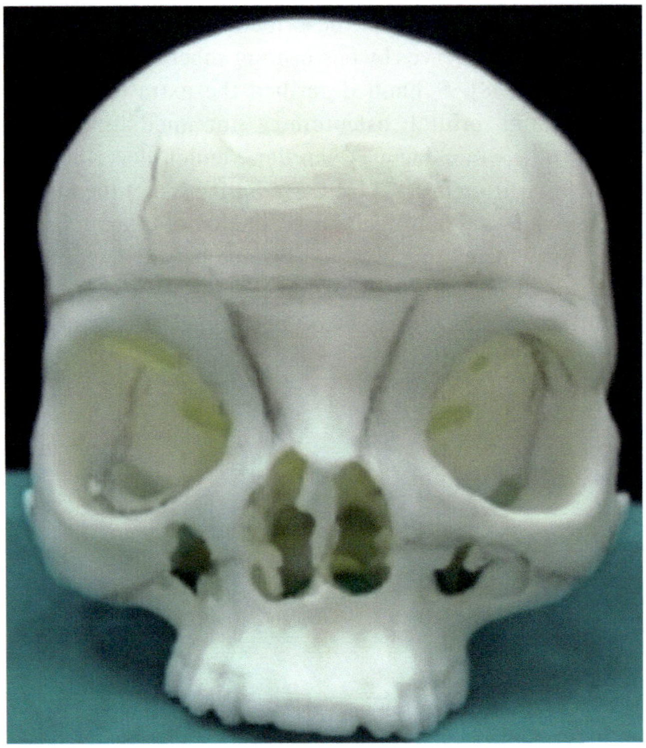

Fig. 77.26 Stereolithographic models—simulation

Pre-op Evaluation

Pre-op evaluation for orbital hypertelorism includes the following:

External facial measurements
Dental casts
Posteroanterior x-ray cephalometry [70]
Modern aids like computed tomographic scan
Three-dimensional imaging and stereolithographic models [71] (Fig. 77.26)

Facial Bipartition

The facial bipartition procedure involves the mobilization and rotation of the entire midface in a monobloc fashion (Fig. 77.27a, b). The osteotomy involves the supra-orbital rims first. It is then continued along the lateral orbital walls in a similar fashion to the LeFort 3 osteotomy and is dropped caudally to involve the dentate segment also in the mobilized segment. The intra-orbital circumferential osteotomies are performed using a combined trans-cranial and trans-facial approach once the hemifacial segments are mobilized, the intervening ethmoids are resected creating space for the upper face to be rotated medially. This causes the maxillary dentate segment and the palate to have a lateral rotation increasing the transverse dimension of the face and correcting the palatal crossbite of the upper posterior teeth. This procedure can also be combined with an advancement of the midface complex by combining it with a LeFort 3 type modification [72].

77.6.3.2 Box Osteotomy (Fig. 77.28a–d)

Correction of orbital hypertelorism done using a box osteotomy may include corrections of associated nasal deformities. Bone and cartilage grafts may be necessary to provide nasal framework. Skin grafts may be required for nasal coverage and may be accomplished by local flaps. The box osteotomy is generally preferred when the dental occlusion is normal.

Van den Elzen et al. (2011) advocated waiting until after age 10 (after eruption of permanent dentition) to perform orbital box osteotomy. Monasterio and Taylor [61] supported the use of orbital translocation after skeletal maturity and have stated that early intervention retards midfacial growth. Tessier (1973) noted that neuro-ophthalmological benefit was increased by correcting hypertelorism at 3 years and psychosocial benefit was heightened by operating at 6 years, before schooling begins, or after 12 years to preserve the dentition. Marchac et al. (1999) also described the use of box osteotomies after 12 years of age.

77.6.3.3 Spectacle Osteotomy (Fig. 77.29a–e)

The spectacle osteotomy is done by performing the trans-frontal craniotomy and preservation of frontal bandeau along with trimming of the bone in the periorbital region and around the pyriform aperture with *medialization* of the orbits.

A lateral canthopexy is an integral part of this procedure [48]. The medial canthi should be recognized and anchored using trans-nasal wires. At times this is performed with a mini-plate anchor for orienting the wires in the right direction [72]. The plate is secured to the thick nasal bone, and the lower hole is kept at the level of the lacrimal crest. The canthi are independently fixed to these holes bilaterally utilizing steel wires (Also refer Chap. 79 on craniofacial syndromes) [73].

77.6.3.4 Soft Tissue Management

The midline cleft lip notch can be successfully treated by holding fast to three noteworthy standards (Fig. 77.30a, b):

1. Excision of the constrictive band on the lip
2. Approximation of the split orbicularis oris muscle at the midline
3. Mucosal lengthening using "Z"-plasties [36, 42, 74–76]

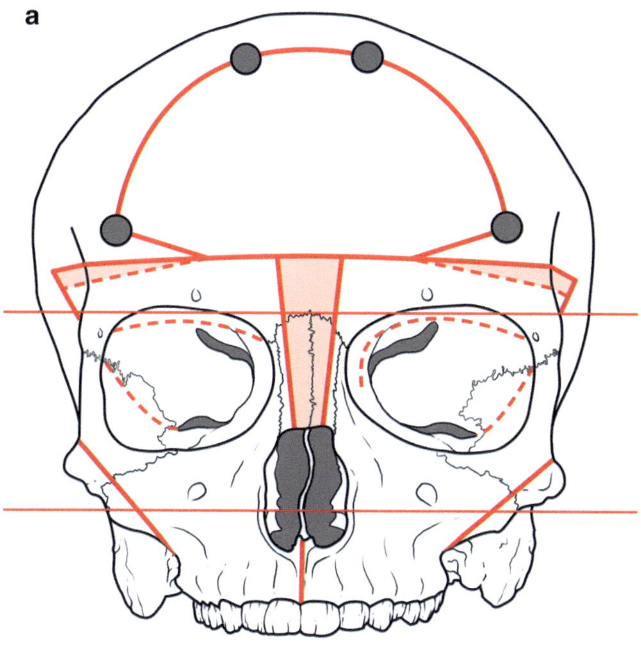

Fig. 77.27 (**a**, **b**) Facial bipartition

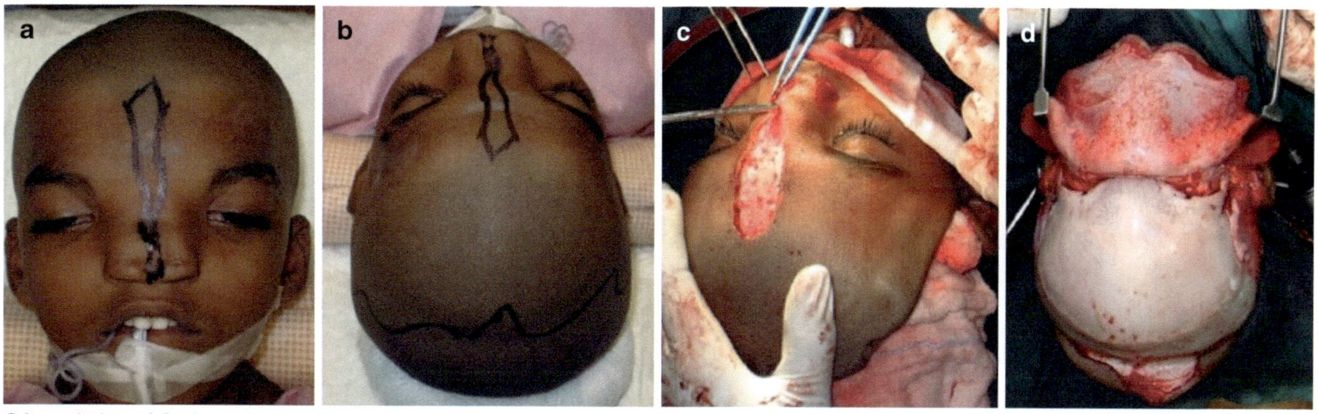

Fig. 77.28 (**a–d**) Box osteotomy—skin incision for the intracranial correction of the orbital hypertelorism consists of bicoronal incision, transfrontal craniotomy sparing the frontal bar, periorbital osteotomy, block bone removed near pyriform area, calvarial bone graft, miniplate fixation and closure

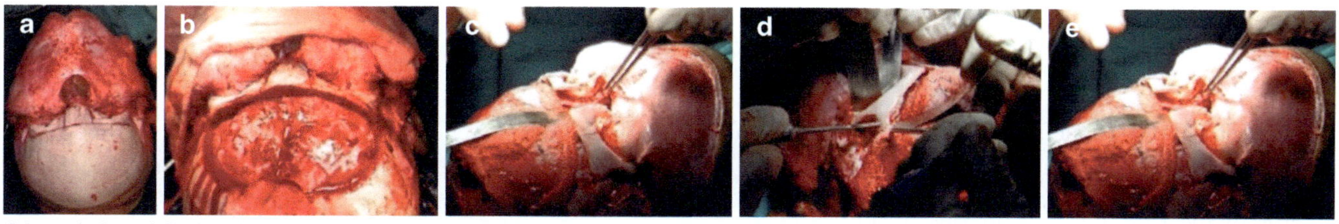

Fig. 77.29 (**a–e**) Spectacle osteotomy

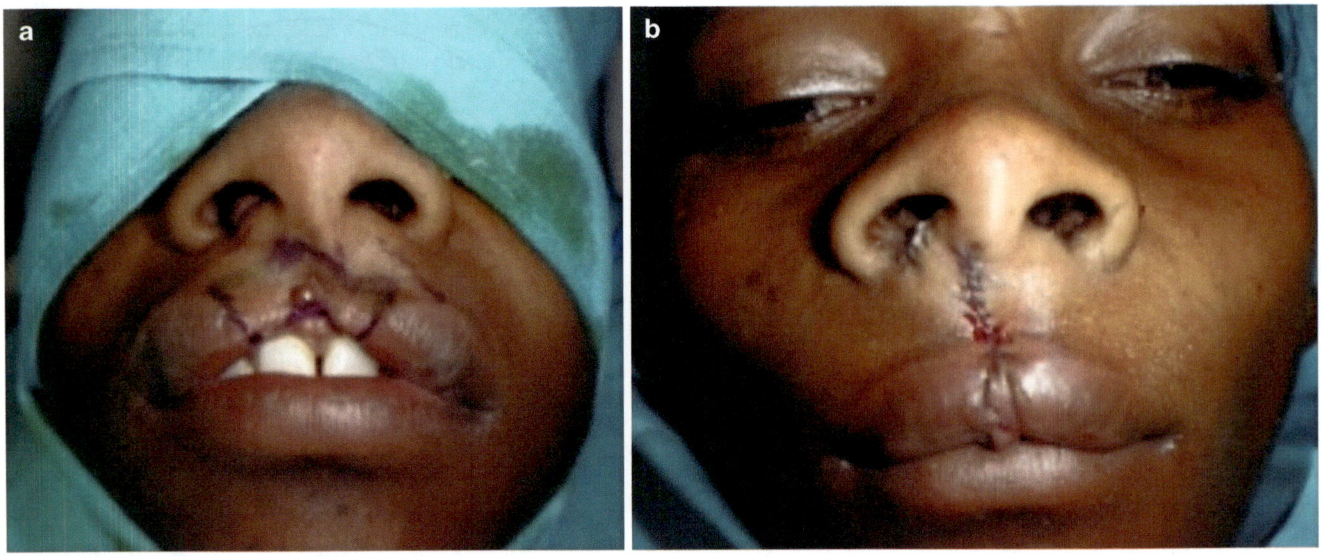

Fig. 77.30 (**a**, **b**) Reconstruction of Cupid's bow and philtrum

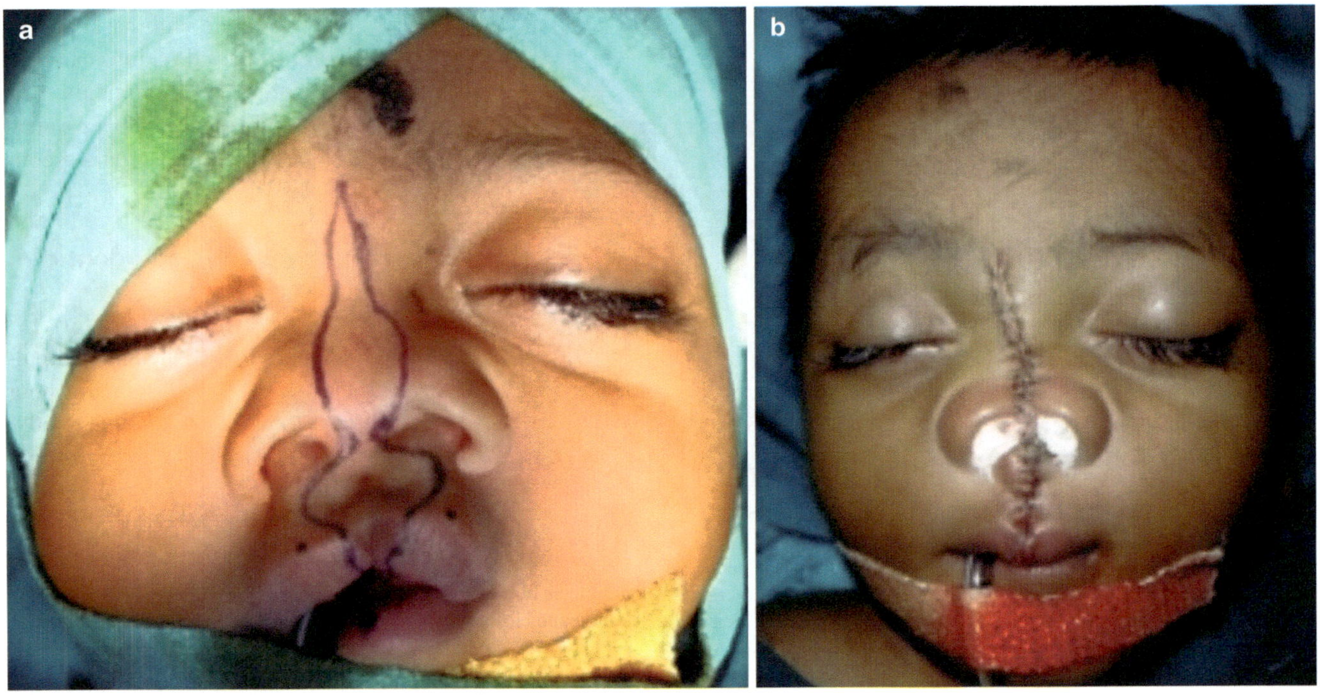

Fig. 77.31 (**a**, **b**) Resection of the excess skin of the nasal dorsum and closing in the midline

In managing the 0–14 cleft, the clinician should be able to diagnose if it is a true or a pseudo occurrence. In cases of a true midline cleft, care should be taken to reconstitute the important components of the lip, external nose, and nasal septum. Resection of excess skin also needs to be planned and performed [36] (Figs. 77.31a, b and 77.32a, b).

Nasal Clefts

Nasal clefts include Tessier no. 2 and Tessier no. 3 clefts.

Principles of surgical management (Fig. 77.33). Because of their rarity and extreme variability, it is not surprising that *standardized* methods of correction have not been established for patients with nasal clefts. Therefore, each case

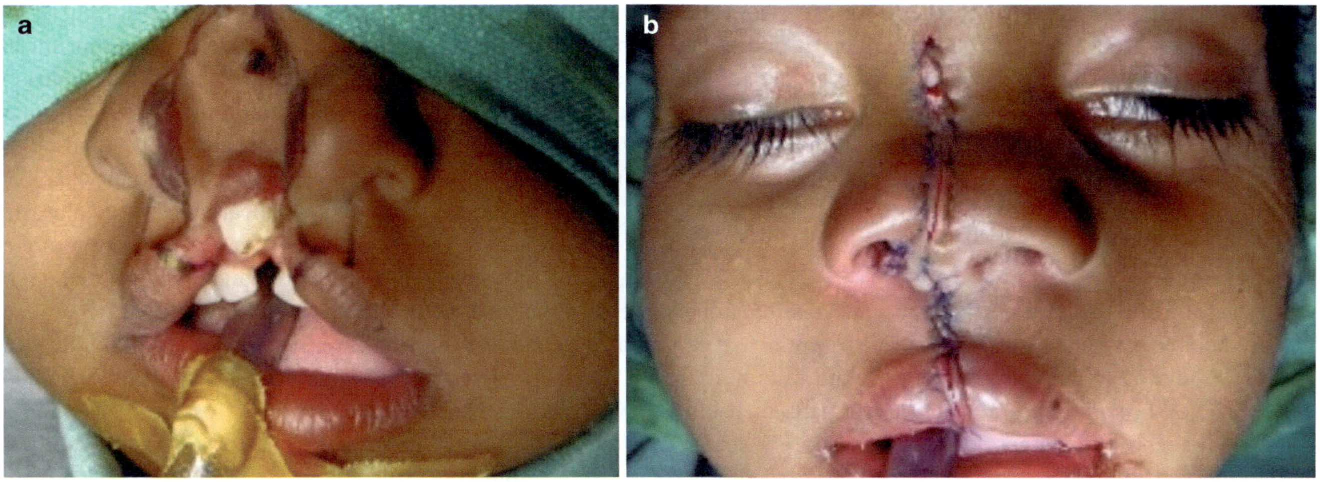

Fig. 77.32 (**a**, **b**) Reconstruction of the lip and resection of the excess skin of the nasal dorsum and closing in the midline

Principles of Management of Complex Nasal Clefts

- ➢ Precise Clinical and Radiographic Diagnosis
- • Physical examination
- • CT/MRI

Inventory of Nasal Components

- ➢ Skin
- ➢ support
  - Cartilage
  - Bone
- ➢ Lining

- • Staged Reconstruction
- ➢ First things first
- ➢ Do not burn bridges

- • Replace Like with Like
- • Re-establish Nasal/Facial Esthetics

Fig. 77.33 Principles of management of complex nasal clefts

must be approached on an individual basis using the basic principles of nasal reconstruction as a foundation.

The fundamental principles and techniques of nasal reconstruction are to assess what is present, what is missing, utilization of available tissue, and importing required tissue as indicated by the deformity.

Inventory of Nasal Components

Each component of the nose, skin, lining, and support (bony and cartilaginous), must be evaluated in a quantitative and qualitative manner. The quality and quantity of external skin and nasal lining are evaluated for deficiency or excess. The integrity of the cartilaginous framework, nasal septum, has to be assessed.

Staged Reconstruction

Patients with complex craniofacial clefts frequently require multiple staged reconstructive procedures. Planning of these procedures must be tailor-made to each patient. Surgical stages must be planned and executed with all subsequent surgical sessions clearly in mind.

Replace Like with Like

Whenever possible absent or deformed tissue should be replaced with identical or similar autogenous material.

Bony defects may be present along the cleft from the alveolus to the orbit. It is essential to reestablish a stable anatomic bony base to ensure adequate support for the soft tissue reconstruction of the nose and orbit. Autogenous split calvarial, rib, and iliac graft are the general preferences.

Cartilage

Free cartilage grafts alone may often suffice to correct small deficiencies of the alar rim, nasal rim, nasal dorsum, or tip. Larger defects of the upper and lower lateral cartilages can be replaced using conchal or septal cartilage grafts. Thin bone from the perpendicular plate of the ethmoid can be used to replace upper lateral cartilage.

Small composite chondro-cutaneous grafts from the concha can be used to replace small defects if additional lining is needed. For larger cartilage defects in the area of the upper laterals, septal hinge flaps can be used. Reconstruction of lower lateral cartilage can be accomplished using conchal cartilages or chondromucosal grafts from nasal septum.

Nasal Lining

Adequate lining to the nose is critical to achieve a functional and predictable aesthetic result. This is also essential to reestablish vascularity to the underlying tissue and to minimize contracture of the soft tissues. Local turnover flaps are useful for small defects, while larger defects may require vascularized tissue transfer.

Skin

Small nasal clefts are amenable with local tissue transfer in the form of rotation flaps from the lateral nasal area. Onus in simple nasal clefts is given to the reestablishment of the alar rim contour [68]. The use of z-plasty techniques and composite grafts helps in achieving additional symmetry [77].

Downward rotation of the cephalically displaced alar rim is the first step in this process. This may require the use of a back cut to rotate the alar margin caudally. The triangular defect produced by the alar rotation is then filled by a transposition flap from adjacent areas having excess skin [78, 79].

Descriptions of a nasal dorsal rotation flap (Figs. 77.34a–d and 77.35a, b) for a Tessier 2 cleft and a brow-eyelid-nasal transposition flap for a Tessier 3 are predictable techniques [80].

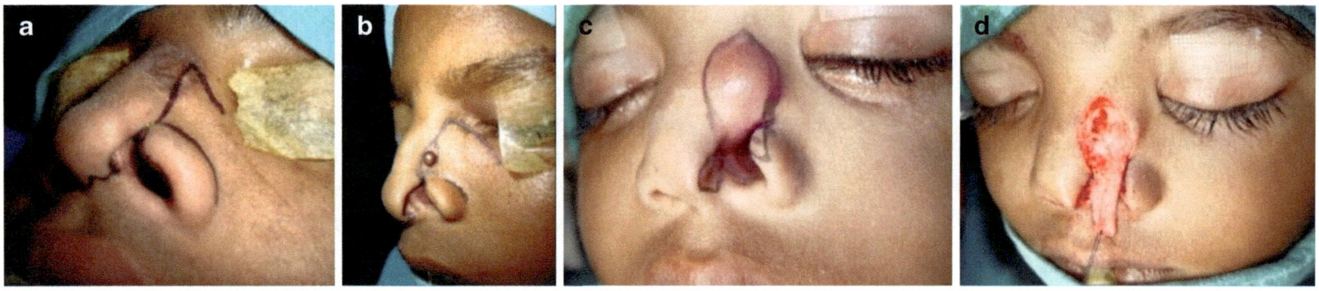

Fig. 77.34 (**a–d**) Design for bilateral Tessier no. 3 cleft—nasal dorsum rotational flap

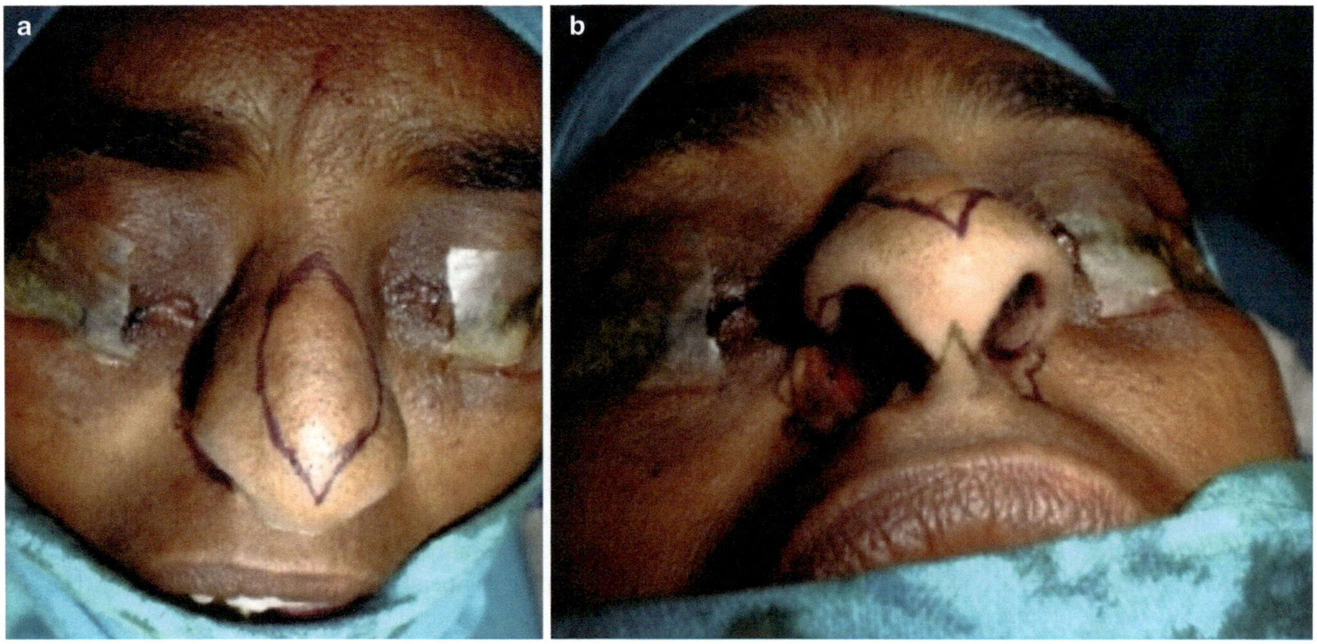

Fig. 77.35 (**a**, **b**) Nasal dorsum rotational flap

The nasal dorsum rotational flap design to correct Tessier no. 2 clefts improves alar symmetry at the cost of reduced nostril size. A notch on the affected ala is a major problem to handle in this technique [80, 81].

The forehead-eyelid-nasal transposition flap (Fig. 77.36) technique involves the use of an inter-eyebrow-forehead flap which is pedicled on the tissue of the nasal bridge. The rotation achieved by the flap gives both the alar and nostril symmetry while reducing the need for revision [80].

Reestablish Nasal/Facial Aesthetics

Optimal reconstruction of the nose should be based on the principle of aesthetic subunits as described by Gonzalez-Ulloa and Castillo (1954) and refined by Burget and Menick (1985). Superior results are better achieved by replacing the entire subunit of the nose rather than simply patching the defect. The achievement of the nasal proportions should be in conjunction with facial proportions though there are many aesthetic and surgical limitations because of associated severe craniofacial deformities. Definitive nasal reconstruction may need to be delayed or staged as explained, until optimal canthal, orbital, and maxillary relationships are obtained.

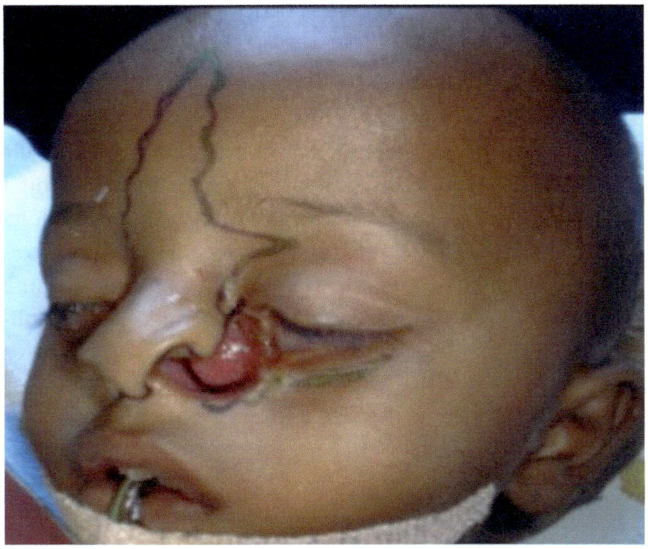

Fig. 77.36 Forehead-eyelid-nasal transposition flap

77.6.4 Tessier No. 4 (Fig. 77.37a, b)

Tessier no. 4 cleft is a rare, complex malformation which has severe implications on both the soft tissue and skeletal structures of the face. As a general rule, priority needs to be given for reconstructing the soft tissue envelop, and the skeletal repair should in the form of osteotomies or bone grafting procedures need to be deferred until the school-going years. This is due to the fact that early intervention to the bony skeleton may hinder the development of the midface and associated (Resnick and Kawamoto 1990; Kawamoto and Patel 1998) [76].

An important clinical indication that necessitates emergency intervention is exposure keratitis of the cornea and resultant blindness. This depends on the gravity of the cleft deformity. In narrow cases of Tessier 4 cleft, the clefting is more toward the medial side of the orbit which retains a large bony component of the lateral orbit. This lends support to the globe and enables reasonable competence of the upper eyelid to cover the cornea. In such instances the early surgical intervention may be avoided [82]. On the other hand in severe cases, there is total absence of the orbital floor causing the globe to sink downward with the cornea facing upward due to a lax supporting structure. This prevents the upper

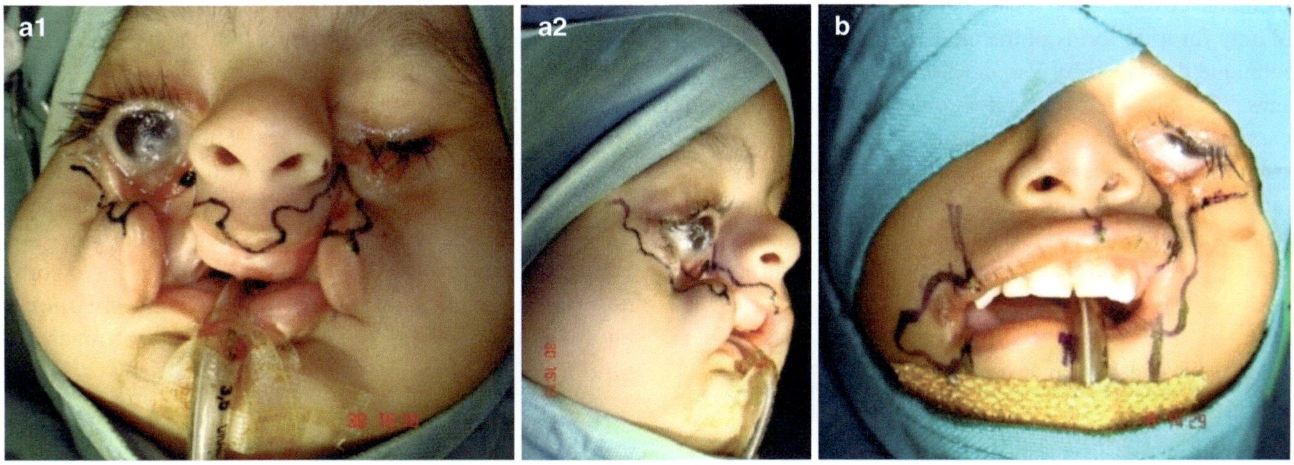

Fig. 77.37 (a) Incision for bilateral Tessier no. 4 (b) unilateral tessier 4 on left side with tessier 7 on right side

eyelid from being able to protect the cornea, with the resultant problem of exposure keratitis and permanent corneal damage. Such instances produce an emergency, and a repair of the orbital support system is mandated. In cases where an early intervention is not possible due to medical and anesthetic implications, emergency intervention at least in the form of a tarsorrhaphy is performed within 2–4 days of birth.

While treating severe deformities like the Tessier no. 3 and Tessier no. 4 clefts, a "split method" of management can be utilized to handle the anatomical regions individually as given below [83].

The affected regions were divided into three segments:

1. Lid segment
2. Lip segment
3. Nasomalar segment

77.6.4.1 Managing the Lid Segment

An ectropion like deformity is commonly present. This can be managed using conventional techniques. They include (a) a back-cut release of the lower eyelid to cheek junction and medial advancement of the lower eyelid with medial canthopexy, (b) lower lid resection with inferior layered tarsal strip, or augmentation of the tarsal plate with spacer grafts. However in cases where there is inadequate tissue locally, tissue must be imported into the lower eyelid for optimal results [83]. Some of the commonly used flaps for this include the median forehead flap and the nasolabial flap. However, free vascularized tissue transfer techniques also may be adopted [84].

Numerous techniques have been described for the management of the Tessier 4 cleft. But most of them result due to the interdigitating scars produce a sub-optimal outcome [33] (Tessier 1976; Kawamoto 1990). Longaker et al. (1997) proposed the superiorly based nasolabial flap that was transposed to the lower eyelid. Though this technique had an advantage cosmetically, it had that limitation that it was useful only for mild forms of the cleft. The cheek advancement technique described by Van der Meulen [4] had the advantages of being useful even for wider clefts and favorable scars along aesthetic facial subunits. Van der Meulen likewise depicted that it was significant for improving the scarring caused by anchoring the cheek flap firmly to the pyriform aperture [85]. However, despite the options available, it is better to understand that a single flap may be insufficient at times to reconstruct the eyelid [86]. To overcome these challenges, the use of tissue expanders and free vascularized transfers have also been advocated [87, 88].

The Veau III method of bilateral lip repair can be used for correcting the lip component. The last area to be addressed is the naso-malar junction [89].

77.6.5 Tessier No. 5–9 Cleft (Fig. 77.38a, b)

> The primary outcomes that are needed for the correction of these clefts include:
>
> - Lower eyelid reconstruction
> - Lateral canthal repositioning
> - Repair of the labio-maxillary cleft
> - Skeletal continuity restoration (this includes the orbital floor) using bone grafts

The principles to be borne in mind in the management of the Tessier 5–9 spectrum have been modified by different surgeons: Tessier (1971) advocated early correction of orbital dystopia – prior to 1 year of age. In all forms of facial clefts that affect the ocular region, priority is given to the preservation of vision by early interventions to prevent exposure keratitis of the cornea. Pre-surgical care includes use of ophthalmic ointments or temporary tarsorrhaphy procedures [48, 89]. Kara and Öçsel (2001) have reported the use of multiple z-plasties for the soft tissue reconstruction as early as 8th day after birth.

77.6.6 Tessier No. 7

Lateral facial cleft or Tessier no. 7 cleft is generally unilateral in presentation, though may also occur bilaterally. The bilateral form produces more gross clinical appearance with the face being amphibious in nature with an expanded mouth and infero-laterally placed commissures.

The condition is often related to syndromes of the first and second branchial arches. The cleft involves the skin, mucosa, and muscles of the oral sphincter (i.e., the orbicularis oris and the buccinator) [89]. In rare instances the cleft may involve the masseter [90]. This is a condition which may be concurrent with a lot of other deformities mandating a very thorough investigation in any patient exhibiting the classical feature of macrostomia [89].

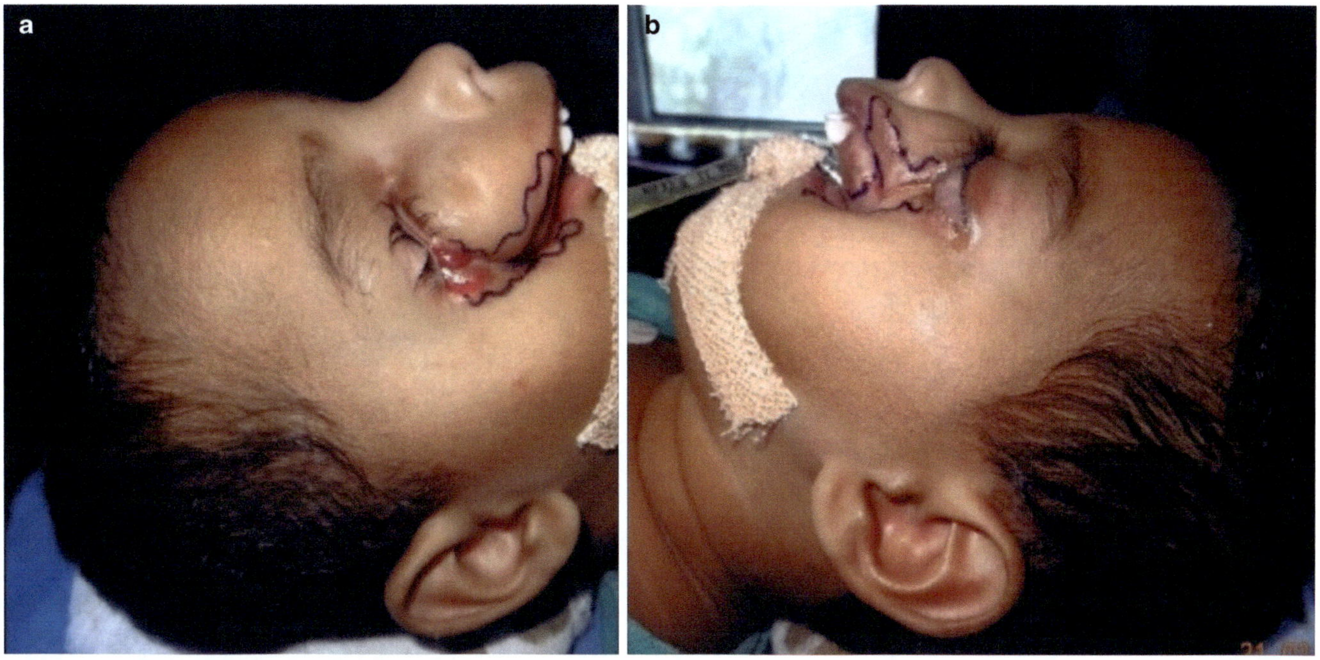

Fig. 77.38 (**a**, **b**) Tessier no 5–9 management

The surgical objectives for the management of the lateral facial cleft have been detailed as follows [90] (Fig. 77.39a–d):

1. Reconstituting the oral sphincter by reconstructing the orbicularis oris and the buccinator
2. Identification and reattachment of the other muscles of facial expression and the masseter in cases
3. Reconstruction of a natural and symmetrical commissure bilaterally
4. Attaining lip symmetry
5. Closure of the defect in layers with the mucosa, muscle, subcutaneous layer and skin [91]

Numerous procedures for the repair of macrostomia have been described in literature; [16, 17, 92, 93, 96, 97] Onizuka 1965; Boo-Chai 1969; Mansfield and Herbert 1972; Skoog 1974; Talukder 1980; Kaplan 1981; Bauer et al. 1982; Fukuda and Takeda 1985; Verheyden 1988; Yoshimura et al. 1992; Torkut and Coskunfirat 1997; Ono and Tateshita 1999.

Maximal care is exercised on the repair of the involved muscles with an overlapping technique [94, 95]. In severe cases other muscles of facial expression like the buccinator and the risorius also need to be repaired (Ono and Tateshita) [93]. This ensures normalization of both form and function of the perioral region [94].

The skin repair consists of two parts: repair of the cheek wall and commissuroplasty. Commissuroplasty denotes the reconstruction of the skin mucosa junction at the corner of the lips. Care is taken to design the repair in such a way that there is no associated contracture in the post-surgical period. There are various descriptions for the commissural repair. The triangular flap repair of Ono and Tateshita [93]. This procedure produced better aesthetics due to the triangular design of the flaps. Kawai et al. in 1998 described an inferiorly based triangular flap taken close to the lower lip to minimize the re-expansion of the commissure in the long term.

Eguchi et al. used the vermillion square flap method for commissuroplasty [96].

Other popular techniques described for the skin repair of the lateral lip element include to direct linear suturing, Z-plasty [94], and W-plasty [96]. The purpose of a Z-plasty is to break the long linear scar. But it is seen that the use of multiple Z-plasty or W-plasty procedures violates the relaxed skin tension lines. Therefore, a single Z-plasty with vertical limb lying in the nasolabial crease is preferred [90].

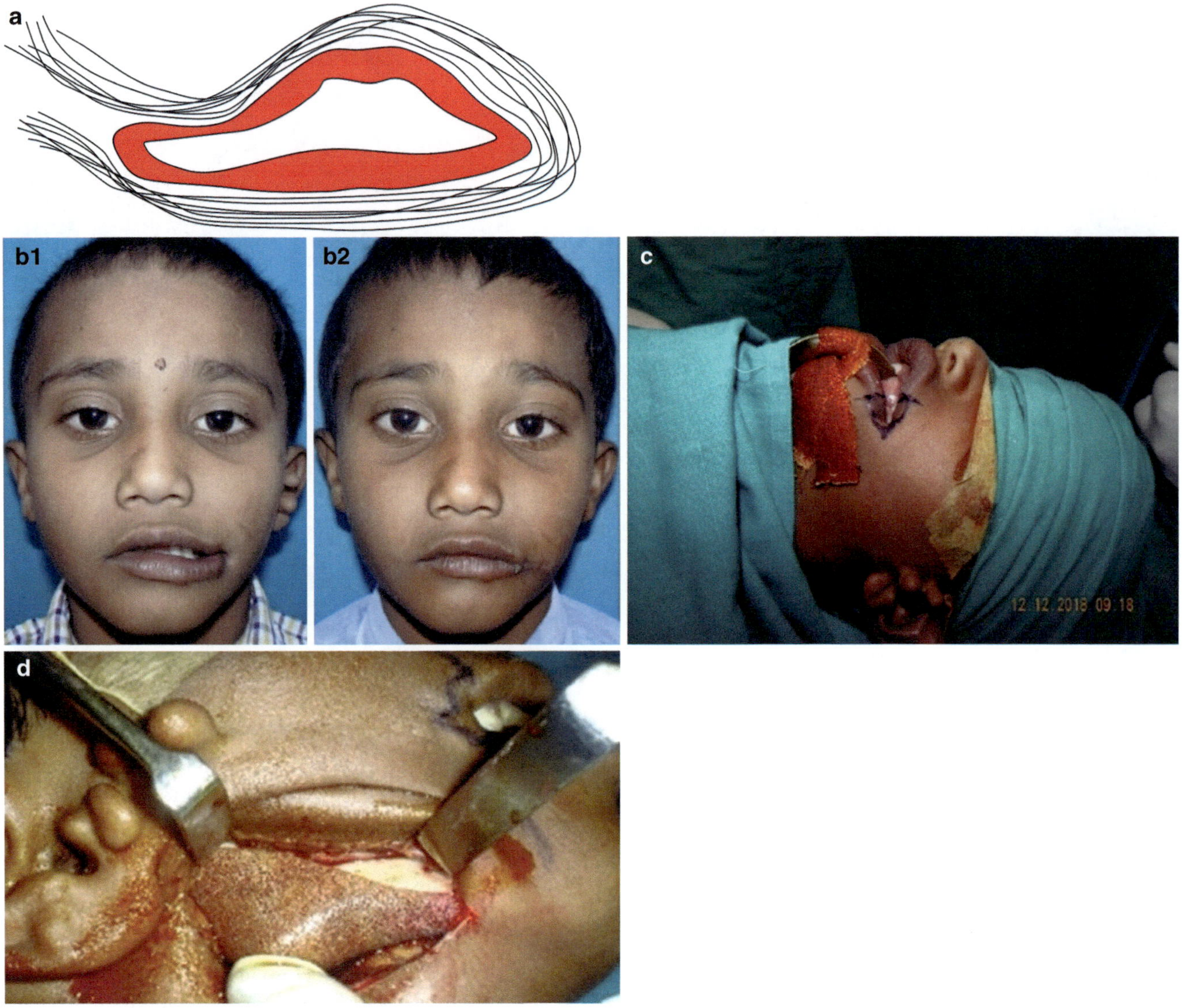

Fig. 77.39 (**a–d**) Tessier no. 7. (**a**) Diagram demonstrating abnormal oral aperture with distorted anatomy of orbicularis oris. (**b1**, **b2**) Clinical presentation of patient with macrostomia. (**c**) Incision marking. (**d**) Angle grafting

77.6.6.1 Bone Grafts

The establishment of normal contour of the soft tissues is never complete without the much needed skeletal support system. The skeletal reconstruction of craniofacial clefts essentially needs the use of bone grafts to fill and bridge both minor and major defects. The consolidation and take of the bone graft in the recipient site happens in two important steps: (i) the bony union of the joints between the grafted bone and the native bone and (ii) graft remodeling and creeping substitution [97]. Bone grafting can be performed at any age and is generally combined with soft tissue reconstruction [97].

Repairs performed in the early years of life can be accomplished with bone stock from the rib or iliac crest. However, the quality of the bone supplied by the ilium is better suited for this work. The cortico-cancellous graft material can be placed as such or carried over titanium cribs. It is important to note that the general consensus for the use of non-vascularized grafts is for defects less than 6 cm [98].

- Iliac crest grafts are the most favored with a good stock of available cortico-cancellous bone. Generally the anterior iliac crest is preferred as the posterior iliac crest requires a change of position to prone and may not accommodate simultaneous work from two teams. Donor site morbidity rate for anterior iliac crest grafts is around 23% and much less for posterior iliac crest. Complications include post-operative pain, iliac or acetabular fractures or instability, persistent hematoma, herniation of abdominal contents, vascular injury, lateral femoral cutaneous nerve injury, and contour defects along the iliac crest [17].

- Occasionally the use of alloplastic materials like Medpor may also be used (Fig. 77.40).
- Calvarial bone is another preferred site and can be freely available when the surgery involves cranial procedures and trans-cranial approaches. It has the lowest rate of resorption among all the bone grafts making it a preferred choice for facial and orbital reconstruction (Fig. 77.41a, b). The parietal calvarium can safely provide up to 8 × 10 cm of the bone for harvesting [99]. The temporoparietal region provides more curved bone suitable for orbital or malar reconstruction. Generally the grafting is performed in strips so that there are no gross fractures and later the strips are joined together to reconstruct larger defects. Calvarium is harvested in three main forms: partial-thickness outer cortex, full-thickness outer cortex, and bicortical grafts. Partial-thickness outer cortex grafts are ideally harvested from children between 4 and 8 years of age, using an osteotome to produce a curling sheet of the bone.
- Calvarial grafts are safe in adults and are the standard indication when simultaneous craniotomy is performed. A bicortical graft is harvested and the graft is split. The inner cortex is used for reconstruction, while the outer cortex is replaced to fill the donor site defect and contour.
- Complications of calvarial grafting include contour defects of the donor site, graft fractures, and rarely dural tears while harvesting bicortical grafts. Dural tears mandate a thorough and formal dural repair to prevent further complications. Intra-cranial hemorrhage is a very rare complication during this procedure but has been documented [100].
- Grafts of ample volume can also be harvested from the anterior tibia both in the form of cancellous bone or in the form of cortical strip from the anterior tibial plateau.
- Rib bone or costochondral grafts can be harvested from ribs 5 to 7 which may be used as full-thickness or split rib grafts. Costochondral grafts are extensively used in the reconstruction of ascending mandibular ramus and condylar defects. Site-specific complications include postoperative pain, injury to the pleura with associated pneumothorax, hemothorax, or pneumohemothorax. Occasionally it may cause exaggerated facial asymmetry due to overgrowth.

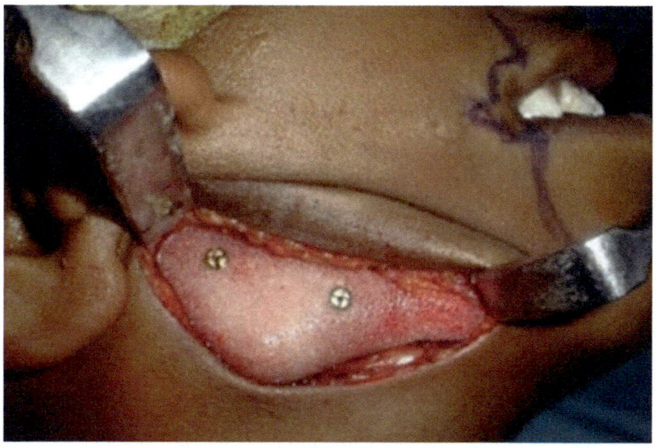

Fig. 77.40 Angle Medpor implant

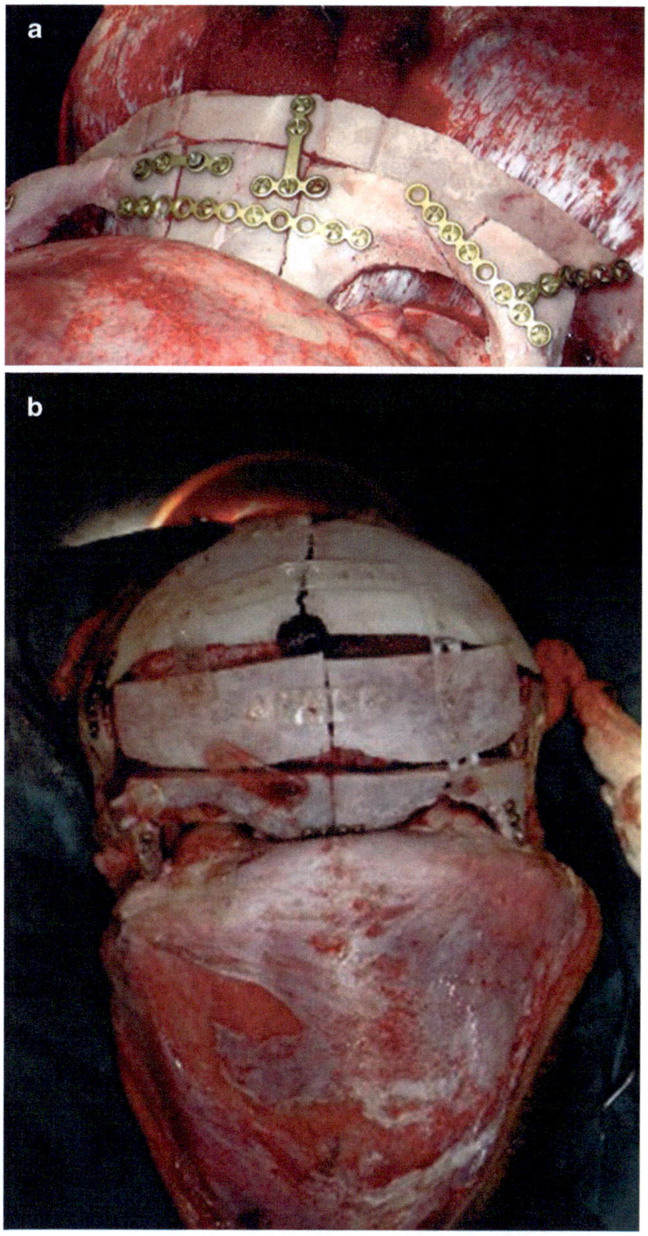

Fig. 77.41 (**a, b**) Calvarial bone graft

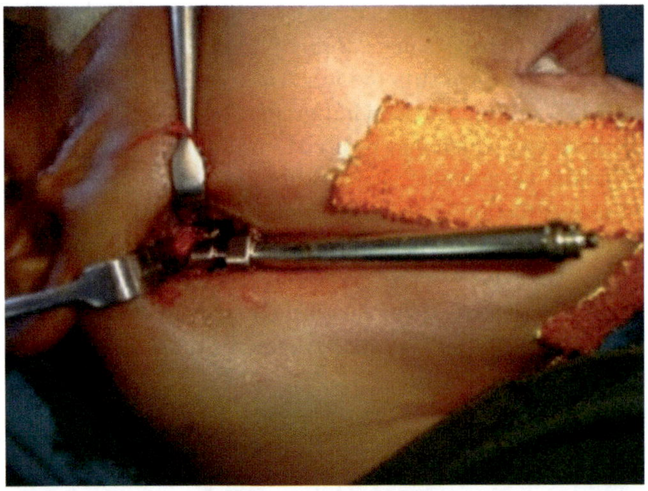

Fig. 77.42 Distraction osteogenesis in the correction of asymmetry

Defects which are larger and demand more complex reconstruction may not be amenable to bone grafting alone and may require well-designed osteotomy techniques [82, 101] or at times, even distraction osteogenesis (introduced by McCarthy and co-workers) [102] to form better contour of the involved skeletal framework and improve function (Refer Chap. 87 on Distraction osteogenesis) (Fig. 77.42).

77.7 Conclusion

The uncommonness of craniofacial clefts has made the accumulation and complete anatomic documentation of this extensive arrangement troublesome. Preoperative and postoperative CT examinations with 3D reproductions will improve the understanding of these complex deformities. The test of managing these monstrous deformities still challenges the skill and experience of many a craniofacial surgeon [35].

This is an effort to bring a comprehensive account on the varied presentation and management techniques employed in the management of craniofacial clefts of the head and face. We also emphasize the utilization of the brilliant and time-tested diagnostic and surgical principles detailed here to establish new protocols for the comprehensive management of these deformities. Moreover we also advocate that more standardization along with structured investigation and planning methods should be utilized to come to sensible yet efficient treatment models that can be utilized by all for the treatment of this unfortunate set of people.

References

1. His WE. Beobachtungen zur Gesichichte und Gamennbildung beim menschlichen Embryo. Kgl Akad Wiss. 1901;
2. Tessier P. Anatomical classification of facial, cranio-facial and laterofacial clefts. J Maxillofac Surg. 1969;4:69e92.
3. Bhattacharya S, Khanna V, Kohli R. Cleft lip: The historical perspective. Indian J Plast Surg. 2009;42(Suppl):S4–s8.
4. van der Meulen JCH. Oblique facial clefts. Plastic Reconstr Surg. 1984;76(2 j); revised January 28, 1985
5. Moore MH. Rare craniofacial clefts. J Craniofac Surg. 1996;7:408–11.
6. Eppley BL, van Aalst JA, Robey A, Havlik JR. The spectrum of orofacial clefting. Plast Reconst Surg. 2005;115:101–14.
7. Wehby GL, Cassell CH. The impact of orofacial clefts on quality of life and healthcare use and costs. Oral Dis. 2010;16(1):3–10.
8. Marcusson A, Akerlind I, Paulin G. Quality of life in adults with repaired complete cleft lip and palate. Cleft Palate Carniofac J. 2001;38(4):379–385.
9. Nagy K, Mommaerts MY. Analysis of the cleft-lip nose in submental-vertical view, Part I—Reliability of a new measurement instrument. J Cranio-Maxillofac Surg 2007; 35:265-277
10. Nollet PJPM, Kuijpers-Jagtman AM, Chatzigianni A, Semb G, Shaw WC, Bronkhorst EM, Katsaros C. Nasolabial appearance in unilateral cleft lip, alveolus and palate: a comparison with Eurocleft. J Craniomaxillofac Surg. 2007;35:278–86.
11. Joos U, Wernker K, Kruse-Löesler B, Kleinheinz J. Influence of treatment concept, velopharyngoplasty, gender and age on hypernasality in patients with cleft lip, alveolus and palate. J Craniomaxillofac Surg. 2006;34:472–7.
12. Carlino F. Modified forked flap for controlling columella length in cleft lip open rhinoplasty. J Craniomaxillofac Surg. 2008;36:131–7.
13. Li Y, Shi B, Song Q-G, Zuo H, Zheng Q. Effects of lip repair on maxillary growth and soft tissue development in patients with a complete unilateral cleft lip, alveolus and palate. J Craniomaxillofac Surg. 2006;34:355–61.
14. Dostal A, Nemeckova J, Gaillyova R. The 18q deletion syndrome and analysis of the critical region for orofacial cleft at 18q22.3. J Craniomaxillofac Surg. 2009;37:272–5.
15. Bütow K-W. Construction of the congenitally missing columella in midline clefts. J Craniomaxillofac Surg. 2007;35:287–92.
16. Berkowitz S. Stare of art of cleft palate orofacial growth and dentistry: A historical perspective. Am J Orthodontics. 1978;74(4):564–76.
17. Ghareeb FM, Hanafy AM. Surgical planning and correction of median craniofacial cleft. Egypt J Plast Reconstr Surg. 2003;27(1):143–52.
18. Bhatt YC. Proboscis lateralis: review of literature and a case report. Internet J Plast Surg. 2008;5:1–11.
19. Carstens MH. Neural tube programming and the pathogenesis of craniofacial clefts, part I: the neuromeric organization of the head and neck. In: Sarnat HB, Curatolo P, editors. Handbook of clinical neurology, vol. 87. London: Elsevier; 2008. Chapter 16.
20. Ishii M, Ishii Y, Moriyama T, et al. Seventeen-year follow-up of a patient with median cleft of the lower lip, mandible, and tongue with flexion contracture: a case report. Cleft Palate Craniofac J. 2002;39(5):555–9.
21. Wyszynski DF, Beaty TH, Maestri NE. Genetics of nonsyndromic oral clefts revisited. Cleft Palate Craniofac J. 1996;33:406–17.
22. Niemeyer MF, van der Meulen J. The genetics of craniofacial malformations. In: Stricker M, Van der Meulen J, editors. Craniofacial malformations. London: Churchill Livingstone; 1990.

23. Reddy SG. Incidence of cleft lip and palate in the state of Andhra Pradesh, South India. Indian J Plastic Surg. 2010;43(2):184–9.
24. Murray JC. Gene/environment causes of cleft lip and/or palate. Clin Genet. 2002;61:248–56.
25. Schuttle BC et al. The many faces and factors of orofacial clefts. Hum Mol Genet. 1999;8(10):1853–9.
26. Prescott NJ, Winter RM, Malcolm S. Nonsyndromic cleft lip and palate: Complex genetics and environmental effects. Ann Hum Genet. 2001;65:505–515
27. Hunt JA, Hobar PC. Common craniofacial anomalies: facial clefts and encephaloceles. Plast Reconstr Surg. 112(2):606–15.
28. Werler MM, Lammer EJ, Rosenberg L, et al. Maternal alcohol use in relation to selected birth defects. Am J Epidemiol. 1991;134:691.
29. Erickson A, Kallen B, Westerholm P. Cigarette smoking as an etiologic factor in cleft lip and palate. Am J Obstet Gynecol. 1979;135:348.
30. Van der Meulen JC, Mazzola R, Stricker M, Raphael B, Kawamoto HK, David JD. Classification of craniofacial malformations . Rare craniofacial clefts. In: McCarthy JG, editor. Plastic surgery. Philadelphia: W.B. Saunders; 1990. p. 2922–2973.
31. Kawamoto HK Jr. The kaleidoscopic world of rare craniofacial clefts: order out of chaos (Tessier classification). Clin Plast Surg. 1976;3:529.
32. Dufresne C, Jelks G. Classification of craniofacial anomalies. In: Smith B, editor. Ophthalmic plastic and reconstructive surgery. Philadelphia: C.V. Mosby; 1987. p. 1185–207.
33. Boo-chai K. The bifid nose. Plast Reconstr Surg. 1965;36:626.
34. Tessier P. Anatomical classification of facial, cranio-facial and latero-facial clefts. J Maxillofac Surg. 1976;4:69–92.
35. Hunt JA, Hober PC. Common craniofacial anomalies: The facial dysostoses. J Craniofac Surg. 2008;110(7):1714-1725.
36. David DJ, Moore MH, Cootes RD. Tessier clefts revisited with a third dimension. Cleft Palate J. 1989;26:163.
37. Da Silva Freitas RI, Alonso N, Shin JH et al. Surgical correction of Tessier number 0 cleft. J Craniofac Surg. 2008;19(5):1348–52.
38. Mullin WR. Management of congenital bilateral cleft nose. Plast Reconstr Surg. 1985;75:253.
39. Edwards WA. Median cleft face syndrome. Am J Ophtalmol. 1971;72:202.
40. Mazzola RF. Congenital malformations in the frontonasal area: their pathogenesis and classification. Clin Plast Surg. 1976;3:573–609.
41. Veau V. Hasencharten menschlicher Keimlinge auf der Stufe 21–23mm SSL. Z Anat Entwiclungsgesch. 1937;108:459.
42. DeMyer W. The median cleft face syndrome: differential diagnosis of cranium bifidum occultum, hypertelorism, and median cleft nose, lip, and palate. Neurology. 1967;17:961–71.
43. Millard DR Jr, Williams S. Median lip clefts of the upper lip. Plast Reconstr Surg. 1968;42:4–14.
44. Ozek C, Gundogan H, Bilkay U, Cankayali R, Guner U, Gurler T, et al. Rare craniofacial anomaly: Tessier no 2 cleft. J Craniofac Surg. 2001;12:355–61.
45. Bradley JP, Kawamoto Jr HK. Craniofacial Clefts. In: Neligan PC. Plastic Surgery. 4ed. St Louis: Elsevier, 2018. p 711–38.
46. Wenbin Z, Hanjiang W, Xiaoli C, Zhonglin L. Tessier 3 cleft with clinical anophthalmia: two case reports and a review of the literature. Cleft Palate Craniofac J. 2007;44(1):1597–05
47. Ewings EL, Carstens MH. Neuroembryology and functional anatomy of craniofacial clefts. Indian J Plastic Surg. 2009;42(2):182–7.
48. Alonso N, da Silva Freitas R, de Oliveira e Cruz GA, Goldenberg D, Dall'Oglio Tolazzi AR. Tessier no. 4 facial cleft: evolution of surgical treatment in a large series of patients. Plast Reconstr Surg. 2008;122:1505–13.
49. da Silva Freitas R, Alonso N, Shin JH, Busato L, Dall'Oglio Tolazzi AR, de Oliveria e Cruz GA. Tessier number 5 facial cleft: surgical strategies and outcomes in six patients. Cleft Palat Craniofac J. 46(2).
50. Van der Meulen JC, Mazzola R, Vermey-Keers C, et al. A morphogenetic classification of craniofacial malformations. Plast Reconstr Surg. 1983;71:560.
51. Longacre JJ, Stevens GA, Holmstrand KE. The surgical management of first and second branchial arch syndrome. Plast Reconstr Surg. 1963;31:507.
52. Grabb WC. The first and second branchial arch syndrome. Plast Reconstr Surg. 1965;36:485.
53. Converse JM, Coccaro PJ, Becker M, et al. On hemifacial microsomia. Plast Reconstr Surg. 1973;51:268.
54. Tessier P, Guiot J, Rougerie JP, et al. Ostéotomies cranio-naso-orbito-faciales. Hypertelorisme Ann Chir Plast. 1967;12:103.
55. Millard Jr, Lehman JA Jr, Deane M, Garst WP. Median cleft of the lower lip and mandible: a case report. Br J Plast Surg. 1971;24(4):391–5.
56. Rosenthal R. Aglossia congenital: Report of a case of the condition combined with other congenital malformations. J Dis Child. 1932;44:383–5.
57. Fearon JA. Rare craniofacial clefts: a surgical classification. J Craniofac Surg. 2008;19(1):110–2.
58. da Silva Freitas R, Alonso N, Busato L, et al. Series of facial cleft number 2-12: strategies for treatment. Rev Bros Cr Craniomaxillofac. 2010;13(4):225–30.
59. da Silva Freitas R, Alonso N, Shin JH. Surgical correction of Tessier number 0 cleft. J Craniofac Surg. 2008;19(5):1348–52.
60. Johnston MC. Embryology of the head and neck. In: McCarthy JG, editor. Plastic surgery. Philadelphia: WB Saunders; 1990.
61. Monasterio FO, Taylor JA. Major craniofacial clefts: case series and treatment philosophy. Plast Reconstr Surg. 2008;122(2):534–43.
62. Jackson IT, Tanner NSB, Hide TAH. Frontonasal encephalocele: "Long nose hypertelorism." Ann Plast Surg. 1983;11:490,
63. Holmes AD, Meara JG, Kolker AR, Rosenfeld JV, Klug GL. Frontoethmoidal encephaloceles: reconstruction and refinements. J Craniofac Surg. 2001; 12(1).
64. Ortiz-Monasterio F, Medina O, Musolas A. Geometrical planning for the correction of hypertelorism. Plast Reconstr Surg. 1990;86:650.
65. Greig DM. Hypertelorism: A hitherto undifferentiated congenital craniofacial deformity. Edinb Med J. 1924;31:560–93.
66. Tessier P. Orbital hypertelorism: I. Successive surgical attempts, material and methods: Causes and mechanism. Scand J Plast Reconstr Surg. 1972;6:135–55.
67. Munro I. Orbito-cranio-facial surgery. The team approach. Plast Reconstr Surg. 1975;55:170.
68. Marchac D, Sati S, Renier D. Deschamps-Braly J, Marchac A. Hypertelorism correction: what happens with growth? evaluation of a series of 95 surgical cases. Plast Reconstr Surg. 2012;129:713–27.
69. Schmid et al. New method for the correction of hypertelorism with preservation of the olfactory nerve. Plast Reconstr Surg. 1996;97:719–25A.
70. Frodel JL. Calvarial bone graft harvesting techniques: considerations for their use with rigid fixation techniques in the craniomaxillofacial region. In: Greenberg A, Prein J, editors. Craniomaxillofacial reconstructive and corrective bone surgery. New York: Springer; 2002. p. 700–712.

71. Van der Meulen JC. Medial fasciotomy. Br J Plast Surg. 1979;32(4):339–42.
72. Sailer HF, Haers PE, Zollikofer CPE, Warnke T, Carls FR, Stucki P. The value of stereolithographic models for preoperative diagnosis of craniofacial deformities and planning of surgical corrections. Int J Oral Maxillofac Surg. 1998;27(5):327–33.
73. Balaji SM. Modified facial bipartition. Ann Maxillofac Surg. 2012; 2(2):170–3.
74. Sharma RK, Makkar SS, Nanda V. Simple innovation for medial canthal tendon fixation. Plast Reconstr Surg. 2005;116:2046.
75. Ramesh K. Sharma hypertelorism. Indian J Plast Surg. 2014;47(3):284–92.
76. Urata MM, Kawamoto H. Median clefts of the upper lip: a review and surgical management of a minor manifestation. Cleft Palat Craniofac J. 2010;47(5):104–6.
77. Wiemer DR, Hardy SB, Spira M. Anatomical findings in median cleft of upper lip. Plast Reconstr Surg. 1978;62(6):866–9.
78. Francesconi G, Fortunato G. Median dysraphia of the face. Plast Reconstr Surg. 1969;43(5):481–91.
79. Bilen BT, Kilinç H. A congenital isolated alar cleft. J Craniofac Surg. 2006;17(3):602–4.
80. Rashid M, Islam MZ, Tamimy MS, Haq EU, Aman S, Aslam A. Rotation-transposition correction of nasal deformity in Tessier number 1 and 2 clefts. Cleft Palate Craniofac J. 2009;46(6):674–80.
81. Jinka JR, Chekuri H, Annavarapu G. Isolated cleft of the ala nasi: A report of seven cases. Indian J Plast Surg. 2012;45(3):512–5.
82. Ortiz Monasterio F, Fuente del Campo A, Dimopulos A. Nasal clefts. Ann Plast Surg. 1987;18(5):377–97.
83. Mishra RK, Purwar R. Formatting the surgical management of Tessier cleft types 3 and 4. Indian J Plast Surg. 2009;42(Suppl):S174–83.
84. Stretch JR, Poole MD, et al Nasolacrimal abnormalities in oblique facial clefts. Br J Plast Surg. 1990; 43(4):463–467.
85. Longaker MT, Siebert JW. Microsurgical correction of facial contour in congenital craniofacial malformations: the marriage of hard and soft tissue. Plast Reconstr Surg. 1996;98(6):942–50.
86. Van der Meulen J, Vaandrager JM. Surgery related to the correction of hypertelorism. Plast Reconstr Surg. 1983;71:6.
87. Tokioka K, et al. Two cases of Tessier no. 4 cleft with anophthalmia. Cleft Palate Craniofac J. 2005;42(4):448–52.
88. Menard RM, Moore MH, David DJ. Tissue expansion in the reconstruction of Tessier craniofacial clefts: a series of 17 patients. Plast Reconstr Surg. 2012;129(6):1337–44.
89. Chen PK, Chang FC, Chan FC, Chen YR, Noordhoff MS. Repair of Tessier no. 3 and no. 4 craniofacial clefts with facial unit and muscle repositioning by midface rotation advancement without Z-plasties. Plast Reconstr Surg. 2012;129(6):1337–44.
90. Pereira FJ, Milbratz GH, Cruz AAV, Vasconcelos JJA. Ophthalmic considerations in the management of Tessier cleft 5/9. Ophthal Plast Reconstr Surg. 2010 ;26(6).
91. Shima Y, Ogawa K, Kuwabara Y, Takechi N, Shin S. Newborn with transverse facial cleft associated with polyhydramnios. J Perinatol. 2002;22:91–2.
92. Yencha M. Congenital macrostomia. Otolaryngol Head Neck Surg. 2001;124:353–4.
93. Tomoaki E, Hirotaka A, Akihiko T, Tsuyoshi T, Kiyonori H. Surgical repair for congenital macrostomia: vermilion square flap method. Ann Plast Surg. 2001;47:629–35.
94. Ono I, Tateshita T. New surgical technique for macrostomia repair with two triangular flaps. Plast Reconstr Surg. 1999;105:688–94.
95. Bauer BS, Margulis A. Invited discussion of surgical repair for congenital macrostomia vermilion square flap method. Ann Plast Surg. 2001;47:328–9.
96. Franco D, Franco T, da Silva FR, Alonso N. Commissuroplasty for macrostomia. J Craniofac Surg. 2007;18:691–4.
97. Eguchi T, Asato H, Takushima A, Takato T, Harii K. Surgical repair for congenital macrostomia: vermilion square flap method. Ann Plast Surg. 2001;47:629–35.
98. Stevenson S, Li XQ, Davy DT, Klein L, Goldberg VM. Critical biological determinants of incorporation of non-vascularized cortical bone grafts. Quantification of a complex process and structure. J Bone Joint Surg Am. 1997;79(1):1–16.
99. Podlesh S, Anthony JP. Alexander A comparison of vascularized and nonvascularized bone grafts for reconstruction of mandibular continuity defects. J Oral Maxillofac Surg. 1997;55(11):1200–6.
100. Nocini PF, Bedogni A, Valsecchi S, Trevisiol L, Ferrari F, Fior A, Saia G. Fractures of the iliac crest following anterior and posterior bone graft harvesting. Review of the literature and case presentation. Minerva Stomatol. 2003; 52(10):441–8.
101. Ortiz-Monasterio F, Medina O, Musolas A. Geometrical planning for the correction of hypertelorism. Plast Reconstr Surg. 1990;86:650.
102. McCarthy JG, Staffenberg DA, Wood RJ, Cutting CB, Grayson BH, Thorne CH. Introduction of an intraoral bone-lengthening device. Plast Reconstr Surg. 1994;96:978–81.

78 Hemifacial Microsomia (HFM) and Treacher Collins Syndrome

Manikandhan Ramanathan

78.1 Introduction

Hemifacial microsomia (HFM) is a three-dimensional congenital deformity of the craniofacial region characterized by abnormal and underdevelopment of the first and second pharyngeal arches. Due to involvement of multiple structures, this disorder has a broad spectrum of involvement with diverse clinical features [1].

The highly variable phenotypes have probably led to variation in its nomenclature as well, alternatives used being craniofacial microsomia (CFM), otomandibular dysostosis, facio-auriculo-vertebral spectrum, oculo-auriculo-vertebral spectrum, first and second branchial arch syndrome, otomandibular-facial dysmorphogenesis, and lateral facial dysplasia [2].

This disorder is characteristically unilateral; however, incidence of bilateral cases is 10–15%. Although this disorder was described first by Carl Ferdinand von Arlt, a German physician in 1881, "hemifacial microsomia" got its name from Gorlin and Pindborg in the early 1960s. Converse et al. proposed the name, craniofacial microsomia, in cases of coexisting cranial deformities where HFM is also associated with vertebral, cardiac, and renal defects, in a condition called as Goldenhar syndrome. It was termed "oculoauriculovertebral dysplasia" (OAVD) by Gorlin. It is also associated with epibulbar dermoids and ear deformities [2, 3].

78.1.1 Epidemiology and Etiopathogenesis

HFM is the second most common congenital anomaly of the face, with a male predilection and which is more common in the right than the left side. The incidence of HFM ranges between 1 in 3500 and 1 in 26,000 live births [4–7].

The cause of HFM remains largely unknown. Poswillo in 1973 reported that hematomas resulting from disruption of embryonic arteries (stapedial artery) in utero produce abnormalities in the development of the structures derived from the first and second pharyngeal arches. The extent of the hematoma and consequent tissue damage during the first 6 weeks of gestation determines the severities of deformities. He was able to produce the CFM phenotype in mice, thus proving his theory. He administered teratogens to produce a hematoma of the stapedial artery and the artery of the second arch which resulted in regional necrosis [4] (Fig. 78.1a, b).

The second widely accepted hypothesis is a change in the migration of neural crest cells (Fig. 78.2). Retinoic acid is believed to influence and alter the migration and distribution of neural crest cells, which may predispose to abnormalities in the pharyngeal arch derivatives. The intake of retinoic acid in humans during the early stages of pregnancy may cause multiple disorders collectively known as "retinoic acid embryopathies" (RAEs); these include variable defects of the jaws and the middle and external ear [3–5]. Apart from retinoic acid, thalidomide, primidone, ethanol and isotretinoin have also been studied as causative agents in HFM through their teratogenic effects [6, 7].

More recent studies have demonstrated an association between HFM and multiple gestations, along with other maternal risk factors such as assisted reproduction, smoking, maternal diabetes mellitus and vasoactive drugs. Moreover, HFM may demonstrate autosomal dominant and recessive Mendelian patterns in families. Positive family history accounts for 50% occurrence of features [8].

Genetic events like duplication of the OTX2 gene (chromosome 14q22.3) have also been researched upon. OTX2 encodes a transcription factor, essential for craniofacial development and anterior brain morphogenesis. Heterogeneity in aetiology along with variable penetrance

M. Ramanathan (✉)
Department of OMFS, Meenakshi Ammal Dental College and Hospital, MAHER University, Chennai, India

Meenakshi Cleft and Craniofacial Centre, Meenakshi Ammal Dental College and Hospital, Chennai, India

K. Bonanthaya et al. (eds.), *Oral and Maxillofacial Surgery for the Clinician*, https://doi.org/10.1007/978-981-15-1346-6_78

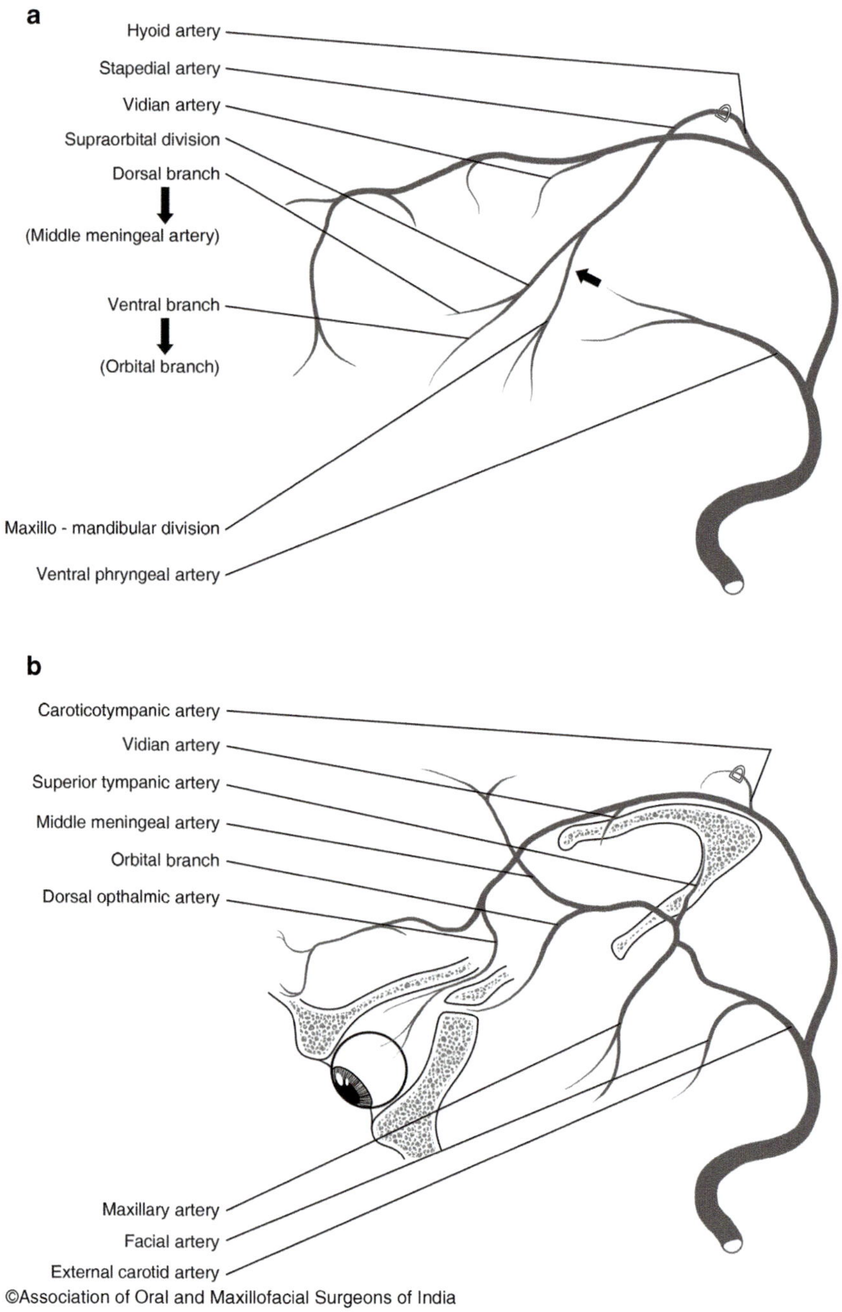

Fig. 78.1 (**a**, **b**) Anatomy of the stapedial artery during embryonic development

and expression is postulated to account for the widely variable phenotypic spectrum of HFM [9, 10].

78.1.2 Classification Systems

Various classifications have attempted to categorize various features of HFM as enumerated below [11–13]:

1. SAT classification.
2. OMENS classification.
3. Kaban-Pruzansky classification.

78.1.2.1 SAT Classification

The skeletal, auricle, and soft tissue (SAT) classification.

The SAT and the OMENS (Tables 78.1 and 78.2) classifications provide an elaborate system covering simple to complex skeletal, soft tissue and neurological involvement. On the other hand, the Kaban-Pruzansky classification explains malformations involving the mandible, masticatory muscles, and TMJ. Therefore, it is more useful for orthodontists and maxillofacial surgeons in reconstruction of the mandible and TMJ. Thus, this classification has become the gold standard. It involves four classes—

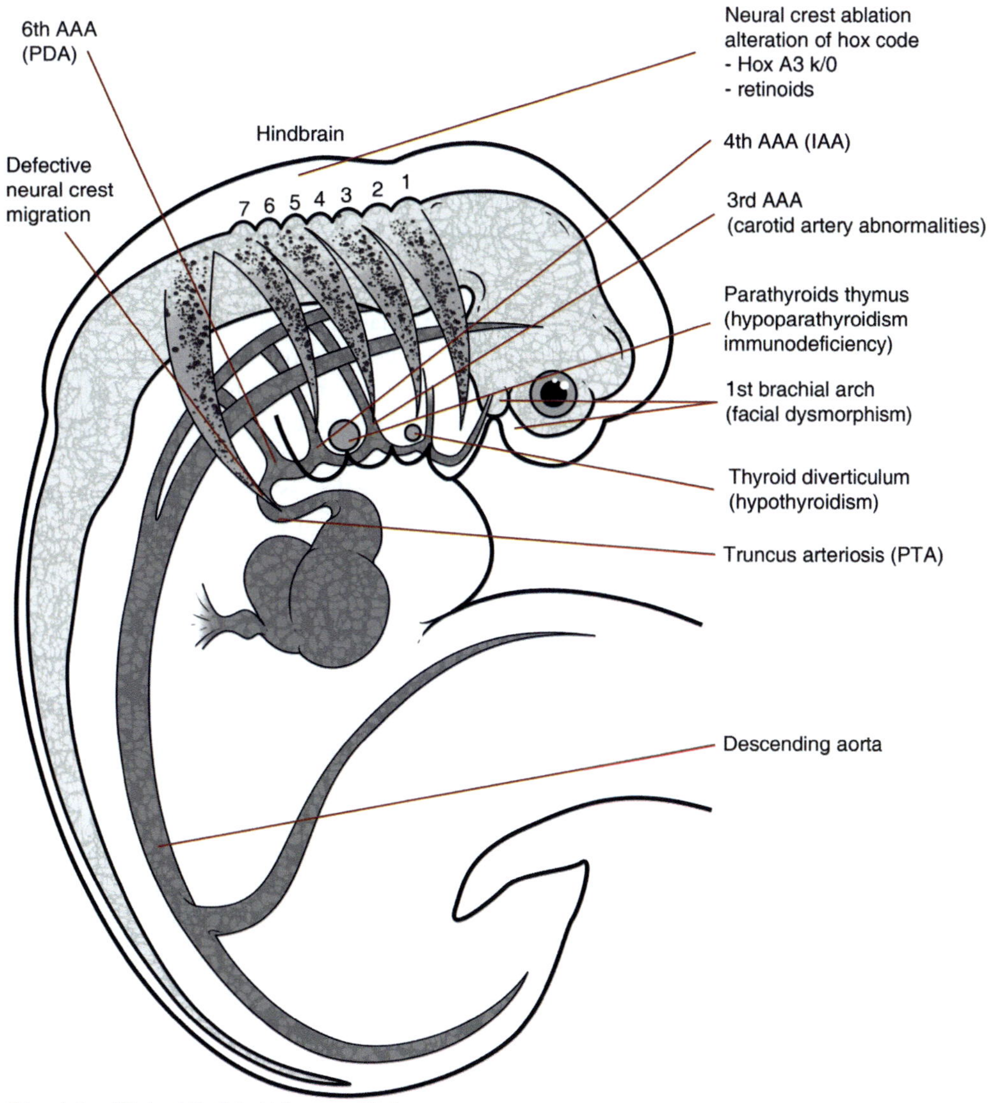

Fig. 78.2 Migration of neural crest cells during embryonic development

Table 78.1 SAT classification of HFM

Skeletal categories (S)	Auricle categories (A)	Soft tissue categories (T)
S1 = small mandible—Normal shape	A0 = Normal	T1 = contour defect minimal—No cranial nerve involvement
S2 = condyle, ramus, sigmoid notch discernible, distorted; mandible remarkably different in size and shape	A1 = small, malformed auricle—With characteristic features	T2 = moderate defect
S3 = severe mandibular deformity, poorly discernible, to agenesis of ramus	A2 = rudimentary auricle with hook at cranial end corresponding to the helix	
S4 = an S3 mandible with orbital involvement, lateral and inferior orbital rims displaced posteriorly	A3 = malformed lobule, pinna absent	
S5 = the S4 defects plus orbital dystopia, hypoplastic, asymmetric, neurocranium and a flat temporal fossa		

Table 78.2 OMENS classification

Orbit	Mandible	Ear	Nerve (cranial nerve VII)	Soft tissue
0 = Normal	Type I	Type I = small ear, the normal structure	0 = Normal	0 = Normal
1 = small size	Type IIA	Type II = severe external ear deformity with a rudimentary auricle	1 = upper branches impaired	1 = mild hypoplasia
2 = poor position	Type IIB	Type III = small rudiment of external ear with no pinna	2 = lower branches impaired	2 = moderate hypoplasia
3 = small size and poor position	Type III	Type IV = Anotia	3 = upper and lower branches impaired	3 = severe hypoplasia

the Type 1, Type 2A, Type 2B, and Type 3 (Fig. 78.3a–d).

Type 1
In this category, the TMJ morphology is normal with adequate bulk and function of masticatory muscles. The mandible is slightly hypoplastic and retruded which may project as a mild asymmetry with deviation of the chin to the affected side (Fig. 78.4a, b).

Type 2A
In this type, the affected side TMJ is shifted anteriorly and medially than its counterpart, but the overall morphology of the condyle and glenoid fossa remains unchanged. The joint is functional associated with moderate muscular hypoplasia. The patient demonstrates moderate hypoplasia of the mandible with occlusal canting or open bite, and the chin is deviated to the affected side.

Type 2B
There is moderate-to-severe involvement of the joint with condyle and the glenoid fossa grossly hypoplastic. The joint exhibits only rotation movement of the condyle and near-normal function. Involvement of other facial bones and deficiency of masticatory muscles are clinically evident. The patient demonstrates severe asymmetry and occlusal canting with or without an open bite (Fig. 78.5a, b).

Type 3
There is gross facial asymmetry with severely hypoplastic or absent muscles of mastication. There is associated severe deformity of the skull and orbito-zygomatic complex as well. The mandible is severely affected with a "floating mandible" appearance due to absence of the condyle and ramus (Fig. 78.6a, b). These patients from birth may often present with signs of a compromised airway due to severe degrees of mandibular retrusion.

78.1.3 Clinical Features

The diagnosis of HFM is challenging owing to its wide phenotypic spectrum. There are no definite diagnostic criteria and classifications. The condition is diagnosed based on its clinical features of phenotype ranging from involving the orbit or ear alone to full-blown hemifacial microsomia under development with jaw malformations. For this reason, certain classification systems have been established to standardize the assessment in an organized manner and formulate treatment plan accordingly. The areas of examination include various components of the face, i.e. external ear, mandible, temporal bone, zygoma, orbit middle ear, facial musculature, facial nerve supply, and other adjacent bony and soft tissues [2, 5, 7, 14] (Fig. 78.7a–d and Table 78.3).

78.1.3.1 Skeletal Defects

Cranio-orbital
The cranial involvement is mainly limited to the squamous part of the temporal bone. Most individuals affected with HFM demonstrate hypoplasia of the zygomatico-maxillary complex. These patients clinically show malar depression with orbital dystopia. The zygomatic bone hypoplasia can lead to alterations in the glenoid fossa.

Maxillomandibular
The maxillomandibular region is primarily affected due to abnormal development of the first and second branchial arches. It presents as unilateral facial deformities with reduced dimensions of facial bones in all three dimensions (3D). This produces varying degrees of gross morphological asymmetry of the face and compensatory changes of the contralateral side. The affected side in HFM may vary in severity and also alters the morphology of the so-called normal contralateral side, resulting in gross deviation in 3D, making it a difficult term as unaffected normal side (Figs. 78.5, 78.7, 78.8a–c and 78.9a–c).

Mandibular growth changes are the earliest manifestations of HFM and are accountable for its classical presentation of facial asymmetry. The ramus of the mandible is either absent or short, with a medial displacement. The contour of the entire mandibular corpus is altered with a shift of the Genium to the affected side. Dental compensations occur for the skeletal discrepancy, which may mask the actual severity of the clinical condition.

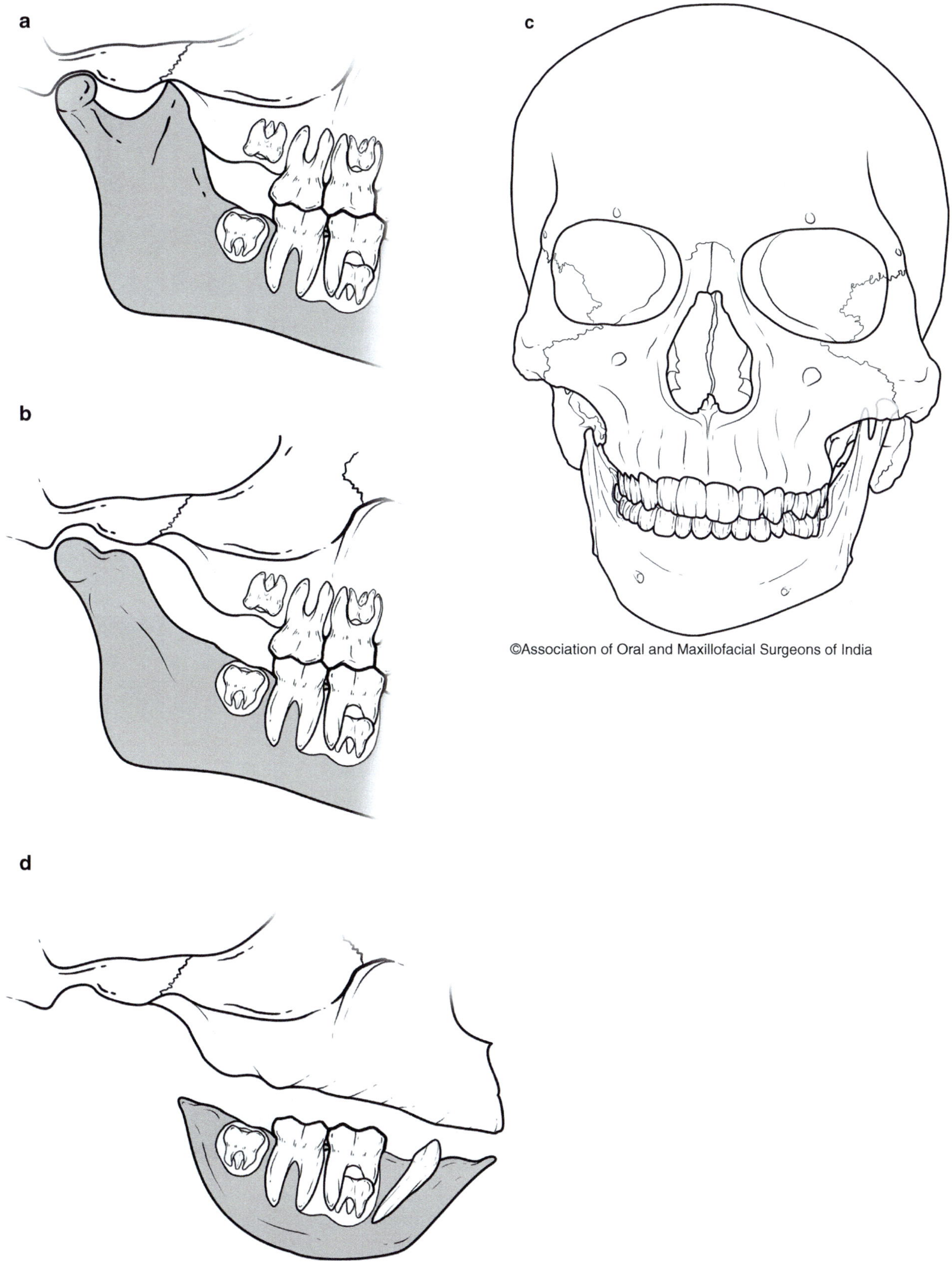

Fig. 78.3 (**a**–**d**) Kaban's modification of Pruzansky's classification for hemifacial microsomia (HFM). (**a**) Type 1, (**b**) Type 2A, (**c**) Type 2B (**d**) Type 3 Note that the temporomandibular joint (TMJ) in Type IIB is medially, inferiorly and anteriorly displaced so as to be operationally equivalent to Type III

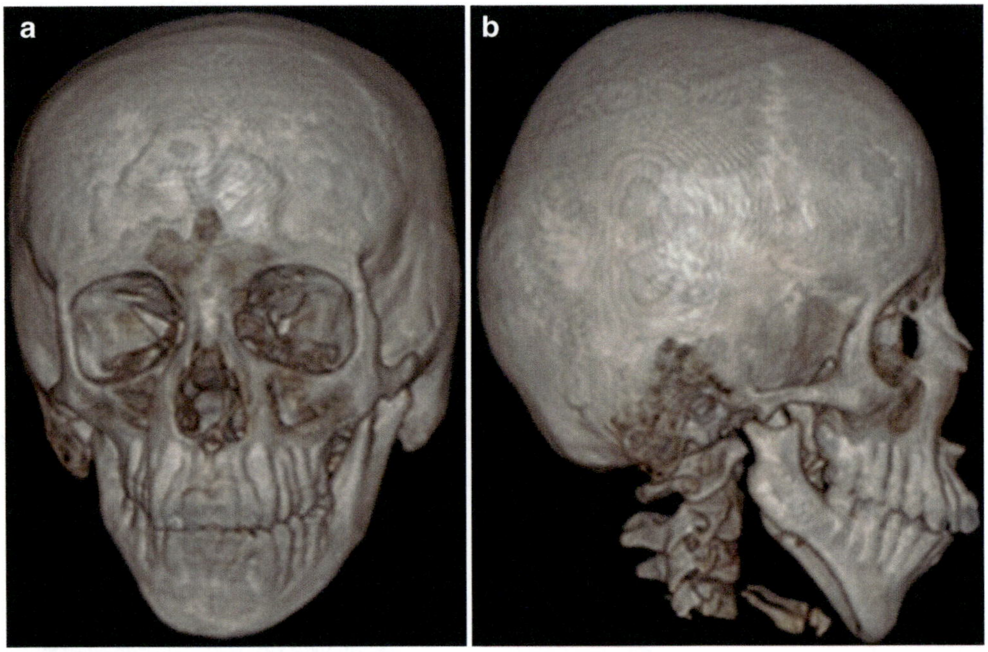

Fig. 78.4 (**a**, **b**) CT scan of patient with left-sided Type 1 Kaban-Pruzansky deformity

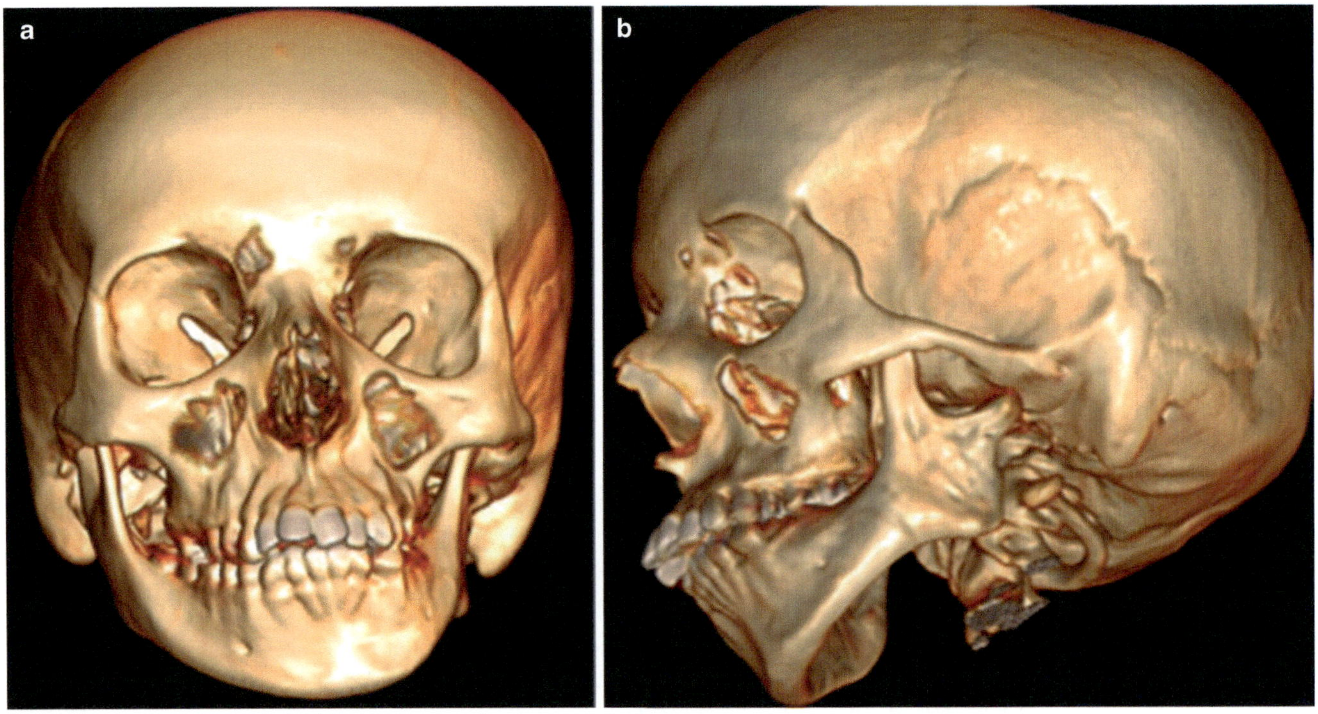

Fig. 78.5 (**a**, **b**) CT scan of patient with right-sided Type 2B Kaban-Pruzansky deformity

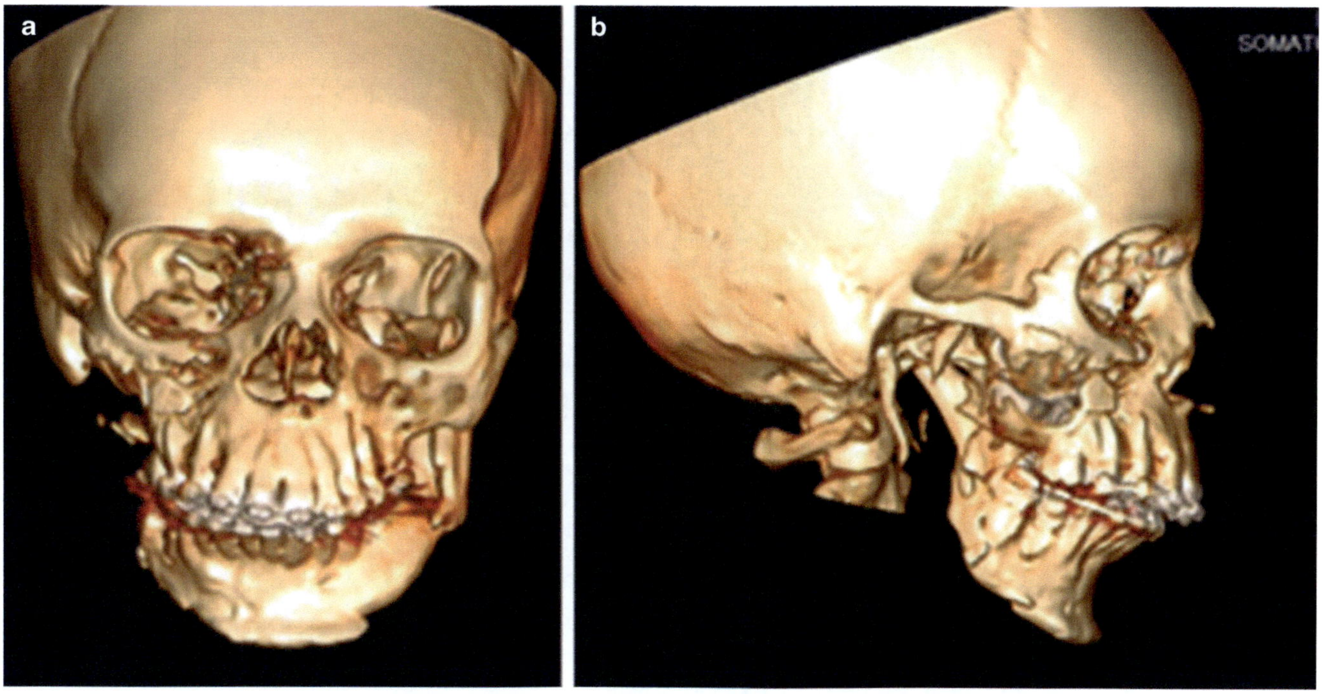

Fig. 78.6 (**a**, **b**) CT scan of patient with right-sided Type 3 Kaban-Pruzansky deformity

78.1.3.2 Soft Tissue Defect

Soft tissue deformities may involve the ear, the seventh nerve and the muscles of facial expression and mastication. Subcutaneous tissues of the face may also be affected to varying degrees. Macrostomia is a common feature along with the presence of skin tags between the tragus and the commissure of the mouth. Lateral facial clefts (Tessiers 6, 7 and 8) may be present involving the soft tissue or hard tissue or both. Function of the cranial nerves, essentially the seventh and rarely the fifth, may be compromised [15, 16]. General soft tissue bulk of the subcutaneous fat and muscles may exhibit deficiency (Fig. 78.7). There may also be compromise in the function of the soft palate.

Skin Tags

Vestigial skin rests also called as auxiliary hillocks or skin tags are usually present along an imaginary line connecting the tragus of the ear to the commissure of the mouth. This is the embryonic line of fusion between the first and second pharyngeal arches. The tags are frequently present in varying numbers and are associated with cartilaginous remnants, blind sinus tracts that may form inclusion cysts if obstructed [4–6] (Fig. 78.7).

Macrostomia

Macrostomia occurs as a result of failure of fusion of the maxillary and mandibular processes, leading to a cleft at the oral commissure including the skin and the underlying orbicularis oris (Fig. 78.10a, b). Sixty-one per cent of patients with HFM exhibit macrostomia as reported by Vento and colleagues [12].

External Ear Deformities

Meurman described a classification for deformities of the external ear which was modified by Marx [17, 18] (Fig. 78.11a–c):

- Grade I: Mild hypoplasia, with all structures present and obvious malformation.
- Grade II: Atresia of the external auditory canal, with a vertically orientated cartilaginous remnant.

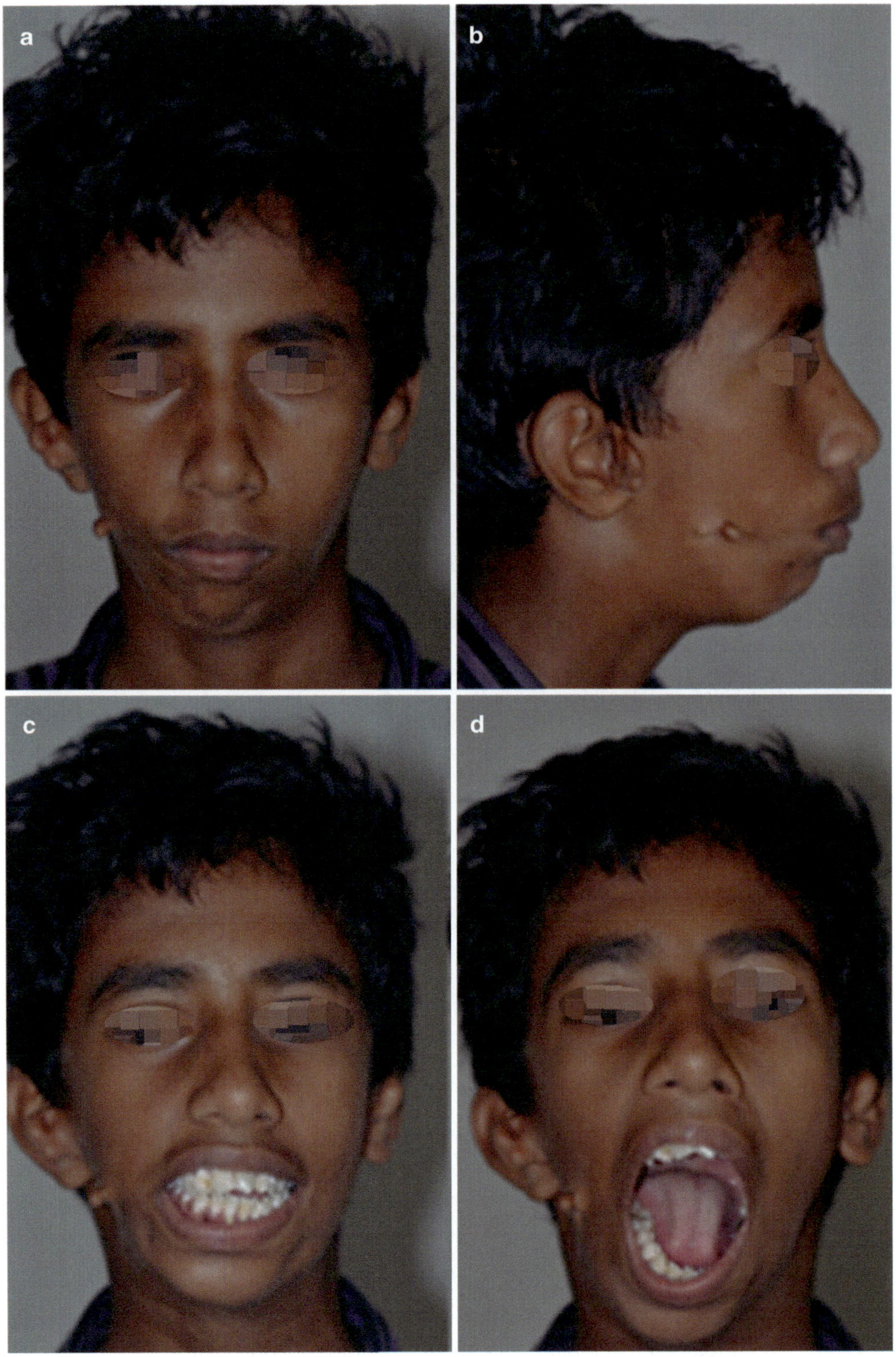

Fig. 78.7 (**a**–**d**) 15-year-old male, frontal and profile view (**a**, **b**) showing features of hemifacial microsomia such as lateral cleft and preauricular skin tags. (**c**) demonstrates macrostomia and maloccusion while (**d**) shows exaggerated oral aperture with deviation of mandible to the right side on mouth opening (Also see Fig. 78.30b)

Table 78.3 Clinical features of hemifacial microsomia and the spectrum of associated anomalies

Head and neck	Associated congenital anomalies
Maxillary and mandibular asymmetry with hypoplasia on the affected side Microphthalmia Hypoplastic adnexal structures Coloboma Zygomatic hypoplasia External ear abnormalities or atresia Internal ear abnormalities Temporomandibular joint hypoplasia or absence Hypoplastic dentition or oligodontia Parotid hypoplasia or agenesis Plagiocephaly Torticollis	Cardiac defects (tetralogy of Fallot, ventricular septal defect, aortic coarctation, patent ductus arteriosus) Lung hypoplasia Renal agenesis, ectopic kidney, multicystic Dysplastic kidney, vesicoureteral reflux, or ureteropelvic junction obstruction Vertebral anomalies Mental retardation, Arnold-Chiari malformation, encephalocele

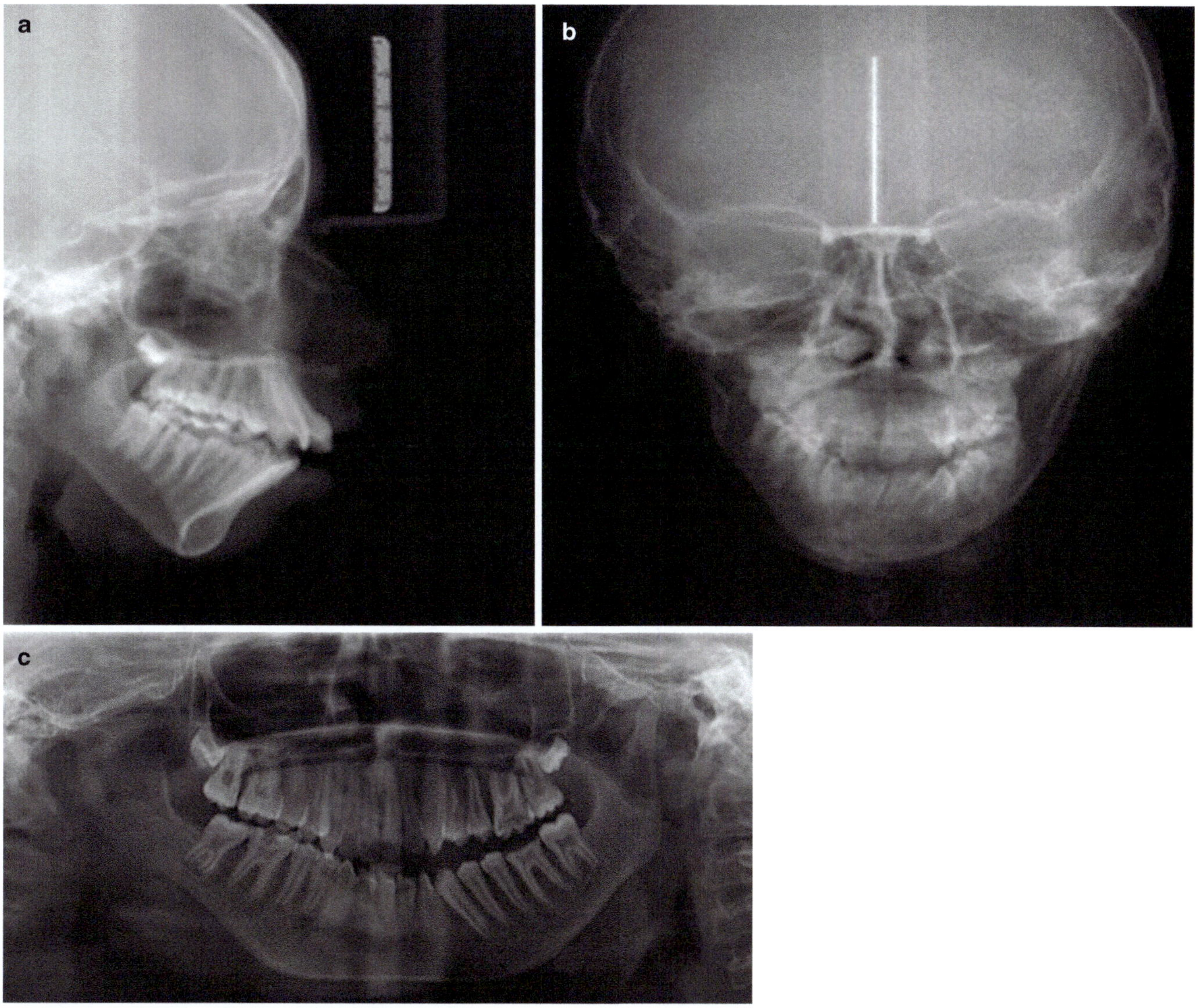

Fig. 78.8 (**a–c**) Radiographs lateral cephalogram (**a**), posteroanterior cephalogram (**b**) and OPG (**c**) showing features of asymmetry. OPG showing deficient body and ramus region

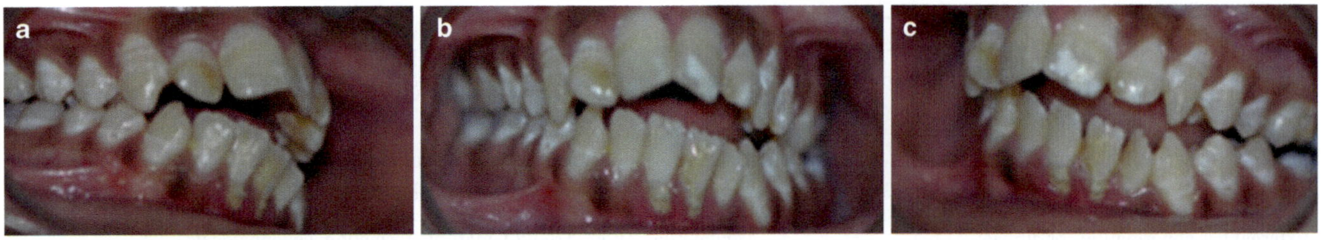

Fig. 78.9 (**a**–**c**) Intraoral views showing malocclusion, asymmetric anterior open bite, canting and crowding

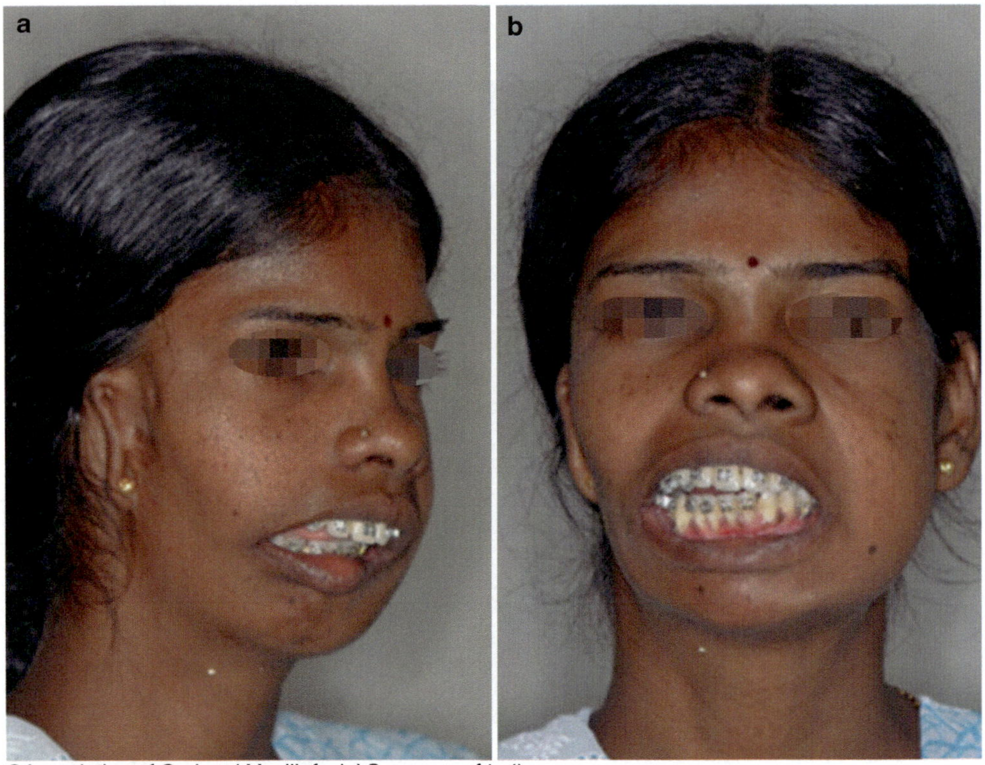

Fig. 78.10 (**a**, **b**) (Left, profile view; right, frontal view): Adult with right-sided hemifacial macrostomia. Note the deviation on mouth opening to the deficient right side. Also note the preauricular skin tags and epibulbar lesions

- Grade III: Absent auricle, anteriorly and inferiorly displaced lobular remnant.
- Radiological assessment using temporal bone CT scans should be used to assess the middle ear structures.

Muscle Deficit

Deficits in the temporalis and the pterygo-masseteric group of muscles may be seen in HFM. This also contributes to the skeletal deficit seen. A hypoplastic temporalis may be associated with a hypoplastic or at times absent ramus-condyle unit (RCU) which includes the coronoid process also; a similar association is also evident with the presentation of the pterygo-masseteric muscles and the ramus of the mandible. With cases of increasing severity, the proximal aspect of the zygomatic arch may also be absent with the aponeurosis of the hypoplastic masticatory muscles filling that space. Lateral pterygoid muscle hypoplasia ranges from mild to complete absence and correlates with the extent of the skeletal defect. Hypoplasia of the muscles and deficiency of the RCU lead to abnormalities of the TMJ and also with absence or altered joint structures. This often leads to deviation of the mandible to the affected side at rest and on mouth opening (Fig. 78.12a).

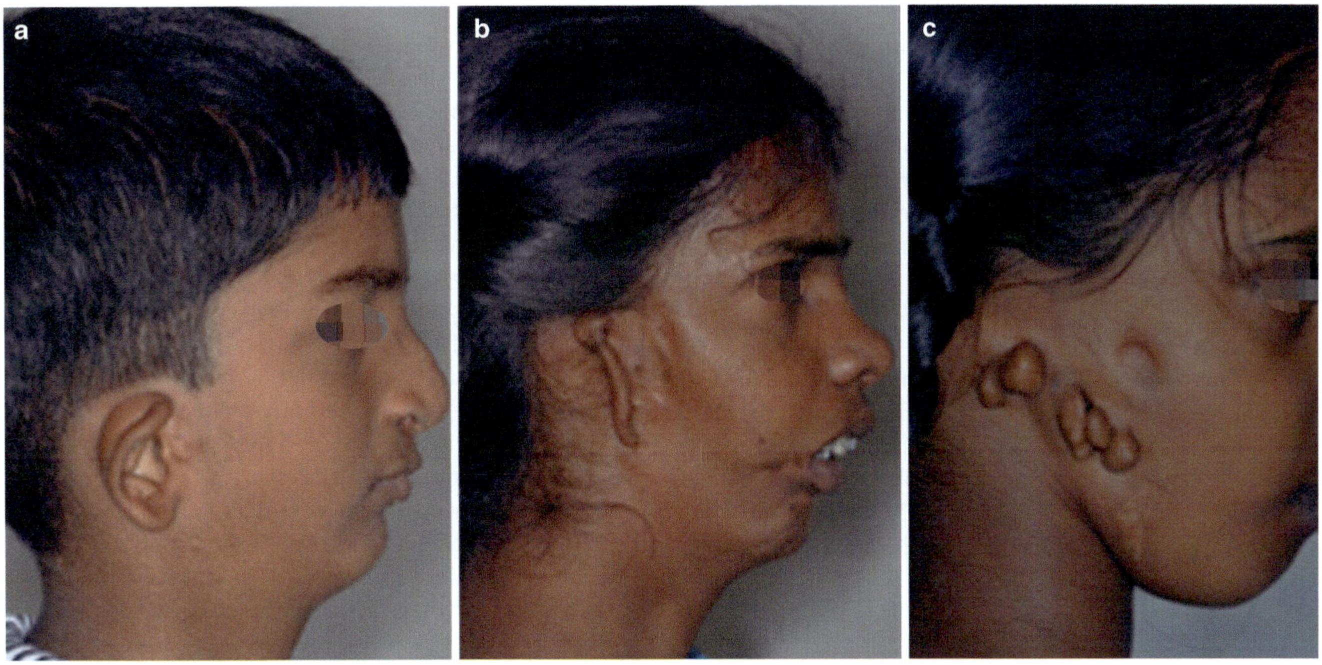

Fig. 78.11 (**a**) Grade 1 mild ear deformity, (**b**) Grade 2 moderate ear deformity, (**c**) Grade 3 severe ear deformity

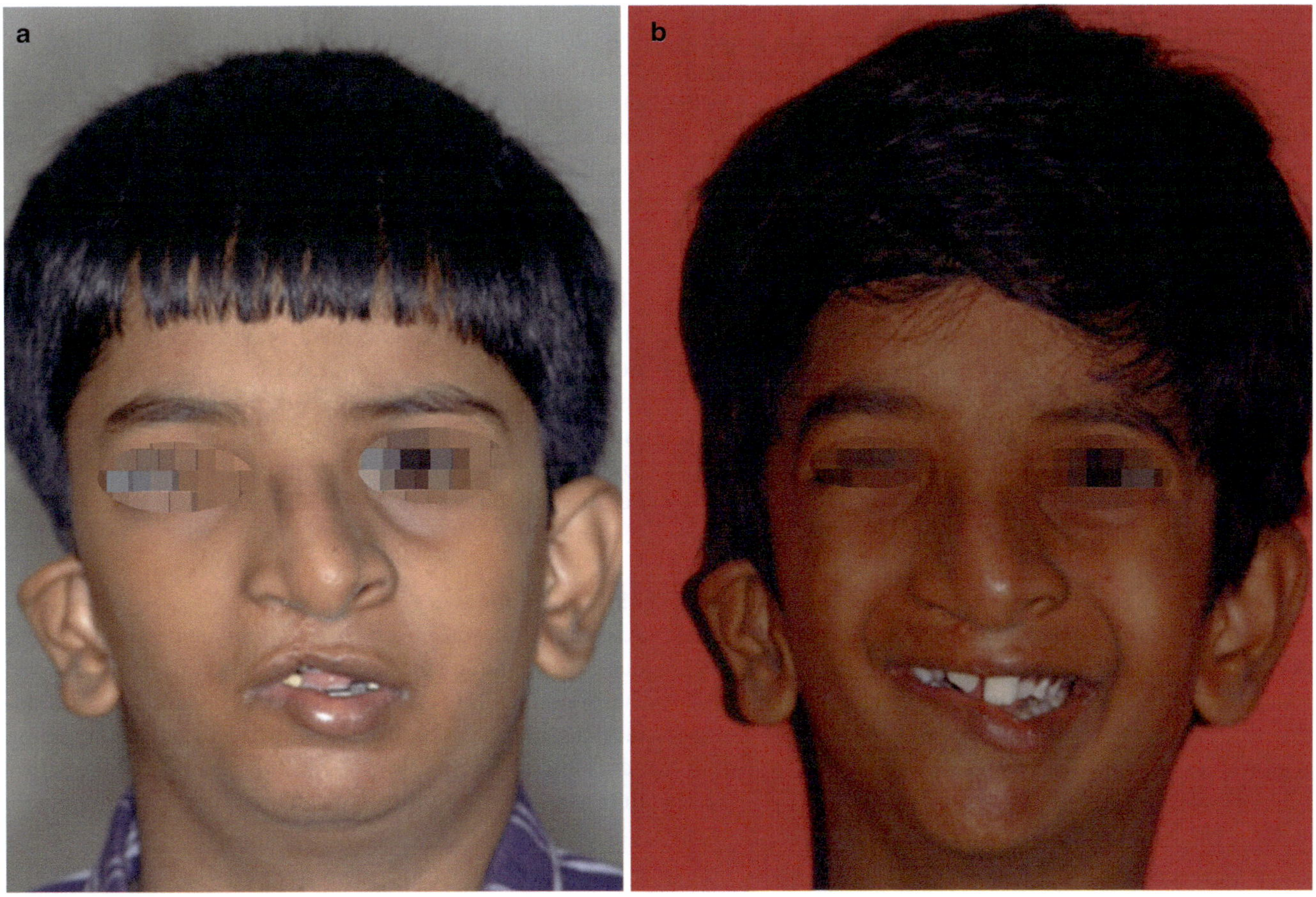

Fig. 78.12 (**a**) Unilateral cleft lip and palate patient with right-sided hemifacial microsomia, Grade 1 ear deformity, right-sided muscle weakness of orbicularis oris, buccinator and orbicularis oculi. (**b**) Deviated smile due to facial nerve deformity

Cranial Nerve Abnormalities

Approximately 25% of the patients with HFM are affected with cranial nerve deficits, resulting in features ranging from nerve weakness to complete paralysis. The marginal mandibular branch is the most commonly affected followed by the frontalis muscle dysfunction. Rarely, there may be a sensory deficit due to trigeminal nerve involvement along with total involvement of the facial nerve [19] (Fig. 78.12b).

Soft Palate Function

The cause for the soft palate deviation (to the normal side) in HFM has long been debated. It is proposed that the deviation may be due to a combination of skeletal asymmetry, neurological deficits, and hypoplastic musculature. Literature shows that patients with HFM are predisposed to velopharyngeal dysfunction, even in the absence of a palatal cleft [20].

78.1.4 Radiological Assessment

Considering the three-dimensional skeletal nature of the deformity, radiological assessment is of paramount importance. Conventional methods of 2D imaging are very helpful and still relevant in assessing the condyle anatomy and extent of asymmetry. Orthopantomogram, posteroanterior cephalogram, and lateral cephalogram should be taken for initial assessment (Fig. 78.9). With the advent of reconstructed 3D imaging, the surgeons can now evaluate the full extent of asymmetry including the cranial base and glenoid fossa (Figs. 78.5, 78.6 and 78.7). Scintigraphy or technetium scan can be done in these cases to rule out apparent hypoplasia due to hyperplasia of one side condyle (Fig. 78.13a, b).

78.1.5 Differential Diagnosis of Hemifacial Microsomia

Patient with HFM must be distinguished from those with Goldenhar syndrome, Treacher Collins syndrome, hemimandibular elongation, Parry-Romberg syndrome, juvenile rheumatoid arthritis, Nager syndrome, traumatic postnatal deformity, postaxial acrofacial dysostosis, muscle dysfunction, branchio-oto-renal syndrome (BOR), and maxillofacial dysostosis. The following is a table of distinguishing features of hemifacial microsomia and other entities (Table 78.4).

Hemifacial Microsomia with Cleft Lip and Palate

The incidence of HFM with concomitant orofacial clefting is a range between 18 and 61%, including presentations of atypical clefts and macrostomia. Fan et al. reported cleft lip with/without cleft palate in 10% of HFM patients. Thus, cleft lip and palate may actually be considered as a part of the HFM spectrum [20, 21]. The laterality and severity of presentation of cleft lip/palate correlate with the severity and side of presentation of HFM. This shows common embryological aetiopathogenesis of HFM and orofacial clefting. However, patients with HFM often present with velar deficiencies, leading to hypernasality and velopharyngeal insufficiency. Patients with HFM have a higher incidence of cleft maxillary hypoplasia than non-syndromic cleft patients. The already present abnormality in maxillary growth in HFM may further influence the midface deficiency seen in HFM patients with CL only.

78.1.6 Principles of Management of Craniofacial/Hemifacial Microsomia

The principles involved in the management of HFM are described below. We have categorized them as per age and the required intervention. Growth considerations are important in formulating treatment plan. Various challenges and treatment methods have been described in literature with focus on the mandible and TMJ reconstruction (Fig. 78.14 and Table 78.5).

78.1.6.1 Neonates and Infants

Due to the morphological severity of the skeletal deformities, severe functional compromise of the infant's airway can happen after birth. Later on, the presence of a compromised airway can also affect the child's ability to swallow. Hence, the primary management in a neonate should be focused on stabilization of the airway and assisted feeding [22].

78.1.6.2 Airway

A grossly compromised airway may necessitate procedures to maintain the patency of the child's airway and facilitate the child to thrive. These procedures are neonatal distraction (early distraction osteogenesis), tongue lip adhesion, or tracheostomy [22, 23]. The neonatal distraction has fallen into disfavour due to future unpredictable

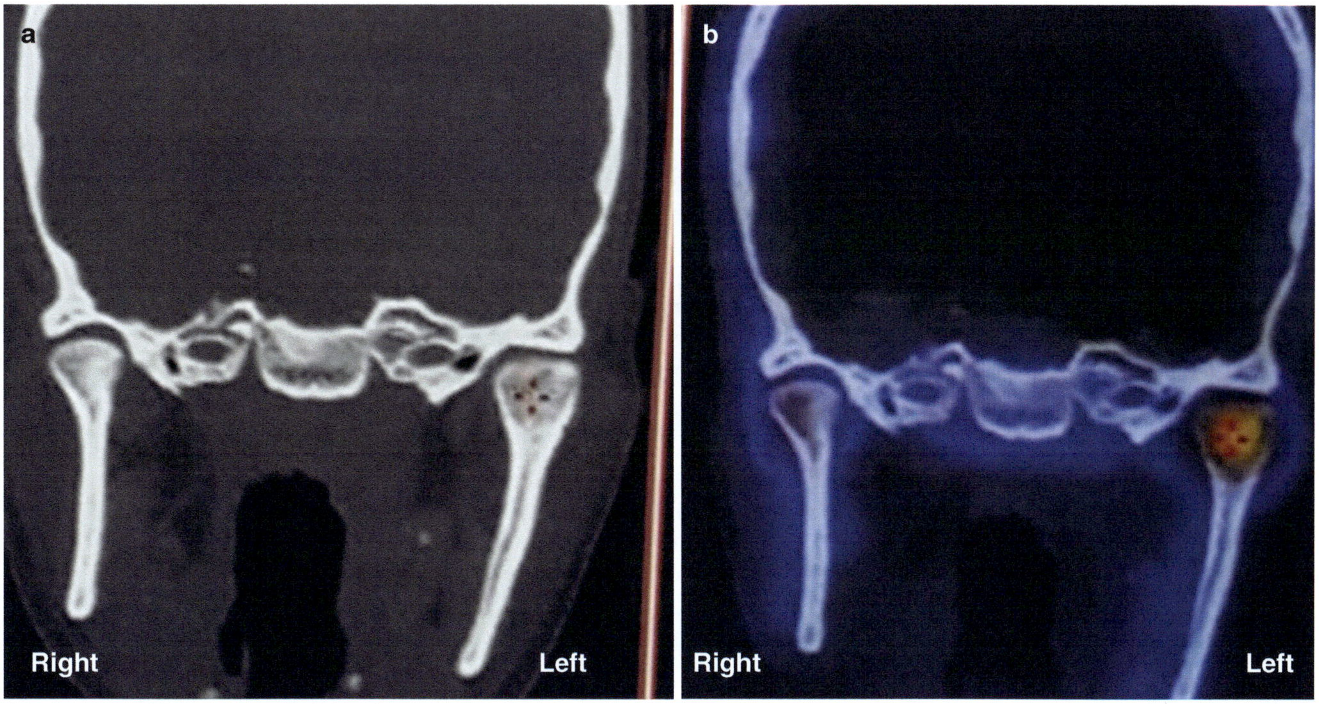

Fig. 78.13 (**a**) SPECT scan in the case of facial asymmetry. (**b**) Note the active uptake on the left side. Technetium scan can be done to rule out asymmetry due to contralateral condylar hyperplasia

Table 78.4 Differential diagnosis of Hemifacial Microsomia

Other entities	Distinguishing features
Treacher Collins	Always bilateral
Old undiagnosed condylar trauma	Condyle and ramus are short, absence of any other soft tissue features and normal ears. History of trauma at birth
Goldenhar syndrome	Vertebral anomalies and epibulbar dermoids and/or eyelid colobomas
Hemimandibular elongation	Mandible deviates to unaffected side. Normal form and size of condyle, slender neck and long ramus Not present since birth, unlike HFM
Juvenile rheumatoid arthritis	Pain and morning stiffness in the affected joint. Multi-articular nature of disease
Parry-Romberg syndrome	Facial atrophy of subcutaneous fat, associated skin, cartilage, and bone which is often unilateral and slow progressing Multisystem involvement in some cases. Presence of coup de sabre Acquired unlike HFM
Nager acrofacial dysostosis	Disorder of facial, limb, and skeletal morphogenesis

growth and possibility of tooth bud damages. Most children presenting with HFM may require assisted feeding using nasogastric tubes or gastrotomy for a few weeks to months.

78.1.6.3 Management of Associated Orofacial Clefting

The incidence of orofacial clefting occurring with HFM is approximately 10%. The most common form of clefting apart from cleft lip is Tessier 7 facial cleft or macrostomia (Fig. 78.15a, b). The cleft is repaired at 3–6 months of age as per the standard protocol [20]. Cleft lip and palate is more severe in HFM and is associated with worse outcomes. There is tissue hypoplasia and neuromuscular deficiency of pharyngeal muscles in patients with HFM. This may be responsible for the development of palatal fistulas and exacerbation of VPI, making management of cleft palate more challenging in such cases.

78.1.6.4 Intermediate Surgical and Orthodontic Management

Management during the growth phase in HFM differs from that of an adult. Intermediate surgical management includes reconstruction of the external ear which may be planned at 6–7 years as the contralateral ear achieves its full growth during this time. Reconstruction of the cranio-orbital region is usually accomplished between 7 and 9 years as calvarial growth is almost complete during this time. A split calvarial graft to reconstruct the lateral orbital rim and zygoma is the

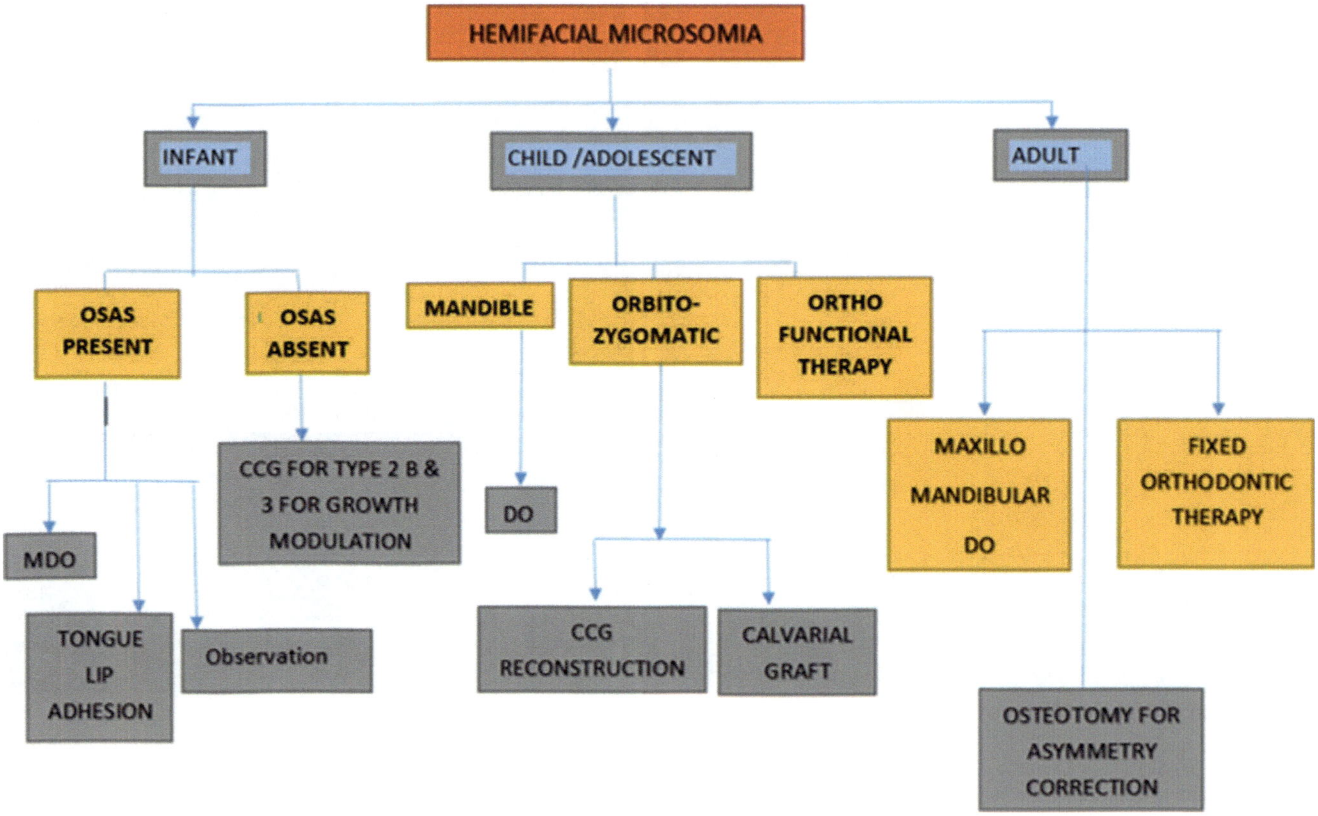

Fig. 78.14 Flowchart depicting algorithm of treatment at various levels according to growth

Table 78.5 Challenges and corrections needed necessary at different ages

Early	Intermediate (during growth)	Delayed (after completion of growth)
• Airway • Swallowing • Vision • Hearing • Cleft lip and palate	• Skeletal correction (DO) • Soft tissue correction (free fat transfer) • Nerve deficit	• Definitive skeletal correction (DO + OGS) • Soft tissue correction (fat/microvascular free flaps)

graft of choice for reconstruction of deficient zygomatico-orbital region. Surgeons have also used temporo-parietal myo-osseous flaps for better bulk, contour and retention of graft in place.

Orthopaedic growth modification can help these patients to correct occlusion in early stage [23–25]. If the patient has growth potential, with the stimulus provided by a hybrid functional appliance and stretching the soft tissue, growth can be increased on the affected side. The child must have at least 20 mm mouth opening to ensure that proper translation of condyles allows mandible growth. An asymmetric functional appliance (hybrid) that guides the mandible to a new postural position, controls the eruption of teeth and inhibits the soft tissue pressure is used [26]. It directs the developmental growth of mandible three dimensionally.

An orthodontist should constantly monitor the eruption of primary and permanent teeth to improve mandibular deficiency and maxillary canting. After the adolescent growth spurt, occlusion can be achieved by means of fixed orthodontic appliances.

78.1.6.5 Correction of Maxillomandibular Complex

Variations in the maxillomandibular complex management range from early intervention (Figs. 78.16a, b, 78.17a, b and 78.18a, b) to late reconstruction after growth completion. Wait-and-watch policy with only dental and orthodontic interventions may be adopted to reduce the impact of the deformity on the dental occlusion and masticatory function. Definitive surgical reconstruction of the maxilla, mandible and TMJ can be taken up after cessation of growth [27–31].

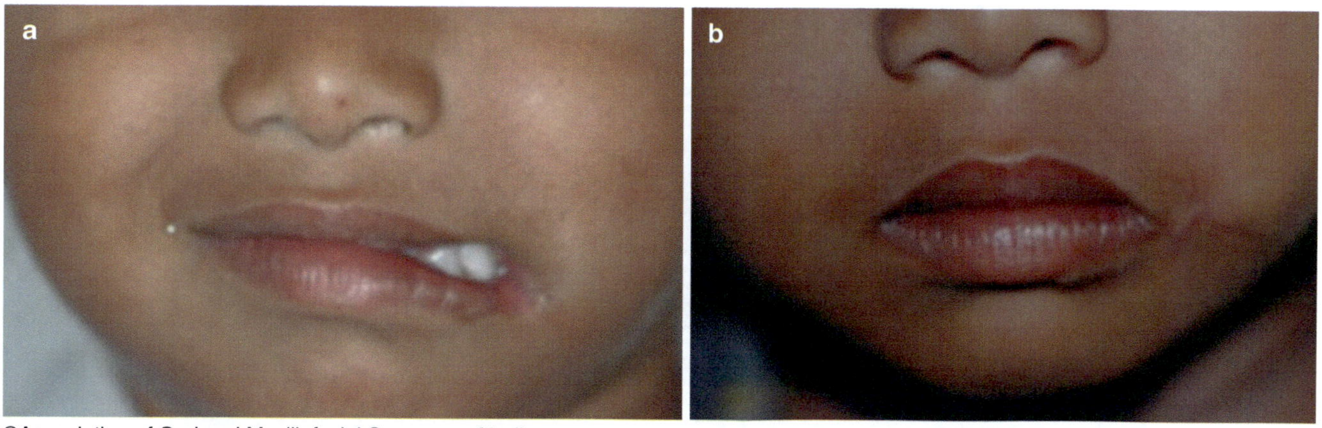

Fig. 78.15 (**a**, **b**) Surgical correction of lateral facial cleft through commissuroplasty. (**a**) pre-operative photo showing macrostomia. (**b**) post-operative photo demonstrating correction with commissure reconstruction

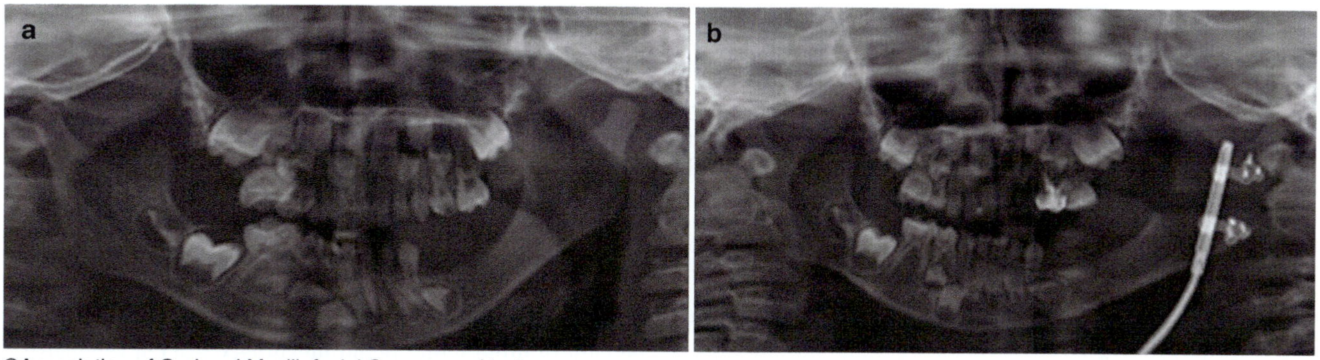

Fig. 78.16 (**a**) Preoperative radiograph-deficient left ramus and body. Note the absence of teeth and tooth buds on the left side. (**b**) Vertical ramus distraction done to achieve symmetry of the mandible and chin

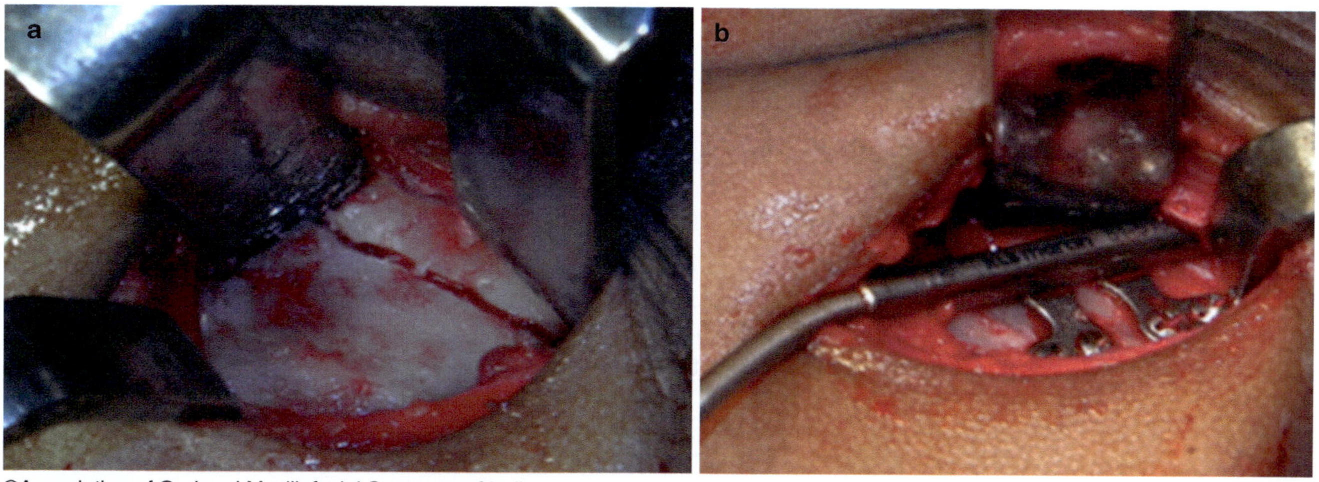

Fig. 78.17 (**a**) Intraoperative photograph of the same patient as in Fig. 78.16, showing the horizontal cut. (**b**) Distractor removal after 3 months showing consolidated anatomic bone formation

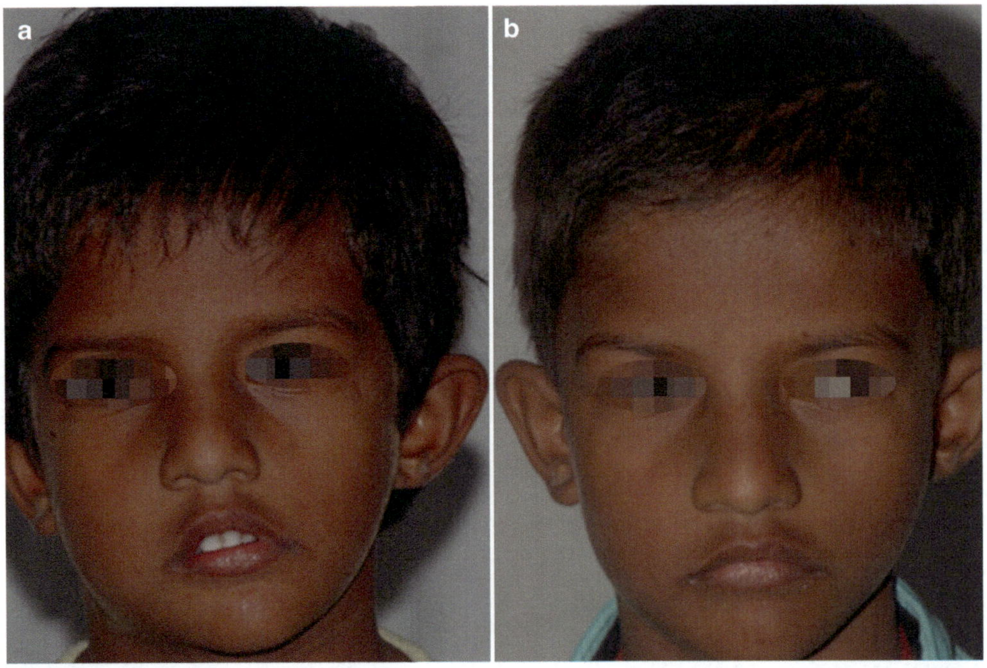

Fig. 78.18 (**a**) Preoperative frontal photo of the same patient in Fig. 78.16 showing left-sided HFM with ipsilateral chin deviation and facial asymmetry. (**b**) Postoperative view showing considerable symmetry of the face

Functional Appliance Therapy

In cases where the ramus-condyle unit (RCU) shows reasonable function to translate into skeletal growth, growth modification with the use of functional appliances does play a role by achieving the following outcomes:

1. To facilitate eruption of the dentition in a favourable pattern.
2. To prevent dentoalveolar compensatory mechanisms from worsening the deformity.
3. To passively guide the growth of the ramus-condyle unit.

The focus of functional therapy is repositioning the affected condyle to a more inferior and anterior position to enable the mandible to grow and catch up for the intrinsic skeletal deficit [29–31].

Ear Reconstruction

Construction of the external ear is a priority in the aesthetic management of HFM patients. Two important factors that affect the ability to construct the ear are the decreased anteroposterior dimension of the upper face and the absence of an adequate platform (i.e. temporal bone cavity). The position and quality of the soft tissue remnants should also be kept in mind while planning surgery. An ear reconstructive surgeon and the maxillofacial surgeon should work collaboratively to determine the most ideal location of the ear relative to the future constructed ramus-condyle unit. Reconstruction options include (1) autogenous rib cartilage, (2) alloplastic options such as Medpore, and (3) tissue-engineered auricular framework. The technique of ear reconstruction is dealt with in detail in Chap. 35 on "Ear Reconstruction".

Though autologous chondral cartilage for reconstruction still remains the best option, it requires a multistage approach to (1) harvest the costal cartilage grafts and create a framework by carving (time-consuming and fixation and retaining of shape challenges), (2) place the graft (positioning as per existing altered morphology), (3) transpose the lobule (soft tissue deficiency—tissue expander may have to be used) and (4) create a post-auricular sulcus (with skin graft and split temporalis graft) (Fig. 78.19a, b).

Various materials have been used for alloplastic ear reconstruction with varied results. Porous polyethylene's inert nature and pore size provide and allow for some tissue ingrowth and are safe to use. The alloplastic materials always carry a risk of rejection and infection and may not have accurate sizes and shapes as they are stock implants with limited sizes.

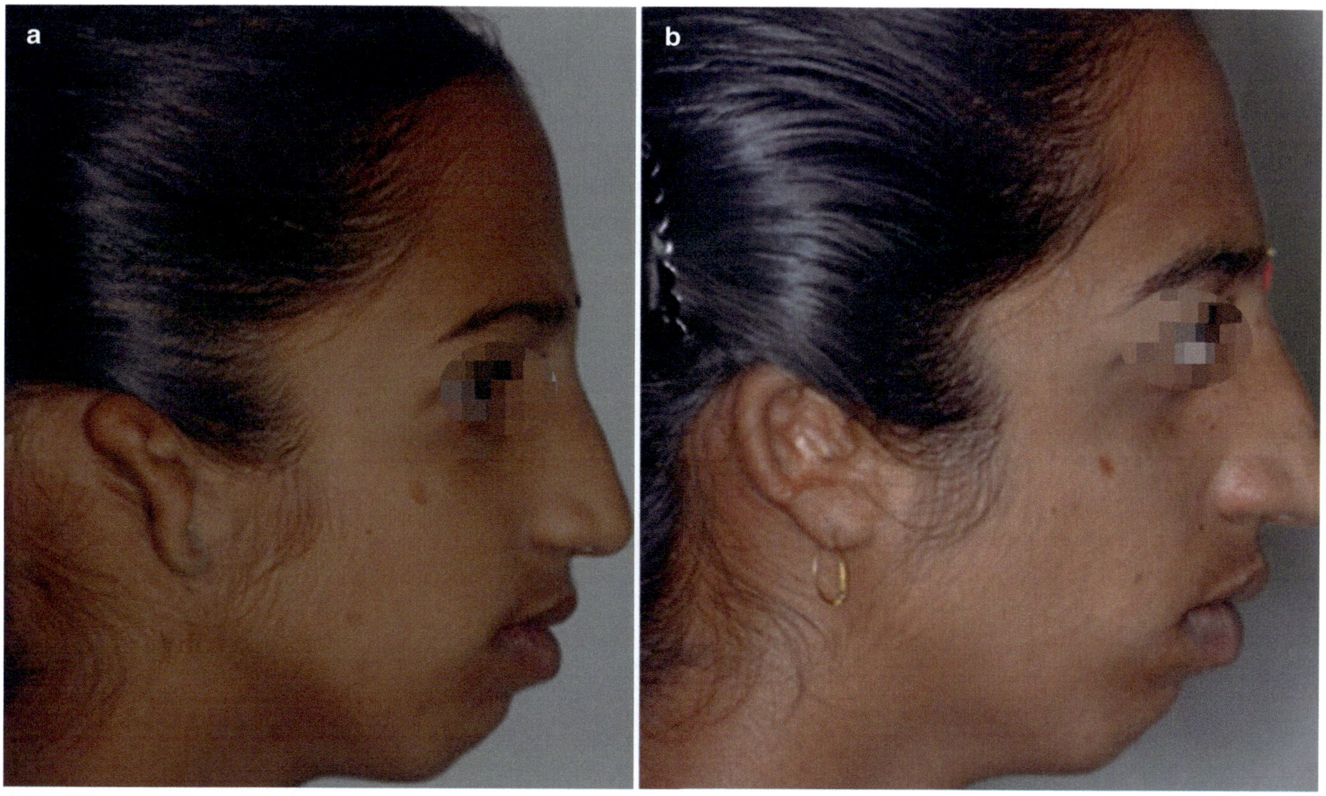

Fig. 78.19 (**a**) Pre- and (**b**) post operative photograph of ear reconstruction using rib graft (Also refer Chap. 35 on Ear reconstruction)

Tissue-engineered 3D cartilage reconstruction and its use in regular clinical practice are under trial in many parts of the world though long-term clinical studies still lack regarding its application and optimal results.

Delayed Management in Adults

Management in adults includes definitive reconstruction for skeletal and residual soft tissue deficits. With the advent of 3D imaging and computer-assisted surgical planning and printing, precise spatial relationship of the cranial structures with maxillomandibular complex can be studied. This printed models give the surgeon extra weapon outside theatre to simulate surgery and make appropriate decisions before going to theatre. Appropriate treatment plan can be virtually executed, and a CAD-CAM splint can be fabricated to facilitate the accurate surgical outcome [32, 33] (Table 78.6).

Table 78.6 Principles of management of the deformed temporomandibular joint

Type of TMJ involvement	Management
Type I	Correction of vertical dimension Adjusting maxillomandibular relationship and facial asymmetry
Type IIa	Augmentation of RCU, preservation of condyle/ glenoid fossa
Type IIb	Neocondyle reconstruction/preservation of glenoid fossa, augmentation of RCU + type I management
Type III	Neocondyle and glenoid reconstruction, augmentation of RCU + type I management Autogenous or alloplastic reconstruction (refer Chap. 89)

Orthodontics for Definitive Skeletal Surgery

Orthodontic preparation before definitive surgical correction of the face is similar to the conventional pre-surgical orthodontic protocols. These include arch levelling and alignments, de-crowding and transverse widening if necessary. Compromise may be necessary in many cases due to the extreme lingual tilt on the affected premolar-molar areas, leaving few options for the orthodontist due to limited bone availability for straightening the teeth [29, 30].

Conventional orthodontic treatment may take longer period and may necessitate the use of anchorage screws for aligning some teeth.

Type 1 and 2A

In types 1 and 2A, the glenoid and condylar components of TMJ are morphologically intact with minimal hypoplasia. There is no specific indication for the reconstruction of the TMJ since the joint exhibits normal movement characteristics, and the patient is able to demonstrate adequate mouth opening and masticatory function. Deviation while mouth opening can be seen towards the affected side.

Teeth eruption and angle of its placement will be hampered even in these two types of situations which will require further definitive treatment. Simultaneous maxillomandibular distraction introduced by Monasterio and Molina is an alternate method for achieving maxillary and mandibular corrections without disturbing the dental intercuspation and occlusal cant [34] (Figs. 78.20a, b and 78.21a, b).

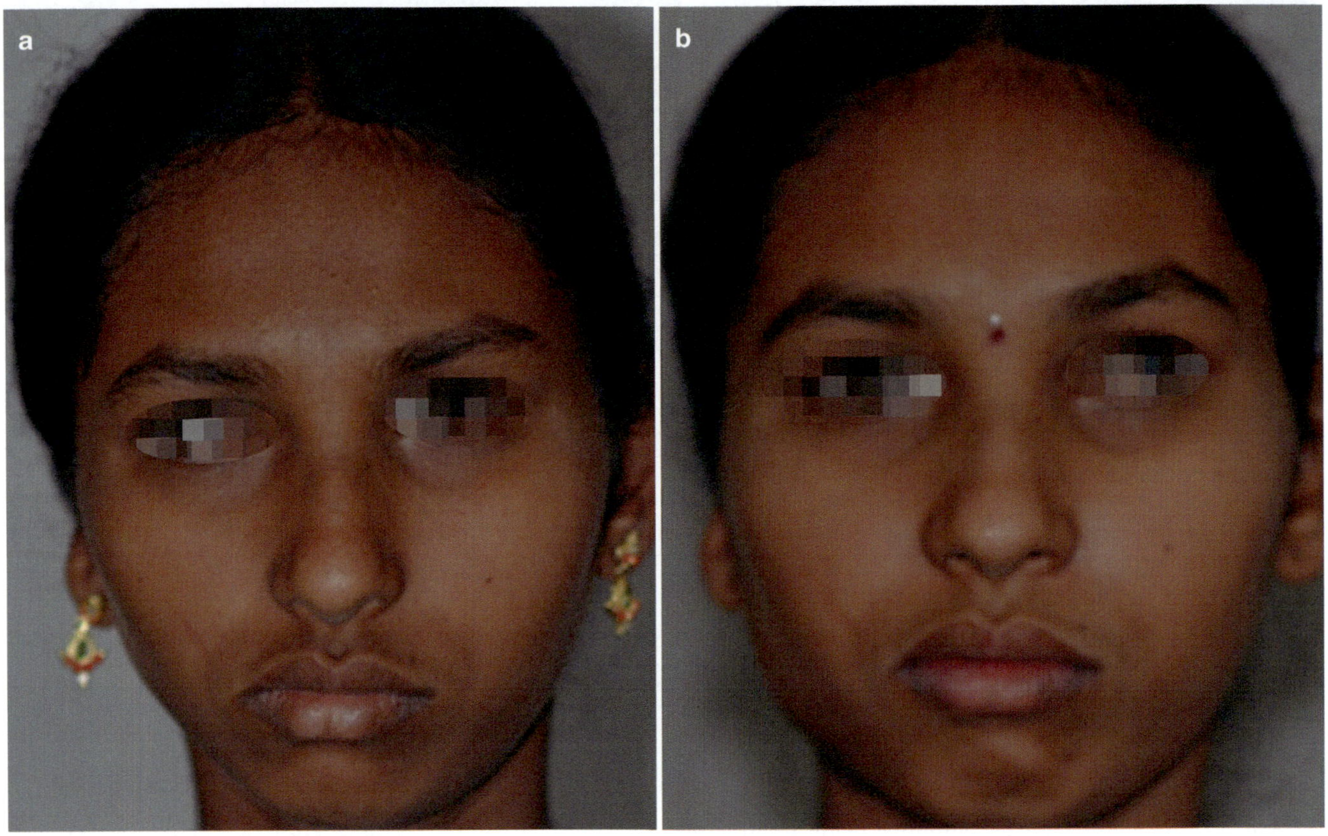

Fig. 78.20 (**a**) Preoperative view showing right-sided maxillomandibular deficiency. (**b**) Postoperative view showing correction of asymmetry following simultaneous maxillomandibular distraction

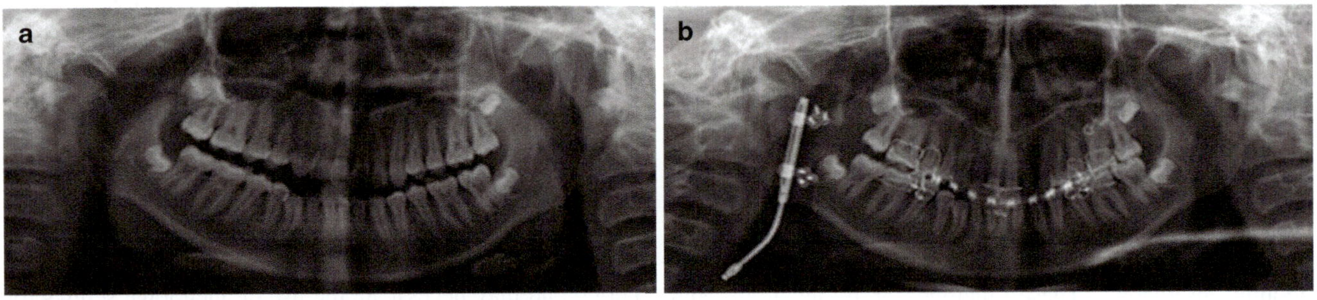

Fig. 78.21 (**a**, **b**) Radiographs of the same patient as in Fig. 78.20 treated with maxillomandibular distraction (Molina's technique). (**a**) Pre-distraction orthopantomogram demonstrating vertically deficient ramus-condyle unit on the right side. (**b**) Post-distraction xray showing lengthening of the right ramus-condyle unit with the distractor in-situ

Type 2B

Type 2B patients exhibit severe hypoplasia of both the condylar and the glenoid elements of the joint, thus causing altered functioning of the joint. This greatly reduces or there is a complete absence of the translatory movement of the joint sparing the rotatory movement. The mandible may completely deviates towards the affected side. The arc of rotation completely shifted, leading to malocclusion and scissor bites sometimes.

Distraction osteogenesis can be used to correct the deficiency of the mandibular body along with reshaping the glenoid and condylar process. The use of osteotomies to correct the dentofacial deformity is also performed either in the same setting or in a staged manner.

Options for reconstruction of the ramal-condylar unit are another concern which can be approached with costochondral grafting and alloplastic joint reconstruction [35]. The costochondral graft for stimulated growth should be used by the age of 7 years, which can be used as an onlay graft on top of the existing ramal segment in the correct position of glenoid fossa. However, large series of cases with success in this technique lacks the scientific evidence of growth similar to the unaffected joint, and reports of under- and overcorrection are plenty in literature.

Type 3

Patients with Type 3 deformities require total reconstruction of the TMJ, i.e. the glenoid-zygomatic complex region and the ramal-condylar unit. For the growing adolescent due to growth completion, glenoid reshaping and costochondral graft reconstruction of the RCU may be undertaken. Total alloplastic joint reconstruction with concomitant orthognathic surgery should be done in adults.

Posterior distraction of existing mandibular segment to create ramal-condylar unit has ended up with limited success due to lack of posterior support of distraction advancing segment and unpredicted movement in 3D dimensions. It was found in authors' experience that the correct direction control of upwardly directing condylar segment is difficult to achieve towards a missing or defective glenoid fossa, and many times the position can alter more medial and anterior than expected rather than posterior towards external auditory meatus.

Management of the Maxillomandibular Complex

Type 1

The minimal asymmetry and deformity associated with a Type 1 HFM may be amenable to minor surgical corrections such as genioplasty (Fig. 78.22a, b). Since the occlusion may

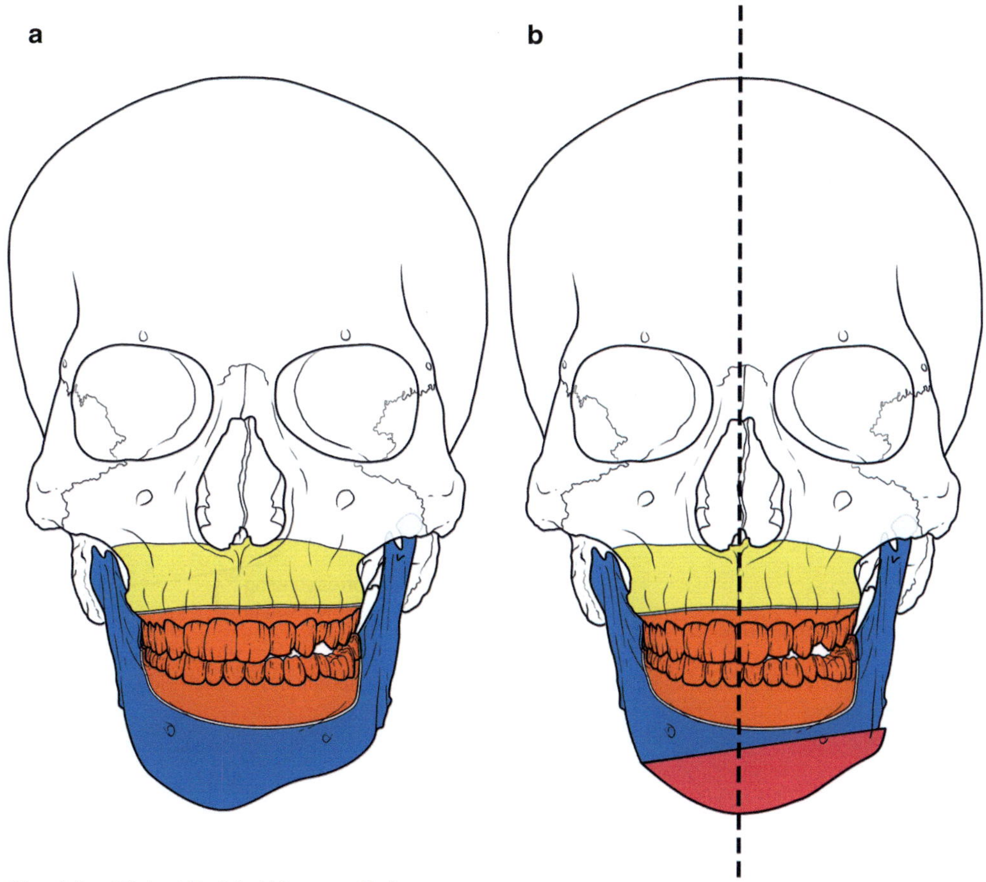

Fig. 78.22 (**a**, **b**) Diagrammatic representation of surgical management of Type 1 Kaban-Pruzansky (**a**) deformity with isolated genioplasty for asymmetry correction (**b**)

be normal or demonstrate minimal occlusal canting, orthognathic surgical correction may not be warranted.

In cases with minimal asymmetry where the patient is not willing to undergo a surgery of the entire maxilla-mandibular complex, it is possible to achieve facial midline symmetry by means of altering the midline chin and mandibular body orientation through an extended operation involving the basal bone of the chin and body of the mandible. It was published by Paul C Salins in 2008 [36]. The author of this chapter was happy to have learned this technique from Salins himself and greatly understood the concept of this 3D movement of genial bone along with body and ramus of the mandible to the unaffected side without altering the occlusal relationship of the maxilla or mandible.

But this technique had obvious disadvantage in the form of significant relapse due to large movements and requirement for multiple points of fixation.

At this juncture, the author of this chapter has designed a distractor which can be placed below the lower border of the mandible to move the genial-body-ramus unit in desired direction by incremental distraction similar to other distraction protocols. This completely eliminated the need for any plate usage, better stability without relapse and more or less excellent unlimited movement in all three directions. This is completely a basal bone distraction which can be either performed in isolation or in combination with other distractions and osteotomies of the maxilla-mandibular skeleton (Figs. 78.23a, b, 78.24a, b, and 78.25a, b).

One of the key advantages of MDO is that the bone movement produces good contour of the chin area along with flat unaffected part of the mandible, and it obviously stretches and accommodates the redundant excess submental-submandibular skin available to a more symmetrical position as shown in Fig. 78.26a, b.

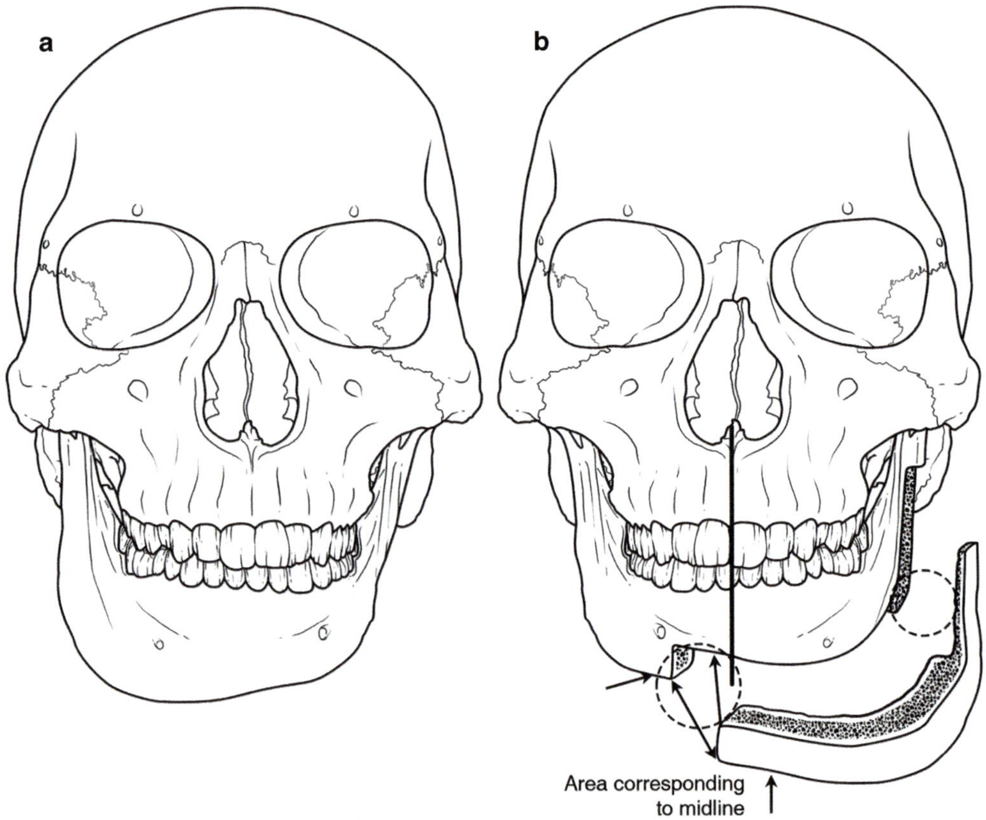

Fig. 78.23 (**a**, **b**) Orthomorphic correction of deficient mandible. (**a**) Diagrammatic representation of a left sided HFM, (**b**) osteotomy design for correction of the left sided deficiency

Type 2A

Patients with Type 2A deformities require planned presurgical orthodontic interventions for definitive orthognathic correction (Fig. 78.27a–d).

Bimaxillary surgery is planned to achieve the following goals:

Maxilla and midface

1. Segmental maxillary procedures for correction of cross-bites.
2. Derotation of the maxilla to achieve midline corrections.
3. Augmentation of the zygomatic complex where necessary.
4. Cant correction.

Mandible

1. Bilateral sagittal split osteotomy procedure to correct the occlusal canting and yaw correction.
2. An inverted "L" or a subsigmoid osteotomy is indicated to achieve elongation of the RCU.

Types 2B and 3

As explained earlier, types 2B and 3 patients require reconstruction of the TMJ as the primary goal. This may be executed either as a Stage 1 correction with only maxillomandibular correction or as Stage 2 with joint reconstruction (Fig. 78.27).

Thus, although skeletal correction improves the dental occlusion and skeletal symmetry, it may accentuate the existing soft tissue discrepancy. Soft tissue augmentation should be taken up after hard tissue correction. Various methods are available such as fat transfer, microvascular free flap for adipose tissue transfer and alloplasts such as Medpore and nanogels to give shape to deficient soft tissue (Fig. 78.28a, b).

78.1.7 Controversies in Surgical Management of HFM

Growth Considerations and Role of Early Mandibular Reconstruction in HFM.

HFM has been reported as a nonprogressive disorder, i.e. proportional deficiency of the face is maintained throughout the growth of the child. Indications for early reconstruction of the RCU during early childhood, especially in types 2B and 3

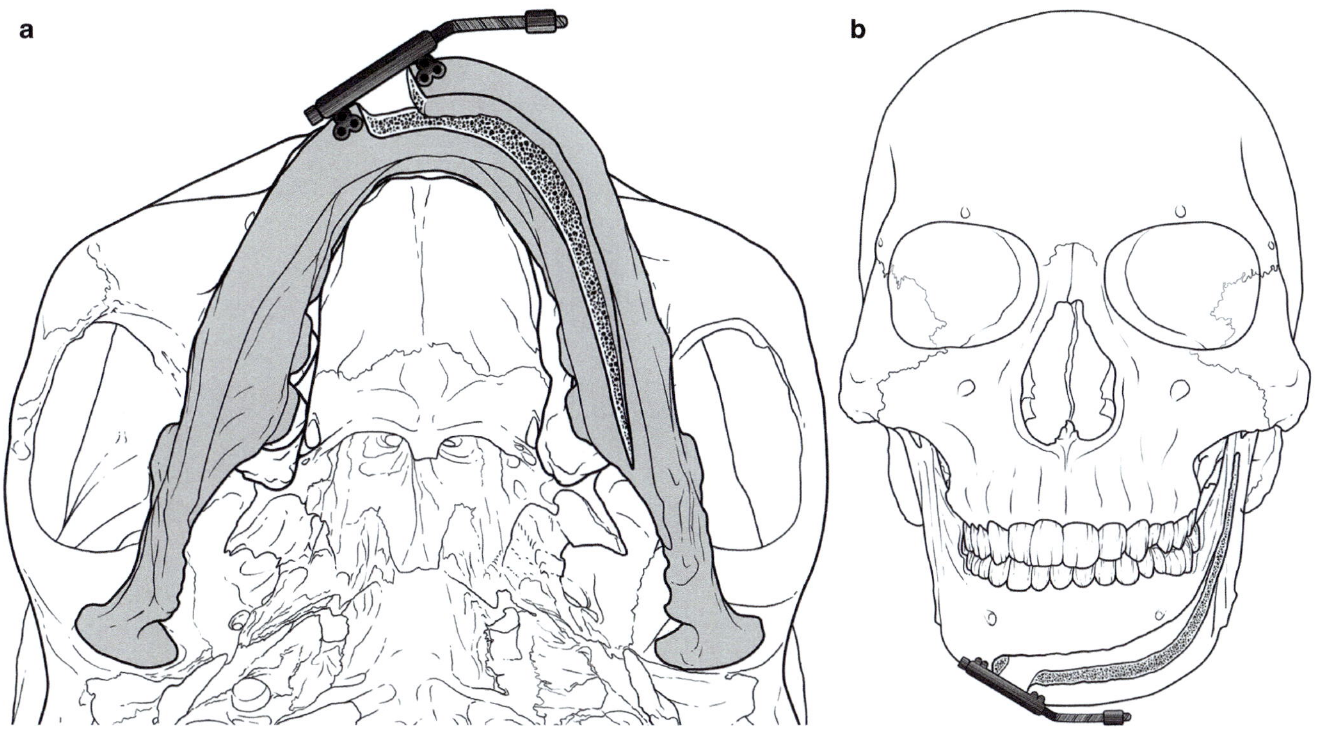

Fig. 78.24 (**a**, **b**) Pictorial view of basal bone osteotomy and orthomorphic distractor placement. (**a**) Basal view showing distractor position for orthomorphic distraction method, (**b**) frontal view of the distractor postion

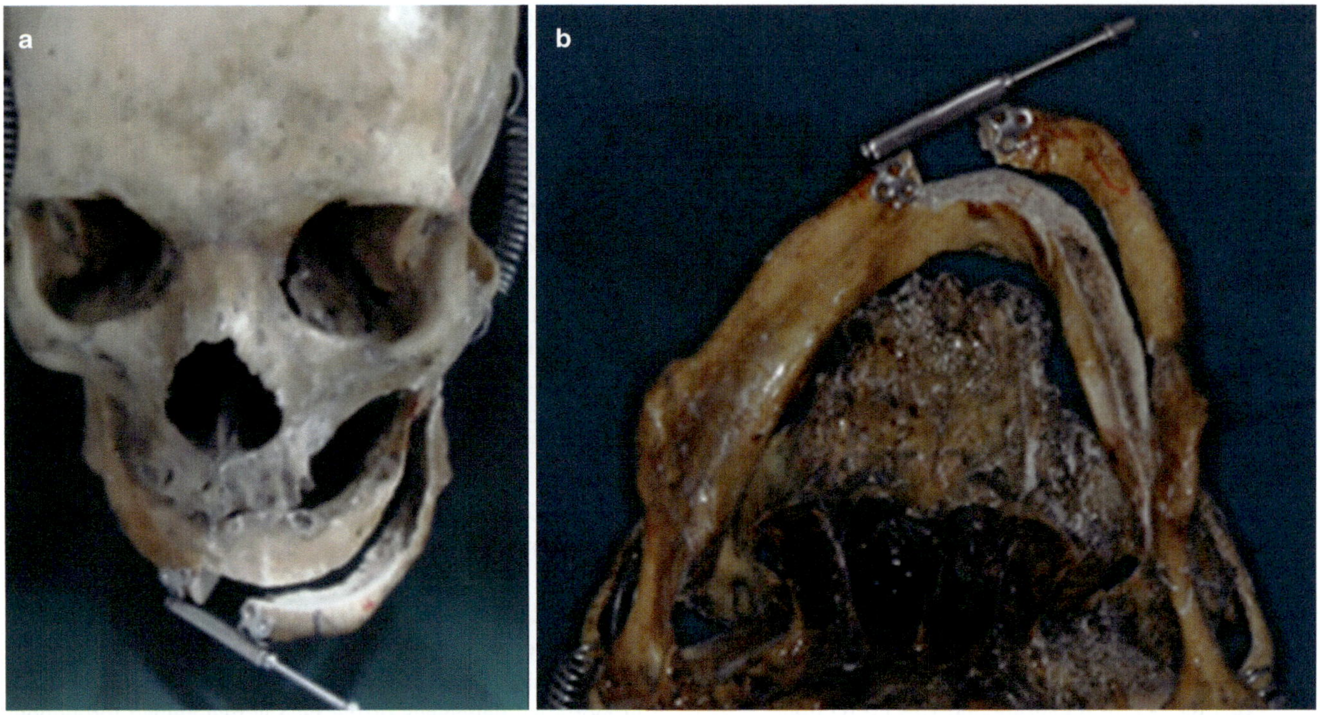

Fig. 78.25 (**a**, **b**) Indigenous distractor made and modified, placement showed in a dry skull mandible. Note the placement of distractor on the basal bone. (**a**) frontal view of distractor placement, (**b**) basal view

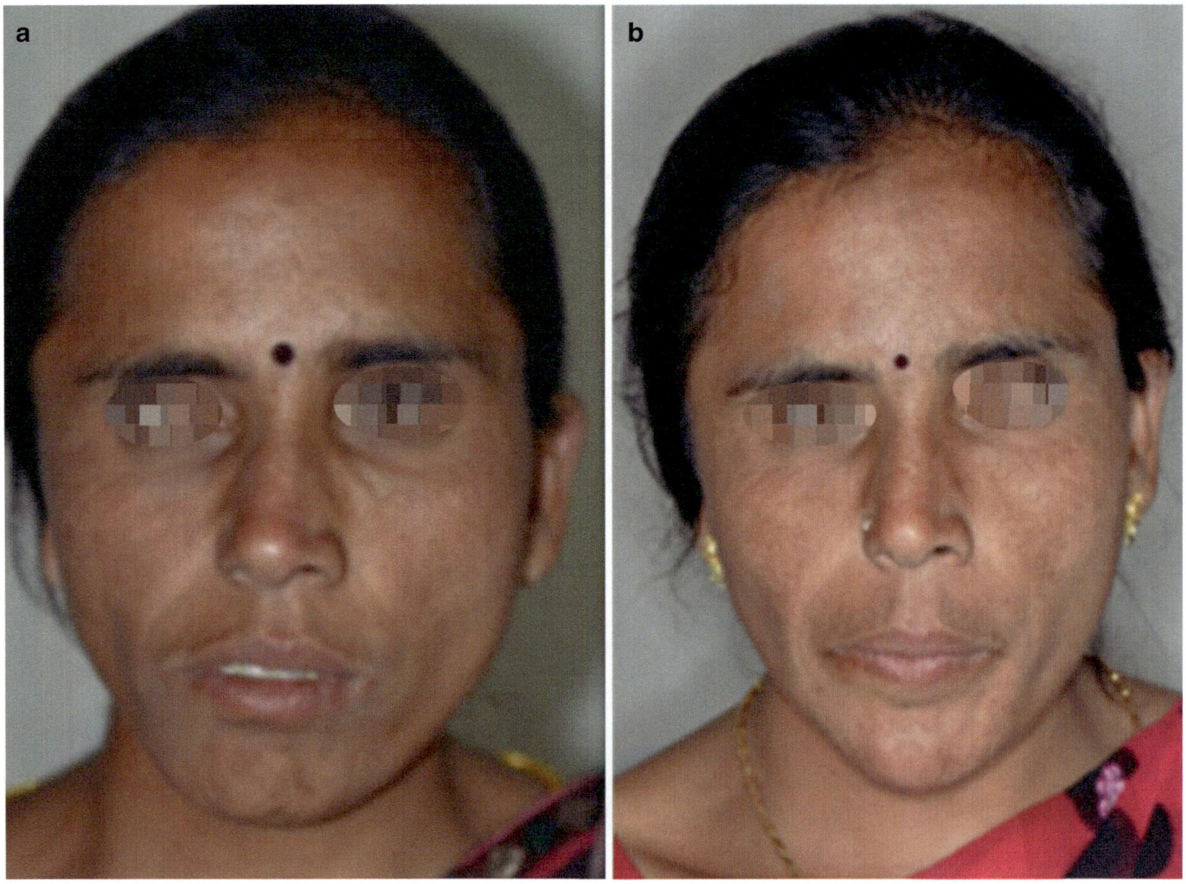

Fig. 78.26 (**a**, **b**) Orthomorphic distraction done in a patient having hemifacial microsomia. (**a**) Pre- and (**b**) postoperative photograph showing achievement of anatomic chin and contour and mandibular asymmetry

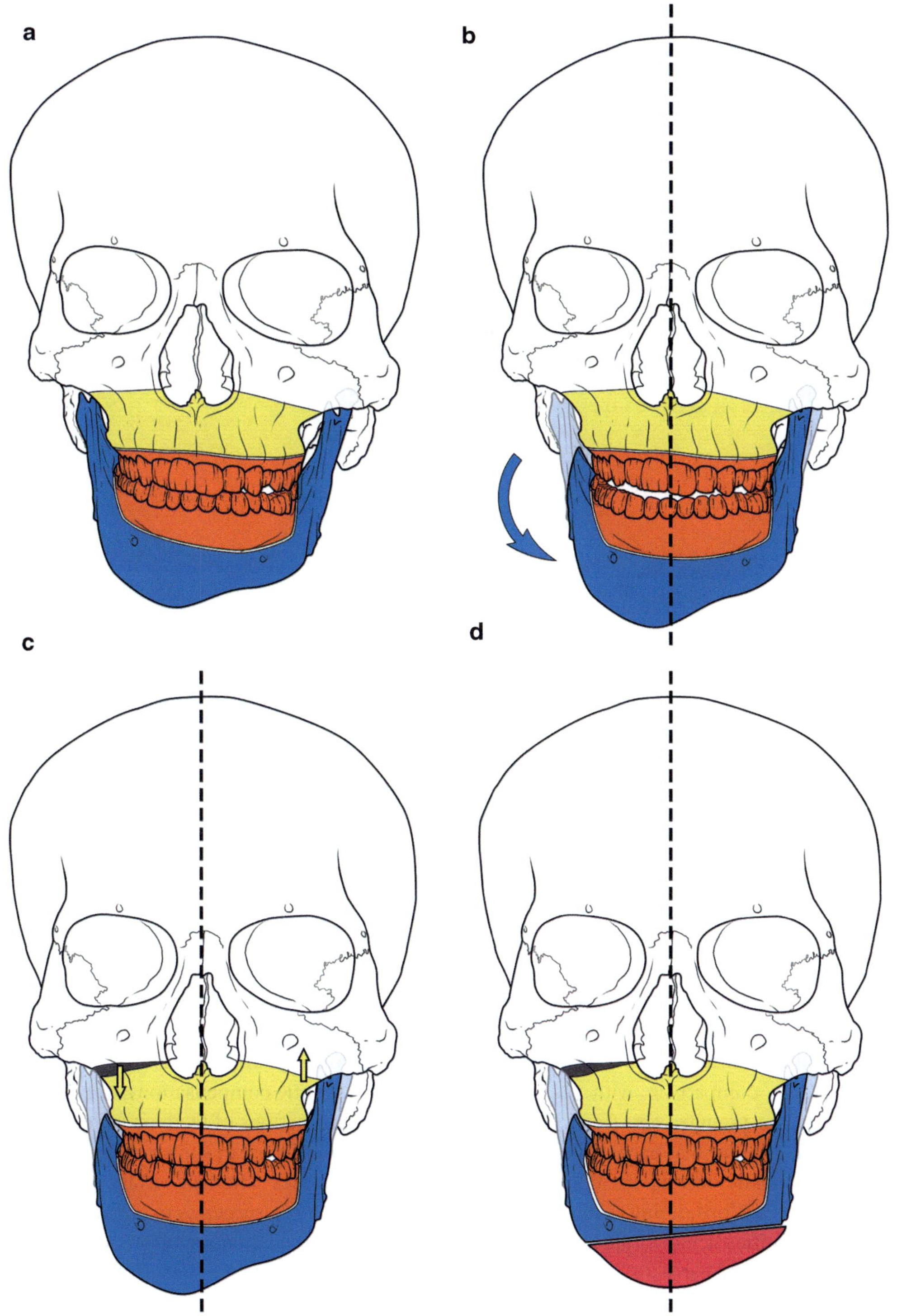

Fig. 78.27 (**a**–**d**) Diagrammatic representation of surgical management of Type 2 Kaban-Pruzansky deformity (**a**). Derotation of the maxilla-mandibular complex by orthognathic surgery (**b** and **c**). Midline skeletal correction with a centring genioplasty (**d**)

classes, has mixed reports of success. Longitudinal studies provide evidence for stable results with early osteodistraction in mild-to-moderate skeletal deformities [20, 33, 34] (Type 1 and Type 2A). However, the role of mandibular distraction may be more relevant in severe deformities. It is also suggested that early intervention makes definitive final correction easier to achieve, since the extent of deformity is reduced.

78.1.8 Long-Term Results

Long-term evaluation of growing HFM patients treated by surgical correction and distraction osteogenesis depends on two main factors: the time of intervention and the severity of the skeletal deformity. According to Hollier et al., by achieving normal mandibular dimensions at a young age, it is

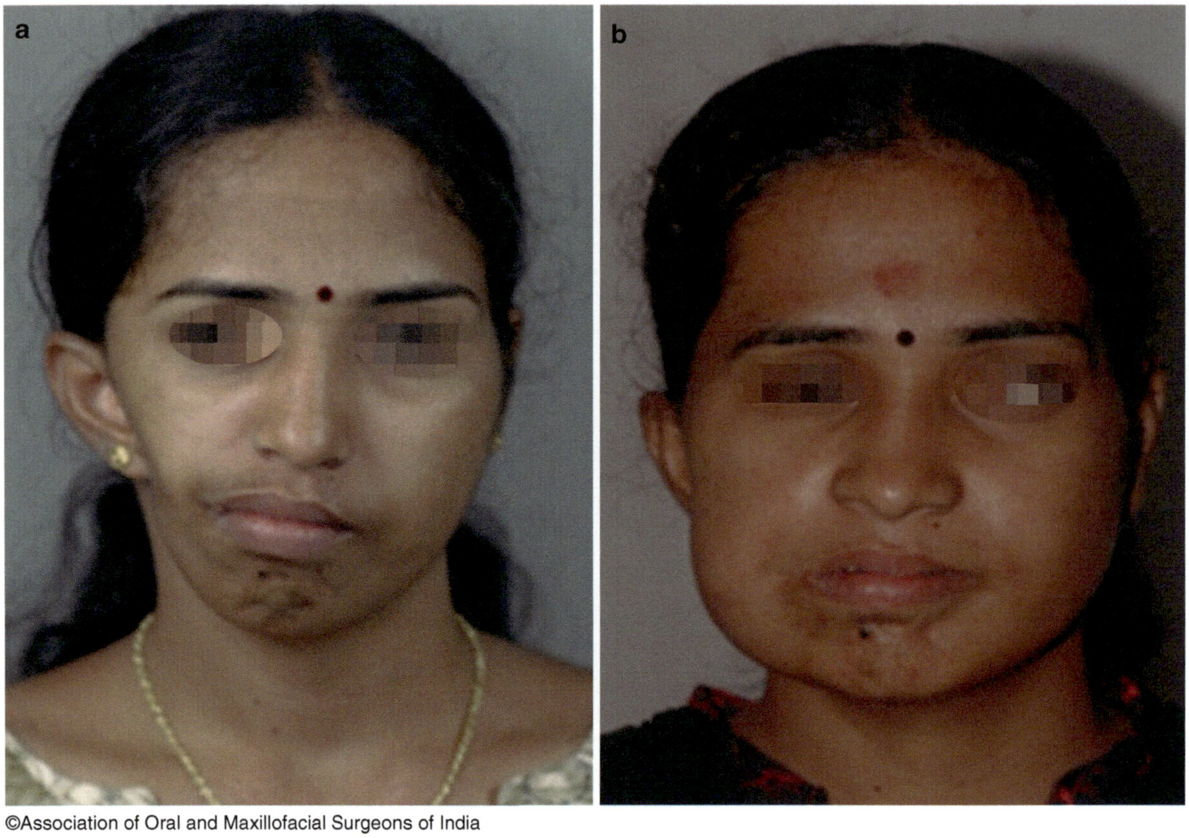

Fig. 78.28 (a, b) Soft tissue augmentation using abdominal autologous fat transplant. (a) pre-surgical frontal view demonstrating severe right sided deficiency in a patient with HFM, (b) frontal view showing soft tissue augmentation

hypothesized that the maxilla, overlying muscle and soft tissue envelope may develop along with a balanced functional matrix [19]. Proponents of mandibular distraction believe that an early intervention would prevent the secondary compensations from taking place or would unravel the compensations at the onset. This means the contralateral and ipsilateral distortions can be reduced in comparison with patients not undergoing distraction in the younger age (Figs. 78.29a, b and 78.30). Clinicians have found that early distraction can also prevent the long orthodontic decompensation phase followed by orthognathic surgery. Considering severity of deformity, the more severe deformities demonstrate less stable and favourable results when attempted early.

The indications for early skeletal correction maybe (1) compromise of airway necessitating immediate mandibular lengthening irrespective of age and (2) negative psychological impact on the child in school-going age.

In authors' experience irrespective of area and direction of distraction in the mandible or in maxilla in younger age, the following findings were concluded in 20 years of clinical follow-up:

1. It is difficult to predict the future growth of already distracted area of bone though claims of growth potential on distracted bone have been debated by many.
2. In majority of the cases, the intensity of the severity of the disease has reduced due to distraction than simply curing the disease as the age advances.
3. The 3D volume achievement in the ipsilateral side is difficult to achieve irrespective of technique of distraction and conventional osteotomies in later ages.
4. Orthodontic compensations, alignment and other associated corrections of teeth on a weak hypoplastic bone are difficult at least in some cases.
5. Many cases after pubertal age needed conventional orthognathic surgeries to achieve symmetry.
6. Soft tissue augmentation was necessary in many patients to balance the soft tissue profile equal on both sides.
7. Compromised occlusions and dental rehabilitation were necessary in some cases especially Type 2B and Type 3 cases and accepted as standard norms to finish orthodontic alignments.
8. The airway disease is not cured to 100% in all cases due to extreme variability treatment outcomes and procedures followed by different surgeons.
9. Expectations of the patient may not be achieved completely, so caution should be given to patient the compromised results outcomes in extreme cases of asymmetry.

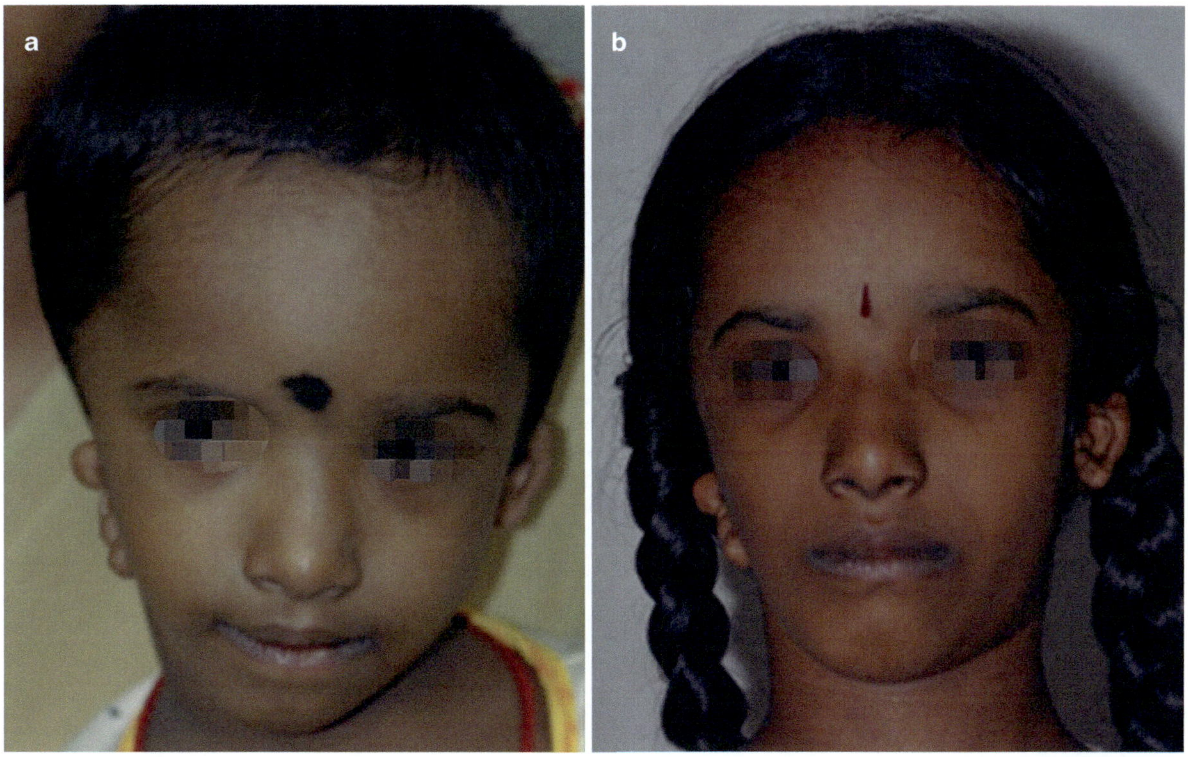

Fig. 78.29 (**a**, **b**) Long-term results of patient treated with mandibular distraction in childhood. (**a**) frontal photo of patient with right sided HFM at, (**b**) frontal photo of patient after 8 years follow up

10. Alloplastic prosthetic condyles should be reserved as a last resort if all other techniques fail to achieve a functionally stable total agenesis of condyles [21].

78.1.9 Recent Advances

The assessment of facial topography using non-invasive methods, such as laser surface scanners, stereophotogrammetry or ultrasonographic measurements, has been recently reported in several studies. Particularly, 3D stereophotogrammetry for the evaluation of soft tissue surface facial asymmetry has been extensively studied [36]. In distraction osteogenesis, recent advancements like automated distraction using battery-operated and hydraulic distractors have been tried. Since hemifacial microsomia involves bone augmentation in a multiplanar fashion, the advent of curvilinear and multiplanar distractors has greatly helped overcome this challenge [37, 38].

Tissue-engineered osteogenic material comprising of culture-expanded mesenchymal stem cells (MSCs) and platelet-rich plasma (PRP) can now be injected at the distraction site to ensure more predictable bone formation. Not only animal studies but also clinical trials have demonstrated that this material can effectively regenerate osseous tissue [39, 40].

78.2 Treacher Collins Syndrome

78.2.1 Introduction

Treacher Collins syndrome (TCS), also called mandibulofacial dysostosis (MFD), is an autosomal dominant disorder of craniofacial development with variable penetrance. It has a worldwide incidence of 1 in 50,000 live births (Gorlin et al. 1990) [41]. Early descriptions were given by Berry (1889), Treacher Collins (1900) and Franceschetti and Klein in 1949. Therefore, this entity is also named as Berry's syndrome and Franceschetti-Zwahlen-Klein syndrome [42, 43]. While 40% of TCS cases have a previous family history, 60% of cases could possibly arise as a result of de novo mutations (Jones et al. 1975) [44].

The TCOF1 gene plays an important role during early embryonic development for tissues derived from the first and second branchial arches, ectodermal clefts and endodermal pouches. TCOF1 gene encodes a nuclear phosphoprotein "Treacle" that may serve as a link between rRNA gene transcription and pre-rRNA processing. TCOF1 mutation leads to abnormal neural crest cell migration or anomalies in the extracellular matrix [45]. Sulik et al. also documented excessive cell death in the maxillary and mandibular processes of the first branchial arch and the apical ectodermal ridge of the limb bud [46]. These deductions have been made on the basis of experimental studies wherein animals were exposed to

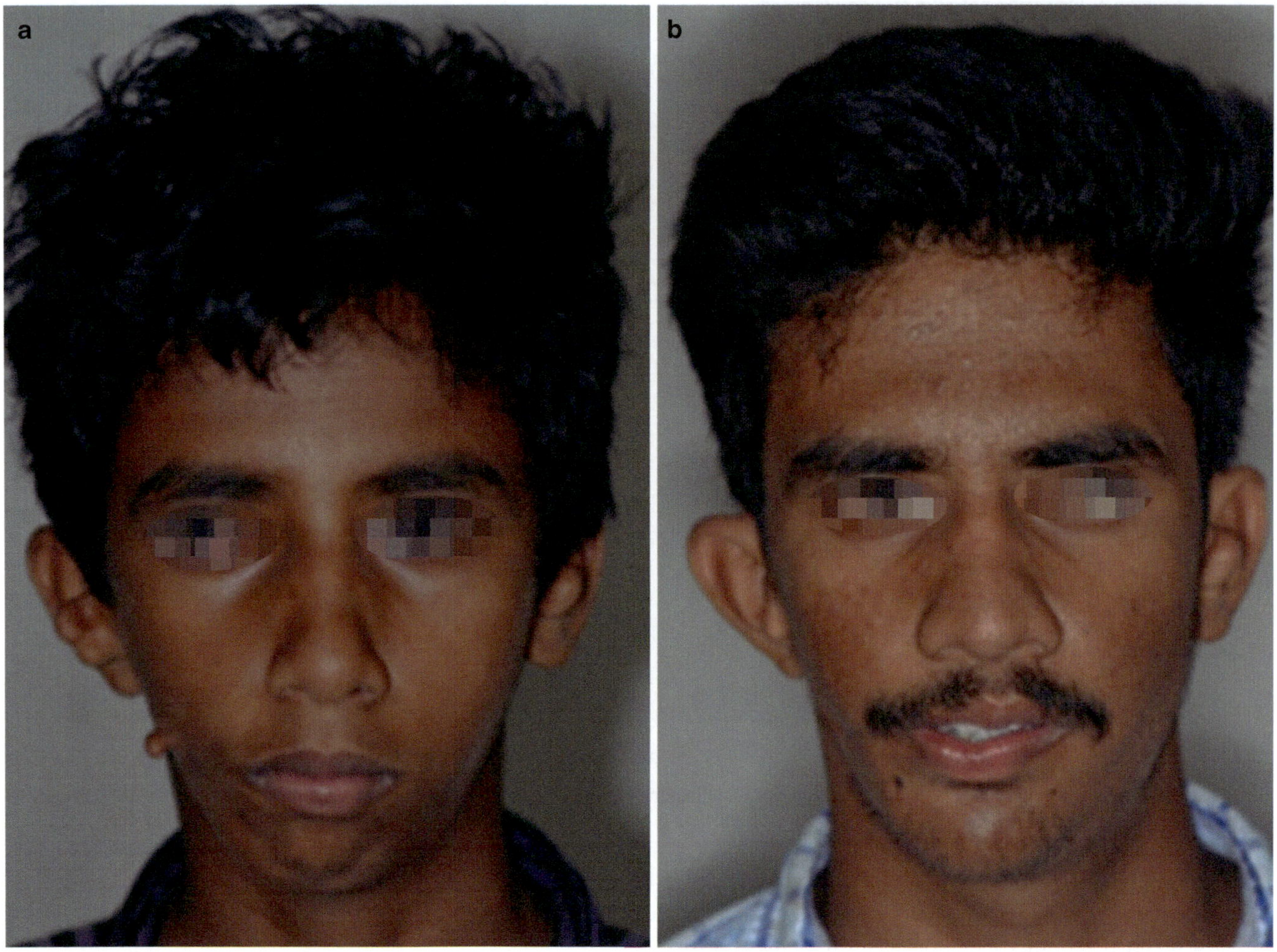

Fig. 78.30 (**a, b**) Definitive skeletal management of patient with HFM. (**a**) Preoperative Frontal photo of patient with right sided HFM at 15 years of age. He underwent mandibular distraction for correction of asymmetry followed by second stage Bi maxillary orthognathic surgery at 18 years of age (Fig. 78.7a). (**b**) Stable skeletal results after a 7 year followup when patient is 25 years of age

teratogenic cis- or trans-retinoic acid during embryonic development. Recently, Dauwerse et al. [47] detected mutations in genes encoding subunits of RNA polymerases I and III in Treacher Collins patients.

Normally, prenatal diagnosis is recommended for families with a history of TCS using fetoscopy or ultrasound imaging [USG]. Prenatal diagnosis using either of these methods can only be performed in the second trimester of pregnancy (approximately 18 weeks). Due to the late nature of the diagnosis, termination of pregnancy can be a particularly traumatic procedure. Imaging with USG has improved immensely in recent years [e.g. 3D sonography], allowing non-invasive prenatal diagnosis to be made. However, mild cases of TCS are still difficult to diagnose. Genetic counselling is highly recommended for affected individuals and their families for prevention of further affected child birth.

78.2.2 Clinical Features and Presentation

The complete spectrum of features which can be present are explained in the table below [48] (Table 78.7).

A case of Treacher Collins syndrome in a 13-year-old female with the following features (Fig. 78.31a, b):

- Eyes: Antimongoloid palpebral fissures are short and slope laterally downwards with either a notch or coloboma of the outer third of the lower eyelid. Lashes are absent medial to coloboma.
- Face: Bilateral and usually symmetric hypoplasia of facial bones is present, e.g. malar and mandibular bones. Depressed cheekbones, receding chin, tongue-shaped process of the hair that extends towards the cheek and large down-turned mouth can be identified.

- Ears: Malformation of the external, middle and inner ear, with low implantation of the auricle which is common. The pinnae are often crumpled and misplaced towards the angle of the mandible. Bat-fan ears, deafness, microtia, extra ear tags and blind fistulas [which may occur anywhere between the tragus and the angle of the mouth] are the other common findings.
- Oral findings: Cleft palate, congenital palatopharyngeal incompetence, high-arched palate and a narrow maxillary and mandibular arch with dental crowding are common (Fig. 78.32a–e).
- Nose: The nose appears larger due to the hypoplastic midface skeletal structures. Hypoplastic alar cartilages, narrow nares and obliteration of the nasofrontal angle are also common.

Table 78.7 Clinical features of TCS

Region	Characteristic feature
Eyes	Antimongoloid slant of palpebral fissures
	Colobomata and hypoplasia of the lower lids and lateral canthi
	Hypertelorism
	Partial absence of eyelid cilia
Ears	Microtia
	Conductive hearing loss
	Hypoplasia of middle ear ossicles
Nose/mouth	Nasal deformity
	Cleft palate with or without cleft lip
	High-arched palate
	Class II or III malocclusion open bite
Facial bone formation	Hypoplasia of the malar bones
	Hypoplastic lateral aspects of orbits
	Hypoplastic maxilla and mandible
	Variable effects on the temporomandibular joints
	Anterior open bite
	A steep occlusal plane

78.2.3 Imaging for TCS

The conventional OPG and the lateral and frontal cephalometric image are pivotal in diagnosing TCS along with clinical correlation. The OPG helps identify the following: hypoplastic condyle with a short condylar neck, absent articular eminence, shortened ramus-condyle unit and severely hypoplastic coronoid process (Figs. 78.33 and 78.34). The lateral cephalogram shows a severely retrognathic mandible with microgenia, clockwise-rotated maxillomandibular complex and a reduced posterior airway space. However, three-dimensional computed tomography [3DCT] is the gold standard in diagnosis as well as treatment planning (Fig. 78.35a–c). The features that are remarkably seen on the 3DCT are hypoplasia of the orbito-zygomatic complex, poorly developed lateral orbital and supraorbital ridges, mandibular hypoplasia and reduced overall facial width. The orbits are hyper-teloric and the infraorbital foramen is usu-

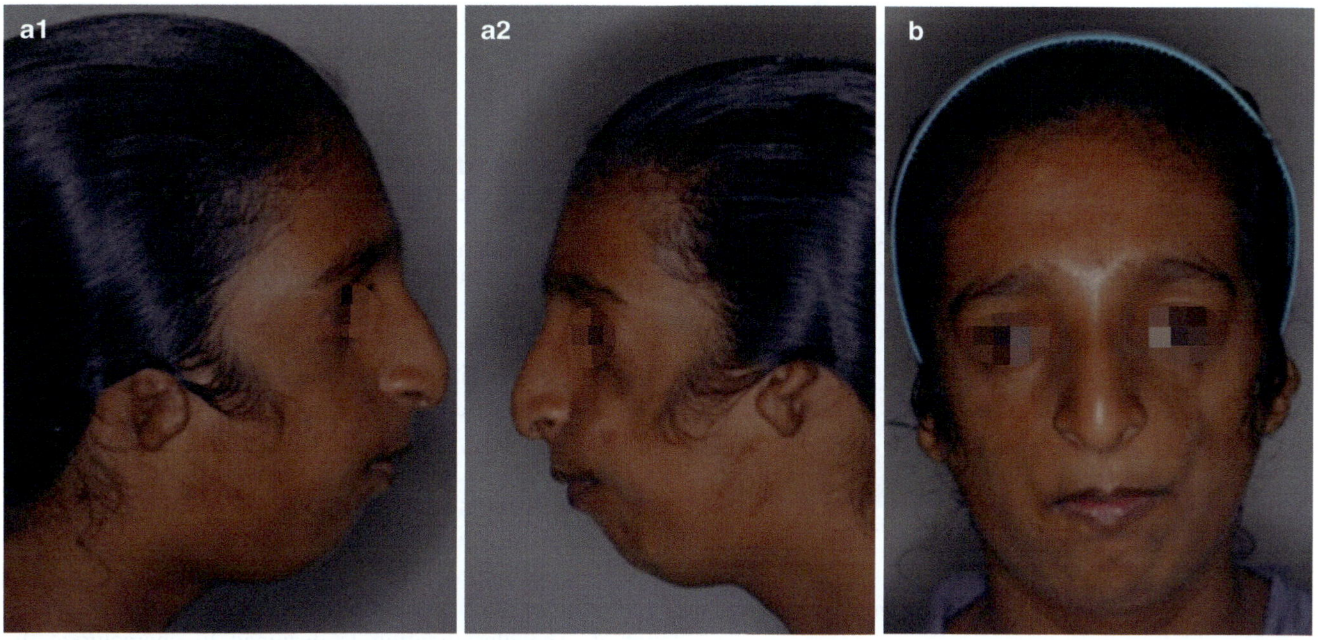

Fig. 78.31 (**a, b**) Case of a 13-year-old female with Treacher Collins syndrome, (**a**) profile and (**b**) frontal photos (Also see Fig. 78.41b)

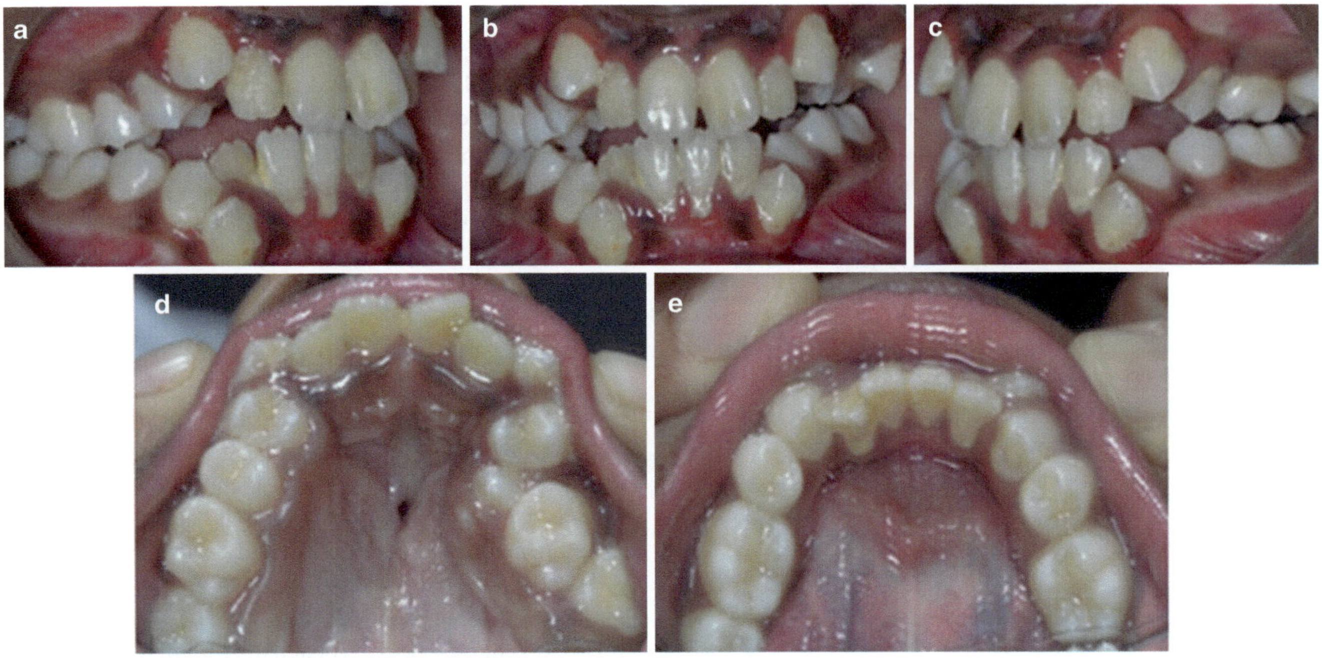

Fig. 78.32 (**a–e**)Intraoral pictures of the same patient in Fig. 78.30 showing operated cleft palate, mixed dentition stage with severe crowding. (**a–c**) frontal and lateral intra-oral dental views, (**d**) maxillary occlusal and (**e**) mandibular occlusal views

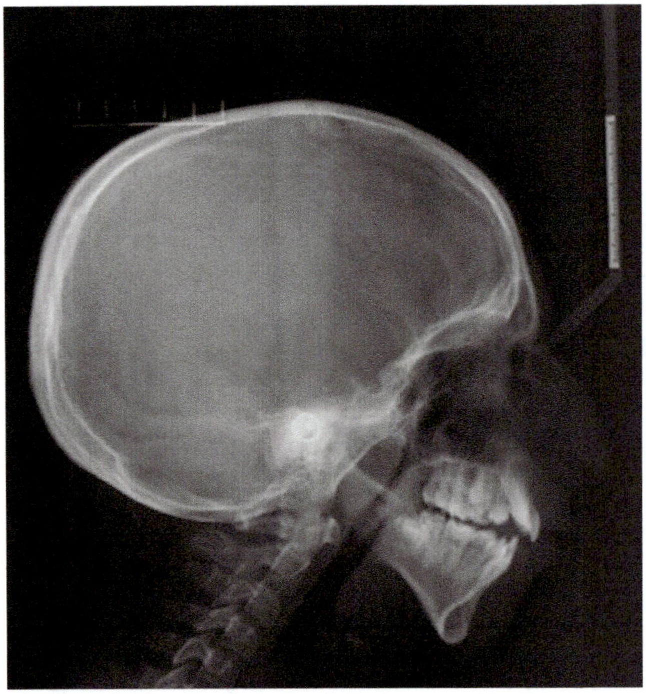

Fig. 78.33 Lateral cephalogram of the same patient in Fig. 78.31 showing reduced posterior airway space, micrognathia and microgenia

ally absent. The paranasal sinuses are often small and may be completely absent. Furthermore, the mastoids are not pneumatized and are frequently sclerotic. The cranial base is also progressively kyphotic [48]. Lastly, these patients require

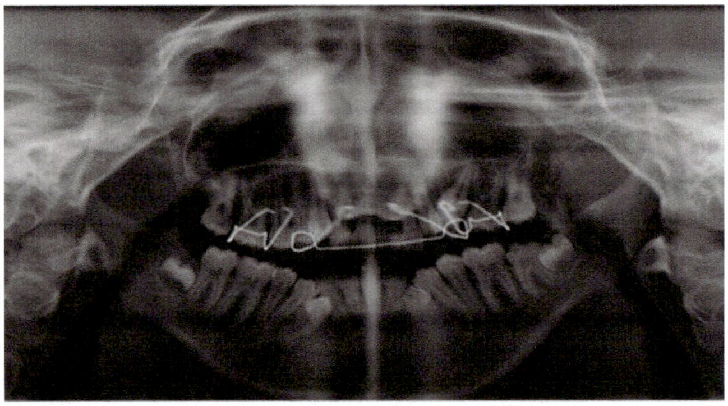

Fig. 78.34 Orthopantomogram of the same patient in Fig. 78.31 showing hypoplastic ramus-condyle unit

long-term follow-up in order to evaluate the effects of mandibular growth, airway dimensions, degree of surgical relapse and the need for additional surgical intervention.

78.2.4 Proposed Classification

A classification system of the orbito-zygomatic skeletal deformities seen in TCS has been proposed by Nikkah D et al. The classification is designed to characterize the degree of deformity and as a guide to the reconstructive planning [49]. Treatment planning becomes complex as TCS can have a variable presentation with respect to the severity of the hypoplasia/dysplasia of the skeletal and soft

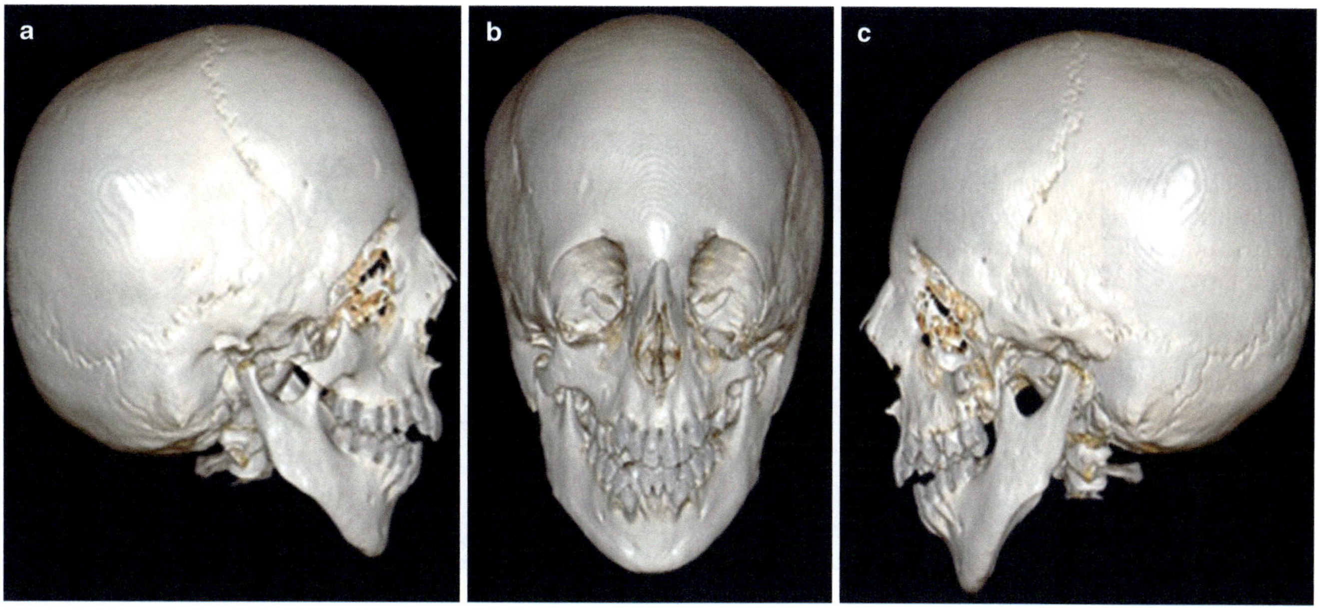

Fig. 78.35 (a–c) 3DCT view of TCS patient showing hypoplasia of orbito-zygomatic complex. (a) Right lateral view demosntrating type 2b deformity, (b) frontal view showing type 2b deformity on the right and type 3 deformity on the left, (c) left lateral view showing type 3 deformity

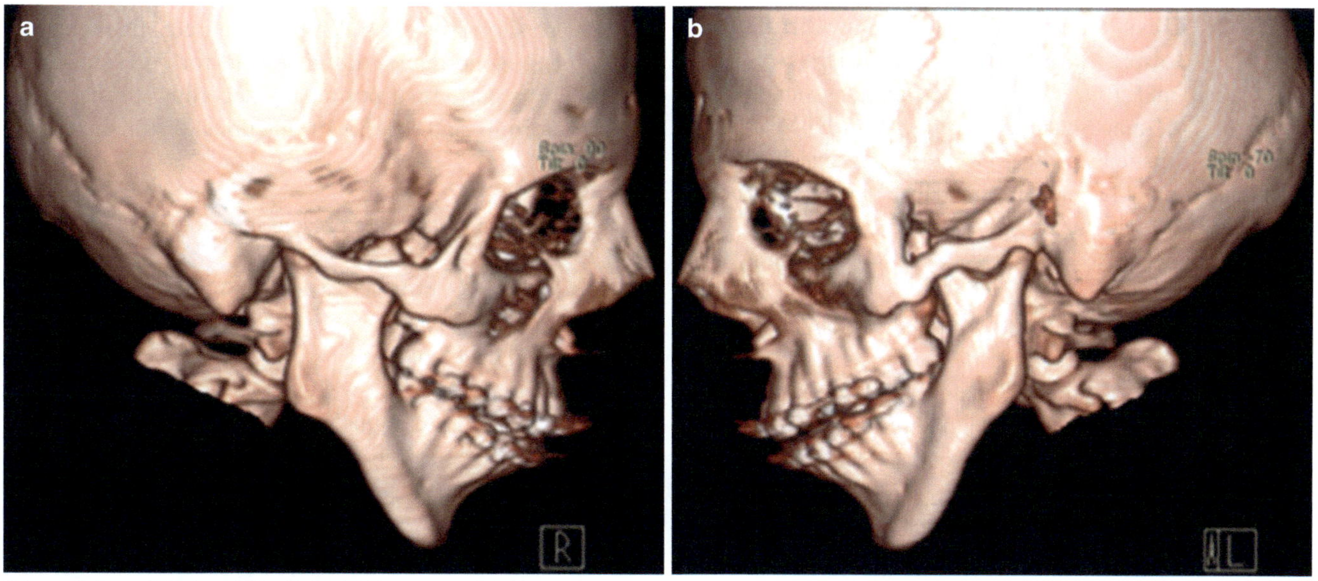

Fig. 78.36 (a, b) Type 1: Patients have the entire orbito-zygomatic complex present but the region is dysplastic and hypoplastic

tissue elements, shape and position of the affected structures and resulting functional deformity. Thus, the challenges faced in treating TCS are similar to those faced in treating HFM.

78.2.4.1 Methods

- *Type 1*: orbito-zygomatic complex present but, dysplastic and hypoplastic (Fig. 78.36a, b).
- *Type 2*: a hypoplastic zygomatic body with a vestigial zygomatic temporal process and a lateral orbital wall that is either dysplastic (2a) or absent (2b) (Fig. 78.35a, b).
- *Type 3:* a hypoplastic zygomatic body and dysplastic orbital wall but with complete absence of the zygomatic temporal process (Fig. 78.35b, c).
- *Type 4*: complete absence of the entire orbito-zygomatic complex (Fig. 78.37a, b).

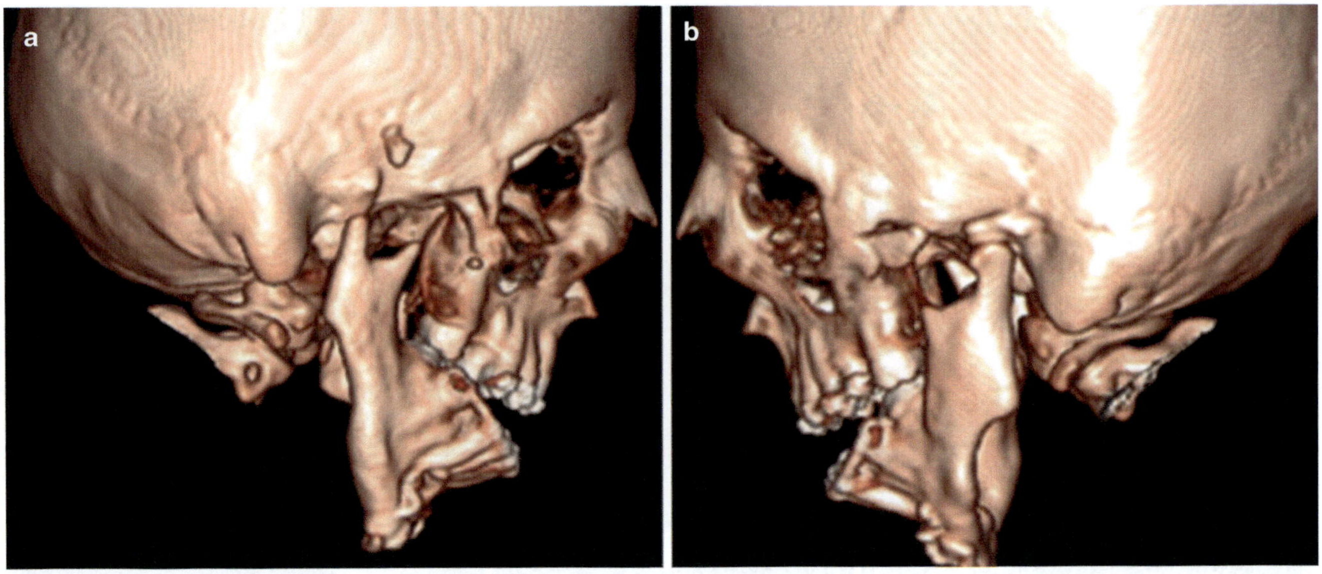

Fig. 78.37 (**a**, **b**) Type 4: Is the most severe with complete absence of the entire orbito-zygomatic complex

There is not always a symmetrical classification as 25% of the TCS demonstrated asymmetry.

78.2.4.2 Classification of Temporomandibular Joint and Mandibular Malformation

The Kaban and Pruzansky classification system for the degree of TMJ-mandibular malformation in HFM is applicable to TCS patients as well [13, 26]. This classification is useful in defining the anomalies and directing reconstruction similar to HFM patients.

78.2.5 Differential Diagnosis

Differential diagnosis of TCS includes acrofacial dysostosis (Nager and Miller syndromes) and oculo-auriculo-vertebral spectrum (hemifacial microsomia and Goldenhar syndrome).

Nager syndrome has facial features similar to that of TCS. In addition, the thumb[s] may be hypoplastic, aplastic or duplicated, and there may be fusion of the radius and ulna. Miller syndrome also has features similar to TCS. Ectropion or outturning of the lower lids is an additional diagnostic feature. Clefting of the lip and palate is more common in this syndrome than in TCS [50]. HFM primarily affects development of the ear, mouth and mandible. Goldenhar syndrome has a spectrum of deformities that include those of HFM in addition to vertebral abnormalities and epibulbar dermoids [51].

78.2.6 Treatment

Though there have been immense medical advances in terms of in utero surgery, stem cell therapy and genetic manipulation, there is currently no treatment for TCS in utero. Treatment is performed postnatally according to the nature of the deformity and severity of functional disturbance [52].

The following issues are present in case of TCS:

1. Airway, i.e. obstructive sleep apnoea.
2. Feeding problems.
3. Brain development.
4. Orbito-zygomatic growth.
5. Mandibular retrognathism with open bite.
6. Dentoalveolar issues including orthodontic alignment.
7. Cleft palate.
8. Hearing issues.
9. Psychosocial development.
10. Deficient soft tissue.

These issues can challenge clinicians from birth to adulthood as concerns vary from aesthetic to functional in nature. Thus, a multidisciplinary approach is indispensable for achieving optimal outcomes.

78.2.6.1 Multidisciplinary Management: Team Members Necessary from Birth to Adult Stage

1. Geneticist.
2. Paediatrician.
3. Anaesthetists.
4. Oral and maxillofacial surgeon.
5. Orthodontist.
6. Paedodontist.
7. General dentist.
8. Paediatric neurosurgeon.
9. Psychiatrist.
10. ENT surgeon.
11. Audiologist.
12. Pulmonologist.
13. Paediatric neuro-physician.
14. Speech therapist.
15. Oculoplastic surgeon.

78.2.6.2 Airway Management

Syndromic patients [e.g. TCS] with micrognathia suffer from OSA frequently due to narrowing of the upper airway [53]. Despite respiratory effort, partial or complete obstruction of the upper takes place, leading to frequent episodes of oxygen desaturation and sleep disruption. In the long term, OSA can harm an individual's physical and mental health, as has been documented recently in the literature [54].

Respiratory compromise is due to two reasons:

(i) Maxillary hypoplasia, constricting the nasal passages and resulting in a degree of choanal stenosis or atresia.
(ii) Mandibular micrognathia and a retro-positioned tongue obstructing the oropharyngeal and hypopharyngeal airway.

Earlier, long-term tracheostomy was the only solution available for severe cases of infantile OSA. However, long-term tracheostomies are commonly associated with morbidities like tracheomalacia, chronic bronchitis, throat tightness and dislocation of the tracheostomy tube [55] (Fig. 78.38a, b). Today, distraction osteogenesis [DO] has become the favoured treatment method for TCS patients with OSA. Mandibular advancement by means of DO helps in increasing the posterior airway space, thus relieving the symptoms of OSA and preventing severe respiratory distress [56]. Due to the unique mandibular and oropharyngeal anat-

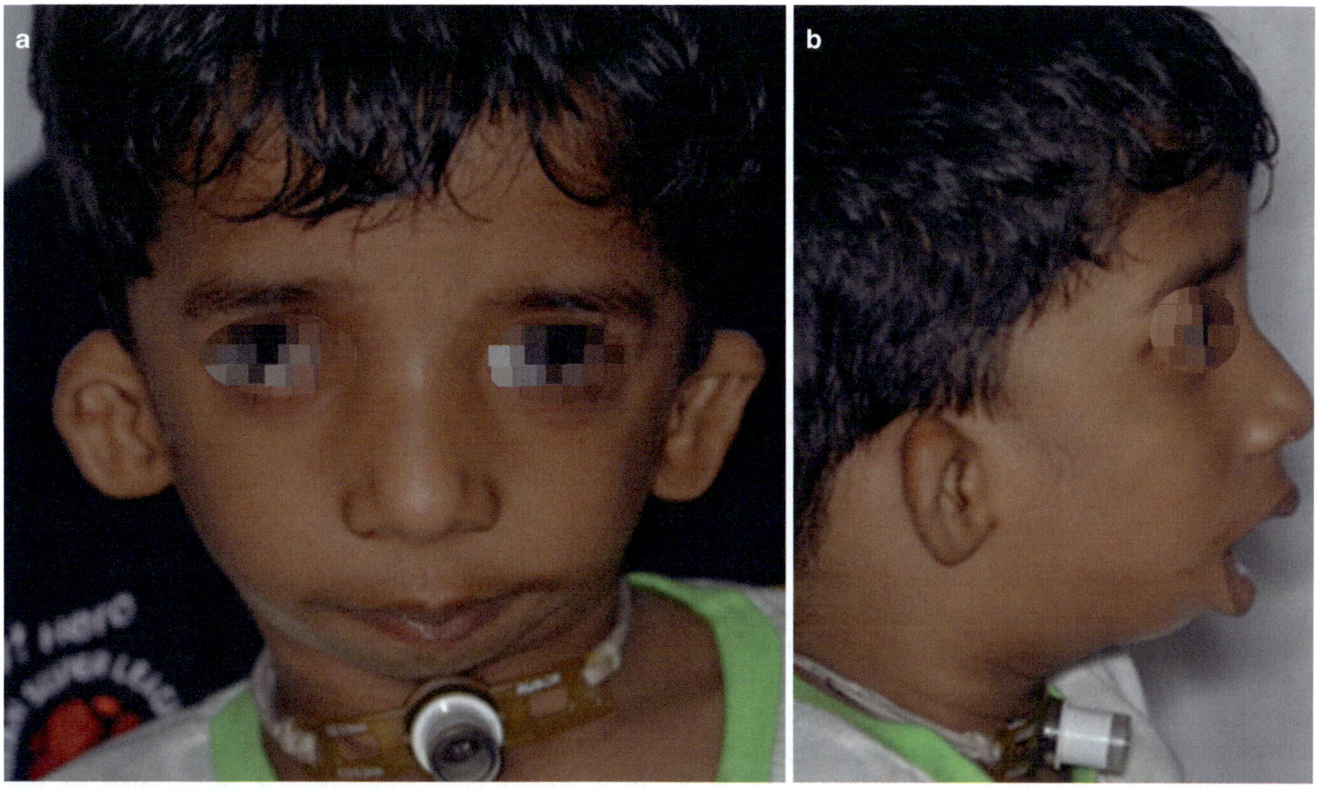

Fig. 78.38 (**a**, **b**) Photograph of a 4-year-old male with TCS. Patient had history of hospitalization due to respiratory distress. Tracheostomy tube in situ since 7 months of age

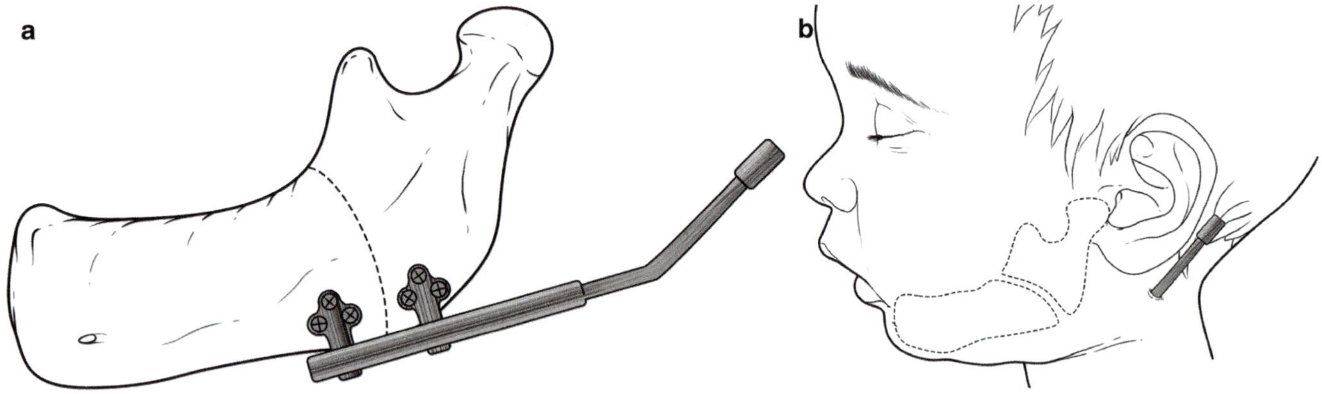

Fig. 78.39 (**a**, **b**) Mandibular advancement using distraction in neonates to increase posterior airway space as a treatment of obstructive sleep apnoea. (**a**) Position of the distractor on the mandible, (**b**) Emergence of activation port in the retromandibular region

omy of TCS patients, a fibre-optic-assisted intubation method similar to that described by Ellis et al. can be successfully used [57].

Paediatric mandibular advancement was initially performed using bilateral external distractors which are advantageous because of their ease of use, manipulation and versatility [58]. However, external devices also create aesthetic [e.g. scarring] and social problems. Another important point to be noted is that retention period of such devices is reduced and an increased relapse rate is seen compared to internal distractor devices [59]. If the child is extremely uncooperative and parents are unable to maintain and monitor the external distractors, an internal distractor should be used (Fig. 78.39a, b).

Recently, paediatric mandibular distraction for OSA has been discouraged in many centres around the world due to concern of permanently damaging the teeth buds. Instead, tongue lip adhesion (TLA) has been popularized by many centres instead of DO as it has significantly lower morbidity. After the airway improves, better feeding and weight gain are expected and cleft palate closure is done. Subsequently, TLA release can be attempted [60]. In comparison to DO, the TLA needs stricter postoperative care in intensive setup as feeding and breathing need to be assessed regularly for a week at the minimum.

78.2.6.3 Feeding Problem

The abnormal or hypoplastic craniofacial issues in TCS can sometimes produce severe feeding problem for infants, leading to weight loss and failure to thrive. Most feeding problems relate to cleft lip and palate, retrognathic jaws and airway problems. Ideally, a craniofacial feeding management team should guide the parents regarding position of feeding, type of nutrition and dietary plan for such children.

Position (holding the baby upright or supporting the cheek and jaw while feeding) is important to avoid aspiration. It is also preferable to do a video-fluoroscopic swallow study (VFSS) to understand the swallowing pattern of the patient and its coordination with breathing [61].

Primary palatoplasty for closure of the cleft palate should be done once the patient gains weight, to assist in normalizing the swallowing pattern without nasal regurgitation.

78.2.6.4 Brain and Psychological Development in TCS

Individuals with TCS have a tendency towards a shorter stature, at least early in life. Intelligence is usually unaffected, but brain and behavioural anomalies such as microcephaly and psychomotor delay have been occasionally reported as part of the condition. Additionally, the facial deformity of this syndrome may affect psychosocial development, school adjustment and other milestones. A psychologist or social worker should be made available for evaluation and counselling if needed.

In the Indian scenario, poor parental awareness, lack of medical advice, social taboos and feeding difficulties lead to failure to thrive among TCS infants and children belonging to lower socio-economic classes. Psychological stress during schooling [e.g. marked out as different by peers] is one of the more challenging issues to be addressed throughout the life of the patient.

78.2.6.5 Management of Cleft Palate

Isolated cleft of the soft palate is the most common form of cleft in TCS. Complete cleft palate up to the alveolus may also be seen. Closure of the soft palate is routinely done at the end of 1 year. Meticulous dissection and suturing of soft palate muscles can produce excellent results, nearing to that of a normal palate. Postoperative maintenance of oral hygiene is necessary and can become challenging in these children for fear of aspiration. Velopharyngeal insufficiency [VPI] is a common issue in these children. VPI can be corrected secondarily with intra-velar palatoplasties or buccal advancement flaps for velar lengthening.

78.2.6.6 Ophthalmological, Auricular and Hearing Issues

Ophthalmological Issues

Eye anomalies include aberrations in the extraocular muscle function, corneal exposure difficulties and visual acuity. Ophthalmologic issues may include vision loss (37%), amblyopia (33%), refractive errors (58%), anisometropia (17%) and strabismus (37%). A thorough paediatric ophthalmological assessment should be done to establish proper management.

Hearing Issues

A 3D CT of the petrous temporal bones should be done to accurately assess the external auditory canal and middle and inner ear anatomy. TCS patients with microtia can have congenital aural atresia and extremely narrow canals, leading to significant conductive hearing loss as the bone blocks passage of sounds to tympanic area and middle ear. Furthermore, exfoliated skin cells and ear wax cannot drain out, leading to otitis media and occasionally form cholesteatoma. Despite hearing loss, these children tend to grow normally. However, the chances of developmental cognitive deficits are not uncommon.

Microtia Correction

Microtia ear correction can be done when the patient is around 6 to 7 years old, an age at which external ear development is complete. The most preferred way of auricle reconstruction is the use of autogenous rib cartilage, in a staged manner. The rib cartilage is harvested from the sixth to the ninth rib. The sixth and seventh rib cartilage are utilized to form the base of the framework. The triangular fossa and scapha are carved in the superior portion of the previously created cartilaginous base. The eighth rib cartilage is then carved to replicate the helical rim. The carved cartilage is then inserted under the skin in the region of the missing ear, with or without skin expansion (Fig. 78.19).

Bone-conduction hearing aids such as the bone-anchored hearing appliance (BAHA) or a middle ear implantable prosthetic device can significantly improve hearing in these patients.

78.2.6.7 Nasal Issues

Nasal deformities can be classified as external or internal in nature. Commonly seen external nasal deformities are the dorsal hump (73%), external deviation (≤55%), bifid or bulbous nasal tip (55%) and columellar septal luxation (55%). Commonly seen internal nasal deformities are nasal obstructions due to septal deviation and presence of spurs. Due to presence of the above structural deformities, functional problems, e.g. snoring and impaired phonation, are commonly present in these patients.

A detailed physical examination along with nasal endoscopy and 3D CT of the nasal and paranasal regions can help identify all the deformities present. The commonly performed procedures that should be paid attention to are dorsal hump reduction, correction of the deviated external osseous deformity, septoplasty and tip plasty.

78.2.6.8 Dentoalveolar Issues and Orthodontic Alignment

- Due to the presence of an anterior open bite and compulsive mouth breathing, there is an increased risk for poor oral hygiene. This is evidenced by the face that up to 60% of TCS patients need dental care [e.g. restorative treatment]. However, the difficulty of performing even simple dental procedures is far higher due to reduced mouth opening, presence of concurrent medical co-morbidities [e.g. congenital heart defects], decreased posterior airway space and hearing loss [61, 62].
- During the late mixed dentition phase, orthodontic treatment aims to increase the transverse dimensions of the constricted maxilla [e.g. quad helix]. In the permanent dentition phase, the fixed therapy is used in order to achieve intercuspation and arch levelling.
- For moderately severe cases, the final goal is to prepare the patient for orthognathic surgical correction of the anterior open bite and skeletal class 2 relationship [63]. Studies have established that bimaxillary orthognathic surgery gives stable long-term results in TCS patients [64]. Sometimes, additional procedures to improve the shape of the chin are required. Figures 78.40a, b, 78.41 and 78.42a, b show double sliding genioplasty done in a patient in early age due to psychological impact owing to the facial appearance.
- For severe cases, DO with external distractors is the ideal surgical intervention wherein gonial angle control is necessary for increase in height of the ramus and lengthening the body of the mandible. In this aspect, multi-vector devices have an advantage with respect to the ability to control the transverse width during distraction (Fig. 78.43a–f).

78.2.6.9 Management of the Adult TCS Patient

Clinical and Cephalometric Features

The adult patient with TCS has a convex facial profile due to severe mandibular retrognathia. However, the horizontal projection of the maxilla to the cranial base remains normal. Over the growth period, the facial convexity angle remains relatively constant, thus confirming that the facial profile morphology of the infant with TCS remains similar to that of the adult.

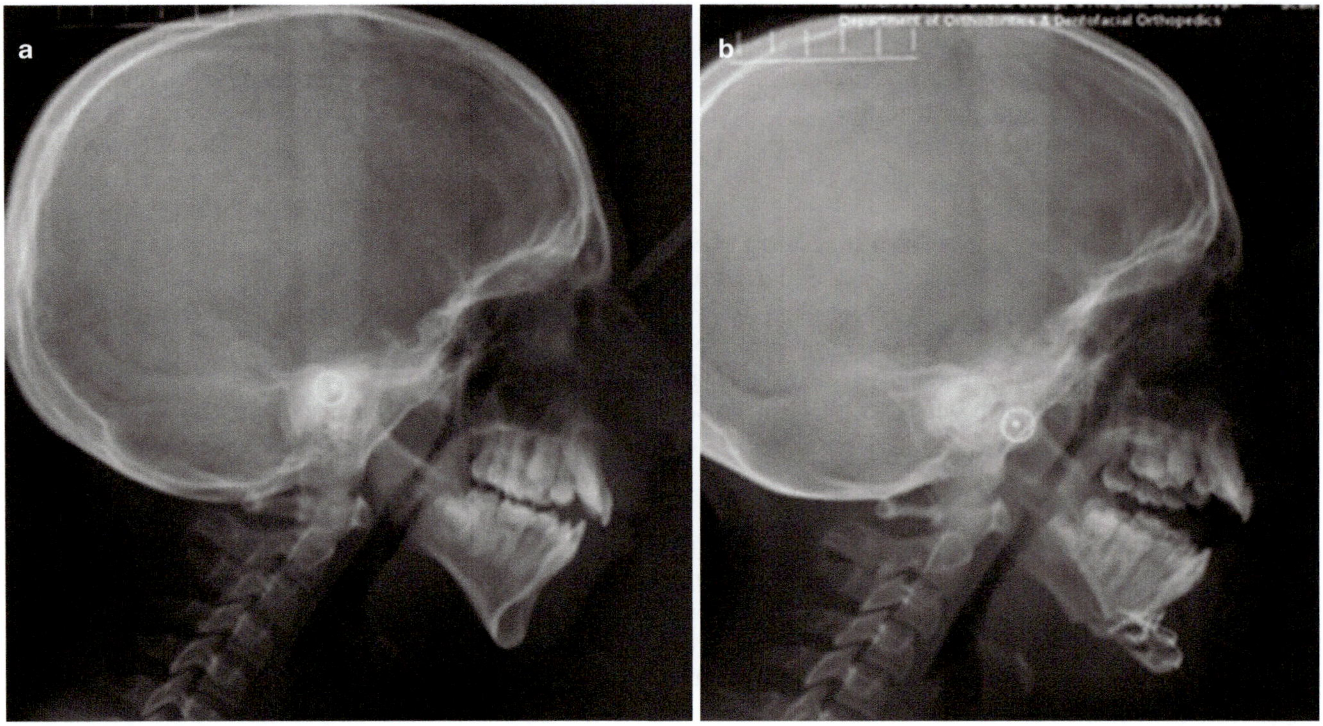

Fig. 78.40 (**a**) Preoperative and (**b**) postoperative lateral cephalogram radiographic view of a patient with Treacher Collins syndrome who underwent double sliding genioplasty

The total facial height is often excessive, with a normal upper facial height. This is due to combination of anterior open-bite malocclusion, mandibular retrognathism and chin dysplasia. Hypoplasia of the orbito-zygomatic complex is a characteristic feature. These hypoplastic facial skeletal features have variable effects on the TMJ, masticatory function and facial soft tissues and expressions.

Both the maxilla and mandible are rotated in a counterclockwise rotation. Thus, the maxillary and mandibular plane angles are excessively steep. Clinically, this translates to a shorter posterior facial height in TCS patients.

The mandible size is evidently decreased in both the ramus height and the body length. The gonial angle is obtuse with anti-gonial notching. The steepness due to clockwise rotation of the maxillomandibular complex along with the anterior and posterior vertical height disproportions and severe horizontal deficiency is reflected in the A-point-to-B-point discrepancy. All of these cephalometric findings explain the clinical facial dysmorphology.

Incidence of cleft palate with or without cleft lip (and choanal atresia of the nasal cavity) is variable. Dental anomalies are present in 60% of individuals such as tooth agenesis enamel, opacities and ectopic eruption of the maxillary first molars.

78.2.6.10 Surgical Management of the Orbito-zygomatic Region

Treatment of the skeletal defect in the orbito-zygomatic region varies according to the severity of the defect. The following classification categorizes the deformities according to severity and their treatment. Since this region attains growth by age of 9, most surgeons postpone definitive reconstruction up to this age.

Type 1 defects: The orbito-zygomatic complex is dysplastic and hypoplastic. Type 1 represents the mildest form of the defect and can be easily treated by autologous fat, either by liposuction and injection or dermis fat graft [65]. The merit of autologous fat grafting is that it is repeatable with minimal donor site morbidity and can be done before growth completion. It is ideal for growing children who are psychologically affected due to a poor facial appearance. The disadvantage of this technique is that it may have to be performed repeatedly to maintain the volume of correction.

Fat transfer can be used alone for correction of minor defects. It has more of an adjunctive role in severe defects after wherein hard tissue augmentation is the preferred intervention.

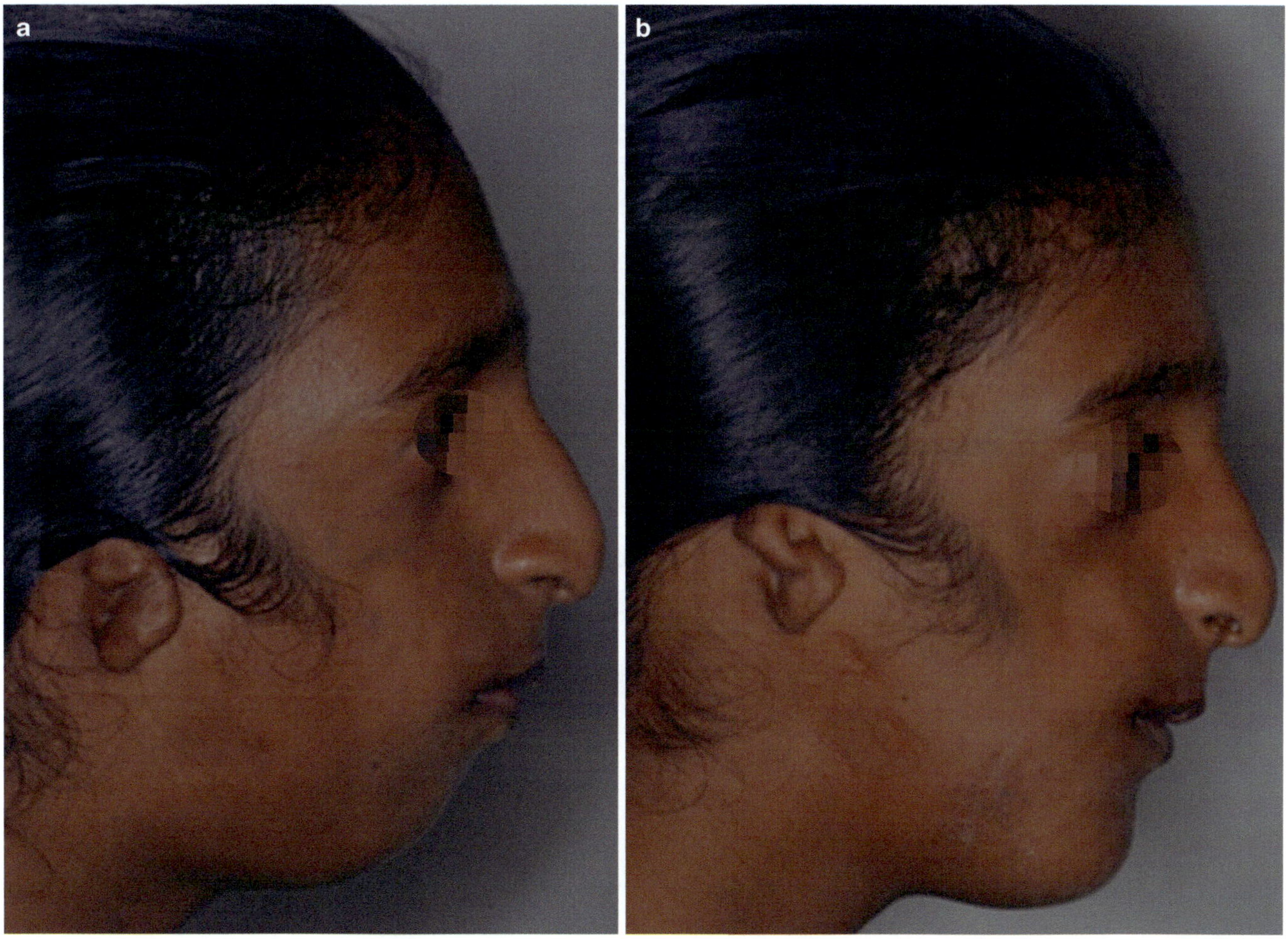

Fig. 78.41 (**a**, **b**) Extraoral profile view showing marked improvement in the lower third of the face. (**a**) Pre-surgical profile photo showing retrogenia (Fig. 78.31a1), (**b**) post-surgical profile photo after a double sliding genioplasty, showing good chin prominence

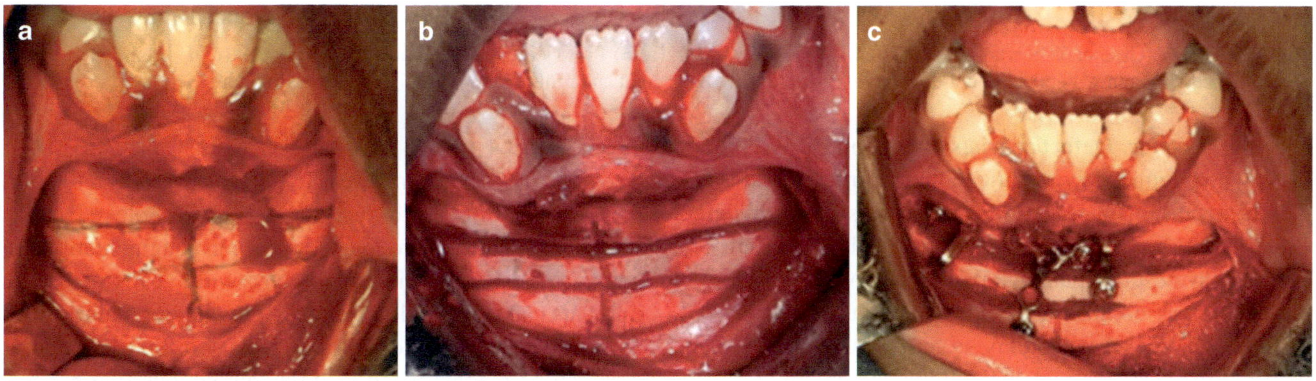

Fig. 78.42 (**a–c**) Intraoperative view of double sliding genioplasty done for the same patient as in Fig. 78.41. (**a**) Surgical exposure of the genium, (**b**) osteotomy design marked on the chin and (**c**) completion of genioplasty with fixation (also see Figs. 68.32 and 68.33 for use of double sliding genioplasty in other clinical situations)

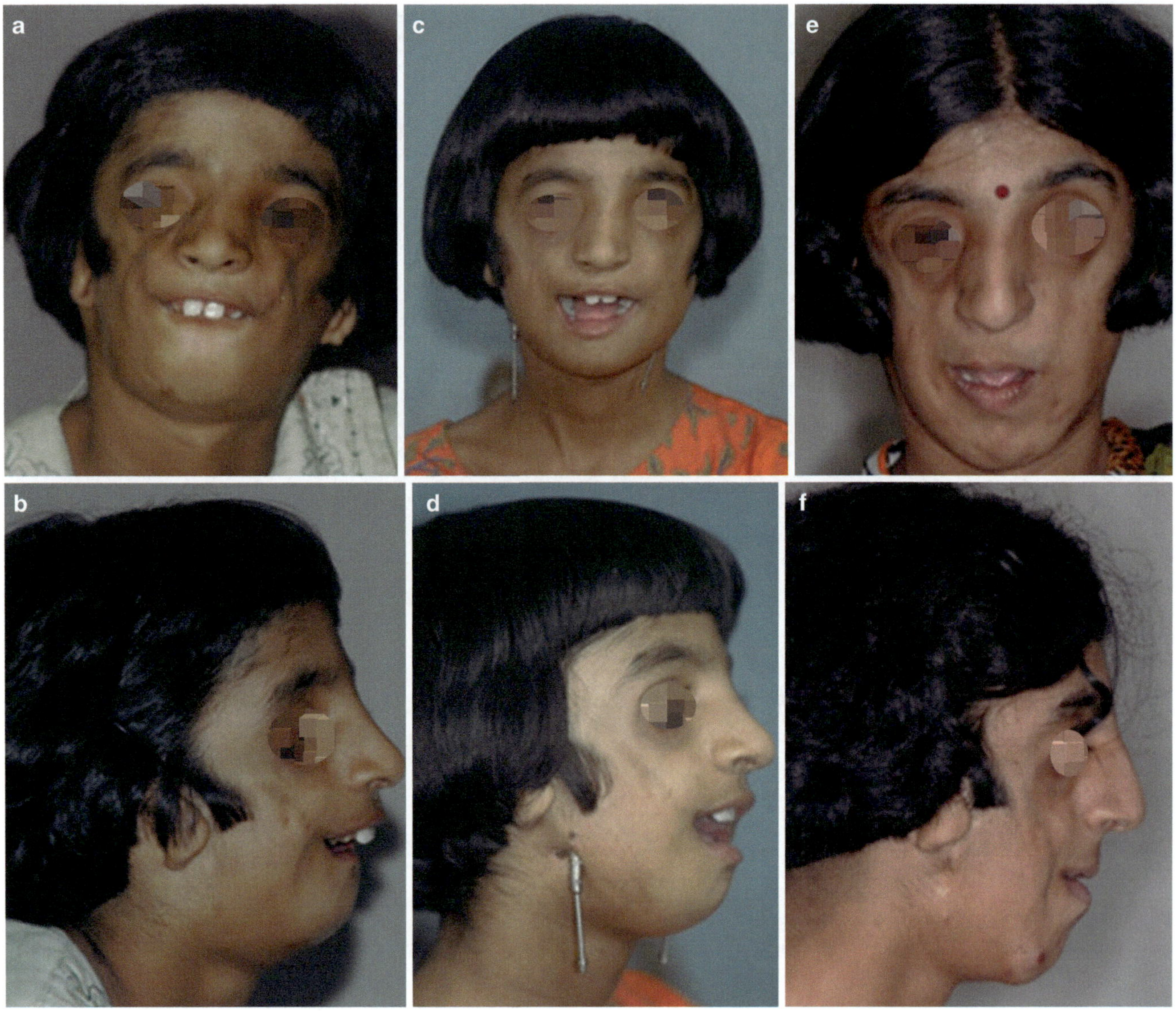

Fig. 78.43 (**a–f**) Case of TCS who underwent early osteodistraction. (**a**, **b**) Pre-operative frontal and profile photos, (**c**, **d**) Frontal and profile photos post distraction with bilateral uni-directional distractors, (**e**, **f**) Frontal and profile views after five years follow-up

Type 2 defects: Defect consists of hypoplastic zygomatic body with a reduced zygomatic temporal process and a dysplastic or absent lateral orbital wall. This class of defect usually requires surgery to address the bony deficiency. Studies have established that a malar osteotomy offers better contour as compared to onlay bone autografting [66]. Though the malar osteotomy is aimed at correcting the width of the midface, it is difficult to augment anteroposterior projection by osteotomy only. It should be noted that this defect is characterized by a deficient vertical dimension as well. Thus, a zygomatic osteotomy is preferably combined with an onlay graft. The Mommaerts zygomatic osteotomy is favoured in some units because it does not alter orbital dimensions. Alloplastic materials [e.g. Medpore] can be very effective alternatives to the traditional onlays [67].

Types 3 and 4

The defects range from severe hypoplasia/dysplasia to complete absence of orbito-zygomatic bony complex. Patients belonging to these groups require bony augmentation. In adults, alloplastic augmentation with patient-specific implants can be considered as they provide optimal results.

In general, the zygomatico-maxillary-orbital bone complex can be reconstructed using an autologous free bone or regional pedicle graft. Non-vascularized autologous bone grafting for larger defects is increasingly prone to loss of graft due to infection and resorption if not fully covered by surrounding soft tissue. Studies have established that resorption occurs due to reduced vascularity and increased functional loads on the graft. Therefore, it is prudent to line the bone grafts by soft tissue on its inner side in the proximity of maxillary sinus and nasal cavity [68].

Calvarial bone grafts have been used for reconstruction of midface in various craniofacial deformities. Full-thickness calvarial grafting outcomes are more stable in the long term due to the dense cortical nature of the graft (Fig. 78.44a, b). Studies [69] have also established that dense membranous bone grafts [e.g. calvarial] are more effective than endochondral grafts [e.g. iliac crest] in the craniofacial skeleton. Calvarial bone grafts have become popular because of their low resorption rates and minimal donor site morbidity for orbito-zygomatic complex reconstruction [70].

78.3 Conclusion

Hemifacial microsomia and Treacher Collins syndrome are both congenital craniofacial anomalies that negatively impact the physiological and psychological wellbeing of an individual [71]. Due to multidimensional nature of the deformity, a multidisciplinary holistic approach is required with proper guidance and counselling of the patients at every level of treatment. However, with the advances in regenerative sciences and genetic engineering, diagnosis and management of such congenital deformities is becoming less challenging. Disclosure Authors have no financial conflicts to disclose.

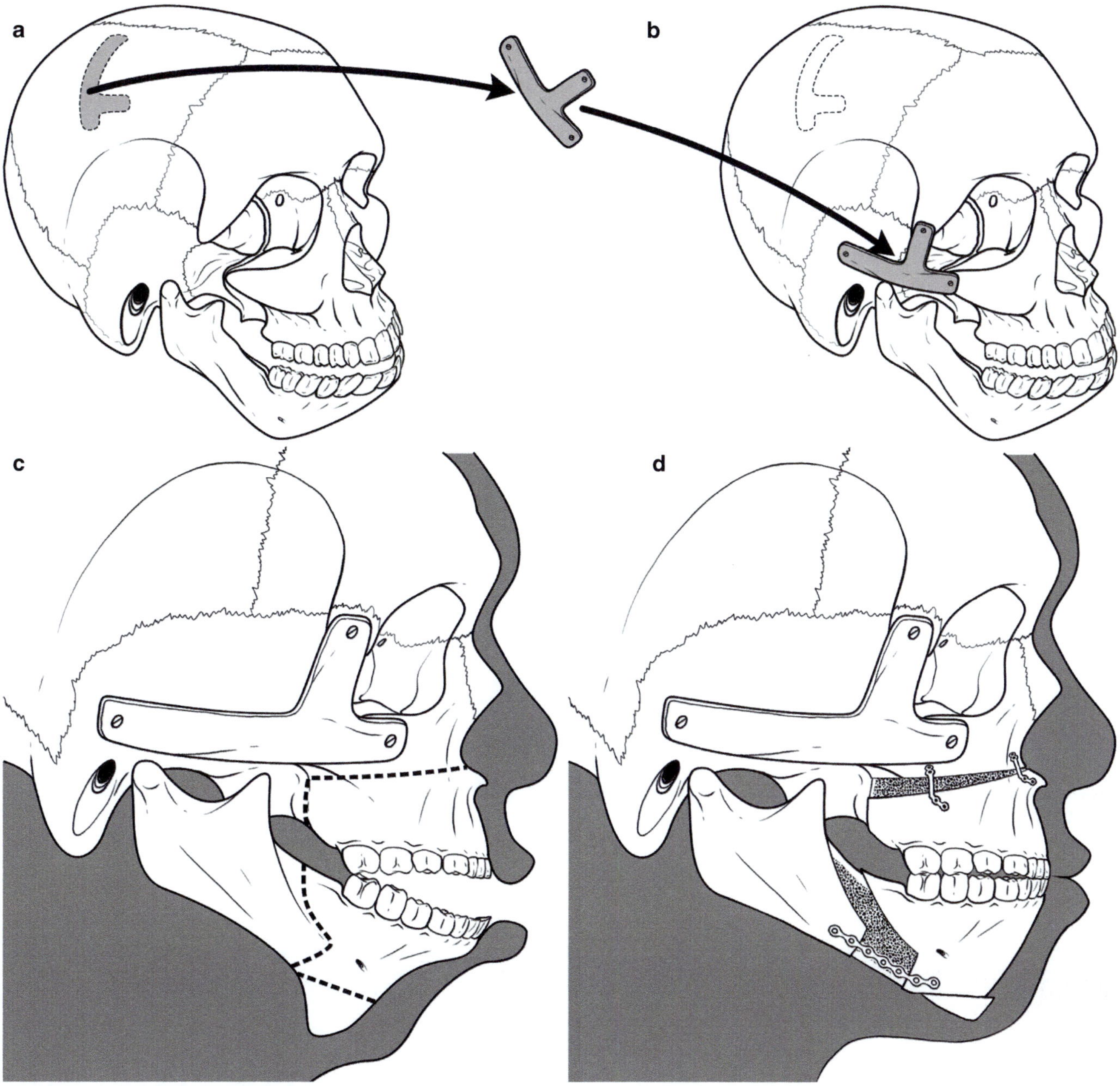

Fig. 78.44 Skeletal correction for TCS. (**a**) Calvarial graft harvest for recsontruction of zygoma, (**b**) graft in place, (**c**) osteotomy design for orthognathic correction with bimaxillary surgery and genioplsty, (**d**) diagram showing post orthognathic final correction

78.4 Case Scenarios

Case 1: Treacher Collins Syndrome (Fig. 78.43a–f)

Case of TCS who underwent early osteodistraction. Note the mandibular advancement using bilateral unidirectional distractors. Follow-up after 5 years. Patient is currently undergoing orthodontic treatment.

Case 2: Hemifacial Microsomia (Figs. 78.45a–e, 78.46a–c, 78.47a, b, 78.48a–c, 78.49a–c, 78.50a, b, 78.51, 78.52a–d, 78.53a, b)

Case of a 20-year-old girl having HFM, undergoing osteotomy for asymmetry correction. Preoperative photographs, radiographs and CT scans showing the extent of asymmetry. Pre-surgical orthodontics for levelling and alignment. Virtual planning to fabricate CAD-CAM splint. Final postoperative

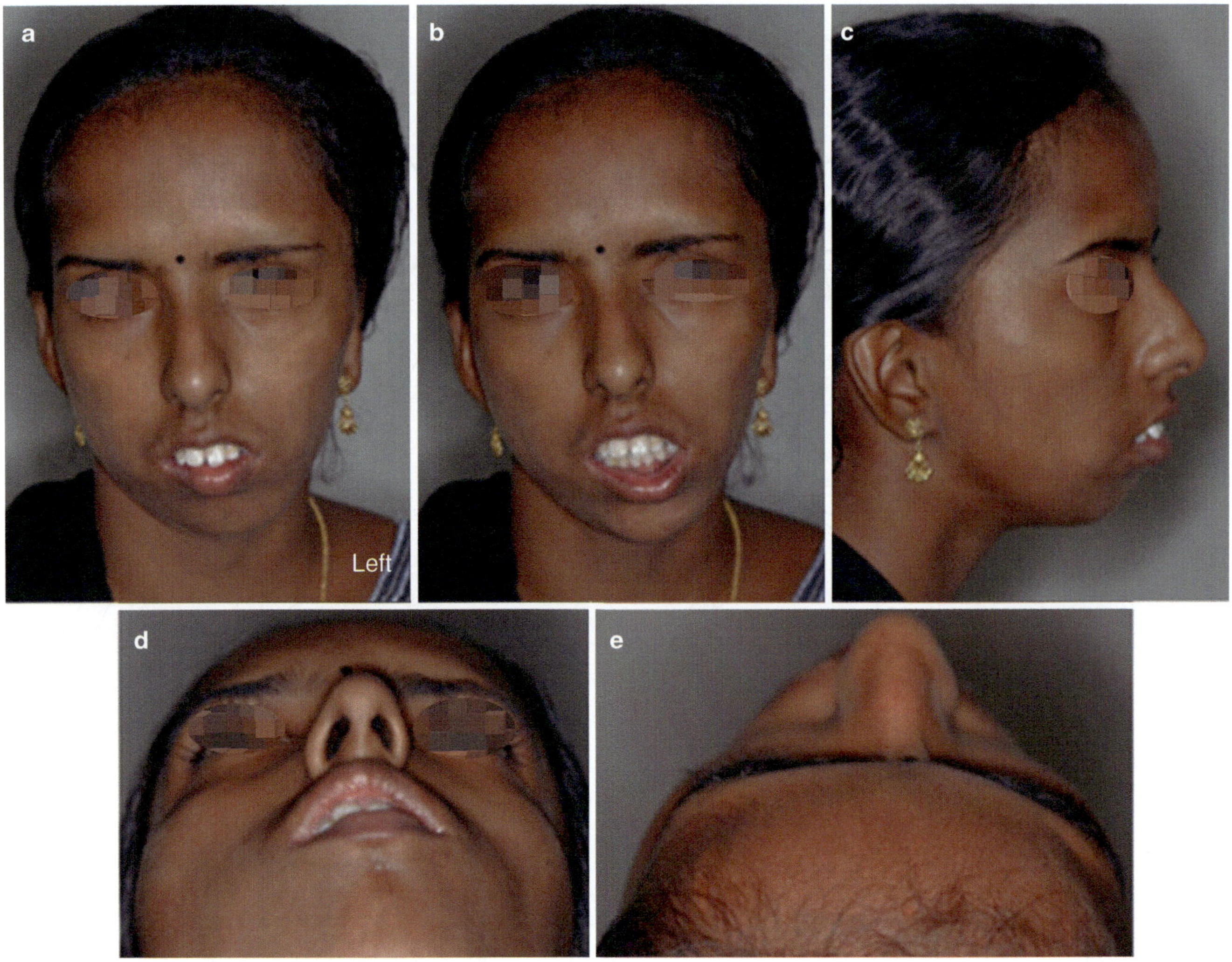

Fig. 78.45 (**a**–**e**) Preoperative views of a female patient with facial asymmetry and deviation towards the left side

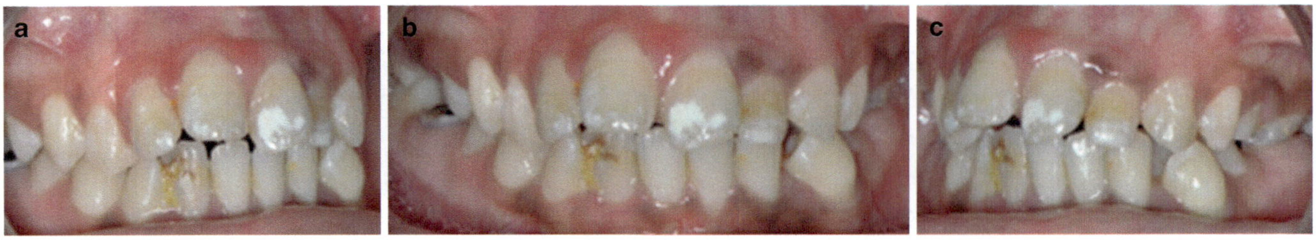

Fig. 78.46 (**a**–**c**) Intraoral view showing malocclusion, crowding and midline deviation

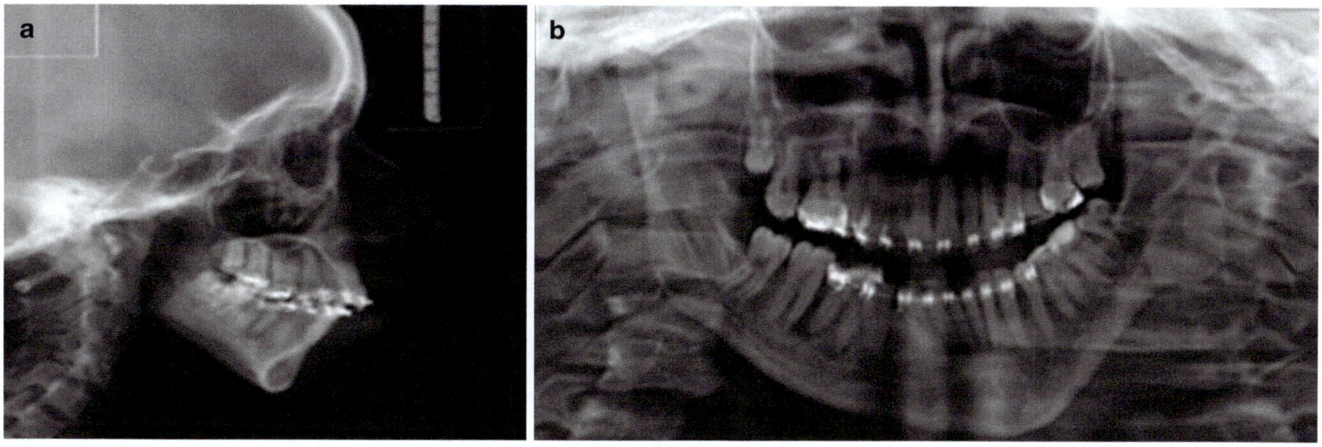

Fig. 78.47 (**a**, **b**) Preoperative (**a**) lateral cephalogram and (**b**) OPG showing Class II skeletal profile with left-sided TMJ deformity

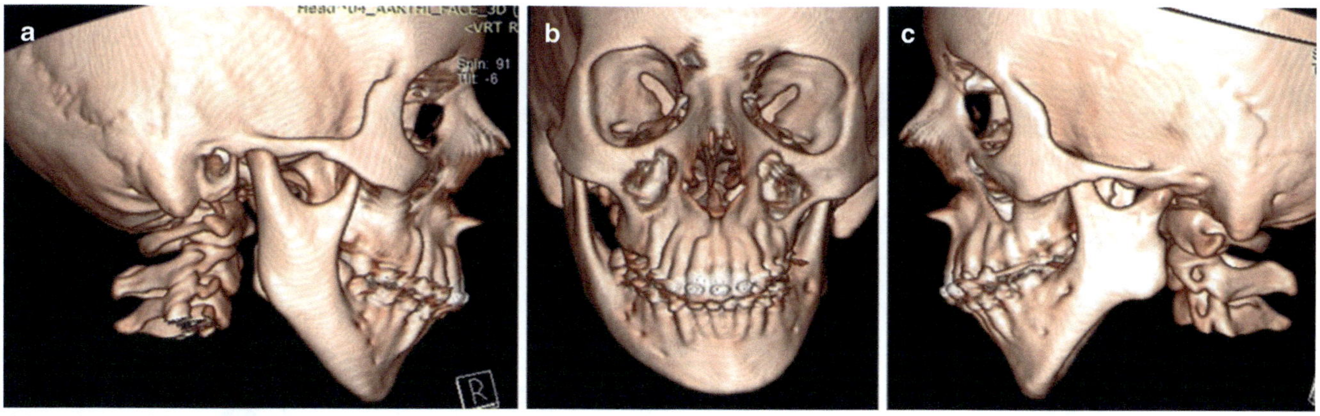

Fig. 78.48 (**a**–**c**) Preoperative CT scans showing TMJ deformity on the left side

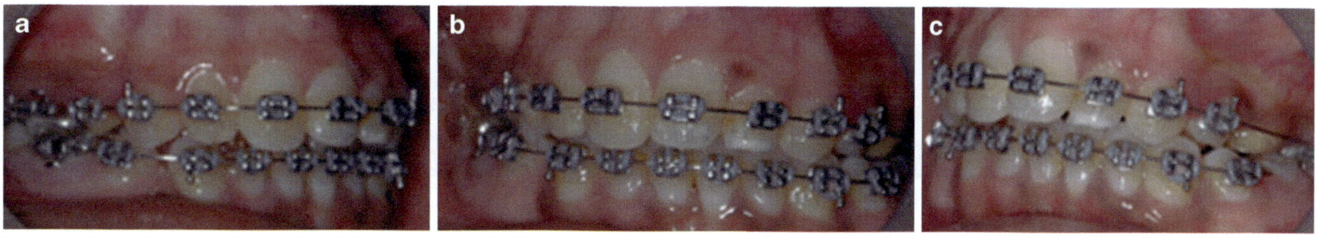

Fig. 78.49 (**a**–**c**) Pre-surgical intermediate orthodontics treatment for alignment and levelling

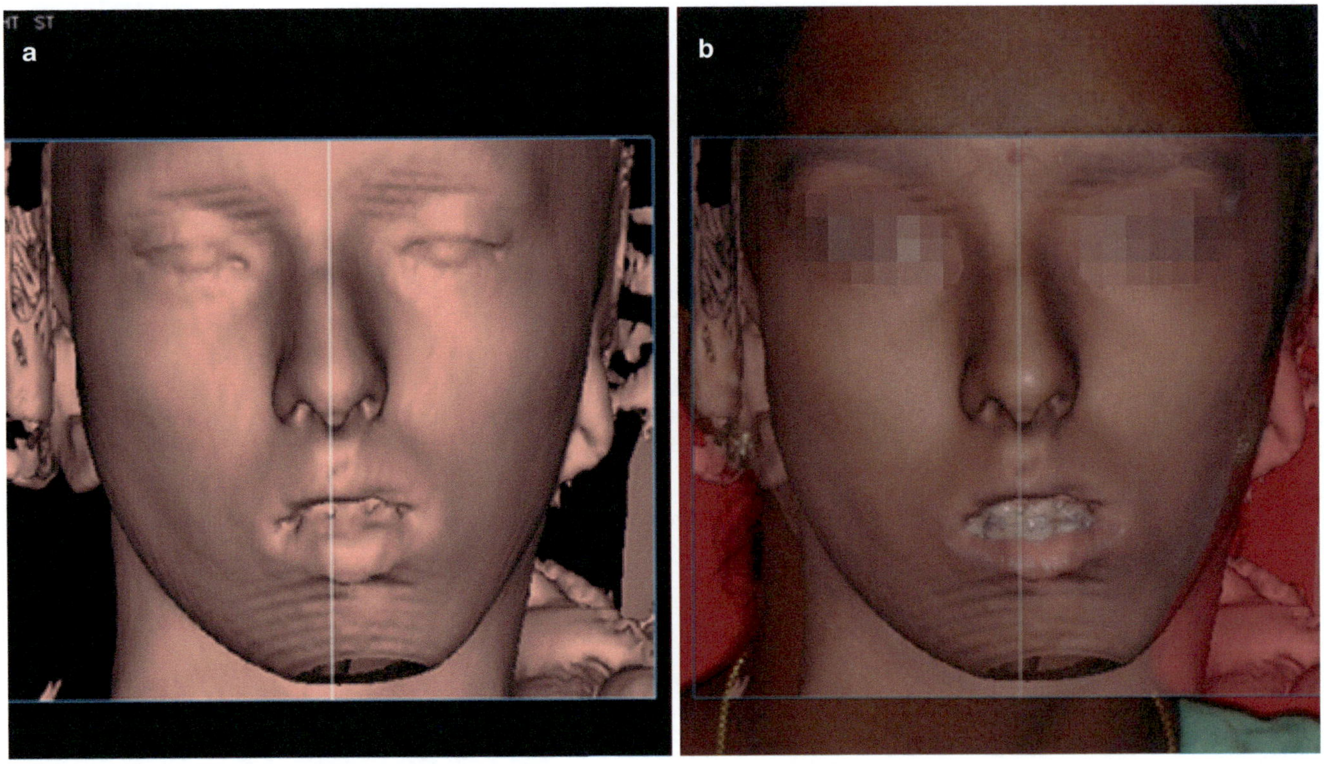

Fig. 78.50 (**a**, **b**) Virtual planning using 3D photogrammetry. (**a**) soft tissue reconstruction from the CT data, (**b**) superimposition of the patients photograph on the CT model

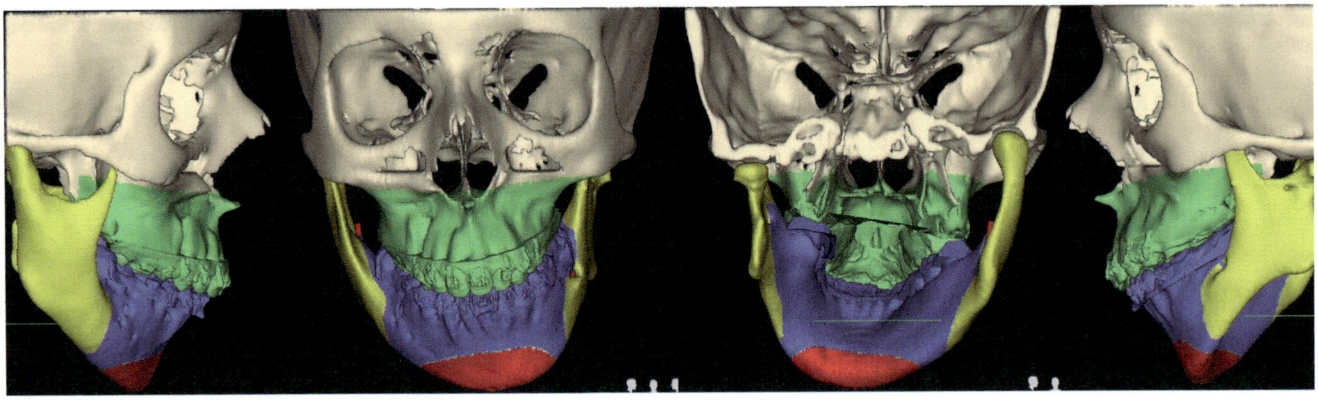

Fig. 78.51 Virtual planning of orthognathic surgery to correct pitching, roll and yaw defect of the maxilla and mandible with genioplasty

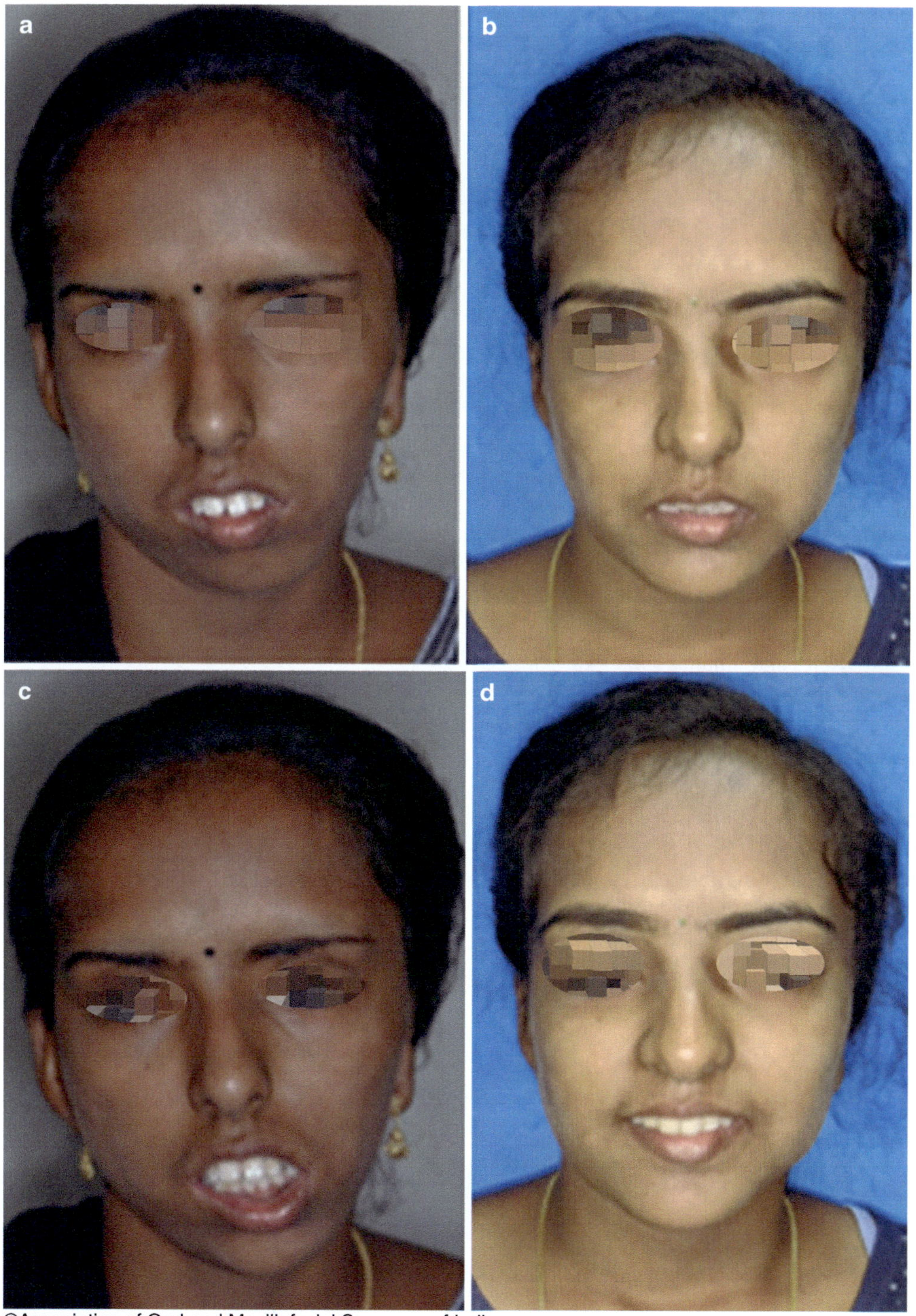

Fig. 78.52 (**a–d**): Pre (**a**, **c**) and post operative (**b**, **d**) photograph showing correction of asymmetry in patient with HFM

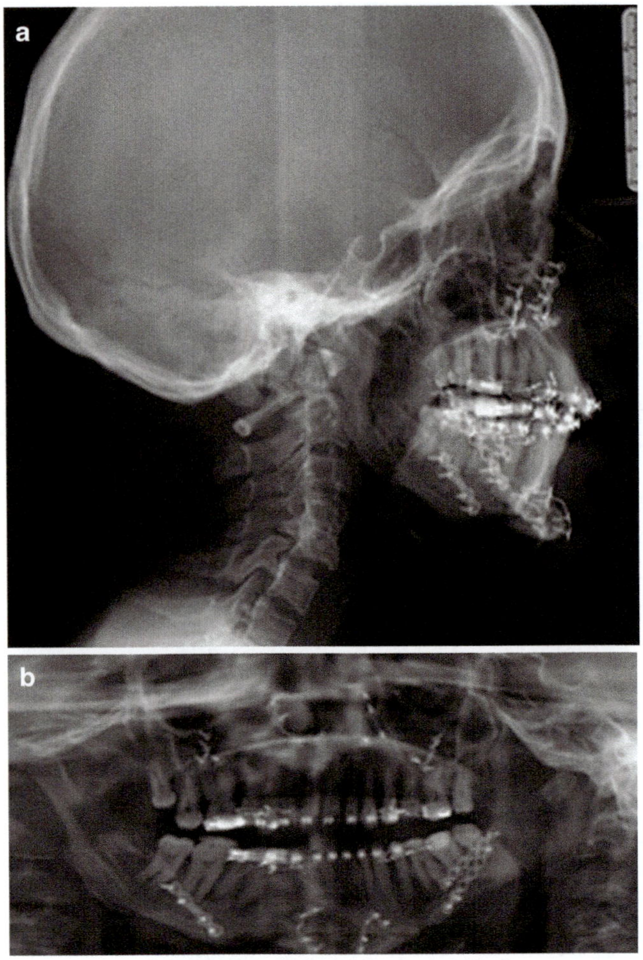

Fig. 78.53 (**a, b**) Postoperative (**a**) lateral cephalogram and (**b**) OPG showing correction of maxillomandibular relation. Refer to Fig. 78.47 for pre-operative xrays

photographs and radiographs showing correction of asymmetry.

References

1. Posnick JC. Hemifacial macrosomia: evaluation and treatment. Principles and practice of orthognathic surgery. St. Louis, Missouri: Elsevier; 2014.
2. Brandstetter KA, Patel KG. Craniofacial Microsomia. Facial Plast Surg Clin North Am 2016 Nov;24(4):495–515. Review.
3. Poswillo D. The aetiology and pathogenesis of craniofacial deformity. Development. 1988;103(Suppl):207–12.
4. Scambler PJ. The 22q11 deletion syndromes. Hum Mol Genet. 2000, Oct 1;9(16):2421–6.
5. Poswillo D. The pathogenesis of the first and second branchial arch syndrome. Oral Surg Oral Med Oral Pathol. 1973;35(3):302–28.
6. Werler MM, Sheehan JE, Hayes C, Mitchell AA, Mulliken JB. Vasoactive exposures, vascular events, and hemifacial microsomia. Birth Defects Res A Clin Mol Teratol. 2004;70(6):389–95.
7. Werler MM, Sheehan JE, Hayes C, Padwa BL, Mitchell AA, Mulliken JB. Demographic and reproductive factors associated with hemifacial microsomia. Cleft Palate Craniofac J. 2004;41(5):494–50.
8. Taysi K, Marsh JL, Wise DM. Familial hemifacial microsomia. Cleft Palate J. 1983;20(1):47–53.
9. Juriloff DM, Harris MJ, Froster-Iskenius U. Hemifacial deficiency induced by a shift in dominance of the mouse mutation far: a possible genetic model for hemifacial microsomia. J Craniofac Genet Dev Biol. 1987;7(1):27–44.
10. Poonawalla HH, Kaye CI, Rosenthal IM, Pruzansky S. Hemifacial microsomia in a patient with Klinefelter syndrome. Cleft Palate J. 1980;17(3):194–6.
11. David DJ, Mahatumarat C, Cooter RD. Hemifacial microsomia: a multisystem classification. Plast Reconstr Surg. 1987;80:525–35.
12. Vento AR, LaBrie RA, Mulliken JB. The O.M.E.N.S. classification of hemifacial microsomia. Cleft Palate Craniofac J 1991;28:68–76. discussion 77.
13. Kaban LB, Mulliken JB, Murray JE. Three-dimensional approach to analysis and treatment of hemifacial microso- mia. Cleft Palate J. 1981;18:90–9.
14. Grabb WC. The first and second branchial arch syndrome. Plast Reconstr Surg. 1965;36(5):485–508.
15. Rollnick BR, Kaye CI. Hemifacial microsomia and variants: pedigree data. Am J Med Genet. 1983;15(2):233–53.
16. Stark RB, Saunders DE. The first branchial syndrome. The oral-mandibular-auricular syndrome. Plast Reconstr Surg Transplant Bull. 1962;29:229–39.
17. Die MH. Missbildungen des ohres. In: Denker AK, editor. Handbuch der Spez Path Anatomie Histologie. Berlin: Springer; 1926. p. 131.
18. Meurman Y. Congenital microtia and meatal atresia; observations and aspects oftreatment. AMA Arch Otolaryngol. 1957;66:443–63.
19. Hollier LH, Rowe NM, Mackool RJ, Williams JK, Kim JH, Longaker MT, Grayson BH, JG MC. Controlled multiplanar distraction of the mandible. Part III: Laboratory studies of sagittal (anteroposterior) and horizontal (mediolateral) movements. J Craniofac Surg. 2000 Mar;11(2):83–95.
20. Fan WS, Mulliken JB, Padwa BL. An association between hemifacial microsomia and facial clefting. J Oral Maxillofac Surg. 2005;63:330–4.
21. Parameswaran A, Ramanathan M. Hemifacial microsomia. J Indian Orthodontic Soc. 2018 Jul 1;52(3):155.
22. Tahiri Y, Viezel-Mathieu A, Aldekhayel S, Lee J, Gilardino M. The effectiveness of mandibular distraction in improving airway obstruction in the pediatric population. Plast Reconstr Surg. 2014;133:352e-9e.
23. Nagy K, Kuijpers-Jagtman AM, Mommaerts MY. No evidence for long-term effectiveness of early osteodistraction in hemifacial microsomia. Plast Reconstr Surg. 2009;124:2061–71.
24. Mishra L, Misra SR, Kumar M, Tripathy R. Hemifacial microsomia: a series of three case reports. J Clin Diagn Res. 2013 Oct;7(10):2383-6.
25. Munro I. Hemifacial micorosmia: the skeletal correction. Oper Tech Plast Reconstr Surg. 1994;1:77–92.
26. Kaban LB, Moses MH, Mulliken JB. Correction of hemifacial microsomia in thegrowing child: a follow-up study. Cleft Palate J. 1986;23(Suppl 1):50.

27. Kaban LB, Padwa BL, Mulliken JB. Surgical correction of mandibular hypoplasia in hemifacial microsomia: the case for treatment in early childhood. J Oral Maxillofac Surg. 1998;56:628–38.
28. Ohtani J, Hoffman WY, Vargervik K, Oberoi S. Team management and treatment outcomes for patients with hemifacial microsomia. Am J Orthod Dentofac Orthop. 2012;141(4 Suppl):S74–81.
29. Silvestri A, Natali G, Iannetti G. Functional therapy in hemifacial microsomia: therapeutic protocol for growing children. J Oral Maxillofac Surg. 1996;54:271–8. discussion 278-80
30. Zanardi G, Parente EV, Esteves LS, Louro RS, Capelli J Jr. Orthodontic and surgical treatment of a patient with hemifacial microsomia. Am J Orthod Dentofac Orthop. 2012;141(4 Suppl):S130–9.
31. Tahiri Y, Chang CS, Tuin J, Paliga JT, Lowe KM, Taylor JA, et al. Costochondral grafting in craniofacial microsomia. Plast Reconstr Surg. 2015;135:530–41.
32. Murra JE, Mulliken JB, Kaban IB. Twenty-year experience in maxillofacial surgery: an evaluation of early surgery on growth function and body image. Ann Surg. 1979;190:320.
33. Ongkosuwito EM, van Vooren J, van Neck JW, Wattel E, Wolvius EB, van Adrichem LN, et al. Changes of mandibular ramal height, during growth in unilateral hemifacial microsomia patients and unaffected controls. J Craniomaxillofac Surg. 2013;41:92–7.
34. Ortiz Monasterio F, Molina F, Andrade L, Rodriguez C, Sainz AJ. Simultaneous mandibular and maxillary distraction in hemifacial microsomia in adults: avoiding occlusal disasters. Plast Reconstr Surg. 1997;100:852–6.
35. Suh J, Choi TH, Baek SH, Kim JC, Kim S. Mandibular distraction in unilateral craniofacial microsomia: longitudinal results until the completion of growth. Plast Reconstr Surg. 2013;132:1244–52.
36. Salins PC, Venkatraman B, Kavarody M. Morphometric basis for orthomorphic correction of mandibular asymmetry. J Oral Maxillofac Surg. 2008 Jul;66(7):1523–31.
37. Weichman KE, Jacobs J, Patel P, Szpalski C, Shetye P, Grayson B, et al. Early distraction for mild to moderate unilateral craniofacial microsomia: long-term follow-up, outcomes, and recommendations. Plast Reconstr Surg. 2017;139:941e-53e.
38. Cassi D, Battistoni G, Magnifico M, et al. Three-dimensional evaluation of facial asymmetry in patients with hemifacial microsomia using stereophotogrammetry. J Craniomaxillofac Surg. 2019;47(1):179–84.
39. Peacock ZS, Tricomi BJ, Faquin WC, et al. Bilateral continuous automated distraction osteogenesis: proof of principle. J Craniofac Surg. 2015;26(8):2320–4.
40. Yamada Y, Ueda M, Hibi H, Nagasaka T. Translational reseach for injectable tissue-engineered bone regeneration using mesenchymal stem cells and platelet-rich plasma: from basic research to clinical application. Cell Transplant. 2004;13:343–55.
41. Gorlin RJ, Cohen MM Jr, Levin LS. Syndromes of the head and neck. 3rd ed. New York: Oxford University Press; 1990. p. 649–52.
42. Franceschetti A, Klein D. The mandibulofacial dysostosis; a new hereditary syndrome. Acta Ophthalmol. 1949;27(2):143–224.
43. Rogers BO. Berry-treacher collins syndrome: a review of 200 cases (mandibulo-facial dysostosis; franceschetti-zwahlen-klein syndromes). Br J Plast Surg. 1964 Apr;17:109–37. Pubmed pmid: 14150863.
44. Jones KL, Smith DW, Harvey MAS, Hall BD, Quan L. Older paternal age and fresh gene mutation: data on additional disorders. J Pediatr. 1975;86:84–8.
45. Posnick JC, Ruiz RL. Treacher Collins syndrome: current evaluation, treatment, and future directions. Cleft Palate Craniofac J. 2000;37:434.
46. Sulik KK, Johnston MC, Smiley SJ, Speight HS, Jarvis BE. Mandibulofacial dysostosis (Treacher Collins syndrome): a new proposal for its pathogenesis. Am J Med Genet. 1987;27:359–72.
47. Dauwerse JG, Dixon J, Seland S, Ruivenkamp CA, van Haeringen A, Hoefsloot LH, et al. Mutations in genes encoding subunits of RNA polymerases I and III cause Treacher Collins syndrome. Nat Genet. 2011;43:20–2.
48. Andrade EC, Júnior VS, Didoni AL, Freitas PZ, Carneiro AF, Yoshimoto FR. Treacher Collins syndrome with choanal atresia: a case report and review of disease features. Braz J Otorhinolaryngol. 2005;71:107–10.
49. Nikkhah D, Ponniah A, Ruff C, Dunaway D. Planning surgical reconstruction in Treacher-Collins syndrome using virtual simulation. Plastic Reconstr Surg. 2013;132:790e–805e.
50. Marszalek B, Wójcicki P, Kobus K, Trzeciak WH. Clinical features, treatment and genetic background of Treacher Collins syndrome. J Appl Genet. 2002;43:223–33.
51. Shete P, Tupkari J, Benjamin T, Singh A. Treacher Collins syndrome. J Oral Maxillofac Pathol. 2011;15:348–51.
52. Waitzman AA, Posnick JC, Armstrong DC, Pron GE. Craniofacial skeletal measurements based on computed tomography: part II. Normal values and growth trends. Cleft Palate Craniofac J. 1992, Mar 01;29(2):118–28.
53. Trainor PA, Dixon J, Dixon MJ. Treacher Collins syndrome: etiology, pathogenesis and prevention. Eur J Hum Genet. 2009;17:275–83.
54. Sher AE. Obstructive sleep apnea syndrome: a complex disorder of the upper airway. Otolaryngol Clin N Am. 1990;23(4):593–608.
55. Hoeve LJ, Pijpers M, Joosten KF. OSAS in craniofacial syndromes: an unsolved problem. Int J Pediatr Otorhinolaryngol. 2003;67.
56. Rachmiel A, Emodi O, Aizenbud D. Management of obstructive sleep apnea in pediatric craniofacial anomalies. Ann Maxillofac Surg. 2012;2:111–5.
57. Ellis DS, Potluri PK, O'Flaherty JE, et al. Difficult airway management in the neonate: a simple method of intubating through a laryngeal mask airway. Paediatr Anaesth. 1999;9:460–2.
58. Morovic CG, Monasterio L. Distraction osteogenesis for obstructive apneas in patients with congenital craniofacial malformations. Plast Reconstr Surg. 2000;105:2324–30.
59. Rachmiel A, Emodi O, Rachmiel D, Aizenbud D. Internal mandibular distraction to relieve airway obstruction in children with severe micrognathia. Int J Oral Maxillofac Surg. 2014;43:1176–81.
60. Diner PA, Kollar E, Martinez H, Vazquez MP. Submerged intraoral device for mandibular lengthening. J Craniomaxillofac Surg. 1997;25:116–23.
61. Hwang DW, Jung KJ, Kim SY, Kim JH. Usefulness of videofluoroscopic swallow study in treacher Collins syndrome with cleft palate: a case report. Ann Rehabil Med 2014 Oct;38(5):707–11.
62. da Silva Dalben G, Teixeira das Neves L, Ribeiro Gomide M. Oral health status of children with treacher Collins syndrome. Spec Care Dentist 2006 Mar–Apr; 26 (2):71–75. quiz 85-7.
63. Okada R, Kuroda T. Orthodontic treatment for a patient with Treacher-Collins syndrome: a case report. World J Orthod 2008 Winter; 9 (4):e37–e47. PubMed PMID:19641756.
64. Hylton JB, Leon-Salazar V, Anderson GC, De Felippe NL. Multidisciplinary treatment approach in Treacher Collins syndrome. J Dent Child (Chic) 2012 Jan–Apr; 79 (1):15–21. Review. PubMed PMID: 22449504.
65. Lim AA, Fan K, Allam KA, et al. Autologous fat transplantation in the craniofacial patient: the UCLA experience. J Craniofac Surg 2012;23(4):1061e6 [Epub 2012/07/11].

66. Posnick JC, Goldstein JA, Waitzman AA. Surgical correction of the Treacher Collins malar deficiency: quantitative CT scan analysis of long-term results. Plast Reconstr Surg. 1993;92(1):12–22.
67. Mommaerts MY, Nadjmi N, Abeloos JV, Neyt LF. Six year's experience with the zygomatic "sandwich" osteotomy for correction of malar deficiency. J Oral Maxillofac Surg Off J Am Assoc Oral Maxillofac Surg 1999;57(1):8e13. discussion 4e5. Epub 1999/01/23.
68. Smolka W, Eggensperger N, Kollar A, Iizuka T. Midfacial reconstruction using Calvarial Split bone grafts. Arch Otolaryngol Head Neck Surg. 2005;131(2):131–6.
69. Freihofer HP. Variations in the correction of Treacher Collins syndrome. Plast Reconstr Surg 1997;99(3):647e57.
70. Marsh JL, Celin SE, Vannier MW, Gado M. The skeletal anatomy of mandibulofacial dysostosis (Treacher Collins syndrome). Plast Reconstr Surg 1986;78(4):460e70. [Epub 1986/10/01].
71. Murray JE, Kaban LB, Mulliken JB. Analysis and treatment of hemifacial microsomia. J Craniofac Surg. 1985;33:377.

Modern Management of Craniosynostosis

79

David Koppel and Jaime Grant

79.1 Introduction

The different presentations of craniosynostosis form the majority of the workload of craniofacial services, and it is important to note that the surgical interventions only form a small part of the overall management of this vulnerable group of patients and their families.

79.1.1 Definition

Craniosynostosis is defined as the premature fusion of one or more of the cranial sutures. This premature fusion can either be an isolated disorder (e.g. sagittal synostosis) or form part of a syndrome (e.g. Apert syndrome). In many cases the resultant head shape is typical of the involved suture such that the Greek/Latin descriptive terms are used synonymously with the description of the affected suture. For example scaphocephaly (boat-shaped head) is used to describe sagittal synostosis; however this approach can lead to confusion as can be seen in the use of the term plagiocephaly (flat head) which may refer to a unicoronal synostosis but also can be used in unilateral lambdoid synostosis, skull base torsion, the deformity resulting from torticollis and positional skull deformities. For this reason it is probably best to avoid the Latin/Greek descriptive terms and identify the affected suture(s) by name.

The majority of craniosynostoses are primary in nature and congenital; however a small proportion are termed secondary—caused by another pathology, usually resulting in reduced brain growth as seen in microcephaly or post-shunting.

D. Koppel (✉)
Consultant Craniofacial/Oral & Maxillofacial Surgeon, Clinical Director Surgery & Gastroenterology, Clinical Lead Scottish National Craniofacial Service for Children and Young People, Royal Hospital for Children, Glasgow, UK
e-mail: davidkoppel@nhs.net

J. Grant
Craniofacial Fellow, Birmingham Children's Hospital, Glasgow, UK
e-mail: jaimegrant@nhs.net

79.1.2 Aetiology

79.1.2.1 Primary Craniosynostosis

In the majority of cases, no cause for the synostosis is identified, but in an increasing proportion (currently about 25%), a mutation is identified. A significant proportion of these mutations are related to six genes FGFR2, FGFR3, TWIST1, EFNB1, TCF12 and ERF, however there is an increasing frequency of additional mutations being identified by more complex genetic analysis.

The incidence of identifying a mutation is much higher in syndromic craniosynostosis cases (69%), but the rate of mutation identification in the non-syndromic cases is increasing (currently 5%) particularly in the bicoronal, multisuture and unicoronal (in decreasing frequency) [1].

These genetic advances have assisted in the diagnosis of these conditions and influence the genetic counselling but have yet to impact on the management of the resultant problems related to the premature suture closure. As the mechanisms of sutural control and homeostasis are elucidated, novel therapies may be introduced.

79.1.2.2 Secondary Craniosynostosis

Microcephaly and babies who have been shunted as well as other systemic conditions such as sickle cell disease, thalassaemia and rickets can lead to synostosis usually affecting all the sutures. In cases of microcephaly, it is important to differentiate between a primary pansynostosis resulting in a small head often with raised intracranial pressure from a secondary synostosis with normal intracranial pressure [2].

K. Bonanthaya et al. (eds.), *Oral and Maxillofacial Surgery for the Clinician*, https://doi.org/10.1007/978-981-15-1346-6_79

79.1.3 Epidemiology

The incidence of craniosynostosis ranges from 1 in 1400 to 1 in 2100 live births worldwide with a slight male preponderance.

The different types of craniosynostosis occur in the following proportions:
- Sagittal 45%.
- Metopic 20%.
- Bicoronal and unicoronal 15%.
- Multiple suture 5%.
- Lambdoid <2% [3].

79.1.4 Classification

The classification of craniosynostosis has, in recent years, changed; the previously utilised terminology of simple and complex, referring to single-suture and multiple suture abnormalities, respectively, has been abandoned. It has little utility and is in fact misleading—the deformity as a result of a unicoronal synostosis is extremely complex and as more is understood about the genetic basis the more complex the condition becomes.

In terms of utility, the craniosynostosis is best classified by the suture(s) involved and whether this is associated with a syndrome (i.e. other abnormalities). See Table 79.1 and Illustrations 79.1, 79.2, 79.3, 79.4, 79.5, 79.6 and 79.7. The condition can be further defined by the genetic abnormalities. In general the syndromic craniosynostosis cases tend to be more severe and have a greater incidence of complicating features.

79.2 Management

The care of babies and children with craniosynostosis is best delivered in a centre with access to a full multidisciplinary team. This team involves the core specialities of paediatric neurosurgery and craniofacial surgery (either OMFS or plastics based) as well as support from paediatricians, neonatologists, geneticists, respiratory specialists, ophthalmologists and ENT surgeons. The input from specialist nurses and psychologists is vital [4].

Table 79.1 Overview of craniosynostoses

Suture affected	Description of shape	Diagram of shape	Description
Metopic	Trigonocephaly	Illustration 79.1a, b	Pointed, protuberant, prow-shaped forehead Reduced intercanthal distance Bitemporal narrowing
Unicoronal	Anterior plagiocephaly	Illustration 79.2a, b	Flattened forehead on affected side with raised eyebrow and shallower orbit Failure of forward growth of the hemiforehead with the ipsilateral ear also posterior
Bicoronal	Brachycephaly	Illustration 79.3a, b	Shortened AP—Coronal dimension Flattening of whole forehead Flattened supraorbital rims
Sagittal	Scaphocephaly	Illustration 79.4a, b	Forehead bossing Occipital bulleting Bitemporal narrowing Increased AP—Coronal dimension
Lambdoid	Posterior plagiocephaly	Illustration 79.5a, b	Bossing of mastoid on affected side Contralateral parietal bossing Ipsilateral ear posteriorised
Pansynostosis	Turricephaly or Oxycephaly	Illustration 79.6a, b	Restricted growth at all or multiple sutures—Upward growth in the region of the Fontanelle Small circumference 'Cone'- or 'turret'-shaped head
Positional	Plagiocephaly	Illustration 79.7a, b	Parallelogramming of the whole head Ears move with the segments No ridging of any sutures

Illustration 79.1 (**a**, **b**) Metopic suture affected in trigonocephaly

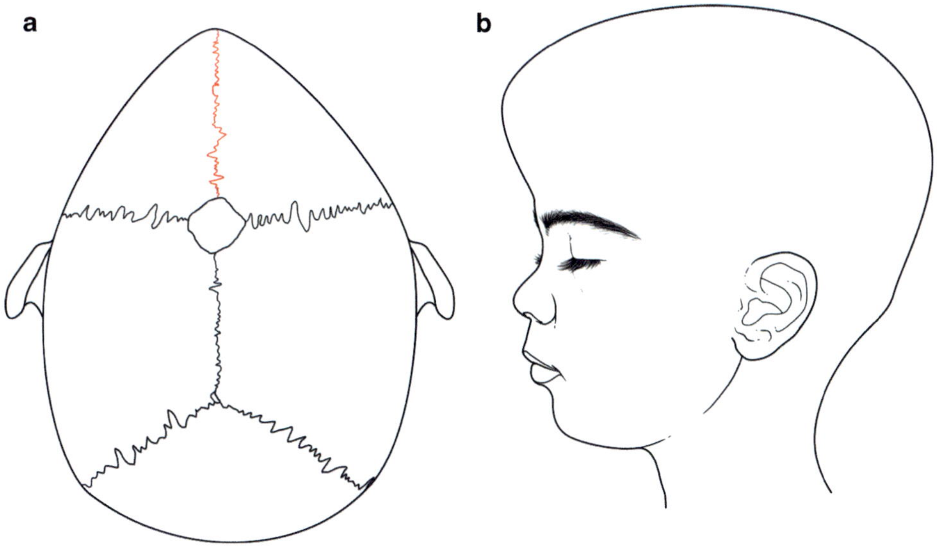

Illustration 79.2 (**a**, **b**) Unicoronal suture affected in anterior plagiocephaly

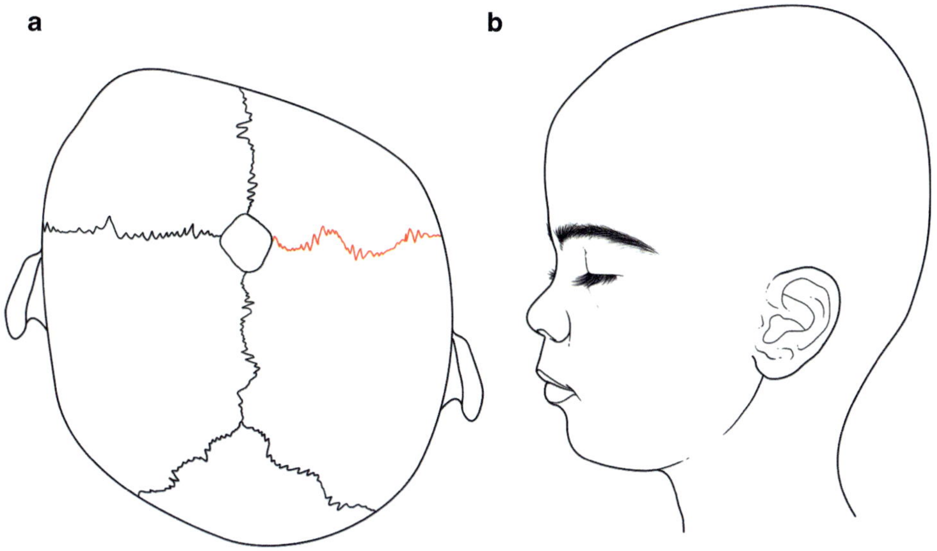

Illustration 79.3 (**a**, **b**) Bicoronal suture affected in brachycephaly

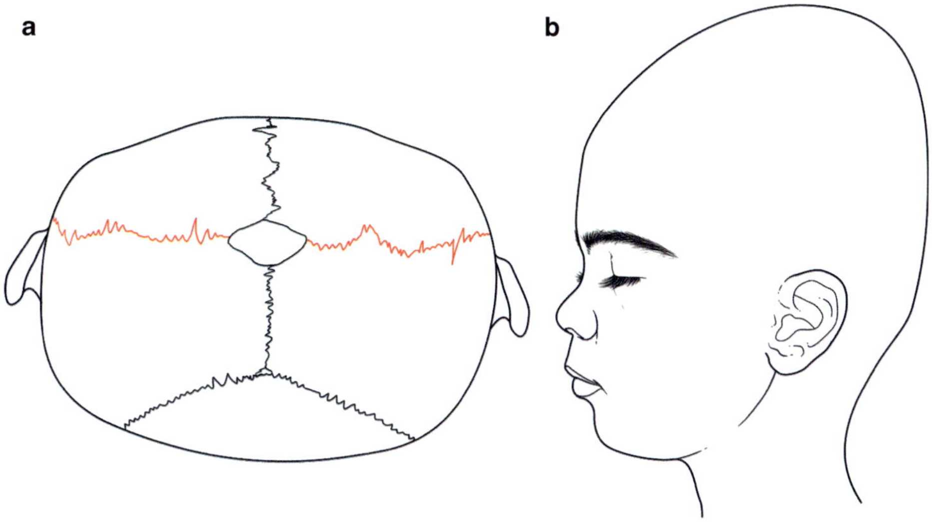

Illustration 79.4 (**a**, **b**) Sagittal suture affected in scaphocephaly

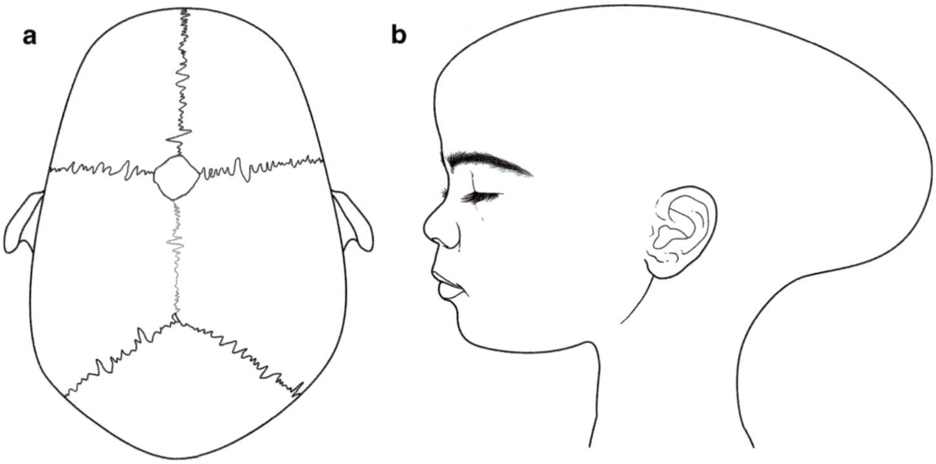

Illustration 79.5 (**a**, **b**) Lambdoid suture affected in posterior plagiocephaly

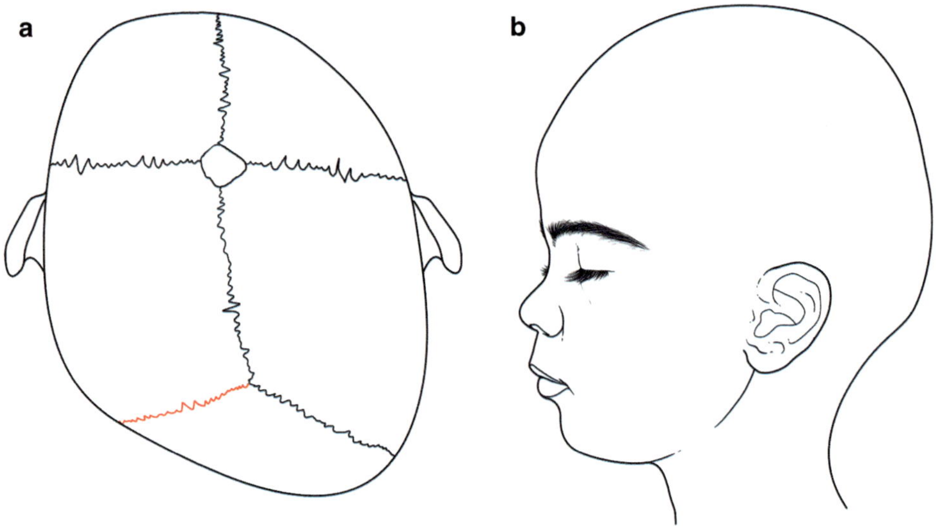

Illustration 79.6 (**a**, **b**) Pansynostosis causing turricephaly or oxycephaly

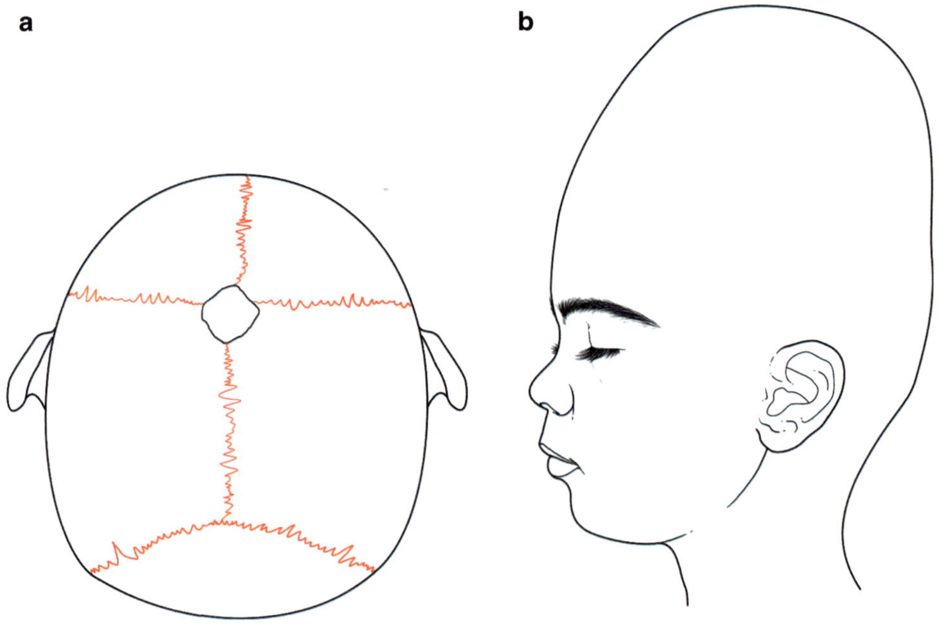

Illustration 79.7 (**a, b**) Positional plagiocephaly

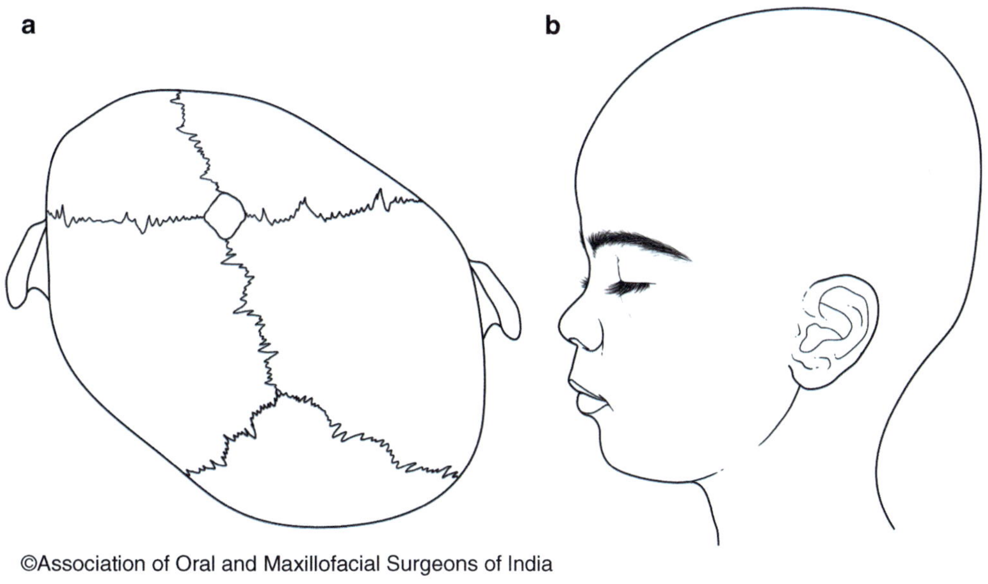

Table 79.2 Treatment options in infancy for complex synostosis problems

Clinical problem	Emergency/urgent treatment options	Definitive treatment options
Upper airway obstruction 2° to midface retrusion	Nasopharyngeal airway Intubation, O_2 support, CPAP, tracheostomy	Transcranial monobloc advancement (± distraction), CPAP, tracheostomy, Subcranial Le fort III advancement
Corneal exposure	Intensive eye care, tarsorrhaphy	Fronto-orbital advancement, Monobloc advancement
Hydrocephalus	External ventricular drain, ventriculo-peritoneal shunt, third ventriculostomy (in selected cases)	Ventriculo-peritoneal shunt
Elevated ICP	Medical treatment with acetazolamide, steroids	Skull vault expansion, fronto-orbital advancement and remodelling (FOAR), monobloc advancement ± implanted telemetric device

79.2.1 Prenatal Diagnosis

The use of high-definition prenatal ultrasound has increased the early diagnosis of both hydrocephalus and craniosynostosis [5]. This facilitates the preparation of parents for the birth of a child who is likely to have additional medical, surgical and emotional needs. In these circumstances parents getting to know the craniofacial team and being better informed of the potential problems often makes supporting them much easier.

79.2.2 Perinatal Care (Table 7.2)

In the perinatal period, care is directed at optimising the airway, ensuring the child is well oxygenated, preventing corneal damage (ocular protection) and confirming the diagnosis. In the majority of single-suture abnormalities, there are often no issues that prompt early intervention; however in the complex syndromic cases, this is not the case. Airway problems due to severe midface retrusion; breathing disturbance due to central problems, often due to posterior fossa crowding and Chiari malformation; corneal exposure secondary to midface and brow retrusion; and associated non-craniofacial anomalies prompt more urgent interventions. The necessity for such interventions is greatest in the syndromic conditions such as Apert, Pfeiffer, Crouzon and Carpenter syndromes. In cases where there is significant midface retrusion, there may also be feeding difficulties [6].

In the severe cases, initial care is supportive. The airway should be assessed and intervention initiated if necessary. It is important to assess the oxygen saturation and the work of breathing and correlate these findings with formal blood gas measurements. This assessment can be augmented with a formal sleep study, and on occasion simultaneous measurement of intracranial pressure may be helpful. Airway support can range from positional nursing, the use of a nasopharyngeal airway, intubation and in some cases tracheostomy. As part of this assessment, when the airway is an issue of concern, consideration should be given to performing a CT scan, and this will be useful to look at cranial anatomy but also the nasal anatomy, particularly to exclude choanal atresia. In assessing the airway, babies often manage satisfactorily but may suddenly decompensate with a minor upper respiratory tract infection or whilst feeding [6].

Surgical intervention in this period is only undertaken when the airway is such that no simple measures are able to overcome the symptoms; often a period of intubation is helpful to allow for a more thorough assessment rather than rushing to either tracheostomy or a monobloc fronto-facial advance. During this period parents and family members have to come to terms with the often unexpected consequences of having a child with additional needs and medical interventions. Early and ongoing support needs to be delivered; this can and should be through multiple avenues. Many such children are born in institutions with little or no experience of the condition(s), and this professional unfamiliarity often adds to parental anxiety. For these reasons early contact with a dedicated craniofacial team is invaluable. Specialist nurses, psychologists and support groups can often ease the stress of this difficult time [7].

79.2.3 Care in Infancy

The management of craniosynostosis in infancy is primarily aimed at addressing the primary consequences of the premature suture closure as well as dealing with the associated problems.

The management of the synostosis has, over the years, evolved considerably and in some respect completed a complete circle. The treatment is aimed at ensuring cranial volume is satisfactory to ensure that there is no elevation of ICP (in the absence of hydrocephalus) as well as attempting to normalise the head shape. The normalisation of head shape is done to maximise the chances of a normal head shape at the completion of growth. Initial treatment introduced in the second half of the last century involved a procedure known as suturectomy [8]. The principle of this was to excise the pathological, prematurely fused suture with the idea that removal of the pathology would allow the skull to continue to grow into a normal shape possibly aided by the continued growth of the brain. This was found to be partially effective especially when done before the age of 18 months [9]. It was however noted that in many cases re-fusion of the suture occurred and a number of surgeons began wrapping the bone edges on either side of the resected suture with silicone edging in an attempt to minimise the chances of re-fusion. Unfortunately this approach did not prevent re-fusion, and this often occurred on the dural side of the silicone edging. In pansynostosis cases the sutures were excised and the remainder of the skull was morselised [9]. These simple techniques have been superseded with more complex reconstructive procedures involving suturectomy and remodelling. (See case series examples (Figs. 79.2, 79.3, 79.4 and 79.5). When the coronal sutures are involved, either unilaterally or bilaterally, and/or the metopic sutures, the mainstay of treatment is a fronto-orbital advancement, with remodelling of the affected bones. When the sagittal suture is involved, the affected suture is excised and the remaining skull remodelled. The extent of remodelling varies from case to case but can involve addressing the frontal bossing, bitemporal narrowing and the occipital bullet [4]. These procedures involve extensive exposure and blood loss with their attendant risks, and for these reasons there has been a move to attempt to correct these abnormalities with less invasive procedures. These less invasive approaches utilise endoscopic suturectomy coupled with active postoperative helmet therapy to mould and harness the ongoing brain and hence skull growth [10]; another approach has used a minimal access suturectomy and specially designed springs to actively separate the affected suture edges [11]. A further technique, particularly in bicoronal or pansynostosis cases, is to utilise distraction osteogenesis; a craniotomy of the occipital bone is performed, and two or three distraction devices are applied; these are then activated over a period of 2–3 weeks, expanding the skull volume and in many cases improving the posterior fossa crowding seen in such cases. For reasons not fully understood, this technique often leads to a significant improvement in the contour of the frontal bones [12].

In terms of timing of surgery, there is considerable variation between different centres. In general elective (not motivated by functional concerns), suturectomy and skull remodelling procedures are performed between the ages of 5 months and 2½ years. The younger the patient, the greater the contribution of normal brain growth in normalising head shape; however the drawback of earlier surgery is the fragility of the skull bones and most importantly the risks of complications—particularly excessive blood loss [13].

During this period patients are generally followed up to monitor for signs of raised intracranial pressure, obstructive sleep apnoea (OSA) and evidence of a significant change in the rate of head growth as indicated by head circumference. Discrepancies between the plots on the growth charts (Fig. 79.1a, b) for length, weight and head circumference as well as plots crossing the centile lines should prompt further investigation.

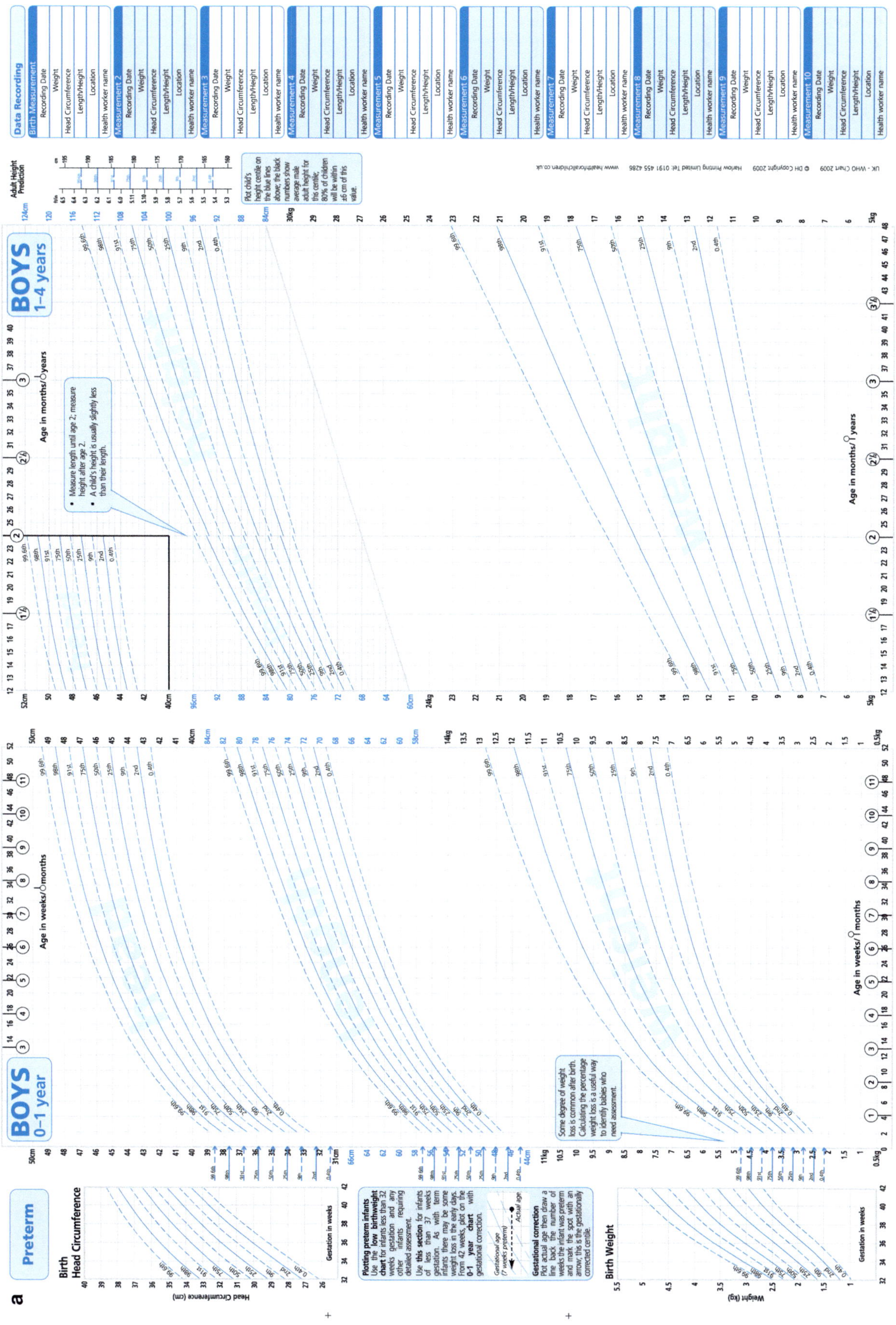

Fig. 79.1 **(a)** (boys), **(b)** (girls) WHO UK growth the chart **(a)** and **(b)** is available Online at https://www.rcpch.ac.uk/resources/uk-who-growth-charts-0-4-years

b

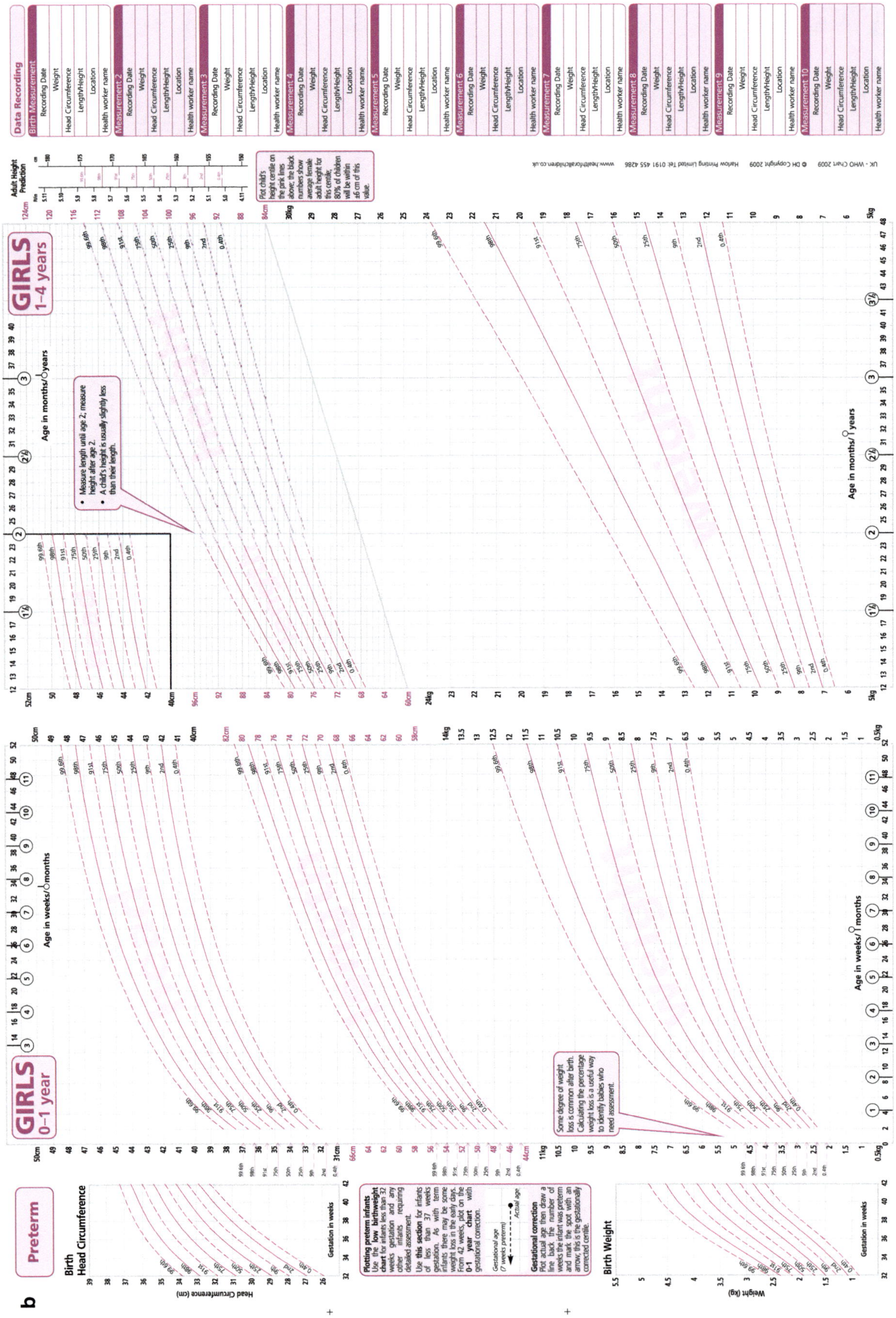

Fig. 79.1 (continued)

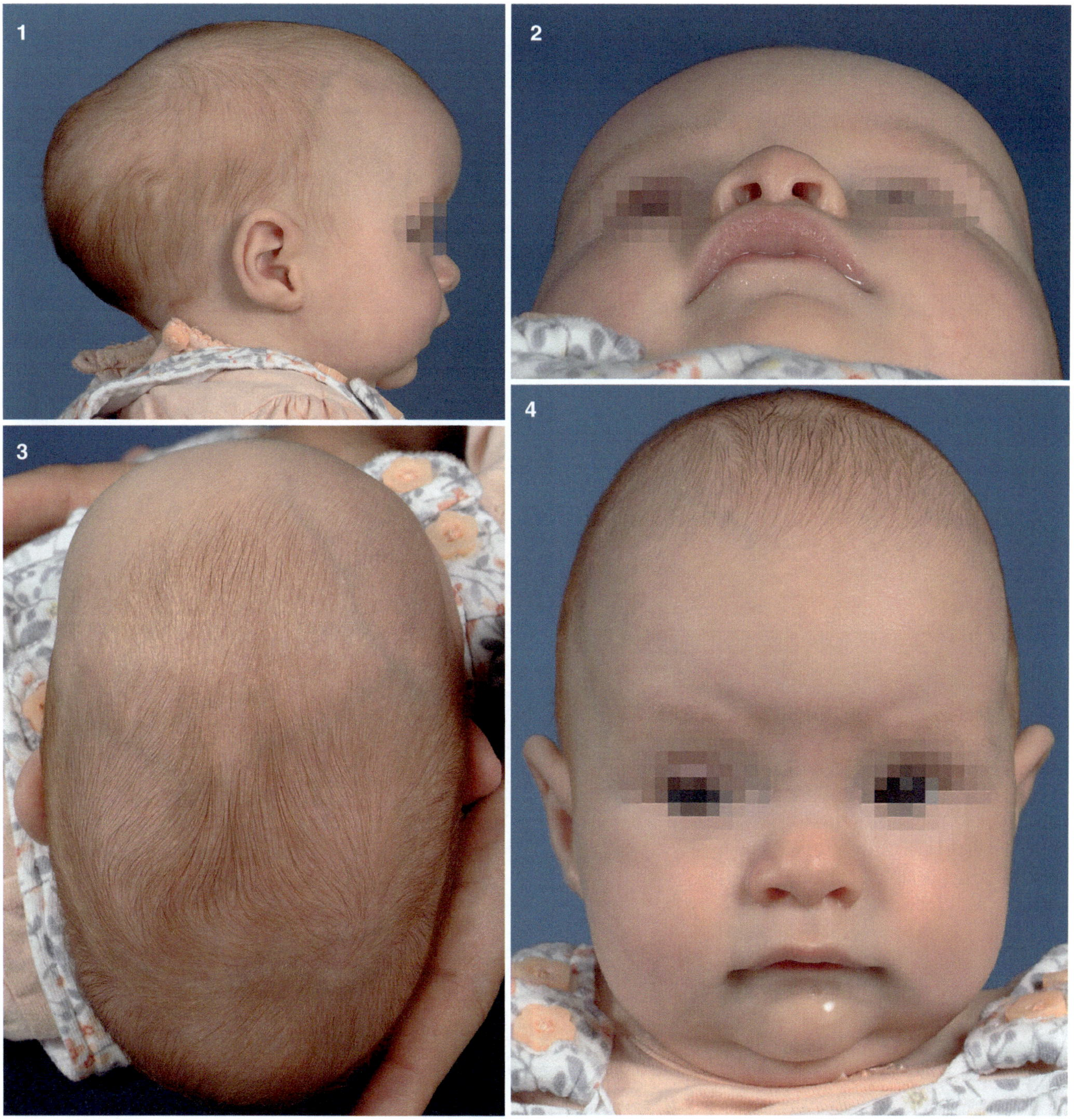

Fig. 79.2 (2.1–2.9) Case series of sagittal synostosis. (2.1–2.4) Preoperative facial views of patient with sagittal synostosis aged 13 weeks. Note elongated A-P dimension and bitemporal narrowing with prominent forehead and occiput. (2.5–2.7) Postoperative facial views of patient with sagittal synostosis after full calvarial remodelling. (2.8 and 2.9) Preoperative CT scan of the same patient with sagittal synostosis

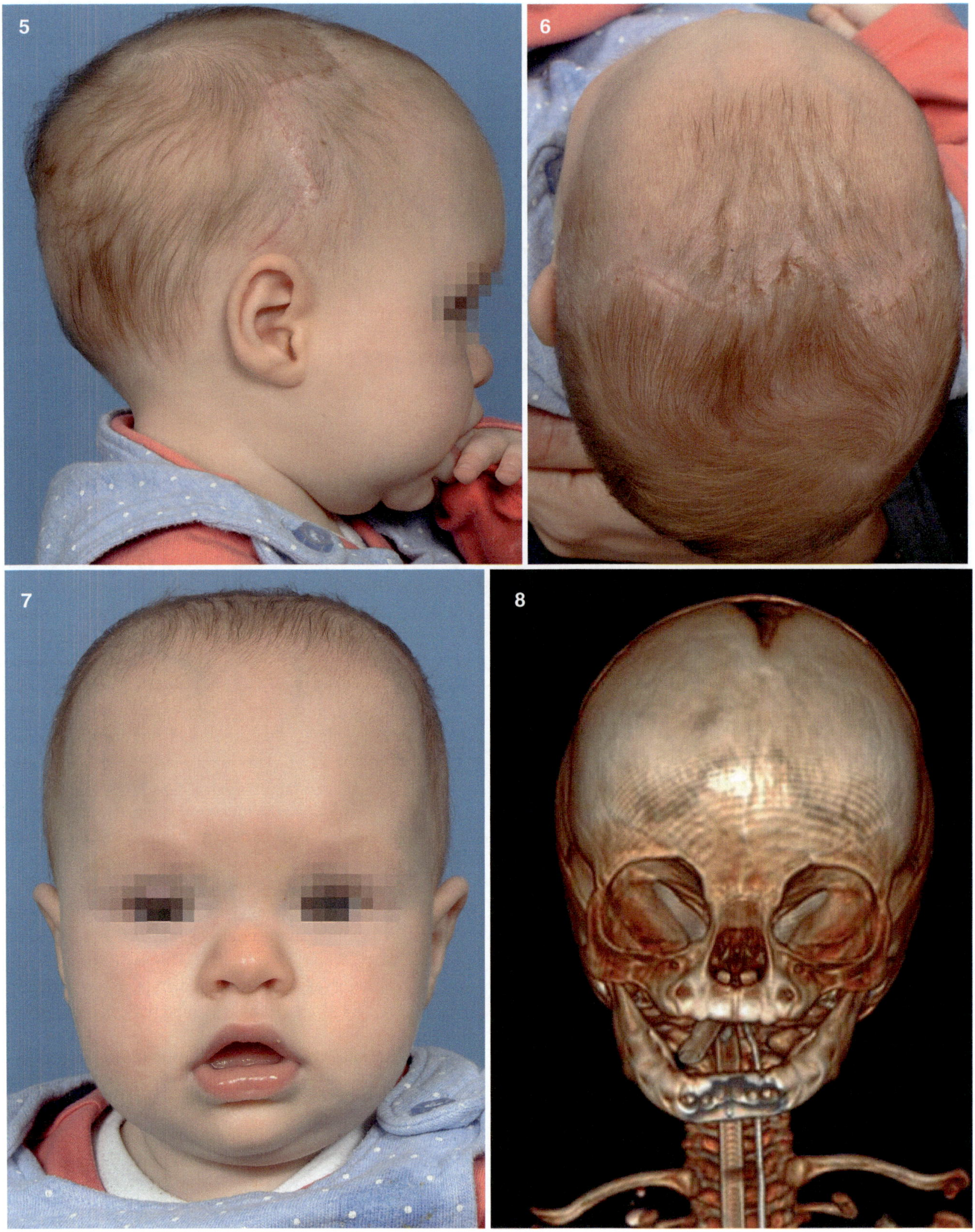

Fig. 79.2 (continued)

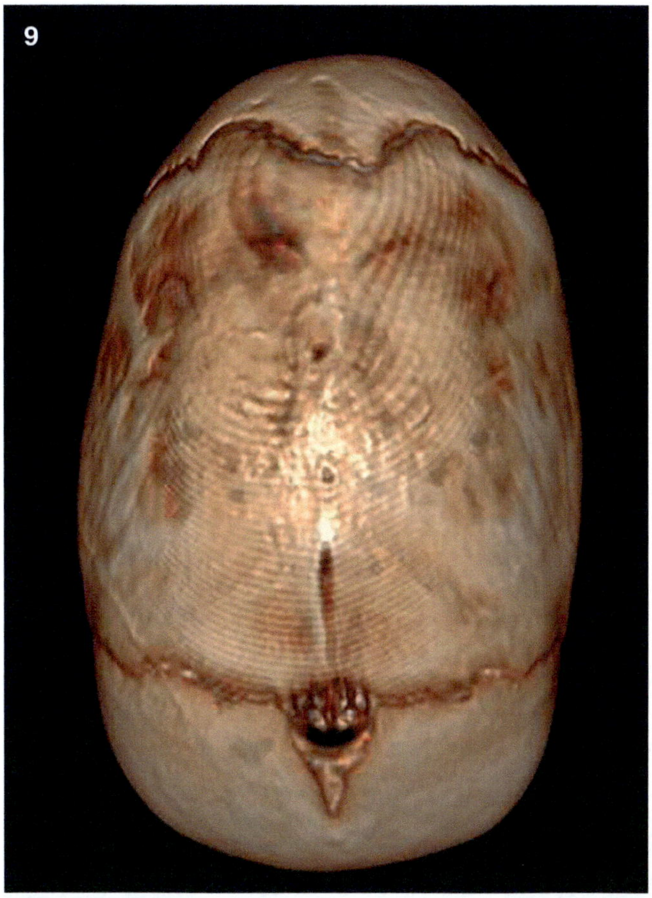

Fig. 79.2 (continued)

Elevated ICP manifests as distressed behaviour, inconsolable crying and headbanging with symptoms being worse at night. When symptoms are combined with papilloedema, urgent intervention is indicated. The absence of papilloedema does not exclude raised ICP, but its presence is of significance. In cases of doubt, formal ICP monitoring can be undertaken. In established cases the use of an indwelling telemetric ICP measurement device may be helpful [14].

Formal ophthalmological assessment should be undertaken and appropriate intervention initiated. Regular assessments are necessary to identify deterioration, particularly to identify corneal exposure and avoid the development of amblyopia.

Routine computerised tomography (CT) cross-sectional imaging is not indicated, and the diagnosis can, in the vast majority of cases, be made on clinical findings alone. In cases where the diagnosis is in doubt or there is the suspicion that there may be posterior fossa crowding, Chiari malformation or craniocervical abnormalities, a CT is indicated. Magnetic resonance imaging (MRI) is indicated to investigate the brain for structural abnormalities. The objective with this very conservative approach to imaging is to minimise the ionising radiation exposure, which has been demonstrated to adversely affect brain development and damage the developing eye [15].

Obstructive sleep apnoea can manifest as noisy snoring, characteristically crescendoing to a maximum followed by a period of silence, representing the apnoeic period with a cyclical restart, or a failure to thrive coupled with daytime tiredness. If OSA is suspected, an initial overnight pulse oximetry study can be undertaken, and if this proves to be suggestive of OSA, a full polysomnogram sleep study should be performed. This can be combined with formal ICP monitoring should there be any concerns about raised ICP. The active management of established OSA requires intervention from the multidisciplinary team, and the respiratory/ENT specialist input is paramount. It is important to establish the causes of sleep disorder and the level(s) of airway obstruction so that the most appropriate intervention(s) can be employed. Further investigations might involve microlaryngoscopy to exclude tracheal abnormalities. Imaging with CT is useful, and interventions should be stepwise with consideration being given to tonsillectomy and adenoidectomy [16].

In the majority of cases of non-syndromic single-suture abnormalities, a single intervention for the surgical correction of the head shape is the norm [4].Whilst there is considerable variation between different units regarding

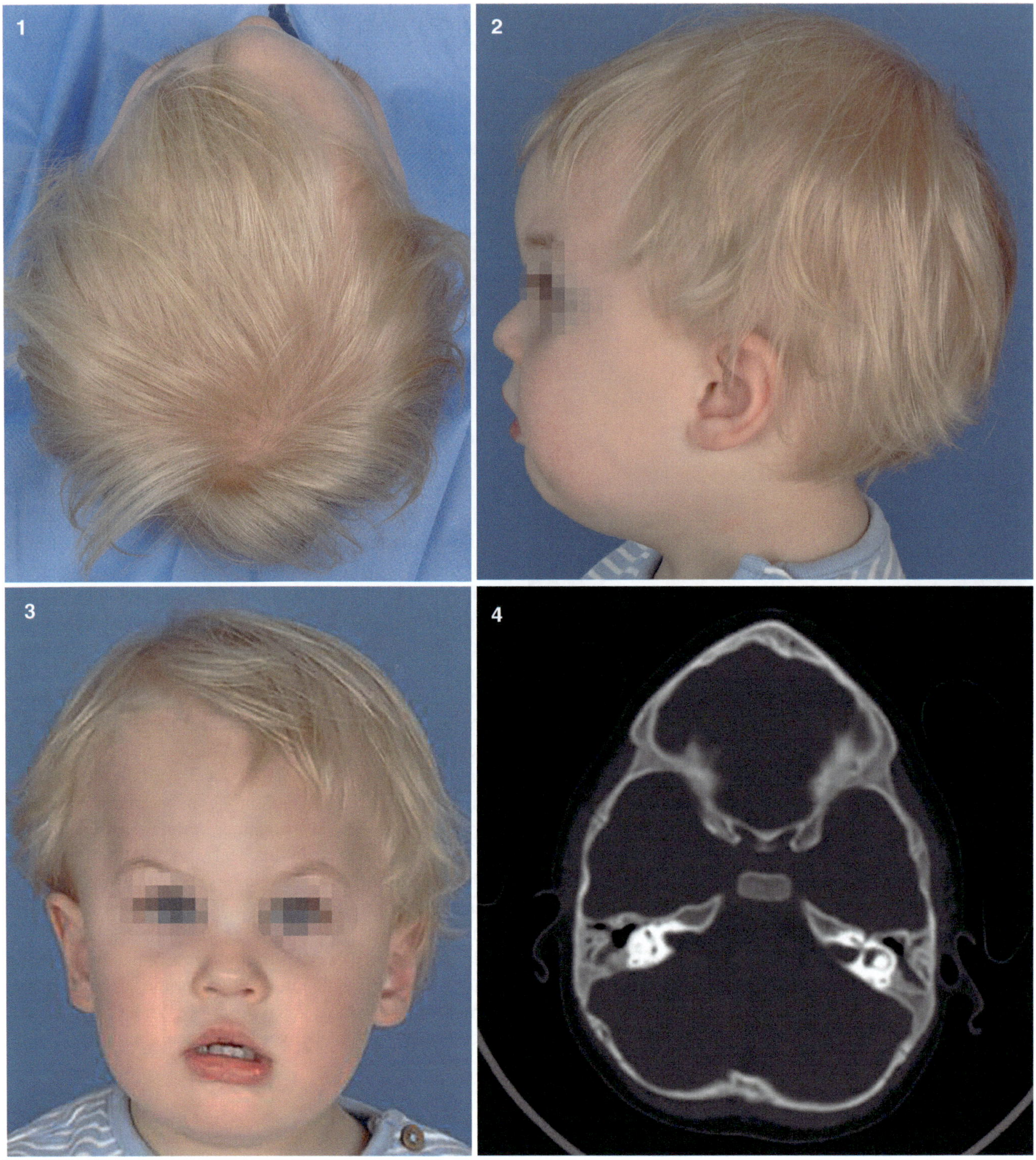

Fig. 79.3 (3.1–3.17) Case series of metopic synostosis. (3.1–3.3) Preoperative facial views of patient with metopic synostosis, age 23 months (late presentation), note pointed brow, triangular-shaped skull and hypertelorism. (3.4–3.6) Preoperative CT scan of the same patient with metopic synostosis—note it is not our usual practice to obtain preoperative CT in metopic synostosis; however this was taken due to the subtle (and late) presentation. (3.7–3.14) Intraoperative views of fronto-orbital remodelling. (3.7) Frontal bar after removal prior to remodelling. (3.8) Frontal bar and fontal bones after removal prior to remodelling. (3.9, 3.10) Frontal bar after remodelling with midline graft to correct hypotelorism. (3.11) Frontal bone osteotomised ready for remodelling. (3.12–3.14) Final views after fixation—fronto-orbital remodelling or anterior two-thirds remodelling. Note use of absorbable plates in load-/tension-bearing areas and absorbable sutures or stainless steel wires in less critical regions. Bone dust and bone dust putty (fibrin sealant mixed with bone dust) are used in resultant bone defects to encourage ossification. (3.15–3.17) Postoperative facial views of patient with metopic synostosis

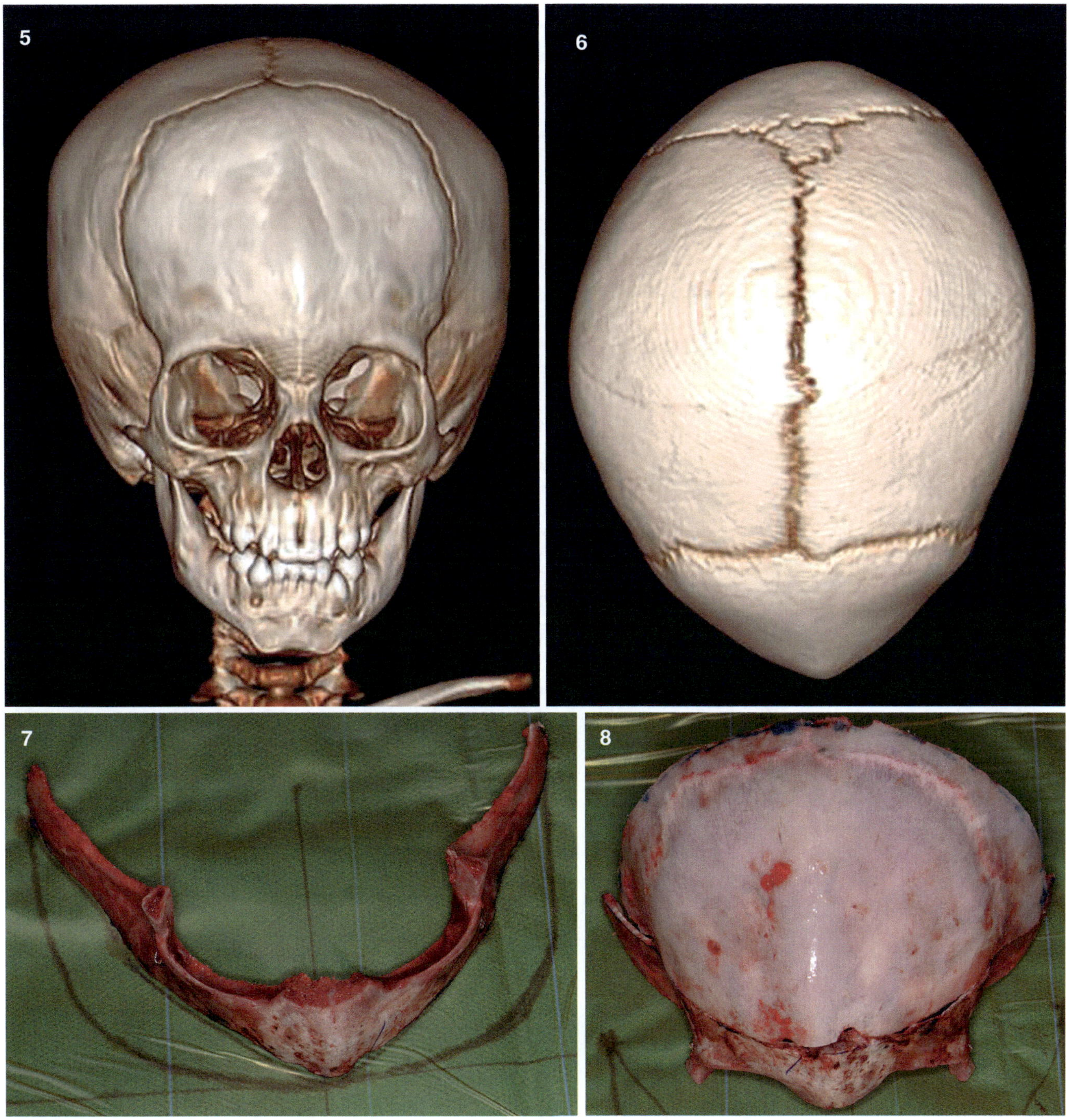

Fig. 79.3 (continued)

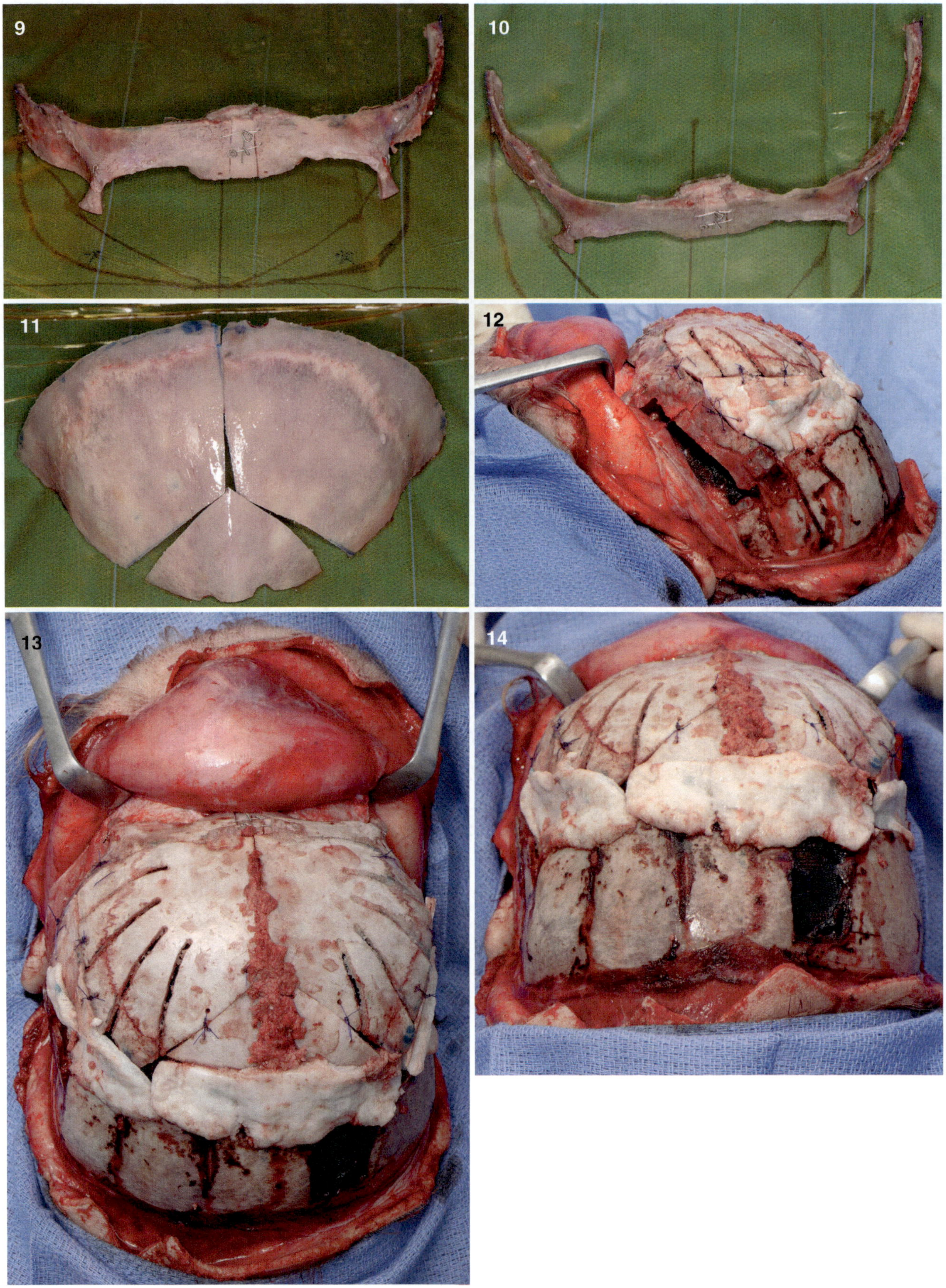

Fig. 79.3 (continued)

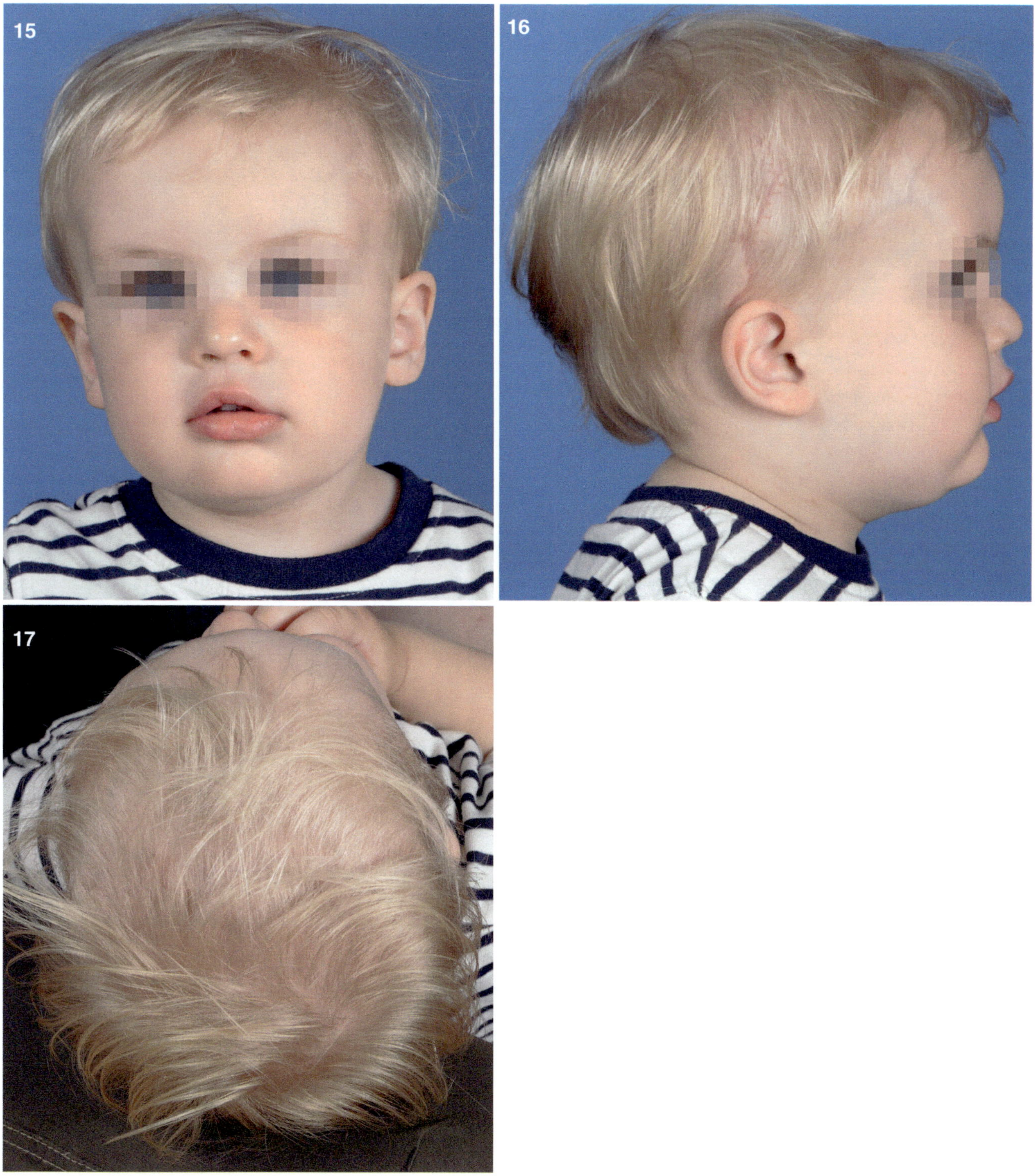

Fig. 79.3 (continued)

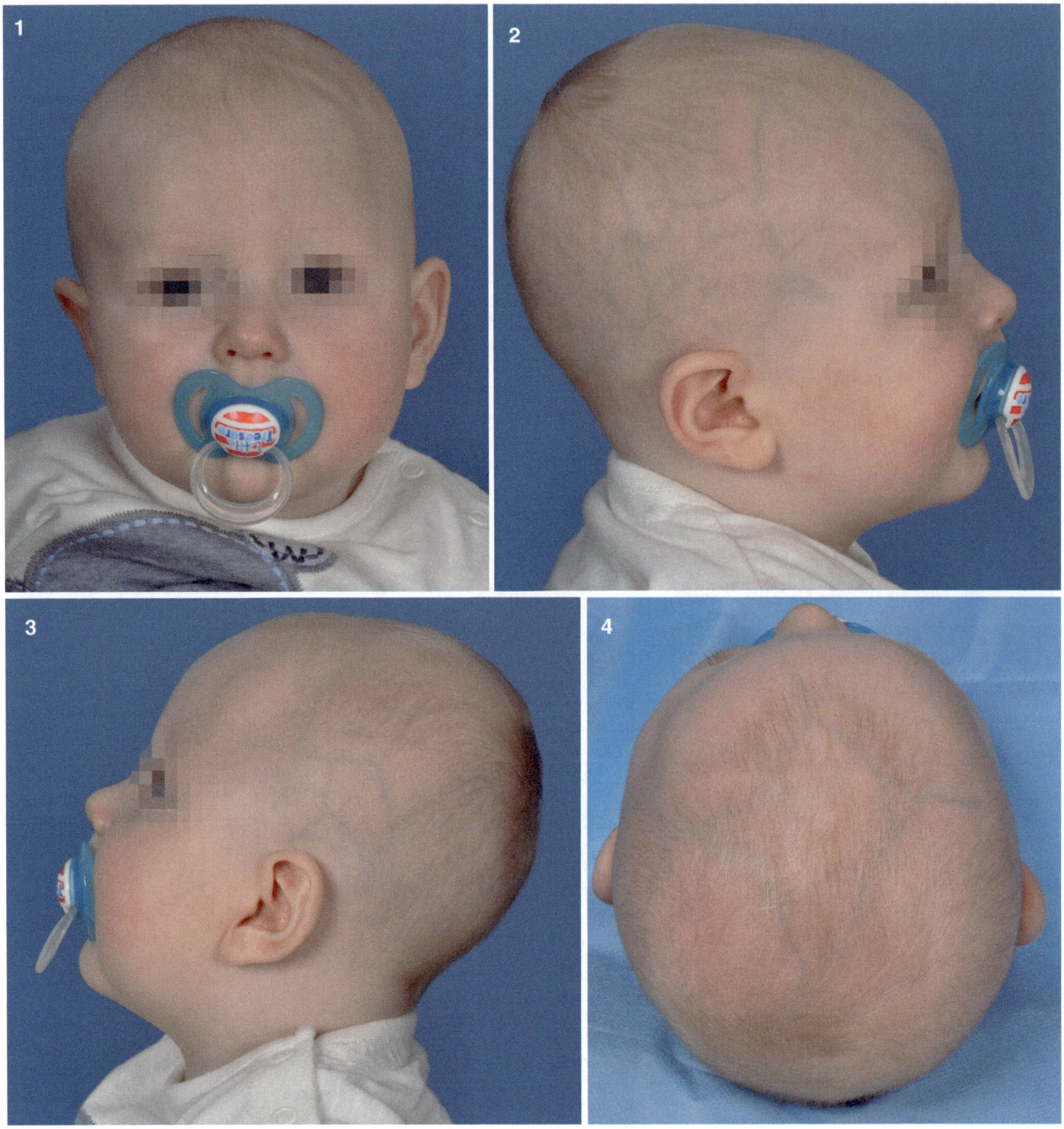

Fig. 79.4 (4.1–4.12) Case series of unicoronal synostosis. (4.1–4.4) Preoperative facial views of patient with unicoronal synostosis, patient aged 31 weeks—left unicoronal synostosis—flattened left brow anterior plagiocephaly when viewed from above and ridging of the involved left coronal suture. (4.5–4.9) Intraoperative views of asymmetric fronto-orbital advance. (4.5) Precraniotomy planning—note the fused left coronal suture. (4.6–4.9) After fixation of the osteotomised segments—asymmetric fronto-orbital advancement; note onlay bone graft to left supraorbital region, fixation with absorbable plates and pins as well as absorbable sutures. (4.10–4.12) Postoperative facial views of patient with unicoronal synostosis

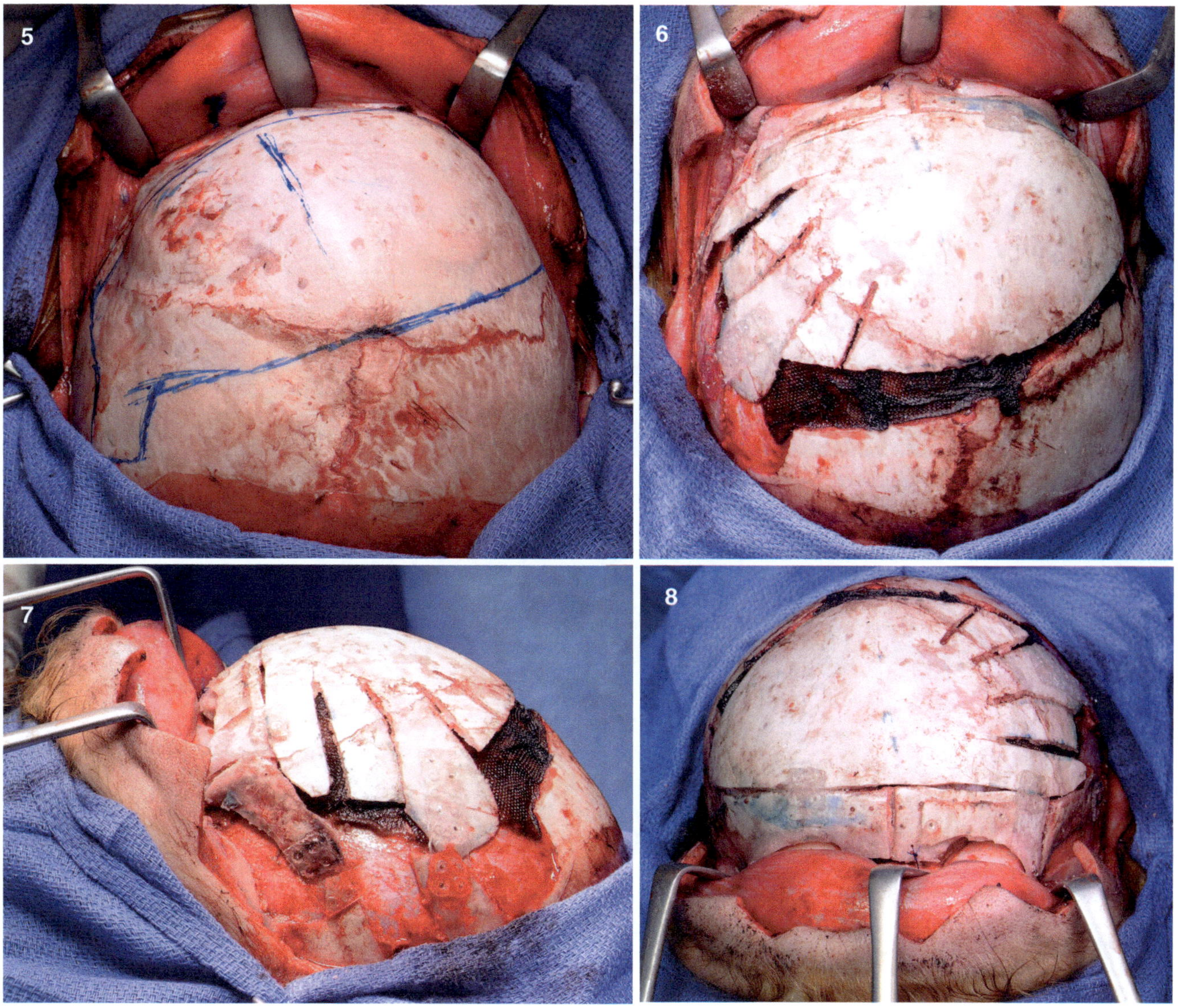

Fig. 79.4 (continued)

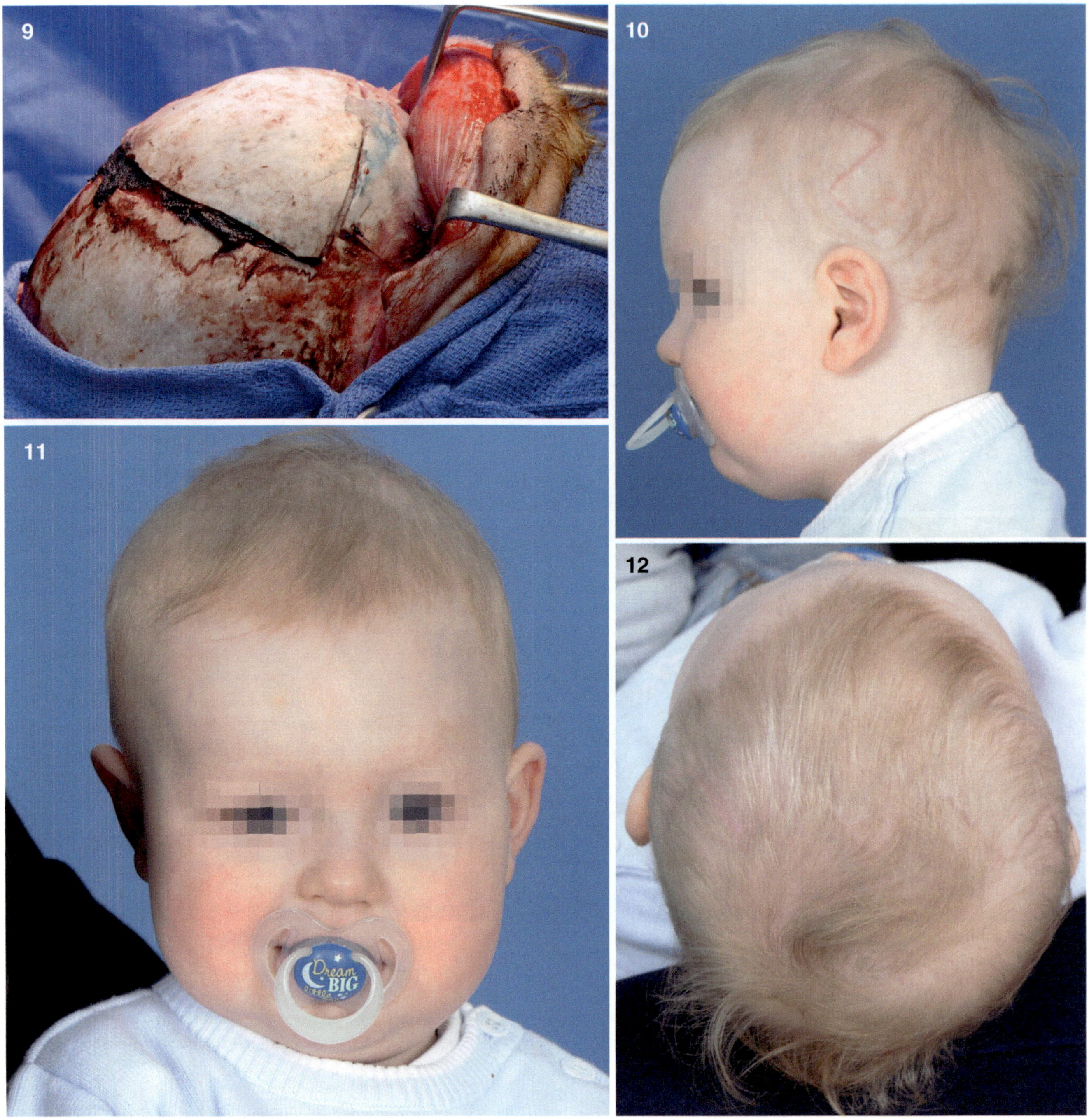

Fig. 79.4 (continued)

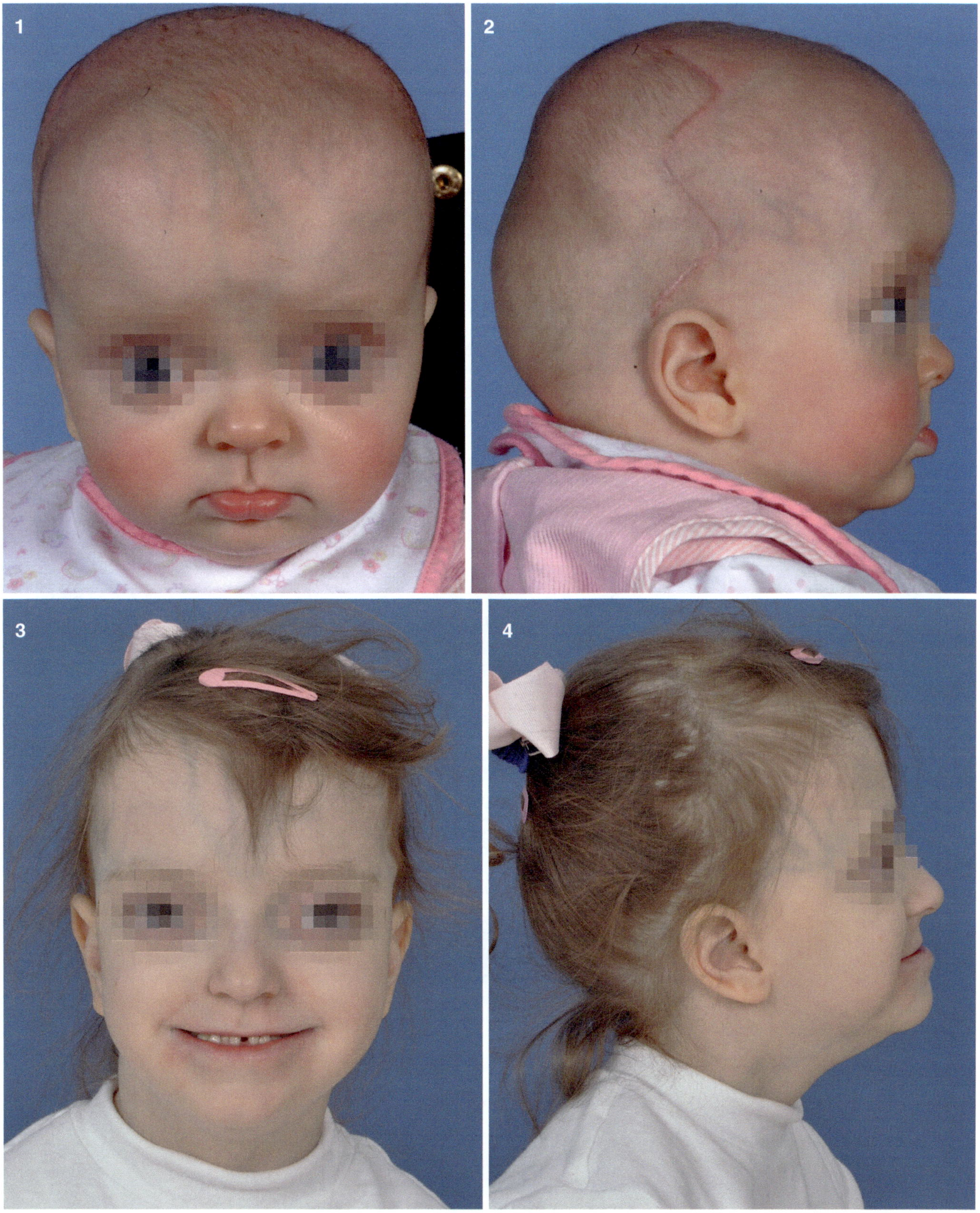

Fig. 79.5 (5.1–5.13) Case series of Crouzon syndrome. (5.1 and 5.2) Patient with Crouzon syndrome after initial calvarial remodelling aged 34 weeks. (5.3 and 5.4) Preoperative facial views of same patient aged 5 with Crouzon's type facies. (5.5–5.7) Postoperative facial views after Le Fort III distraction osteotomies and static fronto-orbital advance with the rigid external distractor (RED frame) and internal distractors in place (day 1 post-op). The use of the internal distractors allows for the early removal of the external device after the active distraction period, acting as fixation devices for the retention period. (5.8–5.9) Final post-operative result immediately after RED frame distractor removal. (5.10–5.11) Late postoperative result following internal distractor removal. (5.12 and 5.13) Pre- and mid-distraction CT images of Le Fort III distraction and static fronto-orbital advance. Note internal distractors engaging zygoma (pushing Le fort III and external RED frame pulling midface). It is not our usual practice to obtain a CT mid treatment, but this was carried out due to concerns around a possible CSF leak. The static fronto-orbital advance is secured with absorbable, radiolucent, plates, but the multiple pin holes are visible

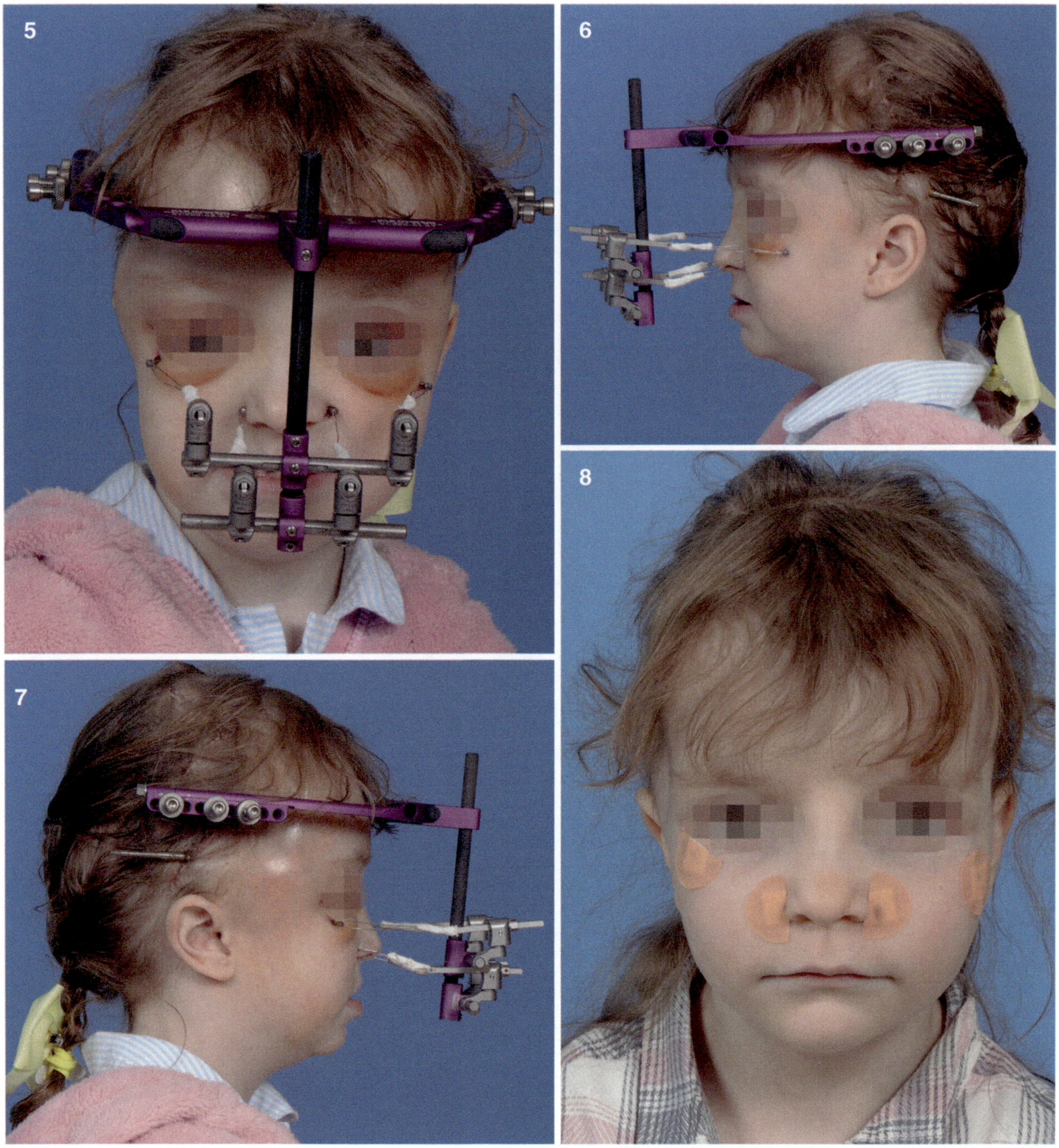

Fig. 79.5 (continued)

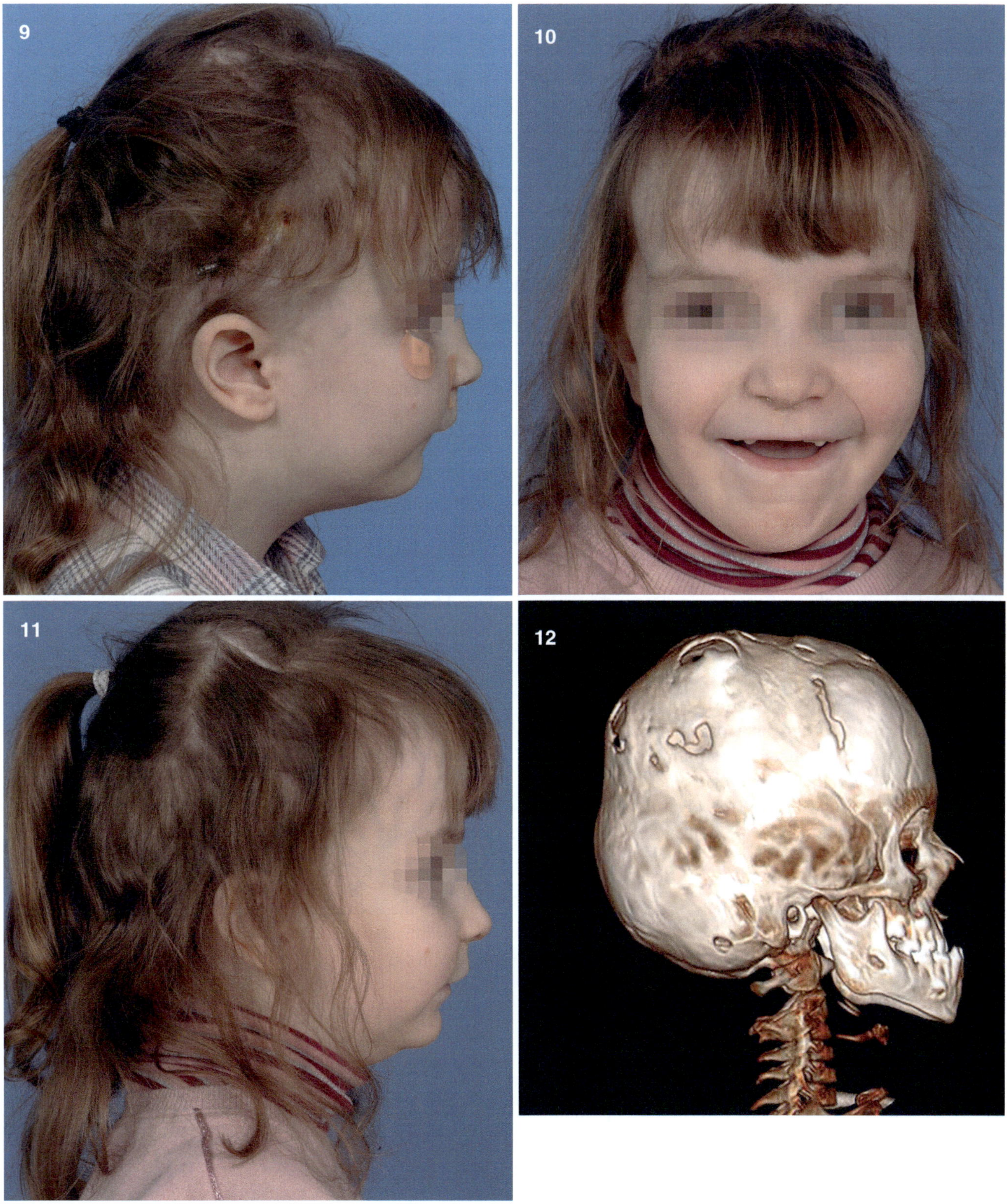

Fig. 79.5 (continued)

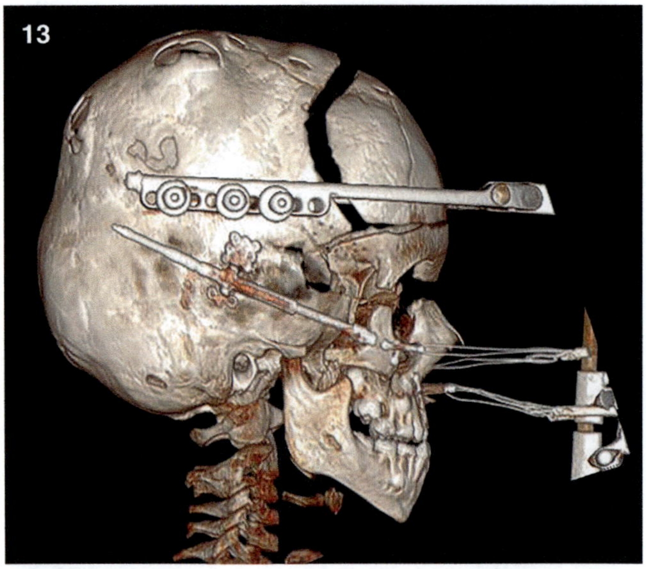

Fig. 79.5 (continued)

timing and actual intervention, the Glasgow craniofacial service protocol is outlined in Table 79.3. See also Table 79.4 for an outline of the surgical procedures commonly carried out and the case series (Figs. 79.2, 79.3, 79.4 and 79.5) for an overview of treatment outcomes.

In the management of the syndromic cases, the treatment has to be more flexible and problem driven. There is considerable variation in the severity and comorbidities in this group of patients. Overall the aim is to minimise the number of surgical interventions; however re-synostosis, systemic problems, corneal exposure, airway obstruction and raised ICP are much more common in the group [14]. In the absence of additional pressing clinical issues, the syndromic synostosis cases can be managed as the non-syndromic cases in terms of the timing and extent of skull surgery.

79.2.4 Management in Early Childhood (3–8 Years)

In this period the management is primarily of observation. The non-syndromic cases are followed up 6 weeks, 6 months and 1 year post-skull vault surgery with growth, particularly head circumference, development and vision being monitored. A final review is usually undertaken immediately prior to the child starting school. Some units have a much longer follow-up period; however we reserve longer follow-up for the small proportion of patients who encounter ongoing development problems or symptoms. This protocol should be modified if there is a less well-developed community-based health surveillance programme.

Table 79.3 Glasgow protocol for the management of non-syndromic synostosis

Condition	Ideal age for intervention	Usual procedure
Sagittal synostosis	5–7 months	Total vault remodelling
Metopic synostosis	10–14 months	Fronto-orbital advancement, anterior remodelling ± hypotelorism correction
Unicoronal synostosis	10–14 months	Fronto-orbital advancement, anterior remodelling—Bilateral
Bicoronal synostosis	5–18 months	Posterior vault distraction
	10–14 months	Bilateral fronto-orbital advancement, anterior remodelling
Lambdoid synostosis[a]	10–14 months	Posterior vault expansion static or with distraction

[a]In the presence of elevated ICP

The syndromic cases are followed up more closely with a minimum of annual reviews. In addition to the parameters noted above, the development of OSA may be insidious, and therefore at every review this should be asked about specifically. Towards the end of this period, consideration can be given to performing either a midface advancement or hypertelorism correction. This decision should be primarily driven by clinical problems rather than purely aesthetics, though teasing, bullying and psychological issues can, and should, play a role in decision-making. The input of child psychologists is often very helpful in developing a treatment plan and choosing the optimal timing [17].

During this period it is also important to monitor dental development and try to optimise routine dental care. In addition, at some time the patient should be referred for a full genetic consultation, though the timing of this can be determined by the needs and desires of the family. Throughout the care of the patient development, psychological, educational, physical and speech and language development should be monitored and intervention initiated when necessary.

Table 79.4 Surgical procedures in craniofacial surgery

Procedure	Access	Technical notes	Illustrations
Fronto-orbital advance and remodelling	– Bicoronal stealth incision in the Alice band region – Anterior dissection to superior orbit for access to frontal bandeau inferiorly (may require osteotomies to free supraorbital nerves/vessels)	1. Design mapped out and bur holes made for access with matchstick craniotome. 2. Frontal bone removed (pre–/post-suture). 3. Frontal bandeau removed—Cuts from anterior cranial fossa with direct vision inferiorly via the superior orbit. 4. Frontal bandeau and frontal bone remodelled as necessary and secured in advanced position.	Illustration 79.8a, b
Sagittal remodelling Total vault remodelling	– Mid-cranial stealth incision for access to anterior and posterior calvarium – Start in prone position with careful eye positioning and intermittent relief and then turn supine – Dissection posteriorly to base of occipit and anteriorly to brow	1. Map out dural sinuses. 2. Draw plan for osteotomies and create bur holes for access with matchstick craniotome. 3. Remove occipital bullet and barrel stave (sun) (bone harvesting as required from inner table). 4. Sagittal suturectomy and lateral barrel staving of mid calvarium/moulding laterally as far anteriorly as permitted whilst prone. 5. Secure occipital portion with PDS. 6. Turn the patient. 7. Frontal craniotomy/remodelling and inner table bone harvesting as required. 8. Complete suturectomy and barrel staving anteriorly. 9. Secure frontal bone (resorbable plates). 10. Fill in areas of bony discontinuity with bone putty (bone dust and tisseal).	Illustration 79.9
Metopic remodelling	– Bicoronal stealth incision in the Alice band region – Anterior dissection to superior orbit for access to frontal bandeau inferiorly (may require osteotomies to free supraorbital nerves/vessels)	1. Design mapped out and bur holes made for access with matchstick craniotome. 2. Frontal bone removed (pre–/post-suture). 3. Frontal bandeau removed—Cuts from anterior cranial fossa with direct vision inferiorly via the superior orbit. 4. Frontal bandeau remodelled with interposing bone graft to increase width and flatten midline prominence. • Internal resorbable strut plate for strength. • Resorbable plates bitemporally ± bone graft in gap from advancement. • Brow resecured in midline (resorbable plate/PDS). 5. Frontal bone remodelling (sectioning and repositioning ± barrel staving). 6. ± barrel staving and moulding of mid calvarium 7. Frontal bone placed and secured (resorbable plates/PDS).	Same as Illustration 79.8b
Unicoronal	– Bicoronal stealth incision in the Alice band region – Anterior dissection to superior orbit for access to frontal bandeau inferiorly (may require osteotomies to free supraorbital nerves/vessels)	1. Design mapped out and bur holes made for access with matchstick craniotome. 2. Frontal bone removed (post-coronal suture). 3. Frontal bandeau removed—Cuts from anterior cranial fossa with direct vision inferiorly via the superior orbit. 4. Frontal bandeau remodelled and secured: • Internal resorbable strut plate for strength. • Resorbable plates bitemporally ± bone graft in gap from advancement. • Brow resecured in midline (resorbable plate/PDS). 5. Frontal bone remodelling (sectioning and repositioning ± barrel staving). 6. Frontal bone placed and secured (resorbable plates).	Asymmetric fronto-orbital advancement for unicoronal synostosis Illustration 79.10

Table 79.4 (continued)

Procedure	Access	Technical notes	Illustrations
Monobloc	– Bicoronal stealth incision in the Alice band region – Anterior dissection (separate pericranial flap) to superior orbit for access to frontal bandeau inferiorly (may require osteotomies to free supraorbital nerves/ vessels) – Dissection to zygomatic arch bilaterally – Intraoral access posterior to hamulus for pterygomaxillary disjunction – Transconjunctival access to orbital floor	1. Design mapped out and bur holes made for access with matchstick craniotome. 2. Frontal bone removed (pre–/post-suture). 3. Access to anterior cranial fossa and superior orbit. 4. Cuts as per frontal bandeau cuts in anterior cranial fossa with direct vision from superior orbit. 5. Cuts at zygomatic arches bilaterally. 6. Inferior orbital cuts from inferior orbital fissure laterally and then superiorly to join superior orbit cuts and medially from inferior orbital fissure running superiorly to join superior cuts. 7. Osteotomes used to achieve pterygomandibular disjunction. 8. Smiths/osteotomes to propagate splits. 9. Fixation may be for: • Static advancement with plates at frontal bandeau butt joint posterior frontal bone bilateral zygomatic arches. • Distraction—Internal distractor at posterior part of frontal process of zygomatic bone and pins for the RED frame in the body of the zygoma and paranasally. • A combination—Static fronto-orbital advancement/remodelling (as for FOAR) with distraction of the Le fort III segment.	Illustration 79.11a, b
Subcranial Le fort III	– Bicoronal stealth incision in the Alice band region – Anterior dissection to superior orbit for access to frontonasal junction (may require osteotomies to free supraorbital nerves/vessels) – Dissection to zygomatic arch bilaterally – Intraoral access posterior to hamulus for pterygomaxillary disjunction ± anteriorly for placement of distractors – Transconjunctival access to orbital floor	1. Cuts in orbital floors avoiding lacrimal apparatus leaving medial canthal tendon attached to bone. 2. Zygomatic cuts may be made from above or below depending on access. 3. Osteotome used to achieve frontonasal disjunction and pterygomaxillary disjunction. 4. Smiths to propagate splits. 5. Fixation may be for distraction as shown (and as per monobloc) or static advancement with fixation at the zygomatic arch, frontozygomatic suture, frontonasal junction and intermaxillary fixation.	Illustration 79.12—subcranial le fort III
Posterior vault distraction	– Mid-cranial stealth incision for access to the posterior calvarium – Posterior dissection to base of occiput – Stealth mapping of dural venous sinuses	1. Posterior bullet osteotomy with matchstick bur and craniotome. 2. Dural mobilisation. 3. Positioning of 2/3 distractors and tunnelling anteriorly to exit either through the wound or anterior to it. 4. May incorporate foramen magnum decompression or insertion of telemetry can ICP monitor if required.	Illustration 79.13—Posterior vault distraction
Facial bipartition/ orbital osteotomies	– Bicoronal stealth incision in the Alice band region – Anterior dissection (separate pericranial flap) to superior orbit for access to frontal bandeau inferiorly (may require osteotomies to free supraorbital nerves/ vessels) – Dissection to zygomatic arch bilaterally – Intraoral access posterior to hamulus for pterygomaxillary disjunction and anteriorly to separate nasal septum and split palate – Transconjunctival access to orbital floor	As per monobloc with additional: 1. Separation of the nasal septum from the palate via an intraoral incision. 2. Midline osteotomy of the palate. 3. Midline removal of bone as required from glabella/nasal region. 4. Secure as per monobloc with additional midline fixation and a palatal splint. Box osteotomies of the orbits to achieve orbital movement separate from the maxillary movement involve the same cuts without disjunction at the Le fort I level	Illustration 79.14a, b

Illustration 79.8 (**a**, **b**) Fronto-orbital advance and remodelling

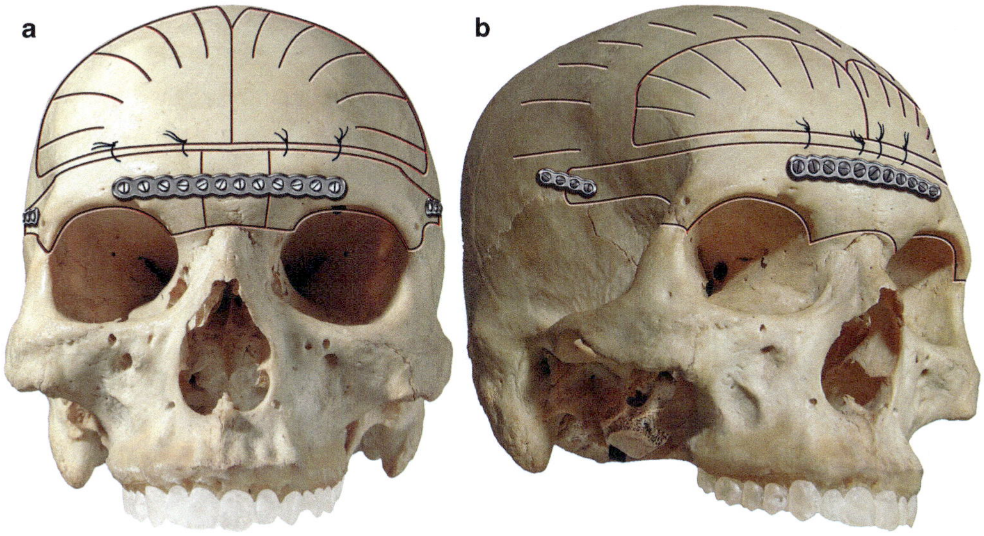

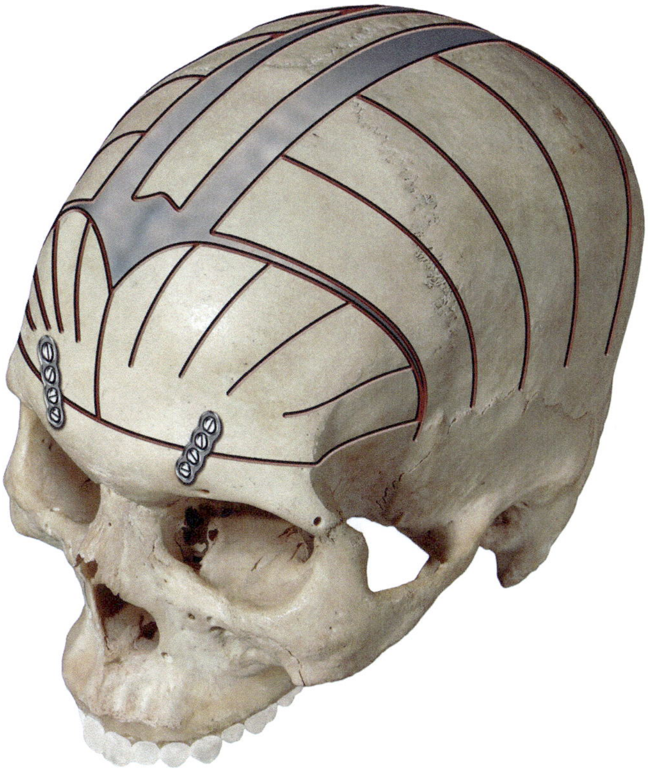

Illustration 79.9 Sagittal remodelling/total vault remodelling

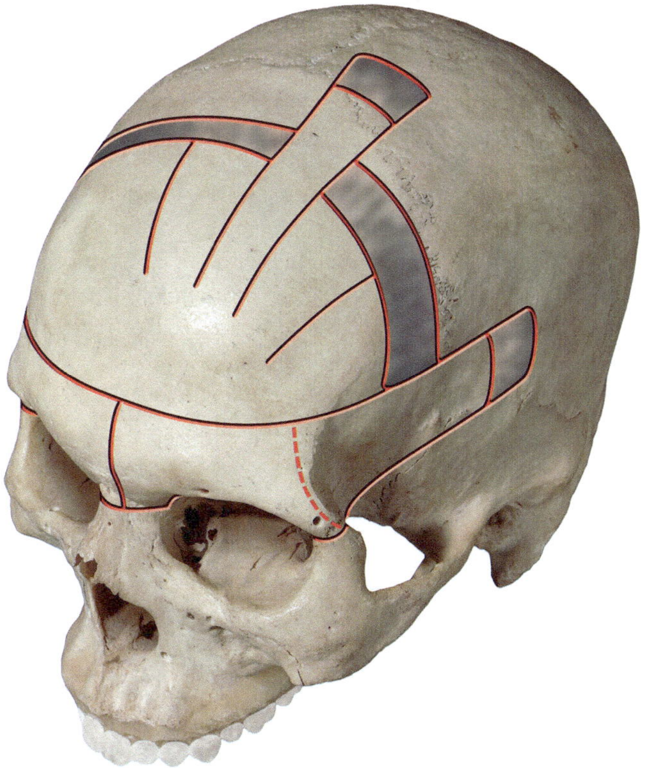

Illustration 79.10 Asymmetric fronto-orbital advancement for unicoronal synostosis

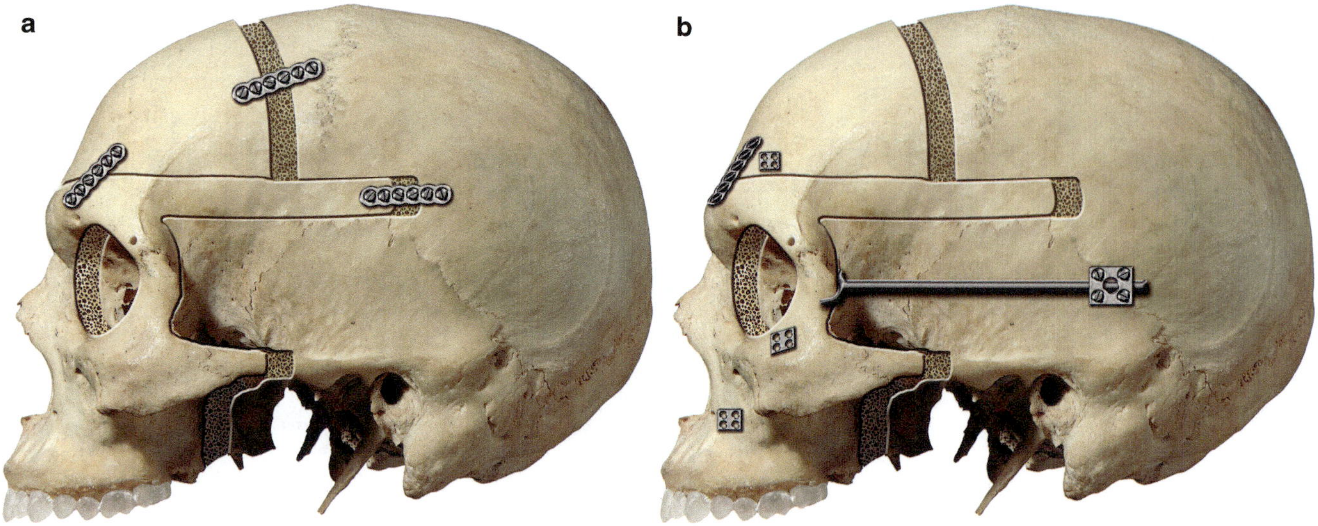

Illustration 79.11 (**a**, **b**) Monobloc advancement

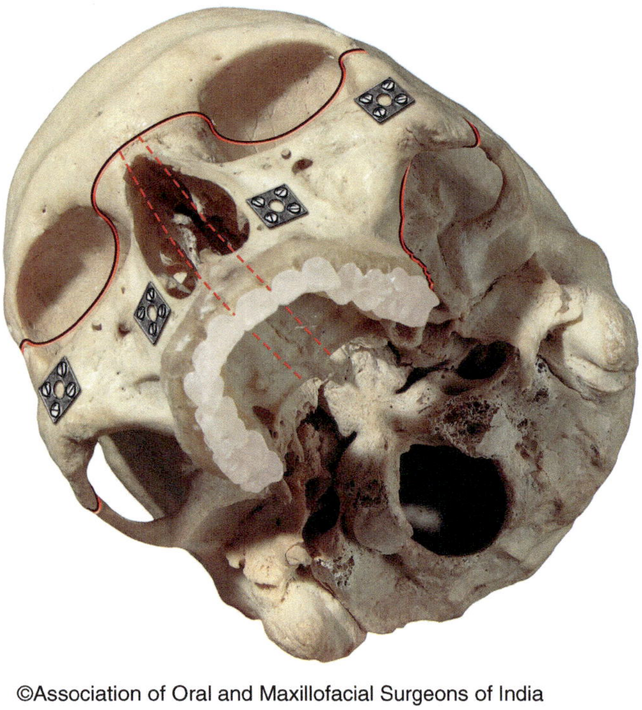

Illustration 79.12 Subcranial Le Fort III

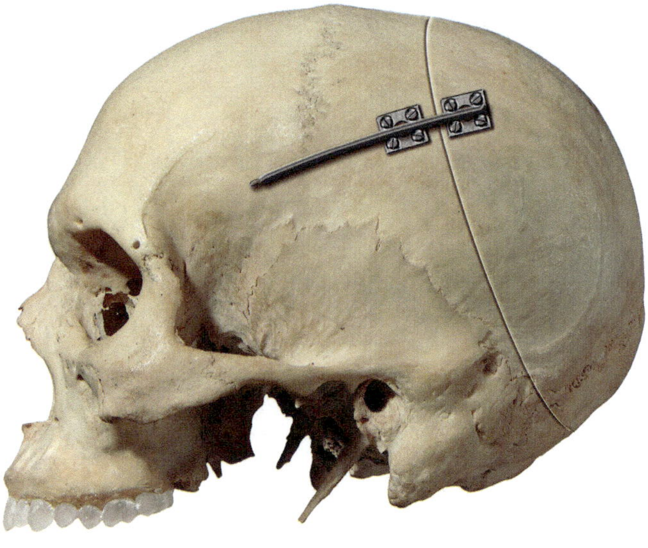

Illustration 79.13 Posterior vault distraction

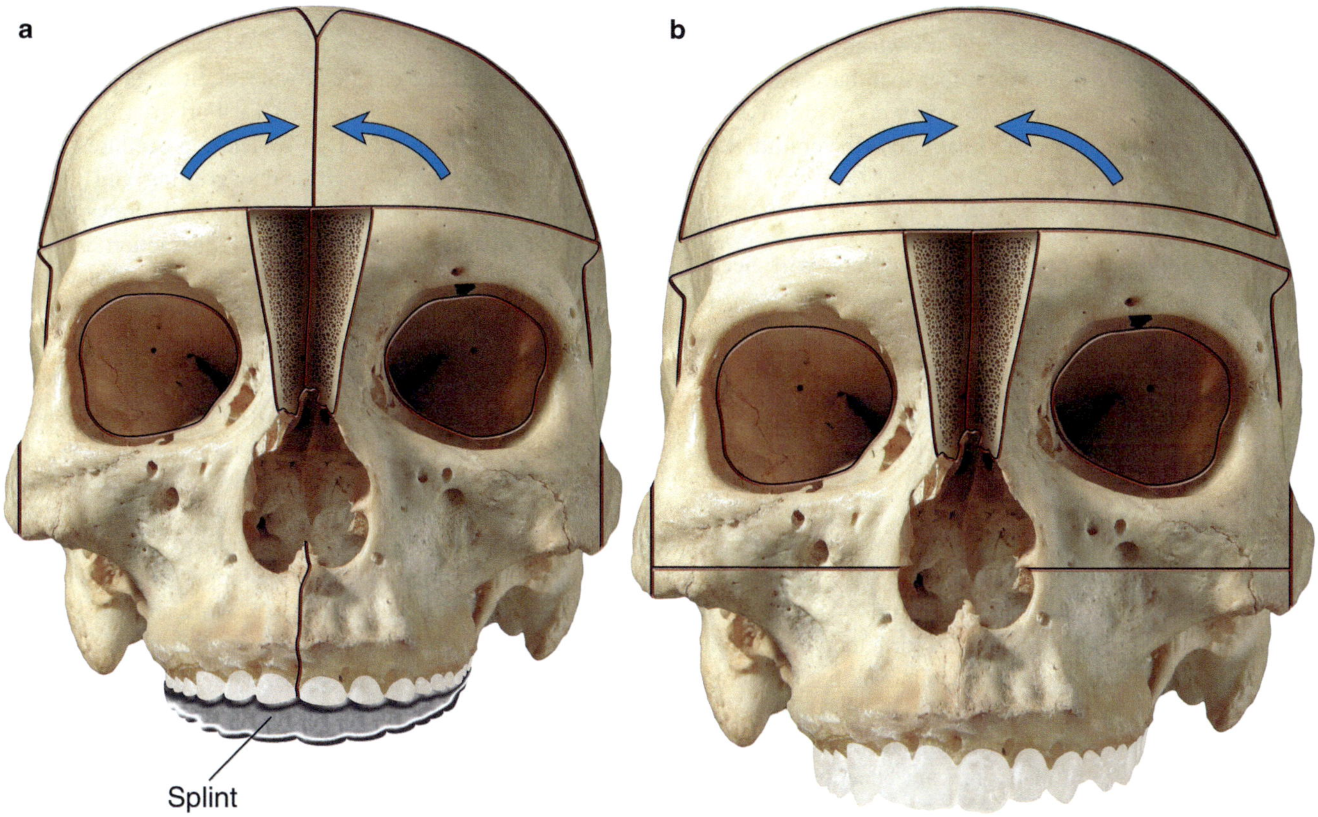

Illustration 79.14 (**a**) Facial bipartition. (**b**) Box osteotomy to correct hypertelorism

79.2.5 Management in Middle Childhood (8–12 Years)

During this period routine monitoring is necessary, and as the face and dentition develop, attention can be turned to managing the midface and occlusion. During the transition from the deciduous to permanent dentition, it is important to have an orthodontic assessment—so that a definitive orthodontic/orthognathic plan can be developed. One of the major factors that may prompt early midface surgery would be the development of OSA; thus regular questioning and targeted investigations at review appointments are necessary. In considering orthodontics it is important to be mindful of the fact that repeated courses of orthodontics will lead to root shortening and also potentially exhaust the tolerance and cooperation of the patient and his/her family [18].

In general, the routine correction of hypertelorism can be safely performed from about the age of 8 years; however this is determined by the chosen technique (facial bipartition vs box osteotomy) (illustration 79.14a, b) and whether an early midface advancement is necessary for the management of OSA [19]. As with all surgery aimed primarily at improving facial appearance, the indications, objectives and expectations of surgery must be discussed at length with the patient and his/her family and a consensus reached. The input from specialist child psychologists is often very helpful. The transition from primary to middle or secondary school is often traumatic, and interventions before this time can be very helpful from a psychological perspective, but it needs to be acknowledged and accepted that further surgery at the completion of growth may well be necessary [18].

79.2.6 Management in Adolescence and after the Completion of Growth

At this stage in development, definitive corrective surgery (when necessary) should be planned and an integrated orthodontic/surgical plan developed. In the syndromic cases, ongoing monitoring for functional and developmental issues is required, and as the child matures, the drive and the responsibility for decision-making will move towards the patient and away from their parents. Many adolescents at this stage are tired of multiple hospital appointments and are not keen on further interventions; in these circumstances it is important to work with the patient and their family to provide care but also respect the patient's wishes and desires. It is better to postpone treatment rather than have a half completed course of orthodontics with poor cooperation and the consequent complications and finally lose the confidence of the patient.

The planning of comprehensive surgery will need assessment in the following areas:

1. Skull shape—irregularities, defects.
2. Orbital position and symmetry.
3. Upper midface morphology.
4. Lower midface morphology.
5. Mandibular morphology.
6. Nasal form.
7. Soft tissue issues.

It is always best to offer and plan for a total correction in the first instance. The discussion around further transcranial surgery is often key to the decision-making. Many patients and families do not want to undertake any further transcranial surgery, in spite of the significant benefits, particularly for hypertelorism or dystopia corrections. None the less these procedures can offer significant improvements in the final result [19].

For residual skull defects of approximately 2 cm diameter or larger, it is usual to offer some form of reconstruction; this could be autologous (usually cranial bone), or alloplastic. Alloplastic reconstructions may be of a variety of materials and can be CAD/CAM designed or shaped intraoperatively. One of the most common residual defects following a fronto-orbital advancement is a degree of temporal hollowing; this can be effectively addressed with the use of mouldable hydroxyapatite synthetic bone material. This technique can be used to satisfactorily address minor skull irregularities and defects, and it is also possible to combine this technique with the use of alloplastic custom-made cranioplasties (e.g. titanium or PEEK) [20].

The assessment of orbital position is critical to deciding on what operative procedure to offer. The combination of hypertelorism and marked maxillary narrowing (particularly if the upper incisors are crossed), as is often seen in Apert syndrome, lends itself to correction with a facial bipartition; this technique can also be used early as the bone cuts do not result in damage to the dentition. The major drawback of this technique is that orbital asymmetries cannot be addressed. The more conventional box osteotomy is used to effect asymmetric movements, hypertelorism and dystopia corrections. The overall aesthetic outcome is often enhanced with nasal augmentation and soft tissue surgery, but the final improvement (particularly in severe hypertelorism cases) unfortunately often does not match the skeletal changes achieved.

The upper midface can be advanced, either as part of the bipartition procedure, transcranial Le Fort III (monobloc), subcranial Le Fort III or Le Fort II. These procedures can be performed conventionally with bone grafting and fixation with either absorbable or titanium plates and screws or with the use of distraction techniques. If distraction is being utilised, the devices can be a halo-based external device or buried devices. It is sometimes helpful to combine external distraction devices with buried devices which facilitate the early removal of the somewhat cumbersome halo device for the retention period [21]. In addition to advancement movements, it is possible to incorporate height changes, but rotatory movements (e.g. to correct the upper dental midline) are very difficult unless the symmetry is equal at all facial levels. Furthermore if the maxillary advancement required has a significant differential between the upper component and dental component, it is possible to combine a Le Fort III (transcranial or subcranial) or a monobloc advance with a simultaneous Le Fort I osteotomy. This additional level of movement allows for differential advancements and/or height changes as well as rotations at the lower level. See case series in Fig. 79.5 of Crouzon syndrome.

The mandible including the chin should be considered as one would for conventional orthognathic surgery, but caution should be exercised in setback procedures as correction of the occlusion to a retrusive maxilla may worsen or precipitate OSA.

Nasal deformity is best dealt with as close to the end of treatment as possible; the range of deformity is considerable; each patient should be treated on their own merits. In cases with severe deficiency, dorsal augmentation with alloplastic or autologous material may be necessary, and this can be refined with nasal tip surgery.

The final phase of surgery is the management of the soft tissues, and again a variety of techniques can be employed to improve the overall aesthetic result. As well as rhinoplasty techniques, facelifting, brow suspension, eyelid surgery, soft tissue augmentation with fillers or fat transfer and soft tissue reduction with direct excision or liposuction all have their place.

See Table 79.2 for an outline of the management of common clinical problems and Table 79.4 for an outline of surgical procedures.

References

1. Wilkie AO, Byren JC, Hurst JA, Jayamohan J, Johnson D, Knight SJ, et al. Prevalence and complications of single-gene and chromosomal disorders in craniosynostosis. Pediatrics. 2010;126(2):e391–400.
2. Bhadkamkar MA, Albright SB, Wolfswinkel EM, Bollo R, Buchanan EP. Posterior cranial vault distraction in the treatment

of shunt-induced craniosynostosis. J Craniofac Surg. 2015 Jan 1;26(1):e70–2.
3. Di Rocco F, Arnaud E, Renier D. Evolution in the frequency of non-syndromic craniosynostosis. J Neurosurg Pediatr. 2009;4(1):21–5.
4. Mathijssen IM. Guideline for Care of Patients with the diagnoses of Craniosynostosis: working group on Craniosynostosis. J Craniofac Surg. 2015;26(6):1735–807.
5. Cornelissen MJ, Apon I, van der Meulen JJ, Groenenberg IA, Kraan-van der Est MN, Mathijssen IM, Bonsel GJ, Cohen-Overbeek TE. Prenatal ultrasound parameters in single-suture craniosynostosis. J Matern Fetal Neonatal Med. 2018 Aug 3;31(15):2050–7.
6. Edmond JC, Nischal K, Forbes B, Katowitz W, Costakos D. Update on the management of patients with craniostenosis. J AAPOS. 2011;15(1):e35.
7. Burokas L. Craniosynostosis: caring for infants and their families. Crit Care Nurse. 2013;33(4):39–50.
8. Mehta VA, Bettegowda C, Jallo GI, Ahn ES. The evolution of surgical management for craniosynostosis. Neurosurg Focus. 2010;29(6):E5.
9. Ingraham FD, Alexander E, Matson DD. Clinical studies in craniosynostosis: analysis of fifty cases and description of a method of surgical treatment. Surgery. 1948 Sep 1;24(3):518–41.
10. Jimenez DF, Barone CM, Cartwright CC, Baker L. Early management of craniosynostosis using endoscopic-assisted strip craniectomies and cranial orthotic molding therapy. Pediatrics. 2002;110(1 Pt 1):97–104.
11. Lauritzen CG, Davis C, Ivarsson A, Sanger C, Hewitt TD. The evolving role of springs in craniofacial surgery: the first 100 clinical cases. Plast Reconstr Surg. 2008;121(2):545–54.
12. Khechoyan D, Schook C, Birgfeld CB, Khosla RK, Saltzman B, Teng CC, Ettinger R, Gruss JS, Ellenbogen R, Hopper RA. Changes in frontal morphology after single-stage open posterior–middle vault expansion for sagittal craniosynostosis. Plast Reconstr Surg. 2012 Feb 1;129(2):504–16.
13. Garza RM, Khosla RK. Nonsyndromic craniosynostosis. Semin Plast Surg. 2012;26(2):53–63.
14. Beez T, O'kane R, Piper I, Koppel D, Sangra M. Telemetric intracranial pressure monitoring in syndromic craniosynostosis. J Craniofac Surg. 2016 Jun 1;27(4):1032–4.
15. Benson ML, Oliverio PJ, Yue NC, Zinreich SJ. Primary craniosynostosis: imaging features. AJR Am J Roentgenol. 1996;166(3):697–703.
16. Gonsalez S, Hayward R, Jones B, Lane R. Upper airway obstruction and raised intracranial pressure in children with craniosynostosis. Eur Respir J. 1997 Feb 1;10(2):367–75.
17. Broder HL. Using psychological assessment and therapeutic strategies to enhance Well-being. Cleft Palate Craniofac J. 2001;38(3):248–54.
18. Evans RD, Bradford R. The dental and orthodontic management of craniosynostosis. In: Bux M, editor. The clinical Management of Craniosynostosis ch 11. London: Mac Keith Press; 2004. p. 211–7.
19. Gonzalez AM, Elahi M, Barakat K, Yavuzer R, Brinkmann B, Jackson IT. Hypertelorism: the importance of three-dimensional imaging and trends in the surgical correction by facial bipartition. Plast Reconstr Surg. 2005 May 1;115(6):1537–46.
20. Feroze AH, Walmsley GG, Choudhri O, Lorenz HP, Grant GA, Edwards MS. Evolution of cranioplasty techniques in neurosurgery: historical review, pediatric considerations, and current trends. J Neurosurg. 2015 Oct;123(4):1098–107.
21. Schulten A, Lim AA, Bruun RA, Hayes C, Mulliken JB, Padwa BL. Combined push-pull distraction for correction of syndromic midfacial hypoplasia. J Oral Maxillofac Surg. 2006 Jan 1;64(1):23–30.

Part XXI

Malignant Pathologies of the Oral and Maxillofacial Region

Premalignant Lesions and Conditions of the Oral Cavity

80

El Mustafa, Sat Parmar, and Prav Praveen

80.1 Premalignant Lesions

It is well established that oral cavity cancer develops in a two-step process and, consequently, that most malignant ulcers are preceded by a precursor lesions [1]. These lesions are typically red or white patches referred to altogether in the 2007 WHO consensus statement as the group of potentially malignant disorders (PMDs) [2] (Table 80.1). Clinical identification of PMDs offers a window for intervention: eliminating diseased mucosa and exclusion of occult invasive cancers. This is important from a clinician's perspective on several fronts. Firstly, it is important to be able to recognise high-risk lesions among a multitude of innocent oral conditions that present with similar features. Some conditions such as oral lichen plans may have a potential for malignant change, but the condition is so prevalent that it becomes impractical to monitor every single patient with the disease. To avoid additional burdens on clinical services, the oral physician or surgeon needs to make a decision as to which patients must be kept under review at a specialist centre and which may be safely referred back for ongoing follow-up in the community. Among those who are reviewed at a specialist practice, ongoing decisions are made at each visit, when to intervene and to what extent one should be aggressive with the treatment plan offered. On a second front are the difficulties of recognition of tumour recurrences following treatment. Surgical treatment and radiotherapy change the tissue appearance and texture irreversibly. Among these patients, it is known that a proportion would develop either a second tumour at the site of surgery or a new tumour in a neighbouring area. It is challenging enough to identify precancerous lesions in nascent tissue, and thus the clinician must be much more vigilant in recognising potentially cancerous new lesions in patients under follow-up posttreatment of head and neck cancer.

E. Mustafa · S. Parmar · P. Praveen (✉)
Department of Oral and Maxillofacial Surgery, Queen Elizabeth Hospital, Birmingham, UK
e-mail: Prav.Praveen@uhb.nhs.uk

Table 80.1 Potentially malignant lesions

Potentially malignant lesions
Leukoplakia (idiopathic)
Proliferative verrucous leukoplakia
Erythroplakia
Oral submucous fibrosis
Oral lichen planus
Chronic hyperplastic candidosis

Further to these concerns, we know that premalignant conditions tend to develop in what is known as field change. This means that for any subsite within the oral cavity at which cellular nuclear damage resulted in a PMD (or even cancer), the adjacent mucosa is almost equally at risk of producing additional PMD lesions even if they appear normal to the naked eye.

Knowledge of the patterns and behaviour of PMDs (premalignant disorder) is thus an essential part of oral medicine and oral surgery practice.

The commonest PMDs are leukoplakia with an overall prevalence of 2.9% in the general population [3] and submucous fibrosis with a prevalence of nearly 11% in high-risk populations [4]. The risk for submucous fibrosis is specific to populations where paan use is prevalent unlike the risk for leukoplakia which is universally applicable. Lesions are considered potentially malignant rather than premalignant. Clinical behaviour is unpredictable; some lesions remain stable; others regress, but in up to 30% of cases, oral malignancy is diagnosed within 5 years of follow-up. Cancer may arise from the lesion itself or at a different subsite within the oral cavity reflecting the concept of 'field cancerisation' explained previously.

It is important to note that a role for primary prevention in patients with leukoplakia is not confirmed. For example, smoking is a risk factor for the development of leukoplakia,

K. Bonanthaya et al. (eds.), *Oral and Maxillofacial Surgery for the Clinician*, https://doi.org/10.1007/978-981-15-1346-6_80

but smoking cessation does not necessarily reduce the risk of developing OCC. There is, however, benefit in screening for potentially malignant lesions, and this was demonstrated in a recent review of the US SEER-Medicare database of head and neck cancer. Yanik et al. [5] reported better treatment and survival outcomes in patients who developed oral cell carcinoma whilst under follow-up for a premalignant lesion [5]. This correlated with the fact that oral cancers were identified at an earlier stage in this patient cohort. Patients without the benefit of such close observation tended to present with more developed or advanced tumour forms. A role for screening patients following treatment for head and neck cancer recurrence is not known, and thus secondary prevention is not currently known to be effective. It is likely, however, that the principle of recognising early tumours and potentially malignant lesions would still result in timely provision of therapy. Table 80.1 enlists premalignant lesions discussed in this chapter.

80.2 Aetiogenesis

Development of a malignancy is a complex multistep process resulting from failures in several regulatory cellular pathways. Dysplasia in oral cancer is usually the first step in the malignant down spiral. Dysplasia is a descriptive term used on microscopic assessment. It indicates that the tissue has accrued a significant population of abnormal cells that display a pattern of nuclear damage that is known to herald cancerous behaviour. These changes are summarised in Table 80.2. Usually but not always, these changes are followed by unregulated hyperplasia (cellular multiplication). The tumour cells have gained autonomy meaning they escaped nuclear and immune mechanisms that limit excess growth and prevent accumulation of damaged cells. The final step is loss of integrity of the basement membrane at the boundary between mucosa and submucosa; the dysplastic cells begin to invade into the surrounding tissues or directly gain access to vascular channels. Each of these steps is controlled by molecular pathways directed by gatekeeper genes and gene products.

Two cellular or microscopic changes broadly define oral premalignancy: *hyperplasia* which results from over activation of the retinoblastoma pathway and the development of various degrees of *dysplasia* due to mutations in the p53 gene. In health and normal physiology, genes along the retinoblastoma pathway activate transcription factors required for taking the cells from the indolent G1 to the active S phase. Overactivation of these genes leads to loss of control of orderly cell division resulting in epithelial hyperplasia. A product of the CDKN2A gene, the p16 protein, usually keeps this stage of cell cycle in check. This protein may become inactivated either because of a mutation/deletion/epigenetic slicing of the parent gene CDKN2A or through direct degradation by a viral product, the E7 protein, of the HPV virus (relevant to the development of oropharyngeal cancer). The retinoblastoma pathway may also be directly upregulated by amplification of the Cyclin D1 gene, a proto-oncogene of the locus 11q13 [6].

With each cell division, there is a probability of errors arising in the nuclear DNA resulting in a defective daughter cell. Most errors are corrected during cell division, or the cells are removed by immune mechanisms. Defective cells that have escaped these reparative measures may still be suppressed by transcription factors that induce apoptosis. Apoptosis is triggered through p53, a tumour suppressor protein. The protein p14 is an alternative reading frame of the CDKN2A gene responsible for initiating the p53 pathway. Direct degradation of p53 by the E6 viral protein (HPV-related cancer) or genetic mutations in the parent gene (in 60% of non HPV cancer) restricts protective physiological apoptosis leading to a shift in cell population and accumulation of dysplastic cells. The premise behind looking out for premalignant disorders is that oral mucosa will change appearance with the onset of dysplastic changes and that the extent of dysplasia does correlate with malignant potential. High-grade dysplastic lesions indicate treatment is required imminently, whereas mild dysplastic lesions may be observed and are even considered a feature of benign chronic inflammation. Dysplasia is classified according to several grading systems summarised in Table 80.3, the most common system in use being the one proposed by the WHO in 2005. Further

Table 80.2 Histological features of cellular dysplasia

Dysplastic changes
Irregular cell shape and orientation
Increased and abnormal mitoses
Nuclear pleomorphism
Coarse and clumped chromatin
Increased nuclear-to-cytoplasmic ratio
Prominent nucleoli
Dyskeratosis

Table 80.3 Grading systems for dysplasia

Definition	WHO 2005	Ljubljana system	Equivalent SIN (squamous intra-epithelial neoplasia)
Increase in the number of normal cells	Squamous cell hyperplasia	Squamous cell (simple) hyperplasia	
Atypical changes confined to the lower 1/3 of the epithelium	Mild dysplasia	Basal/ parabasal cell hyperplasia	SIN1
Atypical changes to the middle 1/3 of the epithelium	Moderate dysplasia	Atypical hyperplasia	SIN2
Changes involve at least 2/3 of the epithelium	Severe dysplasia	Atypical hyperplasia	SIN3

genetic changes are involved in progression towards invasiveness, but these are not as well defined as these are outside the scope of the chapter.

80.3 Leukoplakia

Idiopathic leukoplakia is the most common premalignant disorder. Nearly one in every 10 cases of oral cavity cancer (OCC) is known to arise in leukoplakia (Fig. 80.1), usually within 3 months of diagnosis of the lesion [5]. These lesions are defined as 'white plaques of questionable risk having excluded disorders that carry no increased risk for cancer' [2]. Table 80.4 enlists white lesions without a known malignant potential. These are rare, and thus most persistent white patches are best treated with suspicion until further evaluation.

Clinical variants of leukoplakia include homogenous plaques, nodules, speckled erythroleukoplakia and a distinct subtype discussed separately: proliferative verrucous subtype. Leukoplakia is present in less than 1% of the general population [5] but with greater prevalence reported among those older than 75 years of age and tobacco users of all age groups [7]. Men are twice as much likely to develop leukoplakia compared with women. In the Indian subcontinent, in regions where betel is consumed, prevalence rates approach 5% [8]. The annual risk of malignant transformation is estimated between 1 and 2% [9]. Larger non-homogeneous lesions, particularly those on the tongue and floor of the mouth, are associated with the highest conversion rates to oral squamous cell carcinoma. Table 80.5 lists clinical risk predictors for malignant transformation.

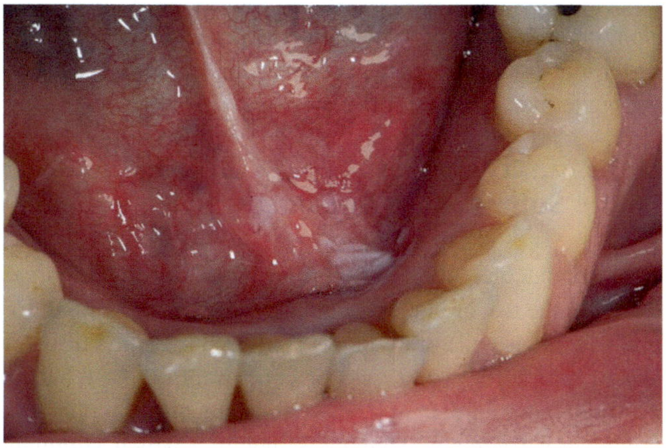

Fig. 80.1 Leukoplakia

Table 80.4 Innocent white patches

White lesions not known to association with oral cancer	
Developmental	Cannon white sponge nevus
Metabolic	Uremic stomatitis
Immune mediated	Benign migratory glossitis
Viral immune suppression	Oral hairy leukoplakia associated with HIV

Table 80.5 Risk predictors for malignant transformation

Risk factors for malignant transformation
Duration
Non-homogeneous type
Size >200 mm squared
Site: Tongue, floor of the mouth
Leukoplakia in a non-smoker
Epithelial dysplasia

Tissue biopsy is required to assess the degree of epithelial dysplasia, an independent and consistently reliable risk factor for malignant transformation. Liu et al., using a binary grading of dysplasia, found that patients with high-risk lesions (moderate/severe dysplasia) eight times as likely to be diagnosed with oral cancer as those with low-risk (no/mild dysplasia) lesions [10]. Histological evaluation may also identify other conditions that are clinically indistinguishable from idiopathic leukoplakia such as hyperplastic candidosis, oral lichen planus variants, lichenoid reactions and discoid lupus.

Categorisation into high- and low-risk lesions is helpful in identifying target areas for surgical removal and those that may be safely observed but closely followed up.

However, in populations with high incidence of oral cancer, studies have shown oral leukoplakia as foci of invasive cancer and have advocated surgical excision of these lesions.

Toluidine blue dye improves visual detection of high-risk mucosa [11] and helps determine the extent of peripheral margins required for complete excision. It is not established whether surgical intervention reduces the risk of subsequent cancer, but a resection specimen may upgrade the histological evaluation or identify areas of occult focal invasion. Recurrence following surgery is observed in 10% of cases [12]. Laser surgery is effective in controlling low-grade leukoplakia, but significantly higher failure rates of up to 9% were reported in high-grade lesions and erythroleukoplakia [13]. Recent reviews have examined photodynamic therapy as a treatment option particularly helpful in controlling widespread and multifocal leukoplakia [14]. Partial and complete response rates as high as 70–100% were reported, but the range of photosensitisers used and photo-irradiation protocols applied varied greatly between individual authors.

Medical treatments for oral premalignancy include systemic vitamin A, systemic beta carotene and topical bleomycin. These were shown to control premalignant lesions, but a 2016 Cochrane review concluded that relapse rates were high and that transformation into oral cancer was not effectively reduced [15].

80.4 Proliferative Verrucous Leukoplakia

Proliferative verrucous leukoplakia (PVL) is a distinct and aggressive form of leukoplakia with one of the highest known malignant transformation rates. It is typically diagnosed in elderly women (4:1 female ration) without a history of tobacco use [16]. Aetiology is thus largely unknown. Lesions often start as isolated flat white plaques but gradually spread to become diffuse and multifocal with a characteristic warty appearance (Fig. 80.2). There typically is no erosive component. The lesions tend to present on the tongue or buccal mucosa or well as the alveolar ridge. They can be mistaken for hyperplastic candidosis or frictional keratosis particularly in denture wearers. Histological appearance is dependent on the stage of the disease ranging from benign hyperkeratosis to dysplastic keratosis merging into verrucous carcinoma. Malignant transformation may also happen simultaneously at multiple foci, and this is one of the clearest manifestations of the field cancerisation concept introduced earlier. Verrucous carcinoma is a squamous cancer with well-differentiated histopathological architecture that displays very little cellular atypia.

PVL is a lesion that benefits from excision biopsy rather than an incisional sample (see biopsy discussion below) for it is estimated that 20% of verrucous lesions, if adequately sampled, would reveal foci of conventional pattern squamous cell carcinoma. Local control is, however, difficult with high recurrence rates following surgical excision and greater malignant transformation rates in excess of 70% [17]. It is also one of the most difficult lesions to follow up, requiring multiple biopsies to monitor behaviour over time.

80.5 Erythroplakia

Erythroplastic lesions (Fig. 80.3) are similarly defined to oral leukoplakia but as red velvety lesions following exclusion of other named entities. It is a rare disorder with prevalence between 0.01 and 0.2% but a much higher transformation rate compared to leukoplakia, reportedly between 51 and 90% [16]. Clinical appearance tends to follow one of three patterns: the homogenous, granular and speckled types [12]. Most common subsides are the palate, the buccal mucosa and the floor of the mouth. Lesions are rarely multicentric and may present a similar clinical appearance to erosive and atrophic oral lichen planus, erythema migrans, stomatitis, candidosis, lymphatic malformations and desquamative gingivitis (e.g. vesiculobullous lesions and gingival lichen planus). Speckled erythroplakia and leukoplakia most likely refer to the same disorder with red appearance correlating to high-risk epithelial dysplasia. Treatment options are surgical excision, laser excision or evaporation as per leukoplakia with a lower threshold for application for wide local excision due to the higher risk of cancer development.

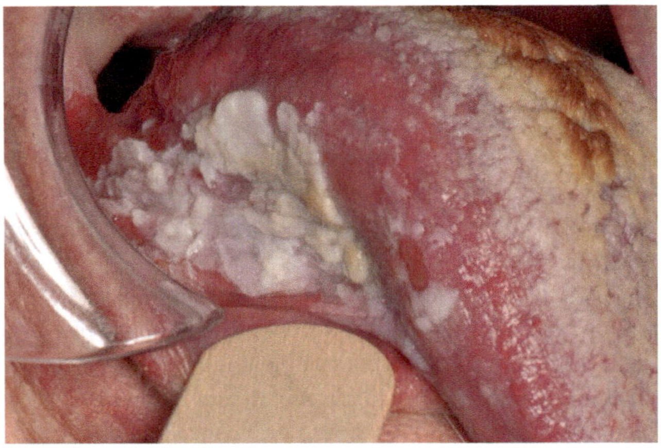

Fig. 80.2 Proliferative verrucous leukoplakia

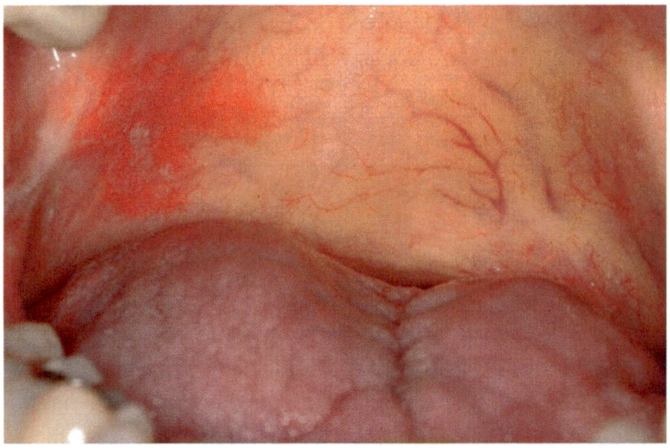

Fig. 80.3 Erythroplakia

80.6 Submucous Fibrosis

Oral submucous fibrosis is progressive scarring disorder linked to the use of betel products (paan). Additional risk for oral squamous cell carcinoma is conferred by the addition of slaked lime to the betel quid or concurrent use of tobacco. The active ingredients in paan include arecoline, copper and polyphenol fragments (flavonols, tannins) which stimulate an intense acute inflammatory response characterised by a polymorphic infiltrate and vascular dilatation. This gives way to a chronic immune response and constrictive vascular changes that end with obliteration of blood vessels in the affected region. Over time, this leads to an epithelial to mesenchymal transition mediated by TGF-β [18]. Fibroblasts are activated, and collagen is deposited steadily replacing the submucous tissues with hyalinised cartilage almost devoid of cellular components. Several genes are known to associate with the risk of developing submucous fibrosis including MMP3 gene promoter region and CYP1A1/CYP2E1 genes,

Table 80.6 Histopathological changes in submucous fibrosis

Very early Stage I	Early Stage II	Moderate advanced Stage III	Advanced Stage IV
• Fine fibrillar collagen and marked oedema.	• Early junta-epithelial hyalinisation	• Moderately hyalinised collagen.	• Completely hyalinised collagen.
• Strong fibroblastic response.	• Moderate fibroblastic response.	• Predominantly fibrocytes, reduced fibroblasts.	• Hyalinised collagen devoid of fibroblasts.
• Acute polymorphic inflammatory cell infiltrate.	• Mononuclear and lymphocytic inflammatory cell infiltrate.	• Lymphocytic and plasma cell inflammatory cell infiltrate.	• Lymphocytic and plasma cell inflammatory cell infiltrate.
• Normal or dilated-congested blood vessels.	• Dilated-congested blood vessels.	• Normal to constricted vessels.	• Markedly constricted or completely obliterated blood vessels.

but the genetic basis for transformation into squamous cell carcinoma is not currently defined. Table 80.6 summarised the histopathological evolution and progression of submucous fibrosis.

Consumption of paan is common in Southeast Asia and the Western Pacific but is now also seen in Europe and North America. It is estimated that more than half a billion persons consume betel worldwide [19]. Early presentation reflects the early histological picture with non-specific inflammatory mucosal changes. The diagnosis becomes clearer when early changes are replaced by the characteristic hypo-vascular blanched appearance with a fibrous texture although these changes may be patchy or reticular causing potential confusion with unrelated mucosal changes (e.g. lichen planus). In general, submucous fibrosis tends to present in young adults (predominantly males) with worsening trismus (37.2% of patients), painful dysesthesia (25.9%), excess salivation (22.5% of patients) and recurrent ulceration. Clinical findings on examination are white patches particularly in the buccal mucosa (20.8%) and the palate (17.7%) followed by the floor of mouth and the retromolar trigone [20]. Clinical signs develop within 3–5 years following commencement of chewing betel preparations. Patients are 19 times as likely to develop oral cancer particularly with betel quid containing tobacco [4]. Malignant transformation rates are reportedly 4–13% [21].

Conservative and medical measures are considered for the early clinical stages. This includes physiotherapy, immune modulators steroids and promoters of blood flow such as pentoxifylline. Many other medical treatments are reported but none with definitive clinical benefit.

Surgical options are limited and complete excision unlikely, but surgery is usually indicated for local release of

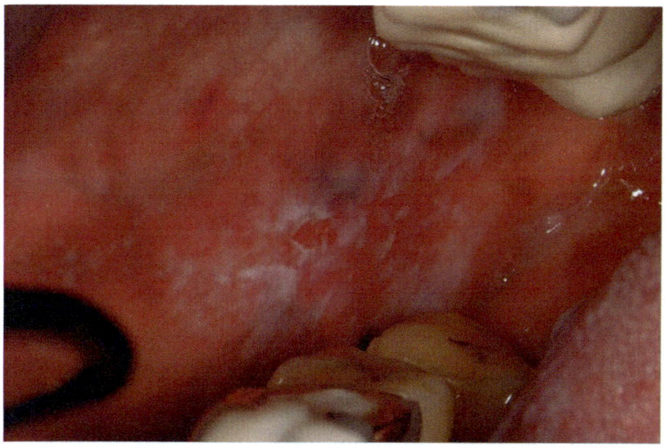

Fig. 80.4 Oral lichen planus

retromolar or buccal scarring to help relieve trismus. Release of trismus is usually necessary at the mouth opening of 25 mm and less and is achieved with incisions, local V–Y flaps and masticator muscle myotomy, resurfacing the defect with the buccal fat pad or other grafts.

80.7 Oral Lichen Planus

Lichen planus (LP) (Fig. 80.4) is a prevalent inflammatory much cutaneous disease affecting 5% of the population worldwide. The pathogenesis is not well understood but is essentially an autoimmune response to the epidermal basal cell layer mediated by cytotoxic T cells. Characteristically, T cells are seen to infiltrate into the lamina propria on microscopy and the damaged basal keratinocytes degrade into apoptotic residues known as civatte bodies (not pathognomonic for LP) [22]. Aetiology is unknown, but it is well recognised that appearances of lichen plans can result from a hypersensitivity reaction to nonsteroidal anti-inflammatories, angiotensin-converting enzyme inhibitors and dental amalgam. These reactions are more commonly referred to as lichenoid mucositis. In rare instances, the disease associates with viral hepatitis (B and C), but in most patients LP, there is no triggering factor. Stress is thought to be a contributing factor.

Commonly, oral lichen planus (OLP) presents as reticular white patterns on the buccal mucosa or the tongue known as Wickham's striae. Many varieties and presentations are recognised such as desquamative gingivitis, plaque form and an unusual form that presents with vesicular bullae. An erosive form is also recognised giving the appearance of the high-risk erythroplakia and mixed red and white lesions [23]. Some authors use the term erosive OLP to refer to the ulcerated type of lesion and erythematous OLP as the commoner type which affects atrophied buccal mucosa (usually seen with reticular lesions). Distribution is usually symmetrical, a feature it shares with discoid lupus.

It is not clear whether oral lichen planus (OLP), a relatively common benign condition, is an independent risk factor for malignancy. A meta-analysis of 7806 patients concluded that just over 1% of patients OLP develop oral cavity cancer [24]. The highest risk subsites were predominantly the tongue (51%) and the buccal mucosa (32%). Malignant transformation was three times as likely in females as it was in men. It is proposed that changes at lower-power magnification of oral leukoplakia resemble lichen planus or that lichenoid changes in epithelial dysplasia are common. Clinically, there is overlap between the clinical appearance of the various types of OLP and between erythroleukoplakia and verrucous leukoplakia. A diagnosis of OLP is more likely in symmetric lesions, but only a biopsy demonstrating epithelial dysplasia would confirm truly high-risk lesions. Correlation between malignant change and certain subtypes of OLP, namely, the erosive and plaque-like forms, has not been consistent. Interestingly a co-existence with proliferative verrucous leukoplakia has been noted by several authors [25, 26].

80.8 Chronic Hyperplastic Candidosis

Candida is present in the oral cavity in between 40 and 60% of healthy individuals. Association between *Candida* infection and cancer is through smoking, an independent risk factor equally for the development of chronic hyperplastic candidosis (CHC) and premalignant mucosal lesions. Once hyperplastic candidosis is established, these lesions manifest and behave similar to homogeneous or speckled leukoplakia with 15% risk of progression to epithelial dysplasia [27]. CHC is usually resistant to antifungal therapy, and thus surgery is indicated particularly for well-defined lesions.

80.9 Premalignant Conditions

Premalignant conditions are a disparate group of rare congenital and acquired disorders of immune regulation, inheritable genetic instability and infectious diseases. Table 80.7 enlists conditions that associate with mucosal SCC followed by Table 80.8 which also provides a summary of clinical features, site distribution and risk probabilities for conditions that associate with the cutaneous type of squamous carcinoma. Reports of malignant transformations are generally few and data concerning the natural history of OCC limited. Conditions that rarely associate with oral SCC such as Plummer-Vinson syndrome are not discussed here.

Table 80.7 Potentially malignant conditions: mucosal SCC

Potentially malignant conditions: mucosal SCC	Aetiology	Clinical characteristics
Dyskeratosis congenita (mucocutaneous variant) [28]	Multigene defects, telomere dysfunction and bone marrow failure. Sporadic de novo, autosomal dominant and X-linked recessive types	Triad: Nail dystrophy, reticular skin pigmentation, oral leukoplakia. Oral leukoplakia in 80% of patients. 40–5% malignant transformation into SCC
Syphilis	Spirochete infection	Verrucous type and speckled leukoplakia in tertiary syphilis. Usually in the lips, tongue or palate. 3–33% risk of transformation
Graft versus host disease	Complication of allogenic stem cell transplantation	Oral lichenoid, erosions and painful ulcers. Few case reports of cancer transformation
Acquired immune deficiency syndrome [29]	HIV virus	HPV positive oropharyngeal SCC. Kaposi sarcoma

Table 80.8 Potentially malignant conditions: cutaneous SCC

Potentially malignant conditions: cutaneous SCC	Aetiology	Clinical characteristics
Actinic cheilitis	Solar radiation	Diffuse, atrophic, ulcerative or keratotic patches in the lower lip. 6% risk of malignant transformation
Xeroderma pigmentosum	Autosomal recessive inheritance	Cutaneous-type SCC on the lower lip observed in young adults, age < 20 years
Discoid Lupus [30]		1.3–6.5% risk of developing SCC and BCC with lighter skin. Risk increased to 22% in discoid lesions. Locally aggressive lesions with high recurrence rates

80.10 Tissue Biopsy

A sample of tissue is required whenever a premalignant disorder is suspected. Dysplasia cannot be visualised on clinical inspection. It is true that some lesions such as the speckled red and white lesions are most likely to harbour dysplastic cells, but it is hard to characterise white patches as dysplastic or not on clinical examination alone. Most sites within the oral cavity are accessible for a biopsy under local anaesthetic. General anaesthetic may well be indicated in some cases depending on tumour site particularly in the oropharynx or in patients not compliant with awake procedures. A biopsy may be obtained either by using a scalpel blade or through a punch biopsy applicator with pre-set width.

A small amount of local anaesthetic is administered locally within the site of the lesion for it provides pain relief and vasoconstriction through the action of an additive. Concentrations of 1:50,000 to 1:200,000 epinephrine are used as vasoconstrictor additives typically to lidocaine. Other vasoconstrictor agents include felypressin typically combined with prilocaine as a local anaesthetic. Care should be taken in patients who take anti-platelets agents or anticoagulant medications. The oral mucosa has a rich blood supply, and bleeding from small biopsy sites may prove to be difficult to control.

Excision of the abnormal patch as a whole may be achievable in smaller lesions, but in large and extensive lesions, an incisional sample is indicated. The site for taking a biopsy in this case is important. A white lesion may contain within multiple foci, and a biopsy from a uniform looking area may miss an area of dysplasia or early invasive cancers. Within a white lesion, it is advisable to take a biopsy from a speckled area, an area where there is induration/thickening and an erosive patch or where there is frank ulceration. When there is ulceration, then removal of tissue from the centre of the ulcer may return tissue that is necrotic and hard for the pathologist to interpret. Thus, it is also advised to take a biopsy from the margin of the ulcer particularly if the margin is elevated or everted. A small extension to incorporate normal looking tissue is helpful to enable the pathologist to visualise pathological transition into normal background architecture and pick up subtle changes that may otherwise be difficult to interpret.

The full thickness of mucosa is required for complete assessment. Invasiveness is impossible to interpret without inclusion of the basement membrane in the tissue biopsy. Traditionally that may not have been crucial for at the highest end of the dysplastic spectrum severe dysplasia is also considered to be at least as intra-epithelial neoplasia and in most cases surgical excision would be indicated. However, recent modifications of the TNM classification system and the work of D'Cruz et al. have highlighted depth of invasion as an independent risk predictor for regional metastasis [31].

Thus a biopsy may not only identify the nature of the lesion and reveal unexpected invasiveness; it may also determine the next step in treatment whether surgical excision of the lesion is enough or whether the threshold for regional surgery (i.e. a neck dissection) is required as well.

Once the sample is removed, haemostasis is required with either bipolar diathermy or, in small sites, chemical cautery with silver nitrate that is useful too. Most biopsy sites lend themselves to primary closure with a resorbable suture, whereas particular sites such as the mucosa overlying the hard palate may be safely left to heal by secondary intent.

80.11 Conclusion

Clinical examination of the oral cavity must include active screening for mucosal changes that are potentially cancerous. This may take place in the primary care setting, in dental practice, for these lesions are mostly asymptomatic and the patients may not be aware of their presence. A high index of suspicion is required for it is well known that although some lesions associate with known risk factors (e.g. oral submucous fibrosis), many lesions do not (e.g. verrucous leukoplakia). Clinical features may be ambiguous with some lesions that are red, erosive or speckled lending themselves to easier recognition compared with faint leukoplakia and subtle early changes in long-standing lichen planus. A low threshold for biopsy is recommended unless the lesion is demonstrably consistent with candidosis (i.e. may be clinically wiped off) or in the case of striated lichen planus that has remained consistent and well defined. Clinical photography is helpful in establishing objective documentation lesions for it is likely that the patient would be reviewed by different clinicians during follow-up. Once identified and histology is characterised, then lesions require stratification into high-risk and low-risk categories in order to determine the long-term plan for the patients, namely, surgical removal versus clinical observation, and the appropriate recall intervals for future follow-up. As discussed above, the treatment options are diverse and are tailored to the size of the lesion and degree of epithelial dysplasia. Although surgical removal does not eliminate the risk of malignant change entirely, early identification and close follow-up of premalignant lesions offer the best chance for achievement of good local control if and when oral cancer develops.

References

1. Reibel J. Prognosis of Oral pre-malignant lesions: significance of clinical, histopathological, and molecular biological characteristics. Crit Rev Oral Biol Med. 2003;14:47–62.
2. Warnakulasuriya S, Johnson NW, van der Waal I. Nomenclature and classification of potentially malignant disorders of the oral mucosa. J Oral Pathol Med. 2007;36(10):575–80.
3. Bánóczy J, Gintner Z, Dombi C. Tobacco use and oral leukoplakia. J Dent Educ. 2001;65(4):322–7.
4. Wollina U, Verma SB, Ali FM, Patil K. Oral submucous fibrosis: an update. Clin Cosmet Investig Dermatol. 2015;8:193–204.
5. Yanik EL, Katki HA, Silverberg MJ, Manos MM, Engels EA, Chaturvedi AK. Leukoplakia, oral cavity cancer risk, and cancer survival in the U.S. elderly. Cancer Prev Res (Phila). 2015;8(9):857–63.

6. Pitiyage G, Tilakaratne WM, Tavassoli M, Warnakulasuriya S. Molecular markers in oral epithelial dysplasia: review. J Oral Pathol Med. 2009;38(10):737–52.
7. Amagasa T. Oral premalignant lesions. Int Clin Oncol. 2011;16:1–4.
8. Gupta PC, Mehta FS, Daftary DK, Pindborg JJ, Bhonsle RB, Jalnawalla PN, et al. Incidence of oral cancer and natural history of oral precancerous lesions in a 10-year follow-up study of Indian villagers. Community Dent Oral Epidemiol. 1980;8:283–333.
9. Brouns ER, Baart JA, Bloemena E, Karagozoglu H, van der Waal I. The relevance of uniform reporting in oral leukoplakia: definition, certainty factor and staging based on experience with 275 patients. Med Oral Patol Oral Cir Bucal. 2012;18(1):e19–26.
10. Liu W, Wang YF, Zhou HW, Shi P, Zhou ZT, Tang GY. Malignant transformation of oral leukoplakia: a retrospective cohort study of 218 Chinese patients. BMC Cancer. 2010;10:685.
11. Chainani-Wu N, Madden E, Cox D, Sroussi H, Epstein J, Silverman S Jr. Toluidine blue aids in detection of dysplasia and carcinoma in suspicious oral lesions. Oral Dis. 2015;21(7):879–85.
12. Lodi G, Porter S. Management of potentially malignant disorders: evidence and critique. J Oral Pathol Med. 2008;37:63–9.
13. Thomson PJ, Goodson ML, Cocks K, Turner JE. Interventional laser surgery for oral potentially malignant disorders: a longitudinal patient cohort study. Int J Oral Maxillofac Surg. 2017;46(3):337–42.
14. Gondivkar SM, Gadbail AR, Choudhary MG, Vedpathak PR, Likhitkar MS. Photodynamic treatment outcomes of potentially-malignant lesions and malignancies of the head and neck region: A systematic review. J Investig Clin Dent. 2018;9(1)
15. Lodi G, Franchini R, Warnakulasuriya S, Varoni E, Sardella A, Kerr AR, Carrassi A, MacDonald LCI, Worthington HV. Interventions for treating oral leukoplakia to prevent oral cancer. Cochrane Database Syst Rev. 2016;7(7):CD001829.
16. Mortazavi H, Baharvand M, Mehdipour M. Oral potentially malignant disorders: an overview of more than 20 entities. J Dent Res Dent Clin Dent Prospects. 2014;8(1):6–14.
17. Munde A, Karle R. Proliferative verrucous leukoplakia: an update. J Cancer Res Ther. 2016;12(2):469–73.
18. Hu Y, Jian X, Peng J, Jiang X, Li N, Zhou S. Gene expression profiling of oral submucous fibrosis using oligonucleotide microarray. Oncol Rep. 2008;20(2):287–94.
19. Nelson BS, Heischober B. Betel nut: a common drug used by naturalized citizens from India, Far East Asia, and the South Pacific Islands. Ann Emerg Med. 1999;34(2):238–43.
20. Pandya S, Chaudhary AK, Singh M, Singh M, Mehrotra R. Correlation of histopathological diagnosis with habits and clinical findings in oral submucous fibrosis. Head Neck Oncol. 2009;1:10.
21. Yaming P, Urs AB, Saxena A, Zuberi M. Roles of CYP1A1 and CYP2E1 gene polymorphisms in Oral submucous fibrosis. Asian Pac J Cancer Prev. 2016;17(7):3335–40.
22. Pranay T, Kumar AS, Chhabra S. Civatte bodies: a diagnostic clue. Indian J Dermatol. 2013;58(4):327.
23. Olson MA, Rogers RS 3rd, Bruce AJ. Oral lichen planus. Clin Dermatol. 2016;34(4):495–504.
24. Fitzpatrick SG, Hirsch SA, Gordon SC. The malignant transformation of oral lichen planus and oral lichenoid lesions: a systematic review. J Am Dent Assoc. 2014;145:45–56.
25. Lopes MA, Feio P, Santos-Silva AR, Vargas PA. Proliferative verrucous leukoplakia may initially mimic lichenoid reactions. World J Clin Cases. 2015;3(10):861–3.
26. Garcia-Pola MJ, Llorente-Pendás S, González-Garcia M, García-Martín JM. The development of proliferative verrucous leukoplakia in oral lichen planus. A preliminary study. Med Oral Patol Oral Cir Bucal. 2016;21(3):e328–34.
27. Shah N, Ray JG, Kundu S, Sardana D. Surgical management of chronic hyperplastic candidiasis refractory to systemic antifungal treatment. J Lab Physicians. 2017;9(2):136–9.
28. Alter BP, Giri N, Savage SA, Rosenberg PS. Cancer in dyskeratosis congenita. Blood. 2009;113(26):6549–57.
29. McLemore MS, Haigentz M, Smith RV, et al. Head and neck squamous cell carcinomas in HIV-positive patients: a preliminary investigation of viral associations. Head Neck Pathol. 2010;4(2):97–105.
30. Bhat MR, Hulmani M, Dandakeri S, Kambil SM, Gatti R. Disseminated discoid lupus erythematosus leading to squamous cell carcinoma. Indian J Dermatol. 2012;57(2):158–61.
31. D'Cruz AK, Vaish R, Kapre N, Dandekar M, Gupta S, Hawaldar R, et al. Head and neck disease management group. Elective versus therapeutic neck dissection in node-negative oral cancer. N Engl J Med. 2015 Aug 6;373(6):521–9.

Oral Squamous Cell Carcinoma: Diagnosis and Treatment Planning

81

Vijay Deshmukh and Kishore Shekar

81.1 Background and Incidence

The incidence of oral and oropharyngeal SCC is on the rise. Each year approximately 263,000 new cases of oral cancer are detected worldwide, and 127,000 people die of the disease [1]. In India it is the third most common cancer and accounts for almost 40% of deaths. Among men it is the second most common site, and in women it is the fourth in India [2]. In 2012, the incidence rate for male was 10.1/1,00,000 and for female 4.3/1,00,000 [3].

81.2 Introduction

Oral carcinoma commonly called as the oral squamous cell carcinoma (OSCC) occurs as an ulceroproliferative lesion of the oral mucosa affecting any site starting from the lips to the oropharynx. The commonest sites are gingivobuccal sulcus of mandible followed by the tongue and floor of the mouth. It should be understood that Indian cancer is much different to other parts of the world. The habit of the tobacco chewing (smokeless tobacco) and pan masala, i.e., a mixture of the tobacco, betel nut, and unknown chemicals used for the color and flavors, is the commonest cause. Classical Indian cancer is the gingivobuccal sulcus (GBS) of the mandible due to the placement and holding of the tobacco-lime mixture, in the area. Over the last three decades, pan masala has become popular, due to the easy availability in pre-mixed packed. This maybe chewed or kept in the oral cavity, i.e., GBS, which leads to continuous action of the contents on the oral mucosa. The constant irritation leads to fibrosis and with time results in submucous fibrosis.

81.3 Etiology of Oral Carcinoma

Etiology of oral SCC is multifactorial. Local irritants contribute significantly to the conversion of a premalignant process to invasive carcinoma. Damage to the epithelial layer followed by the basement membrane and submucosa secondary to chemical and mechanical injury leads to fibrosis of the mucous membrane.

The prominent etiological factors are:

1. Tobacco consumption—All forms of tobacco smoke as well as smokeless have carcinogenic potential. Evidence for smokeless tobacco causing oral and pharyngeal cancer was evaluated and confirmed [4]. India is the third largest producer and consumer of smoked and smokeless forms of tobacco. Tobacco-related cancers account for nearly 50% of all cancers among men and 25% of all cancers among women with the burden of tobacco-related cancers in 2001 estimated to be nearly 0.33 million cases annually. It has been predicted that an incidence of sevenfold increase in tobacco-related cancer is expected between 1995 and 2025 resulting in an increase by 220% of cancer deaths simply related to tobacco use [5]. In India chewable tobacco is consumed in various forms. The traditional form is called the pan (Figs. 81.1, 81.2 and 81.3). Local form of smoking tobacco is called as bidi, which is a crude form of cigarette. This is considered to be more carcinogenic. It commonly causes carcinoma of the palate, oropharynx, and larynx.

Electronic Supplementary Material The online version of this chapter (https://doi.org/10.1007/978-981-15-1346-6_81) contains supplementary material, which is available to authorized users.

V. Deshmukh (✉)
Maxillofacial and Microvascular Surgeon, Deshmukh Institute of Maxillofacial Surgery and Research Centre, Aurangabad, India

Department of Dentistry and Maxillofacial Surgery, JIIU'S Indian Institute of Medical Sciences, Maharashtra, Jalna, India

K. Shekar
Head and Neck Surgeon (OMFS), Ninewells Hospital and Dundee University Medical School, Dundee, UK
e-mail: Kishore.Shekar2@nhs.scot

K. Bonanthaya et al. (eds.), *Oral and Maxillofacial Surgery for the Clinician*, https://doi.org/10.1007/978-981-15-1346-6_81

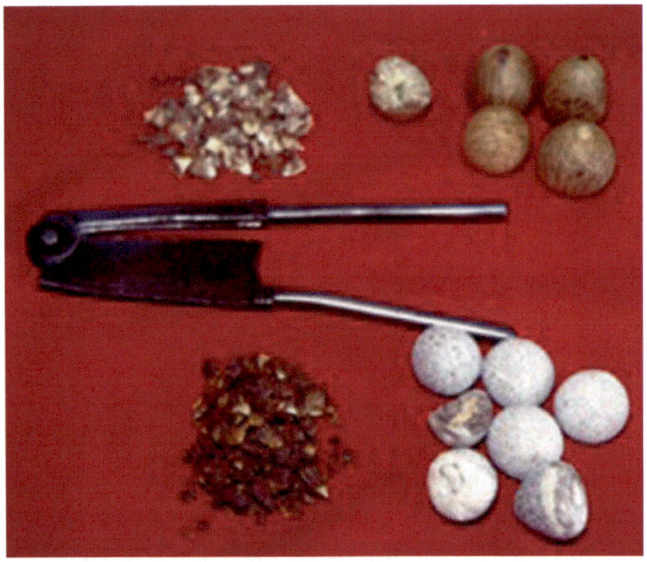

Fig. 81.1 Betel nut (areca nut). Various forms. Raw red in color and roasted white in color. It is broken in pieces with a special cutting device. Pieces are chewed with tobacco-lime mixture or with betel quid (pan)

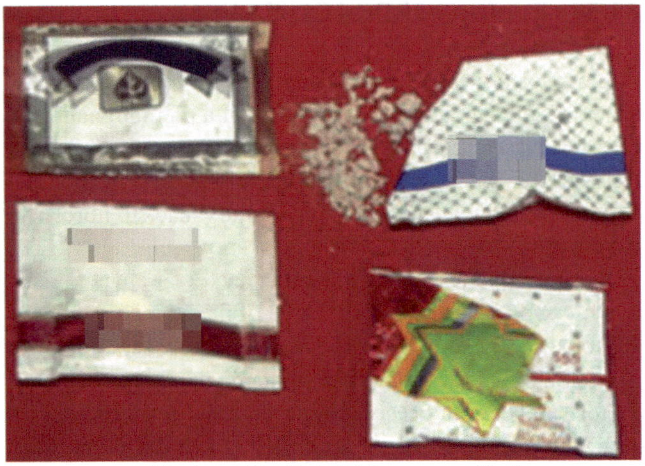

Fig. 81.2 Pan masala (gutkha) pouches. Ready to eat mixture of tobacco, betel nut, lime, catechu, and unknown chemical coloring and flavoring agents

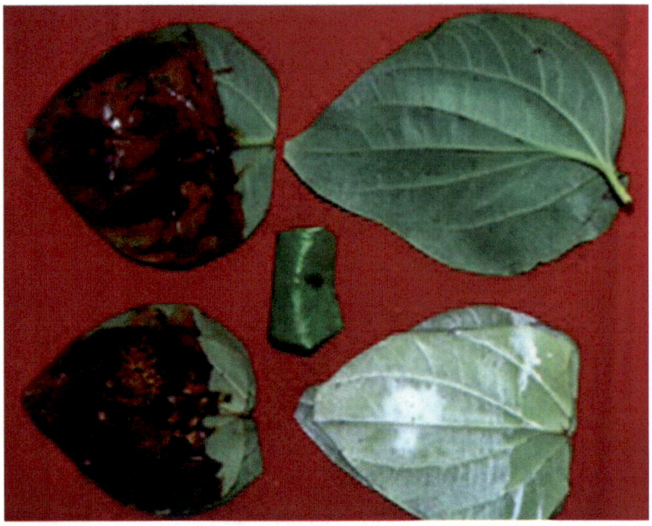

Fig. 81.3 Pan-betel quid. Betel leaf coated with lime-catechu-flavored tobacco-betel nut. It is rolled, wrapped, and pinned with clove. Most commonly chewed in Indian subcontinent

2. Alcohol—Alcohol is considered to be causally associated with oral cancer. As heavy alcohol drinkers are frequently heavy smokers as well, a synergistic effect with cigarette smoking is implicated in oral cancer [6–8]. Excess alcohol consumption is associated with nutritional deficiencies. This acts as an aggravating factor.
3. Betel nut chewing (areca nut)—Chronic chewing of the betel nut leads to abnormal fibrosis of the oral-pharyngeal areas. Betel nut is the endosperm of the fruit of *Areca catechu*. It is consumed in various forms. It is used fresh or dried or may be cured before use by boiling, baking, or roasting. The abrasive mechanical property causes attrition of teeth and physical damage to the mucosa. This sandpaper action makes the mucosa more susceptible to the chemical properties of beetle nut. In India alone 38 different combinations of areca nut with tobacco have been documented (Fig. 81.1). The number of patients with a pan masala chewing habit (68.0%) was higher than the number of patients with betel nut (17.4%) or betel quid chewing habits (14.6%). The chewing of pan masala is associated with earlier presentation of oral submucous fibrosis (OSMF) as compared to betel nut chewing [9]. Pan masala (Fig. 81.2) is the artificial mixture available in small pouches having contents of tobacco, betel nut, spices, coloring and flavoring agents, preservatives, as well as unspecified agents. This has proven to be highly carcinogenic. Consumption of this mixtures leads to OSMF which is a precancerous condition. Development of precancerous lesions like leukoplakia in preexisting fibrosis potentiates carcinoma conversion. Betel nut is also consumed with a pan (Fig. 81.3) a freshly prepared mixture on the betel leaf with tobacco, slaked lime, catechu, and clove. This is chewed over a longer time and remains in contact with oral mucosa causing mechanical and chemical irritation. The important flavonoid components in areca nut are tannins and catechins. These alkaloids undergo nitrosation and give rise to N-nitrosamine which might have cytotoxic effect on cells [10].
4. Nutritional deficiencies—Dietary deficiencies of vitamin A, folate, riboflavin, iodine, and iron add to the risk of cancer. High dietary fiber; vitamins C, E, and A; and selenium offer protection against cancer [11, 12].

5. Poor oral hygiene and traumatic injury of dental origin—Poor oral hygiene is often associated with gingivoperiodontal infections raising bacterial colony count leading to a constant inflammatory response. This together with traumatic tooth injury can lead to a carcinogenic effect.
6. Viral infections—The role of human papillomavirus (HPV) in pharyngeal cancer is well established. However its effect on the oral cavity is still being researched. Globally, HPV infection is relatively more common in OSCC patients [12].

81.4 Precancerous Situations of Oral Cavity

Precancerous situations can be broadly divided into precancerous conditions and precancerous lesions. Precancerous condition's most commonly seen in India are oral submucous fibrosis (OSMF) and oral lichen planus. Precancerous conditions can be associated with the precancerous lesions (please also see Chap. 80 on premalignant lesions and conditions).

81.4.1 Precancerous Conditions

Precancerous conditions make every part of the oral cavity susceptible to cancer conversion as is seen in oral submucous fibrosis (OSMF). The phenomenon simulates field cancerization. Development of a second primary despite adequate treatment of the first is common. Sometimes two primaries at distant anatomical sites are noted in extensive long-standing OSMF.

81.4.2 Oral Submucous Fibrosis (OSMF)

Oral submucous fibrosis is a chronic insidious disease of the oral mucosa characterized by loss of mucosal elasticity and excessive fibrosis (Figs. 81.4, 81.5 81.6 and 81.7). It is always associated with juxta-epithelial inflammation and progressive hyalinization of lamina propria [13]. Oral submucous fibrosis (OSMF) is predominantly seen among betel quid chewers and pan masala chewers in India. OSMF generally starts at the RMT (retromolar trigone), anterior faucial pillars, and the adjoining area of the soft palate. It extends to involve the buccal mucosa, commissure, lips, and rima oris. Resulting trismus is due to mucosal and muscle fibrosis in the masseter and pterygoids. Figures 81.8 and 81.9 shows the traumatic ulcers caused in buccal mucosa and RMT area in OSMF cases mainly due to the limited mouth opening and fibrosis. In such cases early dental intervention or extractions

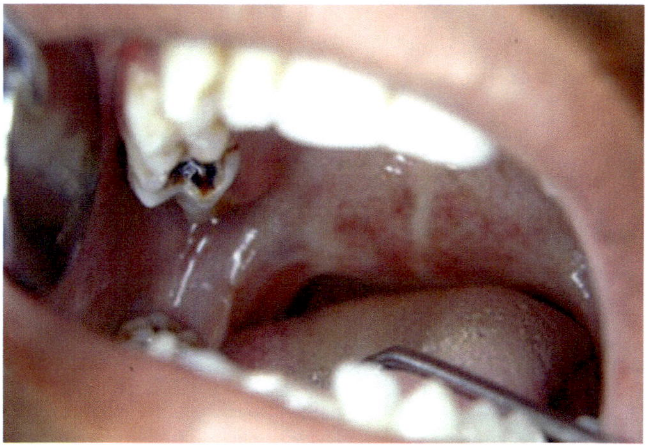

Fig. 81.4 OSMF (oral submucous fibrosis). Note fibrosis affecting RMT, faucial pillars, buccal mucosa, as well as rima oris

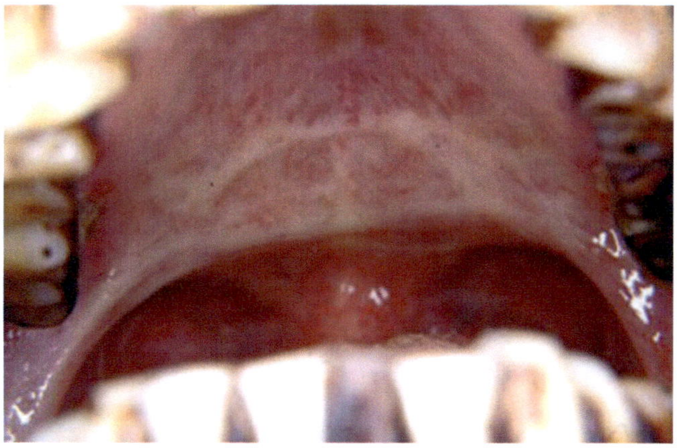

Fig. 81.5 OSMF (oral submucous fibrosis). Note fibrosis affecting RMT, faucial pillars

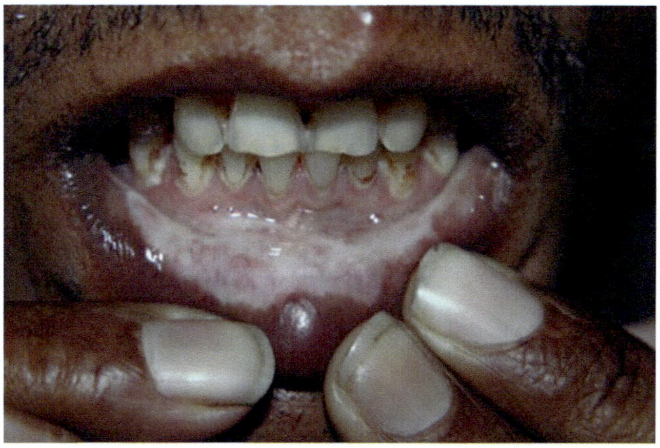

Fig. 81.6 OSMF (oral submucous fibrosis). Note fibrosis affecting lower lip and blanching of mucosa. Note pale nails due to anemia

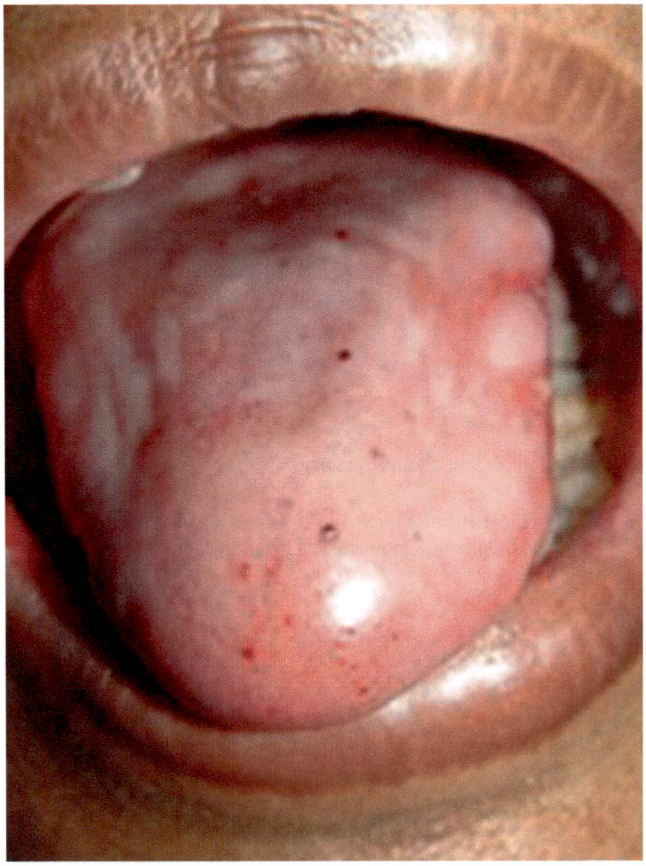

Fig. 81.7 Bald tongue in OSMF. Has high malignant potential

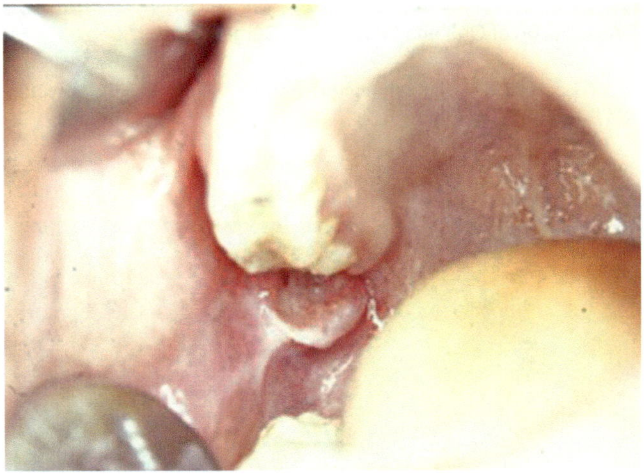

Fig. 81.8 OSMF with traumatic ulceration from last molars

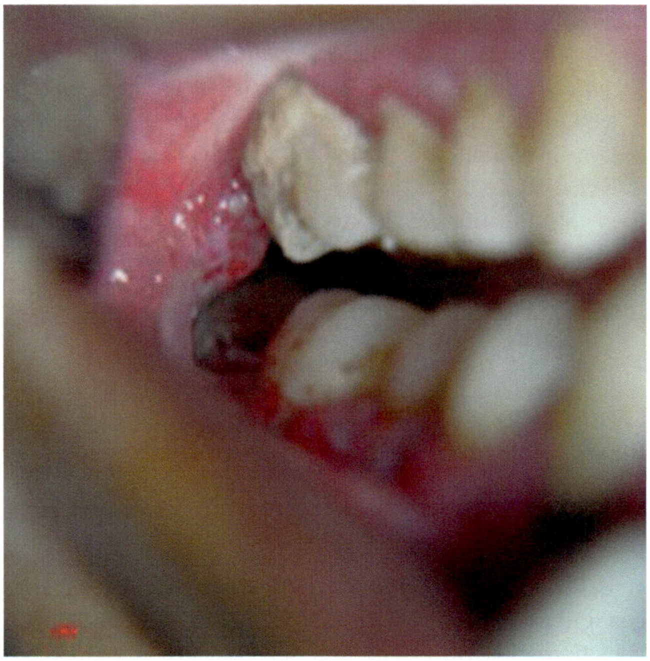

Fig. 81.9 OSMF with traumatic ulceration from last molars

may be delayed due to the difficulty in access to the posterior teeth due to trismus. Such chronic traumatic ulceration may undergo malignant change as seen in Fig. 81.10.

81.4.2.1 Molecular Pathogenesis of OSMF

Time and constant irritation lead to inflammation with mucosal atrophy. It can thus be considered that induction of oral mucosal inflammation by betel quid is a critical event in the pathogenesis of OSMF. Cytokines like interleukin-6 (IL-6), tumor necrosis factor (TNF), interferon-a (INF-a), and growth factors like TGF-b are synthesized at the site of inflammation.

TGF-b1 is a key regulator of extracellular matrix (ECM) assembly and remodeling. TGF-b1 increases collagen production and decreases its degradation [14]. OSMF has characteristic clinical presentation depending on the stage of the disease. The majority of patients have intolerance to spicy food, roughness of oral mucosa, and varying degrees of difficulty in opening the mouth.

OSMF is a well-recognized potentially premalignant condition of the oral cavity. The transformation rate is as high as 7.6% over a period of 10 years [15]. In this group, primary malignancy develops in the buccal mucosa extending to involve the retromolar trigone. This is unique in the context

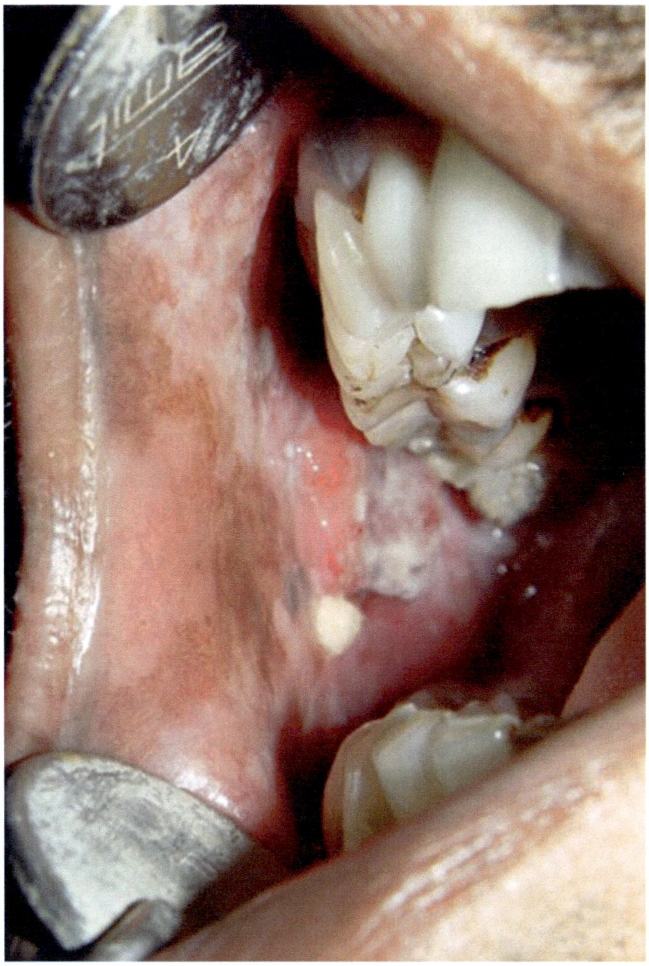

Fig. 81.10 Malignant transformation in posterior buccal mucosa in a case of OSMF, accompanied by chronic trauma form tooth

of the Indian subcontinent, as pure tobacco chewing habit has decreased and is replaced by the gutkha chewing habit. Tobacco-lime preparation used to be kept in the GBS or the floor of the mouth for longer period. This led to leukoplakia and/or erythroplakia, followed by malignant transformation. The current preparation is not constantly placed in the GBS but chewed for long time and swallowed. The chemical effect leads to OSMF and field concretization.

81.4.3 Oral Lichen Planus

Oral lichen planus (OLP) tends to often present bilaterally as white striae on the buccal mucosa. Any mucosal site in the mouth may be involved. Other sites, in decreasing order of frequency, may include the tongue, lips, gingivae, floor of the mouth, and very rarely palate [16].

Six clinical forms of oral lichen planus are recognized [17]: reticular, erosive/ulcerative, papular, plaque-like, atrophic, and bullous. Atrophic/erosive lichen planus is associated with a risk of cancerous transformation [18]. Patients with OLP tend to be monitored closely to detect any potential change early.

The rate of malignant transformation in individual studies ranged from 0 to 3.5%. The overall rate of transformation was 1.09% for OLP.

81.4.4 Precancerous Lesions

Precancerous lesion is a pathology of the oral mucosa which has a tendency to transform into the squamous cell carcinoma. The commonly prevalent lesions are leukoplakia erythroplakia, carcinoma in situ, and smoker's palate.

81.5 Diagnosis of Oral Squamous Cell Carcinoma (OSCC)

Diagnosis of oral squamous cell carcinoma is not a challenging task except in the cases of an unknown primary. History of risk factors, classic clinical appearance of an indurated ulcer, involvement of lymph nodes, and destruction of bone are common features in advanced disease.

81.5.1 Clinical Features of Oral Carcinoma

Oral squamous cell carcinoma often presents as an indurated ulcer, exophytic growth, indurated non-ulcerative patch (endophytic), or a combination of the above appearances. Figures 81.11, 81.12, 81.13, 81.14, 81.15, 81.16, 81.17, and 81.18 shows the various clinical presentation of SCC in tongue. Fig. 81.19 shows multiple primary tumors arising in case of OSMF.

Important parameters to be recorded at the primary site in clinical examination are site of the tumor; size; extension to involve adjacent structures like the skin, muscles, bone of maxilla and/or mandible, and skull base; and extensions into compartments such as the paranasal sinuses, nasal cavity, orbit, pterygoid space, masticatory compartment, and infratemporal fossa. Regional spread to the lymph node basin in the neck needs clinical and radiologic correlation. Evaluation of distant metastasis to lungs and bones forms a part of the staging process.

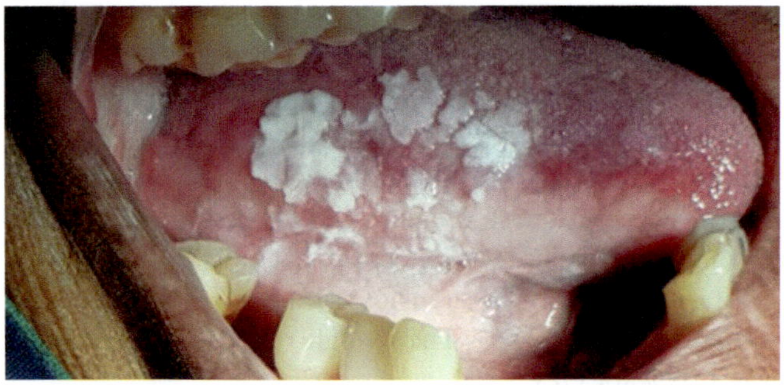

Fig. 81.11 Precancerous lesion of the tongue—diffuse leukoplakia. Lesion has a potential to undergo SCC

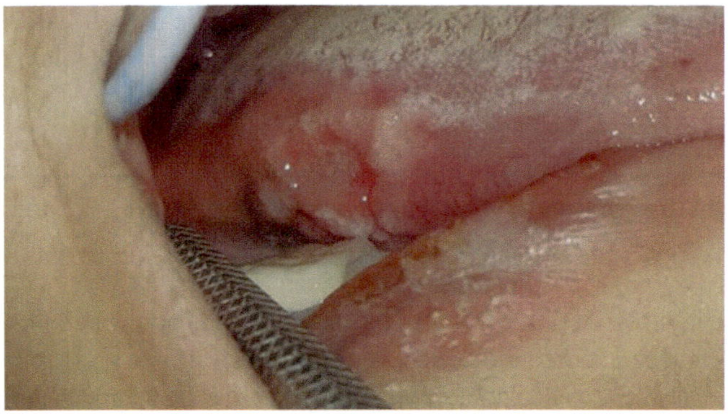

Fig. 81.12 OSCC of the tongue—inverted margins. Lesion not associated with any habit. These lesions often can have genetic predilection and behave aggressively

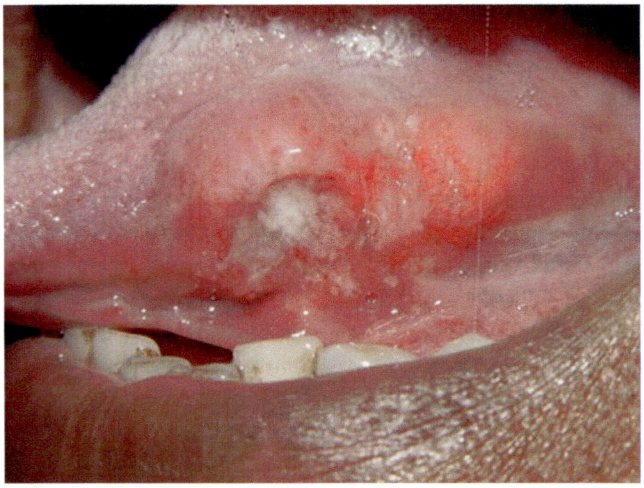

Fig. 81.13 OSCC of the tongue—everted margins. Lesion can behave aggressively often associated with tobacco-related habit

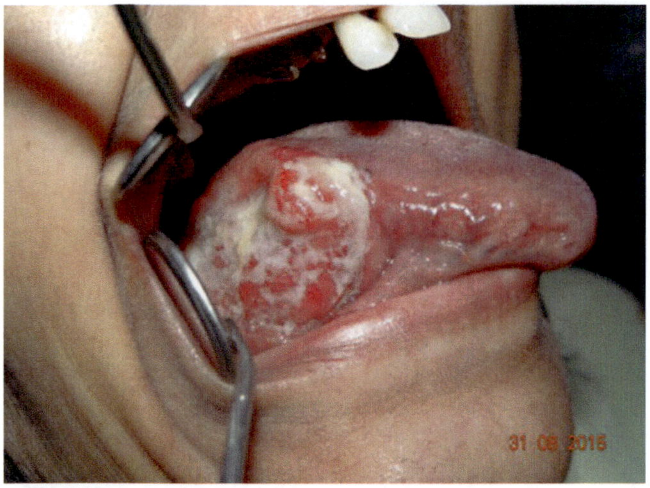

Fig. 81.14 OSCC of the tongue—exophytic growth. Lesions have nonaggressive behavior with better prognosis

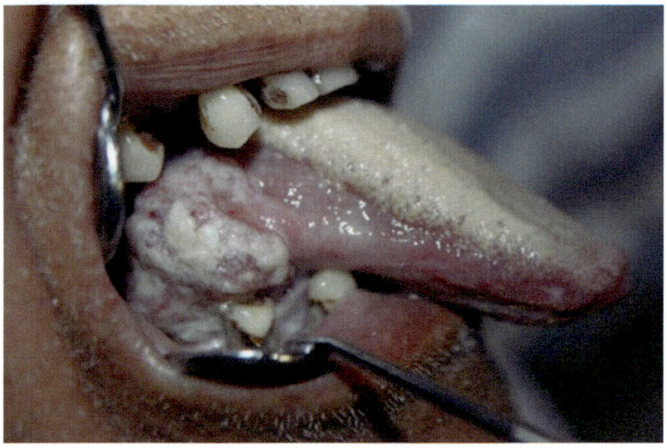

Fig. 81.15 Another case of OSCC of the tongue—exophytic growth. Lesions have nonaggressive behavior with better prognosis

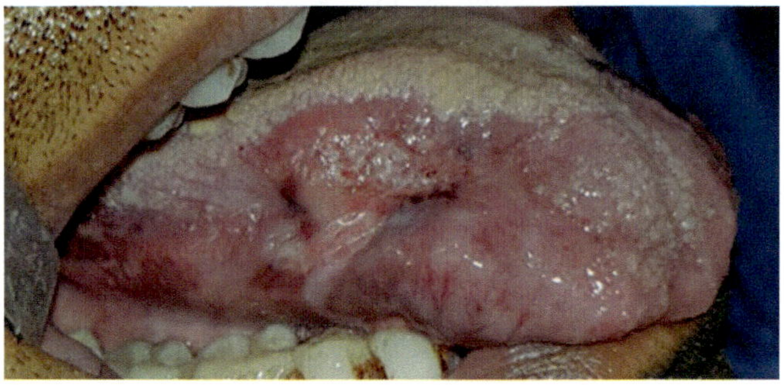

Fig. 81.16 OSCC of the tongue—ulcerative patch. Lesion is not associated with any habit. Genetic predilection

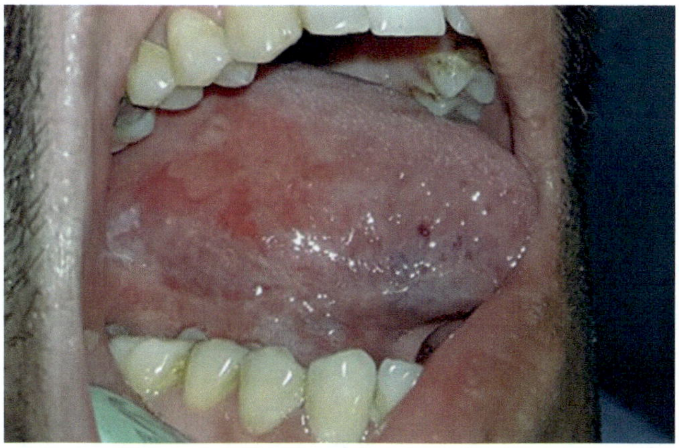

Fig. 81.17 OSCC of the tongue—non-ulcerative patch. Lesion is frequently associated with smoking

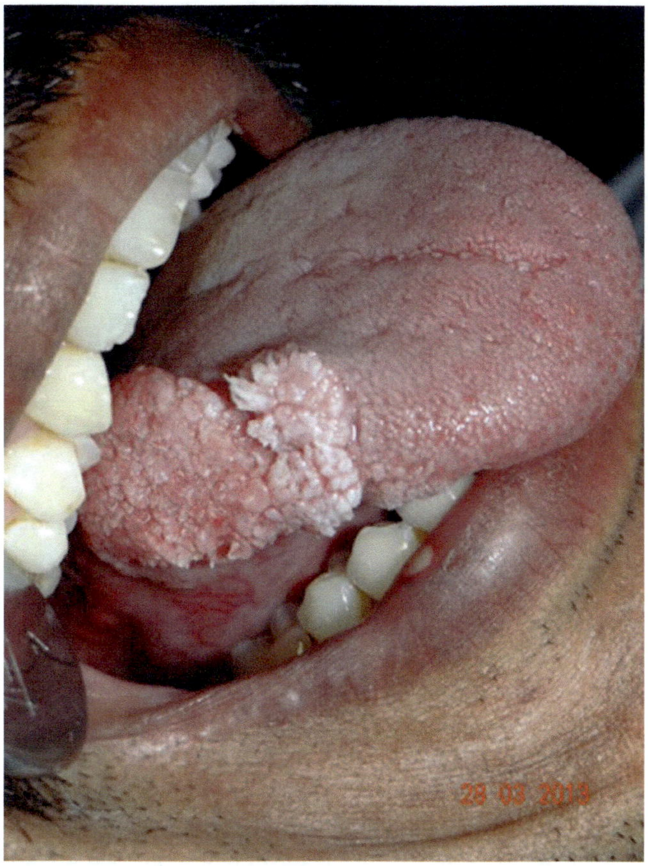

Fig. 81.18 OSCC of the tongue—verrucous growth. Lesion generally has dormant behavior with better prognosis

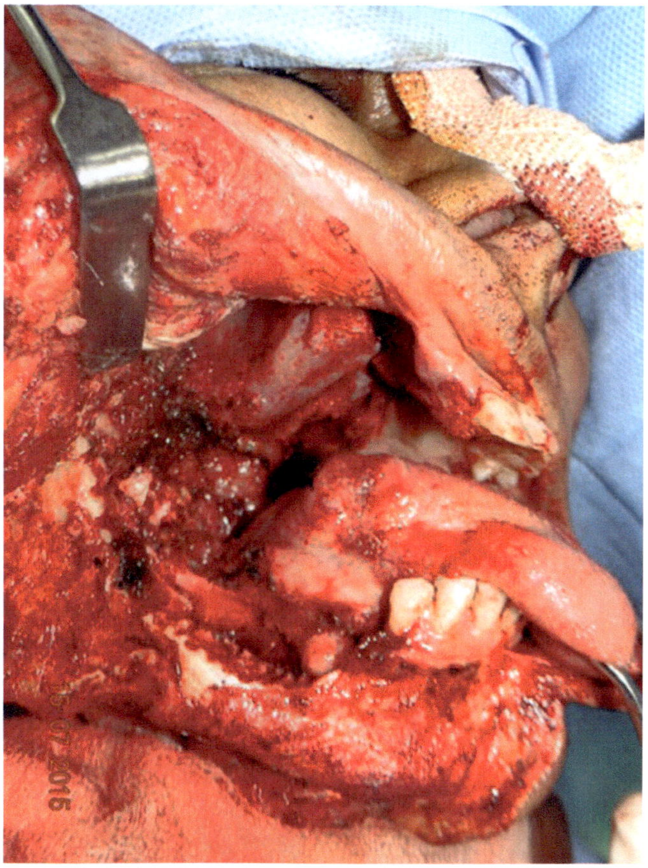

Fig. 81.19 Intraoperative picture. Multiple primary tumors—SCC in OSMF. Rt.GBS/BM—resected, with Tongue-Rt. side. Either of these can be considered as Second Primary Tumour (SPT)

81.6 Imaging in OSCC Diagnosis

The minimum radiologic investigation for the primary site and neck should include imaging from the skull base to the clavicle. Staging of the chest is to detect both metastatic disease and synchronous tumors. MRI and/or CT with contrast is considered to be the gold standard. In poorer socioeconomic background, one could consider ultrasound scan of the neck as a staging modality. This will however not adhere to the current international guidelines. In our units the minimum standard is a MRI of the neck (including the primary) and CT chest. A double-contrast CT of the neck is as valuable as a MRI. Radiologic examination provides a greater accuracy in the staging process. Prognosticators such as depth of invasion and extracapsular spread in lymph nodes can be studied with good accuracy.

Where there is involvement of bone, a MRI and CT will provide better definition for resection. Marrow signal changes can only be evaluated on a MRI. The CT provides

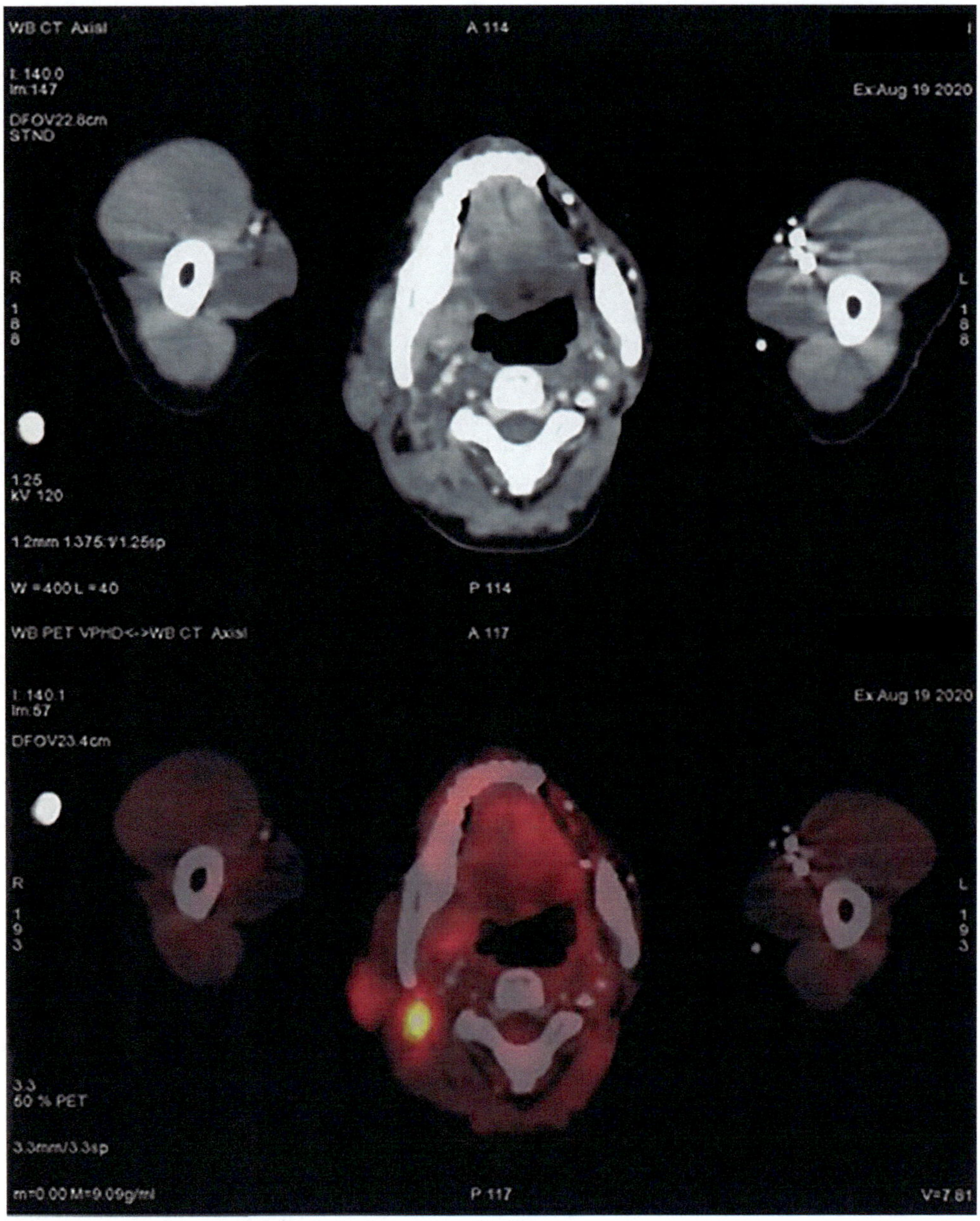

Fig. 81.20 PET-CT-SCC—Contralateral neck metastasis, at IIA, of second primary in Lt. Maxilla

better information on cortical erosion. In addition a thin slice CT helps in 3D planning prior to free flap reconstruction.

The role of a PET-CT is limited. Its primary indication is to detect an unknown primary prior to targeted biopsy. A further role for the PET-CT is in post-radiotherapy evaluation of the neck (Fig. 81.20).

MRI scans offer better accuracy of soft tissue extension of tumor. Studying fat planes between muscle groups allows for compartment resections in T4 tumors.

81.7 Tissue Sampling

Incisional biopsy is the gold standard in the diagnosis of squamous cell carcinoma. FNAC is used for the detection of lymph node metastasis. However with the increased accuracy in MRI and USS reporting, this modality is used less. Biopsy tissue should be taken from the most indurated portion of the tumor. Taking a biopsy from the summit or the center of an ulcer may yield a false-negative result. Scalpel, punch, and low-voltage electrocautery are all good options. Minimum size of the sampled tissue should be ideally 6 mm in all three dimensions. Mapping biopsy from multiple sites may be required at times to evaluate the extent of involvement and to prevent a false-negative result. This is especially the case when a tumor develops in the background of a premalignant lesion.

Deep biopsy is required to get estimation on the depth of invasion (DOI). In cases of exophytic lesions, tumor thickness may cause difficulty in getting deeper tissue; in such cases tumor margin area can be chosen. In order to obtain a good-quality oral biopsy, the clinician should avoid crushing the sample with the tissue-holding forceps, infiltrating anesthetic solution within the lesion, using an insufficient volume of fixing solution and taking insufficient amount of tissue in extension and depth. The specimen should be handled gently, avoiding any crushing, and introduced in the fixing solution such as 10% formalin.

In inaccessible areas, due to the site of tumor or reduced mouth opening, it is good practice to carry out an examination under anesthesia to evaluate the extent of the tumor. This also provides an opportunity for the lesion to be accurately biopsied in a more controlled environment of theaters.

81.7.1 Histopathology

Pathologist is expected to report on the tumor grade—well-differentiated squamous cell carcinoma, Grade 1; moderately differentiated squamous cell carcinoma, Grade 2; or poorly differentiated squamous cell carcinoma, Grade 3. Well-differentiated tumors resemble normal squamous epithelium to a large degree (Fig. 81.21), poorly differentiated tumors exhibiting little or no histologic traits of the squamous phenotype, and moderately differentiated tumors having an intermediate morphology between the two ends of the spectrum. Higher grades have strong potential for recurrence and lymph node metastasis [19].

Several prognostic indicators have consistently demonstrated a correlation with disease-specific survival, local and regional recurrence, and lymph node metastasis in numerous single or multicenter studies. The prognosticators are depth of invasion (DOI), pattern of invasion (POI), perineural invasion (PNI), lymphovascular invasion (LVI), and extranodal extension (ENE).

81.7.2 Depth of Invasion/Tumor Thickness

It is important to differentiate between depth of invasion and tumor thickness. The DOI is a more predictable prognostic factor compared to the latter. It is known that exophytic tumors (verrucous carcinomas being the prototype) or predominantly exophytic tumors have a good prognosis, whereas endophytic or deeply infiltrating tumors are aggressive [20]. Depth of invasion (DOI) is an important independent factor in prognosis with strong effect on disease-free survival and overall survival, correlating with propensity for nodal spread better than tumor size in oral cancer [21–25]. In the floor of the mouth, 1-cm-wide tumor infiltrating at 0.7 cm depth will likely have a worse outcome and carries a higher risk of neck metastasis than a 2-cm-wide tumor with microinvasion or superficial invasion (e.g., less than 2 mm in thickness) [26–28].

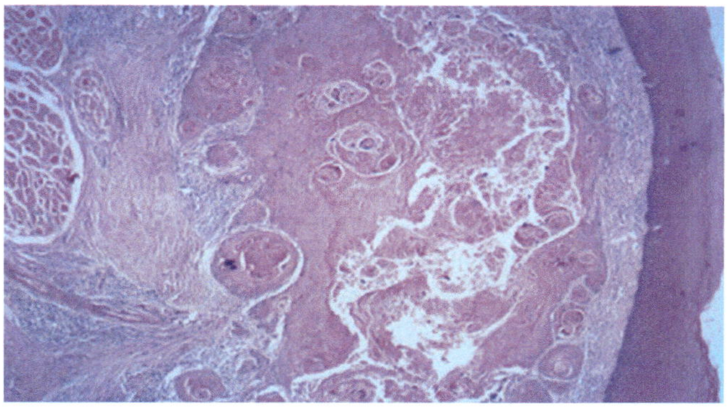

Fig. 81.21 Well-differentiated OSCC. H&E 10x

81.7.3 Pattern of Invasion

Pattern of tumor invasion is an important prognostic factor. Tumor interface abutting deeper tissues has better prognostic value as compared to multiple tumor satellites into the deeper tissues [20].

81.7.4 Perineural Invasion (PNI)

PNI presence is a soft indicator for local recurrence and decreased survival. Multiple studies have shown conflicting results [29]. However it is one of the most important predictors of neck metastasis [30] alongside DOI. PNI increases the rate of occult metastasis [31].

81.7.5 Lymphovascular Invasion (LVI)

Histopathological presence of lymphovascular invasion has poorer prognostic outcome. The presence of LVI is associated with nodal spread or occult metastases [23, 32–34]. Literature review has conflicting evidence regarding the importance of LVI.

81.7.6 Bone Invasion

It is common to see OSCC of GBS and retromolar trigone (RMT) invade the adjoining mandible, maxilla, and pterygoid column. This upstages the tumor to a T4.

The increased risk of local recurrence can be attributed to two factors—tumor character and margin status following resection. Invasion into the pterygoid spaces makes surgical resection difficult. Close margin is expected in these advanced tumors.

Mandible infiltration can be of periosteal fixation, cortical erosion, or medullary invasion. Deeper invasion has poor prognosis [35] (Fig. 81.22).

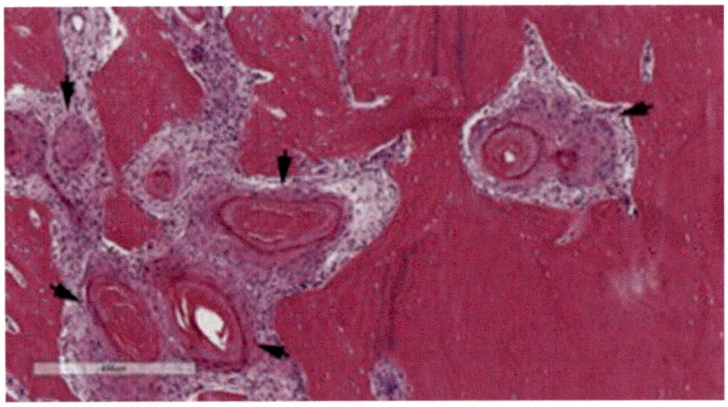

Fig. 81.22 OSCC with bone invasion. H&E 10X

81.8 Neck Assessment in OSCC

A positive neck node is the single most important prognosticator for disease-free survival at 5 years. Size, number of levels involved, fixation to adjacent structures, and extranodal extensions (ENE) are of significance in lymph node assessment of the neck.

In a N0 neck, the pickup rate of a sub-centimeter positive node is less than 50% on clinical examination alone. Use of radiologic examination increases the pickup rate to 90%. A staging neck dissection is the only modality that has a pickup rate greater than 98% [36–38].

A well-lateralized tumor often spreads to the ipsilateral neck. In 5% of patients, the first echelon can be the contralateral neck. Tongue cancers have the propensity for skip metastasis and contralateral spread. For all other regions of the oral cavity, the first echelon spread is at level I/II.

Depending on the literature one reads, the specificity and sensitivity between MRI and CT are confusing. The authors recommend that the radiologist choose the modality he has the greatest confidence in reporting. Ultrasound scan as a screening tool is useful in the outpatient setting.

Radiologic signs of nodal involvement are increases in size of the lymph node, obliteration of the fatty hilum, increased vascularity, an ill-defined outline, and intranodal necrosis. Ten millimeters or more in an axial section are considered positive for nodal involvement in the neck. However, false-positive or false-negative results of 15–20% are noted in the literature [39, 40].

81.9 Distant Metastasis

Distant metastasis needs to be suspected in lungs and vertebrae. Evaluation is done by CT alone or a PET-CT scan.

81.10 TNM Staging System

Cancer staging can be divided into a clinical stage and a pathologic stage. In the TNM (Tumor, Node, and Metastasis) system, clinical stage and pathologic stage are denoted by a small "c" or "p" before the stage (e.g., cT3N1M0 or pT2N0). This staging system is used for most forms of cancer. Accurate staging is critical as treatment is often based on clinical and radiologic stage.

Currently AJCC eighth Edition is used; this includes both the depth of primary tumor invasion and extracapsular extension of lymph node metastases. The AJCC eighth Edition OSCC staging system showed improved disease-free survival discrimination between overall stages and between T categories, while AJCC seventh Edition did not [19].

81.10.1 AJCC Eighth Edition Clinical Staging System

T—Primary tumor.
Tx—Primary tumor cannot be assessed.
Tis—Carcinoma in situ.
T1—Tumor ≤ 2 cm in greatest dimension, ≤ 5 mm depth of invasion (DOI not tumor thickness).
T2—Tumor ≤ 2 cm with DOI > 5 mm or tumor > 2 cm and ≤ 4 cm with DOI ≤ 10 mm.
T3—Tumor > 2 cm and ≤ 4 cm with DOI > 10 mm or tumor > 4 cm with DOI ≤ 10 mm.
T4—Moderately advanced or very advanced local disease.
T4a—Moderately advanced local disease.

Lip: tumor invades through cortical bone or involves the inferior alveolar nerve, floor of the mouth, or skin of the face (i.e., chin or nose).

Oral cavity: tumor invades adjacent structures only (e.g., through cortical bone of the mandible or maxilla, or involves the maxillary sinus or skin of the face). Note: Superficial erosion of bone/tooth socket (alone) by a gingival primary is not sufficient to classify a tumor as T4.

T4b—Very advanced local disease. Tumor invades masticator space, pterygoid plates, or skull base and/or encases internal carotid artery.

Regional lymph nodes (N) ENE—extranodal extension.

Nx—Regional lymph nodes cannot be assessed.

N0—No regional lymph node metastasis.

N1—Metastasis in a single ipsilateral lymph node, ≤ 3 cm in greatest dimension and ENE (−).

N2—Metastasis in a single ipsilateral lymph node, > 3 cm but ≤6 cm in greatest dimension and ENE (−); *or* mets in multiple ipsilateral lymph nodes, ≤ 6 cm in greatest dimen-

Table 81.1 AJCC prognostic staging groups according to the eighth AJCC edition

Clinical group	T	N	M
0	Tis	N0	M0
I	T1	N0	MO
II	T2	N0	MO
III	T3	N0	MO
	T1 T2 T3	N1	MO
IVA	T4a	N0	MO
	T1T2T3T4a	N1, N2	M0
IVB	T4b	Any N	MO
	Any T	N3	M0
IVC	Any T	Any N	M1

sion and ENE *(−); or* mets in bilateral or contralateral lymph nodes, ≤ 6 cm in greatest dimension and ENE (−).

N2a—Metastasis in single ipsilateral lymph node >3 cm but ≤6 cm in greatest dimension and ENE (−).

N2b—Metastasis in multiple ipsilateral lymph nodes ≤6 cm in greatest dimension and ENE (−).

N2c—Metastasis in bilateral or contralateral lymph nodes ≤6 cm in greatest dimension and ENE (−).

N3—Metastasis in a lymph node >6 cm in greatest dimension and ENE *(−) or* metastasis in any lymph node(s) with clinically overt ENE (+).

N3a—Metastasis in a lymph node >6 cm in greatest dimension and ENE (−).

N3b—Metastasis in any lymph node(s) with clinically overt ENE (+).

Distant metastasis (M).

M0—No distant metastasis (no pathologic M0; use clinical M to complete stage group).

M1—Distant metastasis.

AJCC prognostic stage groups are provided in Table 81.1.

81.11 Treatment Planning for the Management of Head and Neck Malignancy

81.11.1 Introduction

The management of head and neck cancer has undergone a sea change since the 1980s. The most important change that has been to the benefit of both patients and clinicians is the emphasis on evidence-based practice, and this has led to the development of the multidisciplinary team (MDT) or the tumor board as it is also known as.

In the more recent past, a new thought process is the practice of realistic medicine. The emphasis is on a more personalized approach to patient care and changing our style to shared decision-making. This is an approach that has been rolled out across Scotland.

81.11.2 MAGIC: Making Good Decisions in Collaboration

The key questions to be asked are:

1. Is this test, treatment, or procedure really needed?
2. What are the potential risks and benefits?
3. What are the potential side effects?
4. Are there alternative simpler, safer treatment options?
5. What would happen if one did nothing?

81.11.3 The Start of Treatment Planning

The beginning of planning treatment starts on the receipt of a referral or patients' attendance. Patients with a history of a neck or salivary gland lump, non-healing ulcer of the oral cavity, bleeding, pain refractory to analgesia, hoarseness, and dysphagia are seen in the clinic within 2 weeks. Clinical examination should include the examination of the tongue base, tonsils, larynx, and nasopharynx with flexible nasoendoscope.

Developing a one-stop clinic helps in avoiding delays, and this has a significant impact on patients' psychological well-being. The one-stop clinic includes a biopsy on the same day for visible lesions and an ultrasound-guided core biopsy of neck lumps. The results of these preliminary investigations should be available in a week, setting up for a second meeting.

81.11.4 The Second Meeting

The second meeting or breaking bad news is perhaps the most important consultation in treatment planning. Patients are invited to attend the clinic with members of their family. Consultation is held in a quiet atmosphere in the presence of a clinical nurse specialist. It is important to be factual and honest. Unrealistic expectations should not be given. One must also bear in mind the impact the diagnosis will have on patients and their families. Empathy is very important. A good rapport with the patient and their family is invaluable.

81.11.5 Staging Scans

The minimum staging scans for head and neck cancer include a MRI and/or CT neck and CT chest. The rationale for staging is localization of the tumor and detection of regional and distant lymph node metastases. This has an importance in both the extent of therapeutic intervention and the disease-specific survival.

81.11.6 Localization of Primary Tumor

The localization of the primary tumor helps in the decision-making regarding the resectability of the lesion with clear margins. Tumor resection with a R1 margin is considered a futile procedure, and at the best it is palliative and at its worst just a "big biopsy." Anatomical areas of interest in localization are the skull base with particular interest to the carotid canal, involvement of the infratemporal fossa, the extent into the orbit, and in the case of tongue tumors proximity to the tongue base and larynx. Involvement of any of the above structure carries a very high risk of a positive or close margins resulting in increased risk of recurrence. Adjuvant treatment would then be inevitable. Functional outcomes are poorer.

MRI of the soft tissues is our preference for localization of the tumor as it helps in planning anatomic resection by determining the depth of infiltration. This can be in the form of compartment resection—medial masticatory compartment resection for retromolar, soft palate, and posterior tongue tumors. Anatomical resections in tongue tumors uses muscle planes to identify margins and vascularity of the remainder tongue. The muscle groups most important to this are the mylohyoid, styloglossus, and stylohyoid. With tumors extending to the infratemporal fossa and skull base, a key landmark is the styloid. Prestyloid resections are considered straightforward, and a R0 margin is to be expected. Tumors in the poststyloid space carry the risk of a close margin.

Tumors involving the mandible and maxilla, in our practice, have a CT and MRI. The MRI helps in determination of marrow signal change and gives an aid to planning resection margins. The CT has a two fold advantage. CT helps localize cortical breach and complements the MRI in planning resection. It has also the added advantage of obtaining 3D models which helps in planning bone reconstruction with a free flap.

For malignancies of the salivary glands, our first line of investigation remains an USS-guided core biopsy followed by a full staging of the neck and chest with MRI and CT, respectively. Tumors of the skull base and infratemporal fossa have both MRI and CT for localization of the primary.

For patients with suspected recurrence, especially under a free tissue flap transfer, the preferred modality is a PET-CT. PET-CT allows for a functional evaluation of the suspect area. In areas of previous surgery, the MRI has higher false-positive rates due to loss of fat planes and the inability to differentiate from scarification. A double-contrast CT scan may give better definition of a recurrence; however both specificity and sensitivity are low. The CT may give better spatial resolution. However false-negative results are high in glottic tumors and in mucosal disease with superficial spread with CT.

The role of PET-CT in our practice is limited to neck lumps with unknown primary, small malignancies and in recurrent SCC. The major drawback for a PET-CT is poor anatomical depiction. Anatomical resection is not possible with a PET-CT alone. PET-CT adds little value in patients who have had recent surgery, i.e., biopsy. This invariably gives rise to a hot spot in inflamed tissue. However, it is more sensitive than CT and MRI in detecting small malignancy. In more than 30% of cases, the PET-CT picks up malignancy not identified by other modalities, and the majority of these are at the tongue base and supraglottic space.

Direct evaluation by examination under anesthesia and pan endoscopy provides probably the most accurate assessment for localization and planning surgery.

81.11.7 Evaluation of the Neck

There are numerous papers regarding the sensitivity and specificity of different evaluation techniques—clinical examination, duplex ultrasound scan, CT scan, MRI, and PET. It is agreed by all that clinical examination of the neck provides the least reliable results of all and an adjunct investigation is necessary. It is the opinion of the authors that both CT and MRI give equally reliable results. The decision to which modality suits an individual team the best is reliant on the expertise of the head and neck radiologist in reporting the scans. In our own clinical practice, we feel that the MRI scan provides a good diagnostic value for staging the neck. In T1 tumors where there is a N0 neck clinically and radiologically, the evidence for staging neck dissection is limited. In cases where the MRI is equivocal, an USS with a FNAC (fine needle aspiration cytology) may be indicated. The USS would evaluate the lymph node for size criteria, presence of necrosis, and the absence of normal hilum. Lymph nodes that are rounded and greater than 1 cm in the neck are regarded to be pathologic until proven otherwise.

The role of USS should not be easily dismissed with the advent of cross-sectional imaging. The USS has many advantages. The spatial resolution of a good USS is better than that of a CT or MRI. Taking account of shape, contour, echogenicity, grouping, internal architecture, necrosis, and pattern of Doppler vascularity enhances the accuracy of US for nodal metastases to greater than 90%.

The USS is a cheap and quick modality that can be used. There is no radiation exposure. Its use as a surveillance scans cannot be surpassed in today's economic constraints. The one major drawback we have noted in our practice is that its sensitivity and specificity are highly operator dependent. It cannot detect retropharyngeal, retrotracheal, and mediastinal lymphadenopathy. In these instances a CT or MRI gives better information.

PET-CT has a limited role in the staging of the neck. PET-CT is a useful tool to look at post-chemoradiation treatment response and to evaluate the neck following radiotherapy with residual neck mass. In the head and neck, misregistration of PET to CT can cause difficulty in reporting and increase false-positive results.

81.11.8 The Role of Sentinel Node Biopsy

The presence of metastatic disease to the neck is an important prognostic factor for disease-free survival in head and neck cancer. Recent papers by Anil D Cruz et al. have shown that patients who had an elective neck dissection fared much better than those on the watchful waiting strategy in both T1 and T2 tumors [29].

Sentinel node biopsy relies on the fact that metastases to the regional lymph nodes follow a predictive pattern in most cases. Migration of cancer cells is often to the first echelon node. It is therefore predicted that if the first echelon node is negative, the more distal node is unlikely to have cancer cell migration. Validation studies involving elective neck dissection have shown that there is 95% detection rate in sentinel nodes. The first echelon node in most oral cancers is at level I or level II. In a well-lateralized tumor, the first echelon node more often than not is on the ipsilateral side.

The indications for a sentinel node biopsy are:

1. T1/T2 tumors which are node negative on staging scans.
2. To assess the need for bilateral neck dissection in tumors close to or just crossing the midline.
3. To clarify the need for contralateral neck dissection in large tumors.

Proponents of SLN biopsy claim the following advantages: reduces the morbidity of elective neck dissection, more accurate staging of the neck, and better prediction in those who have an unpredictable pattern of metastatic disease, therefore guides decision-making, helps identify skip metastases and micrometastases, and saves time and expense.

It is the opinion of the authors that sentinel node biopsy is a very good adjunct. Recent meta-analysis and systematic reviews suggest that high sensitivity, negative predictive value, and accuracy of SNB make this a valid diagnostic tool. NICE (National Institute of Clinical Excellence) guidelines recommend that a SLNB should be offered to all patients with T1 and T2 tumors with a node-negative neck. A word of caution, however, for T1 and T2 tumors with a tumor thickness greater than 5 mm, an elective neck dissection may still be indicated.

81.11.9 The Multidisciplinary Team

Following completion of all diagnostic requisites, the findings are discussed at the weekly MDT or the tumor board meeting. The MDT has a core group of clinicians and healthcare professionals. The MDT comprises of maxillofacial surgeons, ENT surgeons, oncologist, speech and language therapist (SALT), dietician, clinical nurse specialist (CNS), head and neck radiologist, head and neck pathologist, restorative dentist, and cancer audit officer to collect data. We have two clinicians from each of the subspecialties at our MDT. The MDT should not be regarded as a forum to advance individual pride or agenda. This is a group that helps balance evidence base in the management of patients and makes a realistic recommendation of treatment strategy.

The responsibility of the MDT is to protect and facilitate the patients' pathway through cancer treatment. The first and foremost recommendation made by the MDT is the treatment intent—curative or palliative. This is followed by the treatment strategy—surgery or radiotherapy ± chemotherapy (Refer Chap. 84 to read about Adjunctive therapy in oral cancer).

At our MDT, the nature of surgery or the form of reconstruction is rarely discussed. The certainty of achieving tumor clearance and potential morbidity associated with the treatment form the majority of the discussions. Speech and language team assess the need for potential future PEG (gastrostomy) or nasogastric feed. Where there is a high index of suspicion that a PEG feed will be necessary, this is done pre-treatment. Dieticians help in planning feeding regimes both pre- and postoperatively. The restorative dentist offers an opinion on unrestorable teeth that need to be extracted at the time of surgery or prior to chemoradiation to reduce the incidence of future osteoradionecrosis.

81.11.10 Planning Reconstruction

The choice of reconstruction is numerous (Refer Chap. 82 to read about principles of surgical management of oral cancer. Chapter 85 deals with the access osteotomies to maxillofacial region while Chaps. 86 and 88 deals with soft and hard tissue reconstruction respectively). The preferred choice is dependent on the following factors:

- Patient's overall health to withstand long surgery.
- Associated postoperative functional deficit if no reconstruction is carried out.
- Skill of the surgeons.
- Socioeconomic factors.

The best form of reconstruction is to try and substitute like for like. A simple but effective way of looking at reconstruction would be:

- Flaps for lining the defect in T2 defects—radial forearm free flap, anterolateral thigh perforator flap (ALT), medial sural artery free flap, submental flap, nasolabial flaps.
- Flaps that are required for increasing bulk or low volume—anterolateral thigh flap, pectoralis major flap.
- Flaps for major resection which require high volume—rectus flap, latissimus dorsi flap.
- Flaps for lining the pharynx—radial forearm free flap, ALT, pectoralis major flap.
- Skull base defects that require a long pedicle—rectus abdominis flap, ALT, or latissimus dorsi free flap.
- Bone reconstruction—fibula free flap, DCIA (deep circumflex iliac artery) flap, scapula flap.
- Composite defect—combination of the above or scapula flap.

81.11.11 Conclusion

A good functional MDT that practices evidence-based medicine with a realistic approach that is patient centered will be an effective oncology team that will deliver high-quality care for patients.

References

1. Niranjan VR, et al. Oral cancer epidemiology of Aurangabad district (Maharashtra) of India from 2005 to 2014: understanding the burden of disease. Int J Community Med Public Health. 2017 Jul;4(7):2275–81.
2. Gupta B, Ariyawardana A, Johnson NW. Oral cancer in India continues in epidemic proportions: evidence base and policy initiatives. Int Dent J. 2013;63(1):12–25.
3. Park K. Park's textbook of preventive and social medicine. 23rd ed. Jabalpur: M/S Banarsidas Bhanot; 2015.
4. International Agency on Research for Cancer. Smokeless tobacco and some tobacco-specific N-nitrosamines. Monographs, vol. 89. Lyon: IARC; 2007.
5. Murthy NS, Mathew A. Cancer epidemiology, prevention and control. Curr Sci. 2004;86(4):518–27.
6. Gupta PC, Mehta HC. Cohort study of all-cause mortality among tobacco users in Mumbai. India Bull WHO. 2000;78:877–83.
7. Sankaranarayanan R, Duffy SW, Padmakumary G. Tobacco and alcohol as risk factors in the larynx in Kerala. India Int J Cancer. 1990;45:879–82.
8. IARC. Monographs on the evaluation of carcinogenic risk to humans: alcohol drinking, vol. 44. Lyon: IARC; 1988.
9. Kiran Kumar K, Saraswathi TR, Ranganathan K, Devi MU, Elizabeth J. Oral submucous fibrosis: a clinicohistopathological study in Chennai. IJDR. 2007;18:106–11.
10. Anonymous IARC. Tobacco habits other than smoking: betel quid and areca nut chewing and some related nitrosamines. IARC Monogr Eval Carcinog Risk Chem Hum. 1985;37:141–200.
11. Sharma JD, Barman D, Sarma MK, Sharma A, Kalita M, Kataki AC, et al. Burden of head and neck cancers in Kamrup urban district cancer registry of Assam, India: a retrospective study. Int J Res Med Sci. 2014;2:1382–7.
12. Gupta B, Ariyawardana A, Johnson NW. Oral cancer in India continues in epidemic proportions: evidence base and policy initiatives. Int Dent J. 2013;63(1):12–25.
13. Pillai R, Balaram P. Pathogenesis of oral sub mucous fibrosis – relationship to risk factors associated with oral cancer. Cancer. 1992;69:2011–20.
14. Roberts AB, Flanders KC, Kondaiah P, Thompson NL, Van Obberghen-Schilling E, et al. Transforming growth factor beta: biochemistry and roles in embryogenesis, tissue repair and remodeling, and carcinogenesis. Recent Prog Horm Res. 1988;44: 157–97.
15. Neville BW, Damm DD. Allen CM – Oral and maxillofacial pathology. 2nd ed. Philadelphia: WB Saunders; 2002. p. 349–50.
16. Thongprasom K, Carrozzo M, Furness S, Lodi G. Interventions for treating oral lichen planus. Cochrane Database Syst Rev. Jul 6, 2011;7:CD001168.
17. Farhi D, Dupin N. Pathophysiology, etiologic factors, and clinical management of oral lichen planus, part I: facts and controversies. Clin Dermatol. 2010;28(1):100–8.
18. Fitzpatrick SG, Hirsch SA, Gordon SC. The malignant transformation of oral lichen planus and oral lichenoid lesions: A systematic review. J Am Dent Assoc. 2014 Jan;145(1):45–56.
19. Pollaers K, Hinton-Bayre A, Friedland PL, Farah CS. AJCC 8th Edition oral cavity squamous cell carcinoma staging – Is it an improvement on the AJCC 7th Edition. Oral Oncol. 2018 Jul;82:23–8.
20. Moore C, Kuhns JG, Greenberg RA. Thickness as prognostic aid in upper aerodigestive tract cancer. Arch Surg. 1986;121(12):1410–4.
21. Mohit-Tabatabai MA, Sobel HJ, Rush BF, Mashberg A. Relation of thickness of floor of mouth stage I and II cancers to regional metastasis. Am J Surg. 1986;152(4):351–3.
22. Brown B, Barnes L, Mazariegos J, Taylor F, Johnson J, Wagner RL. Prognostic factors in mobile tongue and floor of mouth carcinoma. Cancer. 1989;64(6):1195–202.
23. Woolgar JA, Scott J. Prediction of cervical lymph node metastasis in squamous cell carcinoma of the tongue/floor of mouth. Head Neck. 1995;17(6):463–72.
24. O-charoenrat P, Pillai G, Patel S, Fisher C, Archer D, Eccles S, et al. Tumor thickness predicts cervical nodal metastases and survival in early tongue cancer. Oral Oncol. 2003;39:386–90.
25. Ling W, Mijiti A, Moming A. Survival pattern and prognostic factors of patients with squamous cell carcinoma of the tongue: a retrospective analysis of 210 cases. J Oral Maxillofac Surg. 2013;71(4):775–85.
26. Gonzalez-Moles MA, Esteban F, Rodriguez-Archilla A, Ruiz-Avila I, Gonzales-Moles S. Importance of tumour thickness measurement in prognosis of tongue cancer. Oral Oncol. 2002;38: 394–7.
27. Umeda M, Yokoo S, Take Y, Omori A, Nakanishi K, Shimada K. Lymph node metastasis in squamous cell carcinoma of the oral cavity: correlation between histologic features and the prevalence of metastasis. Head Neck. 1992;14(4):263–72.
28. Kane SV, Gupta M, Kakade AC, D'Cruz A. Depth of invasion is the most significant histological predictor of subclinical cervical lymph node metastasis in early squamous carcinomas of the oral cavity. Eur J Surg Oncol. 2006;32:795–803.
29. Thiagarajan S, Nair S, Nair D, Chaturvedi P, Kane SV, Agarwal JP, D'Cruz AK. Predictors of prognosis for squamous cell carcinoma of oral tongue. J Surg Oncol. 2014;109(7):639–44.
30. Morton RP, Ferguson CM, Lambie NK, Whitlock RM. Tumor thickness in early tongue cancer. Arch Otolaryngol Head Neck Surg. 1994;120(7):717–20.

31. Tai SK, Li WY, Yang MH, Chu PY, Wang YF, Chang PM. Perineural invasion as a major determinant for the aggressiveness associated with increased tumor thickness in t1–2 oral tongue and buccal squamous cell carcinoma. Ann Surg Oncol. 2013;20(11):3568–74.
32. Matsushita Y, Yanamoto S, Takahashi H, Yamada S, Naruse T, Sakamoto Y, Ikeda H, Shiraishi T, Fujita S, Ikeda T, Asahina I, Umeda M. A clinicopathological study of perineural invasion and vascular invasion in oral tongue squamous cell carcinoma. Int J Oral Maxillofac Surg. 2015;44(5):543–8.
33. Sparano A, Weinstein G, Chalian A, Yodul M, Weber R. Multivariate predictors of occult neck metastasis in early oral tongue cancer. Otolaryngol Head Neck Surg. 2004;131:472–6.
34. Close LG, Brown PM, Vuitch MF, Reisch J, Schaefer SD. Microvascular invasion and survival in cancer of the oral cavity and oropharynx. Arch Otolaryngol Head Neck Surg. 1989;115(11):1304–9.
35. Vincent N, Dassonville O, Chamorey E, Poissonnet G, Pierre CS, Nao EE, Peyrade F, Benezery K, Viel D, Sudaka A, Marcy PY, Vallicioni J, Demard F, Santini J, Bozec A. Clinical and histological prognostic factors in locally advanced oral cavity cancers treated with primary surgery. Eur Ann Otorhinolaryngol Head Neck Dis. 2012;129(6):291–6.
36. de Bondt RB, Nelemans PJ, Hofman PA, et al. Detection of lymph node metastases in head and neck cancer: a meta-analysis comparing US, USg FNAC, CT and MR imaging. Eur J Radiol. 2007;64:266–72.
37. Wu LM, Xu JR, Liu MJ, et al. Value of magnetic resonance imaging for nodal staging in patients with head and neck squamous cell carcinoma: a meta-analysis. Acad Radiol. 2012;19:331–40.
38. Kyzas PA, Evangelou E, Denaxa-Kyza D, et al. 18F-fluorodeoxyglucose positron emission tomography to evaluate cervical node metastases in patients with head and neck squamous cell carcinoma: a meta-analysis. J Natl Cancer Inst. 2008;100:712–20.
39. Som PM, Brandwein-Gensler MS. Lymph nodes of the neck. In: Som PM, Curtin HD, editors. Head & neck imaging, vol. 2. 5th ed. St Louis: Mosby; 2011. p. 2287–383.
40. Kuriokose M. Contemporary oral oncology, vol. 1 and 2. Cham: Springer International Publishing; 2017.

Principles of Surgical Management of Oral Cancer

82

Sushma Mehta and Moni Abraham Kuriakose

82.1 Introduction

Management of oral cavity cancers in a curative intent setting mainly involves surgery. The other treatment modalities such as radiotherapy and chemotherapy are most commonly used as adjuvant treatment based on the histopathological features. However, it is to be noted that surgery alone is insufficient to treat oral cancer. Chemotherapy is either concurrent with radiotherapy or in very rare scenario used as induction therapy. The primary cancer treatment and risk factor reduction are of utmost importance to improve effectiveness of the primary treatment and to prevent development of second-primary cancers.

Ablative surgery has evolved over the years with the attempt to extirpate the tumor in its entirety with the understanding of the molecular tumor biology, pattern of tumor invasion of the tumors, as well as availability of better instrumentations.

With the advent of endoscopic assisted and robotic-assisted neck dissection, the branch of oral oncology has truly made progress, thus improving visualization and three-dimensional navigation; however it is still in its infancy and needs further research to understand the benefits over the conventional methods.

This chapter outlines details of ablative surgery and rationale for addressing neck (node positive/node negative) in patients with oral cavity cancers.

Electronic Supplementary Material The online version of this chapter (https://doi.org/10.1007/978-981-15-1346-6_82) contains supplementary material, which is available to authorized users.

S. Mehta
Mazumdar Shaw Cancer Center, Bengaluru, Karnataka, India

M. A. Kuriakose (✉)
Cochin Cancer Research Centre, Kochi, Kerala, India

82.2 Initial Evaluation and Staging

Initial evaluation as for any other medical condition includes history, a clinical examination and investigations to form a diagnosis. The other two important aspects influencing management of oral cavity cancer (mainly squamous cell carcinoma) are habit history and performance status. Table 82.1 describes the performance status scales.

Staging of the disease is particularly important as it helps the clinicians in better communication in a scientific forum and forming a treatment plan for a patient. Various phases in management of oral cancer include accurate diagnosis, appropriate treatment plan, and execution of the advised treatment with relevant reconstruction, rehabilitation, and surveillance. So, to help clinicians in decision-making, there are several guidelines that exist. As these guidelines have a more generalized approach, it is the clinician's knowledge

Table 82.1 Performance status scale: Zubrod scale and Karnofsky scale

Performance Status Scales [1]	
Zubrod scale	Karnofsky scale
"0" normal activity	"100" normal; no evidence of disease
	"90" able to perform normal activities with only minor symptoms.
"1" symptomatic and ambulatory cares for self	"80" normal activity with effort; some activities
	"70" able to care for self but unable to do normal activities
"2" ambulatory >50% of the time; occasional assistance	"60" requires occasional assistance; cares for most needs
"3" ambulatory ≤50% of the time; nursing care needed	"50" requires considerable assistance
	"40" disabled; requires special assistance
	"30" severely disabled
"4" bedridden	"20" very sick; requires active supportive treatment
	"10" moribund

K. Bonanthaya et al. (eds.), *Oral and Maxillofacial Surgery for the Clinician*, https://doi.org/10.1007/978-981-15-1346-6_82

and understanding and experience which will help in tailoring the treatment plan to each individual distinctly. This individualized approach cannot be implemented unless there are multidisciplinary tumor board meetings, which are crucial for clinicians practicing oncology and hence provides team-based practice keeping the patient in mind [2–4]. This is best done before initiating the treatment.

To be able to know the extent of disease and decide the intent and modality of treatment, imaging plays a very important role. Precise imaging information is needed to determine the locoregional extent, erosion, and involvement of underlying bone and marrow space, lymph node involvement and to rule out distant metastasis—especially to the lungs. However the dilemma that most clinicians face is which is the imaging modality of choice for different clinical scenarios. In the following section, we attempt to provide indications of each imaging type available, which probably will help the clinicians in deciding what suits their needs.

Plain radiography is restricted to evaluation of pathological fractures or initial benign lesions. Contrast-enhanced computed tomography (CECT) is considered as the most popular, easily available, and cost-effective diagnostic imaging. It is the imaging modality of choice to know the presence of bone erosion and lymph node characteristic. Bony expansion is usually a feature of slow-growing/benign disease process; however destruction of bone and replacement by the tumor depicts the aggressiveness and hence is a feature of malignant process (Figs. 82.1, 82.2, 82.3 and 82.4).

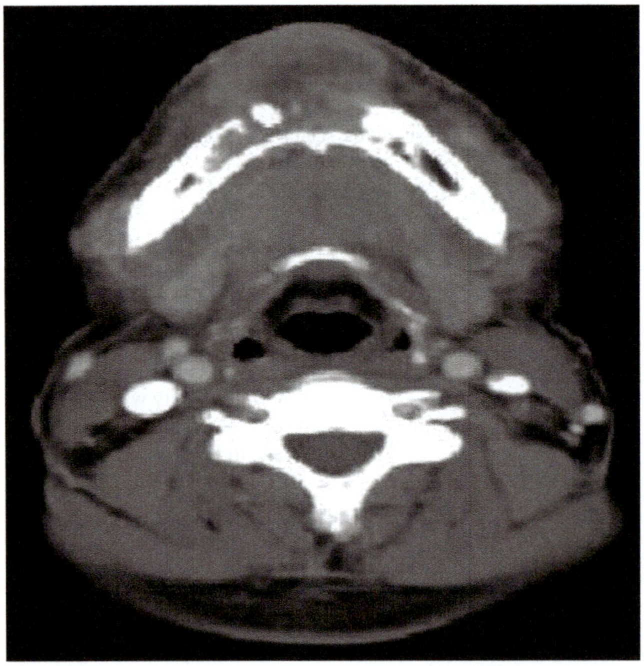

Fig. 82.1 Axial section of contrast enhanced CECT showing an ill-defined heterogeneously enhancing mass lesion along the mandibular alveolus involving the central lateral incisors and canines with erosion of body of mandible

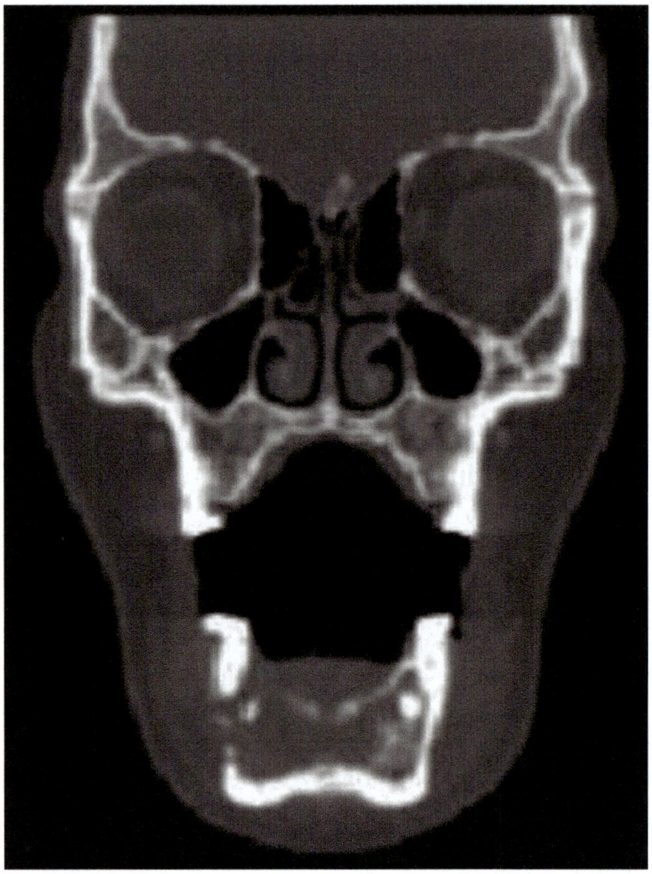

Fig. 82.2 Sagittal section of the patient same as Fig. 82.1 to depict the extent of bony erosion and involvement providing a guide for the osteotomy

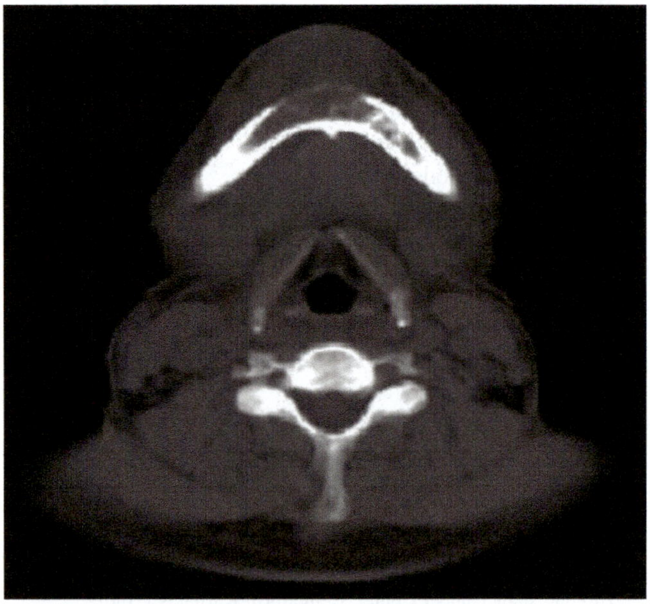

Fig. 82.3 This is axial section in bony window for exact extent of bony erosion

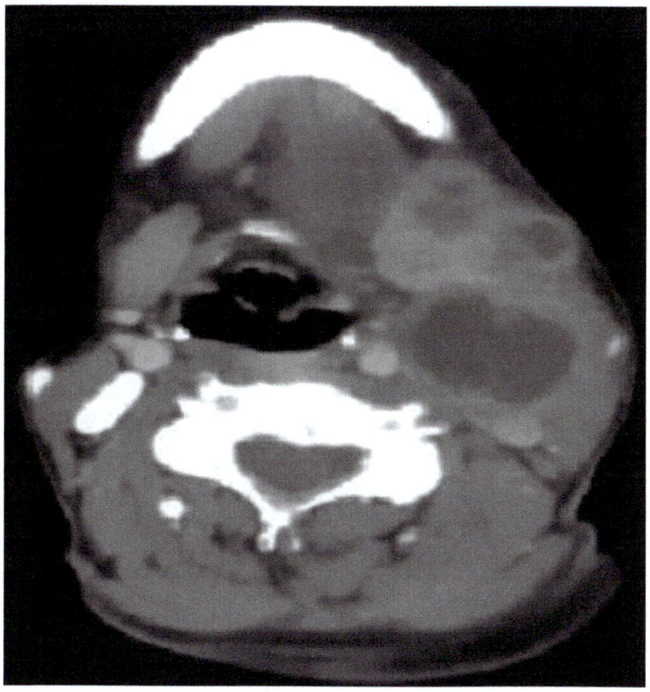

Fig. 82.4 Axial section—contrast-enhanced computed tomography. A heterogeneously enhanced conglomerate of the lymph nodal mass at left level II with cystic areas highly suspicious of metastatic lymphadenopathy. The mass has partially compressed internal jugular vein and pushed it posterolaterally

Magnetic resonance imaging (MRI) is usually indicated as an adjunct as it has better soft tissue delineation. It is also used for assessing dural invasion (linear or nodular), medullary bone involvement, and perineural invasion. Radiographic assessment of tumor extent is invaluable for treatment planning. In case of tongue cancers, MRI has gained popularity for assessment of tongue cancer especially as it is helpful in identifying tumor thickness, involvement of the contralateral side, and involvement of extrinsic muscles. With recent addition of depth of invasion in the AJCC classification for staging, MRI has proven its role. As for buccal mucosa tumors, assessment of masticatory muscles involvement is crucial because it has historically been considered unresectable. However, according to Liao, infranotch lesions are still amenable for resection with favorable oncological outcome.

As oral cancers usually metastasize first to the lung, pre-operative chest imaging is a part of initial pre-operative work-up. This can be in the form of either plain film or 3D imaging such as computed tomography (CT). Fluorodeoxyglucose positron emission tomography (FDG-PET) scan has emerged as the imaging modality of choice in patient with recurrence and high clinical suspicion for distant metastasis (Figs. 82.5, 82.6, 82.7 and 82.8).

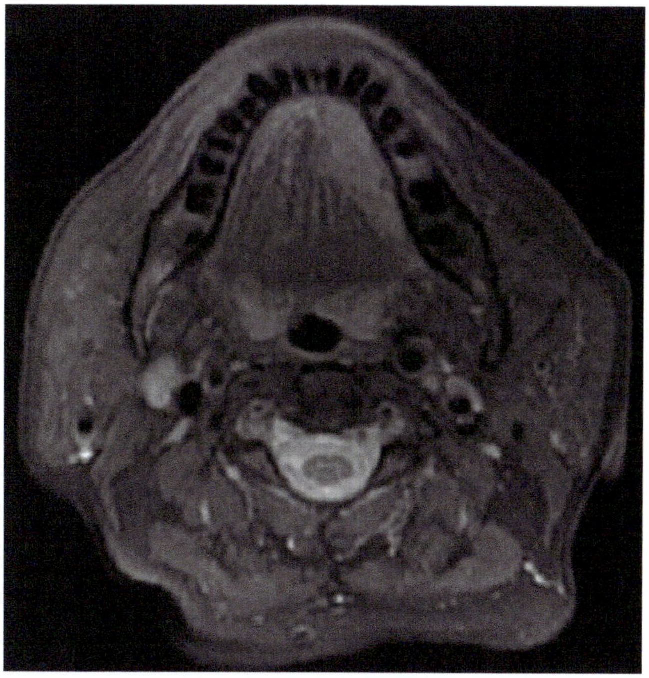

Fig. 82.5 The contrast-enhanced T1-weighted MRI images depicting hyperintensity involving the left lateral tongue with extension till the midline and involving tip of the tongue

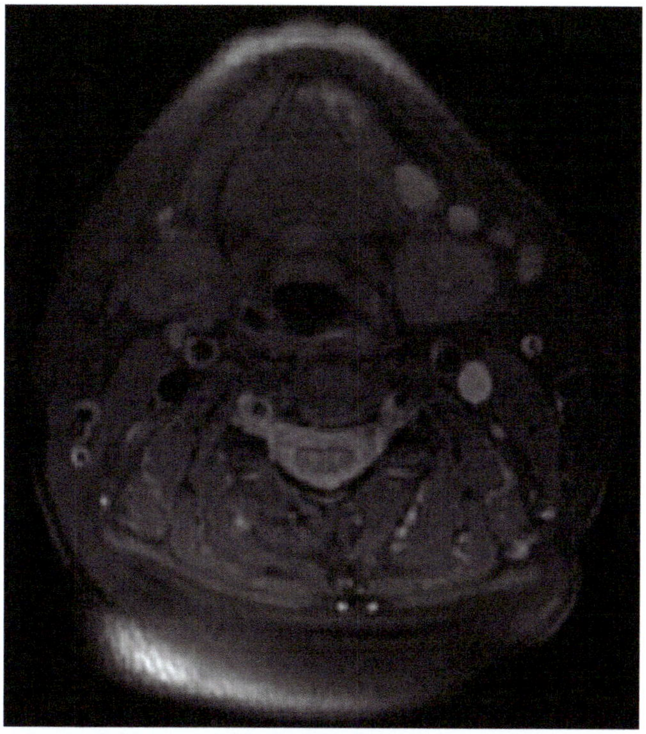

Fig. 82.6 Axial section of an MRI (T2-weighted) showing multiple lymph node metastasis at level IB

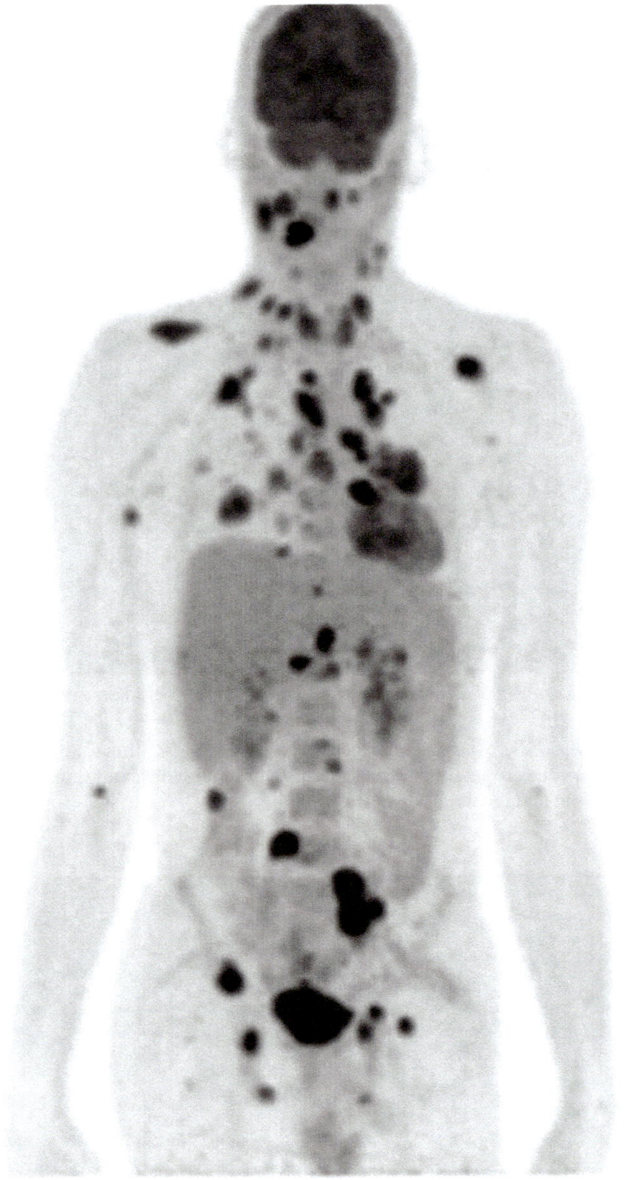

Fig. 82.7 This is the whole body image of PET-CT scan depicting uptake in the multiple areas suggestive of metastatic disease

It is to be noted that any suspicious lesions in PET-CT scan needs to be corroborated with tissue diagnosis (direct or guided) as there are a subset of lesions with false-positive findings; however, PET-CT is considered to have the highest negative predictive value approaching 100%. Although as per the NCCN guidelines, PET-CT has to be advised for all stage III and IV disease, it is usually reserved for patients with recurrent or second primary disease in a resource-constrained setting [5, 6]. Tables 82.2 and 82.3 provide imaging considerations in oral cavity tumors.

Baseline follow-up imaging is usually done after 3 months, and CECT has established its role in ruling out recurrence/residual disease. To avoid misinterpretation, it is important that the concerned imaging radiologist is familiarized with postoperative sequelae of tissue changes or changes that occur following radiotherapy such as nonspecific tissue thickening, edema, or fibrosis and various bony and soft tissue reconstruction methods to facilitate interpretation.

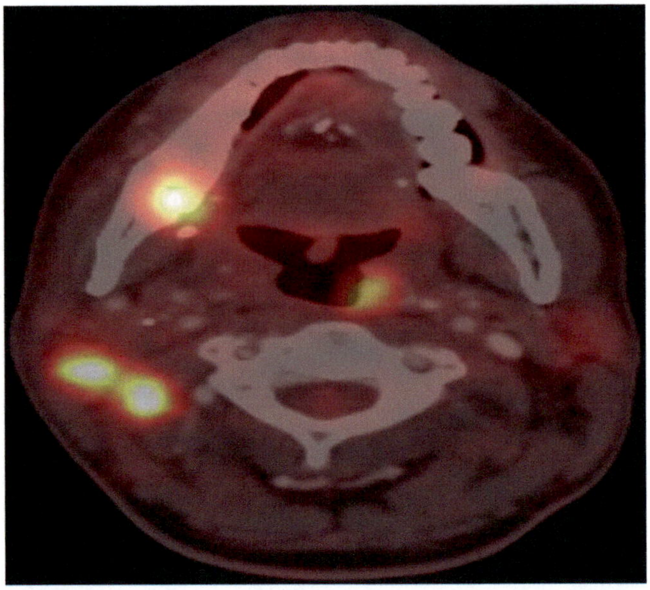

Fig. 82.8 FDG PET-CT images to show FDG avid lesion in the right lower alveolus and ipsilateral level II lymph nodes along with uptake in the right nasopharynx. All the lesion have a similar standard uptake value (SUV) of 15 corresponding to the metabolic activity

Staging the disease is developed to provide ease of communication and helps in understanding the prognosis and planning the treatment. AJCC staging system has been followed for years and provides concise information on size characteristics and extent of primary tumor and involvement of lymph nodes. The recent eighth edition has features like tumor thickness, depth of invasion, and extranodal extension (clinical and pathological).

82.3 Category for Oral Cavity Cancer, Eighth Edition Staging Manual

Table 82.4 provides the categorization for oral cavity cancer [6].

82.4 Principles of Surgical Management

In majority of oral cavity squamous cell cancers, surgery has been the mainstay of treatment, and hence, the need to know intricate surgical aspects has to be emphasized. As there has been improved understanding of disease pattern, biologic behavior of the disease at the molecular level, and the poten-

Table 82.2 Imaging in oral cavity tumors

Radiological means	Indications	Advantages/ Challenges
Computed tomography (CT)	Mainstay for imaging primary disease.	• Bone details. • Obscured to dental artifacts. • Early perineural spread can be missed [7].
Magnetic resonance imaging (MRI)	• Assessment of primarily oral tongue, floor of mouth, and hard palate lesions or bone marrow involvement along with assessment of nasopharyngeal, parotid, sinonasal tumors. • Useful in providing information on encasement of carotid arteries. • Promising results in early detection of perineural extension and detection of dural involvement or intracranial extension.	• Better contrast resolution. Superior detection of tumor spread into bone marrow. • Swallowing artifacts [8].
Ultrasonography (USG)	• To identify lymph node metastases. • For assessment of tumor spread in tongue carcinoma, when MR imaging is contraindicated or unavailable [9].	
Positron emission tomography (PET)	• Diagnosis of an unknown primary tumor, assessment of distant metastasis, response to therapy, surveillance/ detection of recurrence. • Limited role in neck node evaluation.	• Better localization of activity to normal vs abnormal structures, better identification of inflammatory lesions [5].

Table 82.3 Imaging considerations for various sites

Neck nodes	USG-guided FNAC—100% specificity [10, 11]
RMT	• To look for bone erosion—Cortical bone or marrow involvement. • To detect spread of lesion along pterygomandibular raphae.
Palate	• To assess invasion of maxillary sinus, palatal bone, and nasal vault. • Depth of invasion dictates extent of resection.
Infratemporal fossa	• Pterygomandibular raphae provides pathway of spread of lesion into ITF. • CT & MRI are useful.
Tongue	• MRI is preferred; surrounding structure involvement will help in deciding the extent of resection [12, 13].
Bone invasion	• MRI is superior for evaluating medullary space of mandible but inadequate for assessing cortical invasion.

Table 82.4 Category for oral cavity cancer, eighth edition staging manual [6]: Definition of primary tumor (T)

T category	T criteria
TX	Primary tumor cannot be assessed
Tis	Carcinoma in situ
T1	Tumor ≤2 cm with depth of invasion (DOI)* ≤ 5 mm
T2	Tumor ≤2 cm with DOI* > 5 mm Or tumor >2 cm and ≤ 4 cm with DOI* ≤ 10 mm
T3	Tumor >2 cm and ≤ 4 cm with DOI* > 10 mm Or tumor >4 cm with DOI* ≤ 10 mm
T4	Moderately advanced or very advanced local disease
T4a	Moderately advanced local disease Tumor >4 cm with DOI* > 10 mm Or tumor invades adjacent structures only (e.g., through cortical bone of the mandible or maxilla or involves the maxillary sinus or skin of the face) Note: Superficial erosion of bone/tooth socket (alone) by a gingival primary is not sufficient to classify a tumor as T4
T4b	Very advanced local disease Tumor invades masticator space, pterygoid plates, or skull base and/or encases the internal carotid artery

*DOI is depth of invasion and not tumor thickness

T suffix	Definition
(m)	Select if synchronous primary tumors are found in single organ

Definition of regional lymph node (N) clinical N (cN)

cN	Category cN criteria
NX	Regional lymph nodes cannot be assessed
N0	No regional lymph node metastasis
N1	Metastasis in a single ipsilateral lymph node, 3 cm or smaller in greatest dimension ENE(−)
N2	Metastasis in a single ipsilateral node larger than 3 cm but not larger than 6 cm in greatest dimension and ENE(−) Or metastases in multiple ipsilateral lymph nodes, none larger than 6 cm in greatest dimension and ENE(−) Or in bilateral or contralateral lymph nodes, none larger than 6 cm in greatest dimension, and ENE(−)
N2a	Metastasis in a single ipsilateral node larger than 3 cm but not larger than 6 cm in greatest dimension, and ENE(−)
N2b	Metastases in multiple ipsilateral nodes, none larger than 6 cm in greatest dimension, and ENE(−)
N2c	Metastases in bilateral or contralateral lymph nodes, none larger than 6 cm in greatest dimension, and ENE(−)
N3	Metastasis in a lymph node larger than 6 cm in greatest dimension and ENE(−); Or metastasis in any node(s) and clinically overt ENE(+)
N3a	Metastasis in a lymph node larger than 6 cm in greatest dimension and ENE(−)
N3b	Metastasis in any node(s) and clinically overt ENE(+)

Note: A designation of "U" or "L" may be used for any N category to indicate metastasis above the lower border of the cricoid (U) or below the lower border of the cricoid (L). Similarly, clinical and pathological ENE should be recorded as ENE(−) or ENE(+)

N suffix	Definition
(sn)	Select if regional lymph node metastasis identified by SLN biopsy only
(f)	Select if regional lymph node metastasis identified by FNA or core needle biopsy only
U	Metastasis above the lower border of the cricoid

(continued)

Table 82.4 (continued)

N suffix	Definition
L	Metastasis below the lower border of the cricoid
Pathological N (pN)	
pN category	pN criteria
NX	Regional lymph nodes cannot be assessed
N0	No regional lymph node metastasis
N1	Metastasis in a single ipsilateral lymph node, 3 cm or smaller in greatest dimension and ENE(−)
N2	Metastasis in a single ipsilateral lymph node, 3 cm or smaller in greatest dimension and ENE(+) Or larger than 3 cm but not larger than 6 cm in greatest dimension and ENE(−); Or metastases in multiple ipsilateral lymph nodes, none larger than 6 cm in greatest dimension and ENE(−) Or in bilateral or contralateral lymph node(s), none larger than 6 cm in greatest dimension, ENE(−)
N2a	Metastasis in single ipsilateral node 3 cm or smaller in greatest dimension and ENE(+) Or a single ipsilateral node larger than 3 cm but not larger than 6 cm in greatest dimension and ENE(−)
N2b	Metastases in multiple ipsilateral nodes, none larger than 6 cm in greatest dimension and ENE(−)
N2c	Metastases in bilateral or contralateral lymph node(s), none larger than 6 cm in greatest dimension and ENE(−)
N3	Metastasis in a lymph node larger than 6 cm in greatest dimension and ENE(−); Or metastasis in a single ipsilateral node larger than 3 cm in greatest dimension and ENE(+) Or multiple ipsilateral, contralateral, or bilateral nodes, any with ENE(+); Or a single contralateral node of any size and ENE(+)
N3a	Metastasis in a lymph node larger than 6 cm in greatest dimension and ENE(−)
N3b	Metastasis in a single ipsilateral node larger than 3 cm in greatest dimension and ENE(+) Or multiple ipsilateral, contralateral or bilateral nodes any with ENE(+); Or a single contralateral node of any size and ENE(+)
Note: A designation of "U" or "L" may be used for any N category to indicate metastasis above the lower border of the cricoid (U) or below the lower border of the cricoid (L). Similarly, clinical and pathological ENE should be recorded as ENE(−) or ENE(+)	
N suffix	Definition
(sn)	Select if regional lymph node metastasis identified by SLN biopsy only
(f)	Select if regional lymph node metastasis identified by FNA or core needle biopsy only
U	Metastasis above the lower border of the cricoid
L	Metastasis below the lower border of the cricoid

Definition of distant metastasis (M)	
M category	M criteria
cM0	No distant metastasis
cM1	Distant metastasis
pM1	Distant metastasis, microscopically confirmed

tial aggressive nature, the need has arisen for several technical modifications in this era. Hence as surgeons, we have to evolve and adapt to the required changes to improve outcomes of ablative surgery (oncological and functional) in patients with squamous cell carcinoma of oral cavity.

For early-stage oral cavity cancers, especially tongue, it has been proven that both surgery and radiotherapy/brachytherapy offer similar outcome (single modality). For advanced lesions with extensive disease, multimodality treatment is required; surgery being the primary modality and followed by adjuvant radiotherapy +/− chemotherapy (depending on the histopathological evaluation) has been the standard of care.

82.5 Treatment Decision Algorithm [14]

Critical decisions which have to be made are as follows:

1. Intent of treatment—curative vs. palliative treatment.
2. Primary modality—surgical vs. non-surgical treatment.
3. Need for addressing neck in clinically node-negative patients.
4. Type of neck dissection in patients with metastatic lymph nodes.
5. Need for adjuvant treatment.
6. Type of adjuvant treatment.
7. Best supportive care.

Decision 1 Primary intent of treatment: This is the first and most critical decision-making point. All patients other than those with technically unresectable tumors, distant metastasis, poor performance status, and major comorbidities precluding surgery must be considered for treatment with curative intent. However, it is to be noted that surgical excision with positive margins portends poor prognosis. Palliative care is usually when patient has distant metastasis and given only to relieve symptoms and control spread. This is in the form of chemotherapy, radiotherapy or metronomics.

Decision 2 Curative modality of treatment: The primary treatment for patients with oral cavity cancers is surgery. However, in selected scenarios, non-surgical treatment may be considered. This includes primary radiotherapy for tumors of the commissure of mouth and lip tumors where surgery can cause significant esthetic and functional disability. In addition, significant comorbidities that preclude long anesthesia may necessitate the need for primary radiotherapy or chemoradiotherapy. However primary chemoradiotherapy has very limited role in treatment of oral cancers.

Decision 3 Management of neck in N0 stage: Even with no radiographic evidence of significant suspicious lymph-nodes, rate of occult metastasis reaches up to as high as 30% [15]. Presence of lymph node metastasis and the number of lymph nodes involved have a direct relation with the prognosis of the disease; decreasing the overall survival rate by 50%. Moreover, a significant subset of metastatic nodes of less than 1 cm can have extranodal extension [16]. This further worsens the prognosis. There is now level I evidence from a randomized control trial, that addressing the neck surgically irrespective of the lymph node status improves overall survival to about 84% when compared to 69% in patients who were selected for wait-and-watch policy [17]. Therefore, almost all the patients with oral cavity cancer should undergo elective neck dissection. A subset analysis of the same study did not show benefit for primary tumors of depth less than 3 mm. This may be considered in selected patients with cancers of lower nodal metastatic prevalence such as lip and buccal mucosa.

Decision 4 Extent of neck dissection in N+ve oral squamous cell carcinoma: Conventional teaching is that any patients with N+ve neck should undergo modified radical neck dissection covering levels 1–5. This has been questioned by several observational studies. Large cohort of patients who have undergone radical neck dissection for N+ve disease has showed less than 3% incidence of level V nodes [17]. This also was observed only when there were pathologically positive level IV nodes [18]. There are reports of oncologic safety for clearing level I–III lymph nodes for alveolus and buccal mucosal cancers and to clear level IV in addition to levels I, II, and III lymph nodes in patients with oral tongue cancers as they bore high risk of skip metastasis [19]. It is to be noted that when a patient is found to have pathological nodal metastasis, in general, it is recommended for adjuvant radiation that covers all levels of the neck with additional boost in the levels which are positive for metastasis.

Decision 5 Indication for adjuvant radiotherapy: Any patients with more than one of the high risk features should be considered for adjuvant radiotherapy.

This includes (1) nodal metastasis without extracapsular extension, (2) perineural invasion, (3) lymphovascular invasion, (4) poor differentiation, (5) close margin (1–5 mm), and (6) depth of invasion over 1 cm.

But the absolute indication for radiotherapy is stage III and IV disease.

Decision 6 Indication for adjuvant chemoradiotherapy: Meta-analysis of two randomized trials has suggested that in patients with positive surgical margin (<1 mm) and neck nodes with extranodal extension would benefit from adjuvant chemoradiotherapy.

Decision 7 Best supportive care options: This is an important and critical decision. Once the decision for treatment with palliative intent is arrived at, the goal should be made clear with the treating team of doctors and the patient/patient attenders. Ambiguity at this stage may result in loss of trust between the treating team and the patient, causing delay in treatment and possible increase in morbidity. Although this decision is made in the multidisciplinary tumor board, it requires series of meetings with the family to convey the treatment goals. It is also essential to appreciate by treatment group that lack of active treatment does not mean stoppage of care, which needs to be provided by the same team till the end. The quality of death is equally important as quality of life.

The role of best supportive care is to palliate the symptoms the patients may have. In this situation, it is essential to balance the morbidity of treatment versus potential benefit the patient may receive. Often one may have ethical dilemma when faced with young patients with locoregionally advanced tumors. In this situation, temptation of surgery should be tempered. One should consider surgery as palliation to alleviate fungating ulcers or to close a cutaneous fistula. The goal of this surgery must be made very clear to the family. It is essential not to give false hope to the family, which will have deleterious consequence in the patient-physician relationship. In patients with good performance status, especially those who have not received previous radiotherapy, one may consider chemoradiotherapy with curative dose, with the goal to obtain durable palliation. In doubtful situations, induction chemotherapy followed by chemoradiotherapy could also be considered. Local radiation or re-radiation to a limited field may be considered for fungating ulcers. The dose, fractionation, and volume of radiation field need to be tailored for palliative purpose.

In patients with advanced metastatic disease, one needs to be very selective in recommending systemic therapy as the benefit is doubtful. Chemotherapy with targeted anti-EGFr treatment has shown improved survival up to 4 months, with significant morbidity associated with the regimen [20]. An alternate approach is chemotherapy at metronomic dosing regimen, especially the use of methotrexate and celecoxib [21]. Recent evidence of nivolumab, a checkpoint inhibitor, showing improved survival of about 3 months, and acceptable morbidity, is to be considered. However the cost of the treatment is a major deterrent for its wider application. Table 82.5 provides the indications for adjuvant RT and adjuvant CT + RT.

Table 82.5 Indications for adjuvant RT and adjuvant CT + RT

Indications for adjuvant RT		Indications for adjuvant CT + RT
Tumor factors	Nodal factors	
• Perineural invasion. • Lymphovascular invasion +pT3/T4 primary tumor.	• Multiple positive nodes (without ECE). • Positive level IV/V nodes.	• Extra-capsular nodal spread. • Positive margins.
• Bernier J et al. [22]		

82.6 Indications for Adjuvant RT and Adjuvant CT + RT

After various comparative studies, it has been concluded that in adjuvant setting, postoperative IMRT has to be given at dose of 60 Gy in 30 fractions to surgical bed and first echelon nodal stations and the high-risk regions receive a total dose of 66 Gy. It has to be remembered that for salvage surgery cases, concept of re-irradiation should be explained to the patient. A minimum of 12-month duration gap is required prior to re-irradiation to allow for the spinal cord recovery.

In cases with postoperative histopathological features like extranodal extension or positive surgical margins, patients are treated with concurrent chemoradiation (usually 100 mg/m^2 of cisplatin for a maximum of 6 cycles in India). Indication of chemotherapy as described is usually in adjuvant setting in oral cavity cancers.

However role of chemotherapy as induction therapy is evolving. Chemotherapy usually exerts its cytotoxic effects systemically and hence associated with side effects. The major drawbacks of chemotherapeutic agents used commonly are the adverse toxicities and cellular resistance. In an induction setting, most commonly taxanes, platinum, and 5FU are used as 3 cycle regimen (also refer Chap. 84 of this book on Adjunctive therapy in Oral Cancer).

Tumors of oral cavity which are considered technically unresectable are as follows:

- Erosion of skull base, sphenoid bone, and widening of foramen ovale.
- Encasement of internal carotid artery, >270 degree.
- Involvement of mediastinal structures.
- Involvement of prevertebral fascia or cervical vertebrae.

These are considered unresectable not due to surgical technicality but because of the inability to get negative margins and to achieve R0 resection. However, with the superior skills such as endoscopic-assisted surgeries which are associated with less morbidity, and better adjuvant treatment including chemotherapy, an attempt has been made to consider resection of tumors involving muscles of mastication and pterygoid plates especially with the anterior infratemporal fossa involved. Recent studies have shown that surgical resection of these tumors along with adjuvant treatment has shown survival benefit. Also studies from Tata Memorial Hospital, India have shown better outcome in patients who have undergone surgical resection following neoadjuvant chemotherapy.

82.7 Principles of Ablative Surgery

1. Adequate access to the tumor.
2. To achieve negative surgical margins.
3. Utilization of intraoperative frozen section for margin assessment.
4. Wide excision versus compartment resection.

The surgical approaches for tumors of oral cavity depends primarily on the site of tumor (anterior versus posterior), its size, and its proximity to bone (maxilla or mandible). The various approaches frequently used for oral cavity cancers are shown in Figs. 82.9, 82.10, 82.11, 82.12, 82.13, and 82.14 (Also refer Chap. 85 of this book on Access Surgeries and Osteotomies of the Maxillofacial Region).

Types of mandibulotomy is shown in (Figs. 82.15, 82.16a, b) shows marginal mandibulectomy and segmental mandibulectomy.

82.8 Sub-Site-Wise Surgical Management

82.8.1 Tongue and Floor of Mouth

The tongue is a muscular organ which is composed of intrinsic and extrinsic muscles and divided anatomically into the oral tongue (falls in oral cavity cancers) and base of tongue (BOT, sub-site of oropharynx). The tongue is innervated by the hypoglossal nerve, and vascularity is by lingual artery (branch of external carotid artery). Pathway of tumor spread from the oral tongue can be into the floor of mouth, mandible, or/and base of tongue via local extension, the lingual septum being the barrier to tumor spread. For tumors abutting the mandible, marginal mandibulectomy is indicated for negative surgical margin encompassing the tumor and at the same time preserving the mandibular continuity. Segmental mandibulectomy is usually done when there is mandibular erosion or paramandibular spread. Anterior segmental mandibulectomy is more commonly indicated in floor of the mouth cancers.

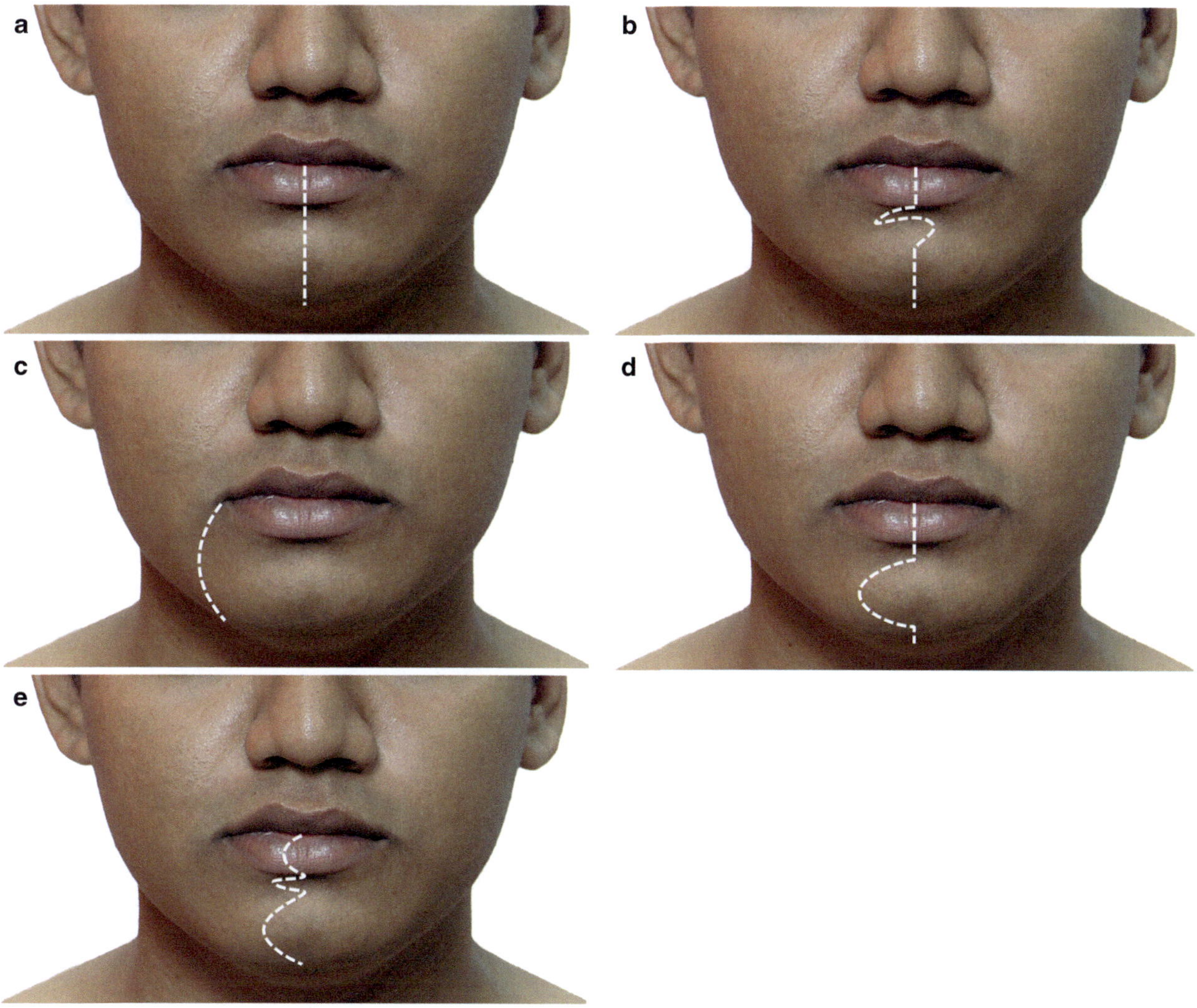

Fig. 82.9 Lip split incisions; (**a**) midline lip split (straight), (**b**) midline lip split with Z-plasty; (**c**) angle/commissure lip split; (**d**) straight midline with chin contour; (**e**) straight midline with chin contour and Z-plasty at vermilion and submental region

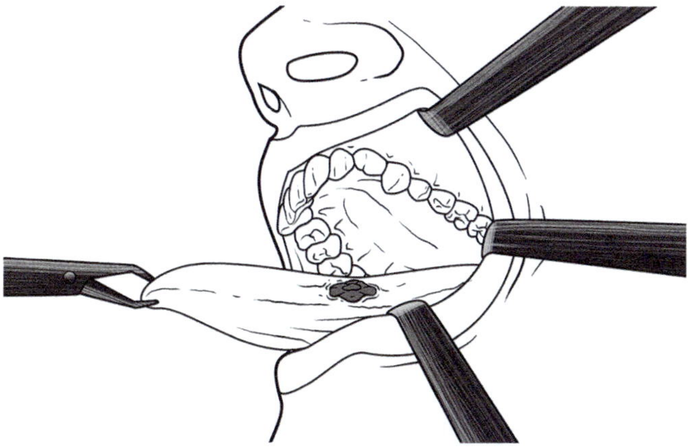

Fig. 82.10 Pictorial representation of excision of lesionally per-orally. This is usually indicated for T1–2 lesion in patients with adequate mouth opening

Lingual artery is an end artery, and hence clinicians have to be careful in resections involving more than two-thirds of tongue mass as this may jeopardize the vascularity and utmost care to be taken to preserve the neurovascular bundle.

There is a recent concept of compartment resection in patients with infiltrative disease where the adjacent extrinsic musculature and neurovascular bundle is excised in continuity to ensure negative margins. This was proposed by Calabrese [23], and all cases underwent access mandibulotomy; hence it is not commonly followed. Tumors of floor of the mouth are usually infiltrative and lymph node metastasis is seen bilaterally. According to Byers, the rate of lymph node skip metastasis at level IV is observed in about 10–15% cases. According to the study by Kowalski [24], tumors of floor of the mouth, tongue cancers crossing the midline, and advanced stage of the disease have a propensity of developing contralateral lymph node metastasis.

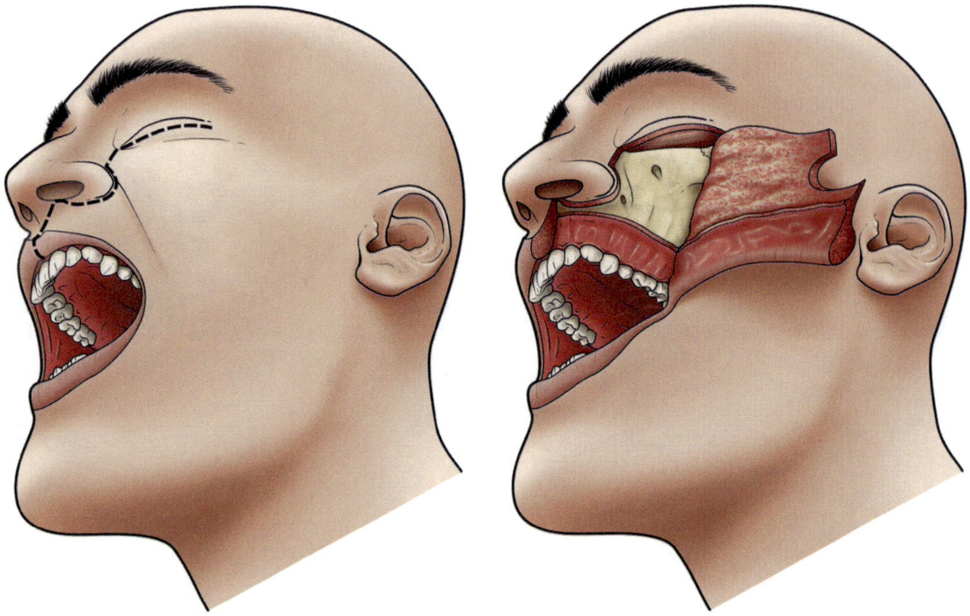

Fig. 82.11 Weber-Ferguson incision for tumors of maxilla not amenable to per-oral excision and not requiring infratemporal fossa access. The upper cheek flap is raised as shown

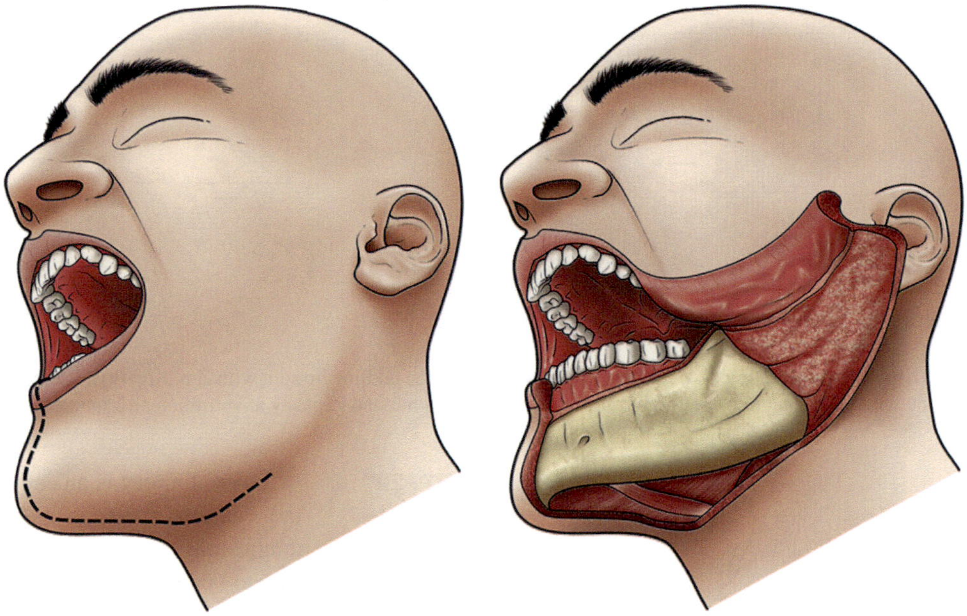

Fig. 82.12 A lower midline lip split incision continued and transverse neck skin crease incision followed by raising of a lower cheek flap. This gives the best access to infra-temporal fossa. The periosteum to be left on the mandible to preserve its periosteal blood supply. The mental neurovascular bundle has to be sacrificed

82.8.1.1 Surgery

Wide local excision (WLE)/adequate glossectomy procedure with adequate surgical margins has been the procedure of choice for early tongue cancers, and this is amenable with per-oral approach. Before planning resection, thorough knowledge about the extent of lesion is important, and palpation of induration provides a guide for the same. Ideal margin for resection of tumour is all 1–1.5 cm all around. Usually it is the deep soft tissue margin which is prone for being close or positive, and this can be avoided by palpation method. In many institutions, it is a useful practice to ligate the lingual artery in the neck before performing WLE for

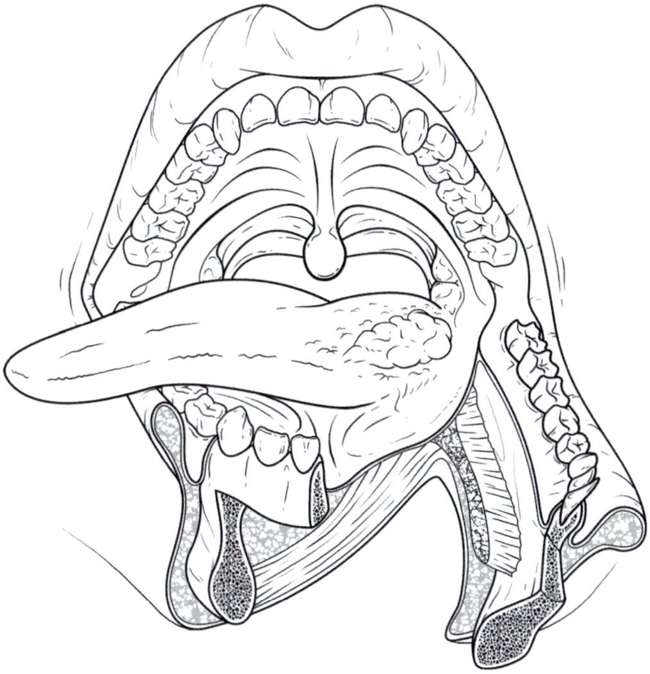

Fig. 82.13 This picture depicts access mandibulotomies for tumors situated in the posterior tongue. The other alternative is pull through approach

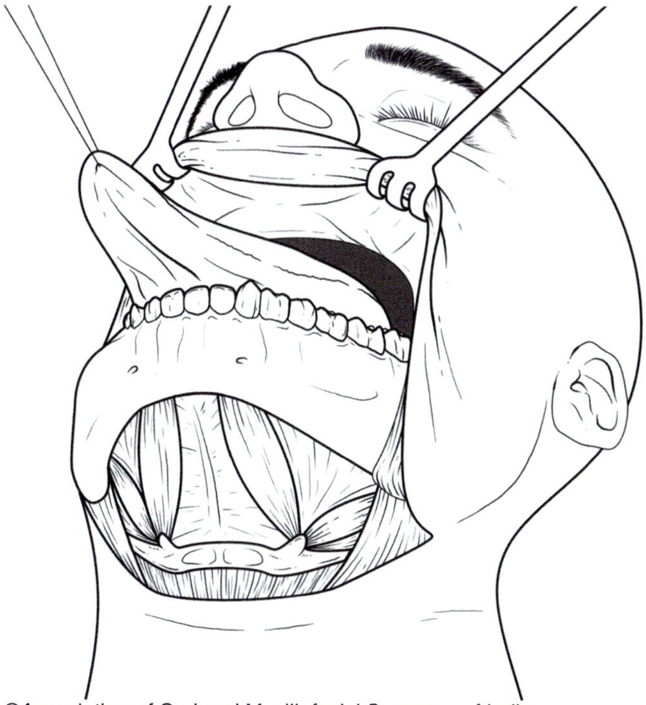

Fig. 82.14 Visor flap provides best access for total and subtotal glossectomy

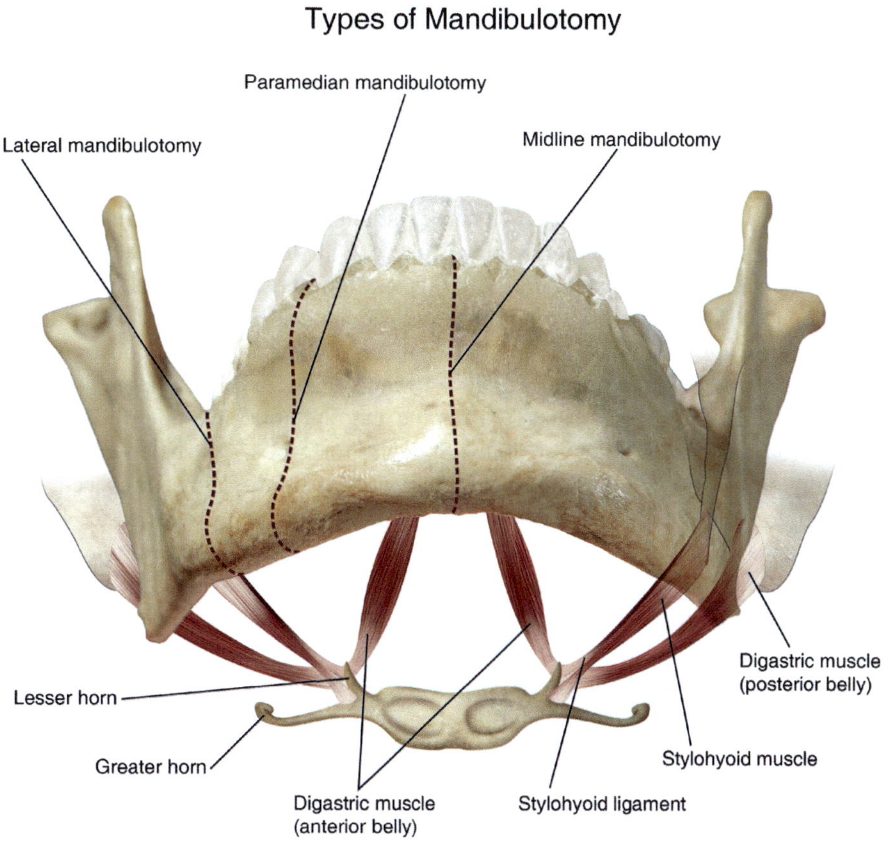

Fig. 82.15 Depiction of various types of access mandibulotomies

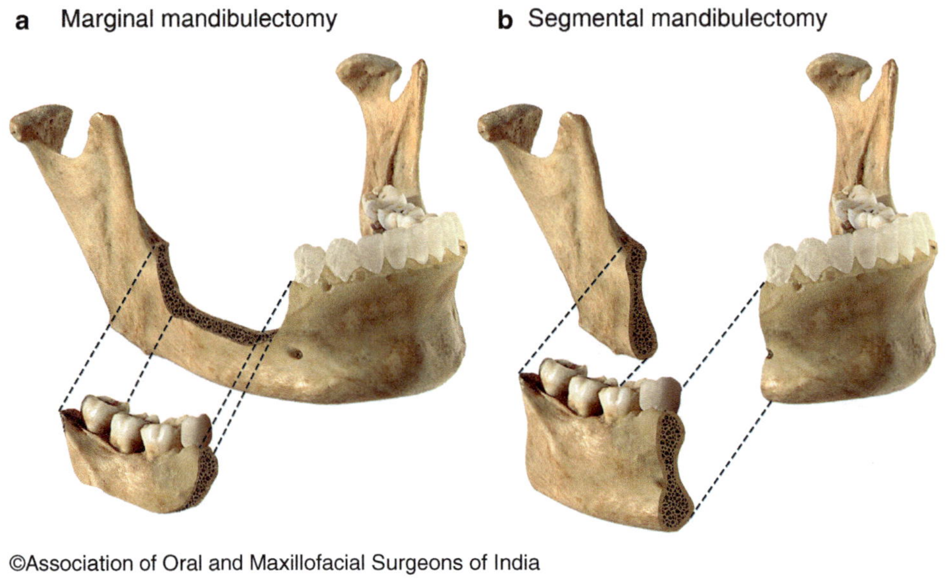

Fig. 82.16 Types of mandibulectomies (**a**) marginal and (**b**) segmental

adequate bleeding control and clean surgical field. The resulting defects of adequate glossectomy for early lesions are usually closed primarily avoiding tethering of the tongue. Excisional biopsy for suspicious lesions is highly discouraged even if the lesion is about 1 cm.

Moderately advanced cancers of the tongue and floor of the mouth (T2–T3) warrant classical hemiglossectomy which sacrifices the tip jeopardizing the tongue mobility resulting in compromised speech and swallowing. Majority of these tumors are excised by combinations of per-oral and pull-through approaches, without the actual need for lip-split or access mandibulotomy. The pull through technique helps in avoiding positive posterior margins as the resection is done under direct vision. All these patients require reconstructive surgery (lining or bulk), along with long-term tracheostomy and feeding tube (ryles tube/PEG) dependence. Free-flap reconstructions have become inevitable following resection of tongue cancers. Locally advanced (T4a) cancers (tumor depth > 20 mm, restricted mobility and hypoglossal palsy) of tongue warrant total glossectomy or near-total glossectomy. Standard total glossectomy procedure involves complete removal of anatomical tongue from mandible to hyoid and from the tip of the tongue upto the vallecula.

The following a is brief outlay of surgical steps: anterior belly of digastric muscle is first divided through the cervical neck incision followed by intra-oral crevicular incision. Then the genioglossus, geniohyoid is divided from the genial tubercle and mylohyoid muscle from the mylohyoid line from the mandible. At the contralateral retromolar region come the division of buccopharyngeal fascia, styloglossus muscle, and the palatoglossus muscle and incision at the vallecula. The same steps are repeated on the other side for total glossectomy. However in near-total/subtotal glossectomy, base of the tongue of uninvolved side is preserved. It is the extent of excision of the base of tongue which determines the postoperative swallowing function.

Tongue and the FOM lesions involving or abutting mandible pose a unique challenge. Resecting the segment of mandible increases morbidity and reconstructive challenge by many times. In such situations an attempt should be made to preserve the mandible whenever possible.

Removal of the level V lymph node is reserved in situations when level IV or V is involved or in N3 nodal disease. According to Kowalski et al., the indications for addressing contralateral lymph nodes are lesions of the tongue crossing the midline, floor of the mouth tumors, and locally advanced T3 and T4 tumors [24].

Reconstruction of the tongue requires a soft tissue flap with large volume to provide the adequate bulk which in turn is believed to aid in swallowing. The drawback of a reconstructed tongue is the impaired mobility resulting in compromised speech. The most commonly used flap is radial forearm free flap and anterolateral thigh free flap. The other uncommon examples for free tissue transfer are lateral arm flap, gracilis flap, and local flap such as FAMM flap and submental flap.

Reconstruction of tongue defect using radial forearm free flap (Figs. 82.17, 82.18, 82.19, 82.20 and 82.21).

Reconstruction of tongue defect with local flap: facial artery myomucosal flap (Figs. 82.22, 82.23, 82.24 and 82.25).

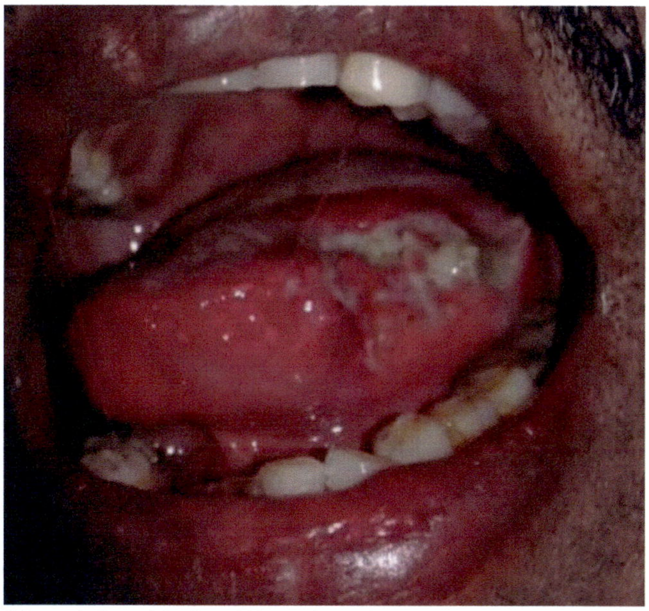

Fig. 82.17 Squamous cell carcinoma of left lateral border of the tongue with induration extending 1 cm short of midline not involving floor of mouth

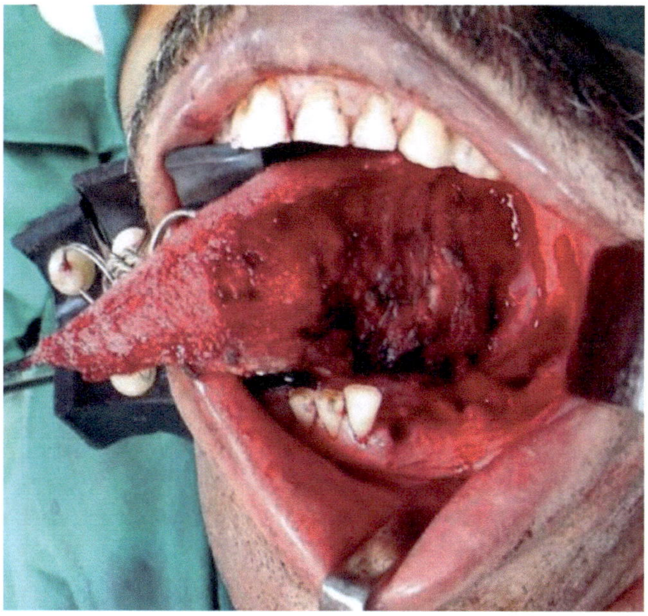

Fig. 82.18 Post-surgical defect following left hemiglossectomy and left marginal mandibulectomy

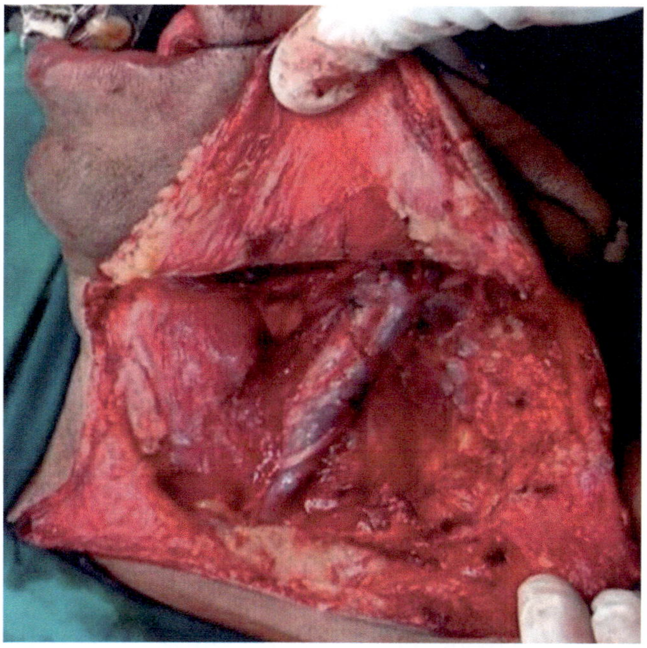

Fig. 82.19 Completed left modified radical neck dissection

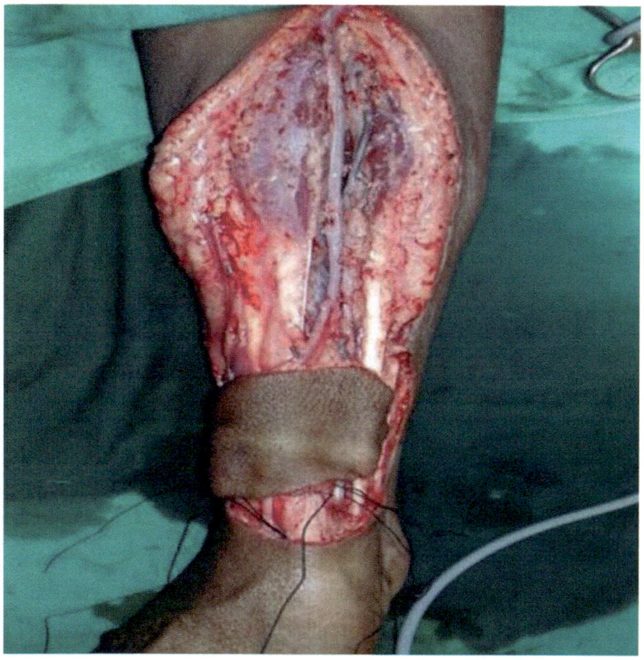

Fig. 82.20 Left radial artery forearm free flap harvested for the defect

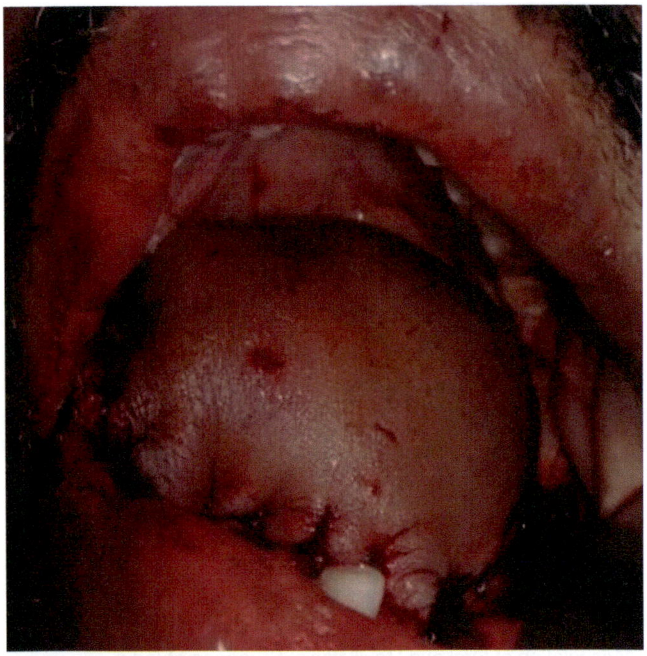

Fig. 82.21 Radial forearm free flap inset into defect and anastomosed to left facial artery and tributory of left internal jugular vein

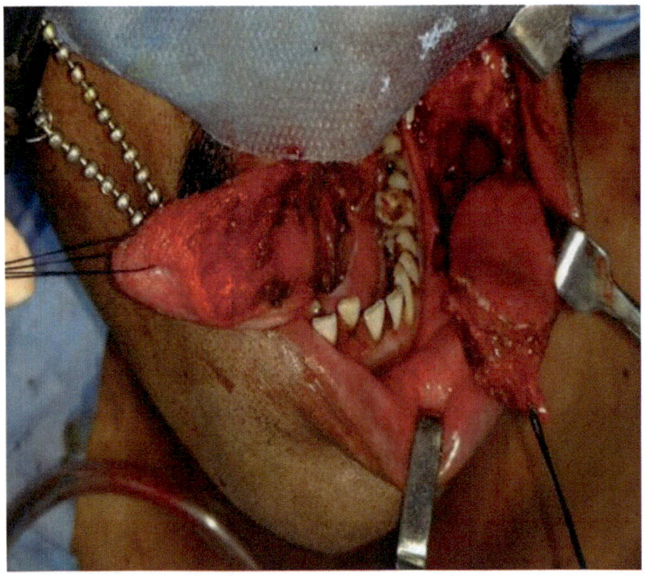

Fig. 82.22 Tongue defect following wide local excision of left lateral border tongue squamous cell carcinoma

82.8.2 Buccal Mucosa

82.8.2.1 T1/T2 Lesions

Surgical Steps: For Early Buccal Cancer Per-oral approach is adequate. It is important to ensure oncologic completeness and appreciate depth. Inadvertent injury to the buccal branch of facial nerve and to the parotid duct should be avoided. Facial artery, facial vein, and parotid duct (if encountered or injured) should be ligated. Mucosal incision around the lesion, with adequate margin, taking the buccinator muscle in specimen forms the deep soft tissue margin. These defects can be reconstructed with split thickness skin grafts/buccal pad of fat/local flaps such as nasolabial flap.

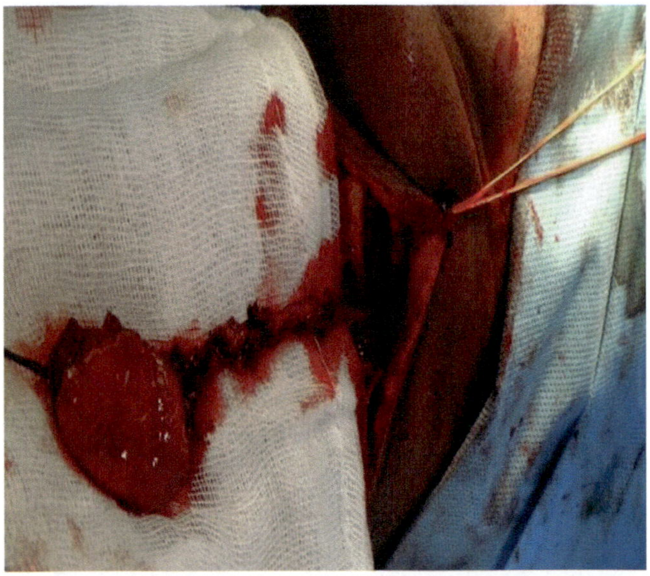

Fig. 82.23 Harvesting of facial artery myomucosal flap (FAMM)

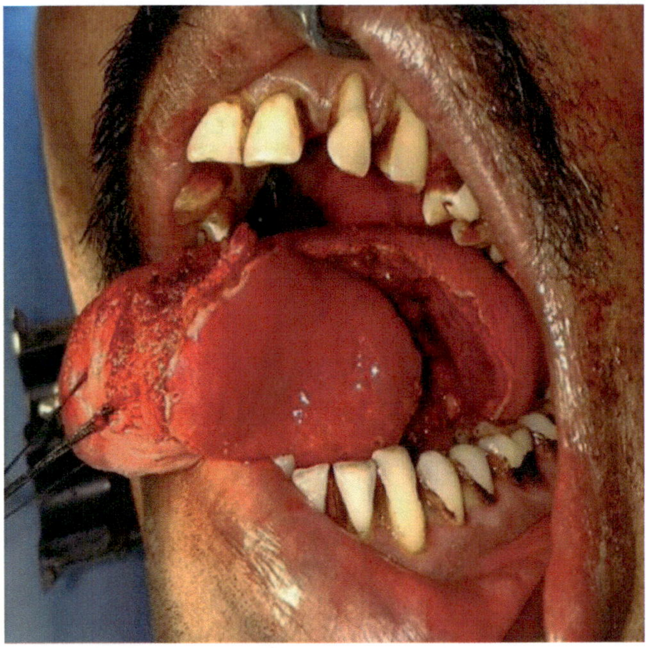

Fig. 82.24 FAMM flap tunneled into the defect and reconstructed

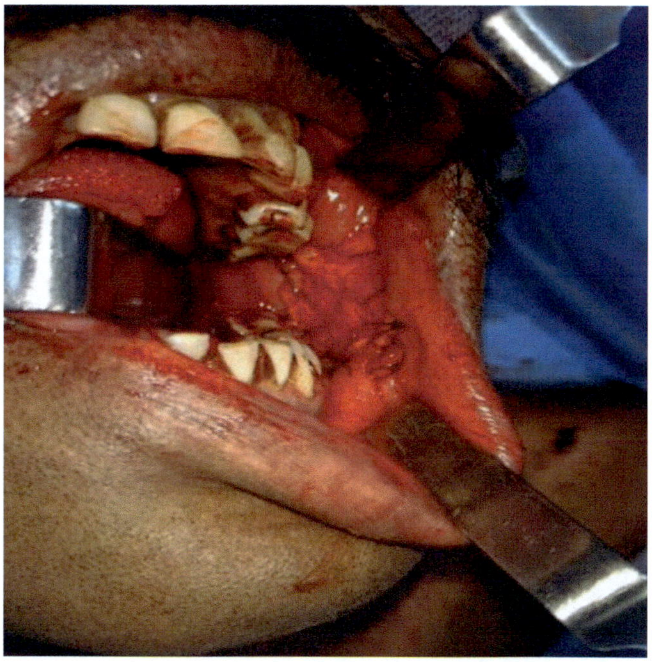

Fig. 82.25 Closure of the donor site

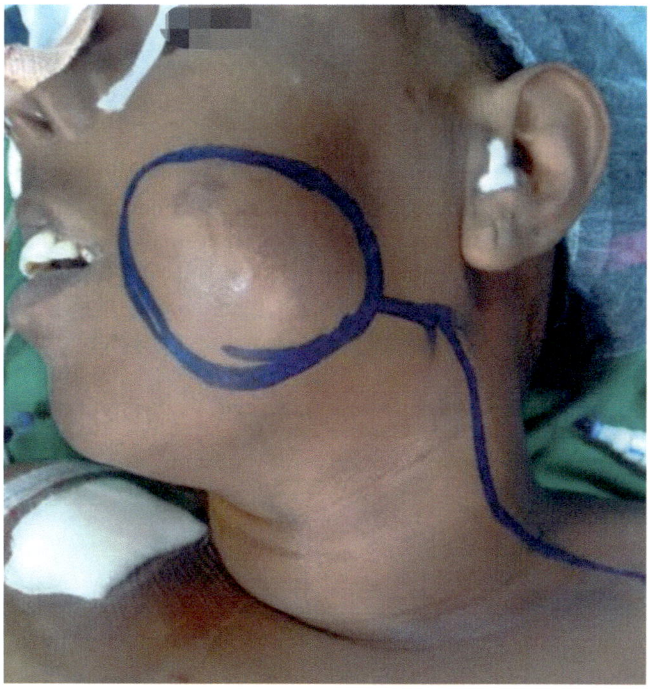

Fig. 82.26 Locally advanced T4a, left buccal mucosa lesion requiring composite resection with excision of the overlying involved skin

Advanced T3/T4 Lesions (Lesions with Skin Involvement/ Bone Involvement/Involvement of Muscles of Mastication) Pre-operative clinical examination revealing a subtle skin puckering and imaging studies shows stranding

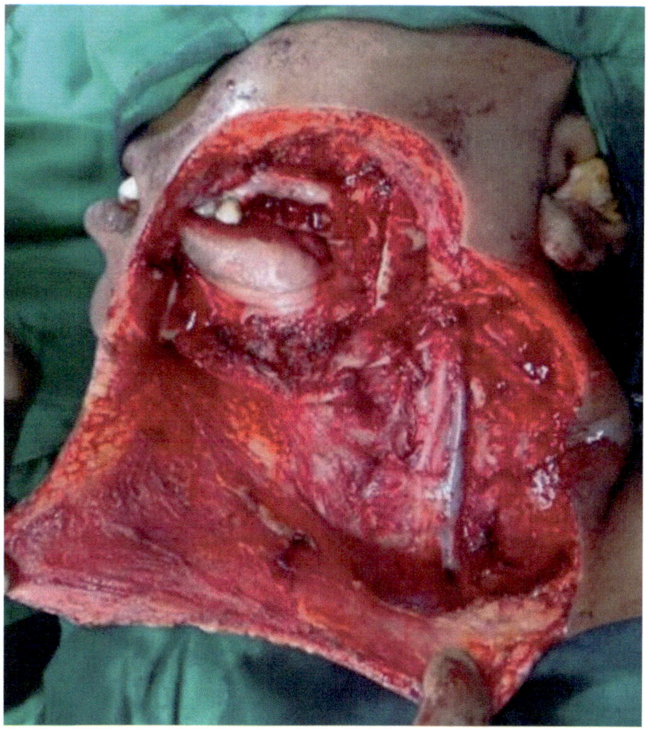

Fig. 82.27 Defect following composite resection and modified radical neck dissection; this defect was reconstructed with anterolateral thigh free flap

of subcutaneous fat that is the early sign of skin involvement. If buccal space involvement is suspected, then buccal fat pad should be included in the specimen.

These advanced lesions require full-thickness cheek resection. The planning of incision may be a midline lip split or angle split, both of which will help in raising a lower cheek flap or when overlying skin is involved, an incision around the skin involved in continuity with the neck dissection incision. The muscle of mastication involvement warrants infratemporal fossa clearance (Figs. 82.26, 82.27 and 82.28).

82.8.3 Gingivobuccal Sulcus

Gingivobuccal sulcus (GBS) tumors are tumors occurring in the upper or lower GBS, usually seen to abut the bone adjacent (Fig. 82.29). These occur almost exclusively in Southeast Asia due to high incidence of chewing tobacco use. Due to the high propensity for local invasion and close proximity of bone, skin, and masticator space, presentation is often advanced, and outcomes are poor. If there is superficial erosion of bone or if the lesion is abutting the mandible, then the resection should include marginal mandibulectomy. Superficial cortical erosion in alveolar tumors is not considered as T4 lesion, and marginal mandibulectomy may still suffice. Although MRI is consid-

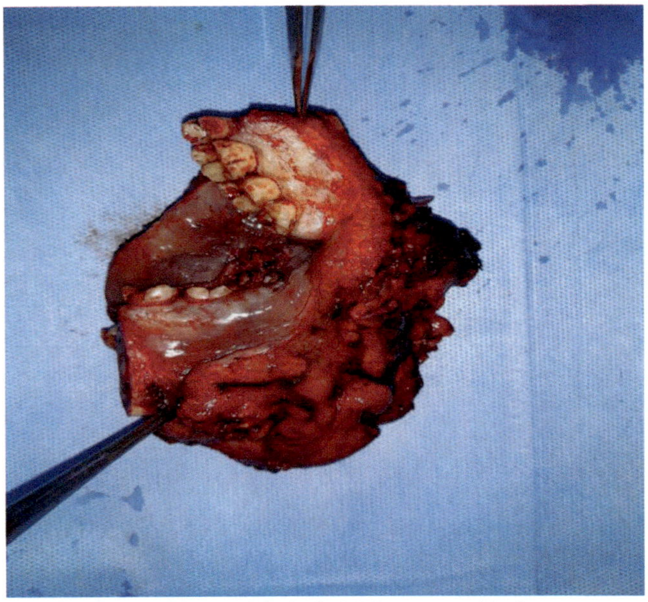

Fig. 82.28 Excised specimen in toto (Same case shown in Figs. 82.26 and 82.27)

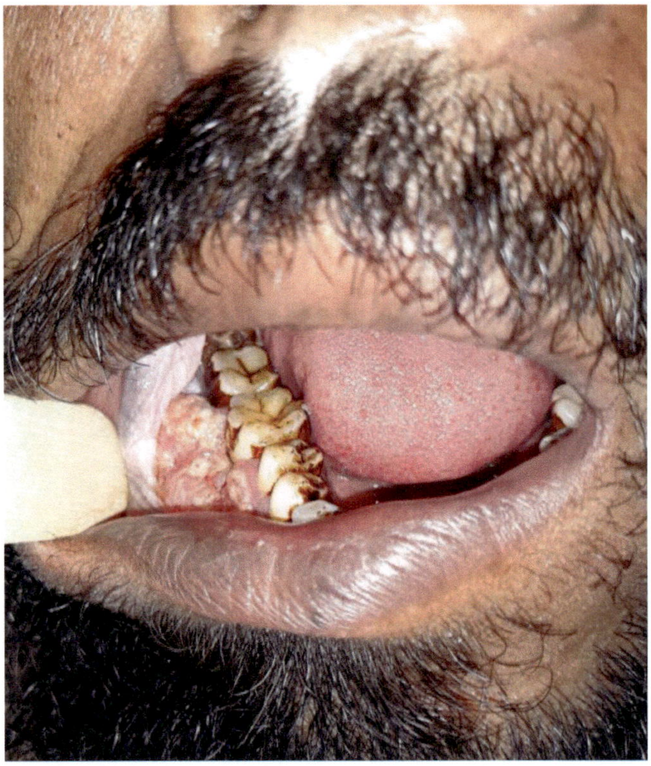

Fig. 82.29 Classic example of a gingivo buccal tumor abutting the adjacent mandible

ered most sensitive imaging modality to determine extent of bony involvement, periosteal stripping is by far the best method to determine extent of bony erosion and helps in decision-making regarding extent of mandibulectomy. GBS tumors usually present at an advanced stage with gross mandibular erosion, paramandibular spread, or overlying skin involvement (skin involvement is never seen in the masseter region as it is a tumor barrier). These findings preclude the use of marginal mandibulectomy, and hence patients often require segmental mandibulectomy and bony reconstruction.

82.8.4 Retromolar Trigone Carcinoma

Retromolar trigone tumors are rare but more aggressive malignancies with poorer outcome. Higher incidence of local recurrence has been reported in squamous cell carcinoma of the retromolar trigone (RMT) and posterior GBS carcinomas. This is attributed to to its higher propensity of infratemporal fossa (ITF) and pterygomandibular fissure involvement. Due to restricted mouth opening at the time of presentation, thorough clinical examination is hindered. For both oncologic and anatomic reasons, tumors with mandibular invasion are best managed surgically by segmental mandibulectomy including coronoid process of the mandible.

> The reason to preserve condyle is as follows: (a) it may be used for secondary reconstruction, and (b) as the condyle lacks medullary bone, it does not act as a pathway of spread and hence can be oncologically safe to preserve it.

As a large proportion of the RMT tumors involve both the upper and lower jaw (Fig. 82.30), excision of ramus of mandible in the form of subsigmoid marginal mandibulectomy with at least an upper alveolectomy and ITF clearance (anterior ITF comprising masseter and medial pterygoid with or without pterygoid plates) is required. Selective neck dissection comprising of level I–V lymph nodes is usually performed electively for all stage cancers for purpose of staging.

82.8.5 Hard Palate

Tumors of the hard palate are less common when compared to tumors of the mandible, tongue, or buccal mucosa and are often of minor salivary gland etiology. Premaxilla provides support for the nose and midface; lesions involving anterior alveolus and hard palate will require bony reconstruction to prevent midface deformity. Lesions of the posterior alveolus and hard palate have a higher tendency to locally invade the orbital floor and skull base or through various neurovascular bundles (greater palatine foramen, sphenopalatine foramen, palatovaginal canal).

Lymph node involvement is very rare for salivary neoplasm of the palate, and neck dissection is reserved only for node-positive disease. However, maxillary alveolar carcinoma has a high propensity for occult lymph node metastasis

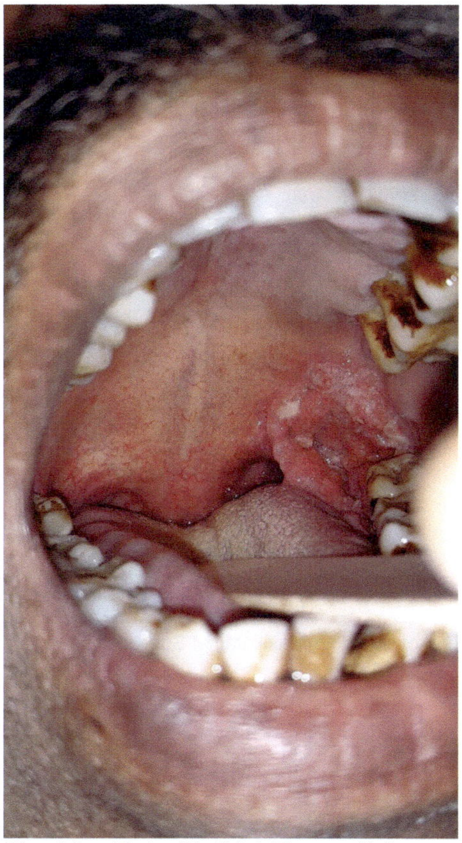

Fig. 82.30 Left retromolar trigone squamous cell carcinoma extending to involve lingual surface of mandible, soft and hard palate ipsilaterally

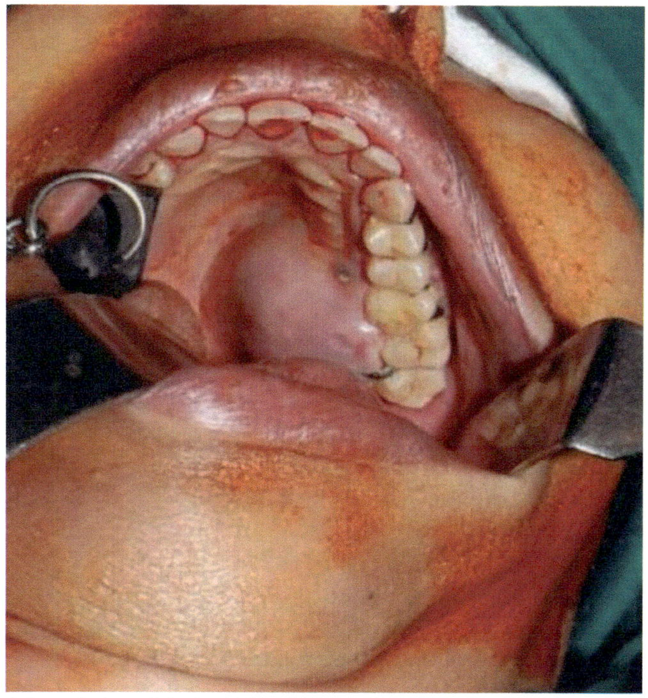

Fig. 82.31 Minor salivary gland tumour of the hard palate

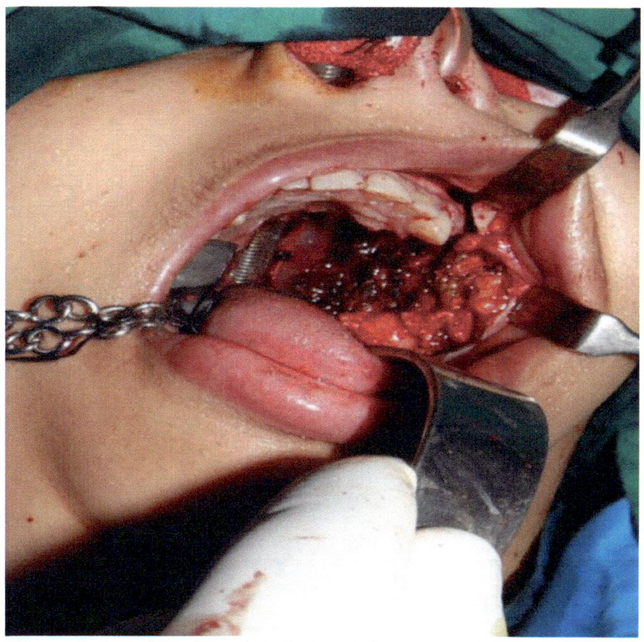

Fig. 82.32 Defect following partial maxillectomy

(15–20%), and also in patients where neck is not addressed, they tend to present with nodal recurrences which are not salvageable in two-thirds of the cases; hence it is wise to consider elective neck dissection. The other point worthwhile and to be noted is that perifacial group of lymph nodes have to be cleared for effective disease control for the upper alveolus (Figs. 82.31, 82.32, 82.33 and 82.34).

82.8.5.1 Brown's Classification System for Maxillary Defects [25] (Fig. 82.35)

Vertical Component

- Class I, maxillectomy with no oroantral fistula.
- Class II, low maxillectomy.
- Class III, high maxillectomy.
- Class IV, radical maxillectomy.

Horizontal Component I, unilateral alveolar maxilla and resection of the hard palate;

(a) resection of less than or equal to half of the alveolar and hard palate, not involving the nasal septum or crossing the midline;

(b) resection of the bilateral alveolar maxilla and hard palate, including a smaller resection that crosses the midline of the alveolar bone, including the nasal septum; and

(c) removal of the entire alveolar maxilla and hard palate.

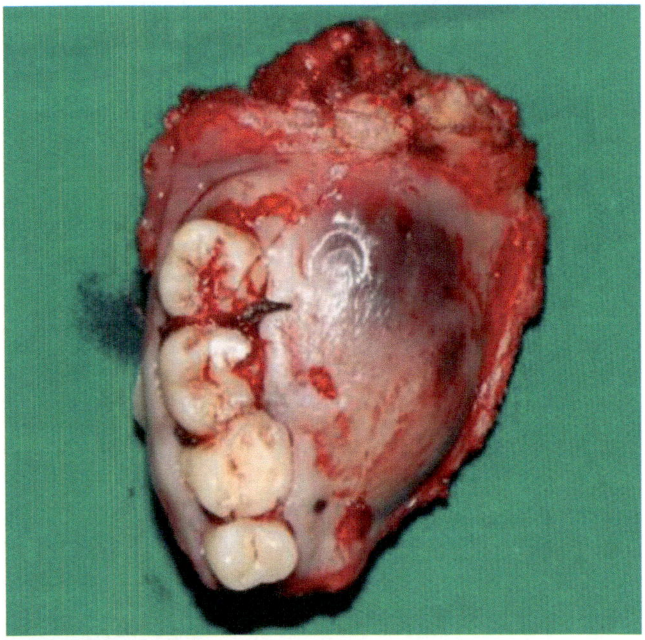

Fig. 82.33 Specimen in toto

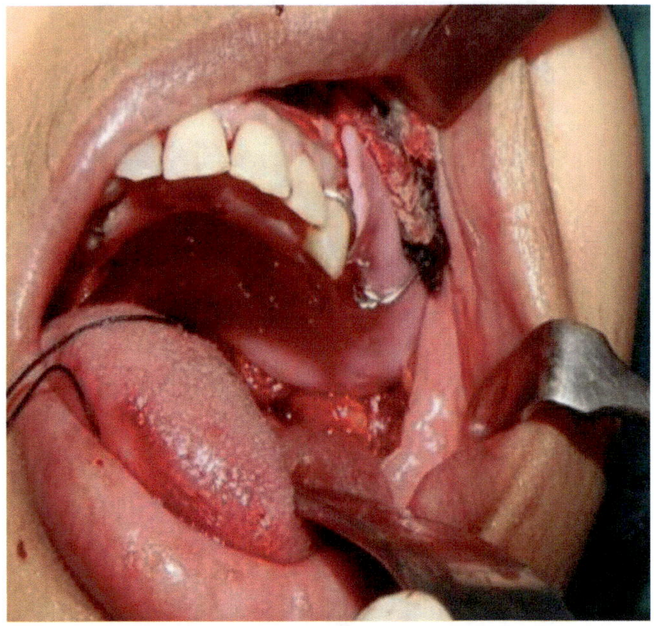

Fig. 82.34 Defect reconstructed with conventional obturator placement

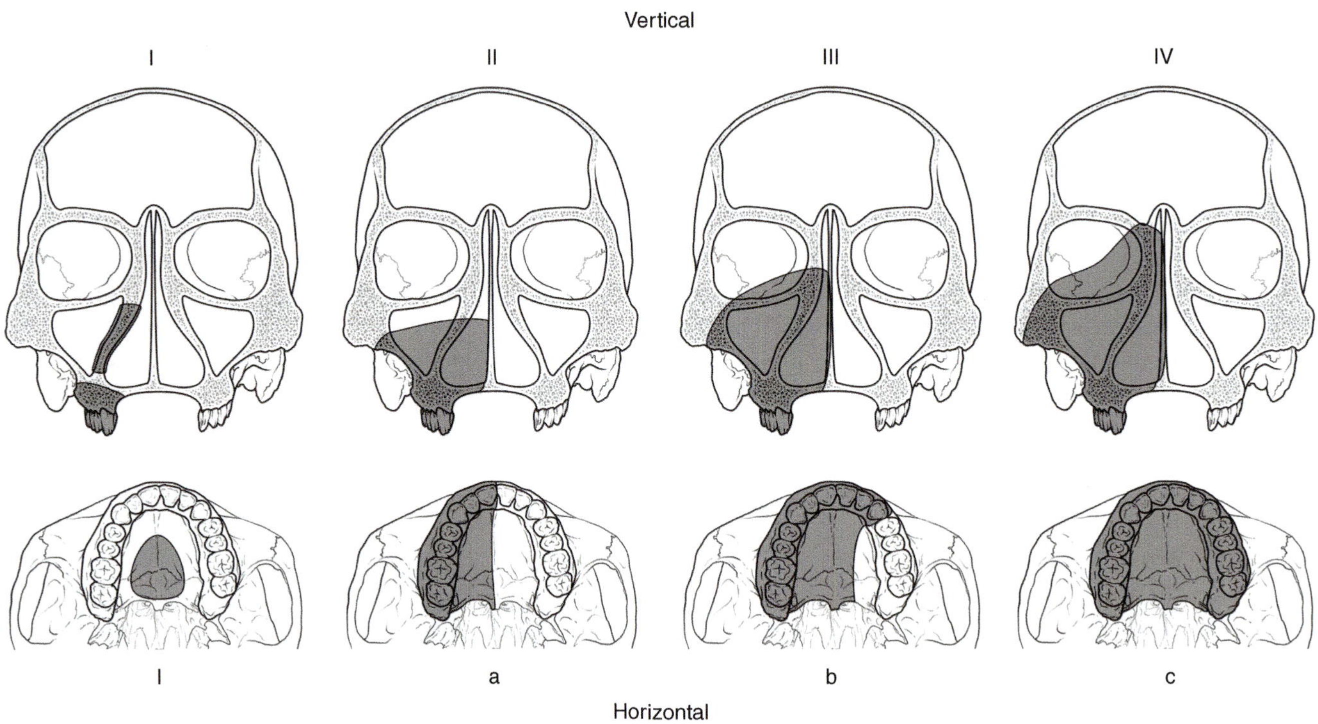

Fig. 82.35 Brown's classification for maxillectomy defects

82.8.6 Lip Carcinoma

Squamous cell carcinoma of the lip is most frequently associated with sun exposure as the risk factor. Lower lip is more commonly involved than the upper lip. Submental and submandibular nodal basins are the primary echelon drainage pathways; regional nodal metastasis occurs in only 10% of patients. Full-thickness excision with up to 1 cm margin is necessary. Lesions that involve less than one-third of the lip are managed with simple wedge excision and primary closure and hence offer acceptable oncologic and reconstructive results. For lesions larger than one-third but less than two-thirds, Abbe-Estlander or

Table 82.6 Treatment modalities of use in oral cancer

T1/T2 N0	Radiotherapy/brachytherapy vs. surgery
T3/T4 N0/ N+	Surgery is mainstay of treatment followed by adjuvant therapy

Karapandzic flap can be utilized (refer Chap. 86 on Soft tissue reconstruction of the Maxillofacial Region). For defects more than two-thirds, free tissue transfer is preferred to achieve better cosmetic result and avoid microstomia and oral incompetence. To ensure oral competence, adjunctive procedures such as fascial sling, palmaris longus sling, or temporalis muscle sling can be used along with the adynamic soft tissue flap.

Table 82.6 describes the treatment modalities of use in oral cancer.

82.8.6.1 Management of the Neck in Oral Cavity

Introduction

Although skip metastasis can occur, lymph node metastasis usually follows a predictable fashion from the first echelon nodes to the second echelon nodes. Tumors of the oral cavity most commonly drain to levels I (submental and submandibular group) and level II (upper jugular group) in the neck. Level IA is between the two anterior belly of digastric muscle, and level IB is between anterior and posterior belly of digastric muscle on either side. The submental triangle drains the anterior portion of the oral cavity and hence can get involved in the tumors of the incisor region, the anterior floor of mouth, or anterior mandibular gingival/alveolar cancers. The level II nodes are found between the level of the hyoid bone inferiorly and anteriorly, the posterior belly of the digastric muscle superiorly, and the posterior border of the sternocleidomastoid muscle (SCM) posteriorly. In the jugular chain, the level III lymph node station is demarcated inferiorly by the omohyoid muscle as it crosses the internal jugular vein (IJV) and contains the mid-jugular lymph nodes particularly the prominent omohyoid node lying in close relationship to the muscle. Level IV (between the omohyoid muscle and the transverse cervical vessels, medially bound by the IJV) and V (between the posterior border of SCM and anterior border of trapezius muscle, further divided into levels A and B by the spinal accessory nerve) nodes are very rarely directly involved by early initial spread of oral SCC. In addition to these classical patterns of spread, buccal cancers may present with parotid nodes, and the posterior maxillary alveolus/hard palate may spread initially to retropharyngeal nodes. Tumors involving/crossing midline and tumors of the floor of the mouth generally require bilateral neck dissection.

82.9 Evaluation and Diagnosis

Evaluation of neck disease for the purpose of staging is best done by USG-guided FNAC, it being both highly sensitive and specific, simple, and cost-effective but observer dependent. Although palpation is most commonly employed, it has a very low accuracy ranging between 50 and 65%. The limitations of palpation method are obese patients or patients with previously treated necks; examination is more difficult. Imaging with CT scan or MR has been said to improve accuracy for metastatic neck disease to approximately 90%. Chaukar et al. found contrast-enhanced CT to give better concordance with histology in the N0 neck than either US or PET/CT.

82.10 Management

Evolution of neck dissection [26, 27]:

- 1906—George Crile described the classic radical neck dissection (RND).
- 1933 and 1941—Blair and Martin popularized the RND.
- 1967—Bocca and Pignataro described the "functional neck dissection" (FND).
- 1975—Bocca established oncologic safety of the FND compared to the RND.

Technique:

- The incision is made through the skin and deepened to divide subcutaneous tissues. Thus exposing the platysma (Thin pink muscle layer) which is incised in a single stroke.
- This is followed by raising of the subplatysmal flaps with the superior limit being the lower border of the mandible; anteriorly it is extends to the midline, posterior border of sternocleidomastoid (SCM) muscle posteriorly, and inferiorly till the clavicle [26].
- Neck dissection can be done either as an antero-posterior fashion or as a postero-anterior approach.
- Firstly the anterior belly of digastric muscle is identified, and mobilization of the fibrofatty tissue begins between the two anterior belly of digastric muscle and hyoid bone.
- In level IB dissection, marginal mandibular nerve is identified and preserved. The next step is to divide the fascia below the submandibular salivary gland, and the gland per se is retracted cephalad. This maneuver exposes the posterior belly of digastric muscle and helps in the identification of the facial artery. It is ligated close to the entry point at the posterior belly of digastric muscle and lower border of mandible. However full length of the facial artery may be preserved in case of full flap reconstruction [27, 28].
- The Sub mandibular gland (SMG), fibrofatty tissue, lymphatics and the prefacial LNs are mobilized off the mylohyoid and hence retracted it anteriorly.
- For the level II–IV lymph node dissection, the fascia over the SCM is raised till the posterior belly of digastric muscle superiorly. Level IIA dissection begins with identification of the Spinal accessory nerve (SAN) and Internal Jugular Vein (IJV) and removal of the LNs, lymphatics, and fibro-

fatty tissue between these structures, the deep limit of dissection being the prepectoral fascia. At any given point on time tractional injury to the SAN has to be avoided.

- This is followed by release of the fascia and tissue along the posterior border of SCM till the clavicle inferiorly; mylohyoid muscle retracted inferiorly and lateral border of IJV identified. Care is taken to preserve deep cervical plexus. Now the level II–IV tissue is retracted anteriorly and peeled off the IJV and continued in the anterior triangle of the neck till the midline, preserved the superior thyroid vessels and tributary of IJV.
- Level IIB is dissected between the posterior belly of digastric and postero-superior to the SAN, posterior limit being SCM.

This completes the selective neck dissection (Figs. 82.36, 82.37, 82.38, 82.39, 82.40, 82.41, 82.42, 82.43, 82.44 and 82.45).

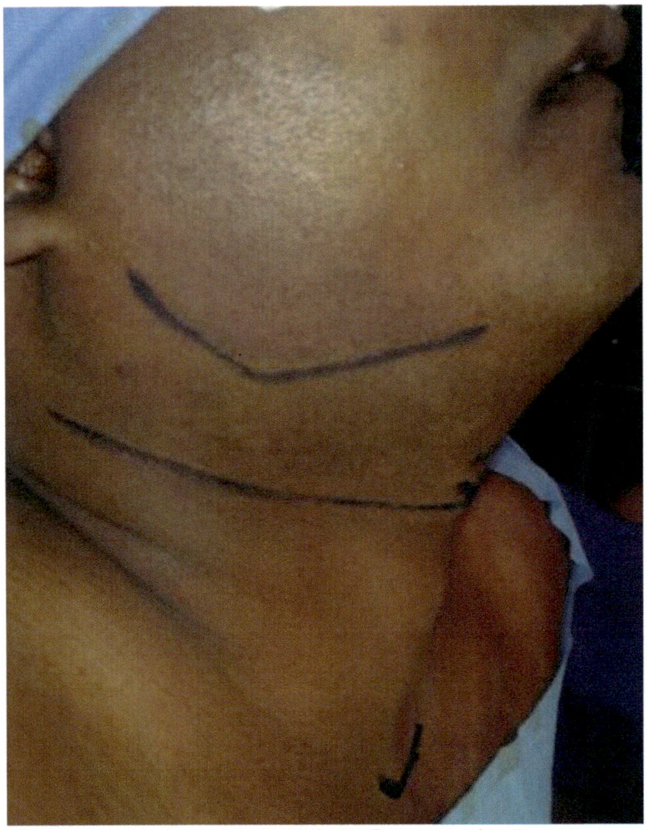

Fig. 82.36 Incision marking for selective neck dissection

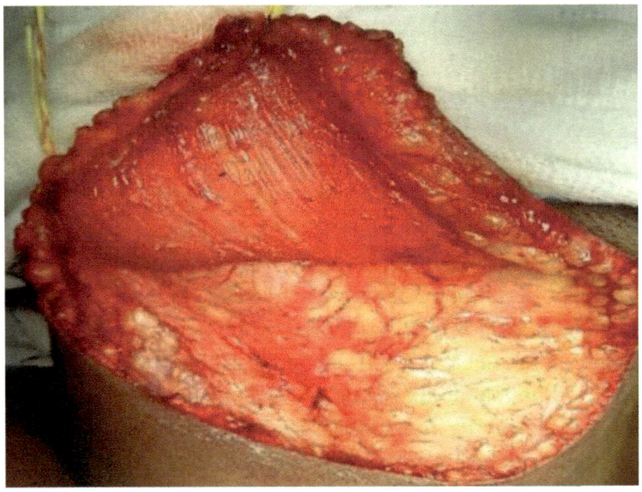

Fig. 82.37 Raising of subplatysmal flap

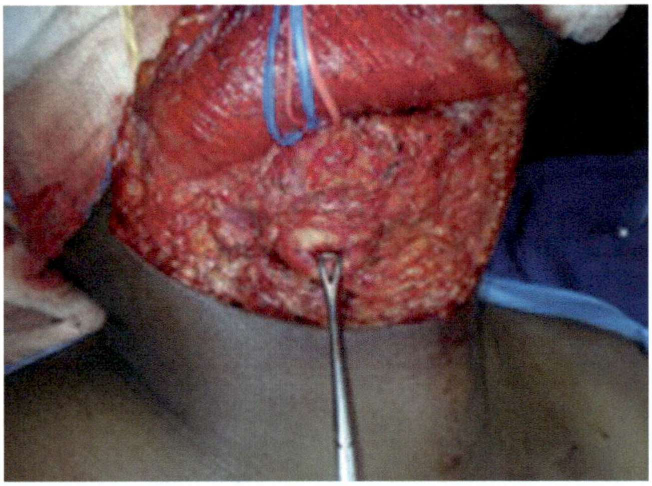

Fig. 82.38 Mobilization of submandibular salivary gland for level I dissection; also seen is isolation of facial vessels

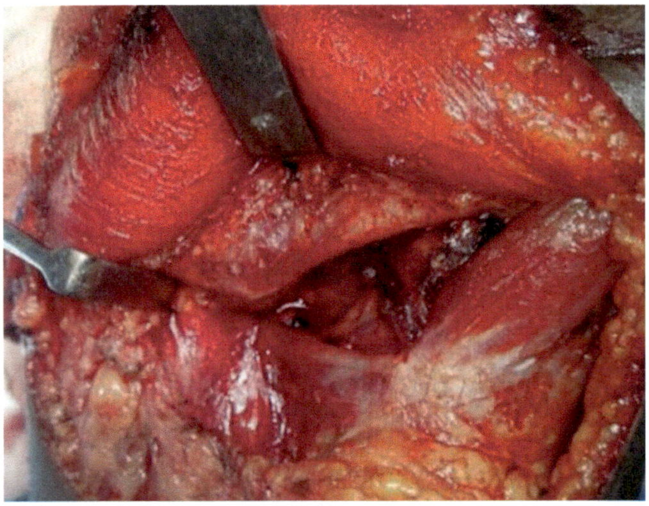

Fig. 82.39 Completed Level Ib dissection, boundaries well appreciated

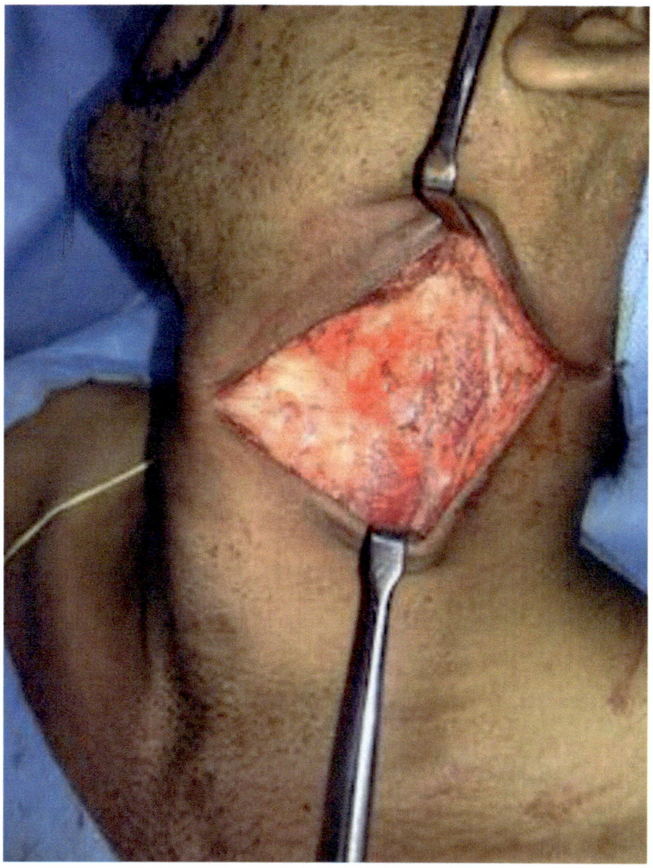

©Association of Oral and Maxillofacial Surgeons of India

Fig. 82.40 Exposed SCM, greater auricular nerve, and external jugular vein can be seen over the SCM

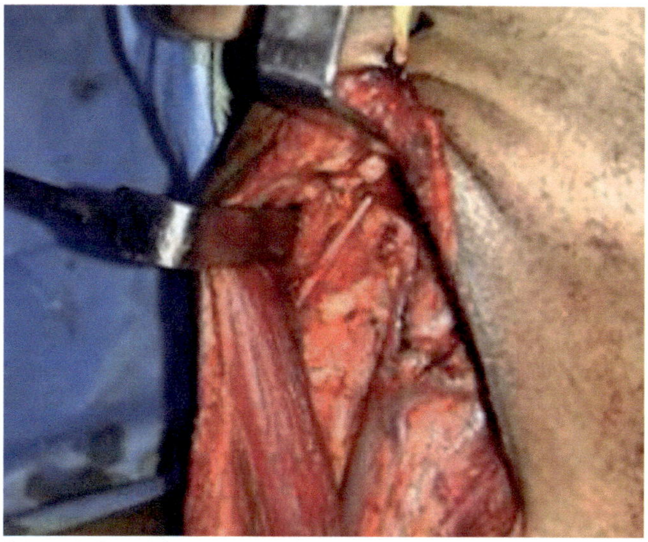

©Association of Oral and Maxillofacial Surgeons of India

Fig. 82.41 Spinal accessory nerve exposed in level II region

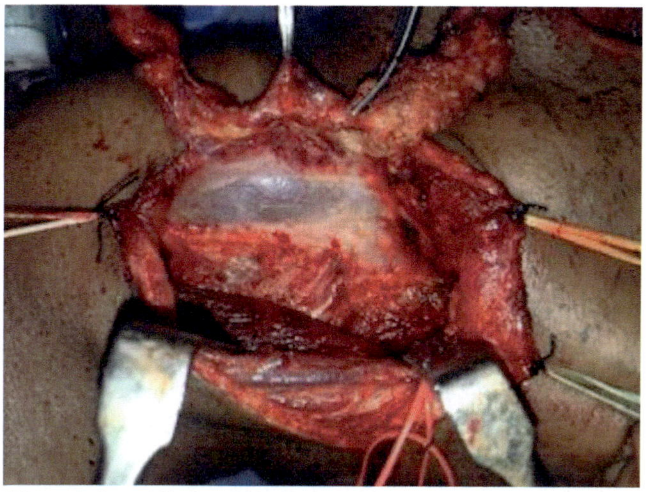

©Association of Oral and Maxillofacial Surgeons of India

Fig. 82.42 Level II–IV Lymph node dissection mobilized over the IJV

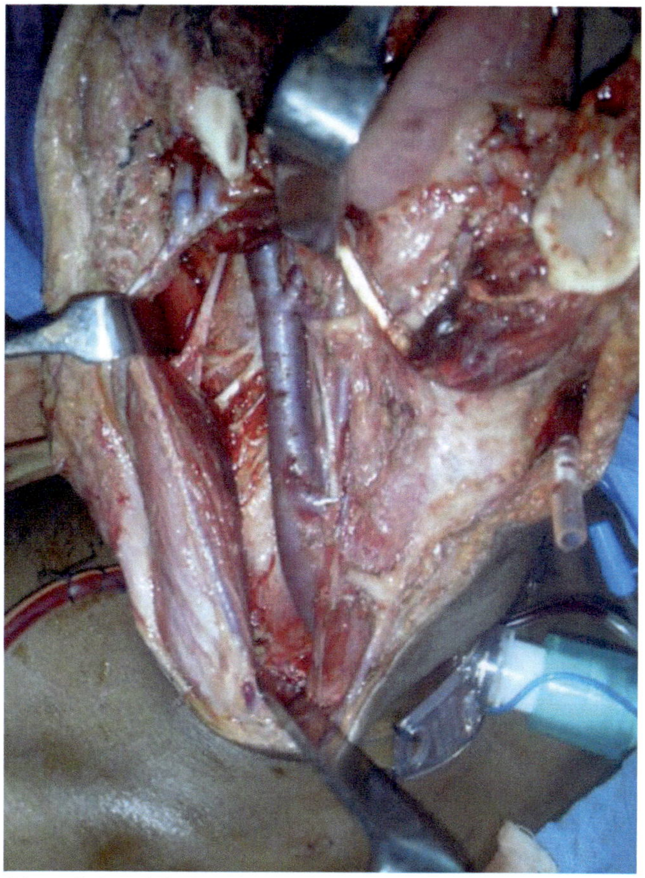

©Association of Oral and Maxillofacial Surgeons of India

Fig. 82.43 Completed selective neck dissection (level I–IV) preserving sternocleidomastoid (SCM), spinal accessory nerve (SAN), internal jugular vein (IJV)

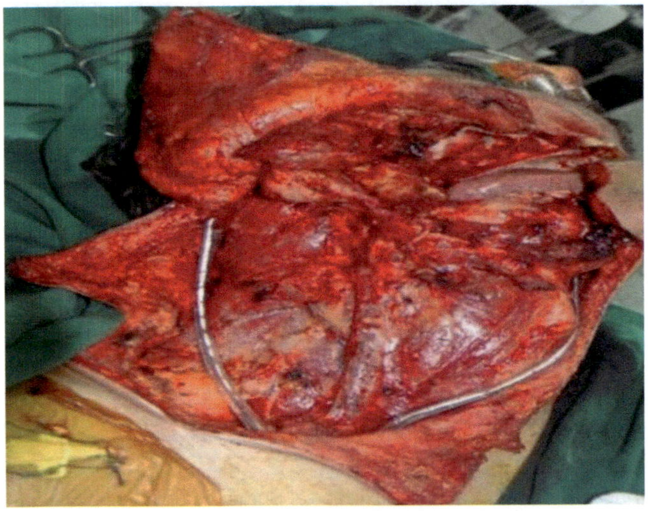

Fig. 82.44 Intraoperative picture depicting right infrastructure maxillectomy, right hemimandibulectomy, modified radical neck dissection (level I–V) preserving only internal jugular vein with suction drains in situ

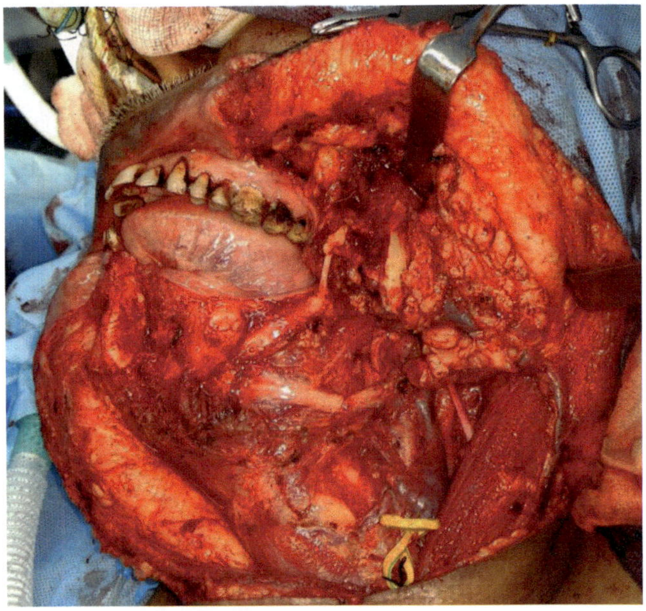

Fig. 82.45 Composite resection with left hemimandibulectomy and selective neck dissection (Level I–IV) preserving the non-lymphatic structure

Table 82.7 Complications of neck dissection [29]

Immediate complications and management	
Hemorrhage	Controlled by ligation or direct cauterization. If hematoma, "milking" the drains may result in evacuation. It is best to return the patient to the operating room and explore the wound if there is suspicion of active bleed and/or there is evidence of hypotension. Blood and blood products to be arranged for blood transfusions. Coagulation profile
Nerve injury	SAN in the level II may be injured either tractional or due to vascular compromise. Vagus, lingual, hypoglossal, and marginal mandibular branch of the facial nerves should be identified and preserved. All attempts should be made to preserve the greater auricular nerve too
Increased intra-cranial pressure	This usually occurs when the internal jugular vein is ligated. When one internal jugular vein is ligated, the pressure rises by three-fold and when both are ligated it increases by five-fold. This usually is temporary and will normalize in 24 h. If it persists, head end elevation, steroids, and mannitol can be used
Pneumothorax	Rare Any tears in the pleura should be identified and closed and their integrity tested
Intermediate complications and management	
Pulmonary	Basal atelectasis and bronchopneumonia may occur in patients who are smokers and have pre-existing chronic obstructive lung disease
Deep vein thrombosis	This is seen in patients in geriatric age group, prolonged duration of surgery, bedridden patients, and patients with previous history of deep vein thrombosis, pulmonary embolism, myocardial infarction and thrombophilia
Chylous fistula	Intra-operative identification can be aided by placing the patient in the Trendelenburg position or adopting a forced Valsalva maneuver. Postoperative leaks are usually identified when feeding is commenced. Multiple approaches to the treatment of an established leak have emerged including nutritional, surgical, and pharmacological therapy
Carotid blowout	Damage to the adventitial layer during surgery may be another contributory factor. If risk of exposure is anticipated, vessels should be covered, e.g., dermal graft, fascia lata or levator scapulae muscle flap. This is particularly important in the post-irradiation subject
Delayed complications and management	
Lymphedema	When both the internal jugular veins are ligated, lymphedema often follows owing to interruption of the lymphatic drainage channels. There are massages advocated as a temporary measure

82.11 Complications of Neck Dissection

Table 82.7 provides a comprehensive view of the complications arising from neck dissection [29].

Disclosure Authors have no conflicts of interest to disclose.

References

1. West H, Jin JO. Performance status in patients with Cancer. JAMA Oncol. 2015;1(7):998.
2. Chen AM, Chen LM, Vaughan A. Tobacco smoking during radiation therapy for head-and-neck cancer is associated with unfavorable outcome. Int J Radiat Oncol Biol Phys. 2011;79:414–9.

3. Hoff CM, Grau C, Overgaard J. Effect of smoking on oxygen delivery and outcome in patients treated with radiotherapy for head and neck squamous cell carcinoma–a prospective study. Radiother Oncol. 2012;103:38–44.
4. Deleyiannis FW, Thomas DB, Vaughan TL, Davis S. Alcoholism: independent predictor of survival in patients with head and neck cancer. J Natl Cancer Inst. 1996;88:542–9.
5. National Comprehensive Cancer Network. Oral cavity cancer (version 2.2014). http://www.nccn.org/professionals/physician_gls/pdf/head-and-neck.pdf. Accessed 19 Dec 2014.
6. Edge SP, Byrd DR, Compton CC, et al., editors. AJCC cancer staging manual. 7th ed. New York: Springer; 2010.
7. Henrot P, Blum A, Toussaint B. Dynamic maneuvers in local staging of head and neck malignancies with current imaging techniques: principles and clinical applications. Radiographics. 2003;23:1201–13.
8. Pentenero M, Gandolfo S, Carrozzo M. Importance of tumor thickness and depth of invasion in nodal involvement and prognosis of oral squamous cell carcinoma: a review of the literature. Head Neck. 2005;27(12):1080–91.
9. Erkan M, Tolu I, Aslan T, Guney E. Ultrasonography in laryngeal cancers. J Laryngol Otol. 1993;17:293–7.
10. Curtin HD, Ishwaran H, Mancuso AA, Dalley RW, Caudry DJ, McNeil BJ. Comparison of CT and MR imaging in staging of neck metastases. Radiology. 1998;207:123–30.
11. Van den Brekel MW, Castelijns JA, Stel HV, Golding RP, Meyer CJ, Snow GB. Modern imaging techniques and ultrasound- guided aspiration cytology for the assessment of neck node metastases: a prospective comparative study. Eur Arch Otorhinolaryngol. 1993;250:11–7.
12. Okura M, Iida S, Aikawa T, Adachi T, Yoshimura N, Yamada T, et al. Tumor thickness and paralingual distance of coronal MR imaging predicts cervical node metastases in oral tongue carcinoma. AJNR Am J Neuroradiol. 2008;29:45–50.
13. Arya S, Chaukar D, Pai P. Imaging in oral cancers. Indian J Radiol Imaging. 2012;22:195–208.
14. Weiss MH, Harrison LB, Isaacs RS. Use of decision tree analysis in planning a management strategy for the stage N0 neck. Arch Otolaryngol Head Neck Surg. 1994;120(7):699–702.
15. Kuriakose MA. Contemporary oral oncology. Cham: Springer Nature; 2017.
16. Huang SH, Hwang D, Lockwood G, Goldstein DP, O'Sullivan B. Predictive value of tumor thickness for cervical lymph-node involvement in squamous cell carcinoma of the oral cavity: a meta-analysis of reported studies. Cancer. 2009;115(7):1489–97.
17. Shah JP. Patterns of cervical lymph node metastasis from squamous carcinomas of the upper aerodigestive tract. Am J Surg. 1990;160:405–9.
18. Pantvaidya GH, Pal P, Vaidya AD, Pai PS, D'Cruz AK. Prospective study of 583 neck dissections in oral cancers: implications for clinical practice. Head Neck. 2014;36(10):1503–7.
19. D'Cruz AK. Elective versus therapeutic neck dissection in node-negative oral cancer. N Engl J Med. 2015 Aug 6;373(6):521–9.
20. Mehanna H, Robinson M, Hartley A, Kong A, Foran B, Lieuw TF, et al. Radiotherapy plus cisplatin or cetuximab in low-risk human papillomavirus-positive oropharyngeal cancer (De-ESCALaTE HPV): an open-label randomised controlled phase 3 trial. Lancet. 2018;393:51–60.
21. Parikh PM, Hingmire SS, Deshmukh CD. Selected current data on metronomic therapy (and its promise) from India. South Asian J Cancer. 2016 Apr–Jun;5(2):37–47.
22. Bernier J, Cooper JS, Pajak TF, van Glabbeke M, Bourhis J, Forastiere A, et al. Defining risk levels in locally advanced head and neck cancers: a comparative analysis of concurrent postoperative radiation plus chemotherapy trials of the EORTC (#22931) and RTOG (# 9501). Head Neck. 2005 Oct;27(10):843–50. https://doi.org/10.1002/hed.20279.
23. Calabrese L. Compartmental surgery in tongue tumours: description of a new surgical technique. Acta Otorhinolaryngol Ital. 2009;29:259–64.
24. Kowalski LP, Bagietto R, Lara JR, Santos RL, Tagawa EK, Santos IR. Factors influencing contralateral lymph node metastasis from oral carcinoma. Head Neck. 1999;21:104–10.
25. Brown JS, Rogers SN, McNally DN, Boyle M. A modified classification for the maxillectomy defect. Head Neck. 2000;22(1):17–26. https://doi.org/10.1002/(sici)1097-0347(200001)22:1<17::aid-hed4>3.0.co;2-2.
26. Robbins KT, Medina JE, Wolfe GT, Levine PA, Sessions RB, Pruet CW. Standardizing neck dissection terminology. Official report of the Academy's committee for head and neck surgery and oncology. Arch Otolaryngol Head Neck Surg. 1991;117:601–5.
27. Medina JE. A rational classification of neck dissections. Otolaryngol Head Neck Surg. 1989;100:169–76.
28. Spiro RH, Strong EW, Shah JP. Classification of neck dissection: variations on a new theme. Am J Surg. 1994;168:415–8.
29. Parnell FW. Complications of radical neck dissection. Arch Otolaryngol. 1968;88(2):180–3.

83 Sarcoma of the Maxillofacial/Head and Neck Region

D' Souza Jacob and Boyapati Raghu

83.1 Introduction

Sarcomas are uncommon malignant tumours with incidence of less than 5% of all head and neck malignancies in adults [1, 2]. They are more common in children, accounting for 30% of head and neck sarcomas [2, 3]. They arise from either soft or hard tissue mesenchyme cells. There is a male predominance and presentation is usually in the third and fourth decade of life in 70% of cases [4, 5].

Metastasis at initial presentation is seen in only 10% of patients, usually from high-grade primary lesions [6–8]. Despite this, prognosis tends to be poor, partly due to the proximity of vital neurovascular structures leading to difficulty in obtaining adequate surgical clearance. Moreover, majority of the sarcomas are poorly differentiated, a poor prognostic marker [9].

Sarcomas tend not be related to the use of tobacco and alcohol. Predisposition to the development of sarcomas is seen in some conditions [4, 8, 10]. Notable examples include association of osteosarcoma in patients with Li-Fraumeni syndrome, angiosarcoma with chronic lymphoedema and Kaposi's sarcoma with HIV infection. Additionally, exposure to chemicals such as vinyl chloride is well-recognised risk factors [10].

83.2 Classification

Broadly speaking, sarcomas can be classified into two categories: soft tissue and hard tissue (bone and cartilage) sarcomas. This, however, is an oversimplification since precise classification is fraught with significant difficulties. For example, fibrosarcoma and malignant fibrous histiocytoma are soft tissue sarcomas that arise in hard tissues [11, 12]. In contrast, chondrosarcomas are classified as soft tissue tumours. Additionally, some hard tissue tumours display extraosseous extension [1–3].

Ten or more main histological types and even more subtypes of sarcomas are described. Osteosarcoma, angiosarcoma and malignant fibrous histiocytoma make up the majority tumours in adults. In children, rhabdomyosarcoma is the most common sarcoma [1–3].

83.3 Staging

Soft and hard tissue sarcomas are staged using different systems (Tables 83.1 and 83.2). The American Joint Committee on Cancer (AJCC) and the International Union Against Cancer (UICC) staging systems are used in most centres [13]. Other systems may be used in selected cases such as the Memorial Sloan Kettering system [14].

83.4 Natural History and Prognostic Factors

Head and neck sarcomas tend to show poorer response to treatment compared to sarcomas affecting the trunk and extremities [5, 6]. This is despite the low rate of lymph node metastasis at presentation (less than 10% of cases) and the modern multimodality treatment with surgery, radiotherapy and chemotherapy [4, 5]. Local and regional nodal recurrence is common and is more likely to result in death than distant metastatic spread [5, 8, 10].

The reasons for treatment failure resulting in disease recurrence are multifactorial. Adequate surgical margins are hard to achieve given the complex anatomy of the maxillofacial and the skull base regions (Fig. 83.1). The morbidity of radical resections is unacceptable, both functional and aesthetic. This is especially true for primary tumour larger than 10 cm at presentation [8, 9, 11]. Resections aimed at minimising morbidity risk positive or involved surgical

D. S. Jacob (✉) · B. Raghu
Maxillofacial Unit, Royal Surrey County Hospital, Guilford, UK
e-mail: dsouzaj@icloud.com; raghusurgdent@doctors.org.uk

K. Bonanthaya et al. (eds.), *Oral and Maxillofacial Surgery for the Clinician*, https://doi.org/10.1007/978-981-15-1346-6_83

Table 83.1 TNM/UICC classification of soft tissue sarcomas

T classification	
Tx	Tumour cannot be assessed
T0	Tumour not evident
T1	Tumour size <5 cm
T2	Tumour size>5cm
N classification	
Nx	Regional lymph nodes cannot be assessed
N0	No regional lymph nodes evident
N1	Regional lymph node metastasis
M classification	
Mo	No distant metastasis
M1	Distant metastasis evident

Histological grading of soft tissue sarcomas

Gx: Grade cannot be assessed

G1: Well differentiated tumour

G2: Moderately differentiated tumour

G3: Poorly differentiated tumour

Staging:

Stage 1: Low grade tumour with no regional or distant lymph node metastasis.

Stage: 2 Intermediate, large or high grade, small tumour with no regional or distant metasta sis

Stage 3: High grade, large tumour or any tumour with regional metastasis.

Stage 4:Distant Metastasis identified

Table 83.2 TNM/UICC staging of bone sarcomas

Stage	Grade	Metastasis
1	Low grade < 8 cm	Absent
1b	Low grade > 8 cm	Absent
2	High grade < 8 cm	Absent
2b	High grade > 8 cm	Absent
3	Any grade, any size	Skip metastasis
4	Any grade, any size	Distant metastasis

margins and are an independent predictor of treatment failure and hence survival [5, 7, 8]. The grade of tumour is another prognostic factor. For example, the 5-year survival rates for high-grade tumours such as malignant fibrous histiocytoma, osteosarcoma and angiosarcoma are in the range of 60%. This is in contrast with low-grade tumours such as chondrosarcoma or dermatofibrosarcoma protuberance which show survival approaching 100% at 5 years [8, 9, 15]. There is optimism, however, with modern combined treatment modalities, for example, patients with rhabdomyosarcomas are showing better survival outcomes. Finally, sarcomas arising in previously irradiate tissues have poor prognosis due to a multitude of factors: delayed diagnosis; high-grade, inadequate surgical margins; limited option of adjuvant radiotherapy; and lack of proven chemotherapy regimens [10, 16, 17].

It is important to interpret the published treatment outcomes and survival rates with caution. Comparison between institutions is unreliable due to different study population, histological subtypes and follow-up regiments. Moreover, lack of standardisation in reporting leads to institutional bias of a selected treatment modality. Reported overall survival for bone sarcomas approach 80% at 2 years and 74% at 5 years [18, 19]. Radiation-induced sarcomas perhaps have the worse survival outcomes, as low as 25% at 5 years [19, 20].

83.5 Principles of Treatment

It is difficult to draw firm treatment guidelines for head and neck sarcomas because they are a rare group of heterogeneous tumours. The treatment philosophies vary between institutions due to multitude of factors as discussed previously in this chapter. Meta-analysis outcomes are therefore controversial and unreliable to draw firm conclusions. Furthermore, there are no randomised controlled trials [20, 21]. Despite this, there is consensus that early surgical resection with appropriately

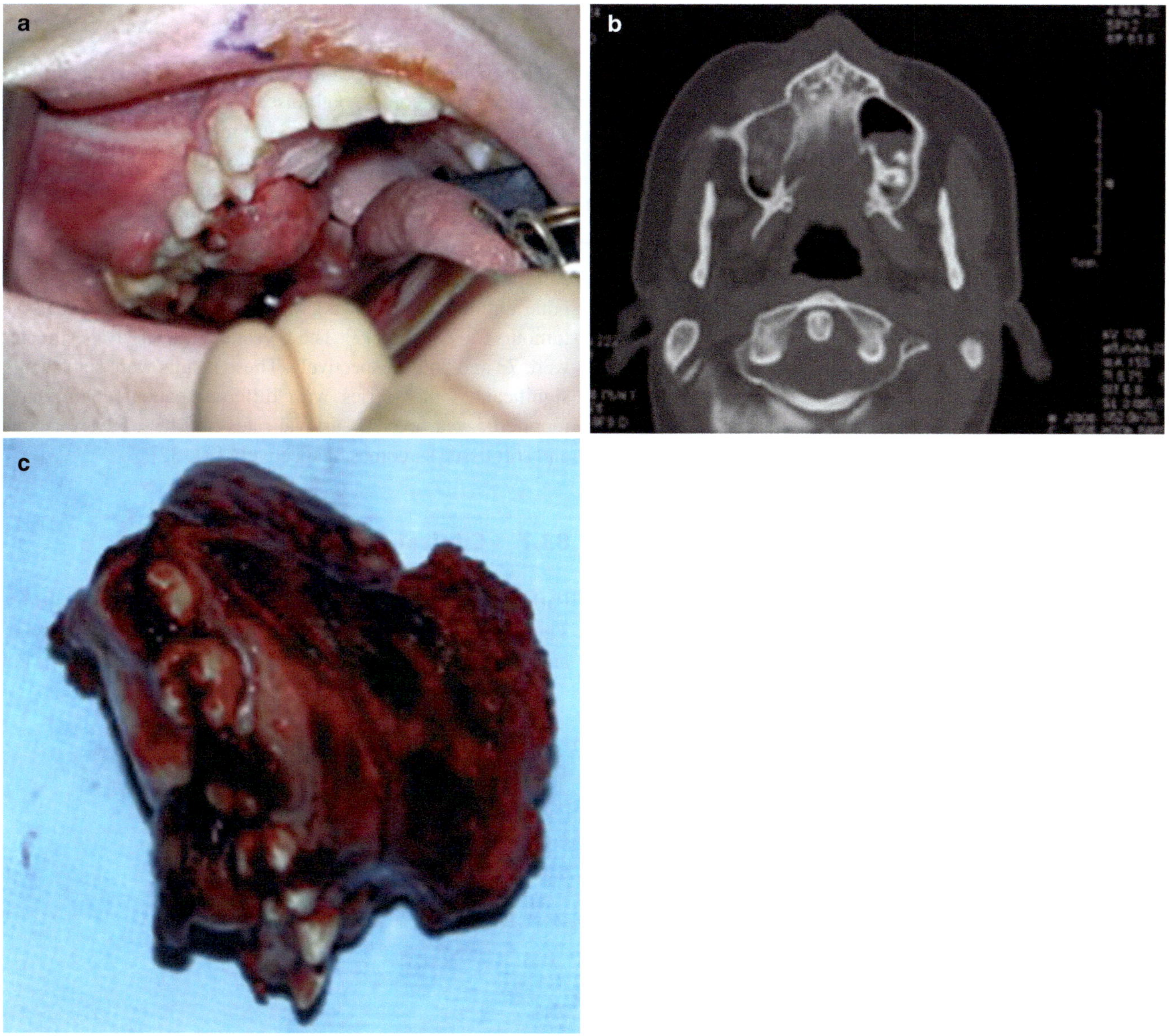

Fig. 83.1 (**a, b, c**) Osteosarcoma of the right posterior maxilla. Photograph showing osteosarcoma of the right maxilla. The extent of bone destruction from the tumour is seen in the scan. The resected specimen confirms the loss of the hemi-maxilla

timed adjuvant therapies can help improve outcomes. Needless to say, the role of multidisciplinary input/tumour board is vital.

Surgical resection of the tumour is the favoured primary treatment modality for patients with sarcomas of the hard tissues [22, 23]. Surgery is often preceded by chemotherapy on a neoadjuvant protocol [19, 22, 23]. The intention is to reduce tumour bulk and hence morbidity by minimising tissue loss. Elimination of micro-metastatic disease, mainly pulmonary deposits, is of added benefit. The role of adjuvant radiotherapy is limited to patients with positive surgical margins who often are not candidates for further resection [19, 24]. Further resections may not be feasible due to anatomical complexity or in those who have undergone complex reconstruction. Note should be made of the evolving role of radiotherapy in Ewing's sarcoma.

The size of the tumour at presentation often restricts the use of surgery in patient presenting with soft tissue sarcoma. Adjuvant radiotherapy is an indication when the resection margins are positive; the tumours are of intermediate or high grade and in cases of recurrent disease [12, 16, 24, 25]. The feasibility of introducing neoadjuvant chemotherapy or preoperative radiotherapy should be considered with diligence in patients with advanced disease at presentation with a view to reduce morbid resections [25, 26]. When surgery is not feasible, the role of palliative radiotherapy alone or in combination with chemotherapy should be considered.

83.6 Principles of Surgery

83.6.1 Hard Tissue Sarcomas

There is a consensus that achieving tumour-free zone of tissue at the resection margins maximises the chance of cure. However, what defines adequate margin remains debated. The current recommendation is resection of the tumour with a 2–3 cm macroscopic margin in patients who receive neoadjuvant chemotherapy aiming to sterilise the microscopic deposits around the main body of the tumour [24–28]. It is important to plan the resection on scans obtained prior to the neoadjuvant chemotherapy. This is because both the tumour-killing effect of the neoadjuvant chemotherapy and tissue shrinkage are unpredictable. Furthermore, one should aim for compartmental excision (Fig. 83.1) that allows for removal of all potentially involved structures beyond the radiographic margins such as intra-osseous extension of the tumour via marrow spaces [2, 19, 24]. Although this approach is radical, for instance, resection of the hemi-mandible to include disarticulation of the condyle in ramus tumours, the chance of surgical clearance can be maximised to 85% or greater [2].

83.6.2 Soft Tissue Sarcomas

Similar to hard tissue sarcomas, adequate surgical margins predict survival outcomes, both disease-free and overall survival. The recommendation is for 1–3 cm macroscopic margins [24, 29, 30]. Achieving this may be limited due to anatomical constrains and an infiltrative pattern of tumour spread that tends to characterise soft tissue sarcomas. One published series reported adequate surgical clearance in 85% of osteosarcomas vs. 64% soft tissue tumours [2]. The 2-year overall survival estimate for bone tumours (51 patients) was 91% vs. 67% for soft tissue tumours (50 patients) [2]. The 5-year overall survival estimates were 73 and 56%, respectively. These results were statistically significant. Other series with different patient cohort have reported 5-year overall survival rates of 74 vs. 57% for bone and soft tissue sarcomas, respectively [31, 32].

83.7 Clinical Assessment

Patients present with a wide range of signs and symptoms. These may range from indolent lumps to rapidly growing and locally destructive lesions (Figs. 83.1 and 83.2). Pain

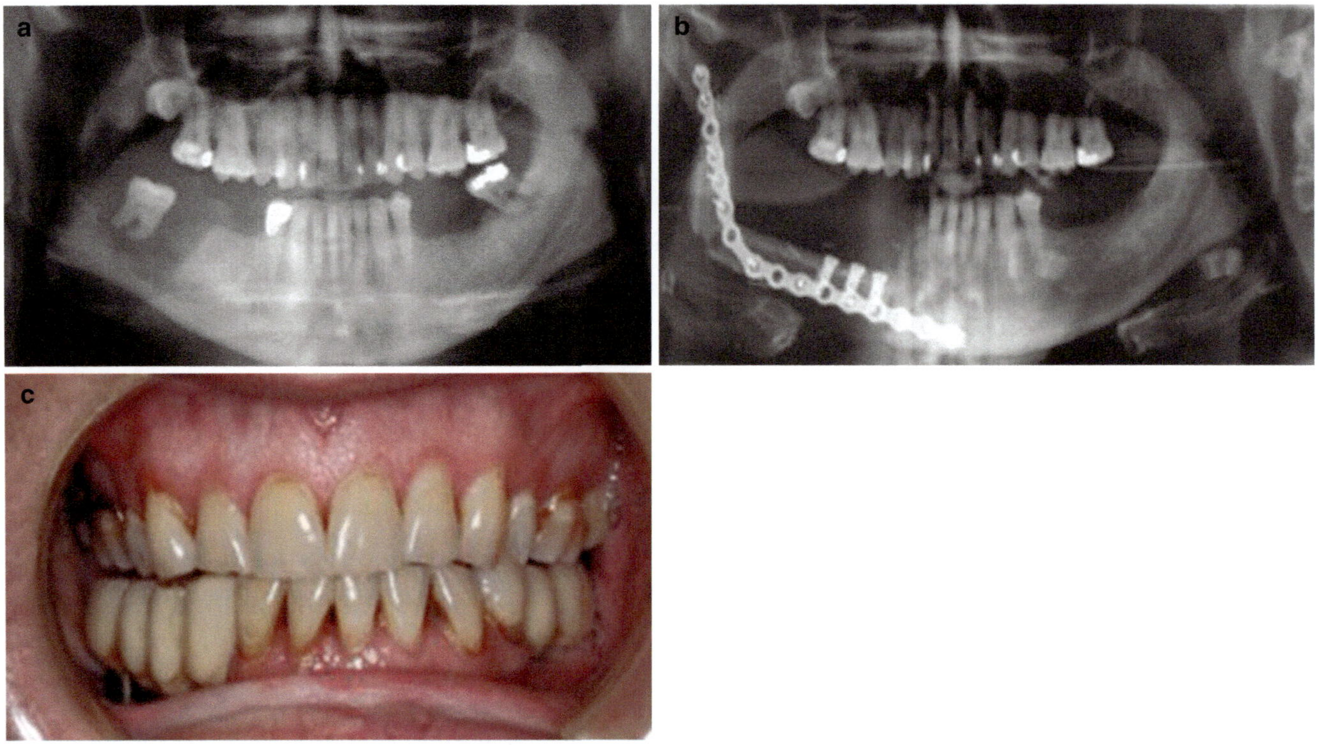

Fig. 83.2 (**a**, **b**, **c**) Osteosarcoma of the right posterior mandible. Plain radiograph showing tumour destruction of the right posterior mandible. A fibula free flap and dental implants are used for rehabilitation

is variable and there is a tendency for nocturnal bone pain [1, 4].

There may be a mass at the primary site, ulceration, sensory change affecting the skin or the mucosa, proptosis, epistaxis or nasal discharge, loosening of teeth and unexplained bleeding.

Involvement of the skull base by direct extension can lead to focal neurology. Metastatic lesions can present with a neck mass. Systemic symptoms tend to be non-specific such as malaise, loss of weight and appetite [8, 23].

83.8 Investigations

Magnetic resonance imaging (MRI) is usually the preferred investigation for primary lesions [30, 33]. They provide information regarding the nature of the primary tumour (solid, cystic, presence or absence of calcifications, internal vascularity, etc.). The relationship of the tumour to adjacent tissues can be accurately defined; this helps plan tumour resection [22, 34, 35]. Computer tomography (CT) scan of the facial bone may be used to complement the MRI scan, especially in patients requiring hard tissue resection and reconstruction (Figs. 83.1 and 83.2). The use of composite flaps with 3-D reconstruction with prefabricated plates is increasingly used in several centres [36, 37]. The use of dental implants has significantly improved outcomes following composite reconstructions (Fig. 83.2). CT scans of the thorax and upper abdomen complete the staging investigations. There is an evolving role for positron emission tomography (PET), both in the initial staging of the disease, the response to treatment and tumour surveillance [38, 39]. Blood tests include comprehensive baseline tests (full blood count, renal and bone profile) and serum alkaline phosphatase. Additional tests may be necessary, often dictated by individual patient profiles. Biopsy for tissue diagnosis must include an appropriate sample that in addition to routing staining provides tissue for immunocytochemistry [4, 12].

83.9 Osteosarcoma

Osteosarcomas are the commonest sarcomas of the bones in adults, representing 1% of all head and neck cancers. They do not show sex predilection. The peak incidence is between 20 and 30 years. However, tumours arising in area of Paget's disease of the bone are seen in older patient 60–70 years of age [25–27]. The mandible is the most frequently affected site, especially the angle/ramus region. In the maxilla, the tumour has a predilection to the alveolar ridge and sinus floor. Notable risk factors include chromosomal abnormalities (deletion of 13q14), germ line mutations (Li Fraumeni syndrome) and dysplasia of bone (Paget's disease and fibrous dysplasia) [25–28]. In some instances, these tumours arise in irradiated bone or de novo.

Patient may present with asymptomatic intra-oral mass, loose teeth and toothache.

Destructive lesions can cause soft tissue cheek swelling, sensory change, proptosis, nasal discharge or bleeding.

Three histological subtypes of osteosarcoma are recognised, namely, osteoblastic, chondroblastic and fibroblastic variants [31, 39].

However, myxoid pattern is the norm (Fig. 83.3). The chondroblastic variant shows binucleated cell characteristic of the lesion (Fig. 83.4) The degree of differentiation classifies them as stage I (well-differentiated and low-grade) to stage IV (poorly differentiated and high-grade). Regional neck metastases at presentation are rare, seen in less than 10% of patients at presentation. Distant metastases are seen in up to 30% of patients at presentation, mostly pulmonary [23, 27, 31]. On rare occasions, patients may present with rapidly progressive, fatal multifocal disease. Imaging reveals local bone. The well-documented finding of subperiosteal bone formation (Codman triangle) is uncommonly seen in head and neck lesions.

Whilst surgery, radiotherapy and chemotherapy are offered as single or multimodality treatments, well-established treatment regimens are lacking in consensus. Various drug combinations have been tried and tested, leucovorin, Adriamycin, cisplatin, ifosfamide and cyclophosphamide, with unpredictable response. One study has shown 2- and 5-year overall survival rates of 100 and 67%, respectively, in those treated with neoadjuvant chemotherapy and surgery. This compares favourably with patient treated with surgery alone showing poorer 2- and 5-year overall survival rates of 66 and 41%, respectively [19, 23, 31]. The role of

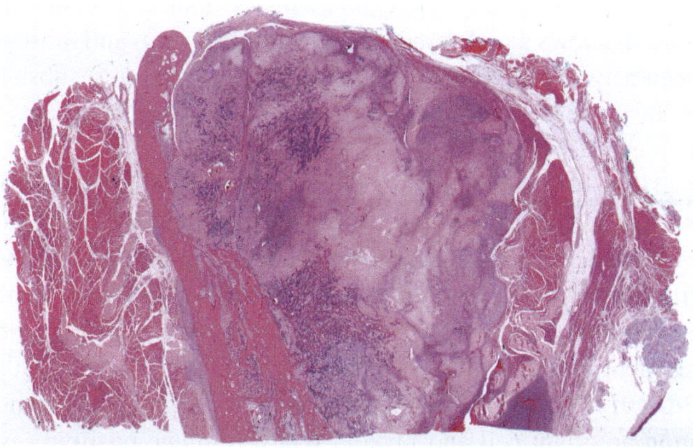

Fig. 83.3 Osteosarcoma-myxoid variant. H&E section of an axial slice through the masseter (far left), ramus of the mandible, tumour, medial pterygoid and palatal mucosa (far right bottom corner)

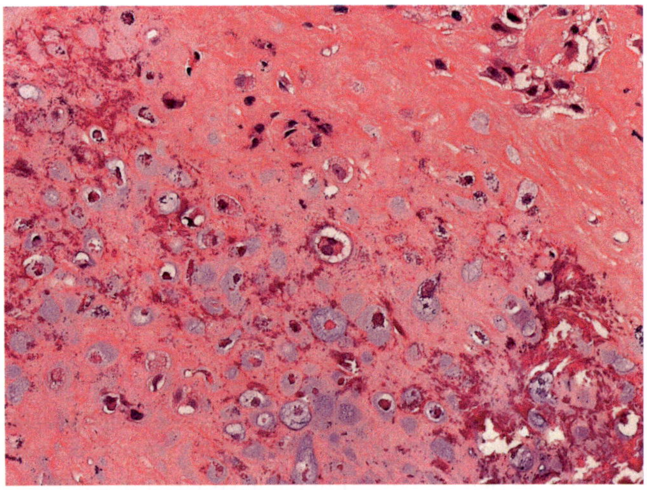

Fig. 83.4 Osteosarcoma-chondroblastic variant. Photomicrograph showing binucleated cells, characteristic of the chondroblastic type

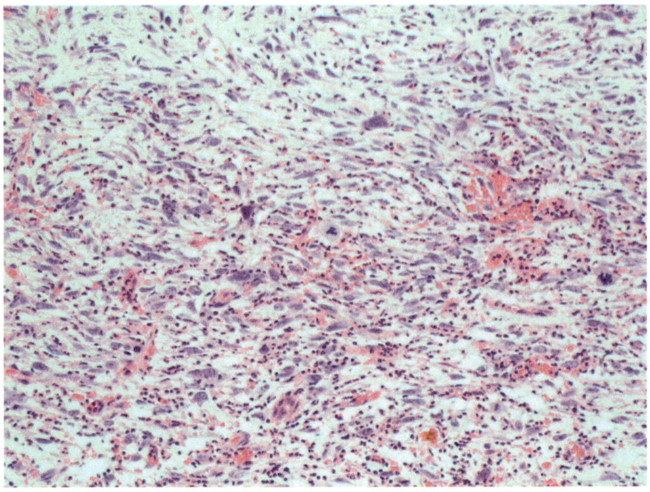

Fig. 83.5 Malignant fibrous histiocytoma. H&E section showing highly pleomorphic tumour cells with atypical mitotic figures amidst dense acute inflammation

adjuvant radiotherapy is applicable in patients with inadequate or positive surgical margins; however, doses in excess of 60Gy are necessary given their radio-resistant behaviours [8, 16, 31].

In addition to high-grade disease and large tumours at presentation, some additional factors have prognostic significance. For example, the expression of the p-glycoprotein confers multidrug resistance negatively impacting on prognosis. Osteosarcomas arising in Paget's disease and elevated alkaline phosphate levels have poorer prognosis [9, 25, 27, 32].

83.10 Malignant Fibrous Histiocytoma

Malignant fibrous histiocytoma is the commonest soft tissue sarcoma affecting the trunks and extremities. However, it is rare in the head and neck region, with less than 3% occurring here. It shows a male predilection with a 2:1 ratio and mostly seen between 40 and 60 years of age. The commonest subsite is the sinonasal tract. There is a strong link to ionising radiation exposure [11].

Histology shows highly pleomorphic fibroblasts mixed with abnormal histiocytes in a storiform pattern with a background dense inflammation (Fig. 83.5). Phagocytised neutrophils with large nuclei/nucleoli are commonly seen. Necrosis is an uncommon feature, but bizarre giant cells or atypical mitotic figures can be seen on most occasions [30, 34, 40]. The commonest subtype is pleomorphic; less common are giant cell and myxoid types. Immune positivity is seen with α-1-antichymotrypsin, vimentin and Ki-67 [11].

Wide surgical resection is the primary treatment, with consideration given to adjuvant chemoradiotherapy [17, 23]. Whist local recurrence is the norm, regional metastases to lymph nodes are rare. Positive margins predict for treatment failure locally and distant spread, usually to the lungs and liver [23, 33].

83.11 Liposarcoma

Although liposarcomas are second most common soft tissue tumours, less than 5% occur within the head and neck region. They show a slight male predominance, most commonly presenting between the ages of 30 and 60. Majority arise de novo rather than developing in a lipoma [24]. Patient may demonstrate risk factors such as repeated trauma, irradiation or genetic abnormality (NF-1 gene). The histological behaviour varies from high-grade (pleomorphic, round) to low-grade (myxoid) tumours. The myxoid variant shows lipoblasts arranged within a chicken-wire vascular network in a dense stroma (Fig. 83.6). The pleomorphic type shows significant numbers of highly atypical fat cells along with lipoblasts (Fig. 83.7). The epithelioid variant can be confused with carcinoma [40].

Whilst surgery remains the primary treatment modality, the role of adjuvant radiotherapy should be considered in patients with high-grade lesions and large tumours with positive resection margins. Published literature supports the use of adjuvant radiotherapy in reducing local recurrence from 60 to 40% [19, 20, 24].

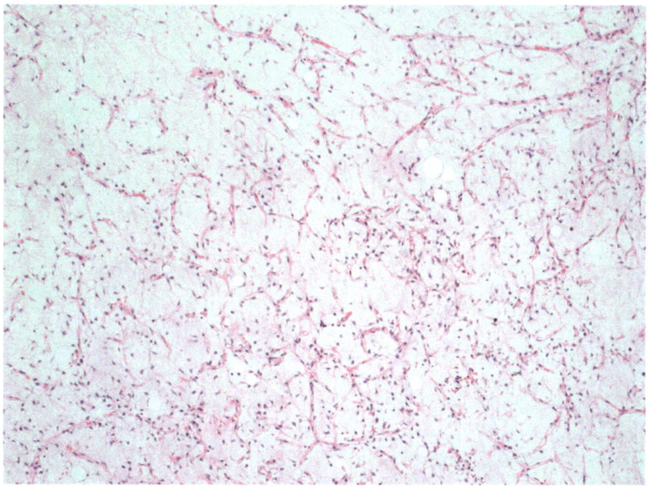

Fig. 83.6 Liposarcoma myxoid variant. H&E section showing myxoid tumour with lipoblasts arranged within a chicken-wire vascular network amidst dense myxoid stroma

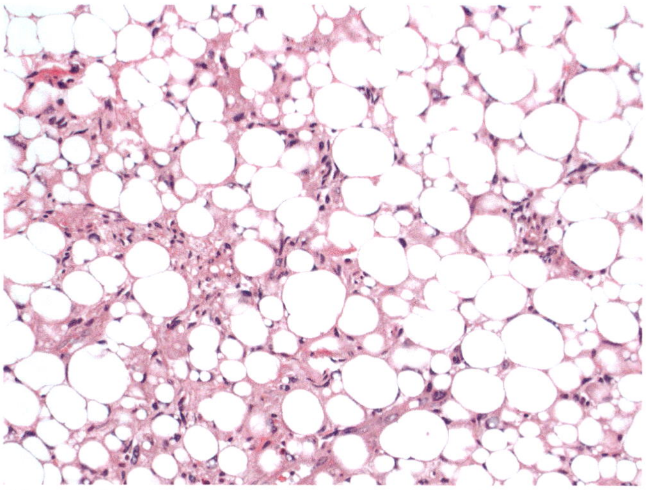

Fig. 83.7 Liposarcoma pleomorphic variant. H&E showing atypical adipocytes along with pleomorphic lipoblasts

83.12 Rhabdomyosarcoma

These are predominantly childhood tumours, usually affecting those below the age of 12 years [2, 4, 5]. They show slight male predilection. In contrast to adult sarcomas, up to half of all rhabdomyosarcomas occur in the head and neck sites. The favoured subsites are the orbits, the nasopharynx and the temporal bones [15].

Histologically, at least 70% of the tumours are of embryonal subtype; less commonly, the alveolar subtypes are seen (Fig. 83.8). Immune positivity to desmin, myoglobin and actin is well documented (Fig. 83.9). Cells show finely granular eosinophilic cytoplasm with cross striations with enlarged nucleus. More differentiated tumours may show elongated rhabdomyoblasts and occasional giant cells. Definitive diagnosis is based on myogenesis, multinucleated myoblasts, individual tumour cells with cross striations and dense eosinophilic cytoplasm [41].

Prognostic indicators include the location of the primary, age at presentation and metastatic disease. The survival rates have shown significant improvement: 71% in 2001 vs. 25% in the 1970s [15, 23, 31]. The orbital tumours show the best prognosis with 5-year survival rates exceeding 90% in children [15]. This contrasts with poor survival rates in adults at approximately 30%.

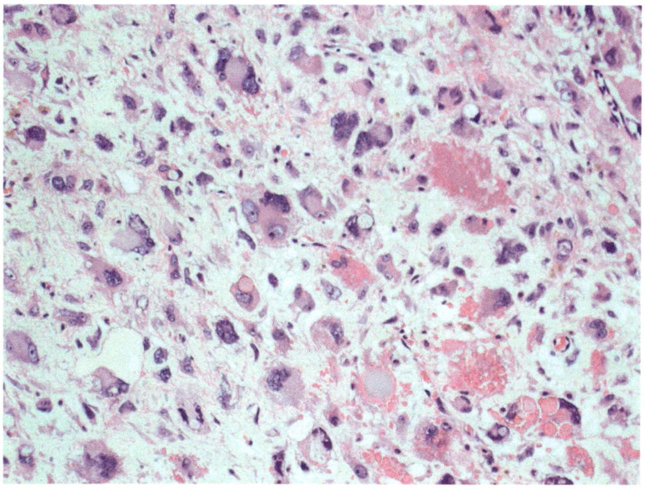

Fig. 83.8 Rhabdomyosarcoma pleomorphic variant. H&E section showing high-grade sarcoma with pleomorphic rhabdomyoblasts

83.13 Chondrosarcoma

Chondrosarcomas are malignant tumours of the bone or cartilage, and 10% are located in the head and neck [2, 8]. The larynx is the most commonly involved subsite, closely followed by the maxilla and mandible. The peak incidence is 30–50 years. At least 80% arise de novo. Secondary tumours arise in abnormal bone in conditions such as Paget's disease and fibrous dysplasia [40]. Rarely, extraosseous tumours are seen due to cartilaginous differentiation of primitive cells. Patient's symptoms depend on location and the extent of local tissue destruction. Despite slow initial progression, multiple metastases can develop rapidly [26]. Radiographic examination may show sunray speculation.

The degree of differentiation can range from well to poorly differentiated tumours. The common subtypes include myxoid and mesenchyme [26]. It is not uncommon for them

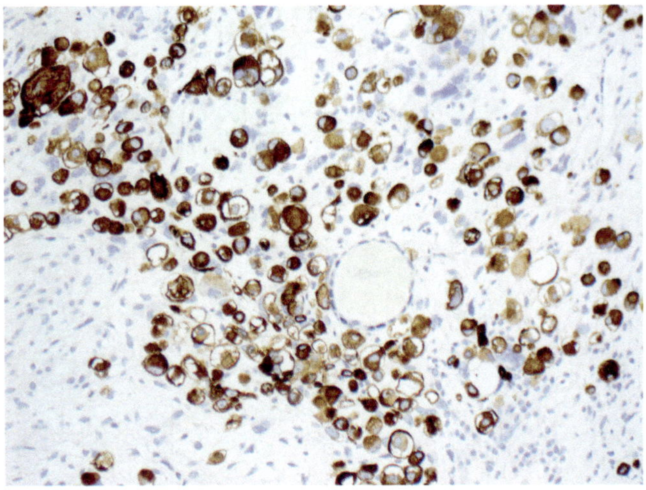

Fig. 83.9 Rhabdomyosarcoma. Showing expression of desmin in rhabdomyoblasts

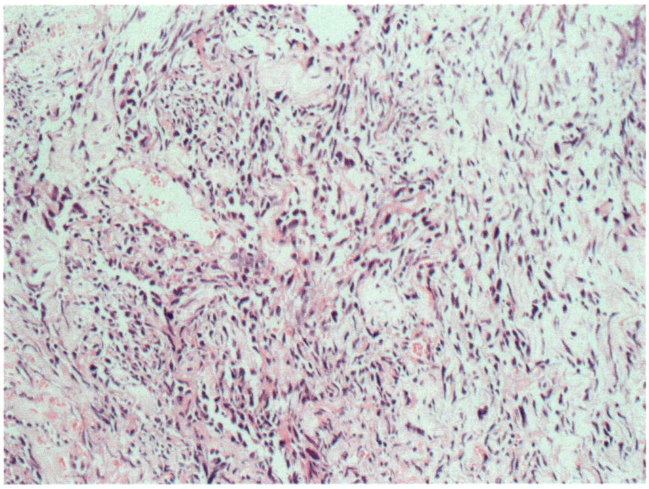

Fig. 83.10 Angiosarcoma. H&E section showing pleomorphic tumour cell lining interconnecting atypical vascular channels

to show histological similarity to tumours such as chondroblastic osteosarcoma and malignant fibrous histiocytoma. Additionally, low-grade tumours may show benign histology such as chondromatosis or osteochondroma.

Surgery remains the primary treatment modality, possibly driven by the belief that these tumours are radio-resistant. Additionally, irradiating areas such as the skull base can be carried out with conventional external beam photon therapy particularly with new techniques like Intensity modulation radiation therapy (IMRT). The role of proton beam therapy delivering high-energy irradiation has shown local control rates of 85–100% at 5 years [42].

The site of the primary tumour has implications for prognosis; for example, laryngeal primaries do better compared to nasopharyngeal primaries. High-grade and dedifferentiation confers poor prognosis due to early local recurrence and distant metastases. The 5-year overall survival rates are less than 50% vs. 80% or greater for high- and low-grade tumours, respectively.

83.14 Angiosarcoma

These tumours arise from the endothelial cells lining the vascular or the lymphatic system. They are most common above the age of 62 years and show male predilection with a ratio of 2:1. They can arise in several different sites given the wide distribution of the endothelium. Some lesions are localised and nodular, whilst others are diffused. Regional metastases are less than 20% of patients at presentation. However, distant metastases may be present in up to 45% of patients at presentation, mostly involving the lungs and liver [6–8]. The tumours show immune positivity for CD31. Histological examination shows anastomosing and infiltrating channels lined by multilayered endothelial cells with variable atypia (Fig. 83.10). Free-floating endothelial cells of 'fish in the creek' pattern with surrounding adnexae and dermal collagen can be a reliable feature [42].

Although surgery is the primary modality of treatment, diffuse lesions can make adequate surgical clearance a difficult task. The reported 5-year survival rates range from 12 to 40%. Predictors of poor survival include location of the primary tumour, size greater than 7 cm at presentation, high-grade and advancing age [1, 20, 23]. Local recurrence is seen in more than 50% of patients with inadequate or positive surgical margins, usually within 2 years. The role of adjuvant therapies is questionable in achieving adequate loco-regional control and improving survival.

83.15 Malignant Schwannoma

These are tumours arising in the nerve: peripheral or cranial. They usually affect the neck, followed by sinonasal areas. Involvement of the maxillofacial skeleton is rare. Although there is an association with von Recklinghausen's disease or neurofibromatosis type 1, sporadic tumours are well recognised [43]. Surgery remains the primary treatment modality. Tracking of the tumour along the nerve sheath limits the resectability, hence the need of adjuvant therapies, be it radiotherapy or chemotherapy.

83.16 Fibrosarcoma

These tumours often present as an asymptomatic painless mass between 30 and 40 years of age. History is positive for previous radiation exposure in at least 10% of patients.

Histological similarities are seen with malignant fibrous histiocytoma [6, 7, 44]. Surgery remains the mainstay of treatment, with adjuvant radiotherapy aimed at those with inadequate surgical margin and lessons that are high-grade. The reported 5-year survival rates are 80% or greater [22, 23].

83.17 Kaposi's Sarcoma

Human herpes virus 8 is implicated in the aetiology of these tumours arising in patients with AIDS. It is worth noting that Kaposi's sarcomas represent up to 80% of oral cavity sarcomas and have poor prognosis [25, 45].

83.18 Synovial Sarcoma

Contrary to the name, synovial sarcomas arise from the pluripotent mesenchymal cells, not the synovial cells. They show a male predilection and a peak incidence between 20 and 40 years. The common head and neck subsites are the hypopharyngeal and retropharyngeal areas. It is worth noting that up to 50% of patients have pulmonary metastases at presentation [5, 7, 15].

All histological subtypes (monophasic, biphasic, poorly differentiated) are high-risk tumours. Up to 90% of patients have chromosomal translocation (tX: 18) [21]. Prognosis tends to be poor with less than 20% of patients with metastasis at presentation alive at 2 years. Increasing age, size greater than 5 cm and poor differentiation predict worst prognosis [18, 22].

83.19 Ewing Sarcoma

These tumours arise in privative neuroectodermal cells and represent 5% of primary tumours. They are second most common malignant tumours of the bone in children. Subtypes include osseous and extraosseous. Metastases at presentation are seen in 20% of patients, mostly involving the lungs [46]. History may be positive of prior childhood malignancies treated with irradiation or chemotherapy. Most patients present with an enlarging mass that may be asymptomatic or painful. Destructive lesions due to osteolysis are evident on radiographs.

83.20 Conclusion

Sarcomas are aggressive tumours, fortunately rare in the head and neck regions except for rhabdomyosarcoma in children, which has shown good, improved outcomes with current treatment regimens. The primary treatment modality is surgery, often preceded by neoadjuvant chemotherapy and followed by postoperative chemoradiotherapy. Large tumours with a risk of positive surgical margins and histologically high-grade tumours are adverse features. Age is an independent prognostic factor in children and adults with sarcomas arising in Paget's disease for bone.

Treatment regiments are often institution-dependent and biased. Given the lack of randomised controlled trials and difficulty in interpreting meta-analysis, close cooperation and data sharing between centres can go a long way in improving treatment outcomes for this diverse group of patients.

References

1. Kevin AP, Tristan G, Marilene BW. Head and neck sarcomas: analysis of the SEER database. Otolaryngol Head Neck Surg. 2014 Oct;151(4):627–33.
2. Vassiliou LV, Lalabekyan B, Jay A, Liew C, Whelan J, Newman L, et al. Head and neck sarcomas: A single institute series. Oral Oncol. 2017 Feb;65:16–22.
3. O'Neill JP, Bilsky MH, Kraus D. Head and neck sarcomas: epidemiology, pathology, and management. Neurosurg Clin N Am. 2013 Jan;24(1):67–78.
4. Meis-Kindblom JM, Kindblom LG. Angiosarcoma of soft tissue: a study of 80 cases. Am J Surg Pathol. 1998 Jun;22(6):683–97.
5. Kraus DH, Dubner S, Harrison LB, Strong EW, Hajdu SI, Kher U, et al. Prognostic factors for recurrence and survival in head and neck soft tissue sarcomas. Cancer. 1994;74:697–702.
6. Young RJ, Brown NJ, Reed MW, Hughes D, Woll PJ. Angiosarcoma. Lancet Oncol. 2010 Oct;11(10):983–91.
7. Sturgis EM, Potter BO. Sarcomas of the head and neck region. Curr Opin Oncol. 2003;15:239–52.
8. Tran LM, Mark R, Meier R, Calcaterra TC, Parker RG. Sarcomas of the head and neck. Prognostic factors and treatment strategies. Cancer. 1992 Jul 1;70(1):169–77.
9. Soliman H, Ferrari A, Thomas D. Sarcoma in the young adult population: an international view. Semin Oncol. 2009 Jun;36(3):227–36.
10. Huang NC, Wann SR, Chang HT, Lin SL, Wang JS, Guo HR. Arsenic, vinyl chloride, viral hepatitis, and hepatic angiosarcoma: a hospital-based study and review of literature in Taiwan. BMC Gastroenterol. 2011 Dec 26;11:142.
11. Enjoji M, Hashimoto H, Tsuneyoshi M, Iwasaki H. Malignant fibrous histiocytoma. A clinicopathologic study of 130 cases. Acta Pathol Jpn. 1980;30:727–41.
12. Beral V, Peterman TA, Berkelman RL, Jaffe HW. Kaposi's sarcoma among persons with AIDS: a sexually transmitted infection? Lancet. 1990;335:123–8.
13. Edge SB, Byrd DR. AJCC cancer staging manual. 7th ed. New York: Springer; 2010. p. 291–8.
14. Shuman AG, Brennan MF, Palmer FL, Kuk D, Moraco N, Singer S, et al. Soft tissue sarcoma of the head and neck: nomogram validation and analysis of staging systems. J Surg Oncol. 2015 May;111(6):690–5.
15. Meazza C, Ferrari A, Casanova M, Massimino M, Luksch R, Spreafico F, et al. Rhabdomyosarcoma of the head and neck region: experience at the paediatric unit of the Istituto Nazionale Tumori. Milan J Otolaryngol. 2006 Feb;35(1):53–9.
16. Parravicini C, Olsen SJ, Capra M, Poli F, Sirchia G, Gao SJ, et al. Risk of Kaposi's sarcoma-associated herpes virus transmission from donor allograft among Italian post transplants Kaposi's sarcoma patients. Blood. 1997 Oct 1;90(7):2826–9.

17. Patel SG, See AC, Williamson PA, Archer DJ, Evans PH. Radiation induced sarcoma of the head and neck. Head Neck. 1999 Jul;21(4):346–54.
18. Bentz BG, Singh B, Woodruff J, Shah PJ, Kraus D. Head and neck soft tissue sarcomas: a multivariate analysis of outcomes. Ann Surg Oncol. 2004 Jun;11(6):619–28.
19. Huber GF, Matthews TW, Dort JC. Soft tissue sarcomas of the head and neck: a retrospective analysis of the Alberta experience 1974 to 1999. Laryngoscope. 2006 May;116(5):780–5.
20. Jernstrom P. Synovial sarcoma of the pharynx; report of a case. Am J Clin Pathol. 1954 Aug;24(8):957–61.
21. Carrillo R, Rodriguez-Peralto JL, Batsakis JG. Synovial sarcomas of the head and neck. Ann Otol Rhinol Laryngol. 1992 Apr;101(4):367–70.
22. Wanebo HJ, Koness RJ, MacFarlane JK, Eilber FR, Byers RM, Elias EG, et al. Head and neck sarcoma: report of the head and neck sarcoma registry. Society of head and neck surgeons committee on research. Head Neck. 1992 Jan–Feb;14(1):1–7.
23. LeVay J, O'Sullivan B, Catton C, Bell R, Fornasier V, Cummings B, et al. Outcome and prognostic factors in soft tissue sarcoma in the adult. Int J Radiat Oncol Biol Phys. 1993 Dec 1;27(5):1091–9.
24. Fletcher CD. Distinctive soft tissue tumours of the head and neck. Mod Pathol. 2002 Mar;15(3):324–30.
25. Fernandes R, Nikitakis NG, Pazoki A, Ord RA. Osteogenic sarcoma of the jaw: a 10-year experience. J Oral Maxillofac Surg. 2007 Jul;65(7):1286–91.
26. Lee SY, Lim YC, Song MH, Seok JY, Lee WS, Choi EC. Chondrosarcoma of the head and neck. Yonsei Med J. 2005;46(2):228–32.
27. Krishnamurthy A, Palaniappan R. Osteosarcomas of the head and neck region: a case series with a review of literature. J Maxillofac Oral Surg. 2018 Mar;17(1):38–43.
28. Clair JM, Arshi A, Abemayor E, John MS. Synovial cell sarcoma of the head and neck: an analysis of 167 cases using the SEER database. JAMA Otolaryngol Head Neck Surg. 2016 Jun 1;142(6):576–83.
29. Gopalakrishnan V, Amini B, Wagner MJ, Nowell EN, Lazar AJ, Benjamin RS, et al. Synovial sarcoma of the head and neck: a single institution review. Sarcoma. 2017 Jun 5;2017:2016752.
30. Breakey RW, Crowley TP, Anderson IB, Milner RH, Ragbir M. The surgical management of head and neck sarcoma: the Newcastle experience. J Plast Reconstr Aesthet Surg. 2017 Jan;70(1):78–84.
31. Marina N, Gebhardt M, Teot L, Gorlick R. Biology and therapeutic advances for paediatric osteosarcoma. Oncologist. July 2004;9(4):422–41.
32. Abdelfatah E, Guzzetta AA, Nagarajan N, Wolfgang CL, Pawlik TM, Ahuja N, et al. Long-term outcomes in treatment of retroperitoneal sarcomas: a 15-year single-institution evaluation of prognostic features. J Surg Oncol. 2016 Jul;114(1):56–64.
33. Dangoor A, Seddon B, Gerrand C, Grimer R, Whelan J, Judson I. UK guidelines for the management of soft tissue sarcomas. Clan Sarcoma Res. 2016;6:20.
34. Gerrand C, Athanasou N, Brennan B, Grimer R, Judons I, Morland B, et al. British Sarcoma Group. UK guidelines for the management of bone sarcomas. Clin Sarcoma Res. 2016 May 4;6:7.
35. O'Sullivan B, Patel S, Sturgis E. AJCC cancer staging manual. In: Amin MB, Edge S, Greene F, Byrd DR, Brookland RK, Washington MK, editors. AJCC cancer staging man. 8th ed. New York: Springer; 2017. p. 1032.
36. Wu J, Wang C, Li M, Luo C, Liu X, Xie L, et al. 3D computed tomography angiography as a novel post-processing approach in diagnosis of paediatric malignant bone tumours. J Xray Sci Technol. 2018;26(1):147–54.
37. Ma L, Zhou Y, Zhu Y, Lin Z, Chen L, Mao C, et al. 3D-printed guiding templates for improved osteosarcoma resection. Sci Rep. 2016 Mar 21;6:23335.
38. Mücke T, Mitchell DA, Tannapfel A, Wolff KD, Loeffelbein DJ, Kanatas A. Effect of neoadjuvant treatment in the management of osteosarcomas of the head and neck. J Cancer Res Clin Oncol. 2014 Jan;140(1):127–31.
39. Liu CY, Yen CC, Chen WM, Chen TH, Chen PC, Yen CC, et al. Soft tissue sarcoma of extremities: the prognostic significance of adequate surgical margins in primary operation and reoperation after recurrence. Ann Surg Oncol. 2010;17:2102–11.
40. Fechner RE, Mills SE. Atlas of tumour pathology. Washington, DC: Armed Forces Institute of Pathology; 1993.
41. Tandon A, Sethi K, Singh AP. Oral rhabdomyosarcoma: a review. J Clin Exp Dent. 2012;4(5):e302–8.
42. Thariat J, Tessonnier T, Bonvalot S, Lerouge D, Mammar H, Vogin G, et al. Proton therapy in soft tissue and bone sarcomas. Bull Cancer. 2018 Sep;105(9):830–8.
43. Sitenga JL, Aird GA, Nguyen A, Vaudreuil A, Huerter C. Clinical features and surgical treatment of schwannoma affecting the base of the tongue: a systematic review. Int Arch Otorhinolaryngol. 2017 Oct;21(4):408–13.
44. Wiener ES. Head and neck rhabdomyosarcoma. Semin Pediatr Surg. 1994 Aug;3(3):203–6.
45. Friedman-Kien AE, Laubenstein LJ, Rubinstein P, Buimovici-Klein E, Marmor M, Zolla-Pazner S, et al. Disseminated Kaposi's sarcoma in homosexual men. Ann Intern Med. 1982;96:693–700.
46. Kridis WB, Toumi N, Chaari H, Khanfir A, Ayadi K, Frikha M, et al. A review of Ewing sarcoma treatment: is it still a subject of debate? Rev Recent Clin Trials. 2017;12(1):19–23.

Adjunctive Therapy in Oral Cancer

84

Amit Dhawan

84.1 Introduction

Oral cancer is the sixth most common cancer in the world, primarily caused by consuming tobacco and its products, alcoholism, nutritional deficiencies, poor oral hygiene, certain strains of human papillomavirus (HPV) and genetic predilection [1, 2]. Considering global incidence of oral cancer, more than 50% of overall head and neck cancer are occurring in Asian subcontinent with India having maximum numbers of these patients. According to some epidemiological studies in Asian Indian population, approximately 80,000 to 1,20,000 new patients of oral cancers are being diagnosed yearly, making oral cancer the third most common cancer in India after lung cancer [1]. Oral cavity cancers are primarily treated surgically owing to gross visual disease, easy accessibility, and less chance of obtaining the R1 resection (resection with positive margins). Retrospectively, all T1 and some of T2 lesions of oral cavity were treated with primary radiotherapy with curative intent, but the results were more promising with upfront surgery followed by some kind of adjuvant treatment depending upon the final histopathology report. Developing countries like India have nonstandardized oral cancer screening protocols due to which most of the oral cancer patients are missed at an early stage and are presented at an advanced stage (stage III–stage IV) with higher T stage (T3–T4) and dissemination of disease in the lymphatics of the neck which further reduces the prognosis for the survivability of the patients. There are other independent predictors on which prognosis of an oral cancer patient depends on like depth of invasion of tumor, involvement of lymph nodes in the neck (lymph node ratio), pattern of invasion of tumor, extranodal extension, and presence of positive margins after surgery. In the recent past, advanced-stage (stage III–stage IV) oral cancer was primarily managed by upfront ablative resection and neck dissection followed by postoperative adjunctive radiotherapy depending upon the other predictors of prognosis. This dual modality approach of followed by radiotherapy has given promising results in advanced-stage cancers, but the overall survival benefit came out to be as low as 40% [2–5].

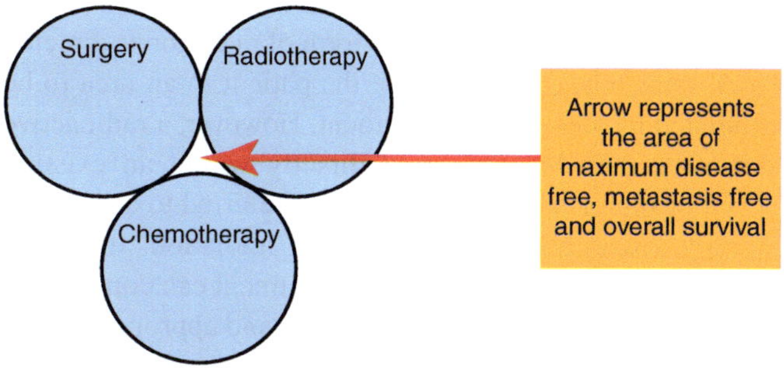

©Association of Oral and Maxillofacial Surgeons of India

Fig. 84.1 The three major treatment modalities available for the treatment of oral cancer

In 2004, two large-scale trials were conducted, Radiation Therapy Oncology Group (RTOG) 9501 in America and European organization for Research and Treatment of Cancer (EORTC) 22,931. The results of these trials had provided the new insights for the management of advanced head and neck squamous cell carcinoma. The evidence from these landmark trials confirms the use of chemotherapy to the adjuvant radiation regime in the treatment of advanced-stage squamous cell carcinoma patients [5, 6].

The addition of chemotherapy may result in better locoregional control, overall survival, and metastasis-free survival in these patients. The three major pillars of treatment for oral squamous cell carcinoma are surgery, radiotherapy, and chemotherapy. To get the maximum survival advantage from these treatment modalities, all the three treatment modalities have to be used as an adjunct to each other [2, 3] (Fig. 84.1).

A. Dhawan (✉)
Department of Oral and Maxillofacial Surgery, SGRD Dental Institute, Amritsar, India

K. Bonanthaya et al. (eds.), *Oral and Maxillofacial Surgery for the Clinician*, https://doi.org/10.1007/978-981-15-1346-6_84

84.2 Basic Principles of Radiotherapy

When the radiation is used for the purpose of treatment, especially in the patients of oral cancer, it is referred to as radiation therapy or radiotherapy. Radiotherapy is frequently used in as an adjunctive therapy or adjuvant therapy, to improve both local-regional control and overall survival. Radiation therapy is thought to kill tumor cells via damage to their DNA. The amount of radiation is typically measured in the unit gray (Gy), which represents joules of energy per kilogram. The following gives the conversion between grays, radiation absorbed dose (rad), and centigrays: 1 Gy = 100 rad = 100 cGy [7, 8].

External beam radiotherapy refers to the treatment, when a targeted beam of energy in the form of radiation is directed from a machine placed outside the patient to an area to be irradiated located within the patient. However, a radioactive substance may be introduced directly within an existing tumor or tumor-bearing area which is referred to as brachytherapy. Arranging for a patient's radiation treatment involves a number of steps before treatment can commence, of which the first is a dental evaluation and appropriate dental care. After consultation, a patient is simulated, which usually involves obtaining a computed tomographic (CT) scan, while the patient is immobilized with a face mask. Afterward, the radiation oncologist outlines the disease on the scan (contouring). Then a medical physicist and dosimetrist devise a method to deliver the radiation safely to the patient while avoiding radiation to normal anatomical structures. At the time of treatment, the radiation therapists verify that the patient lines up appropriately before treatment can begin. Immobilization of the patient is carried out with a predesigned face mask made up of a thermoplastic material. It is to be noted that accurate positioning of the patient without movement and the ability to recreate the same position of the patient every time (up to 6 weeks) are important factors for overall effective radiation treatment of the patient [7–10].

84.2.1 Biology of Radiation Therapy

The current understanding of radiotherapy techniques makes use of radiobiological principles for better treatment planning and outcomes. These principles influence the response of both normal tissues and of tumor clonogens to ionizing radiation, and a basic understanding and application of these principles are vital to improve the narrow therapeutic ratio of tumor versus normal tissue damage.

The 5R' concept of radiobiology is as follows [9, 10]:

- *Reoxygention*: This refers to the process by which surviving hypoxic tumor clonogens become reoxygenated after a period of radiotherapy.
- *Repair*: This refers to the process by which tumor clonogens damaged by radiation may restore cell integrity to its full potential.
- *Redistribution*: Distribution of tumor clonogens to a more even cell age distribution after selective cell killing in certain phases of the cell cycle.
- *Repopulation:* This refers to the process by which tumor clonogens can replenish number of cells following a period of radiation therapy.
- *Radiosensitivity*: This refers to a dosage of radiation required to make a defined level of cell inactivation after radiation exposure.

84.2.2 Primary Radiotherapy

This is also called as radical radiotherapy. The indications of primary radiotherapy only include early-stage oral cancers like carcinoma of lip, ventral surface of tongue, and floor of mouth. According to some reports, primary radiotherapy is indicated for treating T1 and T2 cancers with proliferative character. It is believed that the local control and overall survival of the patients are similar in these cases without upfront surgery with an added advantage of preservation of cosmetic, anatomic, and functional integrity of the head and neck region. The literature supports the use of postoperative radiotherapy instead of preoperative radiotherapy even for small-sized tumors as the locoregional recurrence is reported to be slightly more in primary radiotherapy group as compared to postoperative radiotherapy group, but the survival advantage is not statistically significant.

After radiation therapy, the preferred method for assessment of tumor response, in addition to clinical and endoscopic examination, is a posttreatment positron-emission tomographic (PET)/CT scan at 12 weeks. In most patients with a complete response to therapy and negative PET scan results, routine neck dissection is not recommended in the postoperative setting.

84.2.3 Indications of Adjuvant Radiotherapy

The treatment for the stage III and stage IV oral cancer is complex. According to current National Comprehensive Cancer

Network (NCCN) guidelines, single-modality treatment with either surgery or radiotherapy is recommended for approximately 30% to 40% of initial stage oral carcinoma patients (stage I and II). Both modalities of treatment have resulted in comparable survival benefit in these patients. On the other hand, combined modality treatment is generally recommended for the approximately 60% of patients with locally or regionally advanced disease at diagnosis. The treatment in these individuals depends on factors such as site of the disease, stage, pathological findings, and presence of adverse features in the resected specimen. Several studies have classified the oral cancer patients into low risk, medium risk, and high risk [2, 3].

Postsurgical adjuvant radiotherapy is indicated according to the presence of adverse features on final histopathology.

The adverse features refer to extranodal extension, lymphovascular invasion, and perineural invasion.

Patients who are classified as high or intermediate risk of relapse benefit the most from the addition of postoperative radiotherapy.

The indications of adjuvant radiotherapy after primary ablative surgery in oral cancer patients are as follows:

- Stage III and stage IV oral squamous cell carcinoma patients.
- Positive surgical margins: presence of invasive carcinoma at the border.
- Presence of extranodal extension.
- Involvement of more than two levels of lymph nodes (multiple nodal metastasis).
- Perineural invasion.

Often, radiation to the head and neck involves the selection of different doses depending on the amount of disease in that area. Typically, gross disease receives a dose of 70 Gy. Areas at high risk of microscopic disease often receive a dose of between 60 and 66 Gy. Areas at low risk of microscopic disease typically receive a dose of 50–54 Gy. The areas designated at high risk and low risk will depend on the site of occurrence of disease, the stage, and presence of pathological adverse features. The most common fraction size is 2 Gy of radiation per day [10–13].

84.2.4 Effect of Radiation Treatment Delay

Postsurgical radiation delay has a profound effect on overall survival of patient. Tumati V et al. found an association between treatment delays and oncologic outcomes in patients treated with surgery followed by post-op radiotherapy in a total of 277 patients of oral and oropharyngeal carcinoma. On multivariate analysis it was observed that radiation treatment time had a significant impact on locoregional recurrence in these patients. The authors found out that delays in the postoperative radiation therapy >43 days were associated with statistically significant locoregional recurrences ($p = 0.02$) in patients with non-p16-positive cancers. Many investigators have studies in coherence with the above conclusions. An increase in distant metastasis appears to be the mechanism by which prolonged time to treatment initiation leads to worse overall survival [14].

84.3 Radiotherapy Techniques

Depending upon the indication and treatment plan, there are multiple techniques with which radiation therapy can be delivered to a patient undergoing treatment for oral cancer. The techniques of radiotherapy should deliver the calculated radiation dose to the patient as per treatment plan without much toxic effects to the normal tissues. Some of the radiation techniques are listed below (Table 84.1) [15–19].

Table 84.1 Radiation techniques

Radiotherapy technique	Indications	Advantages
Brachytherapy (a) Interstitial brachytherapy (b) Intraluminal brachytherapy	T1 and T2 tongue and floor of mouth cancers	Radiotherapy source placed directly into the tissues to be irradiated. Less chances of systemic toxicities and treatment interruption.
Conventional radiotherapy	For high-risk oral carcinoma patients	Well established with known pattern of response, local control, and toxicities
Intensity-modulated radiation therapy (IMRT)	Advanced approach to three-dimensional treatment planning and conformal approach. For dose calculated radiation delivery to target volume.	Allows for greater sparing of salivary glands, esophagus, optic nerve, spinal cord, and brain stem. Allows treatment to be delivered in single treatment phase. Offers the possibility of simultaneously delivering higher radiation to regions of gross disease and lower doses to areas of microscopic disease.
Image-guided radiation therapy (IGRT)	Advances in real-time imaging during radiotherapy	Targeted delivery of radiotherapy which spares the vital structures immediately adjacent to high-dose regions

84.3.1 Radiation Dosage and Fractionation Schedule

Radiotherapy schedule, conventionally, is followed for 5–7 days a week with defined breaks in the treatment for reoxygenation and repair of normal tissue cells of the body for target effectiveness of radiotherapy. According to the literature, the tumor cells repopulate in between the radiotherapy regime especially after fourth week, so unscheduled breaks between the course of radiotherapy are not recommended by the radiation oncologists. That's the reason different fractionation schedules have been advocated by the radiation oncologists for successful completion of the treatment without unnecessary treatment breaks which can have a negative impact on the final outcome of the patients [15–19].

- *Conventional fractionation*: Every week for 5 days Monday to Friday.
- *Hyperfractionation*: When more than one fraction of lower radiation dose is delivered to the patient in the same day, it is known as hyperfractionation. The advantage is the treatment can be completed in a shorter time than conventional fractionation, yet the same total dose is delivered with better disease control and without increase in the toxicity.
- *Accelerated hyperfractionation*: More than one fraction of radiotherapy is given everyday or radiotherapy is given more than 5 days per week, the disadvantage is the increase in the toxicity due to no treatment breaks.
- *Continuous hyperfractionated radiotherapy*: When the radiation fraction is delivered thrice daily for the whole week, it is known as continuous hyperfractionated radiotherapy. This uninterrupted radiotherapy regime finishes the total dosage of radiation in 12–14 days.

84.4 Complications of Radiotherapy

Though the dual-modality treatment (surgery and radiotherapy) has become a norm for the treatment of advanced-stage (stage III–stage IV) oral squamous cell carcinoma, there are some unavoidable toxic effects of radiation therapy which can affect the quality of life (QOL) of the patient. Radiotherapy has proved to be very effective in improving the locoregional control and overall survival of the patient, but there are short-term and long-term sequel of radiotherapy which sometimes limit the effectiveness of the therapy due to breaks in the treatment schedule. The intensity of the complications and toxic effects depends upon the dose of delivered radiation and the site exposed to the radiation therapy. Radiation techniques like intensity-modulated radiotherapy IMRT and image-guided radiotherapy IGRT are helpful in controlling the delivered dosage of radiation to the patient, thereby decreasing the rate of complications and increasing the response of the patient toward the therapy.

Depending upon the response to radiation, the complications have been divided into acute toxic effects or short-term sequel and chronic toxic effects or long-term sequel.

IMRT requires that the radiation oncologist outline the tumor, the areas at risk for microscopic spreading, and the critical normal structures on every CT slice (contouring). Outlining the gross disease (gross tumor volume [GTV]) and areas at risk of microscopic spreading (clinical target volume [CTV]) requires a thorough understanding of the anatomy of the region and is significantly more labor-intensive than prior two-dimensional or conventional radiation therapy techniques.

84.5 Acute Toxic Effects

84.5.1 Xerostomia

Xerostomia is also referred to as dry mouth. It is one of the most common acute and chronic side effects of radiotherapy. Xerostomia starts from the first week of radiotherapy and is a more common complaint in the first 2 weeks in those patients in whom submandibular salivary glands have been removed as part of the neck dissection. As far as possible, contralateral submandibular salivary gland should be preserved in uninvolved neck when bilateral neck dissection has to be performed. With the traditional radiographic techniques, parotid gland was not spared which resulted in more profound effects of dry mouth leading to halitosis, stasis of thick saliva, dysphagia, and cervical caries. Stasis of thick saliva leads to dysphagia like symptoms and even aggravation of mucositis earlier in the course of therapy.

Intensity-modulated radiotherapy technique and image-guided radiotherapy have revolutionized the concept of delivery of radiotherapy, thereby minimizing the risks of development of unavoidable side effects like xerostomia leading to more acceptable quality of life. A randomized controlled trial by Nutting et al. confirmed the reduction in postradiation xerostomia significantly. They compared intensity-modulated radiotherapy without taking parotid gland in the radiation field and conventional radiation therapy for all patients. About 83% patients developed grade II or higher xerostomia with conventional radiotherapy as compared to 29% of patients who were adopted for parotid sparing intensity-modulated radiotherapy [19].

Many investigators have assessed the relationship of radiation dosage to parotid and submandibular gland and severity of xerostomia at weekly intervals. The inference from these studies point toward the damage to plasma membrane of secretory granules of glands. Another observation was that the flow of saliva from submandibular and parotid glands considerably decreases up to less than 20% of pretreatment values by the end of the second week of radiation therapy. The recommendations are to use current radiotherapy techniques like intensity-modulated radiation therapy to spare the submandibular and parotid gland with lowest possible exposure. The treatment of xerostomia converges toward the usage of sialagogues, artificial saliva, and fluid therapy along with reassurance to the patient [20, 21].

84.5.2 Oral Mucositis

Oral mucositis due to radiotherapy and other systemic therapies in oral cancer treatment represents a major complication causing a wide spectrum of clinical signs and symptoms. Oral mucositis may hamper the quality of life, resulting from debilitating oral pain and bleeding from oral cavity, dysphagia, infections, and inability to chew food and may interfere with the ongoing radiation treatment, ultimately jeopardizing overall patient outcome. According to certain reports, third week of post-radiotherapy is the most crucial time when the mucositis begins to set in and the severity increases in the subsequent weeks. The severity and agony from mucositis is directly proportional to the total dosage of radiation delivered and the volume of irradiated tissue in a specified interval of time. Mild initial erythema to patchy mucositis (characterized by white patches of fibrinous exudate on an erythematous base) to confluent mucositis (where the exudative patches coalesce) are the presenting symptoms of progression of ongoing mucositis in the oral cavity. On the other hand, if there is an evidence of bleeding to touch from the oral ulcers, it is considered as severe to fulminant mucositis.

Confluent mucositis, common toxicity criteria (CTC) grade 3, is seen in 40–80% of patients receiving more than 60Gy (or equivalent), more frequently in those receiving concurrent chemotherapy or accelerated radiotherapy. The patients should be advised to keep good oral hygiene with 0.12% chlorhexidine gluconate along with sialagogues or artificial saliva which will have protective action for the underlying oral mucosa thus reducing the severity of symptoms and relieve the pain. A narcotic analgesic like tramadol is recommended for pain from mucositis. There are some reports which favor elemental zinc or zinc carnosine complex for relieving the symptoms of severe mucositis.

The role of nonalcohol-based mouthwash has been established by many authors for relieving the debilitating effects of mucositis. Topical steroids had been used in past for the treatment of mucositis in severe stages, but their use is constantly discouraged in the current settings. The radioprotectant drug amifostine has been investigated as a means of reducing the incidence of xerostomia and mucositis. The route of administration of amifostine is intravenous everyday prior to initiation of radiotherapy. Patient should be constantly monitored for hypotension and nausea postoperatively.

Moreover, WHO recommends the constant nutrition support to the patients undergoing radiotherapy which will have a positive effect on the recovery from acute mucositis. If oral route is jeopardized, the nasogastric feeding, PEG percutaneous endoscopic gastrostomy, and parenteral nutrition should be considered based on the severity of mucositis. Recovery of severe mucositis may not begin until 2–3 weeks after treatment completion then take up to 4–8 weeks to regain normal swallowing. The recovery is mostly complete; however, only <5% of patients may remain PEG dependent.

Other known acute toxic effects of radiotherapy are erythema of facial and skin of the neck, lethargy, loss of taste, and smell. Erythema of the skin takes about 7–10 days of complete remission after cessation of radiation therapy; however the skin remains photosensitive even after the completion of therapy [20–22].

84.6 Chronic Toxic Effects

There are multiple chronic toxic effects of radiotherapy enumerated in the literature by different authors and radiation oncologists (Table 84.2). It has been found out that the chronic effects of radiotherapy are more dependent on dosage than the acute effects of radiation.

84.6.1 Osteoradionecrosis of Maxilla and Mandible

Currently, one of the most serious long-term or chronic complications of radiotherapy to the head and neck region is osteoradionecrosis of the jaws. The associated morbidity of this complication and its subsequent treatment will include close observation and/or radical surgical resection followed by reconstruction with free fibula, deep circumflex iliac artery flap (DCIA), or a variety of pedicled and soft tissue free flaps depending upon the severity of necrosis and systemic condition of the patient.

The etiopathogenesis of osteoradionecrosis have been explained on the basis of current theory of Delanian and Lefaix [23]. It states that osteoradionecrosis of the jaws is a radiation-induced fibrosis with histopathological formation of phases which appear similar to those of chronic wounds. There is a histopathological picture of combination of dead or dying osteoblasts without replication of new osteoblasts and excessive proliferation of myofibroblasts. This condition is manifested as loss of trabeculae of existing bone and subsequent decrease in the quality and structure of underlying bone.

Among the risk factors for the development of osteoradionecrosis, total radiation dose delivered to the bone, in a specified period of time, remains the most important and crucial risk factor. The cumulative dose of radiation to the bone will

Table 84.2 Chronic effects of radiotherapy

Chronic toxicity	Risk factors	Prevention strategy
Osteoradionecrosis, mandible, maxilla	Primary bone surgery (marginal mandibulectomy), maxillary osteoradionecrosis is rare. Dentulous patients High radiation dose >65 Gy to the mandible. Traumatic extractions. Women > men. Conventional radiotherapy techniques. Age of the patient.	IMRT, IGRT, calculating the dose to be delivered to mandible. Proper dental consultation and rehabilitation before radiotherapy. Appropriate coverage of remaining bone with free vascularized soft tissue flaps
Trismus	Postoperative radiation to the masseter muscle and pterygoid muscles. Location of the tumor in the oral cavity. In case of maxillary tumors, reconstruction with temporalis flap pose greater risk of developing trismus after radiotherapy	Early institution of radiotherapy within 4–6 weeks of surgery Use of microvascular free flaps for reconstruction which provide extra soft and pliable tissue
Hypothyroidism	Irradiation of thyroid tissue at higher dose. Female patient	Dosage to the thyroid gland should be limited. Use of thyroid shield
Nerve injury (damage to spinal cord, optic nerve, vestibulocochlear nerve)	Radiation dosage >50–54 Gy pose more risk of development of nerve injuries	IMRT, IGRT, calculating the dose to be delivered
Radiation-induced cancers	Radiation-induced tumors are mostly sarcomatous and develop many years after institution of radiotherapy	Regular follow-up of the patient

produce an environment of hypo-cellularity and hypo-vascularity leading to the cause and effect relationship in the underlying bone. Maxillary bone is less susceptible to the development of necrosis than mandible as maxilla has a more porous structure of bone with more vascularity as compared to a single terminal inferior alveolar artery in mandible which undergoes fibrosis after high-dose radiation therapy. Moreover, muscles of facial expression and thick mucoperiosteum in maxilla prevent it from getting hypo-vascular in a shorter period of radiation therapy. Facial artery is notoriously unreliable to produce collateral blood supply to the mandible which is insufficient to prevent osteoradionecrosis. On the other hand, in case of post-neck dissection patients, the facial artery is most of the time ligated in the ipsilateral side during the clearance of level IB (submandibular) group of lymph nodes.

According to a comparative study conducted by Kuhnt et al. [22] on 776 patients with head and neck cancer who underwent intensity-modulated radiotherapy as radical radiotherapy for the treatment of head and neck cancer and as postoperative radiotherapy, the highest cumulative incidence of osteoradionecrosis was found to be 12.4%, and relative frequency was 6.6%. The interesting inference of this study is the actual risk for the development of osteoradionecrosis remains there for a lifetime of the patient and may increase by a factor of two in long-term survivors. There remains a highest risk for the development of osteoradionecrosis in patients who had undergone primary bone surgery during tumor resection (hazard ratio: 5.87 95% confidence interval) and in patients with tumor located in the oral cavity than other sub-sites in the head and neck region. This means the dental treatment including extractions and minor surgical procedures should be performed well before in the patients advised for adjuvant radiotherapy in which mandibular resection (marginal mandibulectomy or segmental mandibulectomy) has been advised. Moreover, it is prudent to cover the marginal mandibulectomy defect with the free flap or a soft tissue pedicled flap to maintain vascularity so as to prevent postradiation chance of osteoradionecrosis.

Gender, dentition (dentulous vs edentulous), and concurrent chemotherapy have no significant clinically relevant influence on the development of osteoradionecrosis. Males are found to have three times more risk for the development of osteoradionecrosis than women. According to a study conducted by Gabriela et al., 25% of patients developed refractory osteoradionecrosis which required some kind of resection and subsequent reconstruction when the radiation dose delivered were more than 66Gy at a daily fraction exceeding up to 2.2Gy as compared to no evidence of osteoradionecrosis at or below 65 Gy of radiation dose [24]. On the other hand, as the daily dose of radiation decreases to 1.8 and 1.9 Gy, and a total dose of 69–75.6 Gy, the rate was 19.6%. Daily dose of radiation is thus considered to be a most significant factor in determining likelihood of developing osteoradionecrosis especially in cases of oral cancer. The close proximity of the cancer to the mandible (with in 1 mm) receiving high dose of radiation remains the other risk factors for the development of osteoradionecrosis.

Prevention is better than the treatment of osteoradionecrosis. One study confirms the effectiveness of hyperbaric oxygen therapy in a very few number of patients. State-of-the-art radiotherapy techniques will limit the total absorbed dose to the mandible and potential sites in the oral cavity thus limiting the incidence of osteoradionecrosis [24, 25].

84.7 Principles of Chemotherapy

The oral cancer is considered as the sixth most common malignancy worldwide accounting up to 1,30,000 cases every year in a developing country like India. Due to poor screening facilities at primary examination level, lack of awareness among patients, and nonstandardization of public health sector, most of the cases are diagnosed when they have attained stage III and stage IV disease.

On the other hand, chemotherapy regimens for oral cancer treatment are evolving. There are multiple methods by which chemotherapy may be offered to the patients for the management of head and neck cancer to improve the overall outcomes in terms of survivability of patients.

Methods of providing chemotherapy for head and neck cancer patients are as follows:

- Single-modality treatment for palliation.
- As concomitant radiation therapy or concurrent chemoradiation (triple modality).
- As adjuvant therapy following surgical resection (dual modality).
- As definitive treatment for locoregionally advanced carcinoma primarily.
- As induction therapy or neoadjuvant therapy (NACT) before definitive treatment for prognostication of the primarily inoperable tumors.

Single-modality treatments usually have low efficacy in terms of locoregional recurrences. On the other hand, chemotherapy with or without radiotherapy poses the patient toward the risk of systemic toxicities and unwanted immunosuppression which may alter the overall result and outcomes of the patient undergoing cytotoxic therapy in any form [25–29].

84.7.1 Cytotoxic Chemotherapeutic Agents

While multiple cytotoxic drugs have been identified for the treatment of oral squamous cell carcinoma in addition to surgery and radiotherapy, some of the chemotherapy agents are listed below (Table 84.3).

84.7.2 Chemoradiation in Oral Cavity Cancers

Earlier it was thought that radiation therapy alone is effective for treating small T1 and T2 lesions of lower lip, floor of mouth, tongue, and palate within the oral cavity. After a decade, many centers adopted surgery alone for smaller lesions of oral cavity as primary treatment. Then a dual-modality approach (surgery followed by radiotherapy) was popularized for locally advanced carcinoma (stage III–stage IV AJCC eighth edition) of oral cavity. Hence, the dual-modality approach emerged as a conventional, widely accepted, and equally effective treatment option for the management of advanced (T3–T4) lesions. Conventionally, the combination of chemotherapy and radiotherapy, as primary treatment modality, had been reserved for those patients with unresectable disease or patients who refuse the surgical treatment.

It has been published by the RTOG trial reports that adjuvant radiotherapy improves the outcome of patients which received the surgical treatment for advanced-stage squamous cell carcinoma arising in the head and neck. At the same time, the disease-free survival and 5-year overall survival came out to be generally between 30 and 40% which is highly nonpromising. These trials also suggested that if the concurrent chemotherapy, using cytotoxic drugs, is added to the conventional postoperative radiotherapy regime, the effects of radiotherapy are intensified. This methodology of adjunctive treatment has significant amount of survival benefit than dual-modality treatment, and the chances of locore-

Table 84.3 Chemotherapy agents used in oral cancer

Chemotherapeutic drug	Mechanism of action	Toxicity and response
Platinum agents: Cisplatin, carboplatin, oxaliplatin	Inhibit DNA synthesis by forming intrastrand and interstrand cross-links between guanine-guanine pairs of DNA	Most active agent with response rates 20–50%. Dose rage is 80–120 mg/m^2 every 3–4 weeks. Renal toxicity, myelosuppression, neurological, and gastrointestinal toxicity (less with carboplatin)
Taxanes: Paclitaxel, docetaxel	Act by promoting the formation of tubulin dimers, stabilizing microtubules during cell division, and thereby leading to arrest of cells in G2/M phase of cell cycle	Particularly severe and life-threatening myelosuppression. Neutropenia, mucositis, and fluid retention Paclitaxel response up to 37% Docetaxel response 22–45%
5- fluorouracil: An antimetabolite	Depletion of nucleotides required for DNA synthesis and repair	Single-agent response is 15% Mucositis, diarrhea, myelosuppression
Methotrexate	Interferes with the use of folate used for DNA synthesis and repair inhibits dihydrofolate reductase (DHFR)	Most commonly used schedule is weekly intravenous bolus regime, using a dose of 40–60 mg/m^2. The objective response rate in this dose range is 10–30%
Cetuximab: a monoclonal antibody against human EGF receptor	It prevents binding of EGFR ligands, results in inhibition of function of the receptor	Significantly improved overall survival in head and neck squamous cell carcinoma patients Consistent severe acneiform skin rash

gional recurrences are likely to be less especially in high-risk patients postoperatively. In the last 10 years of research in the field of head and neck carcinoma treatment, the efficacy of triple-modality therapy has been justified in the literature for postoperative high-risk squamous cell carcinoma patients. Like RTOG a similar trial was conducted in Europe, the EORTC trial. This trial also reconfirmed the addition of adjuvant chemotherapy to the radiotherapy regime. The inference of this trial showed better rates of local control, disease-specific survival, and overall survival and significant decreased incidence of late toxic effects. Both these trials compared the addition of three planned cycles of concomitant cisplatin at 100 mg/m^2 every 3 weeks to radiotherapy (60–66 Gy, over 6–6.5 weeks, standard fractionation) with the same radiotherapy alone in patients with adverse feature of head and neck carcinoma. Therefore the concomitant therapy with cisplatin at 100 mg/m^2 every 3 weeks with adjuvant radiotherapy on day 1, day 22, and day 43 is the regimen of choice. The only limitations of these two trials were that these trials were not oral cancer specific. There are very few studies in the literature who have evaluated the concept of triple-modality therapy yet being site specific to oral cavity. Choi et al. retrospectively reviewed 861 patients with oral carcinoma treated in Korea from 1984 to 1996. Almost 63% of patients had stage III and stage IV cancer, and 36% had T3–T4 lesions. The authors concluded that triple-modality treatment (upfront surgery followed by postoperative chemoradiation) yielded a greater treatment response rate than dual-modality treatment [29]. On the other hand, Zhang et al. conducted a trial in oral cancer patients who received surgery followed by radiotherapy as a primary treatment modality. The trial found out that there is a 3.6 times more incidence to develop distant metastasis in surgery and radiation group as compared to surgery followed by chemoradiation group [3].

Box 84.1 Questions to be answered

Now the question arises.

1. Whether the addition of chemotherapy to the radiotherapy regime will improve the survival outcomes?
2. If the survival benefit is observed, does it have any effect on progression-free survival?
3. Is there any of incidence of chronic toxicities if the chemo radiation is used?
4. Does the technique of administering radiation have any profound effect in the outcome?
5. Whether the patients with adverse features (like: extranodal extension, lymphovascular invasion, and perineural spread) have improved outcomes with chemoradiation?

Explanation for Q1&2: Results of the recent study conducted by Stenson et al. revealed that patients who underwent chemoradiation as primary therapy for advanced-stage oral squamous cell carcinoma had a greater rate of metastasis-free and overall survival benefit with 66.9% disease-free or progression-free survival [30]. One of the recent single-institutional study conducted by Dhawan et al. on 128 patients of advanced-stage high-risk oral carcinoma shows an overall survival benefit of 10% in patients receiving chemoradiation as compared to patients receiving only radiation therapy after primary ablative surgery. This study was conducted in a subset of Asian Indian population to evaluate the benefits of multimodal therapy in the management of stage III/IV oral carcinoma [2]. Zhang et al. in their study showed a survival benefit of 11% in patients receiving chemoradiation as compared to radiation alone [3].

Explanation for Q-3: But the survival benefit doesn't come without a price to the patient. Along with improved survival comes the greater incidence of acute and chronic toxicities due to cytotoxic chemotherapeutic agents. The chances of recurrence always remain high even with the addition of chemotherapy due to the advanced stage and higher volume of the disease being treated. The recurrence potential of the lesion depends on the invasive pattern of tumor invasion at the first place and the presence of cancer stem cells in a given area. According to Pericot et al., high incidence of recurrence is associated with size of the primary tumor (T stage), and the difficulty in obtaining margins free of disease, after surgical resection. So obtaining a positive margin or a close margin (between 1 to less than 5 mm) after resection becomes an indication for administration of concurrent chemoradiation therapy. On the other hand, the development of myelosuppression, neutropenia, mucositis, and xerostomia is inevitable with triple-modality treatment [31].

Explanation for Q-4: The type of radiation (IMRT and routine radiotherapy) also affects the survival outcomes when used concurrently with chemotherapy as IMRT is more effective along with chemotherapy than with conventional radiotherapy.

Explanation for Q-5: Neck node involvement is also considered as an independent predictor of survival in oral cavity cancer. According to the literature, patients with nonpalpable disease in the neck or clinically N0 necks are having greater overall survival rate as compared to subsequent N stages. A recent study by Franceschi et al. found that among patients with involved neck nodes, survival rate was significantly lower when more than two levels of lymph nodes were involved, or when extranodal extension was observed. The adverse features which are found after final histopathological examination of primary as well as neck dissection specimen are currently addressed as extranodal extension, perineural invasion, and lymphovascular invasion. These patients are particularly at higher risk of disease progression and have higher death rates [32]. According to Zhang et al. [3], patients with extranodal extension and perineural invasion had improved disease-specific and metastasis-free survival in the surgery followed by chemoradiation group ($p < 0.05$). In a retrospective study conducted in 2016, authors found out that overall survival was significantly influenced by the type of modality and regional spread of disease. Chemoradiation after primary ablative surgery group had improved overall, disease-specific, disease-free, and metastasis-free survival compared to surgery followed by radiotherapy group even in patients with extranodal extensions, perineural spread, and lymphovascular invasion.

According to RTOG and EORTC landmark trials, there are some absolute indications for postoperative chemoradiation. These studies provided the base for the risk-adapted strategies in postoperative adjuvant therapy and *established extranodal extension and positive surgical margin as the absolute indications for adding concomitant systemic chemotherapy to adjuvant radiation*. However, proper patient assessment preoperatively is mandatory keeping in view the systemic toxicity due to chemoradiation.

Absolute Indications of Adjuvant Chemotherapy in Oral Cavity Cancers

According to RTOG trial, the definition of high-risk patients is as follows:

- Presence of tumor at the surgical resection margins—positive surgical margin.
- Extranodal extension.
- Clinical or radiographic involvement of level IV and level V lymph nodes.
- Stage of pT3 or pT4 with any N except T3N0 of the larynx.
- N2–N3 neck.
- Perineural invasion.
- Vascular embolism.

84.7.3 Induction Chemotherapy Before Surgery

Since 1982, during the days of early clinical trials on chemotherapeutic agents and their clinical advantage in head and neck squamous cell carcinoma, induction chemotherapy was thought to have potential benefits for treating head and neck cancers. Unfortunately, the higher response rates of these chemotherapeutic results have failed to result in statistically significant survival benefit. Induction chemotherapy before surgery is generally instituted in primarily unresectable oral cavity cancers at some centers. The efficacy of induction chemotherapy has yet to be proven in oral cancer treatment with regard to locoregional control and/or overall survival of these patients. The efficacy of induction chemotherapy to downstage oral cavity cancers was observed by a study conducted by Grau et al. in a prospective way with unresectable stage III–stage IV oral cavity cancers. They found out that disease-free survival at 5 years was 26% for patients undergoing resection and 22% for patients who received chemoradiation. Improved outcome is always at an expense of increased toxicity. There are other studies with comparable results which were carried out exclusively in oral cancer patients. Currently, induction chemotherapy cannot be recommended in resectable oral cancer patients for improvement in the survival [33].

84.7.4 Palliative Chemotherapy in Patients with Oral Cancer

Patients with recurrent and metastatic squamous cell carcinoma of head and neck are considered incurable with surgery or radiation. In these patients mainstay of treatment remains the systemic chemotherapy with cytotoxic chemotherapeutic drugs. Chemotherapeutic agents can be used either in combination regimen or as single agent in the management of metastatic oral cavity carcinomas. Radiation therapy with concurrent cetuximab, a monoclonal antibody to epidermal growth factor receptor (EGFR), has been shown to significantly improve overall survival rates compared with radiation therapy alone in the palliative setting. A direct randomized comparison of cetuximab versus platinum-based regimens is underway at many centers in the world. At present, platinum-based regimens (cisplatin, carboplatin) are preferred over other drugs, as long as patients can tolerate the regimen with acceptable complications [34–36].

84.8 Conclusions

Adjunctive therapies are included in the treatment regimen of oral squamous cell carcinoma to improve the disease-free, metastasis-free, and overall survival of the patients. Adjuvant radiotherapy is indicated in high-risk advanced-stage (stage III–stage IV) oral squamous cell carcinoma patients as dual modality. The complications and side effects of radiotherapy can be reduced by adopting advanced radiotherapy techniques like intensity-modulated radiotherapy, image-guided radiotherapy, and stereotactic radiotherapy. Concurrent chemoradiation therapy is adopted as primary treatment in patients with locally advanced oral cavity cancer whose disease is not amenable for surgical resection. Adjuvant chemoradiation is indicated in patients having postresection positive margins and with extranodal extensions or extracapsular invasion as a multimodality treatment. Consider cetuximab synchronously with radiotherapy in patients unsuitable for platinum-based chemoradiation.

References

1. Agarwal AK, Sethi A, Sareen D, Dhingra S. Oral and oropharyngeal squamous cell carcinoma in our population: the clinic-pathological and morphological description of 153 cases. Int J Morphol. 2011;29(3):686–93.
2. Dhawan A, Duggal P, Bhullar RS, Kaur T, Sandhu A, Kaur K. Efficacy of multimodal therapy in the survival outcomes of advanced-stage (stage III-stage IV) oral carcinoma patients: an institutional experience in Asian Indian population. J Maxillofac Oral Surg. 2018;17(1):89–94.
3. Zhang H, Dziegielewski PT, Biron VL, et al. Survival outcomes of patients with advanced oral cavity squamous cell carcinoma treated with multimodal therapy: a multi-institutional analysis. J Otolaryngol Head Neck Surg. 2013;42:30.
4. Cooper JS, Pajak TF, Forastiere A, et al. Precisely defining high-risk operable head and neck tumors based on RTOG #85–03 and #88–24:targets for postoperative radiochemotherapy? Head Neck. 1998;20:588–94.
5. Cooper JS, Pajak TF, Forastiere A, et al. Postoperative concurrent radiotherapy and chemotherapy for high risk squamous cell carcinoma of the head and neck. N Engl J Med. 2004;350:19.
6. Bernier J, Cooper JS, Pajak TF, et al. Defining risk levels in locally advanced head and neck cancers: a comparative analysis of concurrent postoperative radiation plus chemotherapy trials of the EORTC (#22931) and RTOG (#9501). Head Neck. 2005;27:843–50.
7. Liauw SL, Mancuso AA, Amdur RJ, Morris CG, Villaret DB, Werning JW, et al. Postradiotherapy neck dissection for lymph node-positive head and neck cancer: the use of computed tomography to manage the neck. J Clin Oncol. 2006;24(9):1421–7.
8. Fletcher GH. The role of irradiation in the management of squamous-cell carcinomas of the mouth and throat. Head Neck Surg. 1979;1:441–57.
9. Delclos L, Lindberg RD, Fletcher GH. Squamous cell carcinoma of the oral tongue and floor of mouth. Evaluation of interstitial radium therapy. AJR Am J Roentgenol. 1976;126:223–8.
10. NCCN Clinical Practice Guidelines in Oncology (NCCN Guidelines) Head and Neck Cancers. Version I. 2015. Available at: NCCN.org.
11. Chen PY, Chen HH, Hsiao JR, Yang MW, Hsueh WT, et al. Intensity-modulated radiotherapy improves outcomes in postoperative patients with squamous cell carcinoma of the oral cavity. Oral Oncol. 2012;48:747–52.
12. George JR, Yom SS, Wang SJ. Improved outcomes in adjuvant radiotherapy for oral cavity carcinoma at an academic center: a matched-pair analysis. Laryngoscope. 2014;124:1603–8.
13. Kreppel M, Eich HT, Bruggenolte C, Dreiseidler T, Rothamel D, et al. Preoperative vs. post- operative radiochemotherapy in patients with N2 squamous cell carcinoma of the oral cavity. Oral Oncol. 2012;48:1019–24.
14. Tumati V, Hoang L, Sumer BD, Truelson JM, Myers LL, Khan S, Hughes RS, Nedzi L, Sher DJ. Association between treatment delays and oncologic outcome in patients treated with surgery and radiotherapy for head and neck cancer. Head Neck. 2019 Feb;41(2):315–321.
15. Amit M, Yen TC, Liao CT, Chaturvedi P, Agarwal JP, et al. Improvement in survival of patients with oral cavity squamous cell carcinoma: an international collaborative study. Cancer. 2013;119:4242–8.
16. Hartley A, Cheah N. Postoperative radiotherapy in head and neck cancer. Stell and Maran's textbook of head and neck surgery and oncology, 5th edn, 2012.
17. Rowell N. Principles of radiotherapy. Stell and Maran's textbook of head and neck surgery and oncology, 5th edn, 2012.
18. Sher DJ, Thotakura V, Balboni TA, Norris CM Jr, Haddad RI, et al. Treatment of oral cavity squamous cell carcinoma with adjuvant or definitive intensity-modulated radiation therapy. Int J Radiat Oncol Biol Phys. 2011;81:e215–22.
19. Nutting CM, Morden JP, Harrington KJ, et al. Parotid-sparing intensity modulated versus conventional radiotherapy in head and neck cancer (PARSPORT): a phase 3 multi-centre randomised controlled trial. Lancet Oncol. 2011;12:127–36.
20. Overgaard J, Mohanti BK, Begum N, Ali R, Agarwal JP, et al. Five versus six fractions of radiotherapy per week for squamous-cell carcinoma of the head and neck (IAEA-ACC study): a randomised, multicentre trial. Lancet Oncol. 2010;11:553–60.
21. Beitler JJ, Zhang Q, Fu KK, Trotti A, Spencer SA, et al. Final results of local-regional control and late toxicity of RTOG 9003: a randomized trial of altered fractionation radiation for locally advanced head and neck cancer. Int J Radiat Oncol Biol Phys. 2014;89:13–20.
22. Kuhnt T, Stang A, Wienke A, Vordermark D, Schweyen R, Hey J. Potential risk factors for jaw osteoradionecrosis after radiotherapy for head and neck cancer. Radiat Oncol. 2016;11:101.
23. Delanian S, Lefaix JL. Current management for late normal tissue injury: radiation-induced fibrosis and necrosis. Semin Radiat Oncol. 2007 Apr;17(2):99–107.
24. Studer G, Bredell M, Studer S, et al. Risk profile for osteoradionecrosis of the mandible in IMRT era. Strahlenther Onkol. 2016;192:32.
25. Moon SH, Jung YS, Ryu JS, Choi SW, Park JY, et al. Outcomes of postoperative simultaneous modulated accelerated radiotherapy for head-and-neck squamous cell carcinoma. Int J Radiat Oncol Biol Phys. 2011;81:140–9.
26. Posner MR, Hershock DM, Blajman CR, Mickiewicz E, Winquist E, et al. Cisplatin and fluorouracil alone or with docetaxel in head and neck cancer. N Engl J Med. 2007;357:1705–15.
27. Bernier J, Domenge C, Ozsahin M, Matuszewska K, Lefebvre JL, et al. Postoperative irradiation with or without concomitant chemotherapy for locally advanced head and neck cancer. N Engl J Med. 2004;350:1945–1952.
28. Murthy V, Agarwal JP, Laskar SG, Gupta T, Budrukkar A, et al. Analysis of prognostic factors in 1180 patients with oral cavity primary cancer treated with definitive or adjuvant radio- therapy. J Cancer Res Ther. 2010;6:282–9.
29. Choi KK, Kim MJ, Yun PY, et al. Independent prognostic factors of 861 cases of oral squamous cell carcinoma in Korean adults. Oral Oncol. 2006;42:208–17.
30. Stenson KM, Kunnavakkam R, Cohen EEW, et al. Chemoradiation for patients with advanced oral cavity cancer. Laryngoscope. 2010;120:93–9.
31. Pericot J, Escriba JM, Valdes A, et al. Survival evaluation of treatment modality in squamous cell carcinoma of the oral cavity and oropharynx. J Cranio Maxillofac Surg. 2000;28:49–55.
32. Franceschi D, Gupta R, Spiro RH, et al. Improved survival in the treatment of squamous carcinoma of the oral tongue. Am J Surg. 1993;166:360–5.

33. Grau JJ, Estapé J, Blanch JL, Vilalta A, Castro V, Biete A, Daniels M. Neoadjuvant or adjuvant chemotherapy in the multidisciplinary oral cancer stage III and stage IV. Eur J Cancer B Oral Oncol. 1996;32(4):238–41. issn: 0964–1955
34. Bachaud JM, Cohen-Jonathan E, Alzieu C, David JM, Serrano E, Daly-Schveitzer N. Combined postoperative radiotherapy and weekly cisplatin infusion for locally advanced head and neck carcinoma: nal report of a randomized trial. Int J Radiat Oncol Biol Phys. 1996;36(5):999–1004.
35. Bonner JA, Harari PM, Giralt J, Azarnia N, Shin DM, Cohen RB, et al. Radiotherapy plus cetuximab for squamous-cell carcinoma of the head and neck. N Engl J Med. 2006;354(6):567–78.
36. Denis F, Garaud P, Bardet E, Alfonsi M, Sire C, Germain T, et al. Final results of the 94–01 French head and neck oncology and radiotherapy group randomized trial comparing radiotherapy alone with concomitant radiochemotherapy in advanced-stage oropharynx carcinoma. J Clin Oncol. 2004;22:69–76.

85 Access Surgeries and Osteotomies for the Maxillofacial Region

Madan G. Ethunandan

85.1 Bicoronal Scalp Flap

The bicoronal flap was first described by Hartley and Kenyon [1] to access the cranium and popularised by Tessier [2] to provide additional access to the orbits and midface. Various modifications of the flap have been described and include a zigzag (stealth) incision [3], deeper plane of dissection in the temporal scalp region to avoid damage to the facial nerve [4, 5] and strategies to minimise alopecia [6].

The coronal flap provides access to the skull, anterior and middle cranial fossa, upper midface including the nasoethmoid region and orbits and temporal and infratemporal fossa.

The SCALP is an acronym consists of five layers: *S*kin, sub*C*utaneous connective tissue, galea *A*poneurotica, *L*oose areolar tissue and *P*ericranium. The first three layers are firmly attached to each other and are raised as a single layer, superficial to the loose areolar tissue (avascular plane of Merkel). The blood vessels and nerves run within the first three layers. The "perceived" complexity of the layers in the temporal region can be rationalised, if one was to consider the galea aponeurotica as a single layer which extends to the temporal region as the "temporoparietal fascia" (synonym—superficial temporal fascia/supra-zygomatic SMAS) and the pericranium extending as the "temporalis fascia" (synonym—deep temporal fascia) overlying the temporalis muscle. The deep temporal fascia divides about 2–3 cm superior to the zygomatic arch into a superficial and deep layers. The temporoparietal fascia, superficial layer of the deep temporal fascia and the periosteum of the zygomatic arch fuse together on the lateral aspect of the zygomatic arch and contain the frontal branch of the facial nerve. The superficial temporal fat pad is present between the superficial and deep layer of the deep temporal fascia, with the deep layer attached to the deep aspect of the zygomatic arch. Dissection deep to the galea and the temporoparietal fascia affords a relatively bloodless plane and maintains and preserves the blood supply and avoids damage to the nerves, including the frontal branch of the facial nerve. This "safe" plane of dissection can be between the temporalis muscle and the "undivided" deep temporal fascia or (more inferiorly) between the superficial and deep layers of the "divided" deep temporal fascia (Fig. 85.1a).

The frontal branch of the facial nerve crosses the zygomatic arch at least 8 mm (range 8–32 mm) in front of the external auditory meatus, at least 1 cm anterior to the superior attachment of the helix to the scalp, and runs no further than 2 cm above the frontozygomatic suture (Fig. 85.1b).

85.1.1 Procedure

The hair along the incision line can be parted or a small strip shaved. Local anaesthetic containing 1: 200,000 adrenaline is infiltrated above the galea for appropriate haemostasis (you know you are in the right plane if increased resistance is felt. If it is easy to inject, you are in the deeper loose areolar tissue plane). The incision is marked from the anterior attachment of the helix and carried over the vault to the opposite side, inside the hairline (Fig. 85.1c). It can stop at the midline, if only unilateral access is required. If repeated access is likely to be required to the cranial skeleton, it would be useful to incorporate a posteriorly directed "curve", just above the helical attachment to the scalp, to try and avoid injury to the anterior branch of the superficial temporal artery and maintain additional vascularity to the flap. A "bevelled" incision can be made parallel to the hair follicles to minimise alopecia, and a "zigzag" can be incorporated to reduce parting of the hair along a straight incision line. When designing the flap in male patients, the likely influence of male pattern baldness should be taken into account.

The incision commences at the vertex between the superior temporal lines and is made with a blade through the

M. G. Ethunandan (✉)
Consultant Oral and Maxillofacial/Skull Base Surgeon, Honorary Senior Clinical Lecturer, Lead, Head and Neck Cancer, University Hospital Southampton, Southampton, UK

K. Bonanthaya et al. (eds.), *Oral and Maxillofacial Surgery for the Clinician*, https://doi.org/10.1007/978-981-15-1346-6_85

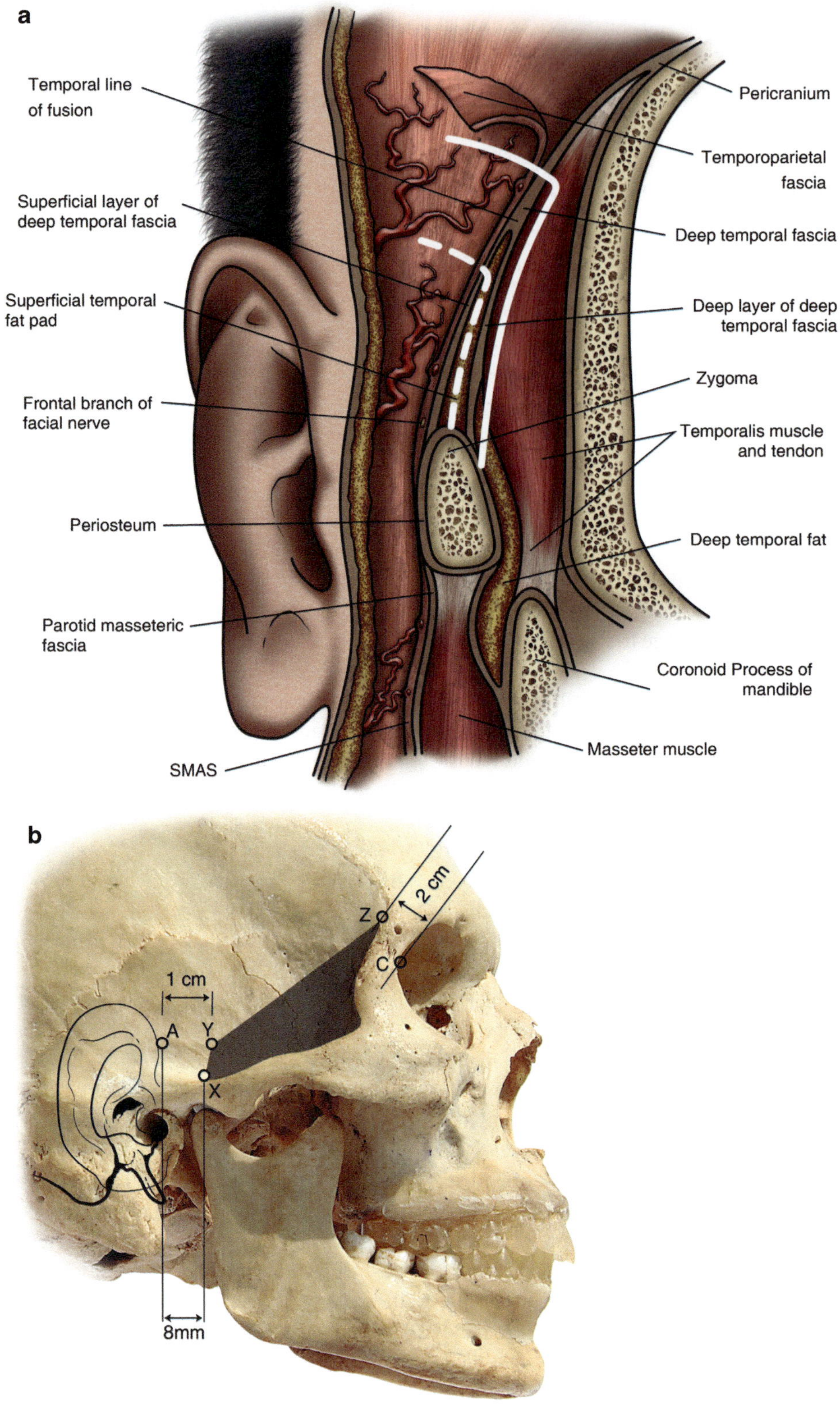

Fig. 85.1 Scalp flap. (**a**) Layers of the scalp in the temporal region. Dotted line—dissection between the superficial and deep layers of the (divided) deep temporal fascia. Solid line—dissection between the (undivided) deep temporal fascia and temporalis muscle. (**b**) Position of the frontal branch of the facial nerve. (**c**) Skin marking for a coronal flap. (**d**) Pericranial flap raised as an extension of the deep temporal fascia incision (note same plane of dissection). (**e**) Incision marked on the undivided deep temporal fascia. (**f**) Periosteal tunnel created along the zygomatic arch, deep to the position of the frontal branch of the facial nerve. (**g**) Exposure of the lateral orbit and zygomatic arch. (**h**) Temporalis muscle retracted to expose the temporal fossa and lateral orbital wall

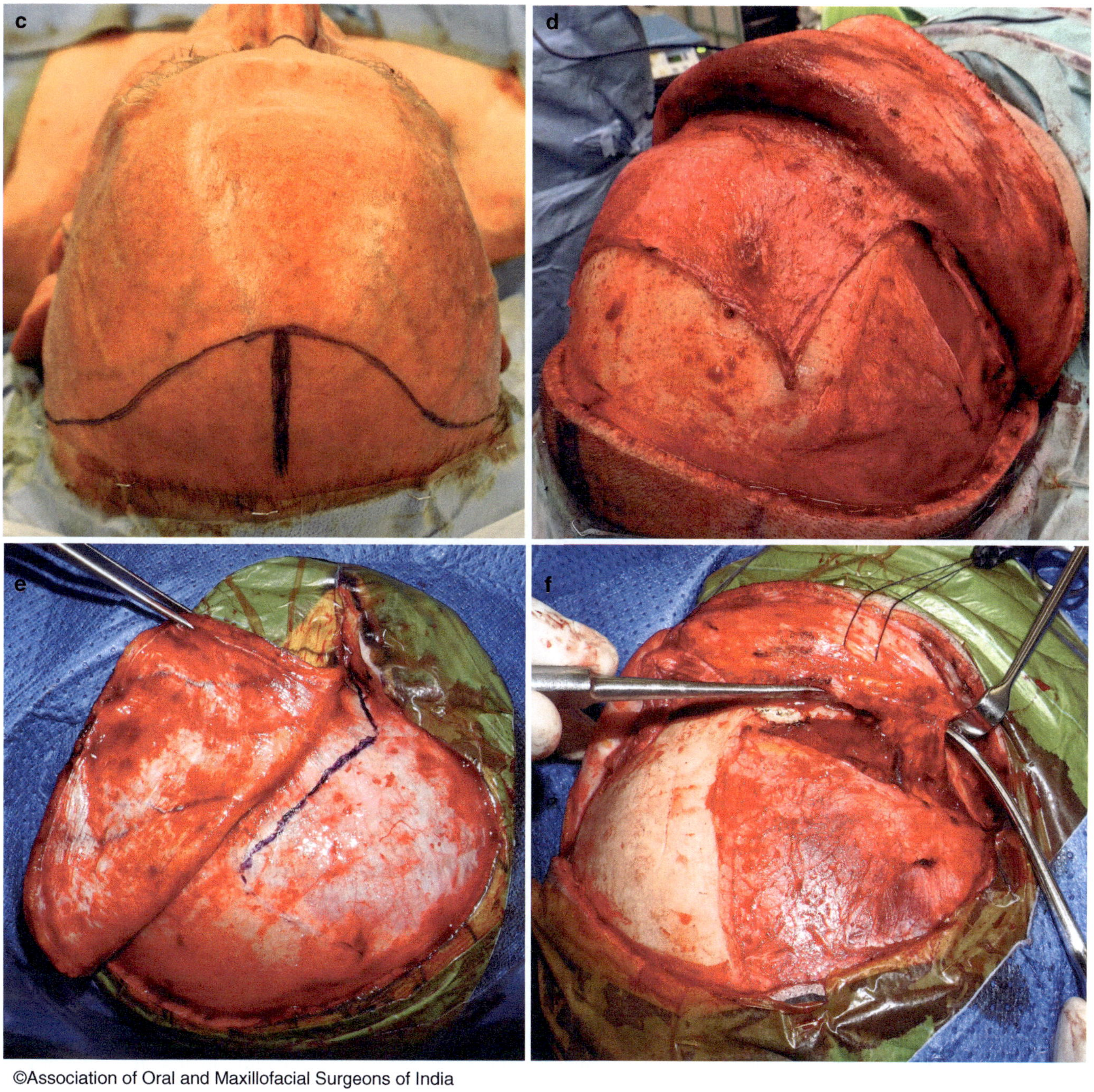

Fig. 85.1 (continued)

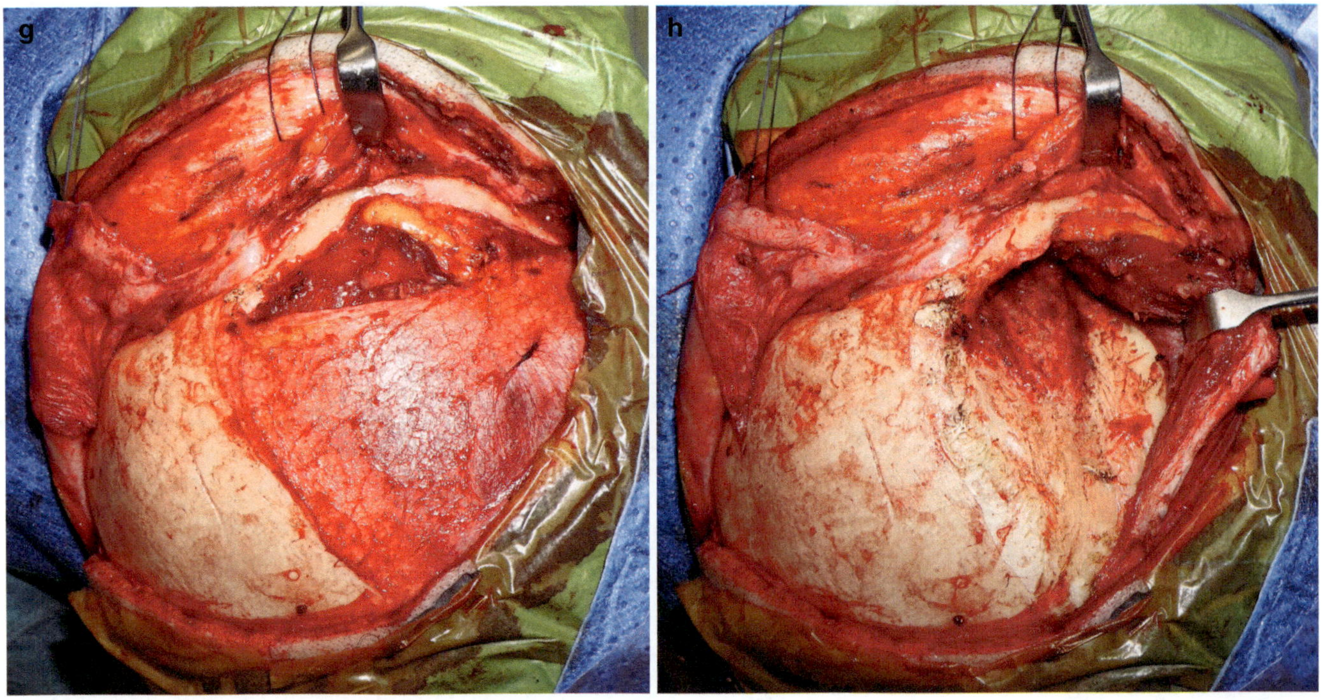

Fig. 85.1 (continued)

galea, up to the loose areolar tissue, and the superficial three layers are raised as a unit. Blunt scissors or a brain retractor can be used to undermine the incision line along this plane, down to the root of the helix, and with the brain retractor in situ, the incision is made down to it. This allows rapid elevation of the flap, without inadvertent damage to the underling temporal fascia/temporalis muscle. Dissection is carried inferiorly in the subgaleal plane. The pericranium is incised approximately 3 cm above the superior orbital rim, and the dissection continued subperiosteally. Resistance can be encountered in the frontozygomatic and frontonasal suture region and around the supraorbital neurovascular bundles. If the supraorbital neurovascular bundle is present within a foramen, rather than a notch, the foramen can be opened with careful use of a fine osteotome (divergent cuts to minimise damage and ease of release).

A pericranial flap could be easily incorporated, by extending the pericranial incision superiorly to the required length, between the superior temporal lines, as an extension of the temporalis fascia incision (Fig. 85.1d). If a pericranial flap is to be utilised, the subgaleal dissection should stop 2 cm above the supraorbital rim, to maintain the vascularity of the pericranial flap.

Exposure of the nasal bones and frontal process of the maxilla can be facilitated by a vertical periosteal releasing incision in the midline. The medial canthal ligaments can be detached from the anterior lacrimal crest, which provides excellent exposure of the medial orbit up to the optic canal and the medial floor up to the infraorbital nerve.

The detached medial canthal tendon must be "tagged" through the periosteum with a unresorbable suture on a round-bodied needle, for subsequent reattachment to a microplate. Subperiosteal dissection medially is now possible as far as the floor of the orbit.

The skin incision is extended inferiorly in a naturally occurring skin crease, to just below the cartilaginous meatus, if exposure of the zygoma, lateral orbit or temporomandibular joint is considered. This could be modified to follow the free edge of the tragus, to make this section less conspicuous. The dissection is carried forward medially following the cartilaginous meatus. At the superior attachment of the helix, the temporalis fascia is incised –1 cm above the zygomatic arch, and angled forwards to join the supraorbital periosteal incision 3 cm above the supraorbital rim (Fig. 85.1e). The incision is extended vertically in along the temporal fascia to the root of the zygomatic arch, which can be felt on palpation above the cartilaginous meatus. A pocket is created at the root of the zygomatic arch, deep to the periosteum and the soft tissues tented with a periosteal elevator to expose the arch. The soft tissues superior to the arch, on the surface of the temporalis muscle, can be transected down to the periosteal elevator to expose the zygomatic arch, zygoma and lateral orbit, without damaging the frontal branch (Fig. 85.1f, g).

Retraction of the temporalis muscle posteriorly provides additional exposure to the temporal fossa and the superior boundary of the infratemporal fossa (Fig. 85.1h).

Closure of the galea and meticulous haemostasis is essential, and drains and/or head dressing can be additionally utilised to prevent haematomas.

85.1.2 Potential Complications and Solutions (Clinical Pearls)

Alopecia: Use a knife for skin incision, meticulous haemostasis with judicious use of bipolar diathermy and tension-free closure.

Frontal nerve damage: Appropriate plane of dissection, care during retraction and the use of diathermy in the temporal/preauricular region.

Supraorbital/supra-trochlear nerve damage: Care during dissection in the supraorbital rim region and judicious use of fine/sharp osteotomes when deroofing the supraorbital foramen.

Clinical Tips

- Inject vasoconstrictor above the galea, make the incision in segments with a blade and use bipolar diathermy to achieve meticulous haemostasis and reduce blood loss.
- Consider making the incision parallel to the hair follicles and use bipolar diathermy "judiciously" to minimise alopecia.
- Start the incision in between the superior temporal lines to "easily" identify the appropriate plane of dissection.
- Stay deep to the galea in the temporal region to avoid injury to the frontal branch of the facial nerve.
- An easier and safer plane of dissection would be between the temporalis muscle and the deep temporal fascia.
- Stop dissection in the subgaleal plane, 2 cm above the supraorbital rims, if a pericranial flap is planned, to preserve its vascularity.
- Place deep sutures along the galea for "tension-free" skin closure but away from the skin surface to minimise "stitch" abscesses.

85.2 Midface Access

A modified Weber-Fergusson approach remains the most popular transfacial approach to the midface. This access was originally described well over 150 years ago by Weber [7] from Germany and Fergusson [8] from the United Kingdom. Various modifications have been incorporated over the years, and the more commonly used ones include the midline lip incision being placed on the philtrum [9], lateral eyelid extension [10] and medial eyebrow extension [11]. The original lateral rhinotomy incision was described by Moure [12], and a modification of the nasal component to lie along the nasal subunits was described by Thankappan [13].

A modified Weber-Fergusson incision provides excellent access to the ipsilateral maxilla and, with appropriate extensions, provides additional exposure to the nasal cavity, orbit and ethmoid (Fig. 85.2a). The "nasal" part of the incision can be utilised for a lateral rhinotomy access.

A Le Fort I down-fracture osteotomy can also be utilised to access the nasal cavity, maxillary antrum, pterygopalatine fossa and clivus. However, with the widespread use of endonasal endoscopic techniques, its use has become limited. The technique is similar to that utilised in orthognathic surgery and is outlined in the orthognathic surgery chapter.

An intraoral vestibular incision can be joined with bilateral piriform fossa and intercartilaginous and septocolumellar transfixion incisions to "deglove" the upper lip, cheek and soft tissues of the nose to provide access to the maxilla and nasal cavity [14, 15].

A maxillary swing procedure can be utilised to access the posterior maxilla, pterygopalatine/infratemporal fossa and nasopharynx. However, with the widespread use of endoscopic techniques, its role has also become limited. Its principal use is in the management of recurrent nasopharyngeal tumours, which cannot be accessed endoscopically [16].

The modified Weber-Fergusson commences with an upper lip split incision that is made along the philtrum and extended along the alar margins. A "V" can be incorporated along the nasal floor to improve localisation of the flap during closure. The incision is carried along the alar margin and extended superiorly at the junction between the nasal side wall and dorsal nasal subunit (Fig. 85.2a).

The intraoral incisions are made along the gingival crevice or buccal vestibule and are principally determined by the location of the tumour. A "V" can be incorporated in the lip mucosa to facilitate accurate approximation during wound closure. The cheek flap is elevated to expose the maxilla (Fig. 85.2b). The plane of dissection is principally determined by the extension of the tumour. A "tonsil" swab can be placed in the nasal cavity and soft tissues along the piriform rim transected to gain access to the nasal cavity and avoid inadvertent damage to the nasal septum.

Lateral extensions can be incorporated, if additional access is required to the orbits and zygoma. This is made along the subciliary/midtarsal skin crease and can be extended laterally along the crow's feet skin crease (Fig. 85.2a). Care is taken to elevate the skin flap "superfi-

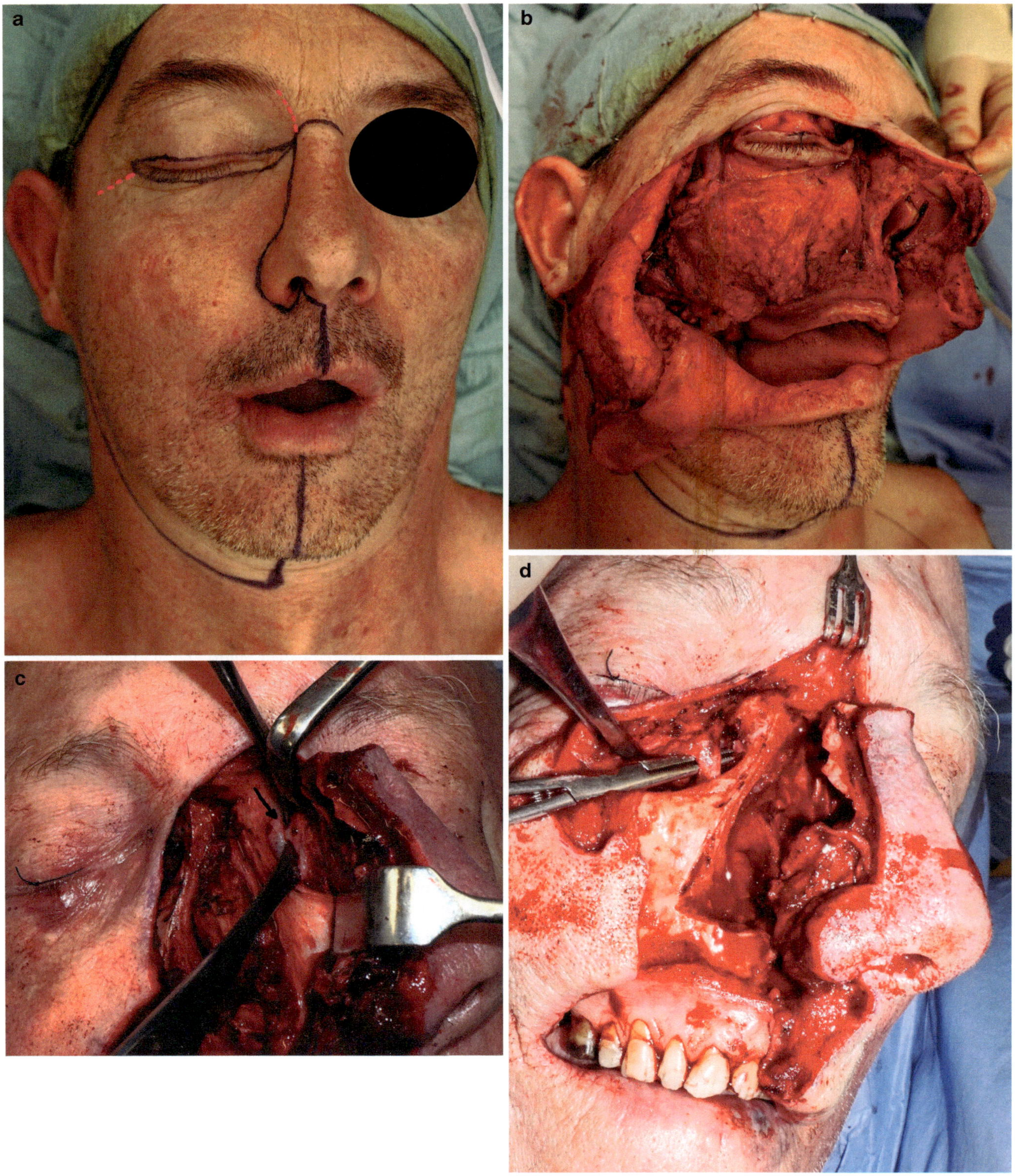

Fig. 85.2 Midface access, (**a**) Marking for a modified Weber-Fergusson incision respecting the nasal subunits. Lateral lower and upper eyelid extensions (for total maxillectomy with orbital exenteration) and medial glabella extension (for additional nasal access). Red dotted lines with Lynch (superior) and crow's feet (lateral) extensions. (**b**) Exposure afforded by the incision. (**c**) Anterior ethmoid artery (arrow), exposed in the medial orbit along the frontoethmoid suture. (**d**) Lacrimal sac/nasolacrimal duct exposed in the lacrimal fossa

cial" to the orbicularis oculi muscle in the eyelid region to preserve function, and it is important to avoid "button holes" in the thin skin of the eyelids.

Superior extension (Lynch [11] modification) can be incorporated, if additional access is required to the medial orbit and ethmoids (Fig. 85.2a). The nasal sidewall incision is extended superiorly along the medial orbit at least, 5 mm medial to the medial canthus, up to the medial end of the eye brow/medial supraorbital rim. The incision deepened down to the bone and the frontal process of the maxilla, anterior lacrimal crest and frontonasal suture exposed. The medial canthal tendon is "formally" identified and detached. It is "tagged" with a 3.0 Prolene suture on a round body needle, for subsequent reattachment. The medial orbit can now be exposed with fine periosteal elevators. The frontoethmoidal suture (FES) in the medial orbit provides an excellent landmark for the position of the anterior and posterior ethmoid vessels and optic canal. These vessels are identified along the suture, skeletonised and ligated/diathermised (Fig. 85.2c). The optic canal lies posteriorly in superomedial orbit, in line with the suture. The number of ethmoidal vessels varies frequently [1–3] and the over-reliance of the distances between the vessels (24 mm, 12 mm, 6 mm) and the optic canal can be dangerous The FES can often lie "above" the cribriform plate, and its relationship to the anterior cranial fossa should be "critically assessed" in the preoperative scans. Osteotomies are best placed below the FES, if "unintentional" intracranial extension is to be avoided.

The lacrimal sac is identified inferiorly in the lacrimal fossa and can be dissected free for retraction or transection (Fig. 85.2d).

A medial extension, along the glabella skin crease, can be incorporated if additional access is required to the nasal bones, roof of the nasal cavity, or if a "nasal" swing is considered (Fig. 85.2a).

The lower eyelid extension can be combined with a similar upper eyelid incision, if a lid-sparing orbital exenteration is planned (Fig. 85.2a).

85.2.1 Potential Complications and Solutions (Clinical Pearls)

Unsightly scar: Use the modified Weber-Fergusson incision along the philtrum, nasal subunits with "v" in the nasal floor and lip mucosa—meticulous layered closure in layers and accurate alignment of the vermillion border.

Delayed bone healing (maxillary swing): Minimal soft tissue elevations along the osteotomy sites, pre-plating prior to completion of osteotomy, use fine saw blades and bur and copious irrigation.

Clinical Tips

- Inject vasoconstrictor, make the incision in segments and use diathermy to minimise blood loss.
- Extend the midline skin incision past the vermillion, prior to incorporating the mucosal "V" to facilitate accurate approximation of the vermillion.
- Tattoo or mark the vermillion, if you feel it would help in later approximation.
- Intraoral incisions and the plane of dissection are dictated by the location of the tumour.
- If a lower eyelid extension is planned, the plane of dissection is ideally above the orbicularis oculi muscle (if eye is preserved).
- Soft tissue "elevation" is kept to the minimum along the osteotomy sites, if a maxillary swing is planned.
- Formal identification and tagging of the medial canthus are necessary for later reattachment.
- Recognise the "orientation" value of the frontoethmoidal suture.
- Beware of using distances between the ethmoidal foramina and optic canal as the "sole" modality during deep dissection of the medial orbit.

85.3 Nasal Swing

This provides access to the nasal cavity, ethmoids and nasal roof and can be considered for bilateral lesions, when the nasal skin/bones can be preserved. Currently, with the widespread use of endoscopic techniques, its role, as a "sole" access to these lesions, is restricted. It is often used for additional access, as part of a wider resection.

A modified Weber-Fergusson incision is made respecting the nasal subunits, and allowance is made for a transverse medial extension along the glabella skin crease (Fig. 85.3a). The soft tissues are retracted laterally and superiorly to obtain exposure of the nasal bones, frontal process of the maxilla and the piriform rims. The soft tissue overlying the nasal bone is left undisturbed. Exposure of the contralateral nasal bones is achieved by undermining in a subperiosteal plane. A fine bur/saw is used to make the bone cuts along the frontal process of the maxilla and across the nasal bones (Fig. 85.3b). The contralateral nasal osteotomy is carried out with fine osteotomes, if necessary, through separate stab incisions. The osteotomy sites are prelocalised with low-profile bone plates, removed and replaced during the procedure. The underlying nasal mucosa and soft tissue along the piriform rim are released with a diathermy. The soft tissue incisions and the bone cuts are stepped or staggered.

The nasal septum restricts complete lateral retraction. The septal cartilage is transected with a cutting diathermy—the damp tonsil swab in the other nostril can prevent accidental injury to the contralateral lateral nasal wall mucosa and the facial skin. The 1 cm strut of nasal septal cartilage is preserved along the dorsum and columella to prevent collapse (Fig. 85.3c). The nasal bones and the soft tissues can now be retracted to the opposite side (Fig. 85.3d).

A soft tissue only and soft and hard tissue nasal swing can be combined with a larger midface/craniofacial resection for pathologies involving adjacent structures. The nasal swing can be linked with a frontal craniotomy for resection of tumours that also involve the central compartment of the anterior cranial fossa (Fig. 85.3e, f).

The plates are replaced, and the wound is closed in layers (Fig. 85.3g).

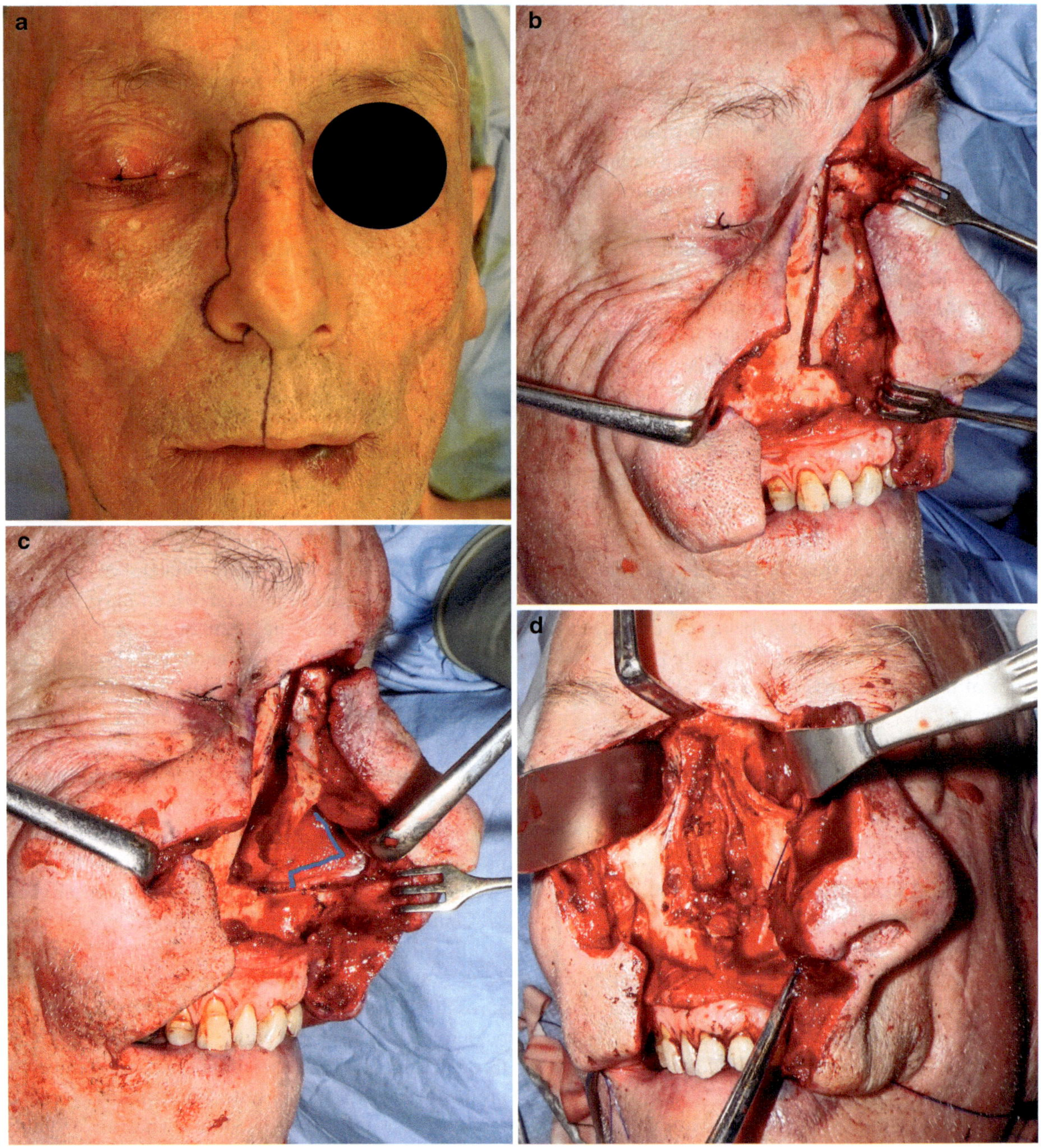

Fig. 85.3 Nasal swing. (**a**) Skin marking, respecting the nasal sub units. (**b**) Bone cuts along the frontal process of the maxilla and nasal bones. (**c**) Marking for septal incision preserving dorsal and caudal strut. (**d**) Exposure of the nasal cavity following retraction of the nose. (**e**) Bone cuts for "nasal/ethmoid clearance" as a part of a craniofacial resection. (**f**) Defect viewed from the cranial aspect following "nasal/ethmoid" clearance. (**g**) Wound closure following nasal swing

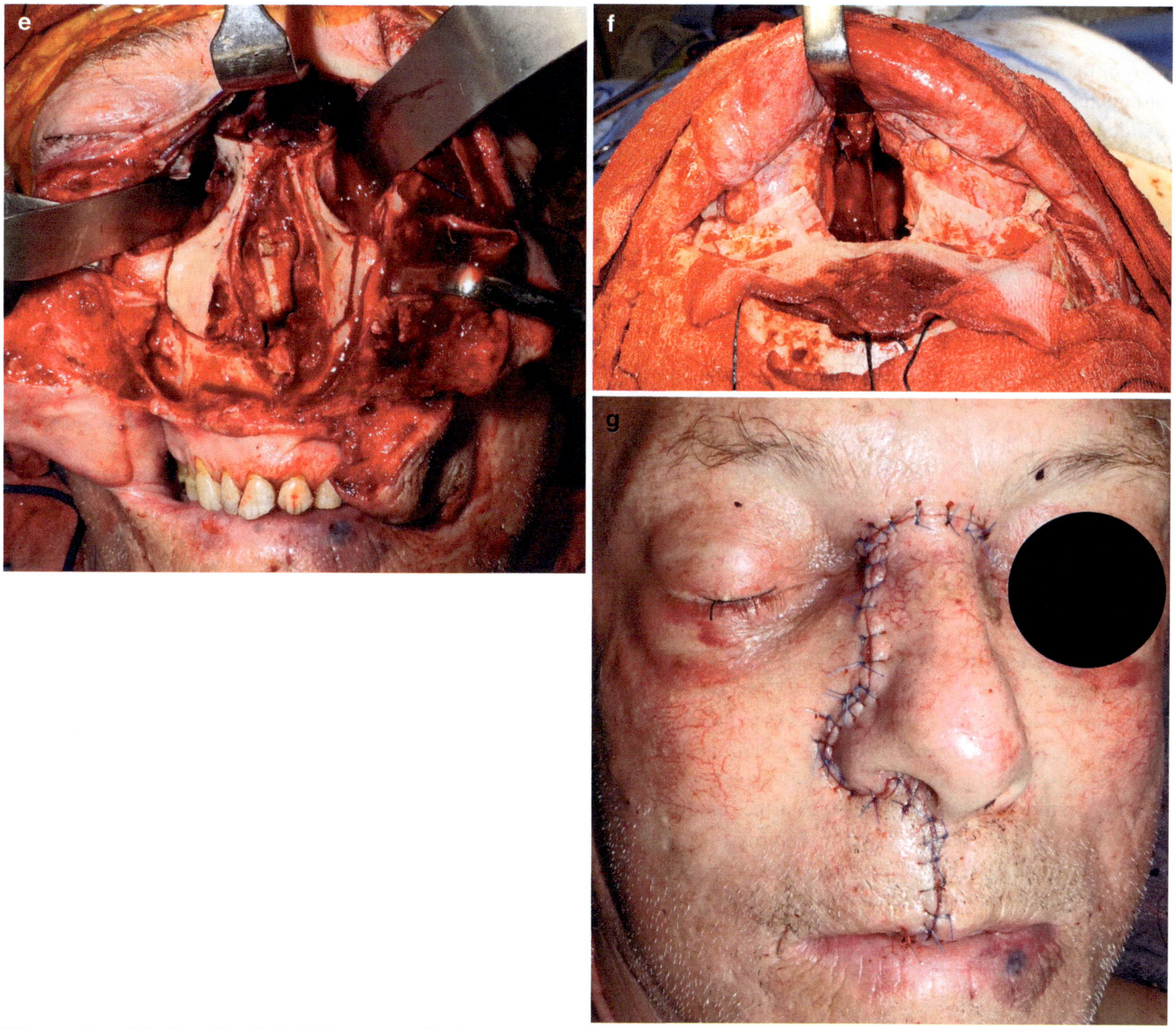

Fig. 85.3 (continued)

85.3.1 Potential Complications and Solutions (Clinical Pearls)

Unsightly scar: Use the modified incision along the philtrum, nasal subunits with "v" in the nasal floor and lip mucosa. Carry out meticulous closure in layers and acheive accurate approximation of the vermillion border.

Delayed bone healing (nasal osteotomy): Minimal soft tissue elevations along the osteotomy sites, pre-plating prior to completion of osteotomy, use fine saw blades, burs and osteotomes and copious irrigation.

Nasal collapse: Attempt to preserve caudal/dorsal septal strut.

Clinical Tips

- The soft tissue dissection is kept to the minimum, overlying the nasal bones.
- The osteotomy is planned along the frontal process of the maxilla, which is mobilised along with the nasal bones.
- Create a contralateral subperiosteal pocket and use "stab" incisions and fine osteotomes to complete the osteotomy.
- Pre-plate the osteotomies prior to completion.
- Preserve at least a 1 cm caudal and dorsal strut of septum to prevent nasal collapse.

85.4 Per Oral Access

A significant proportion of the oral lesions can be accessed and managed per orally. The use of a solely per oral access is dictated by the location and size of the lesion, the mouth opening and status of the dentition. An appropriately sized mouth prop/gag with cheek and tongue retractors and traction sutures can be utilised to provide the necessary access to safely carry out the procedure (Fig. 85.4).

Clinical Tips

- Utilise appropriate retraction to obtain the "best" access.
- "Orthodontic" cheek retractors can be very helpful for additional retraction and protecting the commissures.
- If teeth extractions are planned, these are best carried out prior to the resection to improve access.

85.5 Soft Tissue Lip Split

Lip split incisions to gain additional access to the oral cavity have been in practice for over 150 years. A midline chin incision was described by Roux [17] and subsequently popularised by Trotter [18] in the early 1900s. Further modifications by Macgregor [19] placed the chin component along the mentolabial fold, and Hayter [20] suggested incorporating a chevron in the vermillion and mentolabial area.

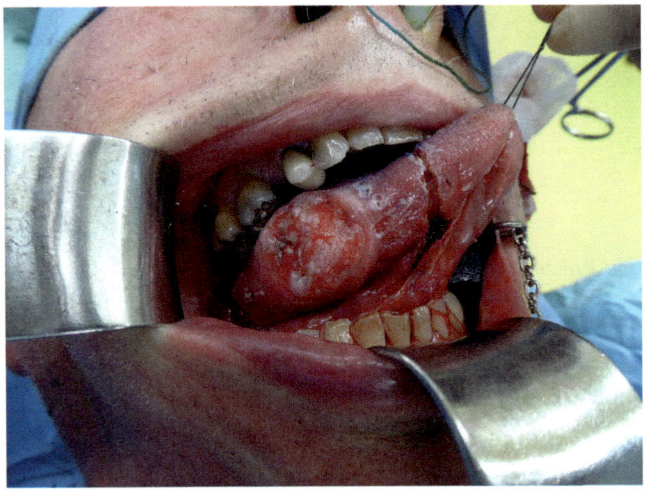

Fig. 85.4 Per oral access. Per oral access for excision of a tongue lesion

Soft tissue only lip split can provide excellent access to the posterior buccal mucosa and mandible, for lesions that cannot be safely excised through a per oral or cervical approach. The principle disadvantage of this approach is the need for lip split scar and likely sacrifice the mental nerve; this must be weighed against improved access. The latter is not a consideration if the inferior alveolar nerve has to be sacrificed in the subsequent resection. A lip split through the commissure would have to be considered for tumours located close to the commissure to avoid devascularising the segment between the midline lip split and commissure. This would also be a consideration for composite resections involving the adjacent skin.

A full-thickness vertical incision is made through the lower lip in the midline and extended inferiorly along the midline of the chin/upper neck (Fig. 85.5a). It continues with an appropriately placed low-neck skin crease incision. A "V" can be incorporated in the mucosal aspect of the lower lip to facilitate accurate approximation. The cosmetic outcome with a midline chin incision is excellent and reduces the risk of numbness and ischemia of the ipsilateral chin, associated with a curvilinear incision along the mental fold.

The neck skin flap is raised in a plane deep to the platysma, up to the lower border of the mandible, taking care to avoid injury to the marginal mandibular branch of the facial nerve. The cheek flap is elevated by detaching the platysma from the lower border of the mandible in the subperiosteal plane. More posteriorly, the dissection can be continued superficial or deep to the masseter muscle (Fig. 85.5b).

Intraoral soft tissue incisions are placed along the gingival crevice or the lower vestibule and are principally determined by the location of the tumour. The wound is meticulously closed in layers, taking care to accurately align the vermillion border.

85.5.1 Potential Complications and Solutions (Clinical Pearls)

Unsightly scar: Accurate alignment of the vermillion border and meticulous layered closure.

Mental and marginal mandibular nerve damage: Appropriate plane of dissection and identification and protection of the nerves.

Lip necrosis: Avoid "additional" midline incision for tumours in the commissure region or composite buccal mucosa resections.

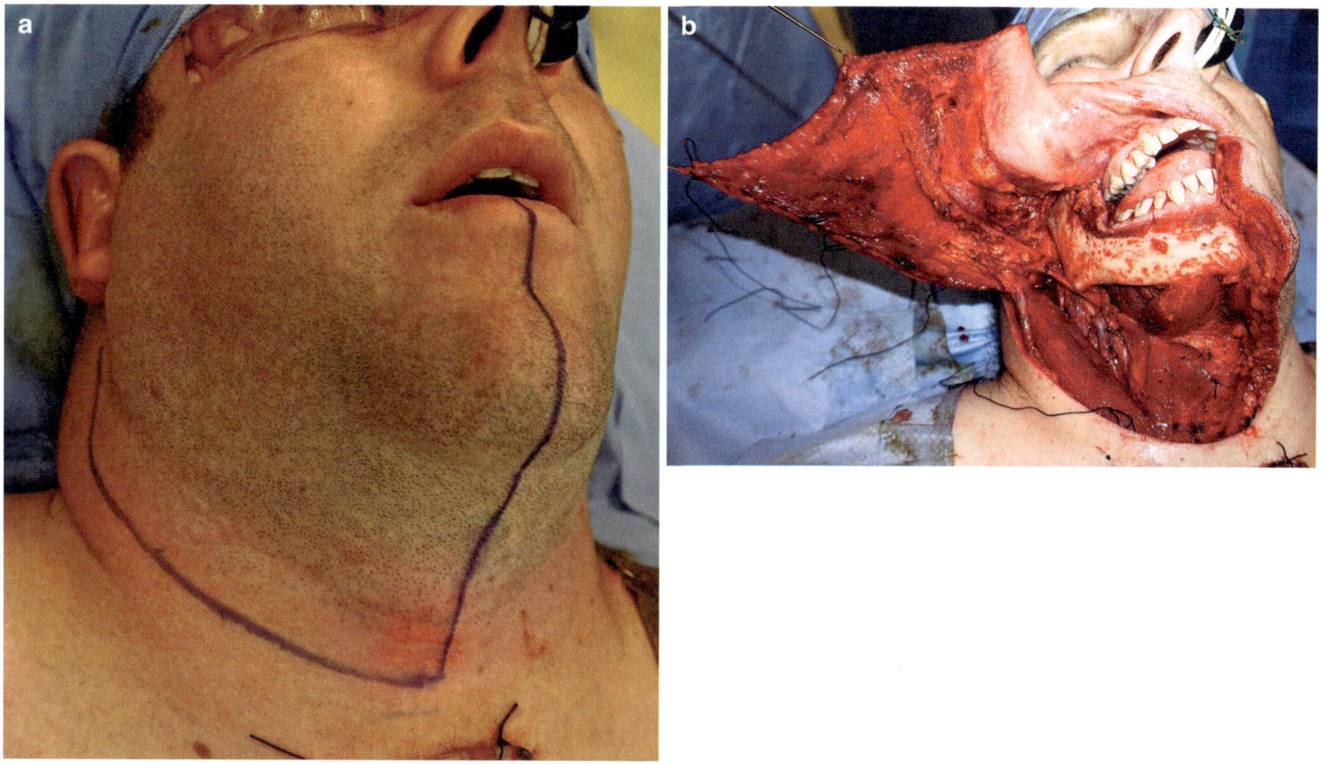

Fig. 85.5 Soft tissue lip split. (**a**) Skin markings for a soft tissue lip split. (**b**) Exposure following flap elevation

Clinical Tips

- Dissection of the anterior mandible is in the subperiosteal plane to minimise injury to the facial and mental nerves.
- Identify the mental nerve and decide if it can be preserved, prior to sacrificing it.
- More posteriorly, the dissection can be superficial or deep to the masseter muscle. If superficial dissection is planned, care must be exercised to prevent injury to the facial nerve branches and parotid duct.
- Avoid midline lip split for tumours adjacent to the commissure and composite resections.

85.6 Visor Flap

A visor flap can be utilised for lesions in the floor of mouth, tongue and mandible and can be combined with bilateral neck dissections. The incision is marked at an appropriate low-neck skin crease and extends from one mastoid tip process to the other (Fig. 85.6a). The skin flaps are raised in the sub-platysmal plane up to the lower border of the mandible, taking care to avoid injury to the marginal mandibular branch of the facial nerve. The periosteum is incised along the lower border of the mandible and a mucoperiosteal flap elevated, taking care to identify the mental nerves. Intraoral mucosal incisions are determined by the location of the lesion, and the mental nerves might have to be sacrificed to obtain further access or adequate margins. The skin flaps are retracted cephalad with "penrose" rubber drains (Fig. 85.6b).

When used as a part of lingual release/pull-through procedure to access a floor of mouth/tongue lesion, the mental nerves and labial/buccal soft tissue can be left undisturbed [21, 22]. Resection of the lesions in the anterior floor of mouth along with the mandible results in detachment of the tongue to the mandible. It is essential that the geniohyoid and genioglossus muscles are reattached to the reconstructed mandible to prevent the tongue from falling back. The wound is closed in layers. An advantage of the visor incision is the avoidance of a lip split facial scar, which needs to be weighed against the risk of bilateral injury to the marginal mandibular branch of the facial and mental nerves.

85.6.1 Potential Complications and Solutions (Clinical Pearls)

Mental and marginal mandibular nerve damage: Appropriate plane of dissection and identification and protection of the nerves.

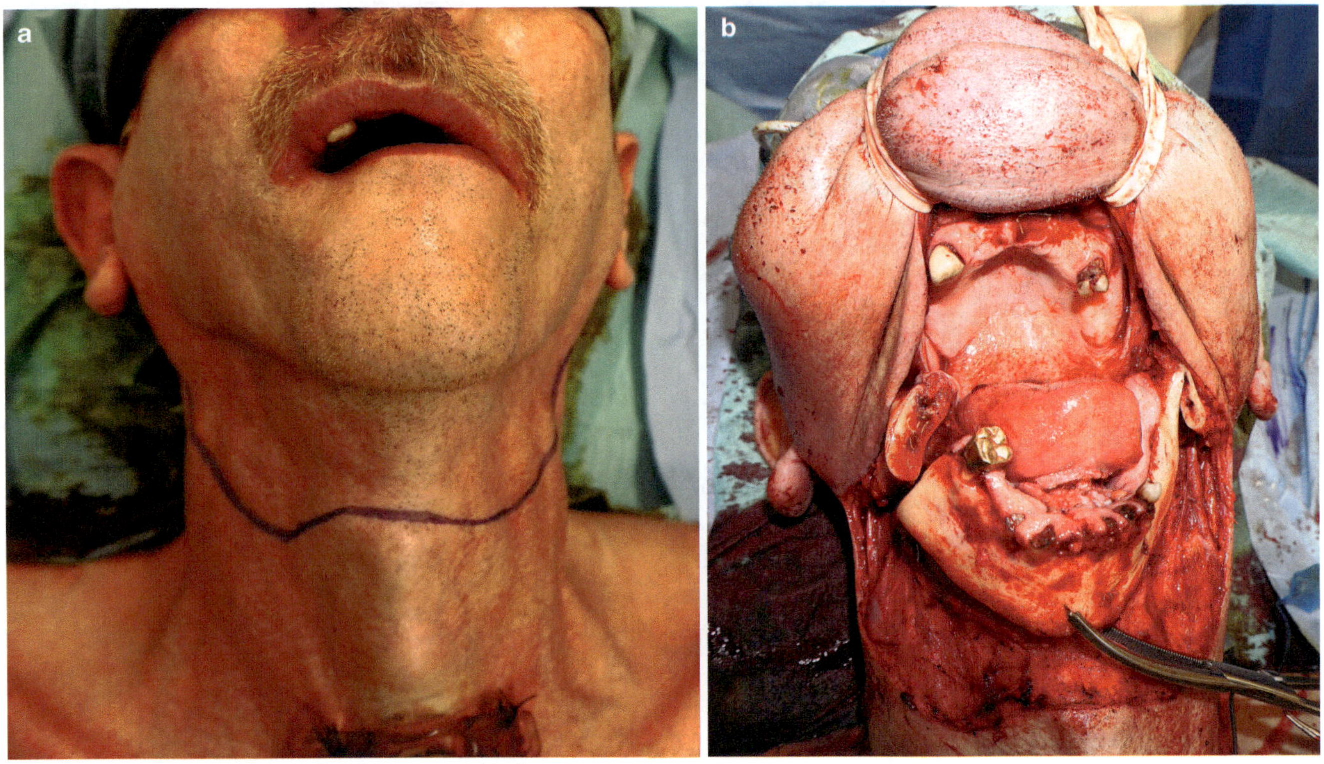

Fig. 85.6 Visor flap. (**a**) Skin markings for a visor flap. (**b**) Exposure following flap retraction with "penrose" rubber drains

Clinical Tips

- Expose the mandible in the subperiosteal plane to identify the mental foramen and minimise damage to the facial nerve.
- The intraoral labial/buccal vestibular incision is determined by the location of the tumour and can be placed along the vestibule or crevicular margins.
- If the tongue and the hyoid apparatus is detached from the anterior mandible, the remnant genioglossus and geniohyoid should be "formally" suspended to the (reconstructed) mandible with non-resorbable sutures.

85.7 Transmandibular Approaches

85.7.1 Mandibular Swing

85.7.1.1 Lip Split Paramedian Mandibulotomy

Mandibulotomy to access oral cavity, oropharynx and skull base has been in use for over 150 years, since its initial description by Roux [17] and Trotter [18]. It was popularised by Spiro [23], who suggested a median mandibulotomy, and McGregor [19] described a paramedian location, anterior to the mental foramen. Though various sites and design of the osteotomy have been described, a straight line paramedian mandibulotomy is currently the most widely used option, as it preserves the attachment of the anterior belly of the digastric, geniohyoid and genioglossus muscles and mental nerve. The availability of rigid fixation and fine saws negate the need for step osteotomies and tooth extractions in most cases.

The lip split with a mandibulotomy provides excellent access to the mid and posterior third of the tongue, floor of the mouth, soft palate, tonsillar fossa, oropharynx/posterior pharyngeal wall and supraglottic larynx. It can be extended posteriorly to provide additional access to the infratemporal fossa and the parapharyngeal space with safe vascular control. It can be considered in three discrete stages; lower lip/chin division, paramedian mandibulotomy and soft tissue elevation on the lingual aspect of the mandible.

A vertical full-thickness incision is made through the midline of the lower lip and extended inferiorly across the midline of the chin/upper neck and continues with an appropriately placed low-neck skin crease incision (Fig. 85.7a). A "V" can be incorporated in the mucosal aspect of the lower lip to facilitate accurate approximation.

The cosmetic outcome with a midline chin incision is excellent and reduces the risk of numbness and ischemia of the ipsilateral chin, associated with a curvilinear incision along the mental fold.

The neck skin flap is raised in a plane deep to the platysma, up to the lower border of the mandible, taking care to avoid injury to the marginal mandibular branch of the facial nerve. Intraorally, the incision through the labial mucosa and

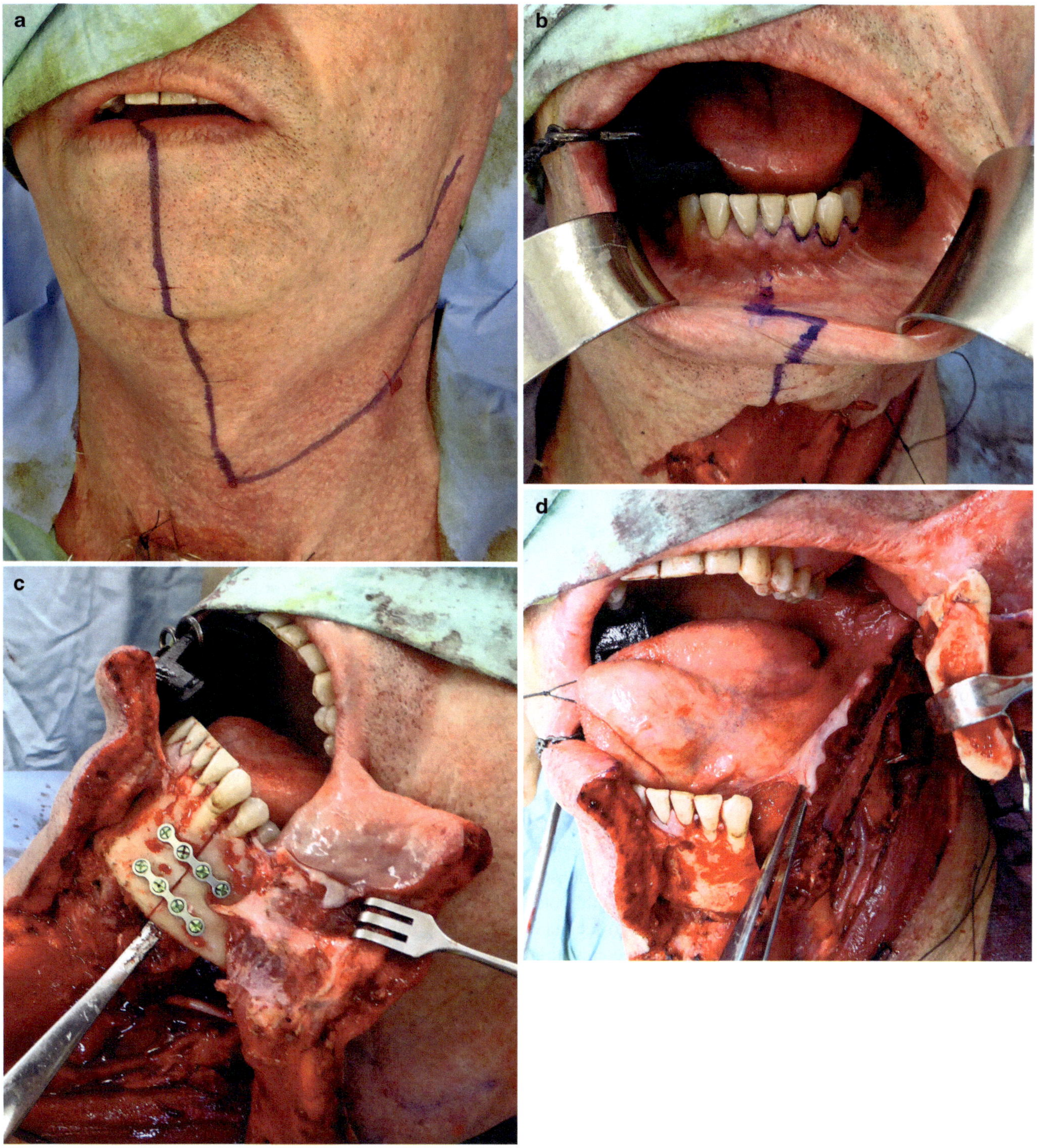

Fig. 85.7 Lip split paramedian mandibulotomy. (**a**) Skin marking for lip split mandibulotomy. (**b**) Mucosal marking for lip split mandibulotomy. (**c**) Lingual subperiosteal tunnel, bone cuts and pre-plating prior to completion of mandibulotomy. (**d**) Lingual crevicular incision and mandible retracted laterally following release of mylohyoid muscle. (**e**) Additional exposure of the infratemporal fossa by tracing the inferior dental and lingual nerves. Defect following maxillectomy and infratemporal fossa clearance (different patients)

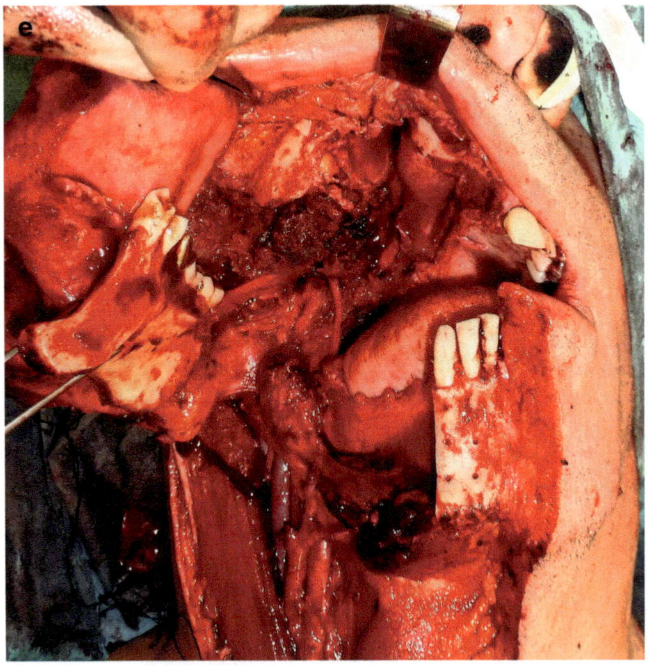

Fig. 85.7 (continued)

attached gingiva is designed (stepped), so that it does not directly overlie the planned osteotomy (Fig. 85.7b). The elevation of the periosteum and mentalis muscle should be restricted to allow identification and protection of the mental nerve and placement of the plates.

A soft tissue pocket is created by elevating the lingual mucosa off the mandible adjacent to the osteotomy. A periosteal elevator is placed in the pocket, and an osteotomy is carried out between the lower lateral incisor/canine or canine/first premolar region (Fig. 85.7c). The mandible is osteotomised with a fine saw, taking care to avoid injury to the tooth roots. Occasionally a tooth would have to be removed to facilitate the osteotomy. The mandible is pre-plated prior to completion of the bone cuts, and these are removed and replaced during the procedure. The osteotomy cuts are in a straight line, as a stepped osteotomy neither aids fixation or bone union and can increase the risk of injury to the teeth apices and mental nerve.

Once the mandible is divided, it is gently retracted laterally, and an incision made along the lingual gingival crevice and the mucoperiosteum elevated off the lingual mandible (Fig. 85.7d). The mylohyoid muscle is detached along its attachment to the mylohyoid ridge. Further soft tissue dissection is dictated by the location of the tumour.

If additional access is required to the infratemporal fossa/parapharyngeal space, it will be necessary to detach the medial pterygoid muscle from the medial ramus of the mandible. In addition, the stylomandibular ligament (at the angle of the mandible) and the sphenomandibular ligament (at the lingula) have to be detached to obtain the best possible access (Fig. 85.7e). The inferior dental and lingual nerve are identified early and protected and can be utilised as roadmaps to the foramen ovale and skull base. The maxillary artery can also be identified entering the infratemporal fossa, at the neck of the condyle by following the posterior border of the mandible. Early identification and ligation can help provide a relatively bloodless field for dissection of the infratemporal fossa.

The lingual gingival crevicular incision facilitates easy closure and avoids placement of the suture line at the depth (sump) of the wound. The mandible is held in occlusion, and the plates are replaced accurately to achieve the premorbid localisation. The wound is meticulously closed in layers.

85.7.2 Potential Complications and Solutions (Clinical Pearls)

Unsightly scar: Accurate alignment of the vermillion and meticulous layered closure.

Mental and marginal mandibular nerve damage: Appropriate plane of dissection and identification and protection of the nerves.

Delayed bone healing: Minimal soft tissue elevations along the osteotomy sites, pre-plating prior to completion of osteotomy, use fine saw blades, burs, osteotomes and copious irrigation. Osteotomy ideally in the canine region.

Damage to adjacent teeth: Design osteotomy where space allows, use fine instruments and consider extraction.

Clinical Tips

- A straight osteotomy in the canine region is ideal and the site pre-plated prior to completion of the bone cuts.
- The soft tissue incision and bone osteotomies are stepped, so that they do not lie on the same plane.
- The lingual soft tissues are retracted following a lingual crevicular incision.
- The medial pterygoid muscle and stylomandibular and sphenomandibular ligaments have to be detached to obtain addition access to the infratemporal fossa.
- The lingual and inferior dental nerves provide excellent landmarks and can be utilised as roadmaps to the skull base and foramen ovale.
- The maxillary artery should be identified at the neck of the condyle, as it enters the infratemporal fossa and ligated early in the procedure to minimise blood loss and improve visibility during infratemporal fossa clearance.

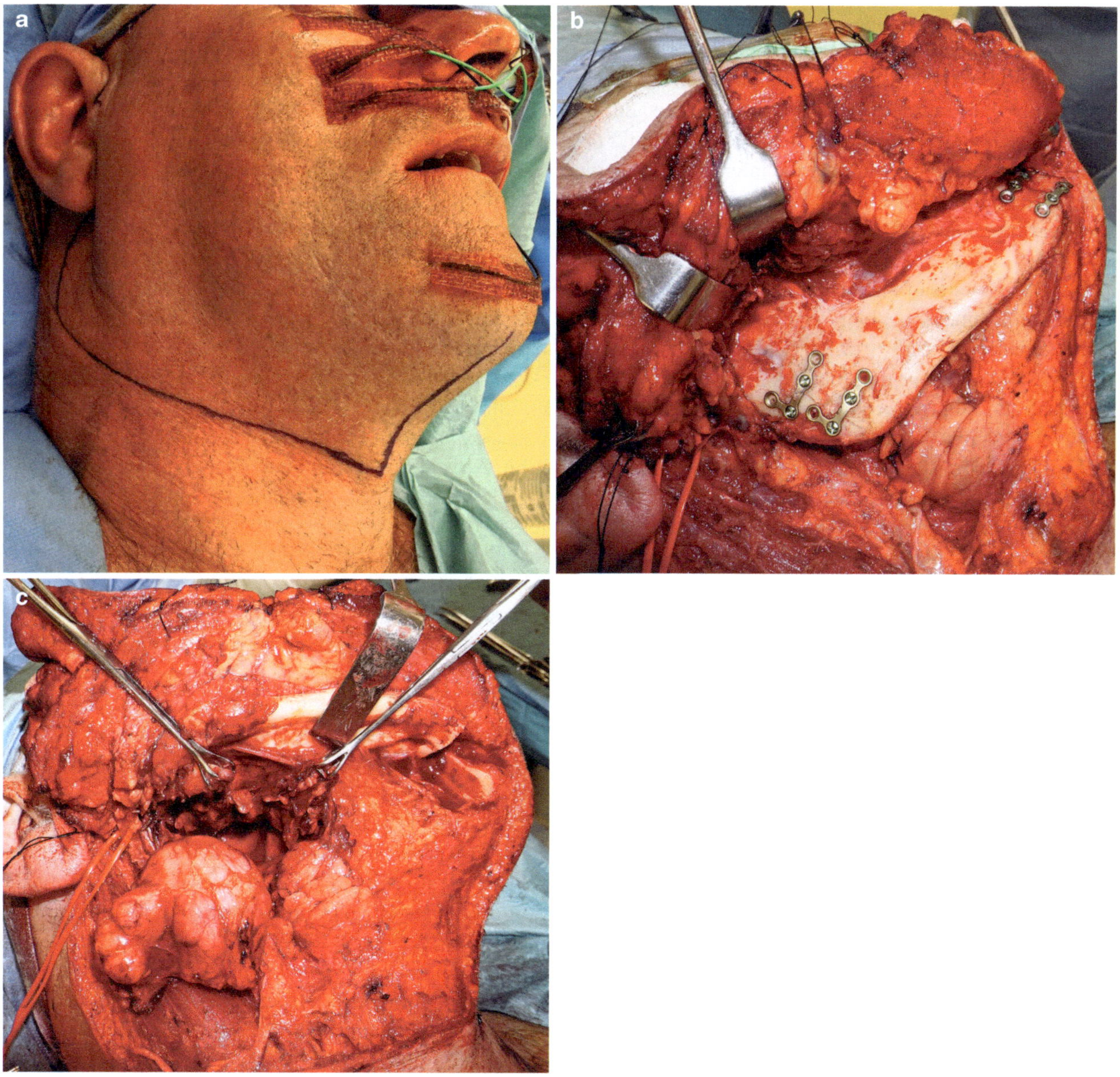

Fig. 85.8 Double mandibular osteotomy. (**a**) Skin markings for double mandibular osteotomy. (**b**) Bone cuts marked and mandible pre-plated. (**c**) Mandibular segment retracted laterally and superiorly to expose deep lobe parotid tumour

85.8 Double Mandibular Osteotomy

Mandibular osteotomies to access the parapharyngeal region can be broadly divided into those involving the oral cavity (lip split mandibulotomy) and those staying out with the oral cavity. Since it was initially popularised by Attia [24] to access parapharyngeal and pterygomaxillary region, several designs of osteotomies have been described, involving one, two and three osteotomies, variously placed in the paramedian and ramus/condylar region [25].

Double mandibular osteotomy provides excellent access to the infratemporal fossa, parapharyngeal space, deep lobe of the parotid and terminal extracranial internal carotid artery adjacent to the skull base, when the oral cavity does not have to be entered.

A low-neck skin crease incision with submental extension is made (Fig. 85.8a), and the neck flap is raised in the subplatysmal plane up to the lower border of the mandible, preserving the marginal mandibular branch of the facial nerve. The lateral mandible is exposed in a subperiosteal plane and the mental nerve identified and protected anteriorly. The masseter muscle is detached from the lateral ramus of the mandible up to the sigmoid notch. The anterior bone cuts are fashioned anterior to the mental foramen, between the canine/lateral incisor or canine/first premolar teeth roots. The posterior bone cut is made from the sigmoid notch to the lower border of the mandible, posterior to the lingula and inferior dental canal (similar to a vertical sub-sigmoid osteotomy). The mandible is pre-plated prior to completion of the bone cuts (Fig. 85.8b). The plates are removed and replaced during the procedure. Following completion of the osteotomy, the segment of the mandible containing the inferior dental nerve is retracted lateral and superiorly to provide wide access to the parapharyngeal and infra temporal areas (Fig. 85.8c).

Further soft tissue dissection is dictated by the necessity to access specific parts of the medial mandibular area.

The stylomandibular ligament can be detached from the posterior "condylar" segment to obtain further exposure of the stylomastoid area. The muscular and ligamentous attachments to the styloid process can be detached, and, if necessary, the styloid process is osteotomised to gain addition access to the "post-styloid" space, terminal extracranial internal carotid and the skull base close to the jugular foramen and lower cranial nerves.

This procedure avoids a lip split scar and helps preserve sensation to the lip while providing access to the more "difficult-to-reach" areas.

85.8.1 Potential Complications and Solutions (Clinical Pearls)

Mental and marginal mandibular nerve damage: Appropriate plane of dissection and identification and protection of the nerves. Osteotomies planned to avoid the course of the inferior dental nerve.

Delayed bone healing: Pre-plating prior to completion of osteotomy, use fine saw blades, burs, osteotomes and copious irrigation.

Damage to adjacent teeth: Design osteotomy where space allows, use fine instruments and consider extraction.

Clinical Tips

- This procedure is considered when intraoral access is "not" required.
- A lip split scar is avoided.
- The lateral mandible is exposed in the subperiosteal plane, and the mental and facial nerve branches are protected.
- The bone cuts are made anterior to the mental foramen and posterior to the mandibular foramen and inferior dental canal.
- The osteotomy site is pre-plated prior to completion of the bone cuts.
- Styloid process and its' attachments can be detached to gain addition access to the post styloid and "stylomastoid" spaces.

85.9 Zygomatic Osteotomy

Facial translocation techniques allow modular craniofacial disassembly of the facial skeleton to access "relatively" inaccessible regions of the skull base and nasopharynx. A variety of osteotomies have been described, but with the increased use of endoscopic approaches, the necessity for extensive procedures continues to diminish. Various modifications of zygomatic and orbital osteotomies in combination with craniotomies has been described since it was popularised by Lesoin [26], Hakuba [27] and Sindou [28] to access skull base lesions.

Zygomatic osteotomy, pedicled on the masseter muscle and its subsequent inferior displacement, provides simultaneous exposure of the temporal and infratemporal fossa and orbit. An additional frontotemporal craniotomy can link the middle and anterior cranial fossa and the middle cranial fossa with the infratemporal fossa. The extent of the "zygomatic" osteotomy and the direction of retraction of the temporalis is determined by the location of the pathology. For subcranial lesions, (temporal/infratemporal fossa/orbit), the temporalis is retracted superiorly following a coronoidectomy. For simultaneous exposure of the anterior/middle cranial fossa and temporal/infratemporal fossa/orbit, the temporalis is reflected inferiorly. The vascularity of the temporalis muscle can be at risk with both superior and inferior retraction.

The zygomatic body, arch and lateral and inferior orbital rims are exposed via a coronal flap (Fig. 85.1e, g). Meticulous subperiosteal orbital dissection is carried out to protect the orbital contents, which are retracted with thin malleable retractors. The temporalis is detached from the lateral orbit in the temporal fossa. The lateral end of the inferior orbital fissure is identified in the temporal fossa and orbit with a blunt hook. The bone cuts are made with a fine saw: superiorly at the frontozygomatic suture, infero-laterally from the lateral infraorbital rim through the body of the zygoma towards the inferior orbital fissure and posteriorly just anterior to the articular eminence. A sagittal bone cut is then made in the lateral orbital wall from the temporal fossa aspect, extending from the frontozygomatic suture osteotomy to the inferior orbital fissure (Fig. 85.9a). A more limited zygomatic arch osteotomy can be utilised, when orbital access is not required (Fig. 85.9b). The osteotomy is preplated, and plates are removed and replaced during the procedure (Fig. 85.9b). The cuts are completed, and the zygoma is mobilised and pedicled inferiorly on the masseter muscle.

Exposure to the infratemporal fossa is limited with a zygomatic osteotomy, which restricts its use to benign pathology, when utilised as a sole means of access. It can however be combined with frontotemporal craniotomy to widely access the anterior and middle cranial fossa, optic canal, superior orbital fissure and for combined middle cranial/infratemporal fossa resections (Figs. 85.1h and 85.9c).

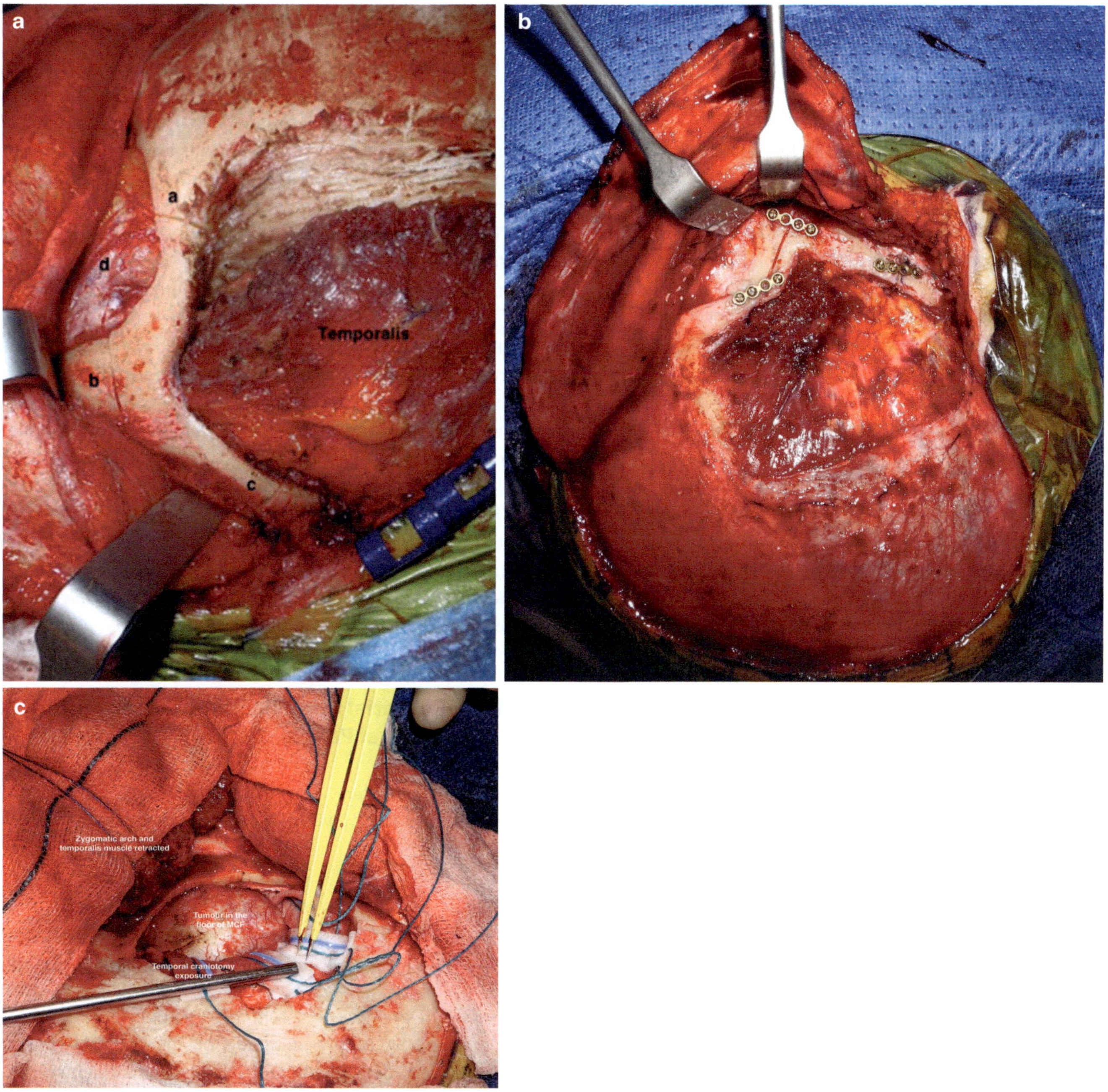

Fig. 85.9 Zygomatic osteotomy. (**a**) Bone cuts marked for a zygomatic osteotomy. (**a**) Osteotomy above frontozygomatic suture, (**b**) osteotomy across body of zygoma, (**c**) osteotomy across zygomatic arch and (**d**) orbital contents. (**b**) Bone cuts marked and pre-plated for zygomatic arch osteotomy (extended to lateral orbital rim due to increased width of orbital rim). (**c**) Tumour exposed in the floor of the middle cranial fossa following temporal craniotomy and retraction of the zygomatic arch and temporalis

85.9.1 Potential Complications and Solutions (Clinical Pearls)

Delayed bone healing: Preserve masseter attachment, pre-plating prior to completion of osteotomy, use fine saw blades, burs, osteotomes and copious irrigation.

Damage to orbital contents: Meticulous intra-orbital subperiosteal dissection and haemostasis, fine malleable retractors for orbital retraction and bone cuts under "direct" vision.

Malposition of lateral canthus: Accurate bone re-approximation with pre-plating. Consider tagging lateral canthus prior to detachment and subsequent reattachment.

Clinical Tips

- The lateral limit of the inferior orbital fissure in the orbit and temporal fossa is an important landmark for orbital and zygomatic osteotomies. A "blunt hook" can help with its safe identification.
- The extent of the osteotomy is determined by the location of the lesion and the need to enter the orbit.
- The attachment of the masseter muscle to the osteotomised zygomatic complex should be preserved.
- The osteotomy along the zygomatic arch should be made anterior to the articular eminence, to avoid disturbing the temporomandibular joint.
- The osteotomy sites are pre-plated, prior to completion of the bone cuts.
- Trismus is often expected and can be minimised by jaw opening exercises.

85.10 Lateral and Superior Orbitotomies

Lateral orbitotomy was initially popularised by Kronlein [29] but with a reverse "C"-shaped incision overlying the temple. A variety of modifications, principally in the design of the skin incisions, have been described subsequently: lateral canthotomy [30, 31] "S"-shaped incision over the orbital rim, upper eyelid skin crease incision and coronal flap.

Superior/lateral orbitotomies, combined with frontal [32] and pterional [33] craniotomies have been extensively used since their original descriptions in the 1980s.

This approach is useful for lacrimal and lateral/superior/inferior extra and intraconal orbital lesions and provides additional access for "lookup" approaches to the anterior and middle cranial fossa and for reconstruction with a temporalis flap following orbital exenteration.

A coronal flap is raised, and the zygomatic complex is exposed as described above for the zygomatic osteotomy (Fig. 85.10a). For isolated lesions, a Stallard-Wright [31] "S"-shaped incision extending from the eyebrow, inferolaterally over the lateral orbital rim to the crow's feet skin crease or an upper eyelid skin crease, can be utilised (Fig. 85.10b). The temporalis muscle is reflected posteriorly to expose the temporal aspect of the lateral orbit, and the orbital periosteum (periorbita) is elevated from lateral orbital wall (Fig. 85.10c). The lateral end of inferior orbital fissure is identified with a blunt hook, both within the orbit and the temporal fossa. Perforating blood vessels are identified and coagulated prior to division.

The orbital contents are protected with a malleable retractor, and the bone cuts are made with a thin saw. Superiorly, just above the frontozygomatic suture; inferiorly, inferior lateral orbital rim along the superior border of the zygomatic arch (the superior border of the zygomatic arch is at the same level as the orbital floor) up to the lateral limit of inferior orbital fissure.

The posterior cut is made with a fine bur/piezo saw in the lateral orbital wall, joining the superior bone cut to the lateral limit of the inferior orbital fissure. This is more easily made from the temporal aspect. The bone cuts are pre-plated prior to removal of the osteotomised segment and plates replaced following completion of the procedure.

The lateral orbitotomy can be combined with a superior orbitotomy and is usually performed in conjunction with a frontotemporal craniotomy. The craniotomy is best performed initially, and the superior orbital wall is delineated from the cranial aspect. With malleable retractors in situ, the superior and lateral orbitotomy can be carried out under direct vision (Fig. 85.10d). This provides excellent exposure of the contents of the superior orbit, superior orbital fissure and optic nerve/canal (Fig. 85.10e). This can also be used for "lookup" approaches to the superior anterior and middle cranial fossa lesions. The bone flaps are replaced (Fig. 85.10f), and the wounds are closed in layers. The medial extent of the superior orbitomy can be limited by the extent of the frontal sinus. The supraorbital neurovascular bundle will have to be protected/retracted.

85.10.1 Potential Complications and Solutions (Clinical Pearls)

Delayed bone healing: Pre-plating prior to completion of osteotomy, use fine saw blades, burs, osteotomes and copious irrigation.

Damage to orbital contents: Meticulous intra-orbital subperiosteal dissection and haemostasis, fine malleable retractors for orbital retraction and bone cuts under "direct" vision.

Malposition of lateral canthus: Accurate bone reapproximation with pre-plating. Consider tagging lateral canthus prior to detachment and subsequent reattachment.

Clinical Tips

- The lateral limit of the inferior orbital fissure in the orbit and temporal fossa is an important landmark for orbital and zygomatic osteotomies. A "blunt hook" can help with its safe identification.
- The extent of the osteotomy is determined by the location of the lesion.
- The superior surface of the zygomatic arch is in line with the orbital floor and is a useful landmark for bone cuts in the lateral orbital rim.
- The osteotomy sites are pre-plated prior to completion of the bone cuts.

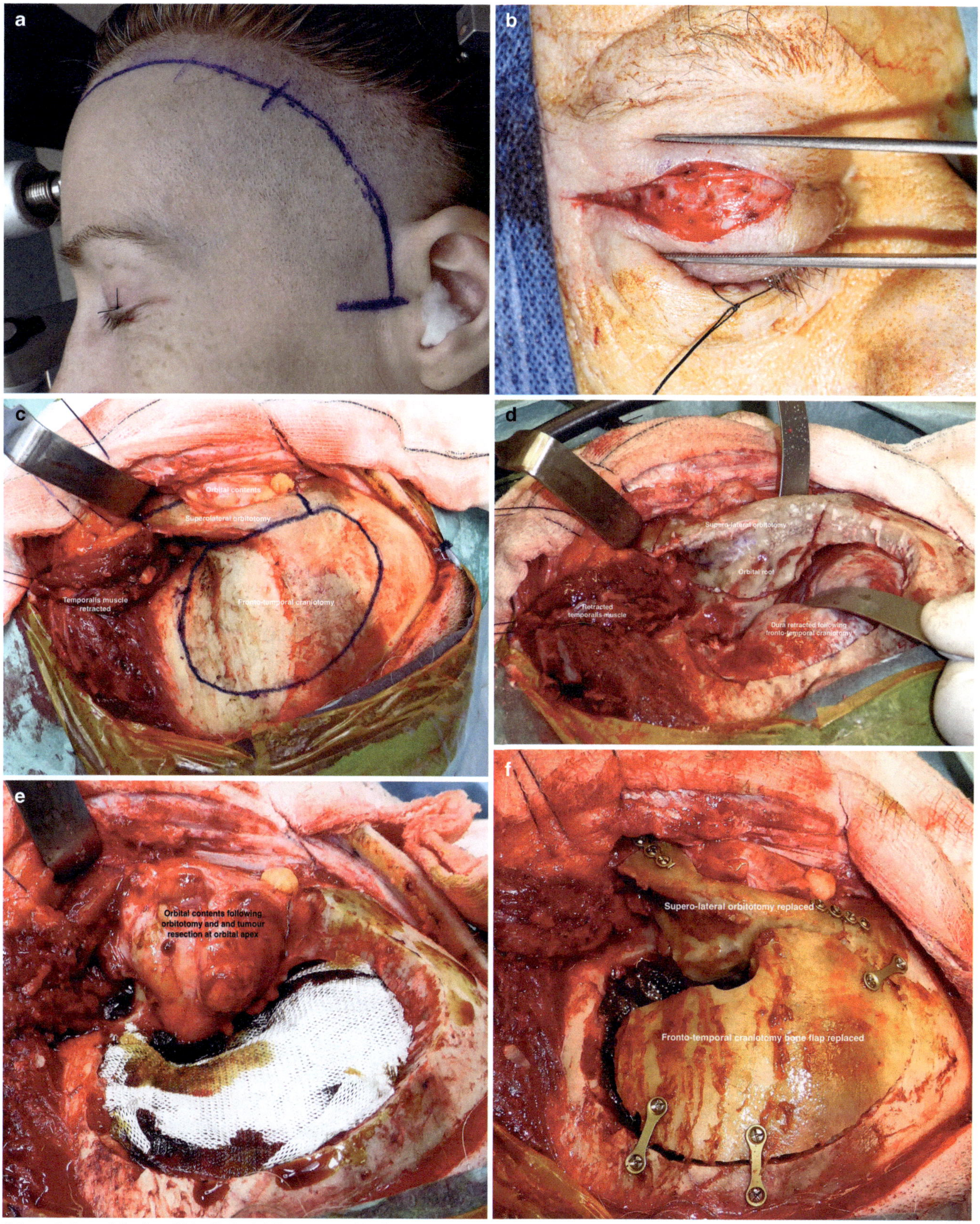

Fig. 85.10 Lateral and superior orbitotomies. (**a**) Skin marking for a hemicoronal flap. (**b**) Upper eyelid skin crease incision for lateral orbitotomy. (**c**) Bone marking for superolateral orbitotomy and frontotemporal craniotomy. (**d**) Superolateral orbitotomy bone cuts following craniotomy. (**e**) Exposure of the orbital contents following orbitotomy. (**f**) Craniotomy and orbitotomy bone flaps replaced

85.11 Conclusion

Multiple routes are available to the clinician to access the pathology in the craniomaxillofacial region. The technical aspects of the individual procedures are described in detail, along with the potential alternatives and a progressive algorithm. An understanding of the relevant anatomy, a critical analysis of the extent of the lesion, exposure required and potential reconstruction helps in determining the most appropriate choice of procedure. There is no substitute to working within well-functioning teams to obtain the relevant clinical experience.

85.12 Algorithms

The following algorithms provide a potential sequence that can be considered for progressive access for pathologies in the head and neck region. The algorithms "exclude" endoscopic approaches that can be used in isolation or in combination with open access for lesions especially in the nose, orbit, anterior skull base and retromaxilla.

1. Access to Buccal mucosa

Per oral access

↓

Soft tissue lip split
(Mid line / commisure lip split)

↓

Composite resection (skin / mucosa involvement)

↓

Compartment resection (skin / mucosa/ bone involvement)

2. Access to Tongue

Per oral access (anterior / lateral tongue)

↓

Lip split mandibulotomy (lateral / posterior tongue / extensive floor of mouth involvement)

↓

Visor / lingual release (extensive bilateral tongue / floor of mouth involvement)

3. Access to Mandible

Per oral access (limited crestal involvement / marginal mandibulectomy)

↓

Transcervical / submental extension (lateral mandible, +/- floor of mouth involvement / segmental mandibulectomy)

↓

Soft tissue lip split (lateral / posterior mandible/ extensive floor of mouth / parapharyngeal involvement / segmental mandibulectomy)

↓

Visor flap (bilateral mandible / floor of mouth involvement)

4. Access to Maxilla*

Per oral access (crestal / infra structure involvement)

↓

Modified Weber-Fergusson (More extensive maxillary involvement, but no significant orbital/ ethmoid or posterior extension)

↓

Modified Weber- Fergusson with Diffenbach extension (Maxillary with significant orbital involvement)

↓

Modified Weber-Fergusson with Lynch extension (Maxillary with significant ethmoid involvement)

↓

Lip split mandibulotomy +/- Modified Weber-Fergusson (posterior maxillary, maxillary with significant posterior extension)

↓

Maxillary swing (posterior maxillary/ postero- medial extension to
Nasopharynx: anterior maxilla can be preserved)

↓

Facial degloving approach (anterior / bilateral maxillary lesion that cannot be accessed with per oral approach and need to avoid facial scar)

*Consider early coronoidectomy to improve access

5. Access to Nasal cavity*

- Per nasal (small anterior lesion)
- ↓ Lateral rhinotomy (ipsilateral nasal lesion)
- ↓ Nasal swing (soft tissue) – Bilateral lesion, able to preserve nasal skin
- ↓ Nasal swing (soft tissue / nasal bone) – Bilateral lesion, able to preserve skin and nasal bone)
- ↓ Facial degloving approach (Bilateral / inferior lesions, able to preserve nasal Skin
- ↓ Lefort 1 osteotomy (bilateral / inferior lesions)
- ↓ *With the wide spread use of endoscopic techniques, the need for open approaches as the "sole" access modality continues to diminish.

6. Access to Orbitotomies

(a) *Lateral orbitotomy (lateral lesions / temporalis reconstruction)*

- Lateral canthotomy
- ↓ Upper eyelid skin crease
- ↓ Hemicoronal

(b) *Lateral / superior orbitotomy (supero-lateral lesions / combined cranio- orbital lesions)*

- Hemi coronal / Bicoronal flap with fronto-temporal craniotomy

(c) *Inferior orbitotomy (inferior lesions)*

- Lower eyelid skin crease incision

7. Access to Parapharyngeal space (deep lobe parotid / post styloid compartment pathology)

- Transcervical
- ↓ Transcervical transparotid
- ↓ Double mandibular osteotomy (no oropharyngeal mucosal involvement)
- ↓ Lip split mandibulotomy (oropharyngeal mucosal involvement)

Common access procedures to the various sites[a]

Access	Procedure
Oral cavity	Per oral
	Soft tissue lip split
	Lip split with access mandibulotomy
	Visor flap
Maxilla	Per oral
	Modified Weber-Fergusson
	Modified Weber-Fergusson with Lynch and eyelid extensions
	Lip split mandibulotomy
	Facial degloving
	Combinations
Infratemporal fossa	Modified Weber-Fergusson with eyelid extension and early coronoidectomy (with maxillectomy)
	Lip split mandibulotomy
	Coronal flap with zygomatic osteotomy
	Maxillary swing
	Combinations
Nasal cavity	Per nasal
	Lateral rhinotomy
	Nasal swing
	Le fort 1 osteotomy
	Facial degloving
Pterygopalatine fossa/ nasopharynx	Maxillary swing
	Transpalatal approaches
	Le fort 1 down fracture ± midline split
Orbit	Various soft tissue incisions
	Lateral orbitotomy
	Superior orbitotomy
	Inferior orbitotomy
	Combinations

[a]Excludes endoscopic approaches, which can be utilised alone or in combination with the open approaches

References

1. Hartley F, Kenyon JH. Experiences in cerebral surgery. Ann Surg. 1907;45(4):481–530.
2. Tessier P. The definitive plastic surgical treatment of the severe facial deformities of craniofacial dysostosis: Crouzon's and Apertt's diseases. Plast Reconstr Surg. 1971;48(5):419–42.
3. Munro IR, Fearon JA. The coronal flap revisited. Plast Reconstr Surg. 1994;93(1):185–7.
4. Al-Kayat A, Bramley P. A modified pre-auricular approach to the temporomandibular joint and malar arch. Br J Oral Surg. 1979;17(2):91–103.
5. Kleinberger AJ, Jumaily J, Spiegel JH. Safety of modified coronal approach with dissection deep to temporalis fascia for facial nerve preservation. Otolaryngol Head Neck Surg. 2015;152(4):655–60.
6. Kadakia S, Badhey A, Ashai S, Lee TS, Ducic Y. Alopecia following bicoronal incisions. JAMA Facial Plast Surg. 2017;19(3):220–4.
7. Weber O. Vorstellung einer kranken mit resection des unterkiefers verhandlungen des naturhist. Med Vereins z Heidelberg. 1845;4:80–2. (in German)
8. Fergusson W. In operation of the upper jaw. A system of practical surgery. Edinburgh: John Churchill; 1842. p. 484.
9. Altemir FH. Transfacial access to the retromaxillary area. J Maxillofac Surg. 1986;14(3):165–70.
10. Dieffenbach JF. Die operative chirurgie. Leipzig: Brockans; 1845.
11. Lynch RC. The technique of a radical frontal sinus operation which has given me the best results. Laryngoscope. 1921;31:1.
12. Moure EJ. Traitment des tumors malignes primitives de l'ethmoide. Rev Laryngol Otol Rhinol (Bord). 1902; 23401–412.
13. Thankappan K, Sharan R, Iyer S, Kuriakose MA. Aesthetic and anatomic basis of modified lateral rhinotomy approach. J Oral Maxillofac Surg. 2009;67:231–4.
14. Conley J, Price JC. Sublabial approach to the nasal cavity and nasopharyngeal cavities. Am J Surg. 1979;38:615–8.
15. Maniglia AJ. Indications and techniques of midfacial degloving. Arch Otolaryngol Head Neck Surg. 1986;112(7):750–2.
16. Wei WL, Lam KH, Sham JT. New approach to the nasopharynx: the maxillary swing approach. Head Neck Surg. 1991;12:200–7.
17. Roux PJ, Butlin HT, Spencer GJ, editors. Diseases of the tongue. London: Cassell; 1900. p. 359.
18. Trotter W. Operations for malignant diseases of the pharynx. Br J Surgery. 1929;16:485.
19. McGregor IA, McDonald DG. Mandibular osteotomy in the surgical approach to the oral cavity. Head Neck Surg. 1983;5:457.
20. Hayter JP, Vaughan ED, Brown JS. Aesthetic lip splits. Br J Oral Maxillofac Surg. 1996;34:432.
21. Stanley RB. Mandibular lingual releasing approach to oral and oropharyngeal carcinomas. Laryngoscope. 1984;94:596–600.
22. Stringer SP, Randall Jordan J, Mendenhall WM, et al. Mandibular lingual releasing approach. Otolaryngol Head Neck Surg. 1992;107:395–8.
23. Spiro RH, Gerold FP, Strong EW. Mandibular swing approach for oral and oropharyngeal tumours. Head Neck Surg. 1981;3:371–8.
24. Attia EL, Bentley KC, Head T, Mulder D. A new external approach to the pterygomaxillary fossa and parapharyngeal space. Head Neck Surg. 1984;6(4):884–91.
25. Smith GI, Brennan PA, Webb AA, Ilankovan V. Vertical ramus osteotomy combined with a parasymphyseal mandibulotomy for improved access to the parapharyngeal space. Head Neck. 2003;25:1000–3.
26. Lesoin F, Pellerian P, Villette L, Autricque A, Jomin M. Value of the mobilisation of the orbito-zygomatico-malar flap. Neurochirurgie. 1986;32(1):90–3.
27. Hakuba A, Liu S, Nishimura S. The orbitozygomatic infratemporal approach: a new surgical technique. Surg Neurol. 1986;26:271–6.
28. Sindou M, Emery E, Acevedo G, Bem-David U. Respective indications for orbital rim, zygomatic arch and orbito-zygomatic osteotomies in the surgical approach to central skull base lesions. Critical, retrospective review in 146 cases. Acta Neurochir (Wein). 2001;143(10):967–75.
29. Kronlein RU. Zur Pathologie und operativen behandlung der dermoidcysten der orbita. Beitr Kilin Chir. 1888;4:149.
30. Berke RN. A modified Kronlein operation. Arch Ophthalmol. 1954;51:609.
31. Stallard HB. A plea for lateral orbitotomy with certain modifications. Brit J Ophthal. 1960;44:718–23.
32. Jane JA, Park TS, Pobereskin LH, Winn HR, Butler AB. The supraorbital approach: technical note. Neurosurgery. 1982;11(4):537–42.
33. Al-Mefty O. Supra-orbital -pterional approach to skull base lesions. Neurosurgery. 1987;21:474–7.

Additional Readings

Ethunandan M, Evans BT, Lang D. Access surgery. In: Langdon J, Patel M, Ord R, Brennan P, editors. Operative oral & maxillofacial surgery. 3rd ed. London: Hodder Arnold; 2017.

Ethunandan M. Infra-temporal fossa and pterygopalatine fossa. In: Brenna PA, Standring S, Wiseman SM, editors. Gray's surgical anatomy. St. Louis, MO: Elsevier; 2019.

Chatni SC, Sharan R, Patel D, Iyer S, Tiwari RM, Kuriakose MA. Transmandibular approach for excision of maxillary sinus tumors extending to the pterygopalatine and infratemporal fossa. Oral Oncol. 2009;45:720–6.

Shahinian H, Dornier MD, Fisch U. Parapharyngeal space tumours: the infratemporal fossa approach. Skull Base Surg. 1995;5:73–81.

Evans BT, Wiesenfeld D, Clauser L, Curioni C. Surgical approaches to the infratemporal fossa. In: Langdon J, BKB B, Moxham BJ, editors. Surgical anatomy of the infratemporal fossa. London: Martin Dunitz; 2003.

Lateral Rhinotomy

Mertz JS, Pearson BW, Kern EB. Lateral rhinotomy. Indications, technique, and a review of 226 patients. Arch Otolaryngol. 1983;109(4):235–9.

Lip Split

Rapidis AD, Valsamis S, Anterriotis DA, Skouteris CA. Functional and aesthetic results of various lip splitting incisions: a clinical analysis of 60 cases. J Oral Maxillofac Surg. 2001;59:1292–6.

Double Mandibular Osteotomies

Kolokythas A, Eisle DW, El-Sayed I, Schmidt BL. Mandibular osteotomies for access to select parapharyngeal space neoplasms. Head Neck. 2009;31(1):102–10.

Flood TR, Hislop WS. A modified surgical approach for parapharyngeal space tumours: use of the inverted "L" osteotomy. Br J Oral Maxillofacial Surg. 1991;29(2):82–6.

Schlieve T, Carlson ER, Freeman M, Buckley R, Arnold J. The double mandibular osteotomy for vascular and tumour surgery of the parapharyngeal space. J Oral Maxillofac Surg. 2017;75:1046–61.

Part XXII

Reconstructive Procedures of the Oral and Maxillofacial Region

86 Soft Tissue Reconstruction of the Maxillofacial Region

Benjamin Turner, John Collin, and Rui Fernandes

86.1 General Considerations

The general precept of reconstructive surgery is to assess what tissue and structures are missing and what is available to replace them, ensuring that where possible 'like should replace like'. Hard tissue defects are best restored with hard tissue and soft, soft tissue. Usually skin closest to the defect will give the best cosmetic match. Hard tissue reconstruction falls outwith the remit of this chapter, but where required it should be performed first to provide the foundation for successful soft tissue reconstruction. Next, muscle and fasciocutaneous tissue should be resuspended from the maxillofacial skeleton to restore muscle function and prevent ptosis of the soft tissues. The aerodigestive tract needs to be isolated from the cranial cavity, deep neck spaces and external skin to reduce the risk of spreading infection, fistula and sinus formation. Finally, the aphorism that form follows function is germane and careful reconstruction of normal anatomy will often meet the dual goals of cosmesis and restoration of function. Anatomical subunits should be respected, and generally if the defect is greater than 50% of a subunit, better results are obtained with removal and reconstruction of the entire subunit such that scars are camouflaged within their boundary lines (Table 86.1).

For any particular defect, the choice of reconstruction can range from simple to complex, along a continuum commonly described as the 'reconstructive ladder'(Table 86.2) [1]. The 'reconstructive matrix' has also been described as a development of this linear concept to take into account technical requirements and potential risks to the patient on additional axes (Fig. 86.1) [2].

Table 86.1 Key concepts of reconstructive surgery

Replace like with like
Hard tissue reconstruction first
Respect anatomical units/subunits
Local skin usually best cosmetic option
Consider options within reconstructive ladder/matrix

86.1.1 Healing by Secondary Intention

Where there has been soft tissue loss and/or the skin is not re-approximated, healing occurs via secondary intention with deposition of granulation tissue (Fig. 86.2). Typically this results in a broader area of scar tissue and is therefore inadvisable at most sites in the maxillofacial region. Superficial defects of concave subsites (e.g. medial canthus, conchal bowl) or mucosa are the exception and may be left to heal by secondary intention with good cosmetic results.

86.1.2 Primary Closure

Primary closure describes the apposition of skin edges to permit healing without granulation tissue formation and minimal scaring (Fig. 86.2). Ideally lines of primary closure should coincide with the boundaries of the anatomical subunits (Fig. 86.3), such that the scar is hidden in a natural skin crease or hairline or mimics the natural highlight of the white roll of the lip, for example. Similarly, for ablative procedures involving 50% or more of an anatomical subunit, it is preferred to remove the entire subunit for these reasons. Obviously reconstruction would then entail some kind of tissue transfer. A further consideration is orientation of closure

B. Turner · J. Collin
Head and Neck Oncologic and Microvascular Reconstructive Surgery, Fellowship, Jacksonville, Florida, USA
e-mail: Benjamin.Turner@jax.ufl.edu; John.Collin@jax.ufl.edu

R. Fernandes (✉)
Professor, Department of Oral and Maxillofacial Surgery, University of Florida, Florida, USA

Division of Head and Neck Surgery, Jacksonville, Florida, USA
e-mail: Rui.Fernandes@jax.ufl.edu

K. Bonanthaya et al. (eds.), *Oral and Maxillofacial Surgery for the Clinician*, https://doi.org/10.1007/978-981-15-1346-6_86

Table 86.2 Reconstructive ladder

Transplantation			**Biomaterials** Decellularised material-Nerve/Bone/Cartilage Dermal matrices Synthetic materials–Hyaluronic acid/Silicone/PTFE Growth Factors
Flaps	Free		
	Pedicled	Distant	
		Regional	
	Local	Axial	
		Random Pattern	
Grafts	Full Thickness	+/ - Tissue expansion	
	Split Thickness		
Primary closure		+/ - plasties	
Secondary Intention		+/ - negative pressure dressings	

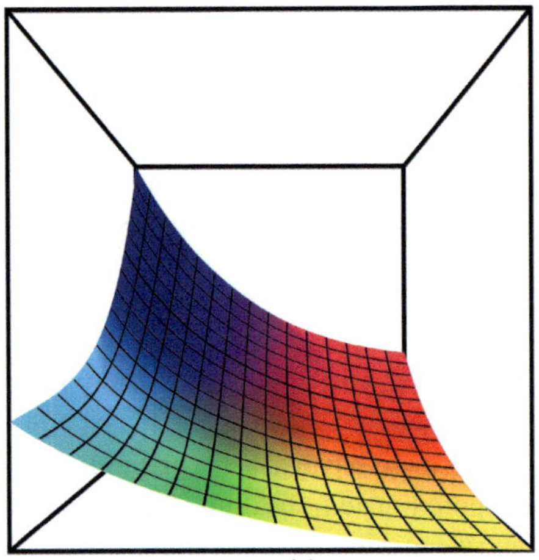

Fig. 86.1 The reconstructive matrix

with respect to the lines of relaxed skin tension that typically run perpendicular to underlying muscle fibres where possible. These two factors may dictate the decision to excise further tissue in a traumatic injury. The temptation to excise and close primarily out with these orientations should be avoided; however, as unless tissue is grossly contaminated or frankly necrotic, a straight surgical scar is usually more prominent than random pattern scars. The generous vascular supply of the face means that it is always best to err on the side of caution and perform minimal debridement such that a maximum of soft tissue is preserved.

Primary closure is appropriate for small defects that can be closed without significant tension or distortion of key areas such as the apertures of the mouth, nares and orbit. The latter is particularly sensitive to these effects and can result in ectropion and ocular sequelae if appropriate care is not taken. Techniques such as a creating a superior lateral canthal curve to the Mustarde flap, canthopexy and Frost sutures can be employed to reduce the risk of ectropion.

86.1.3 Grafts

The third rung of the reconstructive ladder is occupied by grafts, which may be further categorized as simple if composed of a single tissue type—commonly split or full-thickness skin but also mucosal grafts, or composite when containing more than one tissue type. Generally they are autografts, although xenografts and bioengineered material such as porcine collagen (Permacol), Polytetrafluoroethylene, fish skin and dermal matrix (e.g. Integra) have certain utility in maxillofacial reconstruction (Table 86.2).

86.1.4 Flaps

Flaps may be local, pedicled (regional or distant) or free. Local flaps transfer tissue to a defect by advancement and/or rotation and are typically supplied by a random vascular pattern. Axial flaps based on a named vessel can potentially pro-

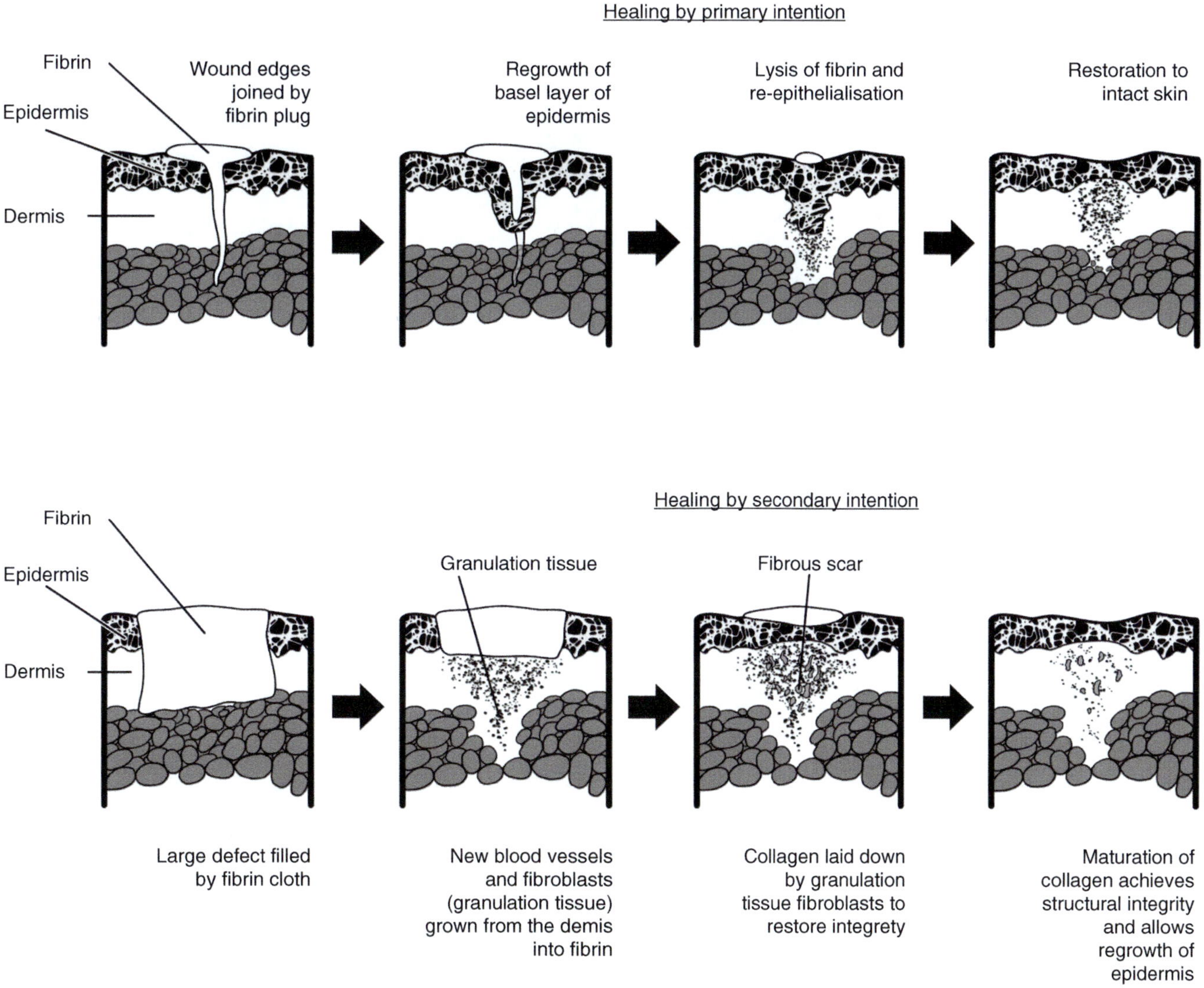

Fig. 86.2 Wound healing by primary and secondary intention

vide a flap of longer length to width ratio. Examples in the head and neck region include the paramedian forehead flap, nasolabial flap and facial artery myomucosal flap.

Regional pedicled flaps are able to provide a far greater area of soft tissue coverage than is possible with local flaps in the maxillofacial region, without requiring the facilities and expertise for microvascular reconstruction. They are generally less technique sensitive and susceptible to failure than microvascular free flaps; however, partial failure can still be problematic. For example, the pectoralis major myocutaneous flap has been reported to have a partial necrosis rate of up to 29% [3, 4]. Furthermore, while pedicled flaps are versatile and can usually provide a good skin match, free tissue transfer can often be a better option.

Free flaps offer many reconstructive options and can provide good cosmetic and functional outcomes. They may be sub-classified according to the tissue they contain and whether the pedicle is a named vessel or from a perforator system. Free flaps are available to reconstruct practically any size of defect in the maxillofacial region. Freedom from a pedicle allows them to be placed in any location, native vessels permitting.

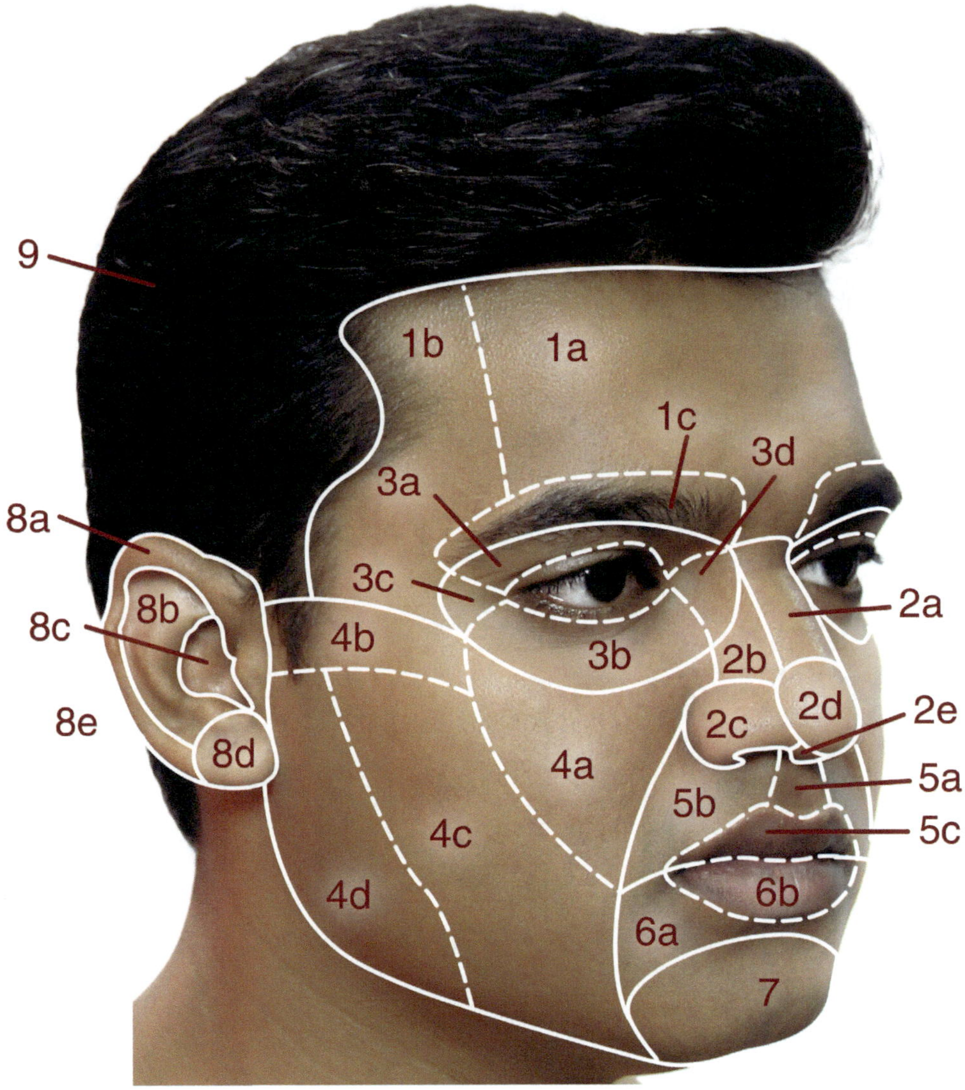

Fig. 86.3 Facial aesthetic units (Also refer Fig. 49.2)

Facial Cosmetic Units

1. Forehead:
   - 1a. Central
   - 1b. Lateral
   - 1c. Brow
2. Nose:
   - 2a. Dorsum
   - 2b. Lateral wall
   - 2c. Ala
   - 2d. Tip
   - 2e. Columella
3. Eyelid:
   - 3a. Superior
   - 3b. Inferior
   - 3c. Lateral canthus
   - 3d. Medial canthus
4. Cheek:
   - 4a. Infraorbital
   - 4b. Zygomatic
   - 4c. Buccal
   - 4d. Parotid-masseteric
5. Upper lip:
   - 5a. Philtrum
   - 5b. Lateral
   - 5c. Vermilion
6. Lower lip:
   - 6a. Central
   - 6b. Vermilion
7. Chin
8. Ear:
   - 8a. Helix
   - 8b. Antihelix
   - 8c. Concha
   - 8d. Earlobe
   - 8e. Retroauricular
9. Scalp

4. Cheek:
4a. Infraorbital
4b. Zygomatic

Disadvantages of flaps include:

- Their cost in resources and expertise.
- Increased operative time.
- Donor site morbidity.
- The risk of partial or complete failure.

86.1.5 Transplantation

Over recent years a number of partial and total facial transplants have been performed successfully. These cases are rare, requiring extremely careful selection and require a huge amount of resources. When indicated, however, this may be the only option to provide a cosmetic and to some extent functional outcome. Additional factors not associated with other reconstructive techniques, including donor selection, psychology, ethics and long-term immunosuppression require thorough consideration.

86.2 Reconstruction of the Oral Cavity

The functional roles of the oral cavity are among the most important in the body and are extremely sensitive to alteration resulting from even an apparently small defect. The coordinated action of structures within a relatively small anatomical region are critical for both nutrition (mastication and deglutition) and social interaction (speech and facial expression), two of the most vital activities that determine a patient's quality of life.

86.2.1 Reconstruction of the Lips

The aim of lip reconstruction should be to restore both function and aesthetics. Careful reconstitution of lip anatomy, such as the white roll, vermilion border and Cupid's bow, are required for a satisfactory cosmetic outcome. Continuity of the orbicularis oris muscle and adequate perioral sensation are needed to maintain lip competence. This is important during mastication and the oral stage of deglutition, particularly with fluids, and to prevent drooling in repose. The size of the reconstructed oral aperture will affect function too. All of these factors will contribute to the aesthetics of the lower third of the face.

The lips are unique in that they represent the transition from cutaneous tissue to keratinized dry and non-keratinized wet mucosa. As a result reconstruction of lip defects is best achieved by using remaining lip tissue when possible. This also often preserves contiguous, innervated orbicularis oris muscle and hence function as explained above.

Table 86.3 Time line of lip reconstruction techniques

Year	Author	Technique
1000 BC	Shushruta	First mention of lip repair
1597 AD	Tagliacozzi	Upper and lower lip repair using forearm flap
1768	Louie	Wedge excision described
1838	Sabattini	Full-thickness switch from lower to upper
1845	Dieffenbach	Cheek advancement for upper lip repair
1857	Von Bruns	Cheek advancement for lower lip repair
1872	Estlander	Upper to lower switch at commissure
1898	Abbe	Lip switch for bilateral cleft lip
1909	Lexer	Tongue flaps for lip repair
1954	Schuchardt	Sliding inferiorly based cheek flaps
1969	Bakamjian	Deltopectoral flap to lower lip defect
1974	Karapandzic	Advancement along nasolabial fold for lower lip defects

Therefore, local rotational, advancement and cross-lip flaps have become mainstays of reconstruction for larger deformities not amenable to direct or sliding lip closure (Table 86.3).

86.2.2 Reconstruction of the Vermillion

Deformity of the vermillion and the white roll of the lips is readily apparent to most observers; therefore careful reconstruction is vital for cosmesis. Small superficial defects that do not involve the underlying orbicularis muscle may be left to heal satisfactorily by secondary intention, although the process is slow (25 days on average) and can result in contracture [5, 6]. For these reasons, primary closure of a small vertically oriented fusiform excision is the preferred option, especially as often the defect will extend just beyond the vermillion, so control of the vermillion border re-approximation is required. Where redundant 'dog ear' mucosal tissue is likely to occur with primary closure of a mucosa only defect, a V-Y island of mucosa can be advanced from the labial mucosa or laterally from adjacent vermillion [7].

Large superficial defects of the upper or lower vermillion are best managed by resection of the entire vermillion subunit (lip shave) and advancement of a flap of labial mucosa. This provides a close cosmetic match, particularly in older patients. Sensation often returns with this approach; however, atrophy and contracture can be apparent particularly if the depth of the flap is not matched carefully to the depth of the defect. Alternatively, transfer of the vermillion of the opposing lip has been described, either as a single or bi-pedicled mucosal flap. Underlying muscle can be included as a myomucosal flap pedicled on the labial vessels [8]. These approaches require division and inset as a second procedure, arguably for minimal benefit compared with mucosal advancement from the labial mucosa. Reconstruction with tongue [9], buccal mucosal or myomucosal flaps can give acceptable results. Finally, anal verge mucosa grafts to the lips has also been described [10].

86.2.3 Reconstruction of the Lower Lip

86.2.3.1 Defects Up to one Half of Lower Lip Width

Depending on the laxity of the lower lip, which is mainly related to the age of the patient, most defects of less than one third to half the width of the lower lip can be closed primarily with excellent cosmetic and functional outcomes. The defect is extended inferiorly along a 'v' or shield shape incision. The point of the 'v' can be curved laterally to follow the labiomental groove to camouflage the scar in wider defects. In even larger defects, this groove can be followed on one or both sides of the base of the resection to aid in tissue mobilization. Some surgeons utilize a 'w'-shaped incision at the base of the defect, but this may result in a less cosmetic scar. Defects that involve the commissure can be more challenging as blunting that results may require a further commissuroplasty procedure.

86.2.3.2 Defects Greater Than One Half Lower Lip Width

Lower lip defects of this proportion are unlikely to be able to be closed primarily without causing unacceptable microstomia.

Lip Switch Flaps

A reverse Abbe flap (see *upper lip reconstruction* below) can be used to reconstruct larger lower lip defects, whereby a segment of upper lip with the same vertical dimension, but around 50% of the width of the lower lip defect is pedicled laterally on the labial artery. To prevent deformity of the upper lip, harvest should only be from lateral to the philtrum. In theory bilateral reverse Abbe flaps can be used, although the two pedicles that result make oral intake difficult until the flaps are inset.

Karapandzic Flap

The Karapandzic flap allows reconstruction of lower lip defects up to 80% of the lower lip width [11], with good preservation of function and aesthetics (Fig. 86.4). Some degree of microstomia and blunting of the commissures is caused, however. Unilateral or bilateral transdermal curvilinear incisions that follow the nasolabial creases allow mobilization and re-approximation of the remaining lower lip [12]. The incision extends through dermis only, preserving the neurovascular supply to the remaining lower lip either side of the defect. This is the main advantage compared with the older advancement flaps such as the Gillie's fan flap (Fig. 86.5), which disrupt underlying neurovasculature due to full-thickness incisions.

86.2.3.3 Subtotal Defects

Cheek Advancement Flaps

Bilateral horizontal cheek advancement flaps where described by Bernard (1852) and von Burow (1853) for reconstruction of large lip defects [13]. Tissue is advanced from the cheek by extending incisions laterally from the commissure and excising three triangles – two lateral Burow's triangles and one triangle around the defect of the lower lip itself. Webster refined this technique for reconstruction of lower lip defects using only partial-thickness incisions along the nasolabial and labiomental creases [14] (Figs. 86.6, 86.7 and 86.8). This concept was further refined

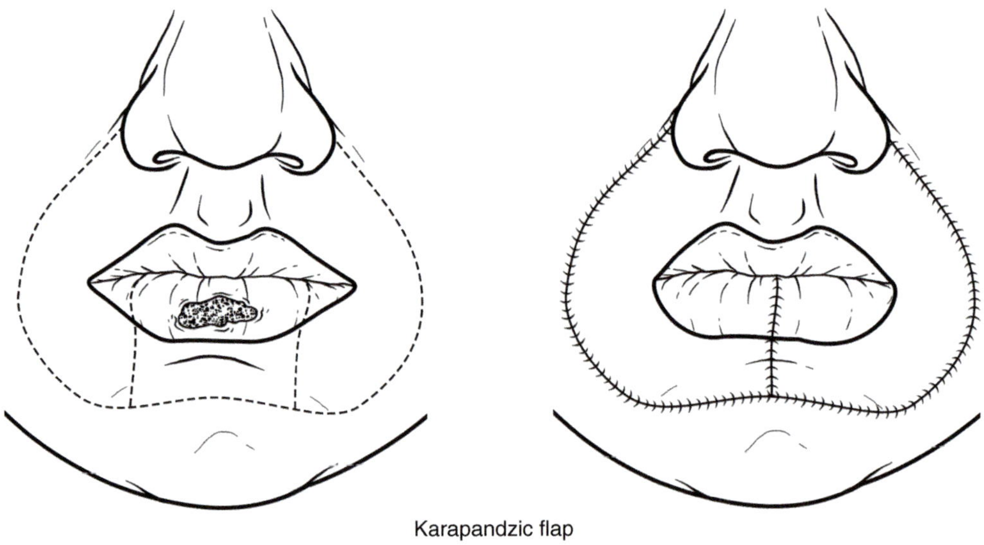

Fig. 86.4 Bilateral Karapandzic flaps for reconstruction of lower lip defect

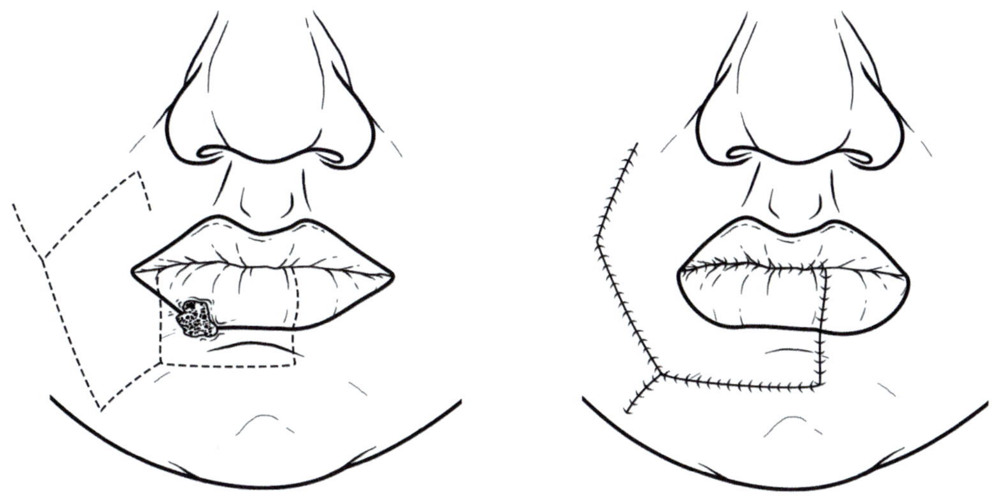

Fig. 86.5 Gillies fan flap for reconstruction of lower lip defects

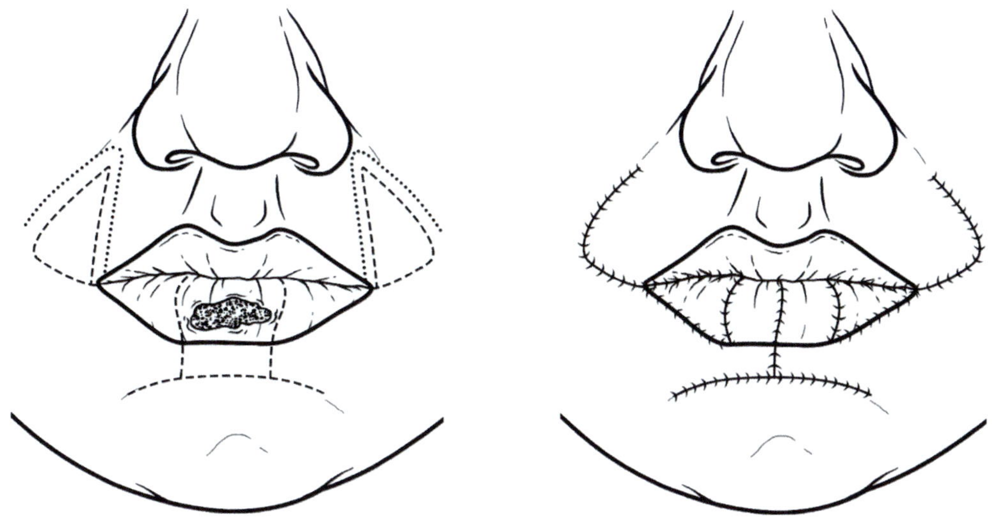

Fig. 86.6 Webster modification of Bernard-von Burow flap for lower lip reconstruction

by Pirgousis and Fernandes for lower lip reconstruction [15] (Figs. 86.9 and 86.10).

Nasolabial Flaps

Fujimori described 'gate' flaps that are effectively nasolabial flaps, which can be combined with a lower labial mucosa advancement flap to reconstruct the entire lower lip [16]. A similar technique allows reconstruct of the upper lip [17] (Fig. 86.11).

86.2.3.4 Reconstruction of the Upper Lip

Primary Closure

Defects of the upper lip are less amenable to primary closure than those of the lower lip. There is relatively less laxity, and asymmetry is more apparent because of deviation or distortion of the philtrum and nasal base. Defects up to around one quarter to one third of upper lip width can still be reapproximated satisfactorily, particularly if laterally situated. The philtrum is less forgiving though and while defects up to around half the width can be closed primarily, there is a tendency for flattening and upwards retraction of the vermillion in this subsite.

Lip Switch Flaps

The first report of a two-stage pedicled 'lip switch' flap was by Sabattini in 1838 [18]. The labial artery-based flap was popularized by Abbe in 1898, however, for use in cases of bilateral cleft lip [19]. The lower lip donor site is designed to be half the width of the upper lip defect (to equalized the horizontal discrepancy between upper and lower lips), equal to the height of the defect, and with a laterally based pedicle.

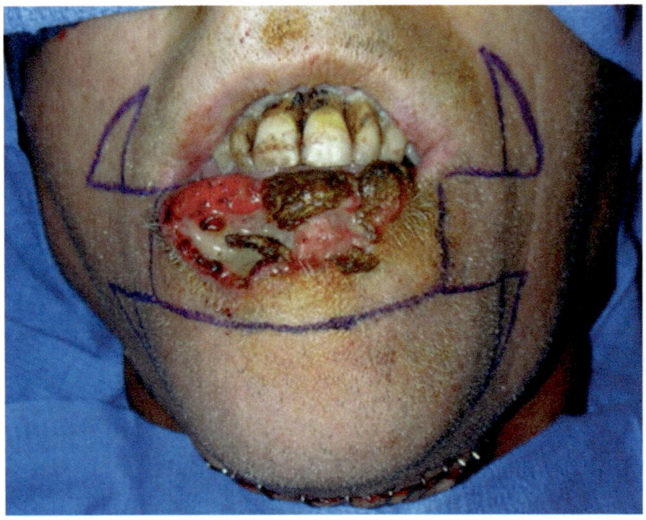

Fig. 86.7 Webster-Bernard-Burrow flap markings prior to lower lip resection

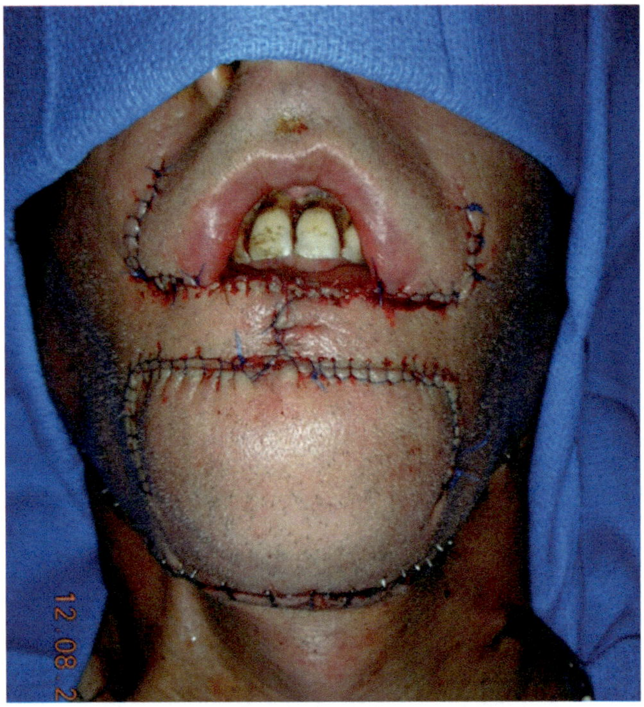

Fig. 86.8 Webster-Bernard-von Burow flap following closure

The central lower lip is the preferred donor site, as it is hair-bearing in males and leaves the least prominent scar. The white roll should be marked prior to incision and potential obscuration due to bleeding, oedema and pallor. The flap is raised including skin, muscle and mucosa but with preservation of the lateral vermilion incorporating the labial vessels. The flap is rotated and inset, taking care to re-approximate

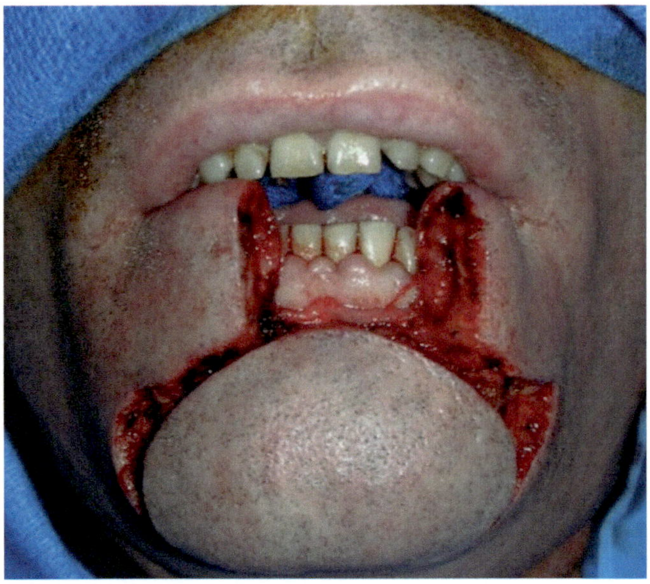

Fig. 86.9 Fernandes flap incisions following lower lip resection

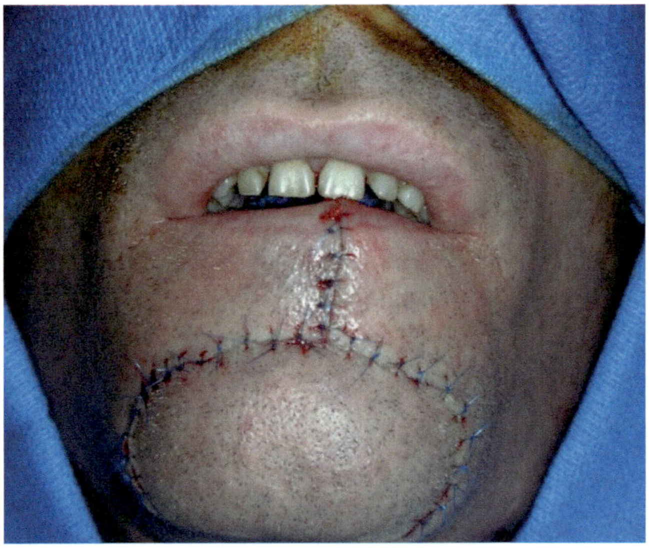

Fig. 86.10 Fernandes flap following closure

the orbicularis oris muscle and align the white roll (Fig. 86.12). After 2–3 weeks, the pedicle is divided and the flap inset. For defects of the commissure, Estlander described a similar flap where the commissure is the rotation point, and therefore no secondary insetting is required (Fig. 86.13).

Perialar Crescentic Advancement

Initially described by Webster [20], a perialar incision can be made unilaterally or bilaterally to recruit lateral tissue for closure of upper lip defects (Figs. 86.14 and 86.15). This technique can also be combined with an Abbe flap to recon-

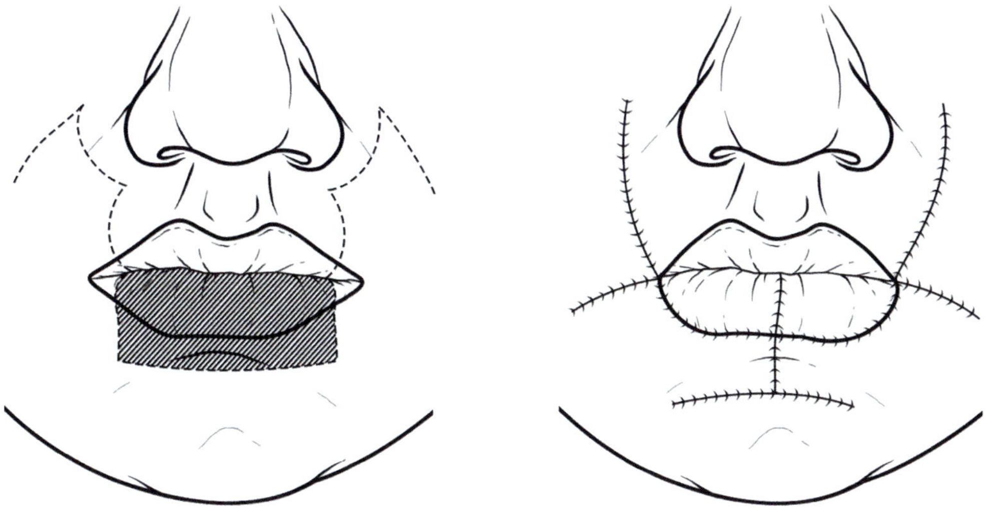
Nasolabial (von bruns) flap

Fig. 86.11 Bilateral nasolabial flaps for lower lip reconstruction

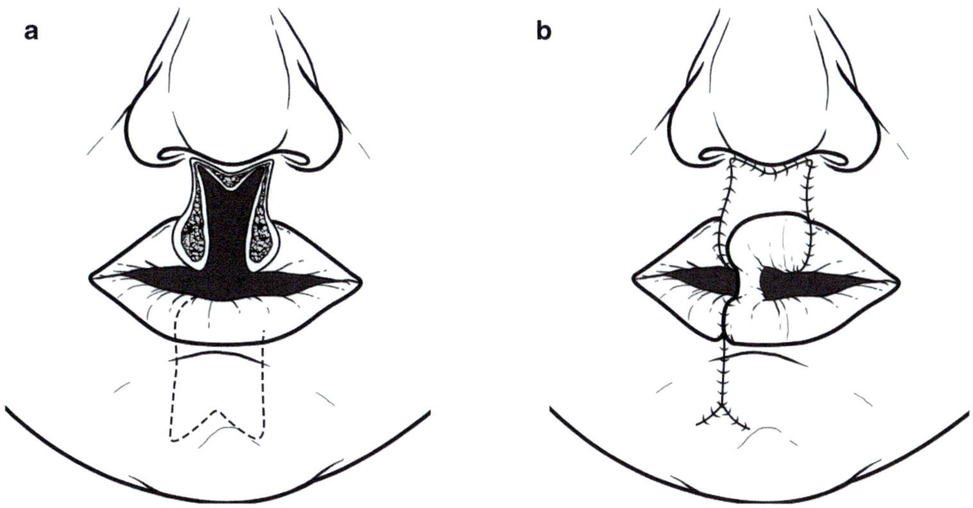

Fig. 86.12 Abbe flap for upper lip reconstruction. (**a**) Defect and flap markings. (**b**) Flap inset prior to division of pedicle

struct the philtrum when defects involve the midline of the upper lip.

Reverse Karapandzic

Incisions following the melolabial groove upwards to join the superior margin of an upper lip defect can be used to advance lateral tissue in a similar fashion as the Karapandzic flap does for closure of lower lip defects.

86.2.3.5 Commissuroplasty

Most of the reconstructive techniques described above result in blunting and rounding of the oral aperture. The simplest way to correct this is to make a horizontal full-thickness incision through the blunted commissure, extending laterally to correspond with the position of the contralateral normal commissure. Epithelium superior and inferior to the incision is excised and labial mucosa advanced from intraorally to recreate the vermilion (Fig. 86.16). An alternative method was described by Gillies and entails excision of a triangular segment of skin lateral to the rounded commissure, to a point comparable with the normal side. A vermilion flap from the opposite lip is then raised and rotated into this and a mucosal flap advanced to reconstruct the vermilion of the donor site (Fig. 86.17).

86.2.3.6 Total Lip Defects

A combination of the techniques presented above can be employed to reconstruct total defects of one or other lip. Increasingly, free tissue transfer is used instead, however. The most commonly used flap for this purpose is the radial free flap (Figs. 86.18 and 86.19). This is mainly due to the thin, soft, pliable tissue offered and reliable, long pedicle.

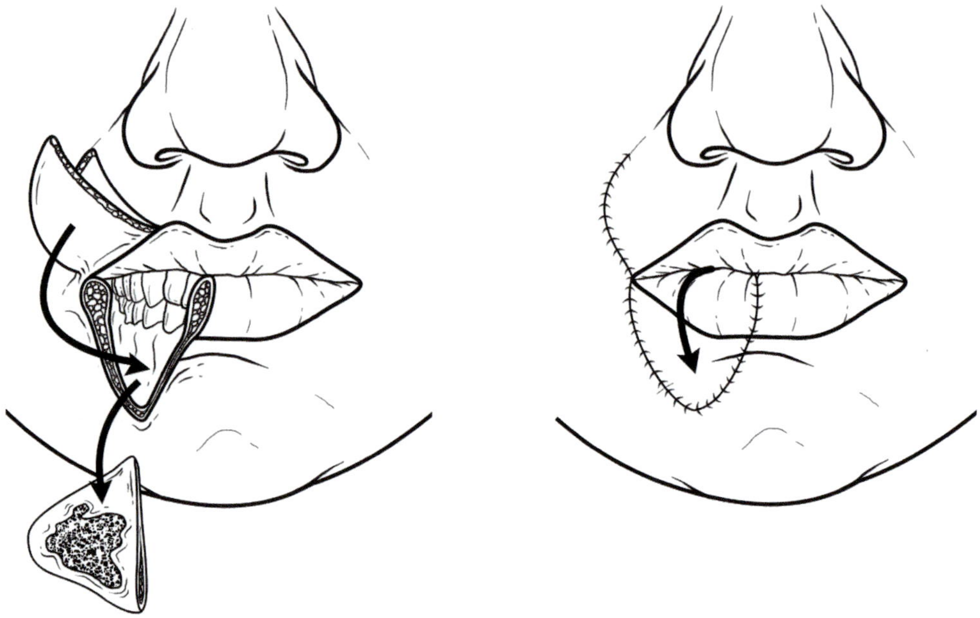

Fig. 86.13 Estlander flap for reconstruction of defect involving commissure. A medially pedicled full-thickness flap half the width of the defect is raised from the upper lip and inset into the lower lip defect

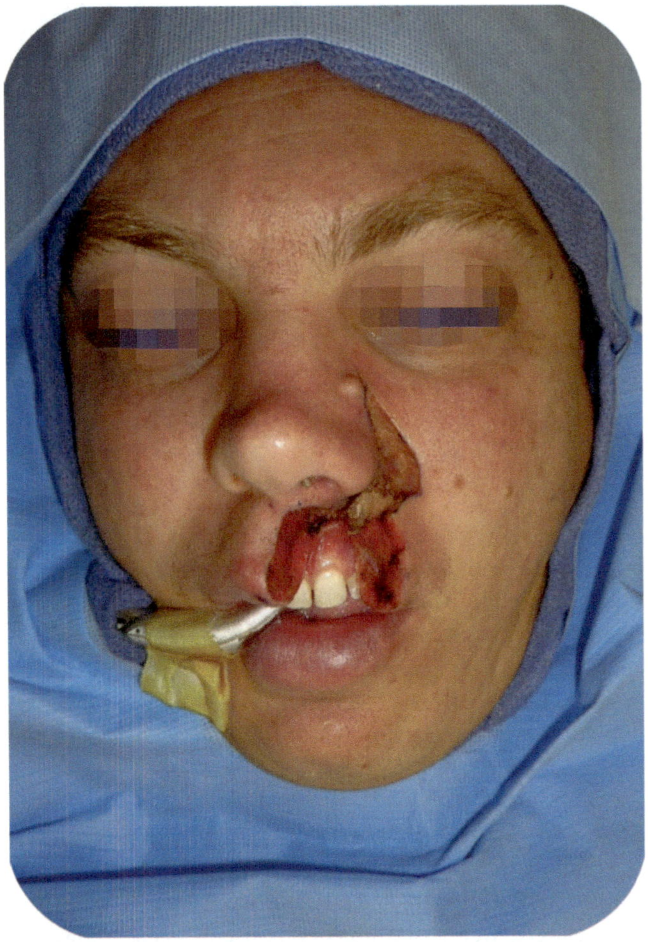

Fig. 86.14 Perialar crescentic flap to reconstruct upper lip defect

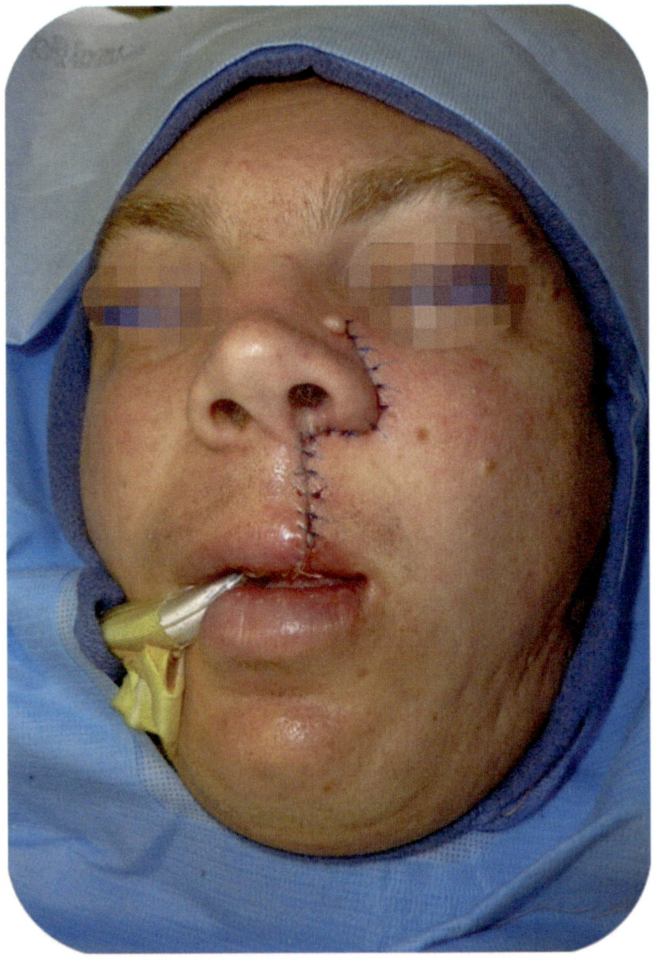

Fig. 86.15 Perialar crescentic flap after closure

Fig. 86.16 (**a–d**) Commissuroplasty. A full thickness incision is made through the blunted commissure and an area de-epithelialised to mirror the normal side (dashed lines, **a**). This is then re-surfaced with mucosal flaps raised from intraorally (**b–d**)

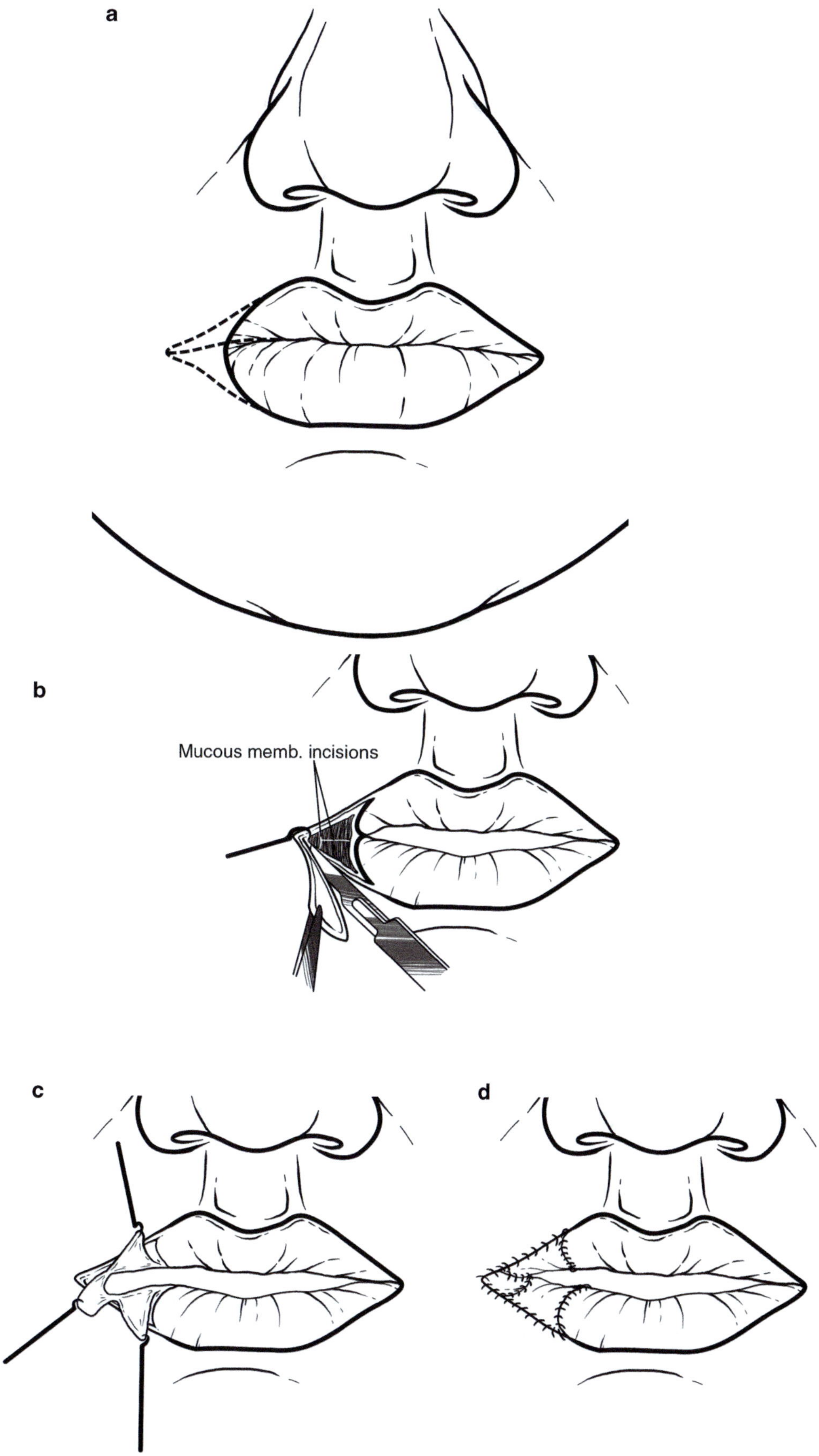

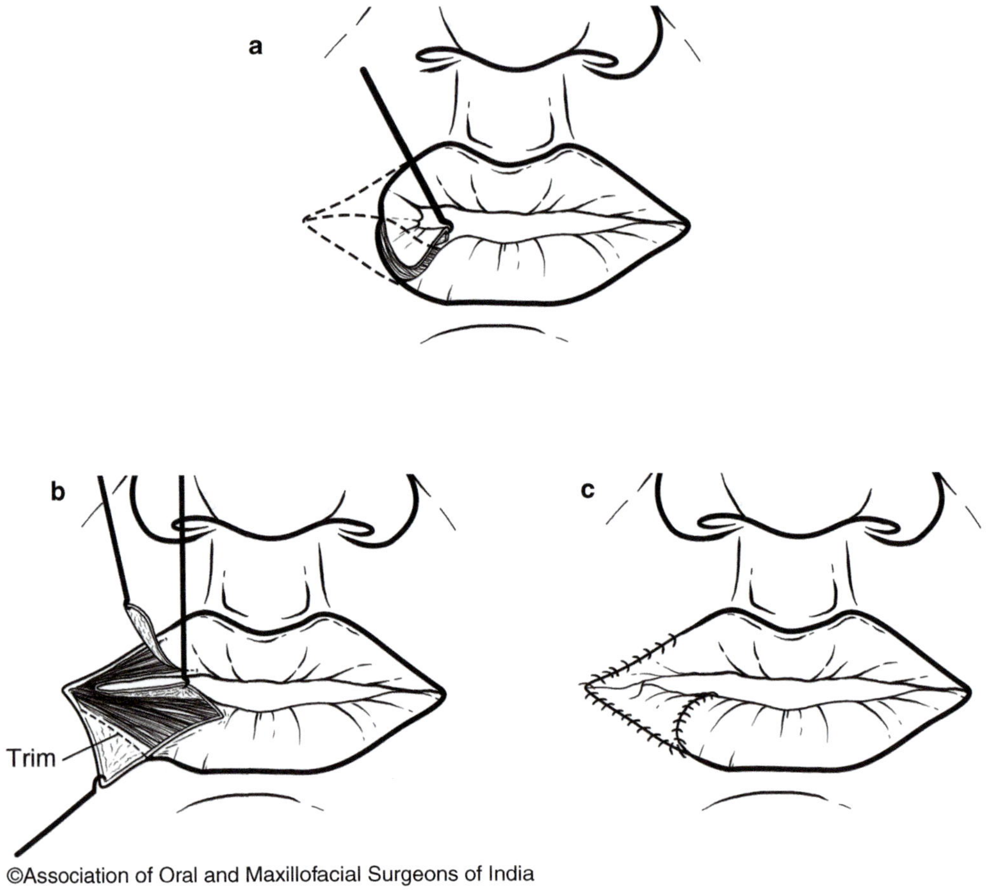

Fig. 86.17 (**a–c**) Gillies commissuroplasty. An area mirroring the normal commissure is de-epithelialised (dashed lines, **a**). Vermillion is raised from the lower lip and inset into the de-epithelialised upper lip (**a**, **b**). The lower vermillion is reconstructed with a mucosal flap raised from the labial mucosa (**b**, **c**)

There is also the option to include palmaris longus tendon harvest [21]. This can be used as a sling between the commissures, or to the malar periosteum to improve lip form and oral competence. Alternatively, the flexor carpi radialis tendon or a nonvascularized fascia lata graft can be utilized for the same purpose. Coaptation of the lateral antebrachial cutaneous nerve to the mental nerve has been described to restore sensation to radial flap reconstruction of the lower lip [22]. Other free flaps that have been employed for total lip reconstruction include the gracilis for the lower lip [23–25] and temporal scalp for upper lip defects [26, 27].

86.3 Buccal Mucosa and Cheek

The main function of the cheek is to hold food between the occlusal surfaces of the teeth during mastication. Inadequate reconstruction can lead to excess tissue that interferes with mastication or insufficient tissue and scarring that results in trismus. Where possible the parotid duct should be repaired and/or re-sited in the buccal mucosa if involved in the defect or reconstruction to prevent obstructive parotitis. Small buccal mucosa defects can be closed primarily, but larger mucosal defects often benefit from reconstruction with a split-thickness skin graft or ipsilateral buccal fat pad [28]. As size and depth of the defect increases, the use of regional flaps described in the part of this chapter that addresses floor of the mouth defects should also be considered. The radial forearm flap is the most commonly used flap for reconstruction of intraoral buccal defects due to its pliability and lack of bulk (Figs. 86.20 and 86.21). Thicker and more extensive defects may benefit from an anterolateral thigh flap, depending on the patient's body habitus. Full-thickness cheek defects often require reconstruction of both the intraoral and extraoral surfaces. A combination of techniques may be employed, for example, a regional or free flap for the skin and a split-thickness skin graft for mucosa, but often it is best to consider reconstructing with a folded or dual paddled flap. Both radial forearm [29] and anterolateral thigh [30] free flaps are well suited for bi-paddled designs. The first is more pliable and thinner; the second can be made larger and confers less donor site morbidity, as it can generally be closed primarily. The portion between the paddles is de-epithelialized where it will lie within the substance of the cheek. Alternatively, if the lip is involved in the defect, the intervening tissue can instead be used to reconstruct the lip. Obviously this will be a static repair and will therefore have an effect on oral competence.

Full-thickness cheek defects often involve the buccal or marginal mandibular branches of the facial nerve, with con-

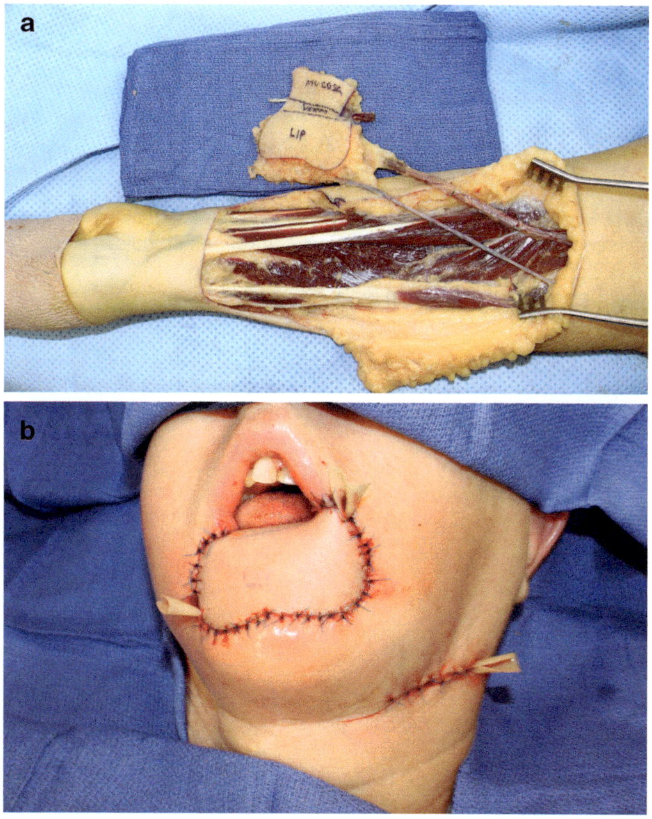

Fig. 86.18 (**a**) Design of RFFF for lower lip reconstruction. (**b**) RFFF after inset to subtotal lower lip defect

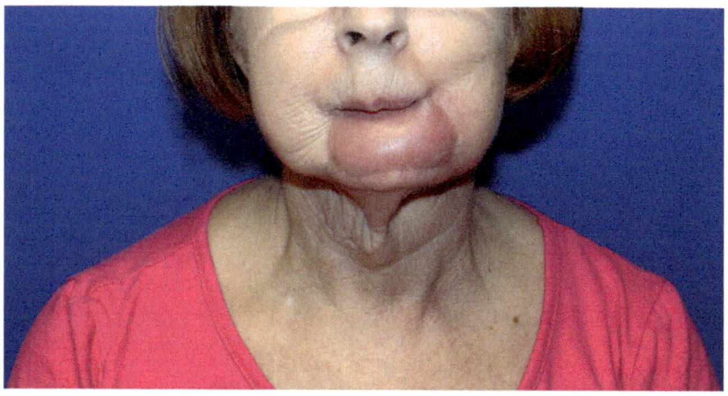

Fig. 86.19 Late postoperative appearance of RFFF reconstruction of subtotal lower lip defect

sequent paralysis of the lower face. A detailed description of facial reanimation is outwith the scope of this chapter; however the methods can broadly be categorized as either static or dynamic. Static reanimation includes gold or platinum weights or springs to aid upper eyelid closure and resuspension of the oral commissure to deep temporal fascia with palmaris longus, fascia lata, acellular dermal matrix, PTFE or polypropylene [31]. Dynamic reanimation involves either

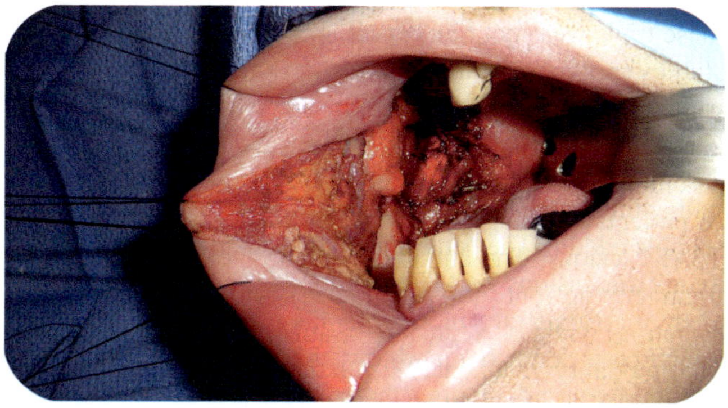

Fig. 86.20 Buccal mucosa defect

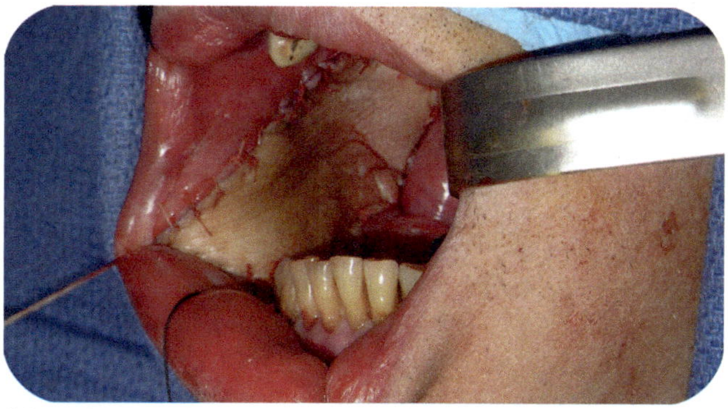

Fig. 86.21 RFFF inset to reconstruct buccal mucosa defect

the reinnervation, usually with nerve grafts or the interposition of innervated muscle, commonly temporalis transposition or a gracilis neuromuscular free flap [32].

86.4 Floor of Mouth

The floor of the mouth comprises the myomucosal diaphragm that extends from the ventral surface of the tongue, bounded anteriorly and laterally by the lingual aspect of the mandibular gingiva and posteriorly by the retromolar trigone. This inferior limit of the oral cavity provides a reservoir for food during mastication, while the muscles are also active during deglutition. The mylohyoid, geniohyoid and anterior digastric muscles raise the aerodigestive tract anterosuperiorly during swallowing, anchoring the tongue and increasing the diameter of the fauces. At rest the same muscles, particularly genioglossus, prevent upper airway compromise by posterior displacement of the tongue: an important consideration when reconstructing this region. Finally, mobility of the tongue during speech, mastication and swallowing depends on adequate anterolateral separation from the mandible, and therefore reconstruction should also aim to recreate the lingual sulcus and prevent ankyloglossia.

One commonly employed method to reconstruct floor of mouth defects is the submental artery island flap, first described by Martin et al. in 1993 [33]. It is easily raised with minimal donor site morbidity to provide a large and reliable paddle. The pedicle is up to 8 cm in length, and cutaneous dimensions up to 7 × 18 cm can be harvested, sufficient to reconstruct most pure floor of mouth defects. It confers less donor site morbidity than the main alternative of a radial forearm flap; often there is even a cosmetic improvement in the patient's soft tissue profile. The main concern with the use of this flap is in the oncological setting is due to potential compromise of nodal dissection in level 1. In one small series, four of nine patients undergoing SIF suffered local or regional recurrence thought to be attributable to incomplete nodal harvest [34]. On the other hand, Howard et al. found that in 50 patients undergoing SIF, all with clinically negative level 1 nodes, none experienced recurrence attributable to the flap [35]. It is generally accepted that the flap is contraindicated in necks with clinically positive nodes, particularly in level I. A history of radiation is a relative contraindication, though good outcomes have been described despite this [36, 37]. Finally, since the submental vessels arise from the facial vessels, the flap cannot be performed in patients who have undergone a neck dissection with sacrifice of the facial vessels. In such patients or where tissue is required outside previous radiation fields, the infrahyoid island flap [38] is an alternative of similar size and character to the SIF. Supraclavicular island (Fig. 86.22) and pectoralis major flaps are also well-proven options that generally lie outside any previously operated or radiated field. They have broad pedicles, which unless skeletonized can introduce excess tissue into the defect or the tunnel from donor site. A radial forearm free flap may therefore be preferred, providing a thin, supple reconstruction with negligible pedicle bulk (Figs. 86.23 and 86.24).

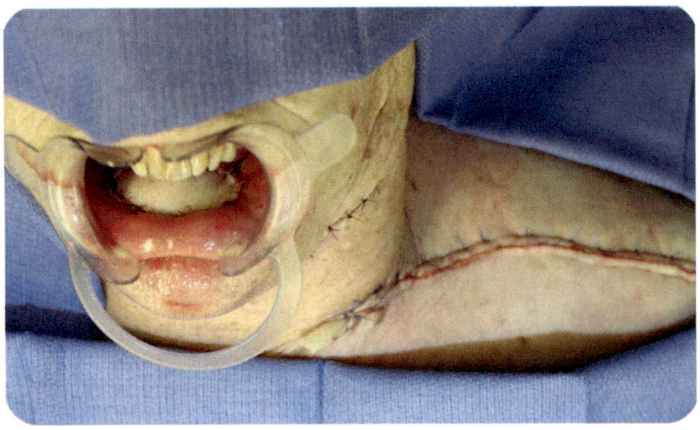

Fig. 86.22 SCIF inset to reconstruct floor of mouth defect

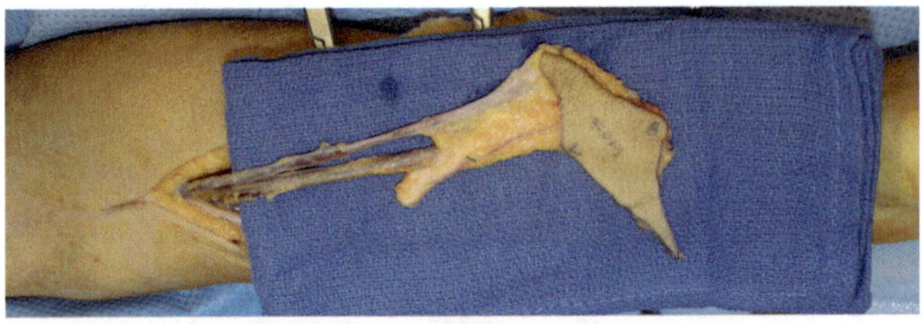

Fig. 86.23 Design of RFFF for floor of mouth defect

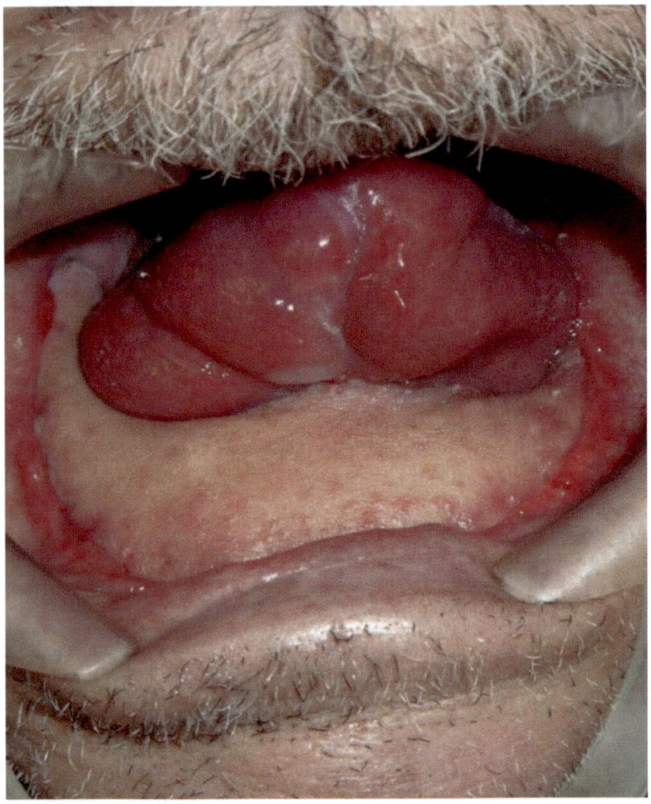

Fig. 86.24 RFFF reconstruction of floor of mouth defect demonstrating good tongue mobility

86.5 Tongue Reconstruction

Adequate tongue function requires interaction between sensory and motor components of both voluntary and involuntary nervous systems to achieve intelligible speech, mastication and swallowing. Therefore tongue defects have a significant effect on quality of life compared with other oropharyngeal structures, proportional to their volume. Tongue reconstruction that recreates the biomechanics of the healthy tongue leads to better function and even cortical adaptation to the neotongue [39]. In terms of speech, the ability for the anterior tongue to contact the palate is particularly important. Speech therapy following tongue reconstruction should be considered as it can improve proprioception of the reconstructed tongue and facilitate cortical plasticity.

86.5.1 Primary Closure

Small volume defects of the free oral tongue can often be closed primarily with satisfactory outcomes (Figs. 86.25 and 86.26). As the area of the defect increases, the option of healing by secondary intention should be considered as this can result in a more natural tongue morphology, while dehiscence is often the natural course for primary closure in any case.

86.5.2 Pedicled Flap Reconstruction

Tongue defects can be reconstructed with a variety of pedicled flaps, often utilized when free tissue transfer is precluded. Prior to development of free tissue transfer, the pectoralis major and deltopectoral flap were common options, with the facial artery myomucosal flap an alternative for smaller volume defects. There has been a renaissance in the use of other regional flaps over recent years, such as the submental (Figs. 86.27 and 86.28), supraclavicular, trapezius and infrahyoid island flaps.

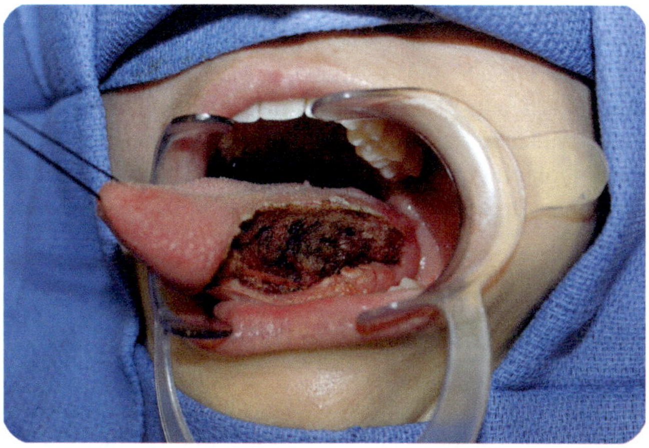

Fig. 86.25 Superficial defect of lateral tongue

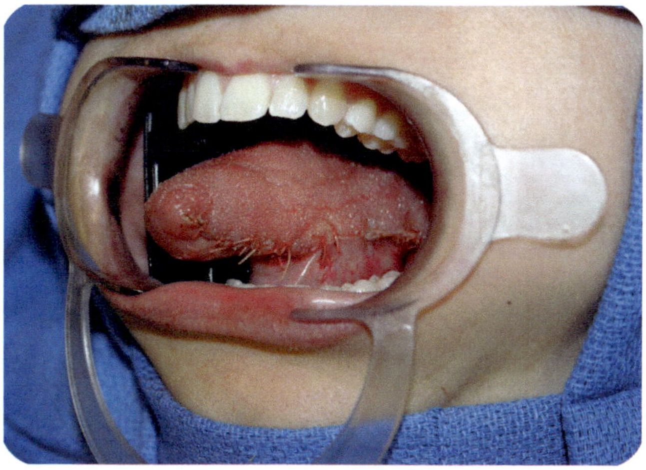

Fig. 86.26 Primary closure of lateral tongue defect

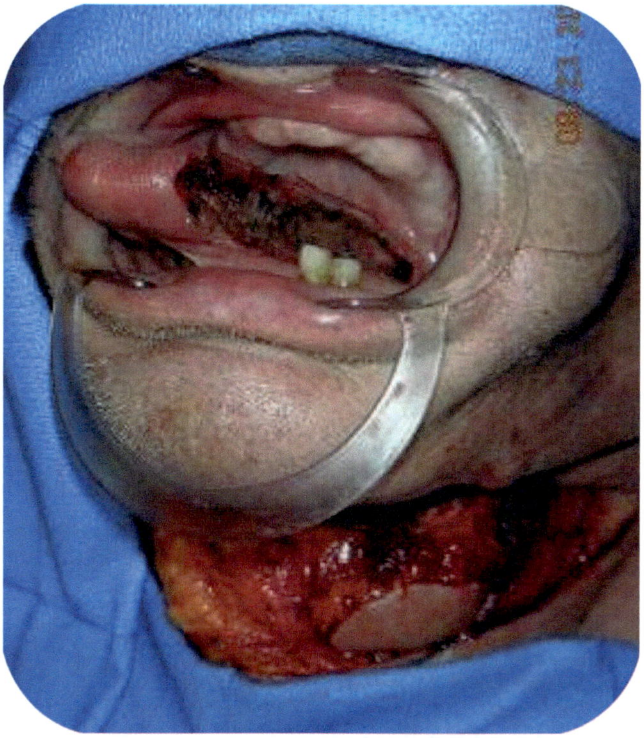

Fig. 86.27 Submental flap prior to reconstruction of lateral tongue defect

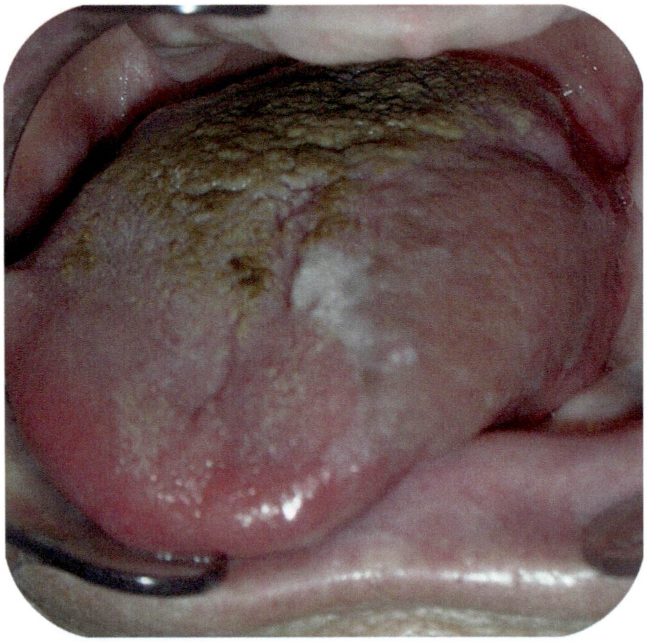

Fig. 86.28 Late postoperative appearance of submental flap reconstruction of left lateral tongue

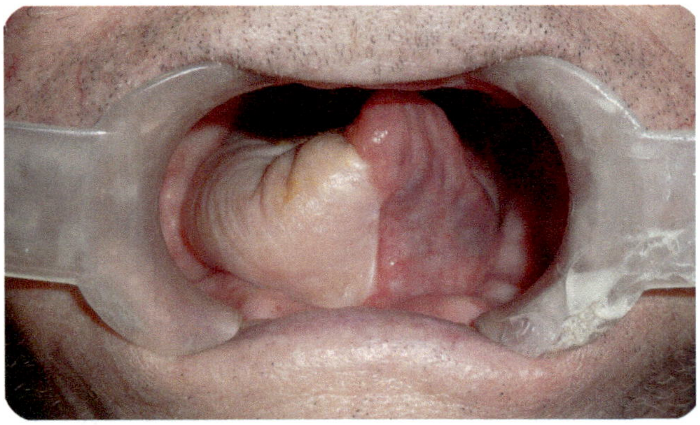

Fig. 86.29 RFFF to reconstruct right hemiglossectomy

86.5.3 Free Flap Reconstruction

Tongue reconstruction with a microvascular free flap is usually recommended to restore form, resist contractures and tethering in defects greater than a quarter of the original tongue size [40]. The flap should be designed to recreate premorbid morphology in all three dimensions as far as possible.

The radial forearm free flap is the workhorse of tongue reconstruction for good reason (Fig. 86.29). It provides thin, pliable, soft tissue and large-calibre vessels of consistent anatomy and excellent length for microvascular anastomosis. Harvest can be simultaneous with resection and presents limited morbidity. The lateral antebrachial cutaneous nerve can be coapted to the lingual nerve to provide a sensate flap with some evidence of improved function and resistance to atrophy [41]. Defects greater than three quarters of the tongue may benefit from reconstruction with tissue of greater substance such as an anterolateral thigh (ALT) or rectus abdominis free flap. ALT harvest results in a more easily hidden scar and potential sensory loss is less troublesome. Total glossectomy reconstruction is particularly challenging. Recreation of three-dimensional morphology is critical, with emphasis on height and a tip protruberance, to facilitate speech and swallowing [42] (Figs. 86.30 and 86.31). A flap that is around one third greater than the defect is recommended to achieve this aim due to inevitable atrophy. Hyolaryngeal suspension should also be considered as an adjunct, to reduce the risk of persistent laryngeal aspiration [43].

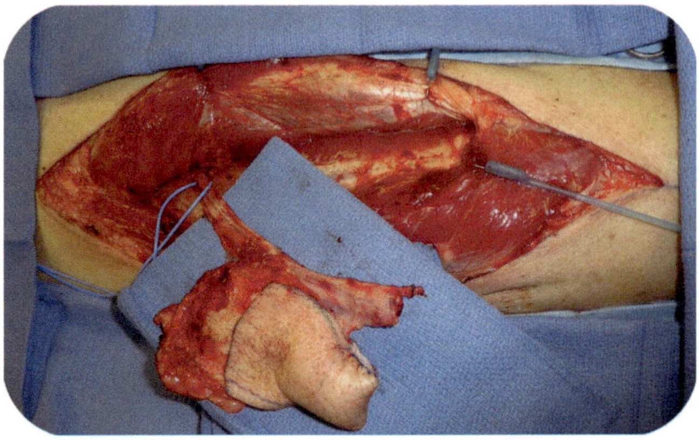

Fig. 86.30 Folded ALT flap for glossectomy reconstruction prior to pedicle division

86.6 Palatal Soft Tissue Defects

Simple mucosal defects overlying the hard palate can be left to close by secondary intention. Although the process is sometimes prolonged, pain and remucosalization can be aided by an acrylic cover plate retained by bone screws or dental cribs. Buccal mucosa with or without buccal fat pad can be advanced to repair palatal mucosa if the adjacent alveolus is edentulous. Palatal mucosal flaps, facial artery myomucosal flaps, temporalis or temporoparietal flaps and tongue flaps are alternatives. Functional reconstruction of the soft palate is difficult, but uvula, posterior pharyngeal wall or folded radial free flaps are options to consider.

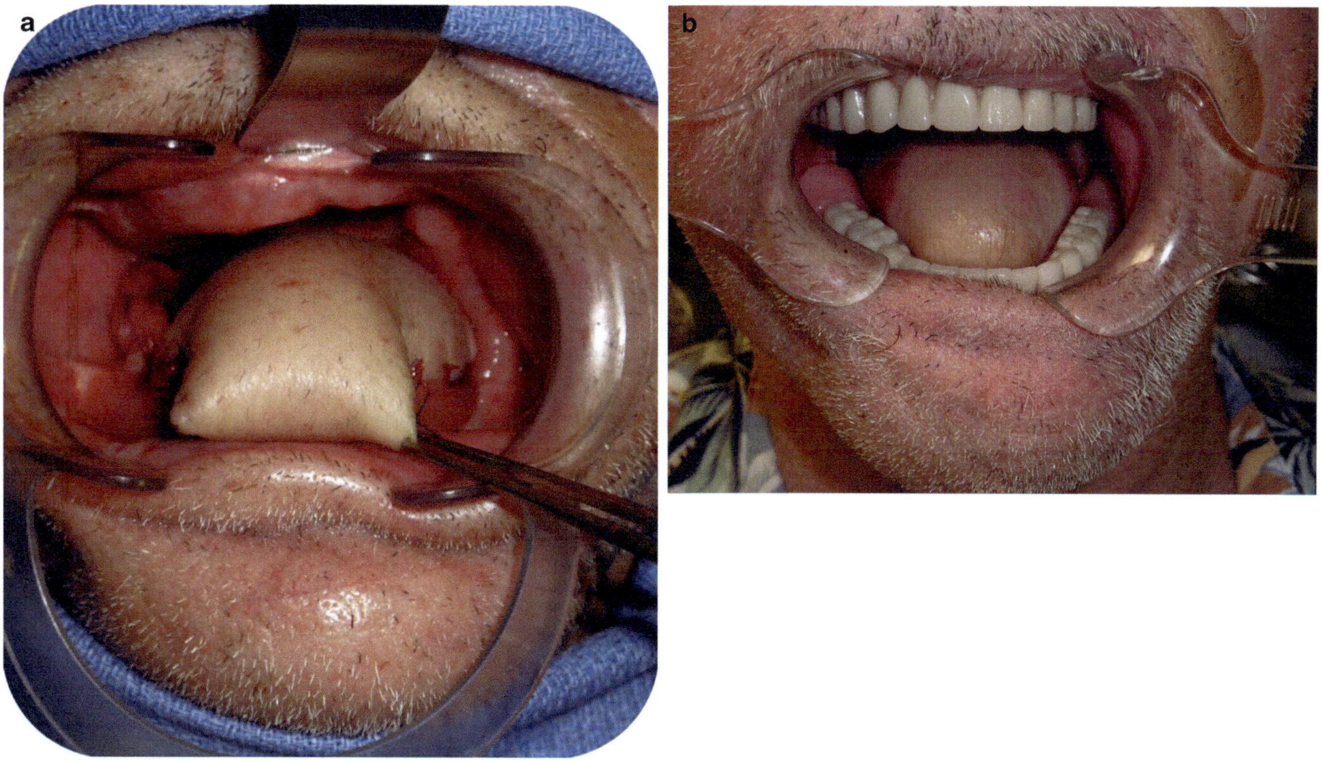

Fig. 86.31 (**a**) ALT flap inset for glossectomy reconstruction. (**b**) Late postoperative appearance

86.7 Facial Reconstruction

The aims of facial reconstruction differ from those of oral reconstruction. While the emphasis in the latter case is on function, without neglecting cosmesis, the priority here is reversed. Besides the disfigurement itself, patients will often suffer significant and irremediable social detriment due to inadequate facial reconstruction. Cosmetically acceptable results require a detailed understanding of facial anatomy. This is best considered in terms of the facial aesthetic units [44] (Fig. 86.3). This approach was first described by Gonzales-Ulloa [45–48], who demonstrated that scars can be hidden in the natural lines dividing units from one another. Menick later discussed the importance of human perception in reconstruction [49].

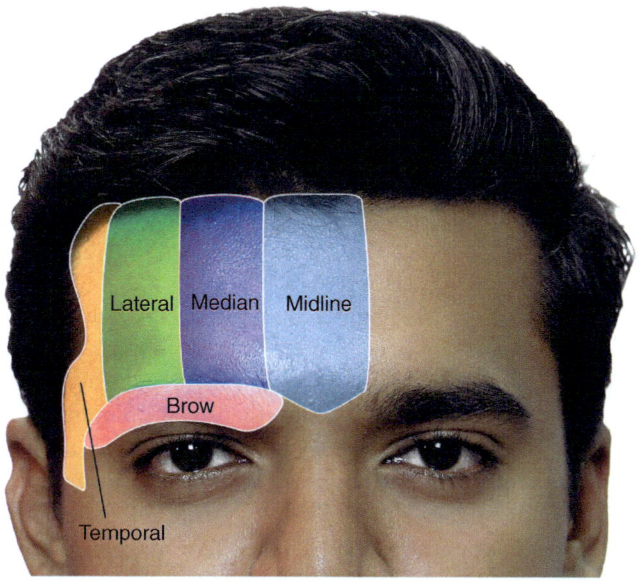

Fig. 86.32 Aesthetic subunits of the forehead

86.7.1 Forehead Reconstruction

The forehead comprises midline and paired median, lateral, temporal and brow subunits (Fig. 86.32). Small defects can be closed primarily parallel to horizontal RSTLs that run perpendicular to the underlying frontalis muscle fibres. The defect can be extended to an ellipse or with terminal M-plasties to achieve this. Midline defects may be closed vertically with acceptable results, particularly in the aged face. Undermining and careful closure of the galeal layer is important when closing larger defects primarily.

Split or full-thickness skin grafts can be used for large defects, although there will be a mismatch with the native skin particularly if split thickness. An alternative is tissue expansion either to provide full-thickness skin from a site such as the supraclavicular fossa or locally to provide tissue for a local flap.

Reconstruction of the forehead with local flaps usually has a better cosmetic outcome than skin grafts. Unilateral or bilateral horizontal 'H' advancement flaps work well, as does an 'A' to 'T' flap at the hairline. Finally, large forehead and scalp defects can be reconstructed with free tissue transfer. With this option, often the best cosmetic results are achieved with a radial flap or latissimus dorsi muscle flap combined with a skin graft.

86.7.2 Eyelid Reconstruction

The eyelids are of critical importance in protecting the globes and preventing loss of vision through exposure keratitis. The main goals of reconstruction are therefore to recreate a lid that lies passively against the globe without ectropion or entropion and permits full eye closure (Table 86.4). Both the upper and lower eyelids have a bilaminar structure, which has relevance to reconstructive options. The anterior lamella is composed of the thinnest skin in the body and underlying preseptal orbicularis oculi muscle. The posterior lamella is comprised of the tarsal plate and conjunctiva. The tarsal plates impart some rigidity to the eyelids and contain meibomian glands to produce the lipid component of tears. They are around 25 mm in width and 1 mm thick, with the upper plate 7–12 mm and the lower plate 3–4 mm in height. The upper tarsal plate is attached to the levator palpebrae superioris (oculomotor innervation) muscle via the levator aponeurosis and sympathetically innervated Muller's muscle. The lower plate is attached to orbital septum rather than an aponeurosis.

The orbicularis oculi muscle has three parts. The preseptal and pretarsal components are active in blinking, promoting lachrymal flow from gland to canaliculi and insert into the canthal tendons. The outermost orbital component is involved in voluntary eyelid closure and does not insert into the canthal tendons. There are two preaponeurotic fat pads present in the upper lid and three post septal fat pads in the lower lid (nasal, central and lateral). They are separated by fibrous septa, plus the inferior oblique muscle between nasal and central lower fat pads.

Table 86.4 Aims of eyelid reconstruction

Reconstruction of anterior and posterior lamellae
Adequate supple skin that permits normal eyelid movements
Avoidance of entropion or ectropion
Non-keratinized mucosa adjacent to globe
Degree of rigidity such that lid is applied to the globe in all areas

86.7.2.1 Healing by Secondary Intention

Small superficial defects limited to the anterior lamella may be left to heal by secondary intention particularly in the medial canthal region where the nasal bones resist scar contracture and therefore ectropion. This approach should generally be avoided in central or lateral lower eyelid defects due to the high risk of cicatricial ectropion.

86.7.2.2 Primary Closure and Grafts

Small defects not involving the ciliary margin can be closed parallel to relaxed skin tension lines if lagophthalmos does not result. For larger defects confined to the anterior lamella, full-thickness skin grafts from the opposing lid are ideal, providing a good match with minimal hair and resistance to the contraction associated with split-thickness grafts.

If the defect involves the ciliary margin, primary closure is possible up to one third of the lid width. Typically a 7/0 resorbable vertical mattress suture though meibomian gland orifices is used to align the ciliary margin, the tarsal plate is closed with 6/0 resorbable sutures and finally skin with 6/0 fast resorbing sutures (Fig. 86.33). Conversion to a pentagonal defect with squaring of the tarsal defect and a slight temporal slant to the anterior lamella portion can be helpful to prevent notching of the ciliary margin. A lateral canthotomy and superior or inferior cantholysis can help recruit lateral tissue. Care must be taken to appose both the tarsus and skin to avoid notching of the ciliary margin.

86.7.2.3 Local Flaps

Full-thickness defects up to 60% of the lower lid width can be repaired with a Tenzel flap [50] (Fig. 86.34), which rotates and advances tissue from the lateral canthus. Alternatively defects of this size can be repaired with a tarsoconjunctival graft and musculocutaneous advancement flap or a Hughes flap [51] (Fig. 86.35). The latter method is a two-stage procedure that involves a pedicled tarsoconjunctival flap from the upper lid covered with skin grafted from one of the upper lids. The pedicle is divided after 4–6 weeks. To prevent entropion of the upper lid, 3–4 mm of tarsus should be preserved. This method in reverse has also been described to repair defects of the upper eyelid [52]. A cervicofacial (Mustarde) flap can also be combined with a Hughes flap, free tarsoconjunctival or palatal mucosa or nasal septal graft to reconstruct lower lid defects.

Defects one third to one half the upper lid width can be repaired with a reverse Tenzel flap or sliding tarsoconjunctival flap (Fig. 86.36) and skin graft. Larger defects can be repaired with a Cutler-Beard flap [53] that transfers an infratarsal full-thickness lower lid flap underneath a bridge of preserved lower ciliary margin (Fig. 86.37). The pedicle is divided after 6–8 weeks. Interposition of a cartilage or dermal matrix graft between the lamellae of the flap can improve the form of the reconstructed upper lid [54] (Table 86.5).

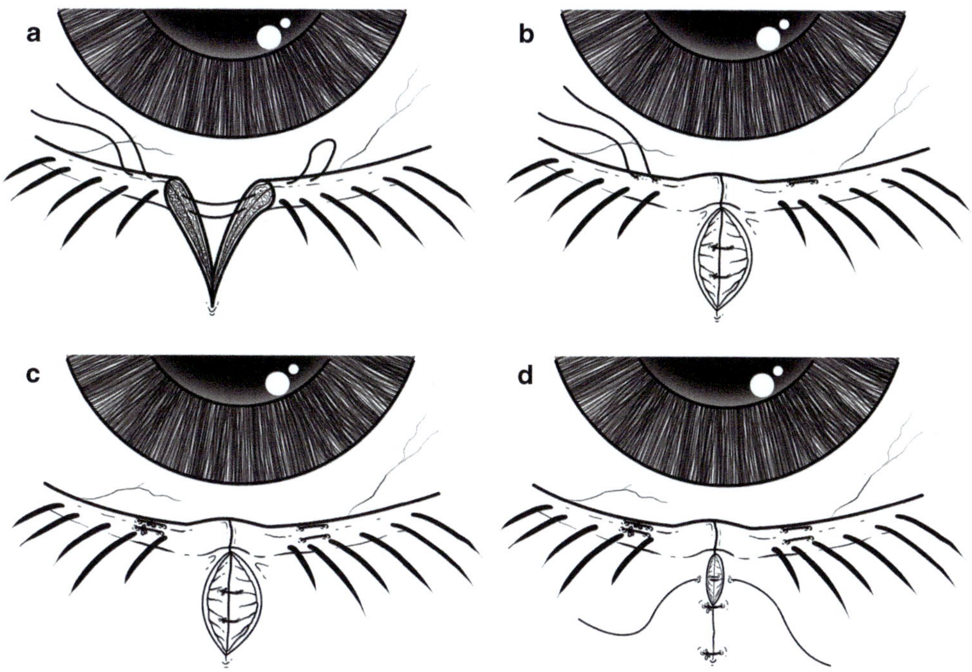

Fig. 86.33 (**a**–**d**) Primary closure for small defects involving the ciliary margin. A vertical mattress resorbable suture is placed through the meiobian duct orifice region (**a**), to oppose the ciliary margin (**b**). The muscle (**c**) and skin (**d**) are then closed in layers

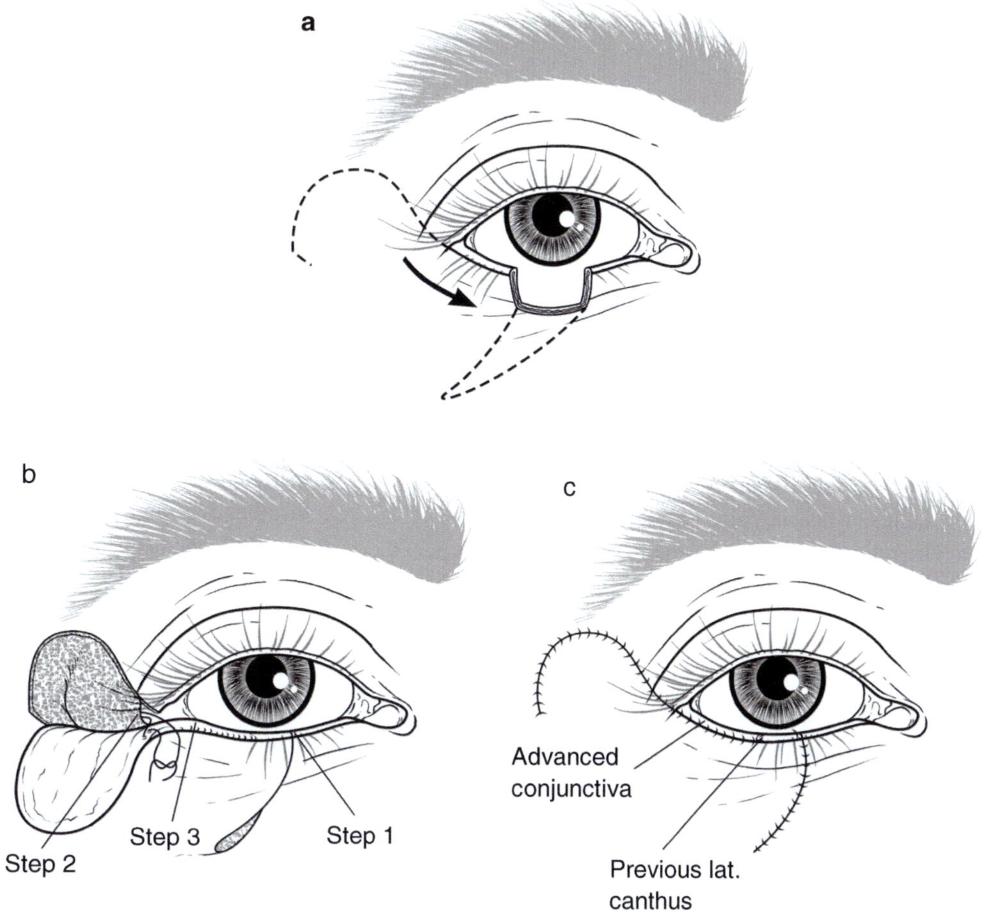

Fig. 86.34 (**a**–**c**) Tenzel flap to advance lateral tissue into lower lid defect. A superiorly curved incision is extended laterally through the lateral canthus (**a**) to allow advancement of a partial thickness flap and remaining lateral lid to close a lower lid defect (**b**). Excess skin inferior to the defect is excised in the manner of a Burow's triangle

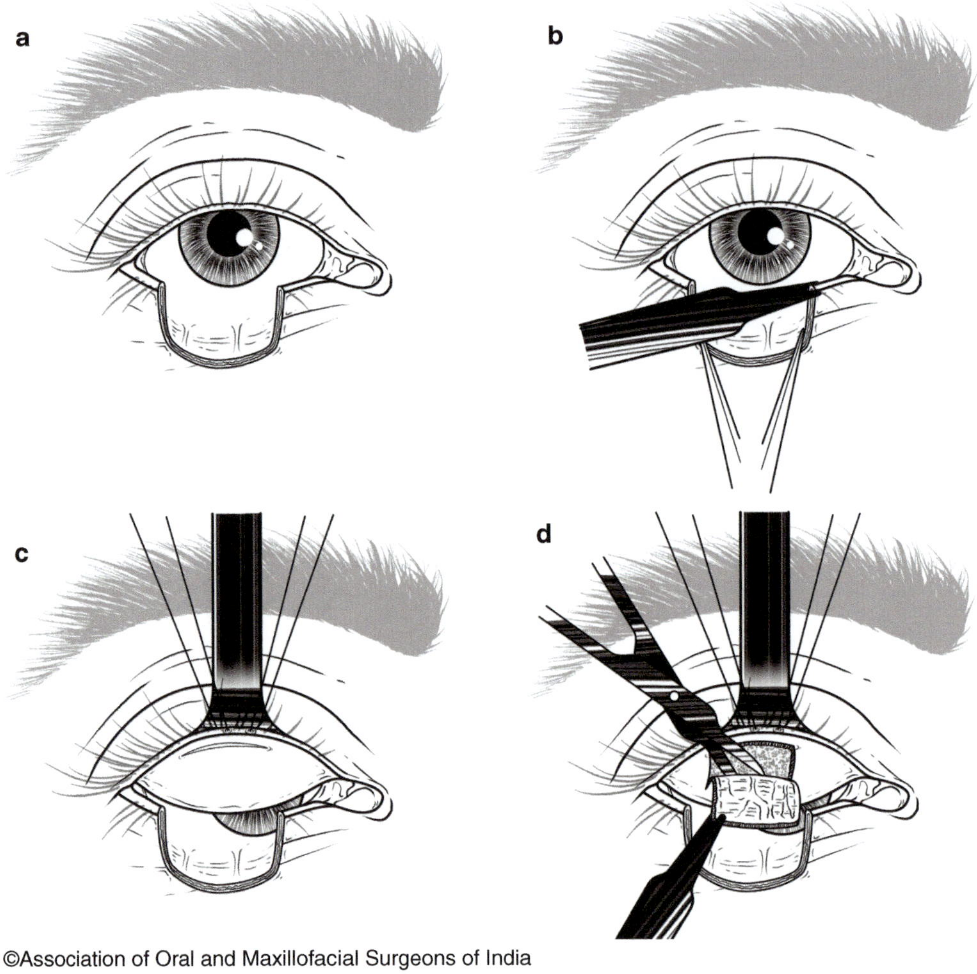

Fig. 86.35 (**a–d**) Hughes tarsoconjunctival flap from upper lid to reconstruct lower lid defect. A lower lid defect (**a**) is reconstructed with a superiorly based tarsoconjuctival flap raised from the deep aspect of the upper lid (**b–d**). The flap is covered with a skin graft from one of the upper lids and the pedicle divided after 4-6 weeks

86.7.3 Ear Reconstruction (Also refer Chap. 35)

The external ear is a relatively isolated aesthetic unit with its own complex subunit anatomy (Fig. 86.38). Reconstruction requires attention to shape, angular orientation with respect to the adjacent skull, and symmetry with the contralateral ear [55]. Of these three points, the last is the most important. Finally, the reconstructed ear should serve as support for spectacles or hearing aids (Table 86.6).

The major constitutive subunits, working from peripheral to central, are the helix, scapha, antihelix and concha (subdivided into cymba and cavum). The tragus, antitragus and lobule are less critical to overall auricular aesthetics, as a defect involving these subunits has minimal effect on the shape of the remainder of the external ear.

Orientation with respect to the skull follows these general guidelines [55]:

1. Auricular height = distance between lateral orbital rim and root of helix at the level of the brow.
2. Approximately 15° deviation from the skull in the vertical axis.
3. Approximately 25–30° deviation from the skull in the horizontal axis.
4. Highest point of helix level with lateral brow.
5. Helical rim protrudes 1–2.5 cm from skull.

The following will concentrate on helical defects, since the helix is the most common site, and many lesions centred in other regions will extend to involve it as well [56]. The classical reconstructive ladder is somewhat modified for defects of the ear. For defects overlying intact perichondrium, a full-thickness skin graft is the optimal technique, rather than primary closure [55]. Alternative approaches must be used when perichondrium has been resected, as denuded cartilage will not support a skin graft. If the defect exposes cartilage in an area where it can be resected without altering the shape of the ear, it should be resected down to the opposing perichondrium, which should be covered with a skin graft [55]. The retroauricular skin is the best colour match, and the scar at the donor site is well hidden by the ear.

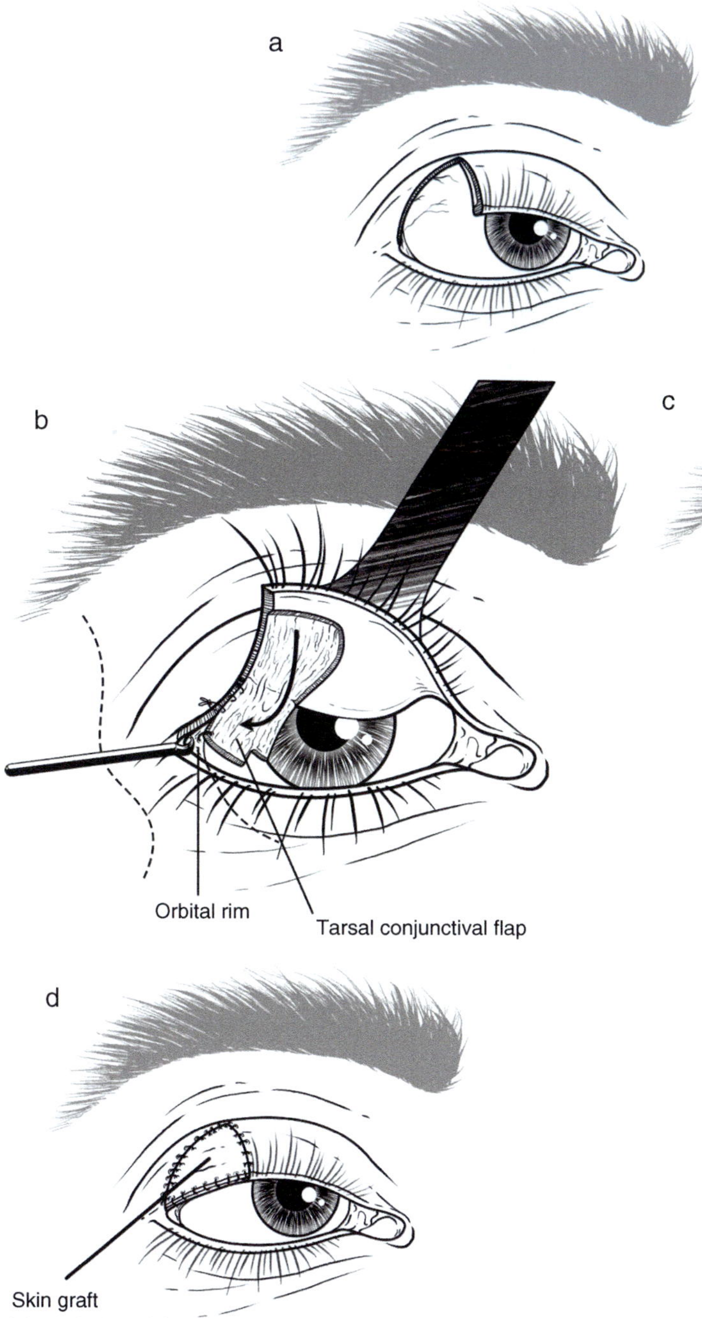

Fig. 86.36 (**a–d**) Sliding tarsoconjunctival flap for upper lid defect repair. An upper lid defect (**a**) is repaired with a superiorly based tarsoconjunctival flap raised from the adjacent remaining lid (**b**). The flap is transposed and inset into the defect (**c**), prior to coverage with a skin graft harvested from another eyelid (**d**)

Resection of shape-determining cartilage requires further subdivision. Small helical defects, ideally less than 1.5 cm, can be closed primarily [57]. Primary closure can be facilitated by the extension of the defect into a wedge excision.

For larger defects, the resulting distortion exaggerates the ear's lateral depth and makes it stand out too far from the skull. Defects between 1.5 and 2.5 cm, or roughly one third of the ear's height, can be closed by means of the helical advancement flap first described by Antia and Buch [57–59] (Fig. 86.39). In this repair, the helical sulcus is incised superiorly and inferiorly through the cartilage, but sparing the posterior perichondrium and skin, which then serves as the vascular supply for the flap. A crescent of skin and cartilage can be resected from the scapha anterior to this incision, in order to decrease the size discrepancy between the helix and antihelix and thereby the degree of cupping in the final repair [57].

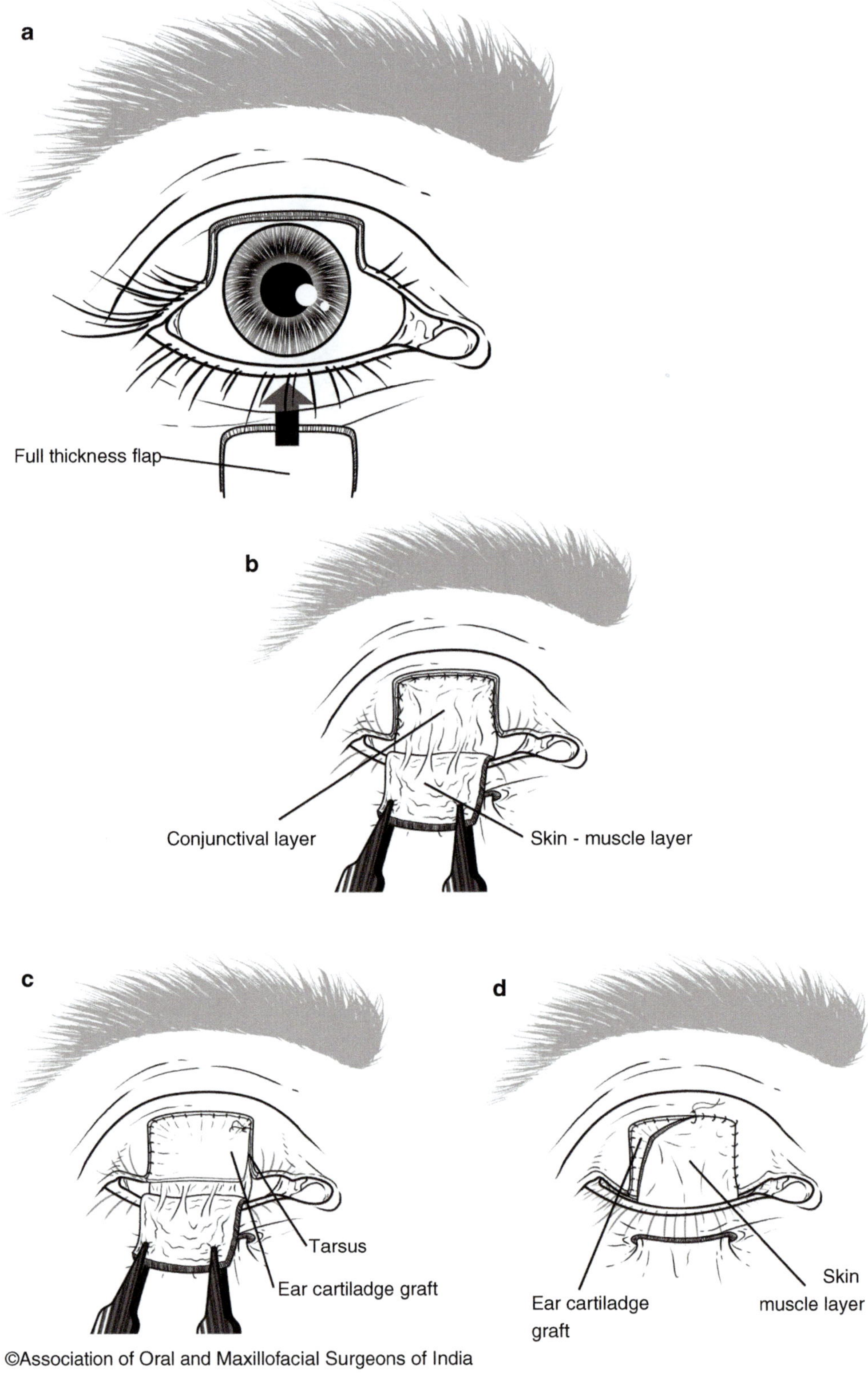

Fig. 86.37 (**a**–**d**) Cutler-Beard full-thickness lower lid flap to upper lid defect

Table 86.5 Options for eyelid reconstruction

Lower eyelid reconstruction
Direct closure (<30–45% defects)
Lateral canthotomy and inferior cantholysis (gains 5 mm)
Tenzel flap (<60% defects)
Tarsoconjunctival graft and musculocutaneous advancement
Hughes flap
Mustarde flap + graft for posterior lamella
Upper eyelid reconstruction
Direct closure
Lateral canthotomy and superior cantholysis
Sliding tarsoconjunctival flap
Cutler-Beard flap (60%–100% defects)

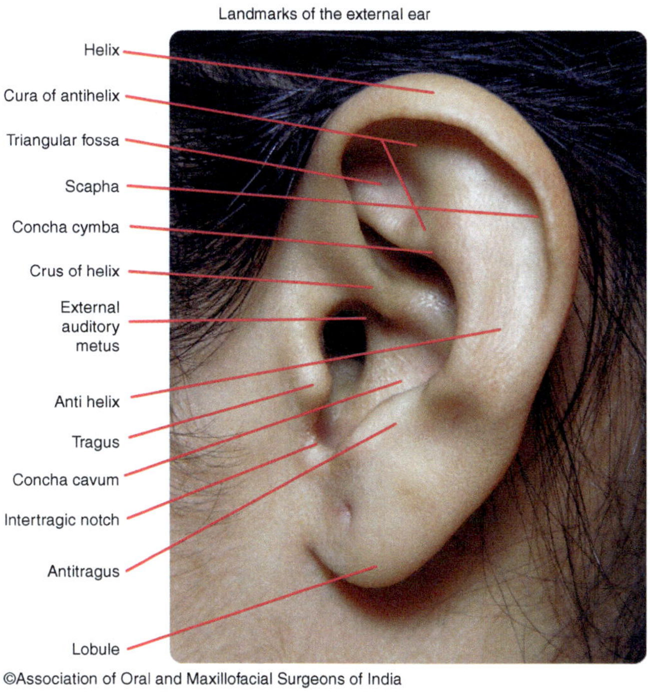

Fig. 86.38 Anatomy of the pinna

Table 86.6 Aims of ear reconstruction

Recreation of natural morphology	
Symmetry with contralateral ear	Height
	Projection
	Size
Support for spectacles/hearing aids	

Some authors suggest that the Antia-Buch approach is not appropriate for larger marginal defects, since it induces excessive microtia [55]. Others advocate a more aggressive Antia-Buch repair [57], arguing that the microtia will only be noticeable in those exceptional viewing situations when both ears are visible at once. Alternate strategies for a larger defect include adjacent tissue transfer such as a staged tubular pedicled graft [60] or retroauricular flap [61].

For near or complete loss of the external ear, the three options are:

1. No reconstruction.
2. Staged autogenous reconstruction.
3. Prosthetic reconstruction.

A patient wishing to avoid repeated surgery, or a poor surgical candidate, might be best served by the first option. Staged autogenous reconstruction was pioneered by Tanzer [62], who described a six-stage approach. This has since been simplified to a three or two-stage approach by the work of Brent [63] and then Nagata [64]. In summary, a cartilaginous framework is fashioned from costal cartilage, sutured to the remainder of the native ear and reposed beneath the skin as stage one. Stage two refashions the posterior aspect of the ear and establishes the correct angulation away from the skull. Exogenous cartilage substitutes can be used for this approach as well.

Finally, the entire external ear can be reconstructed with a prosthesis attached via adhesive or osseointegrated implants [65–67]. This solution is often best for patients in who the surrounding skin is compromised, for example by radiation or burns [55]. Typically implants require a minimum of 4 mm thickness of temporal bone and connect to the prosthesis via magnets.

86.7.4 Nasal Reconstruction

Nasal reconstruction must be considered with respect to aesthetic subunits (Fig. 86.40). The nine nasal subunits are the dorsum, lateral walls, tip, ala, soft triangles and columella. A detailed discussion of nasal aesthetics is beyond the scope of this text, but we will describe the approaches most pertinent to trauma and oncologic reconstruction. Only the smallest nasal defects can be closed primarily. However, the available regional flap options are versatile and highly cosmetically acceptable. Lateral defects can often be closed with a nasolabial flap, providing a good colour match and hiding the donor scar in the nasolabial fold [68]. Some blunting of the nasofacial angle can occur particularly if not resisted with deep sutures. Larger defects (>2 cm.) cannot be closed with the limited volume of tissue available, and the dorsum and tip are not accessible with this flap [69]. Other options are the bilobed rotation flap for sidewall defects or sliding Rintala flap for dorsal and tip defects.

Larger defects, and those centred near the midline, are generally best repaired with a paramedian forehead flap. This approach was first described by Sushruta in the sixth-century BC [70] and has undergone very little change since.

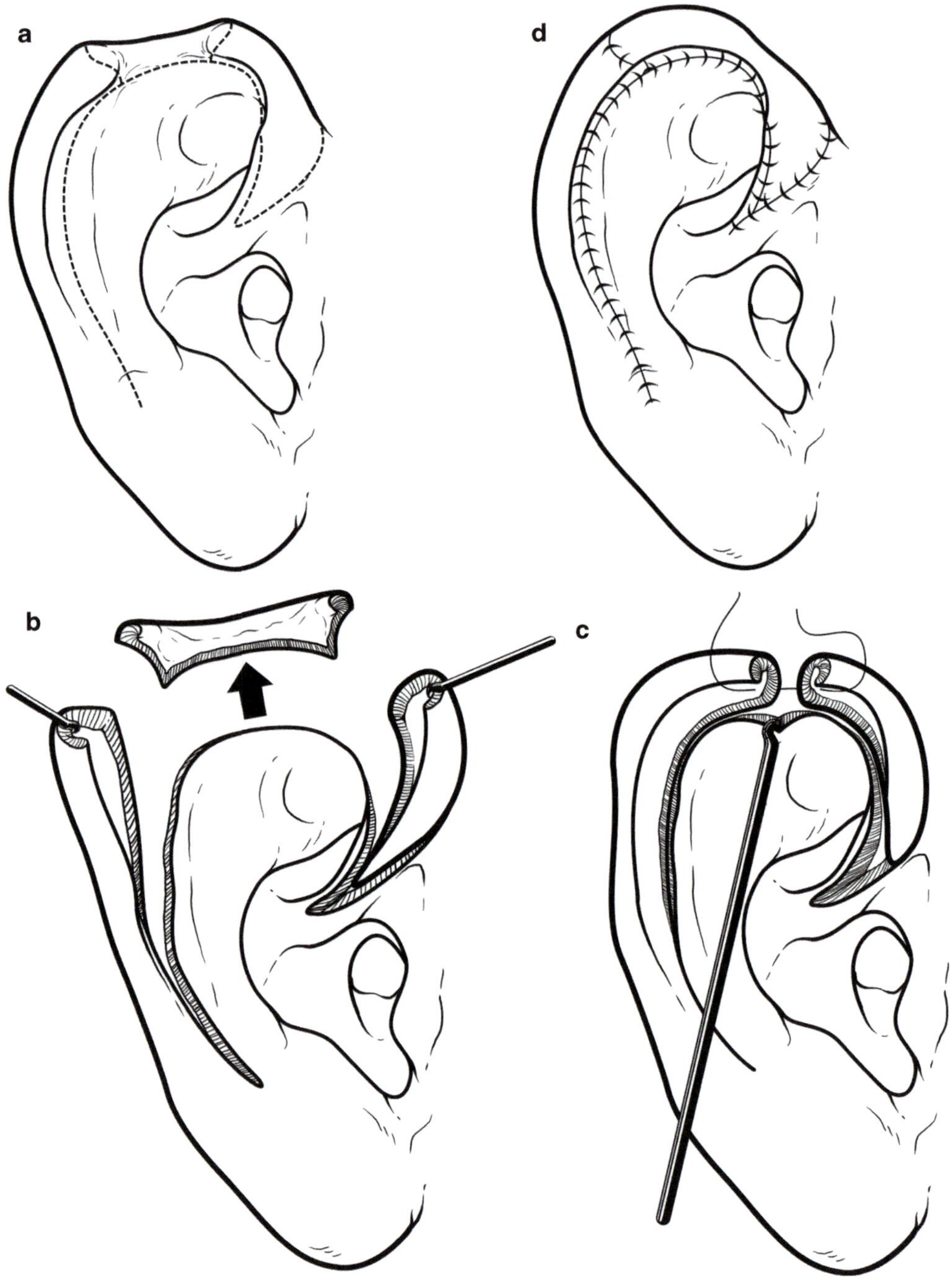

Fig. 86.39 (**a–d**) Antia-Buch helical rim advancement flap. A defect of the helix is repaired by advancement of adjacent helix. Full thickness incisions are made along the inside of the helix +/– a partial thickness incision anterior to the root of the helix (dotted lines, (**a**). A crescent or wedge of scaphal cartilage is excised (**b**) to reduce its circumference and permit approximation of the remaining helix (**c**). Finally, excess skin overlying the scaphal cartilage can be trimmed and the incisions closed (**d**)

The flap provides skin of similar character and sufficient size to replace an entire nasal subunit and also a portion of nasal vestibule for alar defects, potentially improving aesthetic outcome [68, 69]. The first stage involves rotation of a paramedian skin paddle about a narrow pedicle based on the supratrochlear vessels. The flap is generally based on the contralateral vessels, as this produces less torsion of the vessels. The dissection is carried out in the subcutaneous plane at the distal aspect, to provide pliable skin for the repair, but transfers to the subgaleal and ultimately subperiosteal planes as it proceeds proximally towards the pedicle. The paddle is sutured in place, with stents for the nares if necessary. The second stage is carried out approximately 3 weeks after the first, in order to provide for neovascularization. At this stage, the pedicle is divided and the superior edge of the flap inset. A third stage can be carried out to debulk the flap and is often required for ideal aesthetic outcome [69]. In patients with vascular disease, a greater proportion of the flap can be carried out in the subgaleal plane, and a debulking stage performed before division and inset, in order to decrease the chance of flap necrosis [70]. Reconstruction of alar nasal mucosa in full-thickness defects can be achieved with a

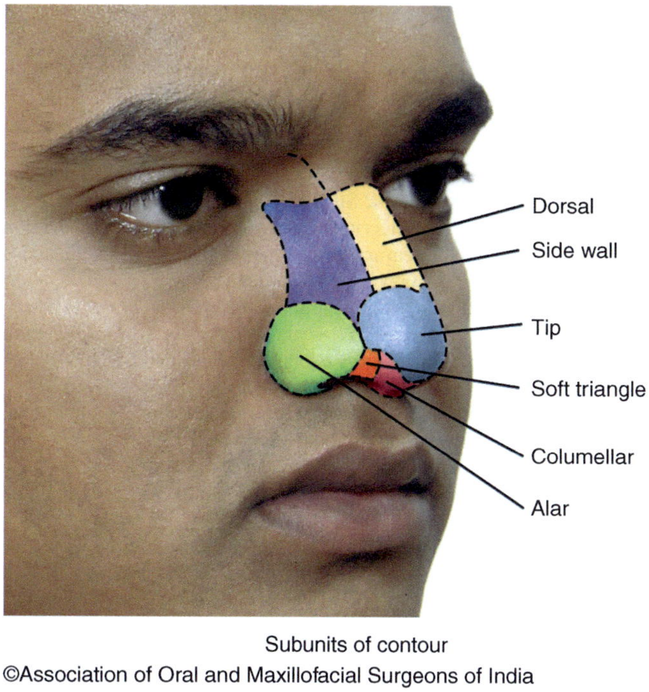

Fig. 86.40 Aesthetic subunits of the nose

hinged nasal septum mucoperichondrial flap. Alar rim defects can also benefit from reconstruction with composite grafts harvested from the lobule or helical rim of the pinna.

Defects involving significant bony or cartilaginous destruction require repair with similar tissue. Small cartilaginous defects can be reconstructed with nasal septal cartilage [68], but only a limited volume can be harvested without impairing septal integrity and tip support. Grafts may also be taken from the ear or rib; the first confers less morbidity and has a favourable contour for alar reconstruction, while the second provides a larger volume of cartilage stock [55]. Many potential donor sites are available for bony defects, including calvarium, mandible, iliac crest and long bones (tibia or radius). The dorsal contour is the most important to reconstruct; this can be accomplished with an osseous strut graft [69].

In total or subtotal nasal defects, reconstruction of the internal and external soft tissue and hard tissue requires consideration. Most commonly a radial forearm free flap is employed and can be harvested with a portion of radial bone for use as a dorsal strut [71]. The best cosmetic outcome is generally achieved with this flap when combined with paramedian forehead flap to reconstruct the external skin. Finally, nasal prostheses require less surgery and can provide an excellent match in appearance to the premorbid nose. They can be retained with adhesive, spectacles or osseointegrated implants. Their chief disadvantage is cost, as they must be replaced every 1 to 2 years [68].

86.7.5 Reconstruction of the Extraoral Cheek

The greater laxity and simpler architecture of the skin of the cheek allows primary closure of most defects, usually by conversion to an ellipse. However, even moderate tension can result in a wide scar or distort adjacent aesthetic units, and ectropion of the lower eyelid is a particular concern here. If primary closure can be achieved to lie along the nasolabial or preauricular creases, this can give an excellent cosmetic outcome. For larger defects, these natural lines can be utilized with cervicofacial rotation flap reconstruction.

References

1. Ray E. Head and neck reconstructive surgery. In: Cancer treatment and research. New York, NY: Springer; 2018. p. 123–43.
2. Erba P, Ogawa R, Vyas R, Orgill DP. The reconstructive matrix: a new paradigm in reconstructive plastic surgery. Plast Reconstr Surg. 2010 Aug;126(2):492–8.
3. El-Marakby HH. The reliability of pectoralis major myocutaneous flap in head and neck reconstruction. J Egypt Natl Canc Inst. 2006 Mar;18(1):41–50.
4. Shah JP, Haribhakti V, Loree TR, Sutaria P. Complications of the pectoralis major myocutaneous flap in head and neck reconstruction. Am J Surg. 1990 Oct;160(4):352–5.
5. Zitelli JA. Wound healing by secondary intention. A cosmetic appraisal. J Am Acad Dermatol. 1983 Sep;9(3):407–15.
6. Leonard AL, Hanke CW. Second intention healing for intermediate and large postsurgical defects of the lip. J Am Acad Dermatol. 2007 Nov;57(5):832–5.
7. Jin X, Teng L, Zhang C, Xu J, Lu J, Zhang B, et al. Reconstruction of partial-thickness vermilion defects with a mucosal V–Y advancement flap based on the orbicularis oris muscle. J Plast Reconstr Aesthetic Surg. 2011 Apr;64(4):472–6.
8. Wagner DJD, Newman DMH. Bipedicled axial cross-lip flap for correction of major vermilion deficiency after cleft lip repair. Los Angeles, CA: Sage; 2017.
9. Ceran C, Demirseren ME, Sarici M, Durgun M, Tekin F. Tongue flap as a reconstructive option in intraoral defects. J Craniofac Surg. 2013 May;24(3):972–4.
10. Levi B, Ricci JA, Donelan MB. Vermillion reconstruction with anal verge transitional epithelium. J Burn Care Res. 2017 May 20;39(2):1.
11. Sood A, Paik A, Lee E. Lower lip reconstruction: karapandzic flap. Eplasty. 2013;13:ic17.
12. Karapandzic M. Reconstruction of lip defects by local arterial flaps. Br J Plast Surg. 1974 Jan;27(1):93–7.
13. Bernard C. Cancer de la levre inferieure opere par un procede nouveau. Bull Mem Soc Chir Paris. 1853;3:357–64.
14. Webster RC, Coffey RJ, Kelleher RE. Total and partial reconstruction of the lower lip with innervated muscle-bearing flaps. Plast Reconstr Surg. 1960 Apr;25(3):360–71.
15. Pirgousis P, Fernandes R. Reconstruction of subtotal defects of the lower lip: a review of current techniques and a proposed modification. J Oral Maxillofac Surg. 2011 Jan;69(1):295–9.
16. Fujimori R. Gate flap for the total reconstruction of the lower lip. Br J Plast Surg. 1980 Jul;33(3):340–5.
17. Aytekin A, Ay A, Aytekin O. Total upper lip reconstruction with bilateral Fujimori gate flaps. Plast Reconstr Surg. 2003 Feb;111(2):797–800.

18. Agostini T. The Sabattini-Abbé flap: a historical note. Plast Reconstr Surg. 2009 Feb;123(2):767.
19. Abbe R. A new plastic operation for the relief of deformity due to double harelip. Plast Reconstr Surg. 1968 Nov;42(5):481–3.
20. Webster JP. Crescentic peri-alar cheek excision for upper lip flap advancement with a short history of upper lip repair. Plast Reconstr Surg. 1955;16(6):434–64.
21. Fernandes R, Clemow J. Outcomes of total or near-total lip reconstruction with microvascular tissue transfer. J Oral Maxillofac Surg. 2012 Dec;70(12):2899–906.
22. Sakai S, Soeda S, Endo T, Ishii M, Uchiumi E. A compound radial artery forearm flap for the reconstruction of lip and chin defect. Br J Plast Surg. 1989;42(3):337–8.
23. Cordova A, D'Arpa S, Moschella F. Gracilis free muscle transfer for morpho-functional reconstruction of the lower lip. Head Neck. 2008 May;30(5):684–9.
24. Sacak B, Gurunluoglu R. The innervated gracilis muscle for microsurgical functional lip reconstruction: review of the literature. Ann Plast Surg. 2015 Feb;74(2):204–9.
25. Gurunluoglu R, Glasgow M, Williams SA, Gurunluoglu A, Antrobus J, Eusterman V. Functional reconstruction of total lower lip defects using innervated gracilis flap in the setting of high-energy ballistic injury to the lower face: preliminary report. J Plast Reconstr Aesthetic Surg. Churchill Livingstone. 2012 Oct 1;65(10):1335–42.
26. Lyons GB, Milroy BC, Lendvay PG, Teston LM. Upper lip reconstruction: use of the free superficial temporal artery hair-bearing flap. Br J Plast Surg. 1989 May;42(3):333–6.
27. Chang K-P, Lai C-S, Tsai C-C, Lin T-M, Lin S-D. Total upper lip reconstruction with a free temporal scalp flap: long-term follow-up. Head Neck. 2003 Jul;25(7):602–5.
28. Dean A, Alamillos F, García-López A, Sánchez J, Peñalba M. The buccal fat pad flap in oral reconstruction. Head Neck. 2001 May;23(5):383–8.
29. Liu F, Wang L, Pang S, Kan Q. Reconstruction of full-thickness buccal defects with folded radial forearm flaps: a retrospective clinical study. Medicine (Baltimore). 2017 Aug;96(32):e7344.
30. Liu Z-M, Wu D, Liu X-K, Liu W-W, Li H, Li Q, et al. Reconstruction of through-and-through cheek defects with folded free anterolateral thigh flaps. J Oral Maxillofac Surg. 2013 May;71(5):960–4.
31. Liu YM, Sherris DA. Static procedures for the management of the midface and lower face. Facial Plast Surg. 2008 May;24(2):211–5.
32. Coyle M, Godden A, Brennan PA, Cascarini L, Coombes D, Kerawala C, et al. Dynamic reanimation for facial palsy: an overview. Br J Oral Maxillofac Surg. 2013 Dec;51(8):679–83.
33. Martin D, Pascal JF, Baudet J, Mondie JM, Farhat JB, Athoum A, et al. The submental island flap: a new donor site. Anatomy and clinical applications as a free or pedicled flap. Plast Reconstr Surg. 1993 Oct;92(5):867–73.
34. Cariati P, Cabello Serrano A, Marin Fernandez AB, Perez de Perceval Tara M, Juliá MA, Ildefonso Martinez Lara M. Is submental flap safe for the oncological reconstruction of the oral cavity? J Stomatol oral Maxillofac Surg. 2018 Jun 27;119(4):284–7.
35. Howard BE, Nagel TH, Donald CB, Hinni ML, Hayden RE. Oncologic safety of the submental flap for reconstruction in oral cavity malignancies. Otolaryngol Head Neck Surg. 2014 Apr;150(4):558–62.
36. Wu Y, Tang P, Qi Y, Xu Z, He Y. Evaluation for submental island flap. Zhonghua Kou Qiang Yi Xue Za Zhi. 2002 Nov;37(6):418–20.
37. Taghinia AH, Movassaghi K, Wang AX, Pribaz JJ. Reconstruction of the upper aerodigestive tract with the submental artery flap. Plast Reconstr Surg. 2009 Feb;123(2):562–70.
38. Deganello A, Manciocco V, Dolivet G, Leemans CR, Spriano G. Infrahyoid fascio-myocutaneous flap as an alternative to free radial forearm flap in head and neck reconstruction. Head Neck. 2007 Mar;29(3):285–91.
39. Mosier K, Liu W-C, Behin B, Lee C, Baredes S. Cortical adaptation following partial Glossectomy with primary closure: implications for reconstruction of the Oral tongue. Ann Otol Rhinol Laryngol. 2005 Sep 28;114(9):681–7.
40. Brown L, Rieger JM, Harris J, Seikaly H. A longitudinal study of functional outcomes after surgical resection and microvascular reconstruction for Oral Cancer: tongue mobility and swallowing function. J Oral Maxillofac Surg. 2010 Nov;68(11):2690–700.
41. Biglioli F, Liviero F, Frigerio A, Rezzonico A, Brusati R. Function of the sensate free forearm flap after partial glossectomy. J Cranio-Maxillofacial Surg. 2006 Sep;34(6):332–9.
42. Kimata Y, Sakuraba M, Hishinuma S, Ebihara S, Hayashi R, Asakage T, et al. Analysis of the relations between the shape of the reconstructed tongue and postoperative functions after subtotal or total glossectomy. Laryngoscope. 2003;113(5):905–9.
43. Weber RS, Ohlms L, Bowman J, Jacob R, Goepfert H. Functional results after Total or near Total Glossectomy with laryngeal preservation. Arch Otolaryngol Neck Surg. 1991;117(5):512–5.
44. Fattahi TT. An overview of facial aesthetic units. J Oral Maxillofac Surg. 2003 Oct;61(10):1207–11.
45. González-Ulloa M. Restoration of the face covering by means of selected skin in regional ⊣sthetic units. Br J Plast Surg Elsevier. 1956 Jan;9:212–21.
46. González-Ulloa M. Regional aesthetic units of the face. Plast Reconstr Surg. 1987 Mar;79(3):489–90.
47. Gonzalez-Ulloa M, Stevens E. Reconstruction of the nose and forehead by means of regional aesthetic units. Br J Plast Surg. 1961 Jan;13:305–9.
48. Gonzalez-Ulloa M, Castillo A, Stevens E, Alvarez Fuertes G, Leonelli F, Ubaldo F. Preliminary study of the total restoration of the facial skin. Plast Reconstr Surg (1946). 1954 Mar;13(3):151–61.
49. Thompson S, Menick FJ. Aesthetic facial reconstruction: blending human perception and the facial subunit theory. Plast Surg Nurs. 1994;14(4):211–6. 224
50. Tenzel RR. Surgical techniques and problems in cosmetic blepharoplasty. Trans Am Acad Ophthalmol Otolaryngol. 1969;73(6):1154–61.
51. McClellan WT, Rawson AE, Wendell L. Hughes' life and contributions to plastic surgery. Plast Reconstr Surg. 2011 Dec;128(6):765e–72e.
52. Mauriello JA, Antonacci R. Single tarsoconjunctival flap (lower eyelid) for upper eyelid reconstruction,(reverse modified Hughes procedure). Ophthalmic Surg. 1994 Jun;25(6):374–8.
53. Cutler NL, Beard C. A method for partial and total upper lid reconstruction. Am J Ophthalmol. 1955 Jan;39(1):1–7.
54. Mandal SK, Fleming JC, Reddy SG, Fowler BT. Total upper eyelid reconstruction with modified cutler-beard procedure using autogenous auricular cartilage. J Clin Diagn Res. 2016 Aug;10(8):NC01–4.
55. Louis PJ, Aponte-Wesson RA, Fernandes RP, Clemow J. Autogenous and prosthetic reconstruction of the ear. Oral Maxillofac Surg Clin North Am. 2013 May;25(2):271–86.
56. Thomas SS, Matthews RN. Squamous cell carcinoma of the pinna: a 6-year study. Br J Plast Surg. 1994 Mar;47(2):81–5.
57. Tay S, Nikkhah D, Teo TC. The antia-buch flap revisited. Clin Otolaryngol. 2017 Aug;42(4):951–3.
58. Antia NH, Buch VI. Chondrocutaneous advancement flap for the marginal defect of the ear. Plast Reconstr Surg. 1967 May;39(5):472–7.
59. Krunic AL, Weitzul S, Taylor RS. Chondrocutaneous advancement flap for reconstruction of helical rim defects in dermatologic surgery. Australas J Dermatol. 2006 Nov;47(4):296–9.
60. Masud D, Tzafetta K. The "double headed slug flap": a simple technique to reconstruct large helical rim defects. J Plast Reconstr Aesthet Surg. 2012 Oct;65(10):1410–3.

61. Cordova A, Pirrello R, D'Arpa S, Moschella F. Superior pedicle Retroauricular Island flap for ear and temporal region reconstruction. Ann Plast Surg. 2008 Jun;60(6):652–7.
62. Tanzer RC. Total reconstruction of the auricle. The evolution of a plan of treatment. Plast Reconstr Surg. 1971 Jun;47(6):523–33.
63. Brent B. Ear reconstruction with an expansile framework of autogenous rib cartilage. Plast Reconstr Surg. 1974 Jun;53(6):619–28.
64. Nagata S. A new method of total reconstruction of the auricle for microtia. Plast Reconstr Surg. 1993 Aug;92(2):187–201.
65. Mevio E, Facca L, Mullace M, Sbrocca M, Gorini E, Artesi L, et al. Osseointegrated implants in patients with auricular defects: a case series study. Acta Otorhinolaryngol Ital. 2015 Jun;35(3):186–90.
66. Granström G, Bergström K, Tjellström A. The bone-anchored hearing aid and bone-anchored Epithesis for congenital ear malformations. Otolaryngol Neck Surg. 1993 Jul;109(1):46–53.
67. Gentile P, Bottini DJ, Colicchia GM, Trimarco A, Cervelli V. Burns: bone-anchored, extra-oral implantology. J Burn Care Res. 2008 Jul;29(4):627–31.
68. Fernandes JR, Pribaz JJ, Lim AA, Guo L. Nasal reconstruction. Ann Plast Surg. 2018 Dec;81(6S Suppl 1):S30–4.
69. Menick FJ. Nasal reconstruction. Plast Reconstr Surg. 2010 Apr;125(4):138e–50e.
70. Shokri T, Kadakia S, Saman M, Habal M, Kohlert S, Sokoya M, et al. The Paramedian forehead flap for nasal reconstruction. J Craniofac Surg. 2018 Dec;30(2):330–3.
71. Koshima I, Tsutsui T, Nanba Y, Takahashi Y, Akisada K. Free radial forearm osteocutaneous perforator flap for reconstruction of total nasal defects. J Reconstr Microsurg 2002 Oct;18(7):585–588. discussion 589–90.

87 Distraction Osteogenesis of the Maxillofacial Region

R. S. Neelakandan

87.1 Introduction

Reconstruction of the facial skeleton is a technique sensitive process for the reconstructive surgeon as the resulting outcome should improve the form and function of the patient. Distraction osteogenesis (DO) can be defined as the biologic process consisting of new bone formation between the bone segment surfaces that are gradually separated by incremental applied traction. It is a technique to which precludes donor site morbidity which is commonly performed to correct long bone deformities but gaining popularity in the maxillofacial reconstructive procedures in the recent times. The recent advancement of DO procedure is the transport distraction osteogenesis (TDO) which involves osteogenesis and histogenesis from the residual host tissues.

Following gradual movement of the transport segment, new bone regenerate formation occurs behind it filling the defect.

Ilizarov and his colleague's classified bone transport techniques as:
Monofocal.
Bifocal.
Trifocal.

The bifocal and trifocal techniques play a major role in regenerating new bone across the continuity defects. TDO involves creating a new bone and soft tissue to cover the defect by moving a segment of bone and new soft tissue formation behind it until the segment docks the receiving host bone. TDO can be achieved by movement of bone segments across the defect (Fig. 87.1a, b, and c).

TDO is of three types:
Bifocal.
Trifocal.
Quadrifocal.

Bifocal distraction is the incremental movement of one viable bone segment, trifocal distraction is the incremental movement of two viable bone segments and quadrifocal distraction is the incremental movement of three viable bone segments.

87.2 History of DO

Distraction osteogenesis (DO), a well-established technique used for several decades by orthopedic surgeons to repair long bone defects has over the past 15 years gained acceptance for correction of various craniofacial deformities. Bone distraction is not a new concept. Distraction was introduced first by Codvilla nearly a 100 years ago and was subsequently popularized during the 1940s by Ilizarov, who developed a single-stage procedure to lengthen long bones without the use of grafting material. The feasibility of applying Ilizarov's principles to different craniofacial deformities was not considered until several decades after his pioneering work in the peripheral skeleton. In the purest sense, the first reports of craniofacial DO were in the early 1960s, when rapid expansion of the palate was carried out in growing patients. This practice, however, involved distraction of a naturally occurring physis. Finally, in 1973, Snyder first described the Ilizarov technique to lengthen a surgical osteotomy of the

Electronic Supplementary Material The online version of this chapter (https://doi.org/10.1007/978-981-15-1346-6_87) contains supplementary material, which is available to authorized users.

R. S. Neelakandan (✉)
Department of Oral and Maxillofacial Surgery, Meenakshi Ammal Dental College and Hospital, MAHER, Chennai, Tamil Nadu, India

K. Bonanthaya et al. (eds.), *Oral and Maxillofacial Surgery for the Clinician*, https://doi.org/10.1007/978-981-15-1346-6_87

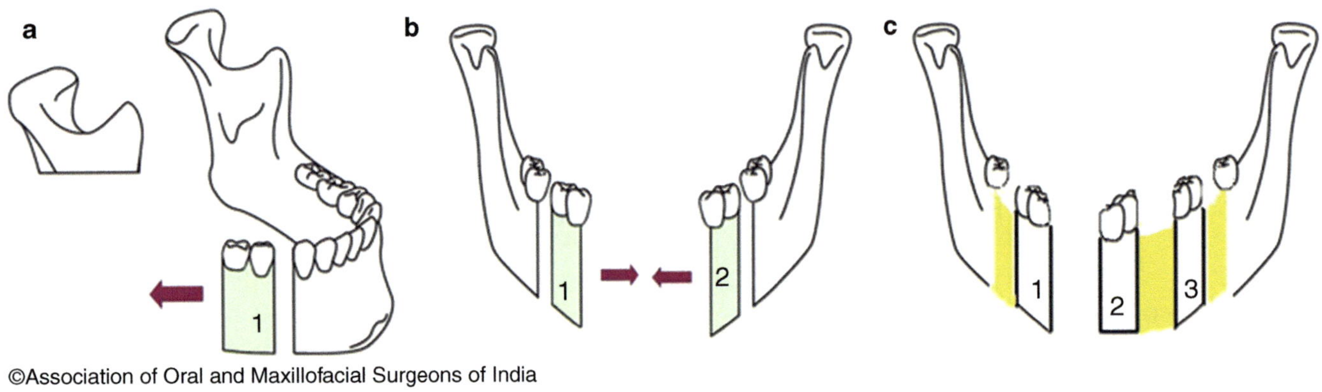

Fig. 87.1 (**a**) Bifocal distraction, (**b**) Trifocal distraction, (**c**) Quadrifocal distraction

canine mandible. Interest in craniofacial distraction at first grew slowly, with sporadic experimental reports appearing over the ensuing two decades. However, in the early 1990s, experimental investigation intensified following reports from New York University on lengthening of dog mandibles and from Constantino and Friedman et al., who used DO to successfully close canine segmental lower jaw defects. Thereafter, several studies on various animal models demonstrated the application of osteodistraction at a number of different sites, including the mandible, midface, and cranial vault. It was Michieli and Miotti who first suggested the protocol for mandibular distraction in humans which included a latency period of 1 week after osteotomy followed by activation rate of 1 mm on alternate days and a minimum of 45 days consolidation period of every 15 mm distraction. In 1992, the first clinical results of craniofacial DO were reported by McCarthy et al. in a small series of patients with congenital mandible deformities. Since then, several larger series with longer follow-up periods have appeared. More recently, the technique has been successfully used for midfacial and upper craniofacial skeletal defects (Table 87.1) [1].

87.3 Biology of Transport Distraction

The adaptive function of bone to mechanical stimuli causing resorption of existing bone and formation of new bone is the continuous remodeling process of the bone tissue and was recognized as the Wolff's law. The principle behind DO is the application of defined mechanical strains to the reparative callus that is formed in the osteotomy gap. It is based on the law of tension stress by which states that gradual traction on living tissues creates stresses that can stimulate and maintain regeneration and active growth of these tissues.

Table 87.1 The history of DO is long and various researchers has contributed to its development, as summarized below

1728	Fauchard	Arch Expansion for accommodation of crowd teeth
1828	Wescott	Palatal arch expansion device
1893	Angel and Goddard	Modified Wescott's device
1905	Codivilla	Femur distraction
1927	Rosenthal	Intraoral tooth borne osteodistraction device for mandible
1937	Kazangian	Over the face appliance and distracted mandible using elastic traction
1948	Crawford	Demonstrated distraction force on a fracture callus
1959	Kole	Used traction to correct anterior open bite
Mid-twentieth century	Ilizarov	Long bone distraction
1973	Synder et al.	Distraction of membranous bone of facial skeleton
1976	Michieli and Miotti	Developed mandibular distraction. First suggested operative protocol for human mandibular distraction protocol
1989, 1992	McCarthy et al.	Used miniature orthopedic device for small bone lengthening. Reported first clinical case of mandibular DO in humans
1990	Constantino et al.	Reported the first bifocal distraction (TDO) of the mandible by using an external custom made distraction device
1997	Fedotov	Designed a semi-circular external distractor, very similar to the present day external distractors. Designed monofocal, bifocal, and trifocal distraction based on the size of the defect to be reconstructed
1987	Wolfson	Designed the first intra oral distractor—Considered as a landmark in TDO But was never used in patients

The sequence of DO is, osteotomy first, followed by latency period, which is the duration from bone division to the onset of traction. The third phase is the distraction phase which is the time when gradual traction is applied and distraction regenerate is formed, followed by the consolidation period which allows maturation and corticalization of the regenerate after traction forces are discontinued. The last stage is the remodeling phase where there is completion of the regenerated bone remodeling [1] (Fig. 87.2a, b).

Sequence of DO

Osteotomy.
Latency period.
Distraction phase.
Consolidation period.
Remodeling phase.

The entire healing process of TDO is similar to that of a fracture healing process. The osteotomy causes discontinuity of the skeletal segment which triggers an evolutionary process of bone repair. It involves recruitment of osteoprogenitor cells, followed by cellular modulation or osteoinduction, and establishment of an environmental template or osteoconduction resulting in a reparative callus. The latency period is the period from bone division to the onset of traction. It represents the time allowed for reparative callus formation. On the fifth day after osteotomy, a mini-cellular network of growing capillary loops is formed in the medullary canal of both proximal and distal segments in the areas adjacent to the fracture line. This is a stage represented by soft callus where granulation tissue is converted to fibrous tissue by fibroblasts starting in the periphery.

During distraction phase traction force is applied to the bone segments and is slowly pulled apart, resulting in formation of new bony tissues which progressively increases the intersegmental gap. The cartilaginous callus is replaced by new bone formation due to various cellular activities, and this stage of hard callus remains for approximately 3–4 months. However, the normal fracture healing process is interrupted by the application of gradual traction to the soft callus. As distraction begins, the fibrous tissue of the soft callus becomes longitudinally oriented along the axis of distraction. In the second week of distraction, primary trabeculae

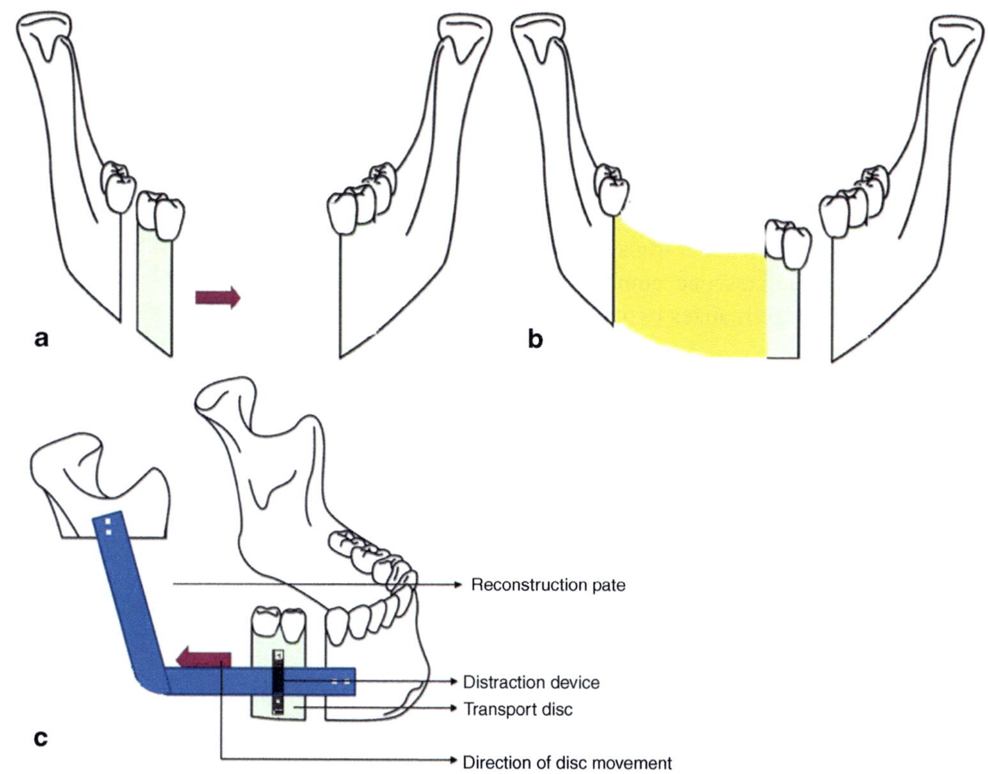

Fig. 87.2 (**a**, **b**) Traction force applied to the bone segments, slowly pulling them apart, resulting in formation of new bone. (**c**) Line diagram depicting process of TDO in a mandible requiring reconstruction for a segmental defect

begin to form and the osteoid begins to mineralize. In TDO both membranous and endochondral processes play an important role in the process of new bone formation.

The consolidation period is defined as the time between cessation of traction forces to the removal of distraction device. It represents the time required for complete mineralization of the distraction regenerate. The remodeling period is the period from the application of full functional loading to the complete remodeling of the newly formed bone. The distraction regenerate is remodeled to mature bone during remodeling at a later stage.

87.4 Biology of Bone Transport

Biologically, bone transport techniques are based on two distinct processes, *distraction osteogenesis* and *transformational osteogenesis*. DO as previously described, is a biologic process of new bone formation between the surfaces of bone segments that are gradually separated by incremental traction. Transformational osteogenesis is a mechanically induced biologic process of pathologic bony tissue transformation into normal bone. Importantly, these two processes occur simultaneously during bifocal bone transport. Distraction osteogenesis occurs between the surfaces of the residual host bone segment and the trailing edge of the transport disc, while transformational osteogenesis occurs between the leading edge of the transport disc and the residual target bone segment (Figs. 87.3 and 87.4a, b).

In TDO the transport segments undergo stress due to compressive forces as well as distraction force. For instance, in bifocal transport, the leading edge realizes compression force, while the trailing edge realizes distraction force, and with trifocal transport, the leading edge of both segments realizes one common compressive force, and the trailing edge realizes two distraction forces one on either side.

87.5 Device Design

The concept of TDO has been increasingly applied to the craniofacial skeleton in the recent years. Initially used in experimental animal models, then gradually it gained popularity in the clinical setup. After encountering failures with avascularized and vascularized grafts in our patients with mandibular continuity defects, this modality of reconstruction was contemplated in our clinical practice. After treating 22 cases with earlier generation distraction devices, there were certain biological and mechanical problems resulting due to lack of vector control and inadequate tension stress effect. For these reasons various modifications were made in

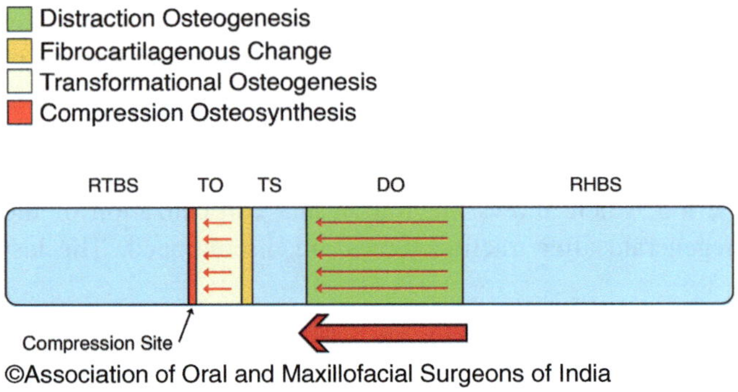

Fig. 87.3 Biology of bone transport. (*DO* distraction osteogenesis, *RHBS* residual host bone segment, *TS* transport segment (transport disc), *RTBS* residual target bone segment, *TO* transformational osteogenesis)

the initial design with an aim to improve the vector control and stability of the device.

> The transport distraction device may be divided into three components:
> - The reconstruction plate for stability.
> - The distractor component for mobilizing the transport segment on activation.
> - The screws for anchorage.

A proper surgical plan and device design should be followed in each case to achieve the desired results. Few factors that are to be considered are the cross-sectional dimension of the transport disc and the length of the defect along with number of teeth in the disc which can be used for prosthetic rehabilitation as well as to monitor the movement of transport disc during the distraction. It is essential to decide if the condyle should be retained or disarticulated to incorporate the condylar component in the device. It is advisable to retain the condyle when possible so as to maintain the natural joint architecture (Table 87.2 and Figs. 87.5, 87.6, 87.7, 87.8, 87.9 and 87.10).

87.6 Biomechanical and Vector Consideration in Mandible and Selection of Device

The success of distraction osteogenesis is based on biological and biomechanical factors. The biological factors are the length and geometric shape of the defect (straight unilateral posterior/curved across midline), cross-sectional area, and

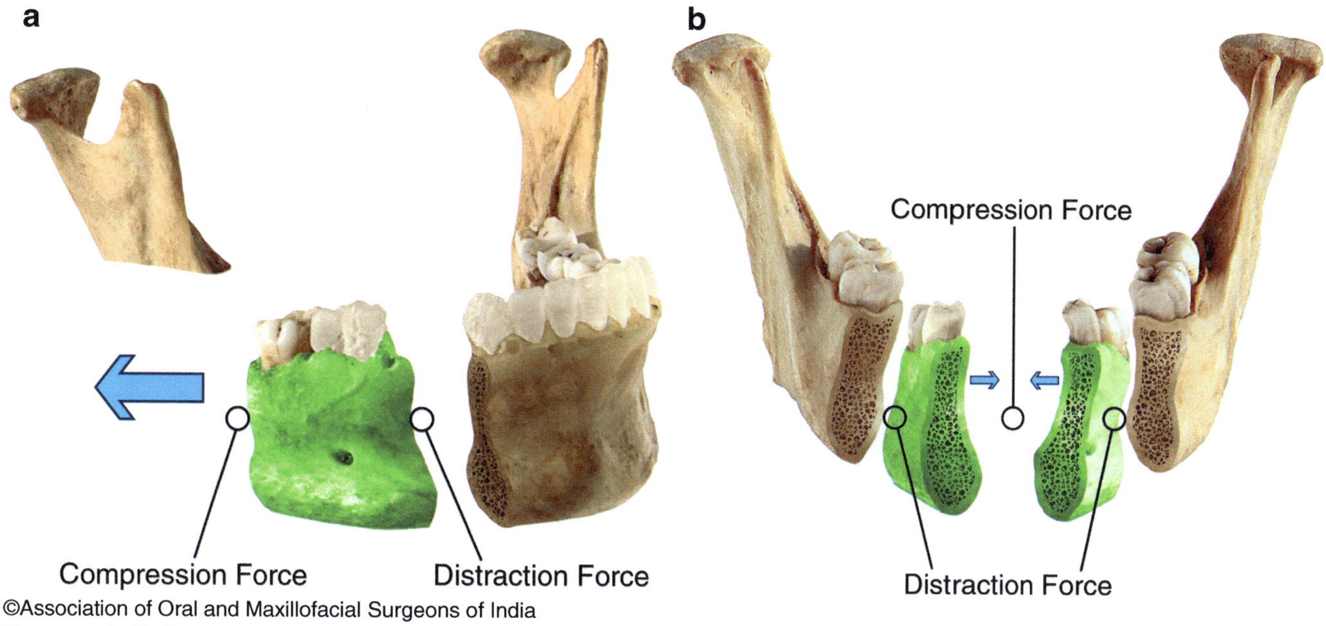

Fig. 87.4 (**a**, **b**) Stress realized by transport segment in bifocal and trifocal distraction

Table 87.2 Generations of transport distraction devices, its merits, and demerits

DO device	Design	Merits	Demerits
1st generation extraoral device (Fig. 87.5a, b, c, d, e)	A single guidance rod with a single anchorage fixator on either side of the cut ends of residual host bone without a reconstruction plate to stabilize the cut ends of the mandible		Unstable residual host bone with inadequate control of the transport segment producing sagittal deviations Pin tract scarring
2nd generation (Fig. 87.6a, b, c)	Reinforced with an additional guidance rod, and the device is anchored to the residual host bone of either side with double anchorage fixators The cut ends of the bone are stabilized with a reconstruction plate	Better control of the transport disc and improved anchorage Reduced incidence of sagittal deviation	
3rd generation cantilever distractor (Fig. 87.7a, b)	Used when there is no proximal bone available for fixing the anchorage fixator All the anchorage fixators are anchored to the available bone, proximal to the transport segment	Used when there is no proximal bone available	
4th generation internal distractor (Fig. 87.8a, b, c)	A straight device- and plate-guided internal distractor with 1 mm calibrated guidance rod with a transport device, attached directly to the reconstruction plate	Better vector control owing Better patient compliance No pin tract scar	Can be used only for straight regeneration
5th generation (Fig. 87.9a, b, c)	An arched device consisting of a reconstruction plate bent according to the contours of the defect and is tissue buried to which a 1 mm calibrated arched guidance rod is attached with a connecting vertical arm	Completely placed intraorally Can be used to regenerate bone across the midline for central defects	
6th generation push ball device (Fig. 87.10a, b)	Push ball device consists of a C-shaped cross-sectional hollow guidance rod with the transport device transfixed to the underlying transport segment that is moved through a series of metal balls within the guidance rod activated through a portal at the free end of the rod	It can be used for both straight and curved defect	Over-riding and clogging of the metal balls can happen

density of the transport disc and tension of the soft tissue envelope. The biomechanical factors are dependent on the length and geometric shape of the defect that dictates the selection of straight or curved device.

Every vector is a one-dimensional entity, whereas the desired movements are in most cases two- or three-dimensional. The base of the mandible is constituted by five linear vectors (Fig. 87.11). Two A-P linear vector running

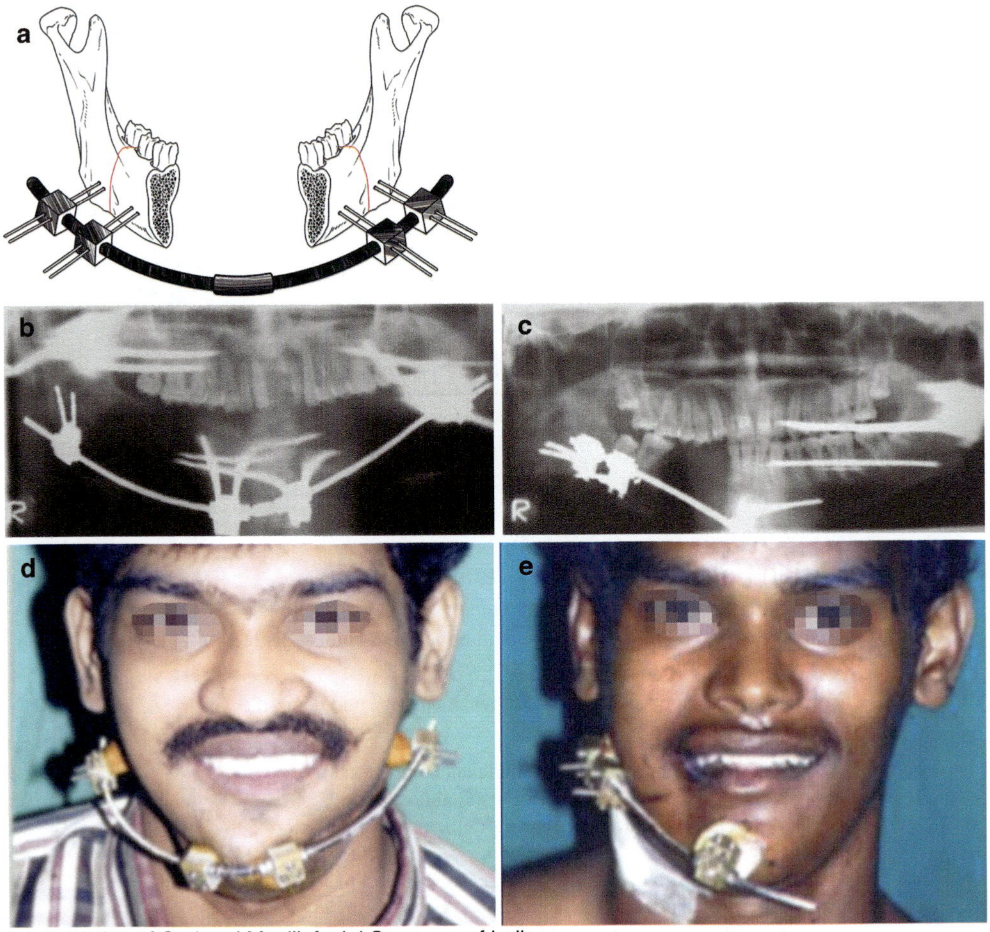

Fig. 87.5 (**a**) first generation extraoral device. (**b**, **c**) Panoramic radiographs showing the placed first generation distractor device. (**d**, **e**) Clinical pictures with the first generation device

parallel to the base of the mandible one on either side in the body region, two A-P linear vector running parallel to the base of the mandible in the parasymphysis region, and one horizontal linear vector running again parallel to the base of the mandible in the mid symphysial region. If the defect is along a single vector, it is best reconstructed with straight regeneration, and if the defect is along more than single vector, it is best reconstructed with arched regeneration.

With the advent of various generations of devices for distraction osteogenesis, it is the author's contention that the straight tissue buried distraction device is preferred for unilateral defects, whereas, for bilateral defects crossing the midline, extraoral transcutaneous pin fixation device, either bifocal or trifocal is preferred, as it provides better vector control.

87.7 Classification of Mandibular Defects in TDO

Mandibular defects for reconstruction purpose are classified as central and lateral defects. Central defects can be either symmetrical or asymmetrical, and lateral defects can be either straight, when the defect is posterior to the second premolar and arched when the defect is from anterior to second premolar (Fig. 87.12a, b).

For reconstruction of central defects, when there is a symmetrical central defect, arched regeneration could be contemplated trifocally with identical transport segment from either side and when there is an asymmetrical central defect arched regeneration could be contemplated quadrifocally with nonidentical transport segments (Fig. 87.13).

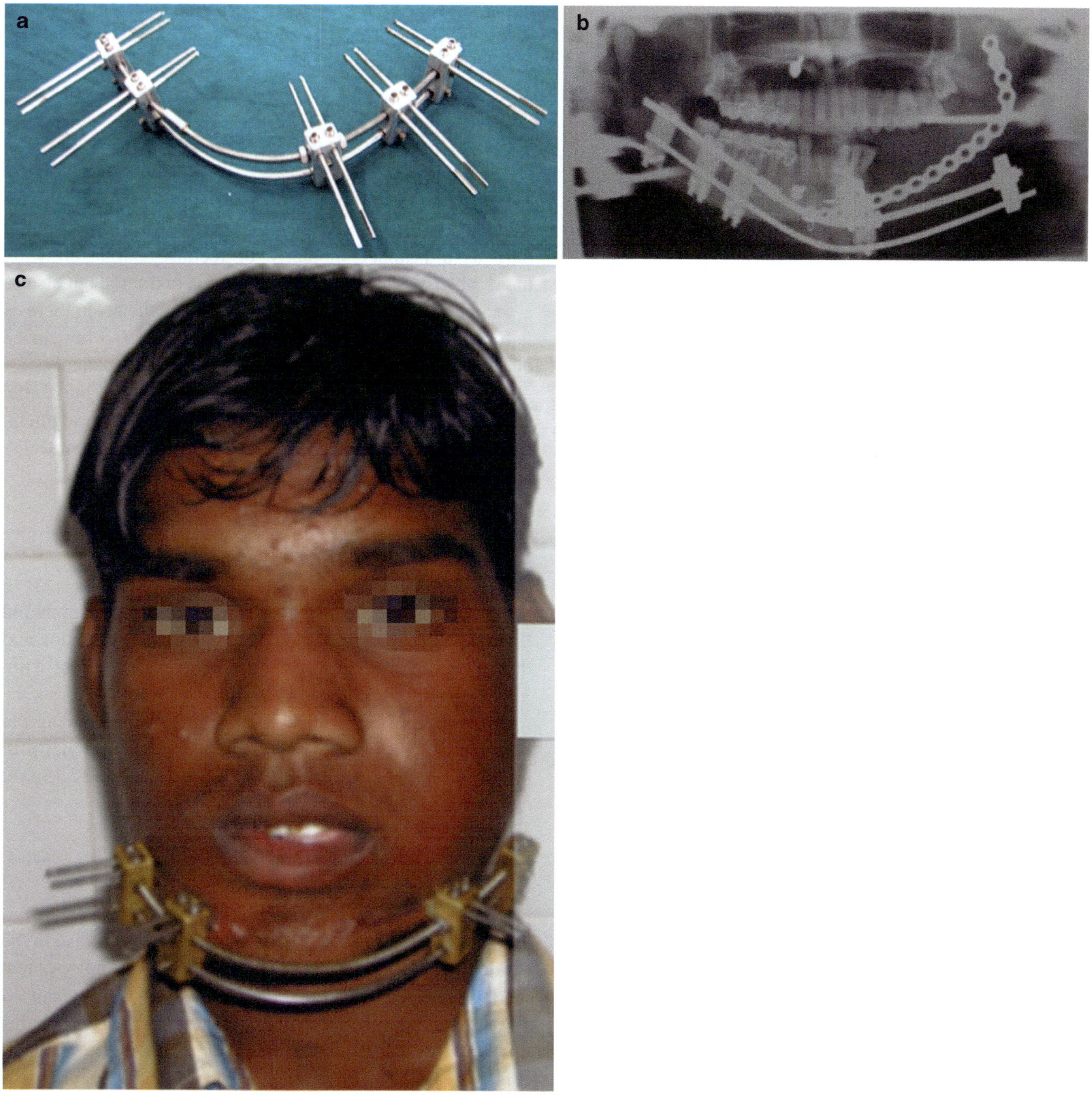

Fig. 87.6 (**a**) second generation transport distraction device. (**b**) Panoramic radiograph showing placement of second generation device with a reconstruction plate. (**c**) Clinical picture showing second generation device

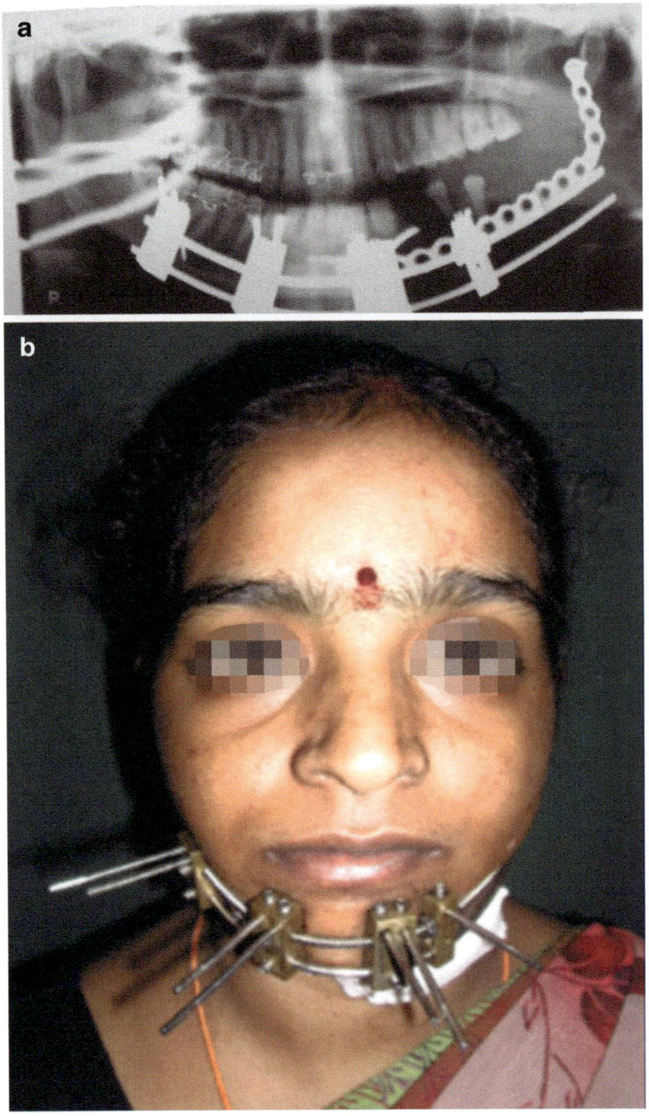

Fig. 87.7 (**a**) Frontal profile view of patient with placement of third generation distractor device. (**b**) Panoramic radiograph showing the presence of third generation distractor device

When it comes to reconstruction of lateral defects, a single-vector defect posterior to the second premolar could be regenerated bifocally, and a two-vector defect anterior to canine could be regenerated either bifocally or trifocally depending upon the availability of horizontal ramus to create transport disc (Fig. 87.14a, b).

The choice of the transport distraction device is dependent upon the site of defect. For defects posterior to second premolar, a straight bar device with or without condylar prosthesis could be used and for defects anterior to first premolar an arched bar device across the midline could be used. However, a curvilinear push ball device could be used for both the types of defects.

87.8 Indications of TDO

Transport regeneration is indicated when there is a continuity defect of mandible due to any cause. It is indicated not only as a primary modality of reconstruction following tumor ablative surgery or bone loss due to trauma but also as a secondary modality of reconstruction whenever there is failure with previous reconstruction. It can also be carried out on pediatric patients and even on irradiated patients.

However, it has a limitation when there are no horizontal rami available on either side to create transport segment. Even in such situation, bone grafting and subsequent transportation can be contemplated.

87.9 Presurgical Investigations

When it comes to investigations, panoramic radiograph and CT will help us to know the exact extension of the lesion and thereby to assume the type of defect we are dealing with. This helps in selection of device.

Stereolithographic 3D models help us in contouring the device exactly along the defect presurgically. This helps in minimizing the working time on the table (Fig. 87.15a, b, c, d).

87.10 Surgical Procedure

Transport distraction involves creating a transport disc in the residual host bone stump, adjacent to a discontinuity defect or a resection site. The transport disk is then advanced 1.0 mm per day to span the discontinuity defect. As this transport disc advances toward the target host bone segment, callus forms at its trailing edge, which gradually matures and calcifies. Once the transport disc reaches the docking site, the segment is held in neutral fixation until a cortical outline is seen in the regenerate. At the time of distractor removal, a small bone graft may need to be positioned between the transport disc and the docking site because the transport disc becomes rounded and encased with a fibrocartilaginous cap on the advancing front. Osseous union between the disc and docking site necessitates removal of this intervening fibrocartilaginous cap.

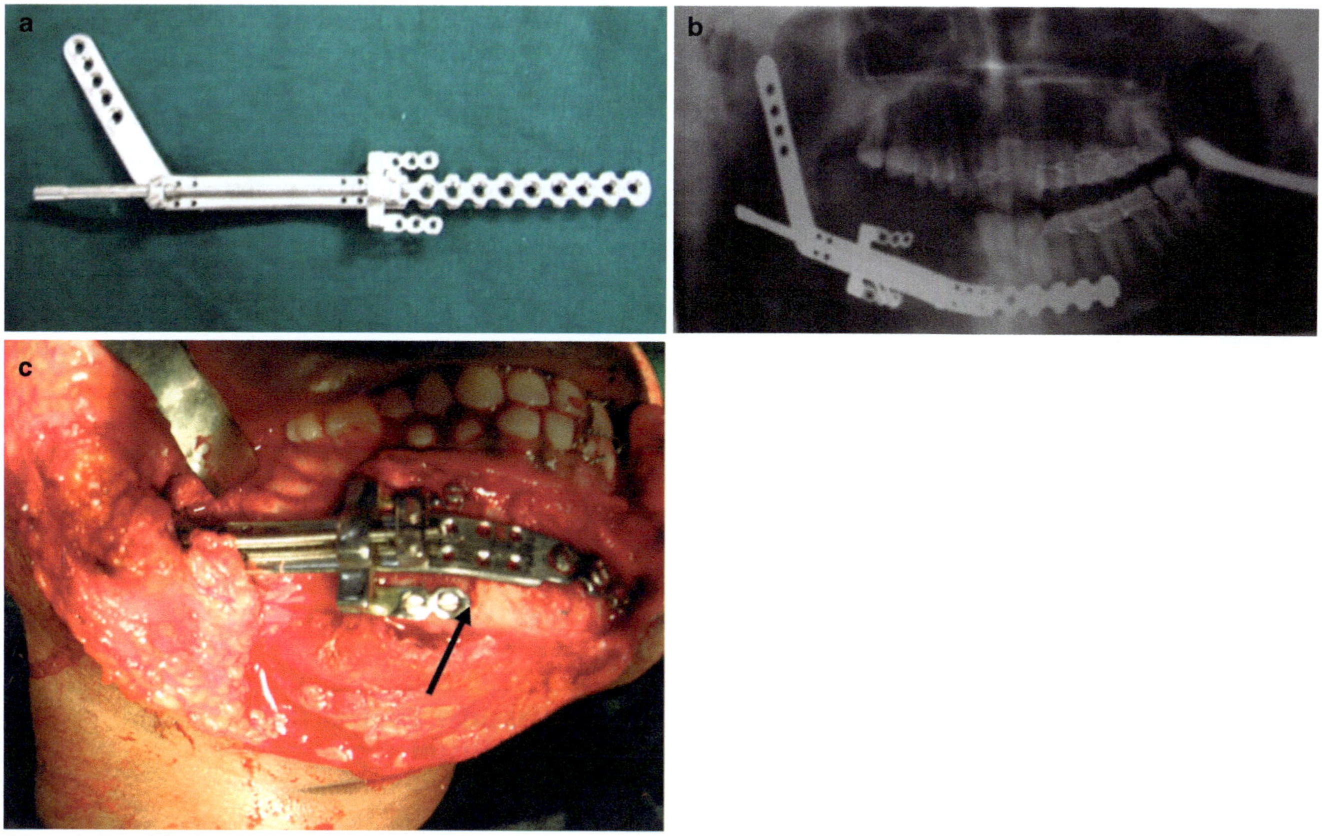

Fig. 87.8 (**a**) fourth generation distractor device with an attached reconstruction plate. (**b**) Panoramic view showing presence of fourth generation device without a condylar component. (**c**) Placement of the device in the mandible after a lip split incision

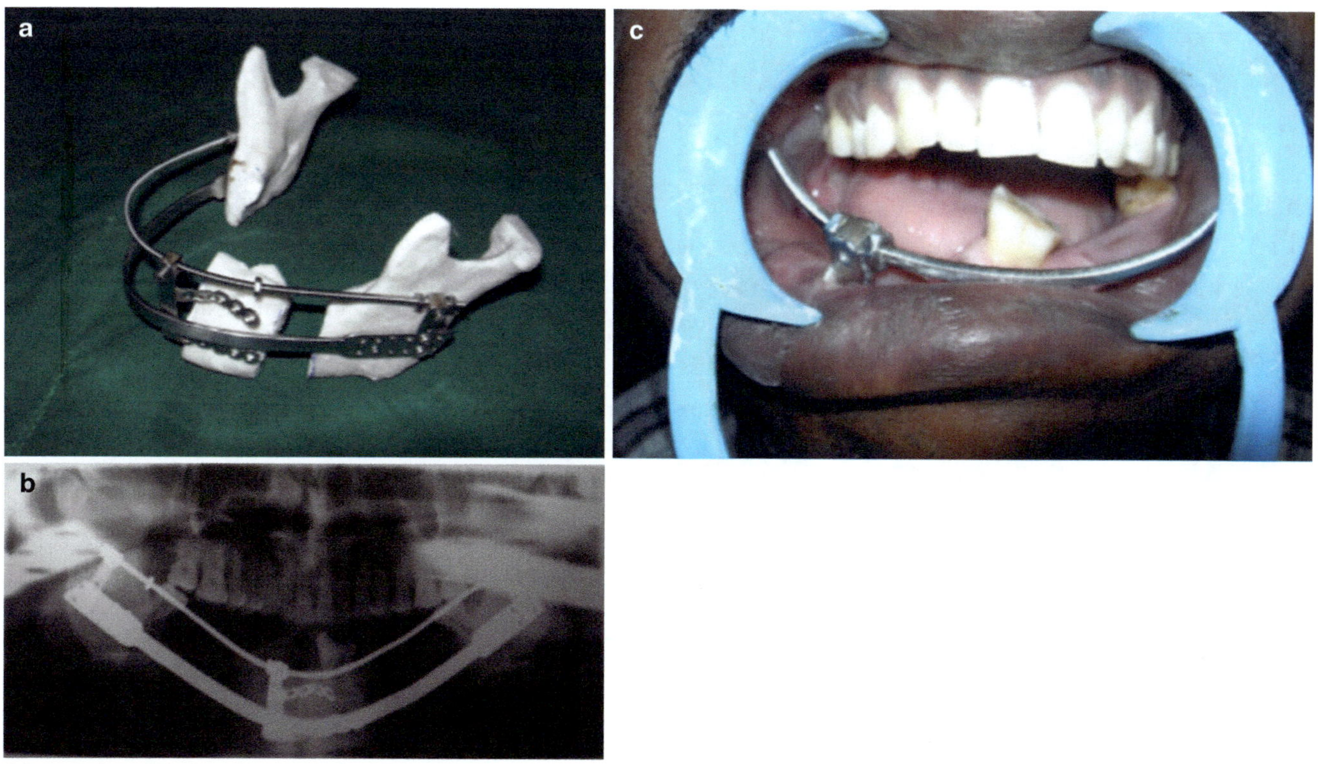

Fig. 87.9 (**a**) fifth generation arc-shaped device, adapted on STL model. (**b**) Panoramic radiograph showing the placement of fifth generation device. (**c**) Clinical picture of fifth generation device

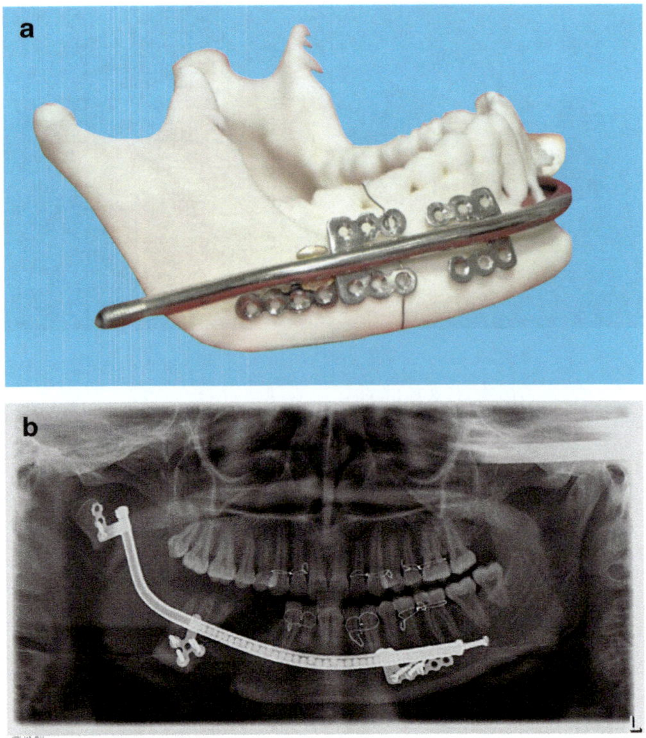

Fig. 87.10 (**a**, **b**) Curvilinear ball device for straight and arched regeneration

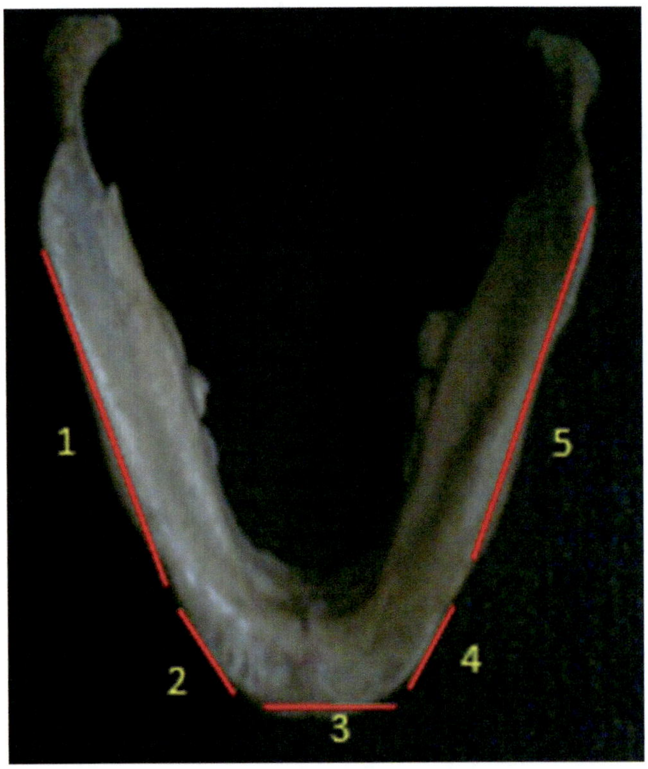

Fig. 87.11 Linear vectors in mandibular reconstruction

87.11 Biological Consideration While Designing Transport Disc

Periosteal preservation is the single most important biologic consideration while designing bone transport, for the transport segment solely depends on periosteal blood supply for its viability. Hence extreme care at every stage—right from making a small incision to minimal periosteal reflection to abundant irrigation and water tight mucosal closure over the transport segment—should be ensured.

While designing the transport segment, parallelism of the cut edges of the residual host bone segment, transport segment, and target bone segment should be ensured to achieve even docking of the transport disc to the cut edges of residual target bone segment. This is carried out by taking the vertical osteotomy cut perpendicular to an imaginary baseline that runs between gonion and menton and parallel to maxillary occlusal plane (Fig. 87.16a–e) followed by implant rehabilitation (Figs. 87.17 and 87.18).

87.12 Vascular, Clinical, Radiological, and Histological Features of the Regenerated Bone

The process of TDO induces tensile stretching of the osteoblast-like cells that alters the local regulation of bone formation and increases the expression of the growth factors. This entire process is vascular-dependent and requires the maintenance of an adequate blood supply. DeCoster et al. in their animal experimental model on transport distraction osteogenesis used injection angiography to study the arterial response of the bone undergoing transport distraction. The angiographic techniques revealed that the transport segment had an intact arterial supply after the osteotomy cut was completed (adhering to surgical principles of TDO) and, also, after transport distraction was activated. They also showed an extensive increase in vessels in distracted limbs of the experimental animals with proximal stretching and distal kinking of the major artery in that limb. Such studies involving major facial vessels during TDO are awaited to be added to maxillofacial literature [2]. Formation of callus can be detected earliest with ultrasonography where it appears as a mixed to hyper echoic area depending upon the degree of maturation. The color Doppler study of the callus demonstrates the quantum of vascularity in the regenerate before maturation [1, 2] (Fig. 87.19).

For radiological examination (Figs. 87.20 and 87.21) regular plain film radiographs remain the mainstay for screening the TDO during active distraction and consolidation period. Panoramic radiograph, submento-vertex view, lateral oblique mandibular projections, and posteroanterior and lateral skull views may all aid in planning and screening the

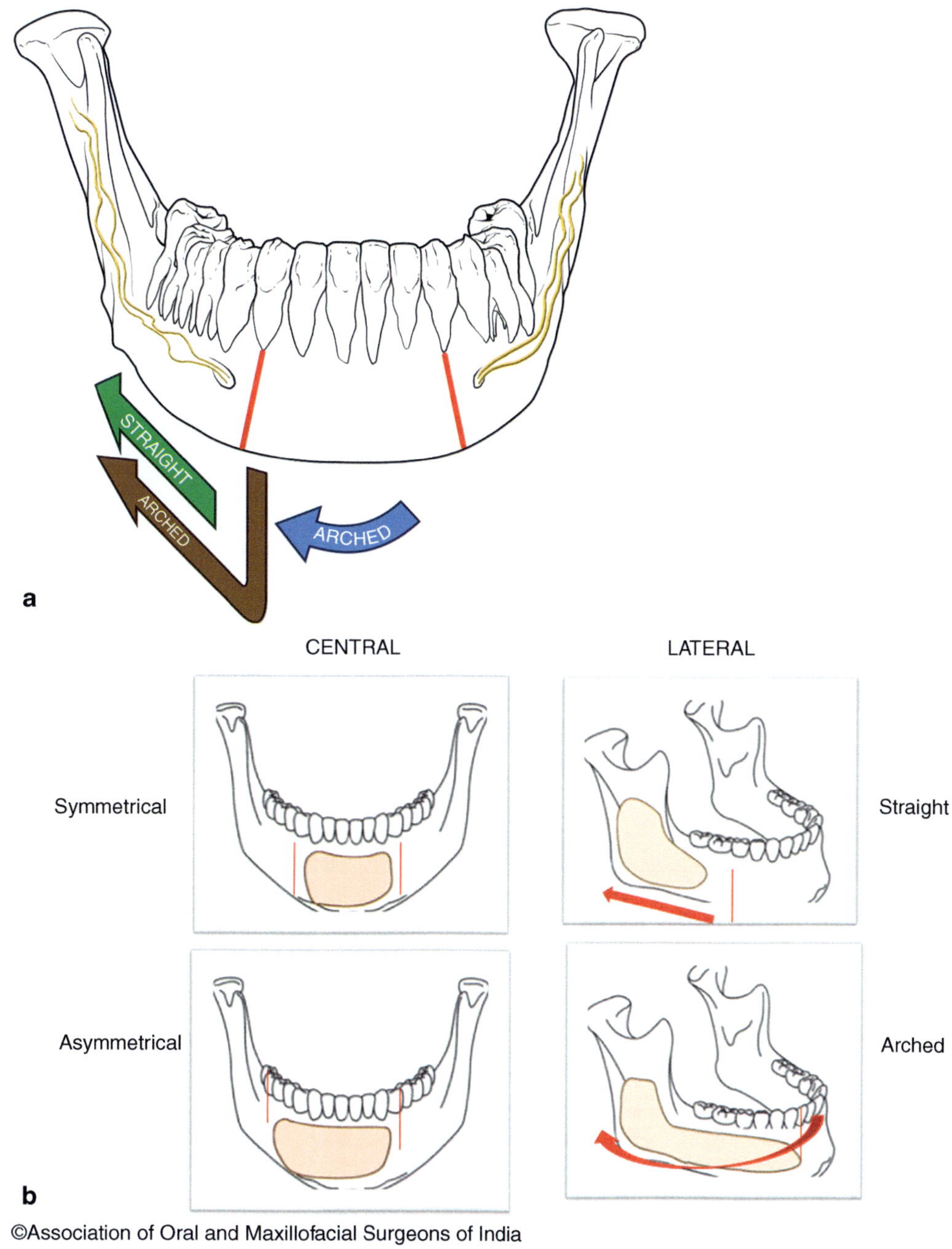

Fig. 87.12 (**a**) Defect posterior to second premolar, straight vector; defect anterior to second premolar, arched vector. (**b**) Classification of mandibular defects

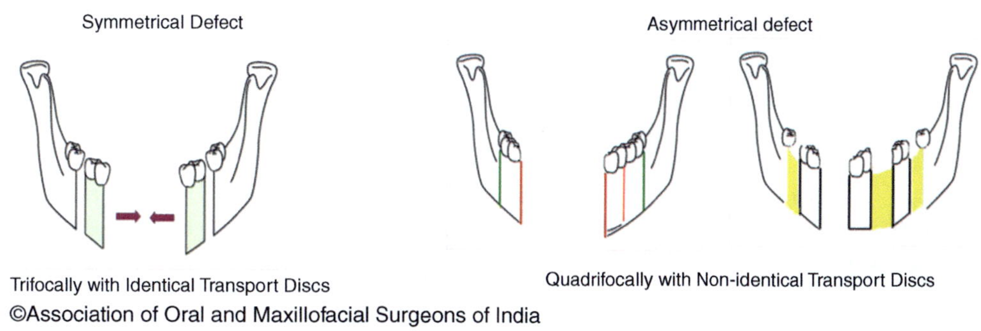

Fig. 87.13 Reconstruction of central defects

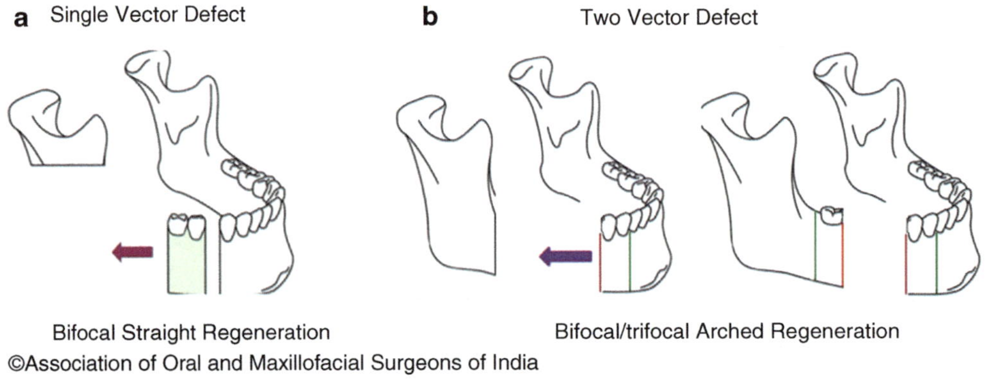

Fig. 87.14 (**a**, **b**) Reconstruction of lateral defects

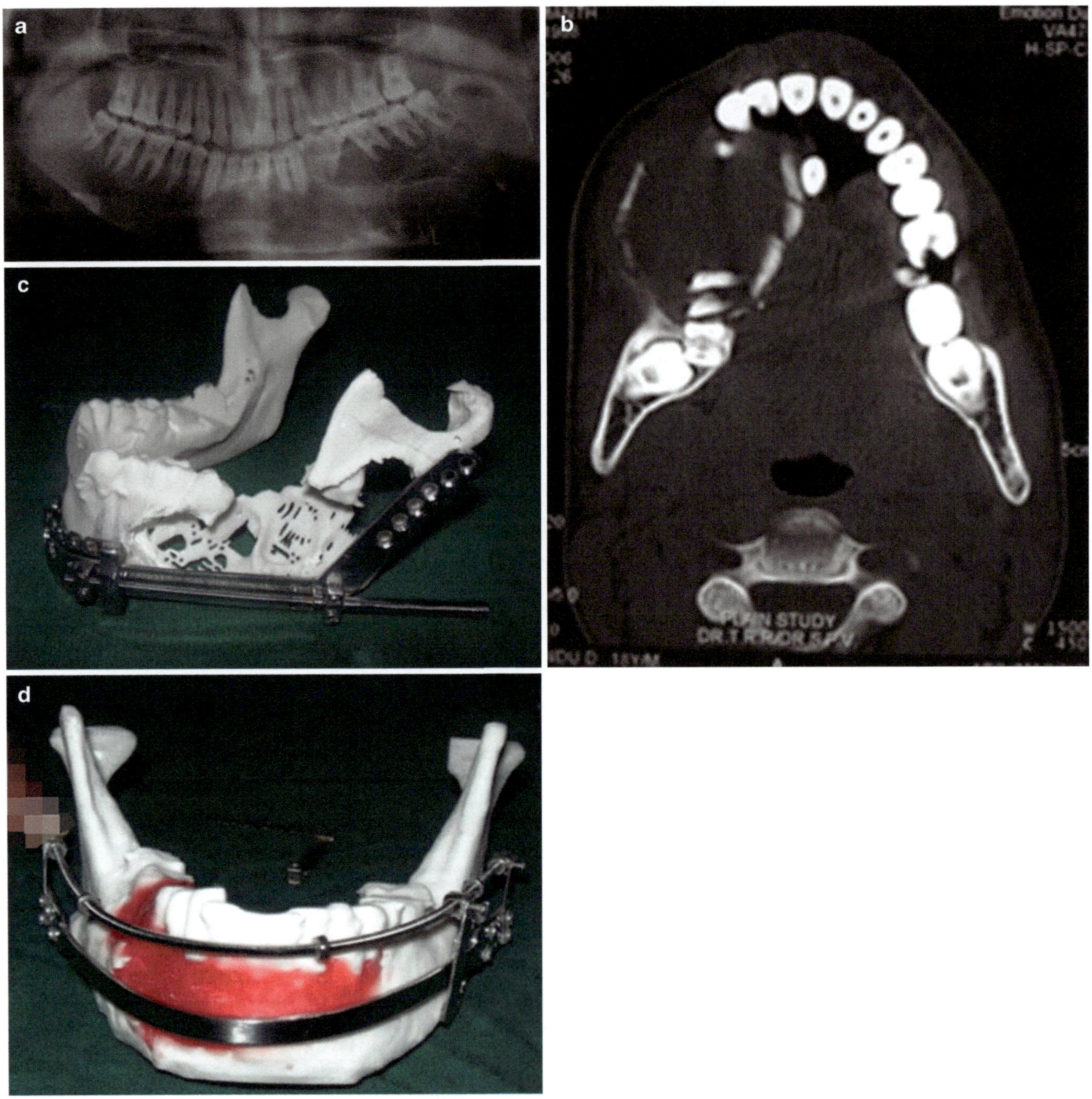

Fig. 87.15 (**a**, **b**, **c**, **d**) Presurgical planning

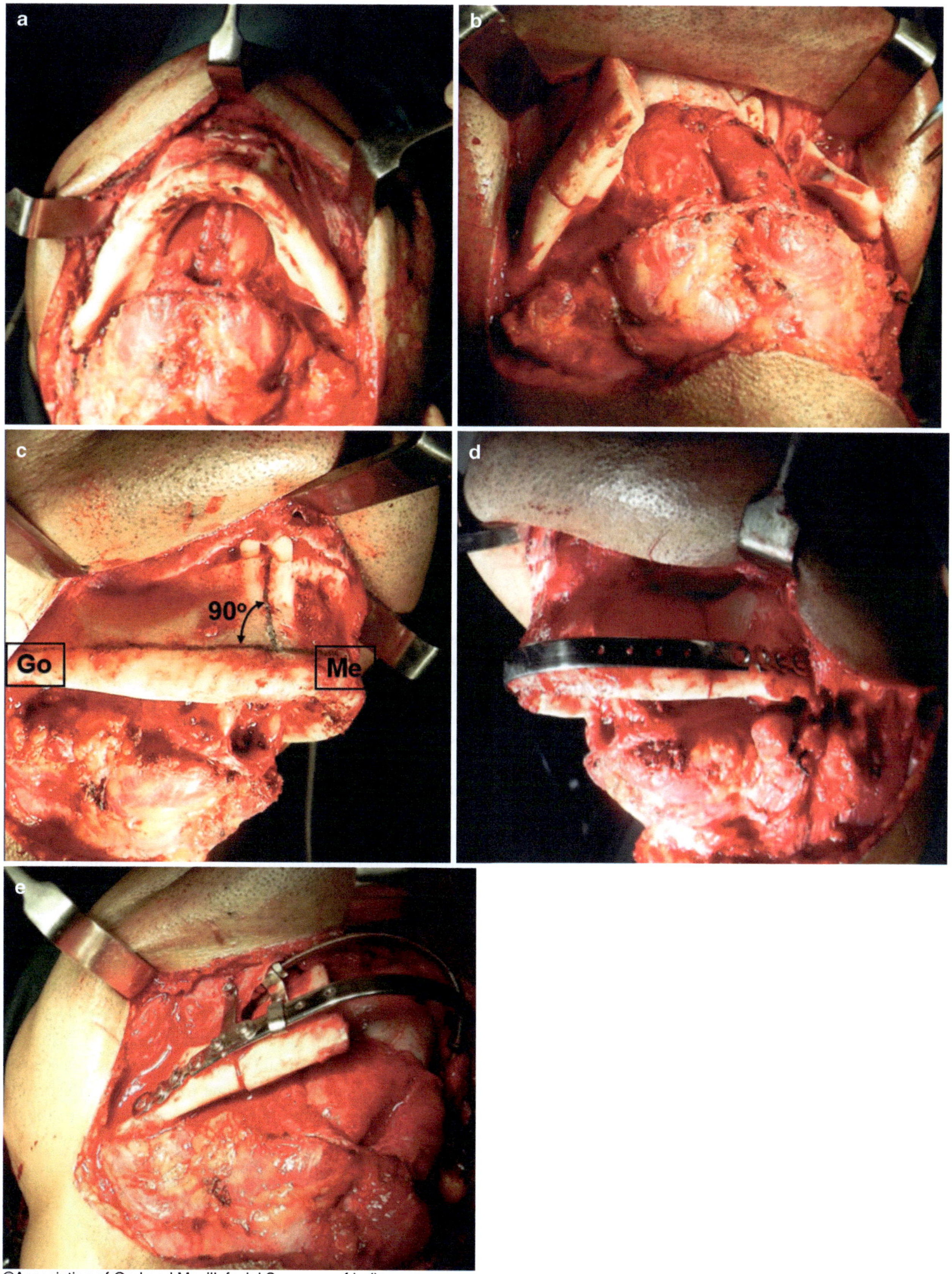

Fig. 87.16 (**a**) Incision extending bilaterally to expose the entire mandible inferiorly after layered dissection. (**b**) The lesion resected with clear margins of the preserved bone. The osteotomy should be kept parallel and free from the lesion. (**c**) Osteotomy cut perpendicular to an imaginary baseline that runs between Go and Me and parallel to maxillary occlusal plane. (**d**, **e**) Placement of fifth generation distractor

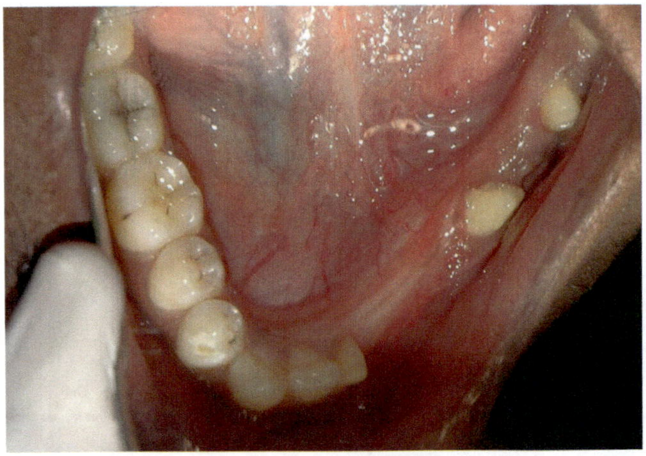

Fig. 87.17 Clinical appearance of regenerate of patient from Fig. 87.16

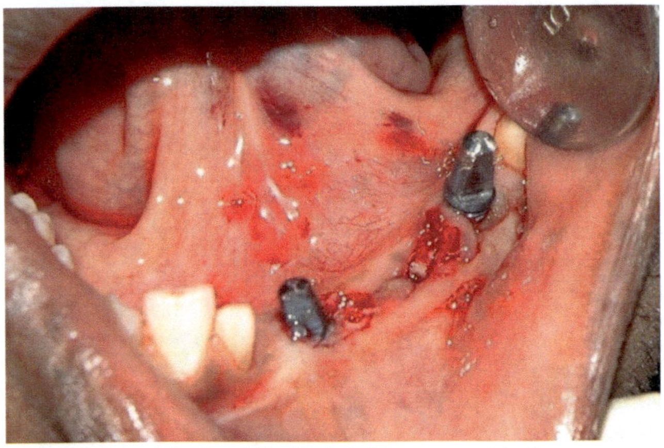

Fig. 87.18 Implants placed on the regenerated bone after 1 year of the same patient from Fig. 87.16

TDO. These radiographs have their limitation of 2D view of the mutivectorial 3D procedure.

Multi-slice-computed tomographic scans provide a better preview but have the limitation of excessive radiation exposure and scatter due to the distraction device when it is in situ. Elsalanty et al. have extensively experimented on cone-beam CT densitometry and three-dimensional histomorphometry in mandibular bone defects reconstructed with bone transport and found that the physical dimensions and architectural parameters of the new bone regenerated remain comparable to the contralateral normal bone in TDO [3]. In their study, the radiographic density comparison was done

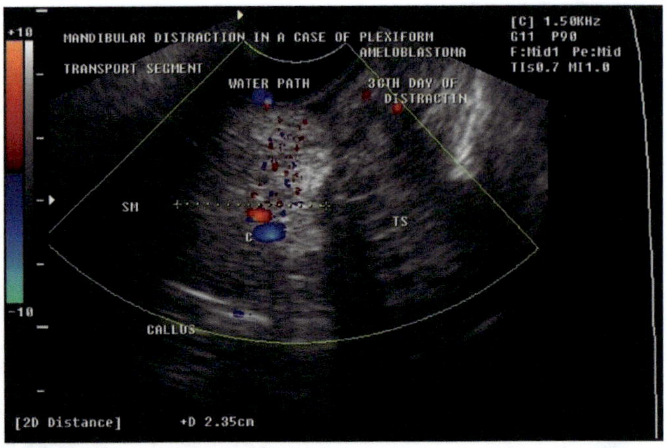

Fig. 87.19 Ultrasound appearance of regenerate

by studying the radiographic attenuation of the regenerate measuring in Hounsfield units (HU) and comparing it to the outer, inner, and inferior cortices of the bone on opposite side of the mandible (normal bone). Their results showed that the density of the distraction regenerate was comparable to the inner and outer cortices of the control bone, whereas the lower border of the control side of the mandible showed higher density than the regenerate at 1 month of consolidation. The Hounsfield unit value of the regenerate by TDO was toward the 2000 mark (2000 HU) after a month of consolidation. Microcomputed tomography-based three-dimensional histomorphometry used to assess percentage of bone volume, bone mineral density, degree of anisotropy, trabecular thickness, trabecular number, trabecular pattern factor, and trabecular separation showed no significant differences between the regenerate and the normal bone after a month of consolidation in all parameters except percent bone volume and the trabecular separation. Percentage bone volume is reported to be significantly less, while trabecular separation is significantly higher in the regenerate (Fig. 87.22a, b).

Garcia et al. studied the histology of the regenerate and docking site in bone transport in the tibial-diaphyseal defect of adult sheep model and concluded that there is a marked difference between the ossification of the docking site and of the regenerate. Intramembranous ossification plays a major role in the regenerate, with bone forming from the host bone segment to the target segment. The ossification of the docking site shows endochondral and intramembranous ossification simultaneously, but the intramembranous ossification is limited to rare and small foci [4].

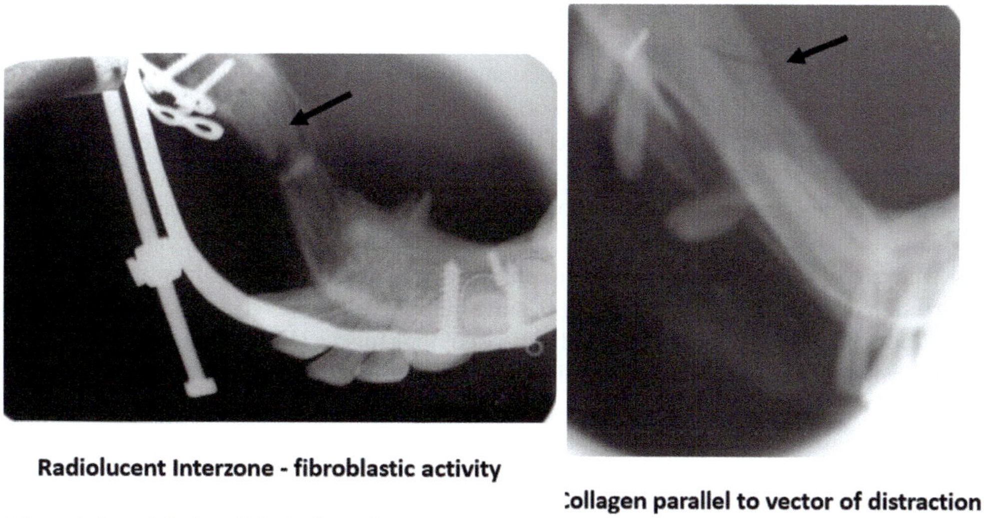

Fig. 87.20 Radiological appearance of regenerate during active distraction

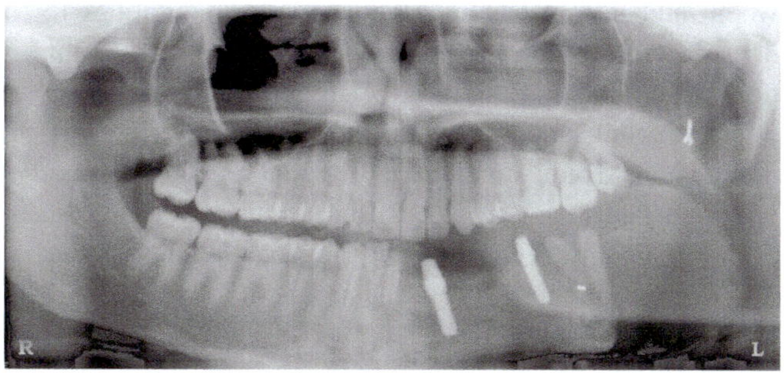

Fig. 87.21 Osseointegrated dental implants in the regenerated bone

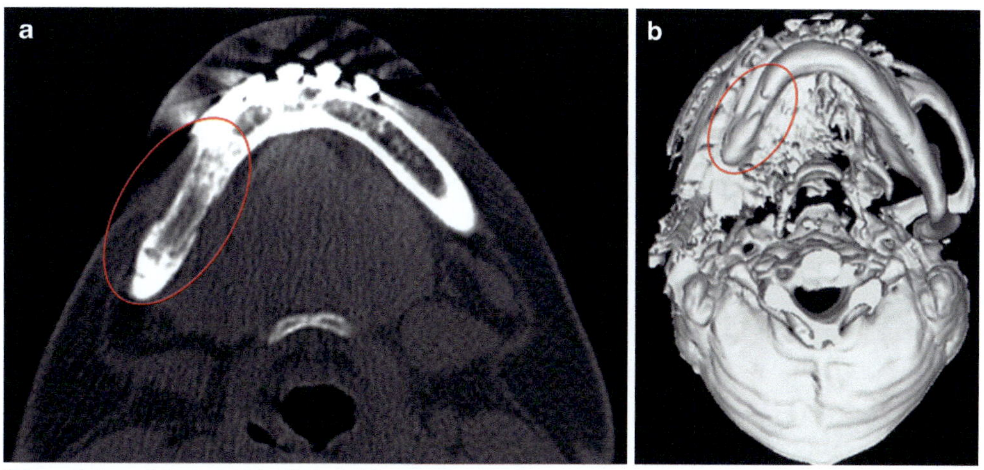

Fig. 87.22 (**a**, **b**) CT appearance of regenerate

Studies done on the architecture and microstructure of cortical bone regenerated with TDO, it has been found that at 12 weeks of consolidation, bone created during bone transport distraction osteogenesis was comparable to native bone in microstructure, architecture, and mechanical properties, and when appropriate time has lapsed, the properties of the regenerate bone were identical to the host bone.

Çakır-Özkan et al. in their study on immunohistochemical analysis of reconstructed sheep mandibles by transport distraction osteogenesis reported strong positive staining for BMP-2, -4, and TGF-β in the cells, and matrix components. These growth factors are believed to enhance the osteogenesis in TDO [5].

87.13 Transport Distraction Osteogenesis in Maxilla

Ever since the concept of transport distraction on long bone was initiated by Ilizarov and then after it was subsequently introduced on the facial skeleton by Constantino, Fodotov, Wolford, and many others, a lot of articles got published in the world literature affirming the possibility of regenerating quality bone for any length of mandibular defects [6]. It has even become a gold standard in comparison to other modalities of reconstruction. So, the question arises whether transport distraction has a role in maxillary reconstruction. [7, 8]

Cheung et al. were the first to publish their work on reconstruction of a maxillectomy defect using transport DO in animal experimental model [9]. Our contention is that when transport distraction has become an accepted norm in the reconstruction of mandibular continuity defects, maxilla with its multiple vascular perfusion, rich periosteal supply, and increased cancellous bone is expected to biologically respond even better to the distraction force [10].

Here are a few cases showing our evolution in transport distraction osteogenesis for reconstruction of maxillary defects.

In our maiden clinical attempt at reconstructing a maxillary defect using TDO a straight distraction device was used. The limitation we had with straight bar device was that they were all buccally directed and not conforming to the posterior maxillary arch (Fig. 87.23a, b, c, d, e, f). Subsequently we have successfully employed bifocal transport distraction (Fig. 87.24a, b, c, d, e, f, g, h, i) and trifocal transport distraction (Fig. 87.25a, b, c, d, e, f, g, h) for reconstruction of maxillary defects. Maxillary TDO has also been successful to treat alveolar clefts of maxilla (Fig. 87.26a, b, c, d, e, f, g).

87.14 Advantages of TDO

Though bone transport may not be possible in all situations, when indicated, it has an edge over other modalities for it doesn't require any specialized hands or equipment, it doesn't prolong the duration of surgery and hence is cost-effective. Since no bone grafting is required, there is no donor site morbidity, and there is recreation of alveolar ridge with attached mucosa, buccal, and lingual sulci, all in near normal anatomy. TDO not only regenerates new bone but also every element of soft tissue around it as well. These are summarized in Table 87.2.

87.15 Complications of Bone Transport

The complications with bone transport in regenerating new bone formation can be discussed under biological and mechanical factors.

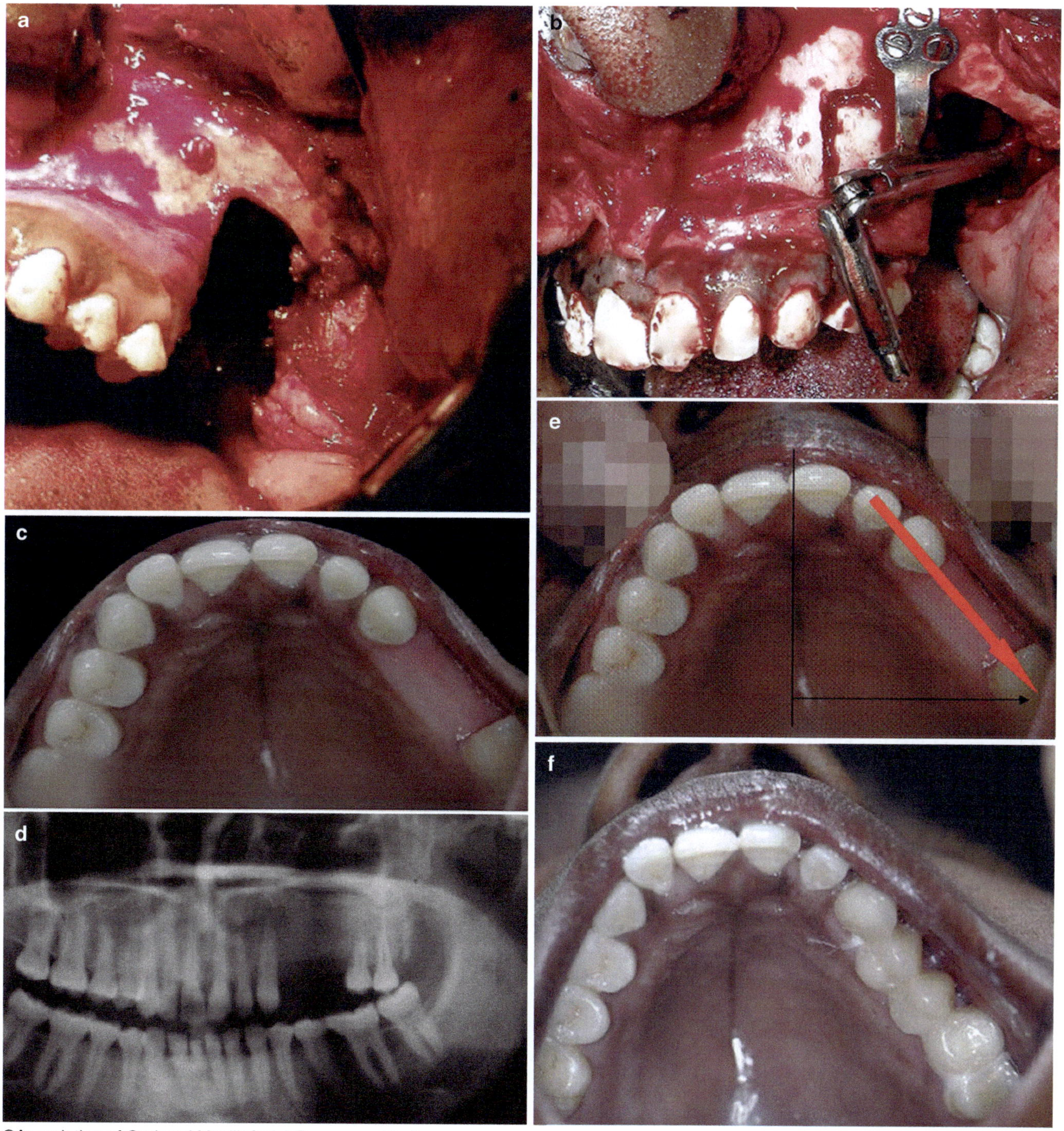

Fig. 87.23 (**a**) Straight transport distraction device post-resection defect. (**b**) Transport disc with device. (**c**, **d**) Evidence of histogenesis and osteogenesis in the clinical picture and OPG respectively, after consolidation phase. (**e**) Buccal deviation of the regenerate. (**f**) Rehabilitation with FPD

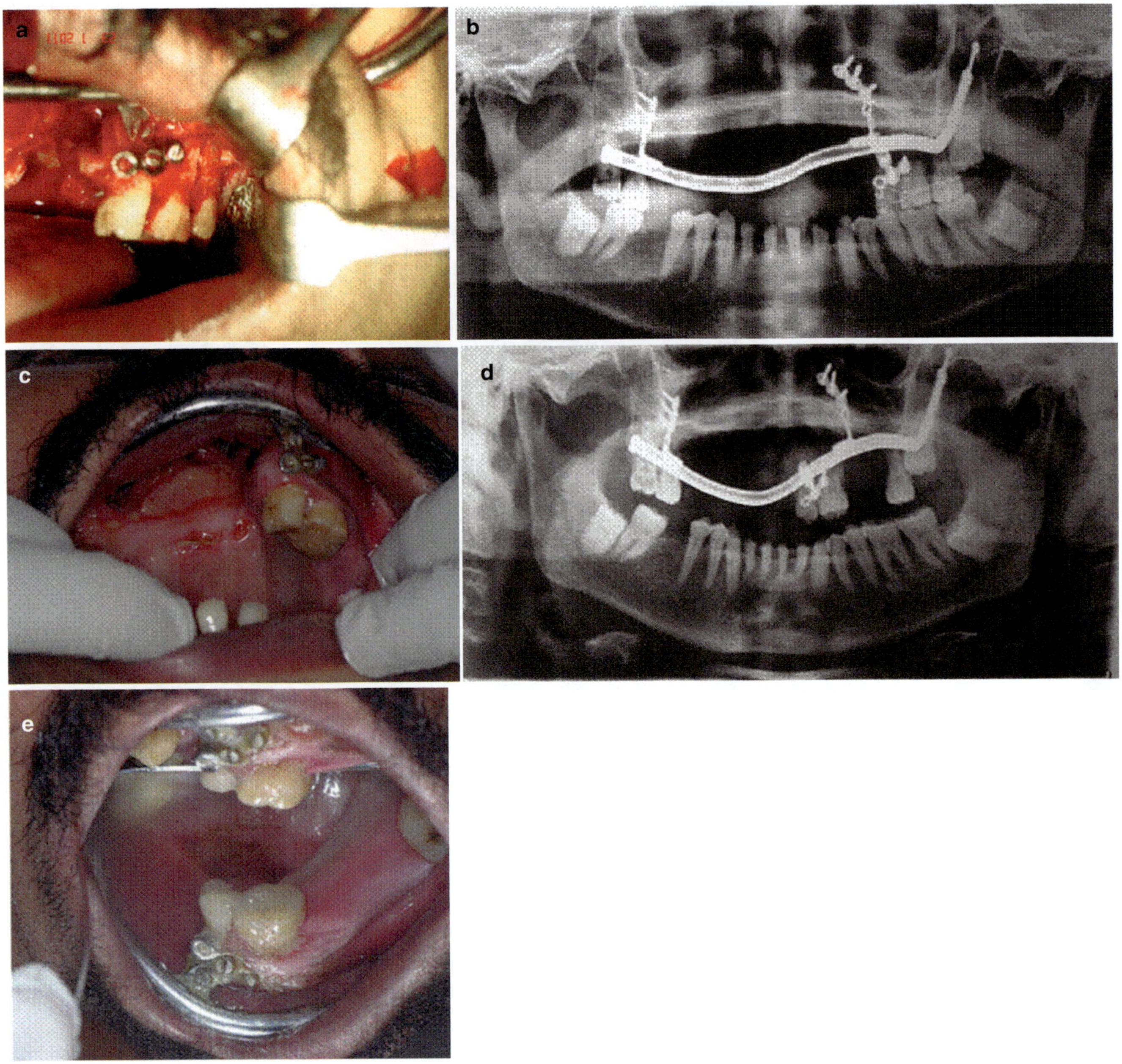

Fig. 87.24 (**a**) Arched bifocal regeneration with push ball device. (**b**) Bifocal push ball device in situ—latency period. (**c**, **d**) Transport distraction in progress on same side. (**e**) Transport distraction in progress across midline. (**f**, **g**) Transport disc on docking and consolidation. (**h**, **i**) Post-consolidation and rehabilitation with complete denture

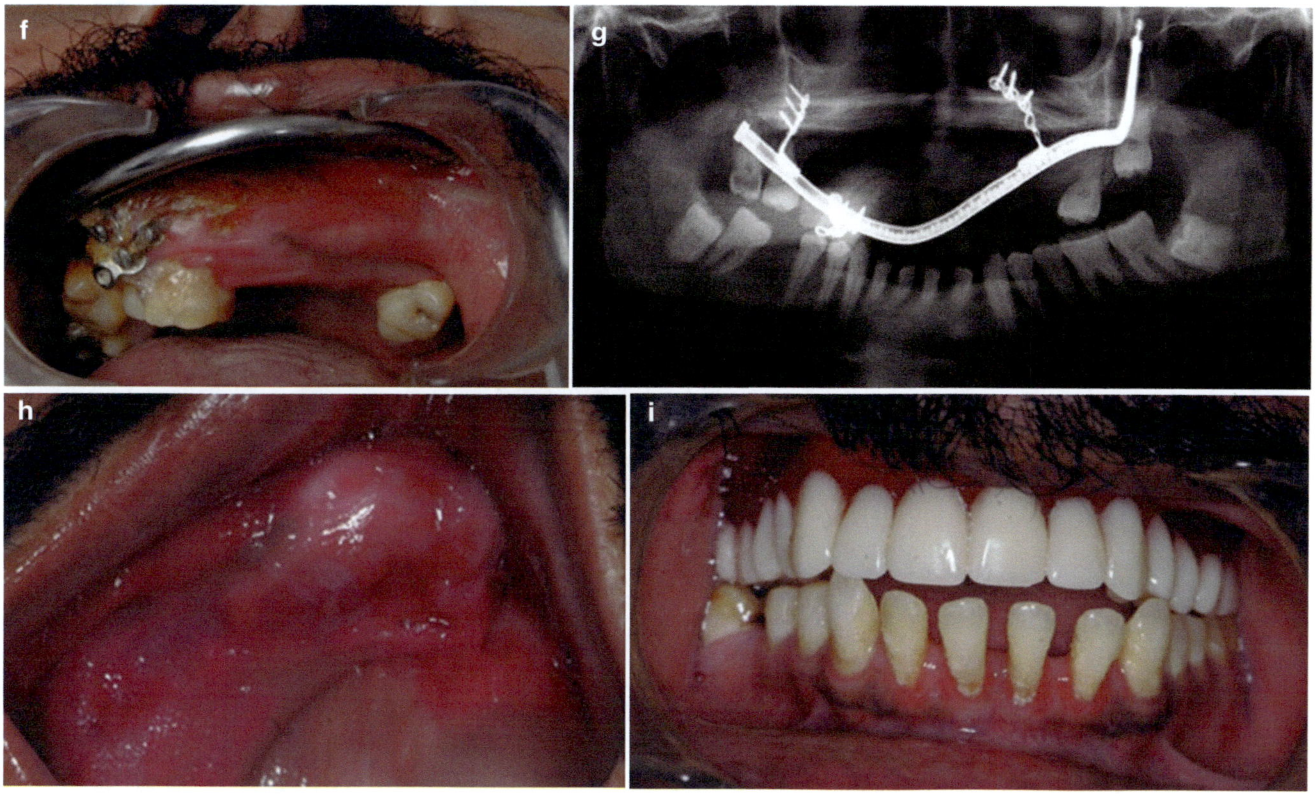

Fig. 87.24 (continued)

The biological factors are the ones which we have very little control over, whereas the mechanical factors of vector control and bodily movement of transport segment across the midline can be successfully carried out by modifying the device (Table 87.3) [11, 12].

87.15.1 Hypertrophic Regenerate

This occurs when a single transport segment is designed to regenerate a lengthy defect, when the collagen fibers are overstretched with the central portion of the callus narrowing representing an hourglass appearance in the radiograph (Fig. 87.27). This phenomenon can also occur when the cross-sectional thickness of the transport segment is not adequate to recreate good volume of bone.

87.15.2 Drifting of Teeth

The teeth in the transport segment and RHBS tend to drift as distraction proceeds due to pull of transseptal fibers across the line of osteotomy. This problem could be overcome by applying a figure of eight wire to stabilize the teeth in each segment (Fig. 87.28a, b, c).

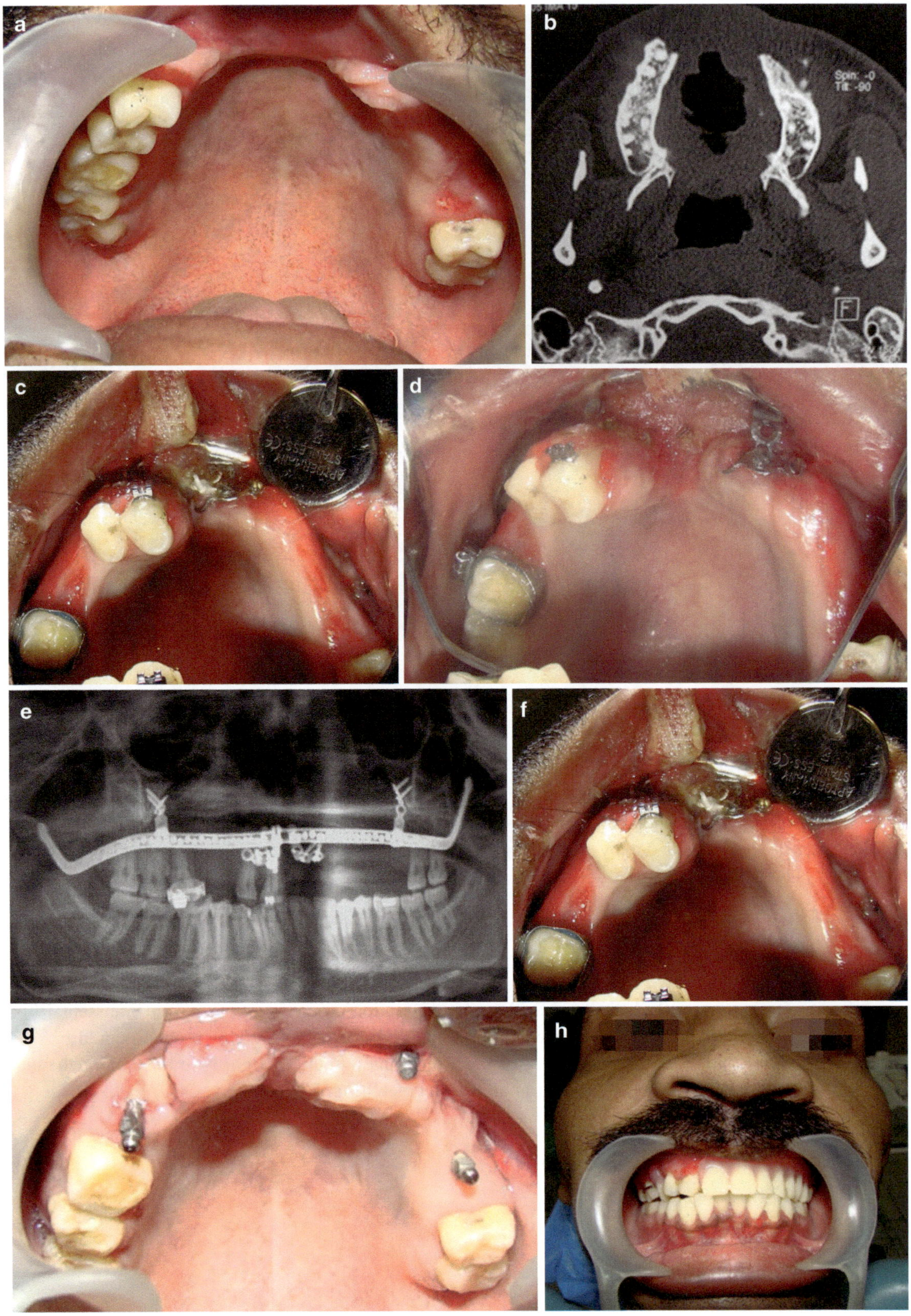

Fig. 87.25 (**a**) A case of continuity defect across midline following gunshot injury in a soldier. (**b**) CT image of case in 25 a. (**c, d**) Trifocal distraction in progress. (**e**) OPG view showing the trifocal distraction in progress. (**f**) Transport on docking and consolidation. (**g**, **h**) Dental rehabilitation using implants post-consolidation

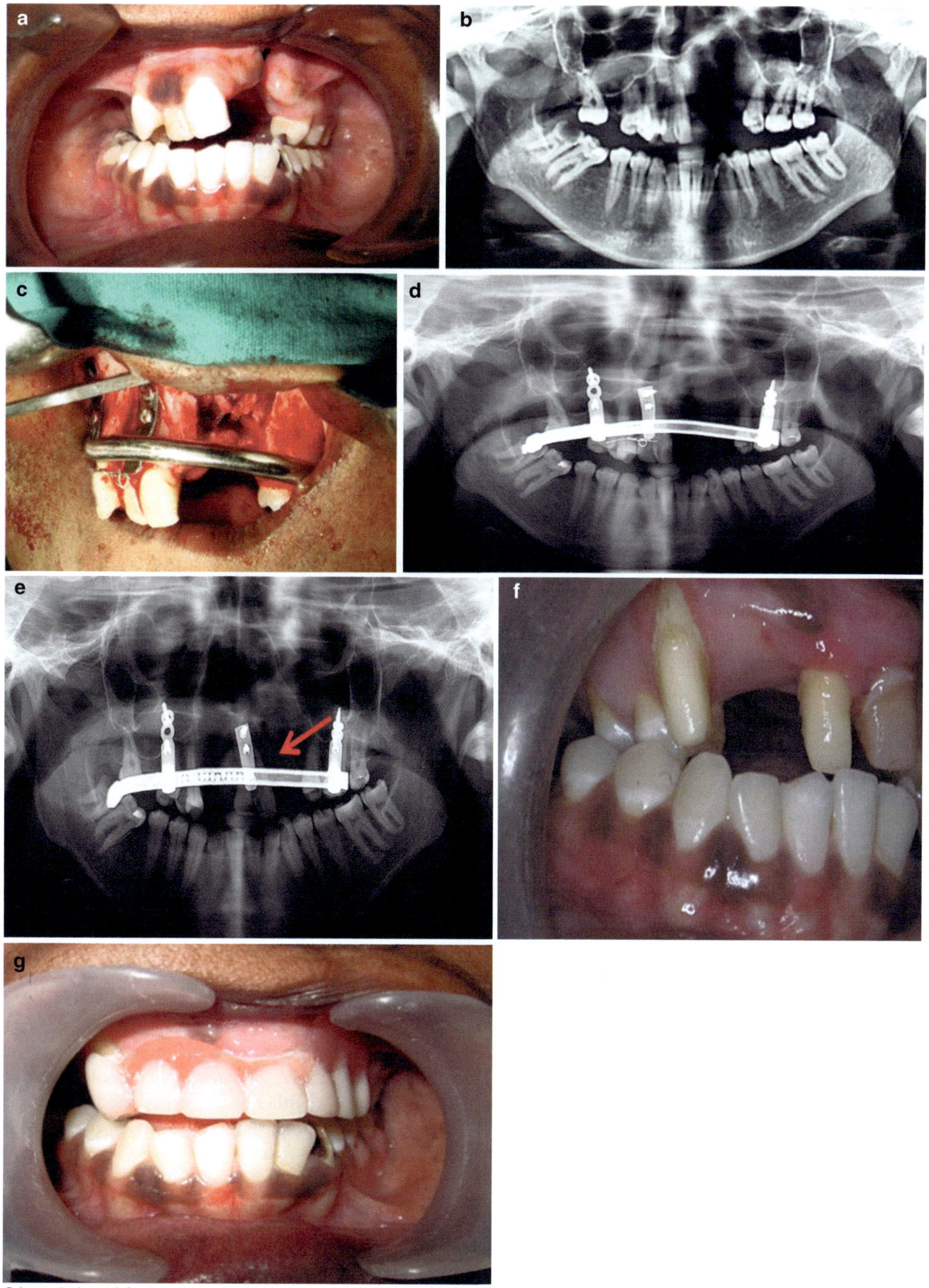

Fig. 87.26 (**a**, **b**) A case of maxillary cleft alveolus. (**c**, **d**) Latency period of 5 days. (**e**) Docking of the transport disk on eighth post-op day. (**f**, **g**) Post-consolidation phase rehabilitation

Table 87.3 Complications of TDO

Biological complications of TDO
• Hypotrophic regenerate. • Drifting of teeth. • Relapse. • Straight regeneration across midline.
Mechanical complications of TDO

• Misdirected vector.
  – Sagittal deviation.
  – Coronal deviation.
• Midline consolidation.

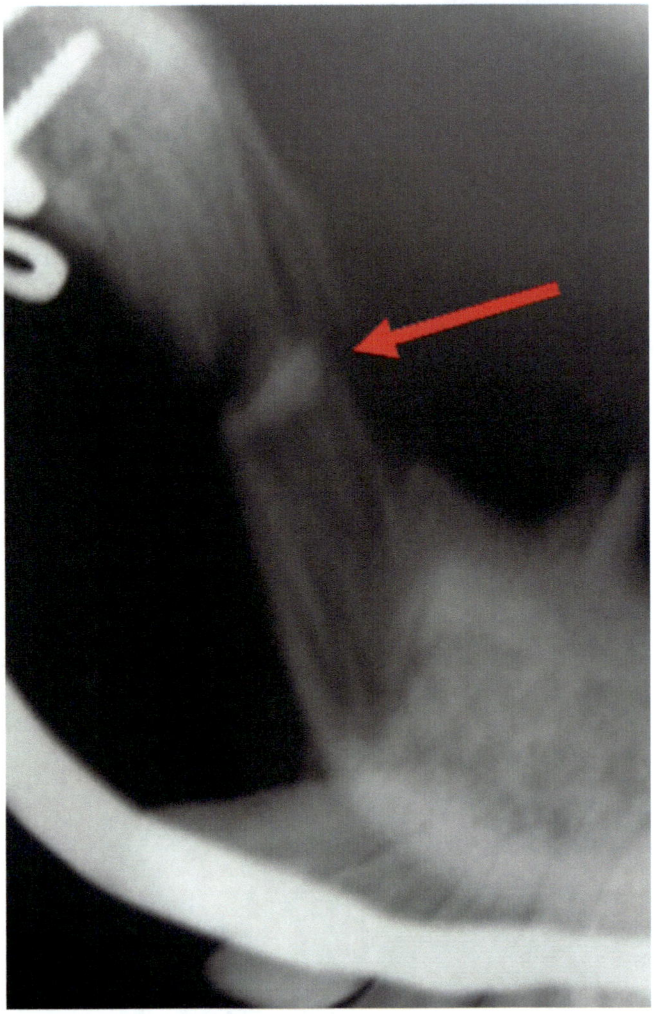

Fig. 87.27 Hourglass deformity

87.15.3 Relapse

Relapse of the new bone regenerate can occur resulting in contracture of the regenerate that could be avoided either by using an acrylic space maintainer or by placing a fixed partial denture immediately after the intended length of bone regenerate is formed across abutment teeth on either segment. It is a wise practice to retain the teeth in the transport disc for this purpose.

87.15.4 Straight Regeneration

Straight regeneration occurs while transporting the disc across the midline because the collagen fibers does not follow arc architecture of the defect in the midline; instead they get stretched in a straight direction, similar to an elastic band (Fig. 87.29a, b).

Misdirected vector in sagittal and coronal plane can occur when the guidance rod is not kept parallel to the occlusal plane. When such misdirection takes place, it can be allowed to proceed in the same vector until the intended length of bone regenerate is achieved, which could be corrected by callus molding before consolidation of the regenerate. The callus is molded by the rate and rhythm of the distraction and plating is done to achieve stability of the device. IMF is done to keep the occlusion intact on the contralateral side (Fig. 87.30a, b, c, d, e, f).

87.15.5 Midline Consolidation

The major limitation that we have with this modality of reconstruction is midline consolidation in both mandible and maxilla with arched regeneration. The transport segment freezes by the time it reaches a point lateral to midline on the opposite side. The concept of midline consolidation is that as the distraction proceeds beyond canine across the midline, the buccal cortex of the transport segment expresses greater movement than the lingual cortex for the same degree of rotation, as with the long and short arm of a clock suggesting lingual cortical tipping movement less than the required 1 mm per day. This results in lingual consolidation. This can be overcome by further re-distracting the transport segment after performing a lingual cortical osteotomy alone (Fig. 87.31a, b, c, d, e).

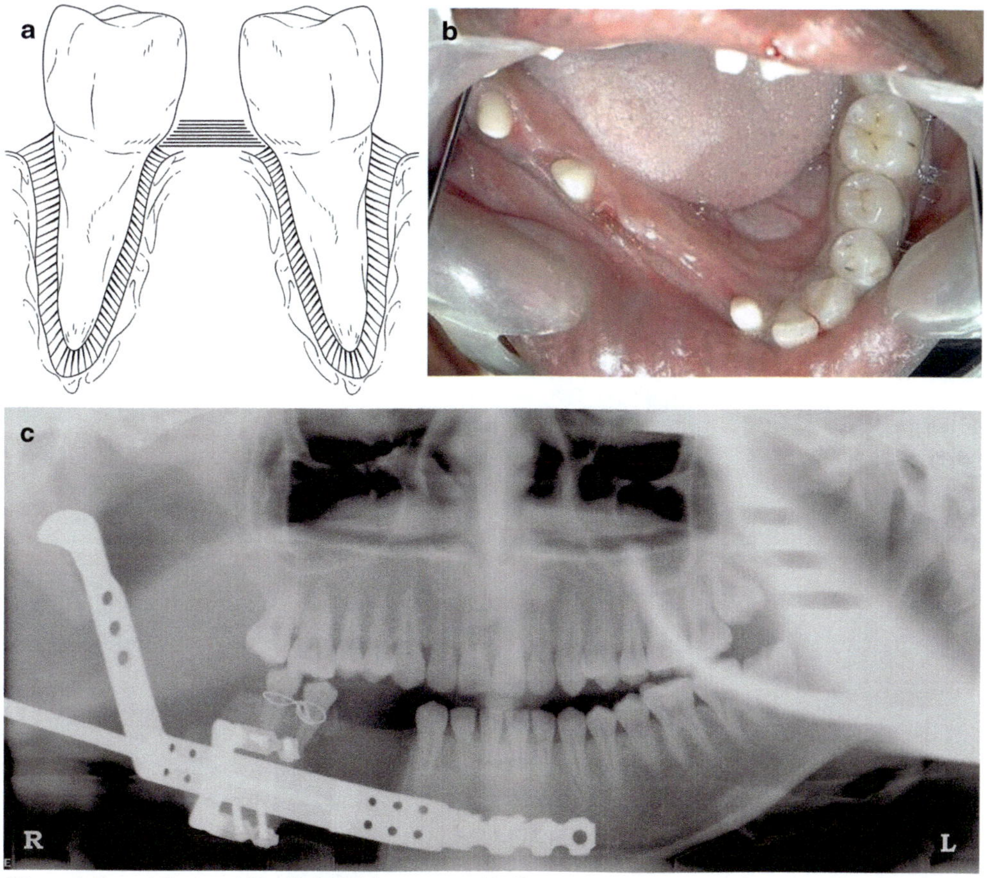

Fig. 87.28 (**a**) Pull of the transseptal fibers. (**b**) Drifting of teeth. (**c**) Figure of 8 wiring

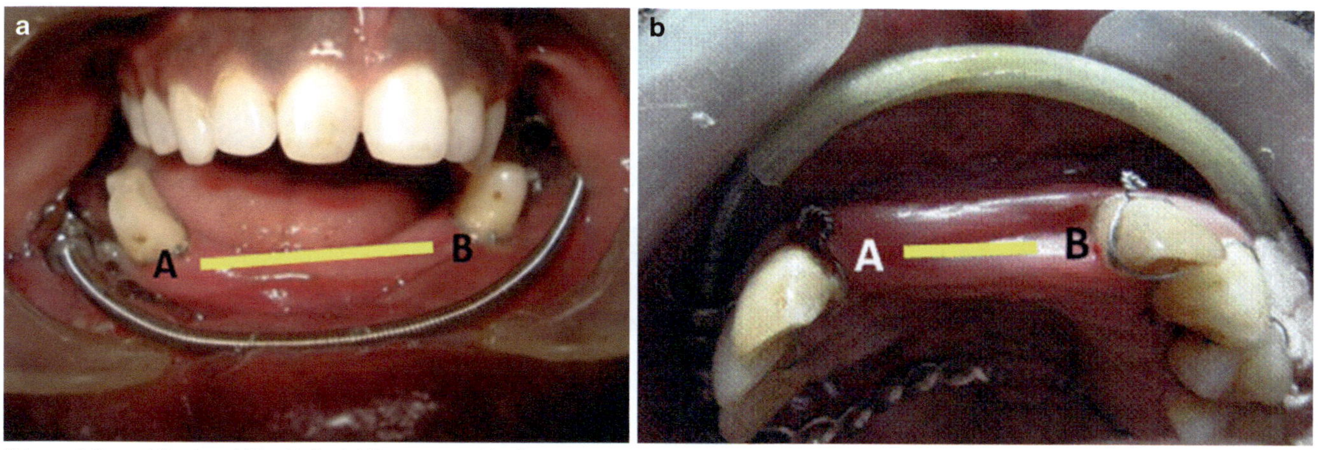

Fig. 87.29 (**a**, **b**) Straight regeneration not conforming the arch form in mandible and maxilla

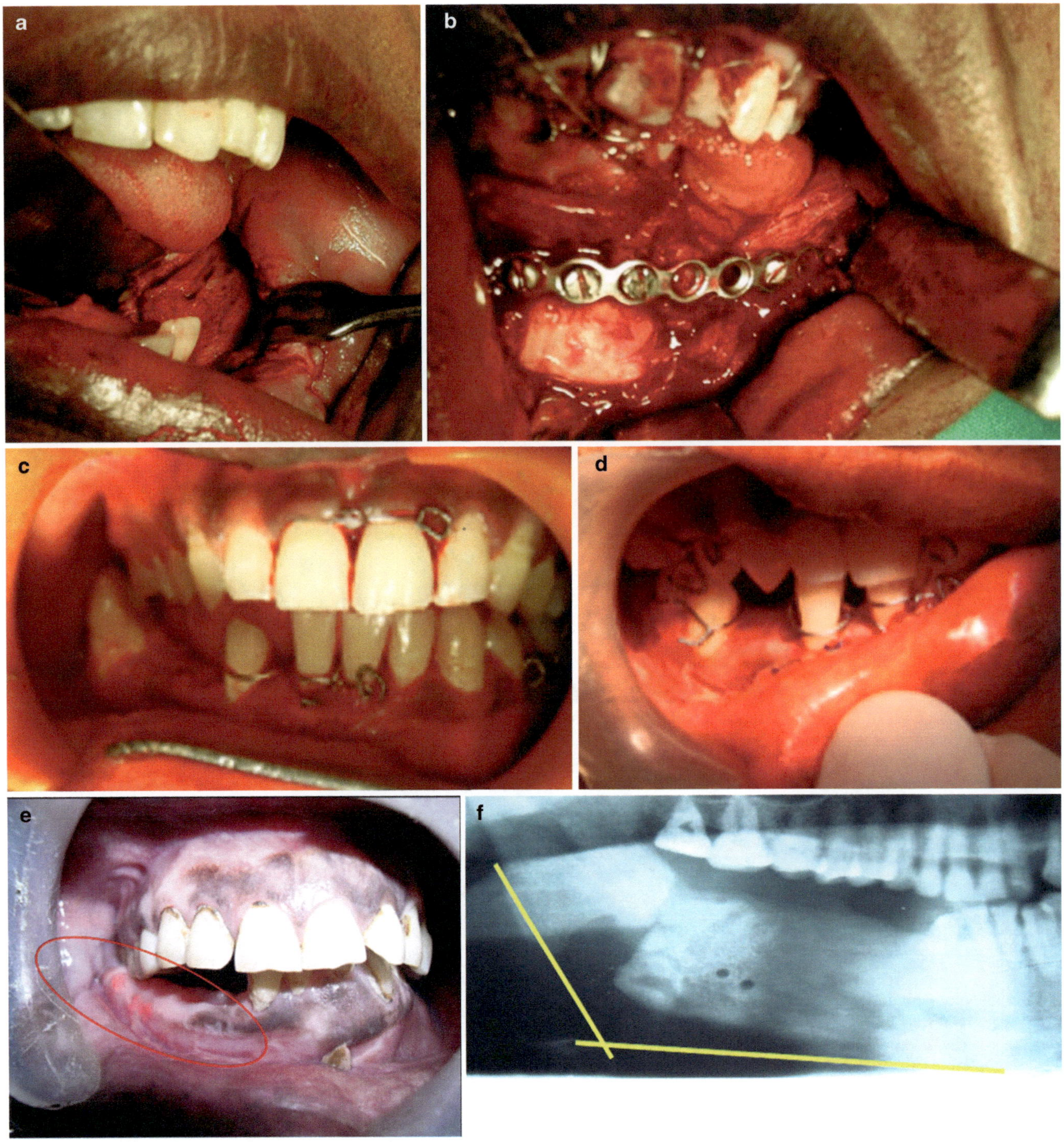

Fig. 87.30 (**a**, **b**) Callous molding and plating done for lingual deviation. (**c**, **d**) Callous molding and IMF done for buccal deviation. (**e**, **f**) Coronal deviation

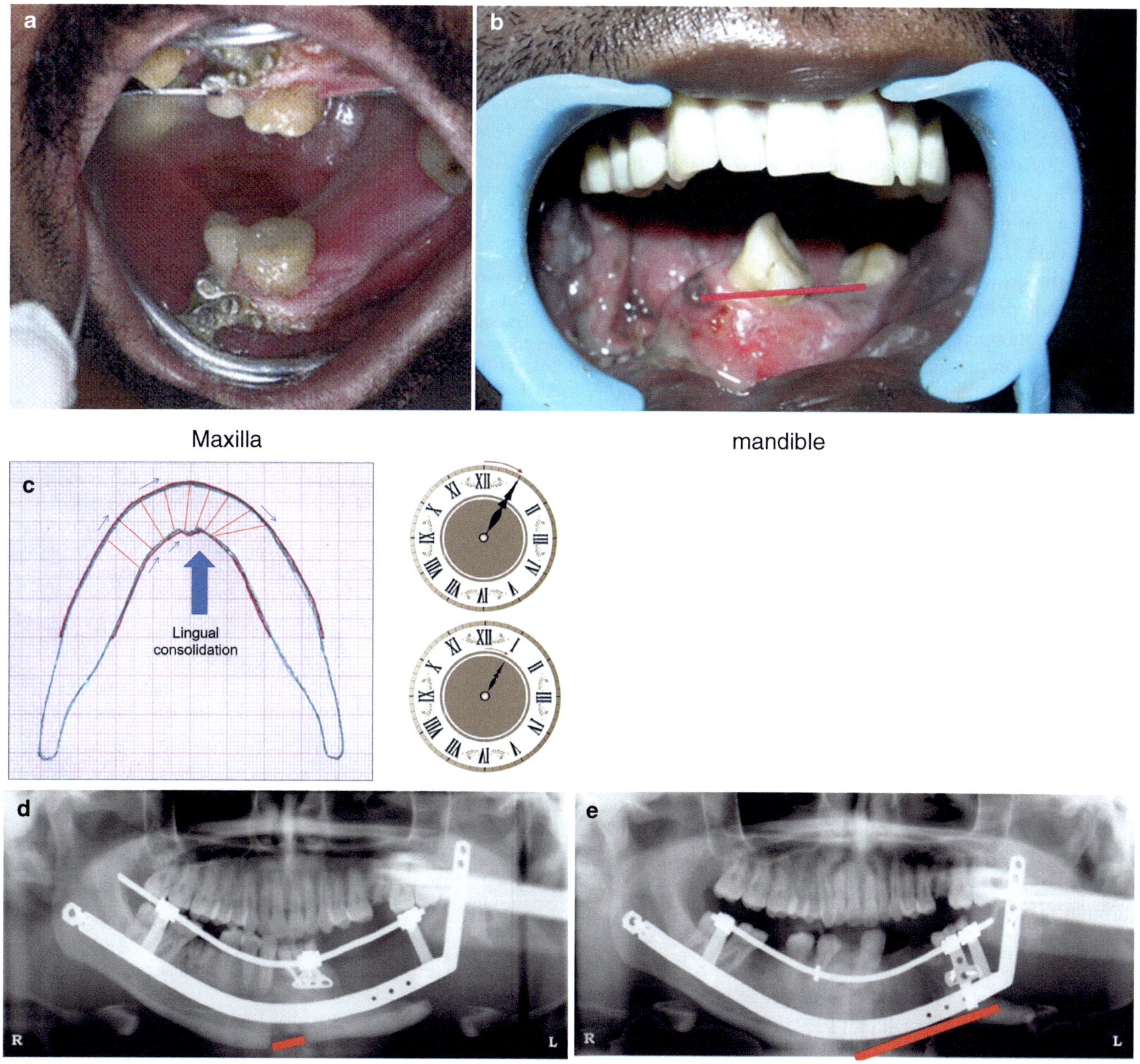

Fig. 87.31 (**a**) Midline consolidation in maxilla (**b**) mandible. (**c**) Lingual consolidation as a result of lingual cortical tipping movement less than the required 1 mm per day (left) similar to the long and short hands of a clock. (**d**) Lingual consolidation (*red line indicates the site where callus will be formed after distraction*). (**e**) Re-distraction after lingual cortical osteotomy (*red line indicates the site where callus will be formed after distraction*)

87.16 Role of Exogenous Growth Factors and Platelet-Rich Plasma (PRP) in TDO

Studies have highlighted that the transforming growth factor-beta, basic fibroblast growth factor, and insulin-like growth factor I are the chief upregulated factors during TDO. These factors are present in the bony matrix, in the cytoplasm of the cells, in osteoblasts, and in a few mesenchymal cells. Distraction at faster rate shows stronger presence of the growth factors but clinically a poor regenerate. An optimum distraction rate, presence of the growth factors, and strict adherence to the biomechanical principles of DO remains the key to successful clinical outcome. Currently, external administration of the exogenous growth factors remains controversial and is a subject of further research, with evidences both for and against it. It may be concluded that the optimum TGF-beta1 is present during the distraction phase in vivo and its exogenous administration may not be recommended based on the evidences from future research. Injection of platelet-rich plasma (PRP) is found to have more favorable clinical outcome to enhance bone healing during distraction osteogenesis. PRP releases platelet-derived growth factor and transforming factors (TGF-1 and TGF-2). Platelet-derived growth factors are the initial growth factors present in a wound and initiate connective tissue healing, bone regeneration, and repair. Platelet-derived growth factors are a cost-effective and safe alternative to enhance mineralization of the distraction chamber.

In our experience with bioregulators, limited to PRP, we have found that injecting PRP into the site of new bone regenerate chamber after achieving the desired length through TDO, we can reduce the time of consolidation phase by one-third compared to consolidation phase without PRP. PRP has proved to hasten the mineralization of the regenerate and we can achieve the quality of bone that is usually expected in 6 weeks without PRP in 2 weeks' time itself, thus reducing the duration of treatment [13].

87.17 Conclusion

As we understand, microvascular surgery is not restricted to a particular specialty and is a technique that can be mastered by any surgeons of any specialty. However, it requires a steep learning curve, whereas bone transport doesn't require any additional training or equipment. It involves only the routine plate bending and fixing. So, to conclude, distraction osteogenesis is a continually evolving field of research and study and an aesthetically and functionally acceptable option for managing extensive maxillomandibular defects and those not amenable to conventional methods. It is akin to "old wine in new bottle" especially brewed to the taste of oral and maxillofacial surgeons, for it is the only contemporary modality of reconstruction that we maxillofacial surgeons can master ourselves and also one that we can call with pride as "our own (Refer Figs. 65.14, 65.15, and 65.17 for TMJ ankylosis cases where distraction osteogenesis has been used as a part of the overall treatment plan)."

Acknowledgments Figures 87.1 (a, b, c), 87.2 (a, b), 87.15c, 87.19, 87.22(a, b), 87.28 (a, b, c) are from Neelakandan RS, Bhargava D. Transport distraction osteogenesis for maxillomandibular reconstruction: current concepts and applications. J Maxillofac Oral Surg. 2012;11(3):291–299. Springer, https://www.ncbi.nlm.nih.gov/pmc/articles/PMC3428445/.

Figure 87.23 (a, b, c, f) from Neelakandan RS, Mathew PC. Intraoral maxillary transport distraction: a casereport. J Oral Maxillofac Surg. 2009 Aug; 67(8):1751–5. PubMed PMID: 19615594. https://doi.org/10.1016/j.joms.2009.03.038. License Number 4613700616915. License date Jun 21, 2019. Licensed Content Publisher Elsevier.

Figure 87.25 (a, c, e) from https://www.ncbi.nlm.nih.gov/pmc/articles/PMC5328860/, https://doi.org/10.1007/s12663-015-0861-7; Rajkumar K, Neelakandan RS, Devadoss P, Bandyopadhyay TK. Reconstruction of a Post Traumatic Anterior Maxillary Defect by Transport Distraction Osteogenesis. J Maxillofac Oral Surg. 2017 Mar;16(1):118–122. Springer.

Figure 87.31 (d, e) from S. Neelakandan, R & Bhargava, Darpan. (2011). Transport distraction along the mandibular midline. International journal of stomatology and occlusion medicine. 4. 123–126. https://doi.org/10.1007/s12548-011-0018-3. (open access).

References

1. Neelakandan RS, Bhargava D. Transport distraction osteogenesis for Maxillomandibular reconstruction: current concepts and applications. J Maxillofac Oral Surg. 2012;11(3):291–9.
2. DeCoster TA, Simpson AH, Wood M, Li G. Biologic model of bone transport distraction osteogenesis and vascular response. J Orthop Res. 1999;17(2):238–45.
3. Kontogiorgos E, Elsalanty ME, Zapata U, Zakhary I, Nagy WW, Dechow PC, Opperman LA. Three-dimensional evaluation of mandibular bone regenerated by bone transport distraction osteogenesis. Calcif Tissue Int. 2011 Jul;89(1):43–52.
4. Garcia FL, Picado CH, Garcia SB. Histology of the regenerate and docking site in bone transport. Arch Orthop Trauma Surg. 2009;129(4):549–58.
5. Çakır-Özkan N, Eyibilen A, Özkan F, Gülbahar MY, Kabak YB. Immunohistochemicalanalysis of reconstructed sheep mandibles: transport distraction osteogenesis versus autogenous bone grafting. J Oral Maxillofac Surg 2011 Apr;69(4):1248–54.
6. Barber S, Carter L, Mannion C, Bates C. Distraction osteogenesis part 1: history and uses in the craniofacial region. Orthod Update. 2018;11(1):14.
7. Neelakandan RS, Mathew PC. Intraoral maxillary transport distraction: a case report. J Oral Maxillofac Surg. 2009;67(8):1751–5.
8. Rajkumar K, Neelakandan RS, Devadoss P, Bandyopadhyay TK. Reconstruction of a post traumatic anterior maxillary defect by transport distraction osteogenesis. J Maxillofac Oral Surg 2017 Mar;16(1):118–22.

9. Cheung LK, Zhang Q, et al. Reconstruction of maxillectomy defect by transport distraction osteogenesis. Int J Oral Maxillofac Surg. 2003;32(2):515–20.
10. Neelakandan RS, Bhargava D. Transport distraction along the mandibular midline: conceptual analysis. J Stomat Occ Med. 2011;4:123–6.
11. Synder CC, Levine GA, Swanson HM, et al. Mandibular lengthening by gradual distraction: preliminary report. Plast Reconstr Surg. 1973;51:516.
12. Ruhaimi KA. Comparison of different distraction rates in mandible: an experimental investigation. Int J Oral Maxillofac Surg. 2001;30(1):216–20.
13. Chin M, Toth BA. Distraction osteogenesis in maxillofacial surgery using internal devices. Review of five cases. J Oral Maxillofac Surg. 1996;54:45–54.

Hard Tissue Reconstruction of the Maxillofacial Region

88

Srinivasa R. Chandra and Vijay Pillai

Abbreviations

ACS	acellular collagen sponge
BFGF	basic fibroblast growth factor
BMP	bone morphogenic protein
IGF-1,2	insulin-derived growth factor 1,2
PDGF	platelet derived growth factor
rh BMP-2	recombinant human bone morphogenic protein-2
TGF-β	transforming growth factor beta

88.1 Introduction

The maxillofacial skeleton can be visualised as a three-dimensional structure, and its integrity is essential for neurovisceral function like vision, airway conduction, nutritional luminal support, etc. The location and the size of the defect determine the hard tissue reconstruction and the donor site selection.

88.2 General Principles [1]

- The bone graft recipient site should have viable vascular and infection free environment.
- Adequate evaluation of the donor site morbidity has to be undertaken.
- Evaluation for vascular versus nonvascularized bone graft has to be done with adequate immobilization and if required vascular anastomosis.
- Comorbidities of the patient and surgical appropriateness have to be prioritized. Smoking, cicatrization, radiation, pain issues and functional status are considerations as well.

88.3 Principles of Reconstruction

- Age is a factor but not a contraindication for reconstruction.
- There is no 'ideal reconstruction' but there is 'optimal reconstruction'.
- Patient comorbidities and future adjuvant radiation should be strongly weighed.
- 'Like to like tissue' reconstruction especially hard tissue substitution is optimal.

88.4 Terminology

Autograft: Transplant between areas within the same individual.
Allograft: Transplant between individuals (same species).
Xenograft: Transplant between individuals of different species.
Isograft: Transplant between monozygotic twins.

Osteoconduction is the phenomenon of bone regeneration which needs a scaffold for ingrowth of capillaries, osteoprogenitor cells and perivascular tissue. The ingrowth of capillaries from the recipient bed causes differentiation of the osteoprogenitor cells and results in the formation of new bone. There are materials which promote osteoconduction as

Electronic Supplementary Material The online version of this chapter (https://doi.org/10.1007/978-981-15-1346-6_88) contains supplementary material, which is available to authorized users.

S. R. Chandra (✉)
Department of Head and Neck Oncology and Reconstructive Microvascular and Oral and Maxillofacial Surgery, UNMC, Omaha, NE, USA

Nebraska Medicine Fred & Pamela Buffett Cancer Center, Omaha, NE, USA

V. Pillai
Department of Head and Neck Surgical Oncology, Mazumdar Shaw Cancer Center, Narayana Health, Bangalore, India

K. Bonanthaya et al. (eds.), *Oral and Maxillofacial Surgery for the Clinician*, https://doi.org/10.1007/978-981-15-1346-6_88

grafts or scaffolds. These can be autologous or alloplastic, homologous, xenogeneic bone particles, bone glass and hydroxyapatite ceramic material.

Osteogenesis is the spontaneous growth of new bone. It can either be *spontaneous* from progenitor cells in the area of the bone defect, or it could be *transplanted* osteogenesis arising from grafted progenitor cells.

Osteoinduction is auto induction by differentiation of mesenchymal cells from the native bed into osteoblastic tissue. This requires inductive stimulation, either from the grafted bone material (there is natural bone morphogenetic protein release with the resumption by osteoclastic activity on the middle matrix) or by the addition of recombinant bone morphogenic protein-2. This results in recruitment from the surrounding bed of mesenchymal cells, which then differentiate. This is mediated by graft-derived factors, viz. recombinant human bone morphogenic protein-2 (rhBMP-2), in situ BMP, TGF-ß, IGF-1 and IGF-2, BFGF, PDGF.

Clinical Pearls

Key concept in bone grafting which is a part of hard tissue reconstruction is the extent of ostial induction, ostial conduction and osteogenesis caused by the graft. The main tenet is that only autologous bone graft grafts can promote osteogenesis due to its volume of biocompetent viable cells. Allo- and xenografts do not have osteogenic potential.

88.5 Bone Grafts [2, 3]

88.5.1 Cortical vs Cancellous Grafts

Cancellous grafts revascularize more rapidly when compared to cortical grafts. For example, cranial bone revascularizes more rapidly than other cortical bone.

Mechanism of healing:

- Cancellous: Apposition and subsequent resorption.
  - Cancellous grafts repair more completely.
  - Cortical bone incompletely resorbed/remodelled
- Cortical: Resorption then apposition.

  50% reduction in strength at 6 weeks–6 months.

88.5.1.1 Considerations in Usage of rhBMP-2 [4]

In March 2007, the US Food and Drug Administration (FDA) approved the use of rhBMP-2 in maxillofacial surgical procedures for intraoral ridge augmentation.

Biologic concept—the mechanism is through osteoinduction by chemotactic osteoprogenitor cellular proliferation and differentiation causing osteoid maturation.

Technique—BMP is carried in the acellular collagen sponge (ACS) to the defect where the formed osteoid matures into an ossicle about 6 months after the cycle of resorption and remodelling. There are multiple case reports of allogenic freeze-dried, crushed cancellous bone with BMP and platelet-rich plasma used in large maxillofacial reconstructions. rhBMP-2 is a lyophilized powder mixed with prepackaged sterile water. Concentration of 1.5 mg/mL of rhBMP-2/ACS is advised. For molecular binding the mixture is kept soaked for 15 minutes. To prevent desiccation and protein loss, rhBMP/ACS mixture must be used within 2 hours. Informed consent, warning of swelling and tension-free closure are important considerations.

Indications: Approved by FDA—spinal fusions (2002), treating open tibial fractures (2004) and oral and maxillofacial sinus and ridge augmentations (2007).

Contraindications and precautions:

- Local health advisory or FDA issued black box warning.
- Pregnancy.
- History of malignancy.
- Active infection.
- Hypersensitivity to BMP or collagen matrix.
- Unknown evidence of safety in children and females of childbearing age.
- Proximity to airway due to severe oedema postoperatively.

88.5.2 Bone Graft Carriers and Fixation Techniques

- Mesh.
- Custom fabricated cribs, implants, plates, etc.
- Titanium plates and screws.
- Lag screws.
- Autologous or allogenic bone cribs (Fig. 88.1).

Autogenous Bone Donor Sources

The choice of donor site depends on:

(a) Quantity.
(b) Quality.
(c) Anatomical contour (height, weight, volume).
(d) Donor site morbidity.
(e) Patient and anatomical access to harvest.
(f) Type of carrier and fixation needed.
(g) Surgical competence.

Common Locations of Autogenous Bone Donor Sites

- Iliac crest (anterior and posterior).
- Costochondral rib graft.
- Cranial bone.
- Tibia.
- Scapula.
- Maxilla.
- Mandible.

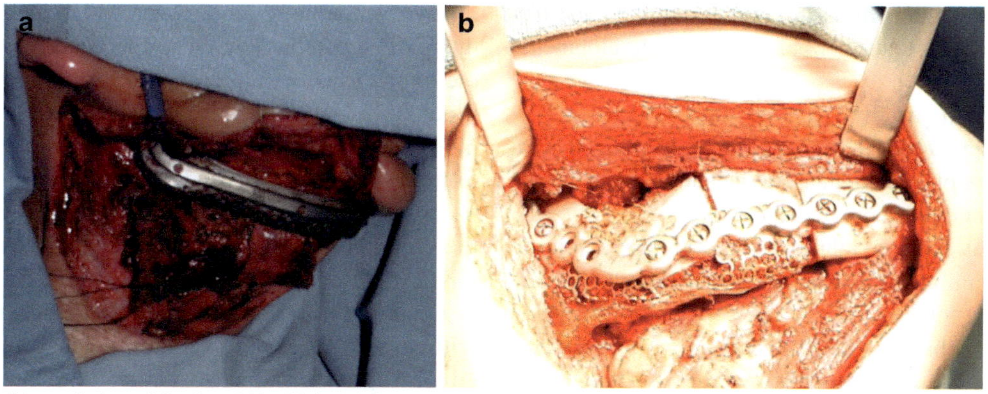

Fig. 88.1 Bone graft carriers and fixation techniques(**a**–**b**) custom made implants compared to stock prosthesis. (**a**) Custom-built bone graft carrier and plate as patient specific implant—note that this can be planned for optimal areas of fixation (anchoring the crib to the plate, the span and width of the screws, etc.). (**b**) The figure shows a reconstruction bar adapted with stock titanium mesh for carrying a non-vascularised iliac bone graf

88.5.3 Costochondral Graft

The costochondral rib graft came into vogue with the concept of transplanting a growth centre to the recipient site in reconstruction. This was initially used for temporomandibular joint arthroplasty and extended to the ramus condyle subunit, as it was a substitute for the growth centre at the condyle and was needed to maintain the growth potential of the joint.

88.5.3.1 Technique

A submammary incision is placed around the 5th–seventh rib, taking care not to extend beyond to avoid a flail segment. The incision is made in the mid-clavicular line, placed more medially if a costochondral graft is needed. It is deepened down to bone, and a circumferential subperiosteal dissection is done with a stripper. If the cartilage is harvested, a sleeve of periosteum is retained. Subperiosteal dissection is done avoiding pleural damage. Once the graft is removed, inspect the cavity with saline and check for any air leaks. A layered closure is performed with a drain.

88.5.3.2 Indications

Laryngotracheal reconstruction, nasal reconstruction, auricular reconstruction, facial augmentation in syndromic disorders.

Clinical Pearls

- Good cartilage yield.
- Superior strength.

Pitfalls

- Inferior pliability.
- High tendency for warpage.
- Subcostal scar, pneumothorax.

88.5.4 Autologous Rib Grafts

Rib grafts are a good source of corticocancellous membranous bone that can be used as onlay bone grafts for the craniofacial skeleton. Being soft and flexible, it is unable to withstand zones of high stress placement.

The harvest is similar to the costochondral graft; however, leaving the periosteum in situ would allow for regeneration of the rib but would reduce the take of the rib graft.

Pitfalls

- Subcostal scar.
- Pneumothorax.
- Atelectasis.
- Higher incidence of resorption if used as onlay grafts due to the higher cancellous component.

88.5.5 Iliac Crest

The ilium is a rich source for cortical, cancellous and a combination of corticocancellous bone grafts.

It is primarily utilized for arthrodesis, bony non-unions and alveolar clefts.

The anatomy of the ilium with the dense cortical bone permits grafts for high stress areas like the long bones and hands and also allows for rigid fixation. The outer table has numerous muscular attachments, thus is not preferred. The inner table is commonly harvested.

The iliac crest allows the harvest of large amounts of cancellous bone.

The cartilaginous apophysis in children must not be disturbed as it contributes to the normal growth and development.

88.5.5.1 Technique

The anterior approach is the most commonly utilized with the incision being placed after careful palpation to ensure the scar lies on the lateral aspect of the crest.

The incision is deepened through the skin, fascia, muscle and periosteum up to the bone. Ideally the inner or medial table is preferred for harvest as it does not cause disruption of the muscle attachments on the lateral side. The bone cuts should be placed preserving the crest so that it is hinged laterally and can be repositioned once the desired bone has been harvested. Maintaining the periosteal attachments of the crest would preserve its blood supply and further fixation would not be needed.

Good haemostasis, meticulous-layered closure with a drain in the subcutaneous tissue can help prevent a postoperative haematoma. It is also common practice to place an epidural catheter into the bed to permit infusion of a long acting local anaesthetic agent for the first 24 hours.

Most of the disadvantages of iliac bone harvest can be circumvent if the amount of bone graft needed is not too excessive by using the trephination technique.

Pitfalls

- Postoperative morbidity depending on the extent of bone harvested.
- Injury to the lateral femoral cutaneous nerve with prolonged post- surgical pain.
- Haematoma.
- Gait disturbances.

88.5.6 Tibia

88.5.6.1 Tibial Autogenous Cancellous Bone Harvest

This was first reported by Catone [5] in 1992 and is used in maxillofacial bone grafting techniques with a harvest volume of about 25–40 cc from a unilateral site. Harvest can be performed under local or general anaesthesia. The anatomical access to the tibial proximal head can be medial or lateral. Paediatric harvest has been reported, but the growth plate of the tibial plateau should be mature for adequate safety. The contraindications for tibial bone harvest cited are metal prostheses, athletes and history of knee trauma.

88.5.6.2 Technique

As mentioned the approach can be medial or lateral to the midline patellar tendon. In the lateral approach—Gerdy's tubercle is the bony prominence which is palpated between the midline patellar tendon and the lateral proximal head of the fibula. This bony prominence has the attachment of the iliotibial fascial tract. In the medial approach, there is no significant bony prominence, and the only overlying structures to the tibial proximal head are just skin and subcutaneous tissue. Accordingly, an incision on either side goes through the skin and subcutaneous tissue and a self-retaining retractor can be used for retraction.

Once the tibial head is identified, using a narrow drill with a postage stamp technique, a window is created either supra or subperiosteally. This cortex can be left attached to the periosteum and repositioned at the end of the harvest if cortical bone is not needed. Cancellous bone can be curetted with adequate care not to perforate the superior tibial plateau entering the knee joint. Adequate haemostasis with local cautery should be used to prevent any postoperative haematomas. Deep and superficial layer closures are performed. No immobilization is recommended, but active weight bearing is avoided for a couple of days. If there is any concern for superior tibial plateau perforation or knee joint violation, an orthopaedic review is mandated.

88.5.7 Cranial Bone [2]

It is well-known through craniofacial surgery that paediatric skull defects less than 1 cm with an intact pericranium can cause adequate bone healing with osseous regeneration. Calvarial bone grafts can be performed as mono- or bicortical harvest based on the surgeon's competence. Cortical bone shavings are commonly utilized. Just off the midline of the skull sagittal plane, parietal cortical calvarial bone is accessed through skin and the scalp layer incision. Adequate retraction is performed with a self-retaining retractor or assistance. The amount of bone needed is identified in the subperiosteal plane and marked with round bur of a narrow diameter. Adequate outer beveling is performed (as depicted in the figure) using a straight fissure bur for a flat osteotomy technique as parallel to the outer surface. Multiple fissuring osteotomies in a parallel fashion can be performed too. The intracortical medulla is carefully traversed through osteotomes and if any small dural perforations are made, they can be covered with artificial allografts or even haemostatic material. A neurosurgical review is needed in case of dural tear. Haemostasis with bone wax or electrocautery and good pericranial adjacent tissue rotational coverage and closure of the scalp layers leads to reduced postoperative haematomas. The bone harvested can be contoured with a crimping forceps as shown in the figure (Fig. 88.2a and b).

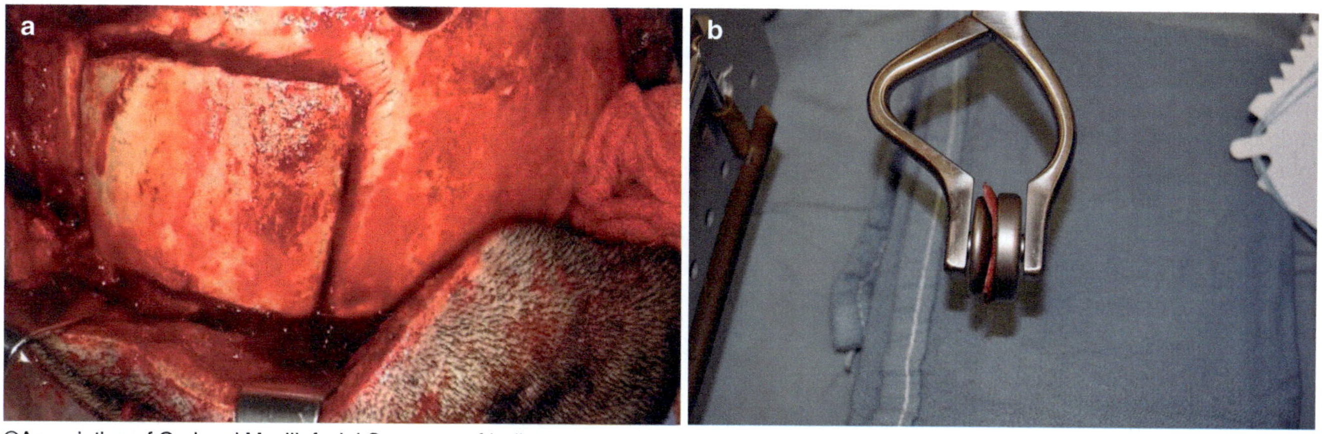

Fig. 88.2 (**a**) Cranial bone graft harvest with circumfrential trough and beveling. It is ideal to harvest this in the parietal area. Narrow strips are ideal for harvest. (**b**) Cranial non vascular bone graft being contoured with pinch forceps

88.6 Microvascular Free Tissue Transfer

Most hard tissue grafting using this technique is a 'composite' bone and soft tissue transfer by arteriovenous anastomosis. This transferred bone is usually held in place by plates and/or screws. There is osteogenesis at the interface of the native and grafted bone interface. Current techniques of vascular free tissue using microvascular anastomosis along with minimal donor site morbidity have a success rate close to 98 percent. There is a potential for failure due to anastomotic complication. The vascularized free transferred tissue is resistant to infection and radiation to a degree of volume. There are concepts of creating a vascular envelope and subsequent allogenic or xenogeneic grafting for better osteoconduction by vascular ingrowth.

88.6.1 Osteocutaneous Radial Forearm Free Flap (OCRFFF)

The popular workhorse fasciocutaneous radial forearm free flap is very well-known for most reconstructive surgeons. Whereas an osteocutaneous variant of this flap is not the 'go to' flap in composite reconstructions. There is significant donor site morbidity with about 70% postharvest strength and an increased fracture risk of the distal radius. Distal radius can be reinforced with a prophylactic plate by internal fixation. Figure 88.3 shows osteocutaneous radial forearm free flap for maxillary reconstruction including the orbital rim. Figure 88.4a and b shows radial forearm flap for reconstruction of maxillary and mandibular defects.

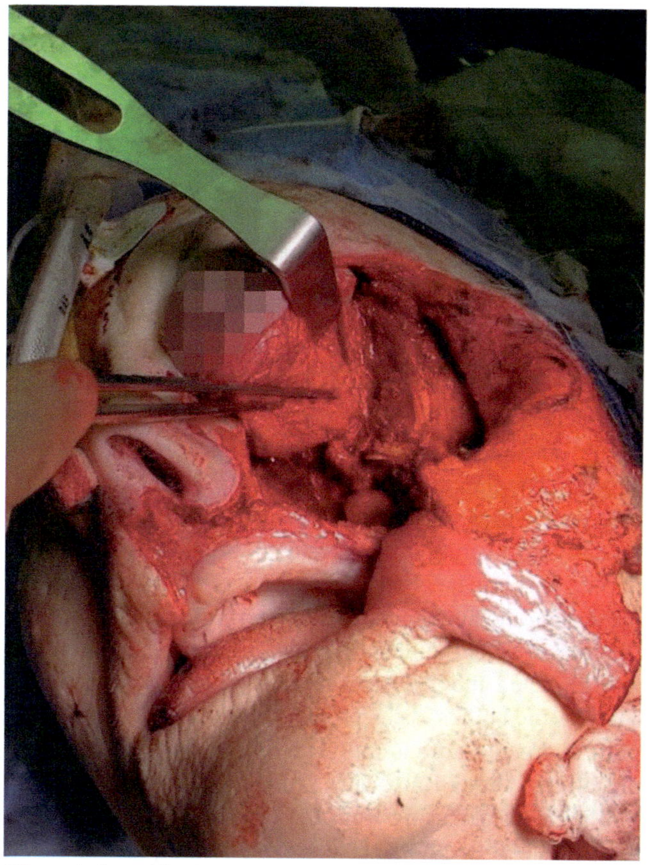

Fig. 88.3 Osteocutaneous radial forearm free flap for maxillary reconstruction including the orbital rim

88.6.1.1 Indications

Periorbital, nasal and maxillary subunit reconstructions are the common indications for an osteocutaneous radial forearm free flap. It is a real alternative if other donor sites are not viable.

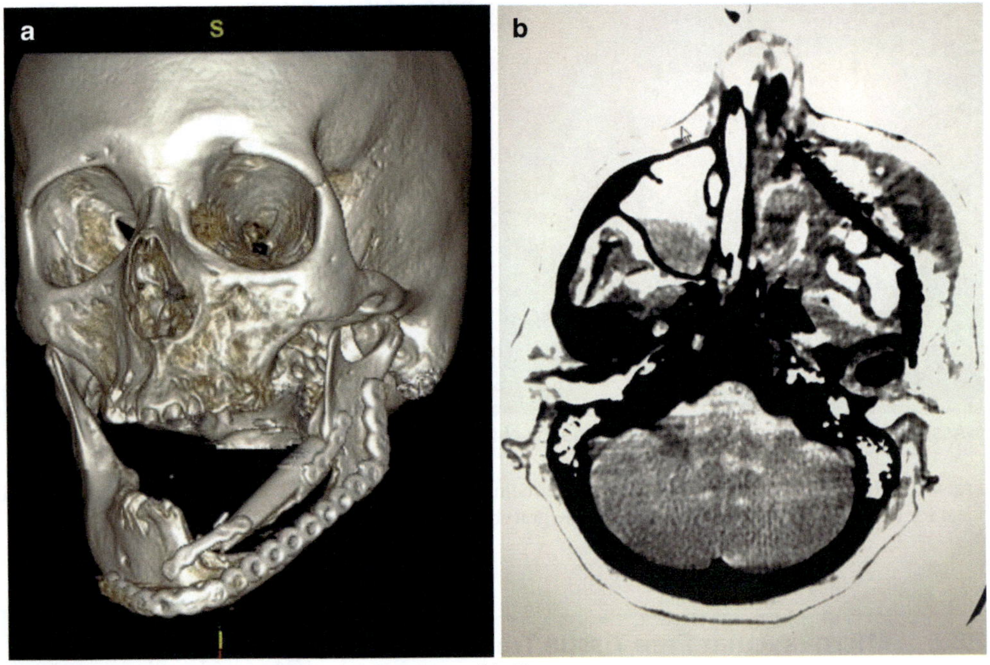

Fig. 88.4 (**a** and **b**) Radial osteocutaneous flap as an alternative in mandible (**a**, 3D rendering) and (**b**) maxillary reconstruction (left maxilla CT)

88.6.1.2 Technique

Surface markings of the soft tissue from the distal wrist skin crease as the horizontal line, the radial pedicle and the cephalic vein are outlined. The osseous part of the anterior lateral radius segment between the insertion of the pronator teres and the brachioradialis is harvested up to 10–13 cm in length and about 40 percent in circumference. The distal styloid aspect of the radius should have at least 2 cm to complete a bone plate fixation after the flap harvest. The fascial and muscular periosteal vascularity is retained in harvest. The flap can be raised from the radial or the ulnar side in a subfascial plane. The brachioradialis is retracted laterally protecting the superficial branch of the radial nerve. A sharp incision is made down to the periosteum preserving the attachment of the intermuscular septum. On the medial side, the flexor carpi radialis muscle is reached and retracted medially so the median nerve is protected. The muscle bellies of the pronator quadratus and the flexor pollicis longus are carefully dissected distal to proximal preserving enough muscular cuff to retain perforators to this segment perfusing from the radial artery in its lateral intermuscular septum. Once the radius periosteum is incised in length noting the curve of radius bone, multiple drill holes are used to outline the osteotomy. A boat-shaped harvest is completed of the cortex protecting the radial vasculature after distal ligation and the muscular perforators to the osseous part. The proximal harvest is completed of the pedicle similar to radial forearm harvest by radial artery and vena comitans ligation. A prebent compression plate is adapted and fixated using bicortical screws across the site of harvest (Fig. 88.5). Osteotomy scan be performed of this donor segment with close attention for orbital rim reconstruction if needed.

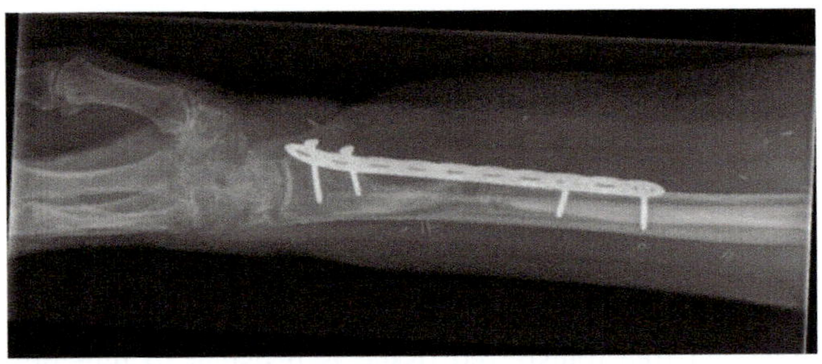

Fig. 88.5 Post-radial osteocutaneous flap harvest with orthopaedic internal bicortical fixation of radius as prophylaxis for prevention of radial shaft fracture

88.6.2 Scapula Free Flap [6]

Theoretical conceptualization of the scapular flap was first described by Saijo in 1978 and popularized by Dos Santos [7] in 1979. This scapular system which got described includes a myriad of options based on the subscapular vessels. It can be used as two types of bony composite flaps with the utilization of angle of the scapula and the lateral border. The major branches of the subscapular system are the circumflex scapular artery and the thoracodorsal artery. Circumflex scapular artery and its associated vein with the lateral border of the scapula are the classical osseous flap. Scapular and parascapular flaps offer the most flexibility with combinations of osseous, muscular, fasciocutaneous free tissue transfer based on the subscapular vascular system. Approximately 10–14 cm of the length with a thickness of 0.5–1.5 cm bone composing the lateral aspect of the scapula and or the angle of the scapula can be harvested.

Figure 88.6 shows the advantage of this flap: independence of soft tissue pedicle in relation to the bone.

It can also be harvested using the angular artery, a branch of the thoracodorsal artery obtaining a longer vascular pedicle and teres major muscle along with the scapular tip. The medial border of the osseous scapular flap has been described; the flexibility of the overlying fasciocutaneous part is not very pliable. The medial border is comparatively narrow even in males for placement of osseointegrated implants.

Tips for donor site confirmation to the defect:
- Contralateral lateral border of scapula for mandibular reconstruction.
- Ipsilateral scapular tip for the palate and maxilla.
- The angle of the scapula can also be used for the mental prominence reconstruction.

Studies have shown good conformance between the scapular tip and the palate. The tip can be used horizontally for a palate and vertically for anterior maxillary reconstruction. There are reports of nonvascular scapular tip being used for orbital floor reconstructions.

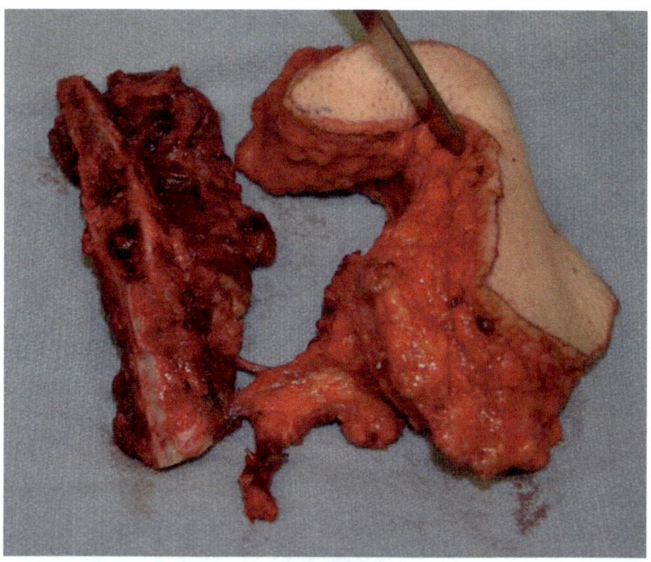

Fig. 88.6 The osteocutaneous scapular free flap. The great advantage of this flap is the independence of the soft tissue pedicle in relation to the bone

88.6.2.1 Indications

Composite and complex midfacial defects of the orbit, maxilla, skull base and mandible can be reconstructed using this chimeric flap.

88.6.2.2 Advantages

- Minimal donor site morbidity.
- Useful in elderly patients with peripheral vascular disease.

88.6.2.3 Disadvantages

- Concurrent flap harvest during ablation is not possible, as patient needs to be in the lateral decubitus or prone position.
- Inadequacy of the bone stock for osseointegrated implants.
- Variation in the anatomy with the circumflex scapular arising from the axillary artery.

88.6.2.4 Technique

Clear understanding of the scapular arteriovenous system and its branches composing the circumscapular, descending branch and parascapular vessel anatomy is essential.

The osseous branch of the circumflex scapular artery to the lateral border runs directly into it along with the vein. There is a gap between this and the cutaneous perforator which provides the flexibility of the skin paddle.

Patient can be positioned in a lateral decubitus or prone position for access between the axilla to the midline spine. The author's choice is use of a beanbag under the ipsilateral side and a protected axilla for the contralateral side. To increase the flexibility of the pedicle in relation to the lateral border of the scapula, a scapular or parascapular skin paddle can be based on the circumflex artery. The triangular space is made by the teres minor superiorly and teres major inferiorly, and the long head of the triceps laterally is identified using a Doppler 2 cm superior to the posterior axillary fold edge. The fasciocutaneous flap elevation is medial to lateral superior to the muscular fascia until the omotricipital triangle is reached. The circumflex vascular pedicle can be followed proximally to the subscapular and axillary arterial system with dissection between the teres minor and major muscles superiorly. The circumflex scapular artery is dissected in the lateral aspect of the scapular border with preservation of the muscular perforators to the bone by medial retraction of the teres minor and inferior retraction of the latissimus dorsi. An incision parallel to the lateral border of the scapula is made through the teres minor and infraspinatus muscle and periosteum. Protecting the vascular pedicle laterally on the glenohumeral joint superiorly osteotomy can be performed using a saw to the desired length with or without the angle of the scapula. Scapular angle can be harvested independently with identification of the angular perforators. Adequate care is taken to protect the underlying subscapularis musculature. Teres major muscle is reattached with multiple drill holes to the new border of the lateral scapula donor site to prevent winging. Perioperative drain and post-operative immobilization of the arm after primary closure of the defect site are commonly utilized along with physiotherapy.

88.6.3 Fibula Free Flap [8, 9]

Taylor et al. first introduced the fibula flap in 1975 for extremity reconstruction but was reintroduced for mandible reconstruction by Hidalgo. Though designed as an osteocutaneous free flap, the initial reports of unreliability of the skin paddle did not find favour in its use as an osteocutaneous flap.

Clinical Pearls

- Ease of simultaneous two team harvest.
- Consistent anatomy.
- Reliable usable bone length of around 24 cms, with the capability of performing multiple osteotomies.
- Variable design as bone only, osteocutaneous or with cuff of flexor hallucis longus or soleus muscle and with accompanying fat and fascia.
- Adequate length of vascular pedicle and suitability of the peroneal vessels for anastomosis.
- Accepts dental implants and osseointegrates.
- Minimal donor site morbidity.

88.6.3.1 Anatomy

The fibula is a triangular bone in cross section, around 40 cm in length and 1.5–2.0 cms in diameter, articulates proximally with the tibia and distally with the tibia and talus and has dense cortical bone with a small amount of cancellous bone.

Blood supply: Dual endosteal and periosteal. The dominant endosteal nutrient pedicle enters posterior to the interosseous membrane at the junction of the upper and middle thirds of the fibula. It is the segmental periosteal blood supply arising from the peroneal artery that permits multiple osteotomies. Average pedicle length depending on the bone length harvested is from 5 to 10 cms with a diameter of 1.8–2.5 mm and venous drainage via paired venae comitantes.

Skin paddle: The skin territory for the flap harvest on the lateral aspect of the leg can be up to 25 cm in length and around 15 cms in width and is supplied by perforators from the peroneal system which can be either septocutaneous or musculocutaneous passing through the flexor hallucis longus and soleus. The number of perforators is around 4–8.

88.6.3.2 Preoperative Assessment

- History of trauma or surgery to the lower limb, any peripheral vascular disease which might coexist.
- Examination of the circulation with the dorsalis pedis and posterior tibial pulse.
- *Imaging*: MR angiography, CT angiography to rule out peronea magna and also identify perforators. If angiographic studies are contraindicated, perform an arterial and venous duplex ultrasound demonstrating the flow pattern.

Figure 88.7 shows the fibula free flap reconstruction for the left mandibule of the body, angle and ramus. Figure 88.8a–c shows the planning and execution for fibula free flap on a stereo lithographic model. The closing osteotomies are made with measurements using a ruler template; the smallest fibula segment is noted as marginally more than 2 centimetres. In Fig. 88.8b, one can see a sterile ruler held at the lateral fibula harvest with pedicle attached proximally and skin paddle. In Fig. 88.8c, the osteotomized fibula is immobilized to a reconstruction plate at the lower extremity donor site with the pedicle flowing intact.

88.6.3.3 Technique

Prepare the whole lower limb circumferentially from the calf downwards and the opposite limb for a skin graft. Perform the surface markings of the fibula, with the design of the skin paddle centred along the posterior border that corresponds to the intermuscular septum. Design the skin paddle after the perforators have been mapped out using a Doppler probe. Preserve at least 4–5 cm bone proximally and distally for the stability of the knee and ankle joint and to avoid injury to the

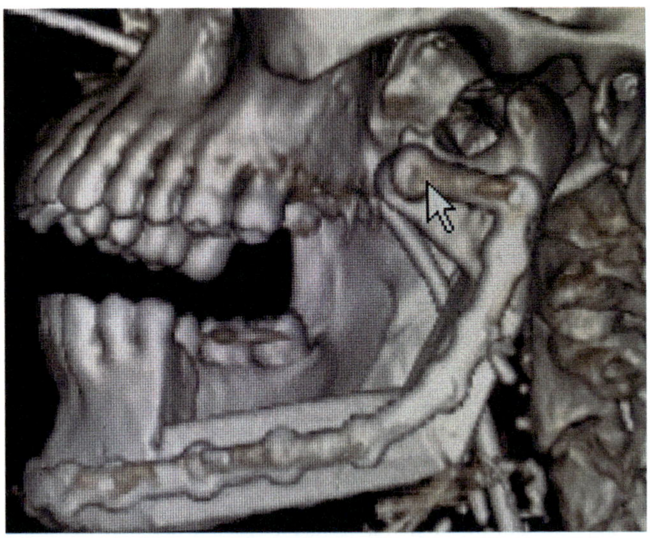

Fig. 88.7 Fibula free flap reconstruction for the left mandible of the body, angle and ramus

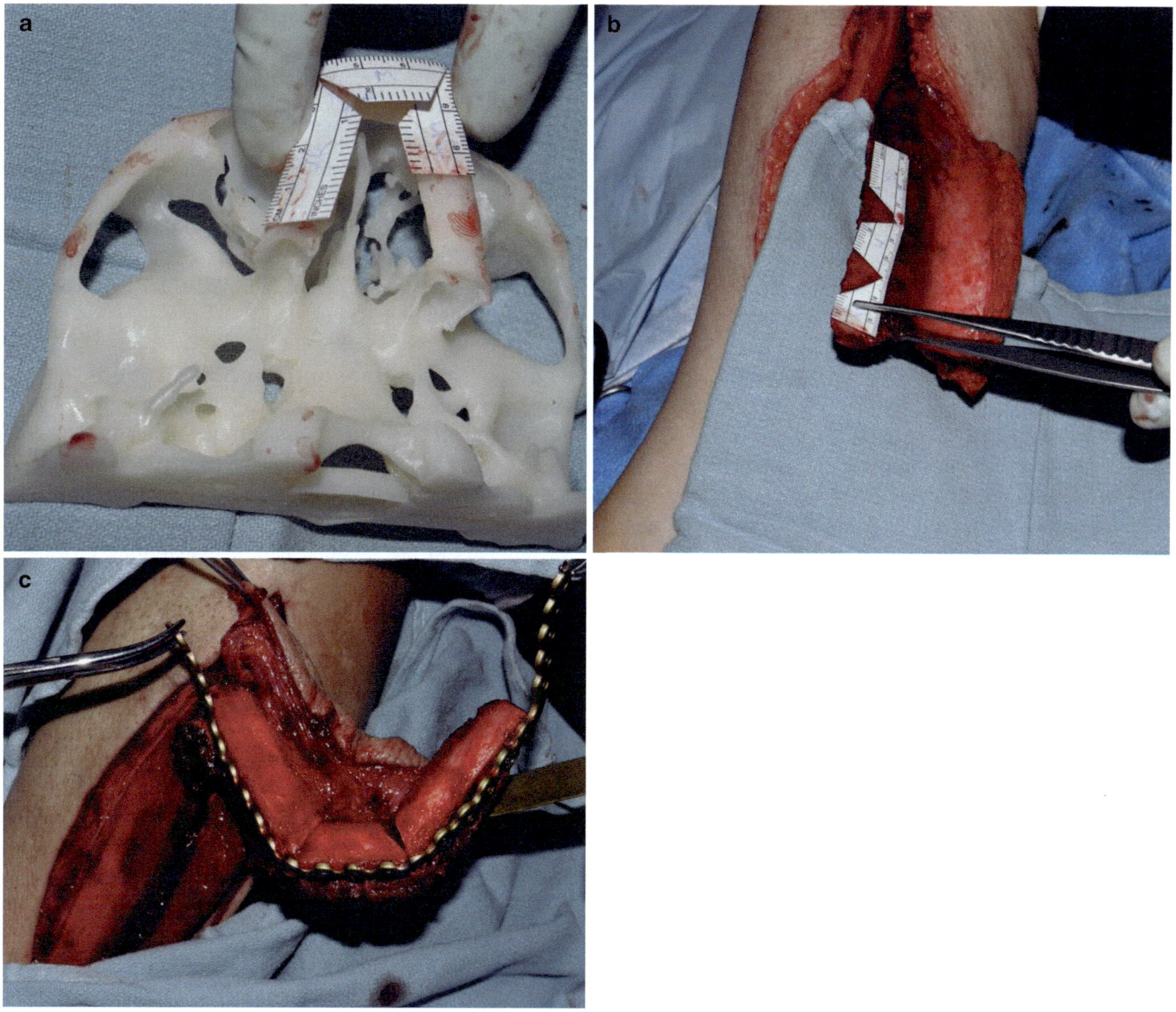

Fig. 88.8 Maxillary reconstruction planning for fibula osteotomies. (**a**) Planning for fibula free flap on a stereo lithographic model. The closing osteotomies are made with measurements using a ruler template; the smallest fibula segment is noted as marginally more than two centimetre. (**b**), the template being transferred to the fibula area for planning the closing osteotomies. You see a sterile ruler held at the lateral fibula harvest with pedicle attached proximally and skin paddle; (**c**) The osteotomized fibula immobilized to a reconstruction plate at the lower extremity donor site with the pedicle flowing intact

superficial peroneal nerve. Carefully apply a tourniquet and exsanguinate the lower limb.

The incision begins anteriorly on the skin paddle deepened into the subfascial plane over the peroneus longus and brevis and dissected to identify suitable perforators. The incision is extended in a curvilinear manner proximally, and dissection in the lateral compartment is done keeping a cuff of peroneus muscle cobblestoned on the bone.

The next step is the dissection in the anterior compartment of the extensor hallucis longus and extensor digitorum longus up to the dense interosseous membrane which is incised. The anterior tibial vessels are seen anterolateral to the fibula and preserved.

Proximal and distal osteotomies are performed using a reciprocating saw, preserving the superficial peroneal nerve superiorly. Distally ligate the peroneal vessel once the bone is osteotomized.

The posterior compartment dissection is performed between the tibialis posterior and flexor hallucis longus which identify the peroneal vessels. Keep a cuff of flexor hallucis or soleus muscle onto the graft depending on the soft tissue requirement and if the skin paddle is centred along the mid bone.

The posterior design of the skin paddle is made in a similar manner deep to the fascia over the soleus and lateral gastrocnemius preserving the saphenous vein and sural nerve.

Identify and preserve the posterior tibial vessels and tibial nerve 1–1.5 cm medial and parallel to the peroneal vessels.

Perforators to the soleus must be ligated, and additional length of the pedicle can be obtained by a subperiosteal dissection or ligation of the lateral posterior tibial vein.

Shaping of the fibula can be done on the benchside or while still connected with the circulation using either a prebent plate, cutting guides with virtual surgical planning. Closing wedge osteotomies are performed and fixation done.

Donor site closure should be meticulous with good haemostasis; suction drains closing the proximal and distal skin incisions and grafting the remaining donor site. Immobilization with a posterior splint with the ankle in 90 degrees flexion is recommended though not routinely practiced.

Postoperative physiotherapy for the lower limb can commence by the second day and with accompanying gradual weight bearing.

Pitfalls

- Vascular anomalies and variations can preclude the use.
- A double barrel segment might be needed due to inadequate bone height.
- The soft tissue component may be inadequate for extensive resections.

88.6.4 Deep Circumflex Iliac Artery-Based Composite Flap or Vascularized Iliac Crest Flap (DCIA)

Similar to the fibula the DCIA can be planned virtually. Opening osteotomies are performed instead of closing osteotomies in maxilla-mandibular reconstruction (Fig. 88.9a, b, c, d).

This flap can be harvested as an osseous or an osseocutaneous with the soft tissue component of the muscle and skin. This flap is based on the deep circumflex iliac artery and vein with the pedicle length as long as 8 cm with a diameter of the vessels between 1.5 and 3 mm. The iliac crest osteocutaneous free flap (ICFF) was described separately by Taylor [10] et al. and Sanders and Mayou in 1979 and popularized by Urken in 1989 for mandibular reconstruction and by Brown [11] in 1996 for maxillary reconstruction and use of internal oblique muscle [11]. The deep circumflex iliac artery and vein vessels arise from the external iliac vessels. The bone quality and quantity are excellent for both the maxillary as well as mandibular reconstruction.

Maxilla and mandibular segments can be reconstructed using the iliac crest bone based on the deep circumflex branch of the external iliac artery. The authors prefer a harvest using the superior approach in reference to the spermatic cord or the round ligament. Donor site morbidity is not significant, and the patient can be supine allowing a two-team approach. Up to 14 cm of bicortical bone with internal oblique muscle can be harvested. The thickness can vary between 0.5 cm and 2.5 cm.

88.6.4.1 Indications and Contraindications

This composite flap offers optimal volume of bone for endosteal implants as well as segmental mandibular defects with need of reconstruction of the dentate contour. Maxillary palatal contour and the regional complex subunits after maxillectomy can be reconstructed. The relative contraindications for this harvest are inguinal hernia, obesity, hip prosthesis and polyparity in women.

88.6.4.2 Vascular Anatomy

Just above the inguinal ligament, the deep circumflex iliac artery (DCIA) branches off the posterolateral aspect of the external iliac artery. As it traverses laterally parallel to the inguinal ligament, the ascending branch takes off 1–2 cm medial to the anterior superior iliac spine. This is located between the internal oblique on the transversalis fascia with penetrating perforators. The DCIA has a diameter averaged at 2 mm and a pedicle length of 5–6 cm. Vena comitans accompanies the artery draining into the external iliac vein. The position of the DCIA is about 2 cm inferior to the surface of the iliac crest at the fusion of the transversalis fascia and iliacus muscle. The two variations reported are the ascending branch takeoff in medial relation to the anterior superior iliac spine (1–2 cm versus 2–4 cm) and multiple ascending branch perforators instead of a single identifiable ascending branch of the DCIA.

88.6.4.3 Technique

With the patient supine, a soft hip support is placed and the skin prepped from the midline pubis laterally to the midaxillary line, superiorly from the subcostal margin to the anterior thigh inferiorly with the greater trochanter included in the field. This includes the planned cutaneous paddle. The cutaneous perforators are concentrated 5 cm lateral to the anterior superior iliac spine and 4 cm superior to the iliac crest midpoint. Only internal oblique musculature for lining of the oral mucosal lining is included. Incision is made in a superomedial elliptical fashion through the Scarpa's and Camper's fascia up to the external oblique musculature. This is identified in its orientation from the lateral to medial direction, and as this is incised, the underlying 90 degree medial to lateral internal oblique muscle is identified. The external oblique musculature is included with the osteocutaneous

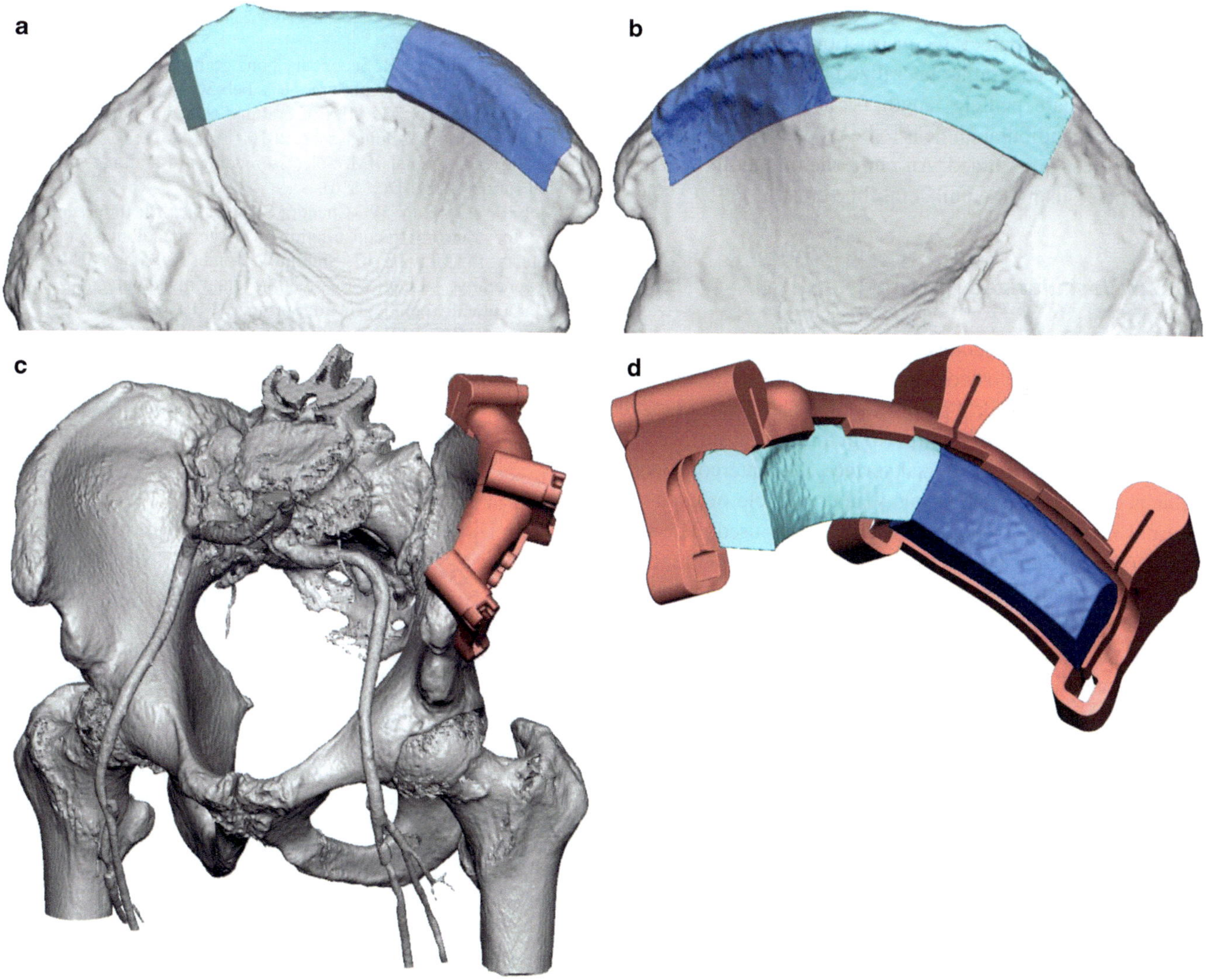

Fig. 88.9 (**a**, **b**, **c**, **d**) Similar to fibula DCIA can be planned virtually. Opening osteotomies are performed instead of closing osteotomies in maxilla-mandibular reconstruction

flap. The external oblique incision extends from the lateral entirety of the whole length up to the border of the inguinal ligament. The superior part of the flap is retracted and the internal oblique muscle exposed, and the amount of this internal oblique muscle inclusion is identified for harvest superior to the iliac crest attachment. The internal oblique and transversalis fascia is dissected sharply from the superior lateral aspect to the inferior lateral direction with superior retraction and access. The ascending branch is visualized and dissection is directed to identify the DCIA itself. The ileacus muscle is visualized and preserved based on the pedicle position and harvesting about 2 cm of it. At least 4 cm of the internal oblique muscle is harvested lateral to medial towards the ilioinguinal ligament. The vein runs over the DCIA medially to the external iliac vein.

The bone harvest is performed after detaching the gluteus medius muscle from the outer aspect of the ilium. The medial bone cut is made depending on the inclusion of the anterior crest of the ilium. The template as shown in the figure (anterior maxillary virtual finding figure) is used for making medial and lateral cuts using an oscillating saw. The medial side should be protected for pedicle integrity and peritoneum. If osteotomies are needed of the bony pedicle, they're performed with adequate care to gently greenstick the components.

The abdomen is closed in layers after adequate haemostasis of the donor osseous margins of the osteotomies. Multiple postage stamp holes are made in the bicortical iliac cortex and the residual muscular layers reattached with thicker non-resorbable sutures. And non-resolvable mesh can be used to reinforce the harvested internal oblique defect, and this can be sutured to the cortical holes as described above. The cutaneous closure is performed over suction drainage with multiple layer closure.

The quality and quantity of the bone of this flap are ideal for maxillofacial defect reconstruction. Maxillary reconstruction may need a rather lateralized bony segment harvest to gain adequate pedicle length for anastomosis into the neck. If the mandibular angle is to be reconstructed, the anterior iliac crest is included. An entire hemimandible can be reconstructed using the unilateral iliac crest.

88.6.5 Vascularized Rib Graft

There are other osteocutaneous flaps which are described like posterior costal osteocutaneous flap similar to the harvest of the costochondral part of the rib. These vascularized grafts can be from the right fifth rib in the ventral surface and up to the ninth rib in the dorsal surface. The intercostal vascular pedicle and subcutaneous venous pedicle or even the internal mammary perforators medially are used. The ribs can also be a part of the pectoralis major osteomyocutaneous flap, latissimus dorsi, serratus and trapezius muscular harvest with their pedicles. Of course the isolated rib graft with or without the costochondral graft has been the work horse for temporomandibular reconstruction for decades. The harvest has been documented well in surgical literature over the years.

88.6.5.1 Lateral Femoral Condyle Free Flap

The choice of this flap is for novelty in maxillofacial surgical needs. Femoral internal condyle with the descending genicular artery and vein as a pedicle can be harvested as free flap. The bony corticocancellous segment measuring up to 8 × 1.5 × 1.5 cm can be harvested [12].

88.7 Conclusion

In conclusion the hard tissue regeneration and reconstruction have been a primary focus in clinical and research interests for all reconstructive maxillofacial surgeons. The techniques and molecular science have ongoing updates persistently for the optimal and ideal technique. The understanding of intercellular and molecular behaviour of regeneration and grafting procedure is sought by biomedical scientists by research. And with virtual surgery and planning with guided navigation, the future of hard tissue reconstruction is poised for technically predictable results.

References

1. Boyne PJ, Sands NR. Secondary bone grafting of residual alveolar and palatal clefts. J Oral Surg. 1972 Feb;30(2):87–92.
2. Marks R, Stevens M. Atlas of oral and extraoral bone harvesting. Hanover Park, IL: Quitessence; 2010.
3. Abubaker O, Oghalai M. Selected readings in oral and maxillofacial surgery. 2001 Dec; 9(6).
4. Melville JC, Shum JW, Chandra SR. Chapter 12: tissue engineering for transoral reconstruction of large mandibular continuity defects. In: Melville JC, Shum JW, Young S, Wong ME, editors. Regenerative strategies for maxillary and mandibular reconstruction: a practical guide. Cham: Springer; 2019. p. 143–54.
5. Catone G, Reimer B, Mcneir D, Ray R. Tibial autogenous cancellous bone as an alternative donor site in maxillofacial surgery: a preliminary report. J Oral Maxillofac Surg. 1992;50:1258–63.
6. Swartz WM, Banis JC, Newton ED, Ramasastry SS, Jones NF, Acland R. The osteocutaneous scapular flap for mandibular and maxillary reconstruction. Plast Reconstr Surg. 1986;77(4):530–45.
7. Dos Santos LF. Un novo retalho livre microcircugio. Rev Bras Cit. 1980;70:133.
8. Taylor GI, Miller GD, Ham FJ. The free vascularized bone graft. A clinical extension of microvascular techniques. Plast Reconstr Surg. 1975;55(5):533–44.
9. Hidalgo DA. Fibula free flap: a new method of mandible reconstruction. Plast Reconstr Surg. 1989;84(1):71–9.
10. Taylor GI, Townsend P, Corlett R. Superiority of the deep circumflex iliac vessels as the supply for free groin flaps. Plast Reconstr Surg. 1979;64(5):595–604.
11. Brown JS. Deep circumflex iliac artery free flap with internal oblique muscle as a new method of immediate reconstruction of maxillectomy defect. Head Neck. 1996;18(5):412–21.
12. Martin D, Bitonti-Grillo C, De Biscop J, Schott H, Mondie JM, Baudet J, Peri G. Mandibular reconstruction using a free vascularised osteocutaneous flap from the internal condyle of the femur British. J Plast Surg. 1991;44:397–402.

Suggested Reading List

1. Langdon JD. Operative Oral and Maxillofacial Surgery. second ed. London: Hodder Arnold: 2009.
2. Coleman III JJ. Plastic Surgery Indications, Operations and Outcomes. Volume Three Head and Neck Surgery. first ed. St Louis: Mosby: 2000.
3. Wolff KD. Raising of Microvascular Flaps. A Systematic Approach. second ed. Berlin: Springer: 2011.
4. Cheney ML. Facial Surgery Plastic and Reconstructive. second ed. FL: CRC Press Taylor & Francis Group: 2015.

GPSR Compliance

The European Union's (EU) General Product Safety Regulation (GPSR) is a set of rules that requires consumer products to be safe and our obligations to ensure this.

If you have any concerns about our products, you can contact us on ProductSafety@springernature.com

In case Publisher is established outside the EU, the EU authorized representative is:

Springer Nature Customer Service Center GmbH
Europaplatz 3
69115 Heidelberg, Germany

Batch number: 10683581

Printed by Printforce, the Netherlands